Fourth Edition

Webb & Higgins' Thoracic Imaging

Pulmonary and Cardiovascular Radiology

Fourth Edition

Webb & Higgins' Thoracic Imaging

Pulmonary and Cardiovascular Radiology

Travis S. Henry, MD
Division Chief, Cardiothoracic Imaging
Professor of Radiology
Duke University
Durham, North Carolina

Karen G. Ordovas, MD, MAS
Chief, Cardiothoracic Imaging Section
Professor of Radiology and Associate
Vice-Chair for Academic Affairs
University of Washington
Seattle, Washington

Wolters Kluwer

Philadelphia • Baltimore • New York • London
Buenos Aires • Hong Kong • Sydney • Tokyo

Acquisitions Editor: Nicole Dernoski
Development Editor: Eric McDermott
Editorial Coordinator: Priyanka Alagar
Marketing Manager: Kirsten Watrud
Production Project Manager: Matthew West
Design Coordinator: Stephen Druding
Manufacturing Coordinator: Lisa Bowling
Prepress Vendor: TNQ Tech

Fourth edition

9 8 7 6 5 4 3 2 1

Printed in Mexico

Library of Congress Cataloging-in-Publication Data

ISBN-13: 978-1-975199-38-8

Cataloging in Publication data available on request from publisher.

shop.LWW.com

QUADM1024

To all the residents, fellows, faculty, family, and friends who challenge me to be a better radiologist and person every day—and make it fun along the way.

and

To my parents, who showed me the joy of academics and fostered my growth as an educator.

—Travis S. Henry

To the many trainees and colleagues with whom I have had the joy of working during my career. To my mentor and friend Charles B. Higgins who inspired my passion for cardiac imaging. To W. Richard Webb whose steadfast dedication showed me the value of a lifetime commitment to teaching.

and

To my beloved husband and kids, and to my parents who have encouraged and supported me along the way.

—Karen G. Ordovas

In Memoriam

In memory of W. Richard "Rick" Webb. 1945-2022.

Contributors

Bradley D. Allen, MD, MS
Assistant Professor
Chief, Cardiovascular and Thoracic Imaging
Department of Radiology
Northwestern University Feinberg School of Medicine
Chicago, Illinois

Dianna M. E. Bardo, MD
Vice-Chair of Radiology - Quality and Safety
Department of Medical Imaging
Ann & Robert H. Lurie Children's Hospital of Chicago
Chicago, Illinois

Benedikt Bernhard, MD
Research Fellow
Division of Cardiovascular Medicine
Brigham and Women's Hospital
Boston, Massachusetts

Sadaf Bhutta, MBBS
Associate Professor
Department of Pediatric radiology
University of Washington
Seattle, Washington

Zahra Chakeri, MD
Postdoctoral Fellow
Department of Radiology
University of Washington
Seattle, Washington

Hamid Chalian, MD
Associate Professor of Radiology
Department of Radiology
University of Washington
Seattle, Washington

Katherine Cheng, MD
Assistant Professor
Department of Radiology, Cardiothoracic Imaging
Duke University Hospital
Durham, North Carolina

Carole Dennie, BSc, MD, FRCPC
Section Head, Cardiac and Thoracic Imaging
Department of Medical Imaging
The Ottawa Hospital, University of Ottawa
Ottawa, Ontario

Tilman Emrich, MD
Attending Radiologist
Department of Diagnostic and Interventional Radiology,
University Medical Center of the Johannes Gutenberg-University
Mainz, Germany

Nicola Fink, MD
Radiology Resident
Department of Radiology
University Hospital, LMU Munich
Munich, Germany

J. David Godwin, MD
Professor of Radiology
Department of Radiology
University of Washington
Seattle, Washington

Michael B. Gotway, MD
Professor and Consultant
Department of Radiology
Mayo Clinic, Arizona
Phoenix, Arizona

Victor Billy Guerra, BS. (CT) (MR) RADIOLOGIC TECHNOLOGY
Senior 3D Imaging Analyst
Department of Medical Imaging
Ann & Robert H. Lurie Childrens Hospital of Chicago
Chicago, Illinois

Avanti Gulhane, MD, DNB, FSCMR
Assistant Professor
Department of Cardiothoracic Imaging, Radiology
University of Washington
Seattle, Washington

Mark M. Hammer, MD
Associate Professor of Radiology
Department of Radiology
Brigham and Women's Hospital
Boston, Massachusetts

Kate Hanneman, MD, MPH
Associate Professor
Department of Medical Imaging
University of Tornoto
Tornoto, Ontario

Charles B. Higgins, MD
Professor Emeritus
Department of Radiology
University of California San Francisco
San Francisco, California

Clinton E. Jokerst, MD
Associate Professor, Cardiothoracic Imaging
Department of Radiology
Mayo Clinic Arizona
Scottsdale, Arizona

Jeff Kanne, MD
Professor of Radiology
Department of Radiology
University of Wisconsin - Madison
Madison, Wisconsin

Eric Krieger, MD
Professor of Medicine
Division of Cardiology, Department of Medicine
University of Washington School of Medicine
Seattle, Washington

Tushar Kumar, MBBS, MD
Fellow
Department of Cardiothoracic Radiology
University of Washington
Seattle, Washington

Kacie Kuykendall, MD
Assistant Professor
Department of Diagnostic Radiology
Mallinckrodt Institute of Radiology
St. Louis, Missouri

Raymond Kwong, MD, MPH, FACC, FSCMR
Director of Cardiac Magnetic Resonance Imaging
Cardiovascular Division, Department of Medicine of Brigham and Women's Hospital
Professor of Medicine, Harvard Medical School
Boston, Massachusetts

Harold I. Litt, MD, PhD
Professor of Radiology and Medicine, Chief Cardiothoracic Imaging Division
Department of Radiology
Perelman School of Medicine of the University of Pennsylvania
Philadelphia, Pennsylvania

Cíntia A. Melo, MD
Cardiac Imaging Medical Coordinator and Assistant
Diagnostic Medicine Department
Beneficência Portuguesa of São Paulo Hospital
São Paulo, Brazil

Seyed Ali Nabipoorashrafi, MD
Post Doctoral Scholar
Department of Radiology
University of Washington
Seattle, Washington

Daniel Ocazionez, MD
Associate Professor of Radiology
Department of Radiology
The University of Texas Health Science Center
Houston, Texas

Rex Parker, MD
Associate Professor
Department of Diagnostic Radiology
University of Kansas School of Medicine
Kansas City, Kansas

Andrada R. Popescu, MD
Assistant Professor Pediastric Radiology
Department of Medical Imaging
Ann & Robert H Lurie Children's Hospital
Chicago, Illinois

Constantine Raptis, MD
Professor
Cardiothoracic Imaging
Mallinckrodt Insitution of Radiology
St. Louis, Missouri

Gautham Reddy, MD, MPH
Professor and Vice Chair for Academic Affairs
Department of Radiology
University of Washington
Seattle, Washington

U. Joseph Schoepf, MD, FACR, FAHA, FSCBT-MR, FNASCI, FSCCT
Professor of Radiology, Medicine, and Pediatrics
Assistant Dean of Clinical Research, College of Medicine
Department of Radiology and Radiological Science
Medical University of South Carolina
Charleston, South Carolina

Felipe S. Torres, MD, PhD
Assistant Professor of Radiology
Department of Medical Imaging
University of Toronto
Toronto, Ontario

Akos Varga-Szemes, MD, PhD
Professor of Radiology, Vice Chair of Research
Department of Radiology and Radiological Science
Medical University of South Carolina
Charleston, South Carolina

Eric Williamson, MD
Diagnostic Radiologist
Department of Radiology
Mayo Clinic
Rochester, Minnesota

Preface

Both of us relied on earlier editions of *Thoracic Imaging: Pulmonary and Cardiovascular Radiology* during our radiology training as "the Bible" of chest and cardiac radiology. Now, we are thrilled to continue the tradition in this fourth edition. Rick and Charley had a vision for this book—to provide a single volume, with a comprehensive but easy-to-digest review of both pulmonary and thoracic cardiovascular imaging—and we aim to continue that approach in this edition. It is intended to provide the fundamentals of thoracic imaging including chest radiography, CT/CTA, and MRI/MRA for Medical Students and Residents and Fellows in Radiology, Pulmonology, Cardiology, and Cardiovascular Surgery.

In this edition, the chapters are grouped in sections, related to key findings or fundamental clinical problems or diagnoses, in the hope that this may guide the reader to an organized understanding of disease and diagnosis. Several new chapters have been added including Thoracic MRI, The Diaphragm, and CTA for Guidance of Structural Heart Disease Procedures. Progress in understanding pulmonary and cardiovascular disease continues, and many entities we discuss in our sections and chapters are newly defined or have been redefined, reclassified, or have had their diagnosis clarified. Hundreds of new/updated images, videos, new tables, and illustrations have been provided to summarize and illustrate these additions and changes. We would like to thank all the experts in the field of cardiothoracic radiology who have contributed to this edition. Enjoy your learning experience!

Travis S. Henry, MD
Karen G. Ordovas, MD, MAS

Contents

SECTION SIX Pleural Abnormalities

SECTION SEVEN Great Arteries

SECTION EIGHT Radiography of Heart Disease

SECTION NINE Acquired Nonischemic Heart Disease

SECTION TEN Congenital Heart Disease

SECTION ELEVEN Ischemic Heart Disease

SECTION TWELVE Cardiac Arrhythmias

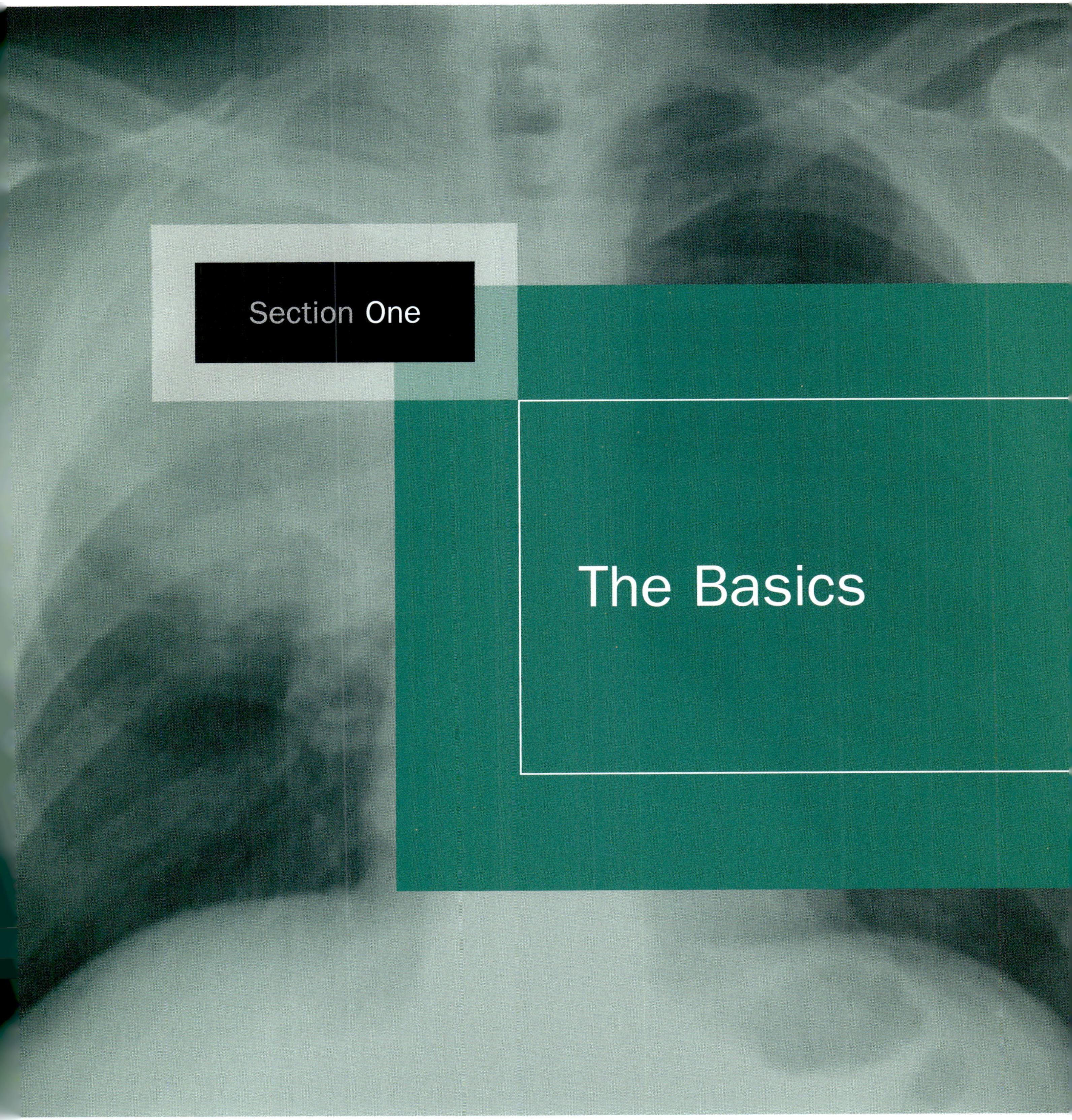

Section One

The Basics

Chapter 1

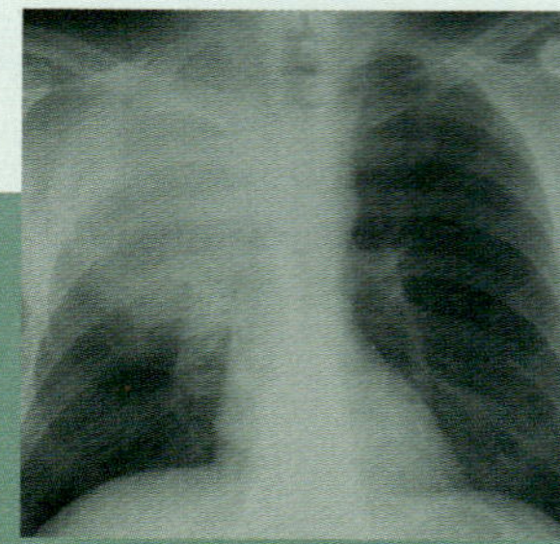

Travis S. Henry

Lobar Anatomy, Air-space Consolidation, the Silhouette Sign, and Atelectasis

LOBAR ANATOMY AND THE INTERLOBAR FISSURES

The lung lobes are separated from each other by interlobar fissures, which may be incomplete in some cases. Accessory fissures, present in some patients, are discussed in Chapter 26.

Major (Oblique) Fissures

On the right, the major (oblique) fissure separates the upper and middle lobes from the lower lobe. On the left, it separates the upper lobe from the lower lobe. The major fissures are not normally seen on a frontal radiograph but are often visible on the lateral projection. The major fissures originate posteriorly above the level of the aortic arch, near the level of the fifth thoracic vertebra, and angle anteriorly and inferiorly, nearly parallel to the sixth rib (Fig. 1.1). Posteriorly, the superior aspect of the left major fissure is cephalad to the right in 75% of cases. They terminate along the anterior diaphragmatic pleural surface of each lung, several centimeters posterior to the anterior chest wall.

On the lateral radiograph, the right and left major fissures may be distinguished in many patients by noting their relationships to the right or left hemidiaphragms or posterior ribs. The hemidiaphragms may be distinguished based on their relative positions or relationship to the stomach bubble and heart or by using the "big rib sign" (see below).

On computed tomography (CT), the orientation of the major fissures is clearly seen. Their positions vary at different levels. In the upper thorax, the major fissures angle posterolaterally from the mediastinum. Within the lower thorax, the major fissures angle anterolaterally from the mediastinum (Fig. 1.2A). The fissure may be seen as a linear opacity on thin slices. Alternatively, on thick slices, the location of the major fissures may be determined by recognizing a 1- to 2-cm-thin, relatively avascular band (lung adjacent to the fissure contains only small vessels) having a typical orientation.

Distinguishing the Major Fissures and Hemidiaphragms (The "Big Rib Sign")

The right hemidiaphragm is most easily identified on a lateral radiograph by its association with the right ribs. The right ribs can be identified on a lateral radiograph because they are projected posterior to the left ribs and because they appear bigger than the left ribs (ie, *the big rib sign*) (Fig. 1.3A). In the standard left lateral projection, the left side of the body is against the detector to minimize magnification of the heart. Therefore, the right ribs, being farther from the x-ray detector, are relatively magnified by the diverging x-ray beam (Fig. 1.3B). Also, the diverging x-ray beam, because of parallax, results in the right ribs being projected posterior to the left ribs, even on a perfectly positioned lateral view. Similarly, on the lateral radiograph, the left hemidiaphragm can be identified by its relationship to the left (more anterior and smaller) ribs (Fig. 1.3A).

If the stomach is filled with air, the left hemidiaphragm may be identified by its close approximation to the stomach bubble. Although not always apparent, the right hemidiaphragm is often visible all the way to the anterior ribs, while the left hemidiaphragm often is invisible anterior to the point it contacts the heart (Fig. 1.3A).

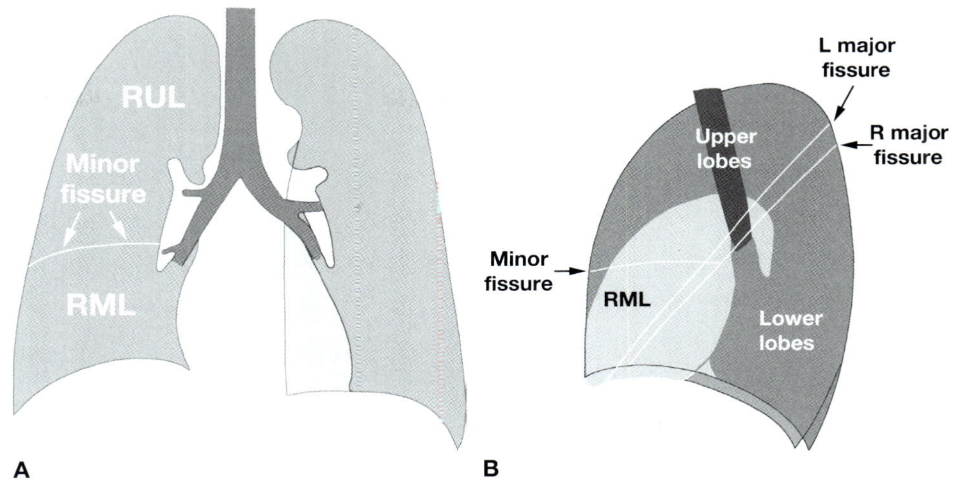

Figure 1.1. Normal appearances of the fissures on chest radiographs. **A:** Frontal projection. The major fissures are not normally visible. The minor fissure is visible in 50% to 80% of cases, appearing as a roughly horizontal line, generally at or near the level of the anterior fourth rib. Medially, it arises at the level of the interlobar pulmonary artery, and its lateral part is often inferior to its medial part. RML, right middle lobe; RUL, right upper lobe. **B:** Lateral projection. The major fissures originate posteriorly above the level of the aortic arch and near the level of the fifth thoracic vertebra. Posteriorly, the superior aspect of the left (L) major fissure is cephalad to the right (R) in 75% of cases. They terminate along the anterior diaphragmatic pleural surface of each lung, several centimeters posterior to the anterior chest wall.

Minor (Horizontal) Fissure

Right-sided consolidation anterior to the major fissure and inferior to the minor fissure involves the right middle lobe.

The minor or horizontal fissure separates the superior aspect of the right middle lobe from the right upper lobe. On frontal (posteroanterior [PA] or anteroposterior [AP]) radiographs, the minor fissure or a portion is visible in 50% to 80% of the cases, appearing as a roughly horizontal line, generally at or near the level of the anterior fourth rib (see Fig. 1.1B). Its contour is variable, but its lateral part is often visible inferior to its medial part. Medially, the fissure usually appears to arise at the level of the right hilum and interlobar

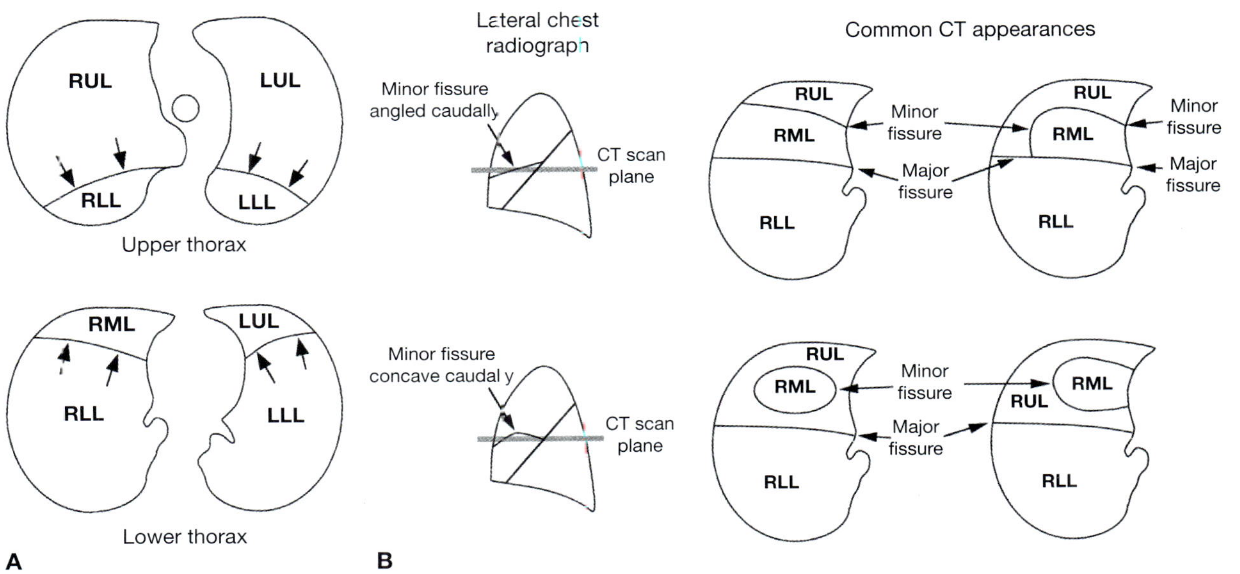

Figure 1.2. Normal appearances of the fissures on CT. **A:** Major fissures. In the upper thorax, the major fissures angle posterolaterally from the mediastinum. In the lower thorax, the major fissures angle anterolaterally. **B:** Minor fissure. The appearance of the minor fissure on CT is related to its orientation as seen on the lateral chest radiograph. LLL, left lower lobe; LUL, left upper lobe; RLL, right lower lobe; RML, right middle lobe; RUL, right upper lobe.

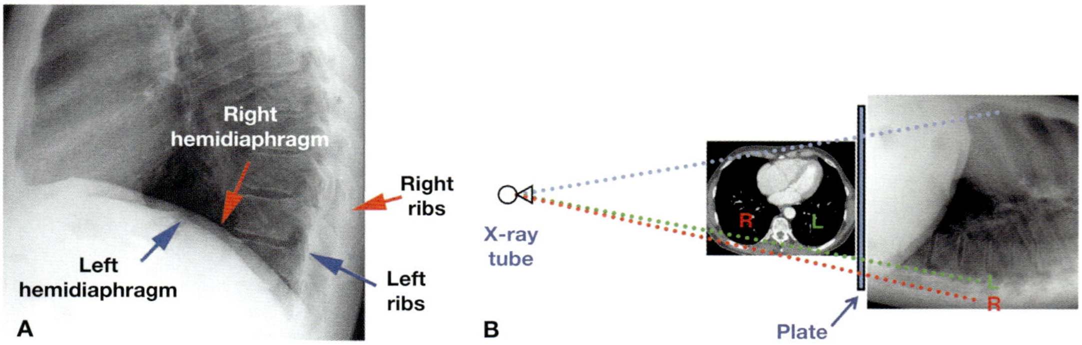

Figure 1.3. The "big rib sign." **A:** Coned-down view of a lateral chest radiograph. The posterior right ribs are projected posterior to and appear larger than the left ribs. The corresponding hemidiaphragms can be identified by their relation to the right and left ribs. Also, note that the right hemidiaphragm is visible anteriorly to the chest wall, while the left hemidiaphragm stops at the heart. **B:** Mechanism of the big rib sign. Because of the diverging x-ray beam, the right ribs being farther from the recording plate are projected posterior to the left ribs, even on a perfectly positioned lateral view, and are more magnified.

pulmonary artery. On the lateral radiograph, the anterior part of the fissure often appears inferior to its posterior part. The posterior part of the fissure may be seen to end at the major fissure or may project posterior to it.

On CT, the minor fissure tends to parallel the scan plane and may be difficult to see with thick slices. In such cases, the position of the minor fissure can be inferred because of a broad avascular region in the anterior portion of the right lung, anterior to the major fissure, and at the level of the bronchus intermedius. With thin slices, the minor fissure may be seen as a discrete line, similar to the appearance of the major fissure.

When visible, the minor fissure is variable in appearance, depending on its orientation. Because the minor fissure often angles caudally, the lower lobe, middle lobe, and upper lobe may all be seen on a single CT scan (see Fig. 1.2B). If this is the case, the major and minor fissures can have a similar appearance, with the major fissure being posterior and the minor fissure anterior; in this situation, the lower lobe is most posterior, the upper lobe is most anterior, and the middle lobe is in the middle.

If the minor fissure is concave caudally, it can sometimes be seen in two locations or can appear ring shaped (Fig. 1.2B), with the middle lobe between the fissure lines or in the center of the ring and the upper lobe anterior to the most anterior part of the fissure.

AIR-SPACE CONSOLIDATION

Air-space consolidation is a common radiographic finding and represents replacement of alveolar air by fluid, blood, pus, cells, or other substances. *Consolidation*, *alveolar consolidation*, and *parenchymal consolidation* are synonyms. Recognizing and localizing consolidation is fundamental to an understanding of pulmonary radiology and also helps in describing lung and lobar anatomy. *Ground-glass opacity* is a similar abnormality but is less specific, and best diagnosed using high-resolution CT (HRCT); it is discussed in a later chapter.

Radiographic and CT Findings of Consolidation

Radiographic and computed tomography abnormalities indicating the presence of air-space consolidation include the following:

- Homogeneous opacity obscuring vessels
- Air bronchograms
- Ill-defined or fluffy opacities
- "Air alveolograms"
- Patchy opacities
- "Acinar" or air-space nodules
- Preserved lung volume
- Extension to pleural surface
- "CT angiogram" sign

Homogeneous Opacity Obscuring Vessels

With complete replacement of alveolar air, homogeneous opacification of the lung results. Vessels within the consolidated lung are invisible (Fig. 1.4A).

Air Bronchograms

In patients with consolidation, air-filled bronchi are often visible on plain radiographs or CT, appearing lucent compared with opacified lung parenchyma (see Fig. 1.4). This finding is termed an *air bronchogram*. The bronchi usually appear normal in caliber, without evidence of displacement of distortion.

With some causes of consolidation, air bronchograms may not be visible. This usually occurs because of central bronchial obstruction (eg, by cancer or mucus) or filling of bronchi in association with the underlying pathologic process. For example, pulmonary infarction often results in consolidation without air bronchograms because of blood filling the bronchi. In patients with bronchopneumonia, bronchi may be filled with mucus or pus.

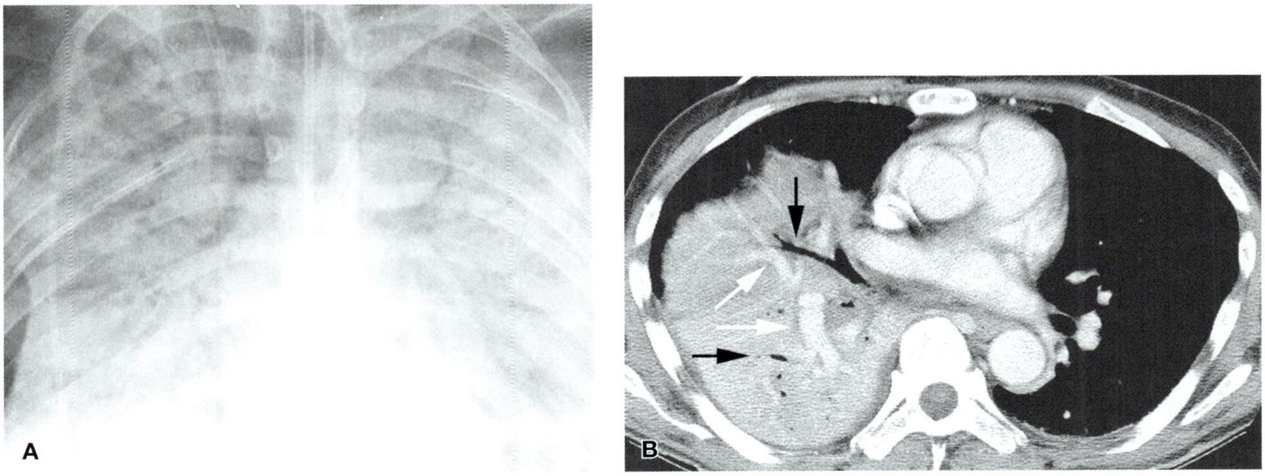

Figure 1.4. Consolidation: homogeneous opacity obscuring vessels, air bronchograms, and the CT angiogram sign. **A:** Right lung consolidation due to pulmonary edema. Air bronchograms are visible bilaterally within the consolidated lung, and pulmonary vessels are obscured. **B:** Enhanced CT in a patient with right middle and lower lobe pneumonia shows homogeneous consolidation, preserved lung volume, air bronchograms (*black arrows*), and opacified vessels (*white arrows*), appearing denser than surrounding consolidated lung (ie, the "CT angiogram" sign).

If air bronchograms are visible within an area of consolidation, bronchial obstruction is unlikely (but not ruled out) as its cause. Although air bronchograms are considered a classic sign of air-space consolidation, they may also be seen in the presence of confluent interstitial disease and sometimes within a mass; in such cases, the bronchi may appear narrowed or displaced.

Ill-Defined or Fluffy Opacities

Consolidation often results in opacities with ill-defined margins (Figs. 1.5 and 1.6), in contrast to the relatively sharp margins usually associated with a tumor or lung mass. Ill-defined margins result from patchy local spread of disease with variable involvement of alveoli at the edges of the

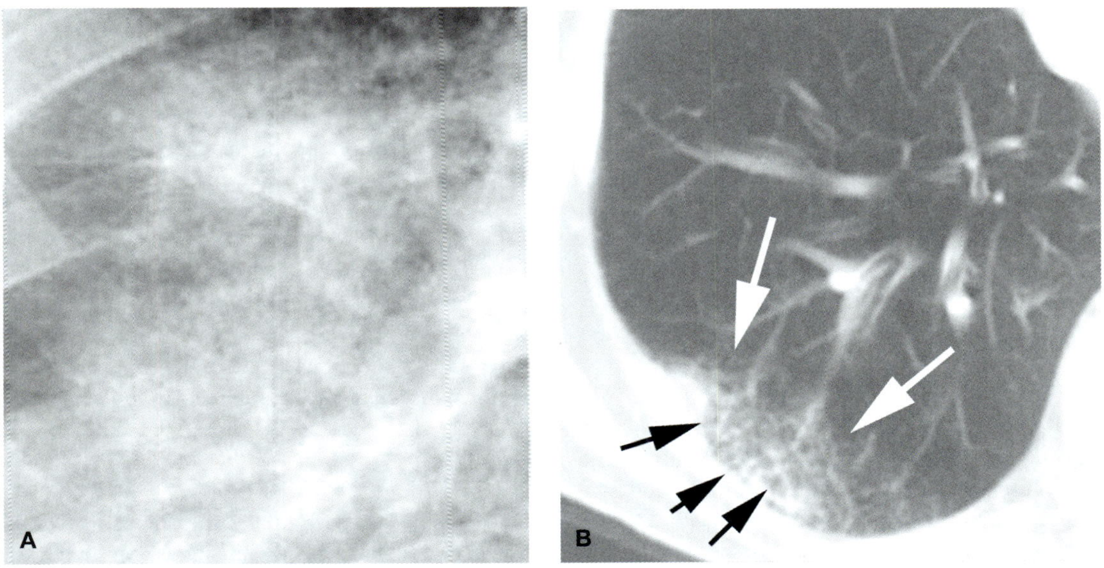

Figure 1.5. Consolidation: ill-defined, fluffy opacities with "air alveolograms." **A:** Detailed view of incomplete right lower lobe consolidation shows fluffy ill-defined opacity containing small rounded lucencies. These lucencies have been termed *air alveolograms*, although they do not correspond to alveoli. **B:** Ill-defined fluffy consolidation (*white arrows*) is visible on CT in a patient with right lower lobe pneumonia. Small focal lucencies (*black arrows*) within the area of consolidation are "air alveolograms."

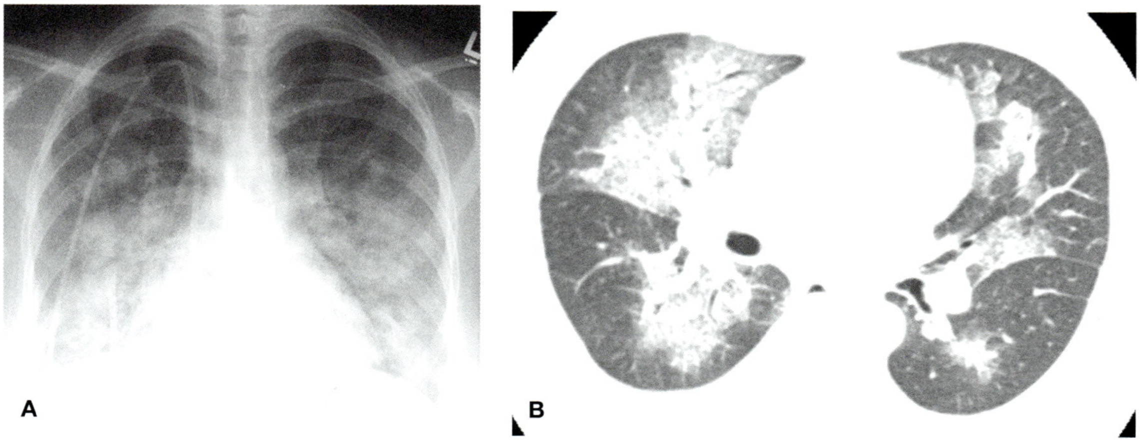

Figure 1.6. Consolidation: patchy opacities. **A:** Chest radiograph in a patient with pulmonary edema due to renal failure shows patchy perihilar consolidation. **B:** Patchy areas of fluffy consolidation are seen on CT. The fluffy margins are due to variable involvement of alveoli at the edges of the pathologic process.

pathologic process. When consolidation is bordered by an interlobar fissure, it may appear sharply marginated.

"Air Alveolograms"

If lung consolidation is not confluent and homogeneous, small focal lucencies representing regions of uninvolved lung may be visible within the abnormal area (see Fig. 1.5). These have been termed "air alveolograms," but this is somewhat of a misnomer as individual alveoli are too small to see radiographically or on CT. However, patchy consolidation surrounding clusters of normal alveoli results in this appearance.

Patchy Opacities

Variable consolidation in different lung regions results in patchy areas of increased opacity (Fig. 1.6). Pulmonary vessels may be obscured or poorly defined.

Patchy consolidation visible on chest radiographs sometimes appears to be lobular or multilobular on CT (ie, involving individual pulmonary lobules; Fig. 1.7). Some lobules appear abnormally dense, while adjacent lobules appear normally aerated.

"Acinar" or Air-Space Nodules

An acinus is the largest unit of the lung in which all airways participate in gas exchange. Anatomically, it is located distal to a terminal bronchiole and is supplied by a first-order respiratory bronchiole. Acini average 7 to 8 mm in diameter.

The terms *acinar nodule* and *air-space nodule* are used to describe poorly marginated rounded opacities, usually 5 to 10 mm in diameter, that occur due to focal consolidation (Fig. 1.8). Although these nodules approximate the size of acini, they are often centrilobular and peribronchiolar rather than acinar. They may be seen as the only finding of consolidation or may be seen in association with larger areas of opacified lung.

These nodular opacities are more easily seen on HRCT than on chest radiographs. On HRCT, their centrilobular location is usually discernible. This appearance is described further in Chapter 10.

Preserved Lung Volume

In the presence of consolidation, because alveolar air is replaced by something else (eg, fluid), the volume of affected lung tends to be preserved (see Fig. 1.4B). Although some volume loss may be seen in patients with consolidation, it is usually of a minor degree. Alternatively, in some patients with consolidation, a lobe may appear expanded.

Extension to Pleural Surfaces

Pathologic processes resulting in consolidation often spread from alveolus to alveolus until reaching a fissure or pleural surface (see Fig. 1.8B). The pleural surface prevents further spread. When extension to a pleural surface occurs, the abnormality may appear lobar, as in lobar pneumonia.

CT Angiogram Sign

A unique finding seen on CT in patients with consolidation is the "CT angiogram" sign. This sign is present if normal-appearing opacified vessels are visible within the consolidated lung following infusion of intravenous contrast (see Figs. 1.4B and 1.9). Although opacified vessels are sometimes seen within a

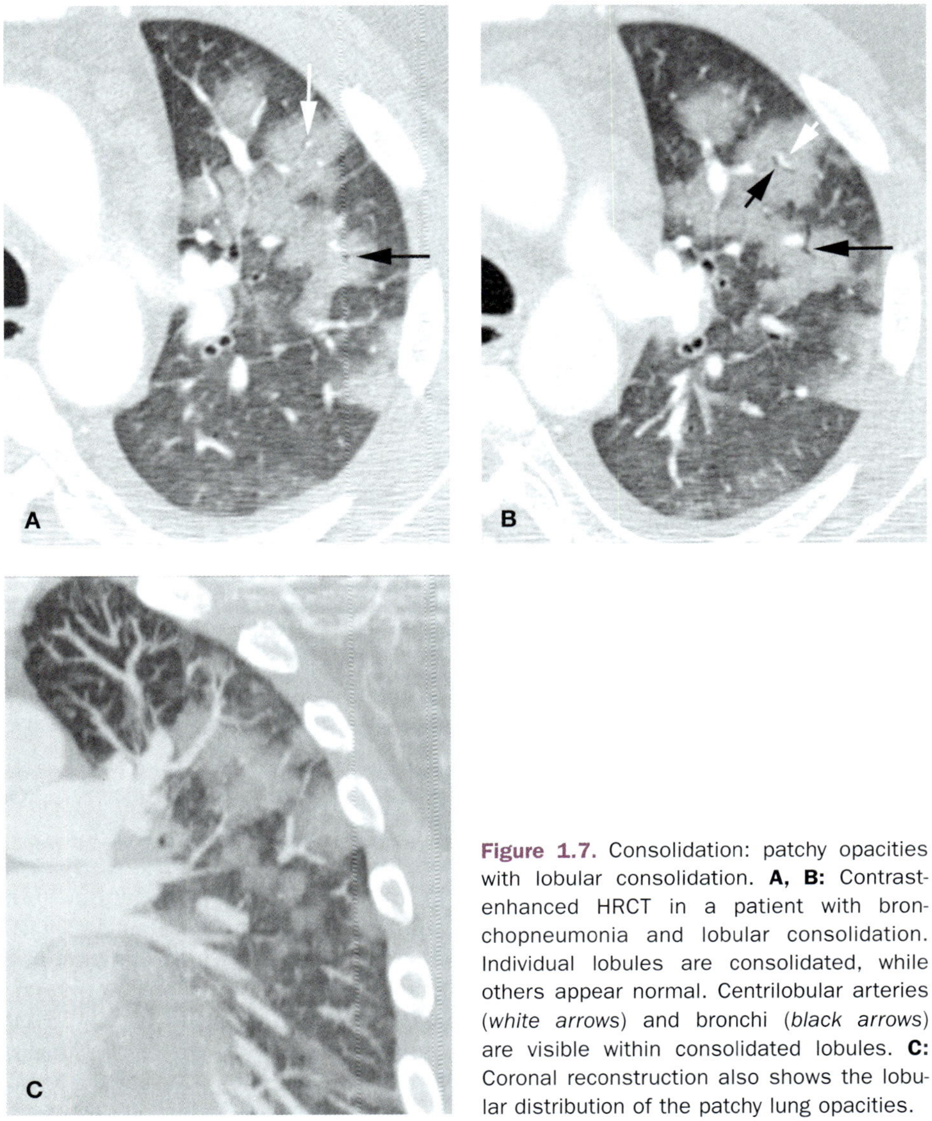

Figure 1.7. Consolidation: patchy opacities with lobular consolidation. **A, B:** Contrast-enhanced HRCT in a patient with bronchopneumonia and lobular consolidation. Individual lobules are consolidated, while others appear normal. Centrilobular arteries (*white arrows*) and bronchi (*black arrows*) are visible within consolidated lobules. **C:** Coronal reconstruction also shows the lobular distribution of the patchy lung opacities.

lung mass, they usually appear compressed or distorted. The CT angiogram sign is the vascular equivalent of an air bronchogram.

Differential Diagnosis of Consolidation

A wide variety of pathologic processes can result in air-space consolidation. In general, the differential diagnosis is based on a consideration of what may be replacing alveolar air:

1. Water (eg, the various types of pulmonary edema)
2. Blood (eg, pulmonary hemorrhage)
3. Pus (eg, pneumonia)
4. Cells (eg, lung adenocarcinoma, lymphoma, eosinophilic pneumonia, organizing pneumonia [OP])
5. Other substances (eg, lipoprotein in alveolar proteinosis, lipid in lipoid pneumonia, aspirated substances)

PATTERNS OF CONSOLIDATION

Based on the radiographic or CT pattern of abnormalities, patients with consolidation may be divided into two primary groups for the purpose of differential diagnosis: those with diffuse or bilateral consolidation and those with focal consolidation.

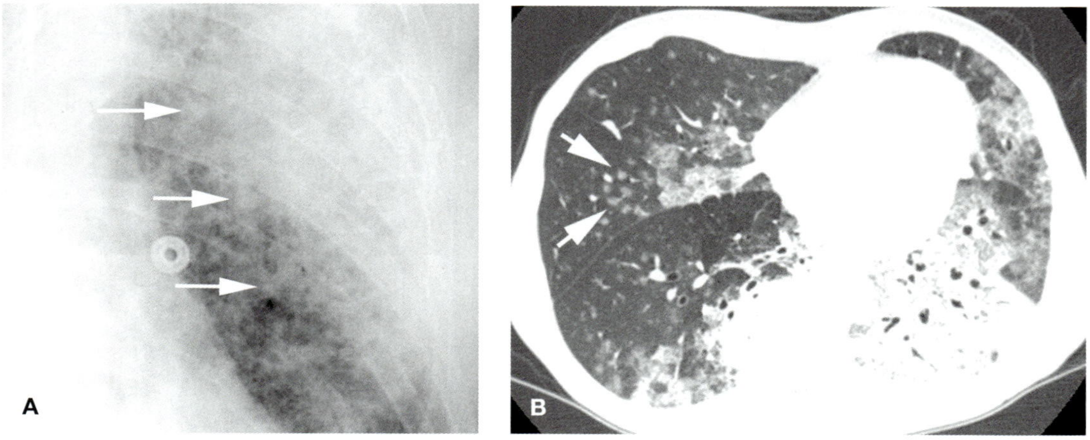

Figure 1.8. Consolidation: acinar or air-space nodules. **A:** Chest radiograph shows a patchy left upper lobe pneumonia. Ill-defined nodular opacities less than 1 cm in diameter (*arrows*) are visible on the edge of the area of denser consolidation. These represent air-space or acinar nodules. **B:** CT (5-mm slice thickness) in a patient with bilateral consolidation. Air bronchograms are visible in the left lower lobe. Patchy consolidation and ground-glass opacities are present. Air-space nodules are visible in the right middle lobe (*arrows*) and the right lower lobe. These nodules are ill defined, 5 to 10 mm in diameter, and centrilobular in distribution.

Diffuse or Extensive Consolidation

Diffuse consolidation has a number of possible causes (Table 1.1), and the clinical history is often more important than the radiographic findings in making the diagnosis. Several patterns or distributions of diffuse consolidation may suggest possible causes.

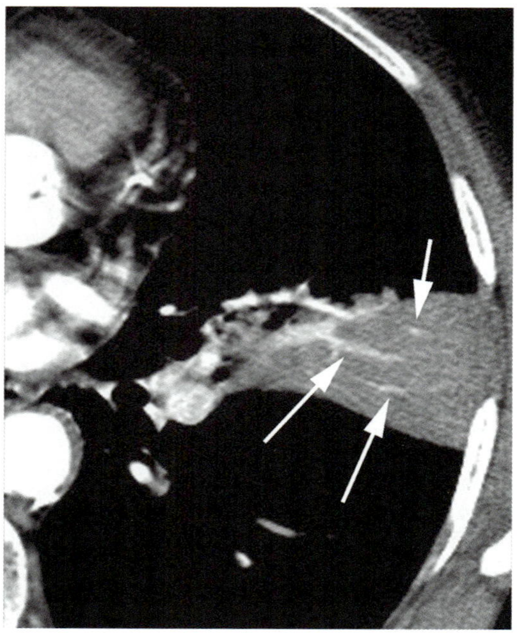

Figure 1.9. Consolidation: the CT angiogram sign. Contrast-enhanced CT in a patient with pneumonia shows focal consolidation. Opacified arteries (*arrows*) appear denser than does consolidated lung (ie, the CT angiogram sign). The consolidation borders on the major fissure posteriorly and appears segmental.

Perihilar "Bat-Wing" Consolidation

Perihilar "bat-wing" consolidation shows central consolidation with sparing of the lung periphery (Figs. 1.10 and 1.11). It is most typical of pulmonary edema (hydrostatic or permeability). This pattern also may be seen with pulmonary hemorrhage, pneumonias (including bacteria and atypical pneumonias such as *Pneumocystis jirovecii* pneumonia [PJP] and viral pneumonia), and inhalational lung injury. In patients with pulmonary edema, a perihilar distribution is most often present when rapid accumulation of fluid has occurred. Relative sparing of the lung periphery has been attributed to better lymphatic clearance of edema fluid in this region, although the exact mechanism is unclear and undoubtedly varies with the disease.

Peripheral or Subpleural Consolidation

Peripheral or subpleural consolidation is the opposite of a bat-wing pattern (ie, a reverse bat-wing pattern). Consolidation is seen adjacent to the chest wall, with sparing of the perihilar regions. It is most often seen in patients with a chronic lung disease (also the reverse of what is true of a bat-wing pattern). It is classically associated with eosinophilic lung diseases, particularly eosinophilic pneumonia (Fig. 1.12A), but may also occur with OP (see Fig. 1.12B), sarcoidosis, radiation pneumonitis, lung contusion, or mucinous adenocarcinoma. Peripheral consolidation need not always appear peripheral on the frontal (PA AP) radiograph; it may be peripheral in the anterior or posterior lung and overlie the parahilar regions.

Table 1.1 Differential Diagnosis of Diffuse Consolidation

Water (Edema) (See Chapter 12)

Hydrostatic (cardiogenic) pulmonary edema
- Heart failure
- Left atrial or pulmonary venous obstruction
- Volume overload
- Low intravascular oncotic pressure
- Hypoalbuminemia
- Liver disease
- Renal failure

Increased permeability (noncardiogenic) pulmonary edema
- With diffuse alveolar damage (acute respiratory distress syndrome [ARDS])
  - Acute interstitial pneumonia
  - Aspiration of gastric acid
  - Drugs
  - Fat embolism
  - Infection and sepsis
  - Near-drowning
  - Pneumonia
  - Radiation
  - Shock
  - Toxic fumes or gases
  - Trauma
- Without diffuse alveolar damage
  - Any cause of ARDS, in a mild form
  - Drug reactions
  - Hantavirus pulmonary syndrome
  - Transfusion reaction

Mixed types of edema
- Air embolism
- High-altitude pulmonary edema
- Neurogenic pulmonary edema
- Posttransplantation edema
- Postpneumonectomy
- Reexpansion edema
- Reperfusion edema
- Tocolytic therapy
- Hydrostatic and permeability edema

Blood (hemorrhage) (see Chapter 19)
- Aspiration of blood
- Bleeding diathesis
  - Anticoagulation
  - Chemotherapy
  - Leukemia
  - Low platelets
- Collagen vascular disease and immune complex vasculitis
  - Systemic lupus erythematosus most common
  - Behçet syndrome
  - Henoch-Schönlein purpura
  - Antiphospholipid syndrome
- Goodpasture syndrome
- Idiopathic pulmonary hemosiderosis
- Trauma
- Vasculitis
  - Granulomatosis with polyangiitis (Wegener granulomatosis)
  - Churg-Strauss granulomatosis
  - Microscopic polyangiitis

Pus (pneumonia)
- Bacterial pneumonia
- Pneumonia in an immunosuppressed patient
- Tuberculosis
- Nontuberculous mycobacteria
- Fungal pneumonia (histoplasmosis, aspergillosis most common)
- Atypical organisms
  - Virus
  - *Pneumocystis*

Cells
- Neoplasm
  - Pulmonary adenocarcinoma
  - Lymphoma and other lymphoproliferative diseases
- Eosinophilic pneumonia or other eosinophilic diseases
- Organizing pneumonia
- Interstitial Lung Disease
  - Nonspecific interstitial pneumonia
  - Desquamative interstitial pneumonia
- Sarcoidosis

Other substances
- Alveolar proteinosis (lipoprotein)
- Lipoid pneumonia (lipid)

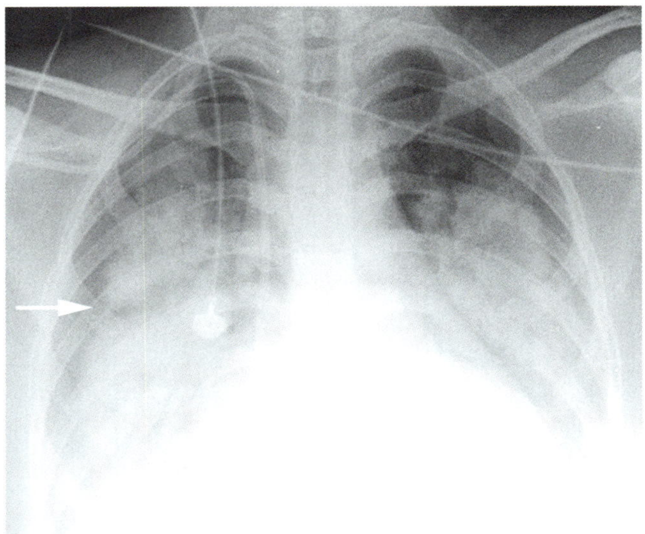

Figure 1.10. Perihilar "bat-wing" consolidation in pulmonary edema. Chest radiograph in a patient with pulmonary edema due to renal failure (note the dialysis catheter in the right atrium) shows a distinct perihilar bat-wing pattern of consolidation. The lung periphery is spared. Note the lucency at the level of the minor fissure (*arrow*) because of sparing of peripheral lung adjacent to the fissure.

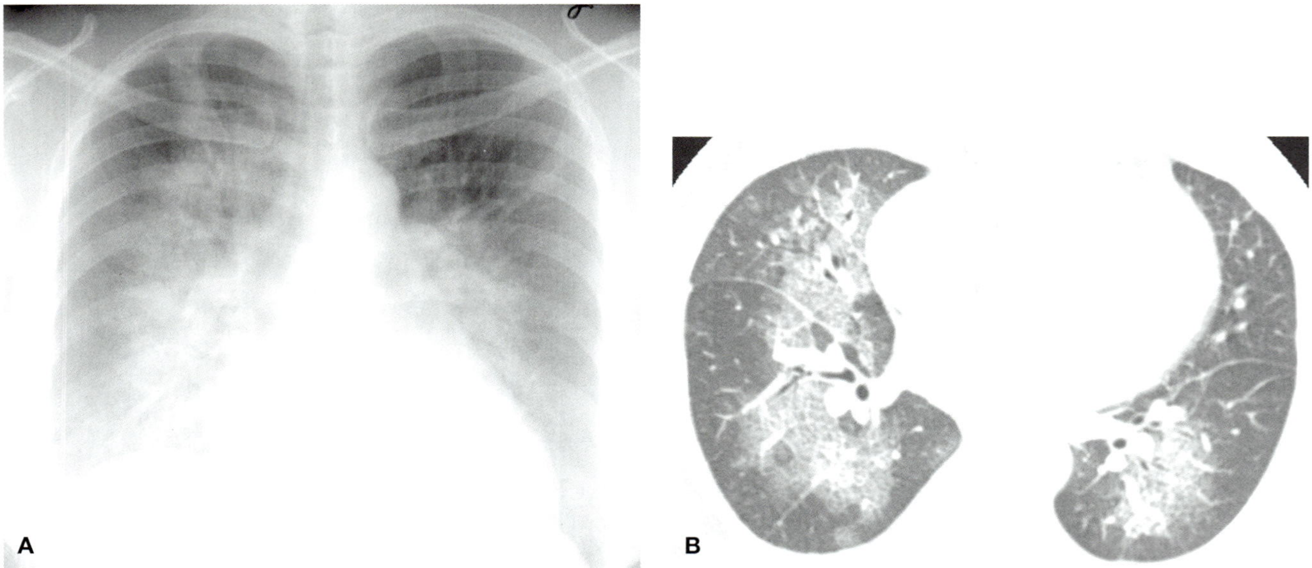

Figure 1.11. Perihilar "bat-wing" consolidation in pulmonary edema. **A:** Chest radiograph shows a distinct perihilar predominance of consolidation. The heart is enlarged. **B:** CT shows sparing of the lung periphery.

Diffuse Patchy Consolidation

Diffuse patchy consolidation (Fig. 1.13) may be seen with any pneumonia (bacterial, mycobacterial, fungal, viral, *Pneumocystis carinii* pneumonia), pulmonary edema (see Fig. 1.6A) (hydrostatic and permeability), acute respiratory distress syndrome (ARDS), pulmonary hemorrhage syndromes, aspiration, inhalational diseases, eosinophilic diseases, and invasive mucinous adenocarcinoma. The patchy opacities may correspond to consolidation of lobules, subsegments, or segments.

Diffuse Air-Space Nodules

Diffuse air-space nodules as a prominent feature of consolidation are typical of endobronchial spread of disease (Fig. 1.14). This appearance is seen in patients with

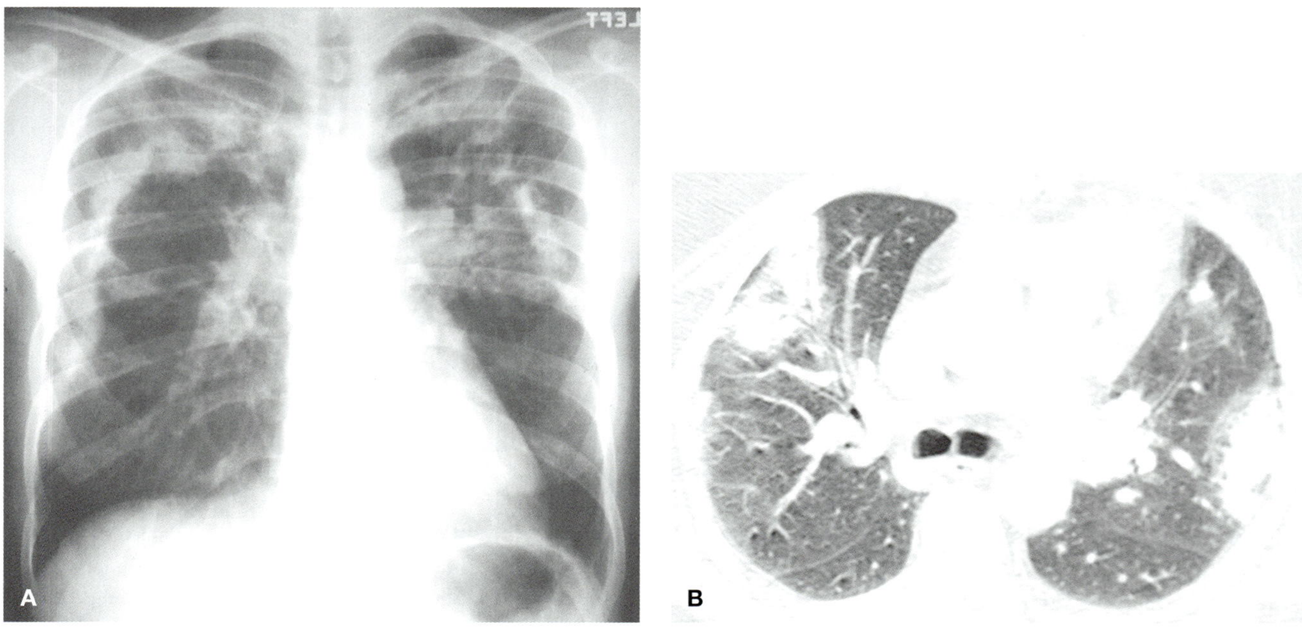

Figure 1.12. Peripheral subpleural (reverse bat-wing) consolidation. **A:** Chest radiograph in a patient with chronic eosinophilic pneumonia shows areas of consolidation in the subpleural lung. The perihilar regions are spared. **B:** CT in a patient with organizing pneumonia shows patchy areas of consolidation in the subpleural lung.

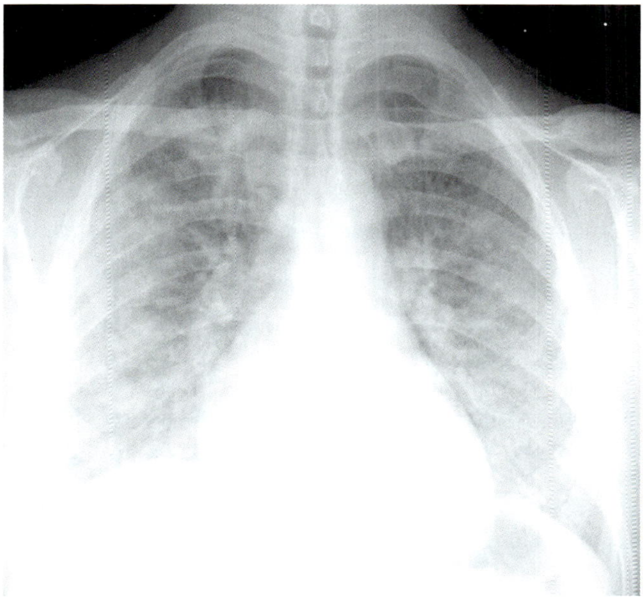

Figure 1.13. Diffuse patchy consolidation in a patient with viral pneumonia.

endobronchial spread of infection such as tuberculosis (TB) or *Mycobacterium avium* complex, bacterial bronchopneumonia, viral pneumonia (cytomegalovirus, measles), invasive mucinous adenocarcinoma with endobronchial spread pulmonary hemorrhage, or sometimes aspiration.

Diffuse Homogeneous Consolidation

Diffuse homogeneous consolidation is most typical in patients with pulmonary edema, ARDS, pulmonary hemorrhage, pneumonias (including viral and PJP), alveolar proteinosis, and extensive atelectasis.

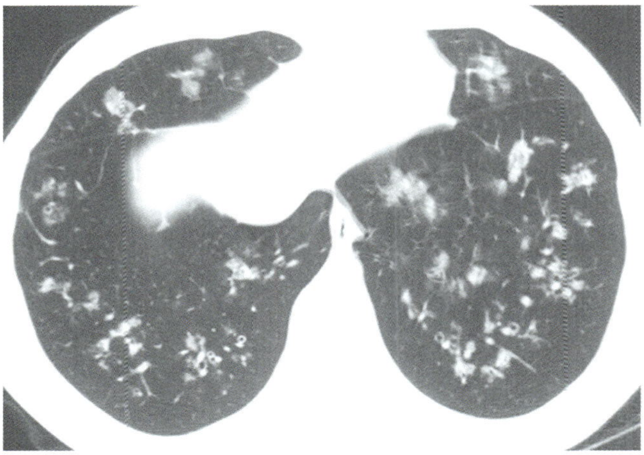

Figure 1.14. Diffuse air-space nodules in bronchopneumonia. Multiple small nodular opacities are typical of spread of infection through the airways. This represented a bacterial bronchopneumonia, but other organisms such as tuberculosis, *Mycobacterium avium* complex, fungus, or viruses may be involved.

Focal or Localized Consolidation

The most likely causes of focal consolidation include pneumonia, atelectasis with or without bronchial obstruction, pulmonary infarction, and neoplasm. Pulmonary edema and hemorrhage are much less likely than in patients with diffuse abnormalities.

Focal consolidation (Table 1.2) may represent pneumonia; postobstructive pneumonia; aspiration; pulmonary adenocarcinoma; lymphoma or other lymphoproliferative disease; infarction; hemorrhage due to trauma, pulmonary embolism, or diseases such as granulomatosis with polyangiitis; pulmonary infarction; radiation pneumonitis; OP; eosinophilic pneumonia; atelectasis; or rarely focal edema. The appearance of focal consolidation may also result from confluent interstitial disease, as in patients with sarcoidosis.

Table 1.2 Differential Diagnosis of Focal Consolidation
Water (Edema) (Uncommon)
Papillary muscle rupture with mitral prolapse (right upper lobe)
Edema in a patient with
Pulmonary artery obstruction (eg, pulmonary embolism)
Hypoplastic pulmonary artery
Swyer-James syndrome
Decubitus position
Reexpansion edema
Pulmonary vein occlusion
Systemic to pulmonary artery shunt (congenital or acquired)
Bland aspiration
Atelectasis with drowned lung
Blood (hemorrhage)
Contusion
Infarction
Aspiration of blood
Vasculitis
Pus (pneumonia)
Bacterial
Tuberculosis or nontuberculous mycobacterial
Fungal
Virus (uncommon)
Pneumocystis (uncommon)
Aspiration pneumonia
Atelectasis with postobstructive pneumonia
Cells
Neoplasm
Pulmonary adenocarcinoma
Lymphoma and other lymphoproliferative diseases
Eosinophilic pneumonia or other eosinophilic diseases
Organizing pneumonia
Sarcoidosis
Other substances
Lipoid pneumonia (lipid)

The appearance or pattern of focal or multifocal consolidation may be helpful in differential diagnosis.

Lobar Consolidation

Consolidation involving a single (or more than one) lobe is most typical of pneumonia (including *Streptococcus pneumoniae*, *Klebsiella* [Fig. 1.15A], *Legionella*, and TB) and abnormalities associated with bronchial obstruction. Consolidation can be localized to one or more lobes if its relationship to a specific fissure or fissures is apparent on either frontal or lateral radiographs, or on CT.

Lobar consolidation with pneumonia often occurs because of interalveolar spread of disease via the *pores of Kohn* (small holes in the alveolar walls). This type of spread continues until a fissure or pleural surface is reached. Organisms associated with spread of pneumonia via the pores of Kohn are characterized by thin secretions (thus passing easily through the pores). The presence of an incomplete fissure may lead to a lobar pneumonia becoming bilobar (or trilobar) (see Fig. 1.15B).

Lobar consolidation resulting from interalveolar spread of disease can also be seen with lymphoma and invasive mucinous adenocarcinoma (see Fig. 1.15B). The term *lepidic growth* is used to describe the local spread of tumors such as nonmucinous or mucinous pulmonary adenocarcinoma, using alveolar walls as a scaffold.

Bronchial obstruction with postobstructive pneumonia or atelectasis also commonly results in lobar consolidation. The differential diagnosis is that of bronchial obstruction and includes neoplasm, lymph node enlargement, inflammatory lesions, stricture, and foreign body.

Lobar consolidation is uncommonly the result of vascular abnormalities. Right upper lobe consolidation representing pulmonary edema may occur in patients with acute myocardial infarction resulting in papillary muscle rupture and mitral valve prolapse; it occurs because a jet of regurgitant blood is directed into the right superior pulmonary vein. Focal pulmonary hemorrhage may lead to a lobar consolidation. Lobar consolidation is uncommon with pulmonary embolism.

Lobar expansion in association with lobar consolidation suggests infection, particularly by *Klebsiella* (see Fig. 1.15A) or *Pneumococcus*, TB, bronchial obstruction with postobstructive pneumonia, or consolidation associated with neoplasm (see Fig. 1.15B).

Lobar consolidation can be localized by attention to the interlobar fissures. Simply stated, consolidation on the right (seen on the frontal view), which is posterior to the major fissure on the lateral view, is located in the lower lobe. Right-sided consolidation anterior to the major fissure may be in the upper lobe or middle lobe, depending on whether it is above (thus involving the upper lobe) or below the minor fissure (involving the middle lobe). On the left, consolidation anterior to the major fissure is in the upper lobe, while consolidation posterior to it is in the lower lobe. The inferior half of the left upper lobe roughly corresponds to the lingula (lingular segments of the left upper lobe).

Round or Spherical Consolidation

Round or spherical consolidation is most typical of pulmonary adenocarcinoma (nonmucinous or mucinous), lymphoma or lymphoproliferative disease, or pneumonia (ie, *round pneumonia*). A round or spherical pneumonia is typical of organisms that spread via the pores of Kohn and progress to being lobar, such as *S. pneumoniae*, *Klebsiella*,

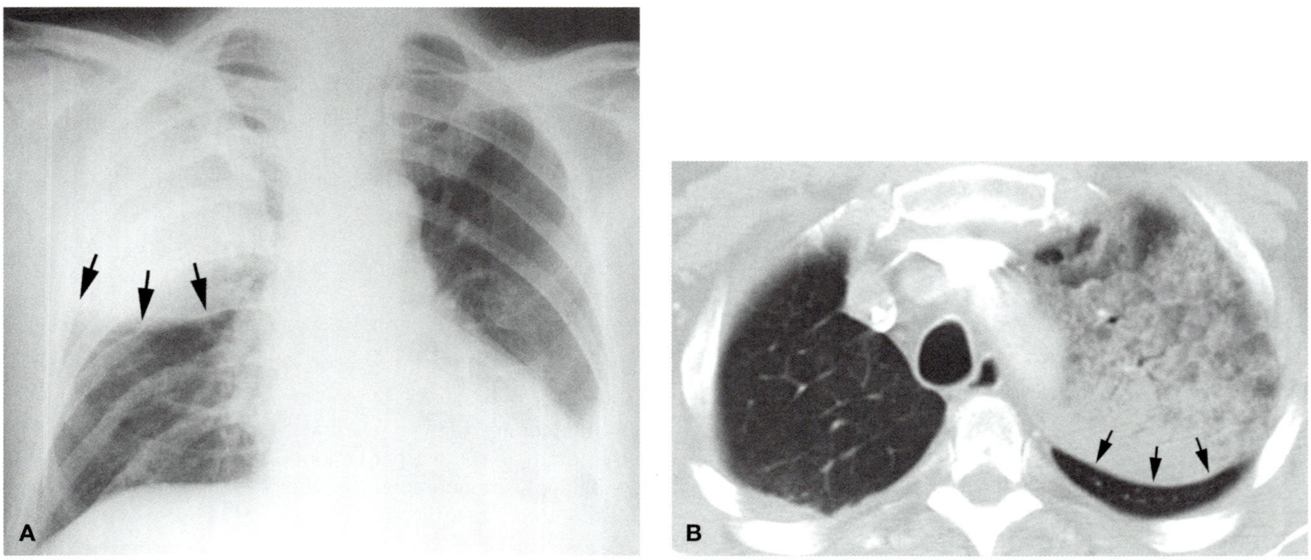

Figure 1.15. Lobar consolidation with expansion. **A:** A patient with right upper lobe consolidation due to *Klebsiella* pneumonia shows downward bowing of the minor fissure (*arrows*) because of lobar expansion. **B:** Invasive mucinous adenocarcinoma involving the left upper lobe with posterior bulging (*arrows*) of the left major fissure.

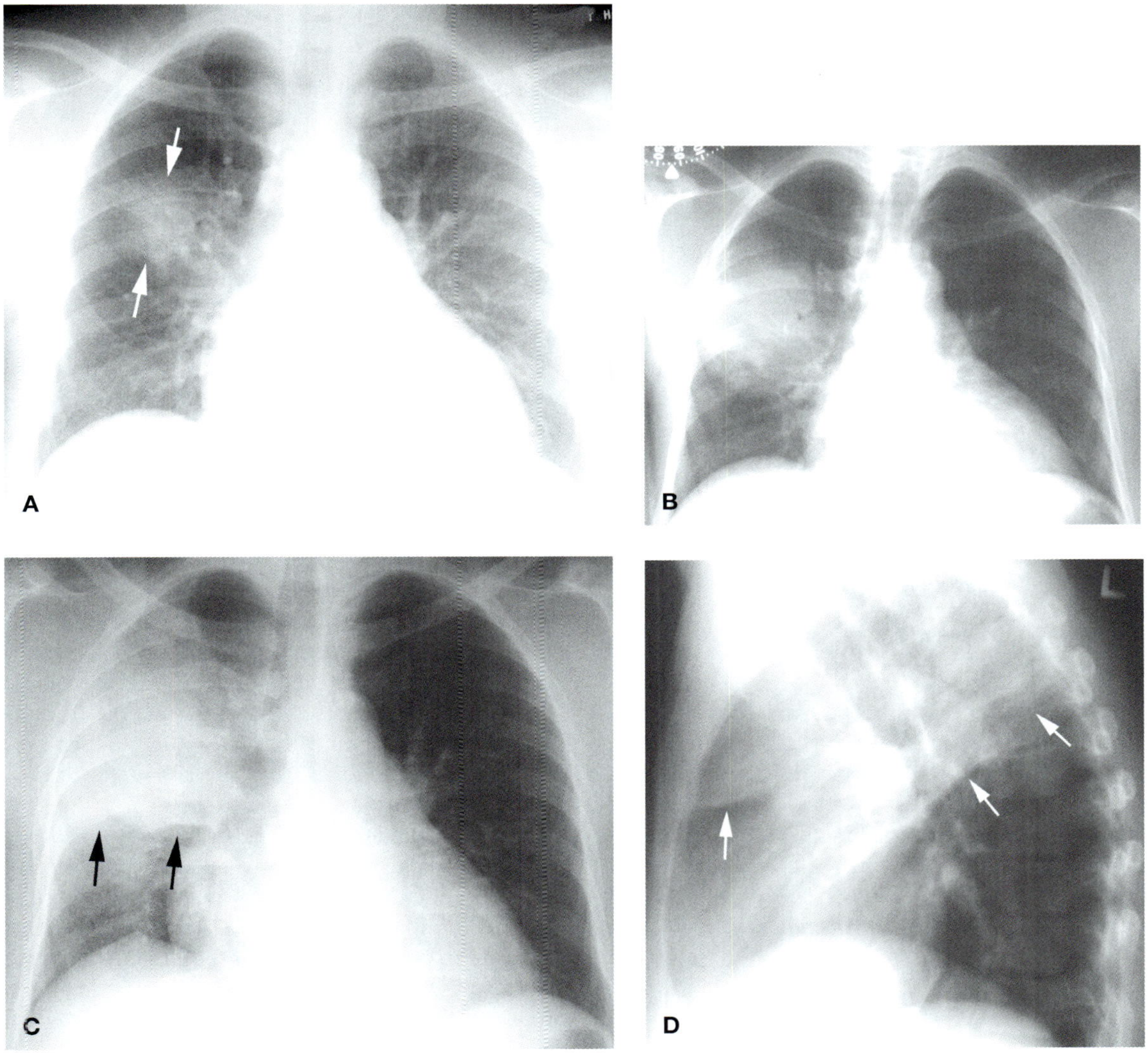

Figure 1.16. Spherical consolidation due to pneumonia. **A:** On the initial radiograph, a patient with *Legionella* pneumonia shows a poorly defined area of consolidation (*arrows*) in the right upper lobe. This may be termed "round pneumonia." **B:** Over the next several days, the spherical consolidation increases in size because of local interalveolar spread. This appearance may be seen in the early stages of lobar pneumonias. **C:** Further progression results in consolidation of the right upper lobe, marginated by the minor fissure (*arrows*). **D:** A lateral view at the same time as (**C**) shows upper lobe consolidation marginated by the major and minor fissures (*arrows*). Partial right middle lobe consolidation is also present.

Legionella, or TB (Fig. 1.16). Such diseases begin at a single site and result in an enlarging ill-defined sphere of consolidation as more and more alveoli become involved. As the growing sphere reaches a pleural surface or fissure and cannot spread further, it becomes lobar.

Segmental (or Subsegmental) Consolidation

Segmental (or subsegmental) consolidation may be diagnosed if a wedge-shaped opacity of more than a few centimeters in size is visible with the apex of the wedge pointing toward the hilum (see Figs. 1.9 and 1.17). This finding suggests an abnormality related to a segmental (or subsegmental) bronchus or artery, such as bronchial obstruction due to mucus or tumor, bronchopneumonia, focal aspiration, or pulmonary embolism with infarction.

Focal Patchy Consolidation

Focal patchy consolidation is typical of pneumonias, endobronchial spread of TB, or endobronchial spread of tumor such as mucinous adenocarcinoma (see Fig. 1.6). CT may show a pattern of lobular consolidation. Centrilobular nodules are seen in some cases (see Fig. 1.7).

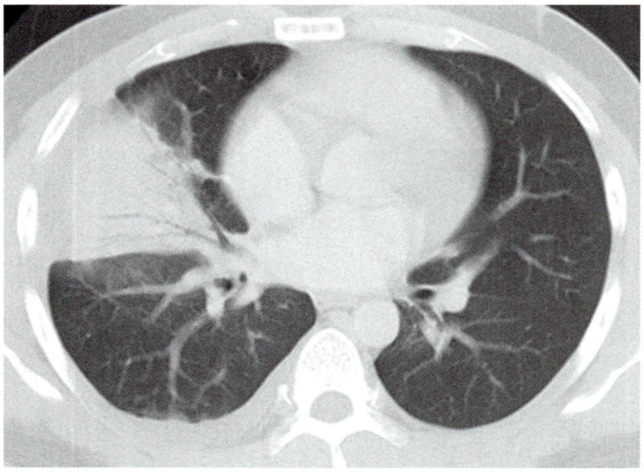

Figure 1.17. Segmental consolidation. A patient with pneumonia shows consolidation of the lateral segment of the right middle lobe. The segmental bronchus is seen within the consolidated lung as an air bronchogram. The medial segment, adjacent to the right heart border, is normally aerated. The consolidated segment borders posteriorly on the major fissure.

Patchy consolidation is typical of bronchopneumonia. Pneumonias associated with this pattern (eg, *Staphylococcus, Haemophilus, Pseudomonas*) are characterized by thick and tenacious secretions and spread via airways rather than the pores of Kohn. Infected secretions are typically present within the bronchi. Bronchopneumonia is also known as *lobular pneumonia* because of its tendency to involve individual lobules. *Mycoplasma pneumonia* often results in this pattern.

Differential Diagnosis of Consolidation Based on Time Course

The time course over which consolidation develops, or the duration of symptoms in a patient presenting with consolidation on radiographs or CT, is important in differential diagnosis. The likely diagnoses associated with acute symptoms or progression of radiographic abnormalities (hours, a few days, or a week or two) are quite different than those associated with a subacute, chronic, or progressive symptoms (a few weeks or months or years).

Rapidly Appearing Consolidation or Consolidation With Acute Symptoms

Rapidly appearing consolidation (a few hours) or consolidation associated with acute symptoms suggests atelectasis with drowned lung, aspiration, pulmonary edema, pulmonary hemorrhage, pulmonary embolism with infarction, or rapidly progressing pneumonia, particularly in an immunocompromised host. Of these, only pulmonary edema and drowned lung may clear quickly. Occasionally, a lymphoproliferative neoplasm progresses within hours.

Long-Standing Consolidation or Consolidation With Chronic Symptoms

Long-standing (chronic) consolidation (4-6 weeks or longer) with little change suggests eosinophilic pneumonia, OP, mucinous adenocarcinoma, lymphoma, lipoid pneumonia, or some indolent pneumonias such as those caused by fungal organisms. Recurrent processes (eg, recurrent pulmonary edema, pulmonary hemorrhage, or aspiration) may appear to be chronic if radiographs are obtained only during the acute episodes. Pulmonary vein stenosis/occlusion is a rare cause of chronic edema localized to one segment or lobe and is most commonly seen in patients who have undergone an ablation procedure for treatment of atrial arrhythmia.

LOCALIZING CONSOLIDATION: THE SILHOUETTE SIGN

The borders of soft-tissue structures such as the mediastinum, hila, and hemidiaphragms are visible on chest radiographs because they are outlined by adjacent air-containing lung. When consolidated lung (or a soft-tissue mass) contacts one of these structures, its border becomes invisible or is poorly marginated. This is termed the "silhouette" sign (although is technically the loss of the silhouette making the interface indistinguishable). The silhouette sign is used on radiographs to diagnose the presence of a lung abnormality (ie, consolidation, atelectasis, mass) and localize it to a specific lobe or lung region. It should be used in conjunction with identification of the interlobar fissures or may be used when the fissures are not clearly seen. However, keep in mind two caveats regarding the silhouette sign: (1) it does not always work and it should be correlated with other findings and (2) the presence of volume loss (ie, atelectasis) may alter specific anatomic relationships.

The Silhouette Sign on the Frontal Radiograph

On the frontal (PA or AP) radiograph, obscuration (in radiologic parlance, "silhouetting") of specific contours may be related to abnormalities (eg, consolidation or mass) involving specific lobes. Obscuration of specific contours and their correspondence to specific lobes are listed below and illustrated in Figure 1.18:

Right superior mediastinum (ie, superior vena cava [SVC]) = right upper lobe (see Fig. 1.19).
Right heart border = right middle lobe (common; see Fig. 1.20) or medial basal segment of the right lower lobe (less common). This appearance may be mimicked by pectus excavatum.
Right hemidiaphragm = right lower lobe (see Fig. 1.21).
Left superior mediastinum (eg, aortic arch) = left upper lobe (see Fig. 1.22B).
Left heart border = lingular segments of the left upper lobe (see Fig. 1.22).

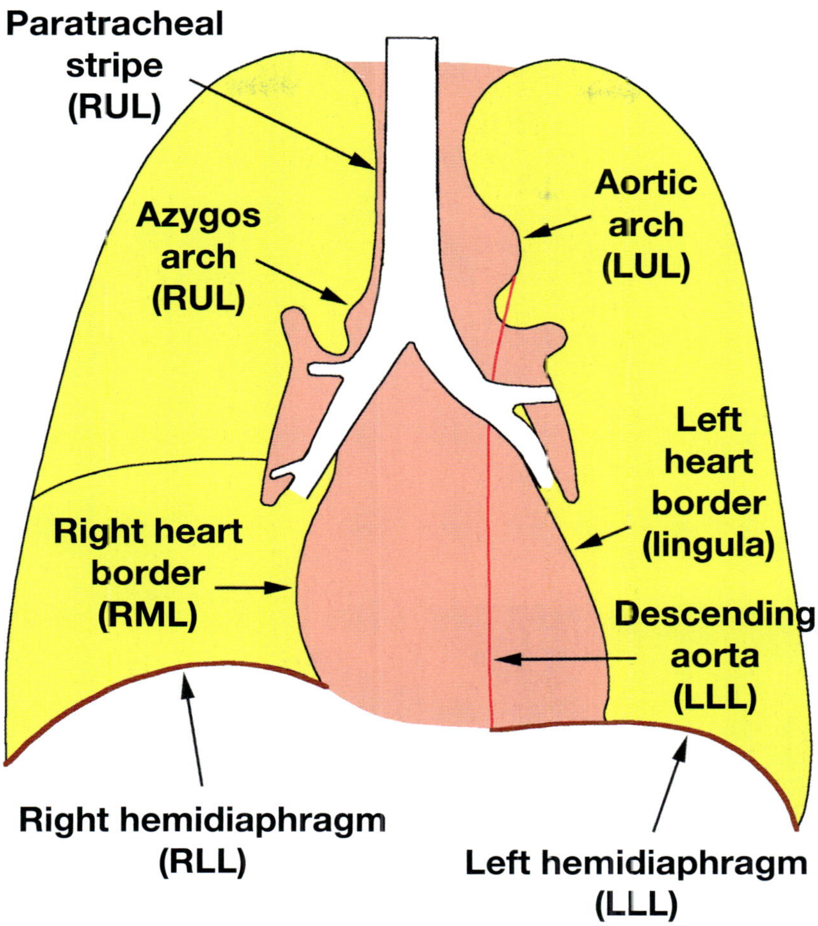

Figure 1.18. Anatomic relationships and the silhouette sign on a frontal radiograph. Obscuration of the borders shown in this diagram is associated with consolidation of the listed lobes. LLL, left lower lobe; LUL, left upper lobe; RLL, right lower lobe; RML, right middle lobe; RUL, right upper lobe.

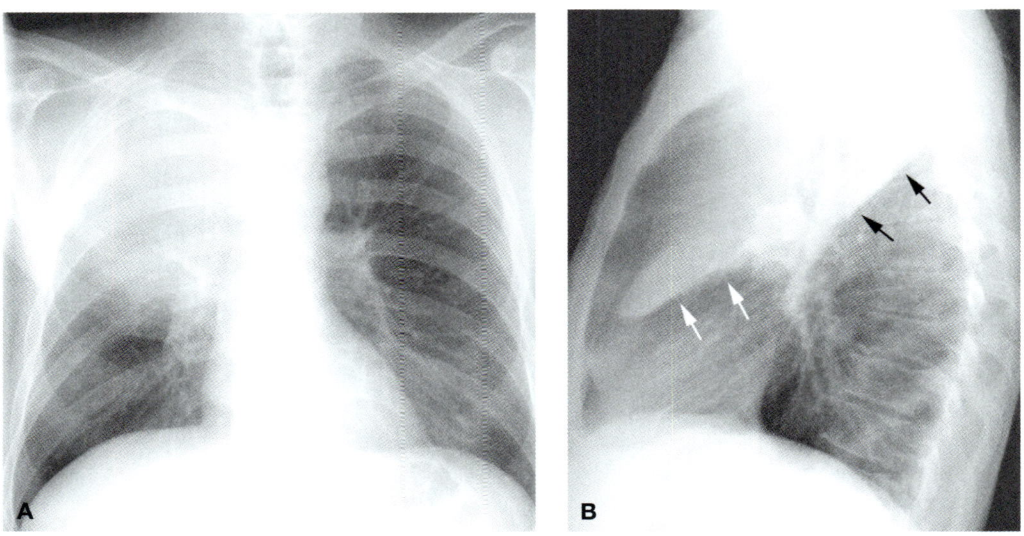

Figure 1.19. The silhouette sign in right upper lobe pneumonia. **A:** Consolidation of the right upper lobe obscures (ie, silhouettes) the border of the right superior mediastinum and superior vena cava. The upper part of the right hilum is also invisible. **B:** On the lateral view, the consolidated upper lobe is outlined superiorly by the upper aspect of the major fissure (*black arrows*). Inferiorly, it is outlined by the minor fissure (*white arrows*).

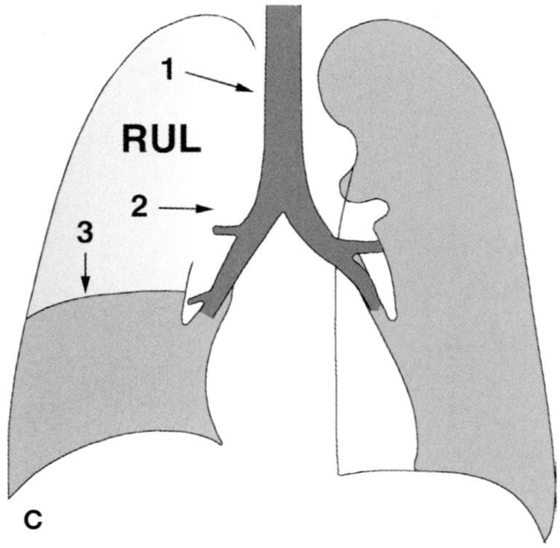

Figure 1.19. *(Continued)* **C:** Typical findings of right upper lobe (RUL) consolidation: (*1*) obscuration of the right superior mediastinum, (*2*) obscuration of the superior right hilum, and (*3*) opacity marginated inferiorly by the minor fissure.

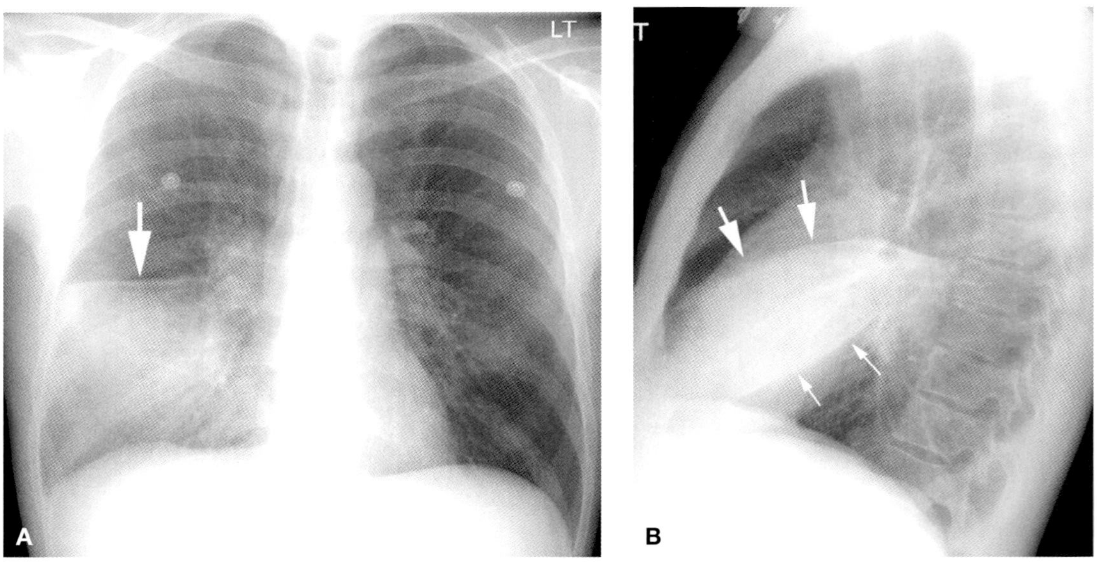

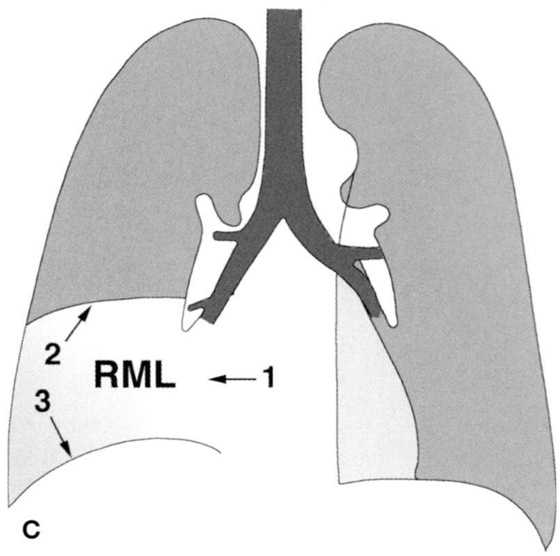

Figure 1.20. The silhouette sign in right middle lobe pneumonia. **A:** Consolidation of the right middle lobe obscures ("silhouettes") the right heart border (ie, it is not clearly seen). In contrast, the left heart border is sharply marginated. The right hemidiaphragm appears sharply marginated. The pneumonia is marginated by the minor fissure (*arrow*). **B:** On the lateral view, middle lobe consolidation is visible, marginated above by the minor fissure (*large arrows*); inferiorly, it is marginated by the major fissure (*small arrows*). **C:** Typical findings of right middle lobe consolidation: (*1*) the right heart border is obscured, (*2*) the opacity is marginated superiorly by the minor fissure, and (*3*) the right diaphragm remains visible.

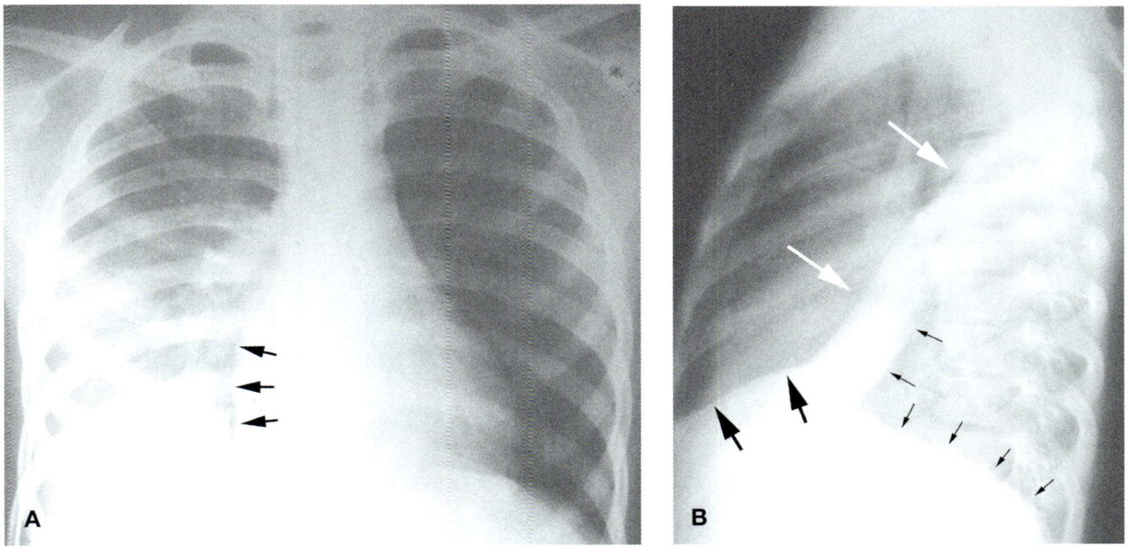

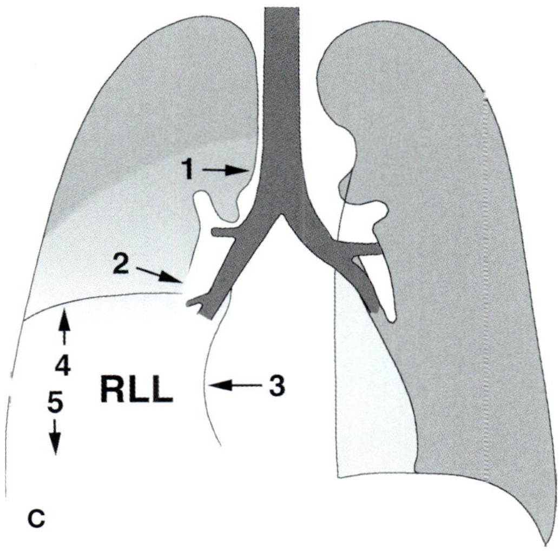

Figure 1.21. The silhouette sign in right lower lobe pneumonia. **A:** The frontal view shows right lower lobe consolidation with obscuration of the diaphragm. The right heart border (*arrows*) remains visible as an edge. **B:** On the lateral view, complete right lower lobe consolidation is visible, outlined anteriorly by the major fissure (*white arrows*). The right hemidiaphragm (*large black arrows*) is sharply marginated anterior to the consolidated lobe but is invisible posteriorly. The posterior left heart border and left hemidiaphragm are sharply marginated (*small black arrows*). **C:** Typical findings of right lower lobe (RUL) consolidation: (*1*) the superior mediastinum is well seen, (*2*) the inferior right hilum is obscured, (*3*) the right heart border remains visible, (*4*) the right hemidiaphragm is obscured, and (*5*) the right minor fissure remains visible as a line.

Left hemidiaphragm or descending aorta = left lower lobe (see Fig. 1.23).

Caveat: The diaphragmatic contour seen on the frontal (PA or AP) radiograph represents the dome, or the highest point, of the diaphragm. The diaphragmatic dome is relatively anterior, and lower lobe consolidation may be posterior to it (see Fig. 1.24); in this case, the hemidiaphragm may remain visible.

The Silhouette Sign on the Lateral Radiograph

The silhouette sign can also be used on the lateral projection (Fig. 1.25). Being able to differentiate the right and left hemidiaphragms is fundamental to its use and is based on several observations.

In some patients, the major fissures can be distinguished on the lateral view, by relating them to the hemidiaphragm that they contact. The right major fissure may sometimes be identified because of its relationship to a visible minor fissure.

Posterior margin of the heart or posterior left hemidiaphragm = left lower lobe (see Fig. 1.23); hiatal hernia may mimic this.

Anterior right hemidiaphragm = right middle lobe.

Posterior right hemidiaphragm = right lower lobe (see Figs. 1.21 and 1.24).

If the border of a specific structure remains visible, absence of the silhouette sign may be used to indicate that an abnormality is *not* in that location. For example, if a lung abnormality is visible at the medial right base but the right heart border remains visible, the lesion is not likely to be in the middle lobe.

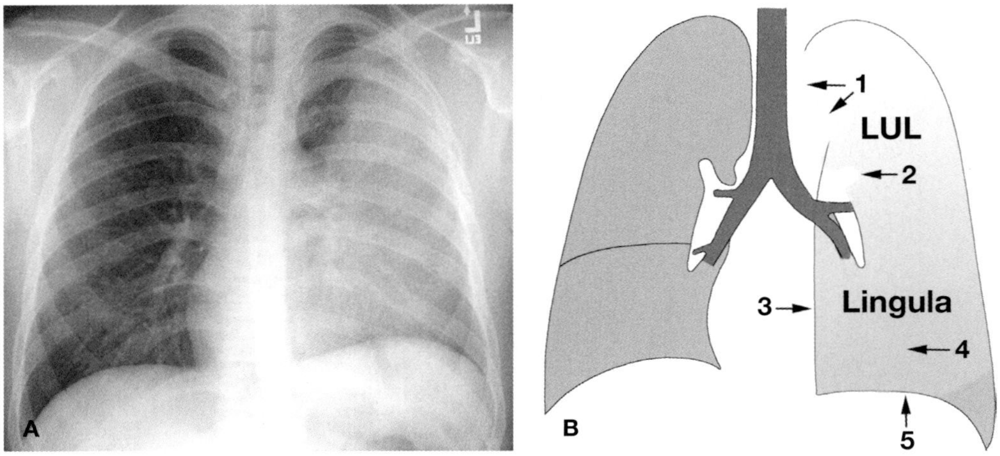

Figure 1.22. The silhouette sign in left upper lobe pneumonia. **A:** The left heart border is obscured because of lingular consolidation. The left superior mediastinum remains sharply marginated because the medial portions of the anterior and apical segments of the left upper lobe remain aerated. **B:** Typical findings of left upper lobe (LUL; and lingular) consolidation: (*1*) the left superior mediastinum and aortic arch are obscured, (*2*) the superior left hilum is obscured, (*3*) the descending aorta remains visible, (*4*) the left heart border is obscured, and (*5*) the left hemidiaphragm remains visible.

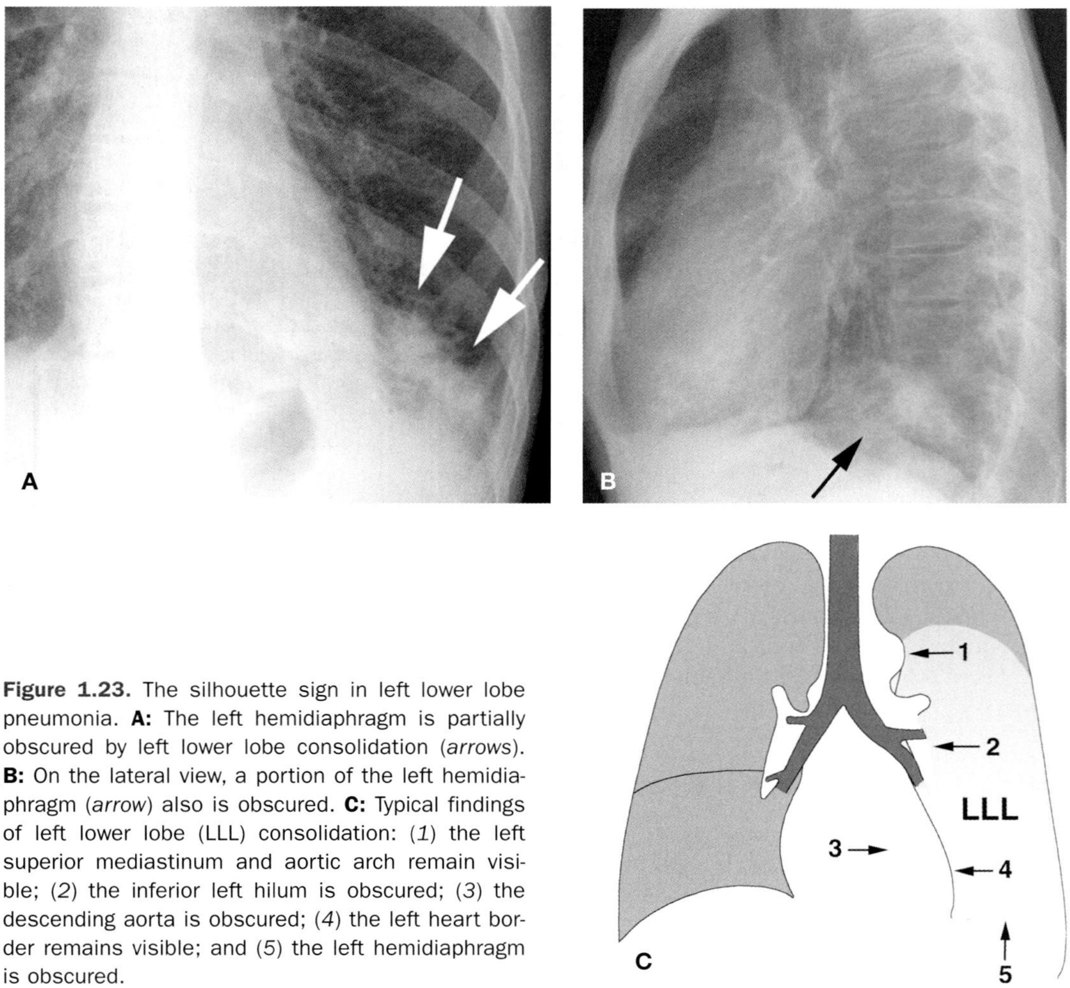

Figure 1.23. The silhouette sign in left lower lobe pneumonia. **A:** The left hemidiaphragm is partially obscured by left lower lobe consolidation (*arrows*). **B:** On the lateral view, a portion of the left hemidiaphragm (*arrow*) also is obscured. **C:** Typical findings of left lower lobe (LLL) consolidation: (*1*) the left superior mediastinum and aortic arch remain visible; (*2*) the inferior left hilum is obscured; (*3*) the descending aorta is obscured; (*4*) the left heart border remains visible; and (*5*) the left hemidiaphragm is obscured.

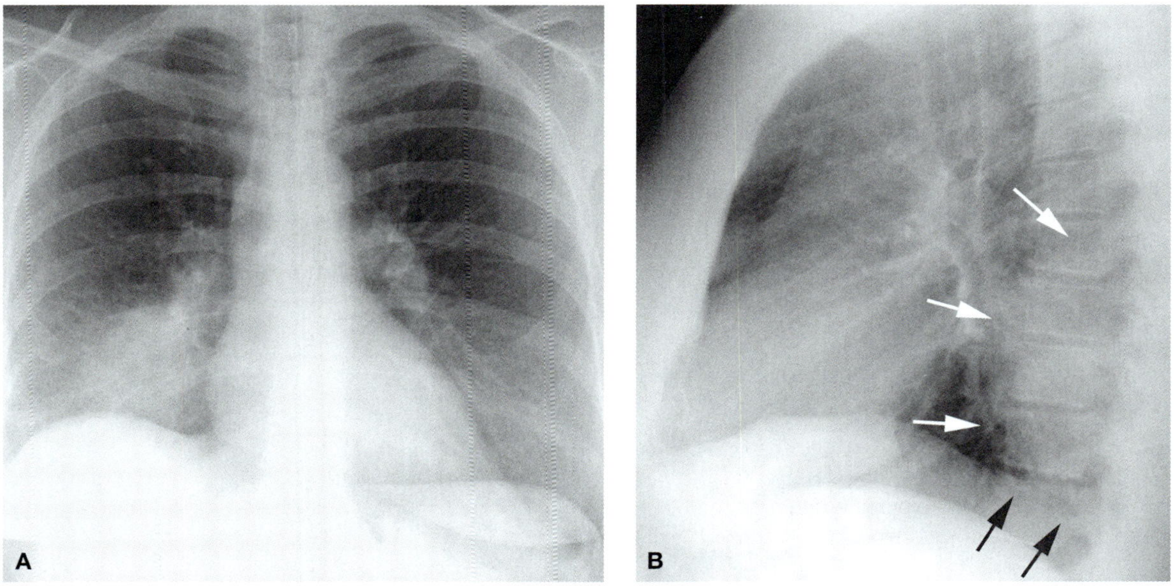

Figure 1.24. The silhouette sign (lateral radiograph) in right lower lobe pneumonia. **A:** There is focal right lower lobe consolidation, which appears to be segmental. The right hemidiaphragm is sharply defined because the consolidated lung is located posterior to the dome of the diaphragm. **B:** The lateral view shows consolidation (*white arrows*) that obscures the posterior aspect of the right hemidiaphragm (*black arrows*). The dome of the right diaphragm (seen on the frontal projection) is sharply marginated.

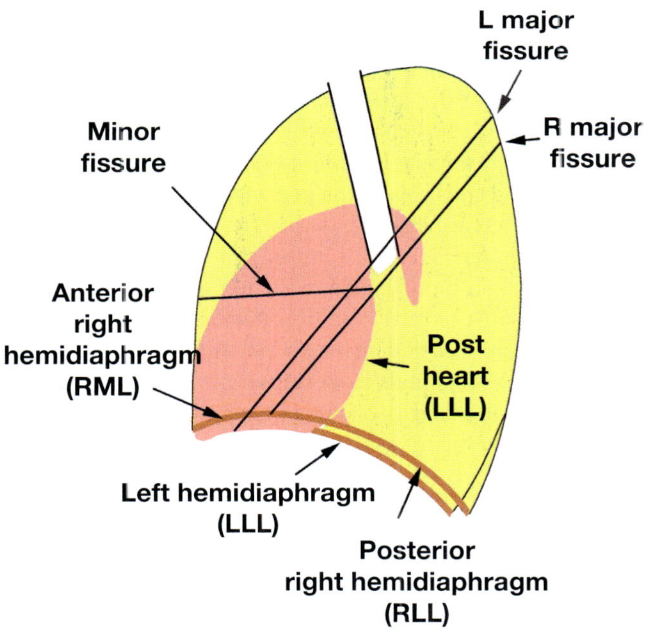

Figure 1.25. Anatomic relationships and the silhouette sign on a lateral radiograph. Obscuration of the borders shown in this diagram is associated with consolidation of the listed lobes. LLL, left lower lobe; RLL, right lower lobe; RML, right middle lobe.

ATELECTASIS

"Atelectasis" means "incomplete stretching" in Greek; in general use, it is synonymous with "collapse." In pulmonary radiology, the term *atelectasis* is used to indicate loss of lung volume, associated with a decrease in the amount of air within alveoli. Atelectasis (loss of lung volume) is usually, but not always, associated with lung consolidation (filling of alveoli by fluid). However, atelectasis and consolidation are separate processes, which may or may not, occur in combination.

The presence of atelectasis, in contradistinction to consolidation, may be important in differential diagnosis, as it may indicate bronchial obstruction by a variety of abnormalities. As with consolidation, atelectasis may or may not be lobar.

Types of Atelectasis

Four different types or mechanisms of atelectasis (lung collapse) are generally recognized (Table 1.3).

Resorption (Obstructive) Atelectasis

Resorption atelectasis occurs when alveolar gas is absorbed by circulating blood and is not replaced by inspired air. It occurs in the presence of airway obstruction. The obstructed airway may be the trachea, main bronchi, lobar bronchi, or multiple small bronchi or bronchioles. Small bronchial or bronchiolar obstruction by mucus resulting in resorption

Table 1.3 Types of Atelectasis

Resorption (obstructive) atelectasis
Caused by airway obstruction and resorption of alveolar gas
Occurs within 24 h
More rapid when breathing oxygen
May result in drowned lung with little volume loss
Collateral ventilation may prevent collapse
With large airway obstruction, air bronchograms are often absent
Relaxation (passive) atelectasis
Atelectasis due to pleural effusion, pneumothorax, or mass
Lung density need not be increased
Adhesive atelectasis
Atelectasis caused by loss of lung surfactant
Typical of respiratory distress syndrome of the newborn, acute respiratory distress syndrome, radiation pneumonitis
Cicatricial atelectasis
Atelectasis caused by lung fibrosis

atelectasis is common after surgery and general anesthesia and some types of pneumonia.

Bronchial obstruction usually results in distal lung becoming airless within 24 hours. Since oxygen is absorbed from the alveoli more rapidly than other inspired gases present in air (eg, nitrogen), resorption atelectasis occurs much more quickly when the patient is breathing pure oxygen; it may occur within minutes. Rapid resorption atelectasis may also occur in the presence of an endobronchial lesion acting as a one-way valve.

In the presence of bronchial obstruction, resorption of gas may be accompanied by rapid transudation of fluid from the circulating blood into the interstitium and alveoli (because of reduced interstitial and alveolar pressure). When this happens, lung may become airless (ie, consolidated) with only a minimal reduction in lung volume (see Fig. 1.26). This occurrence has been termed *drowned lung*. If the bronchial obstruction is relieved, the lung rapidly returns to normal density in most cases. This occurrence is common in ICU patients with mucous plugging or retention of bronchial secretions.

Obstruction of a main bronchus causes atelectasis of an entire lung. Air bronchograms are often absent in an obstructed and collapsed lung (see Fig. 1.26). In a patient with a lung collapse resulting from obstruction of small peripheral bronchi (by secretions), air bronchograms are usually visible. This occurs commonly in postoperative patients.

Obstruction of a lobar or smaller bronchus may or may not result in atelectasis, depending on the absence or presence of *collateral ventilation*. Collateral ventilation represents aeration of a lung lobe or segment because of air flow from adjacent alveoli (usually via the interalveolar pores of Kohn) rather than from its supplying bronchus. Collateral ventilation between adjacent lobes may occur in the presence of incomplete fissures. Collateral ventilation between smaller lung units (eg, segments) occurs more readily. The presence of lung disease, such as pneumonia, may prevent collateral ventilation.

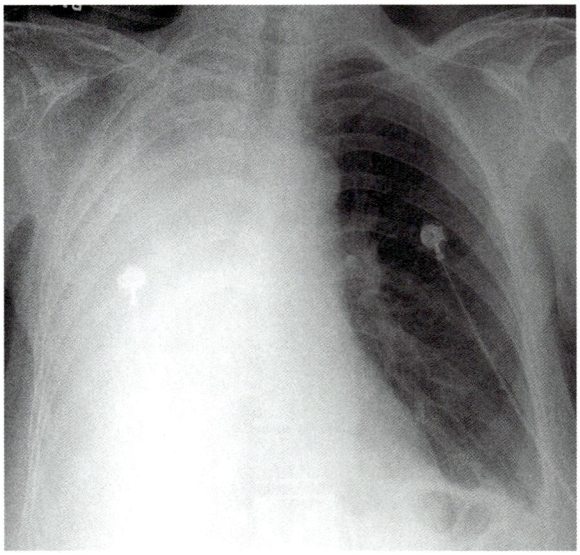

Figure 1.26. Drowned lung in acute bronchial obstruction by mucus. The right lung is nearly airless, but volume loss is minimal. Slight shift of the trachea and mediastinum to the right is visible. Air bronchograms are invisible because of central bronchial obstruction.

Relaxation (Passive) and Compression Atelectasis

The lung is elastic and normally stretches to fill the thoracic cavity because of negative intrapleural pressure. The presence of pneumothorax, pleural effusion, or a mass lesion allows the lung to decrease in volume or *relax* to its natural size, which is smaller than the size of the thoracic cavity. This is termed *relaxation atelectasis* or *passive atelectasis* (Fig. 1.27). The term *compressive atelectasis* can also be used to describe this occurrence, although it implies a reduction in lung volume beyond its normal relaxed state.

When lung collapses in the presence of pneumothorax, a significant increase in lung density (ie, consolidation) need not be visible (see Fig. 1.27B). Approximately half of the density of the lung is blood, and a reduction in lung volume typically results in a reduction in lung perfusion and a decrease in lung density. In patients with pneumothorax, until the lung becomes very small, its density is not usually increased. If increased lung density occurs in association with atelectasis, it is usually due to associated consolidation.

Adhesive Atelectasis

Surfactant reduces the surface tension of alveolar fluid and tends to prevent lung collapse as the alveoli decrease in volume with expiration. Deficiency of surfactant allows alveoli to collapse, the so-called *adhesive atelectasis*. This is most typical of respiratory distress syndrome of the newborn but is also seen in patients with ARDS, acute radiation pneumonitis, or hypoxemia and in the postoperative period.

Cicatricial Atelectasis

This term refers to loss of lung volume occurring in the presence of lung fibrosis. It may be focal, lobar (Fig. 1.28),

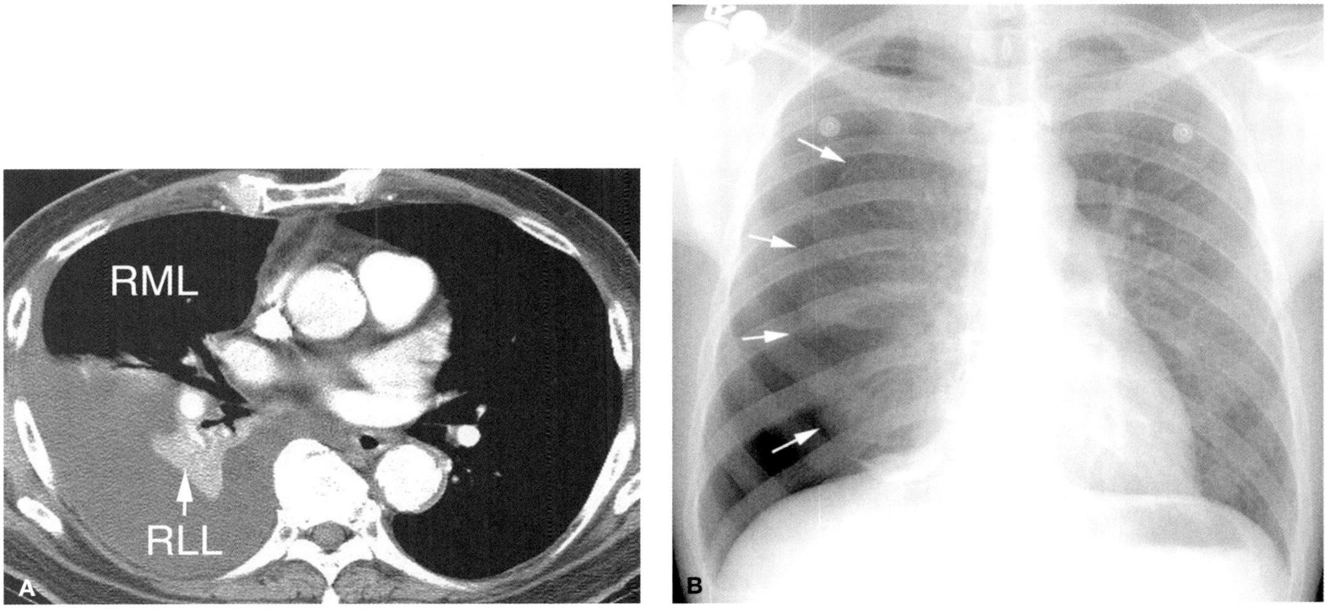

Figure 1.27. Relaxation (compression) atelectasis. **A:** Contrast-enhanced CT in a patient with a right pleural effusion shows right lower lobe (RLL) atelectasis. The right lower lobe is airless. Fluid in the major fissure allows the aerated right middle lobe (RML) to float anteriorly. Little if any mediastinal shift is present because the increased volume of the effusion is compensated for by the decreased volume of the lower lobe. **B:** Right pneumothorax with relaxation atelectasis of the right lung. Despite its reduction in volume (*arrows*), the right lung is not abnormally dense. Vessels in the right lung appear reduced in size compared to those on the left. This reflects reduced lung perfusion. The right lower lobe maintains its contact with the mediastinum because of the inferior pulmonary ligament. Air is seen within the minor fissure, separating the lobes.

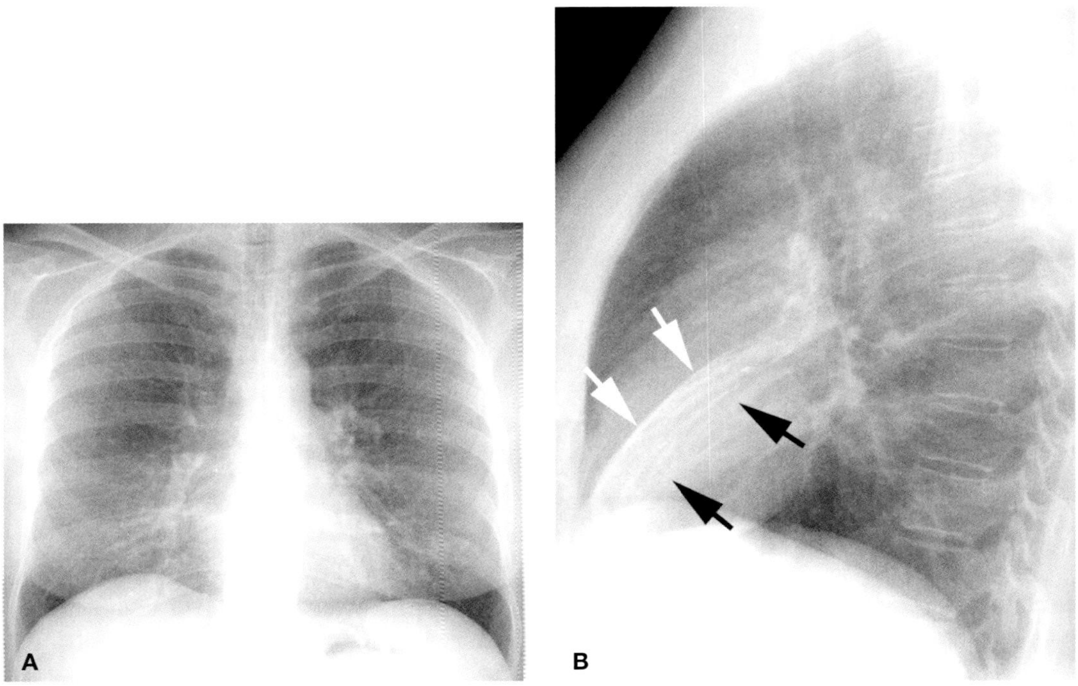

Figure 1.28. Cicatricial atelectasis in a patient with chronic right middle lobe collapse (right middle lobe syndrome) leading to fibrosis. **A:** Frontal chest radiograph shows poor definition of the right heart border, typical of right middle lobe consolidation. There is little increase in opacity at the right base. **B:** Lateral view shows volume loss in the right middle lobe with downward bowing of the minor fissure (*white arrows*) and anterior displacement of the major fissure (*black arrows*). Crowded air bronchograms are visible within the collapsed lobe.

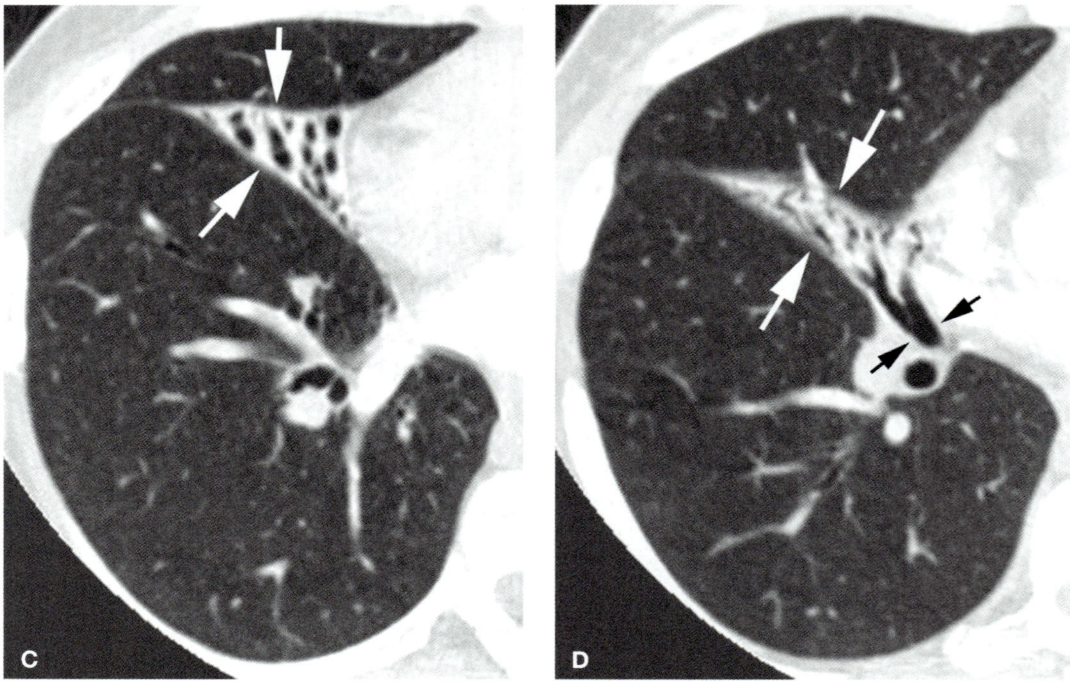

Figure 1.28. *(Continued)* **C, D:** CT scans at two levels show a typical appearance for right middle lobe collapse, having a triangular configuration (*white arrows*). The right middle lobe bronchus (*black arrows*) is patent, and air bronchograms are visible within the collapsed lobe. Collapse in the absence of bronchial obstruction is typical of right middle lobe syndrome. The dilated air bronchograms may indicate reversible bronchiectasis.

or diffuse, depending on the disease responsible. Findings of fibrosis are typically present.

RADIOGRAPHIC FINDINGS OF ATELECTASIS

Radiographic findings of atelectasis are usually considered as direct or indirect (Table 1.4). For practical purposes, the diagnosis is based on a combination of these findings.

Direct Signs of Atelectasis

Direct signs of atelectasis indicate loss of volume within an abnormal lobe.

Table 1.4 Radiographic Signs of Atelectasis

Direct signs: due to lobar volume loss Displacement of fissures Crowding of vessels
Indirect signs: secondary to volume loss Diaphragmatic elevation Mediastinal shift Compensatory overinflation of normal lung Hilar displacement Reorientation of the hilum or bronchi Approximation of the ribs Increased lung opacity Absence of air bronchograms Shifting granuloma sign

Displacement of Interlobar Fissures

Displacement of interlobar fissures is the best direct sign of atelectasis (see Figs. 1.28-1.30), but this finding is not always visible. The appearance of fissure displacement reflects the specific lobe involved. Specific patterns of lobar atelectasis are described below.

Crowding of Vessels or Bronchi

Crowding of vessels or bronchi in a given lobe reflects volume loss and is useful in diagnosis if a shift of fissures is not visible. Crowded air bronchograms may be seen in the presence of collapsed and consolidated lung (see Fig. 1.28B-D). Crowded vessels may be visible on radiographs if volume loss is present without consolidation. Vascular crowding in collapsed and consolidated lung is commonly seen on CT following contrast infusion in patients with atelectasis.

Indirect Signs of Atelectasis

Indirect signs of atelectasis are those not directly due to lobar volume loss but occurring secondary to it.

Diaphragmatic Elevation

Diaphragmatic elevation occurs because of ipsilateral volume loss (see Figs. 1.29-1.31). It is more common with lower lobe atelectasis than upper lobe atelectasis, although it may

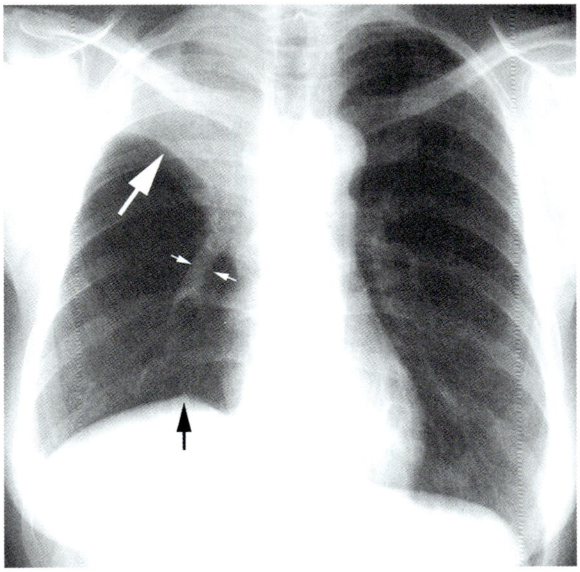

Figure 1.29. Signs of atelectasis in right upper lobe collapse. The right hemidiaphragm is elevated. The minor fissure is displaced and bowed upward (*large white arrow*). The right hilum is elevated compared to the left, and the descending pulmonary artery is rotated outward (*small white arrows*), being more easily seen than normal. The thin triangular opacity at the dome of the right hemidiaphragm (*black arrow*) is a so-called juxtaphrenic peak, which may be seen in upper lobe atelectasis.

be difficult to recognize if the lower lobe is consolidated. Diagnosis is based on knowledge of normal diaphragmatic position or comparison to prior radiographs.

The right hemidiaphragm is up to 2 cm higher than the left in 90% of normal persons. In about 10% of normal persons, the right hemidiaphragm is more than 3 cm higher than the left, the hemidiaphragms are at the same level, or the left hemidiaphragm is higher than the right.

Mediastinal Shift

Mediastinal shift often occurs with lobar atelectasis (see Figs. 1.31 and 1.32A). Shift of the upper mediastinum usually occurs with upper lobe collapse (see Fig. 1.31A) and is most easily recognized by shift of the trachea. Shift of the lower mediastinum predominates with lower lobe atelectasis (see Fig. 1.32A). This may be manifested by shift of the heart, anterior junction line, posterior junction line, or azygoesophageal interface. Shift of normal lung across the midline in a patient with atelectasis is sometimes referred to as lung herniation.

Compensatory Overinflation

Compensatory overinflation of normal lung on the same side as atelectasis appears as increased volume and decreased density of the lung, associated with splaying of vessels. Decreased lung density is easiest to see on CT.

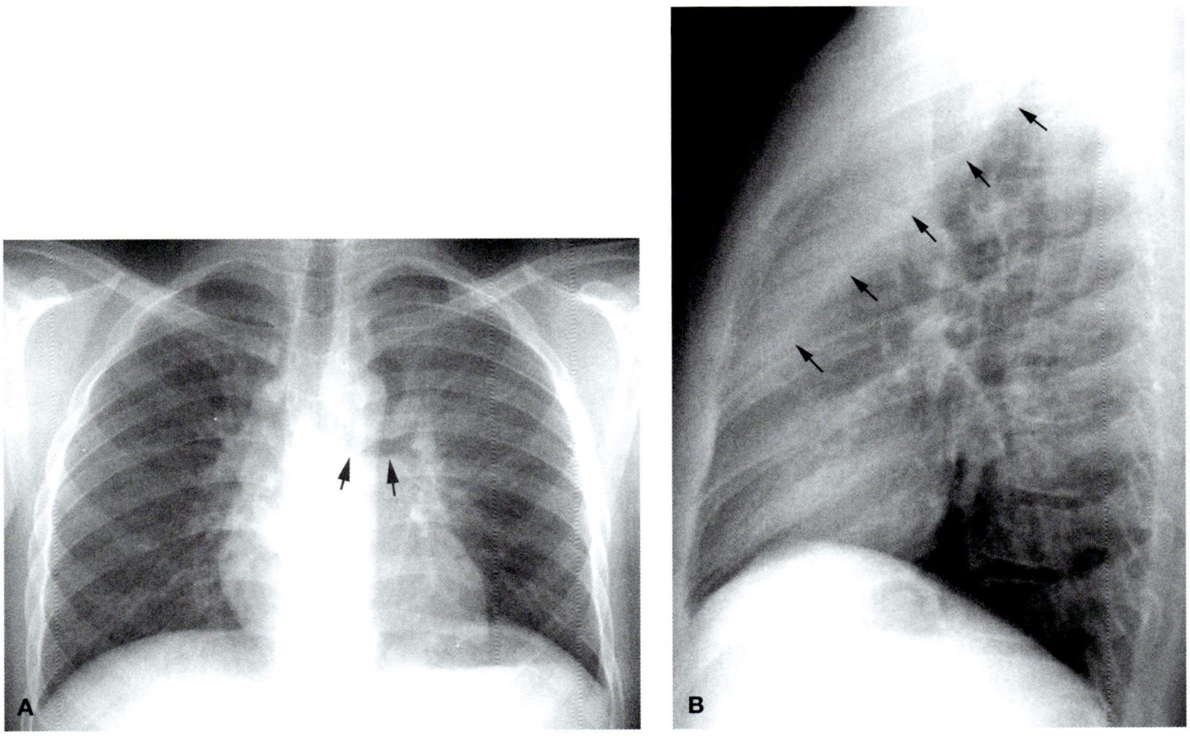

Figure 1.30. Signs of atelectasis in left upper lobe collapse. **A:** The left hilum is elevated. The left main and left upper lobe bronchi (*arrows*) are elevated and appear more horizontal than normal. The left hemidiaphragm is higher than the right, and a slight increase in opacity is seen in the left upper lung. **B:** Lateral radiograph in the same patient as (**A**) shows marked anterior displacement of the major fissure (*arrows*). As the left upper lobe loses more volume, it appears thinner on the lateral view and less dense on the frontal radiograph.

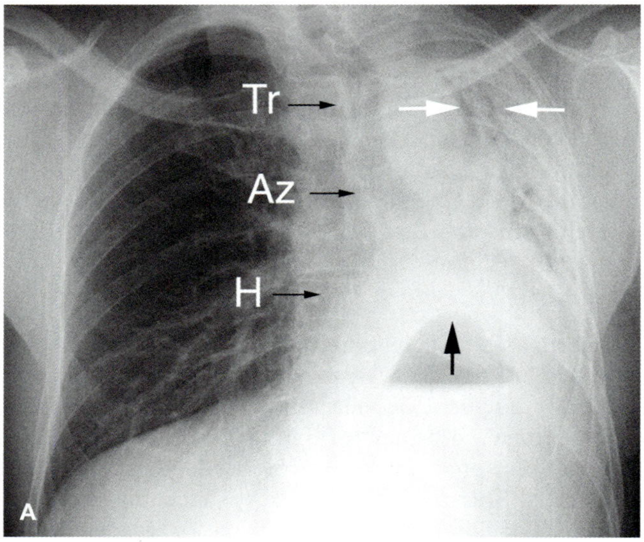

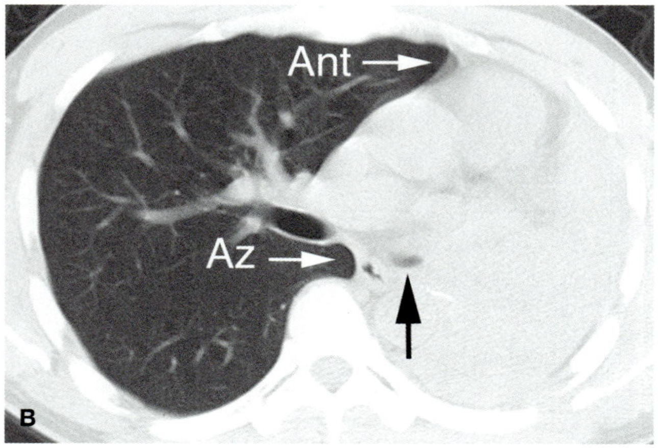

Figure 1.31. Left lung atelectasis due to tuberculosis with bronchostenosis. **A:** The position of the superior aspect of the stomach bubble (*large black arrow*) indicates elevation of the left hemidiaphragm. Marked leftward shift of the trachea (Tr), azygoesophageal recess (Az), and right heart border (H) is present. Air bronchograms (*white arrows*) are visible in the left upper lobe. **B:** CT shows narrowing of the left main bronchus (*black arrow*). The anterior mediastinum (Ant) and azygoesophageal recess (Az) are shifted to the left. Air bronchograms are not visible at this level.

Hilar Displacement

Hilar displacement may occur in the presence of upper or lower lobe atelectasis (see Figs. 1.29 and 1.30). The hilum is elevated in the presence of upper lobe collapse and depressed if lower lobe collapse is present. The left hilum is higher than the right in most normals.

If the hila appear to be at the same level, right upper lobe collapse or left lower lobe collapse may be present.

Reorientation of the Hilum or Bronchi

Reorientation of the hilum or bronchi occurs in association with hilar displacement. With upper lobe collapse, the hilum rotates outward, and the descending pulmonary artery and bronchi are less vertical than normal and more easily seen (see Fig. 1.29). The left main bronchus may appear elevated and more horizontal than normal in the presence of the left upper lobe collapse (see Fig. 1.30A). With lower lobe collapse, the hila are depressed, and the bronchi appear more vertical than normal.

Approximation of the Ribs

The ipsilateral ribs may appear closer together in the presence of ipsilateral volume loss (see Fig. 1.32A). Although this finding may be seen in patients with collapse, other findings of atelectasis will always be seen; never base a diagnosis on this sign alone. Rotation of the patient may mimic this appearance.

Increased Lung Opacity

An increase in lung opacity or attenuation may be seen, but this is nonspecific. It may indicate replacement of alveolar air by fluid (ie, drowned lung) or, when extreme, compressed, and airless lung tissue (see Figs. 1.28-1.32).

Absence of Air Bronchograms

In a patient with lung consolidation, the absence of air bronchograms suggests central bronchial obstruction (see Figs. 1.26 and 1.32). However, air bronchograms are sometimes seen in the presence of an (partially) obstructing central bronchial lesion (see Fig. 1.31A) or resorption atelectasis resulting from small peripheral mucous plugs.

In patients with atelectasis and air bronchograms, air-filled bronchi may appear dilated on plain radiographs or CT because of the collapse, simulating bronchiectasis. This is termed *reversible bronchiectasis* (an oxymoron) as it disappears following reexpansion of the lobe, and bronchiectasis is defined as irreversible bronchial dilatation.

Mucous Bronchograms

In the presence of bronchial obstruction, CT may show low-attenuation mucus within obstructed bronchi (see Fig. 1.32D), equivalent to air bronchograms. Mucus-filled bronchi may appear dilated. This may be due to large mucous plugs or irreversible bronchiectasis.

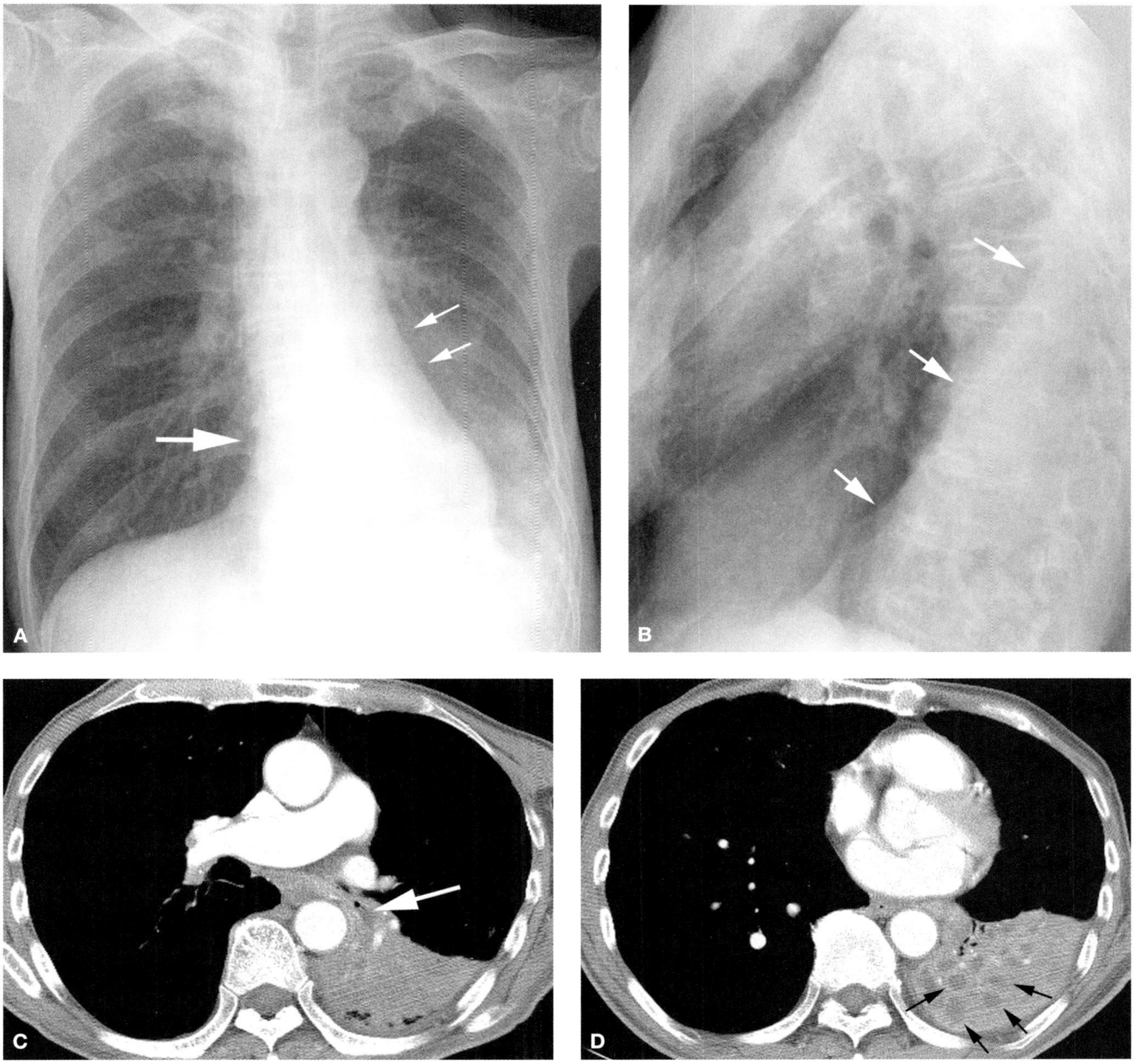

Figure 1.32. Left lower lobe atelectasis due to mucous plugging. **A:** Chest radiograph shows consolidation at the left base with obscuration of the left hemidiaphragm. The heart is displaced to the left (*large white arrow*). The left interlobar pulmonary artery is poorly defined, as is typical in left lower lobe atelectasis. There is flattening of the left heart border (*small white arrows*) due to leftward rotation of the heart and great vessels, termed the "flat waist" sign. The left ribs appear closer together than the right. **B:** Lateral view shows left lower lobe atelectasis with posterior displacement of the major fissure (*arrows*). **C:** Obstruction of the left lower lobe bronchus (*arrow*) is due to mucus. Mucus in the obstructed bronchus appears lower in attenuation than surrounding consolidated lung. Consolidation borders on the major fissure, which is displaced posteriorly. The mediastinum is shifted to the left. **D:** At a lower level, mucous bronchograms (*arrows*) are visible. The mucus-filled bronchi are dilated, but this represents "reversible bronchiectasis."

Shifting Granuloma Sign

Shift in the location of a parenchymal lesion visible on prior films may be seen in the presence of atelectasis.

Indirect Signs Seen With Specific Types of Atelectasis

Other indirect signs of atelectasis associated with specific types of atelectasis are described below and include the following:

Golden S sign: Right upper lobe atelectasis
Juxtaphrenic peak: Upper lobe atelectasis
Luftsichel sign: Upper lobe atelectasis (usually the left upper lobe)
Flat waist sign: Left lower lobe atelectasis
Comet tail sign: Rounded atelectasis

ATELECTASIS OF AN ENTIRE LUNG

Lung atelectasis usually results from obstruction of a main bronchus by an endobronchial lesion or mucous plug (or intubation of the opposite main bronchus), obstruction of small peripheral bronchi by secretions, or large ipsilateral pneumothorax or pleural effusion.

Bronchial Obstruction With Lung Collapse

With bronchial obstruction, common findings include elevation of the ipsilateral diaphragm, shift of both the upper and lower mediastinum to the side of atelectasis, relative apposition of the ipsilateral ribs, and increased lung density in comparison to the opposite side (see Fig. 1.31). The cause of bronchial obstruction may be evident. Absence of air bronchograms suggests a central obstruction; visible air bronchograms suggest peripheral small airway obstruction.

In the presence of bronchial obstruction with acute collapse, alveoli may rapidly fill with fluid, resulting in drowned lung. In this case, little mediastinal shift may be seen (see Fig. 1.26). If complete opacification of a hemithorax occurs acutely with significant mediastinal shift to the opposite side, pleural effusion is the likely diagnosis; if complete opacification of a hemithorax occurs acutely without significant mediastinal shift to the opposite side, drowned lung is the likely diagnosis.

Pneumothorax With Lung Collapse

Pneumothorax causes the lung to collapse centrally toward the hilum and mediastinum. The shape of the collapsed lung usually is maintained (see Fig. 1.27B). Because of the inferior pulmonary ligament, the lower lobe usually maintains its contact with the paracardiac mediastinum and diaphragm.

Until collapse is complete and the lung becomes airless, it may appear normal in density or relatively lucent despite its small size (see Fig. 1.27B). This occurs because of reduced lung perfusion associated with volume loss. Some shift of the mediastinum to the opposite side is typical in patients with a sizable pneumothorax regardless of the presence of tension.

Pleural Effusion With Lung Collapse

Massive pleural effusion results in relaxation or compressive atelectasis of the lung, a variable degree of mediastinal shift to the opposite side (depending on the size of the effusion and the degree of collapse), and variable opacification of the hemithorax (depending on the extent of residual aerated lung).

Large pleural effusion may result in loss of lung volume without complete lung opacification. Because a free effusion in an upright patient predominantly occupies the inferior hemithorax, the lower lobe is usually more compressed, contains less air, and appears denser than the upper lobe.

Collapsed lung is tethered at the hilum, and the lower lobe maintains its relationship with the mediastinum because of the inferior pulmonary ligament (see Fig. 1.27A). However, fluid often separates the peripheral part of the lobe from the chest wall and enters the major fissure or major and minor fissures, allowing adjacent lobes to float apart. These findings are difficult to recognize on chest radiographs unless the lung remains partially aerated. On CT obtained with contrast infusion, collapsed lobes opacify and appear denser than pleural fluid. On unenhanced CT, the collapsed lung usually appears slightly denser than fluid.

LOBAR ATELECTASIS: SPECIFIC APPEARANCES

Specific appearances are associated with collapse of an individual lobe, or lobes in combination. These appearances may be modified by the degree of volume loss, the degree of lung consolidation occurring in association with volume loss, and the presence of pleural effusion or pneumothorax.

Lobar collapse usually results from bronchial obstruction (resorption atelectasis). Lobar cicatricial atelectasis is less common but may be associated with chronic infection. Several general rules apply to lobar atelectasis:

1. Atelectasis usually results in bowing of a fissure toward the collapsed lobe.
2. An atelectatic lobe generally assumes the shape of a triangle or pyramid, with the apex of the triangle or pyramid directed toward the hilum.
3. Unless atelectasis is severe or pleural effusion or pneumothorax is present, a collapsed upper or lower lobe maintains its contact with the costal (peripheral) pleural surface. The middle lobe, on the other hand, commonly loses its costal pleural contact with atelectasis.
4. Because atelectasis is associated with decreased lung perfusion and blood volume, collapse does not result in increased lung density unless the lobe is moderately reduced in volume or air-space consolidation is associated with the volume loss.

5. With total lobar collapse, and in the absence of consolidation or drowned lung, collapsed lobes are small and thin and may be difficult to recognize en face on chest radiographs as an area of increased density.
6. Collapsed and airless lung often appears densely opacified on CT following contrast infusion.
7. Hilar masses causing collapse usually appear less dense than collapsed lung on contrast-enhanced CT.

Right Upper Lobe Atelectasis

Frontal (PA or AP) Radiograph

On the frontal radiograph, the minor fissure bows upward (Table 1.5; see Figs. 1.29 and 1.33A) in the presence of right upper lobe atelectasis. The medial aspect of the lobe maintains its relationship to the hilum, and its lateral aspect (marginated by the minor fissure) rotates upward toward the upper mediastinum in a clockwise fashion.

A collapsed and consolidated right upper lobe obscures the superior mediastinal contours. With complete collapse, the upper lobe is pancaked against the upper mediastinum. It may have a concave margin laterally, representing the displaced minor fissure, or may have a convex lateral edge, mimicking the appearance of mediastinal widening.

In patients with right upper lobe collapse associated with an obstructing lung cancer (the right upper lobe is the most common site for lung cancer) or other mass lesion producing bronchial obstruction, a characteristic appearance may be seen, termed *Golden S sign*. This sign refers to a combination of upward bowing of the lateral aspect of the minor fissure due to volume loss, with downward bulging of the medial fissure due to the presence of a hilar mass (see Fig. 1.33A). This combination results in a shallow reverse S appearance. Although described as a sign of right upper lobe collapse, a similar appearance may be seen in any lobe if the bordering fissure is visible in profile.

Table 1.5 Radiographic Findings of Right Upper Lobe Atelectasis

Frontal radiograph
Ill-defined increase in opacity in the upper thorax
Apparent right mediastinal widening
Silhouetting of the right upper mediastinum
Tracheal shift to the right
Upward bowing and displacement of the minor fissure
Golden S sign
Elevation of the hilum
Outward rotation of the hilum or bronchus
Right-sided juxtaphrenic peak

Lateral radiograph
Upward displacement and bowing of the minor fissure
Anterior displacement and bowing of the upper major fissure

Shift of the trachea toward the right may be seen as a result of right upper lobe volume loss. The hilum is typically elevated, and the bronchus intermedius rotates outward, appearing less vertical than normal (see Fig. 1.29).

With upper lobe atelectasis, a finding termed the *juxtaphrenic peak* may be seen on the frontal (PA or AP) radiograph (see Fig. 1.29). This appears as a small sharp triangular opacity near the dome of the ipsilateral hemidiaphragm. It is related to stretching of an inferior accessory fissure or folds or septa on the undersurface of the lung adjacent to the phrenic nerves or inferior pulmonary ligament.

Lateral Radiograph

On the lateral radiograph, the minor fissure bows upward and rotates superiorly, being anchored at the hilum (see Fig. 1.33B). The superior portion of the major fissure bows anteriorly in a similar fashion, and the lobe assumes the shape of a progressively thinner wedge as it loses volume. The collapsed upper lobe maintains its contact with the anterior chest wall. With marked upper lobe volume loss, a very thin dense wedge may be seen, associated with anterior displacement of the entire major fissure.

Computed Tomography

On CT, the minor fissure rotates anteriorly and medially as the upper lobe progressively flattens against the mediastinum, marginating its lateral aspect (see Fig. 1.33C). The collapsed lobe appears thinner near the hilum than in the apex unless a hilar mass is present. The lobe is usually triangular in cross section. The major fissure outlines the posterior margin of the collapsed lobe and may be bowed anteriorly (see Fig. 1.33D and E). In the presence of a hilar mass, an appearance similar to Golden S sign is visible with posterior bulging of the fissure.

Left Upper Lobe Atelectasis

Frontal (PA or AP) Radiograph

On the frontal radiograph, an ill-defined increase in lung density is typically visible, being most obvious in the upper portion of the hemithorax (Table 1.6). Increased lung opacity is usually associated with obscuration of the left superior mediastinum and left cardiac margin (because of the silhouette sign; Figs. 1.34A and 1.35A). However, with marked collapse, the left upper lobe may become very thin and difficult to recognize as being abnormally dense, and the silhouette sign may not be clearly seen (see Fig. 1.30A and B). If the lingular segments of the left upper lobe remain aerated, the left heart border may remain well defined. On the other hand, if lingular collapse is unassociated with collapse of the apical posterior and anterior segments of the upper lobe, only the left heart border is obscured.

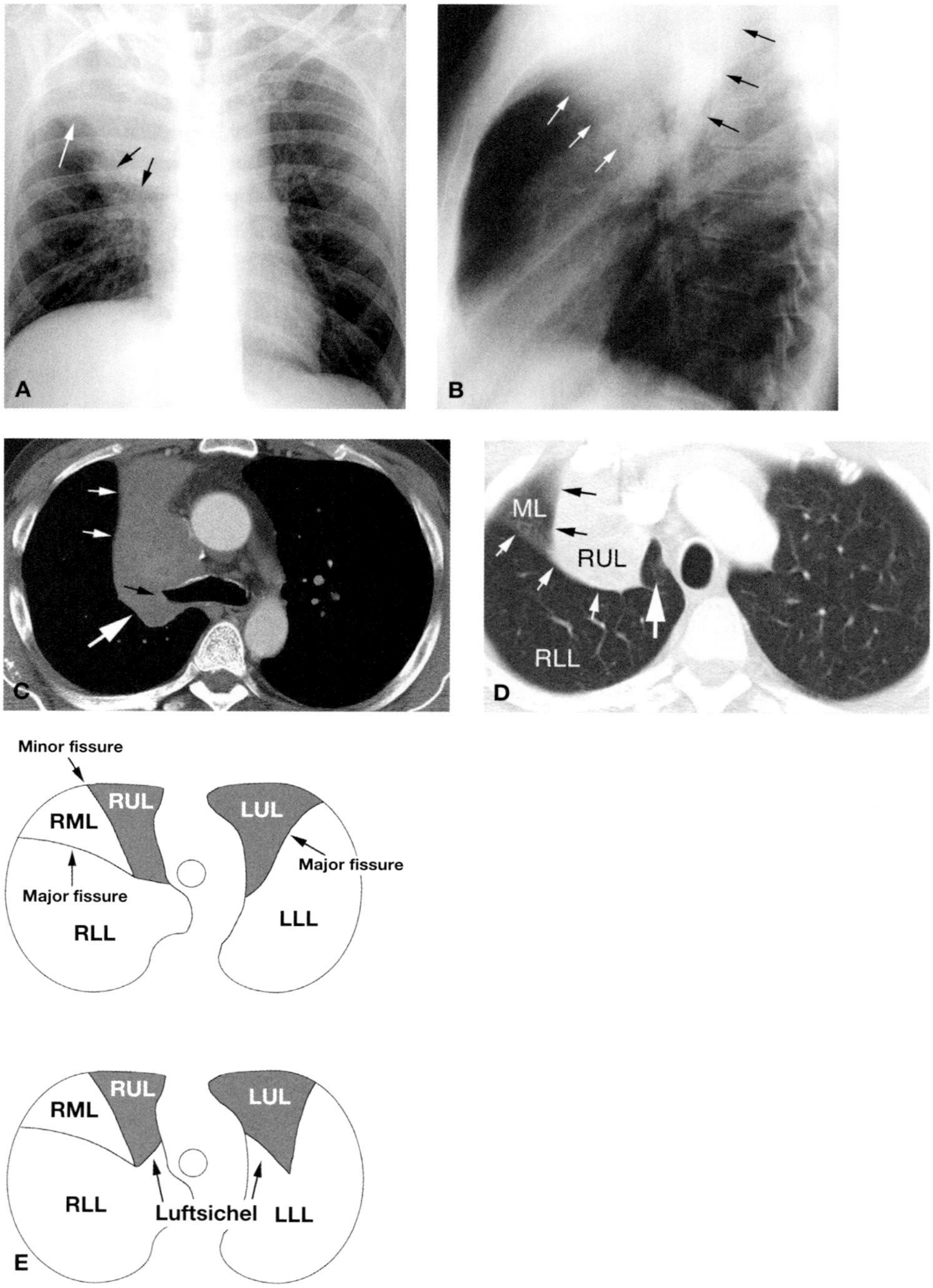

Figure 1.33. Right upper lobe (RUL) collapse with Golden S sign. **A:** PA chest radiograph in a patient with a right hilar carcinoma shows elevation of the lateral aspect of the minor fissure (*white arrow*) due to atelectasis and downward convexity of the medial fissure (*black arrows*) due to the hilar mass. Right upper mediastinal contours are obscured because of adjacent consolidation. The right hemidiaphragm is also elevated. **B:** The lateral view shows upward bowing of the minor fissure (*white arrows*), with the anterior aspect of the fissure being most displaced. There is anterior displacement of the upper portion of the major fissure (*black arrows*). The right upper lobe assumes the shape of a wedge as it loses volume. The collapsed upper lobe maintains its contact with the hilum and anterior chest wall. **C:** CT shows anterior rotation and bowing of the minor fissure (*small white arrows*) outlining the collapsed right upper lobe. The hilar mass results in bulging of the posterior aspect of the major fissure (*large white arrow*), resulting in the CT equivalent of the S sign. The right upper lobe bronchus is obstructed (*black arrow*). **D:** CT with a lung window setting at a higher level shows the collapsed and consolidated upper lobe (RUL) outlined laterally by the minor fissure (*black arrows*) and posteriorly by the anteriorly displaced major fissure (*small white arrows*). A tongue of lung extending medial to the collapsed lobe (*large white arrow*) represents a portion of superior segment of lower lobe. This may result in a luftsichel sign visible on a plain radiograph. ML, middle lobe; RLL, right lower lobe. **E:** Diagram of right and left upper lobe collapse on CT. In some cases, lung extending medial to the collapsed lobe may result in a luftsichel sign, as seen on a chest radiograph. LLL, left lower lobe; LUL, left upper lobe; RLL, right lower lobe; RML, right middle lobe; RUL, right upper lobe.

Table 1.6 Radiographic Findings of Left Upper Lobe Atelectasis

Frontal radiograph

Ill-defined increase in opacity in the upper thorax (decreasing with increased collapse)
Silhouetting of the left upper mediastinum
Tracheal shift to the left
Luftsichel sign
Apical cap
Elevation of the hilum
Outward rotation of the hilum or bronchus
Juxtaphrenic peak

Lateral radiograph

Anterior bowing and displacement of the major fissure

In the presence of upper lobe atelectasis and anterior shift of the major fissure, the superior segment of the lower lobe expands to occupy the apex of the hemithorax. On the frontal radiograph, the superior segment may insinuate itself between the upper lobe and the mediastinum, resulting in an interface where lucent lung contacts collapsed lung. This interface is often crescentic in appearance and has been termed the "luftsichel" *sign* (luftsichel means "air crescent" in German; see Fig. 1.35A). The luftsichel sign is less common with right upper lobe collapse.

If the expanded superior segment does not reach the apex of the hemithorax (usually because upper lobe volume loss is not marked), the airless upper lobe may result in the appearance of a crescentic soft-tissue density shadow over the lung apex (termed an *apical cap*), mimicking apical pleural

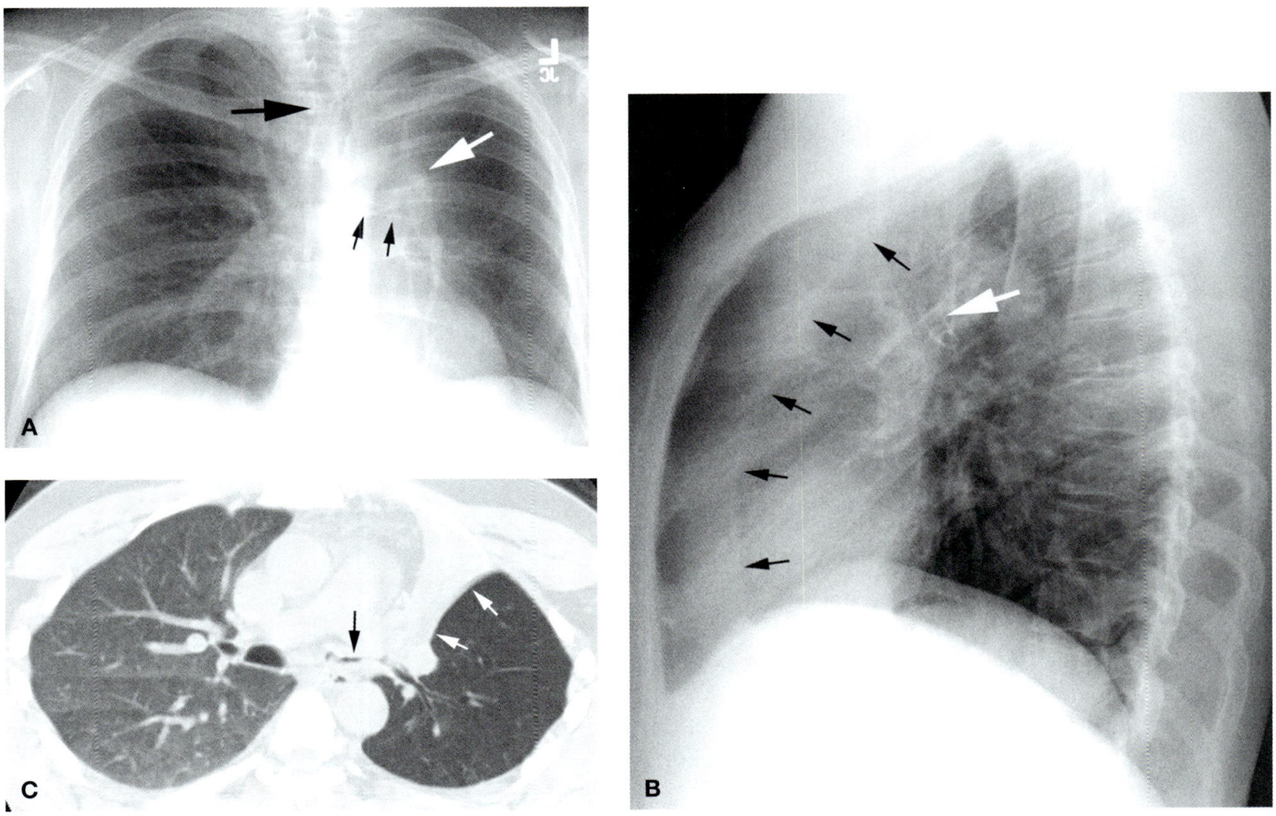

Figure 1.34. Left upper lobe atelectasis associated with bronchostenosis. **A:** The frontal radiograph shows tracheal shift to the left (*large black arrow*), elevation of the left hilum (*white arrow*), an ill-defined increase in lung density, and obscuration of the left superior mediastinum and cardiac border. The edge of the aortic arch, a relatively posterior structure, remains well defined. The left main bronchus (*small black arrows*), faintly outlined by a stent in its lumen, is elevated and appears more horizontal than is normal. The inferior left heart border remains sharply defined because of marked volume loss. **B:** On the lateral view, the left upper lobe is dense and there is anterior displacement of the major fissure (*black arrows*) paralleling the anterior chest wall. The stent within the left main bronchus (*white arrow*) is visible. **C:** CT shows anterior bowing and anteromedial displacement of the major fissure (*white arrows*). The left main bronchus (*black arrow*) is narrowed. A relative decrease in the density of the left lower lobe is due to compensatory hyperexpansion.

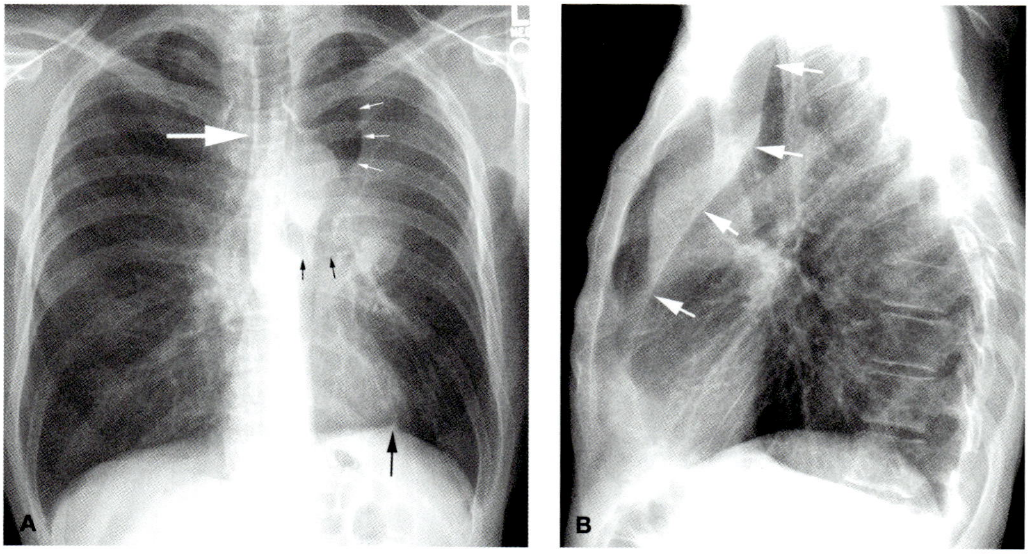

Figure 1.35. Left upper lobe collapse due to lung cancer. **A:** Frontal chest radiograph shows increased density in the left upper lobe region, but a crescentic lucency (*small white arrows*) in the medial aspect of the left lung apex represents insinuation of the aerated superior segment of the lower lobe, the so-called luftsichel sign. Other findings of left upper lobe collapse include tracheal shift (*large white arrow*), elevation of the left main bronchus (*small black arrows*), and a juxtaphrenic peak (*large black arrow*). A left hilar mass represents the carcinoma. **B:** Anterior displacement and bowing of the major fissure (*arrows*) are visible on the lateral view.

thickening or effusion, Pancoast tumor, or an extrapleural fluid collection (Fig. 1.36). This appearance has been termed *peripheral* upper lobe atelectasis. It may also be seen on the right.

As on the right, left upper lobe collapse may be associated with a left-sided juxtaphrenic peak (see Fig. 1.35A). Elevation of the left hilum may be seen; the left main bronchus may appear elevated and more horizontal than normal; and leftward shift of the upper mediastinum and trachea is typically present.

Lateral Radiograph

On the lateral radiograph, left upper lobe atelectasis results in progressive anterior displacement of the major fissure along a line paralleling the anterior chest wall (see Figs. 1.30, 1.34, and 1.35B). Lung anterior to the displaced fissure appears abnormally dense. With complete collapse, a very thin dense band may be seen along the anterior chest wall. The left hilum and bronchi may be displaced anteriorly.

Computed Tomography

On CT, the major fissure rotates anteromedially with upper lobe collapse (see Fig. 1.32C). If lingular segments remain aerated, the appearance closely mimics that of right upper lobe collapse. The luftsichel sign is associated with a V-shaped

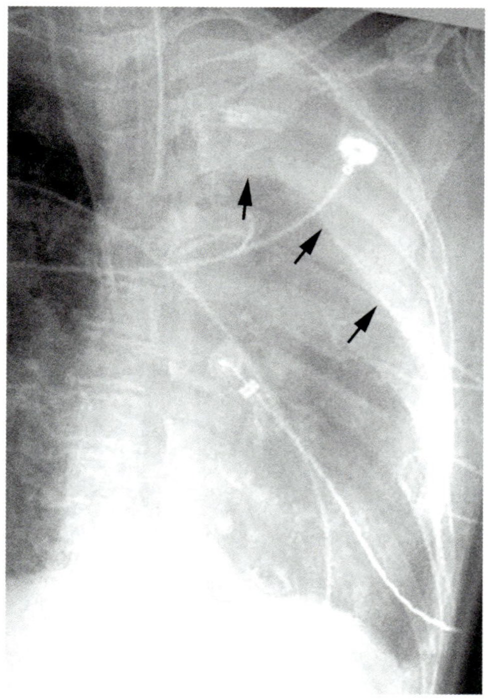

Figure 1.36. Left upper lobe collapse mimicking apical pleural thickening. A crescentic soft-tissue opacity at the left apex represents collapsed upper lobe outlined inferiorly by the aerated superior segment of the lower lobe (*arrows*). This appearance is sometimes termed *peripheral atelectasis*.

appearance at the posterior margin of the collapsed lobe, with the superior segment of the lower lobe extending medial to the collapsed lobe (see Fig. 1.33E).

Right Middle Lobe Atelectasis

Frontal (PA or AP) Radiograph

On the frontal radiograph, the minor fissure is usually invisible in the presence of middle lobe atelectasis; it rotates downward (as shown on the lateral view) and is no longer tangent to the x-ray beam (Table 1.7). Depending on the amount of consolidation and the degree of volume loss, increased lung opacity may be seen, obscuring the right heart border (see Figs. 1.28A and 1.37A). With marked volume loss, increased density may not be visible (see Fig. 1.28A), or the right heart border may appear normal. A lordotic radiograph may be helpful in showing the displaced minor fissure and area of increased density, but this is uncommonly used in clinical practice for making this diagnosis.

With middle lobe collapse, volume loss may not be sufficient to cause hilar displacement or mediastinal shift.

Chronic right middle lobe atelectasis may not resolve even if its original cause is alleviated. The presence of chronic inflammation or infection, bronchiectasis, and fibrosis may prevent reexpansion (ie, cicatricial atelectasis). The occurrence of chronic nonobstructive middle lobe collapse is often termed *right middle lobe syndrome* (see Fig. 1.28). It was originally described as occurring in association with tuberculous hilar lymph node enlargement resulting in transient bronchial obstruction. Typically, the right middle lobe bronchus appears patent, and dilated air bronchograms are visible in the collapsed lobe.

Table 1.7 Radiographic Findings of Middle Lobe Atelectasis

Frontal radiograph
Minor fissure is invisible
Increased lung opacity (decreasing with increased collapse)
Silhouetting of the right heart border
Lateral radiograph
Downward bowing and displacement of the minor fissure
Anterior bowing and displacement of the inferior major fissure
Wedge of consolidated lung anchored at the hilum

Lateral Radiograph

On the lateral radiograph, middle lobe collapse results in upward bowing and displacement of the inferior major fissure and downward displacement of the minor fissure, resulting in a thin wedge-shaped opacity with its apex at the hilum (see Fig. 1.37B).

The appearance of right middle lobe collapse on the lateral view may mimic fluid within the major fissure. However, with fissural fluid, the lower edge of the opacity is often convex downward instead of concave downward, as is typical of middle lobe collapse. If a minor fissure is seen as separate from a similar wedge-shaped opacity, occurring in a normal position, fissural fluid may be diagnosed.

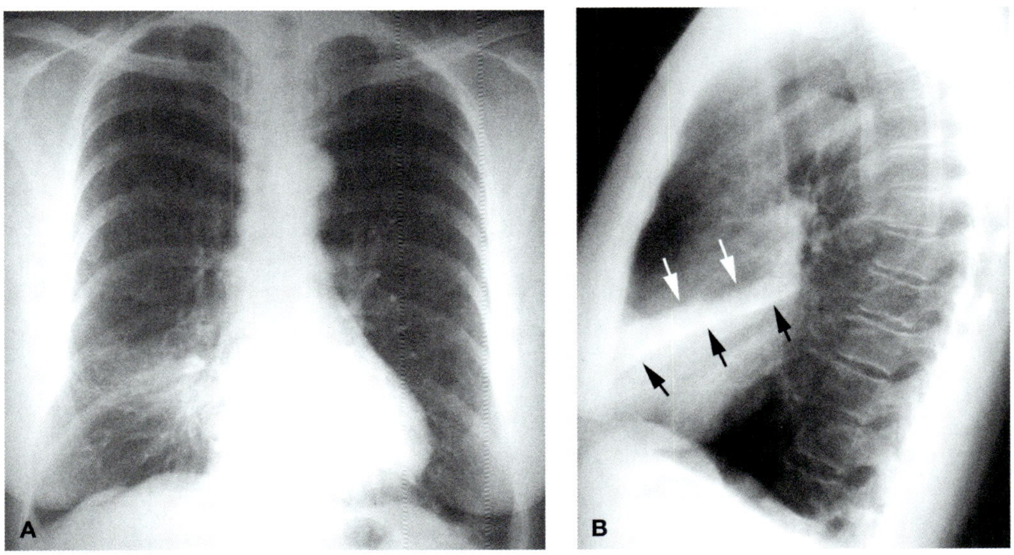

Figure 1.37. Right middle lobe collapse. **A:** On the frontal radiograph, ill-defined middle lobe consolidation obscures the right heart border. **B:** The lateral view shows downward displacement of the minor fissure (*white arrows*) and anterior displacement of the major fissure (*black arrows*). The collapsed middle lobe appears to be a thin wedge-shaped opacity with its apex at the hilum.

Computed Tomography

On CT, as the middle lobe loses volume, the minor fissure, which normally is difficult to see because it lies in the plane of scan, rotates downward and medially and becomes visible on CT. The collapsed lobe assumes a triangular shape, with one side of the triangle abutting the mediastinum and anchored at the hilum (Fig. 1.38). The apex of the triangle is directed laterally. The upper lobe is anterolateral to the collapsed lobe, and the lower lobe borders it posterolaterally (ie, the middle lobe is in the middle). These aerated lobes usually contact each other lateral to the collapsed middle lobe and separate it from the lateral chest wall.

Lower Lobe Atelectasis

Findings of lower lobe collapse are identical on the right and left.

Frontal (PA or AP) Radiograph

With moderate atelectasis, the major fissure may not be visible on the frontal radiograph (see Fig. 1.32A). With further volume loss, the major fissure rotates toward the mediastinum, resulting in the typical triangular or wedge-shaped opacity of lower lobe collapse (Table 1.8; Fig. 1.39A). Often, the upper portion of the major fissure is best seen. The apex of the triangle is at the hilum, and its base is at the diaphragm. Because of the inferior pulmonary ligament, the medial surface of the lower lobe maintains its contact with the mediastinum. With total atelectasis, a thin wedge of consolidated lung may be seen adjacent to the thoracic spine (Fig. 1.40A).

Lower lobe collapse usually results in downward displacement of the hilum (see Figs. 1.39A and 1.40A). The interlobar pulmonary artery is commonly invisible or poorly defined because of adjacent lower lobe consolidation. Obscuration of the diaphragm may be present on frontal or lateral radiographs.

Mediastinal shift is commonly present. Leftward shift and rotation of the heart with left lower lobe atelectasis may result in a straightening of the left mediastinal border, including the left heart margin, aorta, and pulmonary artery. This has been termed the "flat waist" *sign* (see Fig. 1.32A).

Right lower lobe atelectasis may result in downward displacement of the minor fissure seen on the frontal radiograph.

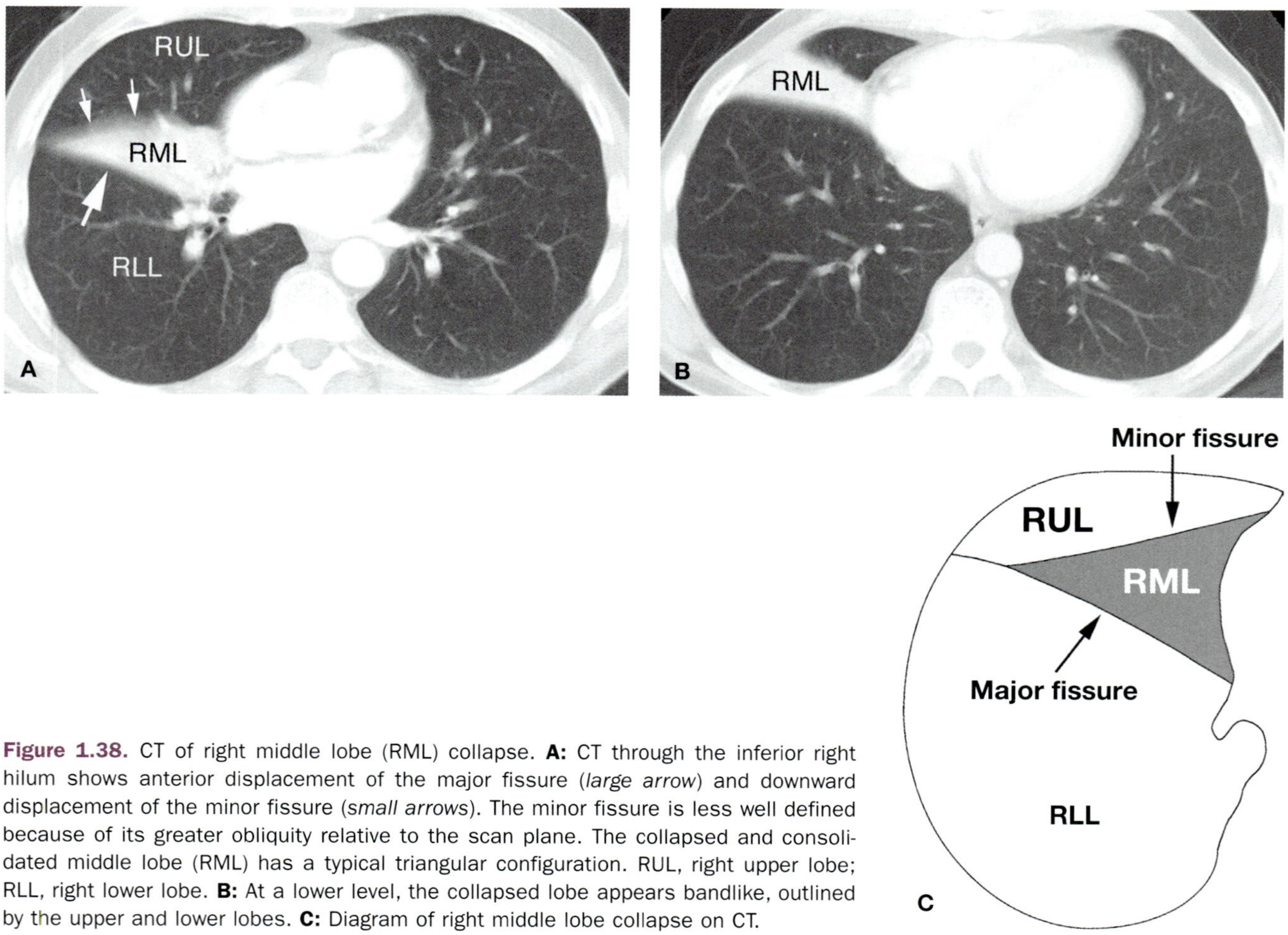

Figure 1.38. CT of right middle lobe (RML) collapse. **A:** CT through the inferior right hilum shows anterior displacement of the major fissure (*large arrow*) and downward displacement of the minor fissure (*small arrows*). The minor fissure is less well defined because of its greater obliquity relative to the scan plane. The collapsed and consolidated middle lobe (RML) has a typical triangular configuration. RUL, right upper lobe; RLL, right lower lobe. **B:** At a lower level, the collapsed lobe appears bandlike, outlined by the upper and lower lobes. **C:** Diagram of right middle lobe collapse on CT.

Table 1.8 Radiographic Findings of Lower Lobe Atelectasis

Frontal radiograph
Major fissure becomes visible (upper portion best seen)
Triangular opacity
Downward bowing of the minor fissure (right lower lobe atelectasis)
Downward displacement of the hilum
Invisibility of the interlobar pulmonary artery
Obscuration of the diaphragm
Shift of the heart
Flat waist sign (left lower lobe atelectasis)

Lateral radiograph
Obscuration of the posterior diaphragm
Posterior bowing of the major fissure
Increased opacity posteriorly (at least in part over the vertebral column)

Lateral Radiograph

In its early stages, lower lobe collapse results in posterior and downward displacement of the major fissure seen on the lateral view (see Fig. 1.32B). However, with more severe atelectasis, the lateral aspect of the major fissure rotates posterior and medially, and the fissure may become invisible on the lateral view (see Fig. 1.40B). Increased density overlying the lower spine may be the only visible abnormality (normally the thoracic spine appears less dense in the inferior chest than at higher levels; this may not be true in the presence of lower lobe atelectasis or consolidation). On the lateral view, the hilum and bronchi may be displaced posteriorly.

Computed Tomography

On CT, the major fissure rotates posteromedially from the hilum with collapse, it may be displaced posteriorly, or both (see Figs. 1.32, 1.39, and 1.40). The collapsed lobe contacts

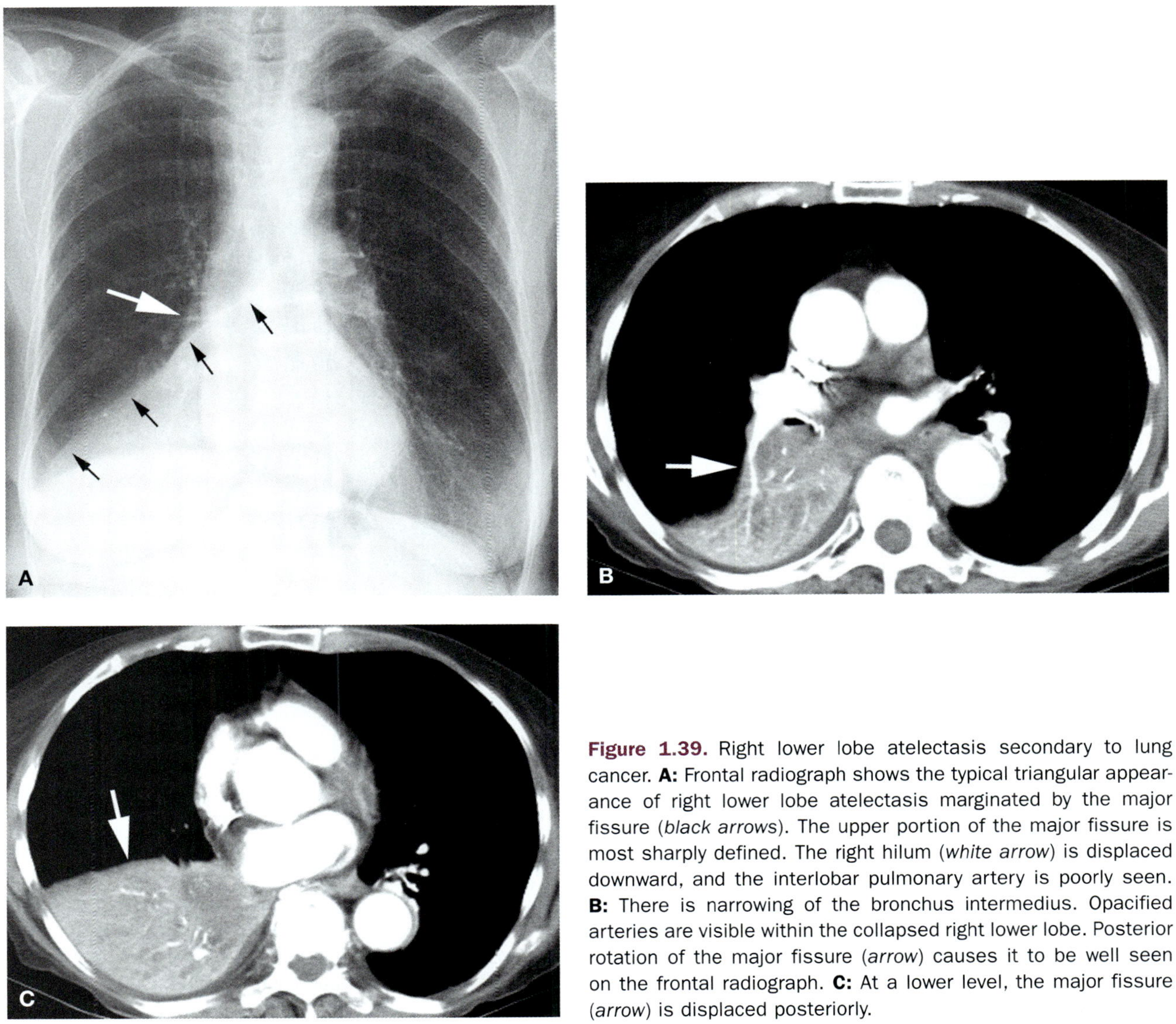

Figure 1.39. Right lower lobe atelectasis secondary to lung cancer. **A:** Frontal radiograph shows the typical triangular appearance of right lower lobe atelectasis marginated by the major fissure (*black arrows*). The upper portion of the major fissure is most sharply defined. The right hilum (*white arrow*) is displaced downward, and the interlobar pulmonary artery is poorly seen. **B:** There is narrowing of the bronchus intermedius. Opacified arteries are visible within the collapsed right lower lobe. Posterior rotation of the major fissure (*arrow*) causes it to be well seen on the frontal radiograph. **C:** At a lower level, the major fissure (*arrow*) is displaced posteriorly.

the posterior mediastinum and posteromedial chest wall and maintains contact with the medial diaphragm.

Combined Collapse of Right Middle and Lower Lobes

This occurs in patients with obstruction of the bronchus intermedius. On the frontal and lateral radiographs, both the displaced major and minor fissures may be variably visible, outlining the consolidated lung. On the frontal view, both the right heart border and diaphragm often appear obscured (Fig. 1.41). This appearance may closely mimic that of right lower lobe collapse associated with an elevated hemidiaphragm or subpulmonic pleural effusion. Absence of a visible minor fissure at a higher level and obscuration of the right heart border favors combined collapse.

Combined Collapse of Right Middle and Upper Lobes

This combination cannot be explained by a single bronchial lesion, an occurrence termed the *double lesion sign*. This most commonly occurs when lung cancer involves the hilum, with invasion of both the upper and middle lobe bronchi, while the lower lobe bronchus remains patent; it may also be seen with multiple isolated bronchial lesions, as in a patient with mucous plugging.

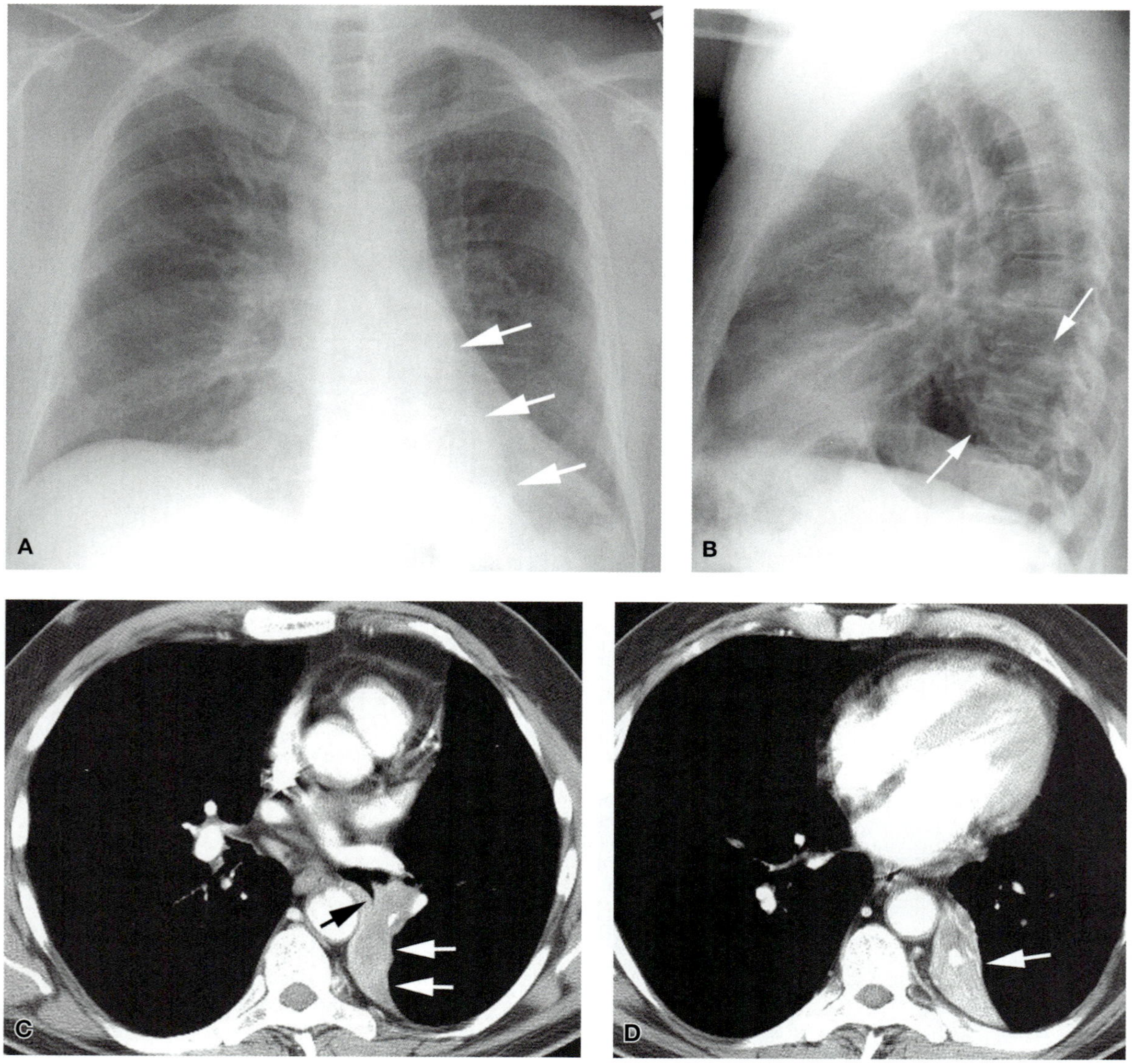

Figure 1.40. Marked left lower lobe atelectasis secondary to lung cancer. **A:** On the frontal radiograph, a thin wedge of consolidated lung (*arrows*) is seen adjacent to the spine. This represents the collapsed lower lobe. The heart is displaced to the left. **B:** Lateral view shows a vague opacity (*arrows*) in the region of the lower lobe. **C, D:** CT shows obstruction of the lower lobe bronchus (*black arrow*) and marked posteromedial rotation of the major fissure (*white arrows*).

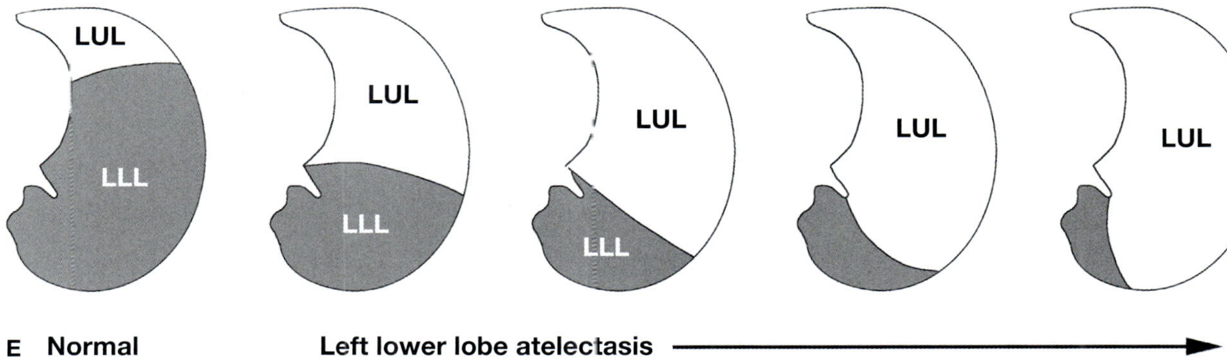

Figure 1.40. *(Continued)* **E:** Diagram of CT appearances of lower lobe atelectasis. With progressive atelectasis (*left to right*), the major fissure rotates posteriorly. LLL, left lower lobe; LUL, left upper lobe.

On the frontal radiograph, right upper lobe opacification obscures the right superior mediastinum, while right middle lobe opacification obscures the right heart border (Fig. 1.42A). Since both lobes anterior to the major fissure are collapsed, the appearance of combined middle and upper lobe collapse on the lateral radiograph is identical to that of left upper lobe atelectasis (see Fig. 1.42B).

SEGMENTAL ATELECTASIS

Segmental (or subsegmental) atelectasis may occur secondary to obstruction of segmental (or subsegmental) bronchi by tumor, mucus, or inflammatory disease. Typically, wedge-shaped opacities are seen radiating outward from the hilum or involving the peripheral lung, with the base of the wedge touching the pleural surface. Indirect findings of volume loss are typically absent because of the small amount of lung tissue involved.

PLATELIKE OR DISCOID ATELECTASIS

Linear areas of atelectasis, a few millimeters to 1 cm thick and at least several centimeters in length, commonly occur in patients with decreased depth of breathing or diminished diaphragmatic excursions. They tend to occur at the lung bases, several centimeters above and parallel to the diaphragm (Fig. 1.43). They cross segmental boundaries. They may also occur in the medial infrahilar regions, typically angled upward from the mediastinum at about a 45-degree angle. They are thought to occur because of decreased ventilation of lung

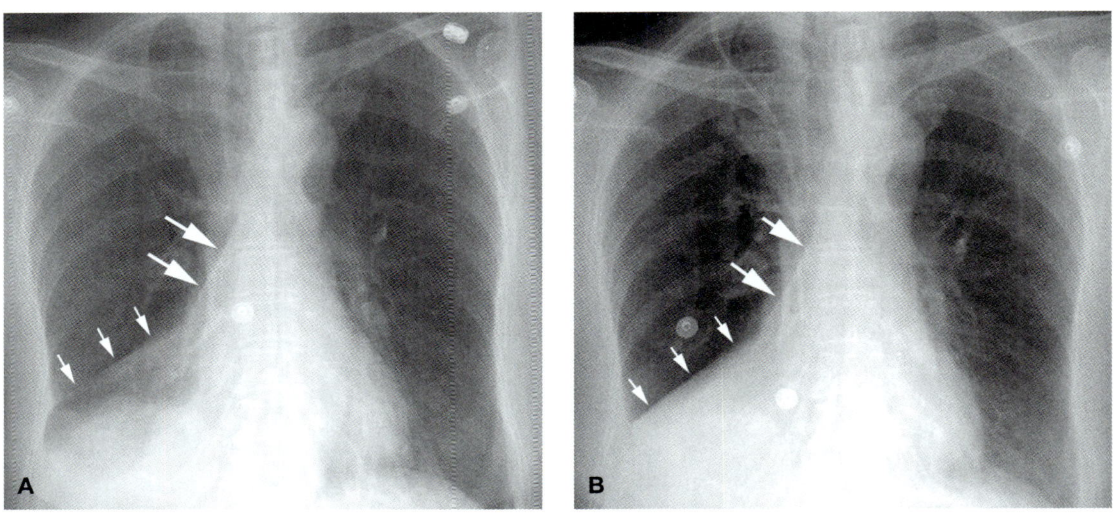

Figure 1.41. Combined right middle and right lower lobe atelectasis. **A:** The superior aspect of the major fissure (*large arrows*) is visible, marginating the collapsed lower lobe. The major fissure merges inferiorly with the minor fissure (*small arrows*), which is displaced inferiorly. The right middle and lower lobes remain partially aerated. **B:** One day later, both the middle and lower lobes are consolidated (drowned lung). The major (*large arrows*) and minor (*small arrows*) fissures sharply marginate the consolidated (drowned) lung. Both the right heart border and diaphragm are obscured.

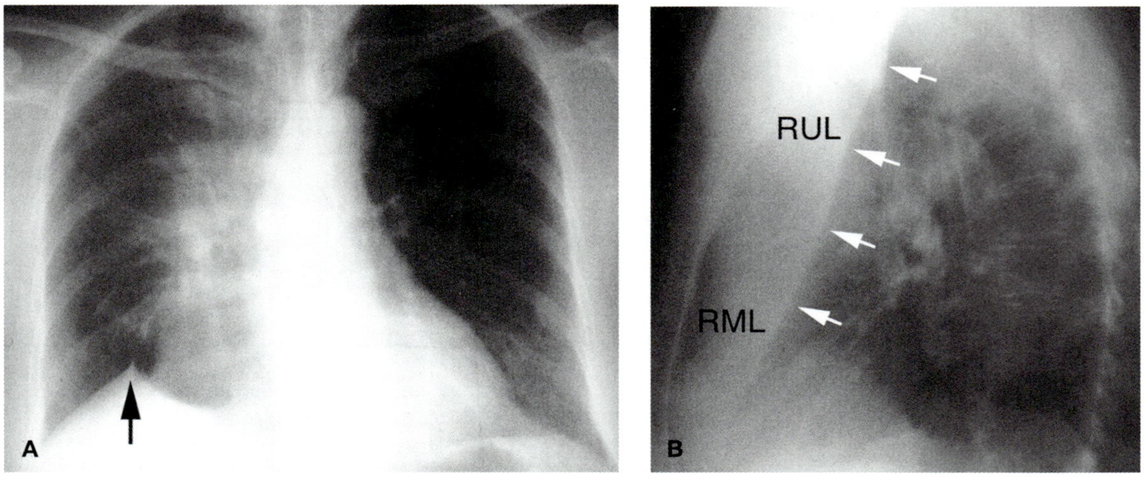

Figure 1.42. Combined right middle and right upper lobe atelectasis in a patient with right hilar lung cancer. **A:** Right-sided volume loss is present with mediastinal shift to the right. The upper mediastinal contour and right heart border are partially obscured and poorly defined. The right hemidiaphragm is elevated, and a juxtaphrenic peak is visible (*arrow*). **B:** The lateral view shows anterior displacement of the major fissure (*arrows*) because of collapse of both right upper (RUL) and middle (RML) lobes. Both lobes are homogeneously consolidated. This appearance mimics that of left upper lobe collapse.

associated with retained secretions. Bronchial obstruction is not a cause. They are of little clinical significance but serve as a marker of poor ventilatory function.

ROUNDED ATELECTASIS

The term "rounded atelectasis" refers to the presence of focal rounded lung collapse. In some patients, it is associated with invagination of the visceral pleura with folding or rolling of the collapsed lung. It usually occurs in the presence of pleural thickening or effusion, and likely results from local restriction of lung expansion. It is most commonly associated with asbestos exposure, empyema, tuberculous effusions, renal failure, and pleural neoplasm but may occur with pleural effusion of any cause. On plain radiographs, rounded atelectasis may mimic neoplasm, but its CT appearance is often characteristic.

To suggest the diagnosis of rounded atelectasis on the basis of chest radiographs or CT, the opacity should be (1) round or elliptical; (2) associated with an ipsilateral pleural abnormality, either effusion or pleural thickening; (3) peripheral in location, having significant contact with the abnormal pleural surface; (4) associated with curving of pulmonary vessels or bronchi into the edge of the lesion (the so-called *comet tail sign*); and (5) associated with volume loss in the affected lobe (Figs. 1.44 and 1.45; Table 1.9). If each

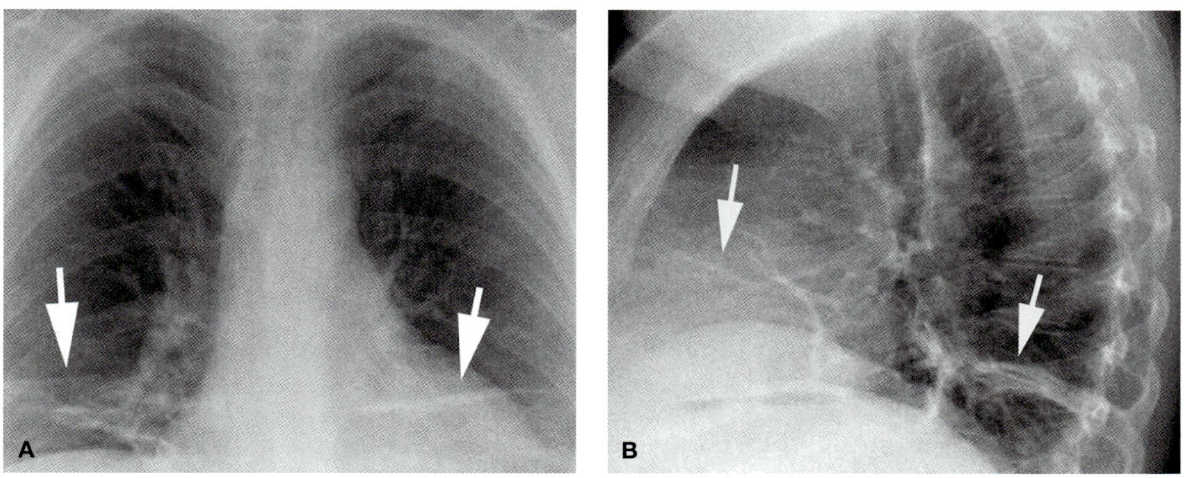

Figure 1.43. Disk atelectasis. Frontal (**A**) and lateral (**B**) radiographs show disk atelectasis (*arrows*) at the lung bases, roughly paralleling the hemidiaphragms.

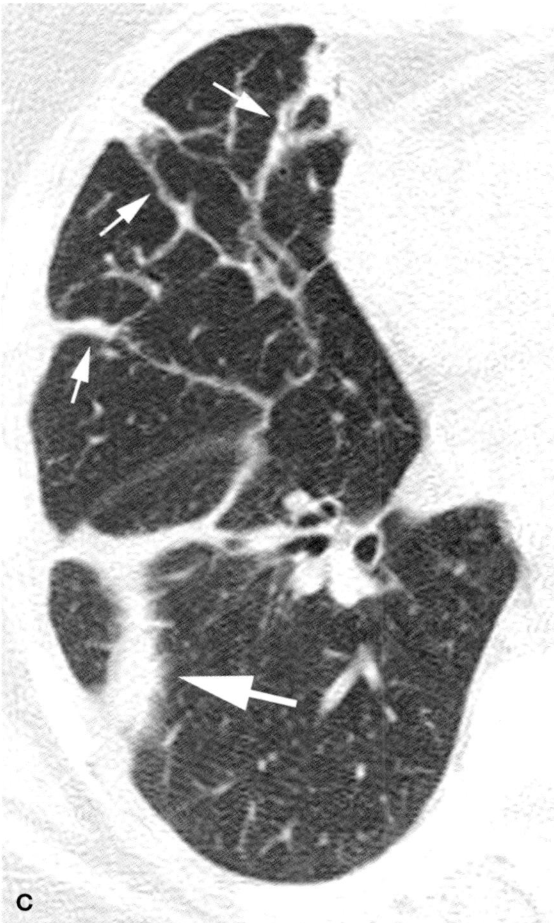

Figure 1.43. *(Continued)* **C:** HRCT at the right base shows linear areas of atelectasis (*small arrows*). When these are oriented parallel to the plane of scan, large areas of opacity may be seen (*large arrow*).

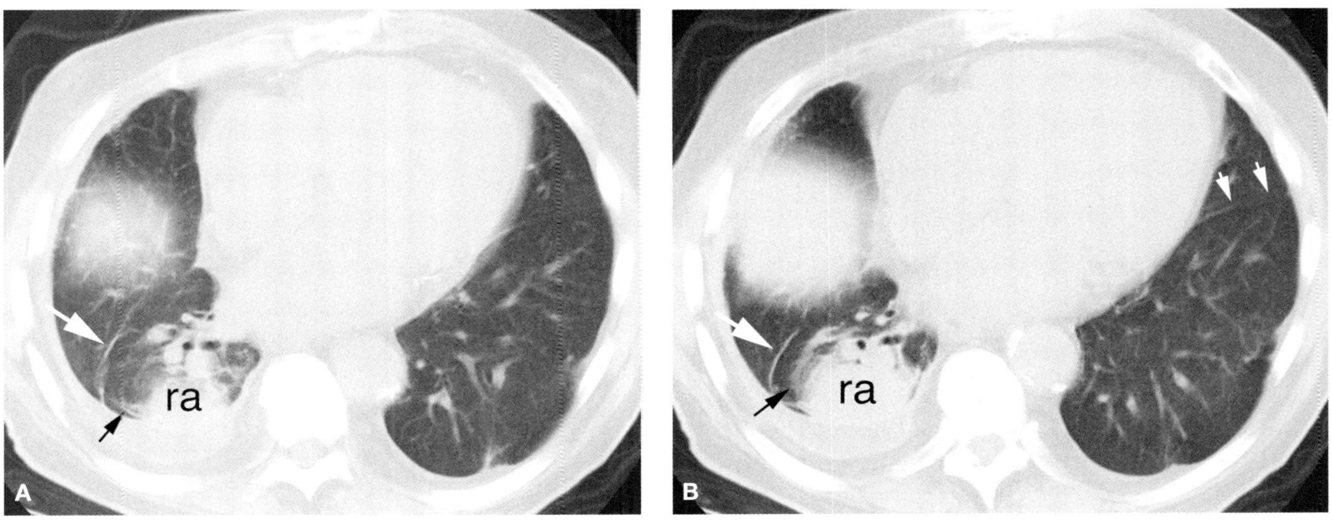

Figure 1.44. Typical rounded atelectasis (ra) associated with pleural effusion. CT scans at two adjacent levels (**A, B**) show characteristic findings of rounded atelectasis. An elliptical opacity is visible (ra), which is peripheral in location and has significant contact with the pleural surface in contiguity with a right pleural effusion. Vessels (*small black arrows*) curve into the edge of the lesion (ie, the so-called comet tail sign). Posterior displacement of the major fissure (*large white arrows*) indicates volume loss in the right lower lobe. For comparison, note the location of the normal left major fissure (*small white arrows*). Because these findings are typical, follow-up should be sufficient.

of these criteria for rounded atelectasis is met, a confident diagnosis can usually be made.

Rounded atelectasis is most common in the posterior lower lobes; this location is typical of patients with free pleural effusion (see Figs. 1.44 and 1.45). In patients with bilateral effusions, it may be bilateral or symmetrical. Rounded atelectasis in patients with pleural fibrosis may be anterior in location (Figs. 1.46-1.48).

On chest radiographs, posteriorly located rounded atelectasis usually appears ill-defined on the frontal projection and well-defined and elliptical on the lateral view, having extensive pleural contact. It is most often seen several centimeters above a blunted posterior costophrenic angle (see Fig. 1.45). Vessels may be seen curving into its inferior edge, representing the comet tail sign.

Rounded atelectasis may have acute or obtuse angles where it contacts the pleura. Since rounded atelectasis represents collapsed lung parenchyma, it can show significant enhancement on CT following the intravenous injection of contrast agents. Air bronchograms may be visible within the collapsed lung.

Atypical examples of rounded atelectasis are often encountered in patients who have pleural thickening and fibrosis rather than pleural effusion (see Fig. 1.47). Such cases may show rounded atelectasis that is irregular in shape, unassociated with the comet tail sign, separated from the pleural surface, or anterior in location.

Table 1.9 CT and Radiographic Findings of Rounded Atelectasis

CT and Radiographic Findings of Rounded Atelectasis
Round or elliptical opacity
Associated with an ipsilateral pleural abnormality
Peripheral in location
Extensive contact with the abnormal pleural surface
Comet tail sign
Volume loss
Posterior, paravertebral lower lobe in patients with effusion
Atypical appearances when associated with pleural fibrosis
Dense opacification on CT after contrast infusion

Rounded atelectasis is seen in as many as 10% of patients with asbestos exposure, usually due to visceral or parietal pleural thickening or plaques, diffuse pleural thickening, or sometimes exudative effusion, and it often appears atypical. Atypical cases of rounded atelectasis may represent a diagnostic problem because lung cancer has an increased incidence in asbestos-exposed individuals. PET-CT and/or needle biopsy may be necessary to exclude carcinoma in cases where not all of the above criteria are met.

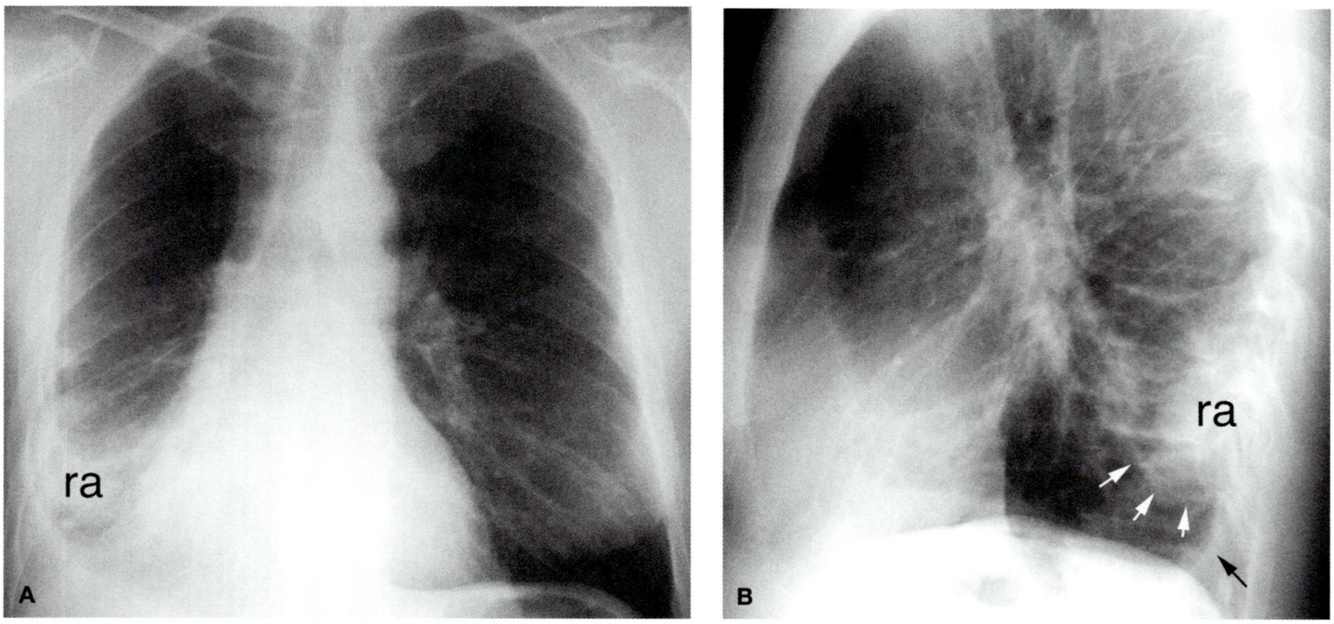

Figure 1.45. Typical rounded atelectasis (ra) associated with pleural effusion. **A:** Frontal chest radiograph shows blunting of the right costophrenic angle due to pleural effusion. An ill-defined opacity (ra) at the right base represents rounded atelectasis. Note the presence of mediastinal shift to the right. **B:** On the lateral view, a well-defined elliptical opacity (ra) is seen posteriorly, having extensive pleural contact. This location, several centimeters above the blunted posterior costophrenic angle (*black arrow*), is characteristic of rounded atelectasis in patients with effusion. Curving of vessels (*white arrows*) into the inferior aspect of the opacity reflects the comet tail sign. The appearance in this case is sufficiently characteristic to allow follow-up.

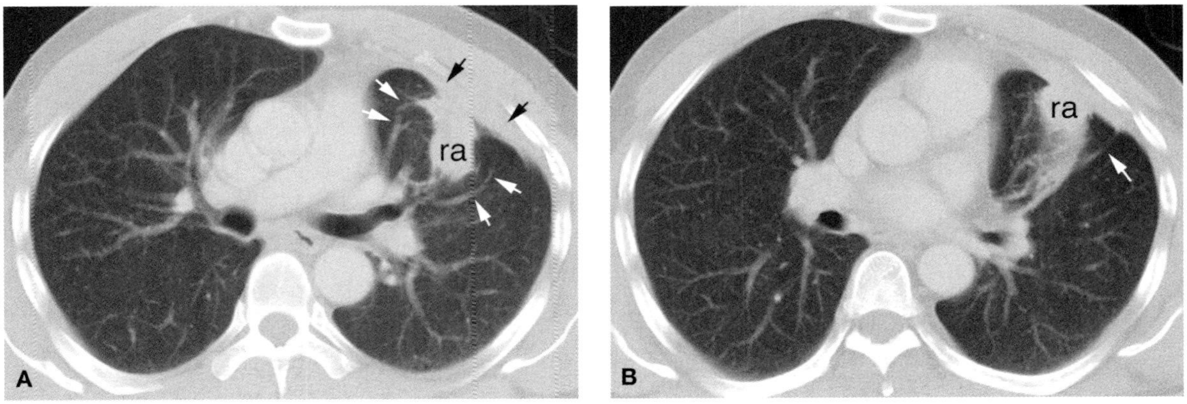

Figure 1.46. Anterior rounded atelectasis associated with pleural fibrosis in a patient with prior tuberculosis. **A:** CT shows left pleural thickening anteriorly (*black arrows*). The area of rounded atelectasis (ra) is irregular in shape but contacts the pleural surface and is associated with the comet tail sign (*white arrows*). **B:** At a lower level, anterior displacement of the major fissure (*white arrow*) indicates volume loss in the upper lobe.

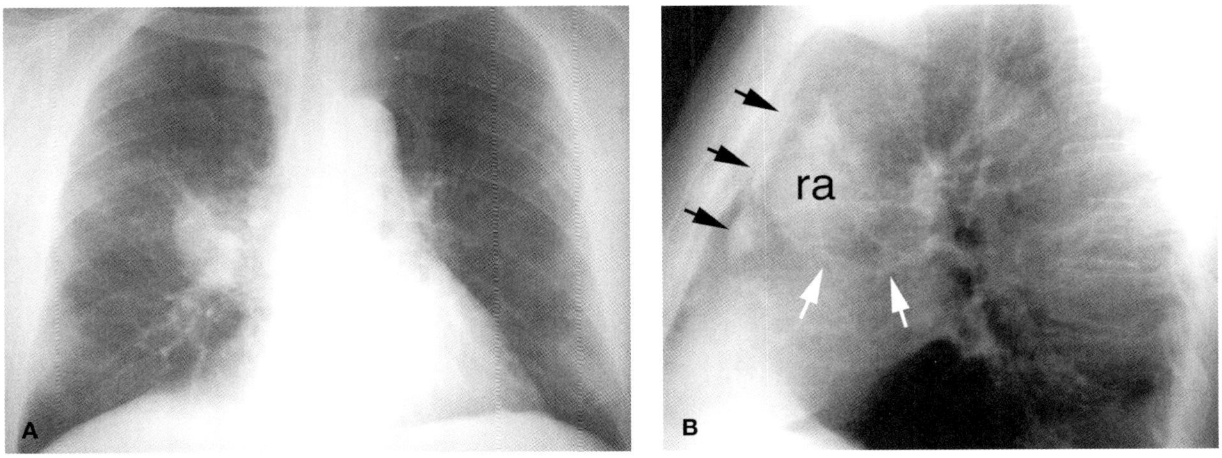

Figure 1.47. Anterior rounded atelectasis in a patient with asbestos-related pleural thickening. **A:** Frontal chest radiograph shows a mass overlying the right hilum. This appearance suggests lung cancer. **B:** Lateral chest radiograph shows anterior pleural thickening and calcification (*black arrows*). A comet tail sign (*white arrows*) is seen adjacent to the area of rounded atelectasis (ra). The area of rounded atelectasis does not appear to contact the anterior chest wall.

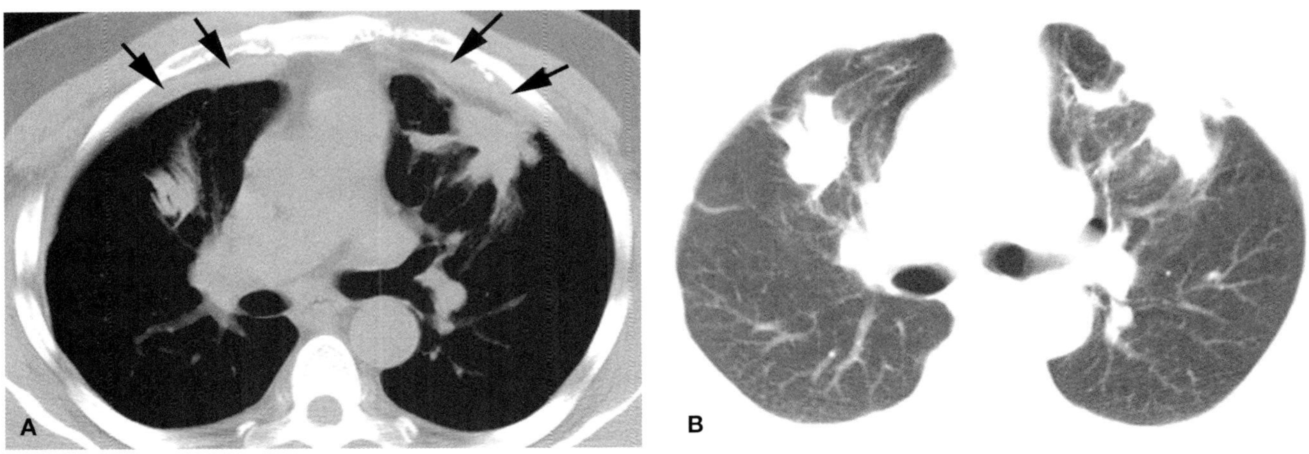

Figure 1.48. Atypical rounded atelectasis in a patient with asbestos-related pleural thickening. **A:** CT using a soft-tissue window shows anterior pleural thickening with calcification (*arrows*). Irregular lung masses are also visible. **B:** CT with a lung window setting shows bilateral masses. Although there is some evidence of the comet tail sign on each side, the right-sided mass does not contact the pleural surface, and the left-sided mass is very irregular in contour. Biopsy of each mass was negative, and follow-up CT showed no change.

SUGGESTED READINGS

Batra P, Brown K, Hayashi K, Mori M. Rounded atelectasis. *J Thorac Imaging*. 1996;11(3):187-197.

Blankenbaker DG. The luftsichel sign. *Radiology*. 1998;208(2):319-320.

Davis SD, Yankelevitz DF, Wand A, Chiarella DA. Juxtaphrenic peak in upper and middle lobe volume loss: assessment with CT. *Radiology*. 1996;198(1):143-149.

Felson B. The roentgen diagnosis of disseminated pulmonary alveolar diseases. *Semin Roentgenol*. 1967;2:3-21.

Genereux GP. Pattern recognition in diffuse lung disease: a review of theory and practice. *Med Radiogr Photogr*. 1985;61(1-2):2-31.

Kattan KR, Wlot JF. Cardiac rotation in left lower lobe collapse: "the flat waist sign." *Radiology*. 1976;118(2):275-279.

Naidich DP, Ettinger N, Leitman BS, McCauley DI. CT of lobar collapse. *Semin Roentgenol*. 1984;19(3):222-235.

Reed JC, Madewell JE. The air bronchogram in interstitial disease of the lungs: a radiological-pathological correlation. *Radiology*. 1975;116: 1-9.

Rohlfing BM. The shifting granuloma: an internal marker of atelectasis. *Radiology*. 1977;123(2):283-285.

Shah RM, Friedman AC. CT angiogram sign: incidence and significance in lobar consolidations evaluated by contrast-enhanced CT. *AJR Am J Roentgenol*. 1998;170(3):719-721.

Westcott JL, Cole S. Plate atelectasis. *Radiology*. 1985;155:1-9.

Woodring JH. The computed tomography mucous bronchogram sign. *J Comput Tomogr*. 1988;12(2):165-168.

Woodring JH, Reed JC. Radiographic manifestations of lobar atelectasis. *J Thorac Imaging*. 1996;11(2):109-144.

Woodring JH, Reed JC. Types and mechanisms of pulmonary atelectasis. *J Thorac Imaging*. 1996;11(2):92-108.

Chapter 2

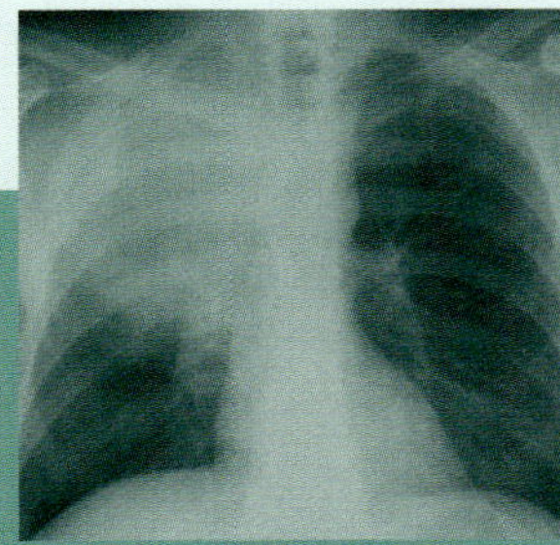

Travis S. Henry

The Normal Mediastinum

INTRODUCTION

The mediastinum is defined as the tissue compartment located between the two lungs, posterior to the sternum, anterior to the vertebral column, and extending from the thoracic inlet to the diaphragm.

CT ANATOMY

The aorta and its branches, the systemic veins, the pulmonary arteries, and the trachea and main bronchi serve as reliable guides to localizing other important mediastinal structures. Different classification schemes have variably divided the mediastinum into either three (anterior, middle, and posterior) or four compartments (the previous three plus the superior mediastinum). The current standard adopted by the International Thymic Malignancy Interest Group (ITMIG) defines a three-compartment model with prevascular (anterior), visceral (middle), and paravertebral (posterior) compartments, which will be discussed in greater detail in Chapter 8.

As an aid to understanding regional anatomy on cross-sectional imaging, the mediastinum can be divided into four compartments, respectively, from superior to inferior: (a) the supra-aortic mediastinum; (b) the region of the aortic arch and aortopulmonary window (APW); (c) the pulmonary arteries, subcarinal space, and azygoesophageal recess; and (d) the heart and paracardiac mediastinum.

Supra-Aortic Mediastinum

Just below the thoracic inlet (Fig. 2.1A and B), the mediastinum is relatively narrow from anterior to posterior. The trachea is centrally located. This is considered part of the visceral compartment in the ITMIG classification scheme.

The *esophagus* lies posterior to the trachea but can be displaced to the left (more common) or right. It is often collapsed and appears as a flattened structure of soft-tissue attenuation. Small amounts of air or fluid may be seen in its lumen.

Other than the trachea and esophagus, the arch branches of the aorta and the brachiocephalic veins are the most apparent normal structures at this level. The *brachiocephalic veins* are the most anterior and lateral vessels visible, lying immediately behind the clavicular heads. Although they vary in size, their positions are relatively constant.

The *right brachiocephalic vein* has a nearly vertical course throughout its length. The *left brachiocephalic vein* is longer and courses horizontally as it crosses the mediastinum (see Fig. 2.1B). The precise cephalocaudal location of this vein is quite variable; although it is most frequently visible at this level, the horizontal portion of the left brachiocephalic vein also can be seen at the level of the aortic arch.

The innominate, subclavian, and carotid arteries lie posterior to the veins and adjacent to the anterior and lateral walls of the trachea. These can be reliably identified by their consistent positions. The *innominate (brachiocephalic) artery* is located in proximity to the anterior tracheal wall, near its midline or slightly to the right of midline in most normals; it is the most variable of all the arch vessels. The *left common carotid artery* lies to the left and slightly posterior to the innominate artery; generally, it has the smallest diameter of the three major arterial branches. The *left subclavian artery* is a relatively posterior structure throughout most of its course, lying to the left of the trachea or slightly posterior to its midline. The lateral border of the left subclavian artery typically indents the mediastinal surface of the left upper lobe. Small vascular branches, particularly the internal mammary veins and vertebral arteries, are often seen in this part of the mediastinum.

In some patients, the *thyroid gland* extends into this portion of the mediastinum, and the right and left thyroid lobes may be visible on each side of the trachea. On CT, the thyroid can be distinguished from other tissues or masses because of its iodine content; its attenuation is greater than that of soft tissue.

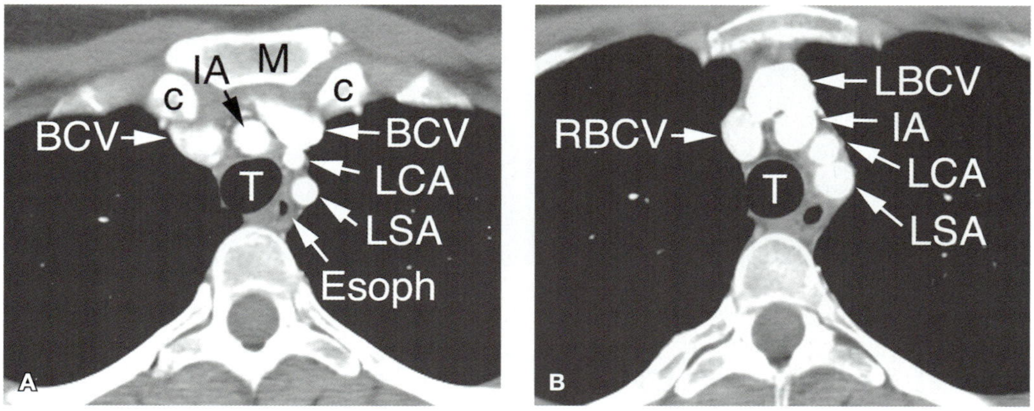

Figure 2.1. Normal CT anatomy. Supra-aortic mediastinum. **A:** *M*, manubrium; *c*, clavicular head; *T*, trachea; *Esoph*, esophagus; *BCV*, brachiocephalic vein; *IA*, innominate artery; *LCA*, left carotid artery; *LSA*, left subclavian artery. **B:** *T*, trachea; *RBCV*, right brachiocephalic vein; *LBCV*, left brachiocephalic vein; *IA*, innominate artery; *LCA*, left carotid artery; *LSA*, left subclavian artery.

Aortic Arch and APW

While the supra-aortic region largely contains arterial and venous branches of the aorta and vena cava, this compartment contains the undivided mediastinal great vessels, the aorta and superior vena cava, and also several important mediastinal spaces and lymph node groups (Figs. 2.2-2.4).

The *aortic arch* has a characteristic but variable appearance (see Fig. 2.2A). The anterior aspect of the arch is located anterior and to the right of the trachea, with the arch passing to the left and posteriorly. The posterior arch usually lies anterior and lateral to the spine. The aortic arch tapers slightly along its length, from anterior to posterior.

The position of the anterior and posterior aspects of the arch can vary in the presence of atherosclerosis and aortic tortuosity; typically, the ascending arch is located more anteriorly and to the right in patients with a tortuous aorta, while the descending aorta lies more laterally and posteriorly, in a position to the left of the spine.

At this level, the *superior vena cava* is visible anterior and to the right of the trachea, usually being elliptical in shape (see Fig. 2.2A).

The *esophagus* appears the same as at higher levels, being posterior to the trachea but variable in position. Often, it lies somewhat to the left of the tracheal midline (see Fig. 2.2A).

The aortic arch on the left, the superior vena cava and mediastinal pleura on the right, and the trachea posteriorly serve to define the paratracheal space (see Fig. 2.2A and B). This fat-filled space contains mediastinal lymph nodes in the anterior paratracheal chains, and is further subdivided into right and left paratracheal spaces with the left lateral wall of the trachea serving as the dividing line. The distinction

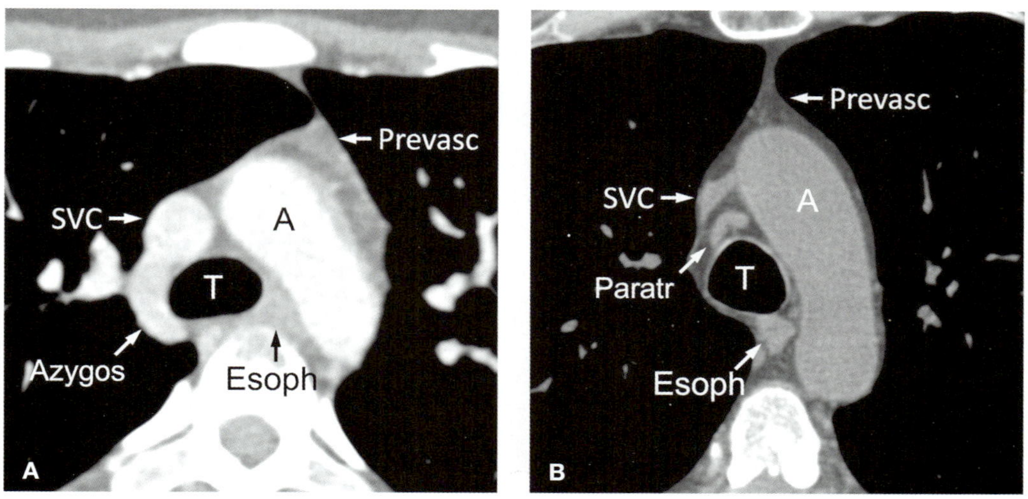

Figure 2.2. Normal CT anatomy. Aortic arch level. **A:** Contrast-enhanced CT at a lower level in the same patient as in Figure 2.1. *T*, trachea; *Esoph*, esophagus; *A*, aortic arch; *SVC*, superior vena cava; *Azygos*, azygos arch; *Prevasc*, prevascular space containing thymus. **B:** Unenhanced high-resolution CT. *T*, trachea; *A*, aortic arch; *SVC*, superior vena cava; *Paratr*, paratracheal space containing normal lymph nodes; *Prevasc*, prevascular space containing thymus replaced by fat.

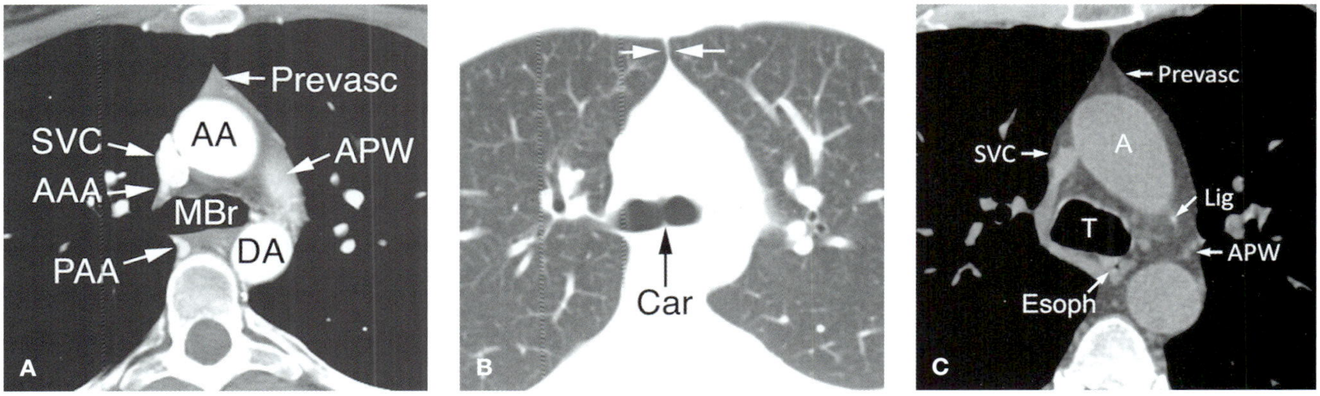

Figure 2.3. Normal CT anatomy. Aortopulmonary window level. **A:** Contrast-enhanced CT at a lower level in the same patient as in Figures 2.1 and 2.2A. *MBr*, main bronchi at the level of the carina; *AA*, ascending aorta; *DA*, descending aorta; *SVC*, superior vena cava; *AAA*, anterior azygos arch; *PAA*, posterior azygos arch; *Prevasc*, prevascular space containing thymus; *APW* aortopulmonary window with volume averaging of superior aspect of the left pulmonary artery. **B:** Lung window scan, same level as (**A**). The tracheal carina (*Car*) is visible. The apex of the triangular prevascular space represents the anterior junction line (*white arrows*). The mediastinal pleural reflections bordering the prevascular space are concave laterally. **C:** Unenhanced high-resolution CT at a lower level than Figure 2.2B. *A*, ascending aorta; *SVC*, superior vena cava; *Prevasc*, prevascular space containing thymus replaced by fat; *APW*, aortopulmonary window containing normal lymph nodes; *Lig*, calcified ligamentum arteriosum; *Esoph*, esophagus *T*, trachea.

of right versus left paratracheal is important in lung cancer staging as will be discussed in Chapter 5. Other mediastinal node groups are closely related to this group both spatially and in regard to lymphatic drainage. It is common to see a few normal-sized lymph nodes in the paratracheal space.

Anterior to the great vessels (aorta and superior vena cava) at this level is another triangular space called the *prevascular space* (see Figs. 2.2 and 2.3). The apex of this triangular space represents the "anterior junction line" (see Figs. 2.2A and 2.3A and B). This compartment primarily contains thymus (described in detail later), lymph nodes, and fat (see Figs. 2.2 and 2.3). The mediastinal pleural reflections bordering the prevascular space may be concave or convex laterally, although a marked convexity suggests a prevascular (anterior) mediastinal mass or thymic enlargement.

At a level slightly below the aortic arch, the ascending aorta and descending aorta are visible as separate structures (Fig. 2.3A and C).

At or near this level, the *trachea* bifurcates into the *right and left main bronchi*. Near the carina, the trachea commonly assumes a somewhat triangular shape (see Fig. 2.2A). The carina is usually visible on CT (see Fig. 2.3A and B).

On the right side, the *azygos arch* arises from the posterior wall of the superior vena cava, passes over the right main bronchus, and continues posteriorly along the mediastinum to lie to the right and anterior to the spine (see Figs. 2.2A and 2.3A). Below the level of the azygos arch, the *azygos vein* is consistently seen in this position. The azygos arch is often visible on one or two adjacent slices and sometimes appears nodular. However, its characteristic location is usually sufficient to

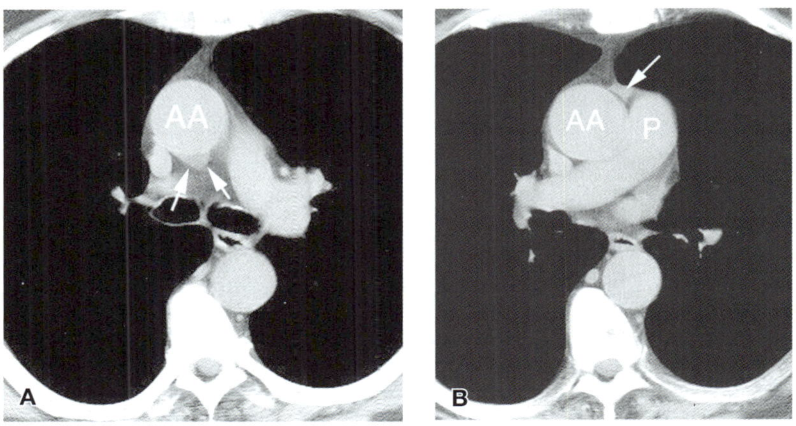

Figure 2.4. Normal superior pericardial recess. Unenhanced CT. **A:** The superior pericardial recess (*arrows*) is visible posterior to the ascending aorta (*AA*) in the precarinal space. **B:** At a lower level, the anterior reflection of the superior pericardial recess (*arrow*) is visible in the groove between the ascending aorta (*AA*) and main pulmonary artery (*P*).

allow its correct identification. When the azygos arch is visible, it marginates the right border of the right paratracheal space.

The *APW* is located on the left side of the mediastinum, caudal to the aortic arch but cephalic to the main pulmonary artery (see Fig. 2.3A and C). The APW contains fat, lymph nodes, the recurrent laryngeal nerve, and the ligamentum arteriosum; the latter two are usually invisible although a calcified ligamentum is occasionally seen especially in older patients. In some patients, the APW is not well seen, with the main pulmonary artery lying immediately below the aortic arch.

The *superior pericardial recess*, containing a small amount of pericardial fluid, is often visible in the paratracheal space immediately behind the ascending aorta (see Fig. 2.4A). Although it is sometimes confused with a lymph node, its typical location, contact with the aortic wall, oval or crescentic shape, and relatively low (water) attenuation allow it to be distinguished from an abnormality. The anterior recess of the pericardial space is sometimes seen anterior to the aortic arch, ascending aorta, and pulmonary artery (see Fig. 2.4B).

Pulmonary Arteries, Subcarinal Space, and Azygoesophageal Recess

At or near the level of the tracheal carina or main bronchi, the *main pulmonary artery* divides into its right and left branches (Fig. 2.5A-C). The *left pulmonary artery* is somewhat higher than

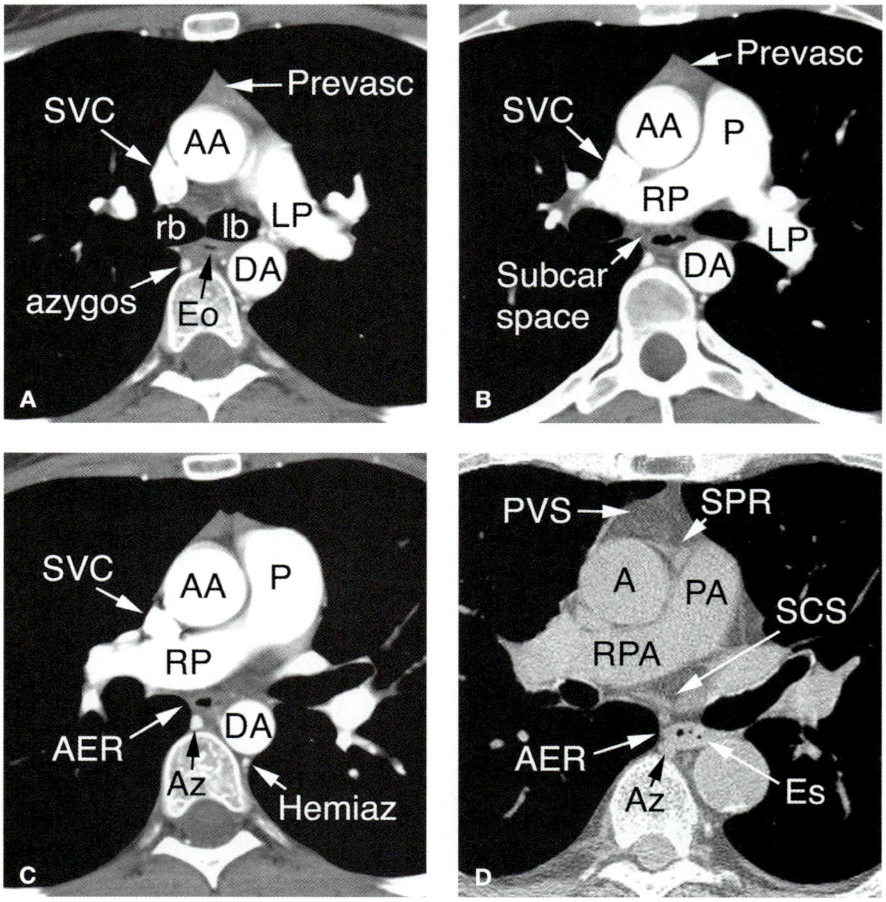

Figure 2.5. Normal CT anatomy. Level of the pulmonary arteries, subcarinal space, and azygoesophageal recess. **A:** Contrast-enhanced CT at a lower level in the same patient as in Figures 2.1, 2.2A, and 2.3A. *rb*, right main bronchus; *lb*, left main bronchus; *AA*, ascending aorta; *DA*, descending aorta; *SVC*, superior vena cava; *azygos*, azygos vein; *Eo*, esophagus; *Prevasc*, prevascular space containing thymus; *LP*, left pulmonary artery. **B:** Contrast-enhanced CT slightly below level shown in (**A**). *AA*, ascending aorta; *P*, main pulmonary artery; *LP*, left pulmonary artery; *RP*, right pulmonary artery; *DA*, descending aorta; *SVC*, superior vena cava; *Prevasc*, prevascular space containing thymus; *Subcar space*, subcarinal space. **C:** Contrast-enhanced CT slightly below level shown in (**B**). *AA*, ascending aorta; *P*, main pulmonary artery; *RP*, right pulmonary artery; *DA*, descending aorta; *SVC*, superior vena cava; *Az*, azygos vein; *Hemiaz*, hemiazygos vein; *AER*, azygoesophageal recess. **D:** Unenhanced high-resolution CT at a lower level in the same patient as (**B**) and (**C**). *A*, ascending aorta; *PA*, main pulmonary artery; *RPA*, right pulmonary artery; *PVS*, prevascular space containing thymus replaced by fat; *SPR*, anterior superior pericardial recess; *SCS*, subcarinal space containing normal lymph nodes; *AER*, azygoesophageal recess; *Az*, azygos vein; *Es*, esophagus.

the right, usually being seen 1 cm above it, and appears as the continuation of the main pulmonary artery, directed posterolaterally and to the left (see Fig. 2.5A and B). The *right pulmonary artery* arises at nearly a right angle to the main and left pulmonary and crosses the mediastinum from left to right, anterior to the carina or main bronchi (see Fig. 2.5B and C). The right pulmonary artery limits the most caudal extent of the paratracheal space and the anterior aspect of the subcarinal space.

The *azygos vein* parallels the esophagus along the right side of the mediastinum and laterally contacts the medial pleural reflections of the right lower lobe, defining the posterior border of the azygoesophageal recess (see Fig. 2.5A-C). On the left side, the *hemiazygos vein* parallels the descending aorta, lying posterior to it (see Fig. 2.5A-C); it is not always visible. The hemiazygos vein generally drains into the azygos vein via a branch that crosses the midline behind the aorta, near the level of the T8 vertebral body. This branch is sometimes seen on CT in normal individuals.

The *subcarinal space* is the region of the mediastinum immediately below the carina, marginated laterally by the main bronchi. It contains a number of lymph nodes and is closely related to the esophagus (see Fig. 2.5B and D).

Below the level of the tracheal carina and azygos arch, the medial aspect of the right lung contacts the mediastinum close to the azygos vein, esophagus, and subcarinal space. This region of the mediastinum is called the *azygoesophageal recess* (see Fig. 2.5C and D). The contour of the azygoesophageal recess is concave laterally in the large majority of normal subjects; a convexity in this region should be regarded as suspicious of mass and the scan examined closely for a pathologic process. However, a convexity in this region may also be produced by a prominent normal esophagus or azygos vein and is particularly common in patients with a narrow mediastinum and in children.

Normal lymph nodes are commonly visible in the subcarinal space, being larger than normal nodes in other parts of the mediastinum and up to 1.5 cm in short-axis diameter (see Fig. 2.5D). The esophagus usually is seen immediately posterior to the subcarinal space, and distinguishing nodes and esophagus may be difficult unless the esophagus contains air or contrast material, or its course is traced on adjacent scans.

Heart and Paracardiac Mediastinum

At the level of the heart, the prevascular mediastinum becomes thin or is obliterated by the heart contacting the anterior chest wall (Fig. 2.6). Little soft tissue is visible anterior and lateral to the cardiac chambers and origins of the main pulmonary artery and aorta. However, posterior to the heart, the azygoesophageal recess remains visible to the level of the diaphragm. As at higher levels, the contour of the azygoesophageal recess is concave laterally, closely opposed to the esophagus and azygos vein. Posterior to the descending aorta, fat, the hemiazygos vein, and small lymph nodes occupy the left paravertebral space. The right paravertebral space is considerably thinner or invisible.

PLAIN RADIOGRAPHIC ANATOMY

On frontal (posteroanterior or anteroposterior) chest radiographs, five important mediastinal structures should be easily identified (Fig. 2.7). In addition to their intrinsic

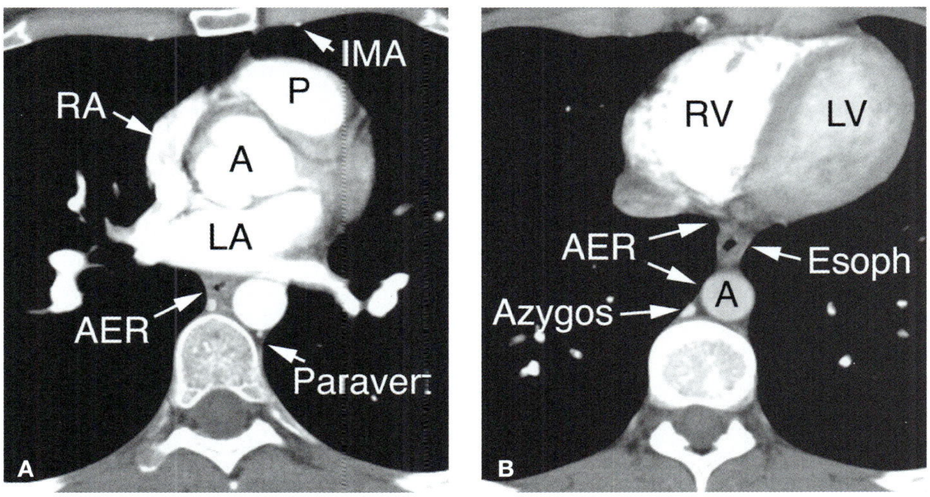

Figure 2.6. Normal CT anatomy. Level of the heart and paracardiac mediastinum. **A:** Contrast-enhanced CT at a lower level in the same patient as in Figures 2.1, 2.2A, 2.3A, and 2.5A-C. *A*, aortic root; *P*, pulmonary outflow tract; *RA*, right atrium; *LA*, left atrium; *AER*, azygoesophageal recess; *Paravert*, left paravertebral space containing hemiazygos vein; *IMA*, internal mammary artery. **B:** Contrast-enhanced CT below the level of (**A**). *RV*, right ventricle; *LV*, left ventricle; *AER*, azygoesophageal recess; *A*, descending aorta; *Azygos*, azygos vein; *Esoph*, esophagus.

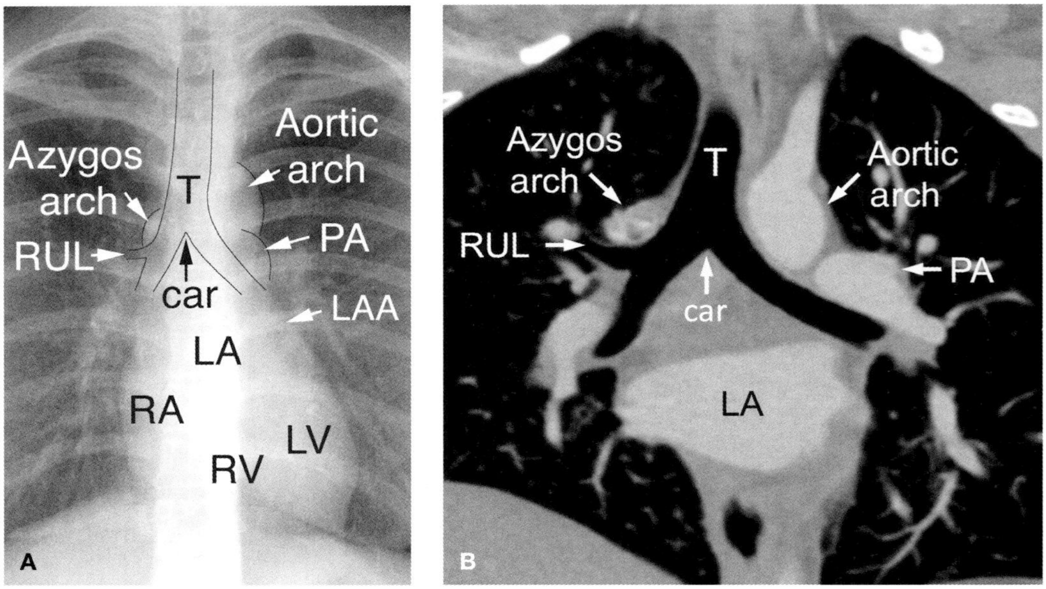

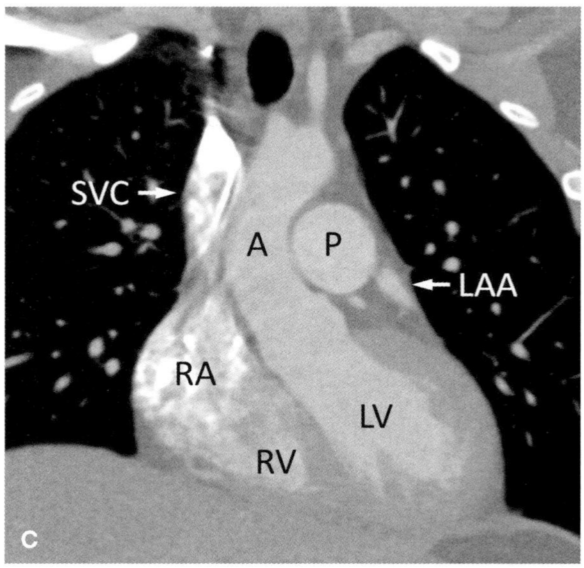

Figure 2.7. Normal structures. **A:** PA chest radiograph. *T*, intrathoracic trachea; *RUL*, right upper lobe bronchus; *car*, carina; *PA*, main pulmonary artery; *LA*, location of left atrium; *LAA*, left atrial appendage; *RA*, location of right atrium; *RV*, location of right ventricle; *LV*, location of left ventricle. **B:** Coronal CT reformation in the same patient through the plane of the trachea and main bronchi. *T*, intrathoracic trachea; *RUL*, right upper lobe bronchus; *car*, carina; *PA*, main and left pulmonary artery; *LA*, left atrium. **C:** Coronal reformation in the same patient at a more anterior level, through the heart. *SVC*, superior vena cava; *A*, ascending aorta; *P*, main pulmonary artery; *LAA*, left atrial appendage; *RA*, right atrium; *RV*, right ventricle; *LV*, left ventricle.

importance in diagnosis, these structures serve to anchor a number of important mediastinal stripes, lines, and interfaces and orient the observer to specific mediastinal regions and compartments that are important in diagnosis. These structures are as follows:

- Trachea, tracheal carina, and main bronchi
- Aortic arch
- Main pulmonary artery
- Azygos vein
- Heart and its chambers

Trachea, Tracheal Carina, and Main Bronchi

The trachea extends from the inferior aspect of the cricoid cartilage to the tracheal carina. It is 10 to 12 cm in length in most individuals. It is divided into extrathoracic and intrathoracic portions at the point it passes posterior to the manubrium (see Fig. 2.7).

The trachea may appear to have a slightly serrated wall because of indentations on the tracheal air column adjacent to the tracheal rings. On the lateral view, serration is seen only along the anterior tracheal wall, as the posterior wall lacks cartilage. Calcification of tracheal cartilages is common in older patients, particularly females. Slight tracheal narrowing with an indentation on the left aortic wall is often seen at the level of the aortic arch.

The tracheal carina is visible at the bifurcation of the trachea into right and left main bronchi. The carina is usually seen near the level of the undersurface of the aortic arch. The right and left main bronchi are usually both visible, with the right main bronchus appearing more vertical than the left. The angle between the inferior walls of the main bronchi, the *carinal angle*, is variable, ranging from about 35° to 90°.

Aortic Arch

The thoracic aorta is usually considered to consist of an ascending segment, a transverse segment or arch, and a descending segment.

The aortic arch begins at the innominate artery and consists of two parts. The proximal part of the arch is the longer and gives rise to the innominate, left carotid, and left subclavian arteries, although variations in the branching pattern of these vessels and their divisions are common. The distal part of the arch, between the origin of the left subclavian artery and the ligamentum arteriosum, is known as the *aortic isthmus*; it is relatively short, measuring 1 to 2 cm in length, and its lumen may be a few millimeters narrower in adults than the aorta immediately distal to the ligamentum. The descending thoracic aorta is distal to the ligamentum arteriosum.

On frontal radiographs, the lateral aspect of the aortic arch (the "aortic knob") is typically visible through about half of its circumference to the left of the trachea (see Fig. 2.7). The lateral edge of the aortic arch visible on radiographs usually represents the edge of the posterior arch. Although it is tempting to measure the aortic diameter as the distance between the edge of the tracheal air column medially and the interface between aorta and lung laterally, these lie in different planes and this measurement is not necessarily valid.

Main Pulmonary Artery

The main pulmonary artery arises at the base of the right ventricle and extends superiorly for a distance of approximately 5 cm before dividing into the right and left pulmonary arteries. The main, right, and left pulmonary arteries are intrapericardial. The main pulmonary artery divides into right and left pulmonary arteries posterior to the ascending aorta and anterior to the main bronchi.

On frontal radiographs, the main pulmonary artery is identified below the aortic arch and above the left main bronchus at the point it appears relatively horizontal. It appears oval, oriented along the superior bronchial wall (see Fig. 2.7). In this location, the visible artery largely corresponds to main pulmonary artery.

Azygos Arch

The arch of the azygos vein is seen in the right tracheobronchial angle, to the right of the distal trachea, above and lateral to the origin of the right main bronchus (see Fig. 2.7). It results in an oval opacity, bordered by air in the trachea medially and air in the lung laterally, and is contiguous superiorly with the right paratracheal stripe. It usually measures 7 mm or less in transverse diameter in normal upright subjects but may be up to 10 mm. Enlargement (more than 10 mm) of this shadow may represent vein dilatation due to deep inspiration or a Mueller maneuver, supine position, pregnancy, increased blood volume, increased central venous pressure, collateral circulation via the azygos vein, azygos aneurysm (rare), or lymph node enlargement.

Heart

The appearance of the heart and its chambers is described in subsequent chapters.

MEDIASTINAL LINES, STRIPES, INTERFACES, AND SPACES

A number of mediastinal lines, stripes, and interfaces have been described on plain radiographs as valuable in the assessment of specific mediastinal structures and spaces. Their visibility and significance vary and are detailed in Figures 2.8-2.25. A *line* is less than 1 mm and represents a structure outlined by air on both sides. A *stripe* is a structure that is generally thicker than a line but still outlined by air on both sides. An *interface* represents a distinct transition between two different densities (eg, lucent lung adjacent to the heart) and often defines the border of spaces. The normal appearances of these lines, stripes, and interfaces is shown using CT reformations, for the large part from the same patient. Figures 2.8-2.22 show the appearances of these on frontal radiographs. In Figures 2.22-2.25, the lines and interfaces visible on the lateral radiograph are described.

Anterior Junction Line

Location: Linear region of contact between the anterior portions of the right and left lungs, posterior to the sternum

Anatomy: Four layers of pleura (visceral pleura covering both lungs and two layers of mediastinal pleura) and a variable amount of retrosternal fat

Appearance:

1. A thin oblique line or sometimes a thicker stripe, beginning at the level of the inferior portion of the manubrium and extending inferiorly and usually slightly to the left, for a variable distance
2. It begins superiorly at the apex of an inverted triangular opacity, usually with concave sides, visible through the manubrium (termed the anterior mediastinal triangle)
3. Inferiorly, the line sometimes is seen to join with the apex of a triangular opacity in the "inferior recesses" of the anterior mediastinum

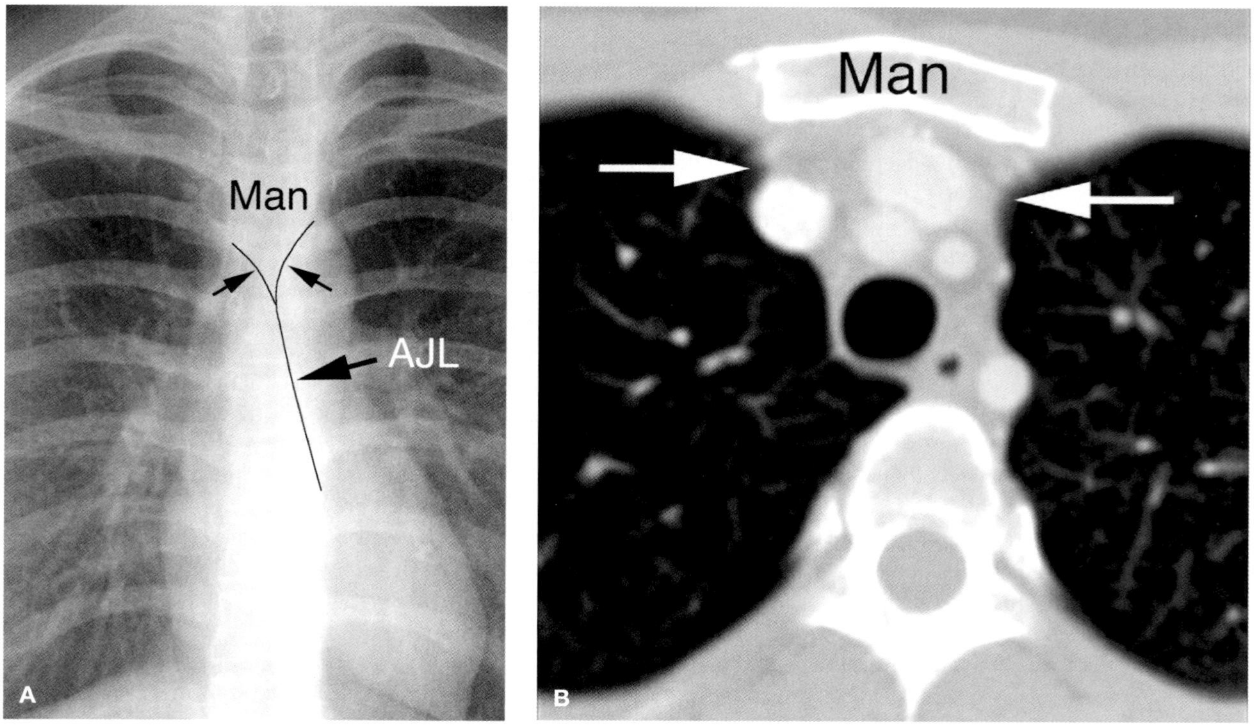

Figure 2.8. Anterior junction line and anterior mediastinal triangle. **A:** PA chest radiograph. The anterior mediastinal triangle (*small black arrows*) is visible through the manubrium (*Man*). AJL, anterior junction line. **B:** CT in the same patient at the level of the manubrium (*Man*). Lung contacting the anterior mediastinum behind the manubrium (*arrows*) results in the anterior mediastinal triangle.

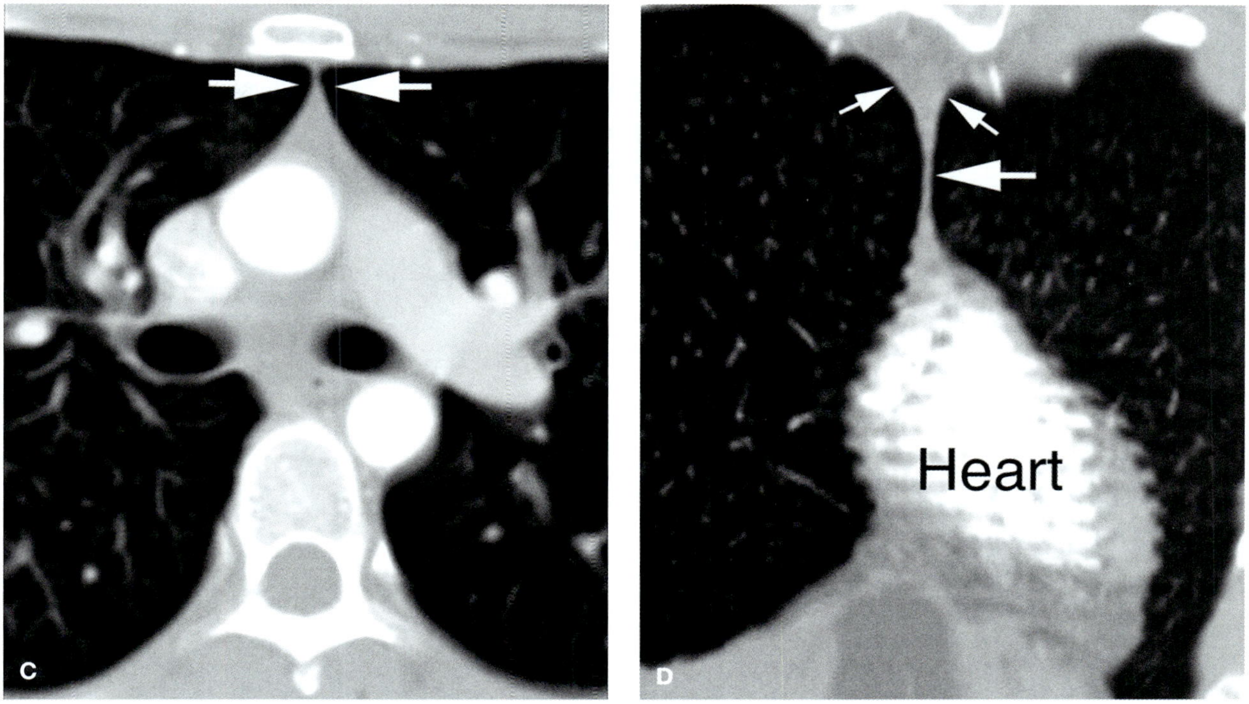

Figure 2.8. (*Continued*) **C:** CT in the same patient at a lower level. Contact between the lungs results in the thin anterior junction line (*arrows*). **D:** CT reformation in the coronal plane shows the anterior mediastinal triangle (*small white arrows*) and anterior junction line (*large arrow*) anterior and superior to the heart.

Anterior Junction Line

Visibility: About 20% of cases; best seen in patients with emphysema because of lung hyperinflation

Significance:

1. May be displaced to the right or left in patients with atelectasis on the same side usually associated with lower lobe volume loss
2. In patients with upper lobe atelectasis and consolidation, the displaced anterior junction line is visible as an interface between the normal aerated upper lobe and the consolidated upper lobe
3. Uncommonly is recognized as focally or diffusely thickened in patients with an anterior mediastinal mass

Cardiophrenic Angles (Right and Left)

Location:	Junction of the anterior hemidiaphragms with the right and left heart borders
Anatomy:	Inferior extent of the anterior mediastinum, containing fat and lymph nodes
Appearance:	Usually concave laterally on both sides; may be convex in the presence of increased mediastinal fat
Visibility:	Very common
Significance:	Convexity or mass may be seen in the presence of (1) large mediastinal fat pad, (2) lipoma, (3) pericardial cyst, (4) enlarged epicardiac lymph nodes, (5) thymic neoplasm or other anterior mediastinal mass, or (6) Morgagni hernia

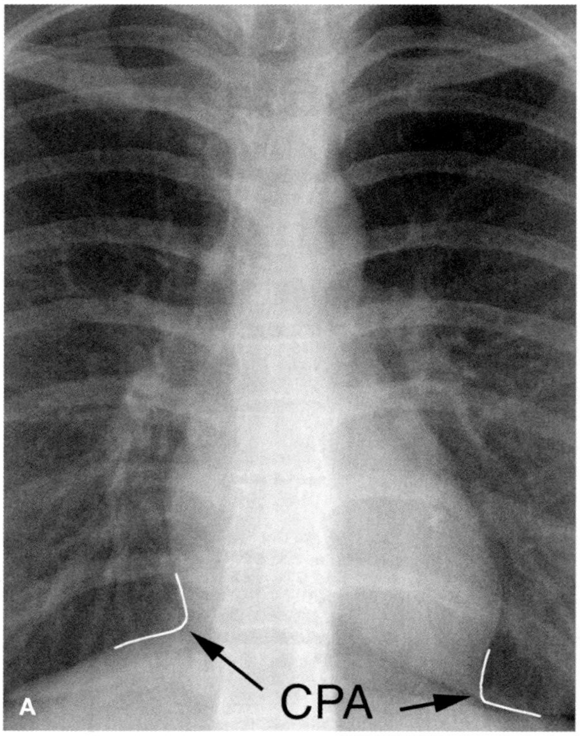

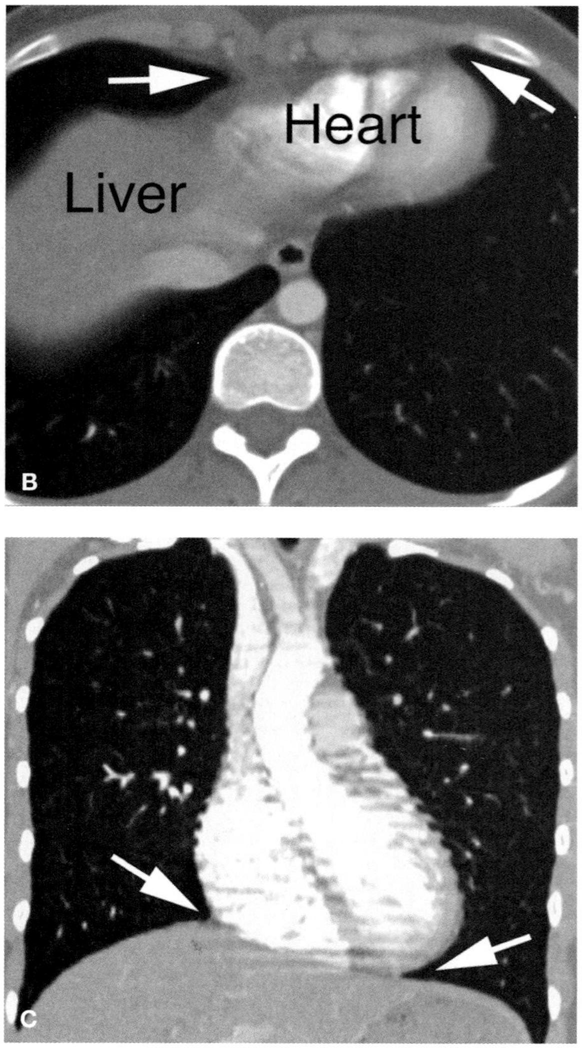

Figure 2.9. Cardiophrenic angles. **A:** PA chest radiograph. The costophrenic angles (*CPA*) are seen at the junction of the anterior hemidiaphragms with the right and left heart borders. **B:** CT in the same patient at the level of the costophrenic angles. These represent contact of the lung with the fat-filled anterior mediastinum (*arrows*) anterior to the heart and liver. **C:** Coronal reformation in the same patient shows the concave costophrenic angles (*arrows*).

Right Paratracheal Stripe

Location: Linear region of contact between the right lung and the right tracheal wall, below the thoracic inlet and above the azygos arch

Anatomy: Tracheal wall, a thin layer of mediastinal fat, two layers of pleura (visceral and parietal)

Appearance: A line or stripe, up to 4 mm thick in normal individuals, seen below the clavicles and blending with the superior aspect of the azygos arch

Visibility: Common, reported to be visible in up to 95% of normal individuals

Significance: Thickening (ie, more than 4 mm) may be due to (1) tracheal wall abnormalities such as tumor or inflammatory disease, (2) pleural thickening or effusion adjacent to the trachea, (3) enlargement of right paratracheal lymph nodes (thickening of the paratracheal stripe occurs in about 30% of patients with right paratracheal lymph node enlargement), or (4) mediastinal infiltration (eg, hemorrhage, infection, neoplasm)

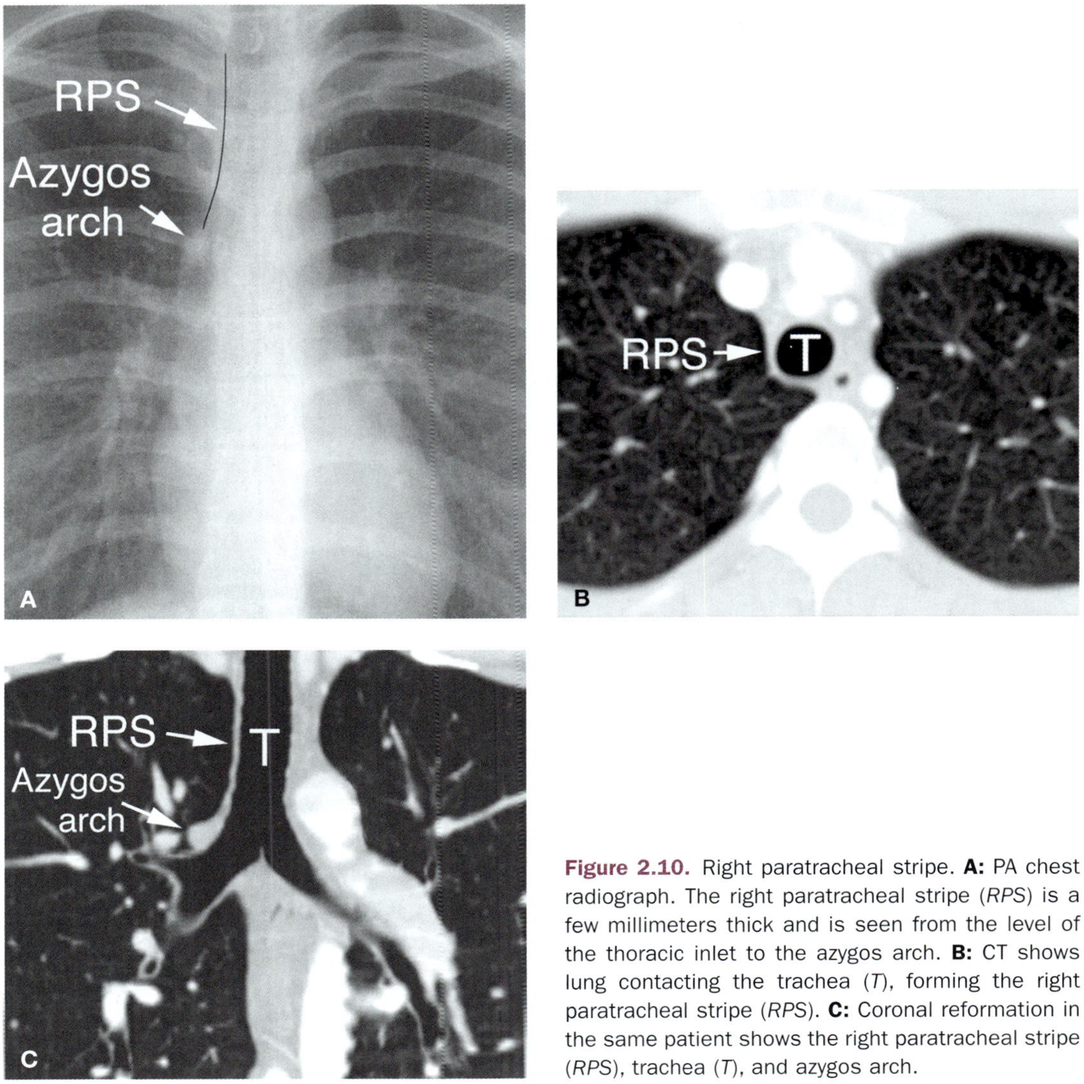

Figure 2.10. Right paratracheal stripe. **A:** PA chest radiograph. The right paratracheal stripe (*RPS*) is a few millimeters thick and is seen from the level of the thoracic inlet to the azygos arch. **B:** CT shows lung contacting the trachea (*T*), forming the right paratracheal stripe (*RPS*). **C:** Coronal reformation in the same patient shows the right paratracheal stripe (*RPS*), trachea (*T*), and azygos arch.

Superior Vena Cava Interface

Location/anatomy:	Interface between the right lung and the right superior mediastinum, above the azygos arch and below the thoracic inlet, lateral to the superior vena cava and right brachiocephalic vein
Appearance:	An interface between lung and mediastinum, slightly concave laterally, above the azygos arch and below the medial right clavicle
Visibility:	Seen in almost all patients
Significance:	Lateral convexity of the superior vena cava interface and increased density of the shadow of the superior vena cava may be seen with (1) dilatation of the superior vena cava (due to deep inspiration or Mueller maneuver [physiologic dilatation], supine position, pregnancy, increased blood volume, increased central venous pressure), (2) lymph node enlargement in the paratracheal space, (3) mediastinal mass, (4) mediastinal infiltration (blood, infection, tumor), or (5) a pleural abnormality

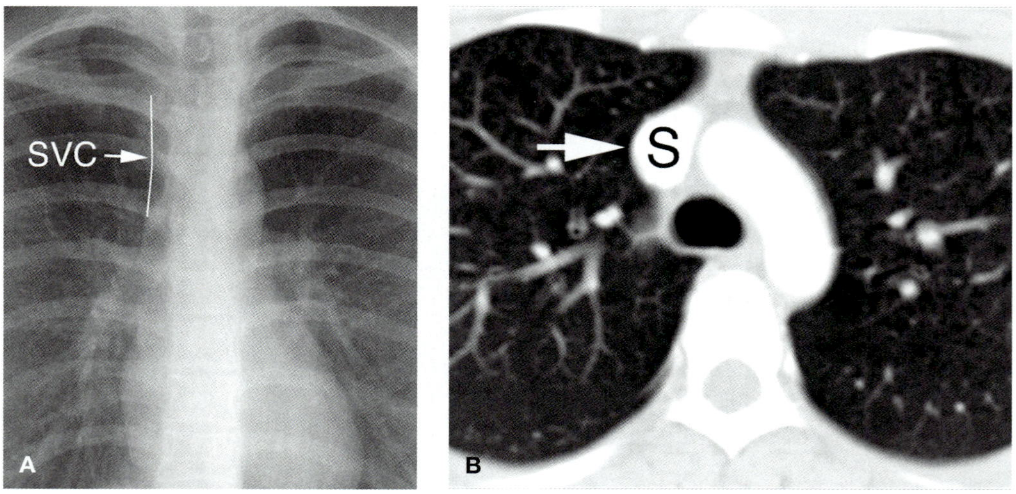

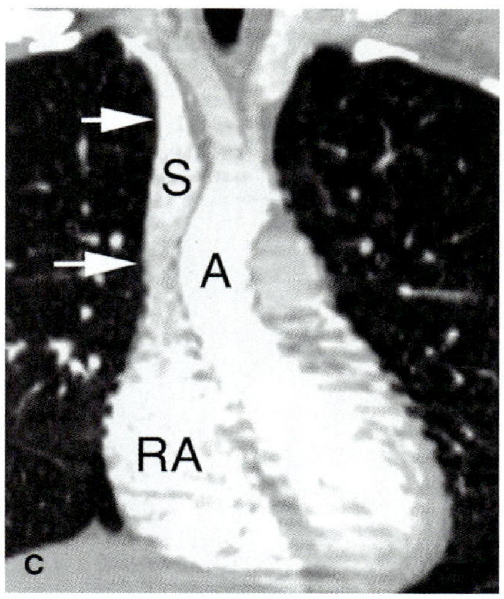

Figure 2.11. Superior vena cava interface. **A:** PA chest radiograph. The right edge of the superior vena cava (*SVC*) is outlined by lung, forming an interface that is slightly concave laterally. It is seen from the thoracic inlet to the level of the azygos arch. **B:** CT in the same patient shows lung contacting the lateral wall of the superior vena cava (*S*). This edge (*arrow*) forms the superior vena cava interface. **C:** Coronal reformation in the same patient shows the superior vena cava interface (*arrows*). *S*, superior vena cava; *A*, aorta; *RA*, right atrium.

Left Paratracheal Stripe or Interface

Location:	Linear region of contact between the left lung and the left tracheal wall and adjacent mediastinal soft tissues, below the thoracic inlet and above the aorta
Anatomy:	Tracheal wall, mediastinal fat, two layers of pleura (visceral and parietal)
Appearance:	A line or stripe of variable thickness seen below the clavicles and above the aortic arch
Visibility:	Uncommonly visible as a thin stripe; in 90%, the left subclavian or carotid artery and mediastinal fat are interposed between the left tracheal wall and aerated lung; what is often perceived as the lateral aspect of the "left paratracheal stripe" usually represents the interface of left subclavian artery or mediastinal fat with lung
Significance:	Thickening is difficult to diagnose because of variability in appearance

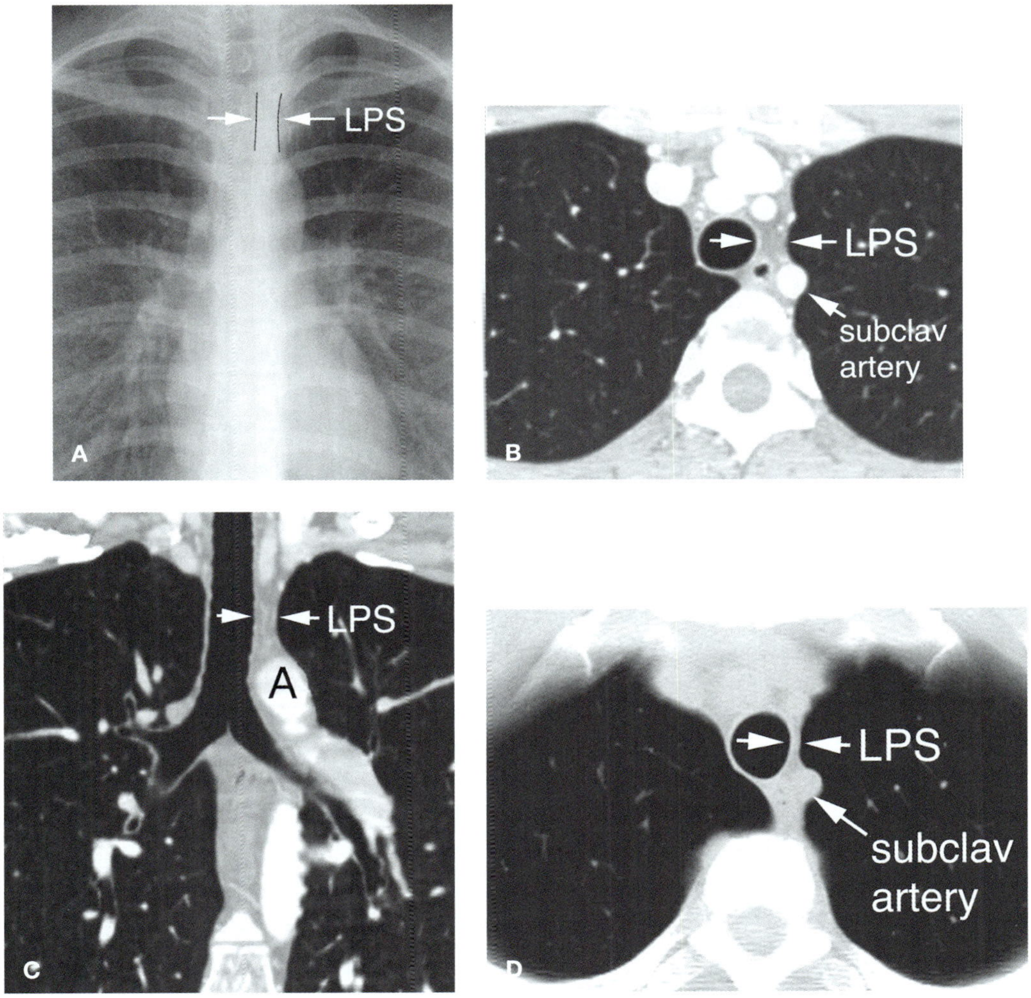

Figure 2.12. Left paratracheal stripe. **A:** PA chest radiograph. The left paratracheal stripe (*LPS*) represents the linear region of contact between the left lung and the left tracheal wall or adjacent mediastinal soft tissues, below the thoracic inlet and above the aorta. It is usually much thicker than the right paratracheal stripe. **B:** CT in the same patient shows lung contacting the lateral wall of the left mediastinum anterior to the left subclavian artery (*subclav artery*). Mediastinal soft tissues along with left tracheal wall make up the left paratracheal stripe (*LPS*). **C:** Coronal reformation in the same patient shows the left paratracheal stripe (*LPS*) above the aorta (*A*). **D:** CT in a different patient shows a thin left paratracheal stripe (*LPS*) corresponding to the left tracheal wall. It is anterior to the left subclavian artery (*subclav artery*).

Left Subclavian Artery Interface

Location:	Interface between the left lung and the left superior mediastinum, above the aorta and below the thoracic inlet
Anatomy:	Pleura outlining the lateral aspect of the left subclavian artery or adjacent mediastinal fat
Appearance:	An interface, usually concave laterally, extending from the shadow of the aortic arch to the level of the medial left clavicle
Visibility:	Common
Significance:	Convexity of this interface indicates (1) subclavian artery dilatation or tortuosity, (2) mediastinal mass or lymph node enlargement, or (3) paramediastinal pleural abnormality

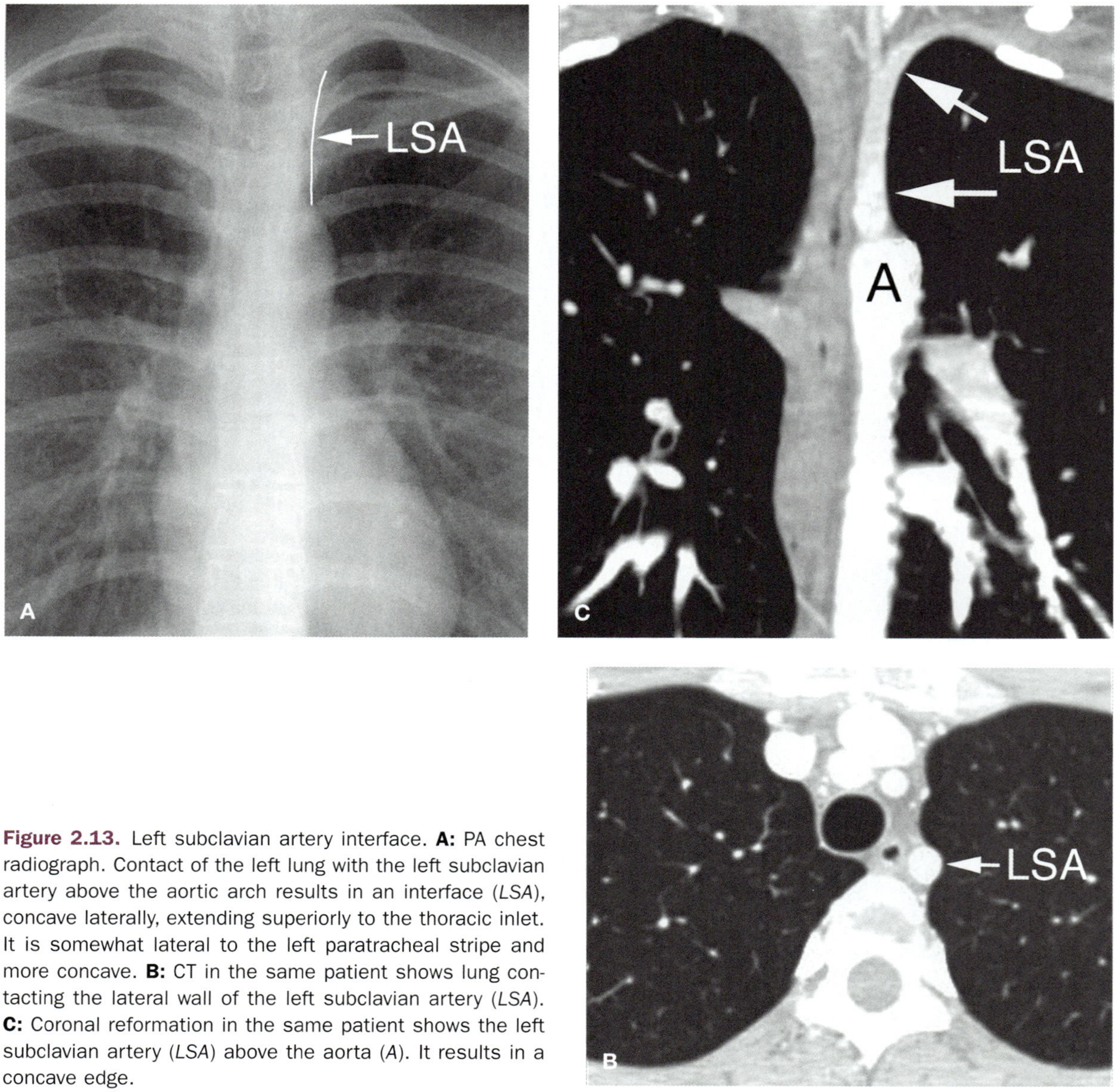

Figure 2.13. Left subclavian artery interface. **A:** PA chest radiograph. Contact of the left lung with the left subclavian artery above the aortic arch results in an interface (*LSA*), concave laterally, extending superiorly to the thoracic inlet. It is somewhat lateral to the left paratracheal stripe and more concave. **B:** CT in the same patient shows lung contacting the lateral wall of the left subclavian artery (*LSA*). **C:** Coronal reformation in the same patient shows the left subclavian artery (*LSA*) above the aorta (*A*). It results in a concave edge.

Vascular Pedicle

Location:	Transverse width of the upper mediastinum
Anatomy:	The overall shadow of the great systemic arteries and veins (ie, the "vascular pedicle" of the heart), mediastinal contents
Appearance:	The width of the vascular pedicle is measured from the point the superior vena cava interface crosses the right main bronchus to a vertical line drawn inferiorly from the point the left subclavian artery arises from the aortic arch; width is variable but measures up to 58 mm in normal subjects
Visibility:	Common
Significance:	Widening may be due to (1) dilatation of the great vessels (due to deep inspiration or Mueller maneuver [physiologic dilatation], supine position, pregnancy, increased blood volume, increased central venous pressure), (2) lymph node enlargement in the paratracheal space, (3) mediastinal mass, (4) mediastinal infiltration (blood, infection, tumor), and (5) a paramediastinal pleural abnormality

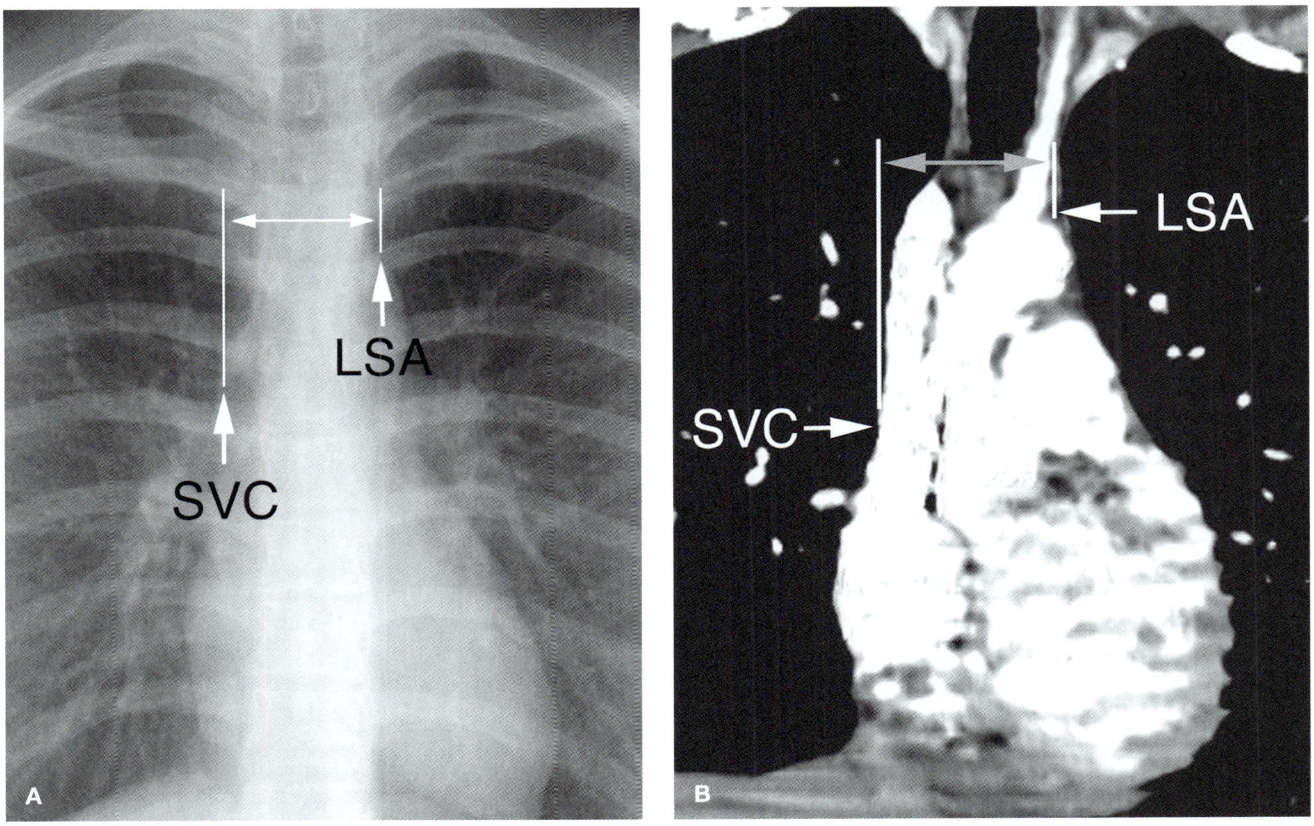

Figure 2.14. Vascular pedicle. **A:** PA chest radiograph. The vascular pedicle (*arrows*) is measured from the point the superior vena cava (*SVC*) interface crosses the right main bronchus to a vertical line drawn inferiorly from the point the left subclavian artery (*LSA*) arises from the aortic arch. **B:** Coronal CT reformation shows the same sites of measurement.

Posterior Junction Line or Stripe

Location:	Linear region of contact between the posterior portions of the right and left lungs in the superior mediastinum, behind the esophagus, and anterior to the upper thoracic vertebral bodies
Anatomy:	Four layers of pleura (visceral pleura covering both lungs and two layers of mediastinal pleura); a variable amount of fat; the esophagus may compose a portion of this line or stripe
Appearance:	Usually seen through or adjacent to the tracheal air column; a straight line or variably concave laterally; it may be seen to reflect onto the superior aspect of the aortic arch or the "middle" portion of the azygos arch; it is of variable thickness depending on the amount of fat included or its relationship to the esophagus, ranging from a few millimeters to nearly 1 cm thick

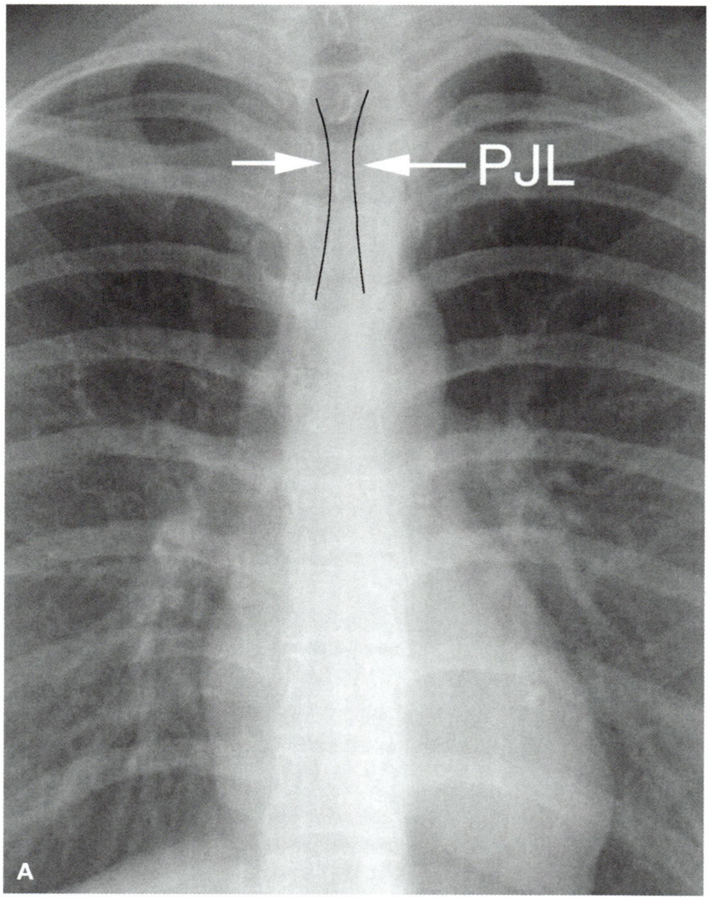

Figure 2.15. Posterior junction line. **A:** PA chest radiograph. The posterior junction line (*PJL*) represents the region of contact between the posterior portions of the right and left lungs in the superior mediastinum, behind the esophagus, and anterior to the upper thoracic vertebral bodies. It is often seen through the tracheal air column and may be straight or variably concave. It is of variable thickness.

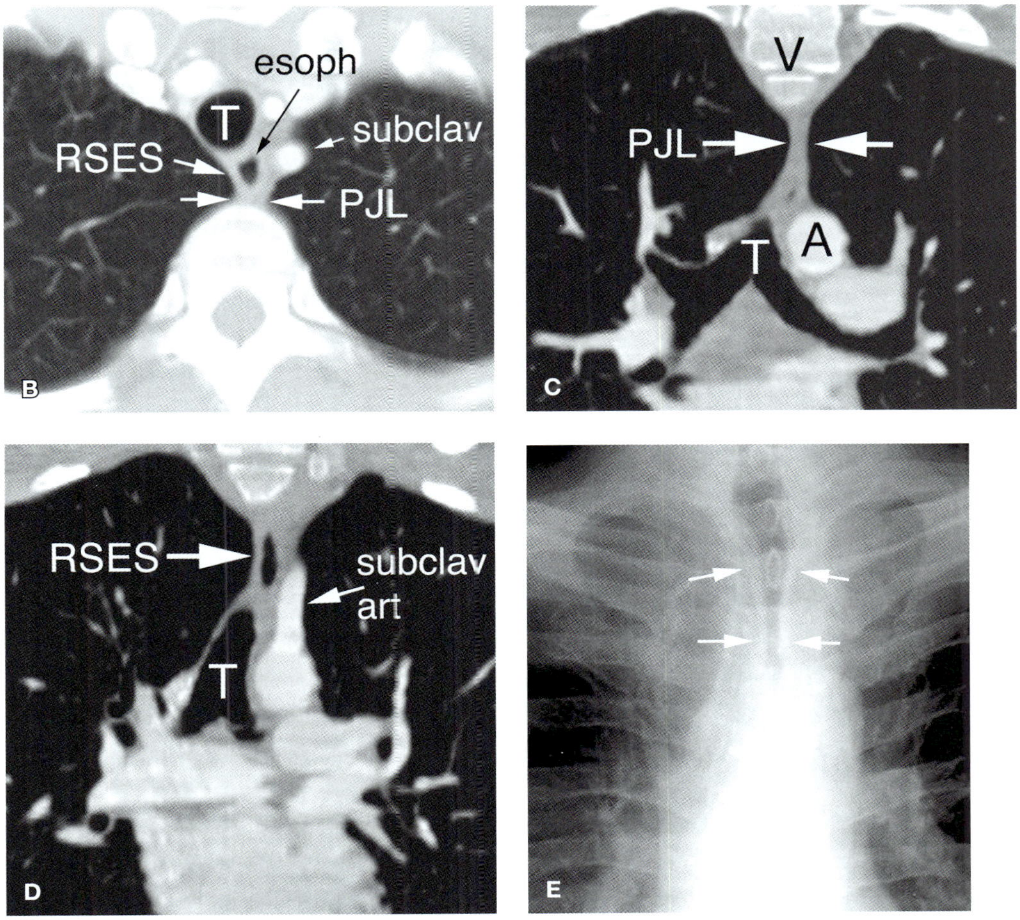

Figure 2.15. (*Continued*) **B:** CT shows lung contacting the right lateral wall of the esophagus (*esoph*). Because of air in the esophageal lumen, this may be seen as the right superior esophageal stripe (*RSES*). The posterior junction line (*PJL*) represents contact of both lungs with the mediastinum. T, trachea; subclav, subclavian artery. **C:** Coronal reformation in the same patient shows the posterior junction line (*PJL*) anterior to the vertebral column (*V*) and cephalad to the aorta *(A)*. *T*, trachea. **D:** Coronal reformation slightly anterior to (**C**) shows the right superior esophageal stripe (*RSES*) outlined by air in the lung and esophageal lumen. *T*, trachea; *subclav art*, subclavian artery. **E:** Right and left superior esophageal stripes (*arrows*) are visible in a patient with intraesophageal air.

Posterior Junction Line or Stripe

Variant: If air is present in the esophagus, two stripes may be visible, each principally representing the right or left esophageal walls; when this occurs, these stripes are referred to as the right and left superior esophageal (or pleuroesophageal) stripes

Visibility: Common; posterior junction line and esophageal stripes each visible in about 40% of normal subjects

Significance: Because of the variability in the appearance of this line or stripe, it is of limited utility in diagnosis; abnormalities are most typically from esophageal thickening or masses in this region

Left Superior Intercostal Vein

Location:	Adjacent to or immediately above the aortic arch shadow
Anatomy:	Left superior intercostal vein drains the left second, third, and fourth intercostal veins into the left brachiocephalic vein; it communicates with the hemiazygos venous system in about 75%

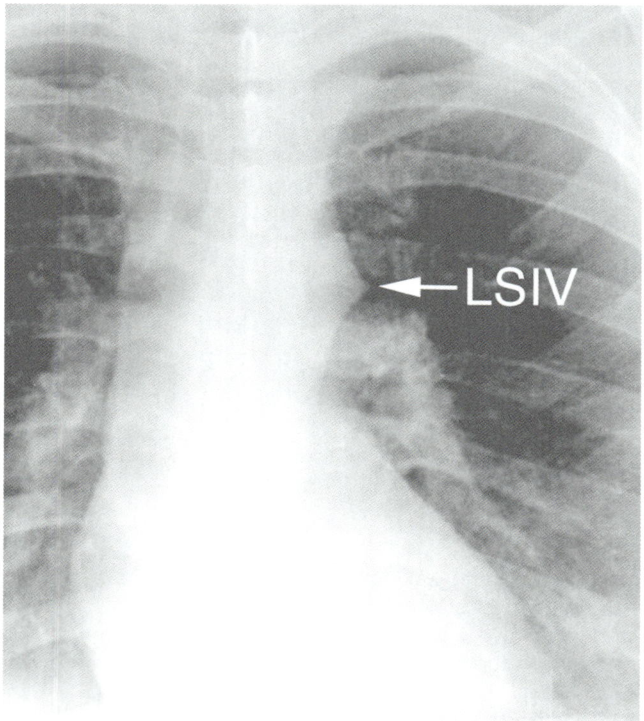

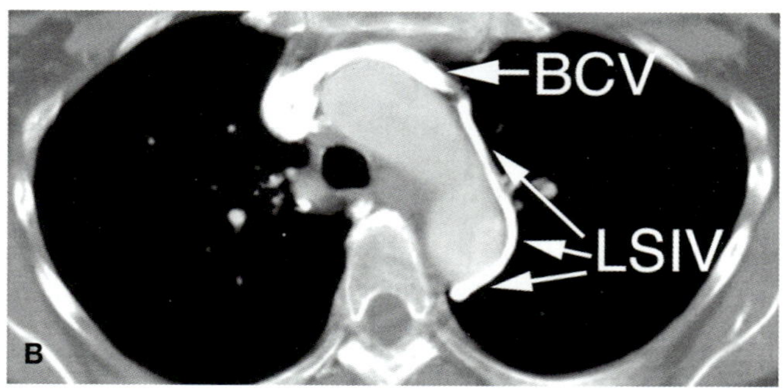

Figure 2.16. Left superior intercostal vein (aortic nipple). **A:** Chest radiograph shows a normal left superior intercostal vein (*LSIV*). **B:** CT in another normal patient shows contrast reflux into the left superior intercostal vein (*LSIV*). It extends posteriorly from the left brachiocephalic vein (*BCV*).

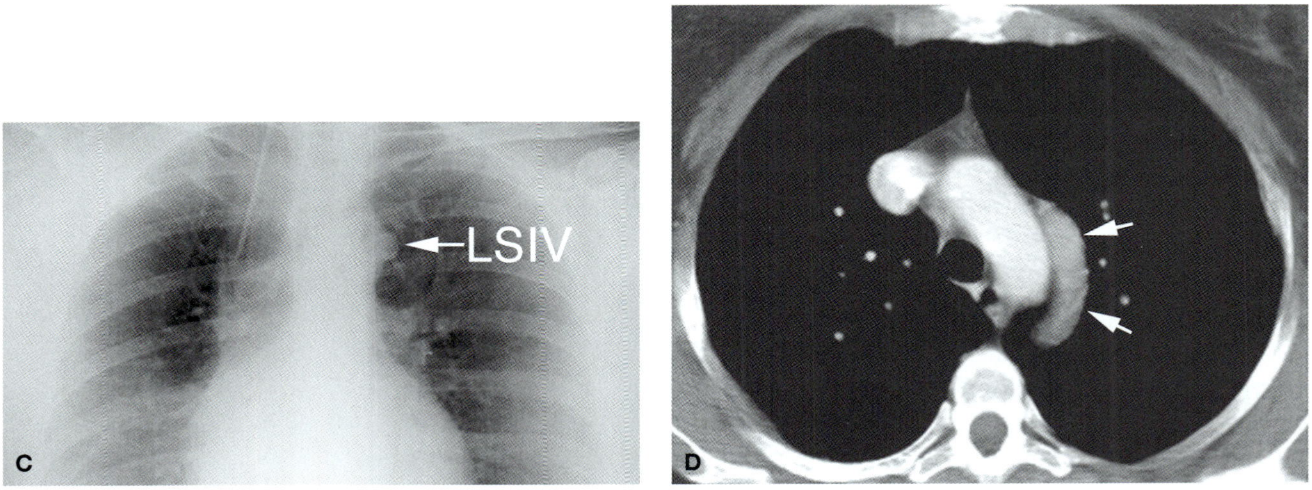

Figure 2.16. (*Continued*) **C:** Radiograph in another patient shows enlargement of the left superior intercostal vein (*LSIV*). It serves as a collateral pathway. **D:** CT in the same patient as (**C**) shows enlargement of the left superior intercostal vein (*arrows*).

Left Superior Intercostal Vein

Appearance: A small round or triangular shadow ("aortic nipple") less than 5 mm in diameter

Visibility: Uncommon; less than 5% of normal subjects

Significance: Dilatation typically occurs as a result of collateral flow through this vein to the hemiazygos and azygos systems; most commonly due to obstruction of the superior vena cava or left brachiocephalic vein

Aortopulmonary Window

Location:	APW is outlined by the left lung between the aortic arch and the left pulmonary artery
Anatomy:	Lateral boundary of the APW is the parietal pleura forming the visible interface; the medial boundary of the APW is the ligamentum arteriosum; the APW largely contains fat and lymph nodes

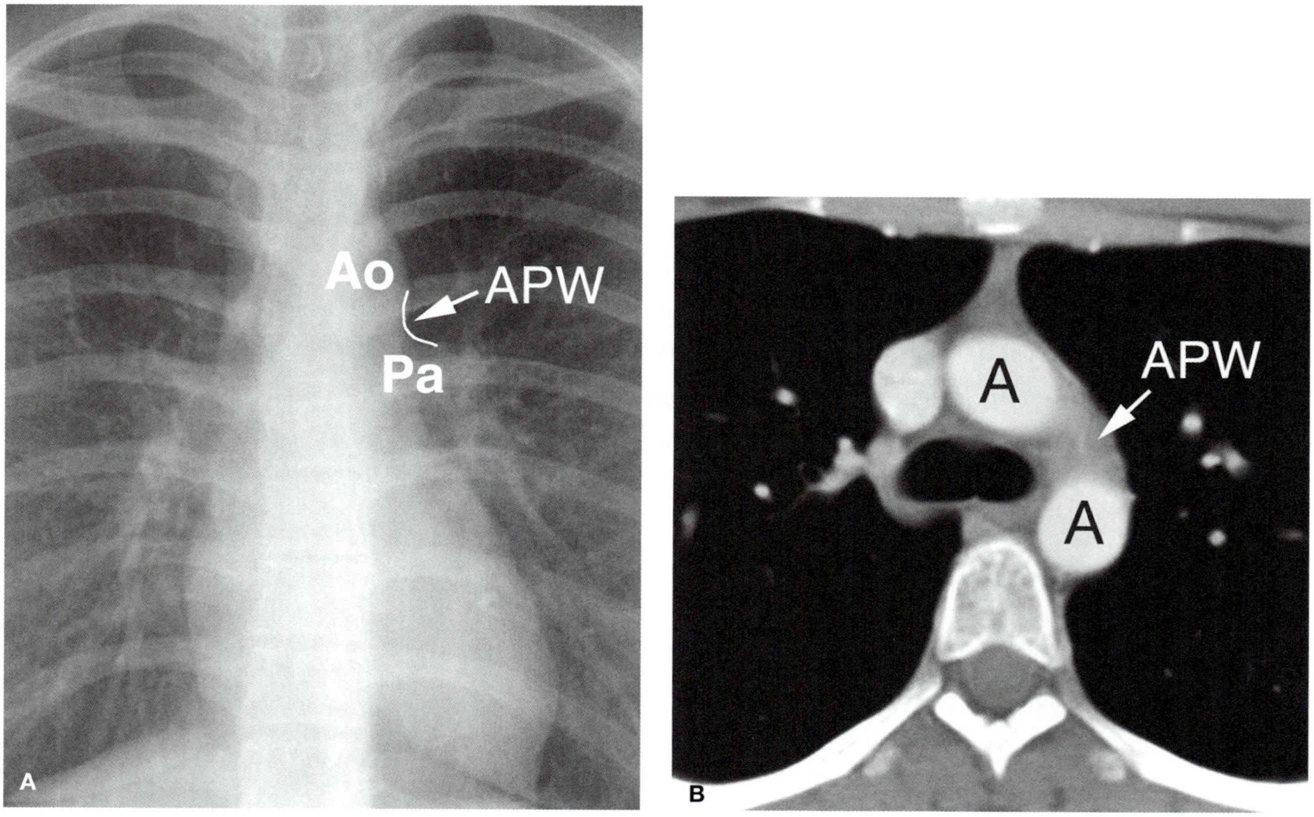

Figure 2.17. Aortopulmonary window. **A:** The aortopulmonary window (*APW*) represents a concave interface between the aorta (*Ao*) and main pulmonary artery (*Pa*). **B:** CT in the same patient shows fat in the aortopulmonary window (*APW*), under the aortic arch (*A*).

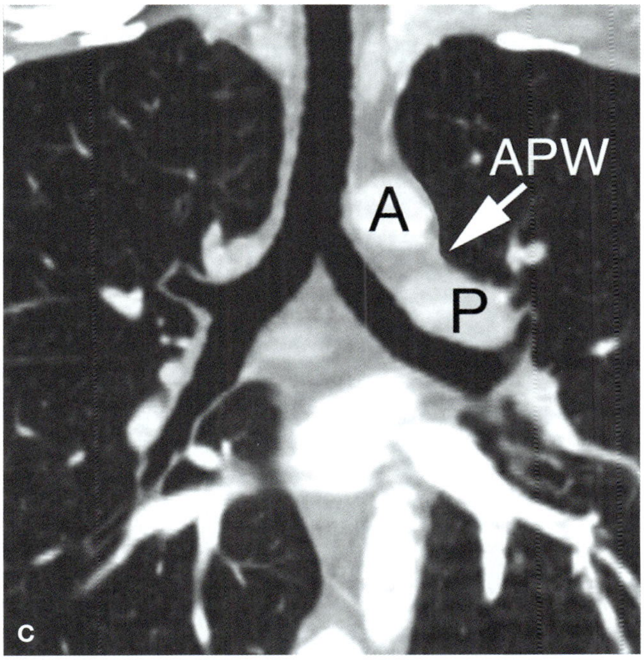

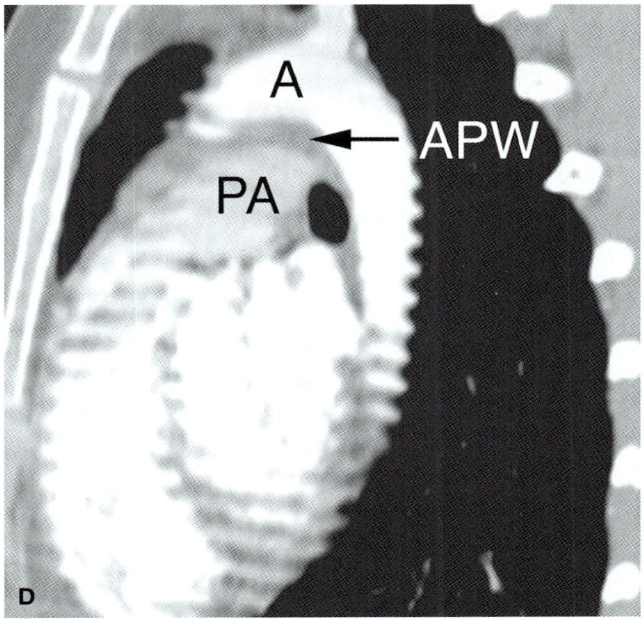

Figure 2.17. (*Continued*) **C:** Coronal reformation in the same patient shows the aortopulmonary window (*APW*) as an interface, concave laterally, between the aorta (*A*) and the pulmonary artery (*P*). This space contains fat and lymph nodes. **D:** Sagittal reformation in the same patient. The aortopulmonary window (*APW*) is located under the aortic arch (*A*) and above the pulmonary artery (*PA*).

Aortopulmonary Window

Appearance: The APW interface is normally concave laterally or straight; it is more concave in the presence of emphysema. However, the appearance of the mediastinal interface in this region is variable, with two common patterns:

1. The interface may be localized to the region below the aorta and above the pulmonary artery
2. The interface may continue inferiorly, overlying the shadow of the left pulmonary artery, merging inferiorly with the left heart border

Visibility: Almost always visible

Significance: Convexity of this interface may indicate (1) lymph node enlargement (most common), (2) mediastinal mass, (3) enlargement of the ductus arteriosus, or (4) aortic aneurysm

Azygoesophageal Recess

Location:	Azygoesophageal recess is a portion of the retrocardiac mediastinum, outlined by the right lower lobe, from the level of the azygos arch above to the level of the diaphragm below
Anatomy:	The azygoesophageal recess contains the posterior azygos vein, esophagus, thoracic duct, and lymph nodes; the superior aspect of the azygoesophageal recess is closely associated with the subcarinal space
Appearance:	The interface between the azygoesophageal recess and the right lung begins at the level of the azygos arch and has a shallow reverse C or reverse S contour, ending at the diaphragm
	In some patients, the superior aspect of the azygoesophageal interface is contiguous with the posterior junction line at the azygos arch, resulting in a shallow three-shaped shadow
Variant:	If air is present in the esophagus, a stripe is commonly visible at the point of contact of right lower lobe and the right esophageal wall; this is referred to as the right inferior esophageal (or pleuroesophageal) stripe; it is most commonly seen immediately under the aortic arch

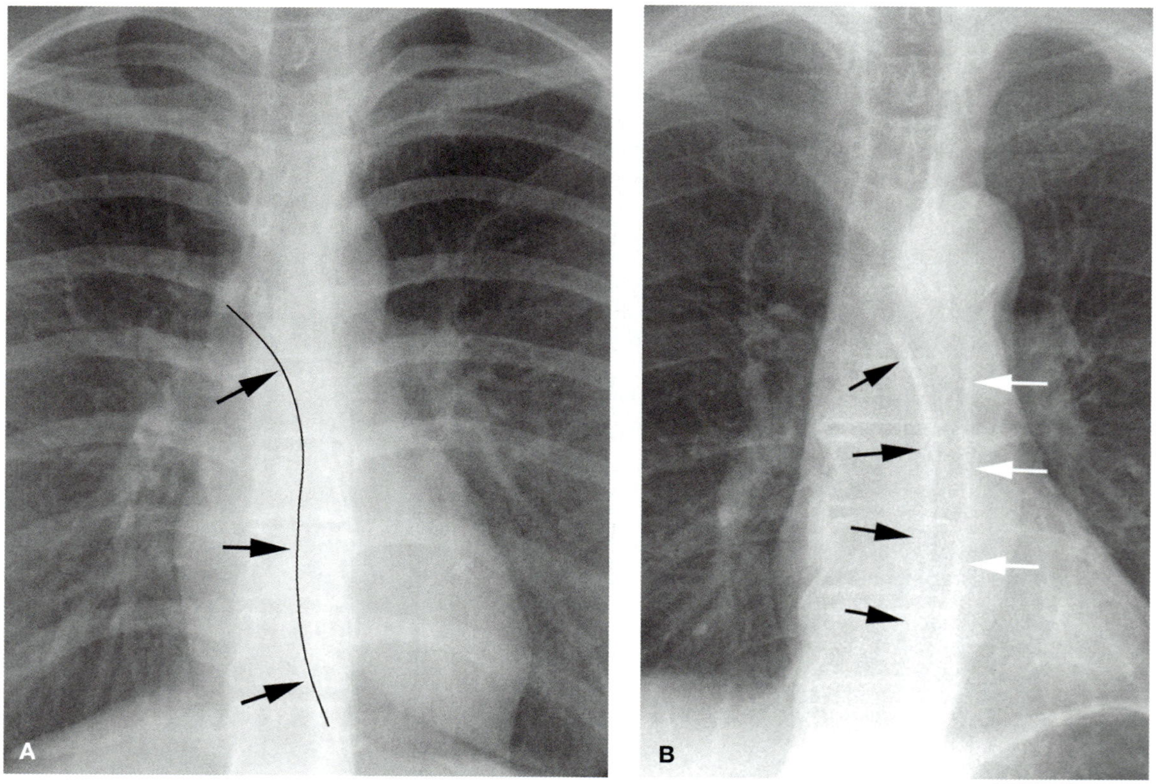

Figure 2.18. Azygoesophageal recess. **A:** PA chest radiograph. The azygoesophageal recess (*arrows*) represents contact between the right lung and the retrocardiac mediastinum, closely related to the locations of the azygos vein and esophagus. It has a shallow reverse C or reverse S contour, ending at the diaphragm. **B:** Right pleuroesophageal stripe in a patient with air in the esophagus. The right pleuroesophageal stripe (*black arrows*) shows the location of the azygoesophageal recess. The left pleuroesophageal stripe (*white arrows*) is also seen, representing contact of the left esophageal wall with the left lung.

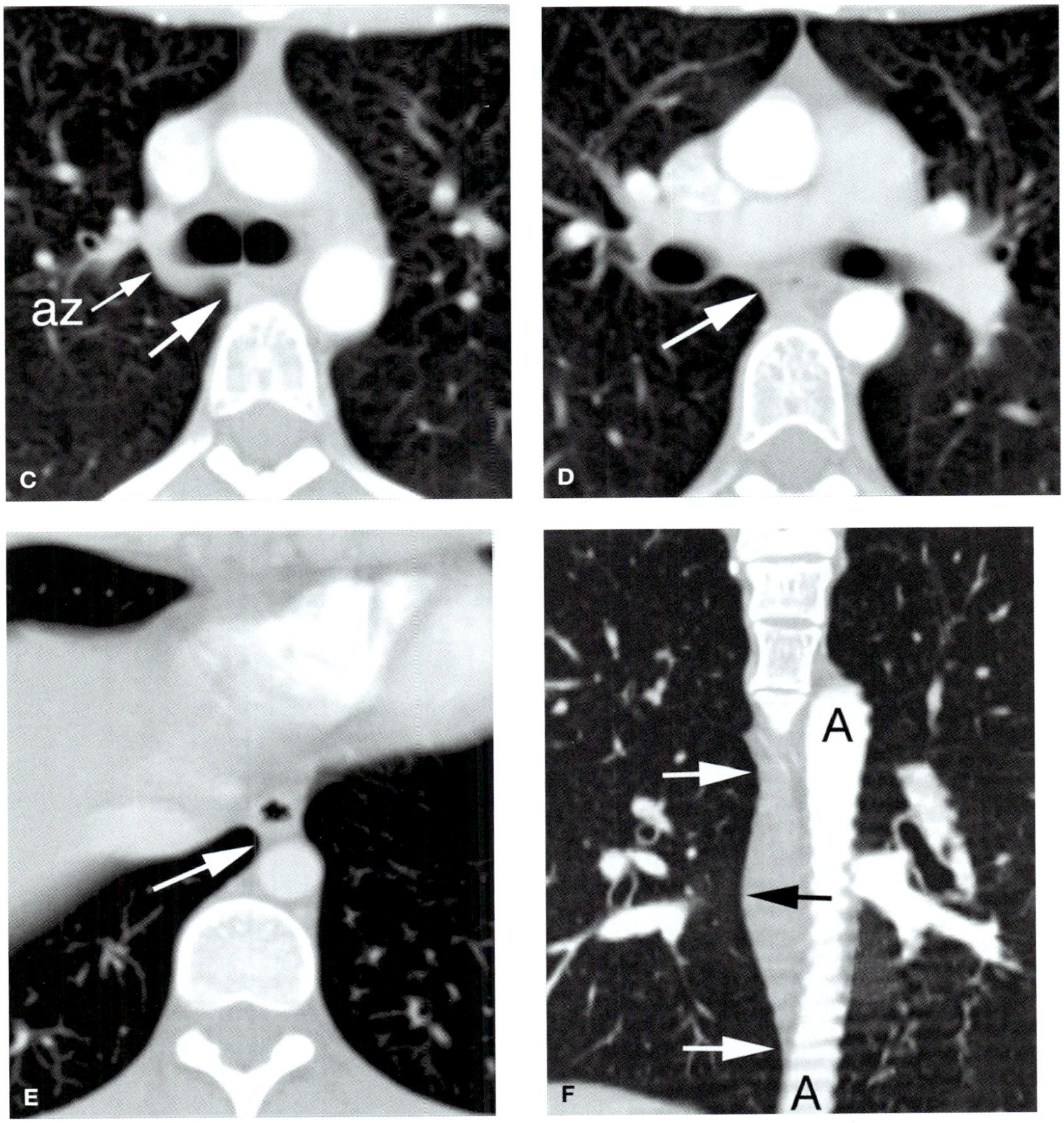

Figure 2.18. (*Continued*) **C-E:** CT at different levels in the same patient as in (**A**) shows the azygoesophageal recess (*arrows*). It begins at the level of the azygos arch (*az*) and ends at the diaphragm. **F:** Coronal reformation in the same patient shows the azygoesophageal recess (*arrows*), with a typical contour. *A*, aorta.

Azygoesophageal Recess

Visibility: Almost always visible on well-penetrated radiographs

Significance: Convexity of the superior aspect of the azygoesophageal recess is most common with (1) subcarinal lymph node enlargement, (2) subcarinal bronchogenic cyst, (3) left atrial dilatation, (4) dilatation of the azygos vein, and (5) esophageal mass or dilatation. Convexity of the inferior aspect of the azygoesophageal stripe is most common with (1) esophageal mass or dilatation or (2) hiatal hernia

Left Paraaortic Interface

Location:	Line of contact between descending aorta and medial left lung
Anatomy:	Descending aorta, adjacent fat, and two layers of pleura
Appearance:	A straight, concave, or convex interface below the aortic arch, parallel to the left paravertebral stripe

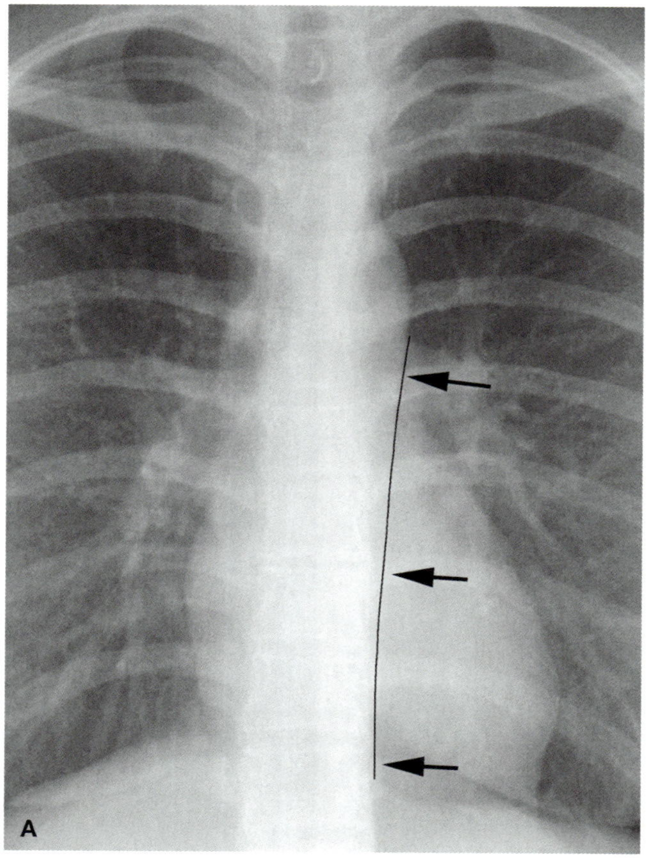

Figure 2.19. Left paraaortic interface. **A:** PA chest radiograph. The line of contact between the descending aorta and medial left lung represents the paraaortic interface. This edge is straight, concave, or convex and is seen below the aortic arch and parallel but lateral to the left paravertebral stripe.

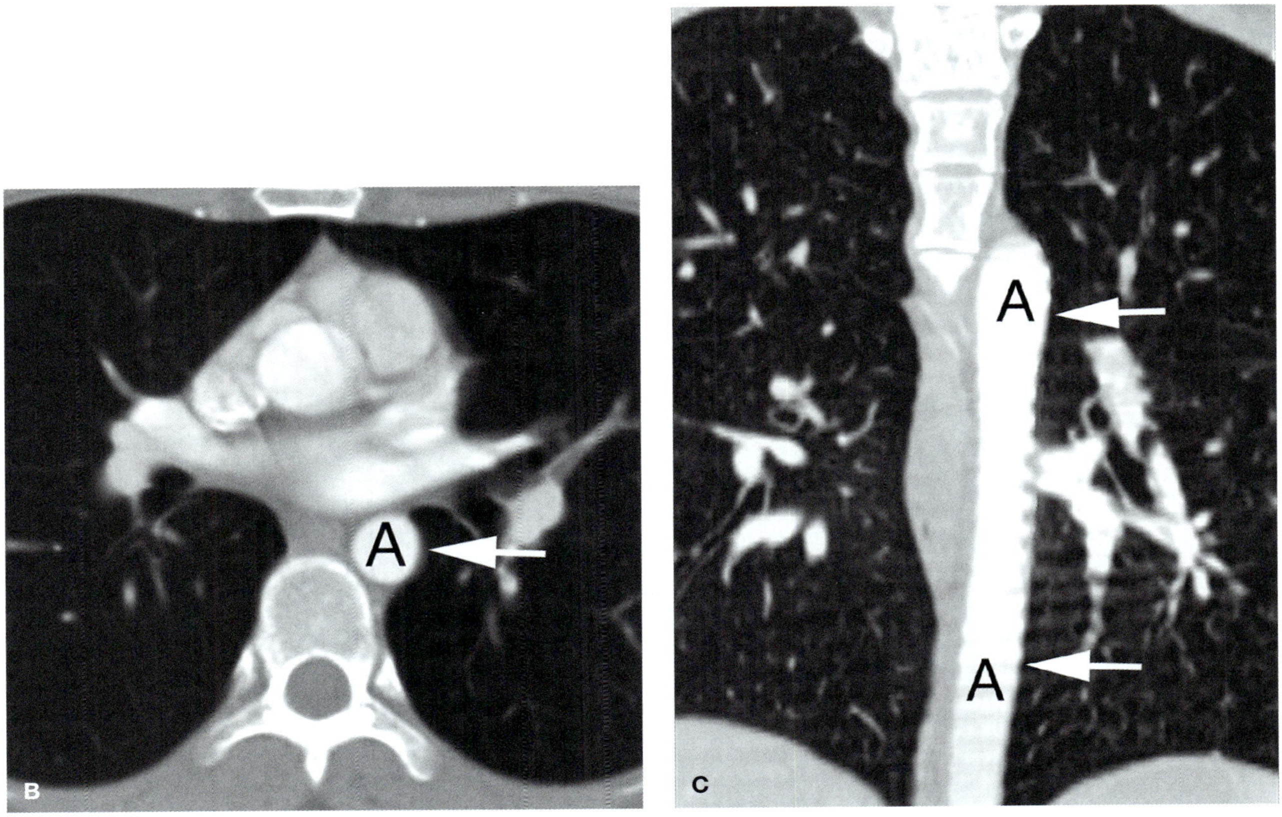

Figure 2.19. (*Continued*) **B:** CT in the same patient. Lung outlines the left lateral wall (*arrow*) of the aorta (*A*). **C:** Coronal reformation in the same patient shows the left paraaortic interface (*arrows*). Its contour is wavy because of pulsations. *A*, descending aorta.

Left Paraaortic Interface

Visibility: Very common

Significance: Increased convexity is related to tortuosity of the aorta or diffuse dilatation (eg, aneurysm or dissection); focal convexity indicates aneurysm, lymph node enlargement, hiatal hernia, or paraaortic mediastinal mass

Preaortic Recess

Location:	Recess in the left mediastinum outlined by the lung, behind the heart, below the aortic arch, and anterior to the descending aorta
Anatomy:	The preaortic recess on the left is analogous to the azygoesophageal recess on the right but is usually thinner and less well seen; the esophagus is variably related to the preaortic recess
Appearance:	This interface is most commonly seen immediately below the aortic arch as the preaortic line, which is usually straight

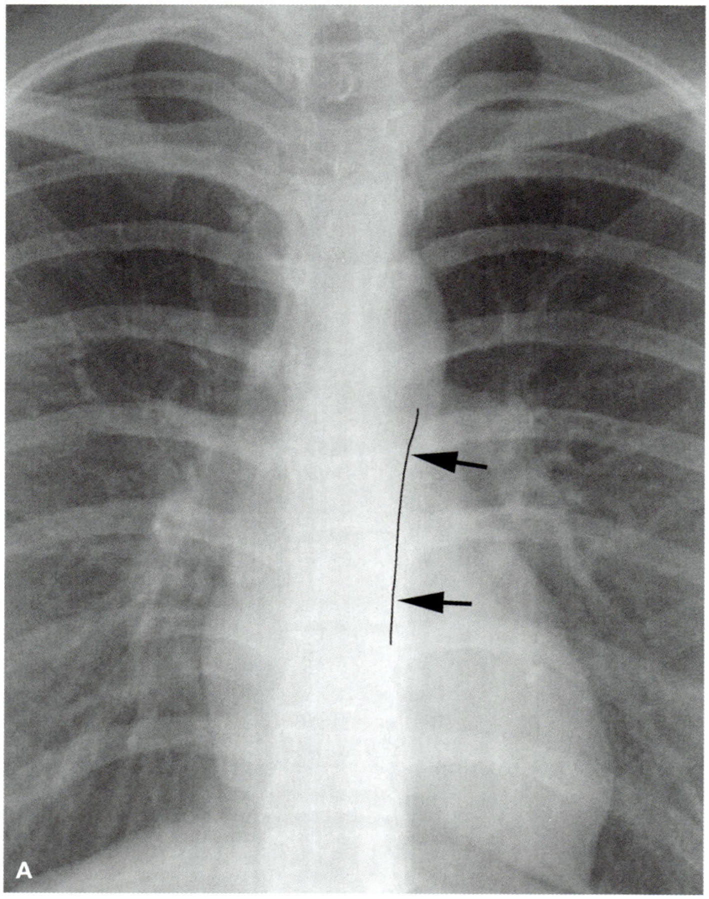

Figure 2.20. Preaortic recess. **A:** PA chest radiograph. The preaortic recess (*arrows*) is outlined by the lung, behind the heart, below the aortic arch, and anterior to the descending aorta. It is seen medial to the descending aorta. It is seen in the left mediastinum and is analogous to the azygoesophageal recess on the right, although it is less well seen.

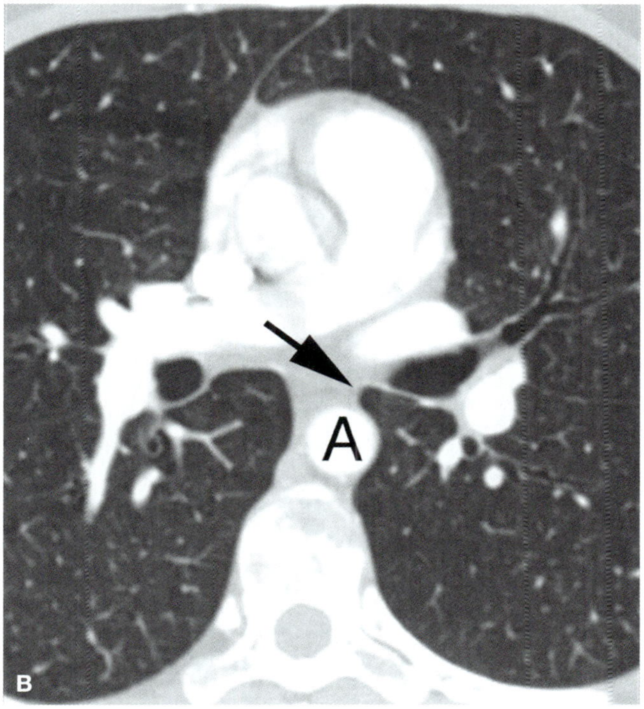

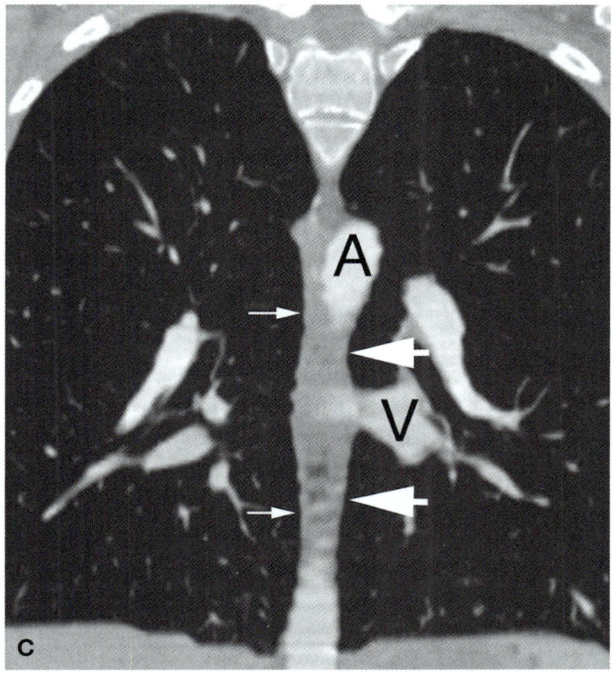

Figure 2.20. (*Continued*) **B:** CT shows the preaortic recess (*arrow*) outlined by the lung, anterior to the aorta (*A*). **C:** Coronal reformation in the same patient shows the preaortic recess (*large arrows*). Its contour is similar to that of the azygoesophageal recess on the right (*small arrows*). *A*, aortic arch; *V*, left pulmonary veins.

Preaortic Recess

Variant: If air is present in the esophagus, a stripe is commonly visible representing the left esophageal wall; this is referred to as the left inferior esophageal (or pleuroesophageal) stripe; it is most commonly seen immediately under the aortic arch

Visibility: Uncommon

Significance: Most useful in diagnosing esophageal or aortic lesions; a lateral convexity in the inferior portion of this line is common with hiatal hernia in association with convexity in the inferior azygoesophageal recess

Paravertebral Stripes or Interfaces (Left and Right)

Location:	Linear regions of contact between the posterior lower lobes and the paravertebral soft tissues adjacent to the spine
Anatomy:	Pleural reflections over paravertebral fat, lymph nodes, and vessels; on the left, the pleural reflection is posterior to the descending aorta and closely related to the hemiazygos vein
Appearance:	Left paravertebral stripe: 1. Commonly visible below the aortic arch, although in obese individuals it may be seen above the arch because of increased paravertebral fat 2. Inferiorly visible below the level of the diaphragmatic dome, merging with the shadow of the diaphragmatic crus 3. Parallels the spine; often seen halfway between the spine and lateral margin of the aorta 4. Usually thin Right paravertebral stripe: 1. Thinner and less often seen than the left paravertebral stripe 2. Visible only adjacent to the lower thoracic spine 3. Inferiorly, it merges with the shadow of the diaphragmatic crus

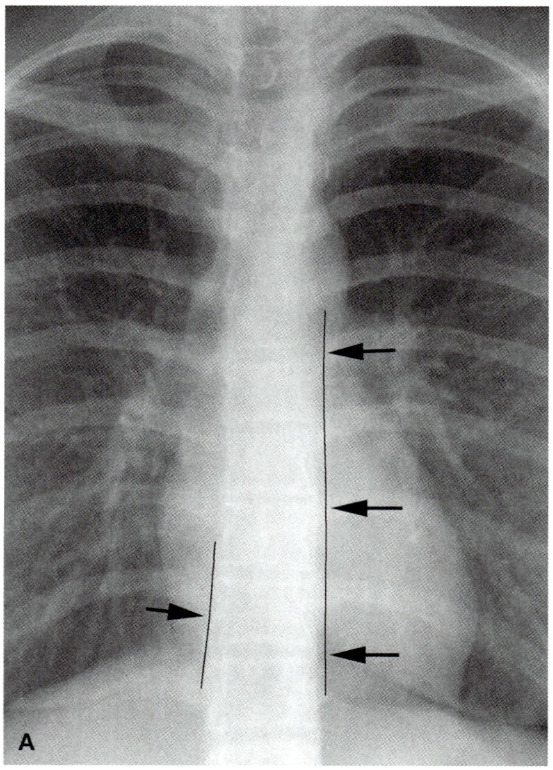

Figure 2.21. Paravertebral stripes. **A:** PA chest radiograph. The paravertebral stripes (*arrows*) represent the linear regions of contact between the posterior lower lobes and the paravertebral soft tissues adjacent to the spine. They parallel the spine. On the left, this stripe is seen medial to the descending aorta. The left paravertebral stripe is usually better seen and seen over a longer course than the right.

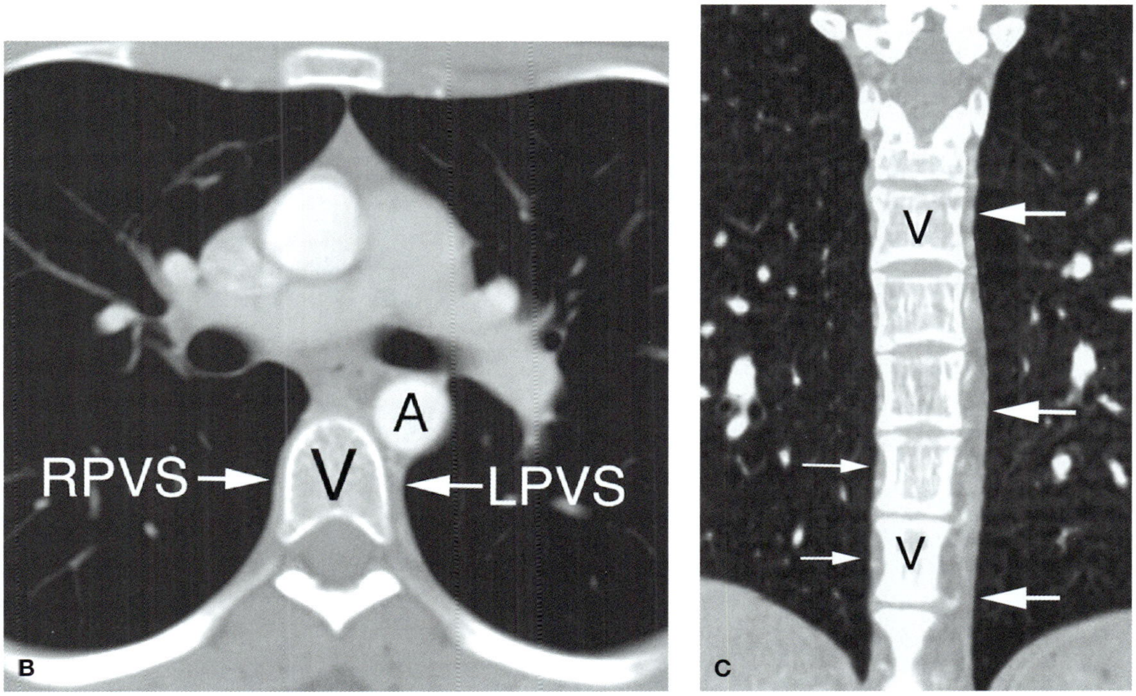

Figure 2.21. (*Continued*) **B:** CT in the same patient shows the left (*LPVS*) and right (*RPVS*) paravertebral stripes (*arrows*) outlined by the lung, lateral to the vertebral body (*V*). The LPVS is thicker and located posterior to the descending aorta (*A*) and medial to its lateral edge. **C:** Coronal reformation in the same patient shows the right (*small arrows*) and left paravertebral stripes (*large arrows*). Their edges parallel the edges of the vertebral column (*V*). Intercostal arteries and veins are visible within soft tissue of the paravertebral stripes.

Paravertebral Stripes or Interfaces (Left and Right)

Caveats:	Left stripe increases in thickness with aortic tortuosity or supine position; right stripe increases in thickness in patients with osteophytes
Significance:	Increased in thickness with (1) pleural effusion, (2) lymph node enlargement, (3) vertebral abnormalities (fracture, infection, neoplasm), (4) paravertebral mediastinal masses, (5) hemiazygos vein enlargement (left stripe), or (6) azygos vein enlargement (right stripe)

Retrosternal Stripe

Location:	The linear region of contact between the anterior lungs and the retrosternal soft tissues
Anatomy:	Retrosternal fat anterior to the lungs associated with the internal mammary lymph nodes and vessels
Appearance:	A smooth stripe of soft tissue, up to 7 mm in thickness in normal individuals, seen posterior to the sternum; inferiorly, the thickness of this stripe increases significantly in relation to the cardiac incisura and is variable in appearance; superiorly, the thickness increases in relation to the brachiocephalic veins and is variable

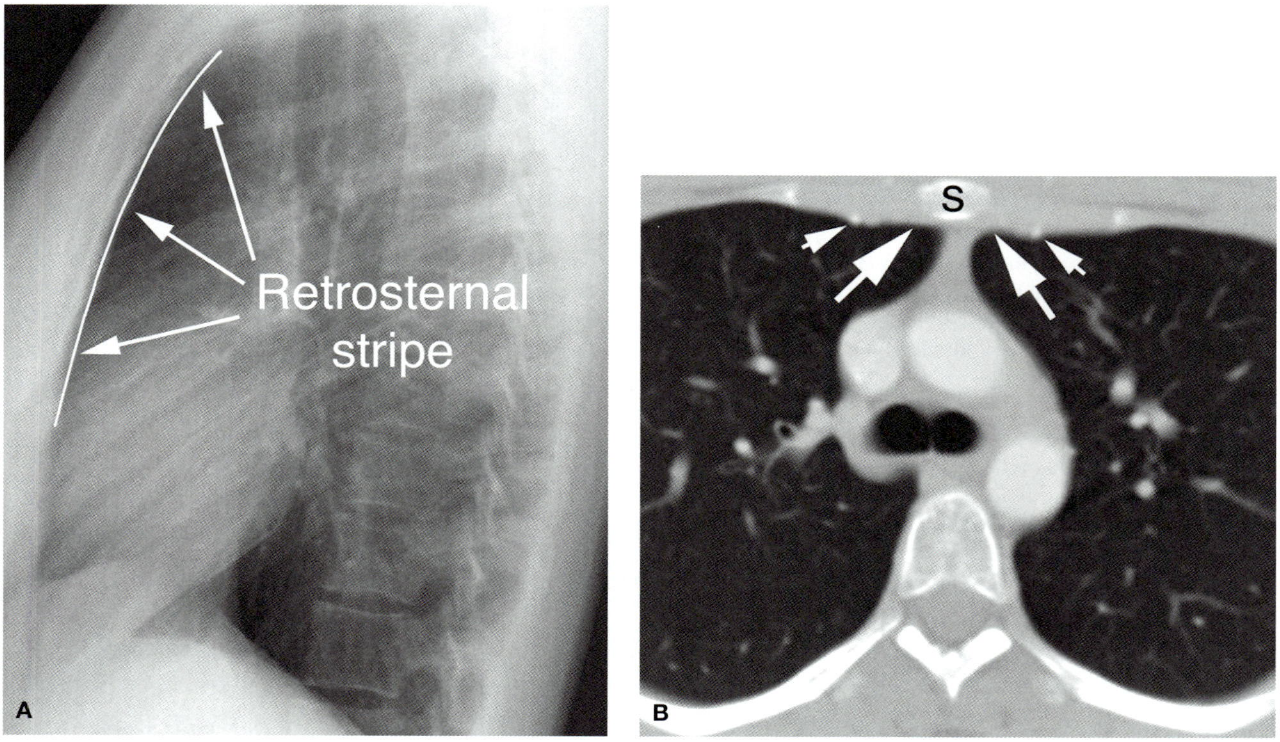

Figure 2.22. Retrosternal stripe. **A:** Lateral radiograph in the same patient as shown in Figure 2.21. The retrosternal stripe is a linear region of contact between the anterior lungs and the retrosternal soft tissues and is visible as a thin line of soft tissue behind the sternum. **B:** CT in the same patient shows soft tissue posterior to the sternum (s) forming an interface with the anterior lung (*large arrows*). The retrosternal stripe may also reflect contact of anterior lung with the region of the internal mammary vessels (*small arrows*) or nodes.

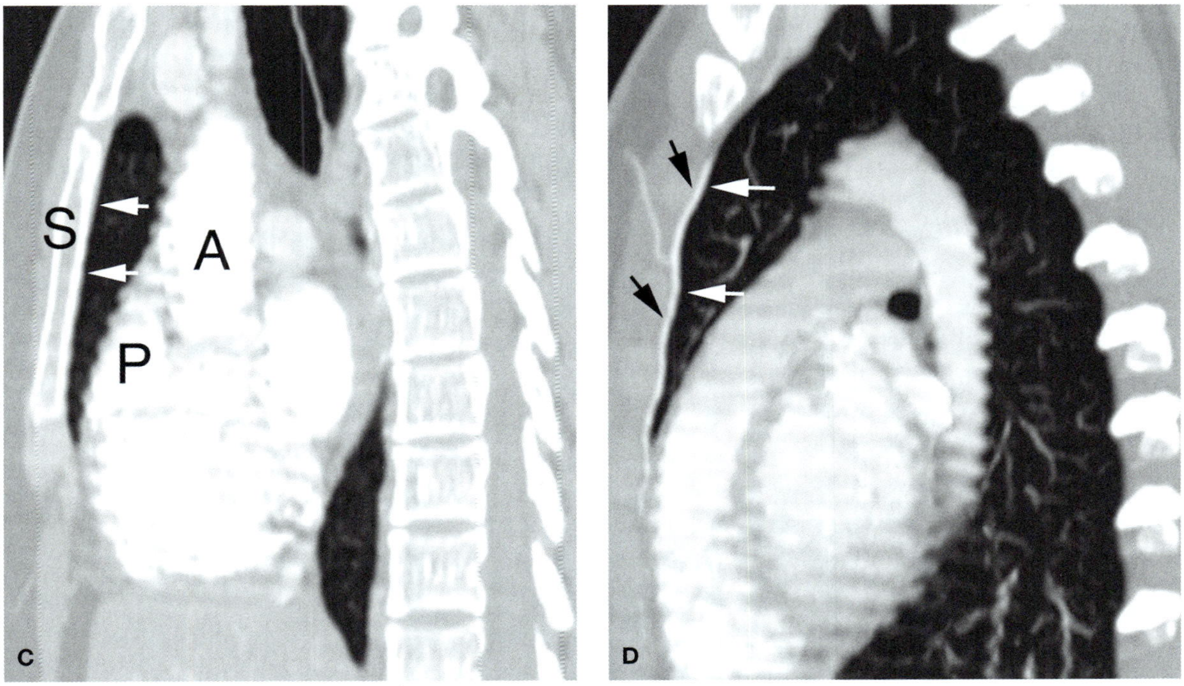

Figure 2.22. (*Continued*) **C:** Sagittal reformation in the same patient shows a very thin retrosternal stripe (*arrows*) posterior to the sternum (*S*). *A*, ascending aorta; *P*, main pulmonary artery. **D:** Sagittal reformation in a more lateral location in the same patient shows a wavy contour of the soft-tissue stripe (*white arrows*). This contour is typically seen with slight rotation. The wavy contour is related to the ribs or costal cartilage. The internal mammary artery (*black arrows*) is visible.

Retrosternal Stripe

Caveat: Slight rotation may project the right or left anterior chest wall posterior to the sternum, mimicking increased thickness of the retrosternal stripe; look for the location of the anterior ribs and costal cartilage before diagnosing an apparent thickening of the retrosternal stripe; a wavy contour of the soft-tissue stripe (related to the ribs) often indicates it is due to rotation

Visibility: Common

Significance: Increases in thickness with (1) internal mammary lymph node enlargement, (2) tortuosity of internal mammary arteries (eg, coarctation), (3) postmedian sternotomy, (4) sternal fractures, or (5) sternal lesions

Retrosternal Clear Space

Synonym:	Anterior clear space
Location:	Region posterior to the sternum; anterior and superior to the heart, main pulmonary artery, and ascending aorta; anterior to the trachea and superior vena cava
Anatomy:	This space corresponds to the prevascular space seen on CT, largely representing thymus and retrosternal tissues
Appearance:	An area of lucency anterior to the heart and great vessels; the anterior margins of the heart and great vessels may or may not be clearly seen

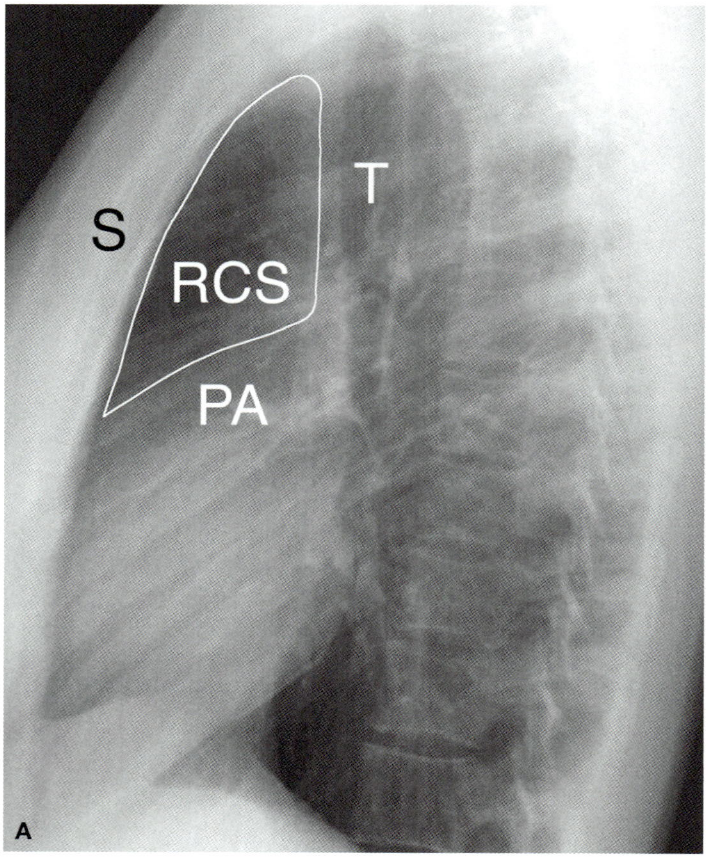

Figure 2.23. Retrosternal clear space. **A:** Lateral radiograph shows an area of relative lucency (*RCS*) posterior to the sternum (*S*), superior to the main pulmonary artery (*PA*), and anterior to the trachea (*T*).

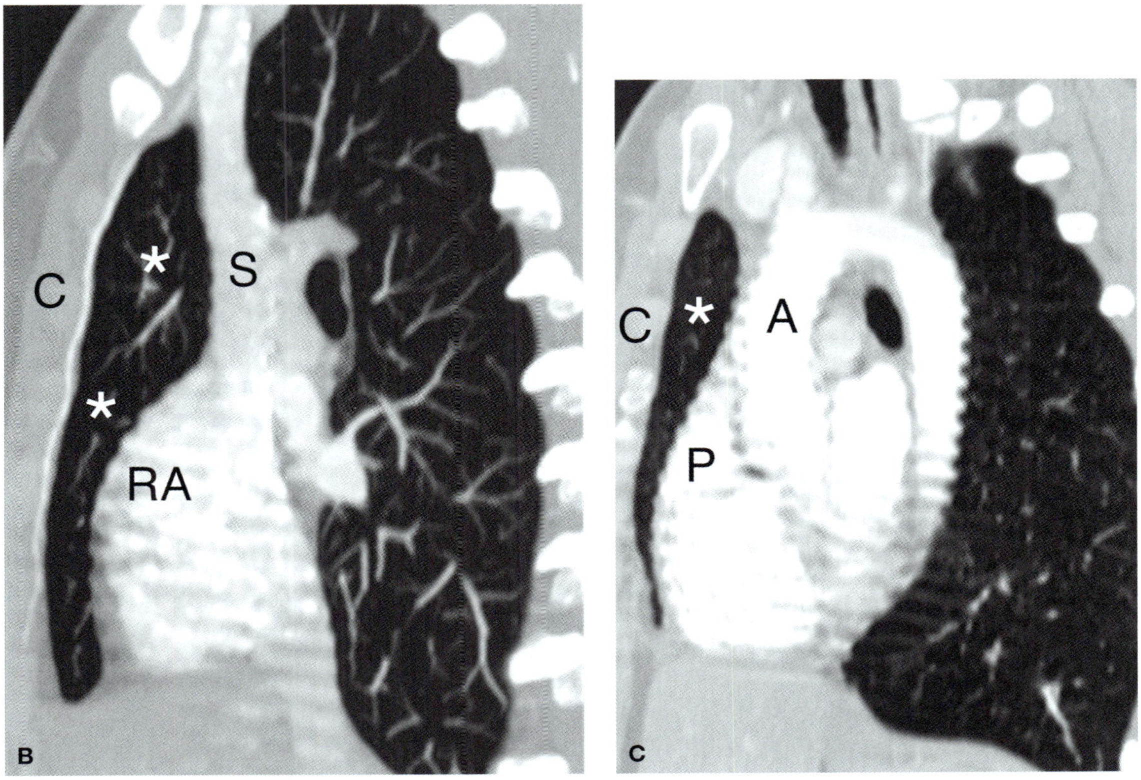

Figure 2.23. (*Continued*) **B:** Sagittal reformation in the same patient to the right of midline shows this area of lucency (*) posterior to costal cartilage (*C*), anterior to the superior vena cava (*S*), and anterior and superior to the right atrium (*RA*). **C:** Sagittal reformation in the same patient to the left of midline shows the retrosternal lucency (*) posterior to the costal cartilage (*C*) and anterior to the aortic arch (*A*) and main pulmonary artery (*P*).

Retrosternal Clear Space

Caveat:	In patients with a large amount of prevascular fat, lucency may be minimal
Visibility:	Common
Significance:	Increase in depth and lucency with emphysema; decrease in depth with right ventricular or main pulmonary artery dilatation; decrease in lucency in patients with prevascular (anterior) mediastinal mass

Posterior Tracheal Band or Stripe

Location: Linear region corresponding to the posterior tracheal wall and sometimes esophagus; below the thoracic inlet and above the tracheal bifurcation

Anatomy: Posterior tracheal wall, a small amount of mediastinal fat, and (variably) one or both esophageal walls, outlined posteriorly by air in lung or the esophageal lumen and outlined anteriorly by air in the tracheal lumen

Appearance: Variable appearance because of variable anatomy:

1. Posterior tracheal wall only: Visible as a very thin line
2. Posterior tracheal wall, esophagus with or without air in the esophageal lumen: A thicker stripe or band

May be seen for the entire length of the trachea; because of variable anatomy, may measure 1 to 6 mm thick in normal individuals

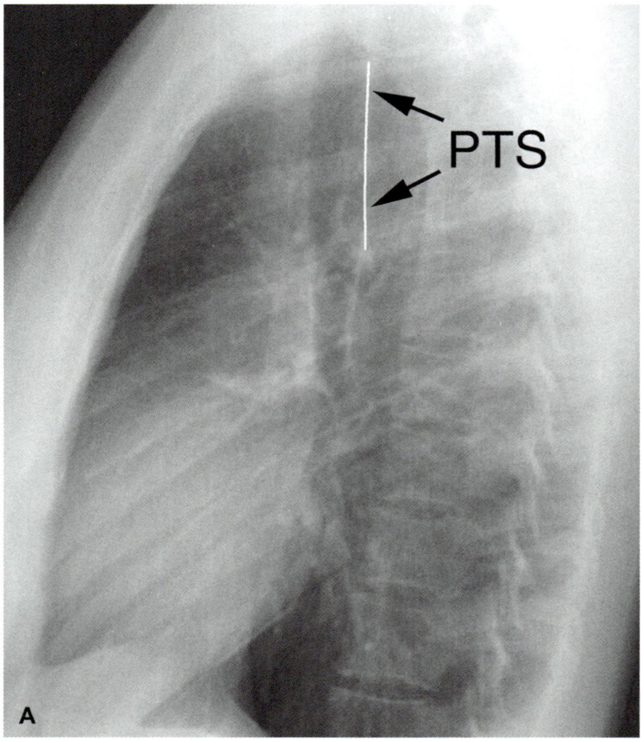

Figure 2.24. Posterior tracheal stripe. **A:** Lateral radiograph. The posterior tracheal stripe (*PTS*) is a linear opacity corresponding to the posterior tracheal wall and sometimes the esophagus, seen below the thoracic inlet and above the tracheal bifurcation. It is of variable thickness.

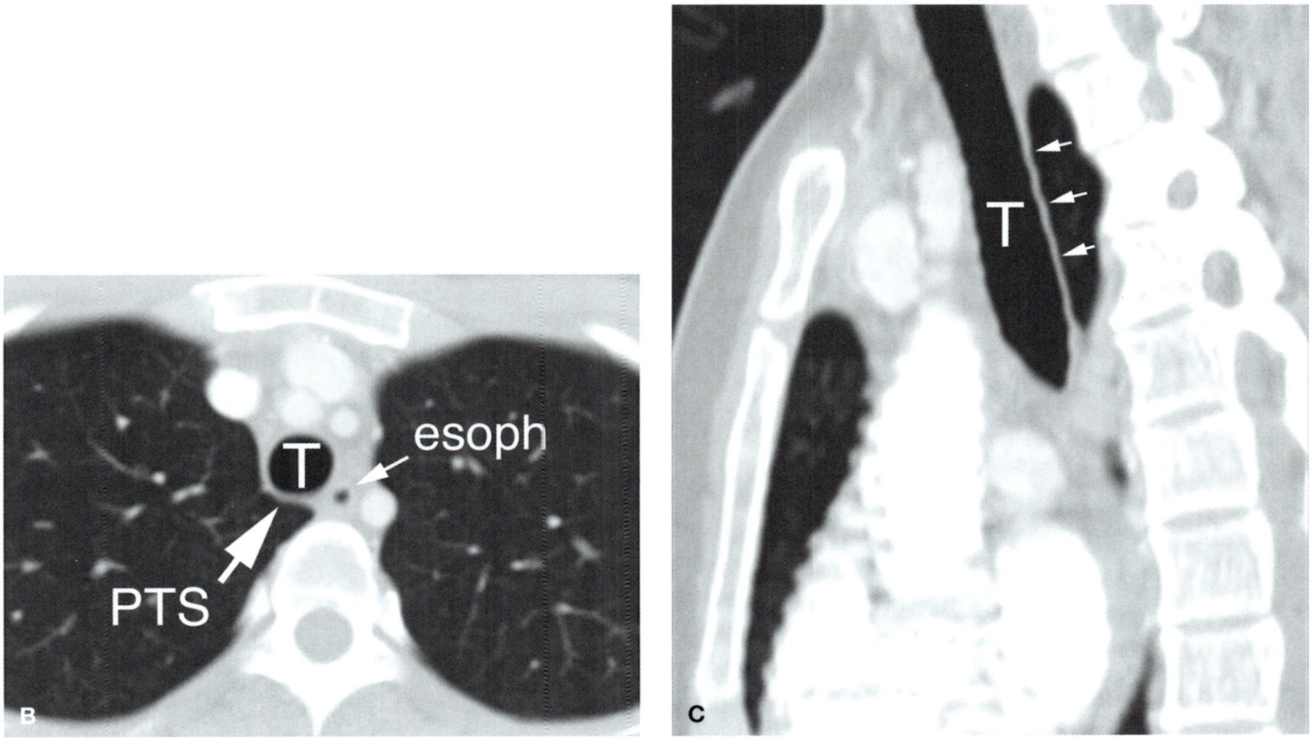

Figure 2.24. (*Continued*) **B:** CT in the same patient shows lung contacting posterior tracheal wall, outlining the posterior tracheal stripe (*PTS*). *T*, trachea; *esoph*, esophagus. **C:** Sagittal reformation in the same patient shows lung outlining the posterior wall of the trachea (*T*), forming the posterior tracheal stripe.

Posterior Tracheal Band or Stripe

Variant: If the stripe also includes anterior esophageal wall (with air in the esophageal lumen) or the entire esophagus, it is termed the posterior tracheoesophageal stripe

Visibility: Common

Significance: Variability in thickness limits usefulness; increased thickness usually indicates (1) esophageal carcinoma, (2) esophageal inflammation/esophagitis, (3) variant arterial anatomy with aberrant subclavian artery, and (4) much less often, tracheal wall thickening

Retrotracheal Triangle

Location:	Region posterior to the trachea, anterior to the spine, and above the posterior aortic arch
Anatomy:	Primarily esophagus with associated lymph nodes; it corresponds to the region of the posterior junction line seen on the frontal film
Appearance:	A relatively lucent region marginated anteriorly by the posterior tracheal stripe and posteriorly by the spine
Visibility:	Common
Significance:	Increased attenuation in this space most common with (1) esophageal lesions, (2) lymph node enlargement, (3) thyroid mass, (4) aberrant subclavian artery, (5) aneurysm, and (6) foregut duplication cyst

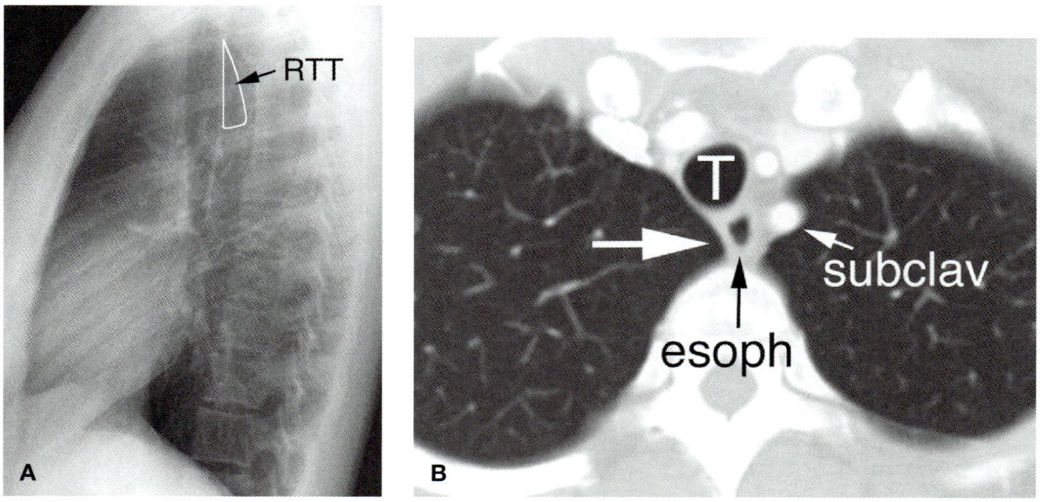

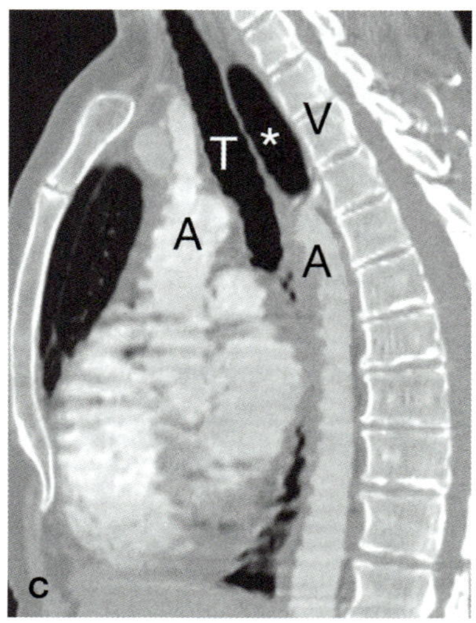

Figure 2.25. Retrotracheal triangle. **A:** Lateral radiograph. The retrotracheal triangle (*RTT*) is a relatively lucent region marginated anteriorly by the posterior tracheal stripe and posteriorly by the spine. **B:** CT in the same patient. The retrotracheal triangle corresponds to the region of the posterior junction line seen on the PA radiograph and reflects a narrowing of the mediastinum (*arrow*) behind the trachea (*T*) and left subclavian artery (*subclav*) and in relation to the esophagus (*esoph*). **C:** Sagittal reformation in the same patient shows the lucent retrotracheal triangle (*), posterior to the trachea (*T*), anterior to the vertebral column (*V*), and above the aortic arch (*A*).

SUGGESTED READINGS

Aronberg DJ, Glazer HS, Madsen K, Sagel SS. Normal thoracic aortic diameters by computed tomography. *J Comput Assist Tomogr*. 1984;8(2):247-250.

Aronberg DJ, Peterson RR, Glazer HS, Sagel SS. The superior sinus of the pericardium: CT appearance. *Radiology*. 1984;153(2):489-492.

Baron RL, Lee JK, Sagel SS, Peterson RR. Computed tomography of the normal thymus. *Radiology*. 1982;142(1):121-125.

Blank N, Castellino RA. Patterns of pleural reflections of the left superior mediastinum. Normal anatomy and distortions produced by adenopathy. *Radiology*. 1972;102(3):585-589.

Breatnach E, Abbott GC, Fraser RG. Dimensions of the normal human trachea. *AJR Am J Roentgenol*. 1984;142(5):903-906.

Carter BW, Benveniste MF, Madan R, et al. ITMIG classification of mediastinal compartments and multidisciplinary approach to mediastinal masses. *Radiographics*. 2017;37(2):413-436. doi:10.1148/rg.2017160095

de Geer G, Webb WR, Gamsu G. Normal thymus: assessment with MR and CT. *Radiology*. 1986;158(2):313-317.

Friedman AC, Chambers E, Sprayregen S. The normal and abnormal left superior intercostal vein. *AJR Am J Roentgenol*. 1978;131(4):599-602.

Gamsu G, Webb WR. Computed tomography of the trachea and mainstem bronchi. *Semin Roentgenol*. 1983;18(1):51-60.

Genereux GP. The posterior pleural reflections. *AJR Am J Roentgenol*. 1983;141(1):141-149.

Gibbs JM, Chandrasekhar CA, Ferguson EC, Oldham SAA. Lines and Stripes: where did they go?—from conventional radiography to CT. *Radiographics*. 2007;27(1):33-48.

Glazer GM, Gross BH, Quint LE, Francis IR, Bookstein FL, Orringer MB. Normal mediastinal lymph nodes: number and size according to American Thoracic Society mapping. *AJR Am J Roentgenol*. 1985;144(2):261-265.

Heitzman ER, Scrivani JV, Martino J, Moro J. The azygos vein and its pleural reflections. I. Normal roentgen anatomy. *Radiology*. 1971;101(2):249-258.

Heitzman ER, Lane EJ, Hammack DB, Rimmler LJ. Radiological evaluation of the aortic-pulmonic window. *Radiology*. 1975;116(3):513-518.

Keats TE. The aortic-pulmonary mediastinal stripe. *Am J Roentgenol Radium Ther Nucl Med*. 1972;116(1):107-109.

Kiyono K, Sone S, Sakai F, et al. The number and size of normal mediastinal lymph nodes: a postmortem study. *AJR Am J Roentgenol*. 1988;150(4):771-776.

Landay MJ. Anterior clear space: how clear? How often? How come? *Radiology*. 1994;192(1):165-169.

McComb BL. Reflecting upon the left superior mediastinum. *J Thorac Imaging*. 2001;16(1):56-64.

Milne EN, Pistolesi M, Miniati M, Giuntini C. The vascular pedicle of the heart and the vena azygos. Part I: the normal subject. *Radiology*. 1984;152:1-8.

Palayew MJ. The tracheo-esophageal stripe and the posterior tracheal band. *Radiology*. 1979;132(1):11-13.

Proto AV, Corcoran HL, Ball JB. The left paratracheal reflection. *Radiology*. 1989;171(3):625-628.

Proto AV. Mediastinal anatomy: emphasis on conventional images with anatomic and computed tomographic correlations. *J Thorac Imaging*. 1987;2:1-48.

Ravenel JG, Erasmus JJ. Azygoesophageal recess. *J Thorac Imaging*. 2002;17(3):219-226.

Savoca CJ, Austin JH, Goldberg HI. The right paratracheal stripe. *Radiology*. 1977;122(2):295-301.

Smathers RL, Buschi AJ, Pope TL, Brenbridge AN, Williamson BR. The azygous arch: normal and pathologic CT appearance. *AJR Am J Roentgenol*. 1982;139(3):477-483.

Chapter 3

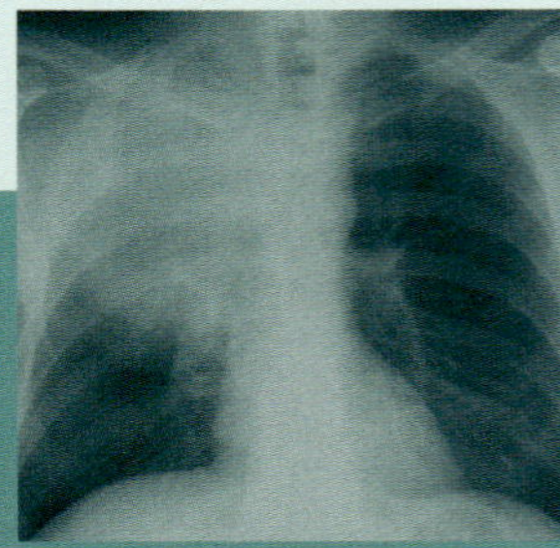

Travis S. Henry

The Pulmonary Hila

CHEST RADIOGRAPHS

In most cases, plain films are adequate for identifying large hilar masses. Small masses or borderline lymph node enlargement can be more difficult to detect because of variation in the radiographic appearances of the normal hila.

Nonetheless, careful evaluation of the hila on chest radiographs can often yield significant diagnostic information. Abnormalities may present as a change in hilar size or density, bronchial wall thickening or narrowing of the bronchial lumen, or an alteration in the hilar contours.

Normal Hilar Contours: Frontal Radiograph

On a frontal (posteroanterior [PA] or anteroposterior) radiograph, the hilar shadows primarily represent the silhouettes of the hilar pulmonary arteries. The left pulmonary artery is situated higher than the right, and consequently, the left hilum appears higher than the right in 97% of cases; in the remainder, they are at the same level. The left bronchus is below the left pulmonary artery (hyparterial), whereas the right bronchus is above the right pulmonary artery (epiarterial).

Right Hilum

The superior portion of the right hilum is made up of the medially located truncus anterior, the artery supplying most of the upper lobe, and the right superior pulmonary vein, which forms the lateral margin of the upper hilum (Fig. 3.1). The anterior segment bronchus of the right upper lobe (RUL) is visible in 80% of patients as a 4- to 5-mm ring shadow in the lateral aspect of the hilum, accompanied by an artery of similar size. The RUL bronchus is sometimes visible.

The lower aspect of the right hilum is made up of the interlobar or descending pulmonary artery laterally and the bronchus intermedius medially. The pulmonary artery typically measures 16 mm or less in thickness lateral to the bronchus (approximately the diameter of a dime) in males and 15 mm or less in females. The interlobar artery tapers inferiorly as it branches, with its lateral aspect appearing straight or slightly convex. Branches of the interlobar artery and segmental bronchi may be seen in the inferior hilum. Occasionally, the lower part of the interlobar artery appears rounded, mimicking a mass or enlarged lymph node. This is most commonly seen when lung volumes are low.

A shallow concave angle is formed at the point where the superior pulmonary vein crosses the interlobar pulmonary artery. This is termed the *hilar angle* (Fig. 3.1).

The right inferior pulmonary vein is located inferior and medial to the hilum and does not contribute significantly to the hilar silhouette.

Left Hilum

The left pulmonary artery passes above the left main and upper lobe bronchus, gives off small upper lobe branches, and descends posterior and lateral to the left upper lobe (LUL) bronchus and lower lobe bronchus. The superior hilar shadow is made up of the superior aspect of the left pulmonary artery, superior pulmonary vein, and small arterial branches (Fig. 3.2). The anterior segmental bronchus of the LUL may be seen in the lateral hilum at this level. As on the right, the interlobar pulmonary artery tapers caudally, but it is less clearly seen and more difficult to measure than the right pulmonary artery. The left inferior pulmonary vein contributes little to the hilar shadow.

Normal Hilar Contours: Lateral Radiograph

The right and left hilar shadows are superimposed on the lateral radiograph, but specific parts of the right and left hila can be seen (Figs. 3.3 and 3.4). Identification of the hilar bronchi should be the first step in analysis of the hila on lateral films.

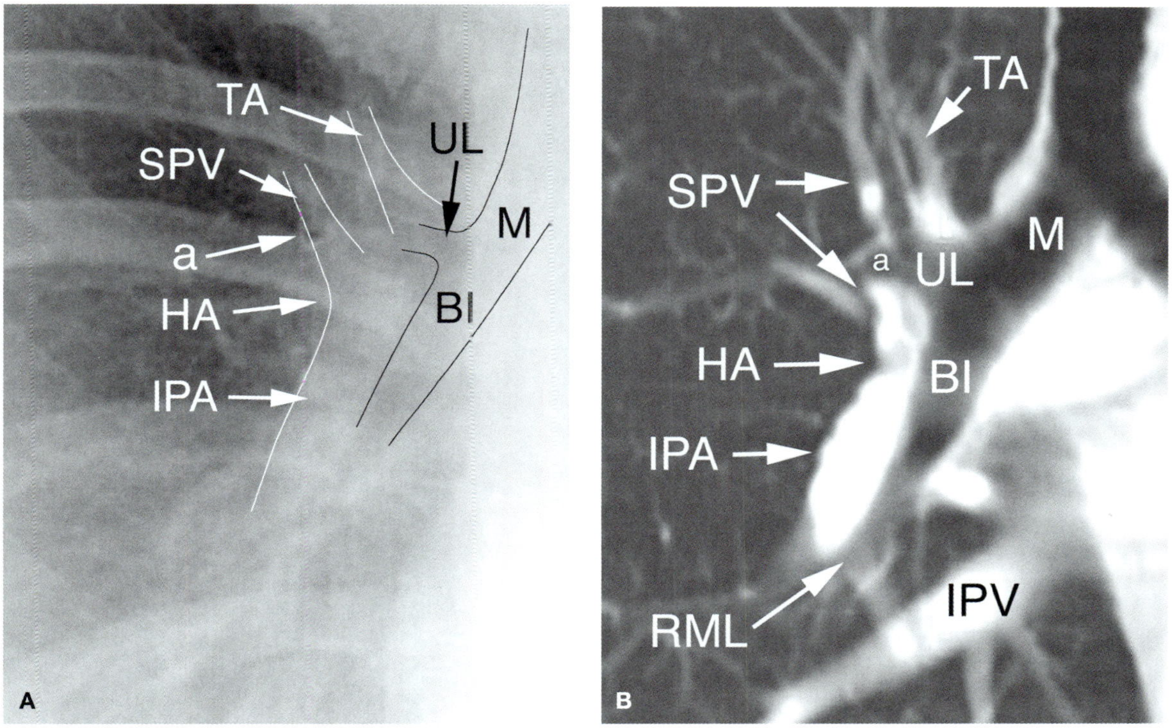

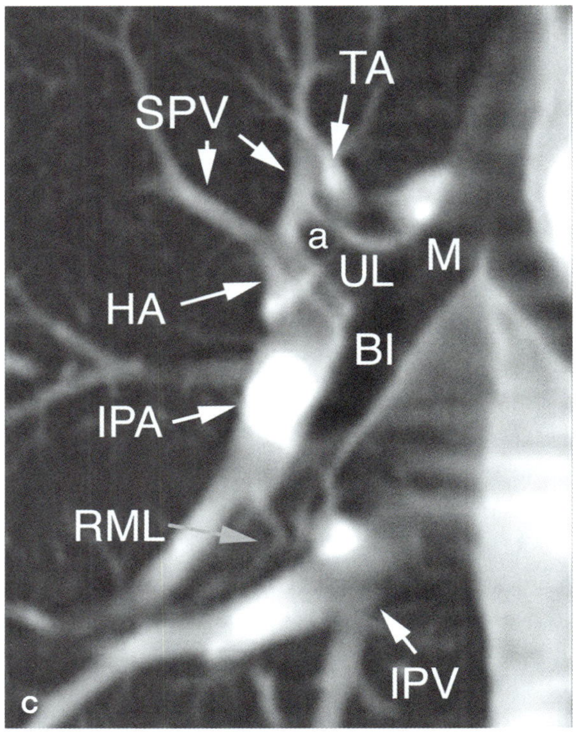

Figure 3.1. Normal right hilum. **A:** Plain radiograph. The large bronchi (*M*, right main bronchus; *UL*, right upper lobe bronchus; *BI*, bronchus intermedius) are visible in the medial hilum. The anterior segment bronchus (*a*) is visible as a ring shadow lateral to the pulmonary arteries. Visible vascular structures include the apical branch of the truncus anterior (*TA*) in the medial superior hilum and the superior pulmonary vein (*SPV*) in the lateral aspect of the superior hilum. The interlobar pulmonary artery (*IPA*) forms the lateral aspect of the inferior hilum and should measure 16 mm or less in men and 15 mm or less in women. A concavity is visible in the lateral hilum at the point the superior pulmonary vein crosses the interlobar pulmonary artery. This is termed the *hilar angle* (*HA*). **B, C:** Coronal CT reformations through the right hilum in two patients. In addition to the structures visible in (**A**), the right middle lobe bronchus (*RML*) is visible inferiorly. The inferior pulmonary vein (*IPV*) lies medial and below the hilar shadow and is difficult to recognize on the chest radiograph because of the heart shadow.

Right Hilum

The location of the tracheal carina and therefore the origins of the main bronchi can be determined by following the tracheal air column inferiorly. The carina is located at the point the air column begins to taper (Fig. 3.3B).

Below this level, a thin line, termed the *intermediate stem line*, is at least partially visible in 95% of patients (see Fig. 3.3). This line may be 5 cm or more in length and measures up to 3 mm in thickness. It corresponds superiorly to the posterior wall of the right main bronchus and more inferiorly to the posterior wall of

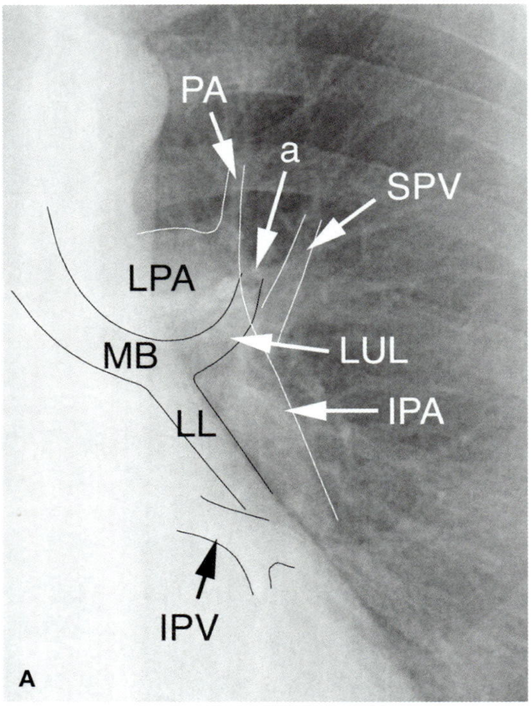

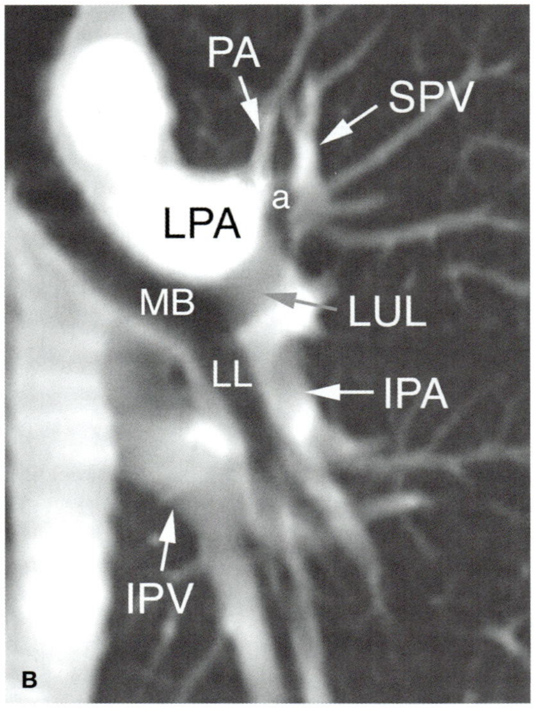

Figure 3.2. Normal left hilum. **A:** PA radiograph. **B:** Coronal CT reformation. *MB*, left main bronchus; *LUL*, left upper lobe bronchus; *LL*, left lower lobe bronchus. The anterior segment bronchus (*a*) is visible as a ring shadow lateral to the main pulmonary artery, overlying the superior trunk of the left upper lobe bronchus. The left pulmonary artery (*LPA*) is visible as an oval opacity above the main and left upper lobe bronchus. The apical branch of the left pulmonary artery (*PA*) arises from the superior aspect of the pulmonary artery and as on the right is located medially. The superior pulmonary vein (*SPV*) forms the lateral aspect of the superior hilum. The interlobar pulmonary artery (*IPA*) forms the lateral aspect of the inferior hilum. The inferior pulmonary vein (*IPV*) may be visible inferiorly.

the bronchus intermedius (PWBI). The RUL bronchus is visible in 50% of patients as a rounded lucency anterior to the upper aspect of the intermediate stem line, but it is seldom seen well.

The anterior wall of the bronchus intermedius is visible as an edge, outlined by the right pulmonary artery and superior pulmonary vein. In combination, these vessels create an oval shadow making up the anterior portion of the hilar silhouette called the *right hilar vascular opacity*. The right middle lobe (RML) bronchus is sometimes seen curving anteriorly below the inferior edge of this oval shadow. In 15% of individuals, the anterior wall of the right lower lobe (RLL) bronchus is visible below this level as a thin straight line, 1 to 2 cm long.

Left Hilum

Below the carina, the left main bronchus is superimposed on the right main bronchus (see Fig. 3.4). A well-defined rounded lucency representing the horizontal portion of the distal left main bronchus and LUL bronchus (LM/LUL continuum) is visible in 80% of subjects several centimeters below the carina. This lucency is more clearly seen, is larger, and is better defined than the rounded lucency representing the RUL bronchus because vessels surround much of its circumference. Localizing the LM/LUL bronchus is an important first step in identifying left hilar structures on the lateral radiograph.

The anterior wall of the left lower lobe (LLL) bronchus is visible below the lucency of the LM/LUL bronchus as a thin curved line, concave anteriorly, in about 45% of cases. It arises tangential to the anterior wall of the LM/LUL bronchus.

The left pulmonary artery forms the roof of the LM/LUL bronchus, a comma-shaped opacity that passes above and then descends posteriorly. Thus, while the right hilar vasculature largely accounts for the soft tissue in the anterior aspect of the combined hilar silhouette, the left pulmonary artery primarily accounts for its posterior aspect.

Plain Film Diagnosis of Hilar Abnormalities: Frontal Radiograph

On a frontal radiograph, patients with a hilar mass or lymph node enlargement may show one of the several findings:

- Hilar enlargement (Fig. 3.5A)
- A focal mass (see Fig. 3.5B)
- Increase in hilar density (see Fig. 3.5C)
- Hilar lobulation (see Fig. 3.5D)
- Convexity of the hilar angle (see Fig. 3.5E)

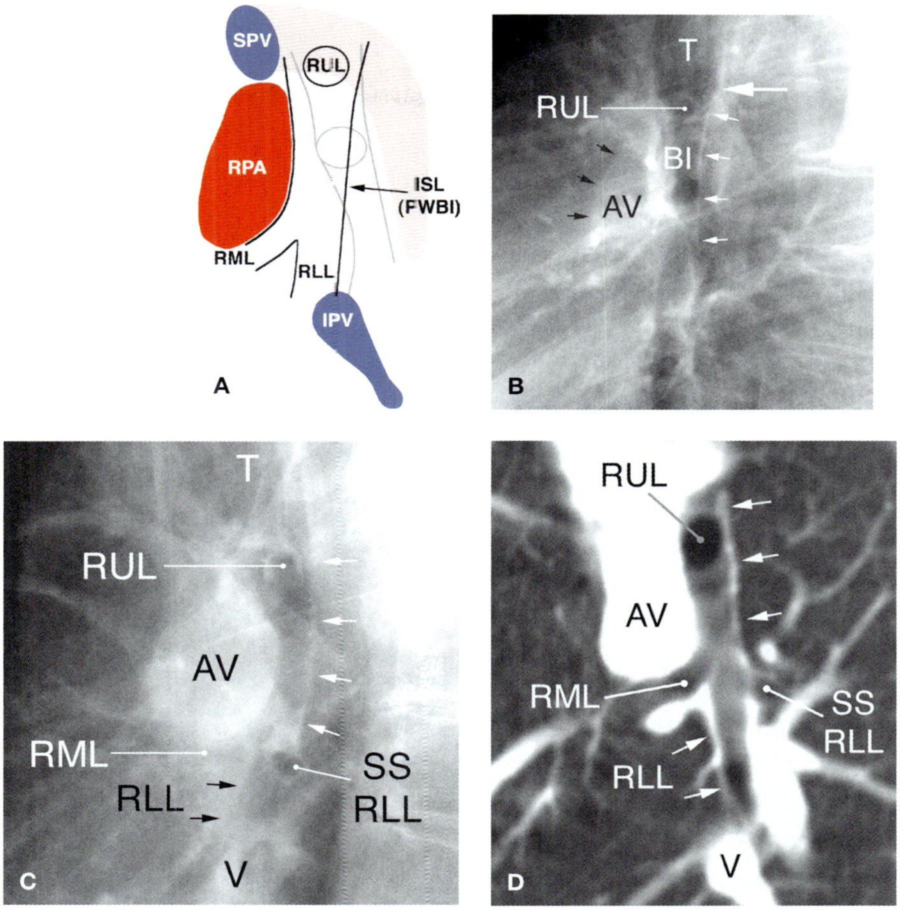

Figure 3.3. Lateral chest radiograph; normal right hilar anatomy. **A:** Diagram of right hilar structures. Anterior is to the left and posterior to the right. Right hilar structures appear dark, and left hilar structures are dimmed. *RUL*, right upper lobe bronchus; *BI*, bronchus intermedius; *RML*, right middle lobe bronchus; *RLL*, right lower lobe bronchus; *ISL*, intermediate stem line; *PWBI*, posterior wall of bronchus intermedius. The interlobar right pulmonary artery (*RPA*) results in an oval shadow anterior to the BI. The superior pulmonary vein (*SPV*), along with the truncus anterior, forms the superior part of the vascular shadow anterior to the bronchi. The inferior pulmonary veins (*IPV*) are inferior. Left hilar structures are described in Figure 3.4A. **B:** Lateral radiograph showing right hilar anatomy. The trachea (*T*) is visible superiorly. The point at which the tracheal air column narrows (*large white arrow*) is the carina; the main and lobar bronchi are seen below this level. The right upper lobe bronchus (*RUL*) may be seen as a rounded lucency within the superior hilar shadow, slightly below the carina. Below the RUL, the bronchus intermedius (*BI*) is visible to the level of its bifurcation. The intermediate stem line or posterior wall of the bronchus intermedius is often visible as a thin white line (*small white arrows*). The oval shadow of the right hilar arteries and veins (*black arrows*; *AV*) is visible anterior to the bronchus intermedius. **C:** Lateral radiograph showing right hilar anatomy in a patient with left pneumonectomy. Only right hilar structures are visible. The trachea (*T*) is visible superiorly. Visible are the right upper lobe bronchus (*RUL*), intermediate stem line (posterior wall of the bronchus intermedius) (*white arrows*), right middle lobe bronchus (*RML*), superior segmental bronchus of the right lower lobe (*SS RLL*), and the anterior wall of the right lower lobe bronchus (*black arrows*; *RLL*). Below the RUL, the bronchus intermedius (*BI*) is visible to the level of its bifurcation. The oval shadow of the right hilar arteries and veins (*AV*) is visible anterior to the bronchus intermedius, and the inferior pulmonary veins (*V*) are located inferiorly. **D:** CT reformation through the right hilum. *RUL*, right upper lobe bronchus; *white arrows*, intermediate stem line (posterior wall of the bronchus intermedius); *RML*, right middle lobe bronchus; *SS RLL*, superior segment bronchus of the right lower lobe; *RLL*, anterior wall of the right lower lobe bronchus; *AV*, right hilar arteries and veins; *V*, inferior pulmonary veins.

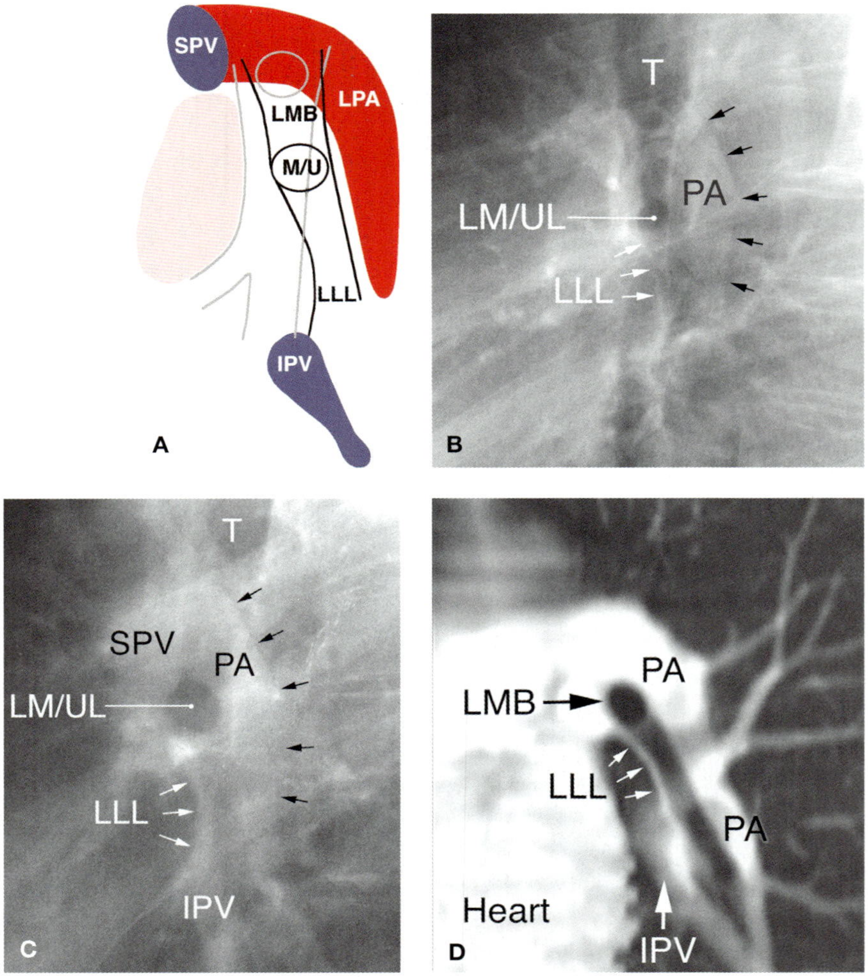

Figure 3.4. Lateral chest radiograph; normal left hilar anatomy. **A:** Diagram of hilar anatomy. Left hilar structures appear dark, and right hilar structures are dimmed. *LMB*, left main bronchus; *M/U*, lucency of the left main and left upper lobe bronchus; *LLL*, left lower lobe bronchus; *LPA*, left pulmonary artery; *IPV*, inferior pulmonary veins; *SPV*, superior pulmonary vein. For right hilar structures, see Figure 3.3A. **B:** Lateral radiograph showing left hilar anatomy; this is the same radiograph as in Figure 3.3B. The trachea (*T*) is visible superiorly. The horizontal portion of the left main and left upper lobe bronchus (*LM/UL*) results in an easily seen oval lucency. Above this level and superimposed on the bronchus intermedius, the main portion of the left main bronchus may be seen. The anterior wall of the left lower lobe bronchus (*LLL*) is visible below the *LM/UL* as a thin white line and typically appears concave anteriorly. *PA*, pulmonary artery. **C:** Lateral radiograph showing left hilar anatomy in a patient with a right pneumonectomy. Only left hilar structures are visible. The trachea (*T*) is visible superiorly. The oval lucency of the horizontal portion of the left main and left upper lobe bronchus (*LM/UL*) is easily seen. Below this level, the anterior wall of the left lower lobe (*LLL*) bronchus is visible as a thin white line, concave anteriorly. The left pulmonary artery (*PA*) is situated above and behind the LMB (*black arrows*). The left superior pulmonary veins (*SPV*) are visible anterior and superior to the LMB, and the inferior pulmonary veins (*IPV*) are located inferiorly. **D:** CT reformation through the left hilum. LMB, left main and left upper lobe bronchus; LLL, anterior wall of the left lower lobe bronchus; PA, left pulmonary artery; IPV, inferior pulmonary veins.

Hilar enlargement is often present in patients with hilar lymphadenopathy (see Fig. 3.5A) or hilar mass (see Fig. 3.5B); it may be unilateral or bilateral. In the large majority of normal patients, the hila appear equal in size on frontal radiographs; comparison of the two hila is helpful in patients with a unilateral abnormality. Measurement of the width of the right hilum lateral to the bronchus intermedius may also be valuable in diagnosis; as indicated above, this measurement should be 16 mm or less in males and 15 mm or less in females.

Masses sometimes produce a unilateral increase in the hilar density on frontal radiographs (see Fig. 3.5A and C).

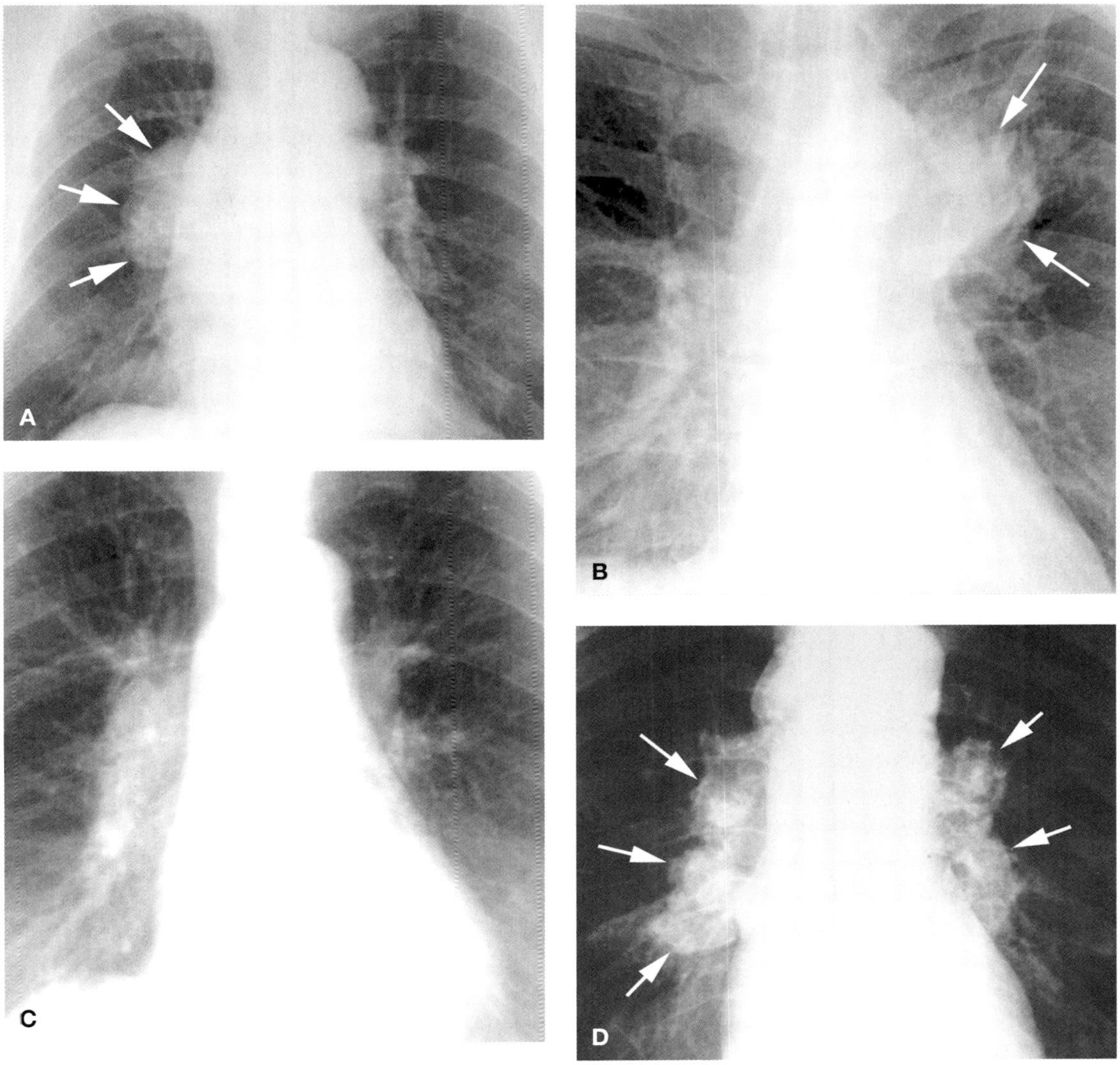

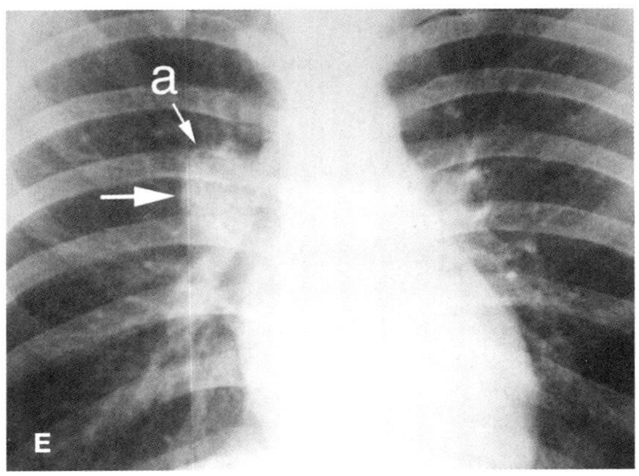

Figure 3.5. Radiographic findings in hilar mass or lymph node enlargement. **A:** Hilar enlargement in a patient with lymph node enlargement due to metastatic renal cell carcinoma. The right hilum (*arrows*) is markedly enlarged and is rounded in contour, without its normal "vascular" shape. **B:** Focal hilar mass in bronchogenic carcinoma. A single, poorly marginated mass (*arrows*) obscures the upper left hilum. This appearance is typical of lung cancer originating in the hilum. **C:** Increase in hilar density due to right hilar carcinoma. The right hilum appears denser than the left. This is often due to mass or enlarged nodes anterior or posterior to the hilum. The right hilum is also enlarged, with a subtle convexity in the hilar angle. **D:** Hilar lobulation due to sarcoidosis. The hila have distinct lobulated contours (*arrows*) typical of lymph node enlargement. Node calcification is also seen. **E:** Convexity of the hilar angle in a patient with Castleman disease involving the right hilum. A mass (*arrow*) is visible in the region of the hilar angle. The mass projects lateral to the anterior segment bronchus (*a*) of the upper lobe.

This generally results when a mass or lymph node enlargement is located in the anterior or posterior hilum and is superimposed on the hilar shadow. In some patients, an increase in hilar density may be the only visible abnormality on the frontal radiograph; in such cases, the mass is often better seen on the lateral radiograph.

Hilar mass results in a focal alteration of the normal hilar contours. Lymph node enlargement may result in a focal abnormality or a more generalized lobulated appearance (see Fig. 3.5A and D). A common site for lymph node enlargement in the right hilum is the normally concave hilar angle; a convexity in this region is abnormal (see Fig. 3.5E).

The normal hila look vascular. The hilar shadows, primarily representing the pulmonary arteries, taper inferiorly with vessels arising from their periphery. Enlargement of the pulmonary artery results in increased hilar size and density, but the hilum retains its "vascular" appearance (Fig. 3.6). The appearance of pulmonary vessels converging on the lateral aspect of the hilum is termed the *"hilum convergence" sign* and is indicative of vascular dilatation as the cause of hilar enlargement. The hilar angle typically retains its normal concave appearance.

Enlargement of hilar arteries occurs most frequently in pulmonary hypertension. In addition to hilar enlargement,

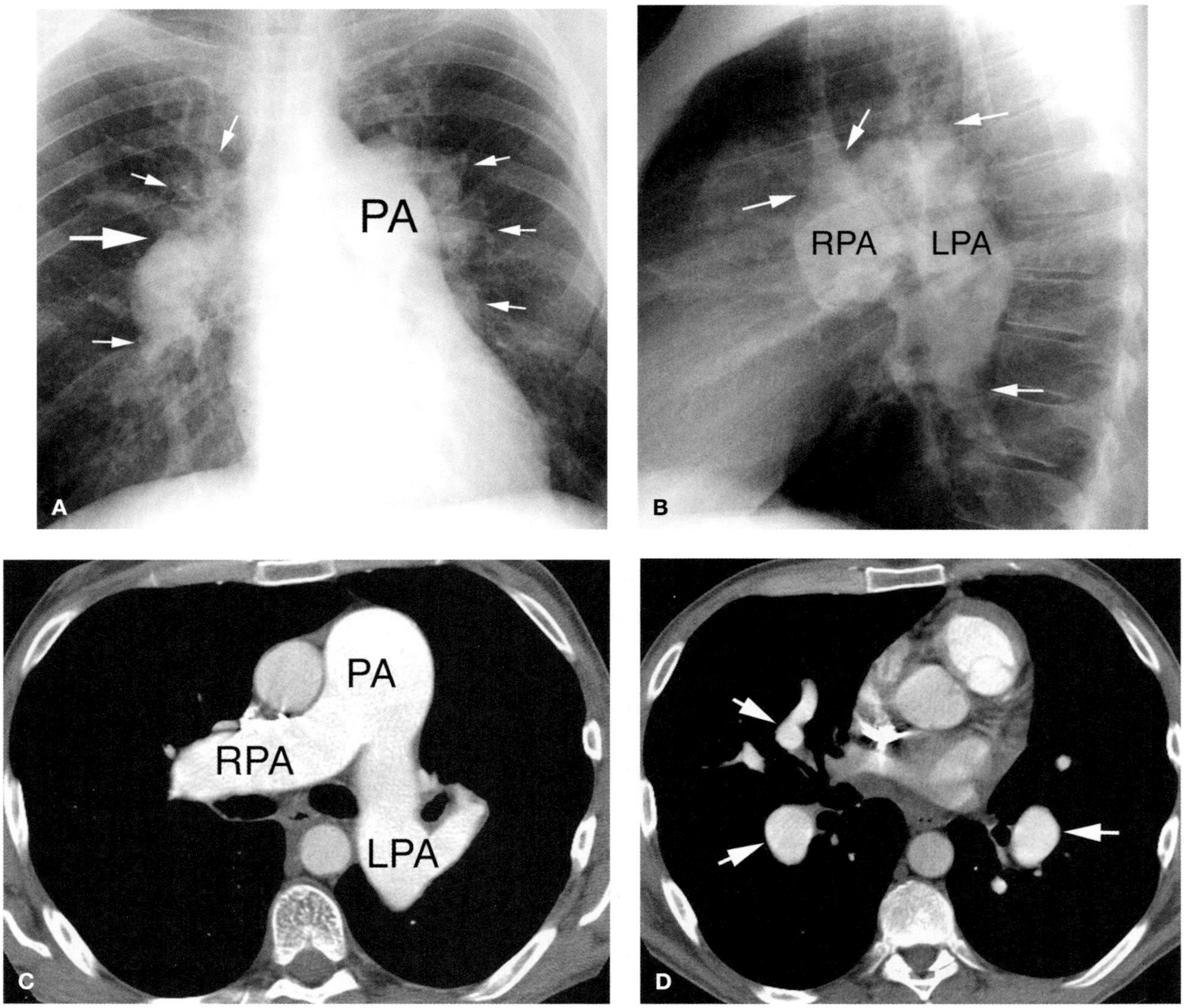

Figure 3.6. Hilar enlargement in pulmonary hypertension. **A:** Enlargement of a pulmonary artery results in increased hilar size and density, but the hilum retains its "vascular" appearance. Vessels (*small arrows*) may be seen arising from the edges of the hilar shadow, the so-called hilum convergence sign, indicating the presence of vascular enlargement. The hilar angle (*large arrow*) remains concave. The main pulmonary artery (*PA*) is also enlarged. **B:** Lateral view. Although increased in size, the right (*RPA*) and left (*LPA*) pulmonary arteries retain their shape. Small branches arising from the edges of the arteries (*arrows*) result in the hilum convergence sign. **C, D:** T shows enlargement of the main pulmonary artery (*PA*), right (*RPA*) and left (*LPA*) pulmonary arteries, and the interlobar and middle lobe branches (*arrows*).

patients with pulmonary hypertension often have an enlarged main pulmonary artery on the PA radiograph, and enlarged main pulmonary artery and right ventricle on the lateral view. Pulmonic stenosis results in enlargement of the main and left pulmonary artery, while the right pulmonary artery usually appears normal in size.

Bronchial narrowing and obstruction associated with a hilar mass are usually difficult to diagnose on plain radiographs unless associated abnormalities such as mucous plugging, atelectasis, or obstructive pneumonia are visible (see Chapter 5).

Plain Film Diagnosis of Hilar Abnormalities: Lateral Radiograph

Enlargement of the oval and comma-shaped shadows of the right and left pulmonary arteries indicates pulmonary artery dilatation (see Fig. 3.6B). As on the frontal radiograph, increased hilar size, focal mass, lobulation of hilar contours, or alteration in the normal oval and comma-shaped shadows can indicate a hilar mass or lymph node enlargement.

Attention to several specific regions visible on the lateral radiograph may also be helpful in diagnosis, including the PWBI, the inferior hilar window (IHW), and the RUL bronchus (sign).

Posterior Wall of the Bronchus Intermedius

The PWBI is seen as a vertical or slightly oblique line or stripe in about 95% of patients (see Fig. 3.3). At its upper extent, the PWBI is contiguous with the posterior wall of the right main bronchus, forming the intermediate stem line described previously. This stripe is normally 0.5 to 3 mm thick. Thickening of this stripe may be seen in patients with neoplasm involving the hilum (Fig. 3.7), hilar adenopathy, interstitial pulmonary edema (Fig. 3.8), or interstitial thickening of various causes. Obliteration of the posterior bronchial wall and the presence of soft-tissue opacity behind it are virtually diagnostic of a mass in the hilum or adjacent lung.

Inferior Hilar Window

On the lateral radiograph, the right hilar vascular opacity is visible in the anterior aspect of the silhouette of the superimposed hila, while the comma-shaped left pulmonary artery occupies its superior and posterior aspect. The inferior hilar shadow contains no large vessels and consequently is termed the *IHW*. The IHW corresponds to an avascular region anterior to both lower lobe bronchi. It appears as a roughly triangular lucency in the anterior and inferior hilar shadow (Fig. 3.9) and mainly corresponds to the subcarinal space on CT and inferior portions of both the right and left hila.

In normal subjects, the IHW appears radiolucent, and the composite hilar silhouette appears as an incomplete oval. Opacity in the IHW may indicate the presence of a hilar and/or subcarinal mass. In abnormals, the addition of an opacity in the inferior hilum (IHW) results in the appearance of a complete oval shadow on lateral radiographs (Figs. 3.10 and 3.11). The side of the mass may be difficult to determine, although the frontal radiograph may help. Also, if a lower lobe bronchus is visible as a linear shadow, the mass must be on the opposite side.

RUL Bronchus (Sign)

Below the tracheal carina, two rounded radiolucencies are commonly seen, one above the other, in line with the tracheal air column and overlying the hilar bronchi. The lower of the two lucencies represents the horizontal portion of the left main and upper lobe bronchus. The upper lucency

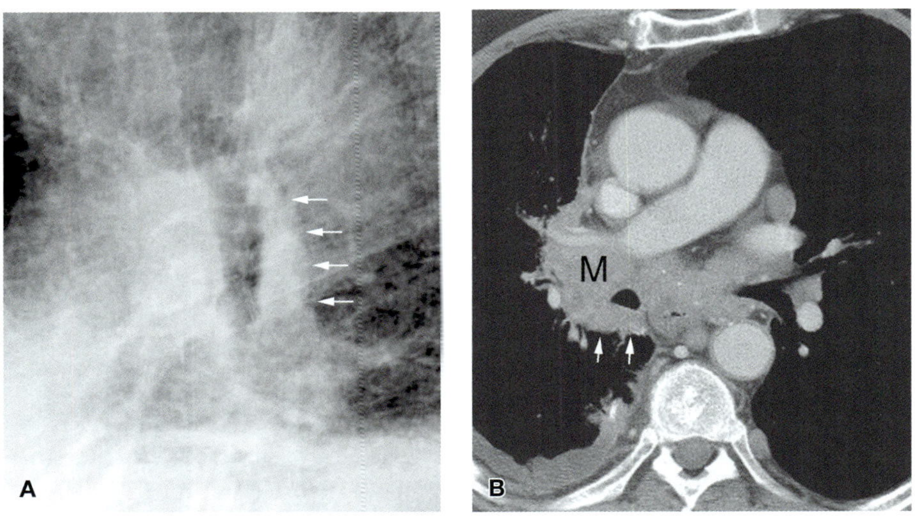

Figure 3.7. Thickening of the posterior wall of the bronchus intermedius in right hilar carcinoma. **A:** Lateral chest radiograph shows marked thickening of the posterior wall of the bronchus intermedius (*arrows*). **B:** CT in this patient shows a right hilar mass (*M*) with infiltration and thickening of the posterior bronchial wall (*arrows*).

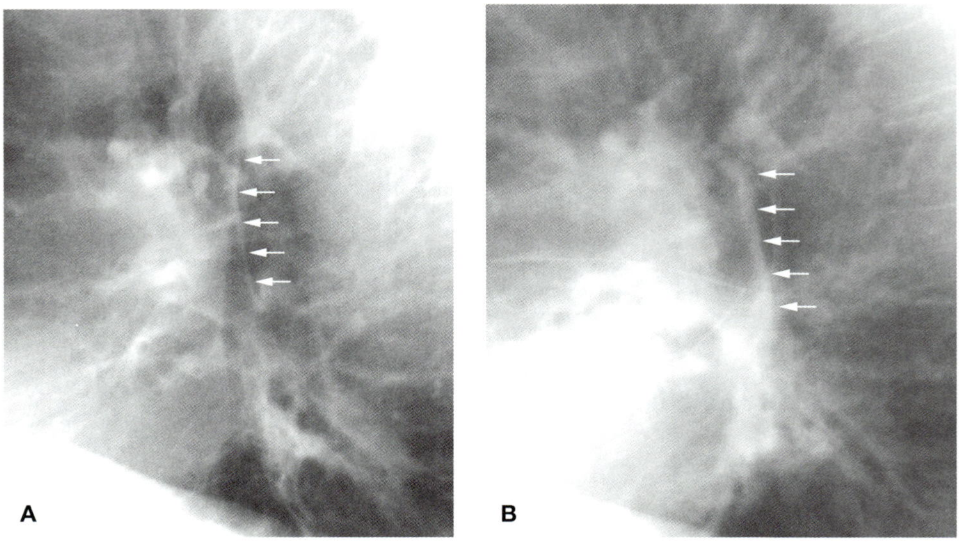

Figure 3.8. Thickening of the posterior wall of the bronchus intermedius in pulmonary edema. **A:** A patient with long-standing renal failure shows a normal posterior bronchial wall (*arrows*). **B:** When the patient is in pulmonary edema, the posterior bronchial wall appears thickened (*arrows*).

represents the RUL bronchus (see Fig. 3.3). It is usually less well seen, as it is not surrounded by vascular structures, but is usually superimposed over the left pulmonary artery.

If the RUL bronchus is sharply marginated throughout its circumference (and more importantly if this represents a change compared to prior radiographs), hilar mass or adenopathy (surrounding and outlining the bronchus) may be present (see Fig. 3.12). This sign can also be helpful in distinguishing hilar vascular enlargement (which does not result in this sign) from hilar node enlargement.

CT OF THE HILA

The pulmonary hila are complex structures made up of the lobar and segmental bronchi, pulmonary arteries and veins, bronchial arteries and veins, soft tissue, and lymph nodes.

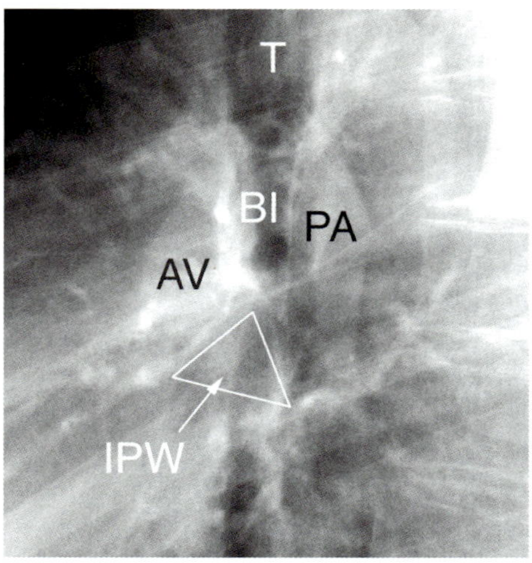

Figure 3.9. The inferior hilar window. Lateral view. This image is the same as that in Figures 3.3B and 3.4B. The right hilar vessels (*AV*) occupy the anterior part of the hilar shadow. The left pulmonary artery (*PA*) is visible posteriorly and superiorly. The inferior hilar window is a roughly triangular lucency (*IPW*) in the anterior and inferior hilar shadow, below these major vascular branches. It represents an avascular region anterior to both lower lobe bronchi. *T*, trachea; *BI*, bronchus intermedius.

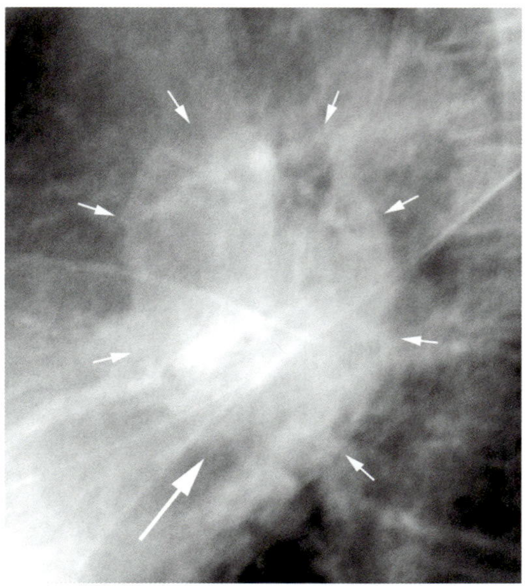

Figure 3.10. Lymph node enlargement in sarcoidosis, with filling in of the inferior hilar window. Enlarged lymph nodes in the inferior hilar window (*large arrow*), when added to the shadows of the pulmonary arteries, result in a complete oval shadow on the lateral view (*small arrows*). This differs from the normal incomplete oval.

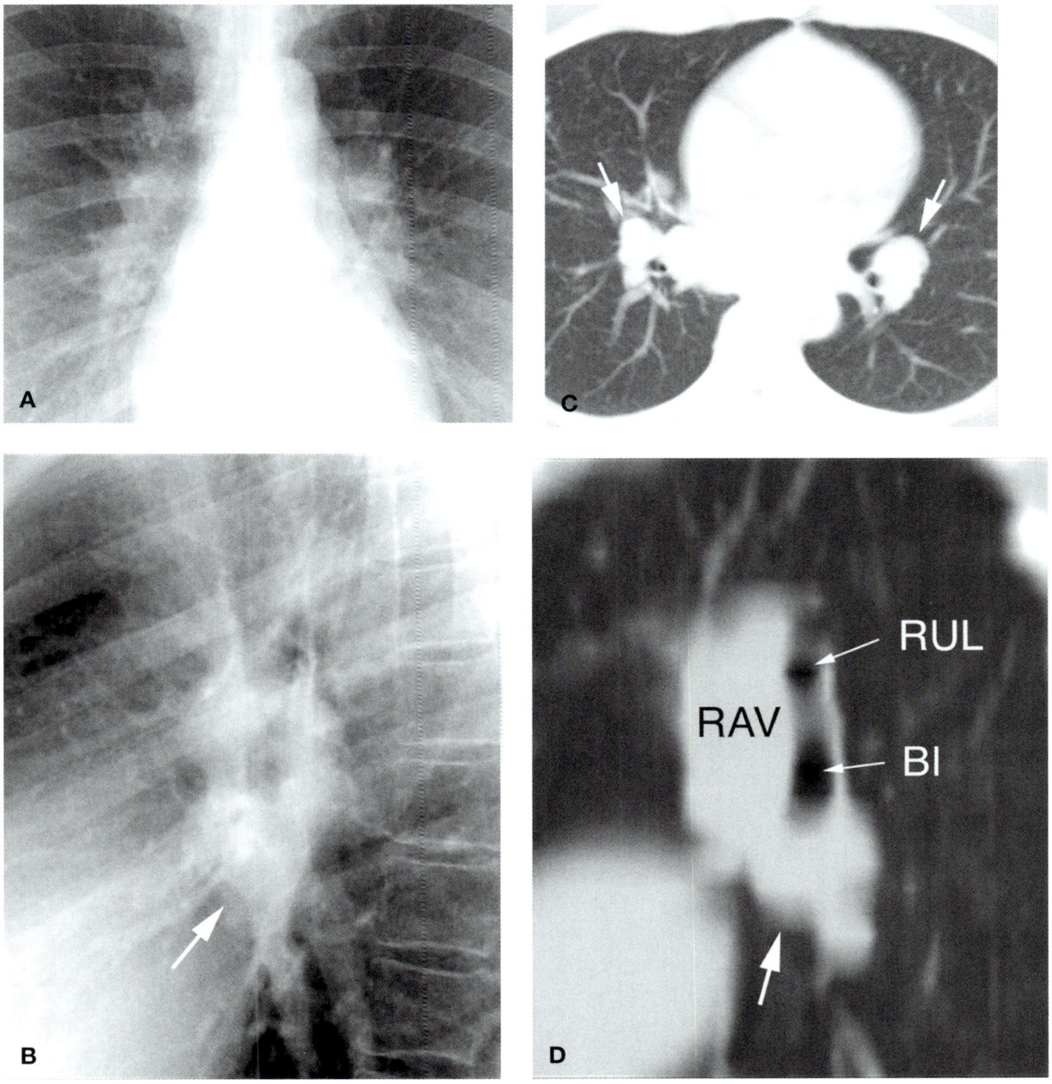

Figure 3.11. Lymph node enlargement in sarcoidosis, with filling in of the inferior hilar window. **A:** PA chest radiograph shows subtle hilar lobulation. **B:** Lateral view shows lobulation of the hilar contours with filling in of the inferior hilar window (*arrow*). The hilar silhouette forms a complete oval. **C:** CT shows lymph node enlargement in the anterior inferior hila (*arrows*), in the space anterior to the lower lobe bronchi. **D:** CT reformation through the right hilum shows lymph node enlargement in the inferior hilar window (*large arrow*), inferior to the right hilar artery and vein (*RAV*). *RUL*, right upper lobe bronchus; *BI*, bronchus intermedius.

The appearances of bronchi, vessels, and nodes and their consistent relationships at different hilar levels allow for reliable identification of these structures. Identification of specific bronchi is the first step in the analysis of the hila. Bronchi are quite consistent in their branching pattern (Fig. 3.13).

CT of the Hilar Bronchi

Using modern CT scanners with a slice thickness of 5 mm or less, all segmental bronchi should be visible. Their appearance depends on their orientation.

Bronchi oriented in or near the scan plane, and therefore seen along their axes as tubular structures, include the RUL bronchus (including both the anterior and posterior segmental bronchi), the LUL bronchus (including the anterior segmental bronchus), a portion of the middle lobe bronchus, and the superior segmental bronchi of both lower lobes.

Bronchi having a vertical course are seen in cross section and appear as circular lucencies. These include the apical segmental bronchus of the RUL, the apical-posterior segmental bronchus of the LUL, and proximal portions of both lower lobe bronchi (below the takeoff of the superior segmental bronchi) and the medial and posterior basal lower lobe segments.

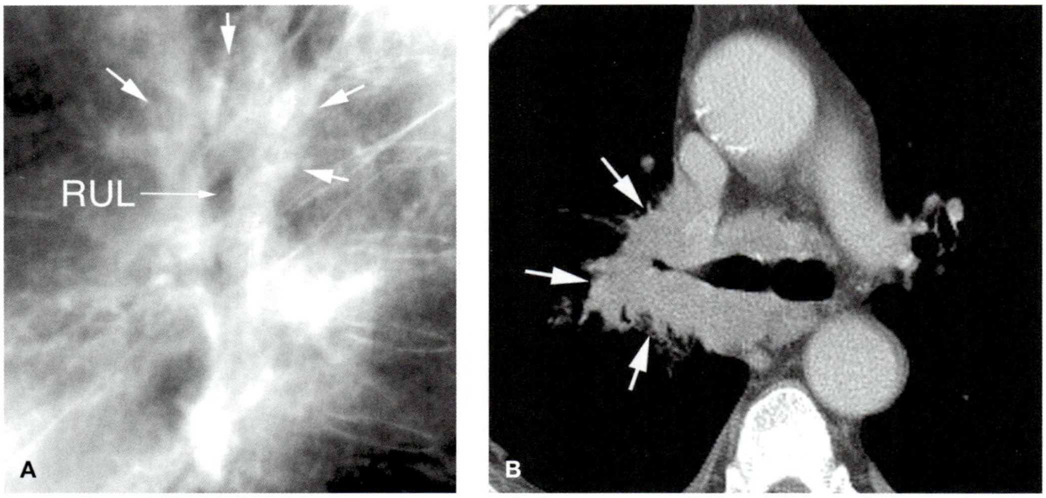

Figure 3.12. Right upper lobe bronchus sign in lung cancer. **A:** Lateral radiograph shows the right upper lobe bronchus (*RUL*) as a lucency surrounded by mass (*arrows*). Thickening of the posterior wall of the bronchus intermedius is also visible. **B:** CT shows a large mass (*arrows*) surrounding the upper lobe bronchus.

The most difficult bronchi to visualize clearly are those oriented obliquely relative to the scan plane, including the superior and inferior lingular bronchi, the lateral and medial segmental bronchi of the middle lobe, and the anterior and lateral basal lower lobe segments. Such bronchi appear elliptical on CT.

Right Bronchial Anatomy

The right main bronchus is relatively short, dividing into the RUL bronchus and bronchus intermedius. Often, the carina, right main bronchus, and RUL bronchus are visible on a single scan.

RUL Bronchus

The RUL bronchus is always found at or just below the carina. The RUL bronchus courses laterally for 1 to 2 cm before dividing into its three segmental branches (apical, anterior, and posterior; Figs. 3.14 and 3.15). Characteristically, the posterior wall of the RUL bronchus is sharply outlined by the lung and is seen as a thin line (see Fig. 3.15). The upper limit of normal for thickness of the posterior wall of the RUL bronchus is 3 to 5 mm. However, the posterior part of the arch of the azygos vein can result in apparent bronchial wall thickening.

The precise branching pattern of the RUL bronchus is variable, primarily due to variation in the site of origin of the apical segmental bronchus.

Apical Segment RUL

The apical segmental bronchus of the RUL is visible above the RUL bronchus itself, usually at or near the level of the distal trachea (see Fig. 3.14). It is seen in cross section as a circular lucency.

Anterior and Posterior Segments RUL

The anterior and posterior segmental bronchi arise as a Y-shaped bifurcation of the RUL bronchus (see Fig. 3.15). The anterior segment bronchus almost always lies in the plane of scan and is more easily seen. The posterior segmental bronchus may have a similar appearance but often angles

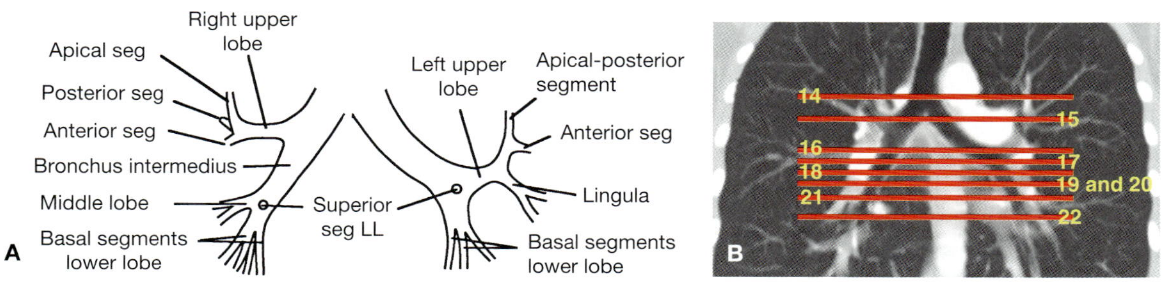

Figure 3.13. Normal bronchial anatomy. **A:** Anatomy of bronchial segments as shown on a PA chest radiograph or CT. *LL*, lower lobe; *seg*, segment. **B:** Levels of CT slices shown in Figures 3.14-3.22, from a two-dimensional reconstruction in the same patient.

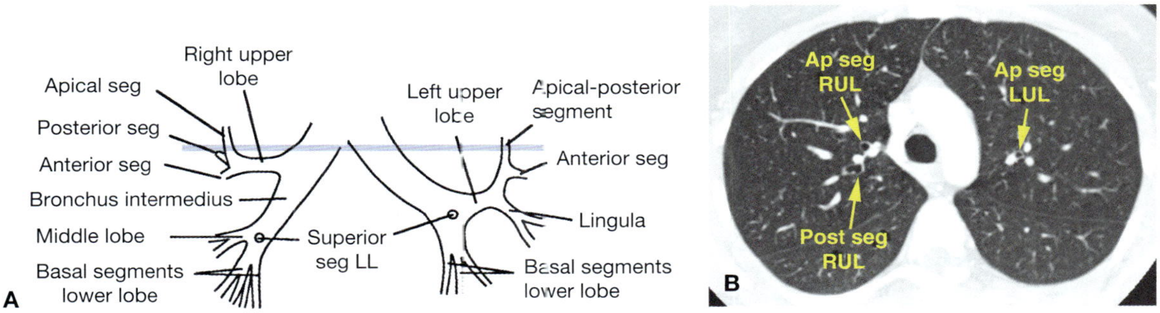

Figure 3.14. Apical and posterior segmental bronchi right upper lobe. **A:** Bronchial anatomy at the level of this scan (indicated in *blue*). *LL*, lower lobe; *seg*, segment. **B:** The apical segmental bronchus (Ap seg RUL) is visible as a ring shadow. A vessel of similar size and shape medial to the bronchus represents the artery to the apical segment. A vein characteristically lies lateral to the bronchus. The posterior segment (Post seg RUL) is also visible. On the left, the apical segment of the left upper lobe (Ap seg LUL) is visible as a ring shadow.

slightly cephalad from its origin and is usually visible at progressively higher levels as it courses posteriorly.

In many patients, a trifurcation of the RUL bronchus is present, with the origin of the apical segment bronchus seen as a rounded area of lucency superimposed on the distal portion of the RUL bronchus, at or just above the origins of the anterior and posterior segments. Major anatomic variants are unusual. The most frequent is a tracheal bronchus, discussed in Chapter 9.

Bronchus Intermedius

The bronchus intermedius is 3 to 4 cm long, beginning at the level of the RUL bronchus. It gives rise to the middle lobe and lower lobe bronchi inferiorly. Because of its length, it is seen on a number of adjacent scans (Figs. 3.16, 3.17, and 3.18B).

The bronchus intermedius appears round or oval in cross section. The PWBI is in contact with the superior segment of the RLL and is sharply outlined. It should appear thin and of uniform thickness, usually measuring no more than 3 mm. A portion of the medial bronchial wall also may be outlined by the lung.

An anomalous bronchus termed the *accessory cardiac bronchus* may arise from the medial bronchus intermedius or lower lobe bronchus, extending medially toward the heart. It supplies a small area of aerated lung or rudimentary (nonaerated) lung tissue (see Fig. 9.3 in Chapter 9).

RML Bronchus

The middle lobe bronchus arises from the anterolateral wall of the bronchus intermedius and extends anteriorly at an angle of about 45°. The origin of the middle lobe bronchus also marks the point of origin of the RLL bronchus (Figs. 3.19B and 3.20B). A thin carina may be seen separating the origins of the RML and RLL bronchi. The middle lobe bronchus lies oblique to the scan plane and appears as an oval lucency. Only a short segment of the RML bronchus may be visible on any one scan, depending on its orientation, the scan thickness, and the degree of volume averaging.

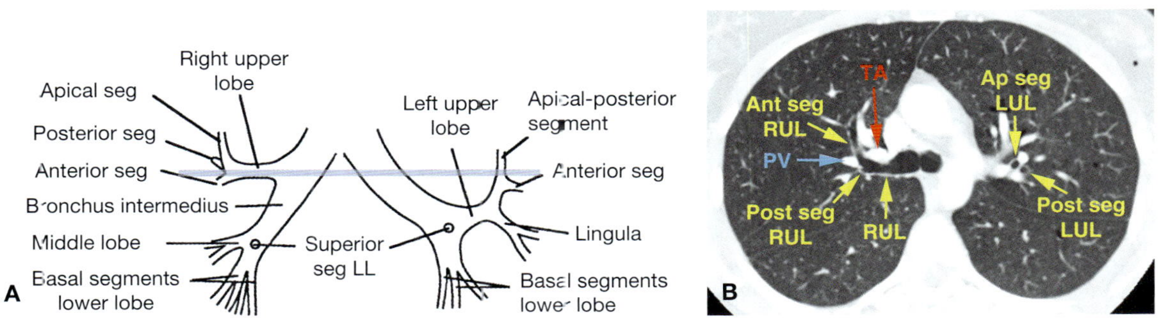

Figure 3.15. Right upper lobe bronchus; apical and posterior segmental bronchi of left upper lobe. **A:** Level of CT. *LL*, lower lobe; *seg*, segment. **B:** Lung window. On the right side, near the carina, the right upper lobe bronchus (*RUL*) is visible along its axis. Its posterior wall is visible as a thin white line. It branches in a Y shape into its anterior (*Ant seg RUL*) and posterior (*Post seg RUL*) segments. The truncus anterior (*TA*) is positioned anterior to the upper lobe bronchus. The posterior vein (*PV*) is typically visible as a rounded structure between the anterior and posterior segmental bronchi. On the left side, the apical segment bronchus (*Ap seg LUL*) and posterior segment bronchus (*Post seg LUL*) are each visible as a ring shadow.

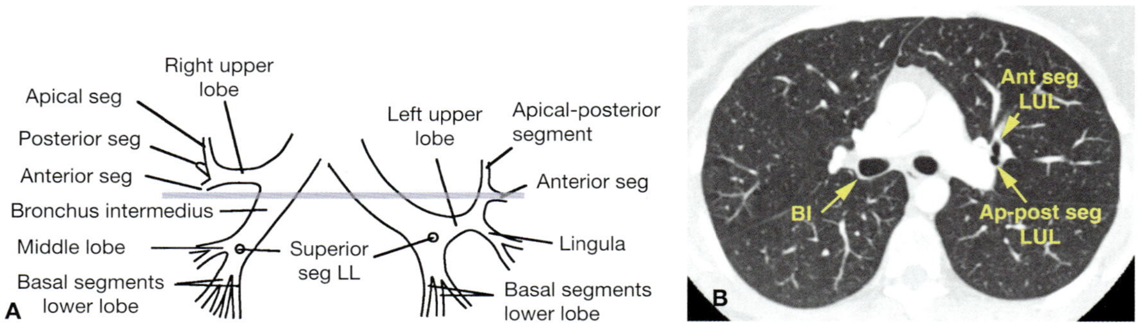

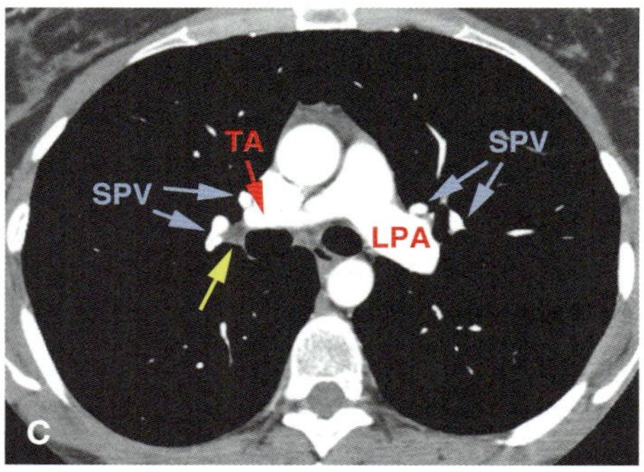

Figure 3.16. Bronchus intermedius; anterior segment left upper lobe (**A**). *LL*, lower lobe; *seg*, segment. **B:** On the right, the bronchus intermedius (*BI*) is visible as an oval lucency. Its posterior wall is sharply outlined by the lung and appears a few millimeters thick. On the left, the anterior segment bronchus (*Ant seg LUL*) of the left upper lobe is seen as it separates from the apical-posterior segment (*Ap-post seg LUL*). **C:** On the right, the right pulmonary artery and truncus anterior (*TA*) are visible anterior to the BI. Two or three branches of the superior pulmonary vein (*SPV*) are visible anterior and lateral to the artery and bronchus. Normal lymph nodes are visible lateral to the pulmonary artery and medial to the SPV (*yellow arrow*). On the left, the left pulmonary artery (*LPA*) is medial. The SPV is anterior and lateral to the bronchi.

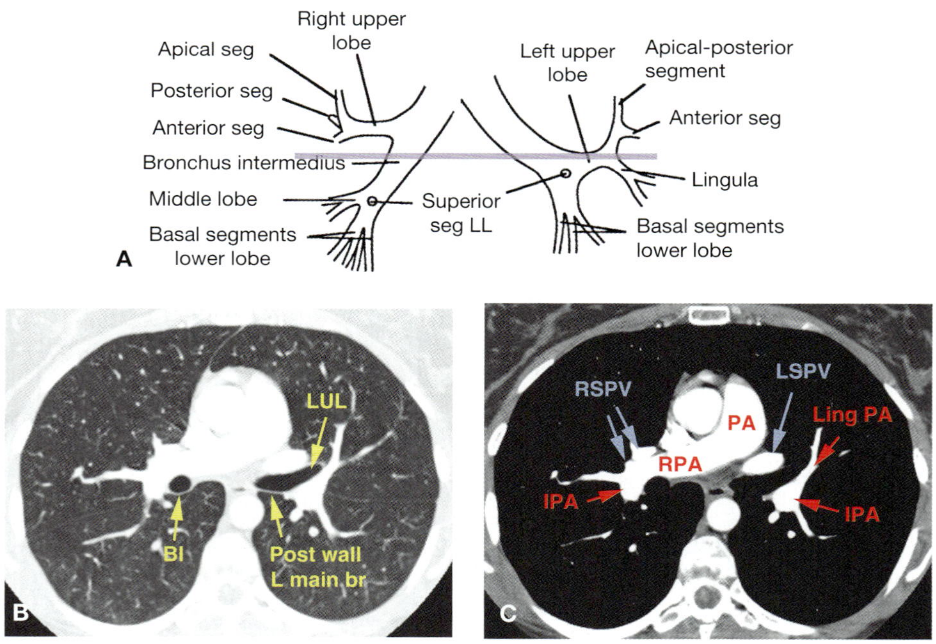

Figure 3.17. Bronchus intermedius; left main bronchus and upper aspect of the left upper lobe bronchus (**A**). *LL*, lower lobe; *seg*, segment. **B:** On the right, the bronchus intermedius (*BI*) appears as an oval lucency. On the left, the posterior wall of the left main bronchus (*Post wall L main br*) is visible as a thin stripe, the left retrobronchial stripe. The superior aspect of the left upper lobe bronchus (*LUL*) is visible. **C:** On the right, the anatomy of hilar vessels is similar to Figure 3.16C. The main pulmonary artery (*PA*) and right pulmonary artery (*RPA*) are anterior. The right interlobar pulmonary artery (IPA) is anterior and lateral to the bronchus, and the right superior pulmonary vein (*RSPV*) branches are visible anterior and lateral to the artery and bronchus. On the left, the interlobar left pulmonary artery (*IPA*) produces a large convexity in the posterior hilum, and the left superior pulmonary vein (*LSPV*) results in an anterior convexity. The lingular artery (*Ling PA*) is visible.

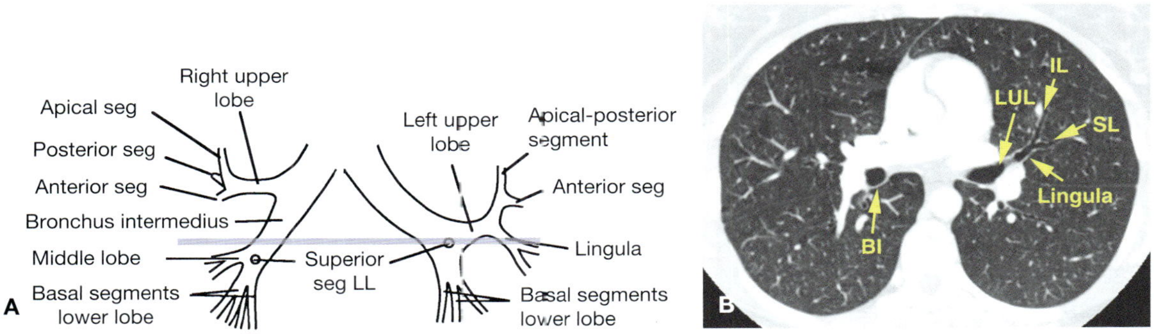

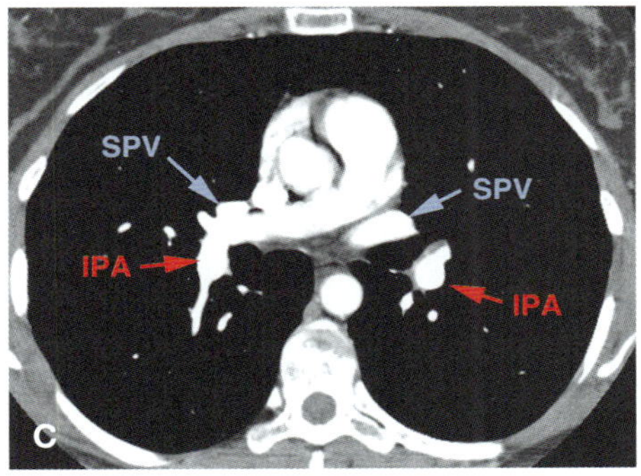

Figure 3.18. Bronchus intermedius; lower aspect of the left upper lobe bronchus and lingular bronchus (**A**). *LL*, lower lobe; *seg*, segment. **B:** On the right, the bronchus intermedius (*BI*) appears as an oval lucency. On the left, the left retrobronchial stripe is again seen, and their inferior aspect of the left upper lobe bronchus is visible, giving rise laterally to the lingular branch (*Lingula*) of the left upper lobe bronchus (*LUL*), with its superior (*SL*) and inferior (*IL*) segments also visible. **C:** On the right, the interlobar pulmonary artery (*IPA*) passes anterior and lateral to the BI. Branches to the superior segment of the lower lobe are directed posteriorly. The combination of the IPA and superior segment branches resembles an elephant's head. The superior pulmonary vein (SPV) is visible anteriorly. On the left, the left IPA is seen in cross section and lies posterolateral to the lingular bronchus. It is round or oval. The SPV passes anterior and medial to the bronchi to enter the left atrium.

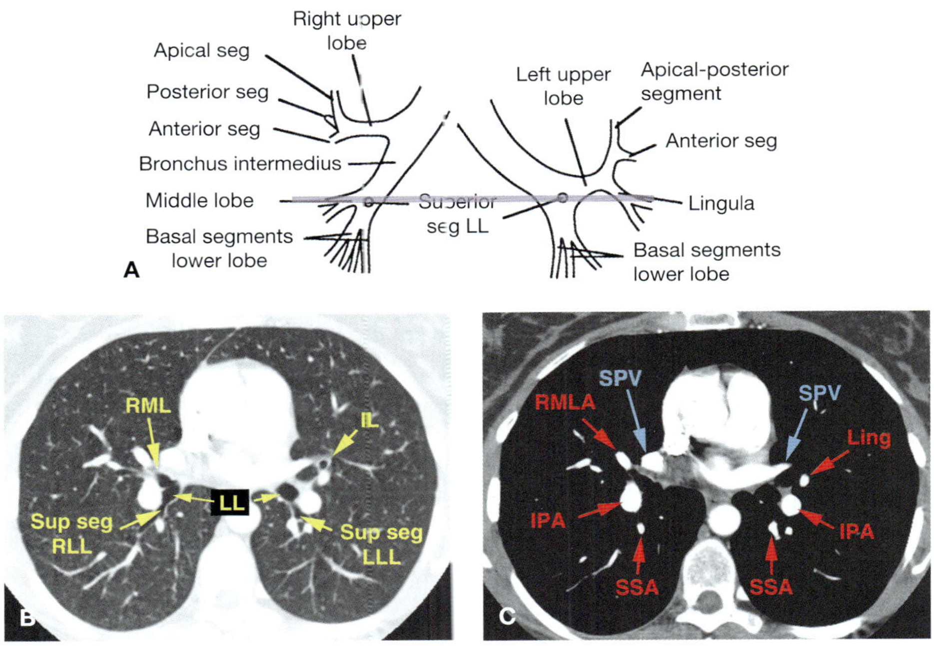

Figure 3.19. Right middle lobe and superior segment right lower lobe; lingular bronchus and superior segment left lower lobe (**A**). *LL*, lower lobe; *seg*, segment. **B:** On the right, the origin of the right middle lobe bronchus (*RML*) is visible. Posterior to it is the lower lobe bronchus (*LL*) and the superior segment of the lower lobe (*Sup seg RLL*). A thin carina separates the middle and lower lobe bronchi. On the left, the inferior segment lingular bronchus (*IL*), lower lobe bronchus (*LL*), and superior segment of the lower lobe (*Sup seg LLL*) have a similar appearance to the right-sided bronchi. **C:** On the right, the interlobar pulmonary (*IPA*) lies lateral to the lateral borders of both the middle and lower lobe bronchi. The right middle lobe artery (*RMLA*) is seen as an anterior branch and the superior segment (*SSA*) of the RLL artery as a posterior branch. The right superior pulmonary vein (*SPV*) passes anterior and medial to the middle and lower lobe bronchi. On the left, the left interlobar pulmonary artery (*IPA*) lies lateral to the lower lobe bronchus. The lingular artery (*Ling*) is anterior.

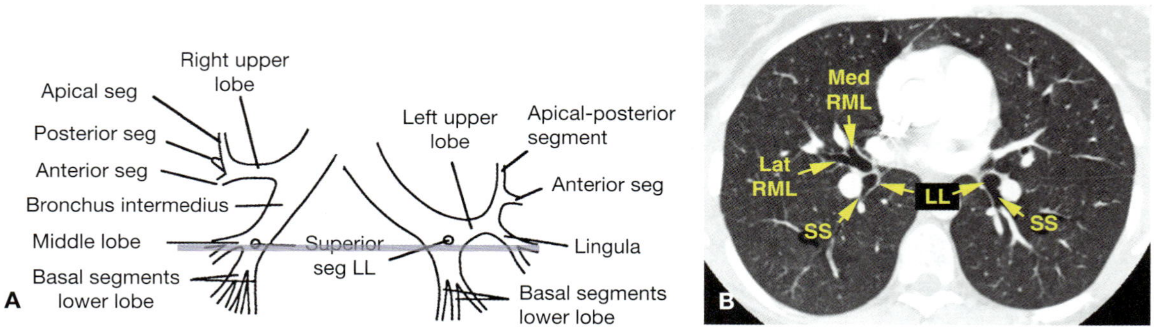

Figure 3.20. Right middle lobe and its segments (**A**). *LL*, lower lobe; *seg*, segment. **B:** On the right, the right middle lobe bronchus and its medial segment (*Med RML*) and lateral segments (*Lat RML*) are visible. The truncus basalis or basal lower lobe trunk (*LL*) and superior lower lobe segmental bronchi (*SS*) are visible on both sides.

Medial and Lateral Segment RML

The middle lobe bronchus extends for about 1 to 2 cm before dividing into its medial and lateral segmental branches. Because of its orientation, the main portion of the RML bronchus and the medial and lateral segments are often seen at level 1 to 2 cm below the origin of the RML bronchus (Fig. 3.20B).

In 60% of cases, the middle lobe bronchus divides into medial and lateral segmental branches of equal size. In most of the remaining cases, the medial segmental bronchus appears larger. Although both middle lobe segmental bronchi are directed inferiorly, the lateral segmental bronchus lies closer to the scan plane and is imaged over a greater distance on each scan.

RLL Bronchus

The undivided lower lobe bronchus is very short. Near its origin, it gives rise to the superior segmental bronchus (see Figs. 3.19B and 3.20B). Distal to the origin of the superior segment, the basal bronchial trunk continues for a short distance (see Fig. 3.21B) before dividing into the four basal segmental branches of the RLL: the medial, anterior, lateral, and posterior segments (Fig. 3.22B).

Superior Segment RLL

The superior segmental bronchus of the RLL may arise at the same level as or slightly caudal to the origin of the RML bronchus (see Figs. 3.19B and 3.20B). In some cases, the

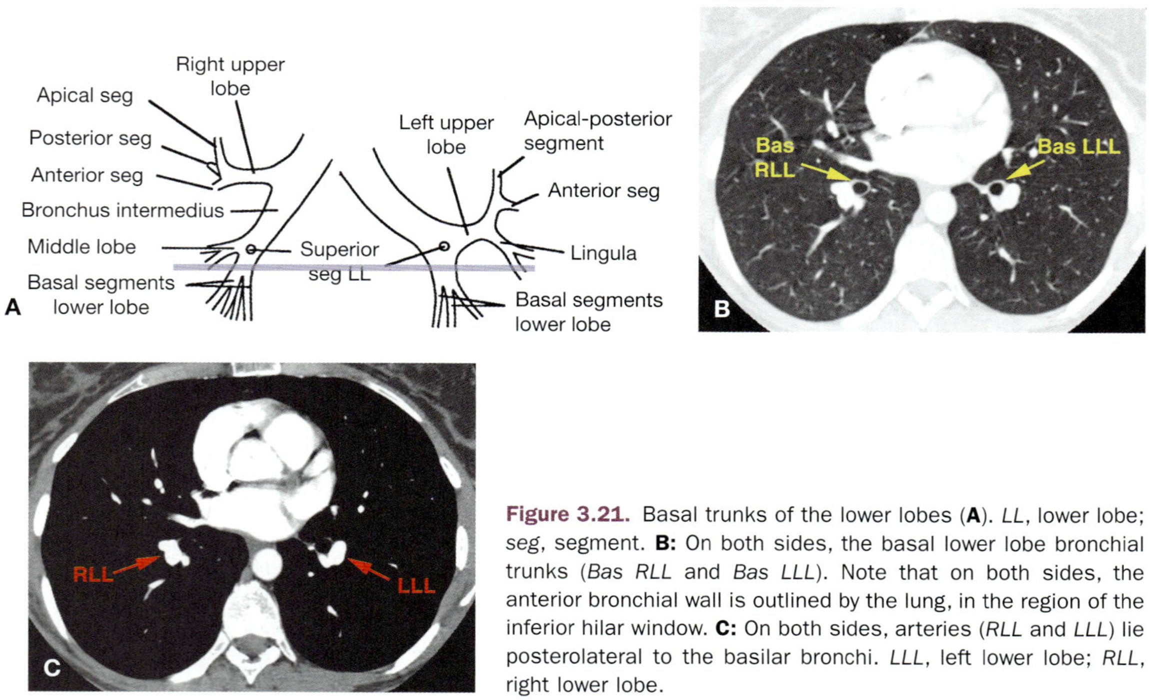

Figure 3.21. Basal trunks of the lower lobes (**A**). *LL*, lower lobe; *seg*, segment. **B:** On both sides, the basal lower lobe bronchial trunks (*Bas RLL* and *Bas LLL*). Note that on both sides, the anterior bronchial wall is outlined by the lung, in the region of the inferior hilar window. **C:** On both sides, arteries (*RLL* and *LLL*) lie posterolateral to the basilar bronchi. *LLL*, left lower lobe; *RLL*, right lower lobe.

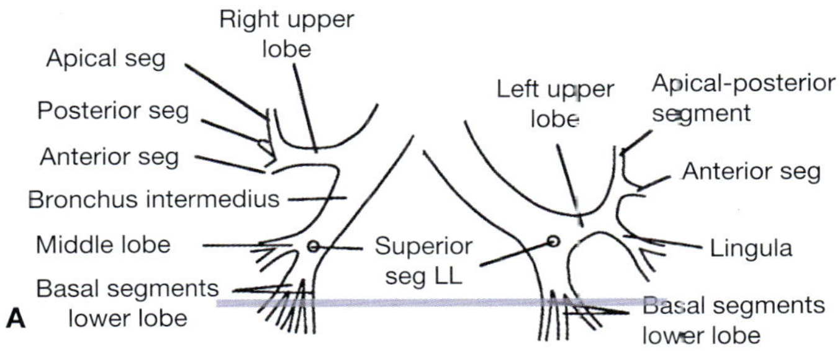

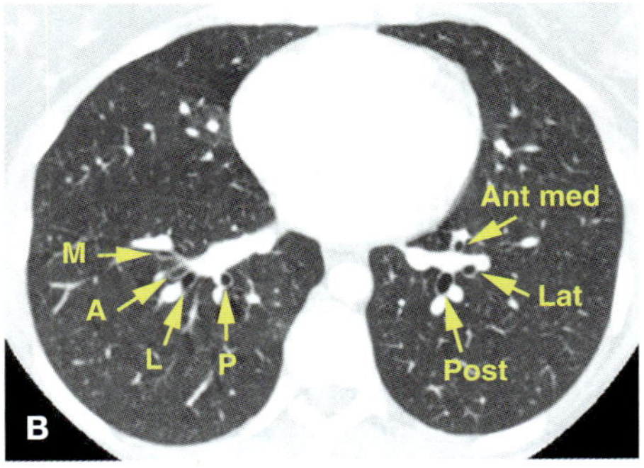

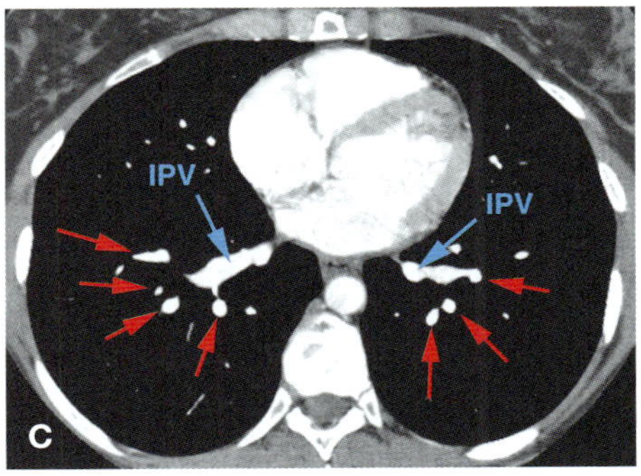

Figure 3.22. Basal segments of the right lower lobe (**A**). *LL*, lower lobe; *seg*, segment. **B:** On the right, the four basal segments are visible. In a counterclockwise direction, these are the medial basal (*M*), anterior basal (*A*), lateral basal (*L*), and posterior basal (*P*), spelling MALP. On the left, three branches are visible, the anteromedial segment (*Ant med*), lateral (*Lat*) segment, and posterior (*Post*) segment. **C:** On both sides, the segmental arteries (*Seg*) lie posterolateral to the proximal portions of the basilar segmental bronchi. The inferior pulmonary veins (*IPV*) pass posterior and medial to the lower lobe bronchi and arteries before entering into the lower portion of the left atrium

superior segmental bronchus arises at a level cephalad to the origin of the RML bronchus.

The superior segmental bronchus, which is about 1 cm in length, arises from the posterior wall of the RLL bronchus and courses posteriorly and laterally within the scan plane (see Figs. 3.19B and 3.20B). The lung often outlines the medial aspect of the superior segment bronchus.

Truncus Basalis and Basal Segments RLL

Below the origin of the superior segmental bronchus, the lower lobe bronchus continues for about 5 to 10 mm as the truncus basalis or basal bronchial trunk, visible as a circular lucency (see Fig. 3.21B). The anterior wall of the truncus basalis is commonly outlined by the lung.

The basal segments have a typical orientation of M-A-L-P, beginning medially and anteriorly and proceeding counterclockwise (see Fig. 3.22B). The medial basal segmental bronchus usually arises as the first branch of the basal trunk, lying just anterior to the inferior pulmonary vein. Although variable in appearance, the anterior, lateral, and posterior basilar bronchi may all be identified because of their positions relative to one another and because they each course toward the segments they supply. In general, the medial and posterior segmental bronchi are imaged more nearly in cross section than the anterior and lateral, which are more obliquely oriented. The medial and lateral segmental bronchi are usually easiest to identify as they abut the mediastinal pleural surface of the RLL. Anatomic variation in the origins of these segments is common.

Left Bronchial Anatomy

The left main bronchus is much longer than the right and is typically seen on several contiguous slices below the carina (see Figs. 3.13, 3.15-3.17). It divides into left upper and lower lobe branches.

LUL Bronchus

The LUL bronchus is 2 to 3 cm long (see Figs. 3.17 and 3.18). In about 75% of patients, the LUL branches into a superior trunk and the lingular bronchus. The superior trunk is about 1 cm in length, giving rise to the anterior and apical-posterior segmental bronchi (Figs. 3.16-3.18). In 25% of cases, the LUL bronchus trifurcates into the apical-posterior segment bronchus, anterior segment bronchus, and lingular bronchus.

At the level of the superior aspect of the LUL bronchus, its posterior wall is smooth and slightly concave (see Fig. 3.17B). At this level, the origin of the apical-posterior segmental bronchus, or the superior bronchial trunk that gives rise to the apical-posterior and anterior segmental bronchi, can be recognized as a rounded area of increased lucency superimposed on the distal portion of the LUL bronchus.

In 90% of cases, the superior segment of the LLL abuts the posterior wall of the left main or upper lobe bronchus, outlining the *left retrobronchial stripe* (see Figs. 3.17B and 3.18B). The bronchial wall should appear similar in thickness to the posterior bronchus intermedius.

Apical-Posterior and Anterior Segments LUL

The anterior segment bronchus of the LUL is usually visible above the level of the LUL bronchus itself (see Fig. 3.16B). It lies roughly in the plane of scan and is oriented almost directly anteriorly; it is usually visible over several centimeters. It is the only LUL branch that has this course.

The apical-posterior segment bronchus is visible as a circular lucency at and above the origin of the anterior segment bronchus (see Figs. 3.14B and 3.15B). If a bronchus is seen in cross section below the anterior segment and above the LUL bronchus, it represents the short superior bronchial trunk; although similar in appearance to the apical-posterior segment and following the same course, it is larger.

Lingular Bronchus

The lingular bronchus arises from the undersurface of the distal portion of the LUL bronchus and courses obliquely downward, in the same manner as the RML bronchus (see Fig. 3.18A). The origin of the lingular bronchus may be distinguished from the origin of the anterior segmental bronchus of the LUL by noting its relationship to the inferior aspect of the upper lobe bronchus or by identifying a thin carina or spur that is usually seen between the lingular bronchus and the LLL bronchus.

Superior and Inferior Lingular Segments

The lingular bronchus extends anteriorly and inferiorly for 2 to 3 cm before dividing into its superior and inferior segmental branches (Figs. 3.18B and 3.19B). The superior segmental bronchus of the lingula is directed more laterally than the inferior segment and lies closer to the scan plane, similar to the pattern of branching of the medial and lateral segments of the RML.

Left Lower Lobe Bronchus

The LLL bronchus usually conforms to the same general branching pattern as the RLL bronchus, although only three basal segments are generally present: the anteromedial, lateral, and posterior.

Superior Segment LLL

The superior segmental bronchus of the LLL arises within 1 cm of the origin of the LLL bronchus and is identical in shape and configuration to the superior segment bronchus on the right side (see Fig. 3.19B).

Truncus Basalis and Basal Segments LLL

The truncus basalis, the lower lobe bronchus giving rise to the basal lower lobe segments, is visible below the origin of the superior segment for a distance of 1 to 2 cm (see Fig. 3.21B). It is generally longer than the truncus basalis on the right. As on the right, the anterior wall of the basal trunk may be outlined by the lung.

The left basilar segmental bronchi are almost mirror images of the RLL basilar bronchi, except that on the left side, the medial and anterior basilar bronchi characteristically originate together as a common trunk (see Fig. 3.22B). Again, the key to the identification of the basal segments is to note the general configuration and position of these bronchi as they course to their corresponding segments. In a clockwise fashion, the relative positions of the bronchi are M-A (in this case named anteromedial)-L-P.

CT of the Hilar Vessels

Bronchi serve as an anatomic framework for the hila. Hilar vessels have a consistent relationship to bronchi, and identifying hilar bronchi is the first step to analyzing the hila. Despite some variation in the branching of segmental hilar arteries, most can be identified by noting their close association with specific segmental bronchi, by following their courses on sequential images, and by determining their sites of origin.

Evaluation of the vascular structures of the hila is simplified by the recognition of specific levels relative to the bronchi (see Figs. 3.16C, 3.17C, 3.18C, 3.19C, 3.20C, 3.21C, and 3.22C). At these levels, the hila have characteristic silhouettes.

Right side:

- Tracheal carina and apical segmental bronchus of the RUL
- RUL bronchus
- Bronchus intermedius
- Middle lobe bronchus
- Lower lobe basilar segmental bronchi

Left side:

- Apical-posterior and anterior segmental bronchi of the LUL
- LUL bronchus
- Lingular bronchus
- Lower lobe basilar segmental bronchi

Vascular Anatomy of the Right Hilum

Tracheal Carina and Apical Segmental Bronchus Level

At or near the level of the carina, a branch or branches of the truncus anterior supplying the apical segment of the RUL and a branch or branches of the right superior pulmonary vein draining the apical segment are visible in cross section, adjacent to the apical segmental bronchus. Typically, the apical segmental artery lies medial to the bronchus and the veins lie lateral to it.

RUL Bronchus Level

At the level of the RUL bronchus, the undivided truncus anterior is usually identifiable (see Fig, 3.15B). This large vessel is the first major branch of the right main pulmonary artery, arising within the pericardium, and characteristically lies just anterior to the RUL bronchus. As a rule of thumb, the truncus anterior usually appears similar in size and shape to the right main bronchus seen at the same level.

Typically, a large branch of the right superior pulmonary vein, the posterior vein, lies within the angle formed by the bifurcation of the RUL bronchus into anterior and posterior segmental bronchi (see Fig. 3.15B). Anterior and medial to the truncus anterior, a small convexity is frequently visible touching the mediastinum, representing another RUL vein, the apical-anterior vein, which is often identifiable without the injection of contrast agent.

Bronchus Intermedius Level

On scans showing the bronchus intermedius, the interlobar pulmonary artery lies anterior and lateral to the bronchus (see Figs. 3.16-3.18). The right superior pulmonary vein lies anterior to the right interlobar pulmonary artery. Frequently, two veins are visible in this location; these should not be mistaken for lymph node enlargement. Infrequently, a small vein branch draining a portion of the posterior segment of the upper lobe passes posterior to the bronchus intermedius; it can be seen to pass medially at successively lower levels to join the inferior pulmonary vein or drain directly into the left atrium (right top pulmonary vein).

Once the interlobar pulmonary artery reaches the lateral border of the bronchus intermedius and enters the major fissure, the artery often resembles an elephant's head (the main portion of the artery) and trunk (the superior segment artery; see Fig. 3.18).

Middle Lobe Bronchus Level

At the level of the origin of the middle lobe bronchus, the lower lobe pulmonary artery lies immediately lateral to the middle and lower lobe bronchi, and the RML artery parallels the RML bronchus (see Figs. 3.19 and 3.20). The lower lobe artery at this point is oriented perpendicular to the scan plane and is thus seen in cross section as an elliptical structure.

The right superior pulmonary vein passes anterior and medial to the middle and lower lobe bronchi and can be seen entering the upper portion of the left atrium. The middle lobe vein is sometimes seen joining the superior pulmonary vein at this level.

Level of the Basal Segmental Bronchi RLL

Below the level of the origin of the middle lobe bronchus, the lower lobe pulmonary artery often bifurcates into two short trunks, which in turn divide into the four basilar segmental pulmonary arteries. These have a characteristic, rounded configuration, lying posterolateral to the proximal portions of the basilar segmental bronchi (see Figs. 3.21 and 3.22). Unlike the basilar pulmonary arteries, which are imaged in cross section, the inferior pulmonary veins are oriented in the transverse plane. They join to form the inferior pulmonary vein, which passes posterior to the lower lobe bronchi and arteries before entering into the lower portion of the left atrium.

Vascular Anatomy of the Left Hilum

On the left side, although characteristic relationships between vessels and airways are also present, there is far more anatomic variation than on the right.

Level of the Apical-Posterior and Anterior Segments of the LUL

The apical-posterior segmental bronchus and associated arteries and veins have a similar appearance to the right apical segmental bronchus and associated vessels. The artery supplying the anterior segment of the LUL is seen medial to the anterior segment bronchus (see Fig. 3.15).

LUL Bronchus Level

At the level of the left upper bronchus, the interlobar left pulmonary artery produces a large convexity in the posterior hilum, and superior pulmonary vein branches are visible medial and lateral to the ascending bronchial trunk or anterior segmental bronchus (see Figs. 3.17 and 3.18).

Lingular Bronchus Level

The lingular bronchus is usually visible at a level near the undersurface of the LUL bronchus. The appearance of the hilar vessels at this level is analogous to that of the right hilum at the level of the middle lobe bronchus. The left interlobar pulmonary artery is seen in cross section and lies lateral to the lower lobe bronchi, posterolateral to the lingular bronchus, and anterolateral to the superior segmental bronchus (see Figs. 3.17 and 3.18). It is round or oval. The superior pulmonary vein passes anterior and medial to the bronchi to enter the left atrium.

Level of the Basilar Segmental Bronchi of the Left Lower Lobe

At the level of the basilar lower lobe trunk and lower lobe segmental bronchi, the anatomy of the inferior portion of the left hilum is nearly a mirror image of that on the right (see Figs. 3.21 and 3.22). Branches of the pulmonary artery to the LLL lie lateral and posterior to the LLL basilar bronchi. The left inferior pulmonary vein passes anterolateral to descending aorta and posterior to the bronchi and arteries to enter the left atrium.

CT of Hilar Lymph Nodes

The use of contrast enhancement usually allows the accurate differentiation of hilar lymph nodes from normal vessels. Hilar lymph nodes are not located randomly but are found in consistent locations. The most important groups are described below in relation to bronchial anatomy.

RUL Bronchus and Left Pulmonary Artery Level

Lymph nodes are common adjacent to the segmental branches of the RUL bronchus but tend to be small (Fig. 3.23). Lymph nodes are commonly seen both medial and lateral to the left pulmonary artery. Lateral nodes are medial to the superior bronchial trunk. These may be mistaken for pulmonary emboli.

Bronchus Intermedius and LUL Bronchus Level

On the right, slightly below the RUL bronchus, lateral to the bifurcation of the main pulmonary artery, anterolateral to the bronchus intermedius, and medial to superior pulmonary vein branches, it is very common in normal subjects to see a large area of unenhanced soft tissue comprising small nodes and fat (see Figs. 3.16B and 3.24). This can range up to 1.5 cm in diameter in some normals. Nodes in this region represent part of the "lymphatic sump" of the right lung. They can be easily mistaken for a hilar mass or thrombus in the right pulmonary artery. Lymph nodes tend to be medial and lateral to the PWBI but not immediately posterior to it. Lymph nodes in this region are in the hilar angle.

At the level of the upper portion of the LUL bronchus, a rim of soft tissue largely representing normal nodes is always seen between the posterior bronchial wall and the pulmonary artery. Lymph nodes are common adjacent to the retrobronchial stripe but are not normally seen.

RML Bronchus and Lingular Level

At the level of the RML bronchus and node group, lymph nodes are commonly seen (70%) lateral to the origin of the middle lobe or lower lobe bronchi and medial to the interlobar pulmonary artery (Fig. 3.25). These can be more than 5 mm in some normal patients. Normal lymph nodes having a similar appearance are also commonly seen on the left, in relation to the lingular bronchus.

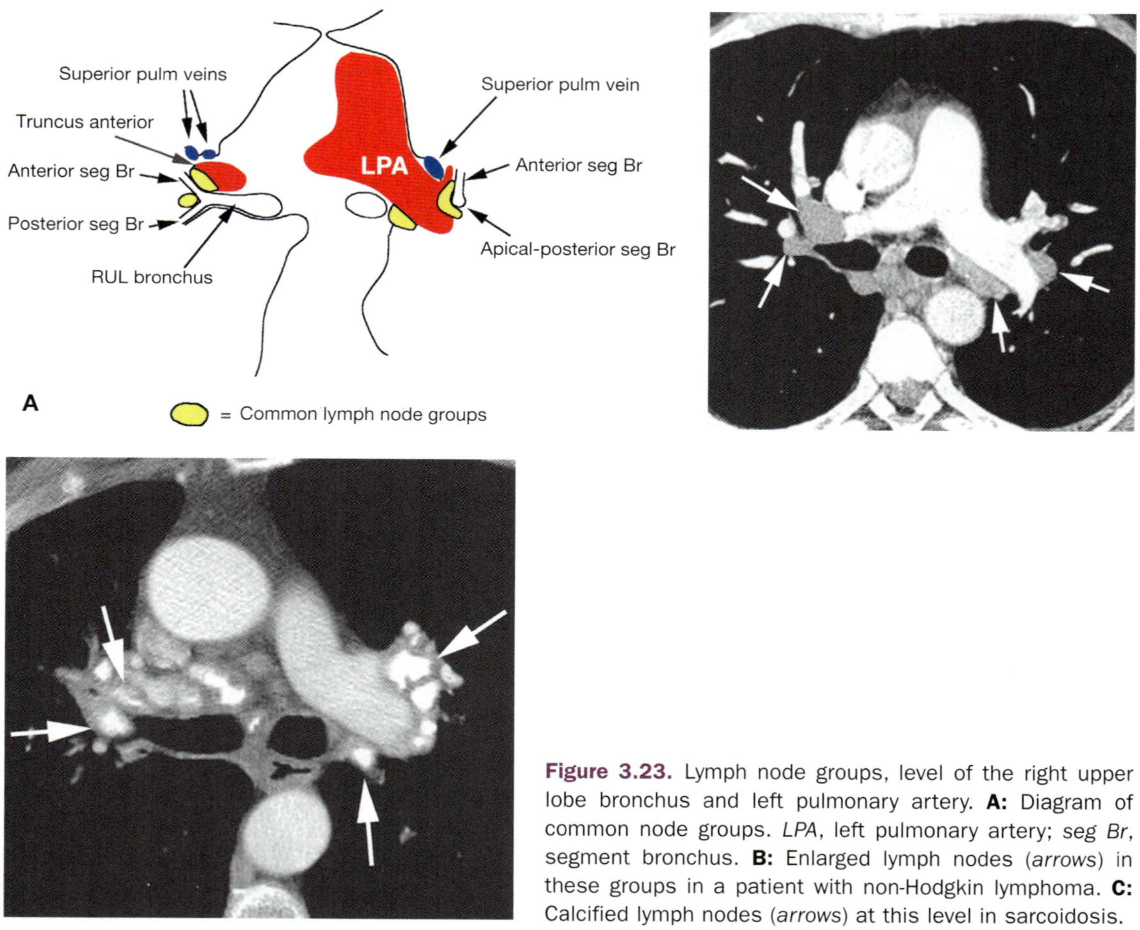

Figure 3.23. Lymph node groups, level of the right upper lobe bronchus and left pulmonary artery. **A:** Diagram of common node groups. *LPA*, left pulmonary artery; *seg Br*, segment bronchus. **B:** Enlarged lymph nodes (*arrows*) in these groups in a patient with non-Hodgkin lymphoma. **C:** Calcified lymph nodes (*arrows*) at this level in sarcoidosis.

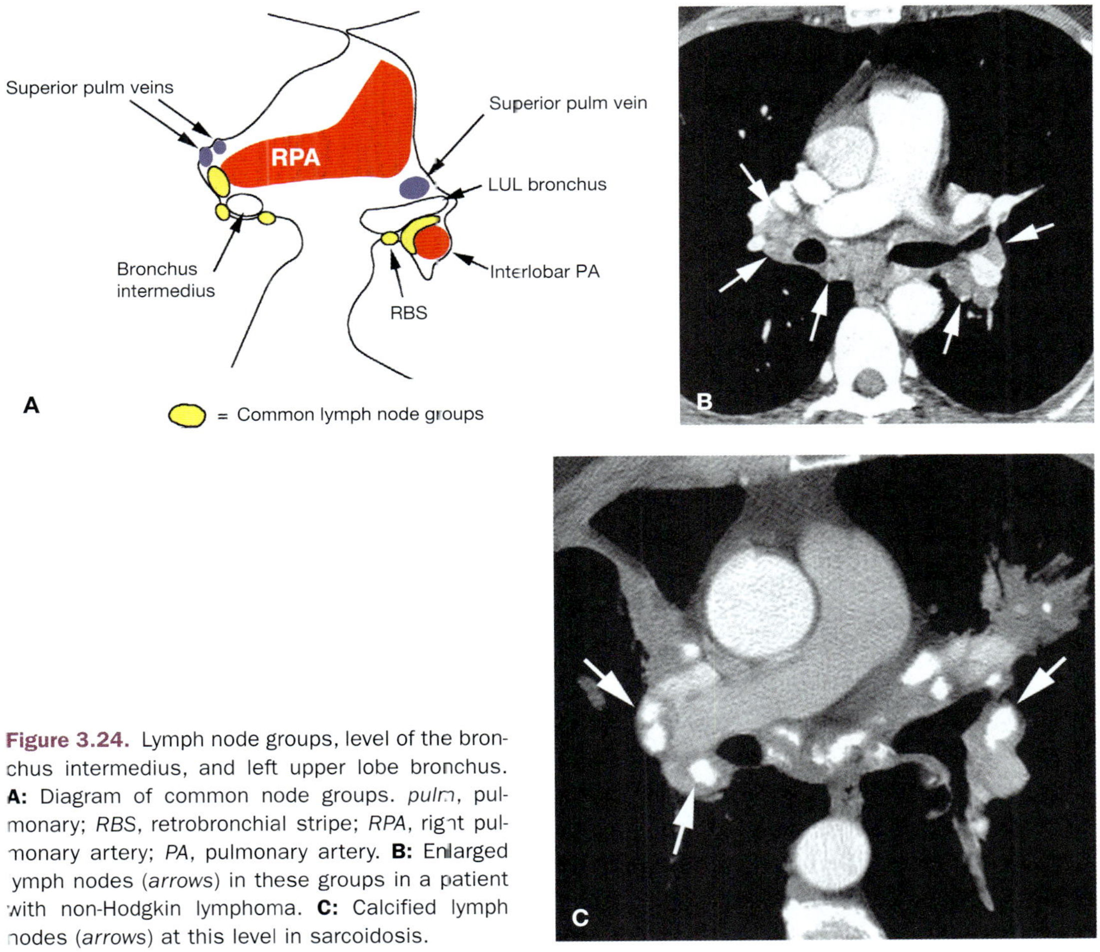

Figure 3.24. Lymph node groups, level of the bronchus intermedius, and left upper lobe bronchus. **A:** Diagram of common node groups. *pulm*, pulmonary; *RBS*, retrobronchial stripe; *RPA*, right pulmonary artery; *PA*, pulmonary artery. **B:** Enlarged lymph nodes (*arrows*) in these groups in a patient with non-Hodgkin lymphoma. **C:** Calcified lymph nodes (*arrows*) at this level in sarcoidosis.

Level of the Lower Lobe Bronchi and the IHW

At the level of the lower lobe bronchial segments, most nodes are interposed between bronchi and pulmonary arteries (Fig. 3.26). Lymph nodes anterior to the truncus basalis and basal lower lobe bronchi are also commonly present, visible in about 15% to 20% of normals. These nodes lie within the region termed the *IHW*.

Normal Hilar Lymph Node Size

In most regions, normal nodes measure only a few millimeters in size as shown on CT, with a short-axis diameter of 3 mm or less. In three locations described previously, however, larger conglomerates of nodes and soft tissue are often visible. These three regions are found at the levels of (1) the bronchus intermedius and bifurcation of the right pulmonary artery, (2) the RML bronchus, and (3) the LUL and lingular and bronchus. In only the first of these, however, can soft tissue exceeding 1 cm in least diameter be seen. Except in this one region, it would seem appropriate to use a short axis node diameter of 10 mm as the upper limit of normal.

CT DIAGNOSIS OF HILAR BRONCHIAL ABNORMALITIES

Generally speaking, scans viewed with a lung window setting (eg, −600/1500 H) are best for identifying normal bronchi and detecting bronchial abnormalities but may overestimate bronchial wall thickness or the degree of bronchial narrowing. Also, a normal bronchus slightly out of the plane of scan and being volume averaged with adjacent soft tissue can appear narrowed on lung window scans. A soft-tissue window is often best for looking at narrowed or obstructed bronchi and associated mass or lymph node enlargement. A wide lung window is a good compromise, providing information about bronchi and soft-tissue masses.

Thin collimation volumetric CT can be of great value in identifying bronchial abnormalities. Although the use of 3D reconstruction techniques may be of some value in the diagnosis of bronchial lesions, their advantage appears to be minimal compared to careful review of the transaxial images and 2D multiplanar reconstructions.

Accurate indicators of bronchial pathology include (1) bronchial wall thickening, (2) endobronchial mass, (3) bronchial obstruction, and (4) narrowing of the bronchial lumen.

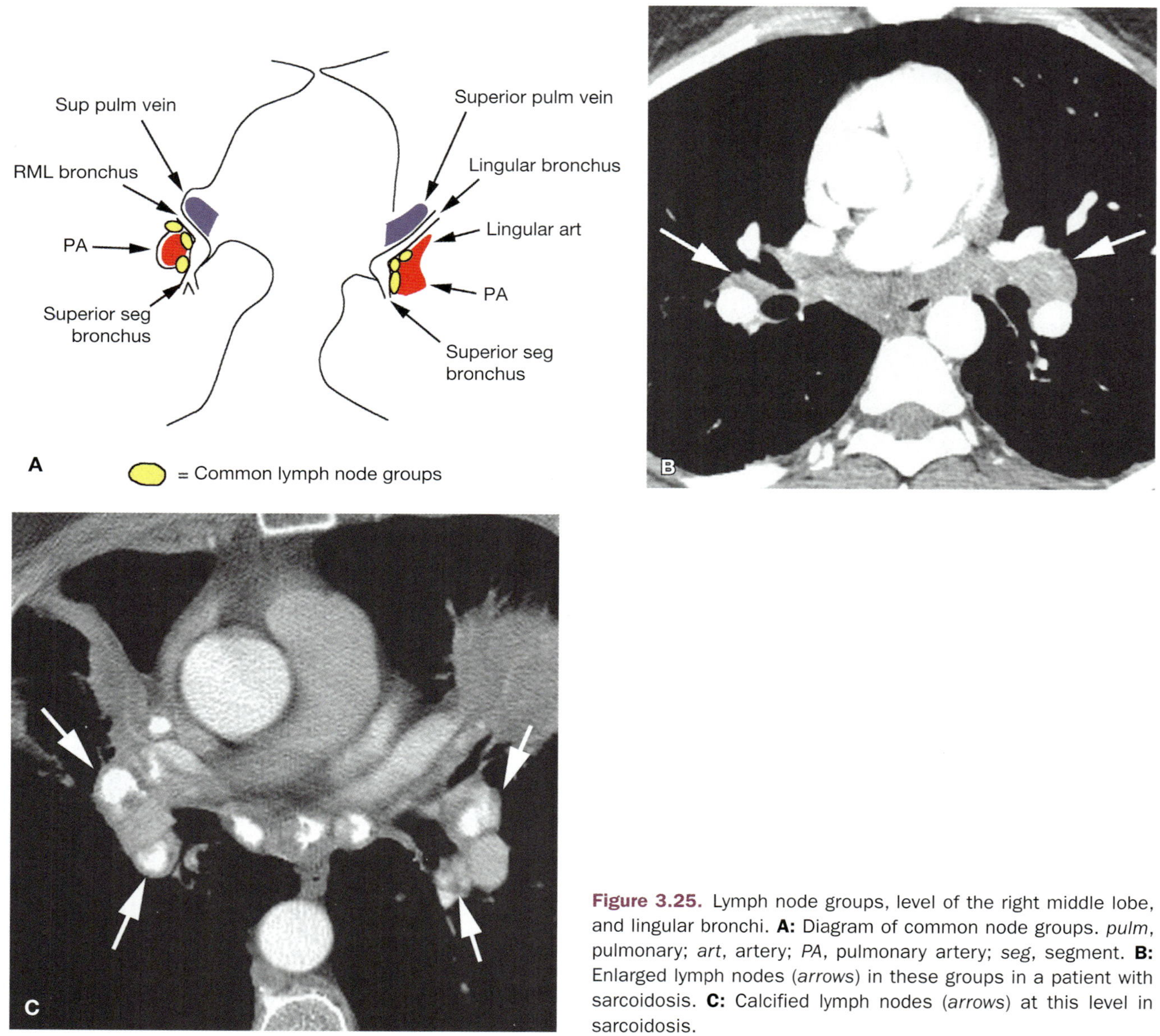

Figure 3.25. Lymph node groups, level of the right middle lobe, and lingular bronchi. **A:** Diagram of common node groups. *pulm*, pulmonary; *art*, artery; *PA*, pulmonary artery; *seg*, segment. **B:** Enlarged lymph nodes (*arrows*) in these groups in a patient with sarcoidosis. **C:** Calcified lymph nodes (*arrows*) at this level in sarcoidosis.

Other findings that may indicate the presence of a bronchial abnormality include mucous plugging, air trapping, atelectasis, or obstructive pneumonia. The differential diagnosis of an endobronchial mass or bronchial obstruction is listed in Table 5.13 in Chapter 5.

Bronchial Wall Thickening

Bronchial wall thickening is most easily assessed for bronchi partially outlined by the lung. Specific bronchi assessed in this manner include the right main bronchus, RUL bronchus, bronchus intermedius, and left main and upper lobe bronchus (left retrobronchial stripe). Smooth bronchial wall thickening can be due to inflammation, edema, or tumor infiltration, while a localized or lobulated thickening usually indicates localized tumor infiltration or lymph node enlargement.

Right Main and RUL Bronchus

The posterior walls of the RML and RUL bronchi are sharply outlined by the lung in normal subjects and should appear quite thin. Generalized thickening suggests tumor infiltration (see Fig. 3.12B).

Posterior Wall of the Bronchus Intermedius

On CT, the PWBI is visible in all patients. Its upper extent is clearly definable by, and is contiguous with, the origin of the RUL bronchus. The inferior extent of the PWBI is obscured by a branch of the inferior pulmonary vein crossing behind the bronchus to enter the left atrium. This usually occurs at the level of the origin of the superior segmental bronchus of the RLL. Thickening or nodularity of the PWBI can be seen with tumor infiltration (see Fig. 3.7B), most commonly

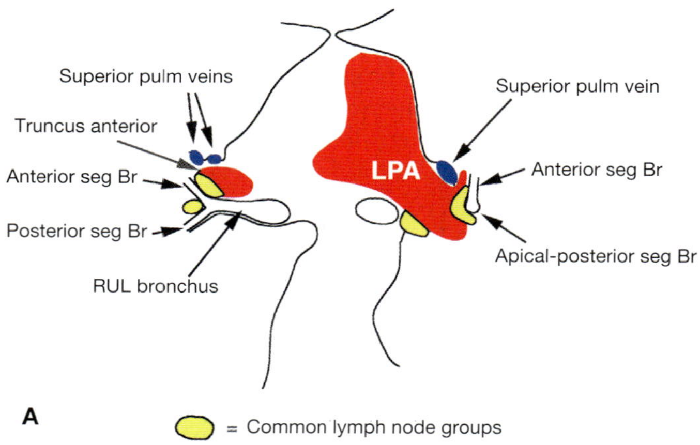

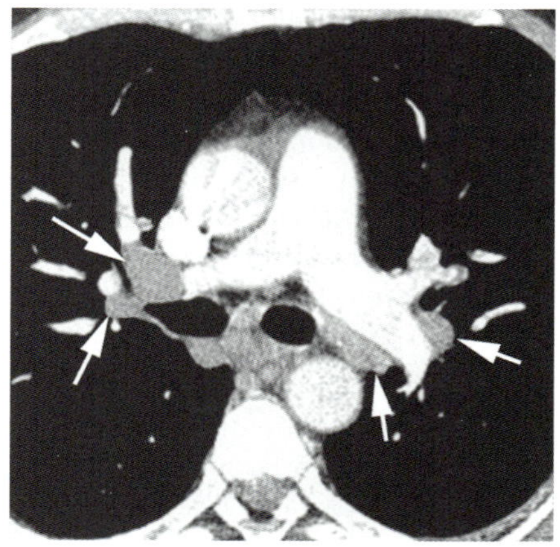

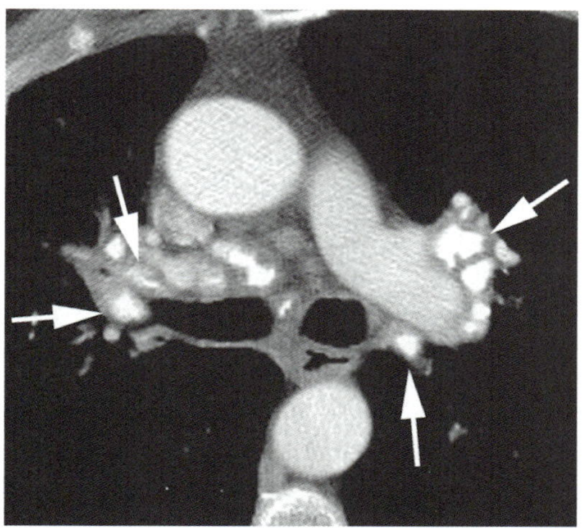

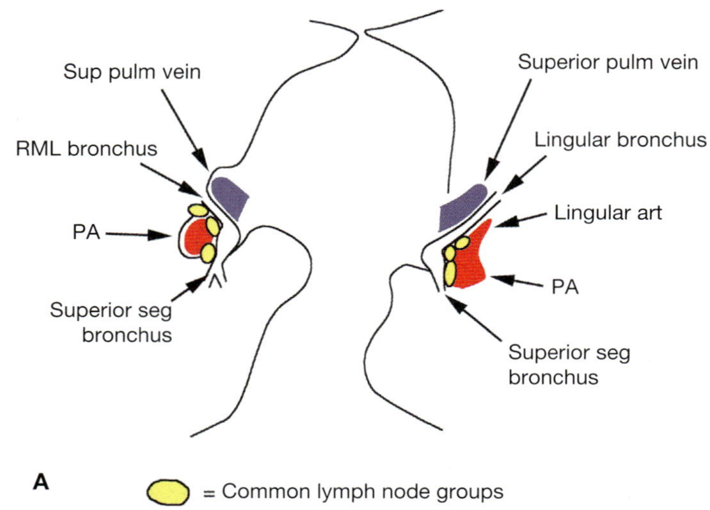

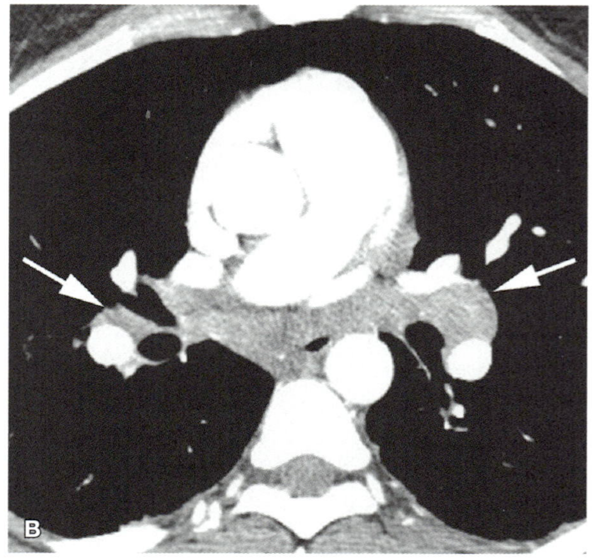

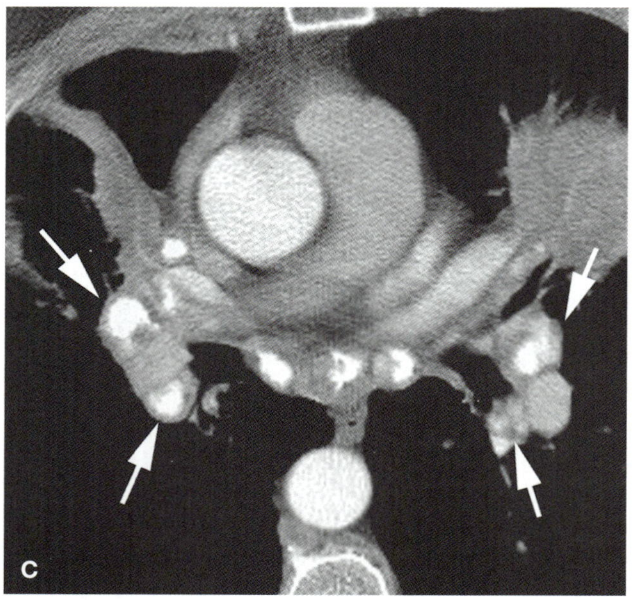

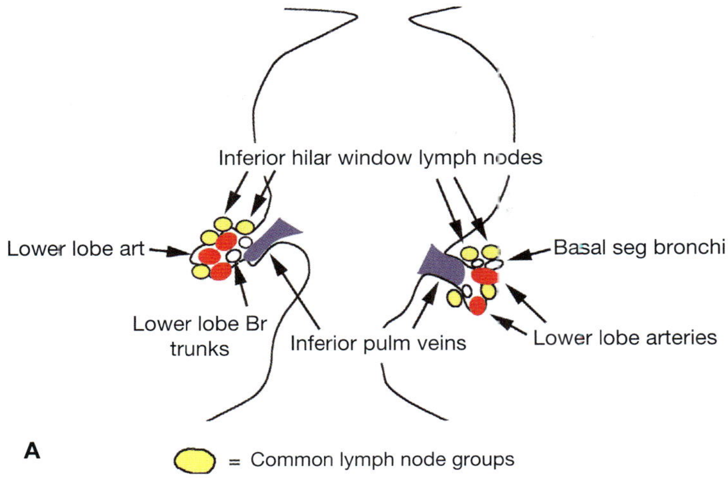

A

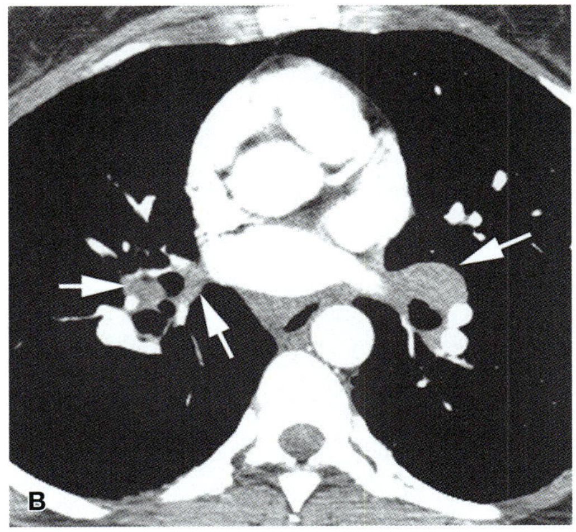

B

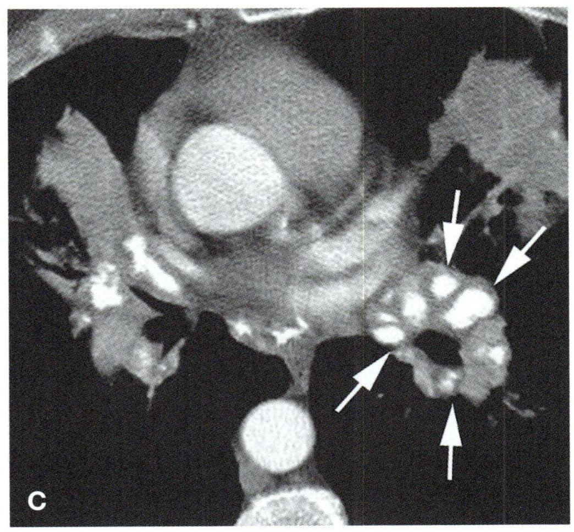

C

Figure 3.26. Lymph node groups, level of the lower lobe bronchi. **A:** Diagram of common node groups. *pulm*, pulmonary; *art*, artery; *Br*, bronchus; *seg*, segment. **B:** Enlarged lymph nodes (*arrows*) in a patient with sarcoidosis. The left-sided lymph nodes are in the region of the inferior hilar window. **C:** Calcified lymph nodes (*arrows*) at this level in sarcoidosis.

by bronchogenic carcinoma, or lymph node enlargement. Slight thickening may be seen in patients with pulmonary edema or interstitial lung disease. Obliteration of the posterior bronchial wall and the presence of soft-tissue densities behind it are virtually diagnostic of a mass in the hilum or adjacent lung.

Left Retrobronchial Stripe

The left posterior bronchial wall is outlined by the lung only at the level of the LUL bronchus. On CT, in approximately 90% of subjects, the lung sharply outlines the posterior wall of the left main or upper lobe bronchus, medial to the descending pulmonary artery, termed the *left retrobronchial stripe* (see Fig. 3.17). Thickening of the left retrobronchial stripe, as seen on CT, indicates lymph node enlargement or bronchial wall thickening, analogous to thickening of the PWBI on the right (Fig. 3.27). In 10% of normal individuals, the lung does not contact the bronchial wall because the descending pulmonary artery is positioned medially, contacting the lateral aorta.

Endobronchial Lesions and Bronchial Obstruction

Endobronchial lesions are sometimes diagnosed because a lesion is visible within the bronchus or focal bronchial obstruction is present in the absence of hilar mass. The differential diagnosis of an endobronchial lesion includes primary malignant and benign bronchial tumors, metastases, lymphoma, stricture, granulomas (infectious or noninfectious), foreign body, broncholith, and mucus (see Table 5.13 in Chapter 5).

Caveats: In patients with a hilar mass, it is difficult to distinguish bronchial compression and obstruction from an endobronchial mass or direct invasion. Endobronchial abnormalities that are primarily mucosal can be missed using CT.

Narrowing of the Bronchial Lumen

Bronchial narrowing in the absence of obstruction may be caused by an infiltrating tumor, inflammation, stricture, or bronchomalacia. Carcinoma often produces a gradual or tapered bronchial narrowing, a so-called rattail appearance.

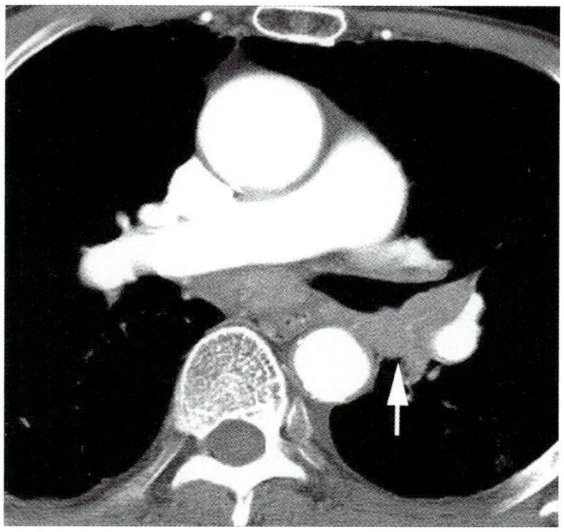

Figure 3.27. Thickening of the left retrobronchial stripe due to metastatic nasopharyngeal carcinoma. Lymph node enlargement posterior to the left upper lobe bronchus (*arrow*) results in thickening of this stripe. Left hilar and subcarinal lymph node enlargement is also seen.

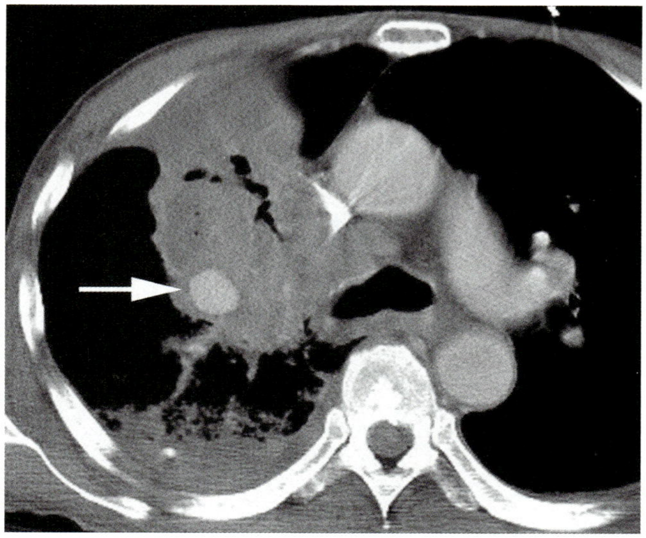

Figure 3.28. False aneurysm in bronchogenic carcinoma. A right hilar carcinoma results in right upper lobe collapse. The right hilar mass is associated with pooling of contrast in a false aneurysm (*arrow*).

because of bronchial wall infiltration by tumor (see Fig. 5.35 in Chapter 5). The presence of an associated mass is important in the differential diagnosis and strongly suggests carcinoma. It is important to look at adjacent scans to confirm that the apparent bronchial narrowing does not reflect an oblique bronchial course or volume averaging.

HILAR VASCULAR ABNORMALITIES

CT is very useful in the diagnosis of pulmonary vascular abnormalities. Pulmonary embolism is discussed in Chapter 28.

Pulmonary Artery Narrowing

Involvement of the pulmonary artery is common in patients with bronchogenic carcinoma involving the hilum or other hilar masses. Usually, artery narrowing or obstruction occurs. Rarely, a false aneurysm is seen in relation to the tumor (Fig. 3.28).

Increased Pulmonary Artery Diameter

A variety of conditions may result in pulmonary artery enlargement (Table 3.1). The most common is pulmonary hypertension with dilatation of the main and hilar pulmonary arteries (see Fig. 3.6). The diameter of the main pulmonary artery on CT—in isolation—is of limited value in identifying pulmonary hypertension. Increasing age, male sex, and body surface area all contribute to larger pulmonary artery diameter. A cutoff of 34 mm in diameter has been proposed for patients considered low risk for pulmonary hypertension, but other factors should also be considered including an increased PA-to-aorta ratio (greater than 1.1:1) and signs of right ventricular remodeling.

Localized enlargement of a hilar pulmonary artery may occur because of pulmonary embolism. In the acute setting, PA enlargement can represent the presence of a large clot impacted in the artery, but chronic thromboembolic pulmonary hypertension may contribute to this appearance.

Enlargement of the main and left pulmonary arteries is seen in patients with pulmonary valve abnormalities including pulmonic stenosis, bicuspid pulmonic valve, or absent pulmonary valve. The pulmonary outflow tract usually appears dilated as well. The right pulmonary artery usually appears normal.

Pulmonary artery intimal sarcoma is a rare neoplasm resulting in an intravascular mass. This may result in

Table 3.1 Pulmonary Artery Enlargement

Pulmonary hypertension (any cause)
Pulmonary arterial hypertension
Pulmonary hypertension due to left heart disease
Pulmonary hypertension due to lung disease/hypoxia
Chronic thromboembolic pulmonary hypertension
Pulmonary hypertension with unclear/multifactorial mechanisms
Pulmonic valve abnormality (stenosis, bicuspid, absent)
Pulmonary artery sarcoma
Pulmonary artery aneurysm/pseudoaneurysm
- Mycotic
- Catheter-related complication
- Takayasu arteritis
- Williams syndrome
- Prenatal varicella
- Pulmonary hypertension
- Behçet syndrome

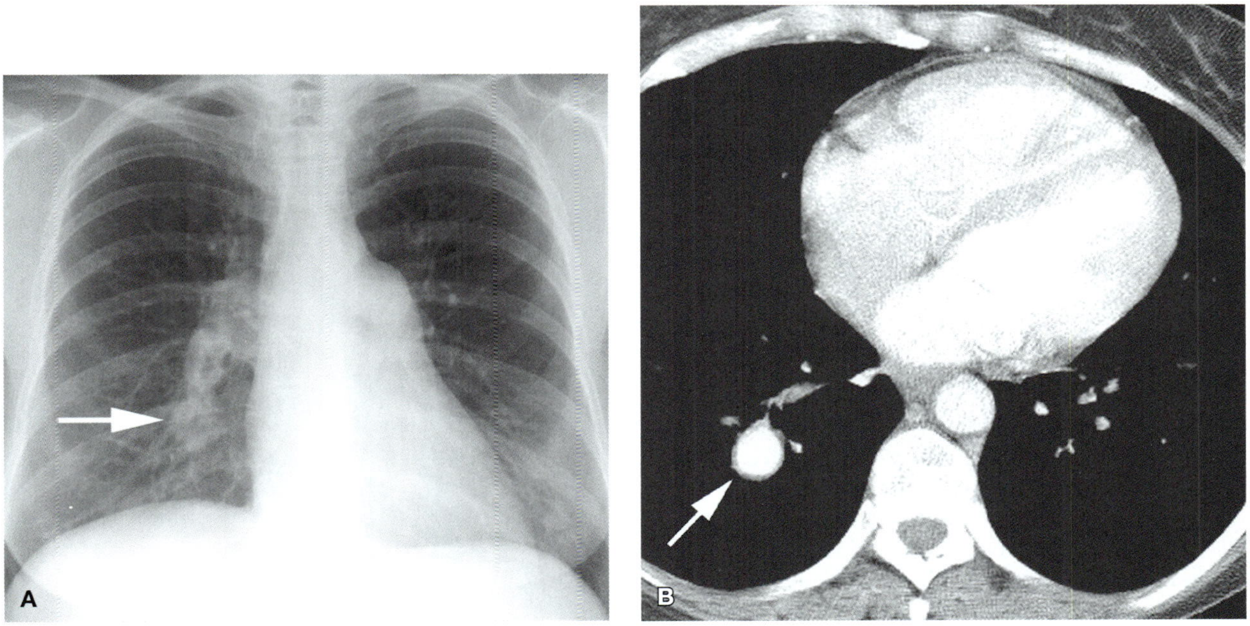

Figure 3.29. Pulmonary artery aneurysm in pulmonary hypertension. **A:** Chest radiograph shows enlargement of the main pulmonary artery (*arrow*) due to pulmonary hypertension. A focal lesion is visible overlying the inferior hilum. **B:** Contrast-enhanced CT shows a focal aneurysm (*arrow*) of a segmental pulmonary artery.

dilatation of the main, right, or left pulmonary arteries. Endovascular metastasis can give the same appearance.

Pulmonary artery aneurysms and pseudoaneurysms are rarely seen (Fig. 3.29); they may be (1) mycotic in origin; (2) due to catheter-related complications; (3) associated with multiple pulmonary artery stenoses or coarctations in patients with Takayasu arteritis, Williams syndrome, and prenatal varicella; (4) associated with pulmonary hypertension; or (5) associated with Behçet syndrome.

Decreased Pulmonary Artery Diameter

Decrease in size of a hilar pulmonary artery has a variety of causes (Table 3.2). It may represent artery or lung hypoplasia, proximal interruption of the pulmonary artery, or conditions resulting in decreased lung perfusion such as chronic pulmonary embolism (Fig. 3.30), chronic collapse, severe unilateral fibrosis or lung destruction, or Swyer-James syndrome. In some patients, enlargement of bronchial arteries or other systemic collaterals is seen on the side of decreased perfusion (see Fig. 3.30). These are best seen with thin slices and rapid contrast infusion.

Table 3.2 Decreased Pulmonary Artery Size

Decreased Pulmonary Artery Size
Hypoplastic lung
Scimitar syndrome
Proximal interruption of the pulmonary artery
Pulmonary embolism
Atelectasis
Swyer-James syndrome
Ipsilateral lung disease

Pulmonary Veins

Pulmonary vein abnormalities are uncommon. Pulmonary vein dilatation (ie, vein varices) occurring in association with chronic elevation of left atrial pressure, mitral valve abnormalities, or anomalous pulmonary vein drainage is most common (see Fig. 10.47 in Chapter 10). In patients with lung cancer or metastatic neoplasm, tumor may invade the pulmonary

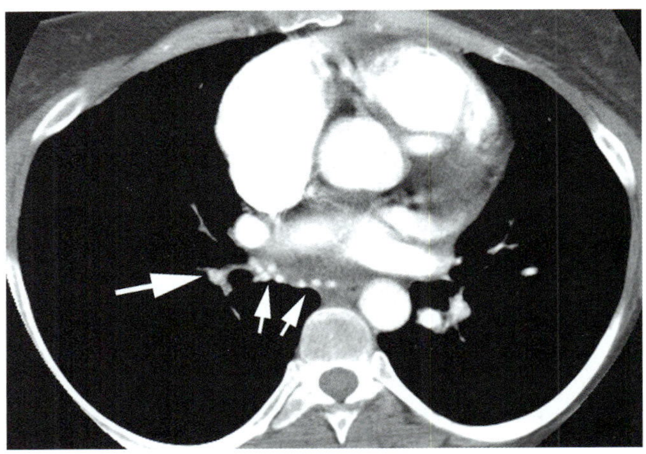

Figure 3.30. Decreased size of pulmonary artery in chronic pulmonary embolism. The right interlobar pulmonary artery is markedly reduced in size (*large arrow*). Bronchial arteries (*small arrows*) are enlarged.

vein, appearing as a filling defect on contrast-enhanced scans. Pulmonary vein stenosis/occlusion is most commonly iatrogenic after left atrial ablation procedures for arrhythmia.

HILAR LYMPH NODE ENLARGEMENT AND HILAR MASSES

There is some value in attempting to distinguish hilar lymph node enlargement from hilar mass, although this is not always possible.

Hilar Lymph Node Enlargement

Hilar lymph node enlargement may be suggested if abnormal soft tissue is localized to node-bearing regions, particularly if more than one node group is involved (see Figs. 3.23-3.27). Nodes usually appear well-defined, smooth, and rounded. Except at the level of the bronchus intermedius, nodes larger than 1 cm may be considered pathologic. Nodes larger than 5 mm are usually abnormal, but these are commonly seen and are likely to be hyperplastic. Very large hilar nodes may result in smooth bronchial compression.

The presence of hilar lymph node enlargement, depending on the clinical situation, suggests hilar metastases from bronchogenic carcinoma, metastatic carcinoma, lymphoma, sarcoidosis, or infection. The differential diagnosis of hilar lymph node enlargement depends on whether it is unilateral or bilateral (Table 3.3).

Table 3.3 Unilateral and Bilateral Lymph Node Enlargement

Unilateral
Bronchogenic carcinoma
Lymph node metastases
Head and neck
Thyroid carcinoma
Melanoma
Renal
Testicular
Breast
Lymphoma
Tuberculosis
Fungal infection (eg, histoplasmosis, coccidioidomycosis)
Bacterial infection
Viral infection
Castleman disease
Bilateral
Sarcoid or berylliosis
Silicosis
Amyloidosis
Collagen vascular diseases
Lymphoma
Lymph node metastases
Pulmonary edema

Hilar Masses

Hilar masses usually are localized to one region, appear irregular in contour, and are often associated with an endobronchial mass or bronchial obstruction (Fig. 3.31). The presence of a mass suggests bronchogenic carcinoma or other primary tumor and makes lymph node diseases less likely. In patients with a hilar mass and bronchial obstruction, collapse or consolidation of the distal lung can obscure the margins of the mass, making it more difficult to diagnose.

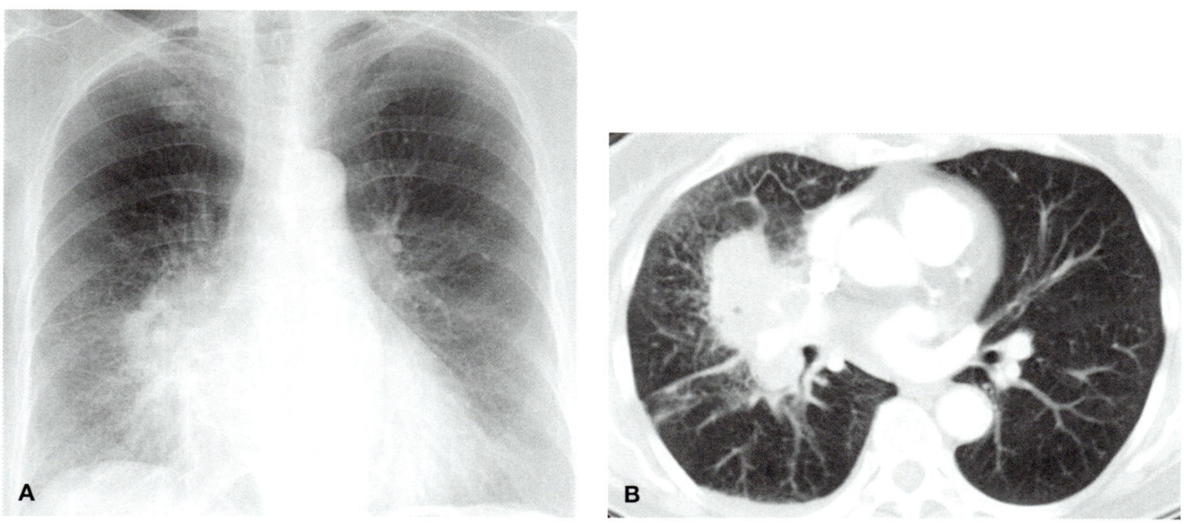

Figure 3.31. Right hilar mass in small cell carcinoma. **A:** A large, ill-defined hilar enlargement is visible on the chest radiograph. This is more typical of hilar mass than lymph node enlargement. **B:** CT shows a large localized right hilar mass associated with obstruction of the right middle lobe bronchus and infiltration of the adjacent lung.

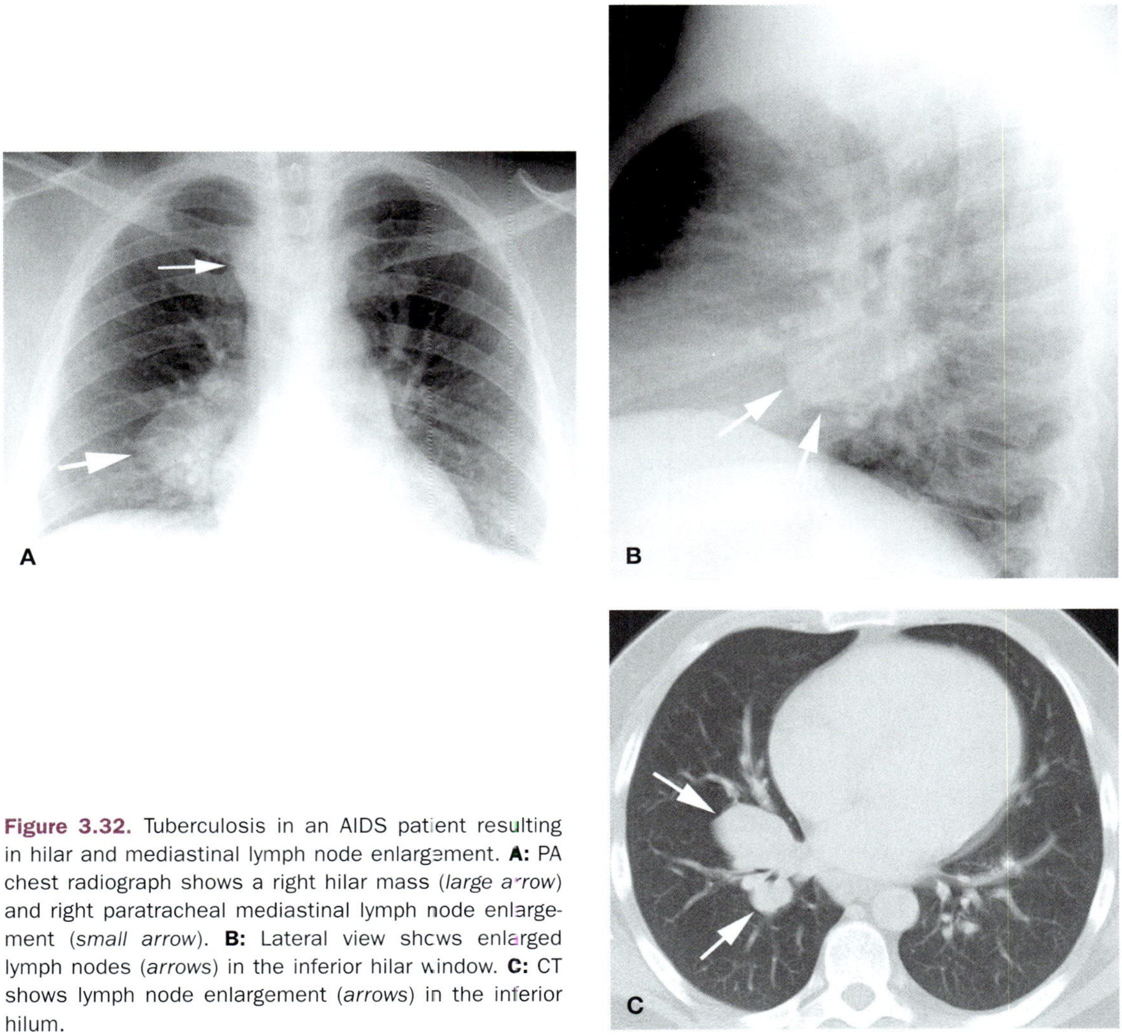

Figure 3.32. Tuberculosis in an AIDS patient resulting in hilar and mediastinal lymph node enlargement. **A:** PA chest radiograph shows a right hilar mass (*large arrow*) and right paratracheal mediastinal lymph node enlargement (*small arrow*). **B:** Lateral view shows enlarged lymph nodes (*arrows*) in the inferior hilar window. **C:** CT shows lymph node enlargement (*arrows*) in the inferior hilum.

Common Causes of Hilar Node Enlargement or Mass

Bronchogenic Carcinoma

The most common cause of hilar mass or lymph node enlargement is bronchogenic carcinoma. The hilar mass can appear irregular because of local infiltration of the lung parenchyma (see Figs. 3.5B, 3.7B, 3.28, and 3.31). In patients with tumors arising centrally (usually squamous cell carcinoma or small cell carcinoma), bronchial abnormalities are commonly visible on CT. When the carcinoma arises in the peripheral lung and the hila are abnormal because of node metastases, the hilar mass or masses may be smoother and more sharply defined than when the hilar mass represents the primary tumor. However, this distinction is not always easily made. Patients with a central mass and bronchial obstruction often show peripheral parenchymal abnormalities.

In patients with hilar node metastases, a bronchial abnormality seen on CT usually reflects external compression by the enlarged hilar nodes, but bronchial invasion may also be present. Hilar node metastases are present at surgery in up to 40% of patients with lung cancer.

Other Primary Bronchial Tumors

Other primary bronchial tumors may be associated with a hilar mass. The most common of these is carcinoid tumor. This malignant tumor arises from the main, lobar, or segmental bronchi in 80% of cases. It tends to be slow growing and locally invasive. A well-defined endobronchial mass is typical, but a large exobronchial, hilar mass is sometimes seen. Carcinoid tumors are very vascular and often enhance following contrast infusion. Carcinoid tumors occasionally calcify. Adenoid cystic carcinoma (cylindroma) and other minor salivary gland tumors can result in a similar appearance.

Benign bronchial tumors, such as fibroma, chondroma, or lipoma, usually appear focal and endobronchial on CT, rather than infiltrative, and do not commonly produce an exobronchial mass. Obstruction is the primary finding on CT. They are relatively rare.

Lymphoma

Hilar adenopathy is present in 25% of patients with Hodgkin lymphoma and 10% of patients with non-Hodgkin lymphoma (see Figs. 3.23B and 3.24B). Hilar involvement is usually asymmetrical. Multiple nodes in the hilum or mediastinum are usually involved. Endobronchial lesions can also be seen, or bronchi may be compressed by enlarged nodes, but this is much less common than with lung cancer. There are no specific features of the hilar abnormality seen in patients with lymphoma that allow a definite diagnosis.

Metastases

Metastases to hilar lymph nodes from an extrathoracic primary tumor are not uncommon. Hilar node metastases may be unilateral or bilateral (see Fig. 3.5A). Endobronchial metastases can also be seen without there being hilar node metastases; these may appear to be focal and endobronchial or infiltrative. Head and neck carcinomas, thyroid carcinoma, genitourinary tumors (particularly renal cell and testicular carcinoma), melanoma, and breast carcinomas are most commonly responsible for hilar or endobronchial metastases.

Inflammatory Disease

Unilateral or bilateral hilar lymphadenopathy can be seen in a number of infectious or inflammatory conditions. Primary tuberculosis usually causes unilateral hilar adenopathy (Fig. 3.32), and the presence of low-attenuation nodes on contrast-enhanced scans strongly suggests this diagnosis. Fungal infections, most notably histoplasmosis and coccidioidomycosis, cause unilateral or bilateral adenopathy. Sarcoidosis causes smooth, lobulated, bilateral, and symmetrical adenopathy in most patients typically involving right paratracheal, bilateral hilar, and subcarinal nodes (see Figs. 3.5D, 3.10, 3.11, and 3.23C).

SELECTED READING

Bankier AA, Fleischmann D, Mallek R, et al. Bronchial wall thickness: appropriate window settings for thin-section CT and radiologic-anatomic correlation. *Radiology*. 1996;199(3):831-836.

Friedman PJ. Practical radiology of the hila and mediastinum. *Postgrad Radiol*. 1981;1:269-304.

Jardin M, Remy J. Segmental bronchovascular anatomy of the lower lobes: CT analysis. *AJR Am J Roentgenol*. 1986;147(3):457-468.

Lang EV, Friedman PJ. The anterior wall stripe of the left lower lobe bronchus on the lateral chest radiograph: CT correlative study. *AJR Am J Roentgenol*. 1990;154(1):33-39.

McGuinness G, Naidich DP, Garay SM, Davis AL, Boyd AD, Mizrachi HH. Accessory cardiac bronchus: CT features and clinical significance. *Radiology*. 1993;189(2):563-566.

Müller NL, Webb WR. Radiographic imaging of the pulmonary hila. *Invest Radiol*. 1985;20(7):661-671.

Naidich DP, Stitik FP, Khouri NF, Terry PB, Siegelman SS. Computed tomography of the bronchi. 2. Pathology. *J Comput Assist Tomogr*. 1980;4(6):754-762.

Naidich et al., 1980 Naidich DP, Terry PB, Stitik FP, Siegelman SS. Computed tomography of the bronchi. 1. Normal anatomy. *J Comput Assist Tomogr*. 1980;4(6):746-753.

Naidich DP, Khouri NF, Scott WW, Jr, Wang KP, Siegelman SS. Computed tomography of the pulmonary hila, 1: normal anatomy. *J Comput Assist Tomogr*. 1981;5(4):459-467.

Naidich et al., 1981 Naidich DP, Khouri NF, Stitik FP, McCauley DI, Siegelman SS. Computed tomography of the pulmonary hila. 2. Abnormal anatomy. *J Comput Assist Tomogr*. 1981;5(4):468-475.

Naidich DP, Zinn WL, Ettenger NA, McCauley DI, Garay SM. Basilar segmental bronchi: thin-section CT evaluation. *Radiology*. 1988;169(1):11-16.

Ng CS, Wells AU, Padley SP. A CT sign of chronic pulmonary arterial hypertension: the ratio of main pulmonary artery to aortic diameter. *J Thorac Imaging*. 1999;14(4):270-278.

Park CK, Webb WR, Klein JS. Inferior hilar window. *Radiology*. 1991;178(1):163-168.

Proto AV, Speckman JM. The left lateral radiograph of the chest. *Med Radiogr Photogr*. 1979;55:30-74.

Quint LE, Whyte RI, Kazerooni EA, et al. Stenosis of the central airways: evaluation by using helical CT with multiplanar reconstructions. *Radiology*. 1995;194(3):871-877.

Remy-Jardin M, Duyck P, Remy J, et al. Hilar lymph nodes: identification with spiral CT and histologic correlation. *Radiology*. 1995;196(2):387-394.

Remy-Jardin M, Remy J, Artaud D, Fribourg M, Duhamel A. Volume rendering of the tracheobronchial tree: clinical evaluation of bronchographic images. *Radiology*. 1998;208(3):761-770.

Remy-Jardin M, Ryerson CJ, Schiebler ML, et al. Imaging of pulmonary hypertension in adults: a position paper from the Fleischner society. *Radiology*. March 2021;298(3):531-549. DOI: 10.1148/radiol.2020203108

Schnur MJ, Winkler B, Austin JHM. Thickening of the posterior wall of the bronchus intermedius: a sign on lateral chest radiographs of congestive heart failure, lymph node enlargement, and neoplastic infiltration. *Radiology*. 1981;139(3):551-559.

Sone S, Higashihara T, Morimoto S, et al. CT anatomy of hilar lymphadenopathy. *AJR Am J Roentgenol*. 1983;140(5):887-892.

Vix VA, Klatte EC. The lateral chest radiograph in the diagnosis of hilar and mediastinal masses. *Radiology*. 1970;96(2):307-316.

Webb WR, Gamsu G. Computed tomography of the left retrobronchial stripe. *J Comput Assist Tomogr*. 1983;7(1):65-69.

Webb et al., 1981 Webb WR, Gamsu G, Glazer G. Computed tomography of the abnormal pulmonary hilum. *J Comput Assist Tomogr*. 1981;5(4):485-490.

Webb WR, Glazer G, Gamsu G. Computed tomography of the normal pulmonary hilum. *J Comput Assist Tomogr*. 1981;5(4):476-484.

Webb WR, Hirji M, Gamsu G. Posterior wall of the bronchus intermedius: radiographic-CT correlation. *AJR Am J Roentgenol*. 1984;142(5):907-911.

Webb WR. Radiologic imaging of the pulmonary hila. *Postgrad Radiol*. 1986;6:145-168.

Chapter 4

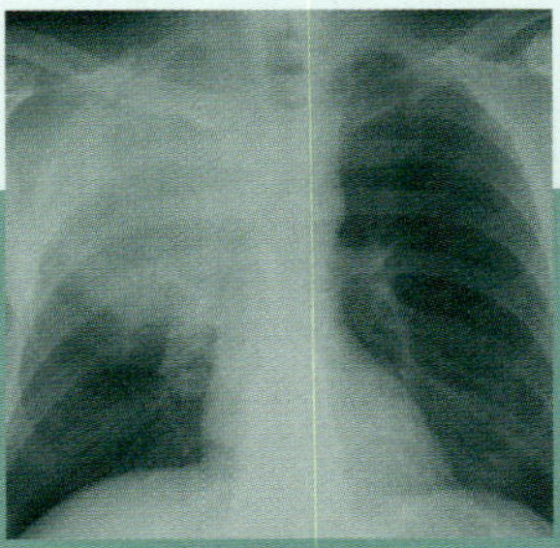

Constantine Raptis • Mark M. Hammer • Rex Parker • Kacie Kuykendall

Thoracic MRI

INTRODUCTION

Rightfully, and as one can determine from flipping through the pages of this textbook, computed tomography (CT) is the primary cross-sectional imaging modality for the evaluation of the thorax. It is widely available, fast, and provides excellent spatial resolution imaging with little technical input from radiologists. Magnetic resonance imaging (MRI) lacks the speed and spatial resolution of CT but provides different advantages, including lack of ionizing radiation, superior contrast resolution, cine-based imaging, and the ability to acquire functional information via diffusion-weighted imaging (DWI) and dynamic contrast enhancement (DCE).

MRI has long had an important role in imaging cardiac and vascular pathologies in the thorax, but its use in evaluating other thoracic pathologies largely remains limited to specific problem-solving applications. Some of these, such as the interrogation of anterior mediastinal soft tissue that may be thymic hyperplasia, recur in clinical practice. Others, such as determining whether a lesion enhances, invades adjacent structures or is composed of macroscopic fat, are questions tailored to a specific patient. As such, MR protocols for imaging the thorax must be able to handle recurring tasks while also being flexible enough to answer additional questions when necessary. In this chapter, we will review a basic approach to noncardiac, non-vascular thoracic MRI protocol creation and present specific case examples to highlight the utility of thoracic MRI.

THORACIC MRI PROTOCOLS

Challenges and Considerations

There are several important challenges encountered when performing MRI in the thorax. First, imaging of the lung parenchyma is difficult, mainly due to low proton density of the lungs. In addition, the air in the lungs results in field heterogeneities that result in further signal loss. As such, the lungs will be black or nearly black on most MRI sequences, and evaluating for parenchymal abnormalities such as fibrosis will be severely limited. Superimposed soft tissue or fluid processes with higher proton density, such as tumors, hematomas, atelectasis, and pneumonia, will typically be visible on the dark lung background.

In part due to these challenges in evaluating lung parenchymal abnormalities, most applications of thoracic MRI in clinical practice focus on the mediastinum or chest wall. Particularly in mediastinal applications, respiratory motion is another important challenge that must be addressed to obtain diagnostic-quality images. The most straightforward way to do this is via breath holding. As most healthy subjects can usually hold their breath for 20 seconds, sequence acquisition time should be less than 20 seconds, preferably as low as possible. In patients who cannot hold their breath for 20 seconds or when performing sequences that cannot be completed in less than 20 seconds, additional strategies can be used. One is to decrease the volume of tissue covered into multiple contiguous stacks of images. Another is to increase the number of concatenations per sequence, allowing for the slices of the original sequence to be distributed over multiple repetition times (TRs), each with their own breath hold.

Respiratory gating is an additional strategy that can be used for longer sequences or in patients with extensive difficulty holding their breath. With respiratory gating, imaging data is only acquired during a designated portion of the respiratory cycle, typically end of expiration. The most commonly used technique for respiratory gating involves employing a sequence that allows the user to select the dome of the diaphragm and then determine an acceptance window wherein data is collected when the diaphragm is in that window. The patient then remains still and breathes normally, obviating the need for breath-holding. The main drawback of respiratory gating is that it results in longer acquisition times, generally 5 to 10 minutes. The length of the sequence is influenced by the width of the acceptance window, as larger acceptance windows will allow data to be collected more often, thus shortening sequence time at the expense of motion reduction. For most applications in the thorax, an acceptance window of 5 mm will suffice, and this can be adjusted based on the smallest structures that need to be imaged, with exams targeting smaller structures potentially requiring a narrower window. Finally, newer sequences with radial k-space acquisition allow for free-breathing postcontrast imaging of the chest at high resolution. These sequences generally have an acquisition time intermediate between breath-holding and respiratory gating.

Cardiac motion can also degrade thoracic MR images, due to blurring of anatomy near the heart and by creating artifacts from cardiac and vascular pulsation. Cardiac motion is mitigated via electrocardiogram (ECG) gating. ECG gating can be prospective or retrospective. In prospective ECG gating, a selected portion of the R-R interval is selected during which data for k-space is acquired. This technique is best suited for obtaining image stacks through a volume of tissue and can be applied to a variety of sequences. In retrospective ECG gating, k-space data is acquired continuously during the entire cardiac cycle and then segmented after the sequence has completed. This is particularly useful in cine imaging in which the data from the segmented R-R intervals can be used to create frames and displayed as a cine loop. ECG gating is not necessary for every thoracic MRI sequence, but it may be of benefit, particularly when the structure being evaluated is near the heart or when the cardiac invasion is questioned.

Additionally, by its nature, the thorax contains a number of air-soft tissue interfaces that cause substantial magnetic field heterogeneity. Thus, chemical (frequency-selective) fat suppression is often inadequate and leads to artifacts or complete lack of fat suppression in the compartment of interest. This can be addressed either with vigilant technologists and/or radiologist monitoring to select the correct fat-suppression frequency on the scanner or, with better effect, by using Dixon-based fat suppression.

Protocol Design

Thoracic MRI sequences can generally be divided into traditional/anatomic, functional, and cine-based. Anatomic sequences depict basic anatomy and tissue intensity characteristics. Basic pre- and post-contrast imaging and chemical shift imaging are included in this category. Most clinical questions in the thorax can be answered with anatomic sequences only. Functional sequences help determine specific tissue parameters, including diffusion-weighted imaging (DWI) to assess cellularity and dynamic contrast enhancement (DCE) to evaluate multicompartment perfusion kinetics. While DWI and low temporal resolution DCE are often obtained in routine practice, high-level analysis of functional sequences, including intravoxel incoherent motion (IVIM) modeling for DWI and kurtosis modeling for DCE are typically not required. Cine-based sequences provide visualization of motion of the structures of the thorax. Cine-based sequences may be ECG gated, which is best suited for evaluating the heart or structures near it, or "real time," which is not ECG gated but allows visualization of the motion of structures during free breathing. "Real time" sequences can be particularly useful in the thorax for evaluating respiratory/diaphragm motion or in determining whether a lesion or structure slides against a pleural surface or is adherent to it.

As with MR of other regions of the body, thoracic MR protocols are designed to answer specific clinical questions. Unlike other parts of the body, however, few nonvascular, non-cardiac exams are performed, and the variety of niche questions that are of interest makes it difficult to develop one-size-fits-all protocols for each indication. As such, thoracic MR protocol design will vary by practice needs and individual patient indications. A potential strategy to address these issues involves developing core protocols that can then be modified with add-ons for specific niche indications. This "building block" approach gives flexibility to radiologists without creating a long list of protocols, many of which will rarely be used. Furthermore, a building block approach can be used to create efficient protocols that remove unnecessary sequences, thus limiting overall exam time. Indeed, keeping overall exam time under 45 minutes, and preferably under 30 minutes, can decrease patient fatigue and improve image quality and patient comfort. Examples of basic mediastinal and pleural MRI protocols are provided in Table 4.1.

EXAMPLE INDICATIONS

There are many potential indications for noncardiac, nonvascular thoracic MRI. Some, such as the evaluation of anterior mediastinal thymic tissue or the evaluation of mediastinal cysts, recur in any practice (see Chapter 8). Others, such as the evaluation of local invasion of a tumor or desire to better characterize an indeterminate lesion, tend to arise as specific questions in individual patients. Centers with more experience may pursue more advanced applications, including using DWI or DCE to characterize lesions. In this section, some basic applications of noncardiac, nonvascular MRI will be presented. These are intended both as a reference and as a means of illustrating the potential of thoracic MRI to be used in other novel situations where it may add valuable information.

Thymic Tissue

The most common recurring indication for thoracic MRI is in the evaluation of anterior mediastinal soft tissue. In normal patients, the thymus is progressively replaced by fat, a process that can have a variable time course but is usually completed by the third decade of life. Some patients may have a later time course of fatty replacement, have an incomplete fatty replacement, or have an inciting factor, such as an infection or chemotherapy, that may result in rebound thymic hyperplasia. In most of these patients, the residual or hyperplastic thymus will

Table 4.1 Sample Basic Mediastinal and Pleural MRI Protocols

Basic mediastinal
Positioning: Phased-array body or cardiac coil, center over mid-chest or lesion of concern
Contrast agent: Single dose at 2 mL/s
Sequences:
- Axial and coronal T2W SSFSE (consider ECG-gating)
- Axial T2W STIR (consider ECG-gating)
- Axial bSSFP (consider ECG-gating)
- Axial T1W dual-echo in- and opposed-phase
  - Can substitute with axial T1W GRE with Dixon fat suppression
- Axial DWI (consider ECG-gating)
  - b = 50, 400, 800 s/mm^2
- Pre-contrast axial T1W GRE
- Post-contrast axial T1W GRE
  - Axial acquisitions at 20-30 s, 60-70 s, 3 min, and 5 min
  - Direct sagittal and coronal acquisitions between the 3 and 5 min axials
- Optional: Real-time bSSFP cine imaging to evaluate for motion of a lesion against another surface

Basic pleural
Positioning: Phased-array body coil, center over mid chest, cover from above clavicles through deep costophrenic sulci
Contrast agent: Single dose at 2 mL/s
Sequences:
- Axial, coronal, and sagittal T2W STIR
- High resolution axial T2W TSE
- Axial and coronal T1W TSE without fat suppression
- Axial DWI, respiratory triggered
  - b = 50, 400, 800 s/mm^2
- Coronal real time bSSFP during normal breath, forced exhalation, and deep inspiration
- Pre-contrast axial T1W GRE
- Post-contrast axial T1W GRE
  - Axial acquisitions at 20-30 s, 60-70 s, 3 min, and 5 min
  - Direct sagittal and coronal acquisitions between the 3 and 5 min axials

Key: bSSFP, balanced steady-state free precession, DWI, diffusion weighted imaging; GRE, gradient recalled echo; SSFSE, single shot fast spin echo, STIR, short tau inversion recovery; TSE, turbo spin echo.

have a characteristic appearance on CT (see also Figs. 8.6 and 8.7), often demonstrating a triangular appearance, frequently with internal macroscopic fat that may have a similar appearance to pancreas tissue. On occasion, the appearance on CT will be equivocal, with an appearance that overlaps with a mass. MRI provides a simple and elegant means of evaluating patients with indeterminate anterior mediastinal soft tissue. This premise for using MRI in this scenario is akin to the evaluation of intravoxel lipid in suspected adrenal adenomas. As with an adrenal adenoma, MRI can detect intravoxel lipid in thymic tissue and allow for differentiation from soft tissue lesions such as thymoma or lymph nodes. In- and opposed-phase sequences are key in this regard. These can be acquired independently or as part of pre-contrast T1W GRE with Dixon technique fat suppression.

Determining the amount of signal loss from in-to opposed-phase is best done by measuring the signal intensity index (SII), which can be obtained when evaluating co-registered dual echo acquired images. First, the reader should place a region of interest on the opposed phase image that includes the largest component of the lesion in question while excluding the peripheral India ink artifact related to chemical shift. Care should be used to avoid cystic, necrotic, or calcified components, which may require correlation with T2-weighted and post-contrast images (and are generally not seen in thymic hyperplasia). Then the same region of interest should be placed in the same location on the corresponding opposed-phase image. SII is then calculated as follows:

$$\text{SIIthy} = \left[(\text{tSIin} - \text{tSIop})/(\text{tSIin})\right] \times 100\%$$

SIIthy of greater than 20% is highly specific for benign thymic tissue as it indicates the presence of intravoxel lipid (Fig. 4.1). When SIIthy is greater than 20%, no further follow-up is indicated. Values between 10% and 20% almost always represent benign thymic tissue. In these cases, a follow-up examination at 6 to 12 months may be of value to confirm stability or regression. Values less than 10% should raise suspicion that the lesion may be a tumor or lymph node rather than benign thymic tissue. Based on the patient's other clinical factors, these can be resected or followed closely (Fig. 4.2).

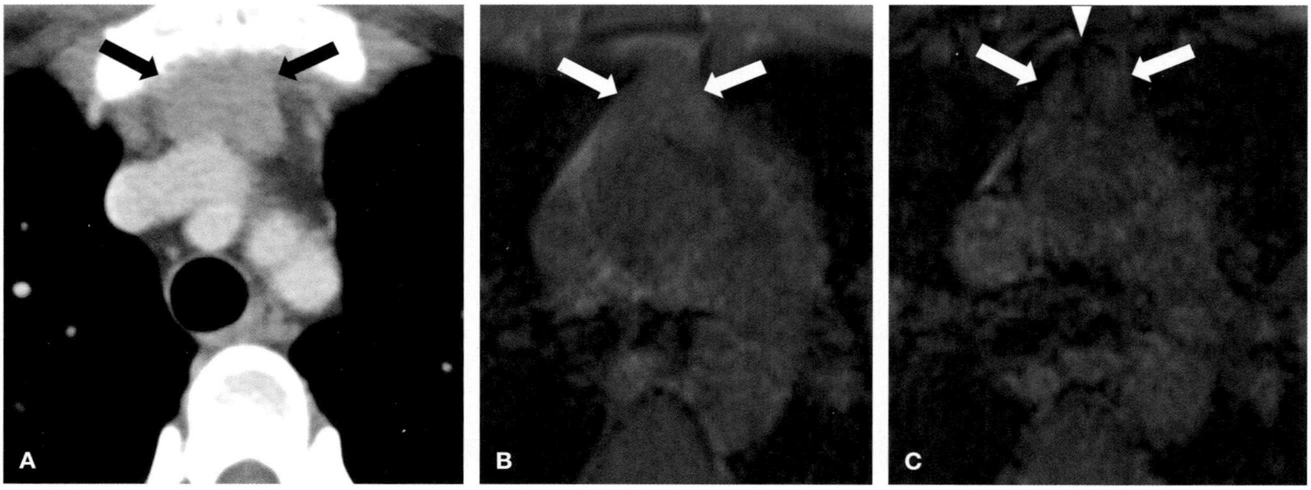

Figure 4.1. 19-year-old with myasthenia gravis. **A:** Axial CT image shows nodular anterior mediastinal soft tissue (*arrows*). Given lobular borders of the more nodular superior portion, the lesion was indeterminate for thymoma and MRI was recommended. **B:** Axial in-phase T1-weighted image shows the anterior mediastinal soft tissue (*arrows*). **C:** Axial opposed-phase T1-weighted image at the same level also shows the anterior mediastinal soft tissue (*arrows*) with surrounding India ink artifact as well as India ink along an internal cleft (*arrowhead*). While there was no definite qualitative loss of signal, measurements of the soft tissue on either side of the cleft demonstrated loss of signal greater than 20%, consistent with thymic hyperplasia.

There are several important pitfalls associated with the interpretation of MRI for the anterior mediastinal thymic tissue. Some patients, particularly young females in their third decade, may have an absence of intravoxel lipid but still have benign thymic tissue. In addition to this demographic information, the tissue in these patients with potential "non-suppressing" thymus may still be triangular in configuration. When this clinical scenario arises, follow-up at 6 to 12 months may be of value. Another pitfall is a thymic cyst, which will not demonstrate signal loss on in- and opposed-phase images. These benign lesions are identifiable based on comparison with other sequences as they will be hypertense on T2-weighted images and demonstrate no enhancement after intravenous contrast (Fig. 4.3). Similarly, anterior mediastinal blood products, which can be post-traumatic or spontaneous, will not demonstrate signal loss on in- and opposed-phase images but will be hyperintense on T1-weighted images and demonstrate no enhancement after intravenous contrast. Finally, it is possible for tumors to develop on a background of benign thymic hyperplasia. Focal areas without signal loss on in- and opposed-phase imaging that demonstrate enhancement should be regarded as suspicious and can be followed or resected.

Mediastinal Cysts

Potential mediastinal cysts are often indeterminate on CT, measuring greater than simple fluid and, therefore, overlapping in appearance with soft tissue lesions such as lymph nodes or masses (see Chapter 8). There are several reasons for this, including proteinaceous or hemorrhagic internal fluid and a lack of a pre-contrast CT phase to evaluate for areas of enhancement. In addition, enhancement, particularly when small in size or mild in degree, may be difficult to appreciate on CT. MRI, by virtue of its superior contrast resolution as well as the ability for pre- and post-contrast subtraction images, can provide a non-invasive assessment of indeterminate potentially cystic mediastinal lesions. This can be of important clinical benefit given that non-infected mediastinal cysts, whether thymic, foregut, or pleuropericardial, do not require surgical resection, whereas soft tissue lesions will require resection or tissue sampling.

Mediastinal cystic lesions are usually T2 hyperintense, although this can be variable as some cysts may have internal blood or proteinaceous contents. In addition to standard T2-weighted sequences, low b-value diffusion sequences can also be used to highlight increased T2 signal. Mediastinal cysts typically do not demonstrate diffusion restriction unless they are infected. Mediastinal cystic lesions are typically unilocular, although some cysts, particularly anterior mediastinal thymic cysts, may have thin septae. Lesions which have previously been infected or bled can also have internal septae and a thicker wall. T1-weighted signal intensity varies from intermediate to hyperintense, inversely related to T2-weighted signal intensity and similarly dependent on the proportion of internal blood products or protein.

Pre- and post-contrast T1-weighted images with subtraction are key in the evaluation of potential mediastinal cysts. To best evaluate for enhancement, the sequences used for this purpose should employ fat suppression, which will increase the conspicuity of enhancement against the background fat. It is also important to ensure that both the pre- and post-contrast acquisitions are obtained with the same parameters to allow for subtraction. When possible, anatomic coverage should be limited to the lesion in question to allow for the shortest scan time and best possible breath

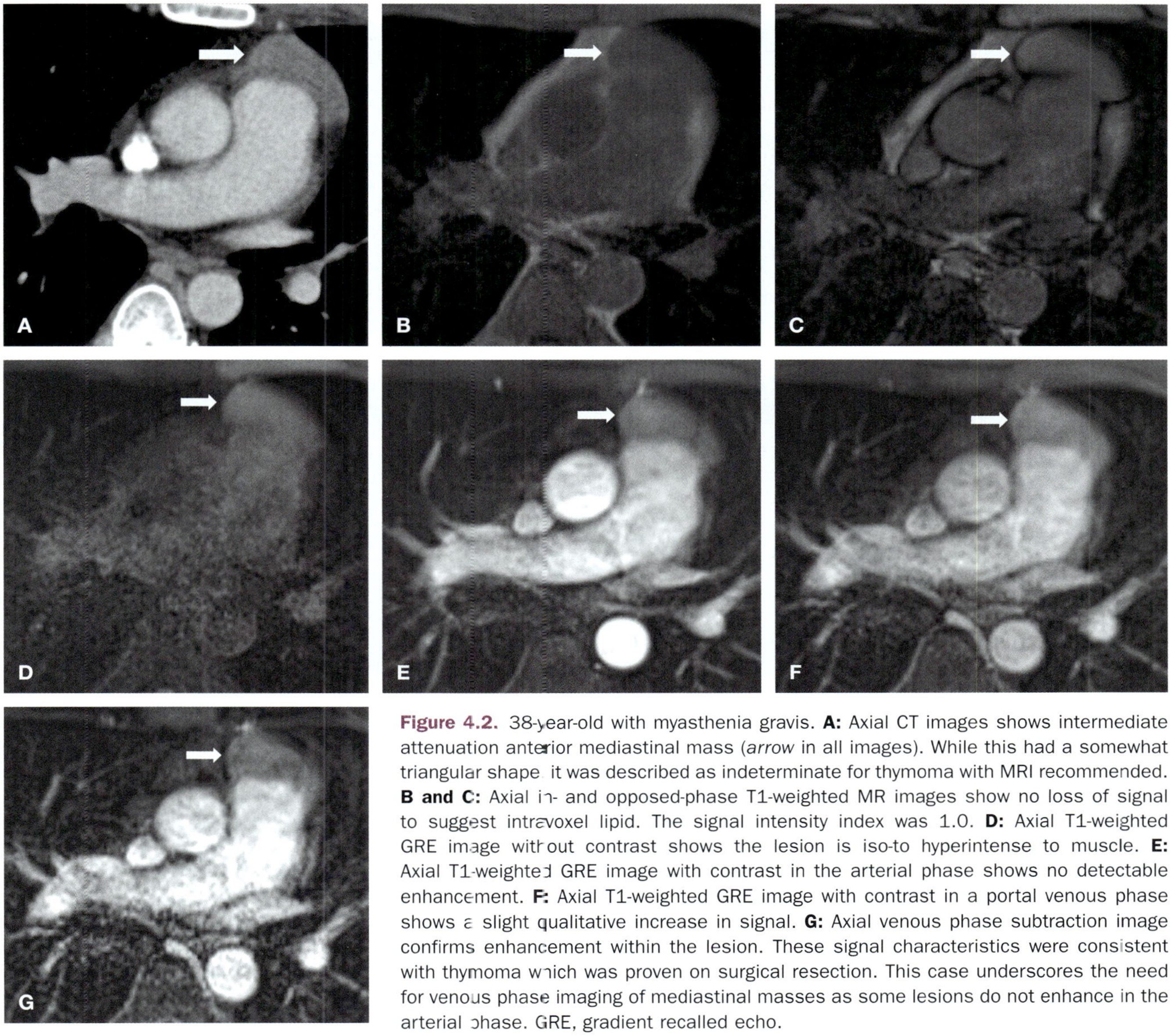

Figure 4.2. 38-year-old with myasthenia gravis. **A:** Axial CT images shows intermediate attenuation anterior mediastinal mass (*arrow* in all images). While this had a somewhat triangular shape it was described as indeterminate for thymoma with MRI recommended. **B and C:** Axial in- and opposed-phase T1-weighted MR images show no loss of signal to suggest intravoxel lipid. The signal intensity index was 1.0. **D:** Axial T1-weighted GRE image without contrast shows the lesion is iso-to hyperintense to muscle. **E:** Axial T1-weighted GRE image with contrast in the arterial phase shows no detectable enhancement. **F:** Axial T1-weighted GRE image with contrast in a portal venous phase shows a slight qualitative increase in signal. **G:** Axial venous phase subtraction image confirms enhancement within the lesion. These signal characteristics were consistent with thymoma which was proven on surgical resection. This case underscores the need for venous phase imaging of mediastinal masses as some lesions do not enhance in the arterial phase. GRE, gradient recalled echo.

hold. While a small amount of misregistration due to respiration motion is common, minimizing this will improve the ability to detect enhancement. Multiple post-contrast phases are also recommended, typically an arterial phase, several venous phases, and a delayed phase at 5 minutes. Some tumors, particularly thymic epithelial neoplasms, will not enhance or only weakly enhance in the arterial phase, thus venous phases are required. In addition, 5-minute delayed phases can be useful for identifying areas of fibrosis, which typically enhance progressively and slowly. Direct acquisitions in coronal and sagittal phases are also recommended for full lesion characterization.

Most mediastinal cysts have no detectable enhancement (Fig. 4.4). Detectable confluent, nodular, heterogeneous, septate, or thick peripheral enhancement typically indicates that a lesion is not a benign mediastinal cyst. These lesions should be biopsied, resected, or followed closely (Figs. 4.5 and 4.6). Thin or smooth peripheral enhancement may be equivocal as this has been reported in some benign mediastinal cystic lesions, particularly those that have had prior complications such as infection or hemorrhage. In these previously complicated mediastinal cysts, the thickened enhancing tissue will be fibrous in origin, and will typically slowly enhance on more delayed phases. The same principles used to evaluate mediastinal cysts can be used to evaluate for enhancement in other lesions, such as potential hematomas or thrombi, that are encountered on CT (Fig. 4.7).

Local Tumor Extent

MRI also has the potential to add important information regarding thoracic tumor extent. Utilization of MRI for this

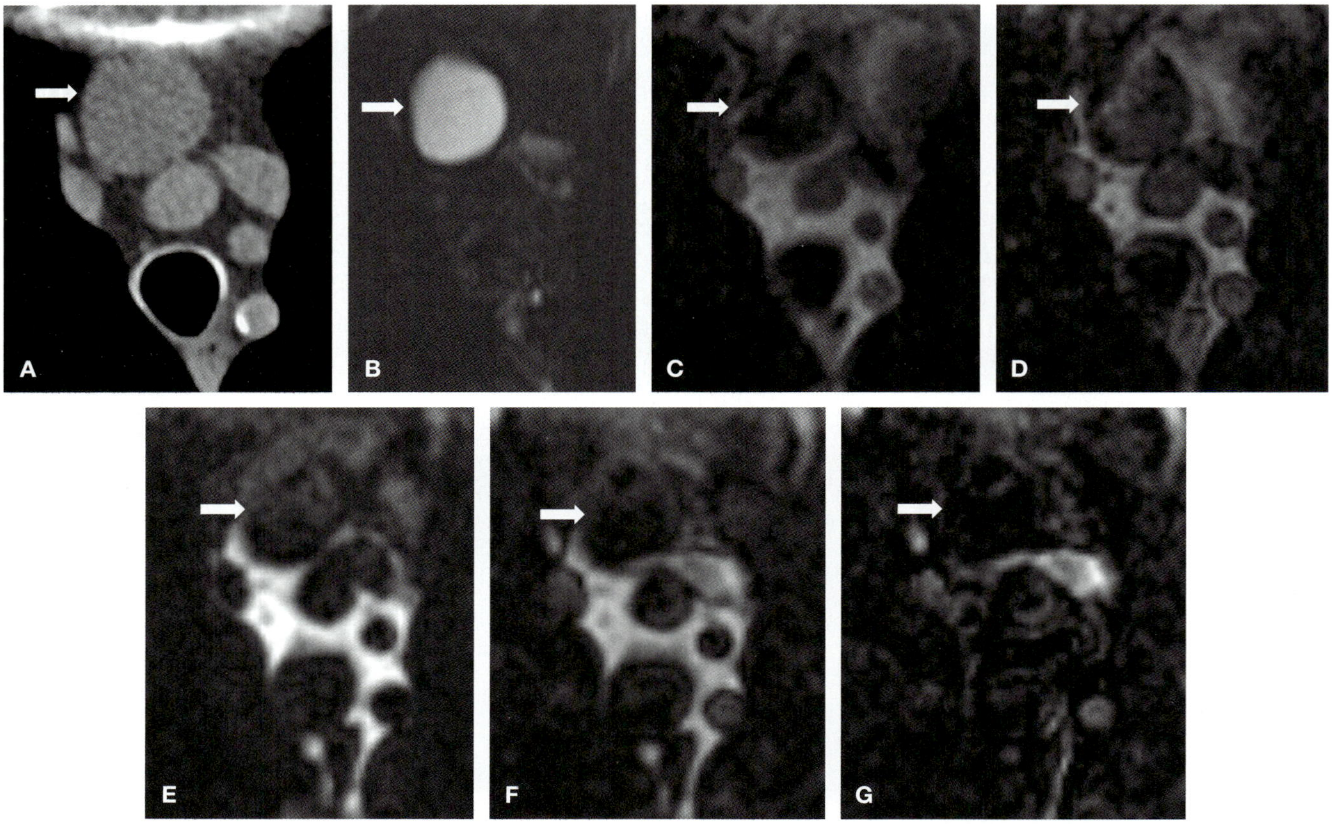

Figure 4.3. 64-year-old presenting for lung cancer screening. **A:** Axial CT image shows a round lesion (*arrows* in all images) measuring approximately 20 HU. This was described as indeterminate for a solid lesion and MRI was recommended. **B:** Axial STIR T2-weighted image shows the lesion is hyperintense, consistent with internal fluid. **C and D:** Axial in- and opposed-phase T1-weighted imaging shows no loss of signal to suggest intravoxel lipid. **E-G:** Axial GRE T1-weighted pre-contrast, portal venous phase post contrast, and portal venous phase subtraction images show no enhancement. Also of note is the failure of fat suppression in the mediastinum. This non-enhancing cystic lesion was consistent with a thymic cyst. GRE, gradient recalled echo; STIR, short tau inversion recovery.

purpose is usually focused on a specific question, but it is also used more routinely in tumors such as mesothelioma or those that involve the superior sulcus. MRI is complementary to CT in most regards, with its main advantage in evaluating tumor extent secondary to superior contrast resolution. This allows for better discrimination between lesions and normal structures (eg, chest wall musculature). Evaluation of invasion typically uses a multisequence approach and relies on evaluation of fat planes, encasement, or direct extension of a tumor into an adjacent structure. Background fat suppression is required, and when an invasion of a specific structure is questioned, multiple planes of their interface should be directly acquired (Fig. 4.8). MRI is of particular value in evaluating tumor within vessels, as tumor can be distinguished from bland thrombus based on the presence of enhancement.

In specific instances, real-time cine MRI, which is not ECG-gated, can be used to determine whether a tumor is adherent to another structure. In a real-time cine sequence, a single slice is repeatedly acquired while the patient breathes, allowing for visualization of the motion of structures. Balanced steady-state free precession sequences are ideal in this regard, as they can be acquired quickly. Typically, the lesion is imaged in multiple planes. If the lesion and adjacent structure slide against each other, they are not adherent, and invasion would be unlikely. If the lesion and adjacent structure move together, it can be assumed they are adherent (Fig. 4.9). Adherence does not definitely mean that the adjacent structure is invaded and additional sequences to determine direct anatomic invasion can be utilized. Ultimately, without evidence of direct anatomic invasion, some lesions may be considered suspicious and require direct surgical and pathologic interrogation for definitive assessment of local invasion.

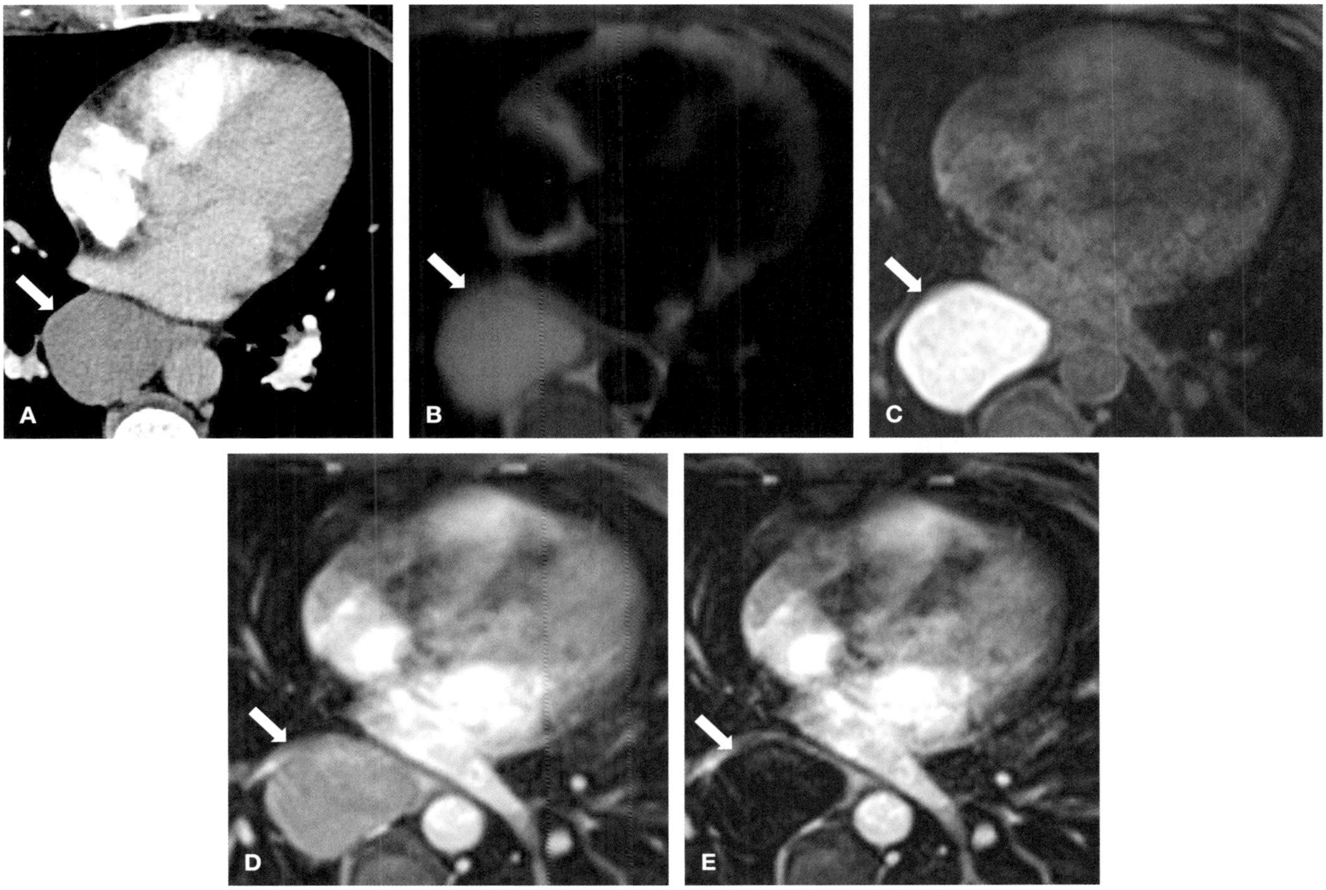

Figure 4.4. 38-year-old with chest pain. **A:** Axial CT image shows round lesion (*arrow* in all images) adjacent to the esophagus measuring 55 HU. MRI was recommended to evaluate for enhancement. **B:** Axial TSE T2-weighted image shows the lesion is T2 hyperintense, consistent with internal fluid. **C:** Axial GRE T1-weighted image without contrast demonstrates T1 hyperintensity, consistent with internal hemorrhage or proteinaceous debris. **D and E:** Axial GRE T1-weighted image with contrast and subsequent subtraction show no enhancement. The signal characteristics of this lesion were consistent with an esophageal duplication cyst. The findings were subsequently reinforced with endoscopy and biopsy. GRE, gradient recalled echo.

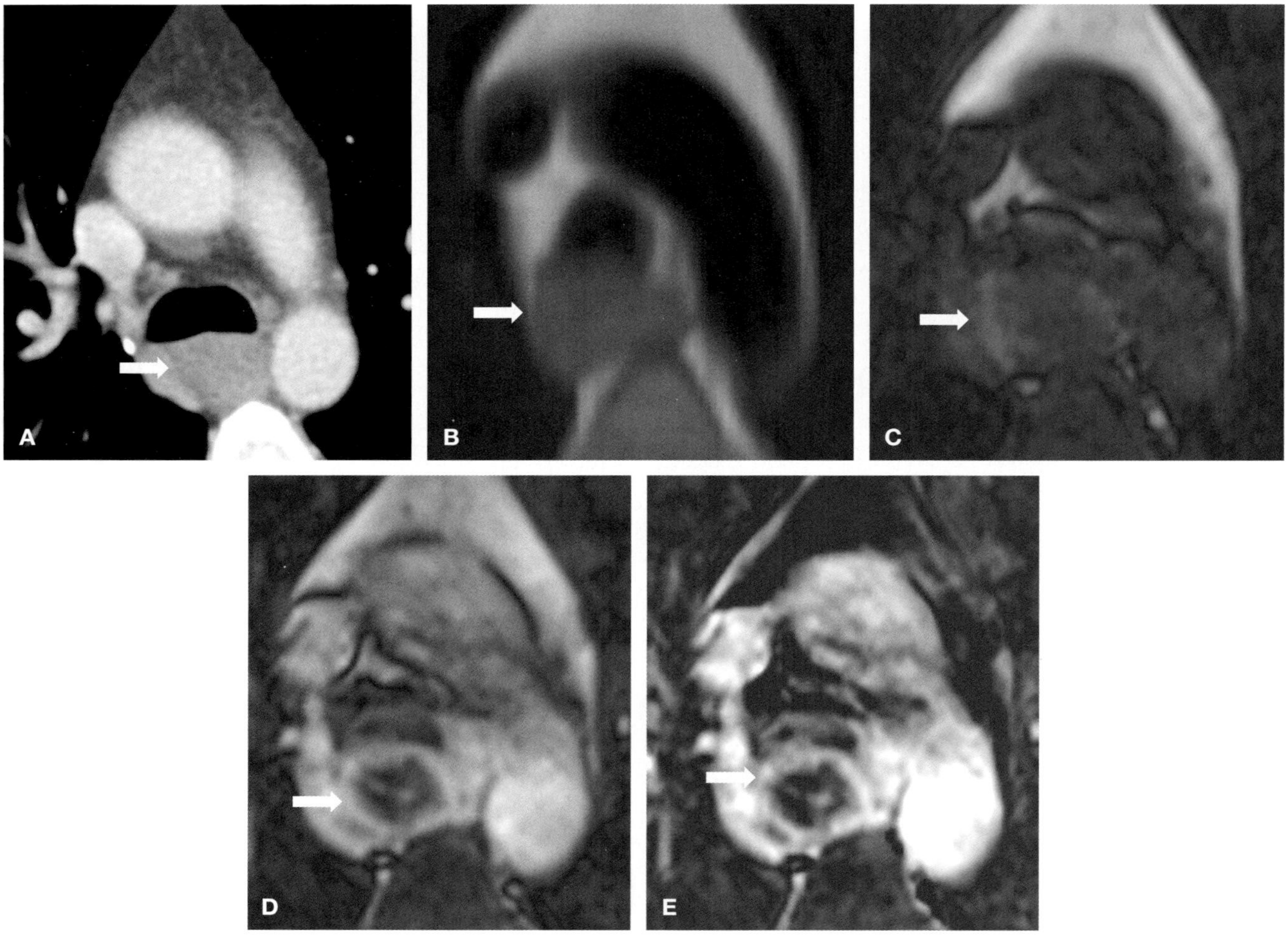

Figure 4.5. 40-year-old with brain mass undergoing evaluation for primary tumor. **A:** Axial CT image with contrast shows a mass measuring approximately 50 HU adjacent to the esophagus (*arrows* in all images). **B:** Axial TSE T2-weighted image shows the lesion is of intermediate signal that is mildly hyperintense to muscle. **C:** Axial GRE T1-weighted image without contrast shows the lesion is hypointense with some peripheral hyperintensity. **D and E:** Axial GRE T1-weighted image with contrast in venous phase with corresponding subtraction demonstrate the lesion has thick peripheral enhancement. A leiomyoma was favored, with a complicated duplication cyst felt to be less likely given the lack of symptoms. The diagnosis of leiomyoma was confirmed with biopsy. GRE, gradient recalled echo.

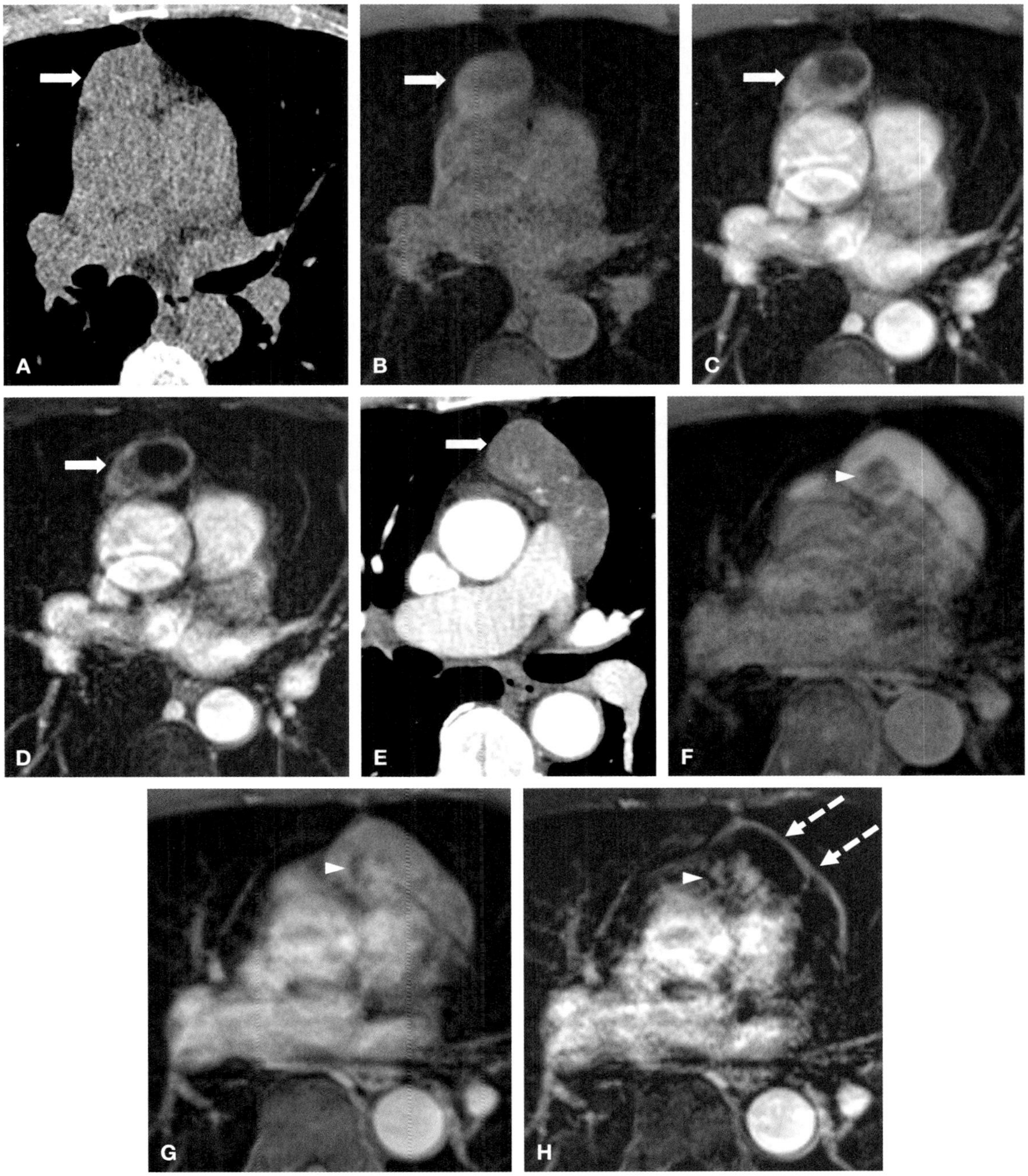

Figure 4.6. Concerning enhancement in two patients with anterior mediastinal cystic lesions. **A-D:** 58-year-old presenting for lung cancer screening. **A:** Axial non-contrast CT image shows an anterior mediastinal lesion (*arrow* in all images) that measures 23 HU. MRI was recommended for definitive characterization. **B-D:** Axial GRE T1-weighted precontrast, portal venous phase postcontrast, and portal venous phase subtraction images confirm the presence of a thick enhancing rim. The signal characteristics of this lesion were consistent with a thymoma. The lesion was resected and was confirmed to be a Type AB thymoma. **E-H:** 72-year-old who presented with cough. **E:** Axial CT image with contrast demonstrates an anterior mediastinal lesion (*arrow* in all images) with a few foci of internal calcium. The non-calcified portions of the lesion measured 25 to 30 HU. The lesion was described as indeterminate and MRI was recommended. **F:** Axial GRE T1-weighted pre-contrast image shows the lesion is predominantly hyperintense with a small nodular focus of decrease intensity (*arrowhead*). **G:** Axial GRE T1-weighted image with contrast in the venous phase shows the focal nodule (*arrowhead*) enhances while the rest of the lesion does not. **H:** Axial subtraction of the post-contrast venous phase further shows the enhancement to advantage (note also smooth misregistration on the left aspect of the lesion (dashed *arrows*)). The nodular enhancement demonstrated on MRI led to cystic thymoma being the favored diagnosis. This was proven at surgical resection as this was a Type A thymoma. GRE, gradient recalled echo.

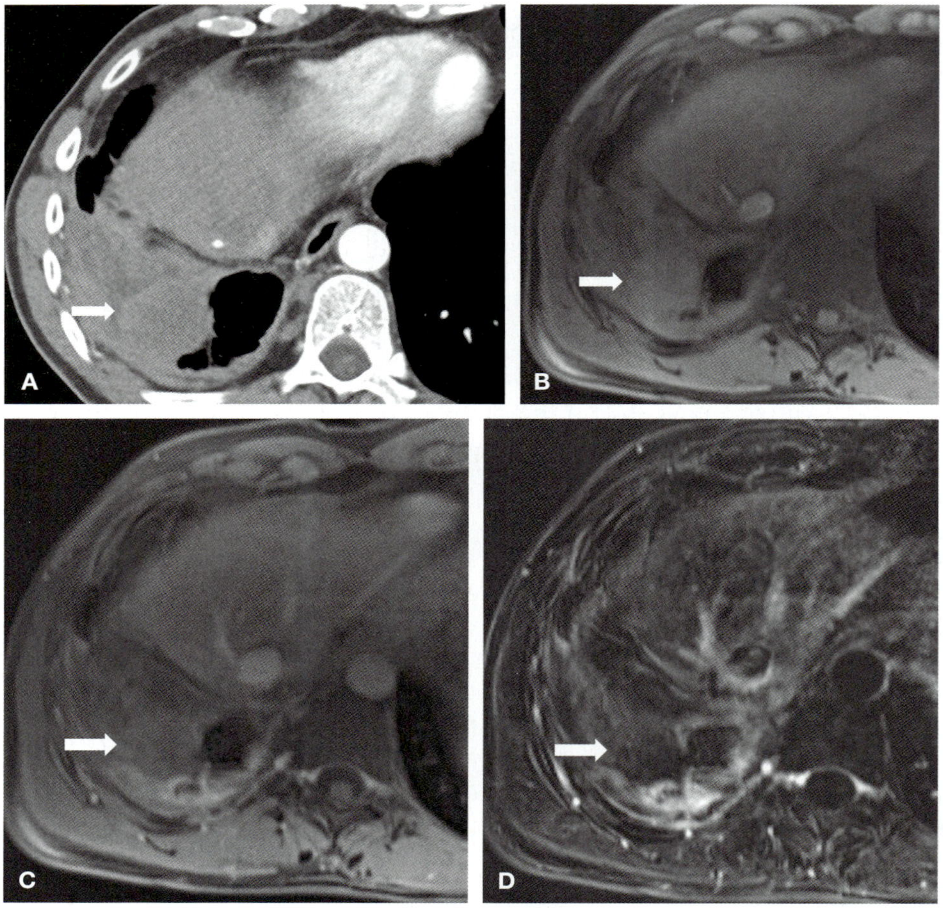

Figure 4.7. 36-year-old with fibrosing mediastinitis. **A:** Axial CT image with contrast showed a rounded area of opacification (*arrows* on all images) at the right lung base, surrounded by pleural thickening. Given the rounded shape, a malignancy was questioned. **B:** Axial GRE T1-weighted image without contrast shows the area of concern is mildly hyperintense. **C and D:** Axial GRE T1-weighted image with contrast in the venous phase with corresponding subtraction demonstrates no enhancement. Note is made of some indistinct increased intensity on the right aspect of the lesion on the subtraction due to misregistration. Given a lack of enhancement, the findings were not consistent with a tumor and the lesion was felt to be an organized hematoma or area of scarring. It was followed and has remained stable for several years. GRE, gradient recalled echo.

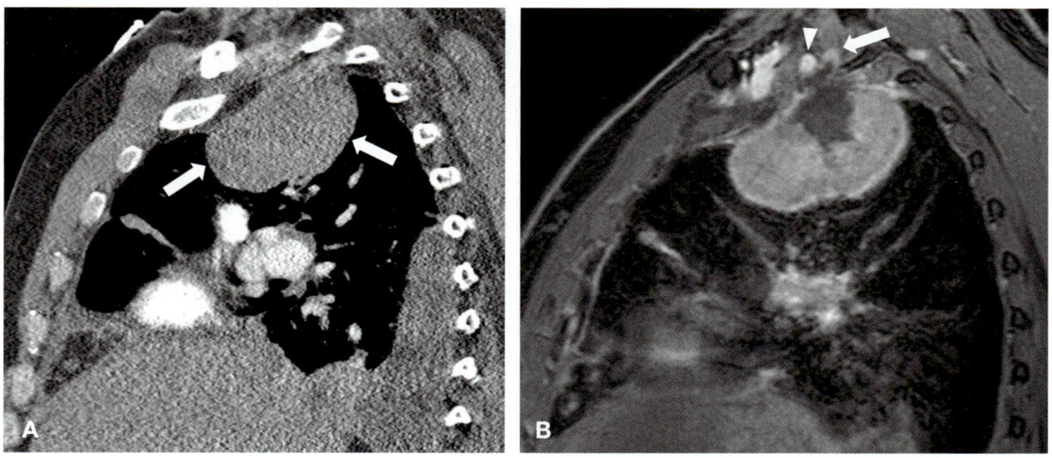

Figure 4.8. 61-year-old with newly diagnosed mesothelioma. **A:** Sagittal CT with contrast shows large mass in the left lung apex (*arrow*). It was difficult to determine whether there was extension in the chest wall on CT. **B:** Sagittal GRE T1-weighted image with contrast shows extension into the supraclavicular space with tumor (*arrow*) partially surrounding the subclavian artery (*arrowhead*). The superior contrast resolution of MRI is of benefit in evaluating local extent of tumors. GRE, gradient recalled echo.

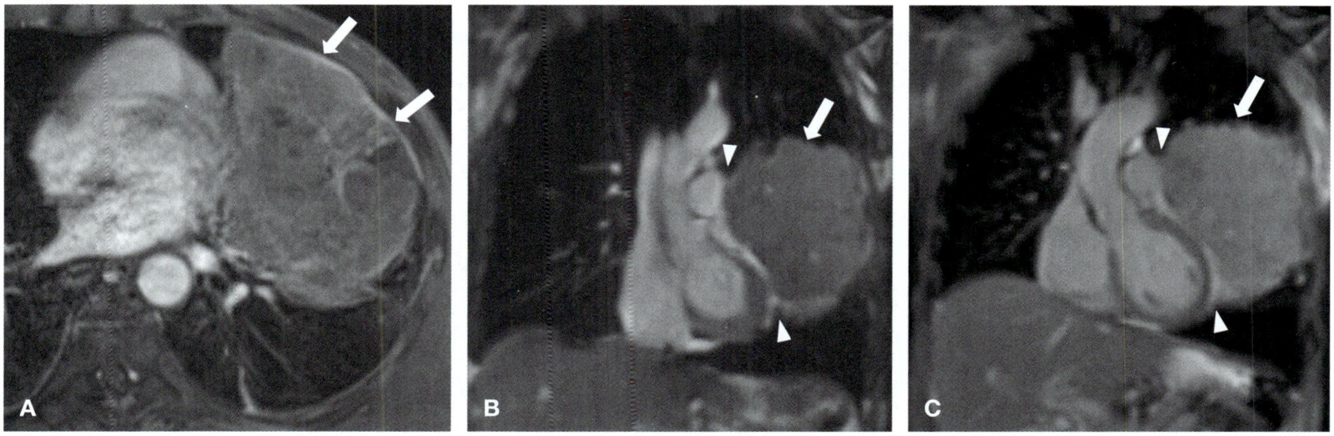

Figure 4.9. 59-year-old with newly diagnosed left upper lobe lung cancer. An MRI was ordered to evaluate for mediastinal invasion. **A:** Axial GRE T1-weighted image shows the large mass (*arrow*) occupying the lingula. There is abutment with segmental loss of the fat plane medially, suspicious for mediastinal pleural involvement. **B and C:** Balanced steady-state free precession free breathing real-time cine images in inspiration and expiration show the mass remains adherent to the mediastinal pleura with fixed relationships at the level of the pulmonary artery and left ventricle (*arrowheads*). GRE, gradient recalled echo.

CONCLUSION

It is important to remember that MRI has an important role as a problem-solving tool in non-cardiac, non-vascular pathologies in the thorax. To best utilize MRI in the thorax, radiologists should create efficient protocols that are focused on providing necessary information to answer clinical questions. While some of these questions, such as the evaluation of anterior mediastinal thymic tissue, recur in clinical practice, many others are specific to a particular patient. These questions may arise while a radiologist is reading another study, typically a CT, or during direct physician consultation on an individual basis or at a tumor board. By recommending and then utilizing thoracic MRI to answer these questions, radiologists can take advantage of this valuable imaging technique, increase its use, and effectively contribute to patient care.

SUGGESTED READINGS

Ackman JB, Gaissert HA, Lanuti M, et al. Impact of nonvascular thoracic MR imaging on the clinical decision making of thoracic surgeons: a 2-year prospective study. *Radiology*. 2016;280(2):464-474.

Ackman JB, Kovacina B, Carter BW, et al. Sex difference in normal thymic appearance in adults 20-30 Years of age. *Radiology*. 2013;268(1):245-253.

Ackman JB, Mino-Kenudson M, Morse CR. Nonsuppressing normal thymus on chemical shift magnetic resonance imaging in a young woman. *J Thorac Imaging*. 2012;27(6):W196-W198.

Ackman JB, Verzosa S, Kovach AE, et al. High rate of unnecessary thymectomy and its cause. Can computed tomography distinguish thymoma, lymphoma, thymic hyperplasia, and thymic cysts? *Eur J Radiol*. 2015;84(3):524-533.

Ackman JB, Wu CC. MRI of the thymus. *Am J Roentgenol*. 2011;197(1):W15-W20.

Ackman JB. MR imaging of mediastinal masses. *Magn Reson Imaging Clin N Am*. 2015;23(2):141-164.

Akata S, Kajiwara N, Park J, et al. Evaluation of chest wall invasion by lung cancer using respiratory dynamic MRI. *J Med Imaging Radiat Oncol*. 2008;52(1):36-39.

Albrecht MH, Varga-Szemes A, Schoepf UJ, et al. Coronary artery assessment using self-navigated free-breathing radial whole-heart magnetic resonance angiography in patients with congenital heart disease. *Eur Radiol*. 2018;28(3):1267-1275.

Biederer J, Hintze C, Fabel M. MRI of pulmonary nodules: technique and diagnostic value. *Cancer Imaging*. 2008;8(1):125-130.

Bilbey JH, McLoughlin RF, Kurkjian PS, et al. MR imaging of adrenal masses: value of chemical-shift imaging for distinguishing adenomas from other tumors. *Am J Roentgenol*. 1995;164(3):637-642.

Bluemke DA, Boxerman JL, Atalar E, McVeigh ER. Segmented K-space cine breath-hold cardiovascular MR imaging: Part 1. Principles and technique. *Am J Roentgenol*. 1997;169(2):395-400.

Boiselle PM, Biederer J, Gefter WB, Lee EY. Expert opinion: why is MRI still an under-utilized modality for evaluating thoracic disorders?. *J Thorac Imaging*. 2013;28(3):137.

Chandarana H, Heacock L, Rakheja R, et al. Pulmonary nodules in patients with primary malignancy: comparison of hybrid PET/MR and PET/CT imaging. *Radiology*. 2013;268(3):874-881.

Chavhan GB, Babyn PS, Jankharia BG, Cheng H-LM, Shroff MM. Steady-state MR imaging sequences: physics, classification, and clinical applications. *RadioGraphics*. 2008;28(4):1147-1160.

Ehman RL, Felmlee JP. Adaptive technique for high-definition MR imaging of moving structures. *Radiology*. 1989;173(1):255-263.

Francis I, Glazer G, Bookstein F, Gross B. The thymus: reexamination of age-related changes in size and shape. *Am J Roentgenol*. 1985;145(2):249-254.

Ginat DT, Fong MW, Tuttle DJ, Hobbs SK, Vyas RC. Cardiac imaging: part 1, MR pulse sequences, imaging planes, and basic anatomy. *Am J Roentgenol*. 2011;197(4):808-815.

Hammer MM, Barile M, Bryson W, Bhalla S, Raptis CA. Errors in interpretation of magnetic resonance imaging for thymic lesions. *J Thorac Imaging*. 2019;34(6):351-355.

Inaoka T, Takahashi K, Mineta M, et al. Thymic hyperplasia and thymus gland tumors: differentiation with chemical shift MR imaging. *Radiology*. 2007;243(3):869-876.

Koyama H, Ohno Y, Seki S, et al. Magnetic resonance imaging for lung cancer. *J Thorac Imaging*. 2013;28(3):138-150.

Lee CH, Goo JM, Kim YT, et al. The clinical feasibility of using non-breath-hold real-time MR-echo imaging for the evaluation of mediastinal and chest wall tumor invasion. *Korean J Radiol*. 2010;11(1):37-45.

Liu M, Luo C, Wang Y, et al. Multiparametric MRI in differentiating pulmonary artery sarcoma and pulmonary thromboembolism: a preliminary experience. *Diagn Interv Radiol*. 2017;23(1):15-21.

McAdams HP, Kirejczyk WM, Rosado-de- Christenson ML, Matsumoto S. Bronchogenic cyst: imaging features with clinical and histopathologic correlation. *Radiology*. 2000;217(2):441-446.

McConnell MV, Khasgiwala VC, Savord BJ, et al. Comparison of respiratory suppression methods and navigator locations for MR coronary angiography. *Am J Roentgenol*. 1997;168(5):1369-1375.

McInnis MC, Flores EJ, Shepard J-AO, Ackman JB. Pitfalls in the imaging and interpretation of benign thymic lesions: how thymic MRI can help. *Am J Roentgenol*. 2016;206(1):W1-W8.

Meier-Schroers M, Homsi R, Schild HH, Thomas D. Lung cancer screening with MRI: characterization of nodules with different non-enhanced MRI sequences. *Acta Radiol.* 2019;60(2):168-176.

Mendelson DS, Rose JS, Efremidis SC, Kirschner PA, Cohen BA. Bronchogenic cysts with high CT numbers. *AJR Am J Roentgenol.* 1983;140(3):463-465.

Murayama S, Murakami J, Watanabe H, et al. Signal intensity characteristics of mediastinal cystic masses on T1-weighted MRI. *J Comput Assist Tomogr.* 1995;19(2):188-191.

Nickell LT, Lichtenberger JP, Khorashadi L, Abbott GF, Carter BW. Multimodality imaging for characterization, classification, and staging of malignant pleural mesothelioma. *RadioGraphics.* 2014;34(6):1692-1706.

Oechsner M, Pracht ED, Staeb D, et al. Lung imaging under free-breathing conditions. *Magn Reson Med.* 2009;61(3):723-727.

Ohno Y, Kauczor H-U, Hatabu H, Seo JB, van Beek EJR, International Workshop for Pulmonary Functional Imaging IWPFI. MRI for solitary pulmonary nodule and mass assessment: current state of the art. *J Magn Reson Imaging.* 2018;47(6):1437-1458.

Priola AM, Priola SM, Ciccone G, et al. Differentiation of rebound and lymphoid thymic hyperplasia from anterior mediastinal tumors with dual-echo chemical-shift MR imaging in adulthood: reliability of the chemical-shift ratio and signal intensity index. *Radiology.* 2015;274(1):238-249.

Puderbach M, Hintze C, Ley S, Eichinger M, Kauczor H-U, Biederer J. MR imaging of the chest: a practical approach at 1.5 T. *Eur J Radiol.* 2007;64(3):345-355.

Rajaram S, Swift AJ, Capener D, et al. Lung morphology assessment with balanced steady-state free precession MR imaging compared with CT. *Radiology.* 2012;263(2):569-577.

Raptis CA, Ludwig DR, Hammer MM, et al. Building blocks for thoracic MRI: challenges, sequences, and protocol design. *J Magn Reson Imaging.* 2019;50(3):682-701.

Raptis CA, McWilliams SR, Ratkowski KL, Broncano J, Green DB, Bhalla S. Mediastinal and pleural MR imaging: practical approach for daily practice. *RadioGraphics.* 2018;38(1):37-55.

Scheffler K, Lehnhardt S. Principles and applications of balanced SSFP techniques. *Eur Radiol.* 2003;13(11):2409-2418.

Scott AD, Keegan J, Firmin DN. Motion in cardiovascular MR imaging. *Radiology.* 2009;250(2):331-351.

Seo JM, Park BK, Park SY, Kim CK. Characterization of lipid-poor adrenal adenoma: chemical-shift MRI and washout CT. *Am J Roentgenol.* 2014;202(5):1043-1050.

Simanovsky N, Hiller N, Loubashevsky N, Rozovsky K. Normal CT characteristics of the thymus in adults. *Eur J Radiol.* 2012;81(11):3581-3586.

Stamatis G. Staging of lung cancer: the role of noninvasive, minimally invasive and invasive techniques. *Eur Respir J.* 2015;46(2):521-531.

Ueda K, Yanagawa M, Ueguchi T, et al. Paradoxical signal pattern of mediastinal cysts on T2-weighted MR imaging: phantom and clinical study. *Eur J Radiol.* 2014;83(6):1016-1021.

Wild JM, Marshall H, Bock M, et al. MRI of the lung (1/3): methods. *Insights Imaging.* 2012;3(4):345-353.

Woodard PK, Li D. *Free-Breathing (Navigator) Coronary MRA: How Do I Do it? Coron Magn Reson Angiogr.* Springer; 2002.

Yi CA, Lee KS, Choe YH, Han D, Kwon OJ, Kim S. Computed tomography in pulmonary artery sarcoma: distinguishing features from pulmonary embolic disease. *J Comput Assist Tomogr.* 2004;28(1):34-39.

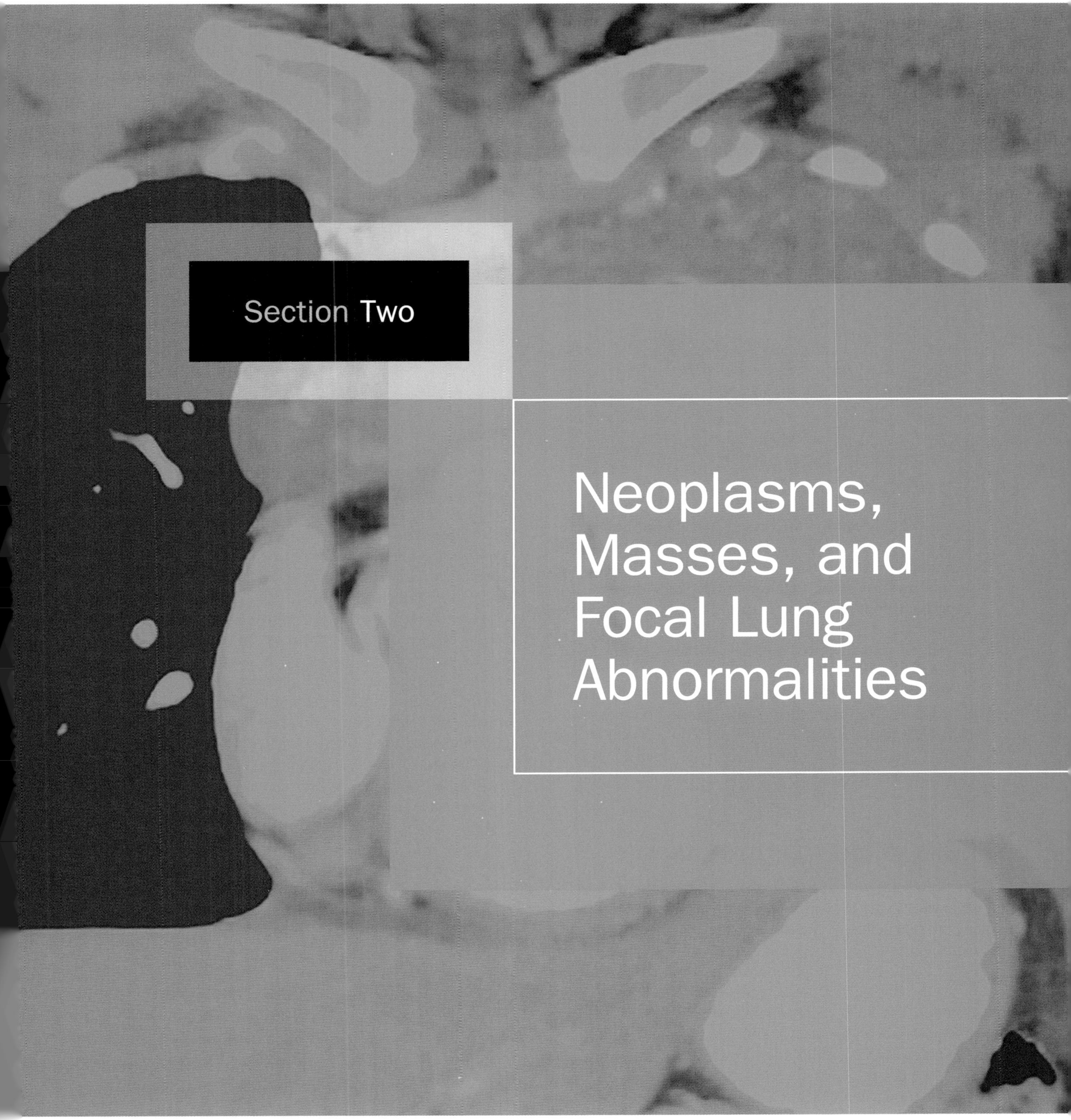

Section Two

Neoplasms, Masses, and Focal Lung Abnormalities

Chapter 5

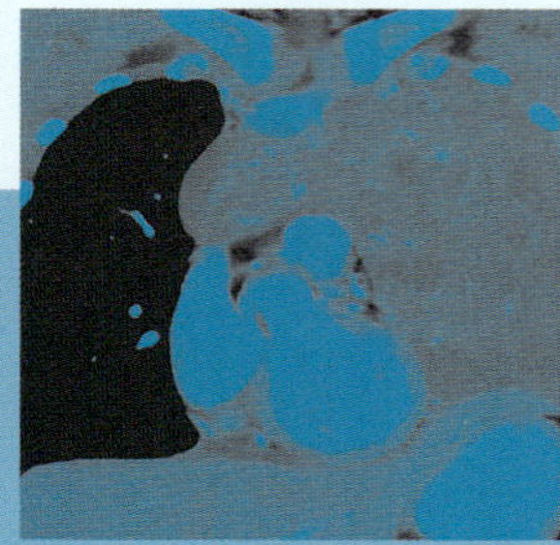

Travis S. Henry

Lung Cancer and Bronchopulmonary Neoplasms

INTRODUCTION

Lung cancer is the most common fatal malignancy in both male and female patients and accounts for about 25% of all cancer-related deaths in the United States. It is estimated that more than 225,000 cases of lung cancer are still diagnosed annually, with at least 125,000 deaths per year. Lung cancer survival has improved in recent years likely due to earlier diagnosis with lung cancer screening and targeted therapies. 5-year survival rates are greater than 90% for stage IA disease but still poor for advanced disease (less than 10% for stage IV disease based on 8th TNM-staging system data).

The number of lung cancers diagnosed yearly is likely to increase as CT screening for lung cancer becomes widely available and more cancers are detected, but with a lesser decrease in lung cancer deaths as some small or indolent cancers detected by CT screening would not have resulted in the patient's death.

RISK FACTORS FOR LUNG CANCER

Tobacco smoking accounts for 80% to 90% of lung cancers. In smokers, the risk of lung cancer correlates with younger age at the onset of smoking, the duration and cumulative amount of exposure, and the depth of inhalation. Heavy smoking is associated with a 20- to 30-fold increase in lung cancer risk compared to nonsmokers. A decrease in risk following smoking cessation has been demonstrated. Well-differentiated squamous cell carcinoma (SCC), small cell carcinoma, large cell carcinoma (LCC), and to a lesser extent adenocarcinoma all demonstrate an increased incidence with increasing cigarette consumption. About 25% of lung cancers in nonsmokers have been attributed to secondhand smoke.

Increasing age is associated with an increased risk of lung cancer. Lung cancers are rare in patients below the age of 30.

Occupational exposures to various substances have been linked to lung cancer; as many as 10% of lung cancer cases may be due to occupational exposure. Agents associated with occupational lung cancer include arsenic, nickel, chromium, asbestos, beryllium, cadmium, chromium, mustard gas, pesticides, and radon or uranium.

Asbestos exposure is the best-recognized occupational risk for lung cancer and is the most frequent exposure in the general population (Figure 5.1). A dose–response relationship between the severity and duration of asbestos exposure and the likelihood of developing lung cancer is well established, although the risk of exposure depends not only on the amount of asbestos to which one is exposed but also the fiber type (increased risk with amphibole fibers), the industrial use of asbestos, the conditions of exposure, and the presence of asbestosis. The risk of lung cancer in a heavily exposed asbestos worker is about five times that of a nonexposed subject. Also, smoking is a synergistic risk in asbestos-exposed subjects: the risk of lung cancer in an asbestos worker who is a heavy smoker is about 20 times that of a nonsmoking asbestos worker and 100 times that of a nonexposed nonsmoker (Table 5.1).

Pulmonary fibrosis has been associated with a 10-fold increase in the risk of lung cancer. In addition, patients with focal lung scarring, particularly as a result of tuberculosis, can develop a carcinoma in association with areas of fibrosis or scarring. Although this is infrequent, cases of carcinoma arising in areas of focal scarring, so-called scar carcinoma, are encountered in clinical practice.

Chronic obstructive lung disease (chronic bronchitis and emphysema) is a risk factor for developing lung

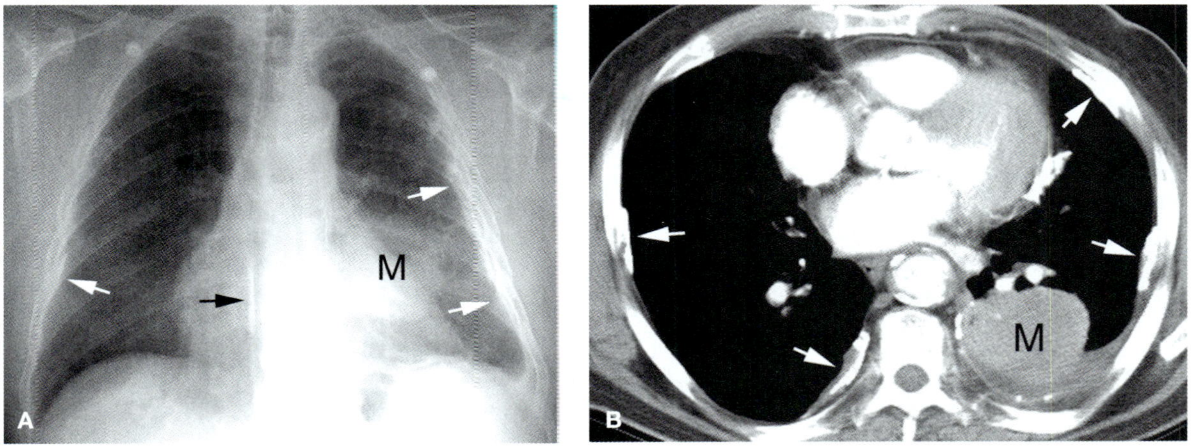

Figure 5.1. Lung cancer associated with asbestos exposure. **A:** Chest radiograph shows a large left lung mass (*M*) representing lung cancer. Bilateral pleural thickening with calcification is also visible (*arrows*). **B:** CT shows a left lung mass (*M*) and bilateral localized calcified pleural plaques (*arrows*) typical of asbestos exposure.

cancer, independent of cigarette smoking. In both chronic obstructive pulmonary disease (COPD) and diffuse pulmonary fibrosis, proposed mechanisms of increased cancer risk include decreased clearance of inhaled carcinogens and epithelial metaplasia. In a recent study, patients with emphysema who had incidental nodules detected on CT were found to have a higher likelihood of cancer than did patients without emphysema.

Genetic predisposition plays a role in the development of lung cancer. In general, relatives of subjects with lung cancer have a higher risk of developing lung cancer (about twofold) than does the general population. An increased risk of lung cancer has been associated with chromosome defects, numerous oncogenes and driver mutations (most commonly EGFR, ALK, KRAS, with an ever growing list of less common mutations), specific HLA antigens, enzyme defects, and defects in proteins normally produced by tumor suppressor genes.

LUNG CANCER SCREENING

In the 1980s and early 1990s, efforts to develop lung cancer screening were focused primarily on chest X-rays and sputum cytology. However, these methods proved to be ineffective in reducing mortality from lung cancer. During the late 1990s, CT technology advanced significantly, and early studies started to indicate that low-dose computed tomography (LDCT) could detect smaller nodules in the lungs than traditional X-rays, suggesting a potential for earlier detection of lung cancer.

The early 2000s saw an increase in research and pilot studies examining the effectiveness of LDCT in lung cancer screening. However, it was the publication of the National Lung Screening Trial (NLST) results in 2011 that marked a turning point. The NLST, conducted in the United States, enrolled over 53,000 participants aged between 55 and 74 years who had at least a 30-pack-year smoking history. The study aimed to compare the effectiveness of LDCT versus standard chest X-rays in reducing lung cancer mortality. After a median follow-up of 6.5 years, the trial found that LDCT screening led to a 20% reduction in lung cancer mortality compared to chest X-ray. This result was groundbreaking and supported the implementation of LDCT as a screening tool for lung cancer. However, the study also reported a high rate of false positives with LDCT.

Following the NLST results, in 2013, the U.S. Preventive Services Task Force (USPSTF) recommended annual screening for lung cancer with LDCT in adults aged 55 to 80 years who have a 30 pack-year smoking history and currently smoke or have quit within the past 15 years. This was a major milestone as it led to the wider adoption of LDCT screening in clinical practice. In 2015, the Centers for Medicare & Medicaid Services (CMS) decided to cover LDCT lung cancer screening for individuals who met the criteria similar to those recommended by the USPSTF. This coverage decision further facilitated access to LDCT screening for a large segment of the high-risk population in the United States.

As more evidence accumulated (such as the NELSON trial in the Netherlands and Belgium), in 2022, the USPSTF updated its recommendations by lowering the age of initiation for LDCT screening from 55 to 50 years and reducing

Table 5.1 Increased Risk of Lung Cancer Associated With Smoking and Asbestos Exposure

Risk Factor	Comparison Group	Relative Risk
Heavy asbestos exposure	No asbestos exposure	5:1
Heavy smoking	Nonsmoker	20:1
Heavy smoking and heavy asbestos exposure	No smoking history and no asbestos exposure	100:1

the smoking history threshold from 30 pack-years to 20 pack-years. This update aimed to expand eligibility and enhance the early detection of lung cancer among high-risk individuals. Unfortunately, screening rates remain low in the United States with less than 10% of eligible patients receiving LDCT.

Lung-RADS is the standardized system developed by the American College of Radiology (ACR) for reporting of LDCT findings and recommendations. The Lung-RADS system was most recently updated in November 2022 and is freely available on the ACR website (see Chapter 10 for more discussion of Lung-RADS).

CLASSIFICATION OF LUNG CANCER AND LUNG TUMORS

In 2021, the World Health Organization (WHO) published a revised classification of lung tumors (Table 5.2), which provides some modifications to the prior (2015) classification. The WHO classification represents a multidisciplinary effort involving pathologists, radiologists, clinicians, molecular biologists, and surgeons. Treatment algorithms for lung cancer are increasingly complex, but a basic understanding is helpful for radiologists.

Primary tumor classification is still based on morphology (eg, squamous cell carcinoma, adenocarcinoma, and small cell carcinoma), which is usually supported by immunohistochemical analysis. A simple designation of "non-small cell carcinoma" is no longer sufficient as therapies are increasingly targeted to not only the histologic subtype but also the presence of driver mutations.

Table 5.2 WHO Classification of Lung Tumors

WHO Classification of Lung Tumors
Epithelial Tumors
Precursor glandular lesions
Atypical adenomatous hyperplasia (AAH)
Adenocarcinoma in situ (AIS)
Adenocarcinoma
Minimally invasive adenocarcinoma (MIA)
Invasive nonmucinous adenocarcinoma (predominant pattern)
Lepidic (predominant) adenocarcinoma (LPA)
Other subtypes (acinar, papillary, micropapillary, solid, etc.)
Invasive mucinous adenocarcinoma (IMA)
Squamous cell carcinoma
Squamous precursor lesions
Squamous cell carcinoma in situ
Squamous cell carcinoma (keratinizing, nonkeratinizing, and basaloid subtypes)
LUNG NEUROENDOCRINE CARCINOMAS
Small cell carcinoma
Large cell neuroendocrine carcinoma
Carcinoid tumors
Typical carcinoid tumor
Atypical carcinoid tumor
Precursor lesion
Diffuse idiopathic pulmonary neuroendocrine cell hyperplasia (DIPNECH)
Large cell carcinoma
Adenosquamous carcinoma
Sarcomatoid carcinomas (multiple cell types)
Salivary gland-type tumors
Mucoepidermoid carcinoma
Adenoid cystic carcinoma (cylindroma)
Less common cell types
Papillomas (squamous, glandular, and mixed)
Adenomas (various cell types)
MESENCHYMAL TUMORS
Pulmonary hamartoma
Chondroma
PEComatous tumors
Lymphangioleiomyomatosis (LAM)
PEComas, benign, and malignant
Diffuse pulmonary lymphangiomatosis
Inflammatory myofibroblastic tumor
Epithelioid hemangioendothelioma
Pulmonary artery intimal sarcoma
Multiple other cell types, similar to soft tissue tumors
HEMATOLYMPHOID TUMORS
Extranodal marginal zone lymphomas of mucosa-associated lymphoid tissue (MALT lymphoma)
Diffuse large B-cell lymphoma
Lymphomatoid granulomatosis
Intravascular large B-cell lymphoma
Pulmonary Langerhans cell histiocytosis and Erdheim–Chester disease
TUMORS OF ECTOPIC ORIGIN
Melanoma
Meningioma
METASTATIC TUMORS

Modified from Nicholson AG, Tsao MS, Beasley MB, et al. The 2021 WHO classification of lung tumors: impact of advances since 2015. J Thorac Oncol. *2022;17(3):362-387. https://doi.org/10.1016/j.jtho.2021.11.003*

Driver mutations can be identified by genotyping, and targeted therapies exist for many specific mutations including epidermal growth factor receptor (EGFR), anaplastic lymphoma kinase (ALK), c-ROS oncogene 1 (*ROS1*), rearranged during transfection gene (*RET*), and others. Some groups have reported detecting mutations in up to 60% of adenocarcinomas, and these numbers are certain to increase as therapy becomes more personalized.

In patients without driver mutations, the expression of programmed cell death ligand 1 (PD-L1) is used to determine whether patients may benefit from checkpoint therapy (immunotherapy) as a single agent or in combination with chemotherapy.

The WHO classification of lung tumors reviews more than 100 types and subtypes of tumors (Table 5.2). In this chapter, only the most common lung tumors and those with specific imaging appearances are reviewed. Reference to the WHO classification, published in book form in 2021, is recommended for those with an interest in this topic. This publication is authoritative, comprehensive, and beautifully illustrated and referenced.

ADENOCARCINOMA

Adenocarcinoma is a malignant epithelial lung tumor characterized by glandular differentiation, pneumocyte marker expression, or mucin production. Adenocarcinoma is the most common cell type of lung cancer, accounting for 40% to 50% of lung cancer cases in the United States (Table 5.3). Its association with smoking is relatively weak, at least when compared to SCC or small cell carcinoma, but nonetheless, an association with smoking exists in recent studies, perhaps related to recent changes in the chemical composition of cigarettes. Adenocarcinoma is thought to arise from bronchiolar or alveolar epithelium and is often characterized by glandular differentiation. Invasion of lung parenchyma is often present. Early metastasis is more common than with SCC, particularly to the central nervous system and adrenal glands.

Multiple genetic abnormalities have been found in adenocarcinoma, and the ever-expanding list of mutations for which specific agents have been approved include EGFR, ALK, KRAS, ROS1, MET, HER2, and NTRK with many others in clinical trials.

Seventy-five percent of adenocarcinomas originate in the lung periphery, presenting as a solitary pulmonary nodule. Adenocarcinoma is most common in the upper lobes. In a few percent of cases, adenocarcinoma originates within a large central airway. Adenocarcinoma may be associated with lung fibrosis (ie, a scar carcinoma or in association with other causes of pulmonary fibrosis) or may result in a desmoplastic fibrotic reaction in the surrounding lung.

Adenocarcinomas often appear as an ill-defined nodule on chest radiographs (see Fig. 5.2A). On thin-slice CT, adenocarcinoma most often appears as a nodule of soft tissue attenuation (*solid*) (Fig. 5.2B), but a nodule of ground-glass opacity (GGO) with some solid components (*subsolid or part solid*) (Fig. 5.3A), a cystic nodule, or a nodule entirely of GGO (*nonsolid*) (Fig. 5.3B) may be seen.

In patients with adenocarcinoma, the presence of GGO on CT results from *lepidic growth*, with tumor spreading as a thin layer of cells using alveolar walls as a framework or scaffold (Fig. 5.3C). Adenocarcinomas appearing as a solid nodule on CT are usually invasive and destroy lung parenchyma as they grow, a pattern termed *hilic* (an uncommonly used term) (Fig. 5.2B). In some cases, they may appear cystic or multicystic, mimicking a benign lesion (Fig. 5.4). Cystic adenocarcinoma may be associated with solid or GGO regions.

On CT, adenocarcinoma appearing as a solid nodule may appear round or lobulated and frequently has an irregular and spiculated margin because of associated lung fibrosis (see Fig. 5.2B). When occurrig in a subpleural location, spiculation may result in pleural retraction with thin linear extensions to the pleural surface (ie, a *pleural tail*; see Fig. 5.2B). Air bronchograms may be visible within adenocarcinoma. Although central necrosis is common histologically, cavitation visible on radiographs or CT is uncommon.

When adenocarcinoma arises from the wall of a central bronchus, it is radiographically indistinguishable from SCC. Of note, some specific CT features in adenocarcinoma have been associated with EGFR (air bronchograms, pleural tail), ALK, or KRAS mutations.

In the 2021 WHO classification, adenocarcinomas are categorized as *precursor glandular lesions*, *minimally invasive*, and *invasive* (Table 5.4). As will be reviewed, these categories have prognostic significance.

Table 5.3 Adenocarcinoma

- 40%-50% of lung cancer cases (most common cell type)
- Weak association with smoking
- Early metastases common
- 75% present as peripheral lung nodule
- Common in the upper lobes
- Often appear speculated
- May be solid, part solid, or nonsolid (ground-glass opacity)
- Appearance correlates with tumor type and survival
- Mucinous and nonmucinous subtypes
- Specific genetic abnormalities described
- Specific drug treatment for tumor mutations in >50% of cases

Precursor Glandular Lesions

Atypical Adenomatous Hyperplasia (AAH)

AAH is a benign or preinvasive lesion characterized by lepidic growth. It represents a pneumocyte proliferation that resembles, but does not meet, the criteria for adenocarcinoma in situ, and it manifests some of the same genetic abnormalities. AAH is typically 5 mm or less in diameter but is sometimes larger; lesions may be multiple.

On CT, AAH appears as a small (usually ≤5 mm) rounded nodule of GGO (Fig. 5.5). It is common, and its incidence ranges from 5% to 20% in the population. AAH is most often found incidentally in pathologic specimens. It may mimic adenocarcinoma in situ on CT, and small GGO nodules appearing to be AAH may represent AIS or even MIA.

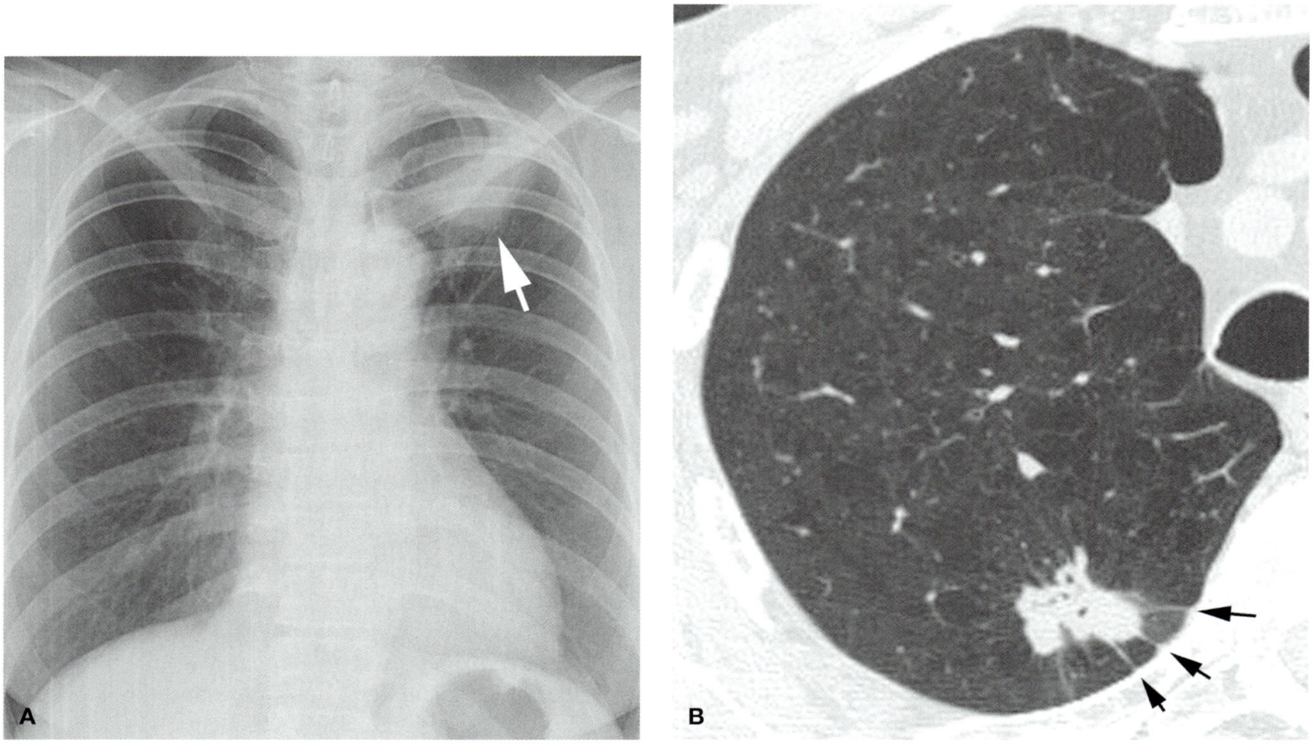

Figure 5.2. Typical appearances of invasive adenocarcinoma. **A:** Chest radiograph in a patient with an invasive adenocarcinoma shows an ill-defined nodule in the left lung apex (*arrow*). Adenocarcinomas often appear ill-defined on radiographs because of their irregular and spiculated edge or because of an associated ground-glass component. **B:** Thin-slice CT in a patient with an invasive adenocarcinoma presenting as a solitary nodule in the posterior right upper lobe. The nodule appears lobulated and spiculated. Extensions to the pleural surface (*arrows*) are termed pleural tails. They result from fibrosis with a puckering of the visceral pleural surface. Air bronchograms are visible within the nodule.

Adenocarcinoma In Situ (AIS)

AIS is defined as a localized, small (≤3 cm) adenocarcinoma consisting of neoplastic pneumocytes growing along alveolar walls (lepidic growth) and lacking stromal, vascular, or pleural invasion. AIS is typically a nonmucinous tumor consisting of type 2 pneumocytes and/or Clara cells; mucinous AIS is rare. A diagnosis of AIS can be made only if the entire tumor is resected and available for pathological examination. In the 2004 WHO classification, AIS was termed BAC, a term that has long since been discontinued but is still occasionally used.

On CT, AIS usually appears as a GGO nodule (Fig. 5.6), but sometimes a small soft tissue component is visible, resulting from focal alveolar collapse. AIS may contain air bronchograms or bubbly lucencies. The bubbly lucencies represent cystic air-filled areas within the tumor and are termed *pseudocavitation*. Some AIS may appear as cystic lesions, with little GGO visible (see Fig. 5.4). Disease-free 5-year survival is 100% following resection.

Minimally Invasive Adenocarcinoma (MIA)

MIA is defined pathologically as a small adenocarcinoma (≤3 cm), with a predominantly lepidic pattern and ≤5 mm invasion (in its greatest dimension). As with AIS, MIA is usually nonmucinous. The term MIA should not be used if the tumor invades lymphatics, blood vessels, or pleura, if tumor necrosis is present, or if the tumor has spread through airspaces (aerogenous spread). As with AIS, this diagnosis can be made only if the entire tumor is resected.

On CT, MIA may appear as a GGO nodule or a GGO nodule with a small (ie, ≤5 mm) solid focus, often near the center of the nodule (Fig. 5.7). As with AIS, air bronchograms or pseudocavitation may be seen. Review of CT may be helpful to the pathologist in evaluating the pathology specimen, because the extent of GGO (usually lepidic) versus solid (usually invasive) patterns can help in determining whether the nodule has been properly measured and/or sampled. MIA is associated with a 5-year disease-free survival near 100%.

Invasive Adenocarcinoma

Invasive adenocarcinoma is present in 70% to 90% of surgically resected lung adenocarcinomas. They are the most common type of adenocarcinoma seen in clinical practice. These tumors typically consist of a complex and heterogeneous mixture of histologic patterns.

Invasive adenocarcinoma subtypes are now classified according to the *predominant* component after performing

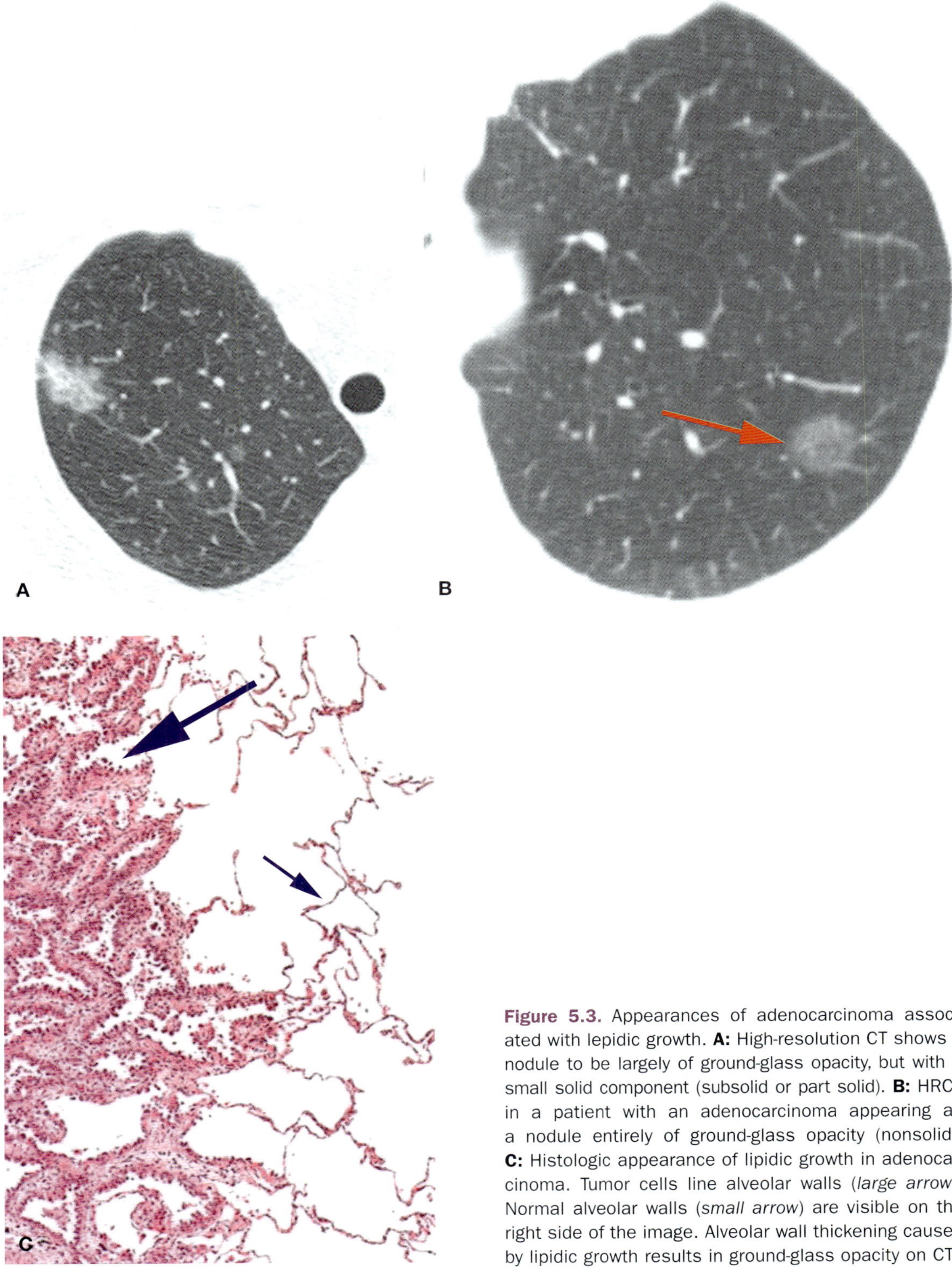

Figure 5.3. Appearances of adenocarcinoma associated with lepidic growth. **A:** High-resolution CT shows a nodule to be largely of ground-glass opacity, but with a small solid component (subsolid or part solid). **B:** HRCT in a patient with an adenocarcinoma appearing as a nodule entirely of ground-glass opacity (nonsolid). **C:** Histologic appearance of lipidic growth in adenocarcinoma. Tumor cells line alveolar walls (*large arrow*). Normal alveolar walls (*small arrow*) are visible on the right side of the image. Alveolar wall thickening caused by lipidic growth results in ground-glass opacity on CT.

comprehensive, quantitative histologic subtyping. In the following discussion, tumors with recognizable imaging appearances are emphasized, specifically lepidic (predominant) adenocarcinoma (LPA or LA), invasive adenocarcinomas appearing as solid nodules, and IMA.

Lepidic (Predominant) Adenocarcinoma

Lepidic predominant adenocarcinoma, or LPA, is a term used in the 2011 IASLC Classification of adenocarcinoma; this tumor is termed *lepidic adenocarcinoma* in the 2021 WHO classification, recognizing that although invasion is present,

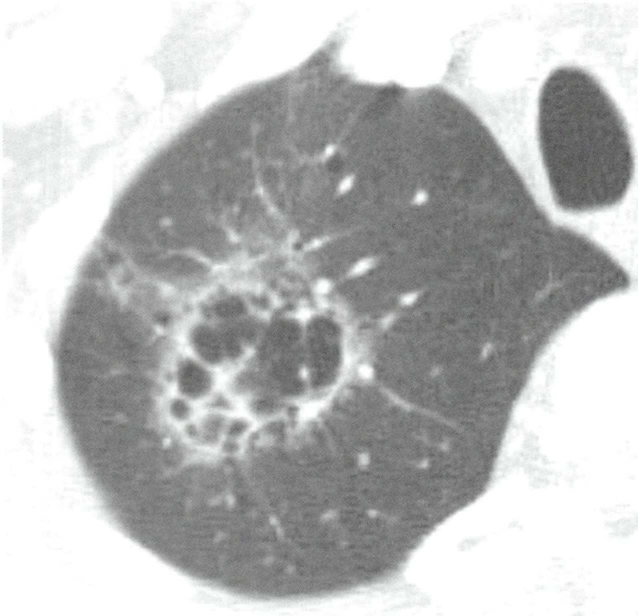

Figure 5.4. Cystic adenocarcinoma. A multicystic mass associated with ground-glass opacity is visible in the right lung apex. Adenocarcinoma with lepidic growth was found on lung biopsy.

a lepidic pattern is predominant. LPA or LA represents a tumor showing a lepidic proliferation of pneumocytes similar to that seen in AIS and MIA, but with invasive adenocarcinoma present in at least one site, measuring more than 5 mm in its greatest dimension. Invasion is defined by the presence

Table 5.4 Classification and Characteristics of Lung Adenocarcinoma

Precursor Glandular Lesions
- Atypical adenomatous hyperplasia (lepidic lesion, usually ≤5 mm)
- Adenocarcinoma in situ (AIS) (≤3 cm, lepidic without invasion)
  - Nonmucinous
  - Mucinous

Minimally invasive adenocarcinoma (MIA) (≤3 cm lepidic predominant with ≤5 mm invasion)
- Nonmucinous
- Mucinous

Invasive adenocarcinoma (characterized by predominant component)
- Lepidic (lepidic with >5 mm invasion) termed lepidic predominant adenocarcinoma (LPA) by IASLC
- Acinar
- Papillary
- Micropapillary
- Solid
- *Invasive mucinous adenocarcinoma (IMA)*
- Colloid
- Fetal
- Enteric

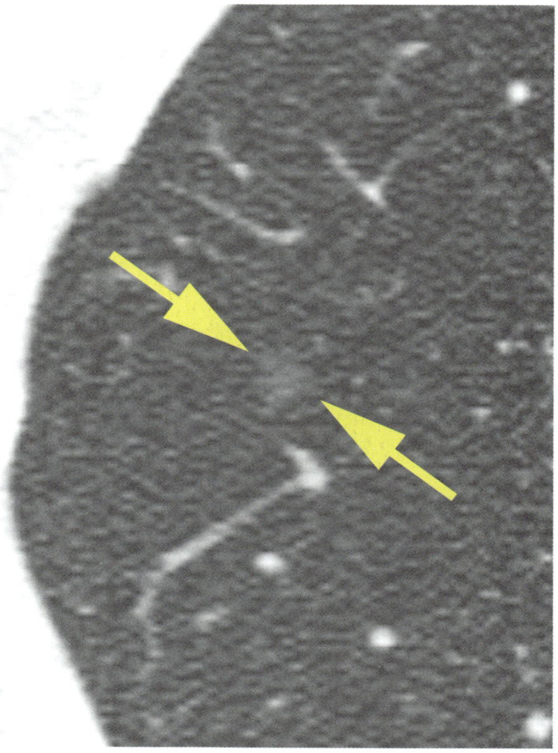

Figure 5.5. Atypical adenomatous hyperplasia (AAH). A small nodule of ground-glass opacity (*arrows*) is visible in the right upper lobe.

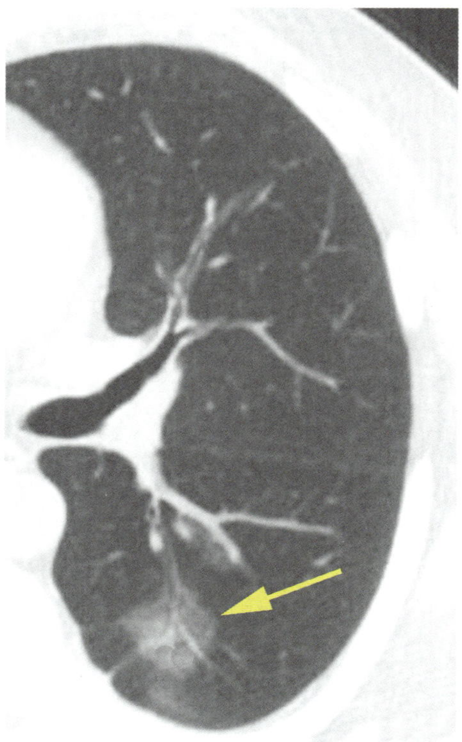

Figure 5.6. Adenocarcinoma in situ (AIS). A nodule entirely of ground-glass opacity (*arrow*) is visible in the left lower lobe. Vessels are visible within the nodule.

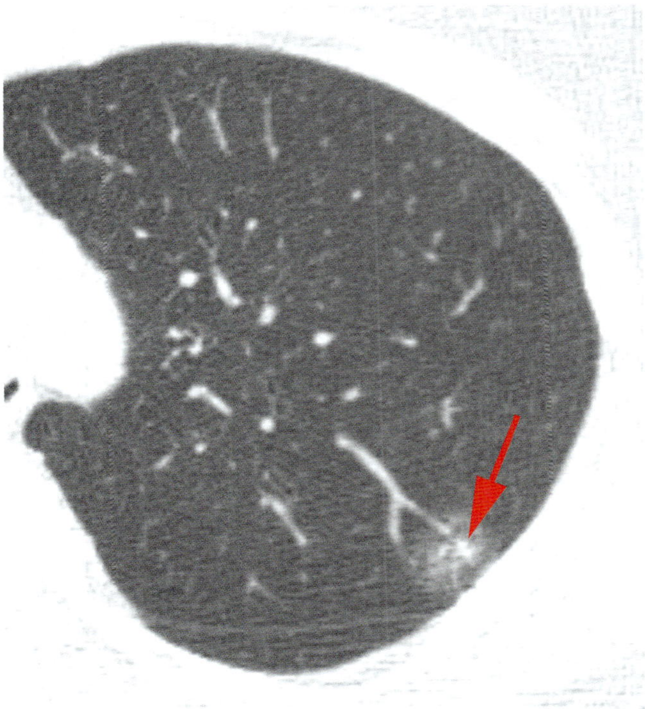

Figure 5.7. Minimally invasive adenocarcinoma (MIA). A nodule primarily of ground-glass opacity with a small solid component (*arrow*) is visible in the left upper lobe.

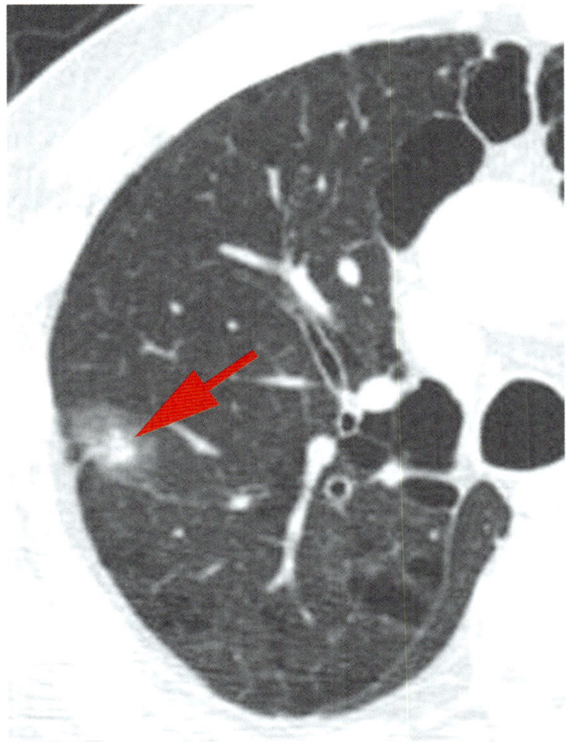

Figure 5.8. Lepidic predominant adenocarcinoma (LPA). A nodule primarily of ground-glass opacity has a central soft tissue component (*arrow*) larger than 5 mm.

of nonlepidic growth (acinar, papillary, micropapillary, and/or solid) and/or myofibroblastic stroma associated with invasive tumor cells. Also, a diagnosis of LPA rather than MIA is made pathologically if the tumor invades lymphatics, blood vessels, or pleura or if it contains regions of necrosis.

On CT, LPA often appears as a GGO nodule with a solid component greater than 5 mm in size (Fig. 5.8), but the solid component may appear smaller than 5 mm on CT in some patients with LPA. In one study, a solid component ≤3 mm was only seen in AIS or MIA, but a solid component between 3 and 5 mm was seen in several invasive adenocarcinomas. Also, a recent study has shown considerable variability in the assessment of the size of the solid component of part solid nodules, even by very experienced thoracic radiologists. Several recent studies of early-stage adenocarcinomas have shown that LPA have a generally favorable prognosis with a 5-year disease-free survival of 86% to 90%.

For lesions suspected of being AIS or MIA that are more than 3 cm in diameter, it is recommended that the term LPA be used, with a comment that an invasive component may be present. As yet, there are insufficient data to show that such patients will have a 100% 5-year disease-free survival, as do AIS or MIA.

Acinar, Papillary, Micropapillary, and Solid Adenocarcinoma

Invasive adenocarcinomas are classified based on their predominant features and graded in 5% intervals. These various histologic types of invasive adenocarcinoma do not have specific CT correlates, although they usually appear as solid nodules (Fig. 5.2B) or may be associated with regions of lepidic growth.

Subtyping of early-stage invasive adenocarcinomas according to their predominant histologic pattern is of prognostic value. In comparison to LPA, micropapillary- and solid-predominant tumors have a poor prognosis (67%-75% 5-year survival), with an intermediate survival for acinar- and papillary-predominant adenocarcinomas (approximately 80% 5-year survival). Other, less common subtypes are also recognized in the 2021 WHO classification.

Invasive Mucinous Adenocarcinoma

IMA represents a tumor consisting of malignant cells having goblet or columnar cell morphology with abundant intracytoplasmic mucin. Similar to nonmucinous tumors, IMA may show a heterogeneous mixture of lepidic, acinar, papillary, micropapillary, and solid tumor growth. These tumors have a strong correlation with KRAS mutation and a lack of EGFR mutations. Prior to 2011, IMA was referred to as diffuse BAC, but that term should no longer be used.

A majority of mucinous adenocarcinomas show invasion, but, rarely, if they meet the appropriate diagnostic criteria, mucinous adenocarcinomas may be considered an AIS or MIA.

IMAs have a propensity for multicentric, multilobar, and bilateral lung involvement likely as a result of aerogenous metastases (metastatic spread via airways). Diffuse or multifocal lung involvement may have the appearance of lung consolidation or multiple ill-defined nodules that are solid or GGO (Figs. 5.9A and B, 5.10). Although lepidic growth is present in such patients, with tumor cells lining alveolar walls, mucin produced by the tumor fills alveoli, resulting in the radiographic appearance of consolidation or a solid nodule (Fig. 5.9C). The CT angiogram sign, in which opacified vessels are visible within the consolidated lung, is often seen if CT is obtained with contrast infusion (see Chapter 1) but is nonspecific. Patients with IMA can present with profuse watery sputum production, termed *bronchorrhea*, as a result of extensive mucin production. IMA has a poor prognosis.

SQUAMOUS CELL CARCINOMA

Precursor Lesions

Squamous Dysplasia and Squamous Cell Carcinoma In Situ

Squamous dysplasia (SD) is a benign squamous lesion with several grades of histologic abnormality. Squamous carcinoma in situ (SCIS) is recognized in the 2021 classification as a preinvasive lesion with differences in cell size and maturation; nuclear features; other histologic characteristics from dysplasia, including distribution of atypical epithelial cells and mitotic figures; and immunohistochemistry. Unlike adenocarcinoma in situ, these lesions are not usually recognizable on CT.

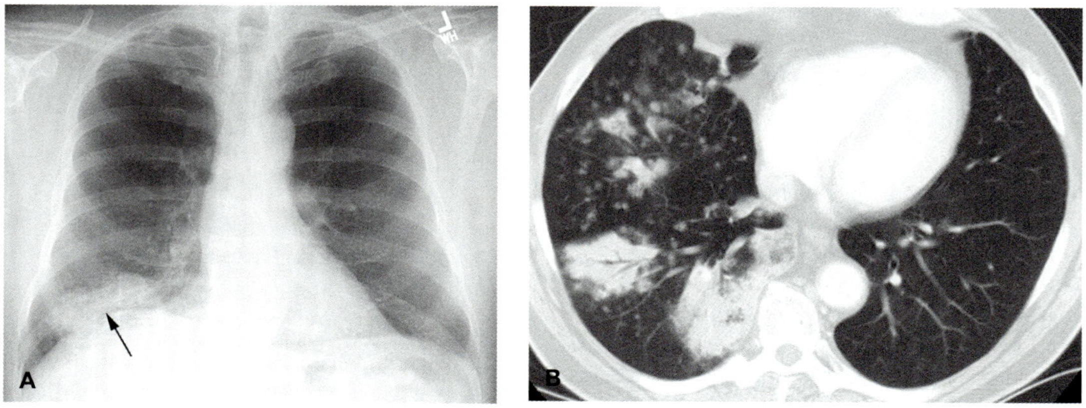

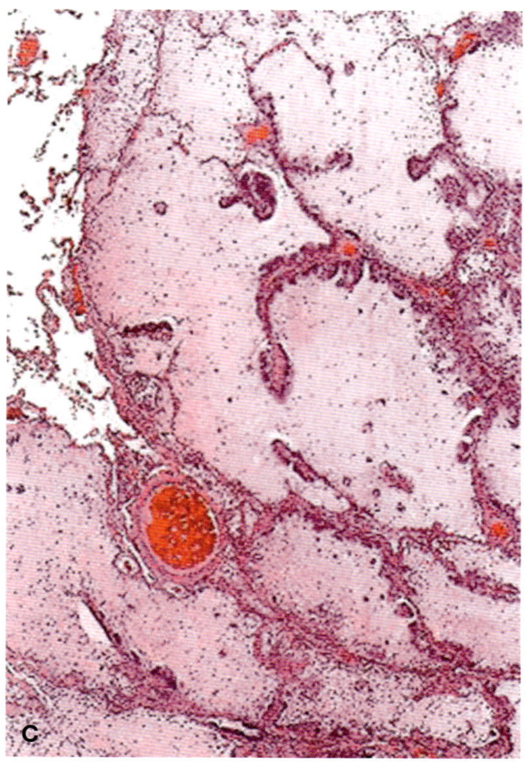

Figure 5.9. Invasive mucinous adenocarcinoma (IMA). **A:** Chest radiograph shows consolidation at the right lung base (*arrow*). **B:** CT with 5-mm slice thickness shows multiple areas of consolidation, with air bronchograms, and numerous ill-defined nodules. These nodules are typically centrilobular and are common in IMA. **C:** Histologic specimen in IMA. Lepidic growth is seen, similar to that in Figure 5.3C. However, note that mucin fills alveolar spaces, visible as a homogenous pink substance. This alveolar filling can result in the appearance of consolidation on CT.

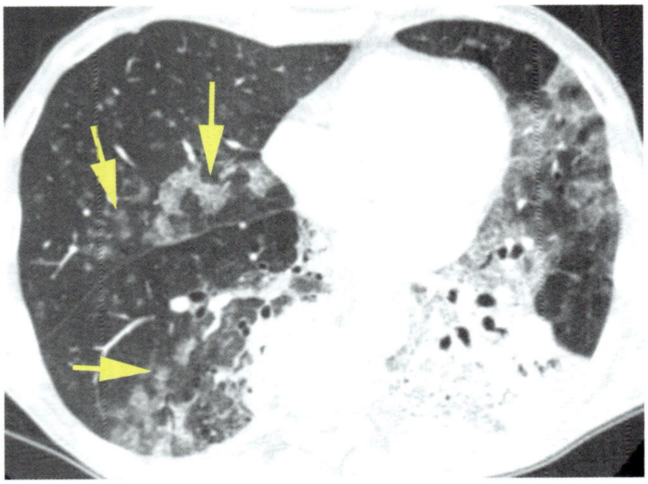

Figure 5.10. Invasive mucinous adenocarcinoma (IMA). Patchy bilateral ground-glass opacity and consolidation are visible. Some areas of involvement are large, and some appear centrilobular or lobular (*arrows*) due to aerogenous spread.

Most bronchi showing SD/SCIS demonstrate a range of abnormalities. The risk of progression of SD/SCIS to invasive SCC is unknown and may take years. Abnormalities may be reversible if exposure to a carcinogen (eg, smoking) stops.

Squamous Cell Carcinoma

Until recently, SCC was the most common cell type of lung carcinoma; it currently accounts for about 20% to 30% of cases. It is strongly associated with cigarette smoking (Table 5.5). Histologically, SCCs show intercellular bridging, squamous pearl formation, and individual cell keratinization. In the 2021 WHO classification, recognized subtypes of SCC are "keratinizing," "nonkeratinizing," and "basaloid." Squamous cell markers (p40, p63, negative for TTF1) are helpful in identifying SCC in small specimens or when typical morphology is lacking. Numerous genetic mutations are common. Survival is primarily related to tumor stage.

Table 5.5 Squamous Cell Carcinoma

- 20% of lung cancer cases
- Strongly associated with cigarette smoking
- 65% arise in main, lobar, or segmental bronchi
  - Endobronchial mass
  - Bronchial obstruction
  - Infiltration of bronchial wall
  - Local invasion
  - Hilar mass
  - Atelectasis and consolidation common
- 30% present as solitary nodule or mass
  - Cavitation relatively common
- Metastasizes late
- Relatively good prognosis

SCC frequently (60%-80%) arises in main, lobar, or segmental bronchi. In this location, tumor growth results in the obstruction of the bronchial lumen, infiltration of the bronchial wall, and invasion of the adjacent lung or vessels. SCC tends to cause symptoms early in its course because of its proximal and endobronchial location and may be detected using sputum cytology before being radiographically visible. Early metastasis is uncommon, and SCC has a relatively good 5-year survival rate.

A polypoid endobronchial mass or bronchial obstruction is frequently seen on CT. Hilar mass is also common due to the central location of the tumor, with local invasion and involvement of hilar lymph nodes (Figs. 5.11 and 5.12). Atelectasis, consolidation, mucoid impaction (mucous bronchograms), and bronchiectasis are common findings, reflecting the presence of bronchial obstruction (see Table 5.5). Less than 20% of SCCs present in the lung periphery as a lung nodule or mass. Central necrosis and cavitation (Fig. 5.13) are more common than other cell types.

NEUROENDOCRINE TUMORS

This category includes high-grade tumors (*small cell lung carcinoma* and *large cell neuroendocrine carcinoma*), intermediate-grade *atypical carcinoid tumor*, low-grade *typical carcinoid tumor*, and precursor lesion *diffuse idiopathic pulmonary neuroendocrine cell hyperplasia* (DIPNECH) (Table 5.6). These tumors are characterized by neuroendocrine morphology and neuroendocrine markers identified using immunohistochemistry. They arise from neuroendocrine Kulchitsky cells associated with respiratory epithelium, contain secretory granules, and can produce active peptides. They are commonly associated with paraneoplastic syndromes.

Neuroendocrine tumors constitute 20% to 25% of invasive lung malignancies. The most common neuroendocrine lung tumor is small cell lung carcinoma (SCLC), which accounts for 15% to 20% of invasive lung malignancies (Table 5.7). In a surgical series, large cell neuroendocrine carcinoma (LCNEC) represents about 3% of lung cancers. Carcinoid tumors represent 1% to 2% of invasive lung malignancies, and only 10% to 25% of these are classified as atypical carcinoid. These tumors reflect a spectrum of abnormalities ranging from typical carcinoid tumor (which has a good prognosis) to SCLC (which has a poor prognosis; Table 5.6).

The neuroendocrine tumors can be divided into two groups based on their genetic abnormalities. Carcinoid tumors (typical and atypical) are characterized by MEN1 and related chromatin modifier mutations, while LCNEC and SCLC are associated with numerous genomic and epigenomic alterations, with RB1 and TP53 gene mutations and characteristic tobacco carcinogen-associated molecular signatures.

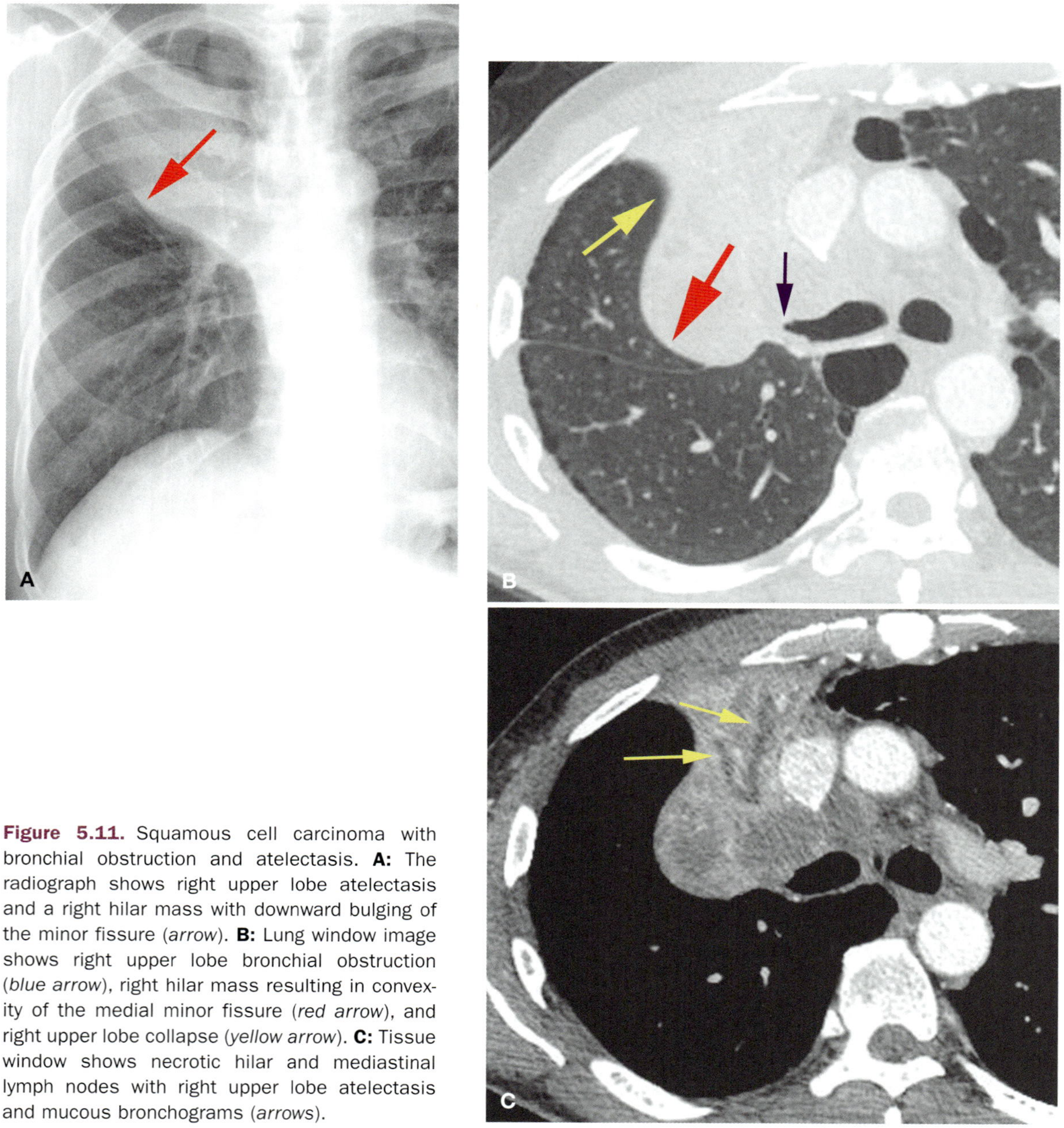

Figure 5.11. Squamous cell carcinoma with bronchial obstruction and atelectasis. **A:** The radiograph shows right upper lobe atelectasis and a right hilar mass with downward bulging of the minor fissure (*arrow*). **B:** Lung window image shows right upper lobe bronchial obstruction (*blue arrow*), right hilar mass resulting in convexity of the medial minor fissure (*red arrow*), and right upper lobe collapse (*yellow arrow*). **C:** Tissue window shows necrotic hilar and mediastinal lymph nodes with right upper lobe atelectasis and mucous bronchograms (*arrows*).

Small Cell Lung Carcinoma

SCLC is the third most common histologic variety of primary lung cancer (15%-20% of cases) and is made up of small cells, similar in size to lymphocytes, which have scant cytoplasm (Table 5.7). SCLC originates from neuroendocrine cells, and electron microscopy shows neurosecretory granules in many cases of small cell carcinoma. Immunohistochemical analysis is helpful in distinguishing SCLC from other tumors.

SCLC is strongly associated with smoking, and its incidence has been decreasing in recent years, as smoking becomes less common in the population. Although it has had a strong male predominance (2.5:1), recent studies have shown a similar incidence in male and female patients.

Small cell carcinoma tends to occur in the main or lobar bronchi and is associated with extensive peribronchial invasion and a large hilar or parahilar mass (Fig. 5.14). Endobronchial tumor masses are less common than SCC, but the large tumor mass frequently compresses bronchi (Fig. 5.15). Atelectasis may be associated. This tumor is commonly associated with marked mediastinal lymph node enlargement (Fig. 5.16). It is a common cause of superior vena cava (SVC) syndrome. Presentation as a solitary lung nodule is very uncommon, accounting for less than 5% of cases.

SCLC is a common cause of endocrine and neurologic paraneoplastic syndromes, including inappropriate antidiuretic hormone secretion, Cushing's syndrome, acromegaly,

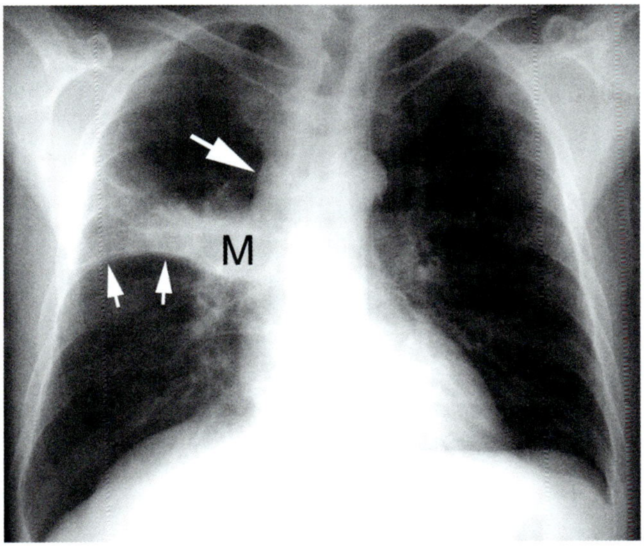

Figure 5.12. Squamous cell carcinoma with bronchial obstruction and right upper lobe atelectasis. Chest radiograph shows a right hilar mass (*M*) with upward bowing of the minor fissure (*small arrows*). This combination results in Golden's S sign. Mediastinal lymph node enlargement is also present (*large arrow*).

autoimmune neuropathy (Eaton–Lambert syndrome), encephalomyelitis, and limbic encephalitis. In patients with SCLC, neurologic symptoms may precede the diagnosis of lung cancer and progress rapidly.

Although the tumor is relatively radiosensitive, its prognosis is very poor because of the frequent presence of distant metastases at the time of diagnosis. Small cell lung cancer is not generally considered amenable to surgical treatment, although the resection of localized pulmonary lesions is often undertaken. Over 90% of cases are stage IV at diagnosis. FDG PET may be very helpful in demonstrating the extent of disease.

Staging of Small Cell Lung Carcinoma

The staging system traditionally used for SCLC-grouped patients into one of two categories: limited-stage (LS) SCLC and extensive-stage (ES) SCLC. In 2018, the 8th TNM stage classification for lung cancer (TNM-8) included SCLC for the first time and should be reported similar to NSCLC. In the TNM system, stages I to III correspond to LS-SCLC and stage IV corresponds to ES-SCLC. Although the use of the TNM system with SCLC does not frequently alter clinical management and is less helpful than simpler systems in assessing prognosis, it allows a more precise description of tumor characteristics. Staging of SCLC using the TNM classification is now common.

Large Cell Neuroendocrine Carcinoma

LCNEC was formerly classified as a subtype of LCC. As with small cell carcinoma, it is high-grade NEC with a high

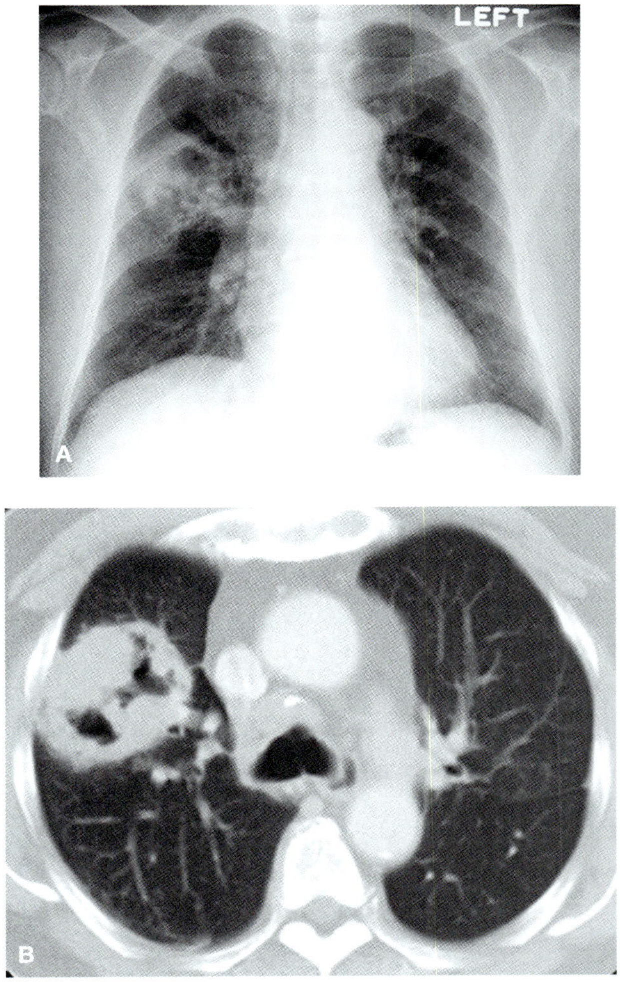

Figure 5.13. Squamous cell carcinoma with a cavitary lung mass. **A:** On a chest radiograph, a large, thick-walled cavitary mass is visible in the right upper lobe. **B:** CT shows the cavity to have a thick and nodular wall. This is typical of cavitary carcinoma. This would be considered a T2 carcinoma.

mitotic rate and a poor prognosis. It is strongly associated with smoking.

LCNEC typically presents as a round or oval nodule or mass, which is most common in the peripheral lung. It may range from 1 to 9 cm or larger in diameter. Typically, tumors are lobulated (80%) and sharply marginated (75%), but spiculation can be seen. Calcification may be present but is uncommon. Heterogeneous enhancement is common following contrast infusion, a finding that correlates with necrosis on pathology. At least 30% of patients have lymph node involvement or distant metastases at time of presentation. Five-year survival averages are about 30%, better than SCLC, but not as favorable as carcinoid tumors or other types of lung cancer.

Carcinoid Tumors

Carcinoid tumors originate from neuroendocrine cells in the bronchial wall. They show relatively few genetic

Table 5.6 Characteristics of Neuroendocrine Tumors

	Typical Carcinoid	Atypical Carcinoid	Large-Cell NEC	Small Cell LC
Demographics				
Typical patient age	40s	50s	60s	60s
Smoking association	None	80%	Strong	Very strong
Male:female ratio	1:1	2:1	4:1	2.5:1
Pathology				
Mitoses per 2 mm^2	<2	2-10	>10 (mean 70)	>10 (mean 80)
Necrosis	No	Focal	Yes	Yes
Imaging Features				
Central:peripheral ratio	4:1	2:1	1:4	10-20:1
Calcification	30%	30%	<10%	20%
Contrast enhancement	Often dense	Often dense	± necrosis	± necrosis
FDG-PET activity	Low	Low	High	High
Clinical Features				
Lymph node metastases	5%-15%	35%-55%	30%	>90%
Distant metastases	5%	15%	35%	60%-70%
5-year survival	90%-100%	45%-85%	15%-55%	5%
Paraneoplastic syndromes	Sometimes	Sometimes	Rare	Common

abnormalities as compared to SCLC and LCNEC. Carcinoid tumors are classified as typical or atypical.

Typical carcinoid tumor is a low-grade malignancy and accounts for a few percent of all primary lung malignancies.

Table 5.7 Small Cell Lung Carcinoma

15%-20% of lung cancers
Strongly associated with smoking
Neuroendocrine carcinoma
Paraneoplastic syndromes commonly associated
Most occur in main or lobar bronchi
Extensive peribronchial invasion
Large hilar or parahilar mass
Bronchial narrowing
Lymph node enlargement
Metastases at diagnosis in >90%
Prognosis very poor

This tumor most often occurs in the central bronchi, resulting in an endobronchial mass, and is locally invasive; it may also present as a lung nodule or mass. Metastases are relatively uncommon.

Atypical carcinoid tumor is a more aggressive, intermediate-grade variant. In comparison with typical carcinoid tumor, it has a higher mitotic rate, is more often associated with metastases, and has a poorer prognosis, intermediate between that of typical carcinoid tumor and high-grade neuroendocrine carcinomas (SCLC and LCNEC).

Typical Carcinoid Tumor

Typical carcinoid tumors are slowly growing and locally invasive. They metastasize to regional lymph nodes in 5% to 15% of cases, and a lesser number of patients have distant metastases.

Typical carcinoid tumors occur most commonly in patients aged 40 to 60 years (mean age, 45-55). However,

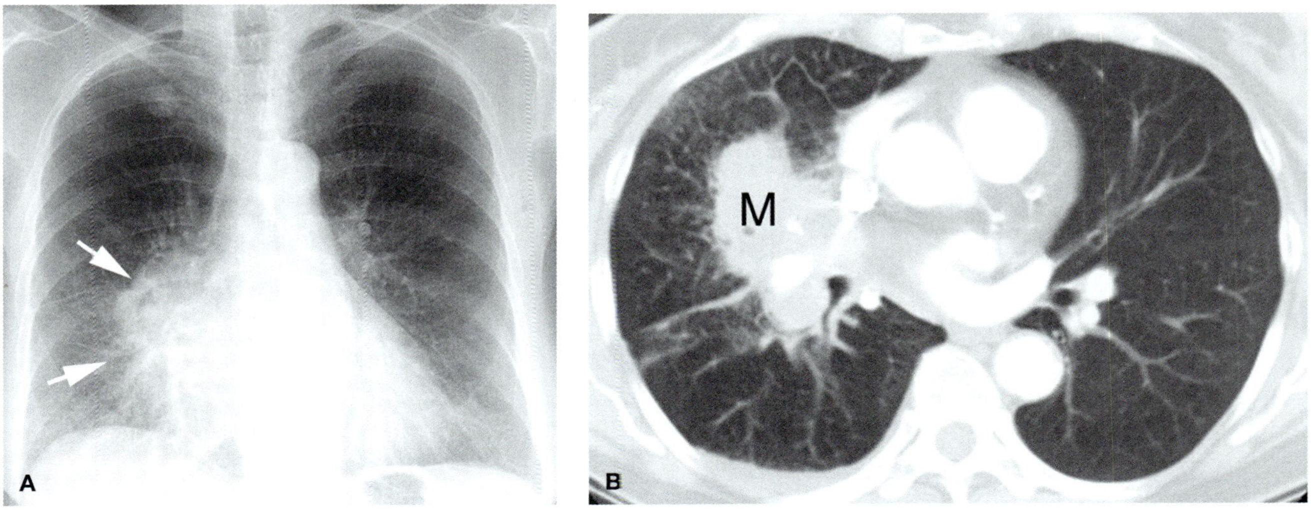

Figure 5.14. Small cell lung carcinoma. **A:** Chest radiograph shows a large right hilar mass (*arrows*). **B:** CT shows the large mass (*M*). Interstitial thickening characterized by interlobular septal thickening in the middle lobe indicates local lymphangitic spread of tumor.

they are not uncommon in patients younger than 20 years, and this tumor tends to occur in a younger population than other lung carcinomas. It is slightly more common in female patients. There is no association with smoking.

Approximately 80% of typical carcinoid tumors occur centrally, in the main, lobar, or segmental bronchi; 1% are intratracheal. Involvement of lobar bronchi (75% of those with airway lesions) is most common (Fig. 5.17). Because of associated bronchial obstruction, symptoms are common and they occur in approximately 75% of cases; the symptoms include cough, fever, and wheezing. These tumors are highly vascular, and hemoptysis is a common presenting complaint. Peripheral carcinoid tumors may be asymptomatic. Patients who have central carcinoid tumors associated with bronchial obstruction tend to present at a younger age than do patients with peripheral lesions.

Nearly half of typical carcinoid tumors are associated with radiographic findings of bronchial obstruction, primarily atelectasis or consolidation, typically limited to a lobe or segment (see Fig. 5.17A). Atelectasis and consolidation are often intermittent, and recurrent episodes of infection can result in bronchiectasis or lung abscess. Bronchiectasis is pathologically present in more than one-third of patients but is less often visible on radiographs. Air trapping related to bronchial obstruction is sometimes seen.

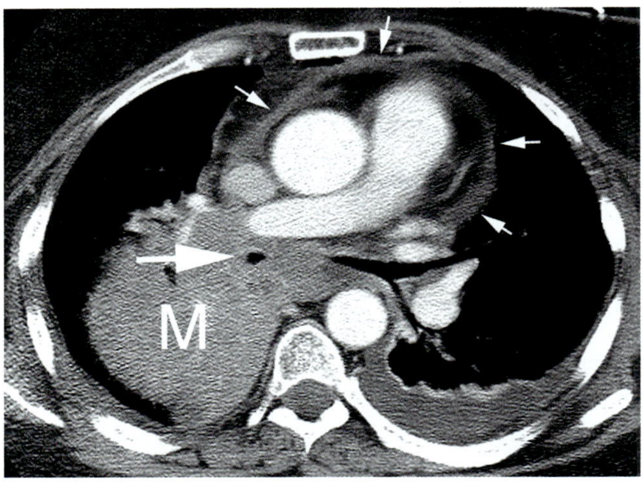

Figure 5.15. Small cell lung carcinoma. Contrast-enhanced CT shows a large hilar mass (*M*). Tumor surrounds and narrows the bronchus intermedius (*large arrow*) and extends into the subcarinal space. Pericardial thickening (*small arrows*) is likely due to local invasion. A left pleural effusion is also present.

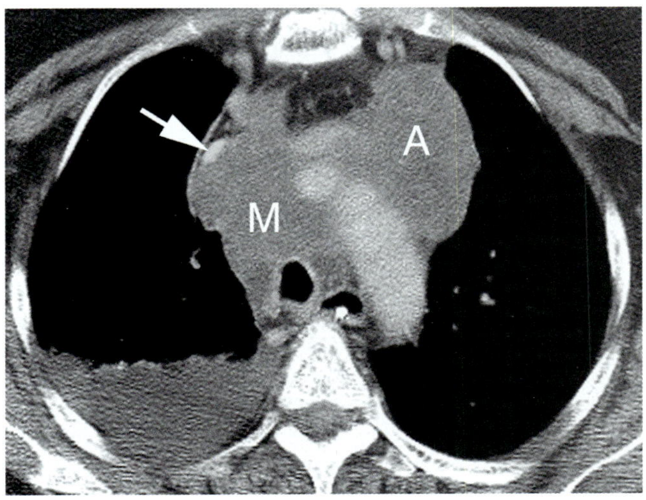

Figure 5.16. Small cell lung carcinoma. CT following contrast infusion shows extensive mediastinal lymph node enlargement typical of small cell carcinoma. The superior vena cava (*arrow*) is displaced anteriorly and markedly narrowed by lymph node mass (*M*) in the right paratracheal space. A large anterior mediastinal lymph node mass (*A*) is also visible. A right pleural effusion is also present.

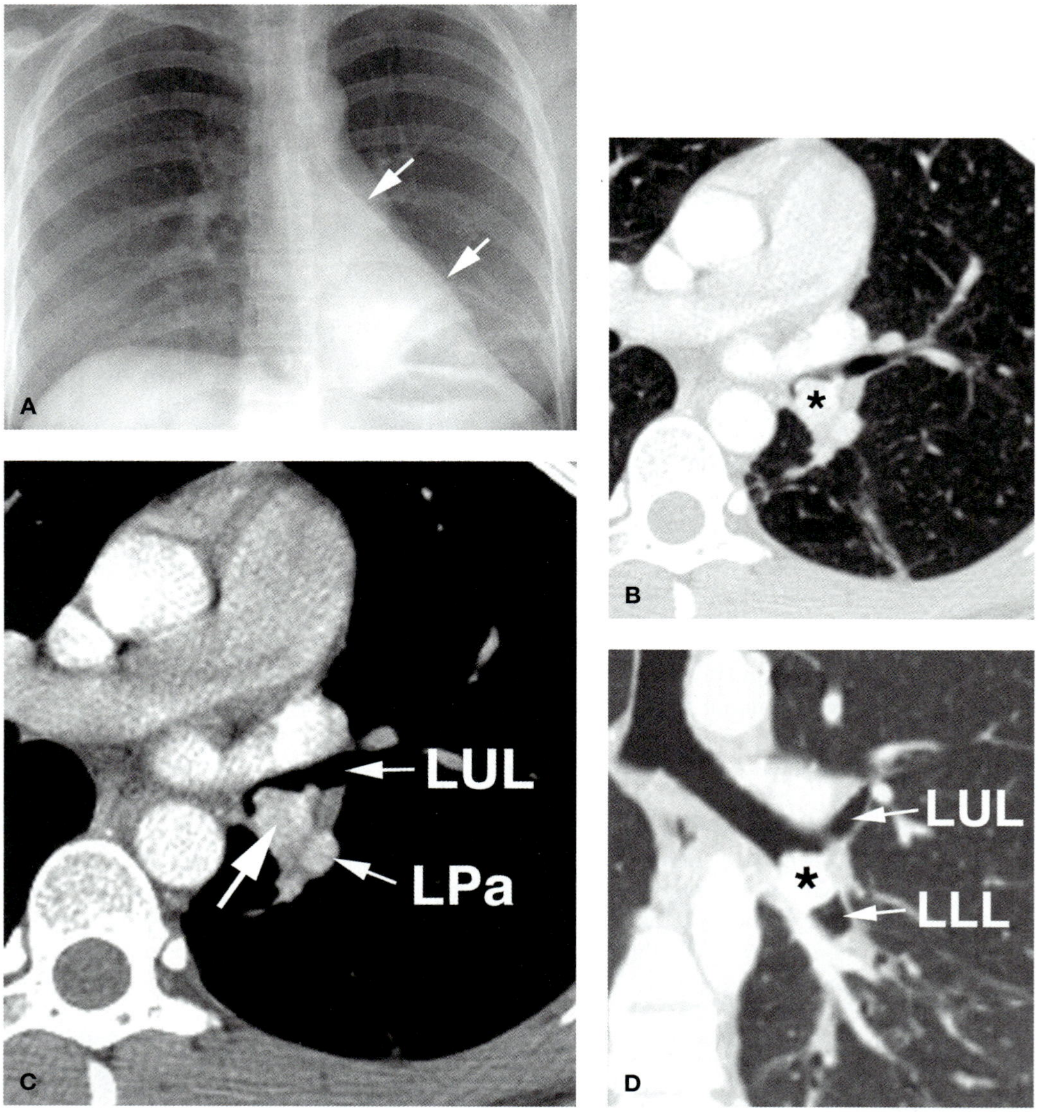

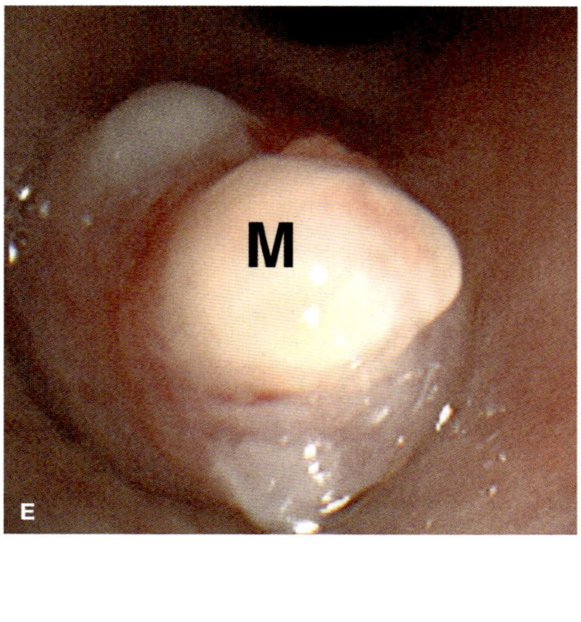

Figure 5.17. Typical carcinoid tumor presenting as an endobronchial mass in a 30-year-old patient with recurrent left lower lobe pneumonia. **A:** Chest radiograph shows left lower lobe atelectasis (*arrows*). **B:** CT at a later date shows a lobulated endobronchial mass (*asterisk*) associated with the obstruction of the left lower lobe bronchus. **C:** Contrast-enhanced CT at the same level shows the enhancement of the tumor (*large arrow*) and its relationship to the left upper lobe bronchus (*LUL*) and the interlobar left pulmonary artery (*LPa*). **D:** Coronal reformation shows the mass (*asterisk*) obstructing the proximal left lower lobe bronchus (*LLL*). The left upper lobe bronchus (*LUL*) is normal. **E:** Bronchoscopic photograph shows the endobronchial mass (*M*) protruding from the left lower lobe bronchus. This mass appeared highly vascular and bled easily.

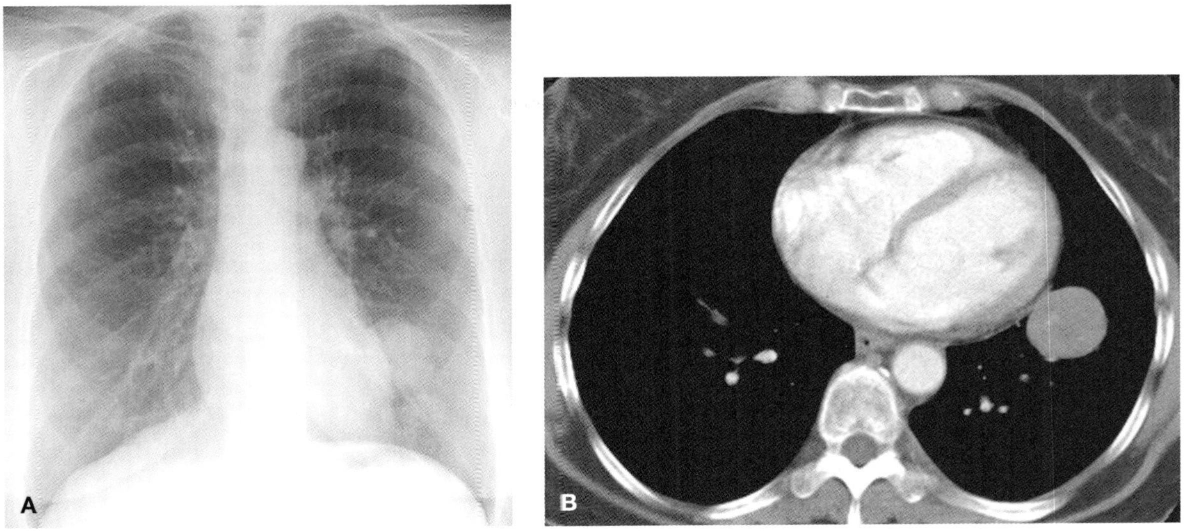

Figure 5.18. Typical carcinoid tumor presenting as a lung mass. A well-defined and sharply marginated rounded mass is visible in the left lower lobe on the chest radiograph (**A**) and CT (**B**).

Central tumors, with or without findings of obstruction may be visible as discrete mass lesions in or near the hila These masses, which are usually less than 4 cm in diameter, can be difficult to recognize without CT. In many cases, these tumors have a large endobronchial component and appear on CT as intraluminal masses (see Fig. 5.17B-D) with a convex margin pointing toward the hilum. Also, lesions that are largely endobronchial can expand the bronchus as they grow, typically resulting in expansion of the bronchial lumen at the point of obstruction. Because they are highly vascular, dense enhancement may be seen on CT (Fig. 5.17C).

A peripheral nodule or mass, not associated with findings of obstruction, is present in approximately 20% of patients (Fig. 5.18). These nodules are often well defined, round or oval, and slightly lobulated.

Calcification and ossification may be seen on plain films in a patient with carcinoid tumor. On CT, calcification of central carcinoid tumors is seen in nearly 40% of cases (Figs. 10.21 and 10.22 in Chapter 10). Calcifications may be large and "chunky."

Radionuclide imaging with somatostatin analogs (eg, octreotide) may be used to localize an occult carcinoid tumor in a patient with Cushing's syndrome or carcinoid syndrome or to diagnose metastases (Fig. 5.19).

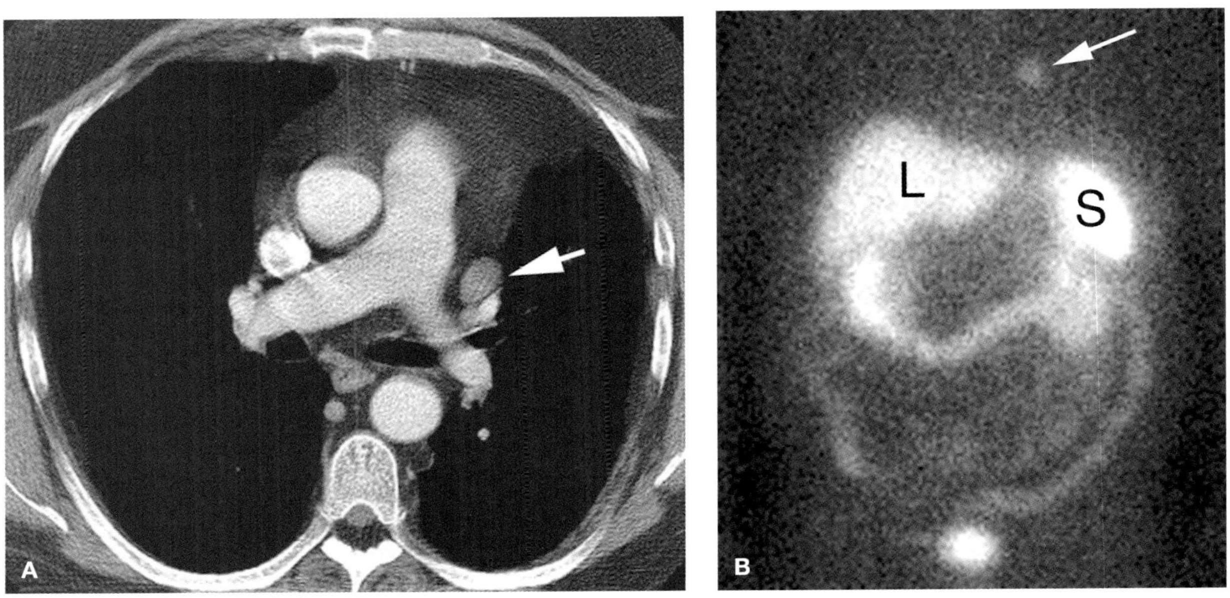

Figure 5.19. Lymph node metastasis in a patient following the resection of a carcinoid tumor. **A:** Chest CT shows an enlarged left mediastinal lymph node (*arrow*). **B:** Octreotide radionuclide scan shows increased activity in the lymph node (*arrow*). The liver (*L*) and spleen (S) are indicated for orientation.

Local extension of typical carcinoid tumors beyond the bronchial wall is common, and endoscopic removal of visible tumor is not usually curative. Surgical resection is the treatment of choice. Peripheral carcinoid tumors can be excised using wedge resection or segmentectomy. For central endobronchial lesions, a sleeve resection may be performed to avoid pneumonectomy or lobectomy. In this procedure, a segment of bronchus containing the tumor is resected and the two bronchial stumps are sutured together.

For patients treated surgically, the prognosis is good. The 10-year survival rate of patients treated with surgery is as high as 90%. Following resection, distant metastasis is more common than local recurrence at the primary site. Bone metastases, either lytic or blastic, can occur.

Atypical Carcinoid Tumor

Approximately 10% to 25% of carcinoid tumors can be classified as *atypical carcinoid tumor* because of histologic features suggesting a more aggressive behavior, including an increased frequency of mitoses and the presence of necrosis. These tumors are considered to be intermediate between typical carcinoid tumor and SCLC in differentiation, the incidence of metastases, and mortality. Lymph node metastases are present in approximately 50% of patients. Patients with atypical carcinoid tend to be slightly older than those with typical carcinoid and male patients outnumber female patients. They are associated with smoking.

Atypical carcinoid tumors tend to present as a lung nodule or mass, round or ovoid, lobulated, and somewhat larger than those seen with typical carcinoid tumor (10 cm or smaller). An endobronchial mass resulting in obstruction and atelectasis is less common than that with typical carcinoid tumor occurring in about 10% of the patients.

These tumors have a worse prognosis than do typical pulmonary carcinoids, and a more aggressive surgical approach is usually employed (lobectomy, sometimes with radiation or chemotherapy). Surgical cures have been reported, and 5-year survival rates range from 50% to 70%. As with typical carcinoid tumor, they can be associated with various paraneoplastic syndromes.

Clinical Syndromes Associated With Carcinoid Tumor

Carcinoid tumors can produce a number of active neuroendocrine peptides, and several clinical syndromes have been associated with this tumor. Typically, metastases are present before these syndromes become manifest; it is unusual for a small localized tumor to produce a sufficient amount of active peptides to result in clinical manifestations.

Carcinoid syndrome occurs in 2% to 5% of patients with pulmonary carcinoid tumor. It is most common in the presence of liver metastases. The carcinoid syndrome consists of flushing, fever, nausea, diarrhea, hypotension, and wheezing; it results from secretion of 5-hydroxytryptamine and other active agents such as bradykinin and prostaglandins. Cardiac valvular lesions and heart murmurs associated with this syndrome may be limited to the left side of the heart because of high concentrations of active substances in the pulmonary venous blood; cardiac valvular abnormalities associated with gastrointestinal carcinoid tumors usually involve the right side of the heart. Some other symptoms are said to help distinguish bronchial carcinoid syndrome from that resulting from intestinal tumors; these include severe flushing, facial edema, lacrimation, salivation, rhinorrhea, and diaphoresis.

Cushing's syndrome can result from the production of ACTH or ACTH-releasing hormone by the tumor. It is uncommon, being seen in about 2% of cases (Fig. 5.20). Approximately 1% of cases of Cushing's syndrome are produced by bronchial carcinoid. Other syndromes associated with bronchial carcinoid tumor include Zollinger–Ellison syndrome, hyperinsulinemia, and acromegaly.

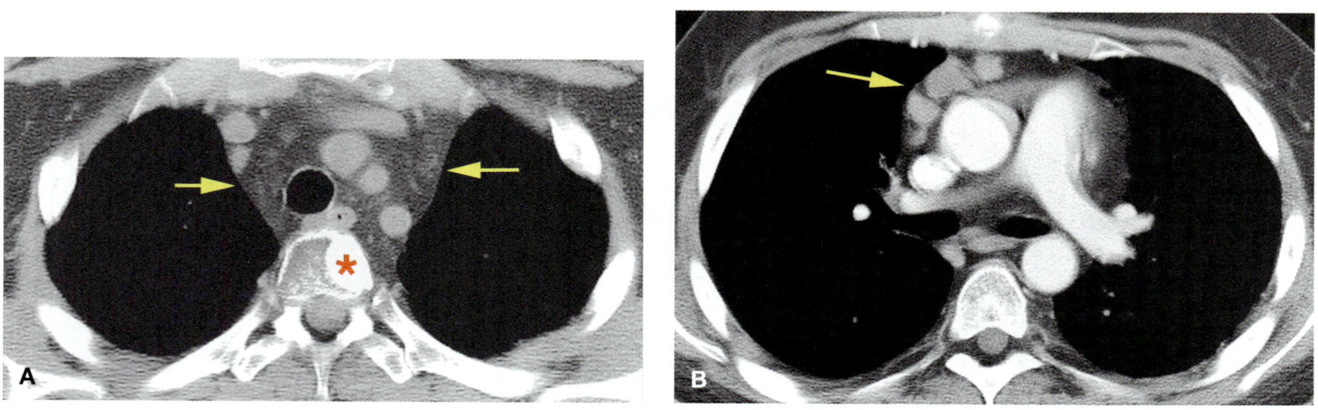

Figure 5.20. Metastatic carcinoid tumor with Cushing's syndrome. **A:** CT shows mediastinal widening and fat deposition (lipomatosis; *arrows*) secondary to Cushing's syndrome. A sclerotic vertebral metastasis (*asterisk*) is visible. **B:** At a lower level, enlarged mediastinal lymph nodes (*arrow*) reflect metastatic tumor.

Precursor Lesion

Diffuse Idiopathic Pulmonary Neuroendocrine Cell Hyperplasia

A benign proliferation of neuroendocrine cells in DIPNECH is typically superficial to the basement membrane and localized to bronchial and bronchiolar epithelium. The term "tumorlets" is used when there is extension of neuroendocrine cell hyperplasia beyond the basement membrane (Fig. 5.21). Nodules 5 mm in diameter or larger are classified as carcinoid tumors, with which DIPNECH is sometimes associated. DIPNECH has also been associated with MEN1 (multiple endocrine neoplasia syndrome, type 1) and Cushing's syndrome. There is a distinct predominance in female patients.

DIPNECH may be asymptomatic, with small nodules being detected on CT obtained for other reasons; it may be localized or diffuse. In some patients, DIPNECH is associated with constrictive bronchiolitis and symptoms of airway obstruction, such as nonproductive cough and dyspnea. Constrictive bronchiolitis may occur in these patients because of the relationship of the neuroendocrine cells to the walls of small airways and perhaps because of their production of fibrogenic cytokines.

In patients with DIPNECH and constrictive bronchiolitis, HRCT shows mosaic perfusion and air trapping on expiratory scans, with or without visible nodules. Bronchiectasis or bronchial wall thickening may also be present. This entity is most common in women who are 50 to 70 years of age. It is typically indolent, although some patients with constrictive bronchiolitis show progressive symptoms; 5-year survival is about 85% in symptomatic patients.

Neuroendocrine cell hyperplasia (NECH), or tumorlets of benign neuroendocrine cells, may also be seen in the walls of small airways in patients with chronic lung diseases such as emphysema, chronic bronchitis, or lung fibrosis. These are considered reactive, while DIPNECH is thought to be a primary proliferation.

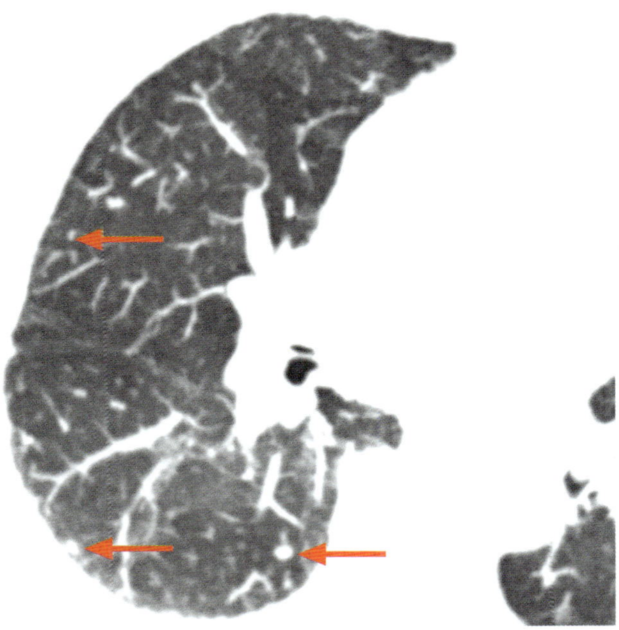

Figure 5.21. DIPNECH. Thin MIP CT image shows multiple small carcinoid tumorlets (*arrows*) and lobules of mosaic attenuation.

LARGE CELL CARCINOMA

In the 2021 WHO classification of lung tumors, the term LCC is used to describe a malignant epithelial neoplasm that does not show squamous, adenomatous, or neuroendocrine differentiation using histology or immunohistochemistry. The incidence of LCC has decreased as improved immunohistochemical analyses have allowed the reclassification of many tumors as poorly differentiated squamous cell carcinoma (p40 expression), adenocarcinoma (TTF-1 expression), and neuroendocrine carcinoma (chromogranin and synaptophysin). As a result, LCC now accounts for only about 5% of lung cancers (Table 5.8). It tends to present as a large peripheral mass; more than 60% are larger than 4 cm at presentation (Fig. 5.22). It is like adenocarcinoma in its radiologic characteristics (except for its large size) and behavior. As with adenocarcinoma, it tends to metastasize early and has a relatively poor prognosis. Survival is primarily determined by tumor stage, but targeted therapy may be used in those patients with specific genetic abnormalities. It is strongly associated with smoking.

ADENOSQUAMOUS CARCINOMA

Adenosquamous carcinoma accounts for a few percent of lung cancer cases. This tumor has mixed histologic characteristics of both adenocarcinoma and SCC, with each cell type constituting at least 10% of the tumor. EGFR and KRAS mutations may be present in both components of the tumor. These tumors usually present as masses in the lung periphery and are indistinguishable from adenocarcinoma or LCC. Metastases are common. Adenosquamous carcinomas are aggressive and have a poorer prognosis than either adenocarcinoma or squamous cell carcinoma.

SARCOMATOID CARCINOMAS

These tumors are rare, accounting for less than 1% of all lung cancers. This disparate group of tumors includes those characterized pathologically by a combination of epithelial and mesenchymal tissues (eg, pleomorphic carcinoma, spindle cell

Table 5.8 Large Cell Carcinoma
5% of lung cancers
Strongly associated with smoking
Reclassified as an undifferentiated carcinoma without markers of another cell type (eg, adenocarcinoma, squamous cell carcinoma, LCNEC)
Usually present as a large peripheral mass (>4 cm)
Metastasizes early
Prognosis poor

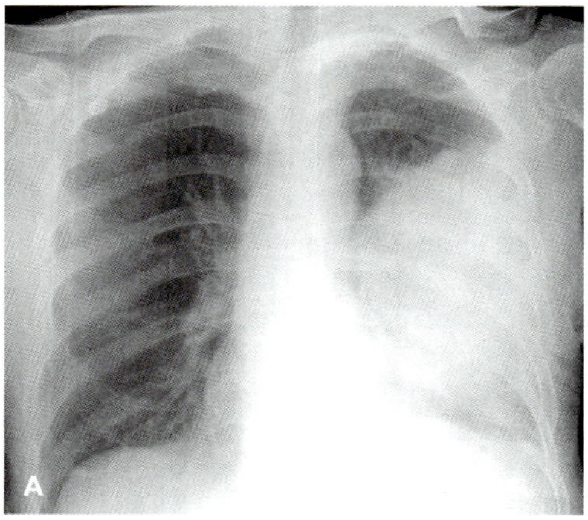

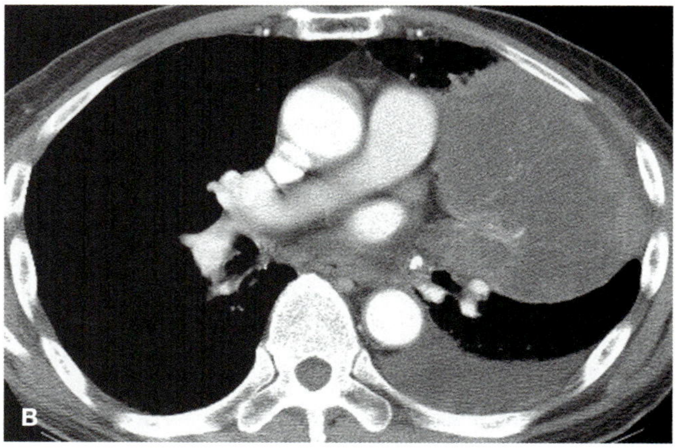

Figure 5.22. Large cell carcinoma. **A:** Chest radiograph shows a large left lung mass. **B:** On contrast-enhanced CT, a large mass occupies the left lung. A left pleural effusion is also present.

carcinoma, giant cell carcinoma, carcinosarcoma, and pulmonary blastoma). They may present as polypoid endobronchial masses or large lung masses. Their prognosis is poor.

Molecular testing for known genetic abnormalities should be performed for histologic components of the tumor with known associations (ie, an adenocarcinoma component should be tested for EGFR mutation and ALK rearrangement). The diagnoses of pleomorphic, spindle cell, or giant cell carcinoma cannot be made on small biopsies or cytology.

SALIVARY GLAND-TYPE TUMORS

Salivary gland-type carcinomas are like salivary gland tumors in their histologic characteristics. They arise from glands in the tracheal or bronchial wall and are also referred to as bronchial gland carcinomas. Salivary gland-type tumors are subdivided into several cell types; adenoid cystic carcinoma (cylindroma) and mucoepidermoid carcinoma (MEC) are the most common; less common cell types are epithelial–myoepithelial carcinoma and pleomorphic adenoma. Bronchial gland tumors account for 0.1% to 0.2% of all lung and bronchial tumors and are one tenth as common as carcinoid tumor.

Adenoid Cystic Carcinoma (Cylindroma)

Adenoid cystic carcinoma is the most common bronchial gland tumor accounting for 75% of cases. The average age at diagnosis is 50; it is not associated with smoking.

Approximately 50% of adenoid cystic carcinomas originate in the main or lobar bronchi (Fig. 5.23), 40% originate in the trachea, and 10% present as peripheral lung nodules. Although adenoid cystic carcinoma is an uncommon neoplasm, it is responsible for as many as 30% to 35% of tracheal malignancies. Although carcinoid is much more common among central bronchial tumors, adenoid cystic carcinoma outnumbers carcinoid in the trachea by 20 to 1.

When it occurs as an endobronchial lesion, adenoid cystic carcinoma presents with symptoms and radiographic findings similar to any cause of bronchial obstruction. The tumor usually protrudes into the airway lumen and may be polypoid or sessile.

When it is endotracheal, this lesion most commonly appears as a sessile mass with obtuse angles where it contacts the tracheal wall; in some patients, it is polypoid. It tends to originate from the posterior or posterolateral tracheal wall (see Figs. 22.5 and 22.6B in Chapter 22). Although CT can be helpful in assessing endotracheal adenoid cystic carcinoma, it tends to underestimate the longitudinal extent of the tumor because of partial volume averaging and the tendency of adenoid cystic carcinoma to grow submucosally. CT, however, accurately demonstrates the extratracheal extension of tumor, which is helpful in planning the surgical approach.

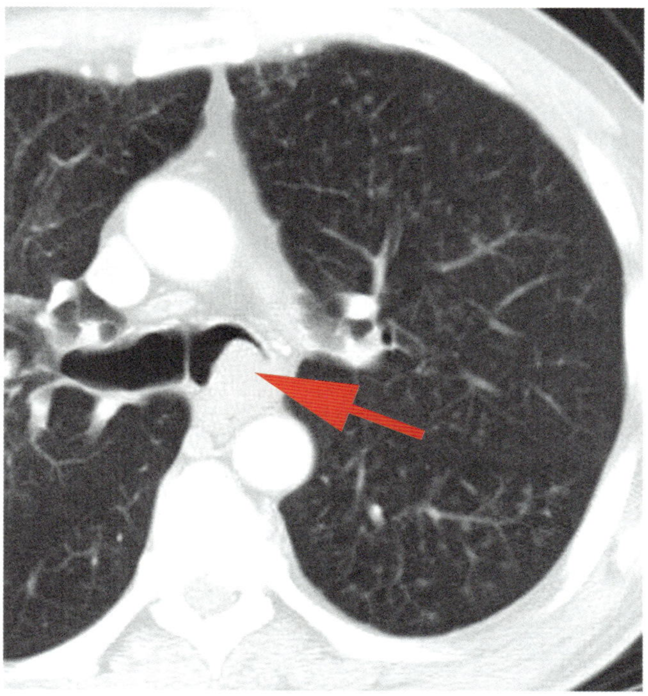

Figure 5.23. Adenoid cystic carcinoma. A polypoid lesion is visible in the left main bronchus (*arrow*).

Adenoid cystic carcinoma has a much better prognosis than do more common forms of lung carcinoma. However, it behaves in a more malignant fashion than does typical carcinoid tumor, is often infiltrative, and metastasizes more frequently.

These tumors are treated using surgical excision but tend to recur locally, as much as 15 years after resection. Recent advances in tracheal resection and carinal reconstruction have made many tracheal lesions resectable. The 5-year survival rate is about 75%.

Mucoepidermoid Carcinoma

MEC is a rare tumor. It may occur at any age, but the mean age at diagnosis is 30 to 40 years, and up to half of cases occur in patients under 30 years. MEC usually arises in the main or lobar bronchi; tracheal or peripheral lesions are uncommon. Low-grade MEC tends to exhibit a more benign course than does adenoid cystic carcinoma or carcinoid tumor, but it may be locally invasive. High-grade MEC has been reported to have a poor prognosis, similar to other non-small cell carcinomas. It is not associated with smoking, and specific gene mutations have been reported.

Presentation and radiographic findings are like those of adenoid cystic carcinoma. Because these tumors are often endobronchial, they result in symptoms and radiographic findings of bronchial obstruction. Surgery is usually curative in low-grade MEC.

PAPILLOMAS

This category includes squamous cell papilloma, glandular papilloma, and mixed squamous and glandular papilloma. Papillomas are most often endobronchial, but they may also occur in the peripheral lung.

Squamous Papilloma and Papillomatosis

A squamous papilloma (SP) consists of a connective tissue core covered by fronds of stratified keratinizing or nonkeratinizing mature squamous cells. SP usually results in a polypoid airway mass. SP may be solitary or multiple; the presence of multiple papillomas is termed *papillomatosis*, with variable involvement of the larynx, trachea, bronchi, and bronchioles.

SP are benign and, when multiple, are almost invariably of viral origin and caused by the human papillomavirus (HPV); less than half of solitary SP are associated with HPV. HPV subtypes 6 and 11 account for more than 90% of all cases. Malignant transformation occurs in about 2% of cases. It has been reported with HPV subtypes 16, 18, and 31/33/35 and may occur in association with mutations in *TP53*.

SP is the most common laryngeal tumor of childhood, and laryngeal papillomas occasionally occur in adults. Laryngeal lesions are often multiple and spread locally. In children, papillomas are successfully treated by surgical excision or regress at puberty.

In 2% to 5% of patients, SP spread distally to involve the tracheobronchial tree, a condition referred to as *tracheobronchial papillomatosis*; the trachea is almost always involved when distal spread occurs. Involvement of the trachea often results in cough or hemoptysis. Hoarseness due to laryngeal lesions may also be present. In most cases, the lesions are multiple and small, ranging from a few millimeters to 1 cm in diameter, but they can be large, resulting in tracheal obstruction. Plain radiographs are rarely of value; CT is usually necessary for diagnosis (Fig. 5.24).

Extension of papillomas to the bronchi, bronchioles, and lung parenchyma is rare. In patients with a history of laryngeal papillomas, the interval between the diagnosis of laryngeal lesions and distal bronchial spread ranges from 1 to more than 30 years. Although laryngeal lesions are most common in children younger than 5, the average age of patients with tumors involving the bronchial tree is 15. Bronchial obstruction results in wheezing, atelectasis, and recurrent pneumonia. Peripheral papillomas arising from small airways may be visible radiographically as nodular mass lesions within the lung, and they often cavitate. Eventually, cavitary lesions may progress to large thick- or thin-walled cysts. Nodules representing papillomas may be seen within cysts (Fig. 5.25). Cystic pulmonary lesions are not usually associated with symptoms.

Bronchoscopic excision or laser treatment of multiple tracheal or bronchial papillomas has been the treatment of choice, but the lesions recur following resection in more than 90% of patients, and instrumentation has been associated with distal spread. In patients with recurrent lesions, interferon alpha or antiviral drug treatment may be used; HPV vaccines may prove beneficial. Tracheostomy may

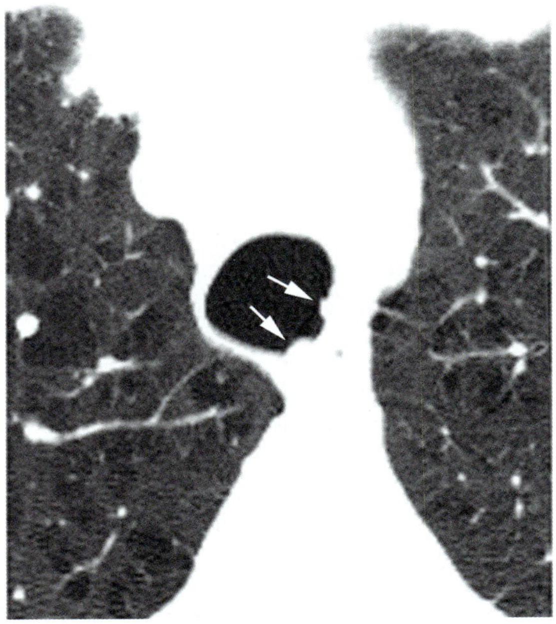

Figure 5.24. Tracheal papillomas. Small nodules (*arrows*) are visible arising from the tracheal wall.

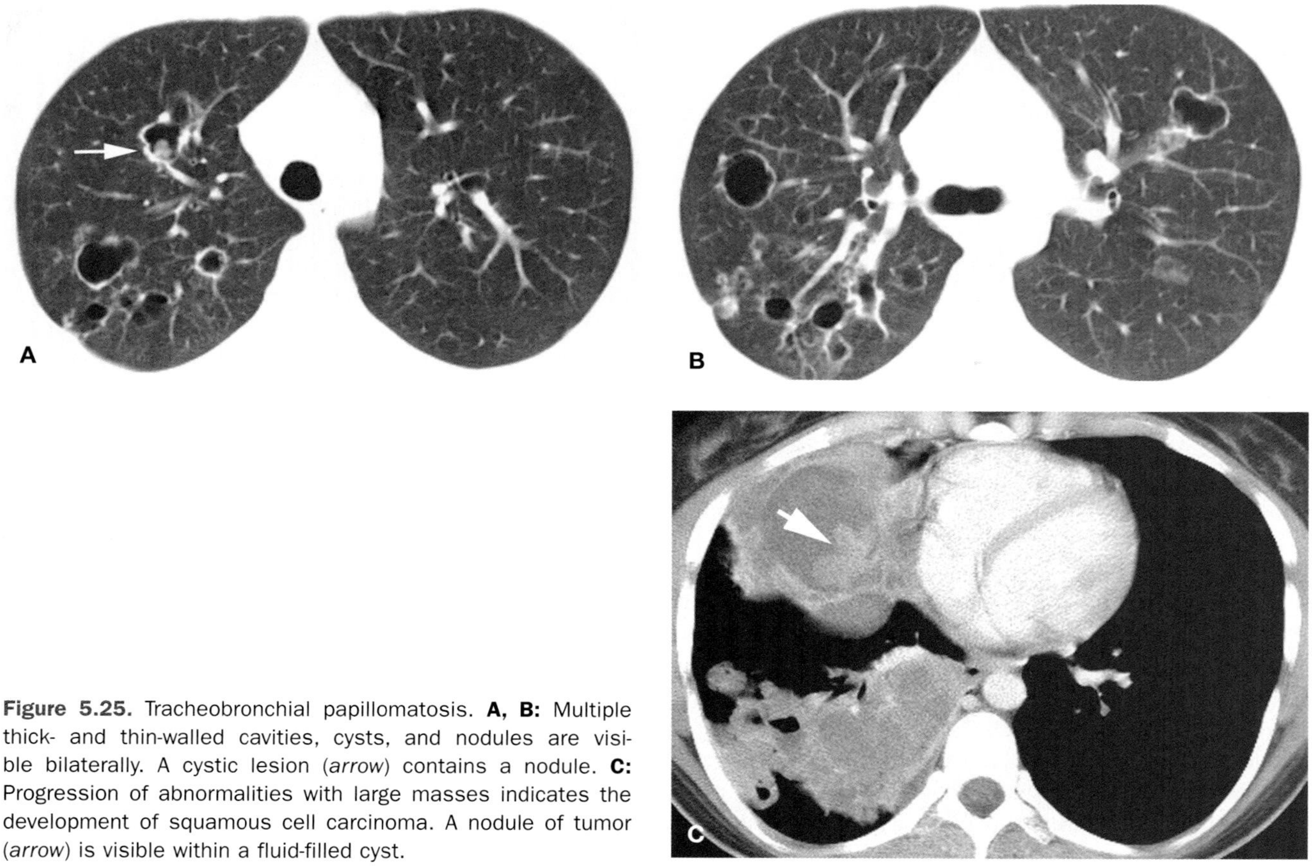

Figure 5.25. Tracheobronchial papillomatosis. **A, B:** Multiple thick- and thin-walled cavities, cysts, and nodules are visible bilaterally. A cystic lesion (*arrow*) contains a nodule. **C:** Progression of abnormalities with large masses indicates the development of squamous cell carcinoma. A nodule of tumor (*arrow*) is visible within a fluid-filled cyst.

be required for associated laryngeal lesions that produce airway obstruction. Malignant degeneration of bronchial or pulmonary lesions may occur, leading to SCC (see Fig. 5.25C).

Solitary papillomas occasionally occur in adults, usually middle-aged men, in the absence of prior laryngeal lesions. They are usually less than 1.5 cm in diameter and most are in a lobar or segmental bronchus. They may result in bronchial obstruction, and symptoms include cough and hemoptysis. Histology is identical to that found in papillomatosis. Most patients are smokers. Solitary SP do not recur after surgical excision, but up to 20% have local tumor recurrence after bronchoscopic removal.

Glandular Papilloma

Glandular papilloma accounts for about 20% of solitary papillomas; it is benign and characterized by pseudostratified or a single layer of ciliated or nonciliated columnar cells admixed with cuboidal cells or mucin-filled cells. Patients are usually in their 50s or 60s at diagnosis. Glandular papillomas tend to arise in lobar or segmental bronchi and present with symptoms of bronchial obstruction (Fig. 5.26). They are benign and do not recur following excision. Mixed squamous and glandular papilloma show an admixture of patterns.

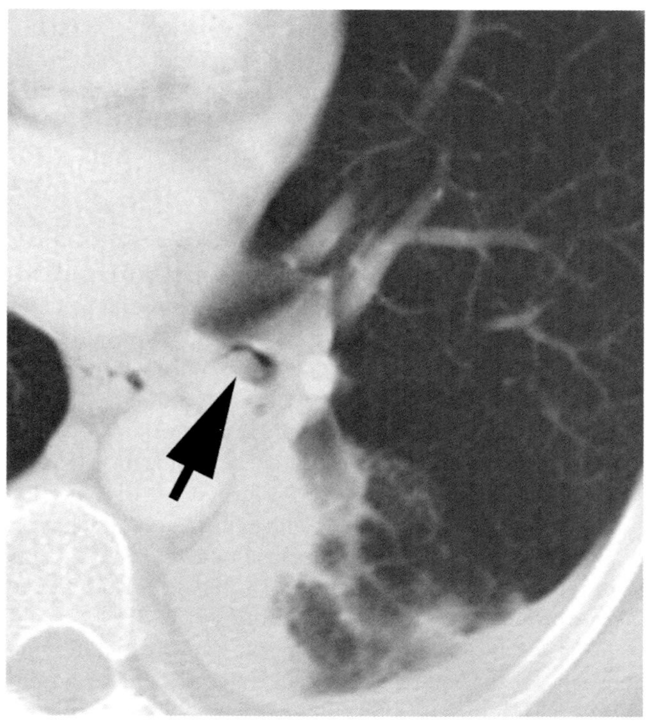

Figure 5.26. Glandular polyp. A polypoid lesion is visible in the left lower lobe bronchus (*arrow*).

ADENOMAS

Types of adenoma include sclerosing pneumocytoma, formerly termed sclerosing hemangioma, alveolar adenoma, papillary adenoma, mucinous cystadenoma, and mucous gland adenoma.

Mucous gland adenoma arises in central bronchi and present with symptoms or signs of bronchial obstruction. A wide age range has been reported. A rounded polypoid endobronchial mass is typically seen on CT. Mucous gland adenoma is benign and bronchoscopic or bronchial sleeve resection is usually appropriate.

Other adenoma cell types arise in the lung periphery, derived from bronchiolar or alveolar epithelium, and usually present as an asymptomatic lung nodule. Nodules are usually homogeneous in attenuation and solid, although rare cases appear cystic or show calcification. Although local invasion and even lymph node metastases have been reported, these tumors behave in a benign fashion after resection.

MESENCHYMAL TUMORS

More than 10 types of mesenchymal tumor are defined in the 2021 WHO classification. Most are very rare and lack specific radiographic findings. In general, mesenchymal tumors may present as a lung nodule or mass, usually detected incidentally on chest radiographs or CT, or as an endobronchial lesion, often rounded or sessile, and associated with symptoms and findings of bronchial obstruction or atelectasis.

Common mesenchymal tumors and those with specific or unique imaging appearances are described below. Mesenchymal tumors listed in the 2021 WHO classification, not discussed in detail, include congenital peribronchial myofibroblastic tumor, pleuropulmonary blastoma, synovial sarcoma, pulmonary myxoid sarcoma, and myoepithelial tumors, both benign and malignant.

Pulmonary Hamartoma

Pulmonary hamartoma is the most common mesenchymal tumor of the respiratory tract and accounts for more than 75% of benign lung tumors (Table 5.9). Pulmonary hamartomas (PH) are neoplasms composed of varying amounts of at least two mesenchymal elements (such as cartilage, fat, connective tissue, and smooth muscle), combined with respiratory epithelium. Because hamartomas in other parts of the body are not generally considered neoplasms, the designation of "pulmonary hamartoma" in the current WHO classification helps emphasize its neoplastic origin. It is characterized by several mutations.

PH are composed predominantly of chondroid or chondromyxoid tissue intermixed with variable proportions of other mesenchymal components, including fat, myxoid fibrous connective tissue, smooth muscle, and bone. Clefts of normal respiratory epithelium are present, being entrapped by the expanding mesenchymal tumor. Endobronchial PH may have a prominent adipose tissue component and overlap with bronchial lipoma described below.

Table 5.9 Pulmonary Hamartoma

75% of benign lung tumors
Patients >50 years of age
Twice as common in men
5%-15% endobronchial
≥85% present as solitary nodule
Usually 1-4 cm
Sharply circumscribed
Round or lobulated
Calcification in 25%
Popcorn calcification
Fat visible on CT in 60%
Slow growth

PH are usually diagnosed in patients older than 50 and are twice as common in men. They are rare in children, and less than 10% occur in patients younger than 40. Prior to the advent of CT (which greatly assists in their preoperative diagnosis), hamartomas accounted for as many as 6% to 8% of resected lung nodules.

In more than 85% of cases, PH appear radiographically as a solitary pulmonary nodule. Peripheral hamartomas are usually 1 to 4 cm in diameter, well defined, sharply circumscribed, and often lobulated. Only 5% to 15% of hamartomas present as an endobronchial mass (Fig. 5.27).

Calcification of cartilage is reported to be visible on plain radiographs in approximately 30% of PH, and the frequency of calcification increases with the tumor's size. Calcification is seen in less than 10% of PH less than 3 cm in diameter but is present in 75% of those 5 cm or larger. On CT, calcification is visible more often than on plain radiographs.

Calcification of PH can be stippled or conglomerate. Conglomerate or "popcorn" calcification is characteristic and is rarely seen with other lesions; it results from calcification of nodules of cartilage (Fig. 5.28). Accumulations of fat can produce lucent or low-attenuation areas within the tumor, usually visible only on CT. Rarely, cystic, air-filled PH have been reported.

CT with thin slices is valuable in diagnosing PH. Nearly 65% of hamartomas may be diagnosed using thin-slice CT because of visible fat (see Figs. 5.27 and 5.29), either focal or diffuse (CT numbers ranging from −40 to −120 HU), or a combination of fat and calcium. A nodule containing fat has a very limited differential diagnosis; lipoid pneumonia is another but much less common cause of this finding. Pulmonary teratoma could also show fat, but this tumor is extremely rare.

In most cases, PH grow slowly, increasing in diameter from 0.5 to 5 mm/year (Fig. 5.30). Rapid growth can occur, however, causing PH to be confused with lung carcinoma. Endobronchial lesions can be resected bronchoscopically unless infection has caused the destruction of the distal

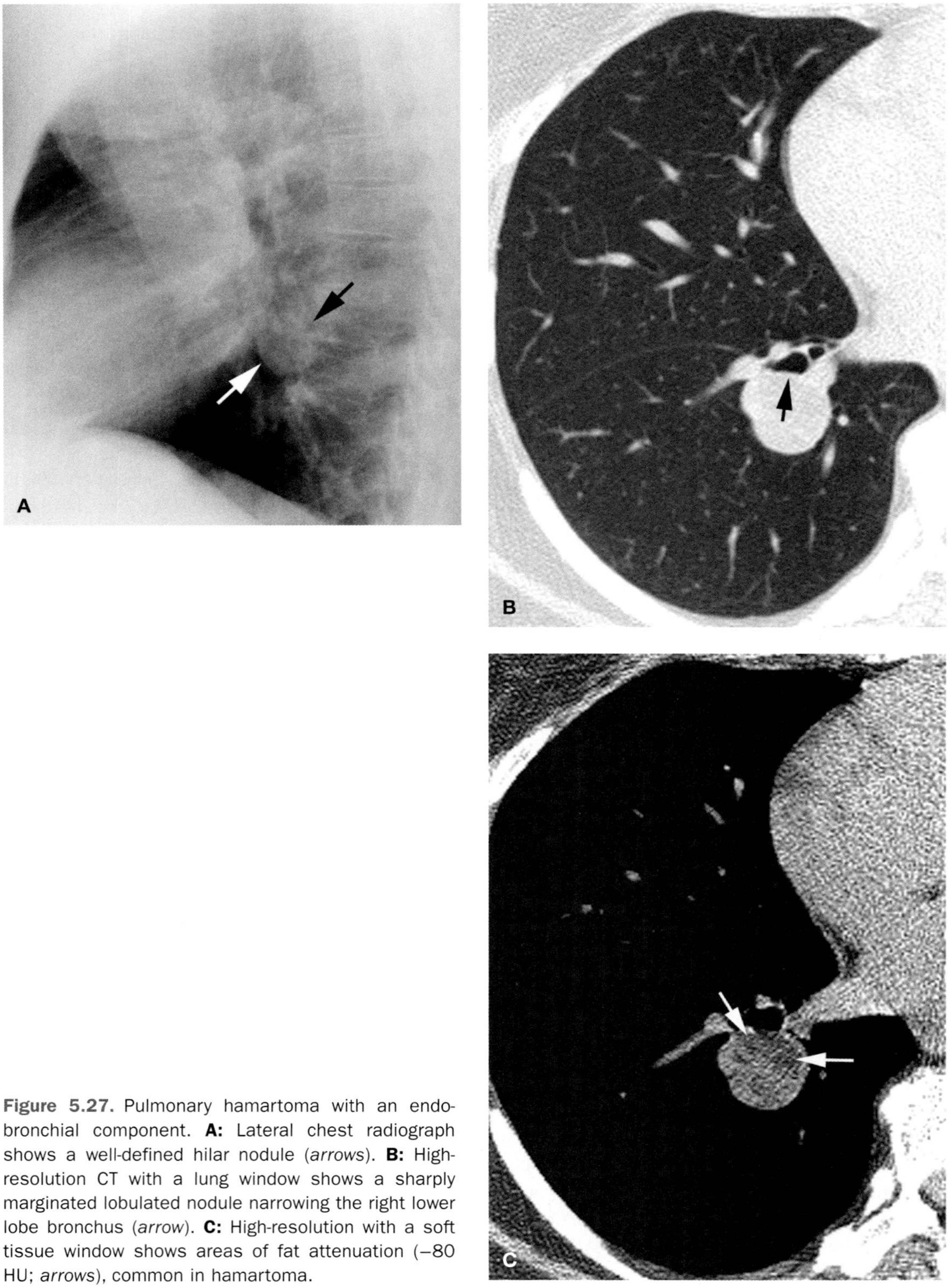

Figure 5.27. Pulmonary hamartoma with an endobronchial component. **A:** Lateral chest radiograph shows a well-defined hilar nodule (*arrows*). **B:** High-resolution CT with a lung window shows a sharply marginated lobulated nodule narrowing the right lower lobe bronchus (*arrow*). **C:** High-resolution with a soft tissue window shows areas of fat attenuation (–80 HU; *arrows*), common in hamartoma.

lung. Needle biopsy can be diagnostic in some cases, but peripheral tumors may require excision for diagnosis. Recurrence following resection and malignant transformation are rare.

Chondroma

True chondromas, containing only cartilage, are exceedingly rare. Unlike hamartoma, they lack epithelial clefts or other tissue elements. They may occur as an endobronchial lesion

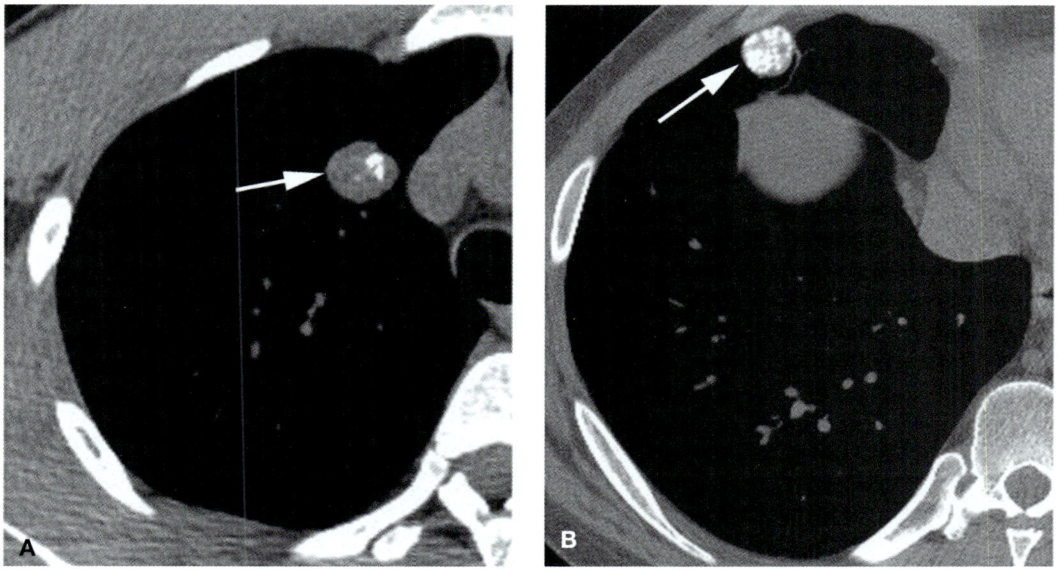

Figure 5.28. Calcified pulmonary hamartoma in two patients. **A:** Hamartoma (*arrow*) with focal calcification. The nodule is round and sharply defined. **B:** Hamartoma (*arrow*) with popcorn calcification. This appearance results from the calcification of nodules of cartilage in the tumor.

or a well-defined solitary nodule. Calcification occurs in about 30%.

Chondromas typically occur as part of *Carney's triad*. This unusual entity is characterized by the combination of multiple pulmonary chondromas, gastric epithelioid leiomyosarcoma, and extra-adrenal paraganglioma. In some cases, only two of the three manifestations are present. This syndrome is most common in female patients less than 30; only 10% of cases occur in male patients. Sporadic cases of chondroma are very rare, usually occurring in middle-aged men.

Chondrosarcoma is also very rare. This tumor occurs much more commonly as a pulmonary mass lesion than as a mass within the trachea or bronchial lumen. They have a very poor prognosis.

PEComatous Tumors and Lymphangioleiomyomatosis

PEComatous tumors are characterized by the presence of perivascular epithelioid cells (PEC), which do not exist in normal subjects. They are classified by WHO as (1) lymphangioleiomyomatosis (LAM), (2) benign PEComa and clear cell tumor, and (3) malignant PEComa. Benign and malignant PEComas usually appear as a lung mass.

Historically, LAM has been considered an interstitial lung disease, but recent findings have resulted in its classification as a low-grade destructive, metastasizing neoplasm. LAM cells usually have growth-promoting biallelic mutations in the tuberous sclerosis gene *TSC2* and show evidence of clonal origin. Genetics and immunohistochemistry in LAM and other PEComas show consistent similarities. Rarely, a diffuse proliferation of PEC with overlapping features between LAM and clear cell tumor may be seen, termed *diffuse PEComatosis*. LAM is described in detail in Chapter 25.

Diffuse Pulmonary Lymphangiomatosis

This entity represents a diffuse proliferation of lymphatic spaces and smooth muscle along otherwise normal lymphatics in the lung and mediastinum. It is typically diagnosed in the neonatal period or in childhood and is characterized by progressive respiratory failure and eventual death. In adults, it may present with wheezing, chylous effusions, and progressive respiratory failure. CT or radiographs may show interstitial thickening characterized by interlobular septal thickening, peribronchial interstitial thickening, mediastinal widening and infiltration, and pleural effusion. There is no effective treatment.

Inflammatory Myofibroblastic Tumor

This tumor is characterized by myofibroblastic spindle cells with an inflammatory infiltrate consisting of plasma cells and lymphocytes. Historically, it has had many names, which should no longer be used, including inflammatory pseudotumor, plasma cell granuloma, fibrous histiocytoma, and invasive fibrous tumor.

Inflammatory myofibroblastic tumor may occur in both children and adults. Although half of the patients are asymptomatic, symptoms include fever, cough, chest pain, and hemoptysis. Tumors may appear as well-marginated peripheral lung nodules or masses, may resemble pneumonia, or may involve the trachea or bronchi. Calcification or regions of necrosis may be present. Involvement of the mediastinum or pleura is uncommon. Inflammatory myofibroblastic

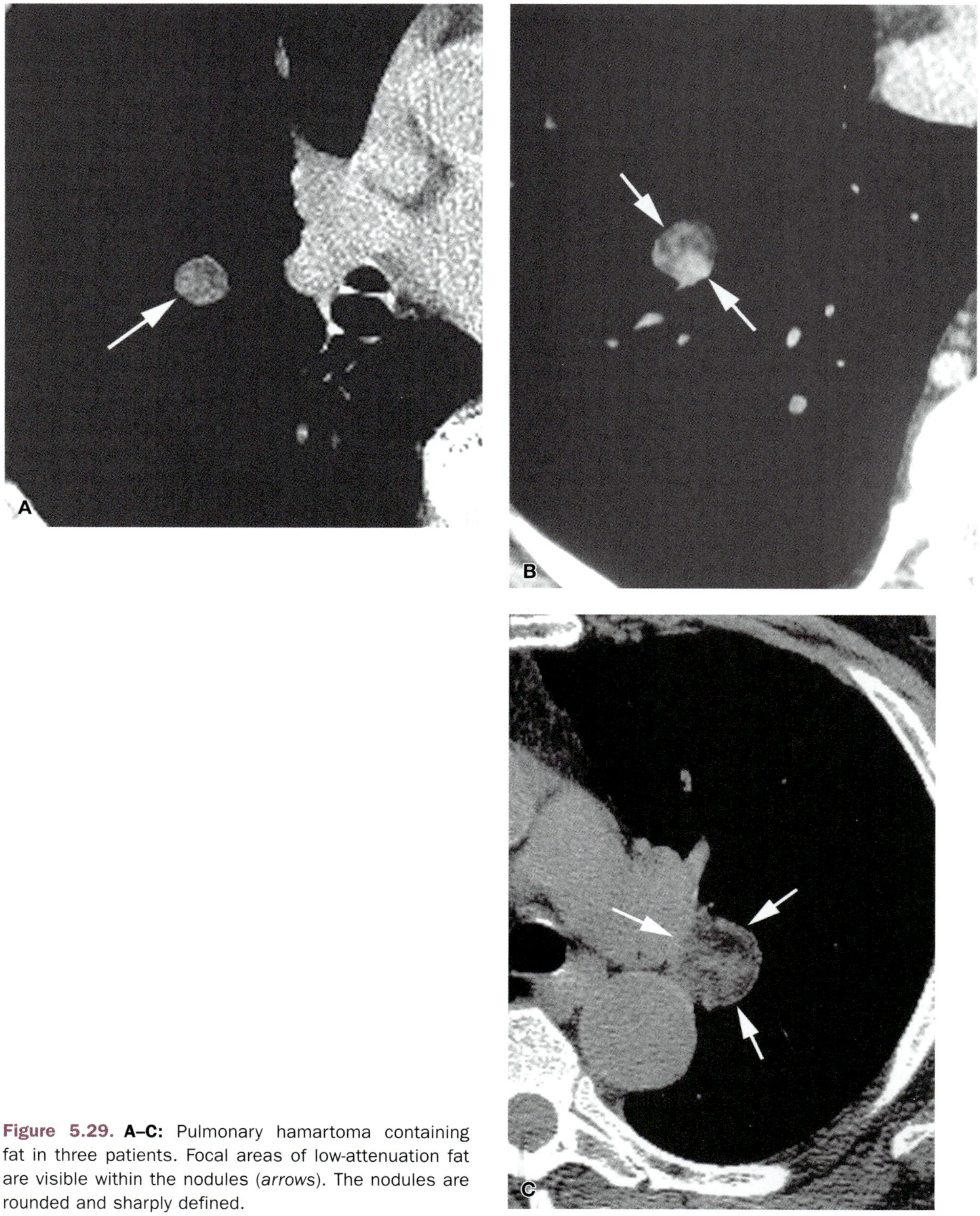

Figure 5.29. A–C: Pulmonary hamartoma containing fat in three patients. Focal areas of low-attenuation fat are visible within the nodules (*arrows*). The nodules are rounded and sharply defined.

tumor behaves in an indolent fashion, but recurrence or metastasis may occur following incomplete resection, particularly for large tumors.

Epithelioid Hemangioendothelioma

Epithelioid hemangioendothelioma is a rare multifocal pulmonary neoplasm. Multiple genetic abnormalities are present. In more than 60% of cases, it is manifested by multiple well-defined or poorly defined lung nodules up to 2 cm in diameter, mimicking the appearance of metastases. Solitary masses up to 5 cm have also been reported. Nodules may calcify or cavitate. Eighty percent of cases occur in female patients, often less than 40 years old. The tumors may be asymptomatic or associated with cough, hemoptysis, or systemic symptoms. This entity is thought to represent a low-to

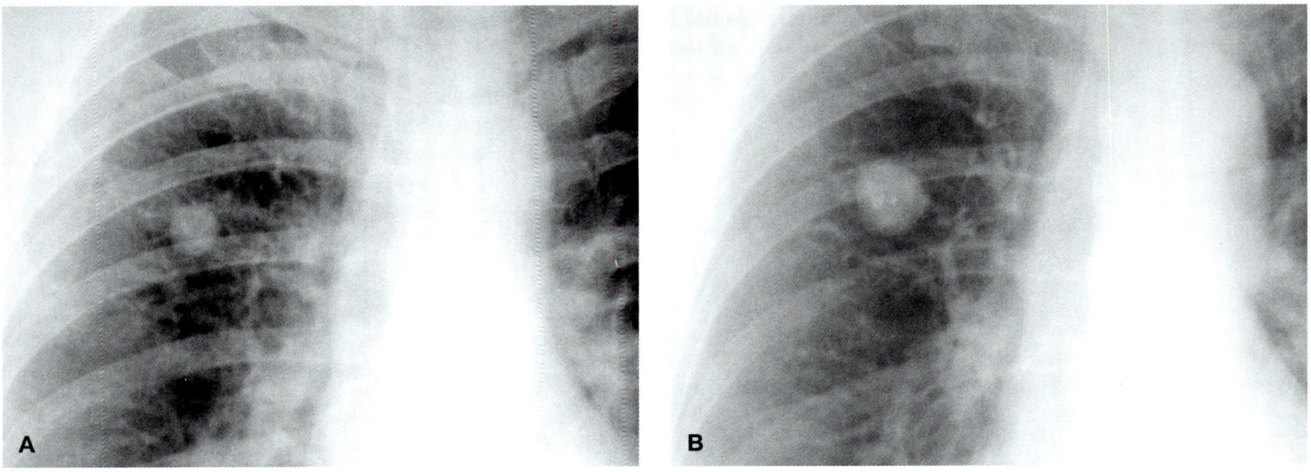

Figure 5.30. Pulmonary hamartoma with growth. **A:** Chest radiograph shows a well-defined upper lobe nodule measuring 1 cm. **B:** Radiograph 3 years later. The nodule now measures 2 cm in diameter. Several foci of calcification are visible within the nodule. The doubling time of this nodule is 1 year.

intermediate-grade vascular tumor, and metastases may sometimes occur. Liver involvement or involvement of other sites may be associated, representing metastases or synchronous development in multiple sites. Five-year survival is about 60%.

Pulmonary Artery Intimal Sarcoma

Pulmonary artery intimal sarcoma, also termed *pulmonary artery sarcoma*, originates from the intima of elastic pulmonary arteries. Clinically, it is commonly misdiagnosed as acute or chronic pulmonary embolism because symptoms mimic this diagnosis. It has been found in a few percent of pulmonary thromboendarterectomy specimens in patients with chronic thromboembolic pulmonary hypertension. The average age at presentation is 50 to 60 years.

Pulmonary artery intimal sarcoma involves the proximal elastic pulmonary arteries (main, right, or left), from the pulmonary valve to lobar branches. On CT, a large intraluminal filling defect is typically seen, which may be irregular, often expansile, and is adherent to the artery wall. This appearance may closely mimic that of chronic pulmonary embolism. However, pulmonary artery intimal sarcoma is often unilateral or predominates on one side, an atypical finding for central pulmonary embolism. Intimal sarcomas grow on serial follow-up exams and the diagnosis may not be recognized until after patients fail anticoagulation therapy.

Delayed enhancement with contrast-enhanced CT or MRI, or increased uptake on FDG-PET may be helpful in distinguishing sarcoma (or endovascular metastases, which may have the same appearance) from pulmonary embolism.

Miscellaneous Mesenchymal Tumors

Mesenchymal tumors may arise from any mesenchymal tissue normally present in the lung and bronchi. These tumors have similar characteristics to those described for tumors when arising in soft tissue and are classified separately by WHO. Several are reviewed below.

Lipoma and Liposarcoma

Lipoma and liposarcoma originate in collections of fat found in the walls of cartilage-containing airways. Lipoma overlaps with fatty hamartoma; liposarcoma is very rare. They may occur in patients of any age, usually ranging from 30 to 65, and nearly 90% occur in men.

Lipomas are most common in the main or lobar bronchi and typically are found in the bronchial lumen. Endobronchial lesions are usually oval, measuring several centimeters in length. They uncommonly occur in the peripheral lung. Symptoms and radiographic findings of bronchial obstruction are common, and obstructive pneumonitis and bronchiectasis are often present. Occasionally, a lipoma extends in a dumbbell fashion to lie primarily outside the bronchus. CT can be diagnostic, showing uniform low attenuation indistinguishable from a fat-containing hamartoma.

Leiomyoma and Leiomyosarcoma

Leiomyoma is thought to arise from smooth muscle found in the walls of the bronchi or perhaps blood vessels. The average age at diagnosis is 50 years, but it occurs in patients ranging from 5 to 65 years; females are more frequently affected. Leiomyoma may occur as a lung nodule (slightly more common) or an endobronchial lesion. Pulmonary parenchymal leiomyomas are usually asymptomatic and detected incidentally. They appear radiographically as well-defined, lobulated, peripheral mass lesions and range up to 20 cm in diameter. Calcification is rare and cavitation does not occur. Endobronchial lesions usually occur in the main or lobar bronchi. Symptoms are common and often due to obstructive pneumonia. In such patients, radiographic findings are usually limited to signs of airway obstruction. CT may show an endobronchial mass.

Leiomyosarcoma is more common than leiomyoma. Patients are usually symptomatic. Radiographs demonstrate a pulmonary mass in most cases, and in general, tumors are larger than leiomyomas. Cavitation may occur. Endobronchial obstruction with atelectasis occurs in about a third of patients.

Multiple pulmonary "leiomyomas" associated with benign smooth muscle tumors of the uterus in females have been termed *benign metastasizing leiomyoma* (Fig. 5.31). The smooth muscle tumors have been found to be clonal and identical to the patient's uterine tumors but with benign histology. Some genetic differences, seen in only a few percent of uterine leiomyomas, have been found. The etiology of benign metastasizing leiomyoma is unclear; suggestions include (a) pulmonary metastases from a low-grade, and undiagnosed, uterine leiomyosarcoma, (b) "metastases" from benign uterine tumors associated with specific mutations or perhaps spread in a manner similar to endometriosis, and (c) a primary pulmonary or generalized leiomyomatosis. Single or multiple lung masses are usually seen on radiographs or CT. They may be quite large, may calcify, and grow slowly (Fig. 5.31). Thin-walled air- or fluid-filled cysts may be associated, best seen on CT (Fig. 5.32).

Fibroma and Fibrosarcoma

Fibroma can involve the lung or tracheobronchial tree and is rare. Pulmonary parenchymal lesions are most common and are usually asymptomatic. Tracheal or bronchial lesions produce symptoms and signs of obstruction.

Fibrosarcomas, regardless of their location, are usually symptomatic. They more often appear as a nodule or mass rather than as an endobronchial lesion. Endobronchial lesions are most common in children and young adults, while pulmonary masses are found in patients of middle age. Pulmonary lesions are usually round and well defined, measuring up to 20 cm in diameter.

HEMATOLYMPHOID TUMORS

Hematolymphoid tumors, as classified by WHO in 2021 (Table 5.2), include (1) extranodal marginal zone lymphomas of mucosa-associated lymphoid tissue (MALT lymphoma), (2) diffuse large B-cell lymphoma, (3) lymphomatoid granulomatosis, (4) intravascular large B-cell lymphoma, (5) pulmonary Langerhans cell histiocytosis, and (6) Erdheim–Chester disease (ECD).

The lymphomas and lymphomatoid granulomatosis are discussed in Chapter 7. Pulmonary Langerhans cell

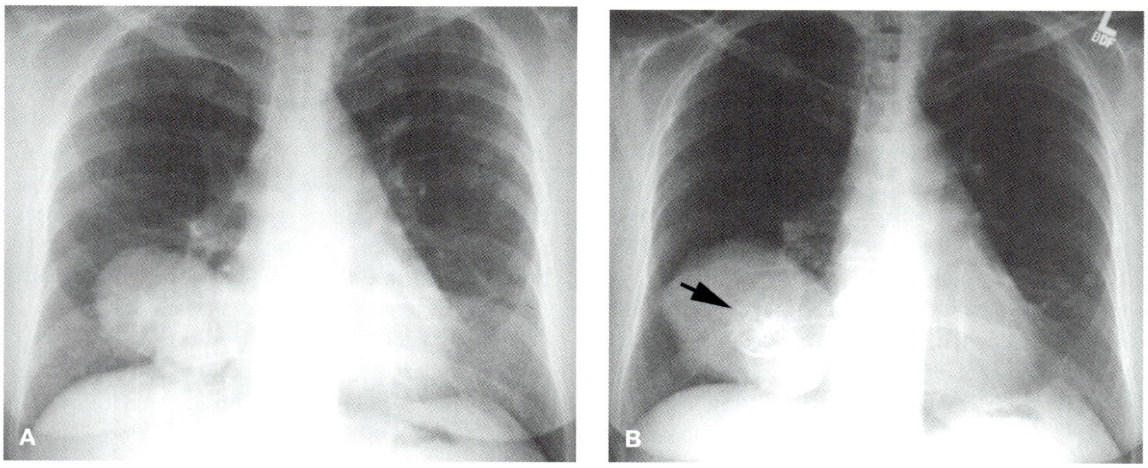

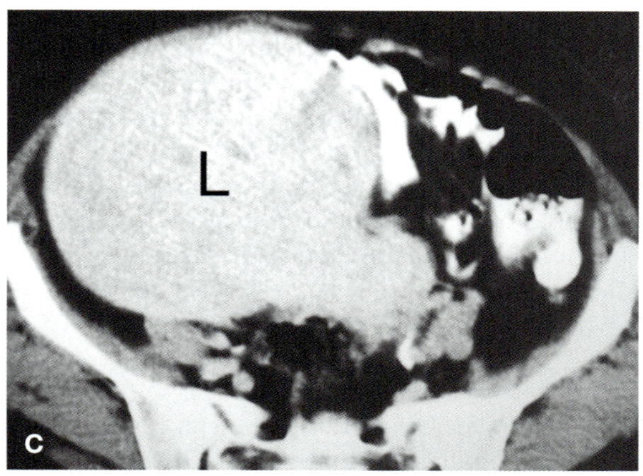

Figure 5.31. Benign metastasizing leiomyoma. **A:** Chest radiograph shows a large right lower lobe mass. **B:** Ten years later, the mass has increased in size. Some central calcification is visible (*arrow*). **C:** CT at the time of prior hysterectomy shows a large uterine mass, representing a low-grade leiomyosarcoma (*L*).

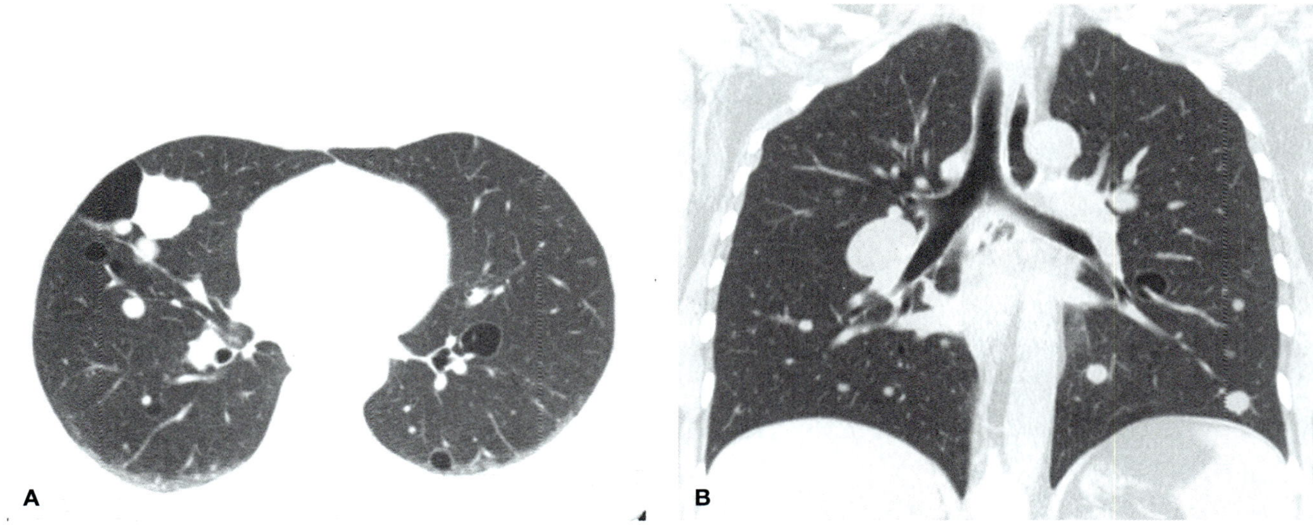

Figure 5.32. Benign metastasizing leiomyoma. **A, B:** In a female patient with proven BML, solid and thin-walled cystic lesions are visible. Some solid lesions were of fluid attenuation.

histiocytosis is discussed along with cystic lung diseases in Chapter 25. ECD is discussed below.

Erdheim–Chester Disease

ECD is a very rare xanthogranulomatous histiocytosis characterized by organ infiltration by lipid-laden (foamy) histiocytes. Some studies suggest it is clonal and specific (V600E) genetic mutations of the BRAF gene in more than half of the cases. EDC affects the skeleton, kidney, heart, and central nervous system, and the lungs are involved in 20% to 30% of cases. Lung involvement consists of interstitial infiltration by histiocytes with resulting fibrosis. Pulmonary symptoms are nonspecific, consisting of cough and dyspnea. Other symptoms include bone pain, fever, weight loss, weakness, exophthalmos, and cardiac or neurological symptoms. In some studies, pulmonary involvement is associated with a poor prognosis. However, targeted therapy with vemurafenib (a BRAF enzyme inhibitor) has been valuable in providing a rapid clinical response.

CT manifestations of thoracic involvement include mediastinal infiltration, right atrial wall infiltration with narrowing of the atrial lumen, pericardial thickening or effusion, and pleural effusion. Lung abnormalities show a perilymphatic distribution, with interlobular septal and subpleural interstitial thickening, poorly defined centrilobular nodules, GGO, and lung cysts. Perinephric and retroperitoneal soft tissue masses are common and may be seen at the inferior aspect of a chest CT.

TUMORS OF ECTOPIC ORIGIN

Tumors usually associated with other sites of origin, occurring in the lung, include germ cell tumors, neurogenic tumors, intrapulmonary thymoma, melanoma, and meningioma. These are exceedingly rare.

Germ Cell Tumors

Germ cell tumors arise from a mix of various germ cells. Most pulmonary germ cell lung tumors are teratomas consisting of tissues derived from one or more embryonic germ layer, with the exclusion of a gonadal or other primary site of origin. They are very rare.

Neural Tumors

Neurogenic tumors of the lung and tracheobronchial tree, both benign and malignant, are rare. They are thought to arise from sympathetic nerve fibers accompanying arterioles or bronchioles. Among benign tumors are neurofibroma, schwannoma, paraganglioma, and meningioma. Neurofibrosarcoma is less common. These most often present as well-defined solitary nodules within the lung parenchyma, but endobronchial lesions have been reported. Neurofibroma, schwannoma, and neurofibrosarcoma may be associated with neurofibromatosis, particularly when multiple.

METASTATIC TUMORS

Metastatic tumors are considered in Chapter 6.

RADIOGRAPHIC APPEARANCES OF LUNG CANCER AND LUNG TUMORS

Although lung tumors can manifest themselves in a variety of ways, a short list of radiographic abnormalities is commonly seen, regardless of the cell type. These abnormalities reflect the location and manner in which lung tumors arise and the common sites to which they may spread. Such abnormalities include the presence of a lung nodule, evidence of bronchial

Table 5.10 Plain Radiologic Findings in Lung Cancer by Cell Type[a]

Finding	Squamous (%)	Adenocarcinoma (%)	Small Cell (%)	Large Cell (%)
Peripheral nodule or mass	30	**75**	5	**65**
Atelectasis	**40**	10	20	15
Consolidation	20	15	20	25
Hilar enlargement	**40**	20	**80**	30
Mediastinal mass	<5	<5	**15**	**10**
Pleural effusions	5	5	5	5
No abnormalities	5	<5	0	0
Multiple abnormalities	35	30	65	45

[a]*Boldface findings are those most helpful in differentiating cell types. Percentages are approximate.*

obstruction with collapse or consolidation of a lobe or lung, a hilar or mediastinal mass, and benign or malignant pleural effusion.

Although the frequency of these findings varies according to the cell type of the tumor (Table 5.10), each of the major cell types of lung carcinoma (adenocarcinoma, SCC, neuroendocrine carcinoma, LCC, salivary gland-type tumors, etc.) can show similar findings. Common or unique imaging findings associated with specific tumors are also discussed in the section devoted to the particular tumor.

Solitary Pulmonary Nodule or Mass

Approximately one-third to one-half of lung cancers present radiographically as a solitary pulmonary nodule or lung mass. A solitary pulmonary nodule (see Figs. 5.2-5.8) is usually defined as being visible as a focal opacity on chest radiographs or CT and is

1. Relatively well defined
2. At least partially surrounded by the lung
3. Roughly spherical
4. 3 cm or less in diameter
5. Solid, of GGO, or both

Similar lesions larger than 3 cm in diameter are usually referred to using the term *mass* (see Figs. 5.1, 5.13, 5.18, and 5.22). This measurement is also used to distinguish T1 carcinomas (3 cm or less in diameter) from a carcinoma classified as T2 or higher (larger than 3 cm).

Among lung cancers presenting as a solitary nodule or mass, the most common cell types are adenocarcinoma (50%-70% of cases) (see Figs. 5.5-5.7) and SCC (15%-20% of cases). LCC, LCNEC, small cell carcinoma, and carcinoid tumors each account for a few percent of lung nodules. LCC and LCNEC typically present as a large mass (see Fig. 5.22), averaging nearly twice the diameter of adenocarcinomas.

Lung cancers presenting as a solitary pulmonary nodule may have specific radiographic appearances that strongly suggest the diagnosis (Table 5.11); if a combination of radiologic, clinical, and laboratory information is used, malignant pulmonary nodules can be diagnosed in over 90% of patients. The radiographic assessment of a solitary pulmonary nodule is a common and important problem; this topic is discussed in greater detail in Chapter 10. The differential diagnosis of a solitary nodule is reviewed in Table 10.1.

Table 5.11 Radiographic Characteristics of a Solitary Pulmonary Nodule That Suggests Lung Cancer

Diameter >2 cm
Upper lobe
Ill-defined, irregular, or spiculated margin
Lobulated or irregular in shape
Solid, ground-glass opacity with a solid component or pure ground-glass opacity
Containing air bronchograms or bubbly lucencies (pseudocavitation)
Cavitation with a thick (>15 mm) and nodular wall
Cavitation without an air–fluid level
Calcification absent or not typical of a benign pattern
Enhancement of ≥15 HU following contrast infusion
Doubling time of 30-200 d (although adenocarcinoma associated with lepidic growth may be very slow growing, ie, doubling time >1000 d)

Superior Sulcus (Pancoast) Tumor

Tumors arising at or near the lung apex are termed *superior sulcus carcinoma, thoracic inlet carcinoma*, or simply *apical carcinoma*. The term *Pancoast tumor* is best reserved for patients with some (although not necessarily all) manifestations of the Pancoast syndrome. Approximately 3% to 5% of lung cancers occur in the superior sulcus; any cell type may be responsible, but adenocarcinoma predominates.

Superior sulcus tumors are commonly associated with symptoms because of their propensity to invade structures in the thoracic inlet, including the brachial plexus, cervicothoracic sympathetic ganglia, subclavian artery and vein (Fig. 5.33), and vertebral column. *Pancoast syndrome* results from the involvement of the brachial plexus and sympathetic ganglia and consists of the combination of

1. Pain in the shoulder
2. Radicular pain along the distribution of the eighth cervical and first and second thoracic nerves, sometimes associated with wasting of the small muscles of the hand
3. Horner's syndrome, consisting of ptosis, miosis, and hemifacial anhidrosis

Classic Pancoast syndrome is uncommon. Most superior sulcus tumors present with shoulder or scapular pain that radiates down the arm and may be associated with ulnar neuropathy. Horner's syndrome is present in only about 25% of patients; atrophy or weakness of the hand muscles is uncommon. Rib or vertebral body invasion is common in patients with superior sulcus tumors.

Radiographic findings include an apical mass (60%), unilateral or asymmetrical apical pleural thickening ("apical cap," 40%), and bone destruction (25%) (Fig. 5.33A). Asymmetry in the thickness of an apical cap exceeding 5 mm is considered suggestive. The presence of an apical cap may reflect diseases other than carcinoma (Table 5.12).

Superior sulcus carcinomas, even if invasive, can often be treated using a combination of pre- or postoperative radiation, chemotherapy, and en bloc resection of the tumor and adjacent chest wall; 5-year survival rates as high as 30% to 50% have been reported using this approach. Contraindications to this therapy generally include (1) tumor involvement of the great vessels above the lung apex, principally the subclavian artery or vein; (2) extensive brachial plexus invasion; (3)

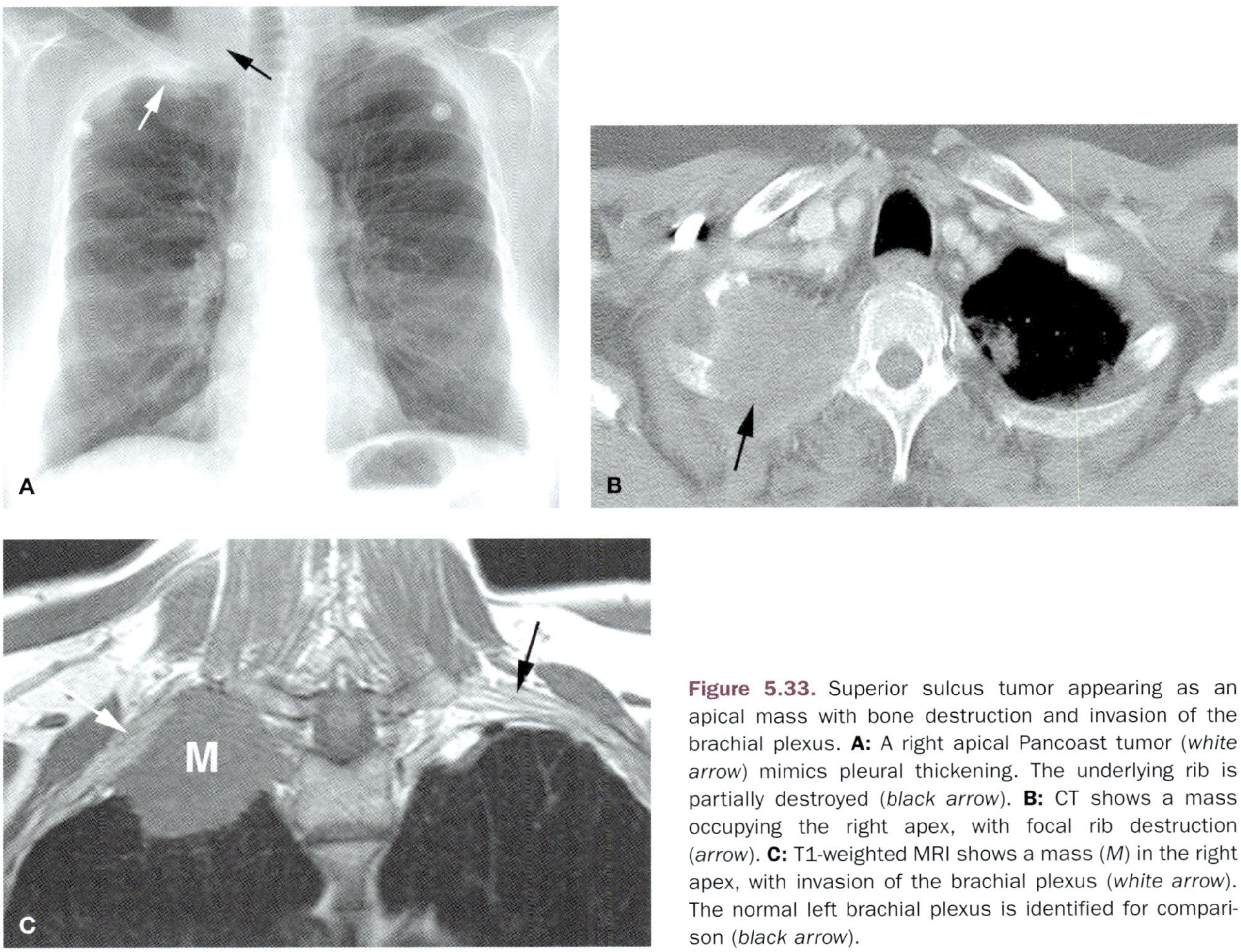

Figure 5.33. Superior sulcus tumor appearing as an apical mass with bone destruction and invasion of the brachial plexus. **A:** A right apical Pancoast tumor (*white arrow*) mimics pleural thickening. The underlying rib is partially destroyed (*black arrow*). **B:** CT shows a mass occupying the right apex, with focal rib destruction (*arrow*). **C:** T1-weighted MRI shows a mass (*M*) in the right apex, with invasion of the brachial plexus (*white arrow*). The normal left brachial plexus is identified for comparison (*black arrow*).

Table 5.12 Differential Diagnosis: Apical Cap/Apical Mass

Normal apical cap: Unilateral or bilateral apical caps, usually <5 mm in thickness, are each seen in 10% of normals on chest radiographs. These represent apical lung scars unassociated with tuberculosis, although their etiology is unclear.

Extrapleural fat: Extrapleural fat deposition can result in smooth, symmetrical apical caps. This can be seen in normals, obese patients, and patients with Cushing's syndrome or those receiving steroids.

Inflammatory disease (tuberculosis): Apical caps associated with inflammatory disease (particularly TB) are rarely the only abnormality visible. Associated upper lobe fibrosis, volume loss, lung destruction, or other evidence of inflammatory disease is usually present. The cap is often quite irregular in appearance because of adjacent lung abnormalities and in one study ranged from 5 to 27 mm in thickness (mean 16.5 mm). In patients with TB, thickened extrapleural fat accounts for most of the apical cap, variably associated with thickening of the pleura and atelectatic lung.

Superior sulcus carcinoma

Neural tumor or other posterior mediastinal mass: These are typically localized masses.

Mesothelioma: Diffuse pleural thickening is often seen.

Mediastinal hemorrhage: Mediastinal blood can dissect laterally in the extrapleural space over the lung apex, resulting in a smooth apical cap. This can be seen with traumatic aortic rupture and is more common on the left.

Radiation fibrosis: Radiation therapy can result in apical lung fibrosis mimicking an apical cap. This is most common following head and neck or supraclavicular node radiation.

Peripheral upper lobe collapse: Peripheral upper lobe collapse is said to be present when the peripheral part of a collapsed upper lobe is pancaked against the apical pleural surface (see Fig. 2.34). It has been reported in a variety of conditions, including inflammatory diseases and bronchial obstruction.

extensive vertebral body or spinal canal invasion; (4) clinical evidence of recurrent laryngeal nerve or phrenic nerve involvement; (5) involvement of the mediastinum, including the trachea or esophagus; and (6) distant metastases. Some patients may have restaging of an extensive tumor following chemotherapy to determine whether resection is possible. In patients with unresectable tumors, chemotherapy and radiation may prolong survival.

Volumetric three-dimensional imaging is of great value in demonstrating tumor extent and its relationship to vital structures. MRI in the sagittal or coronal planes is particularly advantageous and is more accurate than CT in diagnosing apical chest wall invasion and its extent. MRI is often obtained preoperatively in patients with superior sulcus carcinoma to define the relationship of the tumor to great vessels and the brachial plexus (Figs. 5.33 and 5.34). The radiographic assessment of chest wall invasion and superior sulcus tumor is discussed in detail in the section on lung cancer staging below.

Airway Abnormalities

Airway abnormalities are common in lung cancer. The segmental bronchi are most often involved by the primary tumor, followed in frequency by the lobar bronchi and the main bronchi. The trachea is rarely involved as the site of origin.

Radiographs or CT can show evidence of bronchial narrowing or obstruction or abnormalities secondary to bronchial obstruction, such as mucous plugging, air trapping, atelectasis, or obstructive pneumonia. Although lung cancer is a common cause of bronchial obstruction, the differential diagnosis is long and should be kept in mind (Table 5.13).

Bronchial Abnormalities

Bronchial abnormalities sometimes can be recognized on chest radiographs in patients with lung cancer, but CT is much more sensitive. Abnormalities include

1. Narrowing or tapering of the bronchial lumen, a finding that reflects the tendency of lung carcinomas to infiltrate along the bronchial wall (Fig. 5.35A); a tapered narrowing, or "rat-tail," appearance of the bronchial lumen is highly suggestive of carcinoma.
2. Sharp cutoff of the bronchial lumen (see Fig. 5.35B).
3. An endobronchial mass, sessile, irregular, or polypoid in appearance (see Fig. 5.35C).
4. Bronchial wall thickening, most easily seen involving the posterior wall of the right upper lobe bronchus or bronchus intermedius (see Fig. 5.35D).
5. Smooth luminal narrowing caused by bronchial wall infiltration or bronchial compression by an extrinsic mass (see Fig. 5.35D and E).

CT is commonly used to identify bronchial abnormalities in patients with lung cancer in conjunction with bronchoscopy. CT can serve to identify the bronchi involved by the mass, thus guiding bronchoscopy, and can better assess the presence and degree of tumor extension outside the bronchus.

Generally speaking, the CT findings of an endobronchial lesion, an abrupt bronchial occlusion, or bronchial wall irregularities correlate closely with what is seen at bronchoscopy, but the appearances of smooth luminal narrowing or tapered bronchial occlusion can be seen with either endobronchial disease or extrinsic mass.

Mucous Plugging

Rarely, an obstructing or partially obstructing tumor causes retention of mucus distal to the obstruction, while the lobe remains aerated because of collateral ventilation. This can

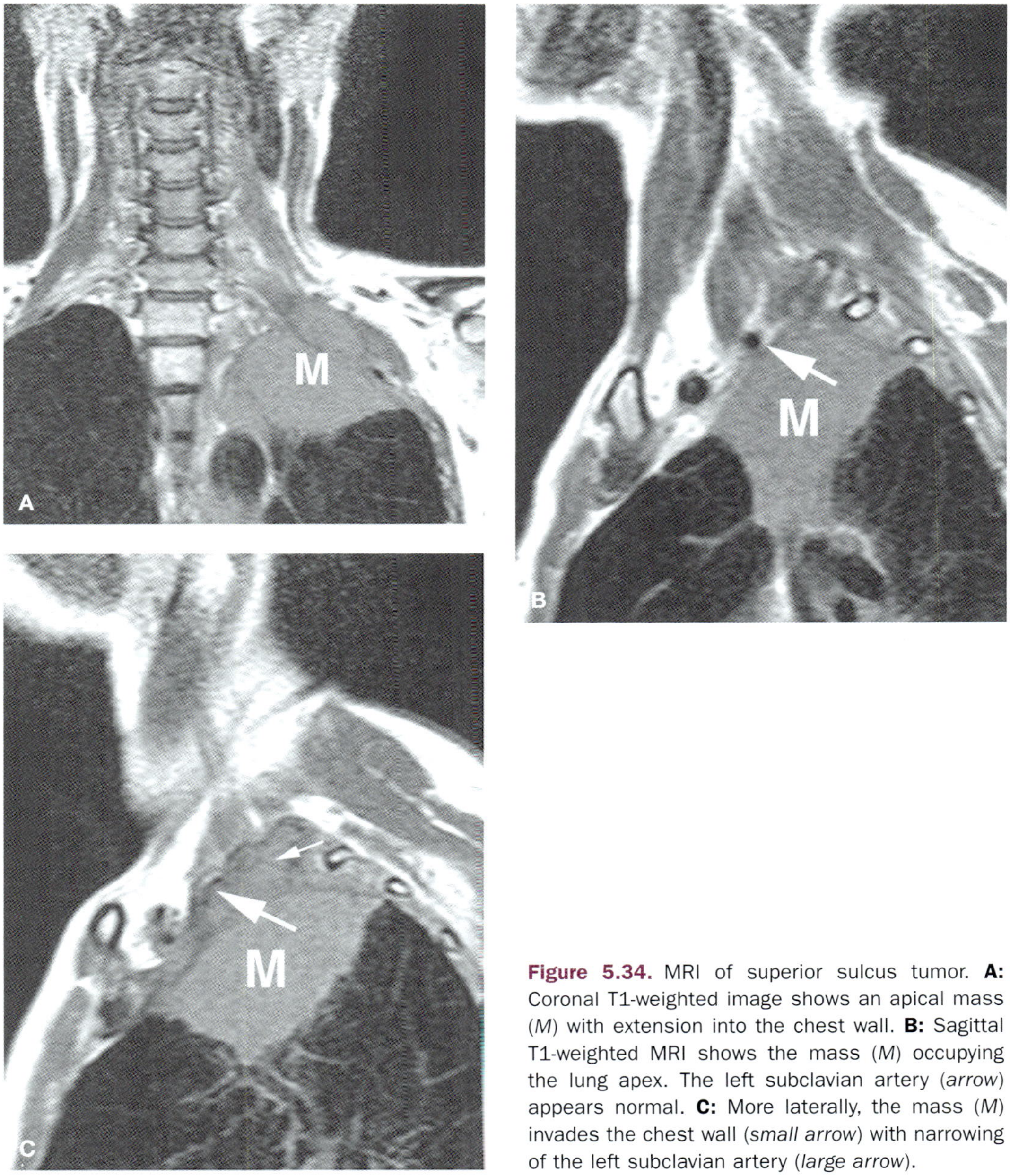

Figure 5.34. MRI of superior sulcus tumor. **A:** Coronal T1-weighted image shows an apical mass (*M*) with extension into the chest wall. **B:** Sagittal T1-weighted MRI shows the mass (*M*) occupying the lung apex. The left subclavian artery (*arrow*) appears normal. **C:** More laterally, the mass (*M*) invades the chest wall (*small arrow*) with narrowing of the left subclavian artery (*large arrow*).

result in a mucous plug or plugs visible on radiographs or CT (Fig. 5.36). It can be recognized on plain film or CT by its typical branching, "finger-in-a-glove," or clustered-grape appearance. On CT, mucous plugs often appear low in attenuation.

More common causes of mucous plugging include asthma, allergic bronchopulmonary aspergillosis, and cystic fibrosis. In patients with these diseases, however, mucous plugs are usually multiple and bilateral. In a patient with focal mucous plugging, bronchoscopy is advisable to rule out an obstructing lesion. In addition to lung cancer, focal mucous plugging can result from benign tumors, strictures, or congenital bronchial atresia.

Air Trapping

An obstructing or partially obstructing carcinoma rarely causes air trapping within the lung distal to the tumor. If a lobar bronchus is involved, the volume of the lobe may be increased. If the lesion involves a main bronchus, the distal lung is of normal or slightly decreased volume on inspiration, but on expiration, air trapping will be recognized. In some patients, bronchial obstruction and air trapping can be detected because of hypovascularity of the involved lobe or lung; poorly ventilated lung tends to be poorly perfused.

Table 5.13 Differential Diagnosis of Bronchial Narrowing or Obstruction

Congenital (bronchial atresia, bronchogenic cyst, cartilage deficiency)
Primary malignant tumor
- Lung carcinoma
- Carcinoid and atypical carcinoid
- Salivary gland-type carcinoma
- Sarcoma

Metastatic tumor
Lymphoma
Benign bronchial tumor (eg, hamartoma)
Papilloma or papillomatosis
Granulomas
- Infectious (eg, tuberculosis, fungal infection)
- Noninfectious (eg, sarcoidosis, granulomatosis with polyangiitis [Wegener's granulomatosis])

Inflammatory stricture (many causes)
Malacia
- Postinflammatory

Polychondritis
Foreign body
Mucous plug
Infiltrative diseases (eg, amyloidosis)
Compression by enlarged lymph nodes (many causes)
Broncholithiasis
Traumatic hematoma or bronchial fracture
Postoperative (eg, lung transplantation)

Tracheal Carcinoma

Less than 1% of lung carcinomas arise in the trachea. SCC and carcinomas of mucous gland origin (adenoid cystic carcinoma) are most common, with SCC being more common in most studies. SCCs arise most commonly in the distal trachea (Fig. 5.37), near the carina, and may cause the obstruction of a main bronchus; adenoid cystic carcinoma is most common in the proximal trachea and often arises from the posterior or lateral tracheal wall.

Radiographic studies may be important in suggesting the diagnosis, because symptoms are often late and nonspecific. Radiographic findings are similar to those seen with tumors affecting the bronchi. However, findings of obstructive pneumonia or air trapping are not seen unless there is secondary involvement of a main bronchus. Focal tracheal narrowing associated with thickening of the right paratracheal stripe, a focal endotracheal lesion, or mediastinal mass is most common on radiographs (Fig. 5.38A). CT may show a polypoid mass, sessile mass, or focal or diffuse tracheal wall thickening. Invasion of the mediastinum may occur, best seen using CT. If the mass extends posteriorly, esophageal obstruction can result (see Fig. 5.38B). Surgery can be curative if the diagnosis is made prior to mediastinal invasion. Tracheal tumors are also discussed in Chapter 22.

Atelectasis, Consolidation, and Diffuse Parenchymal Involvement

Obstructive Atelectasis and Consolidation

Many lung cancers demonstrate atelectasis and/or consolidation as a result of obstruction of a lobar, main, or segmental bronchus or bronchi. Atelectasis is common; a segment, lobe, or entire lung may be involved (see Fig. 5.11). Infection with pneumonia or lung abscess can also result.

The degree of volume loss associated with obstructive atelectasis is variable. The affected lung may be completely airless and reduced to its minimum volume. Alternatively, the

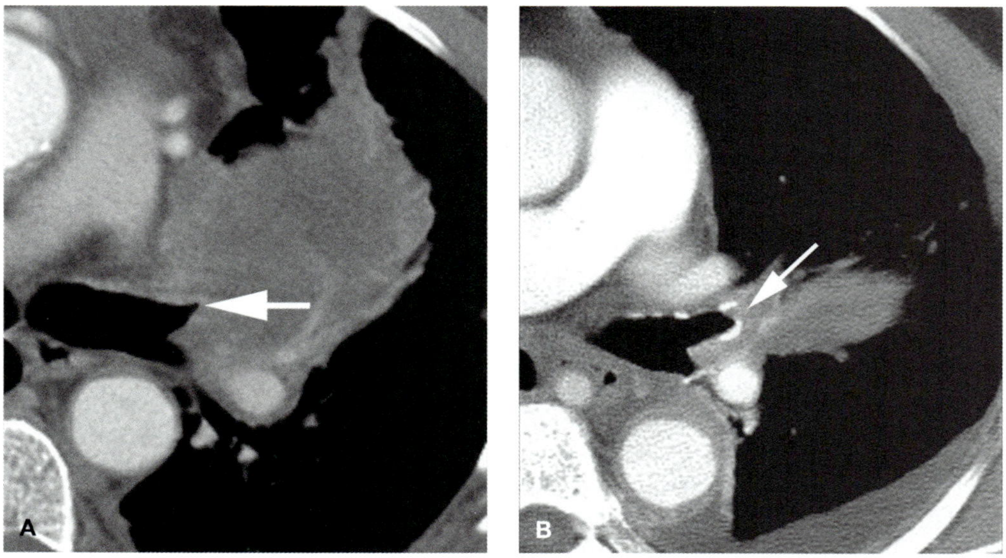

Figure 5.35. Bronchial abnormalities in lung cancer. **A:** The left upper lobe bronchus is obstructed and shows a tapered narrowing or rat-tail appearance (*arrow*). Left upper lobe atelectasis is also present. **B:** Left upper lobe carcinoma (*arrow*) associated with sharp cutoff of the bronchial lumen.

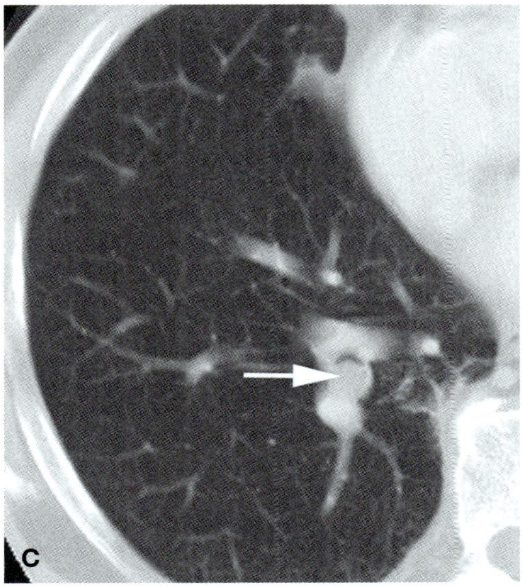

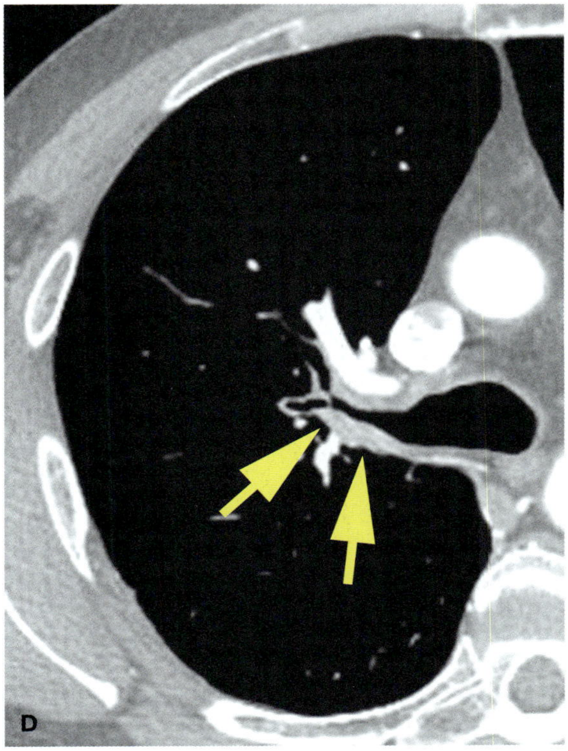

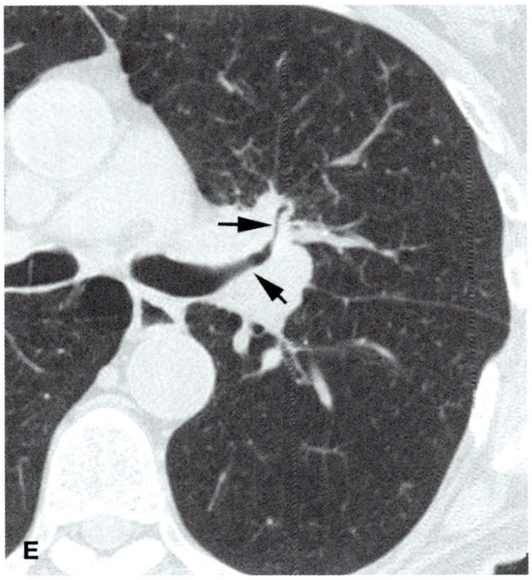

Figure 5.35. (*Continued*) **C:** A polypoid carcinoma (*arrow*) is visible in the right lower lobe bronchus, outlined by a crescent of air. **D:** Thickening of the posterior wall of the right upper lobe bronchus (*arrows*). This usually indicates bronchial infiltration by tumor. **E:** Narrowing of the left upper lobe and anterior segment bronchi (*arrows*) by a left hilar carcinoma. This may be caused by tumor infiltrating the bronchial wall or compression by an extrinsic mass.

obstructed lobe or lung may become filled with desquamated material, mucus, and fluid and lose little of its volume. In both instances, the absence of air bronchograms in the presence of atelectasis and consolidation is suggestive of bronchial obstruction (see Chapter 1). On the other hand, air bronchograms are sometimes visible in the presence of a partially obstructing central bronchial lesion. Low-attenuation mucus-filled bronchi ("mucous bronchograms") are often seen on CT in the presence of bronchial obstruction and lung collapse, particularly when contrast infusion is used (Fig. 5.39).

Obstructive pneumonia is a common manifestation of bronchial obstruction in lung cancer and is visible in about 35% of patients with SCC. This term refers to the presence of obstructive atelectasis, bronchial dilatation and mucous plugging, fibrosis, and parenchymal consolidation by lipid-filled macrophages and inflammatory cells. This entity is sometimes referred to as *endogenous lipoid pneumonia* or "golden pneumonia" because of its yellow color at gross pathology. Infection need not be present. On chest radiographs, lung consolidation and volume loss are typically present. On CT, bronchial obstruction by tumor, lung consolidation, and mucous bronchograms within the consolidated lung are often visible. Areas of necrosis within the tumor mass or lung are sometimes visible using CT.

Typically, a lung carcinoma involves a single bronchus, resulting in the collapse of the segment, lobe, or lung distal to the lesion. It has been suggested that the collapse of two segments or lobes that cannot be explained by the presence of a single endobronchial lesion (eg, the right upper and middle lobes, with the lower lobe being normal) indicates that a benign process is much more likely than lung cancer. This association of two or more endobronchial lesion with benign disease has been termed the "double-lesion sign" (see Fig. 1.42 in Chapter 1). Rarely, a hilar lung carcinoma produces a double-lesion sign by arising in one bronchus and invading or compressing another. In any patient with persisting

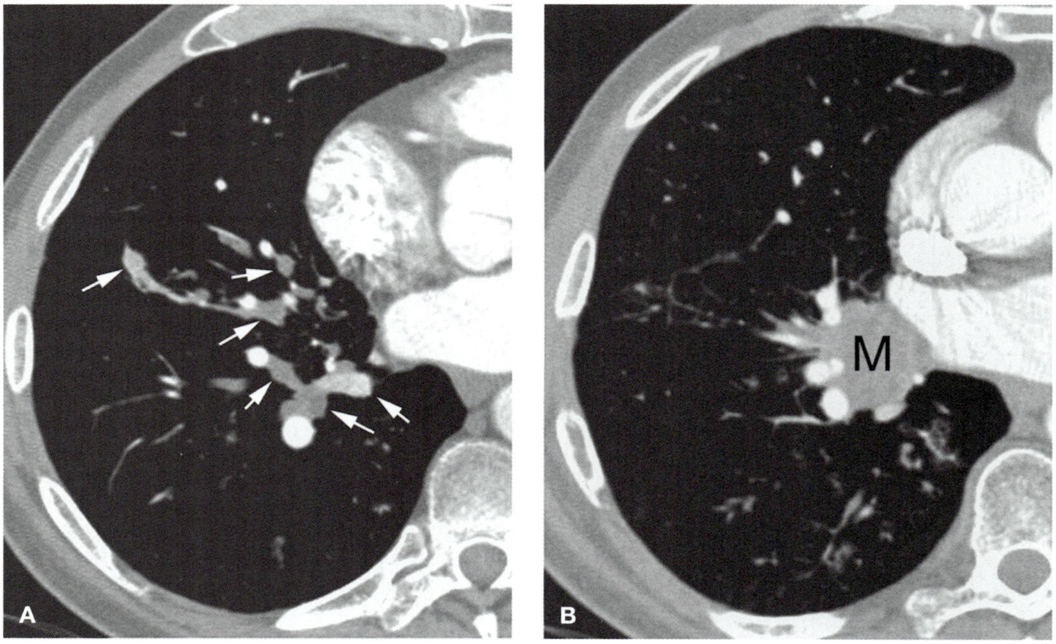

Figure 5.36. Mucous plugs in a patient with carcinoma and bronchial obstruction. **A:** Mucous plugs (*arrows*) fill lower lobe bronchi. Note that the mucus-filled bronchi lie adjacent to opacified pulmonary arteries. The distal lung remains aerated. **B:** At a higher level, a hilar mass (*M*) is associated with the obstruction of the right lower lobe bronchus.

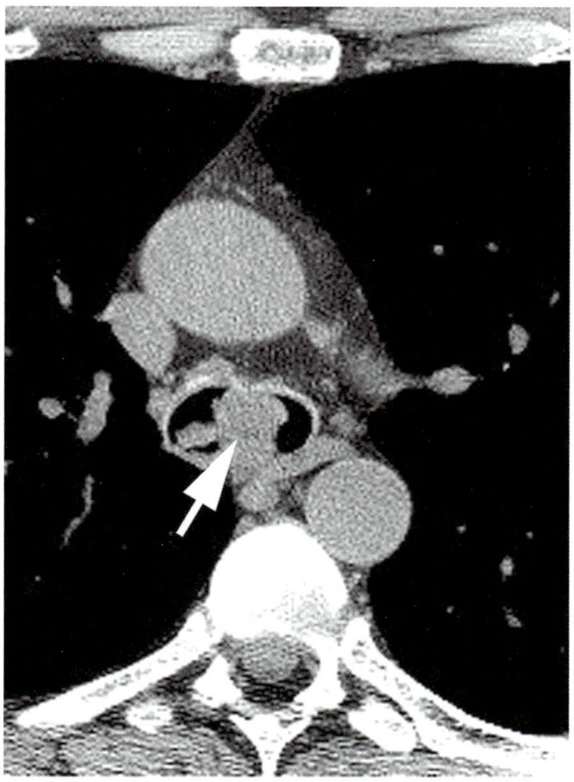

Figure 5.37. Polypoid squamous cell carcinoma of the trachea. A rounded mass (*arrow*) is visible at the level of the carina.

bronchial obstruction, regardless of what segments or lobes are involved, CT and bronchoscopy are advisable.

Consolidation in Invasive Mucinous Adenocarcinoma

IMA, described in detail above, may result in lung consolidation because of mucin produced by the tumor cells. Most patients with IMA show a combination of findings. These include

1. Patchy, lobar, or diffuse consolidation, with air bronchograms (60%; see Figs. 5.9, 5.10, and 5.40A)
2. Multiple ill-defined nodules (30%; see Figs. 5.9, 5.10, and 5.40B and C), which may appear centrilobular
3. Patchy, lobar, or diffuse GGO (10%) (Fig. 5.10)
4. Multilobar or bilateral distribution, although asymmetry is often present (Figs. 5.9, 5.10, and 5.40B)

Consolidation in patients with IMA is often indistinguishable from pneumonia on plain films. On CT, the consolidation seen in patients with IMA is typically low in attenuation or appears as GGO; this largely reflects the presence of watery fluid and mucin produced by the tumor. If a contrast-enhanced CT is obtained, enhancing pulmonary vessels can be seen within areas of consolidation; this has been termed the "CT angiogram sign" and reflects the low density of the consolidated lung (see Figs. 1.4B and 1.9 in Chapter 1). The CT angiogram sign is typical of IMA and should alert you to the possibility of this diagnosis, but it can also be seen with any other cause of consolidation. In IMA,

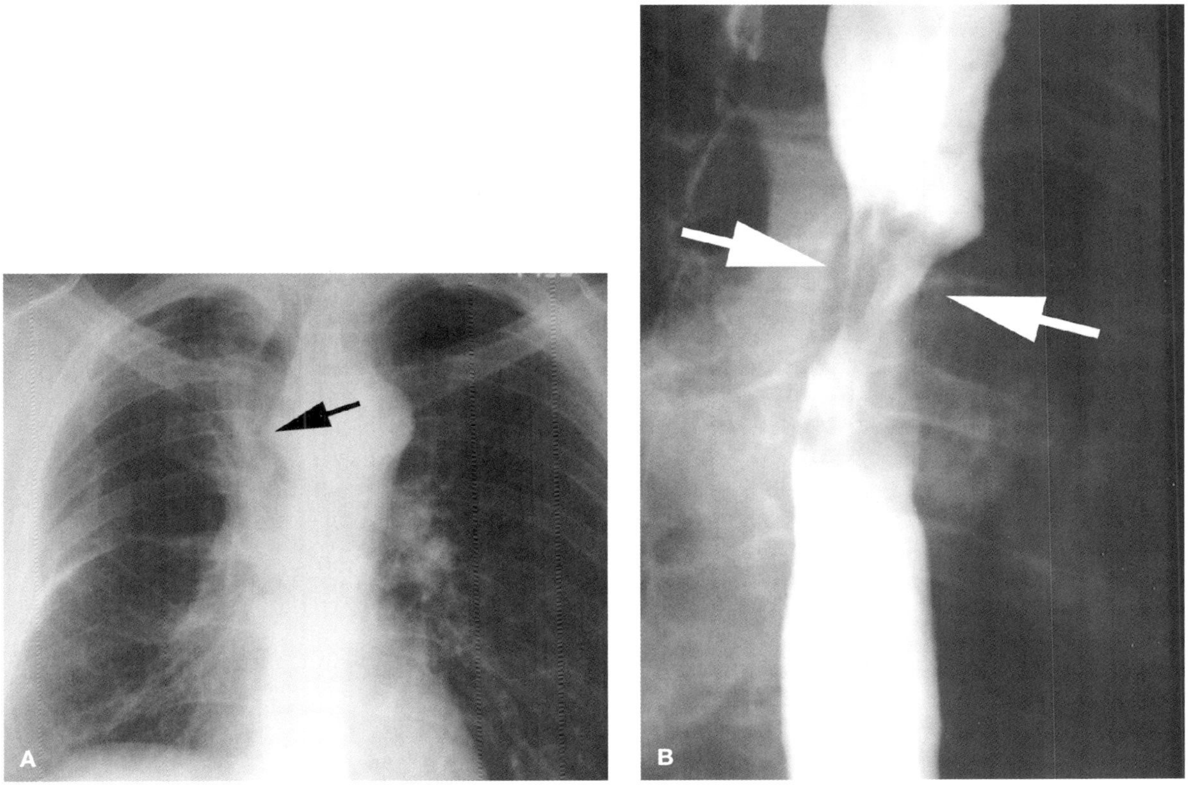

Figure 5.38. Squamous cell carcinoma of the trachea with mediastinal invasion and esophageal involvement. **A:** Plain radiograph shows tracheal displacement to the right by a large mediastinal mass (*arrow*). Focal tracheal narrowing by an endobronchial mass is present. **B:** Esophagogram shows esophageal compression and narrowing (*arrows*) because of invasion by the tumor.

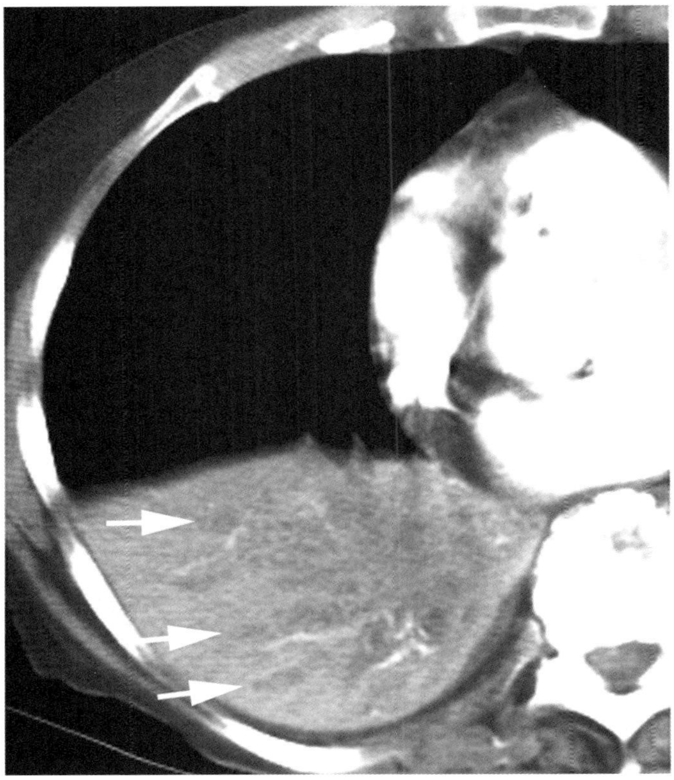

Figure 5.39. Obstructive pneumonia with mucous bronchograms. In a patient with a right hilar carcinoma, right lower lobe consolidation is associated with minimal volume loss. This is typical of obstructive pneumonia. Mucous bronchograms (*arrows*) are visible.

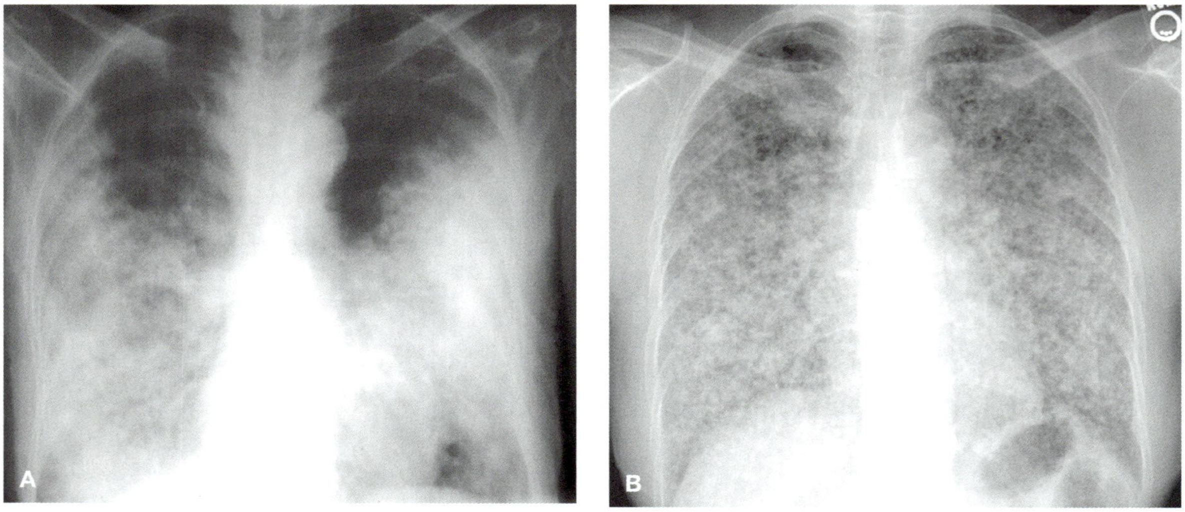

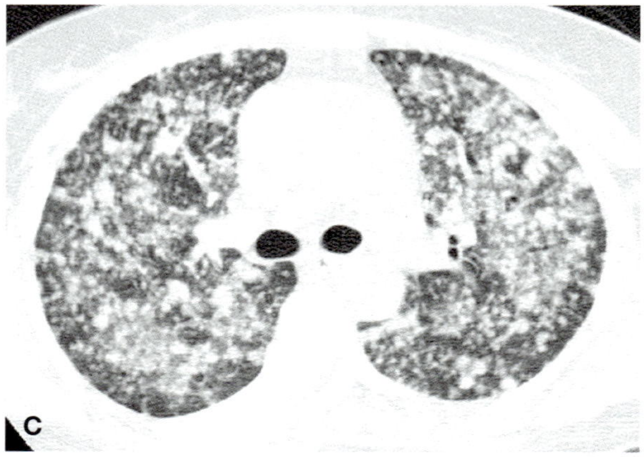

Figure 5.40. Invasive mucinous adenocarcinoma (IMA). **A:** IMA with bilateral lung consolidation. **B:** IMA in another patient with bilateral small ill-defined nodules. **C:** High-resolution CT in the same patient as in (**B**) shows diffuse small nodules.

lung consolidation is not associated with bronchial obstruction; however, air bronchograms may be absent because of fluid within the bronchi.

Ill-defined nodules associated with IMA reflect focal areas of consolidation and have characteristics typical of air-space nodules (see Figs. 5.9, 5.10, and 5.40B). They usually measure from 5 mm to 1 cm in diameter but can be larger. On CT, they are usually centrilobular in location.

Lymphangitic Spread of Tumor

Lung carcinoma commonly spreads via the lymphatic system or interstitium. Diffuse involvement of the pulmonary lymphatics or interstitium results in the appearance of lymphangitic spread of carcinoma, often in association with hilar node enlargement and pleura effusion. The classic plain film appearance is a unilateral or asymmetrical increase in pulmonary interstitial markings, which may be associated with Kerley's B lines; however, atypical appearances are common. High-resolution CT typically shows interlobular septal thickening (Fig. 5.41), thickening of the peribronchovascular interstitium, and thickening of fissures.

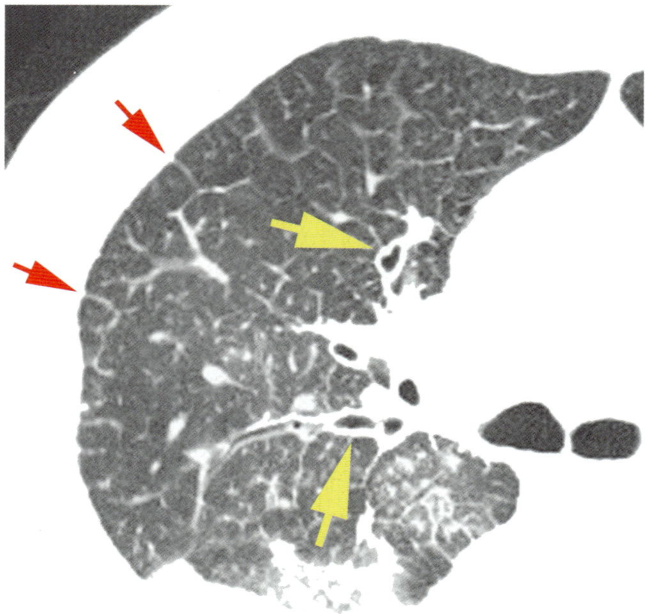

Figure 5.41. Lymphangitic spread of lung carcinoma. High-resolution CT shows typical findings of unilateral interlobular septal thickening (*red arrows*) and thickening of the peribronchovascular interstitium (*yellow arrows*). A right pleural effusion is also present.

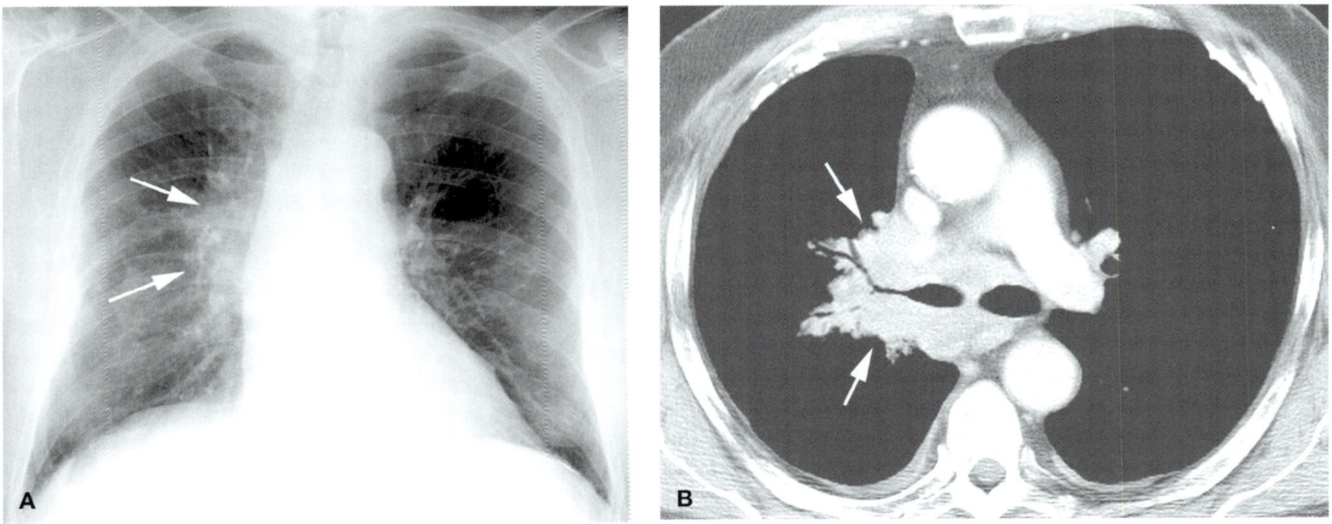

Figure 5.42. Right hilar carcinoma in a patient with asbestos exposure. **A:** Chest radiograph shows an ill-defined right hilar mass (*arrows*). This is typical of carcinoma originating in the hilum. Pleural thickening and calcification typical of asbestos exposure are visible. **B:** A large, poorly marginated right hilar mass (*arrows*) surrounds and narrows the right upper lobe bronchus. This appearance is most typical of small cell carcinoma.

Lymph Node Enlargement

Hilar and mediastinal node enlargement is detected radiographically or on CT in up to 35% of lung cancers at diagnosis, although 50% have evidence of node metastasis at surgery. The diagnosis of hilar and mediastinal mass and lymph node enlargement is discussed in detail in other chapters.

Hilar Mass or Lymph Node Enlargement

Hilar enlargement visible on radiographs can reflect the primary tumor arising in a central location (usually, this results in a poorly marginated hilar mass that may be large; Fig. 5.42) or metastases to hilar lymph nodes from a peripheral lung primary (usually a well-defined hilar mass; Fig. 5.43).

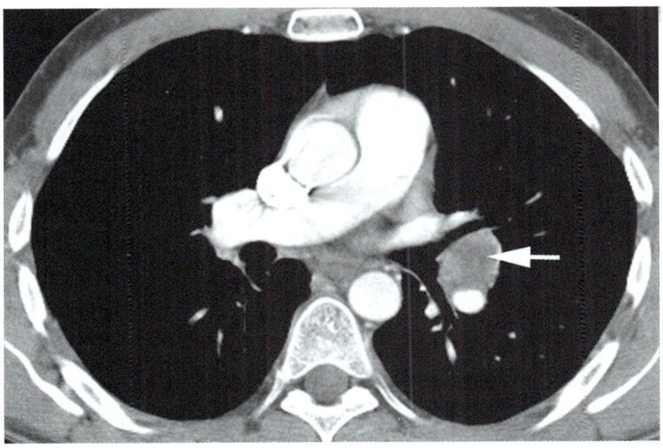

Figure 5.43. Left hilar lymph node enlargement (*arrow*) due to metastasis from a peripheral cancer. The hilar mass is sharply marginated.

Hilar mass is common in SCC. Enlargement of hilar lymph nodes in association with a central mass is characteristic of small cell carcinoma. Hilar enlargement is the first detectable radiographic finding in 10% to 15% of cases of lung cancer. Airway abnormalities (narrowing or obstruction) are common, but not invariably, and are seen in patients with a hilar mass or lymph node enlargement.

Mediastinal Mass or Lymph Node Enlargement

Mediastinal lymph node metastases are common in patients with lung carcinoma, occurring in up to 40% of patients at diagnosis, depending on the size, location, and cell type of the primary tumor. In patients with a small lung nodule as the only presenting finding, mediastinal metastases are found in approximately 20%. CT is most accurate in making this diagnosis.

Mediastinal lymph node enlargement is an uncommon plain film abnormality at initial presentation (see Table 5.10). When visible radiographically, lymph node enlargement is usually limited to the middle mediastinum and is associated with a visible lung or hilar mass. The most common sites of mediastinal node enlargement seen on plain radiographs are the right paratracheal mediastinum for right-sided tumors and the aorticopulmonary window for left-sided tumors. The subcarinal lymph nodes are also commonly involved but are difficult to recognize on plain radiographs unless they are quite large. It is unusual for mediastinal lymph nodes to be involved radiographically without the involvement of the hilum.

In some patients with lung carcinoma, a mediastinal mass may be the first and only presenting abnormality, occurring in the absence of a visible lung mass. Isolated mediastinal masses are usually associated with small cell carcinoma or poorly differentiated carcinoma.

Pleural Abnormalities

Pleural Effusions or Masses

Small pleural effusions are common in patients with lung cancer; pleural effusion occurs in 5% to 15% of patients. They can result from pleural metastases, lymphatic obstruction in the hilum or mediastinum, or inflammatory lung disease associated with bronchial obstruction. The term *malignant effusion* should be reserved for effusions containing malignant cells. The presence of a pleural effusion, particularly when bloody, indicates a poor prognosis in lung cancer, but only a malignant effusion rules out surgical treatment.

Decubitus radiographs, ultrasound, and CT are sensitive methods of detecting pleural effusion. On CT, the presence of pleural thickening or nodularity in association with effusion should be considered highly suspicious for malignancy. However, malignant effusions commonly occur without visible pleural thickening. Extensive involvement of the pleural space mimicking malignant mesothelioma is sometimes seen, particularly in patients with adenocarcinoma.

The presence of pleural nodules or masses, appearing denser than pleural fluid on unenhanced or enhanced CT, predicts the presence of pleural metastases. Small fissural nodules may be seen in the presence of pleural metastases.

Pneumothorax

Spontaneous pneumothorax is rare with primary lung cancer and usually results from direct invasion of the visceral pleura or cavitation (Fig. 5.44). Occasionally, airway obstruction due to a proximal endobronchial lesion causes rupture of a subpleural bulla, producing a pneumothorax.

Pneumothorax ex vacuo is an unusual occurrence in lung cancer. It occurs in the presence of acute lobar collapse due to bronchial obstruction. A sudden decrease in intrapleural pressure around the collapsed lobe results in gas being drawn from blood and tissues into the pleural space. Radiographs or CT scans show a crescentic gas collection localized to the pleural space surrounding the collapsed lobe (Fig. 5.45). It is most common with right upper lobe tumors and resolves with alleviation of the obstruction.

Missed Lung Cancer

Lung cancers presenting as a solitary nodule may be difficult to see on chest radiographs. The *conspicuity* of a lesion is determined by (1) the sharpness of its edge, (2) the visual complexity of the region in which it is seen, (3) its size, and (4) its density. Cancers are usually missed on chest radiographs because of their poor conspicuity, being ill-defined, located in areas that are complex and difficult to evaluate (eg, in the lung apex, in the perihilar lung regions, in the posterior costophrenic angle, and projected below the dome of the diaphragm), or small.

Lung cancers smaller than 5 mm are very difficult to see on chest radiographs, but many missed cancers are not small. Missed cancers average about 1.5 cm in diameter but may be more than 3 cm. On chest radiographs, most (80%) missed cancers are in an upper lobe, with the right upper lobe being the most common site (50% of missed cancers). Lateral radiographs may show the lesion better than frontal films.

Cancers may be missed when films are interpreted prospectively but visible in retrospect. This does not imply malpractice. The detection rate on plain films for nodules 1 cm in diameter ranges from 40% to 90%. In patients with inconspicuous lesions, as many as 25% of visible lung cancers are missed by experienced observers, even if they know a cancer is present.

Cancers may also be missed using CT, even when the purpose of the scan is lung cancer screening and the reader's suspicion is high. Missed cancers may be small and endobronchial or may present as solitary nodules. Missed solitary

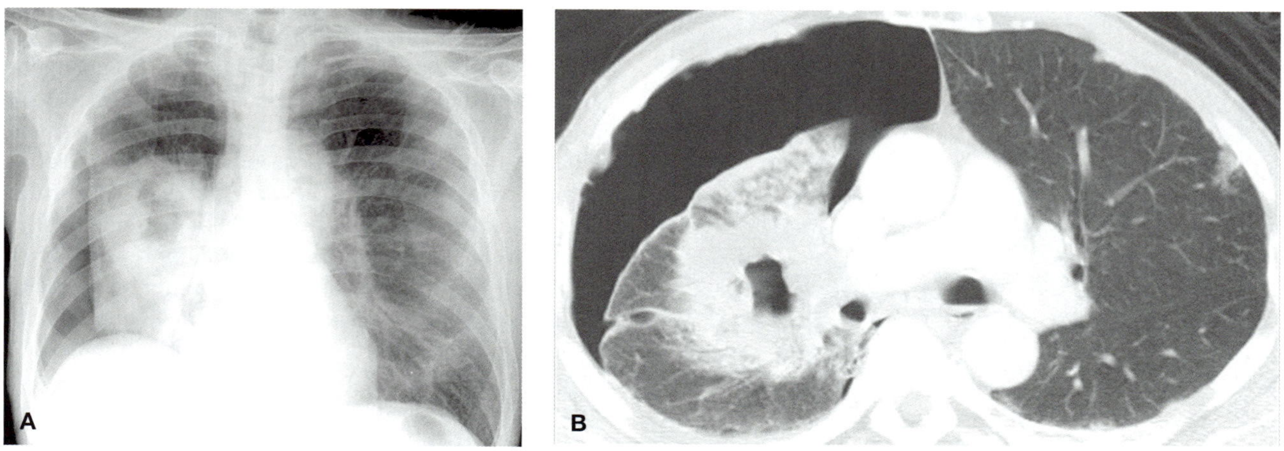

Figure 5.44. Cavitary squamous cell carcinoma with pneumothorax shown on chest radiograph (**A**) and CT (**B**).

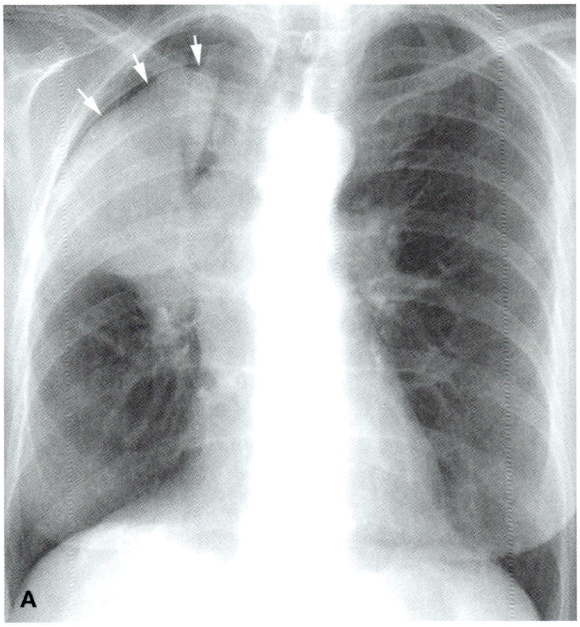

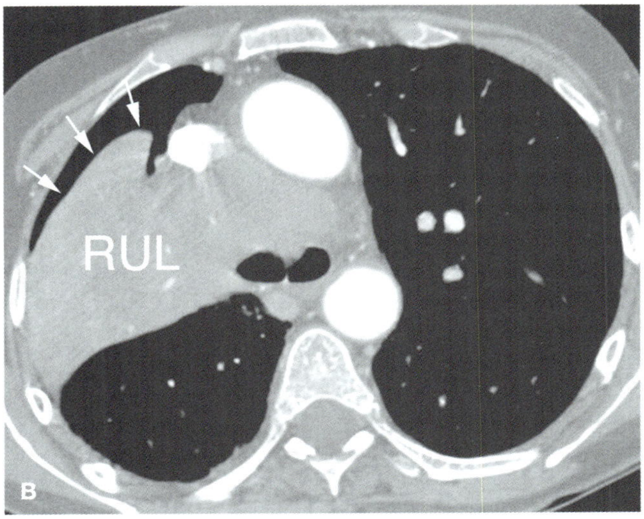

Figure 5.45. Pneumothorax ex vacuo in small cell carcinoma obstructing the right upper lobe bronchus. **A:** Chest radiograph shows a right hilar mass and right upper lobe collapse associated with an apical pneumothorax (*arrows*). **B:** CT shows right upper lobe (*RUL*) collapse capped by a pneumothorax (*arrows*). The right upper lobe bronchus is obstructed and invisible. This appearance is typical of pneumothorax ex vacuo.

nodules are usually small (often less than 3 mm), indistinguishable from adjacent vessels or other lung disease (eg, old tuberculosis), and poorly defined and of GGO or may mimic air-space consolidation or pleural thickening. Cancers missed on CT are often present in a lower lobe. The presence of other significant abnormalities on the CT scan may distract the observer. Missing something because the reader sees something else that is more obvious is termed *satisfaction of search*.

CLINICAL MANIFESTATIONS OF LUNG CANCER

Lung cancer is more common in men and most frequently presents in patients in their 50s and 60s. It is uncommon in patients less than 30 years of age. The clinical manifestations of lung carcinoma result from the following:

1. Local tumor growth
2. Intrathoracic metastases
3. Extrathoracic metastases
4. A paraneoplastic syndrome

Local Tumor Growth and Intrathoracic Metastases

Symptoms associated with lung cancer are largely nonspecific and are present in a minority of patients when the tumor is first detected radiographically (Table 5.14). Most patients with cancer are smokers and have a history of chronic cough; any change in their pattern of cough or sputum production should be considered significant.

Symptoms are most common in patients with central carcinomas involving large bronchi or mediastinal structures and in patients with tumors metastatic to hilar or mediastinal lymph nodes. Symptoms of central carcinoma can include the following:

1. Bronchial obstruction with cough, hemoptysis, wheezing, dyspnea, or fever due to postobstructive pneumonia
2. Hoarseness from the involvement of the recurrent laryngeal nerve
3. SVC syndrome resulting from mediastinal invasion or metastases

Table 5.14 Symptoms in Patients With Lung Cancer

Symptom	Patients With Symptom (%)
Cough	75
Dyspnea	60
Chest pain	45
Hemoptysis	35
Hypertrophic pulmonary osteoarthropathy	10
Hoarseness	10
Wheezing	2

4. Dysphagia from esophageal invasion or compression
5. Chylothorax from the involvement of the thoracic duct
6. Diaphragmatic paralysis from the involvement of the phrenic nerve

Peripheral lung cancers can be associated with pleural or chest wall invasion, resulting in chest pain, dyspnea, or cough. At autopsy, about 10% of patients with lung cancer have chest wall involvement by direct extension. Peripheral carcinomas in the superior sulcus can produce Pancoast syndrome.

Superior Vena Cava Syndrome

Obstruction or narrowing of mediastinal vessels because of mediastinal invasion or lymph node metastases is a relatively common manifestation of lung cancer. Because of its location and relatively thin wall, the SVC is particularly susceptible to involvement by tumor. SVC obstruction is associated with the *SVC syndrome*. About 65% to 85% of cases of SVC syndrome are caused by lung carcinoma. Symptoms and signs of SVC syndrome include the following:

1. Facial fullness, flushing, and cyanosis
2. Headache
3. Edema of the upper extremities
4. Prominent veins on the face and upper chest

Other common causes of SVC syndrome include granulomatous diseases such as histoplasmosis or tuberculosis involving the mediastinum (fibrosing mediastinitis) and venous thrombosis.

Extrathoracic Metastases

Small cell carcinoma grows rapidly and tends to metastasize early. Adenocarcinoma may grow slowly but metastasizes early. SCC may grow rapidly but tends to metastasize late.

Hematogenous spread to many sites has been reported with lung cancer, but the central nervous system, bones, liver, and adrenal glands are most commonly involved. Such metastases preclude successful surgical resection. The use of imaging studies to detect distant metastases in lung cancer patients is discussed below.

Paraneoplastic Syndromes

Paraneoplastic syndromes are disorders associated with malignant neoplasms but not directly related to the physical effects of the primary tumor. Such syndromes are present in 10% of patients with lung carcinoma (20% of those with small cell carcinoma) and result from the production of hormones or peptides by the tumor, antigen–antibody interactions resulting from tumor products, or neurovascular mechanisms. They may precede pulmonary findings by months or even years. A large variety of manifestations have been reported.

Hypertrophic Pulmonary Osteoarthropathy

Digital clubbing and hypertrophic pulmonary osteoarthropathy (HPO) are the most common cutaneous disorders. Eighty percent of cases of HPO in adults are due to lung cancer. SCC is most commonly associated with HPO; HPO is uncommon with small cell carcinoma. Relief of symptoms typically follows resection of the primary neoplasm. Pulmonary osteoarthropathy may precede discovery of the lung neoplasm by up to 2 years.

Vascular Disorders

Thrombophlebitis has an increased incidence in lung cancer patients and is most common with adenocarcinoma.

Endocrine Disorders

Cushing's syndrome, resulting from tumor secretion of ectopic adrenocorticotrophic hormone (ACTH), consists of weakness, hyperglycemia, polyuria, and hypokalemic alkalosis; in patients with lung cancer, it is typically of rapid onset and progression. It can be associated with any cell type of tumor. Cushing's syndrome is most common in patients with carcinoid tumor, and approximately 30% of patients with an ectopic cause of this syndrome have a bronchial carcinoid tumor. Small cell carcinoma is associated with Cushing's syndrome in less than 5% of cases, at least partially because of the short life expectancy of patients with this tumor.

Hypercalcemia associated with lung cancer is most common with SCC. Occasionally, it is associated with bone metastases, but it is more often due to the production of a peptide similar to parathyroid hormone. Other mediators such as prostaglandin have also been implicated in hypercalcemia.

Inappropriate antidiuretic hormone secretion, resulting in hyponatremia, is usually associated with small cell carcinoma. Although 50% of patients with small cell carcinoma have elevated levels of antidiuretic hormone, only 10% to 15% have hyponatremia and less than 5% of patients have symptoms attributable to this syndrome.

Neuromuscular Syndromes

Neuromuscular syndromes associated with lung cancer may result from immunologic mechanisms. Small cell carcinoma is most commonly responsible. Symptoms may precede the diagnosis of the tumor or may be the first sign of recurrence.

Eaton–Lambert syndrome is characterized by proximal muscle weakness similar to myasthenia gravis, with the exception that muscle strength increases (rather than decreases) with use. Hyporeflexia and autonomic dysfunction are also parts of this syndrome. Small cell carcinoma is the most common malignant tumor associated with Eaton–Lambert syndrome; it can also be seen with extrathoracic tumors, and approximately 50% of cases are not associated with a detectable tumor. This syndrome apparently results from the production of anti-calcium channel antibodies, which impairs the release of acetylcholine.

Peripheral neuropathy is associated with small cell carcinoma and less often with SCC and adenocarcinoma. Antineuronal nuclear antibodies are likely involved. Chronic intestinal pseudo-obstruction, limbic encephalitis, necrotizing myelopathy, and visual paraneoplastic syndrome also occur with small cell carcinoma and are associated with antineuronal nuclear antibodies. Symptoms from neuropathy may precede the discovery of the carcinoma by years; however, in most cases, advanced disease is present.

Other neuromuscular manifestations include subacute cerebellar degeneration (ataxia, vertigo, and incoordination) and dementia.

STAGING OF LUNG CANCER

In patients with lung cancer, the cell type of the tumor, tumor genetics and markers, and the tumor extent affect treatment and prognosis and survival following treatment. However, the anatomic extent of the tumor at diagnosis is of primary importance in determining what therapeutic approach will be chosen. Imaging studies play a fundamental role in determining the extent of tumor or, in other words, its anatomic stage.

Lung cancer is staged using a TNM classification, which is based on a combination of findings: the location and morphologic characteristics of the primary tumor (T); the presence or absence of hilar, mediastinal, or other lymphadenopathy (N); and the presence or absence of distant metastases (M). Lung cancer is staged using the TNM Classification System, most recently revised in 2017 (8th TNM), shown in detail in Tables 5.15 and 5.16 and in Figure 5.46A. Using this classification, excellent correlations can be made between tumor stage and survival after treatment (see Fig. 5.46B).

Table 5.15 TNM Staging of Lung Cancer (TNM 7, 2009)

T	**Primary tumor**
T0	No evidence of primary tumor
T1	A tumor that is a. 3 cm or less in greatest dimension **T1a** ≤ 1 cm in greatest dimension **T1b** > 1 cm but ≤2 cm **T1c** > 2 cm but ≤3 cm b. Surrounded by lung or visceral pleura c. Without invasion proximal to a lobar bronchus (ie, not involving main bronchus)
T2	A tumor with any of the following features: a. Larger than 3 cm and ≤5 cm in greatest dimension **T2a** > 3 cm but ≤4 cm **T2b** > 4 cm but ≤5 cm b. Invades the visceral pleura c. Involves a main bronchus (regardless of distance to carina) d. Associated with atelectasis or obstructive pneumonia
T3	A tumor with any of the following features: a. Larger than 5 cm and ≤7 cm in greatest dimension b. Tumor of any size involving any of the following: parietal pleura, chest wall (including superior sulcus), phrenic nerve, or parietal pericardium c. Tumor of any size with satellite nodule(s) in the same lobe
T4	A tumor of any size with any of the following features: a. Larger than 7 cm in greatest dimension b. Tumor of any size involving any of the following: mediastinum, diaphragm, heart, great vessels, recurrent laryngeal nerve, carina, trachea, esophagus, spine c. Tumor of any size with satellite nodule(s) in a different ipsilateral lobe
N	**Regional lymph nodes**
N0	No regional lymph node metastases
N1	Metastases to ipsilateral pulmonary or hilar lymph nodes
N2	Metastases to ipsilateral mediastinal nodes or subcarinal nodes
N3	Metastases to contralateral hilar or mediastinal lymph nodes, or scalene or supraclavicular lymph nodes (either side)
M	Distant metastases
M0	Metastases absent
M1	Metastases present
M1a	Intrathoracic metastases, with either a. Tumor nodule(s) in the contralateral lung b. Tumor with pleural or pericardial nodules or malignant pleural or pericardial effusion
M1b	Single extrathoracic metastasis
M1c	Multiple extrathoracic metastases (two or more foci in a single organ, or at least one focus in multiple organs)

Table 5.16 Lung Cancer Staging Groups (TNM8, 2017)

Stage Groups	Tumor	Node	Metastasis
IA1	T1a	N0	M0
IA2	T1b	N0	M0
IA3	T1c	N0	M0
IB	T2a	N0	M0
IIA	T2b	N0	M0
IIB	T1a-c	N1	M0
	T2a	N1	M0
	T2b	N1	M0
	T3	N0	M0
IIIA	T1a-c, T2a-b	N2	M0
	T3	N1	M0
	T4	N0, 1	M0
IIIB	T1a-c, T2a-b	N3	M0
	T3, T4	N2	M0
IIIC	T3, T4	N3	M0
IVA	Any T	Any N	M1a-b
IVB	Any T	Any N	M1c

Modified from Detterbeck FC. The Eighth Edition TNM stage classification for lung cancer: what does it mean on main street? J Thorac Cardiovasc Surg. *2018;155(1):356-359. https://doi.org/10.1016/j.jtcvs.2017.08.138*

The TNM system is most commonly used for patients with non-small cell lung cancer (NSCLC). Small cell carcinoma has a very poor prognosis regardless of tumor stage and is often associated with metastases at the time of diagnosis. However, staging of early small cell carcinoma using the TNM classification is now recommended as described above.

Treatment of lung cancer is fundamentally based on the tumor stage, although treatment may vary in individual cases, depending on a variety of factors such as the histology and genetics of the tumor, and is subject to continued reassessment in clinical trials. Stage I and II tumors are usually treated by resection, sometimes with adjuvant chemotherapy; stage IIIA tumors are often treated by radiation or chemotherapy followed by resection (if anatomically possible); stage IIIB and higher is usually inoperable and treated by radiation, chemotherapy, or both; and stage IV by chemotherapy (Table 5.17).

In radiologic lung cancer staging, it is most important to determine which patients have localized disease and are likely to benefit from surgical resection and, alternatively, which patients have extensive disease not amenable to surgical treatment. In general, tumors are considered to be unresectable if they are classified as T4, N3, or M1. An exception is invasive T4 carcinomas without or with hilar lymph node metastases; such tumors are often restaged after chemotherapy or radiation and treated surgically if significant reduction in tumor volume and extent makes resection possible.

Different surgeons have different anatomic criteria for considering a tumor to be unresectable, and a careful and detailed discussion of the radiographic findings with the surgeon is necessary. Generally, an imager should be reluctant to make a dogmatic statement about resectability solely based on the radiographic findings (which in themselves may be nonspecific). The results of imaging studies must be considered in the framework of what diagnostic or therapeutic options are available.

Primary Tumor (T Descriptor)

The primary tumor is classified using one of four T designations. Each designation delineates criteria for tumors originating in, or involving, the lung or bronchial tree. The greatest diameter of the tumor is used for measurement.

T1 Carcinoma

A T1 carcinoma usually presents as a small peripheral nodule (defined as ≤3 cm) surrounded by lung or the visceral pleura (Figs. 5.7-5.9). In the 2017 staging system, T1 tumors presenting as a lung nodule are subclassified into those ≤1 cm (T1a), those greater than 1 cm but ≤2 cm (T1b), and those greater than 2 cm but ≤3 cm (T1c). A tumor limited to a lobar bronchus is also considered to be T1 (see Fig. 5.34D). T1 tumors are usually resectable.

T2 Carcinoma

A lung mass larger than 3 cm, but 5 cm or less in diameter (see Fig. 5.13), is classified as T2, as is a tumor invading the visceral pleura. In the 2017 system, T2 carcinomas presenting as a mass are subdivided into those greater than 3 cm but ≤4 cm (T2a) and those greater than 4 cm but ≤5 cm (T2b). Tumor involving a main bronchus regardless

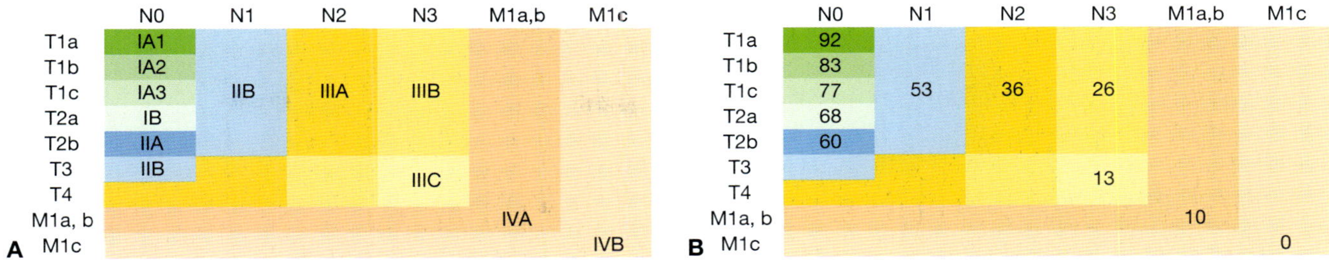

Figure 5.46. Revised lung cancer staging classifications (TNM8). **A:** Lung cancer stage related to combinations of T, N, and M. To determine the stage, find the correct T class and go across the square until reaching the appropriate N class. M1 indicates stage IV regardless of T or N. **B:** Five-year survival rates according to combinations of T, N, and M determined clinically (rather than pathologically). Survival decreases from the top left to bottom right of the diagram.

of the distance from the carina or associated with atelectasis or obstructive pneumonia extending to the hilum is also classified as T2. Presentation as a lung mass and bronchial lesion are both common. T2 tumors are also usually resectable.

T3 Carcinoma

In the 2017 staging system, a tumor greater than 5 cm, but 7 cm or less in diameter is classified as T3, as is a tumor associated with small tumor nodule(s) (ie, satellite nodules) in the same lobe (Fig. 5.47). Tumors that invade parietal pleura, chest wall (including superior sulcus tumors), phrenic nerve, or parietal pericardium are considered T3 regardless of size (Fig. 5.48). These tumors are resectable with difficulty in many cases.

T4 Carcinoma

In the 2017 staging system, a tumor greater than 7 cm is classified as T4. Additionally, satellite nodule(s) in different lobes of the same lung or invasion of any of the following are classified as T4 regardless of primary tumor size: mediastinum, diaphragm, heart, great vessels, trachea, recurrent laryngeal nerve, esophagus, vertebral body, or carina.

Table 5.17 Lung Cancer Treatment Related to Stage

Stage	Common Treatment
I	Resection
II	Resection
IIIA	Radiation or chemotherapy followed by resection
IIIB	Radiation and/or chemotherapy
IV	Chemotherapy

Resectability of the Primary Tumor: Radiographic Assessment

When determining the primary tumor extent and T classification, several key observations need to be made, including the size of the tumor, its location within a bronchus, and its association with atelectasis or consolidation. However, of most importance in determining resectability is the assessment of the specific features that indicate a T4 lesion.

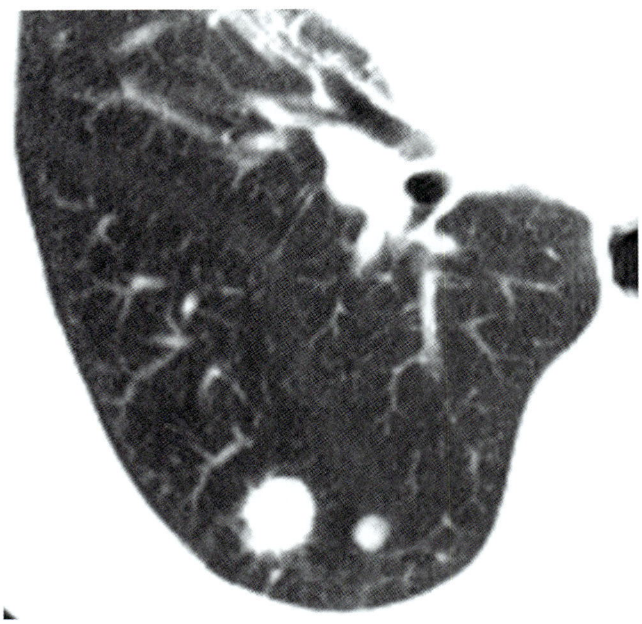

Figure 5.47. Right lower lobe carcinoma with a satellite nodule. This is classified as T3.

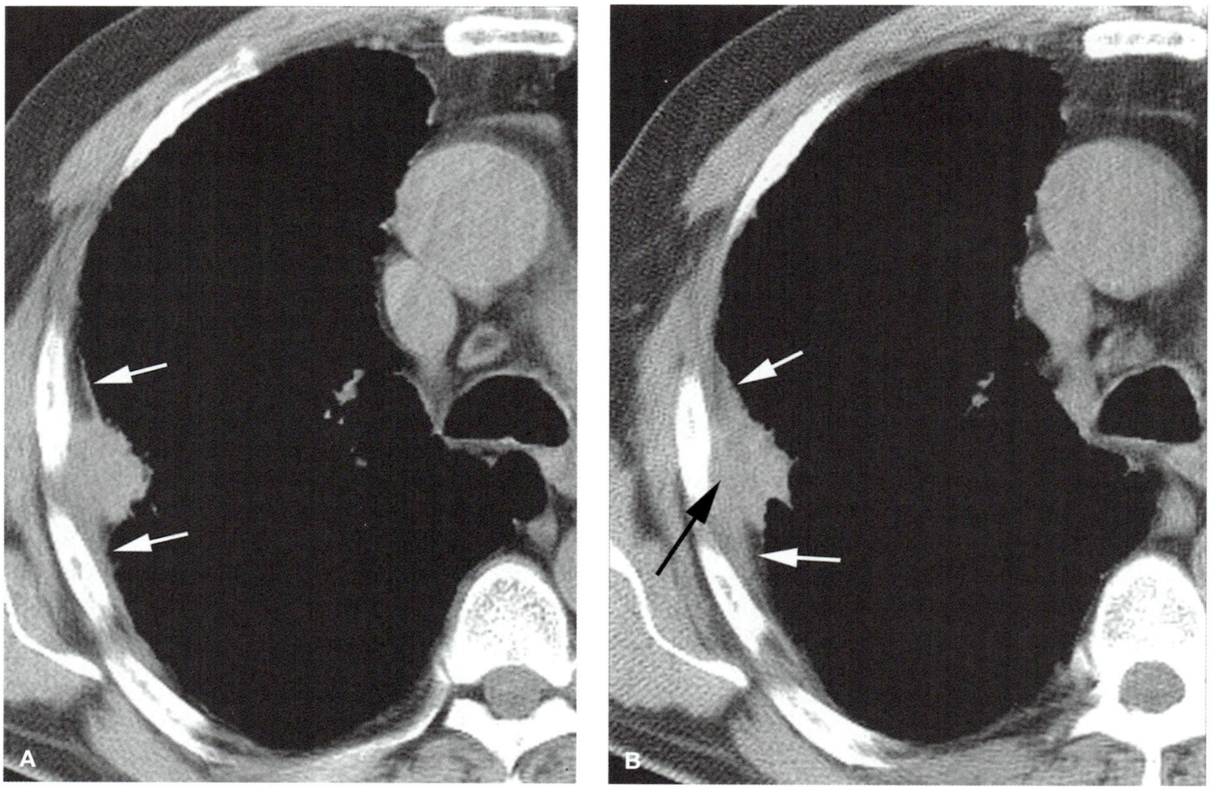

Figure 5.48. Chest wall invasion classified as T3 in the lung cancer staging system. **A, B:** A small peripheral carcinoma is associated with pleural thickening (*white arrows*). The tumor has an obtuse angle at the point it contacts the pleura. These findings suggest chest wall invasion, but their specificity is limited. Also, tumor can be seen invading and thickening extrapleural soft tissues (*black arrow* in **B**).

Chest Wall Invasion

Direct invasion of the pleura and chest wall by a peripheral lung carcinoma may or may not indicate that the tumor is unresectable. Only extensive chest wall invasion rules out surgery.

Unless obvious rib destruction is present, the diagnosis of chest wall invasion on plain radiographs is difficult. However, several plain film findings suggest invasion. Pleural thickening adjacent to a lung mass suggests invasion but is nonspecific. Tumors with extensive contact with the pleural surface are more likely invasive than those with minimal contact. A tumor that appears to flatten out against the pleura (ie, it appears sessile, lenticular, or crescentic in profile) may be invasive.

The accuracy of CT in diagnosing chest wall invasion is 70% to 80%, although sensitivity and specificity values vary from 40% to 90% in different studies. CT findings of value in the diagnosis of chest wall invasion (Figs. 5.49 and 5.50) include the presence of the following:

1. Obtuse angles or pleural thickening at the point of contact between tumor and pleura
2. More than 3 cm of contact between tumor and the pleural surface (5 cm of contact is more specific but less sensitive)
3. A ratio of the tumor diameter to the length of pleural contact by the tumor exceeding 0.5 (the higher this ratio, the more specific this finding)
4. Invisibility of extrapleural (chest wall) fat planes at the point tumor contacts chest wall
5. A mass involving the chest wall
6. Rib destruction

The only definite findings of chest wall invasion include rib destruction or chest wall infiltration of mass. Otherwise, invisibility of the extrapleural fat plane (sensitivity 85%, specificity 85%) and a ratio of tumor diameter to pleura contact exceeding 0.9 (sensitivity 85%, specificity 80%) are most accurate in predicting invasion (Table 5.18; see Fig. 5.40).

The demonstration of motion of the tumor relative to the chest wall during respiration indicates that no invasion is present; alternatively, the absence of motion during respiration suggests that invasion is present. This may be assessed using fluoroscopy, sonography, or dynamic CT or MRI.

The extent of chest wall invasion adjacent to a lung tumor may be better shown using MRI than CT because of the better contrast between tumor and chest wall fat and muscle that can be obtained using MRI.

In patients with superior sulcus tumors, vertebral body invasion (Fig. 5.51A) and invasion of the great vessels above

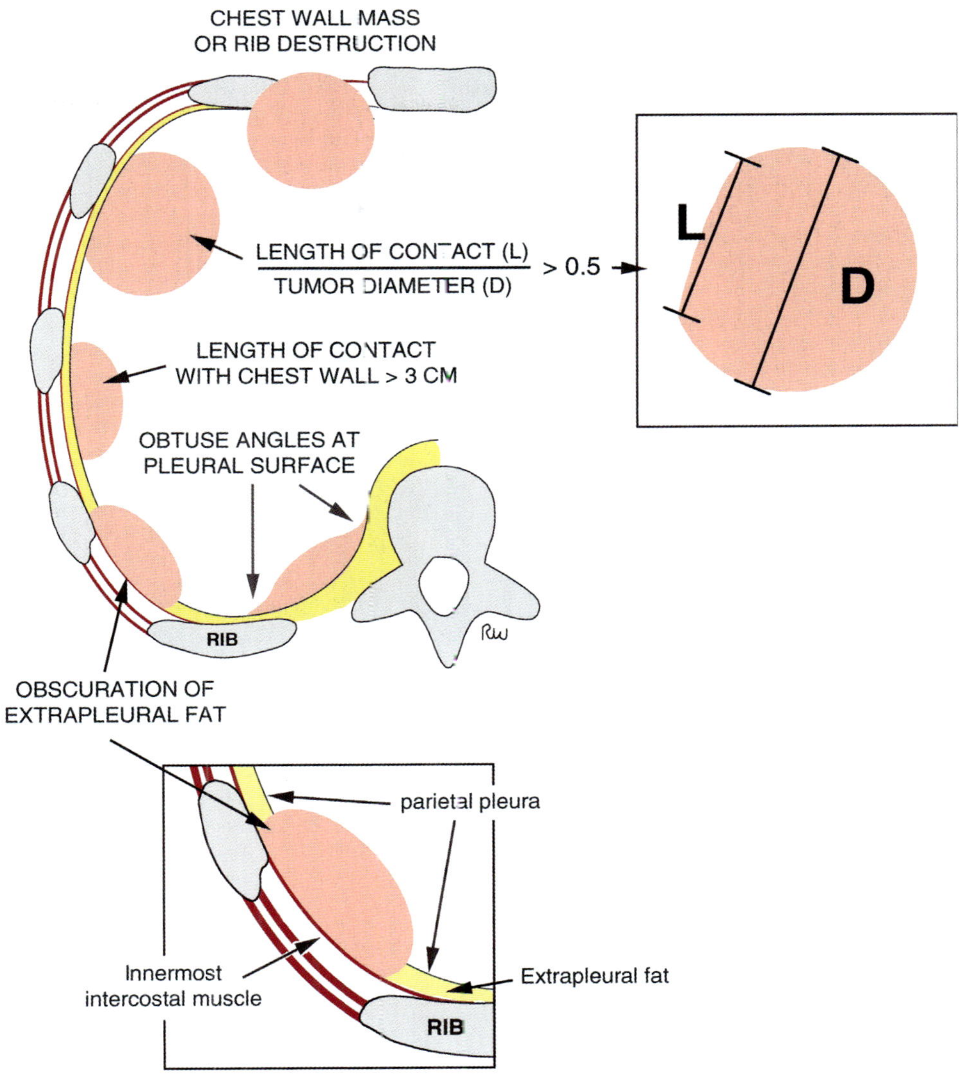

Figure 5.49. CT findings of chest wall invasion.

the lung apex (see Fig. 5.34) generally prevent surgical resection, although patients with such abnormalities may be restaged after radiation or chemotherapy. MRI in the sagittal or coronal planes can be advantageous in imaging apical tumors and is more accurate than CT in diagnosing chest wall invasion and its extent in this region. In patients with a superior sulcus tumor who are being considered for resection, MRI is recommended to determine the extent of chest wall invasion and possible involvement of the subclavian artery (Fig. 5.34) or brachial plexus (see Figs. 5.33 and 5.51B).

Mediastinal Invasion

Contiguous invasion of the mediastinum by tumor, with involvement of the carina, heart, great vessels, trachea, or esophagus, generally precludes resection as does significant invasion of mediastinal fat. Invasion of the mediastinal pleura or parietal pericardium or limited fat invasion does not prevent resection.

On plain radiographs, findings that suggest mediastinal invasion include the presence of a mediastinal mass, extensive contact of tumor with the mediastinum (Fig. 5.52A), or diaphragmatic paralysis, which in turn implies the involvement of the phrenic nerve.

CT is more accurate than plain radiographs in assessing mediastinal invasion. However, some caution in interpreting CT is necessary. Contiguity of tumor mass with the mediastinal pleura or thickening of the mediastinal pleura does not necessarily indicate mediastinal invasion. Also, not all findings indicative of mediastinal invasion indicate unresectability.

CT findings (Fig. 5.53A) usually regarded as indicating "definite" or "gross" mediastinal invasion and unresectability (although they are not 100% accurate) include the following:

1. Extensive replacement of mediastinal fat by soft tissue mass (see Figs. 5.52B and 5.54)

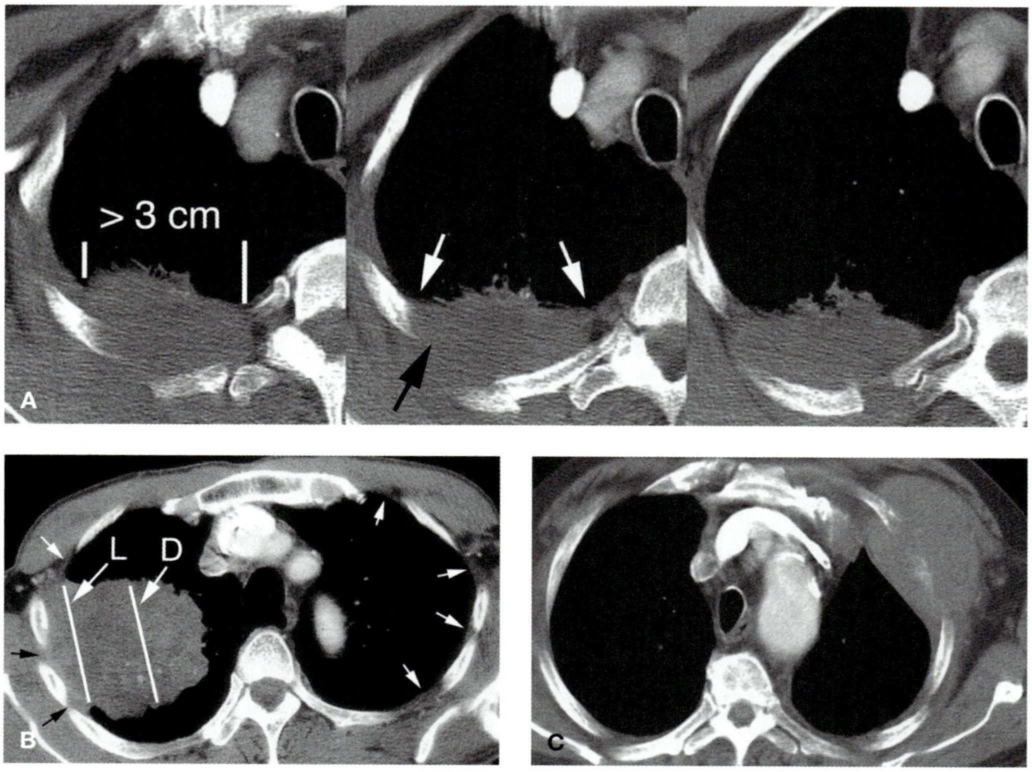

Figure 5.50. CT findings of chest wall invasion in three patients. **A:** CT at three adjacent levels shows a lenticular mass having more than 3 cm of contact with the chest wall, obtuse angles at the point it contacts the chest wall (*white arrows*), and rib destruction (*black arrow*). **B:** There is extensive pleural contact, with the length of contact (*L*) being 5 cm. The tumor diameter (*D*) equals the length of pleural contact (ie, their ratio is 1). Normal fat is seen in intercostal spaces (*small white arrows*), while these fat planes are invisible where the tumor contacts the chest wall (*small black arrows*). **C:** Chest wall invasion by lung cancer with rib destruction and a large chest wall mass.

2. Mass surrounding mediastinal vessels, trachea, or esophagus
3. Mass resulting in obvious invasion of one of these structures (see Fig. 5.54)

In lung cancer patients who do not have gross mediastinal invasion, additional CT findings may be of value in predicting that invasion of the mediastinum and mediastinal structures is present. These CT findings (see Figs. 5.53B and 5.55) include the following:

1. Tumor contact of more than 3 cm with the mediastinum
2. Tumor contact with more than one fourth (90°) of the circumference of the aorta or other mediastinal structures
3. Obliteration of the fat planes that are normally seen adjacent to the aorta or other mediastinal structures
4. Compression of mediastinal structures by a mass
5. Mediastinal pleural or pericardial thickening

The first three findings are highly sensitive but have poor specificity (Table 5.19). Because of the high sensitivity of these three findings, if they are all absent, the tumor will likely be resectable, even if mediastinal invasion is present.

Tracheal and Central Bronchial Lesions

Although tumor masses that cause total lung collapse or consolidation or involve the proximal bronchus may be difficult to treat surgically, they are not generally considered unresectable unless they involve the tracheal carina or trachea (Figs. 5.37 and 5.56). In this situation, it is difficult to perform a pneumonectomy, resect the tumor, and surgically close the remaining airway. However, some surgeons may excise tumors that involve the carina or even the distal trachea, reanastomosing the tracheal stump to the remaining bronchus or bronchi.

In some patients, CT can demonstrate the relationship of a proximal tumor mass to the main bronchus, carina, or trachea (Fig. 5.37). CT findings that suggest carinal involvement include bronchial wall thickening that extends to the carina or carinal thickening, blunting, or nodularity. However, bronchoscopy is more accurate in making this diagnosis. On bronchoscopy, minimal mucosal involvement of the tumor can be diagnosed, while on CT or plain radiographs, only discrete masses are visible. Bronchoscopic confirmation of an apparent carinal or tracheal tumor is usually necessary unless the findings are gross.

Table 5.18 Accuracy of CT Findings for Diagnosing Chest Wall Invasion

CT Finding	Sensitivity (%)	Specificity (%)
Obtuse angles at pleural surface	60	75
Length of contact with chest wall		
>3 cm	95	40
>4 cm	90	55
>5 cm	75	70
Ratio of length of contact/tumor diameter		
>0.5	100	35
>0.7	90	60
>0.9	85	80
Obliteration of chest wall fat plane	85	85
Chest wall mass	33	100
Rib destruction	16	100

Modified from Ratto GB, Piacenza G, Frola C, et al. Chest wall involvement by lung cancer: computed tomographic detection and results of operation. Ann Thorac Surg. *1991;51:182-188.*

Nodules in the Ipsilateral Lung

The presence of satellite tumor nodules in a different ipsilateral lobe than the primary tumor indicates T4 but does not prevent resection. Since benign nodules are common, it should not be assumed that any nodule seen on CT represents a tumor. Also, a second primary lung cancer in a different lobe (a synchronous primary tumor) does not indicate T4.

Lymph Node Metastases (N Descriptor)

Descriptors of lymph node metastasis remain unchanged in the 8th TNM staging system. N0 indicates the absence of lymph node metastases. Radiographs are much less sensitive than cross-sectional imaging for the detection of nodal metastases. On CT, using a short axis cutoff of 1cm sensitivity and specificity range between 51% to 64% and 74% to 86%, respectively. Lymph nodes greater than 2 cm are almost always involved.

The accuracy of CT in predicting the presence or absence of nodal metastases based on node diameter is limited by two factors. On the one hand, the sensitivity of CT in diagnosing lymph node metastases is reduced due to the common occurrence of microscopic lymph node metastases not resulting in increased lymph node size; on the other hand, specificity is reduced due to the presence of enlarged benign hyperplastic lymph nodes, particularly in patients with SCC.

PET/CT with fluorine 18 fluorodeoxyglucose (FDG) can improve sensitivity and specificity particularly for lymph node staging (and distant metastatic disease) as compared to CT (Fig. 5.57). PET/CT has a reported sensitivity of 58% to 94% and a specificity of 76% to 96% for the detection of mediastinal lymph node metastasis although false positives from infection, anthracotic nodes, or noninfectious disease like sarcoidosis does occur.

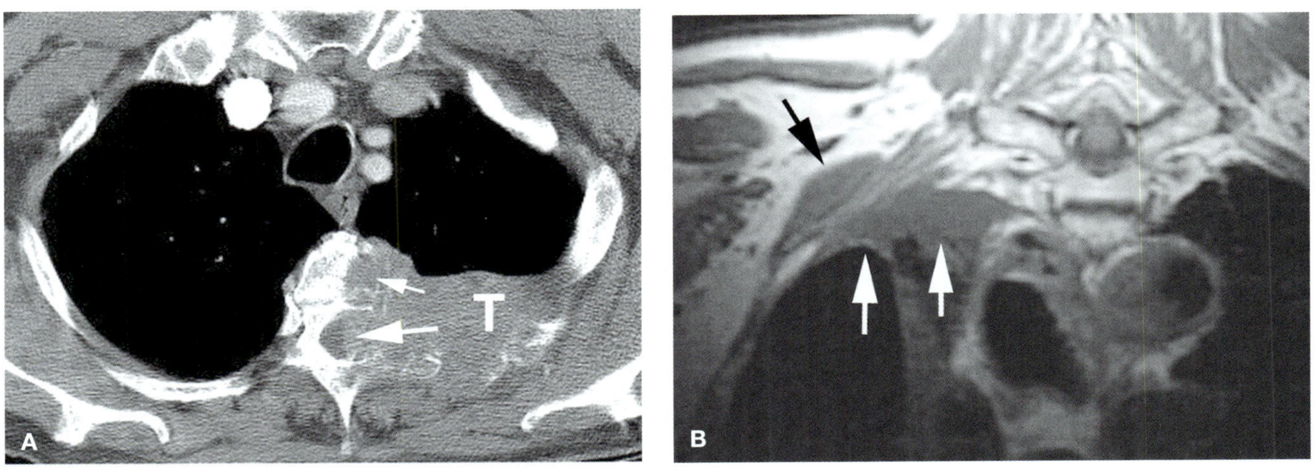

Figure 5.51. CT and MRI diagnosis of chest wall invasion. **A:** Vertebral invasion by lung carcinoma is shown using CT. Tumor (*T*) invades the vertebral body (*small arrow*) and spinal canal (*large arrow*). **B:** T1-weighted MRI shows brachial plexus invasion by a superior sulcus tumor (*white arrows*). Tumor (*black arrow*) surrounds the brachial plexus.

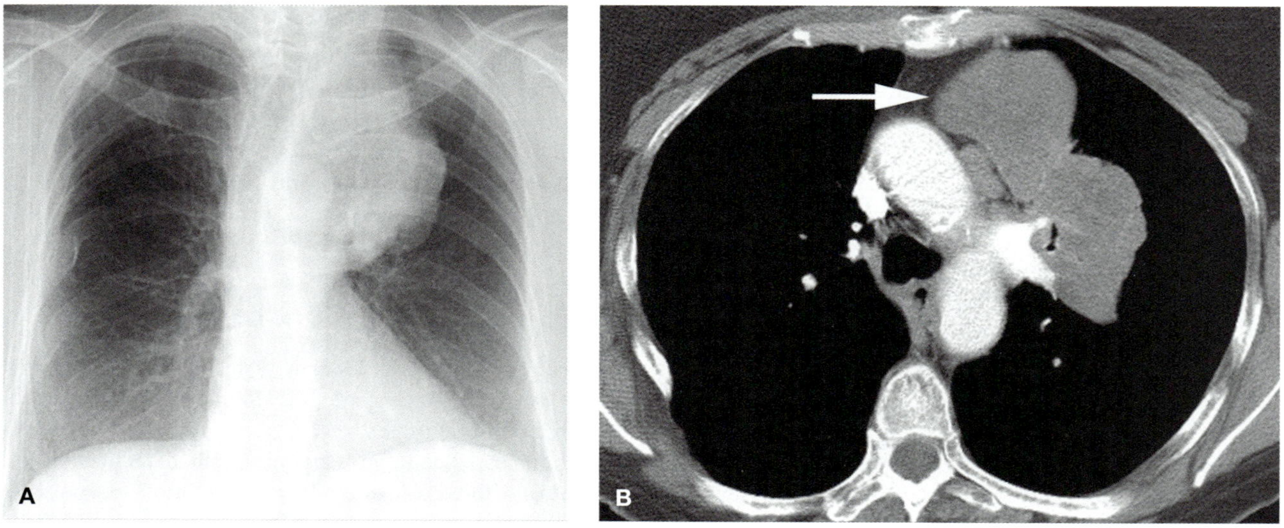

Figure 5.52. Mediastinal invasion by lung cancer. **A:** Chest radiograph shows extensive contact of tumor with mediastinum. **B:** CT shows extensive contact of tumor with mediastinum and a mediastinal mass (*arrow*) contiguous with the lung tumor, with soft tissue replacing mediastinal fat.

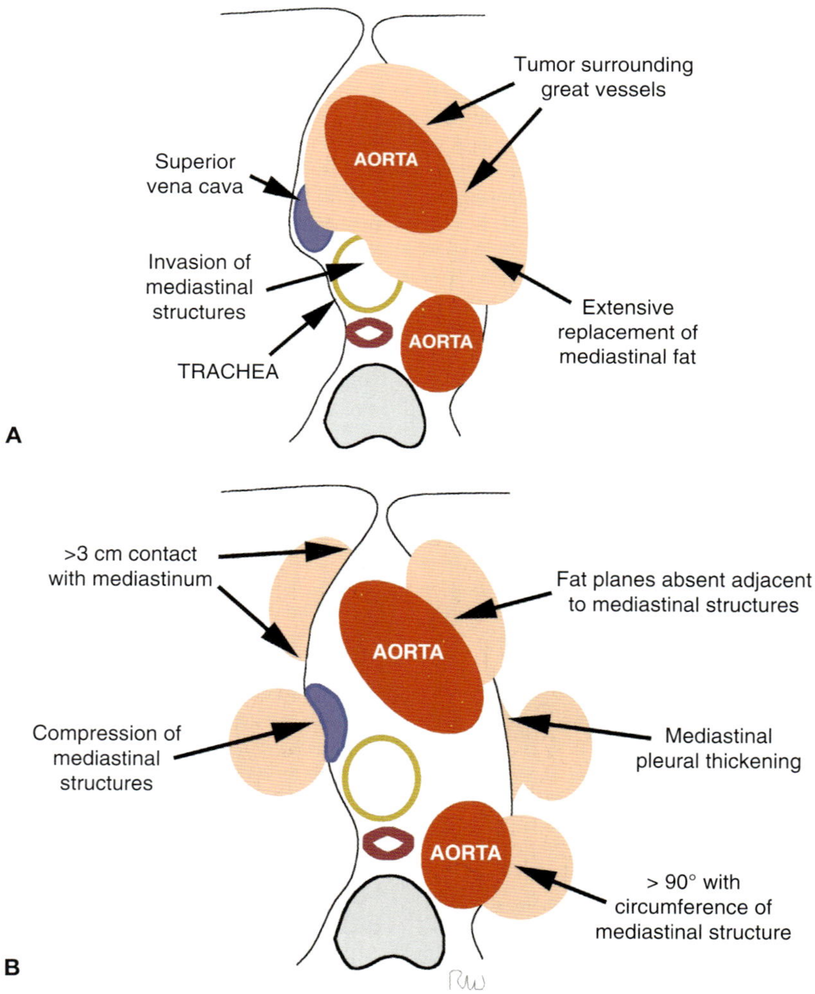

Figure 5.53. CT findings of mediastinal invasion. **A:** Definite findings of mediastinal invasion. **B:** Less specific findings of mediastinal invasion.

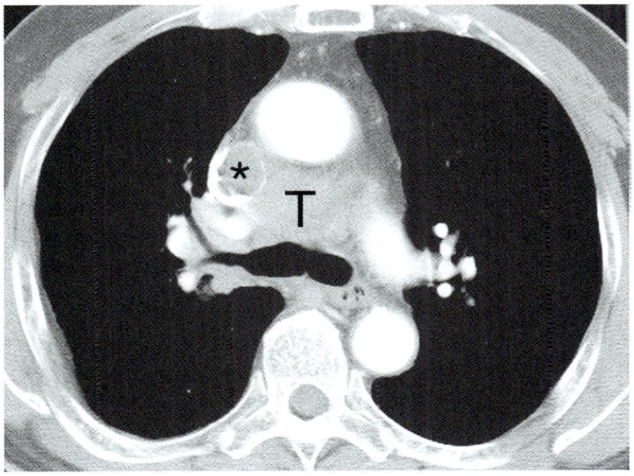

Figure 5.54. Mediastinal and superior vena cava (SVC) invasion by lung cancer. Tumor (*T*) has invaded mediastinal fat anterior to the carina. Invasion of the SVC with a tumor thrombus (*asterisk*) in its lumen is also visible.

Hilar Lymph Node Metastases

The presence of a hilar mass on radiographs or CT may reflect a primary bronchial tumor with local extension (T1-T4 depending on its location) or hilar lymph node metastases (N1; see Fig. 5.43). Hilar involvement by a carcinoma does not generally affect resectability. However, the presence of hilar tumor often means that a pneumonectomy rather than lobectomy needs to be performed. In patients with poor respiratory function who cannot tolerate a pneumonectomy, the presence of hilar metastases may make them inoperable even if the tumor itself is technically resectable.

CT is superior to plain radiographs in evaluating the pulmonary hila. CT findings of bronchial obstruction or narrowing correlate closely with bronchoscopic findings (see Fig. 5.35). CT is quite accurate in showing hilar lymph enlargement; as described above, PET/CT may increase sensitivity particularly for small lymph node metastases less than 1 cm.

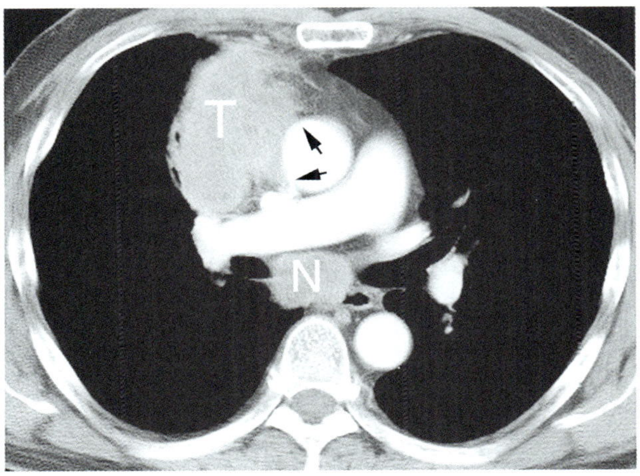

Figure 5.55. Mediastinal invasion by lung cancer. A right upper lobe tumor (*T*) shows more than 3 cm of contact with the mediastinum, replaces mediastinal fat, obliterates the fat plane adjacent to the aorta, and contacts more than one fourth of its circumference (*arrows*). An enlarged subcarinal lymph node (*N*) is also seen.

Table 5.19 Accuracy of CT Findings for Diagnosing Mediastinal Invasion

CT Finding	Sensitivity (%)	Specificity (%)
Contact with mediastinum >3 cm	80	55
Contact with aorta >1/4 circumference	85	75
Absent mediastinal fat plane	90	10
Compression of mediastinal structure	35	75
Mediastinal pleural or pericardial thickening	40	80

Data from Glazer HS, Kaiser LR, Anderson DJ, et al. Indeterminate mediastinal invasion in bronchogenic carcinoma: CT evaluation. Radiology. *1989;173:37-42.*

Assessment of Mediastinal Lymph Nodes

Because large or bulky mediastinal masses in patients with lung cancer are considered unresectable by most surgeons, a patient who has a mediastinal mass visible on plain

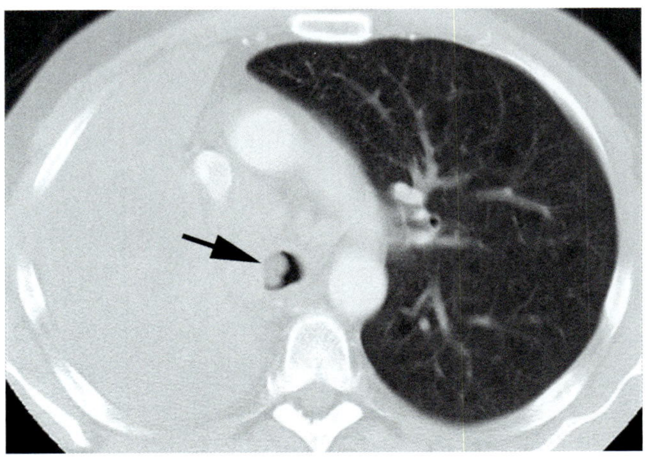

Figure 5.56. Tracheal invasion by a right hilar carcinoma. Right lung atelectasis is due to a carcinoma arising in the right main bronchus. Tumor invades the trachea (*arrow*), precluding resection.

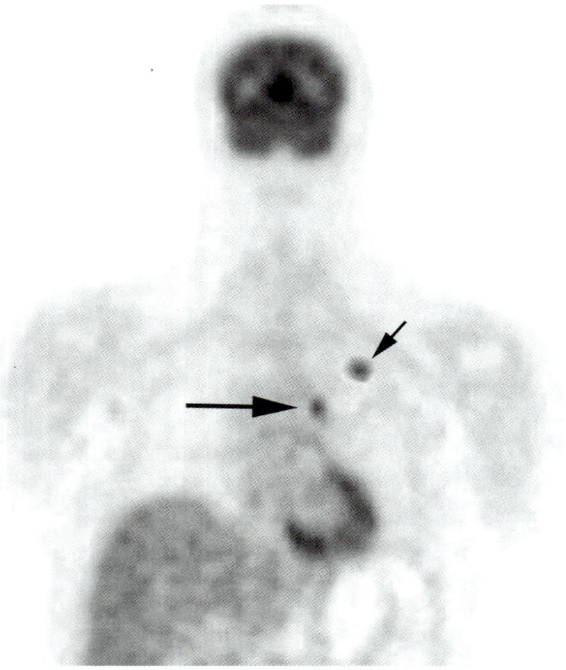

Figure 5.57. Mediastinal lymph node metastasis diagnosed using FDG-PET. A metabolically active left upper lobe carcinoma (*small arrow*) is associated with a lymph node metastasis (*large arrow*) in the aortopulmonary window. High activity is also seen in the myocardium and brain.

radiographs (indicating its large size) is not likely a surgical candidate. In such patients, CT followed by mediastinoscopy or biopsy is generally performed to confirm the presence of mediastinal disease (Fig. 5.58).

Stage and Resectability

Ipsilateral mediastinal or subcarinal node metastases are classified N2 and are considered potentially resectable, usually following preoperative chemotherapy, but this remains the subject of investigation and depends to some extent on tumor histology. Contralateral hilar or mediastinal node metastases or supraclavicular or scalene lymph node metastases on either side are considered N3 and unresectable (see Fig. 5.58). Treatment usually includes chemotherapy.

CT and Mediastinoscopy

Preoperative imaging with CT and/or PET/CT is helpful in determining which patients should have mediastinoscopy prior to surgery. In general, patients who have suspicious mediastinal lymph nodes seen on imaging (either enlarged or metabolically active) have mediastinoscopy prior to surgery; patients without suspicious nodes often have surgery without mediastinoscopy. This approach, however, varies among institutions and some perform mediastinoscopy routinely.

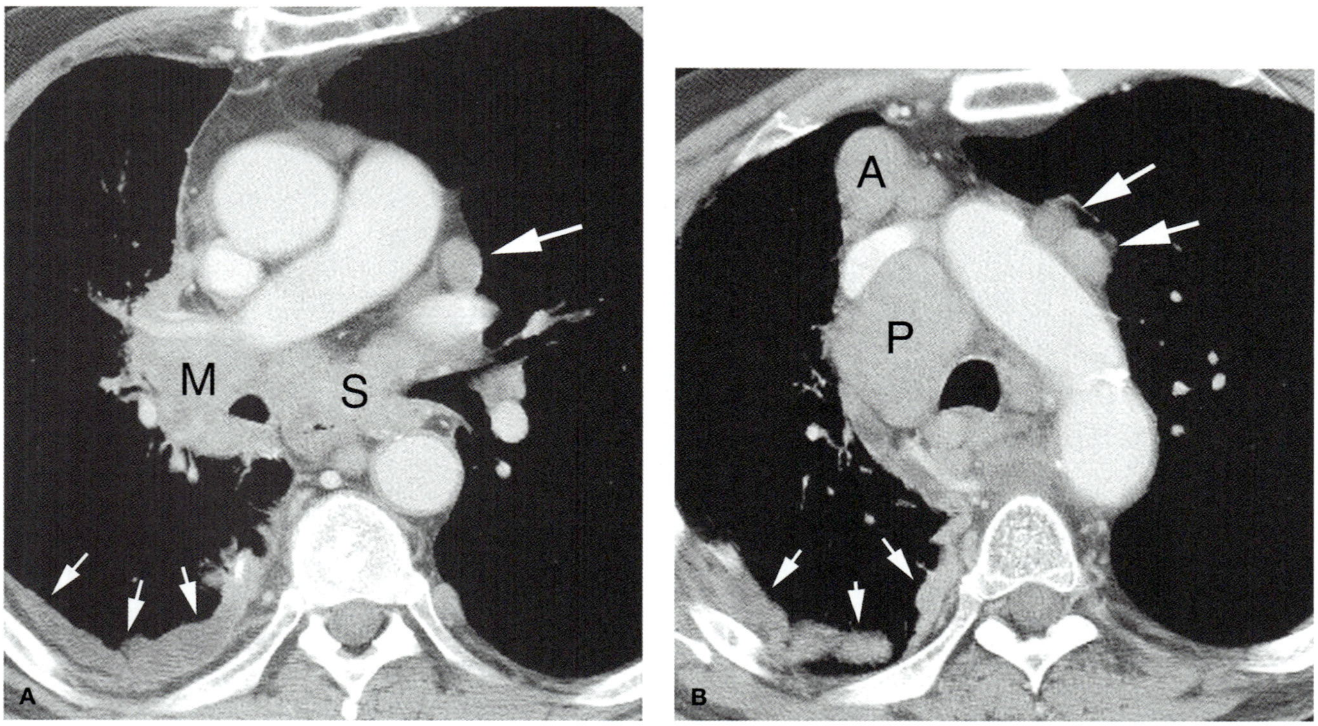

Figure 5.58. Mediastinal lymph node metastases from small cell carcinoma. **A, B:** A large right hilar mass (*M*) is associated with lymph node enlargement in the subcarinal space (*S*), right paratracheal space (*P*), anterior mediastinum (*A*), and the contralateral mediastinum (*large arrows*). Right pleural thickening, pleural nodules, and effusion (*small arrows*) are due to pleural metastases. The large bulky mediastinal nodes and contralateral nodes (N3) preclude resection.

CT is also used as a guide for invasive procedures performed before an attempt at curative resection. Although mediastinoscopy is generally regarded as the gold standard of preoperative mediastinal evaluation, routine mediastinoscopy through a suprasternal incision does not evaluate all mediastinal compartments or lymph node groups. A significant percentage (up to 30%) of patients with lung carcinoma who have a negative mediastinoscopy prove to have mediastinal nodal metastases at surgery.

Routine mediastinoscopy can evaluate paratracheal lymph nodes, nodes in the anterior subcarinal space, and lymph nodes extending anterior to the right main bronchus (Fig. 5.59A). Lymph nodes in the prevascular (anterior) mediastinum, aortopulmonary window, more posteriorly (eg, posterior subcarinal space, azygoesophageal recess) are generally inaccessible using this technique (see Fig. 5.59B), although some of these can be evaluated using a left parasternal mediastinoscopy (Chamberlain procedure). CT or PET/CT can serve to guide the mediastinoscopist to the most suspicious lymph nodes. It may also suggest that needle aspiration biopsy, transbronchoscopic needle aspiration biopsy, or parasternal mediastinotomy would be appropriate.

Metastases (M Descriptor)

M0 indicates the absence of metastases. In the 2017 system, metastases (M1) are subclassified as either intrathoracic or extrathoracic (distant). Intrathoracic metastases, subclassified as M1a, include (a) tumor nodule(s) in the contralateral lung and (b) pleural or pericardial metastases (either nodules or malignant effusion). Distant metastases are subclassified as either M1b (a single extrathoracic metastasis) or M1c (multiple extrathoracic metastases). The distinction between M1b and M1c is new in TNM-8 as survival differs between the groups. Distant metastases are present at diagnosis in 10% to 35% of patients with NSCLC; they are most common with adenocarcinoma or LCC.

Tumor Nodules in the Contralateral Lung

As with nodules in the same lobe as the primary tumor or the same lung, contralateral pulmonary nodules seen on CT may be benign and cannot be assumed to represent metastases. Also keep in mind that a contralateral lung tumor may represent a synchronous primary lung cancer.

Malignant Pleural or Pericardial Disease

In a patient with lung carcinoma, pleural effusion can occur for a variety of reasons, including pleural invasion, obstructive pneumonia, and lymphatic or pulmonary venous obstruction by the tumor. Although the presence of effusion indicates a poor prognosis, only patients who have tumor cells in the pleural fluid (ie, a *malignant effusion*) or on pleural biopsy are considered to have unresectable disease. Patients with other causes of effusion are considered to have resectable lesions despite their poor prognosis; nonmalignant effusion has no effect on stage classification.

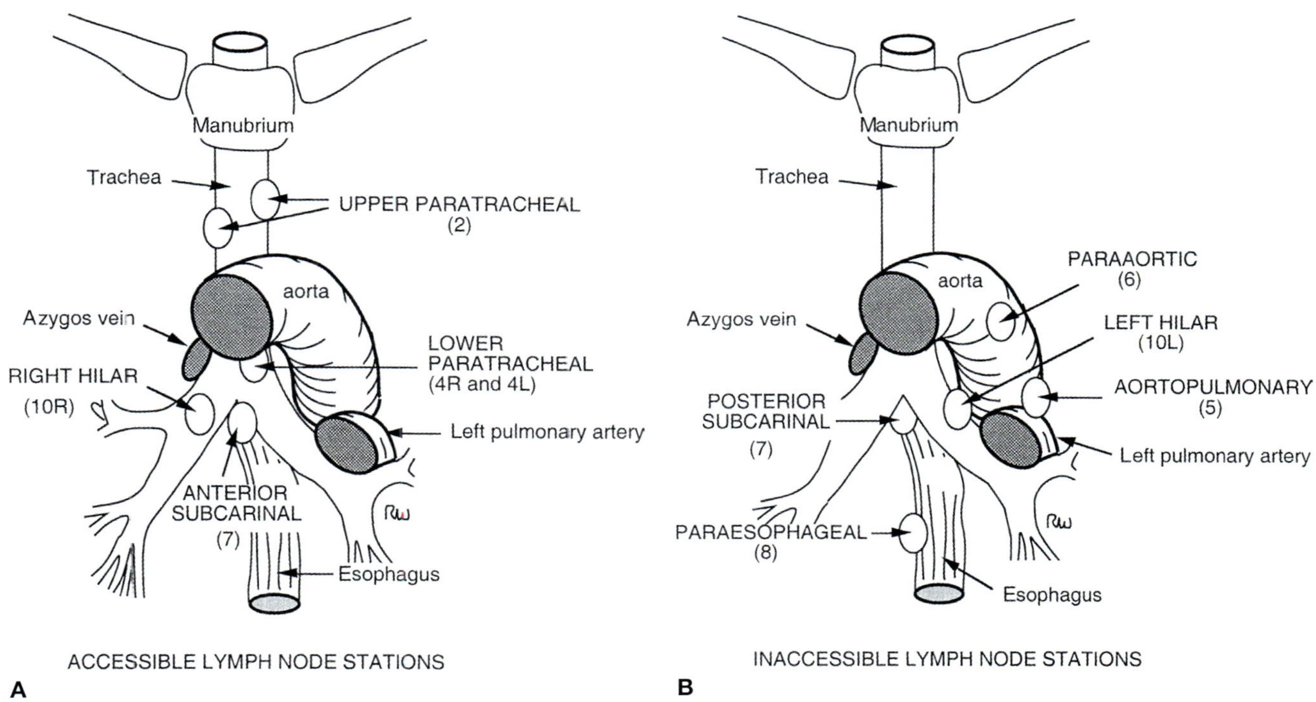

Figure 5.59. Mediastinal nodes accessible (**A**) and inaccessible (**B**) at routine mediastinoscopy performed through a suprasternal incision, as viewed from the front. Numbers indicate the corresponding AJCC/UICC lymph node stations (see Chapter 8).

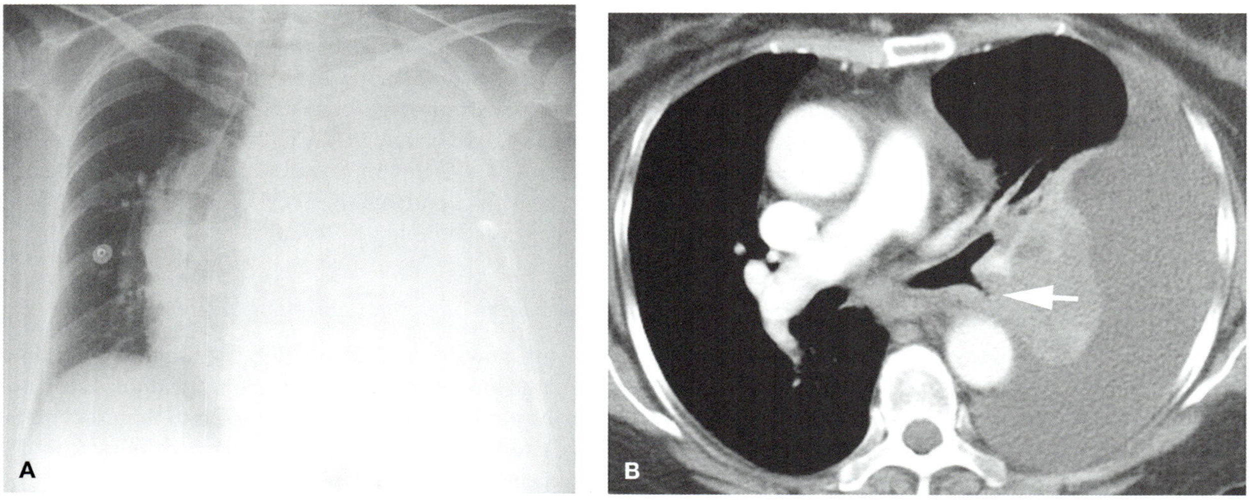

Figure 5.60. Malignant effusion in lung cancer. **A:** Chest radiograph shows a large left pleural effusion with mediastinal shift to the right. **B:** CT shows a tapered obstruction (*arrow*, rat-tail appearance) of the left lower lobe bronchus associated with left lower lobe collapse. There is no evidence of pleural thickening.

Usually, plain radiographs are sufficient for the diagnosis of pleural effusion, leading to thoracentesis or pleural biopsy. On CT, the presence of pleural thickening or pleural nodules in association with pleural effusion should be considered highly suspicious for malignancy (see Chapter 26). However, malignant effusions can occur without pleural thickening (Fig. 5.60), and pleural thickening can be seen in many cases of benign exudative pleural effusion.

In patients with a lung cancer involving the pleural surface, small pleural nodules may indicate the presence of pleural dissemination. They may be seen in the peripheral pleural space or within a fissure and with or without a pleural effusion.

The same is true for the pericardium—patients may have pericardial effusions for a variety of reasons. The presence of discrete pericardial masses or nodules is highly suggestive of pericardial involvement; pericardiocentesis or surgical biopsy may be necessary for the confirmation of metastatic disease if it affects staging.

Distant Metastases

Historically, about half of the patients with lung cancer have distant metastatic disease at time of presentation although this stands to decrease with wider adoption of lung cancer screening. Distant metastases rule out surgery in almost all cases; patients are treated with chemotherapy and have a poor prognosis with 5-year survival of less than 10%.

Common sites of extrathoracic spread in patients with NSCLC include the adrenal glands, liver, bone, and brain.

History, physical examination (including a detailed neurologic evaluation), and blood tests (including liver function tests and serum calcium and alkaline phosphatase determinations) are used to suggest possible metastatic sites but are limited in accuracy. Imaging studies including radionuclide bone scanning with technetium-99m methylene diphosphonate, contrast-enhanced brain and abdominal CT, brain and abdominal MRI, abdominal ultrasound, and FDG-PET or PET/CT are used to confirm organ-specific involvement as suggested by the clinical findings, although recommendations vary. Whole-body PET scanning is particularly useful in assessing distant metastases, except for those involving the brain (because of the high background activity of the brain).

Adrenal metastases are present in up to 20% of patients with NSCLC at diagnosis and are often the only site of extrathoracic spread. Because of this, a chest CT in patients with lung cancer should be extended to encompass the upper abdomen. However, adrenal adenomas are common (3% to 5%) in the general population, and as many as 65% of small (less than 3 cm) adrenal masses in patients with lung cancer represent an adrenal adenoma rather than a metastasis. Although CT without contrast infusion and enhanced CT with delayed images can be helpful in distinguishing benign and malignant adrenal lesions, they may be nonspecific. Other methods of evaluating an adrenal mass include FDG-PET (which is highly accurate), chemical-shift MRI, and biopsy.

Liver metastases are present in 5% to 15% of cases. Their appearance on routine staging CT is often nonspecific and difficult to distinguish from cysts, hemangiomas, or other lesions without further imaging. However, isolated liver metastases are uncommon. CT, MRI, or FDG-PET may be used for diagnosing liver metastases.

Skeletal metastases are present at diagnosis in 5% to 20% of patients with lung carcinoma; they are present at autopsy in up to 30% of patients. SCC and LCC tend to cause osteolytic lesions, while small cell carcinoma and adenocarcinoma produce osteolytic or osteoblastic metastases. The bones most commonly involved are the vertebrae, pelvic bones, and proximal long bones. Metastases to the distal extremities are unusual, but lung carcinoma is the most common cause of distal metastases. Radionuclide imaging should be reserved for patients with symptoms or biochemical abnormalities and has a high false-positive rate (40%). FDG-PET scanning also allows the detection of metastases and has a lower false-positive rate.

Central nervous system metastases are common and are often symptomatic (although the symptoms may be vague). However, asymptomatic brain metastases occur in up to 15% of patients with NSCLC and have a higher incidence with adenocarcinoma and LCC than with other cell types. Consequently, routine brain CT or MRI is recommended in asymptomatic patients with these tumors. With other cell types, imaging is usually limited to patients with symptoms. PET/CT is less valuable due to the high background metabolic activity.

SUGGESTED READINGS

Benson RE, Rosado-de-Christenson ML, Martinez-Jimenez S, Kunin JR, Pettavel PP. Spectrum of pulmonary neuroendocrine proliferations and neoplasms. *Radiographics*. 2013;33(6):1631-1649.

Bepler G. Lung cancer epidemiology and genetics. *J Thorac Imaging*. 1999;14(4):228-234.

Brun AL, Touitou-Gottenberg D, Haroche J, et al. Erdheim-Chester disease: CT findings of thoracic involvement. *Eur Radiol*. 2010;20(11):2579-2587.

Bruzzi JF, Komaki R, Walsh GL, et al. Imaging of non-small cell lung cancer of the superior sulcus: part 1—anatomy, clinical manifestations, and management. *Radiographics*. 2008;28(2):551-620.

Bruzzi JF, Komaki R, Walsh GL, et al. Imaging of non-small cell lung cancer of the superior sulcus: part 2—initial staging and assessment of resectability and therapeutic response. *Radiographics*. 2008;28(2):561-572.

Carter BW, Glisson BS, Truong MT, Erasmus JJ. Small cell lung carcinoma: staging, imaging, and treatment considerations. *Radiographics* 2014;34(6):1707-1721.

Carter BW, Lichtenberger JP, Benveniste MK, et al. Revisions to the TNM staging of lung cancer: rationale, significance, and clinical application. *Radiographics*. 2018;38(2):374-391. doi:10.1148/rg.2018170081

Chong S, Lee KS, Chung MJ, Han J, Kwon OJ, Kim TS. Neuroendocrine tumors of the lung: clinical, pathologic, and imaging findings. *Radiographics*. 2006;26(1):41-58.

Dales RE, Stark RM, Raman S. Computed tomography to stage lung cancer: approaching controversy using meta-analysis. *Am Rev Respir Dis*. 1990;141(5 pt 1):1096-1101.

Detterbeck FC, Boffa DJ, Tanoue LT. The new lung cancer staging system. *Chest*. 2009;136(1):260-271.

Detterbeck FC. The eighth edition TNM stage classification for lung cancer: what does it mean on main street? *J Thorac Cardiovasc Surg*. 2018;155(1):356-359. doi:10.1016/j.jtcvs.2017.08.138

El-Sherief AH, Lau CT, Wu CC, Drake RL, Abbott GF, Rice TW. International association for the study of lung cancer (IASLC) lymph node map: radiologic review with CT illustration. *Radiographics*. 2014;34(6):1680-1691.

Flieder DB, Koss MN, Nicholson A, Sesterhenn IA, Petras RE, Travis WD. Solitary pulmonary papillomas in adults: a clinicopathologic and in situ hybridization study of 14 cases combined with 27 cases in the literature. *Am J Surg Pathol*. 1998;22(11):1328-1342.

Forster BB, Müller NL, Miller RR, Nelems B, Evans KG. Neuroendocrine carcinomas of the lung: clinical, radiologic, and pathologic correlation. *Radiology*. 1989;170(2):441-445.

Gimenez A, Franquet T, Prats R, Estrada P, Villalba J, Bagué S. Unusual primary lung tumors: a radiologic–pathologic overview. *Radiographics*. 2002;22(3):601-619.

Glazer HS, Duncan-Meyer J, Aronberg DJ, Moran JF, Levitt RG, Sagel SS. Pleural and chest wall invasion in bronchogenic carcinoma: CT evaluation. *Radiology*. 1985;157(1):191-194.

Glazer HS, Kaiser LR, Anderson DJ, et al. Indeterminate mediastinal invasion in bronchogenic carcinoma: CT evaluation. *Radiology*. 1989;173(1):37-42.

Goldstraw P, Chansky K, Crowley J, et al; International Association for the Study of Lung Cancer Staging and Prognostic Factors Committee, Advisory Boards, and Participating Institutions, International Association for the Study of Lung Cancer Staging and Prognostic Factors Committee Advisory Boards and Participating Institutions. The IASLC lung cancer staging project: proposals for revision of the TNM stage groupings in the forthcoming (eighth) edition of the TNM classification for lung cancer. *J Thorac Oncol*. 2016;11(1):39-51. doi:10.1016/j.jtho.2015.09.009

Heelan RT, Demas BE, Caravelli JF, et al. Superior sulcus tumors: CT and MR imaging. *Radiology*. 1989;170(3 pt 1):637-641.

Kakinuma R, Ohmatsu H, Kaneko M, et al. Detection failures in spiral CT screening for lung cancer: analysis of CT findings. *Radiology*. 1999;212(1):61-66.

Kandathil A, Kay FU, Butt YM, Wachsmann JW, Subramaniam RM. Role of FDG PET/CT in the eighth edition of TNM staging of non–small cell lung cancer. *Radiographics*. 2018;38(7):2134-2149. doi:10.1148/rg.2018180060

Little BP, Junn JC, Zheng KS, et al. Diffuse idiopathic pulmonary neuroendocrine cell hyperplasia: imaging and clinical features of a frequently delayed diagnosis. *AJR Am J Roentgenol*. 2020;215(6):1312-1320. doi:10.2214/AJR.19.22628

Martin MD, Kanne JP, Broderick LS, Kazerooni EA, Meyer CA. Lung-RADS: pushing the limits. *Radiographics*. 2017;37(7):1975-1993. doi:10.1148/rg.2017170051

McLoud TC, Bourgouin PM, Greenberg RW, et al. Bronchogenic carcinoma: analysis of staging in the mediastinum with CT by correlative lymph node mapping and sampling. *Radiology*. 1992;182(2):319-323.

Mountain CF. Revisions in the international system for staging lung cancer. *Chest*. 1997;111(6):1710-1717.

National Lung Screening Trial Research Team; Aberle DR, Adams AM, Berg CD, et al. Reduced lung-cancer mortality with low-dose computed tomographic screening. *N Engl J Med*. 2011;365(5):395-409. doi:10.1056/NEJMoa1102873

Nicholson AG, Tsao MS, Beasley MB, et al. The 2021 WHO classification of lung tumors: Impact of advances since 2015. *J Thorac Oncol*. 2022;17(3):362-387. doi:10.1016/j.jtho.2021.11.003

Nickell LT Jr, Lichtenberger JP III, Khorashadi L, Abbott GF, Carter BW. Multimodality imaging for characterization, classification, and staging of malignant pleural mesothelioma. *Radiographics*. 2014;34(6):1692-1706.

Park CM, Goo JM, Lee HJ, Kim MA, Lee CH, Kang MJ. Tumors in the tracheobronchial tree: CT and FDG PET features. *Radiographics*. 2009;29(1):55-71.

Patel AM, Peters SG. Clinical manifestations of lung cancer. *Mayo Clin Proc*. 1993;68(3):273-277.

Pennes DR, Glazer GM, Wimbish KJ, Gross BH, Long RW, Orringer MB. Chest wall invasion by lung cancer: limitations of CT evaluation. *AJR Am J Roentgenol*. 1985;144(3):507-511.

Rami-Porta R, Crowley JJ, Goldstraw P. The revised TNM staging system for lung cancer. *Ann Thorac Cardiovasc Surg*. 2009;15(1):4-9.

Rami-Porta R, Bolejack V, Crowley J, et al; IASLC Staging and Prognostic Factors Committee, Advisory Boards and Participating Institutions. The IASLC lung cancer staging project: proposals for the revisions of the T descriptors in the forthcoming eighth edition of the TNM classification for lung cancer. *J Thorac Oncol*. 2015;10(7):990-1003. doi:10.1097/JTO.0000000000000559

Ratto GB, Piacenza G, Frola C, et al. Chest wall involvement by lung cancer: computed tomographic detection and results of operation. *Ann Thorac Surg*. 1991;51(2):182-188.

Rosado de Christenson ML, Abbott GF, Kirejczyk WM, Galvin JR, Travis WD. Thoracic carcinoids: radiologic–pathologic correlation. *Radiographics*. 1999;19(3):707-736.

Salvatierra A, Baamonde C, Llamas JM, Cruz F, Lopez-Pujol J. Extrathoracic staging of bronchogenic carcinoma. *Chest*. 1990;97(5):1052-1058.

Scott IR, Müller NL, Miller RR, Evans KG, Nelems B. Resectable stage III lung cancer: CT, surgical, and pathologic correlation. *Radiology*. 1988;166(1 pt 1):75-79.

Siegelman SS, Khouri NF, Scott WW, et al. Pulmonary hamartoma: CT findings. *Radiology*. 1986;160(2):313-317.

Staples CA, Müller NL, Miller RR, Evans KG, Nelems B. Mediastinal nodes in bronchogenic carcinoma: comparison between CT and mediastinoscopy. *Radiology*. 1988;167(2):367-372.

Travis WD, Garg K, Franklin WA, et al. Evolving concepts in the pathology and computed tomography imaging of lung adenocarcinoma and bronchioloalveolar carcinoma. *J Clin Oncol*. 2005;23(14):3279-3287.

Travis WD, Brambilla E, Noguchi M, et al. International association for the study of lung cancer/American Thoracic Society/European Respiratory Society international multidisciplinary classification of lung adenocarcinoma. *J Thorac Oncol.* 2011;6(2):244-285.

Travis et al., 2015 Travis WD, Brambilla E, Burke AP, et al. *WHO Classification of Tumours of the Lung, Pleura, Thymus and Heart.* WHO Press; 2015.

Travis WD, Brambilla E, Nicholson AG, et al. The 2015 World Health Organization classification of lung tumors: Impact of genetic, clinical and radiologic advances since the 2004 classification. *J Thorac Oncol.* 2015;10(9):1243-1260.

Travis WD. Advances in neuroendocrine lung tumors. *Ann Oncol.* 2010;21(suppl 7):65-71.

UyBico SJ, Wu CC, Suh RD, Le NH, Brown K, Krishnam MS. Lung cancer staging essentials: the new TNM staging system and potential imaging pitfalls. *Radiographics.* 2010;30(5):1163-1181.

Web Reference: American College of Radiology. *Lung CT Screening Reporting & Data System (Lung-RADS).* https://www.acr.org/Clinical-Resources/Reporting-and-Data-Systems/Lung-Rads.

Webb WR, Gatsonis C, Zerhouni EA, et al. CT and MR imaging in staging non–small cell bronchogenic carcinoma: report of the Radiologic Diagnostic Oncology Group. *Radiology.* 1991;178(3):705-713.

White CS, Salis AI, Meyer CA. Missed lung cancer on chest radiography and computed tomography: imaging and medicolegal issues. *J Thorac Imaging.* 1999;14(1):63-68.

Whitesell PL, Drage CW. Occupational lung cancer. *Mayo Clin Proc.* 1993;68(2):183-188.

Zwiebel BR, Austin JHM, Grimes MM. Bronchial carcinoid tumors: assessment with CT of location and intratumoral calcification in 31 patients. *Radiology.* 1991;179(2):483-486.

Zwirewich CV, Vedal S, Miller RR, Müller NL. Solitary pulmonary nodule: high-resolution CT and radiologic–pathologic correlation. *Radiology.* 1991;179(2):469-476.

Chapter 6

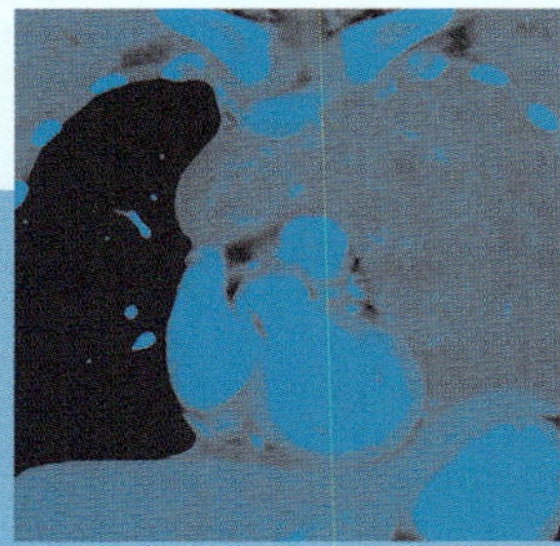

Travis S. Henry

Metastatic Tumor

INTRODUCTION

Nearly every part of the thorax can be involved in patients with metastatic neoplasm, and the chest is often the first site in which metastases are detected.

MECHANISMS OF SPREAD

Metastatic tumor may involve thoracic structures in several ways:

Direct extension from the primary tumor with secondary involvement of the lung, pleura, or mediastinal structures. This mode of spread is most common with thyroid tumors, esophageal carcinoma, thymoma and thymic malignancies, lymphoma, and malignant germ cell tumors.

Hematogenous spread of tumor emboli to pulmonary or bronchial arteries. This usually results in the presence of lung nodules and is most common with primary tumors that have a good vascular supply. Rarely, macroscopic metastases may be visible within pulmonary arteries mimicking pulmonary embolism.

Lymphatic (lymphangitic) spread to involve the lung, pleura, or mediastinal lymph nodes. The lung may be diffusely involved by tumor following lymphatic or lymphangitic spread of cells from hematogenous metastases, hilar lymph node metastases, or upper abdominal tumors. Lymphatic spread of extrathoracic tumors to mediastinal lymph nodes also may occur via the thoracic duct, with retrograde involvement of hilar lymph nodes and the lung parenchyma. Tumors that commonly metastasize in this fashion include carcinomas of the breast, stomach, pancreas, prostate, cervix, and thyroid.

Spread within the pleural space due to pleural invasion by a local tumor (eg, thymoma) or lung carcinoma.

Endobronchial (aerogenous) spread of cells from an airway tumor. This mechanism of metastasis is uncommon, except in patients with invasive mucinous adenocarcinoma. It is also thought to occur in patients with tracheobronchial papillomatosis.

MANIFESTATIONS OF METASTATIC TUMOR

Lung Nodules

Lung nodules are the most common thoracic manifestation of metastasis. In most cases, they are hematogenous in origin (Table 6.1). They tend to predominate in the lung bases, which receive more blood flow than the upper lobes.

Nodules tend to be sharply marginated in most cases and round or lobulated in contour (Fig. 6.1). Poorly marginated nodules may be seen in the presence of surrounding hemorrhage or local invasion of the adjacent lung (Fig. 6.2). In some cases, individual metastases are seen to have a relationship to small vascular branches, suggesting a hematogenous origin. This is termed the "feeding vessel" sign (Fig. 6.3). Nodules may be small or large. Using computed tomography (CT) with thin slices, metastasis as small as 1 to 2 mm may be visible.

Cavitation of metastases is not as common as with primary lung carcinoma, but it occurs in about 5% of cases. It may be seen even with small nodules (Fig. 6.4). The likelihood of cavitation varies with histology. Cavitation is most common with squamous cell tumors and transitional cell tumors but also may be seen in adenocarcinomas, particularly from the colon, and in some sarcomas.

Calcification of metastases occurs most commonly with osteogenic sarcoma, chondrosarcoma, synovial sarcoma, thyroid carcinoma, and mucinous adenocarcinoma (Fig. 6.5). Calcification (or ossification) may be dense, particularly with osteogenic sarcoma, mimicking a granuloma. Calcification may persist following successful chemotherapy despite resolution of the tumor.

CT is considerably more sensitive than plain radiographs in detecting lung nodules in patients with metastatic tumor,

Table 6.1 Nodular Metastases

Nodular Metastases
Hematogenous spread
Multiple nodules typically of different sizes
Basal predominance in size and number
Feeding vessel sign
Macroscopic intravascular tumor
Diffuse or "random" distribution
Poorly marginated nodules
Hemorrhage or invasion
Small nodules
Thyroid carcinoma
Melanoma
Adenocarcinoma
Sarcomas
Cannonball metastases
Renal cell carcinoma
Testicular carcinoma
Colon carcinoma
Cavitation
Squamous cell
Transitional cell
Adenocarcinoma (eg, colon)
Sarcomas
Calcification
Osteogenic sarcoma
Chondrosarcoma
Synovial sarcoma
Thyroid carcinoma
Mucinous adenocarcinoma
Solitary metastases
Colon carcinoma
Renal cell carcinoma
Testicular carcinoma
Sarcomas
Melanoma

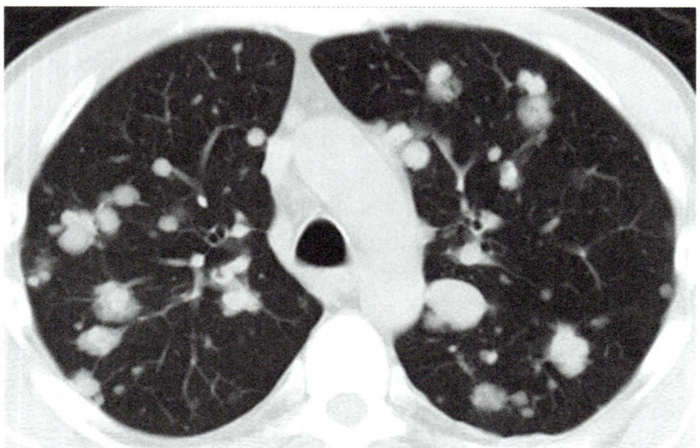

Figure 6.1. Metastatic salivary gland carcinoma with rounded and lobulated metastases. Nodules vary in size; this is typical with metastatic tumor and is less common with benign diseases.

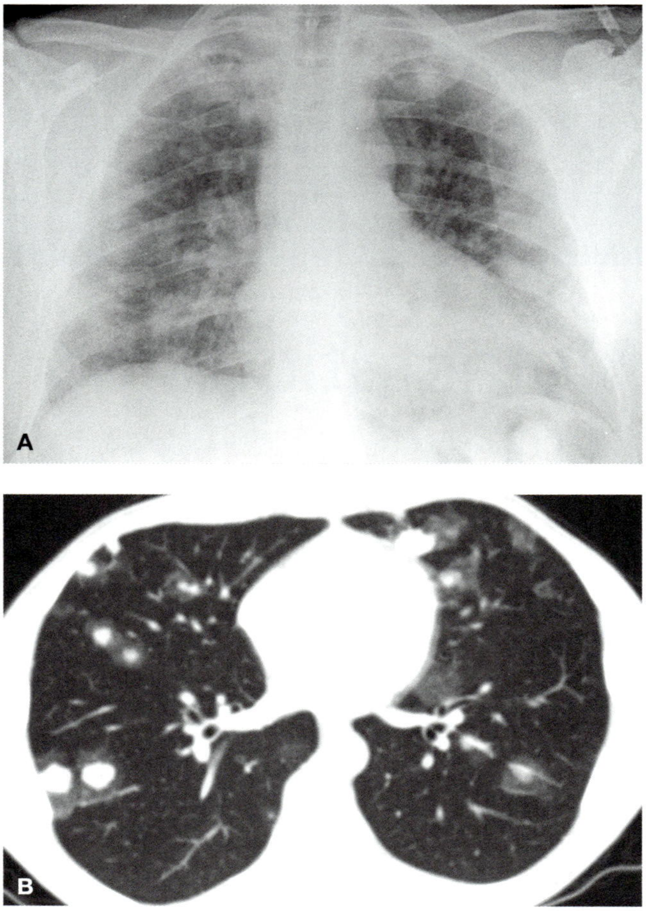

Figure 6.2. Metastases from choriocarcinoma. **A:** Chest radiograph shows multiple ill-defined lung nodules with a preponderance at the lung bases. **B:** CT shows rounded and lobulated nodules, many of which are surrounded by ground-glass opacity (ie, the halo sign). This appearance results from hemorrhage and is common with choriocarcinoma and other vascular tumors. It also may reflect invasion of the adjacent lung.

although the sensitivity of CT varies with slice thickness. The sensitivity of chest radiographs for detecting nodules in patients with lung metastases is about 40% to 45%, although this varies with the size of the nodules. Using CT with 5-mm slice thickness, a sensitivity of more than 80% has been reported for detection of nodular metastases 5 mm or less in diameter; the sensitivity of CT in detecting metastases larger than 5 mm is 100%.

On the other hand, lung nodules seen on CT in patients with a known tumor often represent something other than metastases. Granulomas, focal areas of infection, scarring, and intrapulmonary lymph nodes are all very common and mimic metastases on CT. These are generally small, measuring a few mm in diameter. Intrapulmonary lymph nodes often contact the pleural surface and are triangular in shape and/or have concave margins.

Nodules larger than a few mm, particularly when rounded and sharply defined, are more likely to represent metastatic

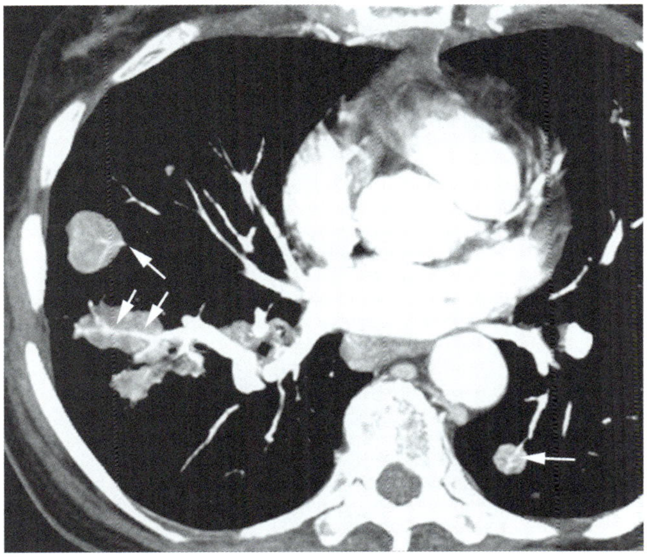

Figure 6.3. The feeding vessel sign. Vascular supply of lung metastases (*arrows*) in a patient with bladder carcinoma is shown using a maximum-intensity projection image obtained with 1.25-mm slice thickness after contrast infusion.

tumor. If small nodules are seen on CT in a patient with a known tumor, obtaining a follow-up CT at approximately 3 months is appropriate. Nodules representing metastases typically show growth; benign nodules usually show no growth, decrease in size, or resolve.

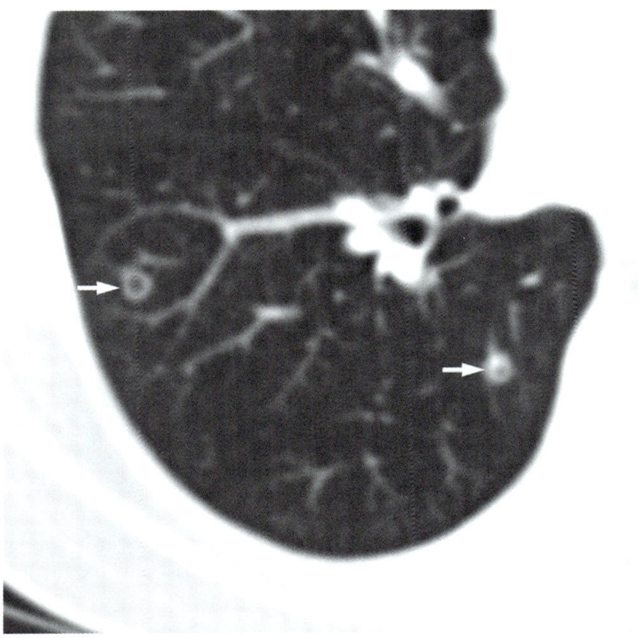

Figure 6.4. Cavitary metastases in metastatic colon cancer. Despite small size, distinct central cavities are visible in both nodules (arrows) within the right lower lobe on this image.

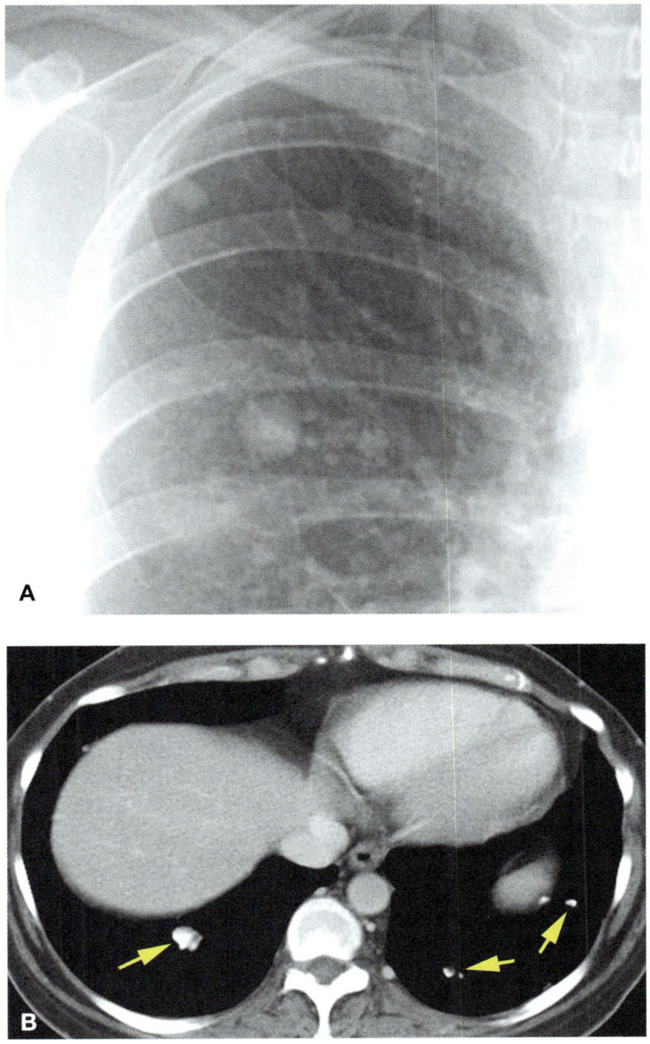

Figure 6.5. Ossified metastases secondary to osteogenic carcinoma. **A:** Chest radiograph shows dense nodules. **B:** CT shows dense calcification of nodules (*arrows*), which is typical of this tumor.

Multiple Nodules

Nodular metastases usually are multiple. The nodules often vary in size, representing multiple episodes of tumor embolization or different growth rates (see Figs. 6.1, 6.2, and 6.6); this appearance is less common with benign nodular disease, such as sarcoidosis. Occasionally, all of the nodular metastases are of the same size. When there are numerous nodules, they tend to be distributed throughout the lung (Fig. 6.7). When the metastases are few in number, they may be predominantly peripheral/juxtapleural.

On CT, numerous nodules tend to involve the lung in a diffuse fashion without regard for specific anatomic structures, a distribution termed "random" (see Figs. 6.7B and 6.8B). This pattern is described in detail in Chapter 11.

The size and number of nodules vary greatly. Nodules may be small (ie, miliary) and very numerous (Fig. 6.8);

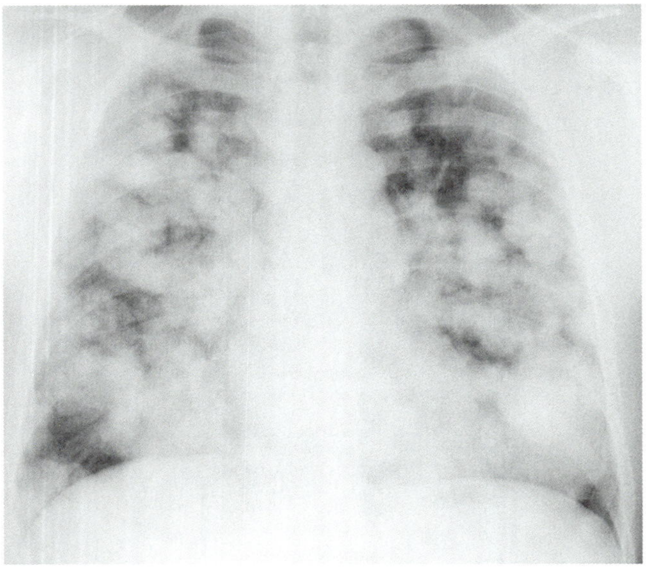

Figure 6.6. Metastatic testicular carcinoma. Nodules vary in size and appear more numerous and larger at the lung bases. A basal preponderance is typical of metastases. Large nodular metastases are sometimes called "cannonball" metastases.

this appearance often is seen with very vascular tumors (eg, thyroid carcinoma, renal cell carcinoma, adenocarcinoma, sarcomas) and presumably reflects a single massive shower of tumor emboli. Fewer, larger metastases also may be seen; when these are well defined, they are referred to as "cannonball metastases" (see Figs. 6.6 and 6.9). This type of metastasis is seen most commonly with tumors of the gastrointestinal or genitourinary tract.

Most patients (80%-90%) with multiple metastases have a history of neoplasm. In some patients, however, there is no history of a primary tumor at the time of diagnosis; in others, the primary tumor may never be found.

Solitary Nodule

Metastatic tumor occasionally presents as a solitary nodule (Fig. 6.10). About 5% to 10% of solitary nodules represent solitary metastases. Solitary metastases are most common with carcinomas of the colon, kidney, and testis, and with sarcomas and melanoma. It must be emphasized that many patients who appear to have a solitary metastasis visible on chest radiograph are discovered to have multiple pulmonary nodules on CT, with one nodule being dominant.

A solitary metastasis is more likely to have a smooth margin than is primary lung carcinoma (see Fig. 6.10), but this finding on its own is not sufficient to permit a reliable distinction between primary and metastatic tumors. Solitary metastases may appear spiculated, and primary carcinomas may be smooth. A solitary metastasis is more likely when the tumor is located at the lung base; primary carcinoma is more common in the upper lobes.

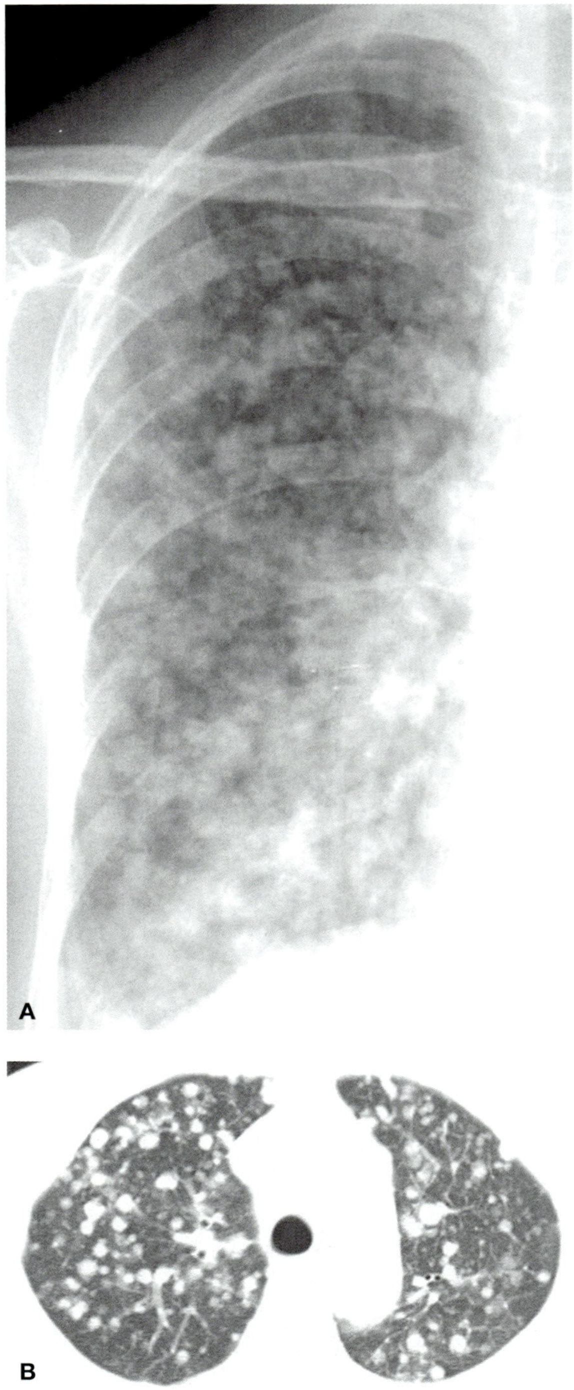

Figure 6.7. Metastatic adenocarcinoma. **A:** Chest radiograph shows numerous small, diffusely distributed nodules. Nodules appear more numerous and larger at the lung bases. **B:** CT shows a diffuse distribution of nodules. This pattern is termed "random," because it involves the lung randomly relative to lung structures. Some nodules typically are seen to involve the pleural surface with a random pattern.

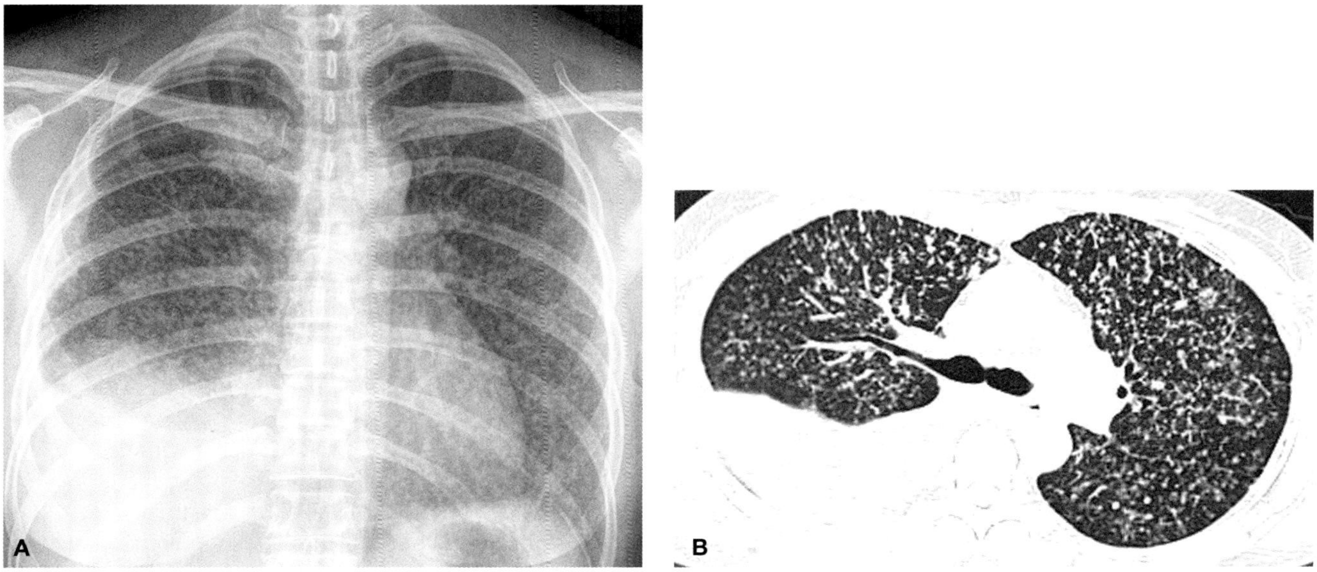

Figure 6.8. Metastatic lung carcinoma. **A:** Chest radiograph shows innumerable small nodular (miliary) metastases. **B:** CT shows a diffuse distribution of small lung nodules, having a random pattern. A right pleural effusion is also present.

In a patient with a known extrathoracic tumor and a solitary nodule detected radiographically, the likelihood that the nodule is a metastasis (as opposed to primary lung cancer) varies with the cell type of the primary tumor. Patients with carcinomas of the head and neck, bladder, breast, cervix, bile ducts, esophagus, ovary, prostate, or stomach are more likely to have primary lung carcinoma than lung metastasis (ratio, 8:1 for patients with head and neck cancers; 3:1 for patients with other types of cancer). Patients with carcinomas of the salivary glands, adrenal gland, colon, parotid gland, kidney, thyroid gland, thymus, or uterus have fairly even odds (ratio, 1:1). Patients with melanoma, sarcoma, or testicular carcinoma are more likely to have a solitary metastasis than a lung carcinoma (ratio, 2.5:1).

Lymphangitic Spread of Tumor

Lymphangitic spread of tumor refers to tumor growth in the lymphatic system of the lungs (Table 6.2). It occurs most commonly in patients with carcinomas of the breast,

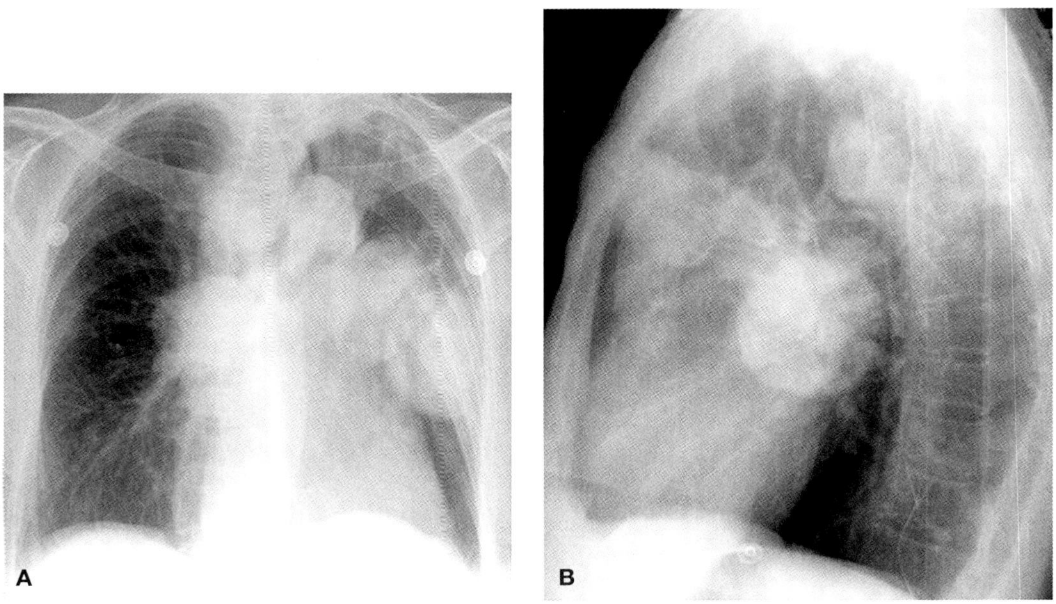

Figure 6.9. Cannonball metastases in metastatic vaginal carcinoma. Frontal (**A**) and lateral (**B**) radiographs show several large, well-defined metastases.

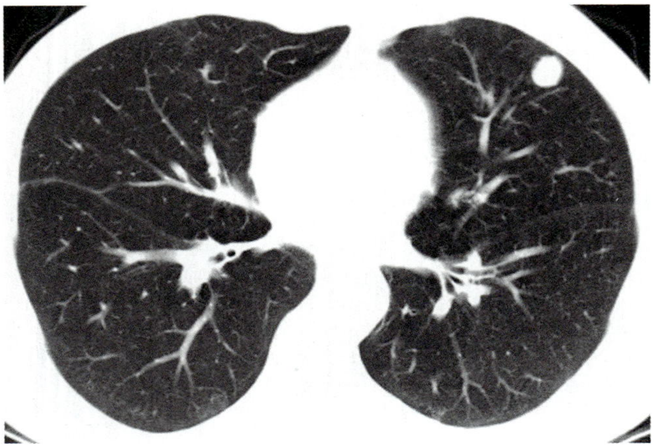

Figure 6.10. Solitary metastasis shown on CT at the lung base. No other nodules were visible. This nodule is sharply marginated. Biopsy showed the same cell type as the primary tumor.

lung, stomach, pancreas, prostate, cervix, or thyroid and in patients with metastatic adenocarcinoma from an unknown primary site; about 80% of cases are due to adenocarcinoma. It usually results from hematogenous spread to the lung, with subsequent interstitial and lymphatic invasion, but also can occur because of direct lymphatic spread of tumor from mediastinal and hilar lymph nodes. Symptoms of shortness of breath are common and can predate radiographic abnormalities.

The radiographic manifestations of pulmonary lymphangitic carcinomatosis include reticular or reticulonodular opacities, Kerley lines, hilar and mediastinal lymphadenopathy, and pleural effusion (Fig. 6.11A and B). The appearance of unilateral or asymmetrical Kerley lines is particularly suggestive. However, these findings are nonspecific. In some patients, the chest radiograph is normal.

On high-resolution CT, lymphangitic spread of tumor typically shows (1) smooth thickening of the interlobular septa, (2) smooth thickening of the peribronchovascular interstitium surrounding vessels and bronchi in the perihilar lung (ie, "peribronchial cuffing"), and (3) smooth subpleural interstitial thickening (ie, thickening of the fissures; see Fig. 6.11C). Less often, nodular thickening of these structures is visible (Fig. 6.12). This pattern of nodules is termed "perilymphatic" (see Chapter 11).

In about 50% of patients, the abnormalities of lymphangitic spread appear focal, unilateral, or asymmetrical rather than diffuse on CT (see Fig. 6.11C). Hilar lymphadenopathy is visible on CT in only 50% of patients with lymphangitic spread. Mediastinal lymph node enlargement also can be seen. Lymph node enlargement can be symmetrical or asymmetrical. Pleural effusion is common.

Table 6.2 Lymphangitic Spread of Neoplasm

Results from:
Hematogenous metastasis with lymphatic invasion
Spread from hilar node metastases
Direct spread from upper abdominal tumors
Findings:
Interlobular septal thickening (ie, Kerley lines)
Thickening of the peribronchovascular interstitium
Thickening of the fissures
Perilymphatic nodules
Abnormalities asymmetric or unilateral in 50%
Common causes:
Breast carcinoma
Lung carcinoma
Stomach carcinoma
Pancreas carcinoma
Prostate carcinoma
Cervical carcinoma
Thyroid carcinoma
Adenocarcinoma from an unknown site

Airway Metastases

Metastatic tumors may involve the tracheal or bronchial wall because of local spread from adjacent mediastinal structures (eg, esophagus), lung, or lymph node metastases or because of hematogenous spread (Table 6.3).

Involvement of the airway wall because of aerogenous spread from other endobronchial tumors is less common but does occur (Fig. 6.13). This pattern of metastasis occurs commonly with tracheobronchial papillomatosis (see Figs. 5.24 and 5.25 in Chapter 5) and invasive mucinous adenocarcinoma (Fig. 6.14).

Airway metastasis may present with symptoms or findings of airway obstruction and atelectasis (Fig. 6.15). If this occurs in the presence of multiple nodular metastases, the diagnosis is not difficult. However, if no other findings are present, or if other findings include lymphangitic spread or hilar lymph node enlargement, it is difficult to distinguish between metastasis and primary lung cancer. In some patients, airway obstruction may be the first manifestation of the extrathoracic neoplasm.

Radiographs or CT may show a tapered narrowing of the airway lumen ("rattail" appearance) due to local invasion, bronchial obstruction, or a sessile or polypoid endobronchial mass, often due to hematogenous spread to the airway wall (Figs. 6.15-6.18). Airway wall metastases are most common in melanoma, thyroid carcinoma, renal cell carcinoma, testicular carcinoma, breast carcinoma, and sarcomas.

Vascular Metastases

Most tumor emboli associated with hematogenous metastasis are microscopic. In occasional patients, tumor emboli are large enough or numerous enough to result in symptoms or findings of vascular occlusion as a primary manifestation

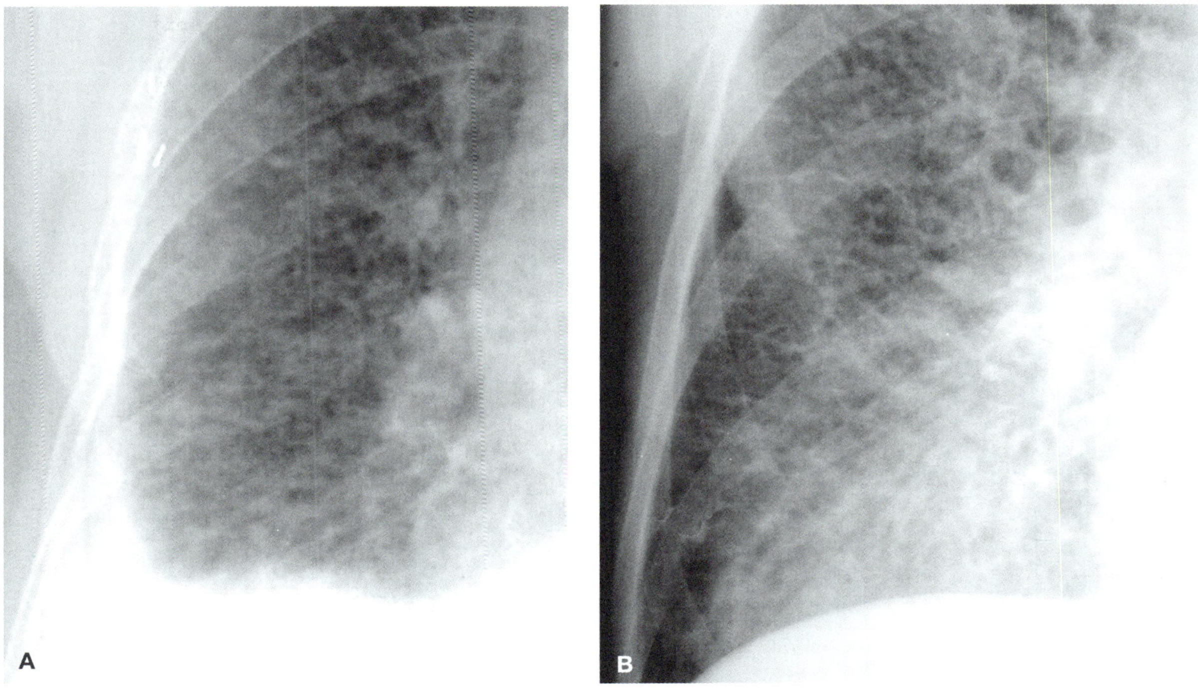

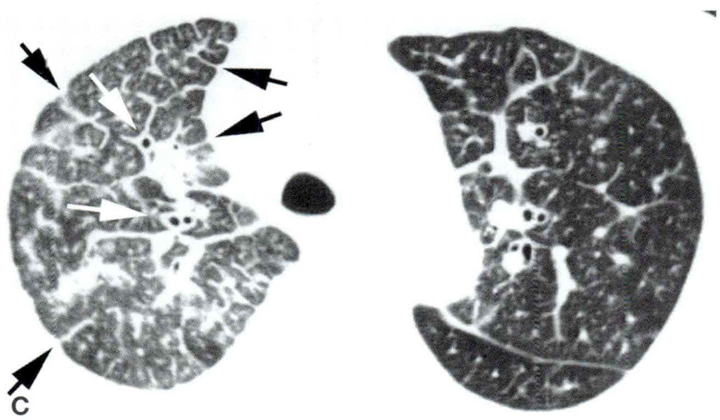

Figure 6.11. Lymphangitic spread of breast carcinoma. **A:** Coned-down radiograph showing that the right lower lobe demonstrates an abnormal reticular pattern and a right pleural effusion. **B:** Coned-down radiograph in another patient shows distinct Kerley B lines. **C:** High-resolution CT in a patient with breast carcinoma. There is asymmetric lung involvement characterized by smooth interlobular septal thickening (*black arrows*) and thickening of the peribronchovascular interstitium surrounding vessels and bronchi in the perihilar lung (ie, "peribronchial cuffing"; *white arrows*). Slight thickening of the left major fissure also is seen.

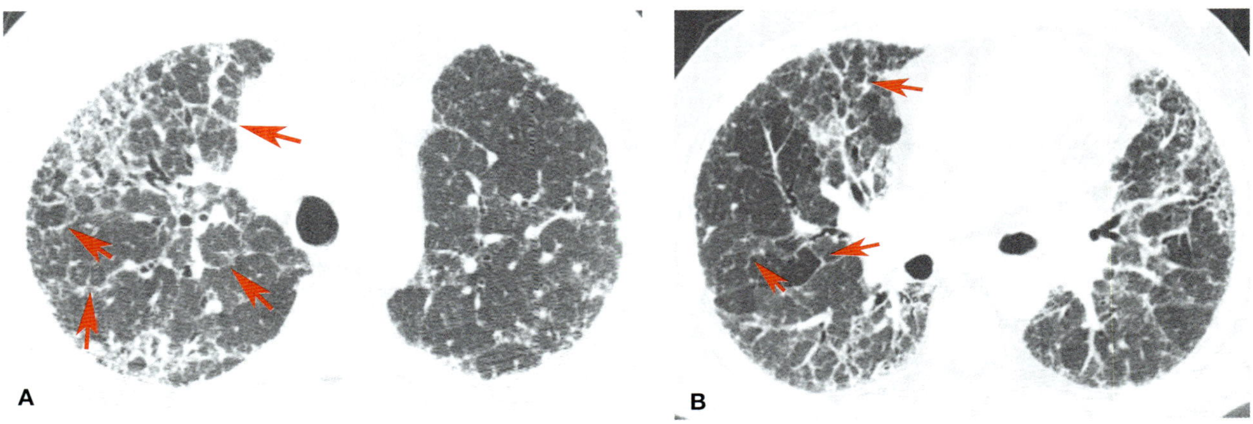

Figure 6.12. Nodular interlobular septal thickening in lymphangitic spread of colon cancer. **A-C:** Septal thickening is visible with some subtle areas of nodularity (*red arrows*, **A**, **B**; *yellow arrows*, **C**). There is some pre-existing fibrosis (*red arrows*, **C**).

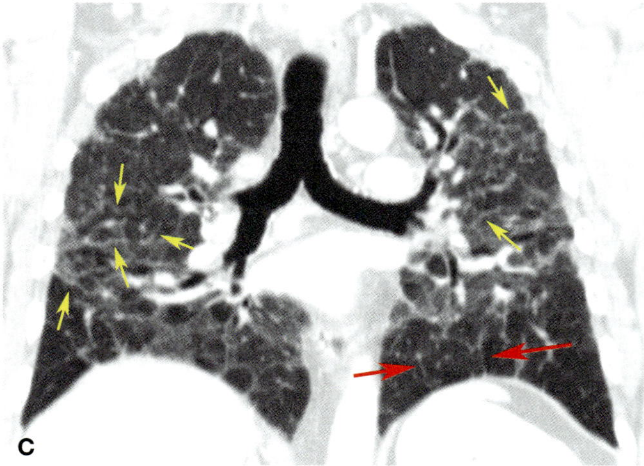

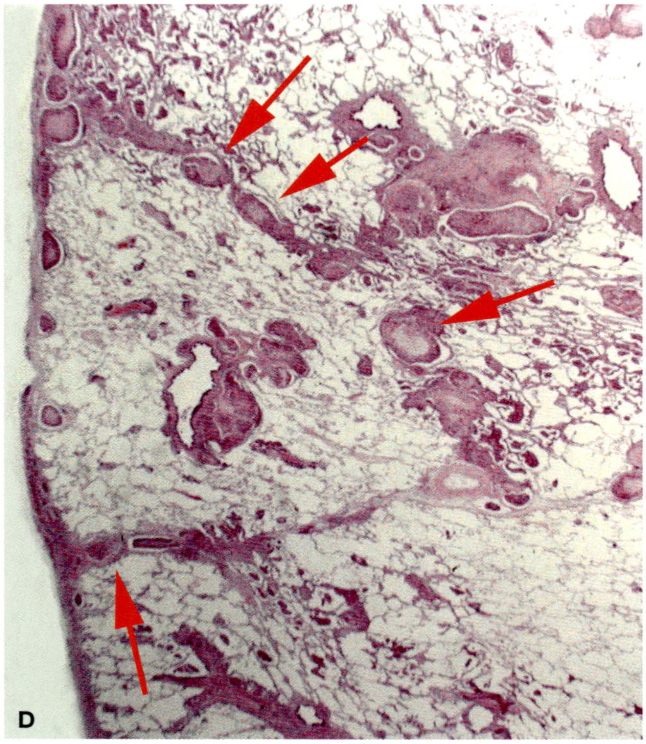

Figure 6.12. (*Continued*) **D:** Nodular thickening of interlobular septa by tumor (*arrows*), shown on histology. (Courtesy of Kirk Jones.)

(Table 6.4). Vascular metastases may mimic pulmonary infarction (large tumor emboli) clinically and radiographically or pulmonary hypertension (large or numerous tumor emboli). Vascular metastases may occur with or without other findings of metastatic tumor.

CT findings include (1) visible tumor emboli mimicking the appearance of pulmonary emboli on contrast-enhanced scans (Fig. 6.19), (2) findings of pulmonary infarction, (3) a nodular or beaded appearance of peripheral pulmonary arteries due to smaller tumor emboli (Fig. 6.20), and (4)

Table 6.3 Airway Metastases

Result from: Local spread from adjacent lung or lymph node metastases Hematogenous spread to bronchial wall Endobronchial spread
Common causes: Melanoma Thyroid carcinoma Renal cell carcinoma Testicular carcinoma Breast carcinoma Invasive mucinous adenocarcinoma (IMA) Papillomatosis
Findings: Mimics primary lung cancer with bronchial obstruction Bronchial narrowing or polypoid endobronchial mass Centrilobular nodules and consolidation (IMA) Nodules, cysts, and cavities (papillomatosis)

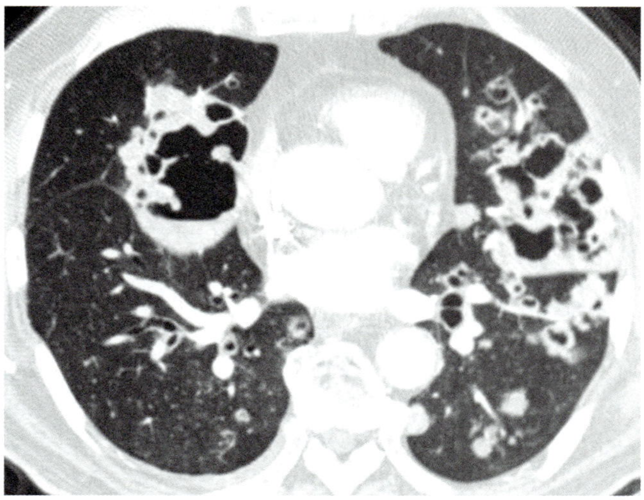

Figure 6.13. Endobronchial spread of squamous cell carcinoma. In a patient with a squamous cell carcinoma involving the right upper lobe, extensive bilateral nodular and cavitary masses are visible. Some lucent lesions likely represent airways. Extensive endobronchial tumor was present.

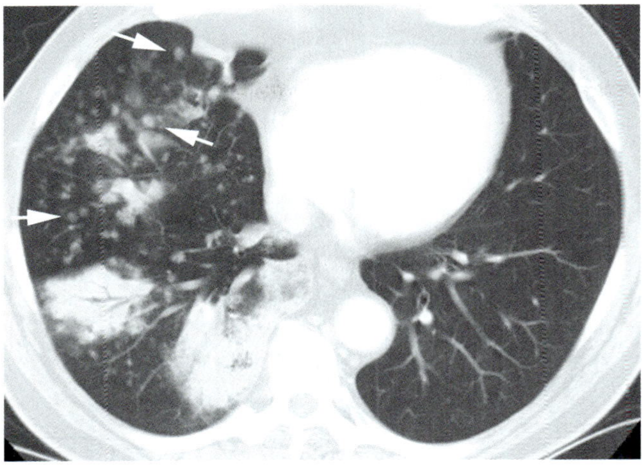

Figure 6.14. Invasive mucinous adenocarcinoma. Patchy areas of consolidation and centrilobular nodules (*arrows*) are visible. This appearance in mucinous adenocarcinoma is due to endobronchial (aerogenous) spread. Focal airway lesions do not occur with this tumor.

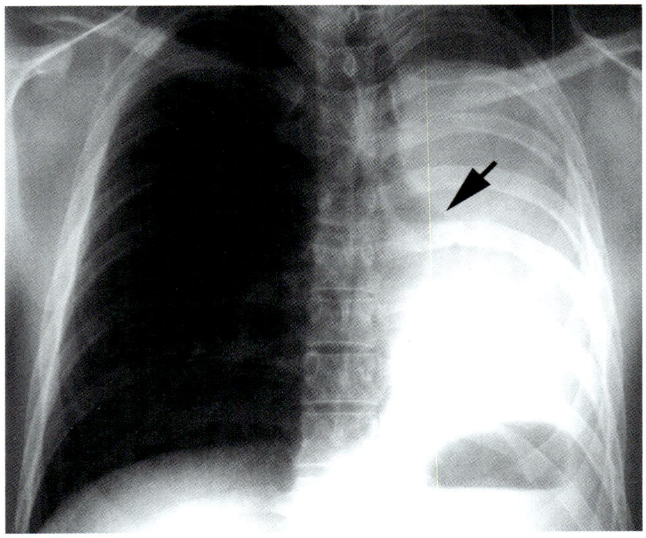

Figure 6.15. Metastasis to the left main bronchus (*arrow*) from testicular carcinoma. There is obstruction of the left main bronchus with left lung atelectasis.

pulmonary artery dilatation due to large tumor emboli or pulmonary hypertension.

Large tumor emboli are most common with tumors resulting in invasion of large systemic veins or the right heart, most often renal cell carcinoma, hepatocellular carcinoma, right atrial myxoma, and angiosarcoma. Numerous small emboli resulting in pulmonary hypertension and cor pulmonale may occur with very vascular primary tumors. In addition to those listed, these include choriocarcinoma and adenocarcinoma.

Lymph Node Metastases

Metastases to mediastinal or hilar lymph nodes from extrathoracic malignancies are uncommon, occurring in less than 3% of cases. The extrathoracic tumors most likely to metastasize to the mediastinum and hila are carcinomas of the head and neck (including thyroid tumors), genitourinary tract (eg, renal and testicular carcinoma), breast, and melanoma (Table 6.5). Enlarged lymph nodes may be unilateral or bilateral and symmetrical or asymmetrical. In distinction to hilar masses occurring in lung cancer, which may be quite irregular and ill-defined due to local invasion, hilar node enlargement in patients with metastases is often sharply marginated (Figs. 6.21 and 6.22).

Most metastatic tumors result in lymph node enlargement without distinguishing characteristics. However, enhancing nodes may be seen secondary to metastatic renal cell carcinoma, papillary thyroid carcinoma, lung cancer, sarcomas, melanoma, and some other tumors (Fig. 6.23). Calcified lymph node metastases are most typical of thyroid carcinoma, mucinous adenocarcinoma, and sarcomas.

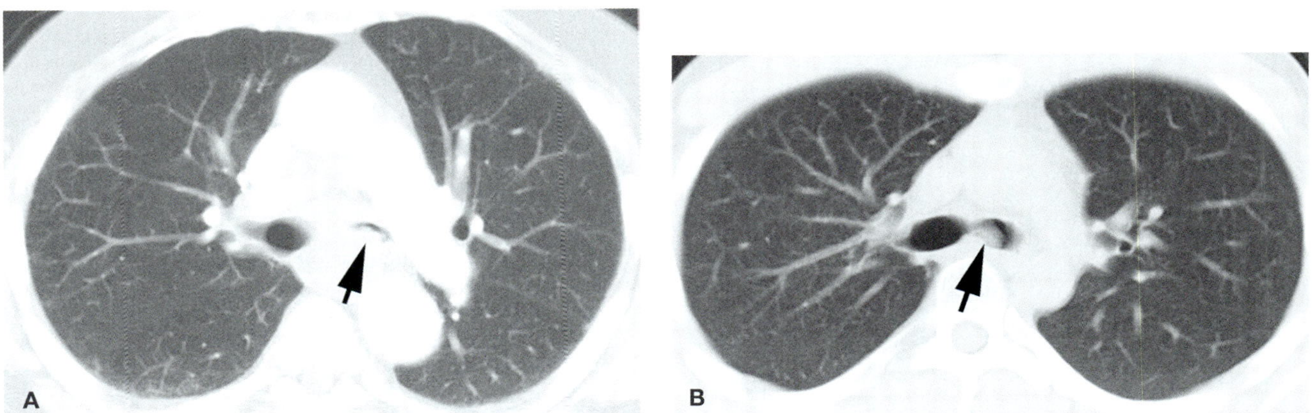

Figure 6.16. Endobronchial metastases. **A:** Metastasis to the left main bronchus from a head and neck carcinoma. A polypoid mass (*arrow*) is seen within the left main bronchus. **B:** Polypoid endobronchial mass (*arrow*) in metastatic melanoma.

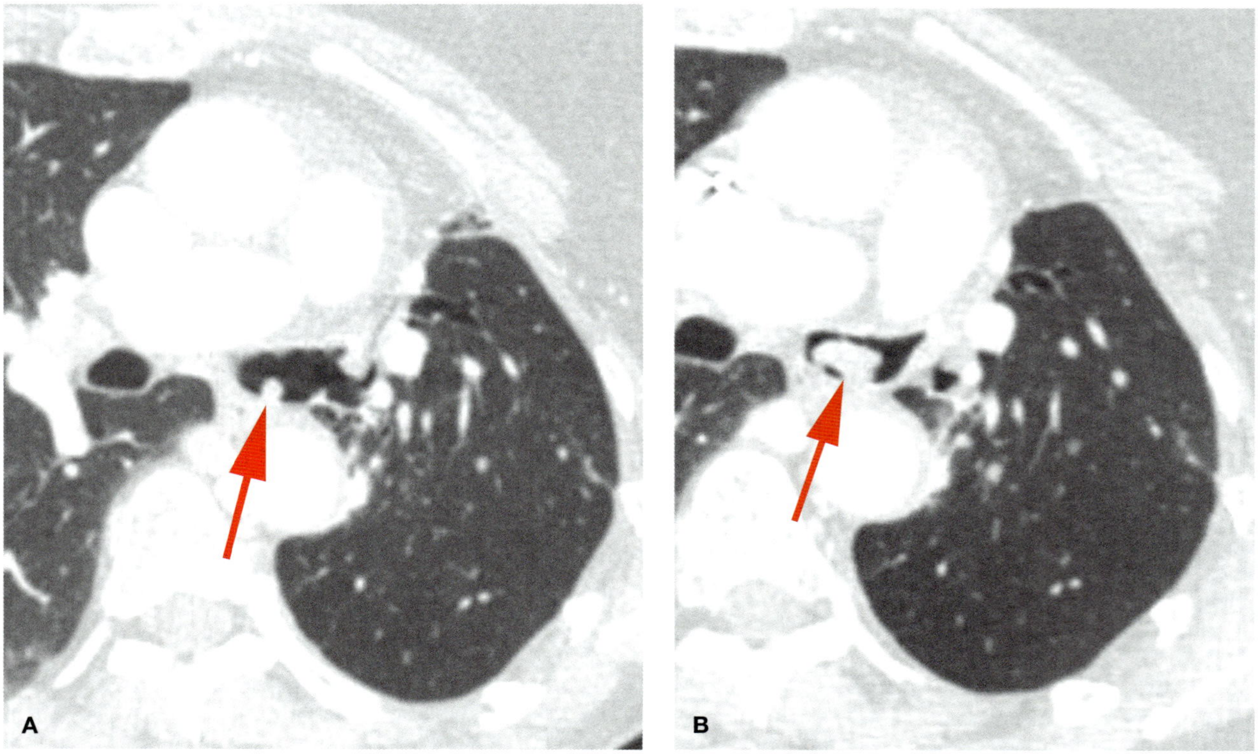

Figure 6.17. Endobronchial metastasis in colon carcinoma. **A:** CT shows a small nodule (*arrow*) arising from the posterior wall of the left upper lobe bronchus. **B:** Follow-up 3 months later shows marked increase in size of the polypoid metastasis (*arrow*).

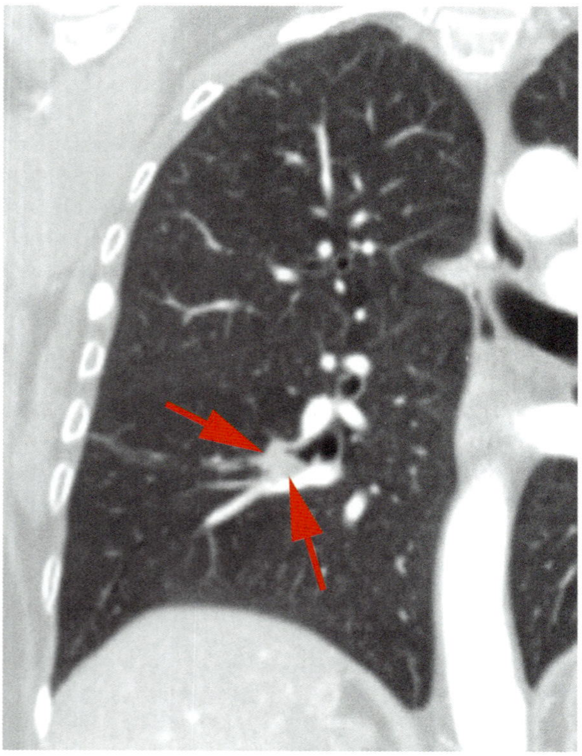

Figure 6.18. Endobronchial metastasis in breast carcinoma. Coronal CT reconstruction shows a small metastasis (*arrows*) obstructing a right lower lobe segmental bronchus.

Calcification of treated metastases also may occur (Figs. 6.24 and 6.25). Necrotic, rim-enhancing, or low-attenuation lymph nodes also may be seen (Fig. 6.26); these are common in testicular carcinoma, renal cell carcinoma, breast cancer, and lung cancer.

The location of enlarged nodes sometimes is suggestive of the primary tumor site.

Superior mediastinal lymph node involvement suggests a head and neck tumor (see Fig. 6.22).

Posterior mediastinal or paravertebral lymph node enlargement suggests an abdominal location for the primary tumor (see Fig. 6.23) or tumors metastasizing via

Table 6.4 Vascular Metastases

Tumor embolism
Findings:
- Vascular filling defects mimicking pulmonary embolism
- Pulmonary infarction
- Beaded vessels
- Pulmonary artery dilatation

Common causes:
- Renal cell carcinoma
- Hepatocellular carcinoma
- Right atrial myxoma
- Angiosarcoma

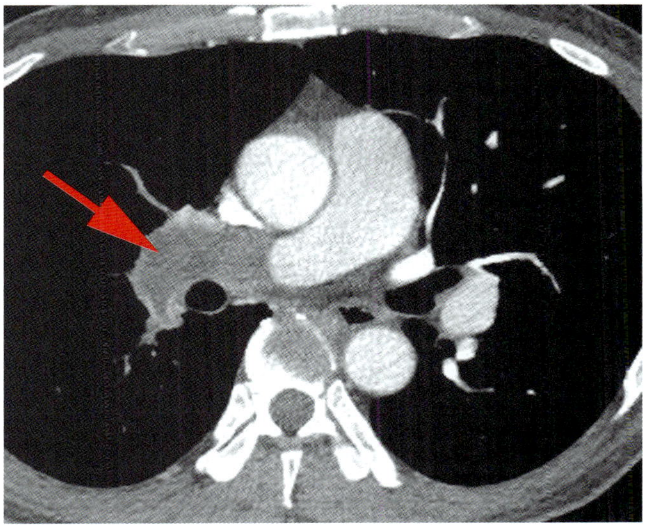

Figure 6.19. Vascular metastasis from hepatocellular carcinoma mimicking pulmonary embolism. Enhanced CT shows a large filling defect (*arrow*) obstructing the right pulmonary artery.

retroperitoneal lymph nodes, such as testicular carcinoma. Retrocrural lymph node enlargement often is an associated finding.

Internal mammary lymph node metastases are most likely due to breast carcinoma (Fig. 6.27). They may be associated with cardiophrenic node enlargement.

Cardiophrenic (epiphrenic) lymph node enlargement may occur as a result of metastasis from abdominal or thoracic tumors, in approximately equal numbers; most common are carcinomas of the colon, lung, ovary, and breast (Fig. 6.28).

Pleural Metastases

The appearance of pleural metastases is discussed in detail in Chapter 26. Pleural metastasis may result from local spread, hematogenous spread, or lymphatic spread. It is most common with adenocarcinoma (Table 6.6).

In patients with pleural metastases, plain films usually show pleural effusion or pleural thickening, which may be lobulated, nodular, or concentric (ie, surrounding the lung). The presence of pleural effusion in patients with neoplasm is nonspecific; it may result from lymphatic obstruction (ie, lymphangitic spread of tumor, hilar or mediastinal node metastases, thoracic duct obstruction) rather than pleural metastases. CT may show pleural effusion with or without pleural thickening, pleural masses and nodular pleural thickening (see Fig. 6.28), or concentric pleural thickening. Nodular pleural thickening or pleural masses in a patient with known malignancy strongly suggest pleural metastasis.

Pneumothorax

Spontaneous pneumothorax may result from metastases involving the visceral pleural surface. The pleural metastases

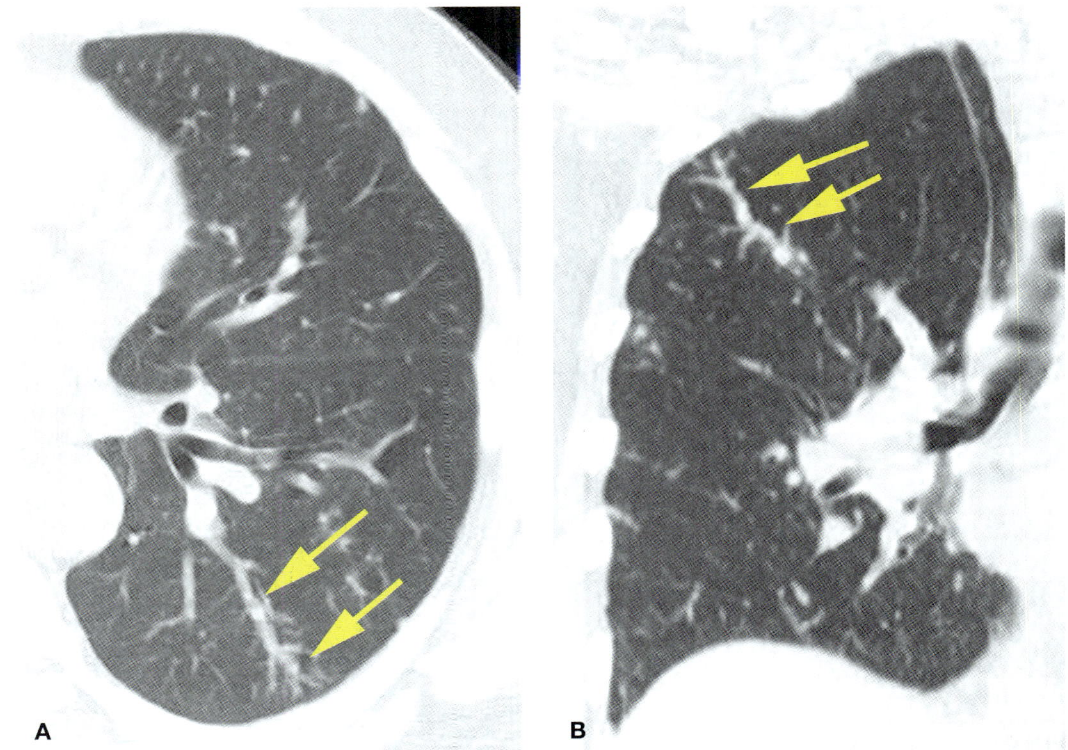

Figure 6.20. Vascular metastasis from transitional cell carcinoma. **A, B:** CT shows dilated and beaded peripheral vessels (*arrows*) due to intravascular metastases. This is a typical appearance.

Table 6.5 Lymph Node Metastases

Result from:
- Spread via the thoracic duct
- Spread to lymph nodes from hematogenous lung metastases

Unilateral or bilateral

Sharply marginated node masses

Common causes:
- Head and neck tumors
- Thyroid carcinoma
- Renal cell carcinoma
- Testicular carcinoma
- Breast carcinoma
- Melanoma

Enhancing lymph node metastases common causes:
- Thyroid carcinoma
- Renal cell carcinoma
- Testicular carcinoma
- Breast carcinoma
- Melanoma

Calcified lymph node metastases common causes:
- Thyroid carcinoma
- Mucinous adenocarcinoma
- Sarcomas

Superior mediastinal lymph nodes common causes:
- Head and neck tumor
- Thyroid carcinoma

Internal mammary lymph node metastases common cause:
- Breast carcinoma

Posterior mediastinal lymph node metastases common causes:
- Abdominal tumors

Cardiophrenic lymph node metastases common causes:
- Colon carcinoma
- Lung carcinoma
- Ovarian carcinoma
- Breast carcinoma

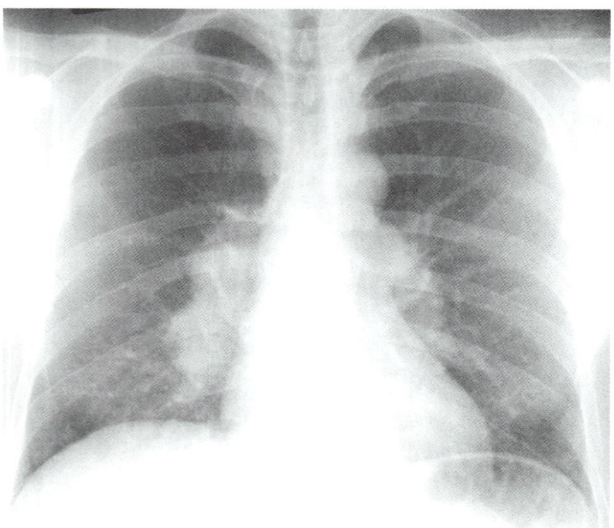

Figure 6.21. Hilar lymph node metastases from renal cell carcinoma. Well-defined, lobulated hilar masses are visible bilaterally.

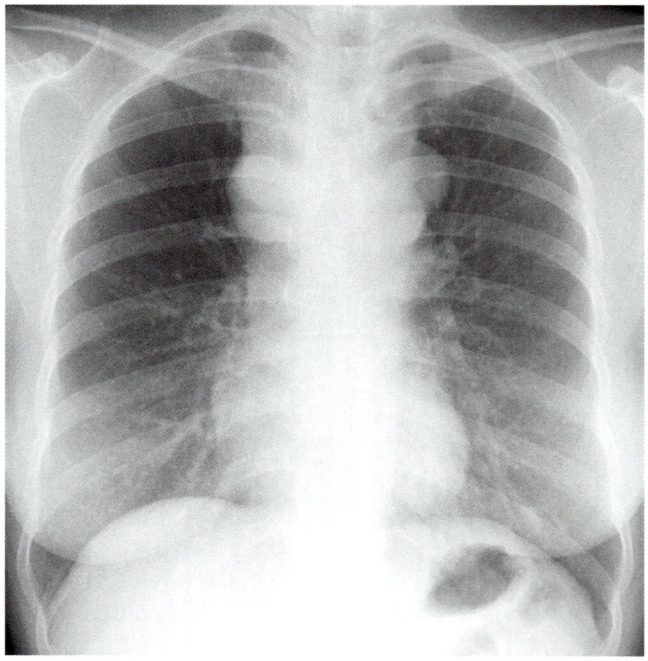

Figure 6.22. Mediastinal lymph node metastases from papillary thyroid carcinoma. Bilateral superior mediastinal and paratracheal masses are visible. The hila appear normal.

may appear necrotic or cavitary, or they may appear solid, with pneumothorax presumably resulting from other mechanisms of pleural disruption or airway obstruction with air trapping (Fig. 6.29). Pneumothorax is most typical of metastatic sarcoma and may be the first symptom of metastasis.

KAPOSI SARCOMA

Kaposi sarcoma (KS) is a tumor derived from primitive vascular tissues, occurring in (1) patients with AIDS or having had transplantation, who may have a poor prognosis and (2) elderly individuals, in whom the disease primarily involves

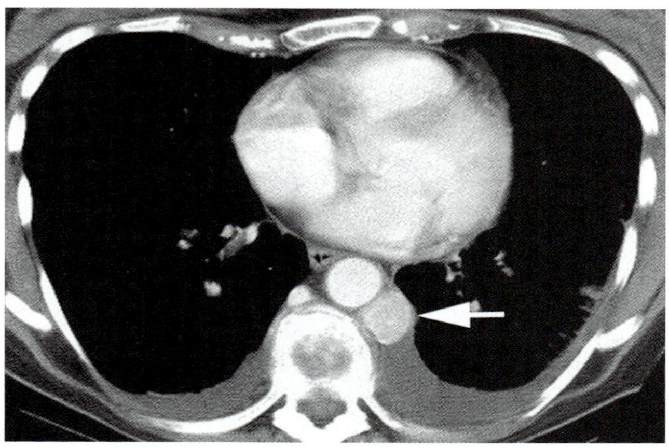

Figure 6.23. Enhancing lymph node metastasis with metastatic paraganglioma. A left paraaortic lymph node (*arrow*) is densely enhancing.

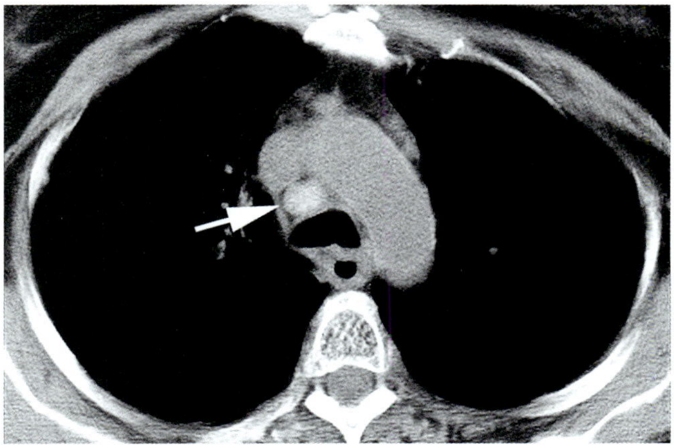

Figure 6.24. Calcified lymph node metastasis in thyroid carcinoma. A faintly calcified and enlarged right paratracheal lymph node (*arrow*) is visible. Lymph node calcification is characteristic of tumors that calcify at their primary site.

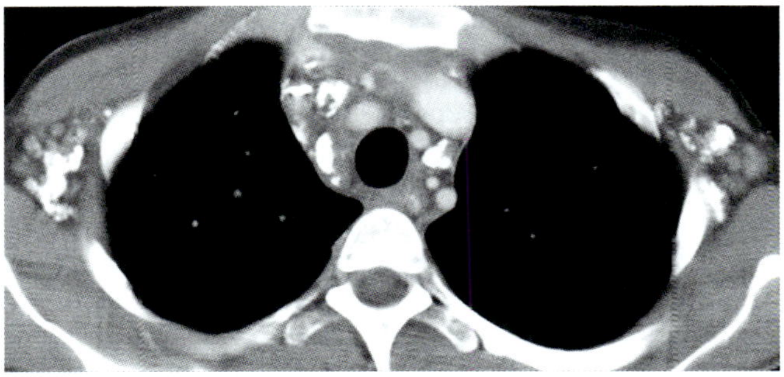

Figure 6.25. Calcified lymph nodes following treatment of metastatic gastric cancer. Multiple densely calcified axillary and mediastinal nodes are visible.

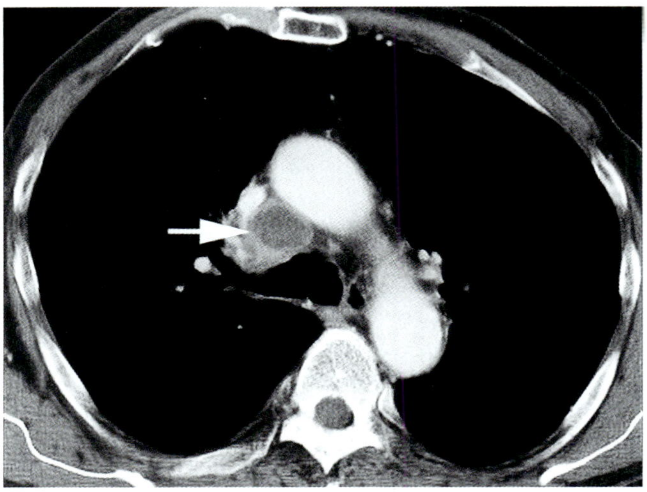

Figure 6.26. Necrotic lymph node in metastatic renal cell carcinoma. An enlarged right paratracheal lymph node (*arrow*) shows a low-attenuation center and rim enhancement.

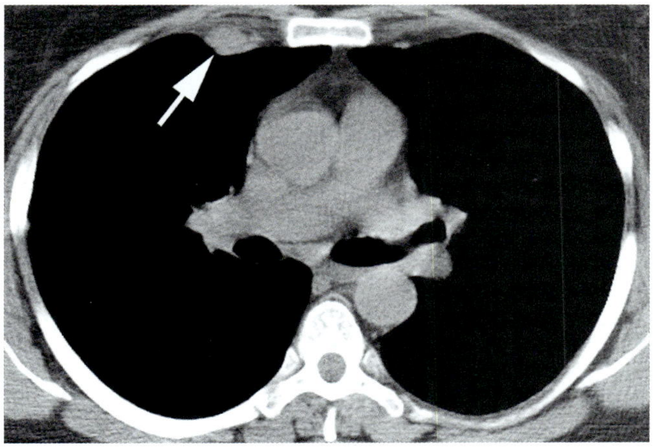

Figure 6.27. Internal mammary lymph node metastasis in breast cancer. An enlarged node (*arrow*) is visible on the right.

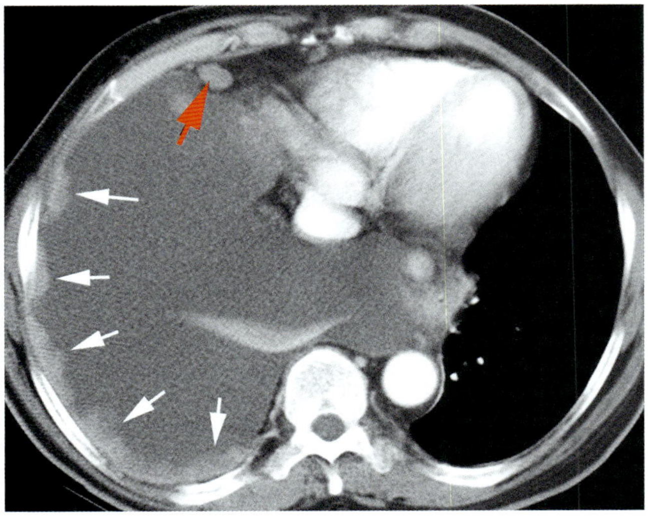

Figure 6.28. Metastatic colon carcinoma with cardiophrenic lymph node enlargement and malignant pleural effusion. Cardiophrenic lymph node enlargement (*red arrow*) is present. Multiple pleural nodules (*white arrows*) are highly suggestive of pleural metastases.

Table 6.6 Pleural Metastases

Result from:
- Local spread
- Hematogenous spread
- Lymphatic spread

Pleural effusion, nonspecific

Findings suggesting neoplasm:
- Nodular pleural thickening
- Concentric pleural thickening

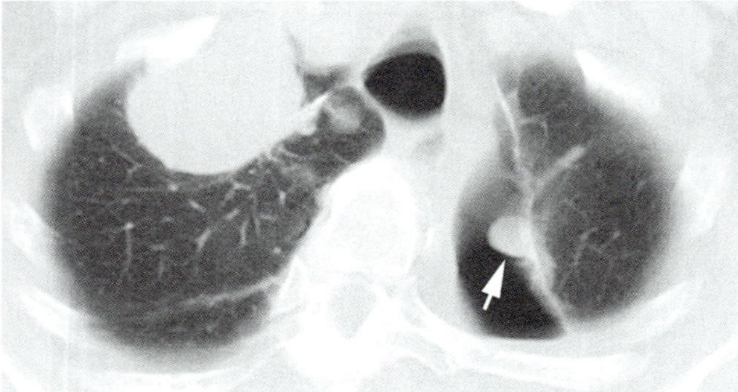

Figure 6.29. Metastatic melanoma with pneumothorax. A solid-appearing metastasis (*arrow*) involving the visceral pleural surface of the left lung is associated with a pneumothorax. A large metastasis is also visible at the right apex.

Table 6.7 Kaposi Sarcoma

Most common in HIV infection and transplantation
Caused by a herpesvirus infection
Pulmonary involvement in 20%-50%
Usually preceded by cutaneous involvement
Airway lesions visible at bronchoscopy
Coarse reticular opacities at the lung bases
Ill-defined or spiculated (flame-shaped) nodules
Parahilar or peribronchovascular distribution
Interlobular septal thickening
Pleural effusion
Lymph node enlargement

the skin and in whom the prognosis is good. The incidence of KS associated with AIDS has decreased significantly because of current aggressive treatments of HIV infection. It is associated with infection by the KS–associated herpesvirus (KSHV), also known as human herpesvirus 8.

Formerly, KS developed in 15% to 20% of patients with AIDS, and it remains most common in patients with HIV infection (Table 6.7). About 1 in 200 transplant patients in the United States get KS; most were infected with KSHV before transplantation.

Pulmonary involvement occurs in 20% to 50% of AIDS patients with KS and usually, but not always, is preceded by cutaneous or visceral involvement. Endobronchial lesions detected at bronchoscopy tend to predict the presence of pulmonary disease. Pathologically, pulmonary involvement in KS is patchy, but it has a distinct relationship to the peribronchovascular interstitium in the perihilar regions and to the pleura.

Chest radiographs typically show bilateral, diffuse abnormalities characterized by the presence of (1) coarse reticular opacities or ill-defined consolidation in the perihilar regions or lower lobes (90% of cases; Fig. 6.30), (2) poorly defined nodules up to several centimeters in diameter (Fig. 6.31A), and (3) focal ill-defined areas of consolidation. A basal predominance of abnormalities is common, and the earliest abnormalities recognized often include thickening of the peribronchovascular interstitium at the lung bases (see Fig. 6.30). Kerley lines may be seen. Pleural effusions, usually bilateral, are seen in 30% of cases. Hilar or mediastinal lymph node enlargement is apparent on the chest radiograph in approximately 10% of patients (see Fig. 6.30B). The chest radiographic appearance is somewhat analogous to that of lymphangitic spread of carcinoma.

Early CT findings include thickening of the peribronchovascular interstitium, particularly at the lung bases, mimicking the appearance of infectious AIDS-related airway

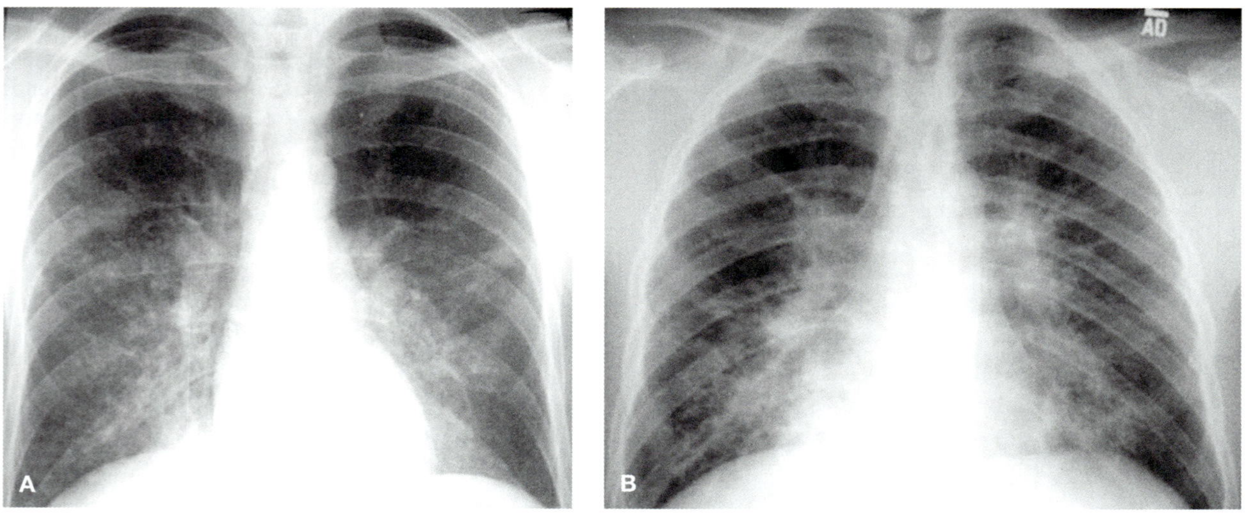

Figure 6.30. Radiographic appearances of Kaposi sarcoma (KS) in two AIDS patients. **A:** Coarse, ill-defined opacities and consolidation are visible in the perihilar regions and lower lobes. This is typical of KS. Several nodules are also visible. **B:** Streaky opacities are visible in the lower lobes. Hilar lymph node enlargement is also visible.

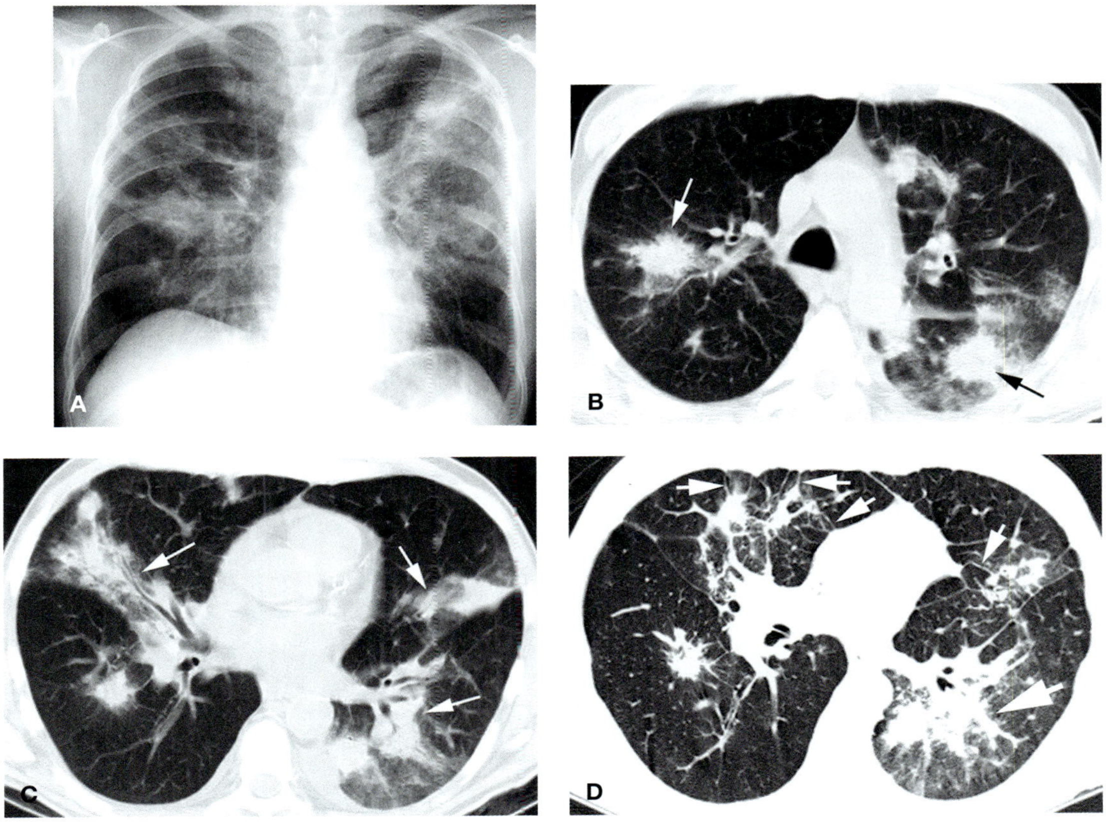

Figure 6.31. Kaposi sarcoma (KS) in an AIDS patient with a CD4 count of 41. **A:** Chest radiograph shows ill-defined nodular opacities and an increase in streaky opacity at the right base. **B:** CT with 5-mm slice thickness shows ill-defined and spiculated nodules (*arrows*). These are typical of the later stages of KS. **C:** CT with 5-mm slice thickness at a lower level shows involvement of the peribronchovascular regions (*arrows*) typical of KS. **D:** High-resolution CT shows spiculated nodules, peribronchovascular infiltration (*large arrow*), and interlobular septal thickening (*small arrows*). Areas of ground-glass opacity may represent associated pulmonary hemorrhage.

disease. Typical CT features of KS in more advanced cases include (1) irregular and ill-defined or spiculated (flame-shaped) nodules, often predominating in the peribronchovascular regions (see Fig. 6.31B-D), (2) peribronchovascular interstitial thickening (see Fig. 6.31D), (3) interlobular septal thickening (see Fig. 6.31D), (4) pleural effusion, and (5) lymphadenopathy. Although a number of infections and tumors in AIDS patients may present radiographically with lung nodules, CT findings of irregular nodules, larger than 1 cm, with a perihilar distribution usually allow KS to be distinguished from other thoracic complications.

SUGGESTED READINGS

Aquino S. Imaging of metastatic disease to the thorax. *Radiol Clin North Am.* 2005;43(3):481-495.

Chou SHS, Prabhu SJ, Crothers K, Stern EJ, Godwin JD, Pipavath SN. Thoracic diseases associated with HIV infection in the era of antiretroviral therapy: clinical and imaging findings. *Radiographics.* 2014;34(4):895-911.

Davis SD. CT evaluation for pulmonary metastases in patients with extrathoracic malignancy. *Radiology.* 1991;180:1-12.

Diederich S, Semik M, Lentschig MG, et al. Helical CT of pulmonary nodules in patients with extrathoracic malignancy: CT-surgical correlation. *AJR Am J Roentgenol.* 1999;172(2):353-360.

Edinburgh KJ, Jasmer RM, Huang L, et al. Multiple pulmonary nodules in AIDS: usefulness of CT in distinguishing among potential causes. *Radiology.* 2000;214(2):427-432.

Goldsmith SH, Bailey HD, Callahan EL, Beattie EJ. Pulmonary metastases from breast carcinoma. *Arch Surg.* 1967;94:483-488.

Gruden JF, Huang L, Webb WR, Gamsu G, Hopewell PC, Sides DM. AIDS-related Kaposi sarcoma of the lung: radiographic findings and staging system with bronchoscopic correlation. *Radiology.* 1995;195(2):545-552.

Hartman TE, Primack SL, Müller NL, Staples CA. Diagnosis of thoracic complications in AIDS: accuracy of CT. *AJR Am J Roentgenol.* 1994;162(3):547-553.

Janower ML, Blennerhassett JB. Lymphangitic spread of metastatic cancer to the lung. A radiologic-pathologic classification. *Radiology.* 1971;101(2):267-273.

Johkoh T, Ikezoe J, Tomiyama N, et al. CT findings in lymphangitic carcinomatosis of the lung: correlation with histologic findings and pulmonary function tests. *AJR Am J Roentgenol.* 1992;158(6):1217-1222.

McGuinness G, Gruden JF, Bhalla M, Harkin TJ, Jagirdar JS, Naidich DP. AIDS-related airway disease. *AJR Am J Roentgenol.* 1997;168(1):67-77.

McLoud TC, Kalisher L, Stark P, Greene R. Intrathoracic lymph node metastases from extrathoracic neoplasms. *AJR Am J Roentgenol.* 1978;131(3):403-407.

Munden RF, Pugatch RD, Liptay MJ, Sugarbaker DJ, Le LU. Small pulmonary lesions detected at CT: clinical importance. *Radiology.* 1997;202(1):105-110.

Munk PL, Müller NL, Miller RR, Ostrow DN. Pulmonary lymphangitic carcinomatosis: CT and pathologic findings. *Radiology.* 1988;166(3):705-709.

Naidich DP, McGuinness G. Pulmonary manifestations of AIDS: CT and radiographic correlations. *Radiol Clin North Am.* 1991;29(5):999-1017.

Naidich DP, Tarras M, Garay SM, Birnbaum B, Rybak BJ, Schinella R. Kaposi sarcoma: CT-radiographic correlation. *Chest*. 1989;96(4):723-728.

Peuchot M, Libshitz HI. Pulmonary metastatic disease: radiologic-surgical correlation. *Radiology*. 1987;164(3):719-722.

Quint LE, Park CH, Iannettoni MD. Solitary pulmonary nodules in patients with extrapulmonary neoplasms. *Radiology*. 2000;217(1):257-261.

Ren H, Hruban RH, Kuhlman JE, et al. Computed tomography of inflation-fixed lungs: the beaded septum sign of pulmonary metastases. *J Comput Assist Tomogr*. 1989;13(3):411-416.

Restrepo CS, Martınez S, Lemos JA, et al. Imaging manifestations of Kaposi sarcoma. *Radiographics*. 2006;26(4):1169-1185.

Seo JB, Im JG, Goo JM, Chung MJ, Kim MY. Atypical pulmonary metastases: spectrum of radiologic findings. *Radiographics*. 2001;21(2):403-417. doi:10.1148/radiographics.21.2.g01mr17403

Stein MG, Mayo J, Müller N, Aberle DR, Webb WR, Gamsu G. Pulmonary lymphangitic spread of carcinoma: appearance on CT scans. *Radiology*. 1987;162(2):371-375.

Chapter 7

Travis S. Henry

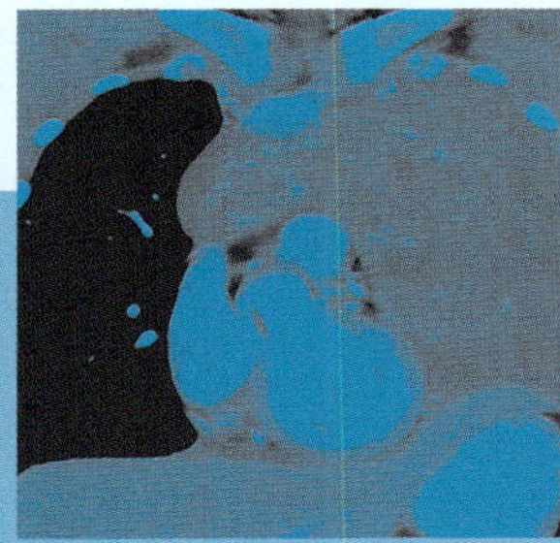

Lymphoma and Lymphoproliferative Disease

CLASSIFICATION OF LYMPHOMAS AND LYMPHOPROLIFERATIVE DISEASE

In this chapter, neoplasms of hematopoietic and lymphoid tissues, as classified by the World Health Organization (WHO), are reviewed. The 5th edition was published in 2022, which replaces the 4th (2008) and Revised 4th (2016) editions. A second classification system of hematologic malignancies was also published in 2022 by the International Consensus Classification. The differences in these classification systems are beyond the scope of this text, and use of either system is appropriate.

The classification of hematologic malignancies is increasingly complex with hundreds of different diagnoses now listed, and the list is certain to grow in subsequent iterations. In the simplest terms, hematologic malignancies are classified by morphology (histology), acuity (acute vs chronic), clinical attributes (cytopenias/cytoses), lineage (immunophenotype), and cytogenetic/molecular mutations (Table 7.1).

In the WHO classification, neoplasms are considered in four groups, primarily based on cell type and genetic differences. These groups include B-cell lymphoid proliferations and lymphomas, T-cell and NK-cell lymphoid proliferations and lymphomas, myeloid proliferations and neoplasms, and histiocytic/dendritic neoplasms. Posttransplant lymphoproliferative disorders (PTLDs) fall under the umbrella of B-cell category and have been further subdivided from the prior classification system.

A number of possible risk factors or etiologies have been recognized as associated with lymphomas and lymphoproliferative disease. Immunosuppression from any cause is a well-known risk factor. Multiple infectious agents have been linked to development of lymphoma and lymphoproliferative disease, including human immunodeficiency virus (HIV), human T-cell lymphotropic virus (HTLV), Epstein-Barr virus (EBV), and hepatitis C virus. Genetic mutations have been linked to multiple lymphoma subtypes, although these have not been fully explored.

In this chapter, for simplicity, lymphomas are considered in two primary groups, Hodgkin lymphoma (HL) and non-Hodgkin lymphoma (NHL). Only those neoplasms that are most common, or commonly result in thoracic manifestations, are reviewed in detail. Although HL is the less common of the two types, representing about 25% to 30% of cases, it is more common as a cause of thoracic and mediastinal disease.

With the exception of Erdheim-Chester disease (discussed in Chapter 5) and pulmonary Langerhans histiocytosis (discussed in Chapter 25), this chapter also reviews the primary pulmonary *lymphohistiocytic disorders* defined by WHO in 2022 (see Chapter 5), including extranodal marginal zone lymphomas of mucosa-associated lymphoid tissue (MALT lymphoma), diffuse large B-cell lymphoma (DLBCL), and lymphomatoid granulomatosis (LG).

STAGING OF LYMPHOMA

The Ann Arbor staging system for lymphoma, first introduced in 1971 and revised in 1989 to include the "Cotswolds modifications," has been applied to both HL and many (although not all) NHLs. Using this system, stage is based on the extent of involvement of nodal groups: stage I, single lymph node group; stage II, multiple lymph node groups, ipsilateral to the diaphragm; stage III, involvement of lymph node groups, both above and below the diaphragm; and stage IV, noncontiguous extranodal involvement (eg, liver,

Table 7.1 WHO Classification of Tumors of Hematopoietic and Lymphoid Tissues: Common Types

Mature B-cell neoplasms (85% of NHL)
Pre-neoplastic and neoplastic small lymphocytic proliferation
Chronic lymphocytic leukemia/small lymphocytic lymphoma
Lymphoplasmacytic lymphoma
Marginal zone lymphoma
Extranodal marginal zone lymphoma of mucosa-associated tissue
Follicular lymphoma
Cutaneous follicle center lymphoma
Mantle cell lymphoma
Transformation of indolent B-cell lymphomas
Large B-cell lymphoma
Diffuse large B-cell lymphoma
Primary mediastinal large B-cell lymphoma
Lymphomatoid granulomatosis
Burkitt lymphoma
KSHV/HHV8-associated B-cell lymphoid proliferation and lymphomas
Primary effusion lymphoma
Lymphoid proliferation and lymphoma associated with immune deficiency and dysregulation (including PTLD)
Hyperplasias arising in immune deficiency/dysregulation
Polymorphic lymphoproliferative disorders arising in immune deficiency/dysregulation
Lymphomas arising in immune deficiency/dysregulation
Plasma cell neoplasms and other diseases with paraproteins
Monoclonal gammopathies
Monoclonal gammopathy of undetermined significance
Diseases with monoclonal immunoglobulin deposition
Immunoglobulin-related (AL) amyloidosis
Monoclonal immunoglobulin deposition disease
Heavy chain disease
Plasma cell neoplasms
Plasmacytoma
Plasma cell myeloma
Mature T-cell and NK-cell Neoplasms (15% of NHL)
Mature T-cell and NK-cell Leukemias
Anaplastic large cell lymphoma
Nodal T-follicular helper cell lymphoma
Other peripheral T-cell lymphomas
EBV-positive NK/T-cell lymphomas
EBV-positive T- and NK-cell lymphoid proliferations and lymphomas of childhood
Hodgkin lymphoma
Classic Hodgkin lymphoma
Nodular lymphocyte predominant Hodgkin lymphoma
Dendritic cell and histiocytic neoplasms
Plasmacytoid dendritic cell neoplasms
Langerhans cell and other dendritic cell neoplasms
Langerhans cell histiocytosis
Langerhans cell sarcoma
Histiocytic neoplasms
Juvenile xanthogranuloma
Erdheim-Chester disease
Rosai-Dorfman disease
ALK-positive histiocytosis
Histiocytic sarcoma

EBV, Epstein-Barr virus KSHV/HHV8, Kaposi sarcoma herpesvirus/human herpes virus 8; NHL, non-Hodgkin lymphoma; NK, natural killer; PTLD, posttransplant lymphoproliferative disorder.

Modified and abbreviated from Khoury JD, Solary E, Abla O, et al. The 5th edition of the World Health Organization classification of haematolymphoid tumours: myeloid and histiocytic/dendritic neoplasms. Leukemia. *2022;36(7):1703-1719. doi:10.1038/s41375-022-01613-1.*

lung, or bone marrow). Subclassification as A and B was used, based on the absence or presence of symptoms, including fevers to greater than 101°F (38.3°C), weight loss, and night sweats. X was used to describe bulky disease.

Revisions to the staging system used for lymphomas were recommended in 2011 at the 11th International Conference on Malignant Lymphoma in Lugano, Switzerland, and published in 2014 as the "Lugano Classification" (Table 7.2). These revisions recognized the important role of CT in staging and the use of positron emission tomography (PET) as routine in the initial evaluation and as a baseline for assessment of treatment response in most lymphomas. PET is used in HL and fluorodeoxyglucose (FDG)-avid NHL (almost all cell types except chronic lymphocytic leukemia [CLL]/small lymphocytic lymphoma [SLL], lymphoplasmacytic lymphoma/Waldenström macroglobulinemia, mycosis fungoides, and marginal zone NHL). PET improves the accuracy of staging compared with CT for both nodal and extranodal sites. It leads to change in stage in 10% to 30% of patients, more often an upstaging, although alteration in management occurs in fewer patients, and there has not been a demonstrated impact on overall outcome. However, improving staging accuracy using PET-CT ensures that fewer patients are undertreated or overtreated and is particularly important for staging before consideration of radiation therapy.

In the Lugano Classification, a modification of Ann Arbor and Cotswold terminology is used for a description of disease extent. Patients are now more simply categorized as having "limited disease" (previously Ann Arbor stage I or II) or "advanced disease" (previously Ann Arbor stage III or IV) disease. A fifth category, stage II bulky, may be considered limited or advanced depending on histology and other prognostic factors. The current definition of "bulky" disease in HL is retained (a mass greater than

Table 7.2 Lugano Staging Classification for Nodal Lymphoma

Stage[a]	Definition
Limited	
I	Involvement of a single lymph node region (I) or a single extralymphatic organ or site (I_E)
II[b]	Involvement of two or more lymph node regions on the same side of the diaphragm (II) or localized involvement of an extralymphatic organ or site and of one or more lymph node regions on the same side of the diaphragm (II_E)
Advanced	
III	Involvement of lymph node regions on both sides of the diaphragm or nodes above the diaphragm with involvement of the spleen
IV	Additional noncontiguous extralymphatic involvement

[a]*In Hodgkin lymphoma, the absence or presence of fever, night sweats, and/or unexplained loss of 10% or more of body weight in 6 months is denoted by the suffix A or B, respectively.*

[b]*Designation of "bulky" disease if a single lymph node is greater than 10 cm or greater than 1/3 of transthoracic diameter.*

10 cm or one-third of the transthoracic diameter), and the associated "X" modifier is no longer applied to HL or NHL. It is recommended, however, that the longest diameter of a mass visible on computed tomography (CT) is recorded for staging purposes in both HL and NHL. The modifiers A and B are only used in patients with HL, as they correlate poorly with outcome in NHL.

LYMPHOMA FOLLOW-UP AND ASSESSMENT OF RECURRENCE

In 1999, the International Working Group recommended that the evaluation of clinical response of lymphoma be based on CT findings. Subsequent modifications in 2007 and 2009 ("the Deauville criteria") defined response on the basis of metabolic activity using PET/CT, and these recommendations were adopted in the Lugano Classification.

One goal of the Lugano Classification is the simplification and standardization of response assessment and reporting. Simply stated, FDG-PET/CT has been incorporated as an essential part of staging and response assessment of FDG-avid lymphomas, as described previously. CT staging remains appropriate for lymphoma types with low or variable FDG uptake, and a diagnostic contrast-enhanced CT should still be performed in the initial staging of lymphoma, to provide optimal anatomic assessment.

Four categories of lymph node response using CT have been defined: (1) *complete radiologic response*, all nodes ≤1.5 cm in longest diameter or disappearance of all CT findings of lymphoma; (2) *partial response*, 50% or greater decrease in disease burden; (3) *stable disease*, less than 50% decrease in disease burden; and (4) *progressive disease*, new or increased adenopathy or new extranodal lymphoma. Disease burden is defined as the sum of the product of lymph node or mass diameters (two perpendicular diameters for each node), for up to six measurable nodes or masses or extranodal sites.

Response assessment using FDG-PET/CT is based on metabolic activity as determined by FDG uptake. The standardized uptake value serves as a marker of metabolic activity, and response assessment is based on the visual assessment of FDG uptake as compared to baseline and is categorized with a simple "five-point scale." The five-point scale includes the following categories: (1) no FDG uptake above background, (2) FDG uptake ≤ mediastinum, (3) FDG uptake > mediastinum ≤ liver, (4) FDG uptake moderately > liver, (5) FDG uptake markedly > liver and/or new lesions. Response criteria for PET are (a) *complete metabolic response*, score of 1, 2, or 3 in nodal or extranodal sites with or without a residual mass; (b) *partial metabolic response*, a score of 4 or 5 with reduced uptake compared with baseline and residual mass(es) of any size; (c) *no metabolic response*, a score of 4 or 5 with no obvious change in FDG uptake; and (d) *progressive disease*, a score 4 or 5 in any lesion with an increase in intensity of uptake from baseline and/or new FDG-avid foci consistent with lymphoma.

The paper by Johnson et al, referenced at the end of this chapter, provides a detailed review of this subject.

HODGKIN LYMPHOMA

HL or Hodgkin disease occurs at all ages, but its peak incidence is in the third and eighth decades; it accounts for about 0.5% to 1% of all newly diagnosed malignancies and 10% of all lymphomas (Table 7.3). It is more prevalent in males, with a male-to-female ratio ranging from 1.4 to 1.9. Intrathoracic HL usually is associated with disease elsewhere; cervical lymph nodes are commonly involved. Constitutional symptoms may be present. HL is characterized histologically by the presence of Reed-Sternberg cells. It is associated with EBV infection in about half of cases. It may occur in association with acquired immunodeficiency syndrome (AIDS) or may be a manifestation of PTLD.

Four histologic types of HL were originally recognized in the Rye classification: nodular sclerosis HL (accounting for 50%-80% of adult HL cases), lymphocyte-predominant HL, mixed cellularity, and lymphocyte depletion. In the 2022 WHO classification, classic definitions of HL are largely retained. Recognized types of HL include nodular sclerosis classical HL, nodular lymphocyte-predominant HL, lymphocyte-rich classical HL, mixed cellularity classical HL, and lymphocyte-depleted classical HL.

Table 7.3 Hodgkin Lymphoma

- Peak incidence in the third and eighth decades
- Characterized by Reed-Sternberg cells
- Nodular sclerosis cell type accounts for 50%-80% of adult cases
- Staged using Ann Arbor system
- Thoracic involvement in 85% of cases at diagnosis
- Lymph node involvement in nearly all with thoracic involvement
    - Superior mediastinal node enlargement in 98%
    - Multiple node groups involved in 85%
    - Nodes show low attenuation in 10%-20%
    - Residual mediastinal masses common after treatment
    - Calcification of lymph nodes common after treatment
- Lung disease
    - 10% have lung involvement at diagnosis
    - Nearly always associated with enlarged nodes
    - Direct infiltration, lung nodules, or consolidation
    - Air bronchograms and cavitation may be seen
    - Lung recurrence may occur without enlarged nodes
- Pleural effusion in 15%, usually due to lymphatic obstruction

HL has a predilection for thoracic involvement. Up to 85% of patients with HL have thoracic involvement at the time of diagnosis; nearly all of them have mediastinal lymph node enlargement.

Lymph Node Involvement

HL most often involves superior mediastinal (ie, prevascular, paratracheal, and aortopulmonary) lymph nodes. These node groups are abnormal in as many as 85% of patients with HL and 98% of those with thoracic involvement (Figs. 7.1 and 7.2); if these nodes appear normal on CT, intrathoracic adenopathy is unlikely to represent HL.

Other sites of involvement in patients with thoracic disease are as follows: the hilar nodes, in about 35% of patients; the subcarinal nodes, in about 25%; the paracardiac (cardiophrenic angle) lymph nodes, in 10%; the internal mammary nodes, in 5%; and the posterior mediastinal (ie, paravertebral, para-aortic, and retrocrural) nodes, in 5% (see Figs. 7.2 and 7.3).

Multiple node groups are involved in 85% of those HL patients who have thoracic node involvement. Enlargement of a single node group can be seen in some patients with HL,

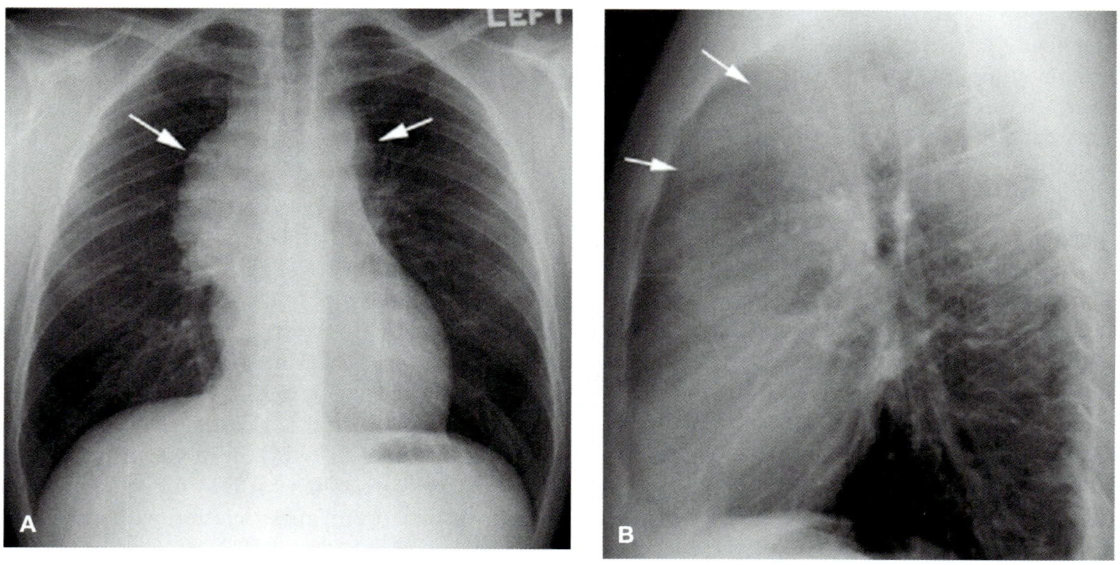

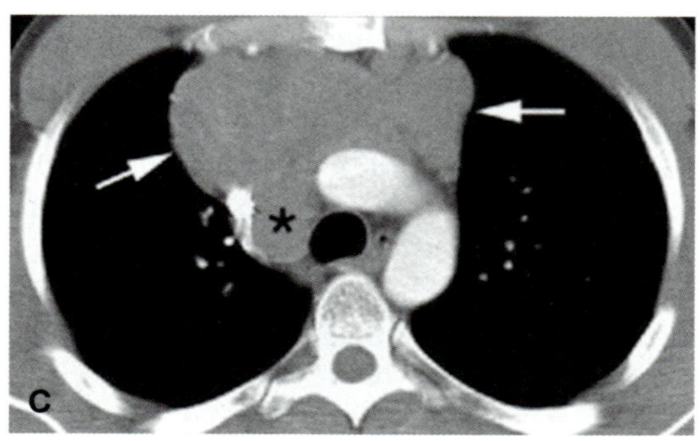

Figure 7.1. Hodgkin lymphoma (HL) involving superior mediastinal lymph nodes. **A:** PA chest radiograph shows bilateral lobulated superior mediastinal masses (*arrows*). **B:** The lateral view shows an anterior mediastinal mass (*arrows*). **C:** Contrast-enhanced CT scan shows prevascular anterior mediastinal lymph node enlargement (*arrows*) and paratracheal lymph node enlargement (*). Lymph node enlargement in these regions is typical of HL.

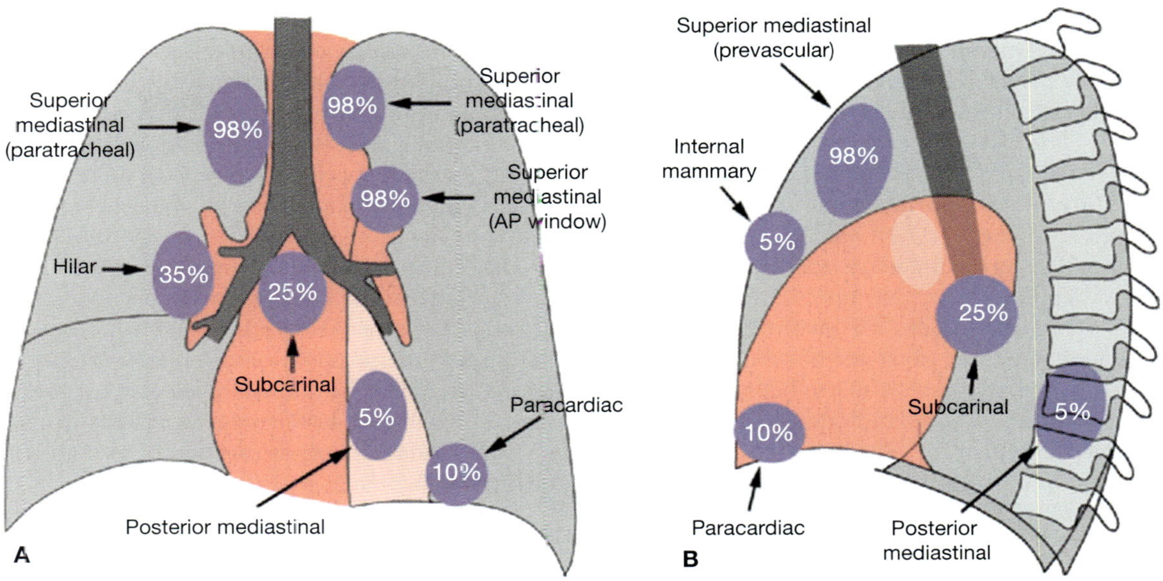

Figure 7.2. Involvement of mediastinal lymph node groups in Hodgkin lymphoma, illustrated as a percentage of patients with thoracic disease. Lymph node groups as shown on the PA (**A**) and lateral (**B**) radiographs.

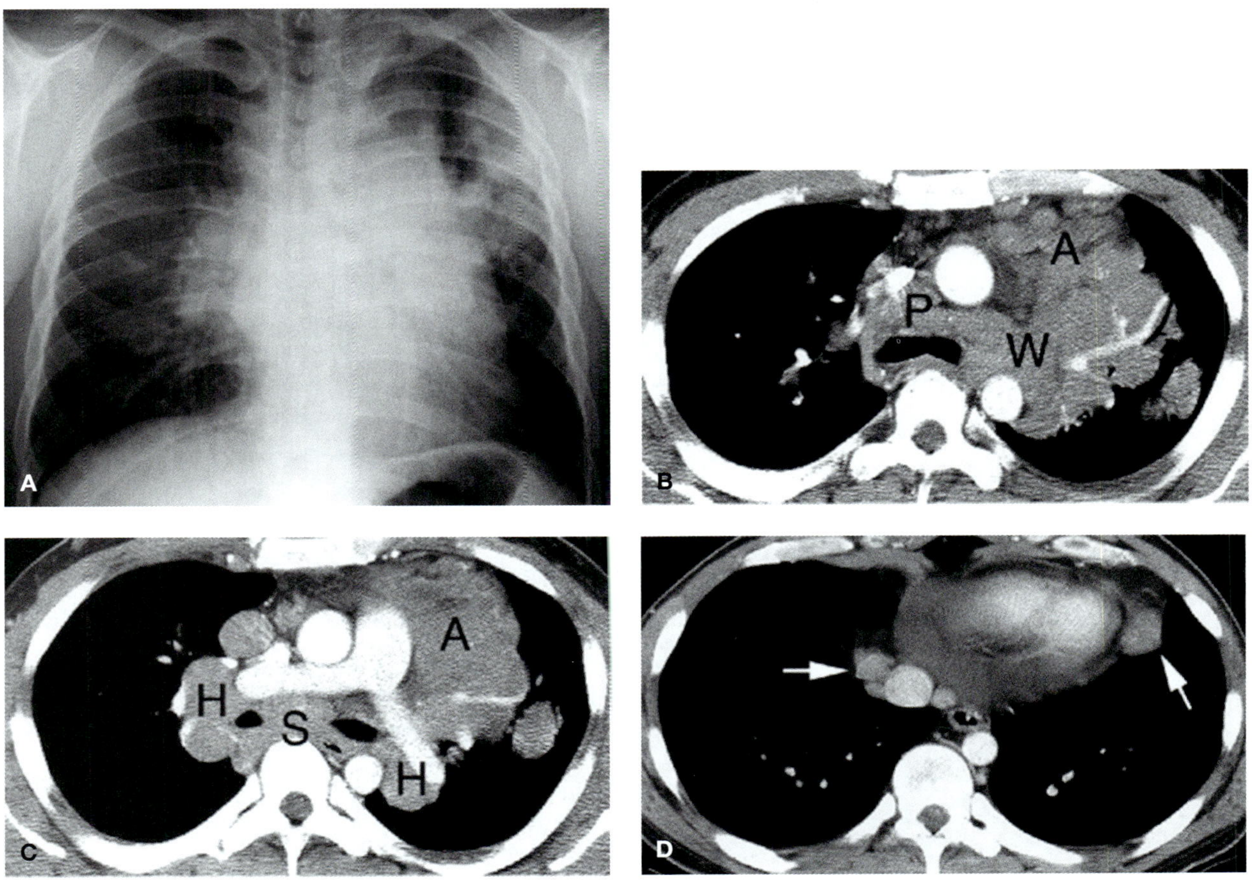

Figure 7.3. Hodgkin lymphoma with involvement of multiple lymph node groups. **A:** PA chest radiograph shows superior mediastinal widening, hilar enlargement, and nodules in the left upper lobe. **B, C:** Large lymph nodes are visible in the prevascular anterior mediastinum (*A*), paratracheal space (*P*), aortopulmonary window (*W*), subcarinal space (S), and both hila (*H*). Some discrete lymph nodes are visible, but other enlarged node masses appear matted together, with fat planes between them being invisible. **D:** Paracardiac lymph node enlargement (*arrows*) is visible at a lower level on CT.

but it is uncommon, occurring in only 15% of cases with node involvement. Anterior (prevascular) lymph nodes are most often involved as a single group (Fig. 7.4), and this appearance usually indicates the presence of nodular sclerosis HL.

On plain radiographs, anterior mediastinal lymph node enlargement may result in a unilateral or bilateral mediastinal abnormality (see Figs. 7.1A and 7.3A). Enlargement of paratracheal or aortopulmonary window nodes often results in a unilateral or asymmetrical abnormality. Because multiple lymph nodes are involved, mediastinal masses in HL often appear elongated or lobulated in contour. Roughly, spherical masses also can be seen (Fig. 7.5). Poor definition of the mass can indicate invasion or extension into adjacent lung.

CT is advantageous in showing abnormalities of mediastinal lymph nodes in patients with HL. Although it is uncommon for CT to show evidence of mediastinal adenopathy if the chest radiograph is normal, in cases in which the radiograph shows lymph node enlargement, CT detects additional sites of adenopathy in many patients. Findings shown only on CT may change the treatment plan in as many as 10% of patients. CT is most helpful in diagnosing subcarinal, internal mammary, and aortopulmonary window node enlargement that is not visible on radiographs.

On CT, abnormal lymph nodes may appear well defined and discrete (Fig. 7.6), may appear matted (with intervening fat planes poorly seen; see Fig. 7.3B and C), or may be associated with diffuse mediastinal infiltration (with individual lymph nodes being invisible; see Fig. 7.5C and D). Most often, enlarged lymph nodes are of homogeneous soft-tissue attenuation, but in 10% to 20% of cases, lymph node masses show areas of low attenuation or necrosis following contrast enhancement (Fig. 7.7). Inhomogeneity without obvious necrosis also may be seen (see Fig. 7.5D). Invasion of mediastinal structures such as the superior vena cava, esophagus, or airways may occur.

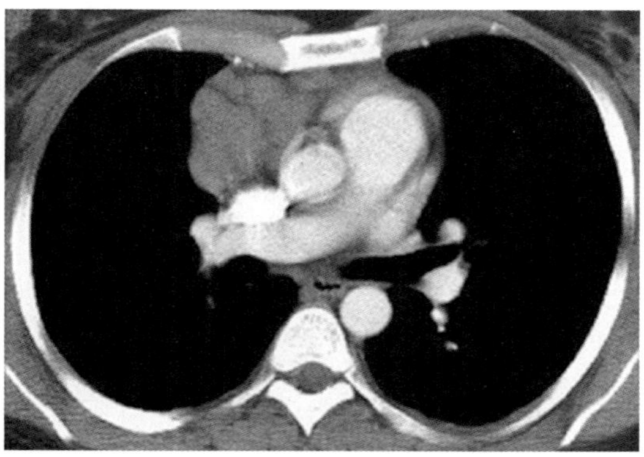

Figure 7.4. Anterior mediastinal lymph node enlargement in nodular sclerosis Hodgkin lymphoma (HL). CT shows lymphadenopathy localized to the anterior mediastinum, which is typical of nodular sclerosis HL.

Rarely, untreated patients show fine, stippled lymph node calcification. Lymph node calcification is much more common following treatment, with a stippled, confluent, or, less often, "eggshell" appearance (Fig. 7.8). Calcification usually occurs after radiation; calcification after chemotherapy is less common.

HL also has a predilection for involvement of the thymus in association with mediastinal lymph node enlargement. Thymic enlargement is seen in 30% to 40% of cases but may be difficult to distinguish from an anterior mediastinal lymph node mass unless the normal thymic shape is preserved (see Figs. 7.5E and 7.9). In the presence of thymic involvement, a visible mediastinal mass can project to both sides of the mediastinum.

HL is believed to be unifocal in origin, spreading to involve contiguous lymph nodes. It is unusual for HL to skip lymph node groups, and if nodes contiguous with the mediastinum, such as the lower neck or upper abdomen, are not involved by HL, it usually is not necessary to scan more distant regions, such as the pelvis.

However, in patients with mediastinal HL, scanning always should be extended to include the upper abdomen. Intra-abdominal para-aortic adenopathy can be found in 25% of patients with HL, and the spleen and liver are involved in 35% and 10% of patients, respectively.

The magnetic resonance imaging (MRI) appearance of lymph node masses in HL varies with the histology. In nodular sclerosis HL, large amounts of fibrous tissue typically are interlaced with malignant cells. Patients typically show a heterogeneous pattern with mixed high and low signal intensities on T2-weighted images. Low signal intensity areas on T2-weighted images are related to regions of fibrosis in the tumor, and high-intensity regions represent tumor tissue or cystic regions. HL also may demonstrate homogeneous high signal intensity similar to that of fat on T2-weighted images.

Lung Involvement

Lung involvement by HL is seen in 10% of patients at the time of presentation. It is almost always associated with mediastinal (and usually ipsilateral hilar) adenopathy (Fig. 7.10). In previously untreated patients, lung disease is uncommon in the absence of radiographically demonstrable lymph node enlargement; however, lung recurrence can be seen without node enlargement in patients with prior mediastinal radiation (see Fig. 7.11).

A variety of manifestations of lung involvement may be seen, but the most common are (1) direct involvement of lung contiguous with abnormal nodes and (2) isolated single or multiple lung nodules, masses, or areas of consolidation. Direct invasion and the presence of nodules or masses occur with about equal frequency.

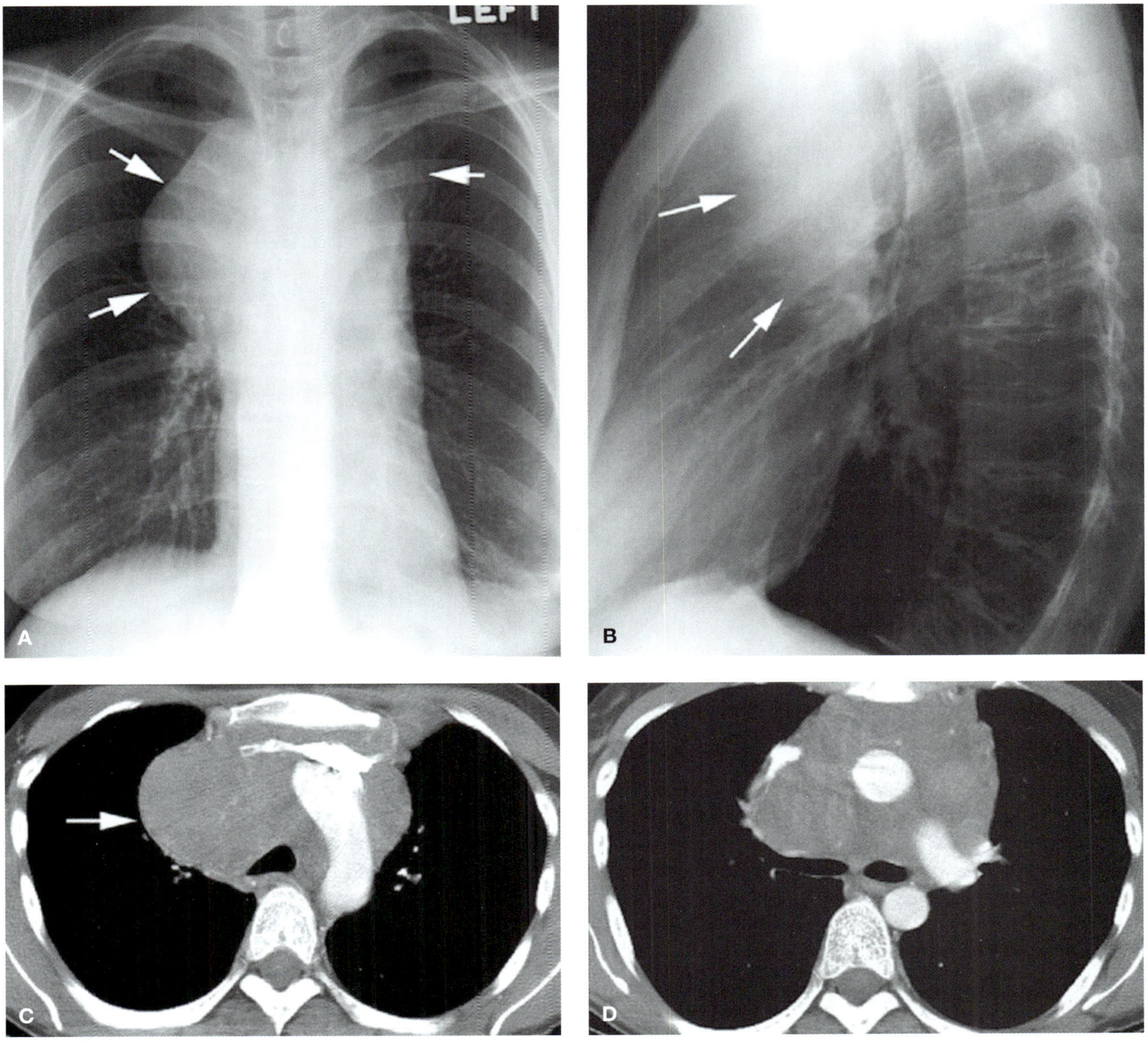

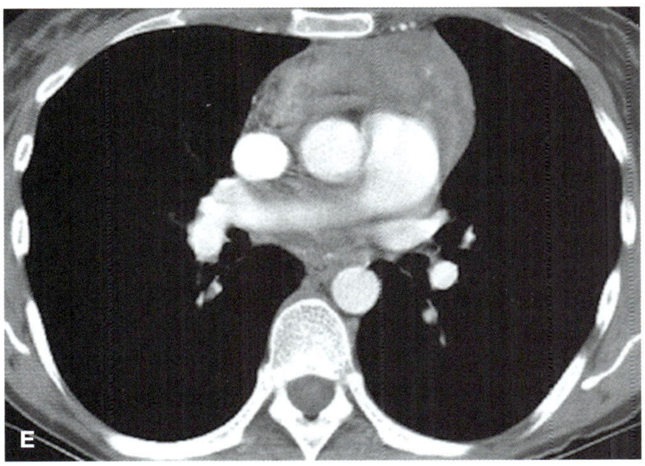

Figure 7.5. Large mediastinal mass in Hodgkin lymphoma. **A:** The PA radiograph shows a large spherical mass projecting to the right, with a smaller left-sided component (*arrows*). **B:** The lateral view shows the mass to be anterior (*arrows*). **C:** At the level of the aortic arch, CT shows a large, rounded mass that largely involves the paratracheal mediastinum (*arrow*). The opacified brachiocephalic veins are displaced anteriorly. Discrete nodal masses are not visible; the mediastinum appears infiltrated by tumor, and no mediastinal fat is visible. **D:** At the level of the left pulmonary artery, CT reveals that the mass occupies the prevascular anterior mediastinum and the precarinal space. The superior vena cava is displaced anteriorly and is compressed. At this level, the mass appears somewhat inhomogeneous in attenuation. Discrete, enlarged lymph nodes are not seen. **E:** At the level of the right pulmonary artery, anterior mediastinal mass appears to represent thymic involvement.

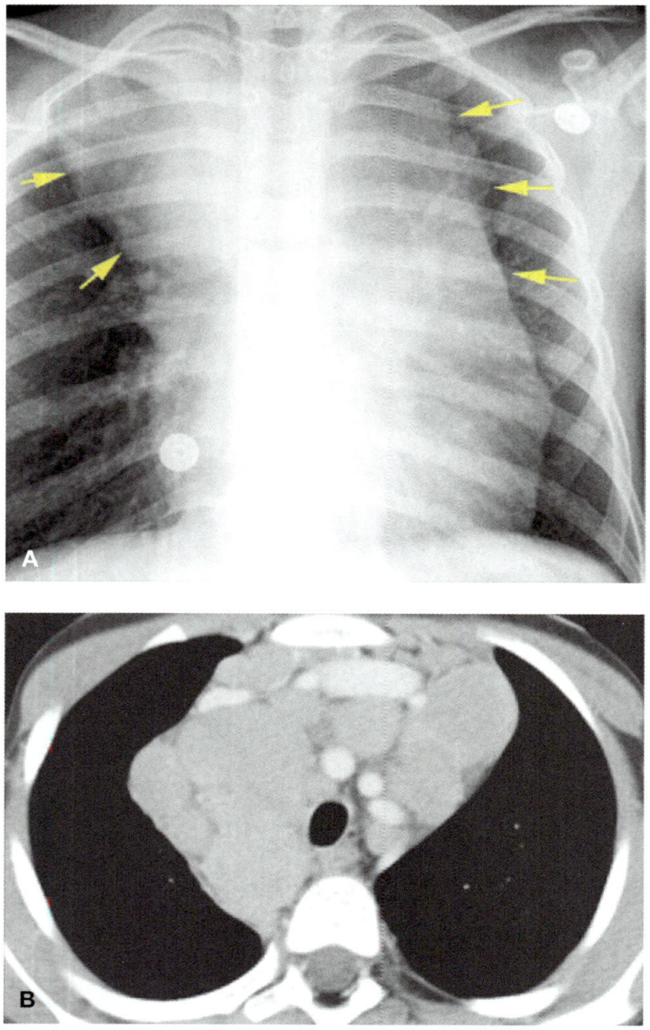

Figure 7.6. Hodgkin lymphoma in a 9-year-old child. **A:** Chest radiograph shows bilateral superior mediastinal masses (*arrows*). **B:** On CT, multiple discrete, enlarged lymph nodes are visible in the middle and anterior mediastinum.

Direct extension from hilar or mediastinal nodes results in coarse linear or streaky opacities radiating outward into the lung, corresponding on CT to thickening of the peribronchovascular interstitium. Interlobular septal thickening may be associated. In some patients, the appearance may mimic that of lymphangitic spread of carcinoma.

Discrete, single or multiple, well-defined or ill-defined, large or small lung nodules or masslike lesions or localized areas of air-space consolidation associated with air bronchograms may be seen (Figs. 7.10 and 7.11). These can cavitate, with thick or thin walls. Peripheral, subpleural masses are relatively common (Fig. 7.12).

HL occasionally involves bronchi with endobronchial masses or bronchial compression associated with atelectasis (Fig. 7.13).

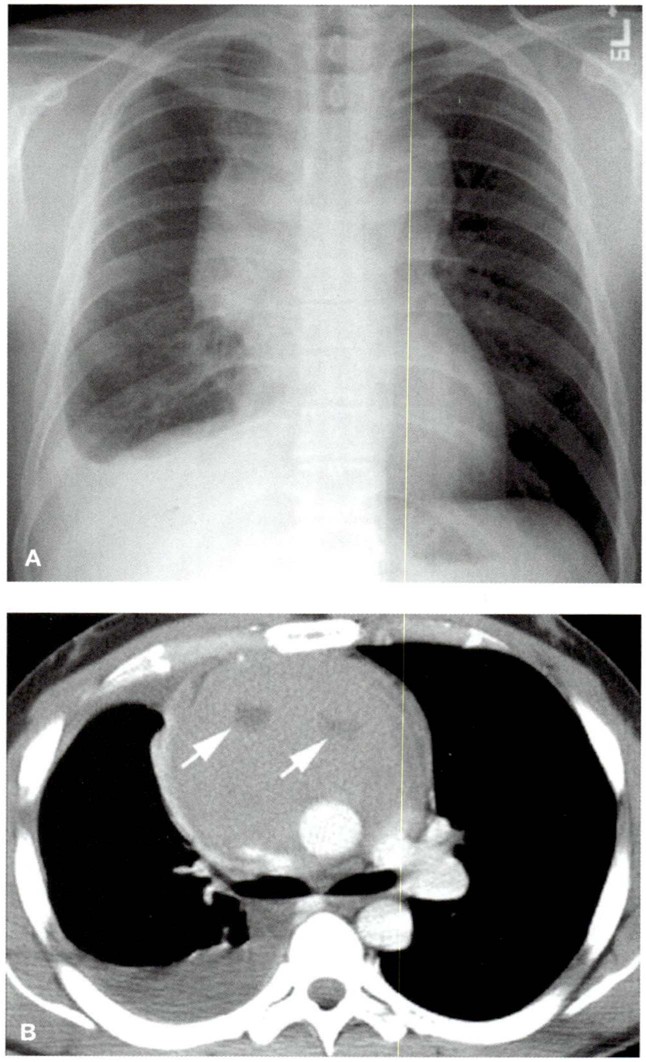

Figure 7.7. Lymphoma with necrosis. **A:** Chest radiograph shows a large bilateral mediastinal mass and right pleural effusion, a portion of which is subpulmonic. **B:** Contrast-enhanced CT scan shows an anterior mediastinal mass containing an area of low attenuation (*arrows*). This finding is seen in 10% to 20% of patients with Hodgkin lymphoma.

Pleural and Pericardial Effusion

Pleural effusion is present in about 15% of patients at diagnosis and usually reflects lymphatic or venous obstruction rather than pleural involvement by tumor (see Fig. 7.7). Effusions tend to resolve following local mediastinal or hilar radiation. However, about 20% to 25% of patients with HL who have effusion have CT findings of pleural or extrapleural tumor or lymph node enlargement. Pericardial effusion, present in 5% of patients, usually indicates direct involvement of the pericardium.

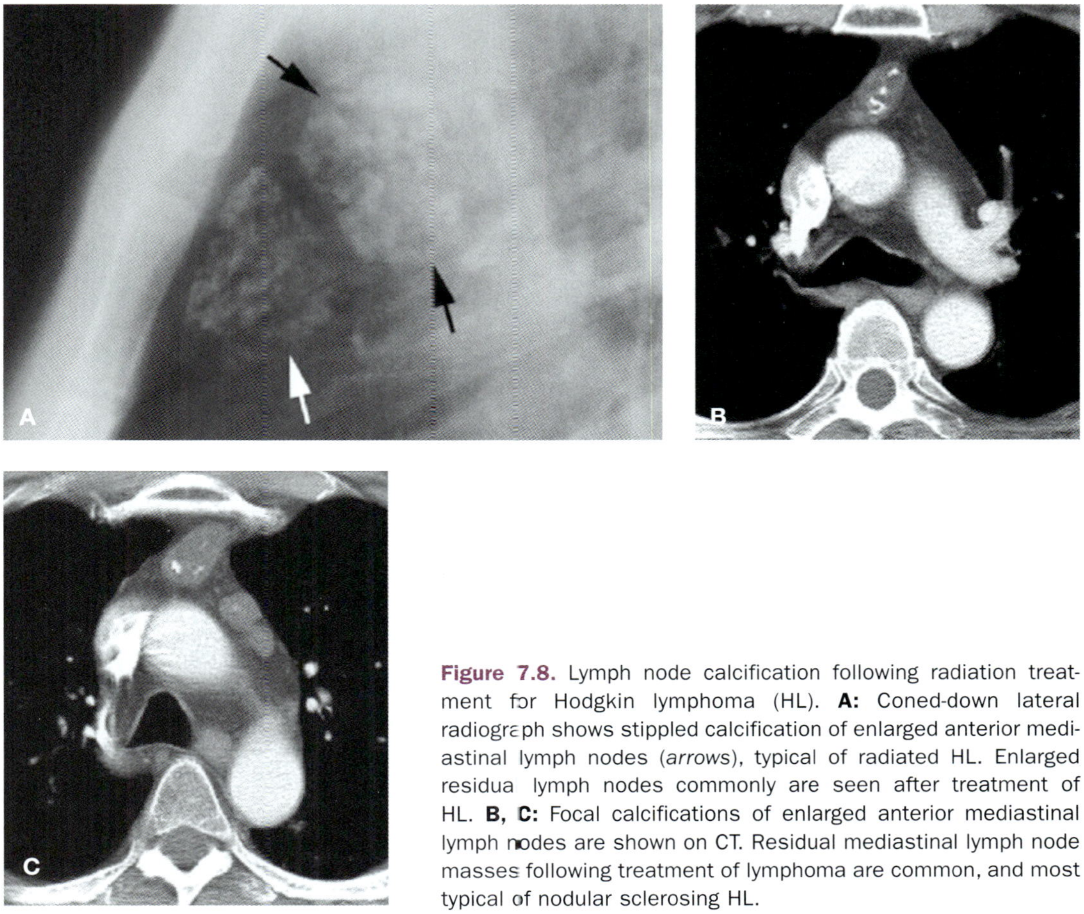

Figure 7.8. Lymph node calcification following radiation treatment for Hodgkin lymphoma (HL). **A:** Coned-down lateral radiograph shows stippled calcification of enlarged anterior mediastinal lymph nodes (*arrows*), typical of radiated HL. Enlarged residual lymph nodes commonly are seen after treatment of HL. **B, C:** Focal calcifications of enlarged anterior mediastinal lymph nodes are shown on CT. Residual mediastinal lymph node masses following treatment of lymphoma are common, and most typical of nodular sclerosing HL.

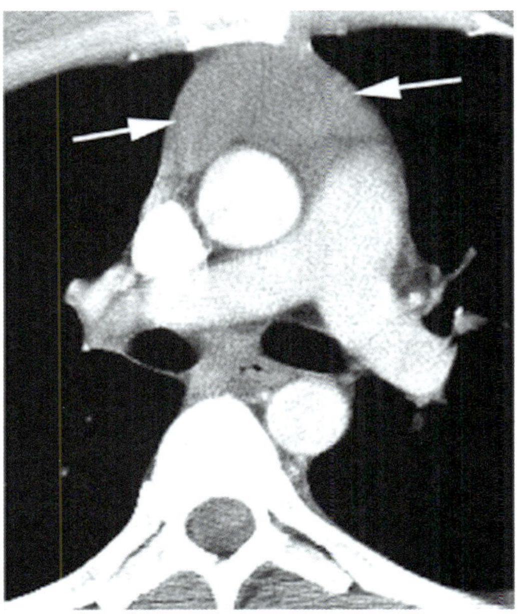

Figure 7.9. Thymic involvement in Hodgkin lymphoma. The thymus is enlarged but maintains a normal shape (*arrows*).

Chest Wall Involvement

Invasion of the chest wall contiguous with mediastinal or lung masses occurs in about 5% of cases. Tumor may involve ribs, sternum, or vertebral bodies and typically results in lytic bone destruction. Involvement of the skeleton because of dissemination often results in mixed lytic and blastic lesions (eg, "ivory vertebra").

Staging, Treatment, and Follow-Up of HL

The Lugano Staging Classification (ie, modified Ann Arbor staging system) is used to describe the anatomic extent of disease at the time of diagnosis and correlates well with prognosis (Table 7.2). Staging and follow-up, as reviewed previously, typically involve CT and PET/CT. FDG-PET usually shows high uptake. Although MRI has been used to assess treatment response, it has been replaced by PET/CT.

Cure is the goal in patients with newly diagnosed HL, and this is achievable in the large majority of cases. Among patients with early-stage HL, treatment usually consists of combination chemotherapy, with or without consolidative radiation therapy. For advanced-stage HL, combination chemotherapy

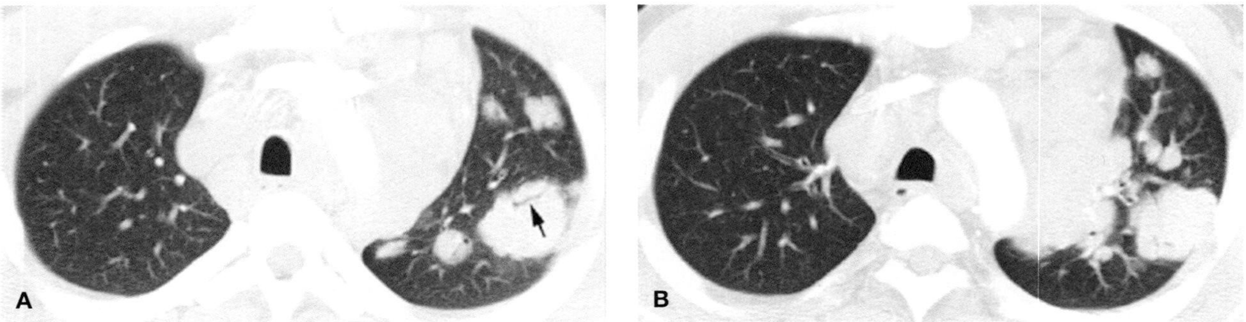

Figure 7.10. Lung involvement in Hodgkin lymphoma in the same patient shown in Figure 7.3. **A, B:** Large lobulated nodules are visible in the left lung. Some are associated with small bronchi or contain air bronchograms (*arrow*). Extensive mediastinal and hilar lymph node enlargement is present.

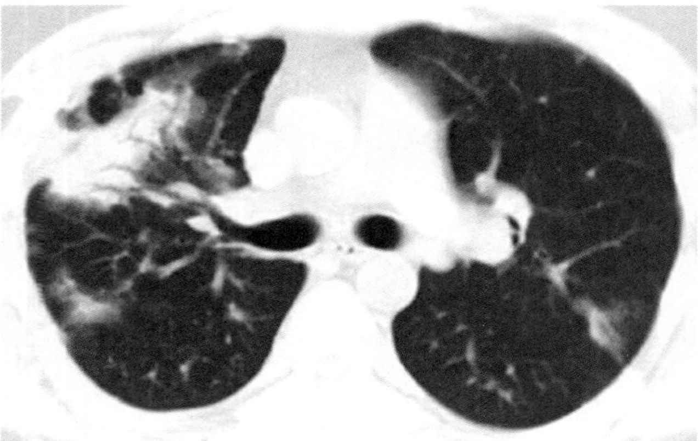

Figure 7.11. Lung involvement in recurrent Hodgkin lymphoma. Poorly defined nodules and areas of consolidation are visible. The large area of consolidation on the right contains a number of air bronchograms. There is no obvious lymph node enlargement.

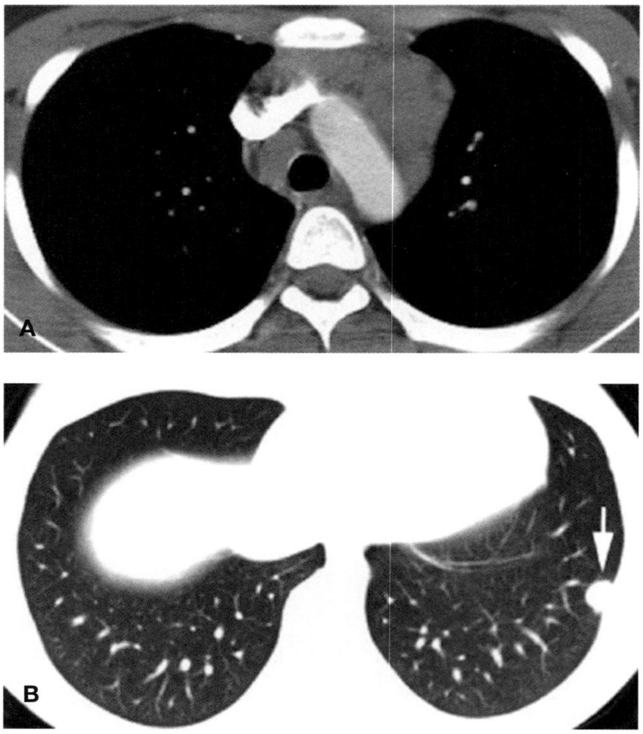

Figure 7.12. Peripheral lung nodule in Hodgkin lymphoma (HL). **A:** CT shows paratracheal and prevascular lymph node enlargement. **B:** A small, well-defined subpleural nodule is visible in the left lung. This was found at biopsy to represent HL.

has been the standard of care, with consolidative radiation therapy considered in patients with bulky disease, although this is evolving with the introduction of immune checkpoint inhibitors. Minimization of radiation fields, as achieved with involved-nodal or involved-site radiation therapy with minimal margins, limits exposure. For patients in whom HL is refractory to initial treatment, or in whom there is relapse, treatment with second-line chemotherapy and, for those who respond, consolidative high-dose therapy with autologous stem cell transplantation are employed. Radiation therapy may be incorporated if not delivered as part of first-line therapy. Treatment of early-stage HL is associated with disease-free survival of more than 90%, while for advanced-stage HL, survival is 60% to 90%.

On CT, reduction of tumor bulk is always seen in patients with adequately treated tumor. Patients who show complete resolution of lymph node masses on CT usually are considered to have a complete response. However, residual mediastinal mass or lymph node enlargement often is seen in cured patients following treatment (see Figs. 7.8 and 7.14). This is particularly common in patients with treated nodular sclerosis HL; residual masses represent fibrous tissue components of the tumor itself, which change little with treatment or posttreatment fibrosis. Residual mediastinal masses can be seen in as many as 88% of patients with HL and 40% of patients with NHL. In most patients, masses remain unchanged on follow-up. In some patients, residual masses continue to decrease in size or resolve over a period ranging from 3 to 11 months.

Most patients with thymic enlargement resulting from HL show a return to normal thymic size following treatment, although residual thymic enlargement may be seen in about 30% of cases.

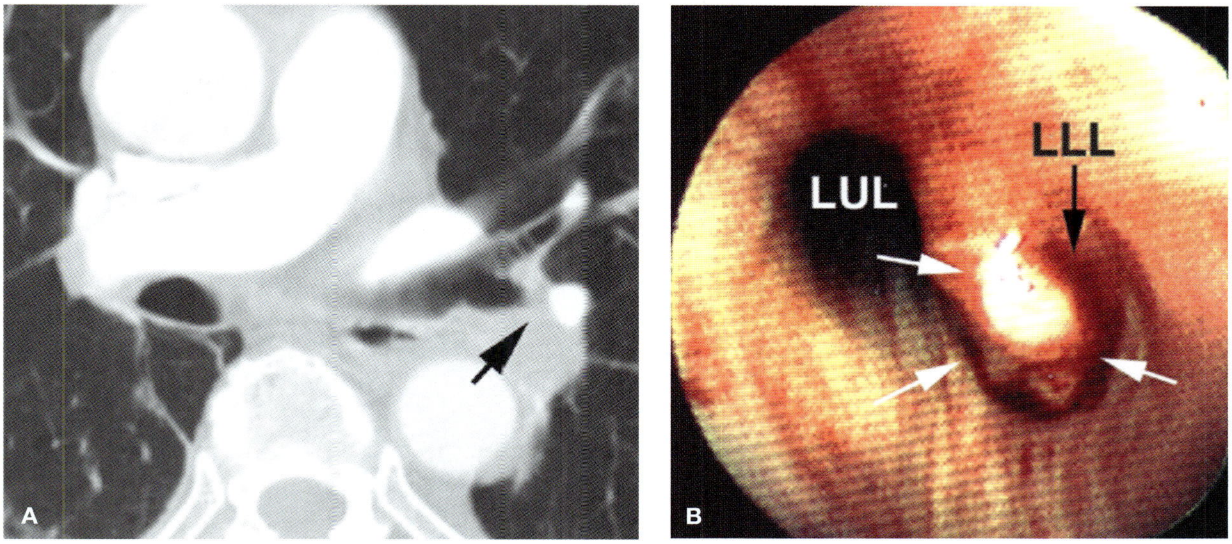

Figure 7.13. Endobronchial Hodgkin lymphoma. **A:** The left lower lobe bronchus is narrowed (*arrow*) by a polypoid endobronchial mass. **B:** Endoscopic photograph showing the left upper lobe bronchus (*LUL*) and a polypoid mass (*white arrows*) filling the left lower lobe bronchus (*LLL*).

It should be kept in mind that patients treated in the past for HL using hilar and mediastinal (mantle) radiation are commonly seen in clinical practice. Recurrent HL does not commonly involve previously irradiated (ie, in field) intrathoracic lymph nodes. However, so-called in-field recurrence is seen in a small percentage of cases. Large masses and masses in the anterior mediastinum generally are considered to carry an increased risk of recurrence.

Common sites of recurrent HL include the upper mediastinum and lung, both seen in about half of cases with recurrence. Lymph node recurrence also may involve paracardiac lymph nodes, which usually are excluded from the treatment field because of their close relation to the heart (to avoid radiation pericarditis). Lung recurrence usually is associated with central or peripheral lung nodules, masses, or areas of focal consolidation, any of which may show cavitation. Lung recurrence is uncommonly associated with visible lymph node enlargement on chest radiographs, although it is visible on CT in about half of cases. Pleural effusions or masses and chest wall involvement also are common.

NON-HODGKIN LYMPHOMA

The term non-Hodgkin lymphoma refers to a diverse group of neoplasms, varying in histology, clinical presentation, radiologic findings, course, and prognosis (Tables 7.1 and 7.4). NHL accounts for about 3% of malignancies in adults.

The National Cancer Institute Working Formulation originally classified NHL into low, intermediate, and high grades based on histology and prognosis. In 1994, the International Lymphoma Study Group developed a consensus list of lymphoid neoplasms, which was published as the Revised European-American Classification of Lymphoid Neoplasms (ie, the REAL classification). The WHO classification of lymphoid malignancies has subsequently been developed, using an updated REAL classification (Table 7.1). A large number of specific tumor types make up this classification and a distinction among cases as low, intermediate, or high grade is not generally employed. Nonetheless, these terms remain in use in describing NHL.

B-CELL NHL

B-cell lymphomas make up most (85%) of NHL. There are numerous cell types. The most common, and those most commonly affecting the thorax, are reviewed briefly.

Diffuse Large B-Cell Lymphoma

DLBCL is the most common type of NHL (30% of cases). It can affect any age group but occurs primarily in older subjects (the average age is mid-60s). About one in three cases of DLBCL is localized when diagnosed. Primary mediastinal B-cell lymphoma is a subtype of DLCBL (see later discussion).

Genetic analysis has shown that there are different subtypes of DLBCL, despite a similar histologic appearance. These subtypes have different responses to treatment and prognosis. DLBCL is fast growing but often responds well to treatment. Overall, about 75% of patients have no signs of disease after the initial treatment, and many are cured with therapy.

Follicular Lymphoma

About 20% of NHLs are follicular lymphoma. The average age at presentation is 60. Usually, it occurs in many lymph node sites and in bone marrow. Follicular lymphomas are often slow growing and respond well to treatment. Over time, about one in three follicular lymphomas become a diffuse B-cell lymphoma.

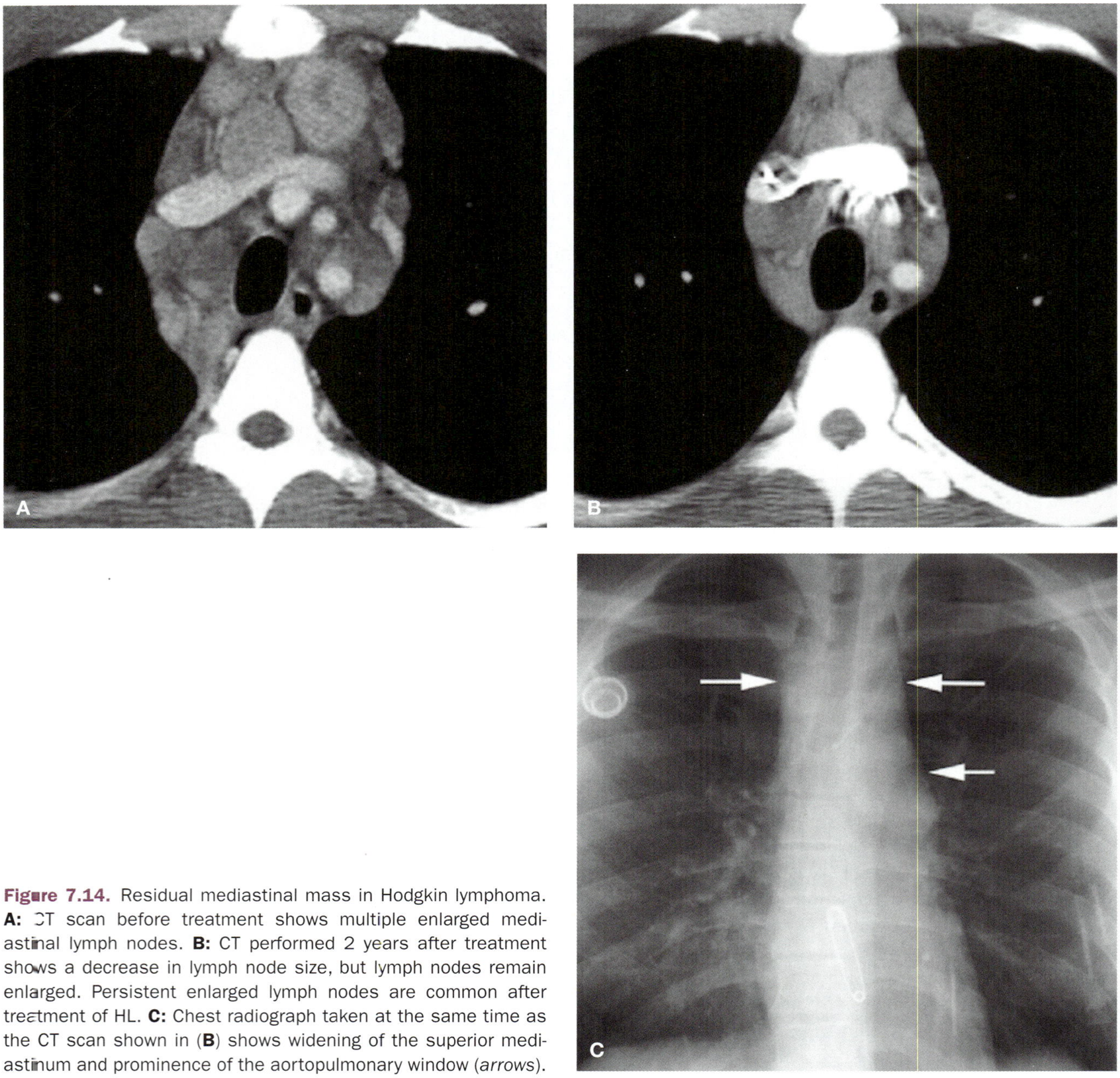

Figure 7.14. Residual mediastinal mass in Hodgkin lymphoma. **A:** CT scan before treatment shows multiple enlarged mediastinal lymph nodes. **B:** CT performed 2 years after treatment shows a decrease in lymph node size, but lymph nodes remain enlarged. Persistent enlarged lymph nodes are common after treatment of HL. **C:** Chest radiograph taken at the same time as the CT scan shown in (**B**) shows widening of the superior mediastinum and prominence of the aortopulmonary window (*arrows*).

Chronic Lymphocytic Leukemia/Small Lymphocytic Lymphoma

The same cell type is seen in both CLL and SLL. In CLL, abnormal cells predominate in blood and bone marrow. In SLL, abnormal cells are primarily present in lymph nodes and spleen. About 5% to 10% of all lymphomas are SLLs (see later discussion).

Both CLL and SLL progress slowly, although CLL, which is much more common, is more indolent. They are usually not curable with standard treatments, but depending on the stage and growth rate of the disease, most patients live longer than 10 years.

Mantle Cell Lymphoma

Mantle cell lymphoma represents about 5% of NHL. Men are affected most often; the average age at presentation is 60. When this MCL is diagnosed, it usually involves lymph nodes, bone marrow, and often the spleen.

Marginal Zone B-Cell Lymphoma and MALT Lymphoma

Marginal zone lymphomas account for about 5% to 10% of NHL. *Extranodal marginal zone B-cell lymphoma of mucosa-associated lymphoid tissue (ie, MALT lymphoma)* is an important subtype.

Table 7.4 Non-Hodgkin Lymphoma

Diverse group of neoplasms
Two tumor types classified by WHO
B cell
T cell and NK cell
Numerous subtypes
More common than HL
Mean age 55 y; more common than HL in children
Associated with immunodeficiency and various infections
Prognosis related to cell type
Staging less important than with HL
Thoracic involvement in 40%-50%
Lymphadenopathy in 75% with thoracic disease
Superior mediastinal lymph nodes involved in nearly all
Involvement of a single node group common (40%)
Posterior mediastinal lymph nodes relatively common
Lung involvement (30%) more common than with HL

MALT lymphomas arise in the stomach, lung, skin, thyroid, salivary glands, and tissues surrounding the eye. Usually, MALT lymphoma is confined to the organ in which it originates. Many MALT lymphomas have been linked to infections with bacteria or viruses. The average age of patients with MALT lymphoma is about 60. It is slow growing and is often curable in its early stages.

Lymphoplasmacytic Lymphoma (Waldenström Macroglobulinemia)

Waldenström macroglobulinemia accounts for 1% to 2% of lymphomas; monoclonal IgM gammopathy is present. Bone marrow infiltration, hepatosplenomegaly, and peripheral lymph node enlargement are common manifestations. Lung or mediastinal involvement is uncommon. Radiographs or CT may show lung consolidation or interstitial infiltration, mediastinal lymph node enlargement, or pleural effusion (see Fig. 7.26).

T-CELL AND NK-CELL NHL

T-cell lymphomas make up less than 15% of NHLs. There are many types of T-cell lymphoma, but most are uncommon.

T-Cell Lymphoblastic Lymphoma/Leukemia

This disease accounts for about 1% of all lymphomas. It can be considered either a lymphoma or leukemia, depending on how much of the bone marrow is involved.

This lymphoma often originates in the thymus, resulting in a large mediastinal mass.

Patients are often young adults, with males being affected more often than females. This lymphoma is fast growing but may be cured with chemotherapy.

Adult T-Cell Leukemia/Lymphoma

This lymphoma is caused by infection with a virus called *HTLV-1*. It is rare in the United States and much more common in Japan, the Caribbean, and parts of Africa, where HTLV-1 is more common. It may be associated with pulmonary abnormalities or lymph node enlargement.

Angioimmunoblastic T-Cell Lymphoma

This has been reclassified as a subtype of nodal T-follicular helper cell lymphoma, angioimmunoblastic-type and accounts for about 3% of all lymphomas. It is more common in older adults. It tends to involve the lymph nodes as well as the spleen or liver, which can cause them to be enlarged. Patients usually have fever, weight loss, and skin rashes and often develop infections. This lymphoma often progresses quickly. Treatment is often effective, but the lymphoma tends to recur.

Approximately 50% of cases show extensive mediastinal and hilar lymph node enlargement, and 35% of cases show lung involvement. Interstitial infiltration in the lower lobes associated with septal thickening or patchy consolidation is typical. Pleural effusion may be present. Enlarged lymph nodes may be seen to enhance if CT with contrast infusion is used.

Anaplastic Large Cell Lymphoma

Anaplastic large cell lymphoma accounts for 2% of lymphomas. It is more common in young people (including children), but it does occur in people in their 50 and 60s. It usually starts in lymph nodes and can also spread to the skin. This type of lymphoma tends to be fast growing, but many are cured with aggressive chemotherapy.

CHARACTERISTICS OF NHL

NHL usually occurs in older persons (40-70 years of age; mean, 55 years) than does HL. NHL also is more common than HL in children (Table 7.5). The incidence of NHL is significantly higher in immunodeficient patients. NHL is associated with congenital immunodeficiency syndromes, HIV infection, and immunosuppressive therapy. These tumors differ somewhat from those that occur spontaneously in immunocompetent patients, as they usually are polyclonal rather than monoclonal and usually involve extranodal sites (eg, central nervous system, lung, gastrointestinal tract).

Thoracic involvement is about half as common as with HL, occurring in 40% to 50% of cases. Although different cell types of tumor can result in different radiographic appearances, some general characteristics of NHL are reviewed and are compared to those seen in HL.

Table 7.5 Comparison of Hodgkin Lymphoma (HL) and Non-Hodgkin Lymphoma (NHL)

	HL	NHL
Incidence	0.5%-1% malignancies	3% malignancies
Age at presentation	Peaks in third and eighth decades	Peaks at age 40-70 y; more common than HL in children
Thoracic involvement	85% of cases	40%-50% of cases
Node involvement		
Mediastinal nodes	Nearly all cases with thoracic involvement	75% of cases with thoracic involvement
Multiple node groups	85% of patients with lymph node disease	60% of patients with lymph node disease
Single node group	15% of patients with lymph node disease	40% of patients with lymph node disease
Superior mediastinal nodes	98% of cases with thoracic lymph node enlargement	75% of cases with thoracic lymph node enlargement
Posterior mediastinal nodes	5% of cases with thoracic lymph node enlargement	20% of cases with thoracic lymph node enlargement
Skips lymph node groups	Uncommon	Common
Lung involvement	10% of cases	30% of cases
Staging	Important (Ann Arbor classification)	Less important (histology more valuable)

Lymph Node Involvement

As with HL, mediastinal lymph node involvement is the most common thoracic abnormality in patients with NHL, but this varies with the cell type of the tumor. Lymph node enlargement is present in more than 75% of patients with intrathoracic disease. Enlargement of paratracheal or anterior mediastinal (superior mediastinal) lymph nodes is the abnormality seen most often; 75% of patients with an intrathoracic abnormality (and 35% of all cases) have prevascular or paratracheal node involvement (Figs. 7.15 and 7.16). Subcarinal lymph node enlargement is present in about 30% of patients with an intrathoracic abnormality (15% of all cases; Fig. 7.17). Other sites of lymph node enlargement (expressed as a percentage of patients with intrathoracic disease) include the hila (20%); posterior mediastinal para-aortic, paravertebral, and retrocrural nodes (20%); and paracardiac nodes (10%).

The pattern of lymph node disease is different than that seen in HL. Involvement of a single node group is much more common in patients with NHL (see Figs. 7.17 and 7.18); 40% of patients with NHL and thoracic involvement have involvement of only one node group, whereas this is seen in only 15% of patients with HL. In addition, the involvement of paravertebral/posterior mediastinal nodal

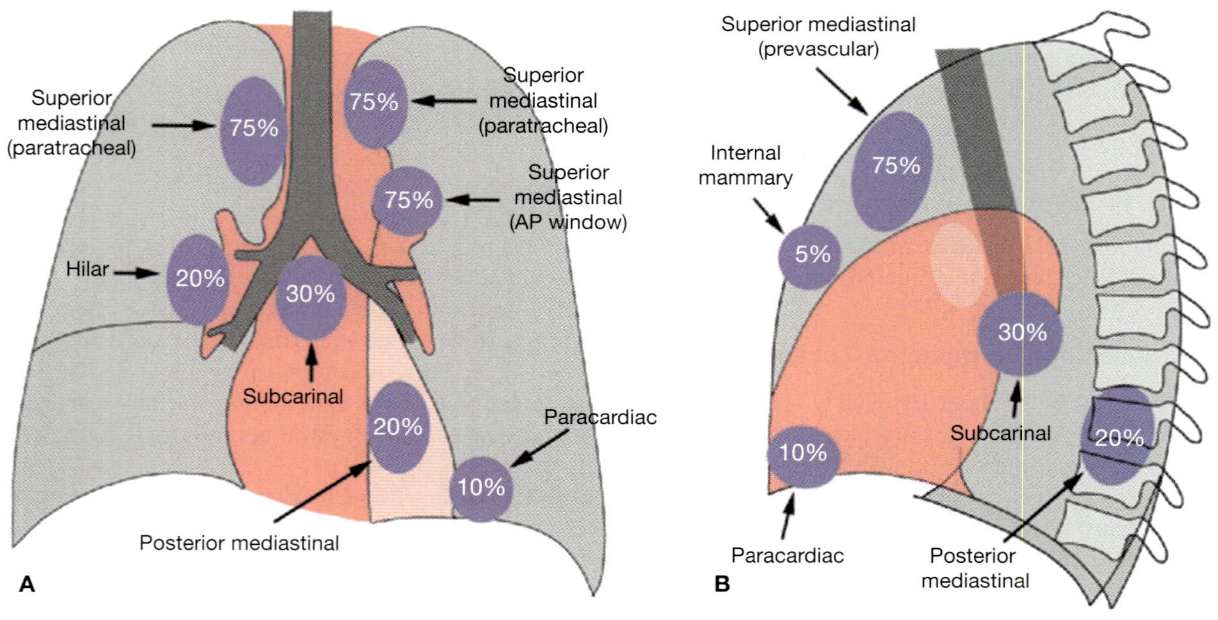

Figure 7.15. Involvement of mediastinal lymph node groups in non-Hodgkin lymphoma, as a percentage of patients with thoracic disease. Lymph node groups as seen on the PA (**A**) and lateral (**B**) radiographs.

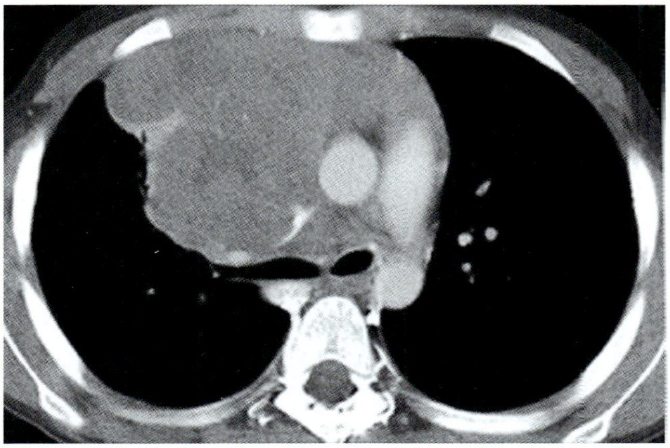

Figure 7.16. Mediastinal lymph node enlargement with non-Hodgkin lymphoma (NHL). Bulky lymphadenopathy is seen in the prevascular mediastinum with compression of the superior vena cava. Enlarged lymph nodes also are seen in the precarinal region. Nearly 75% of patients with NHL and an intrathoracic abnormality have prevascular or paratracheal node involvement.

groups is relatively more common with NHL than with HL; paravertebral lymph node masses often are contiguous with upper abdominal node enlargement (see Fig. 7.17).

Enlarged lymph nodes or mediastinal masses may appear low in attenuation due to necrosis or may be cystic (Figs. 7.19 and 7.20). Calcification of nodes or masses is rare.

As with HL, CT is more sensitive than chest radiographs in detecting lymph node enlargement in patients with NHL. It is most helpful in detecting subcarinal, posterior mediastinal, and paracardiac lymph nodes.

On MRI, lymph node masses in NHL appear homogeneous on T1-weighted images. They may demonstrate homogeneous high signal intensity similar to that of fat on T2-weighted images, because tumors may be composed almost entirely of malignant cells without significant fibrous tissue. However, areas of necrosis may be seen on T2-weighted images or with contrast enhancement (see Fig. 7.20).

Extranodal Disease

Extranodal involvement is much more common with NHL than it is with HL, but this varies with cell type. Extranodal disease seen in patients with a thoracic abnormality includes lung involvement in 30% of patients, pleural effusion or mass in 45% of patients, pericardial effusion or mass in 15% of patients, and chest wall involvement in 10% of patients.

Lung involvement may appear as discrete nodules or masses (Fig. 7.21), air-space consolidation, infiltration contiguous with enlarged lymph nodes or masses (Fig. 7.22), or interstitial thickening resembling lymphangitic spread of carcinoma (Fig. 7.23). In some patients, lung infiltration may be rapid, mimicking pneumonia. Bronchial narrowing or obstruction may occur because of compression by hilar mass (Fig. 7.24A) or bronchial involvement by tumor (see Fig. 7.24B). Some pulmonary NHLs are primary to the lung.

As with HL, pleural effusion most likely reflects lymphatic obstruction. Pleural effusion may be associated with gross pleural or extrapleural (chest wall) tumor (Figs. 7.25 and 7.26).

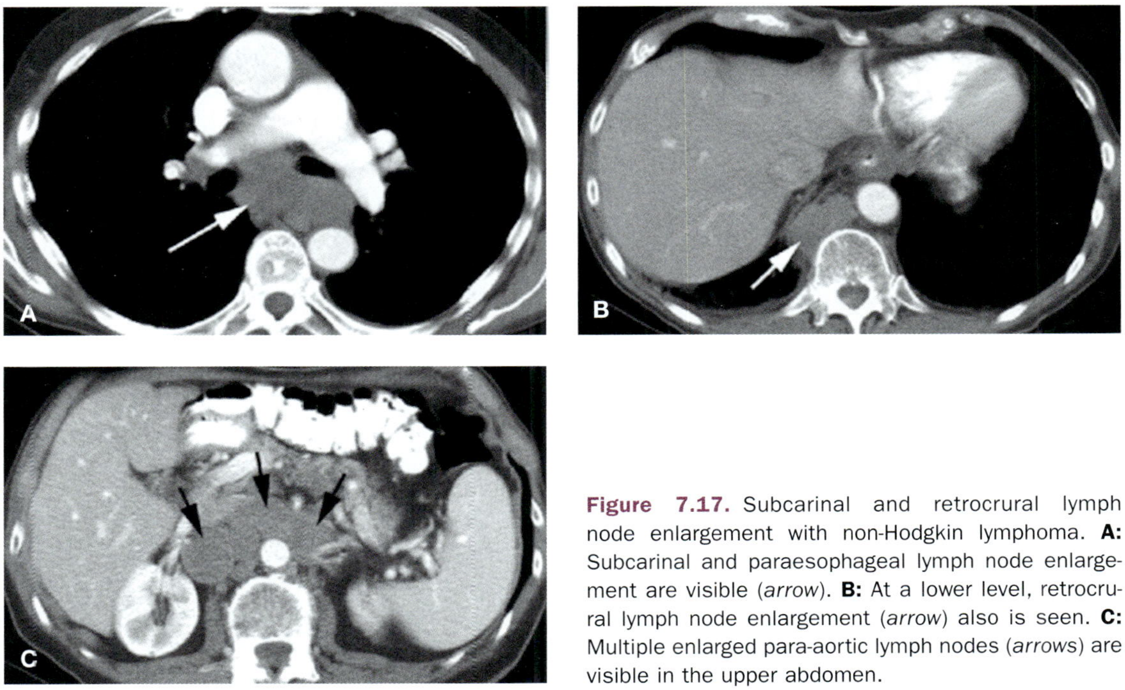

Figure 7.17. Subcarinal and retrocrural lymph node enlargement with non-Hodgkin lymphoma. **A:** Subcarinal and paraesophageal lymph node enlargement are visible (*arrow*). **B:** At a lower level, retrocrural lymph node enlargement (*arrow*) also is seen. **C:** Multiple enlarged para-aortic lymph nodes (*arrows*) are visible in the upper abdomen.

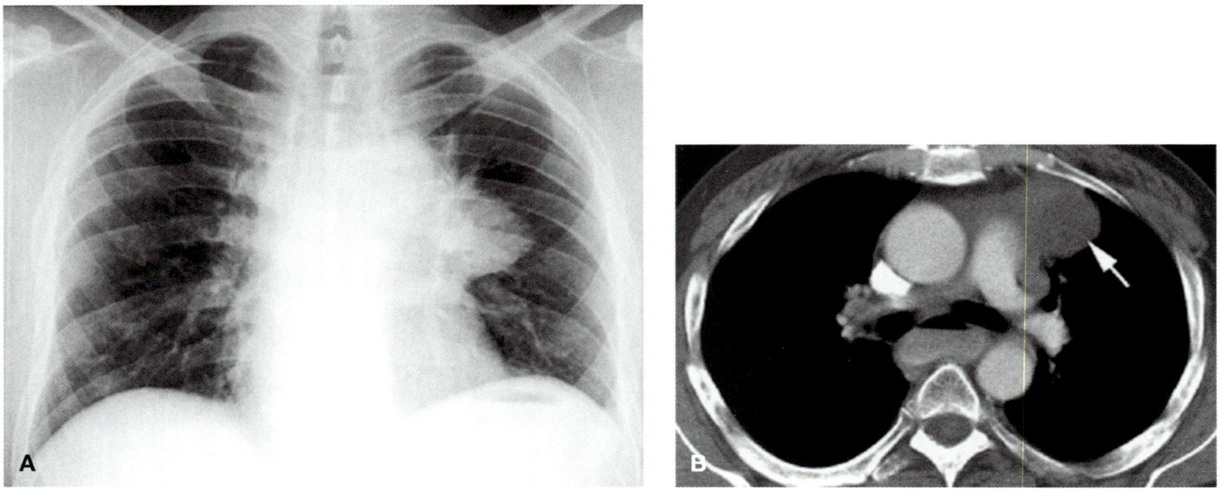

Figure 7.18. Anterior mediastinal lymph node enlargement with non-Hodgkin lymphoma (NHL). **A:** Left mediastinal mass is visible on the PA radiograph. Elevation of the left hemidiaphragm may reflect left diaphragmatic paralysis related to invasion or compression of the left phrenic nerve. **B:** Lymphadenopathy is limited to the prevascular mediastinum (*arrow*). Involvement of a single lymph node group is much more common in patients with NHL than in those with Hodgkin lymphoma.

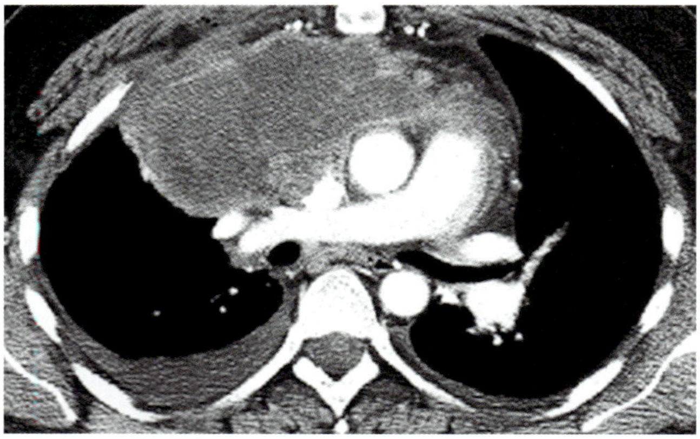

Figure 7.19. Non-Hodgkin lymphoma with a low-attenuation anterior mediastinal mass. The mass appears cystic due to necrosis. Bilateral pleural effusions also are present.

Staging, Treatment, and Follow-Up of NHL

In about 20% of patients with intrathoracic disease, CT shows abnormalities that are not recognized on plain radiographs. CT also shows more extensive intrathoracic disease in 75% of patients with abnormal chest radiographs. FDG-PET/CT should be obtained in staging patients having tumors that are typically FDG avid. The likelihood of thoracic lymph node or lung involvement varies with the cell type. MRI is appropriate for evaluating the central nervous system.

In contrast to HL, NHL is often disseminated. The abdomen, pelvis, and neck must be scanned in patients with NHL, because noncontiguous spread is common. Depending on the cell type, abdominal involvement is more common than in patients with HL, and a variety of findings may be present: intra-abdominal para-aortic adenopathy is found in about 50% of patients with NHL (see Fig. 7.17C); the spleen is involved in 40% of patients, and the liver in 15% of patients. CT of the abdomen and pelvis results in an upgrading of the clinical stage in about 30% of patients with NHL and may detect unsuspected active disease in 40% of patients thought to be in remission.

Treatment of NHL depends on the cell type of the tumor and is rapidly evolving. Treatments include watchful waiting with indolent tumor types, combination chemotherapy, antiviral drugs, radiation, monoclonal antibodies, antibody drug conjugates, small molecule inhibitors of critical oncogenic pathways, radioimmunotherapy, and stem cell transplantation. Survival is variable, but cure may be expected in some cell types.

SPECIFIC TYPES OF THORACIC LYMPHOMA

Primary Pulmonary NHL

Pulmonary NHL is considered to be primary to the lung if it shows no evidence of extrathoracic dissemination for at least 3 months after the initial diagnosis (Table 7.6). Less than 1% of pulmonary lymphomas are primary. Primary pulmonary lymphoma, arising in pulmonary lymphoid tissue, is usually either DLBCL or extranodal marginal zone B-cell lymphoma arising from bronchial-associated lymphoid tissue (BALT), a subtype of MALT lymphoma or MALToma; both are rare. CT findings in pulmonary lymphoma are variable and may include multiple ill-defined solid or ground-glass opacity nodules or masses, focal or multifocal consolidation with air bronchograms, and interlobular septal thickening.

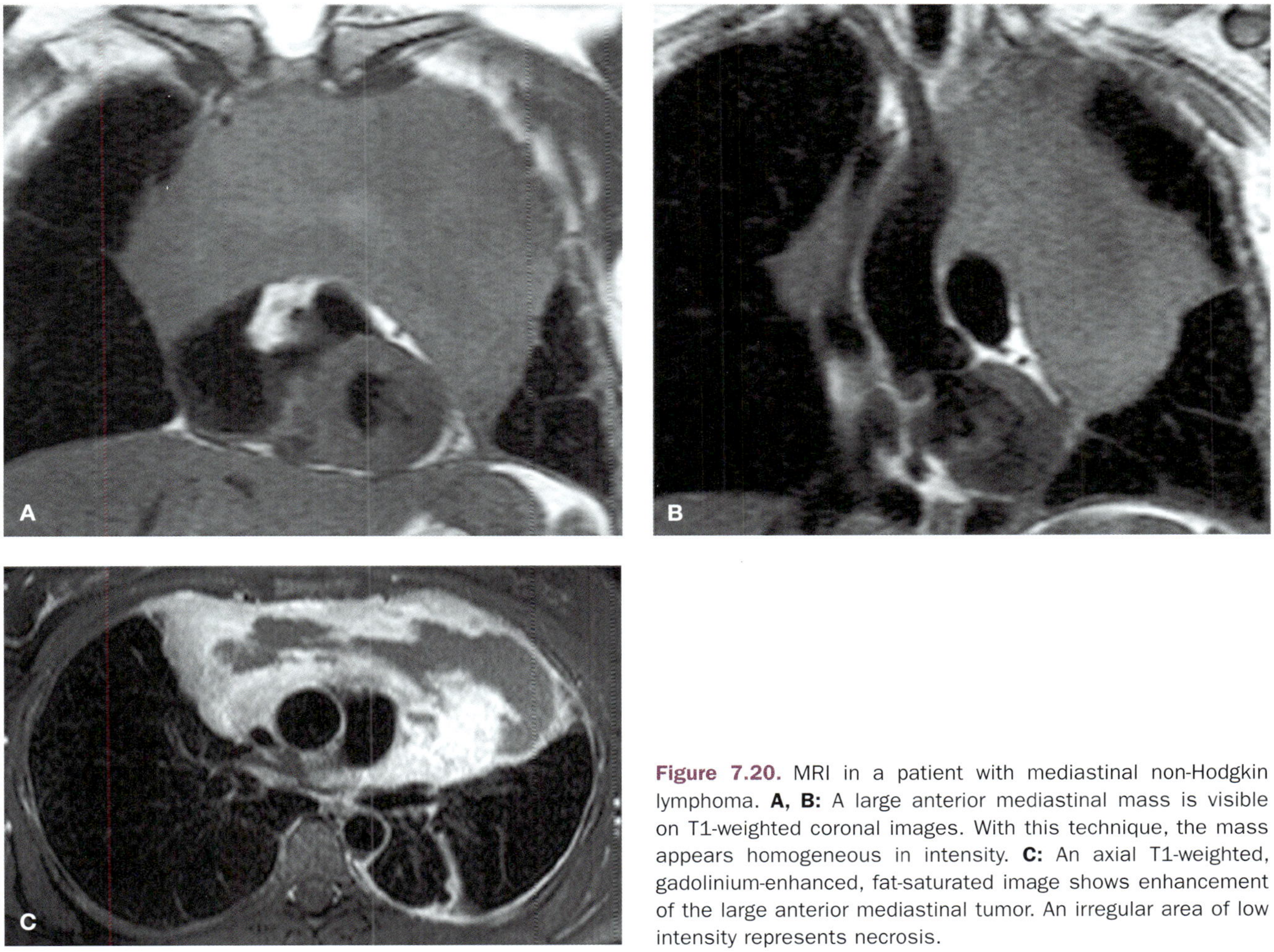

Figure 7.20. MRI in a patient with mediastinal non-Hodgkin lymphoma. **A, B:** A large anterior mediastinal mass is visible on T1-weighted coronal images. With this technique, the mass appears homogeneous in intensity. **C:** An axial T1-weighted, gadolinium-enhanced, fat-saturated image shows enhancement of the large anterior mediastinal tumor. An irregular area of low intensity represents necrosis.

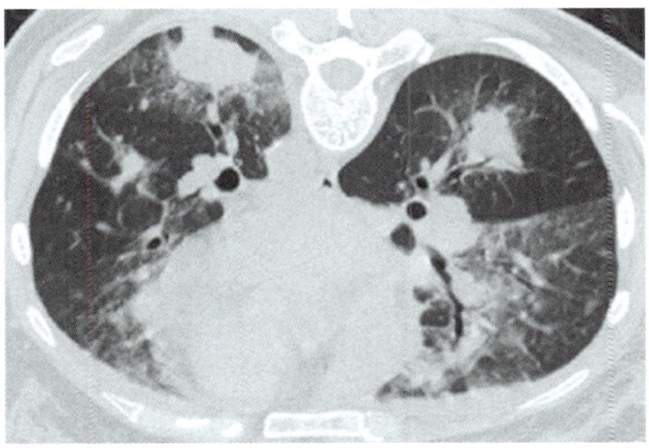

Figure 7.21. Lung involvement with non-Hodgkin lymphoma. HRCT in the prone position shows focal masses. This appearance is common when the lung is involved.

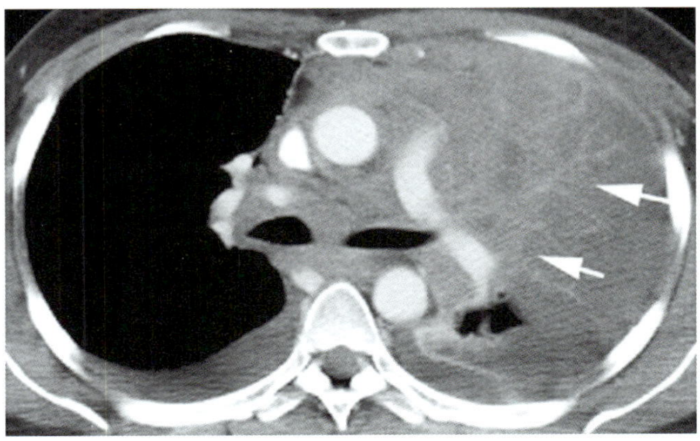

Figure 7.22. Lung infiltration contiguous with mediastinal mass. Enhanced CT shows invasion of the lung (*arrows*) adjacent to a large mediastinal mass. Bilateral pleural effusions also are present.

MALToma

MALToma accounts for 70% to 90% of primary pulmonary lymphomas, but less than 0.5% of all primary lung tumors. These are derived from MALT, hence the term *MALToma* or *MALT lymphoma*, which commonly is used to describe this entity. These tumors are indolent, and patients with primary pulmonary B-cell MALT lymphoma have a good prognosis. These tumors are thought to arise because of chronic antigenic stimulation associated with smoking, autoimmune disease (particularly Sjögren syndrome), or infection. They respond to surgery if localized, chemotherapy and radiation,

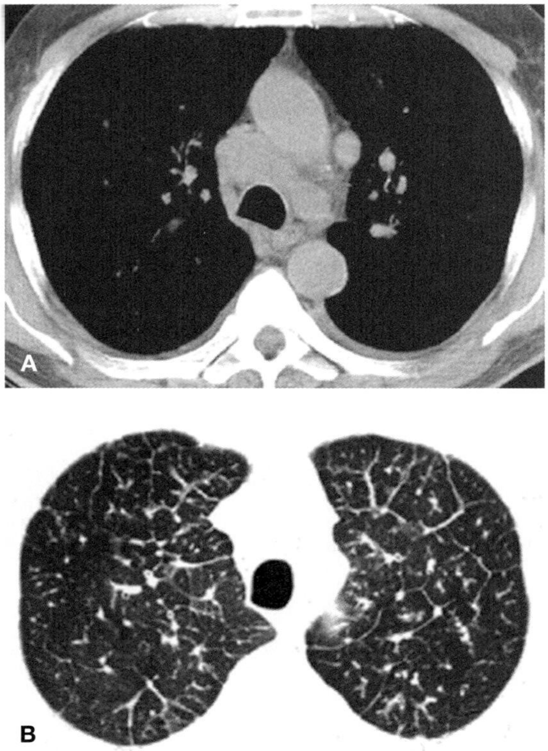

Figure 7.23. Lymphangitic spread of non-Hodgkin lymphoma. **A:** HRCT at a soft-tissue window shows enlarged mediastinal lymph nodes. **B:** HRCT shows diffuse lung infiltration with interlobular septal thickening and some nodularity closely mimicking the appearance of lymphangitic spread of carcinoma.

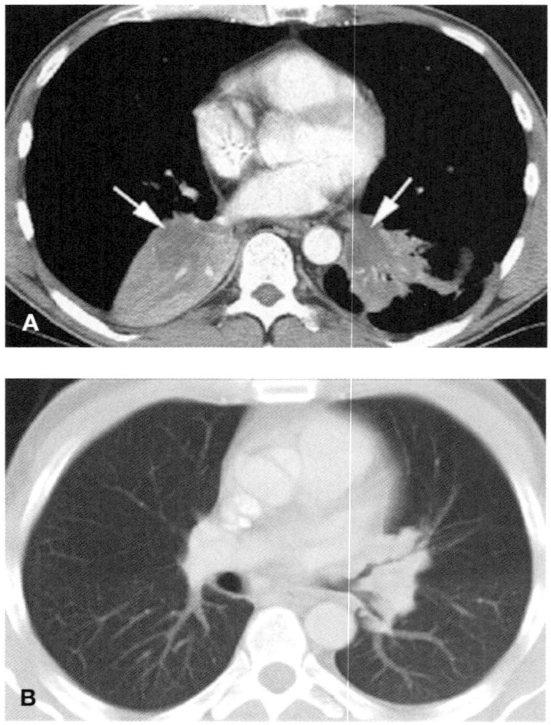

Figure 7.24. Airway abnormalities in mantle cell non-Hodgkin lymphoma (NHL). **A:** Bilateral hilar masses with bronchial obstruction and atelectasis. The masses (*arrows*) appear lower in attenuation than the collapsed lung. **B:** Airway involvement by NHL in a patient with AIDS. There is irregular narrowing of the left bronchi because of tumor involvement of the bronchial wall.

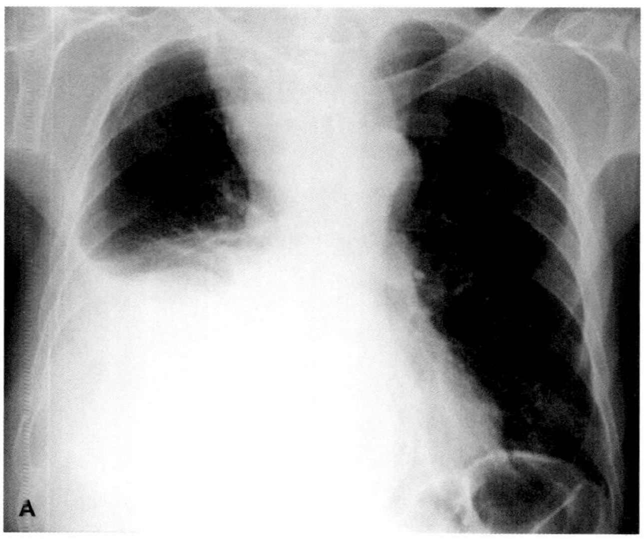

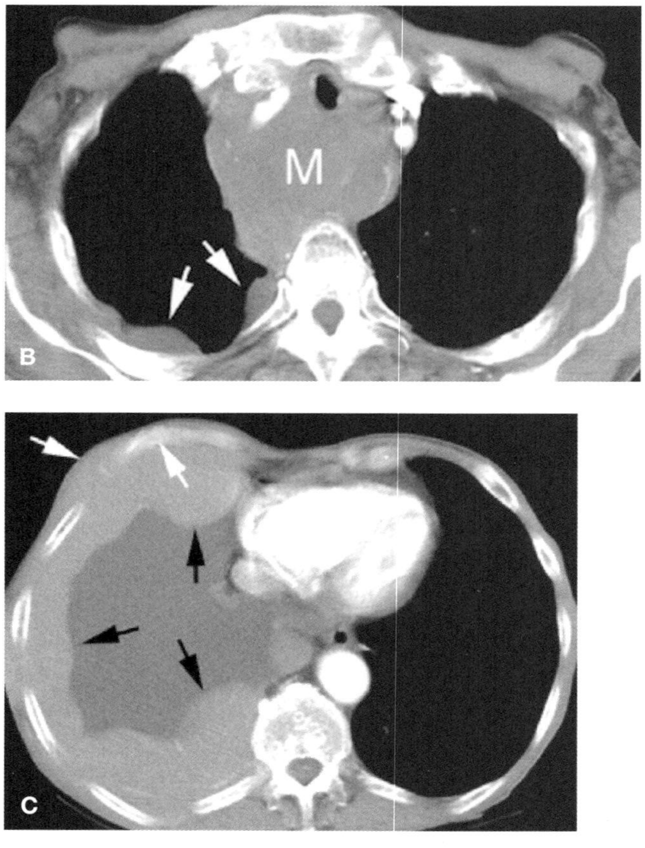

Figure 7.25. Non-Hodgkin lymphoma with pleural effusion and pleural and extrapleural tumor. **A:** Chest radiograph shows a right superior mediastinal mass and a large right pleural effusion. **B:** CT shows a large mass (*M*) posterior to the trachea and associated pleural or extrapleural masses (*arrows*). **C:** At a lower level, a large pleural effusion is visible, with extensive infiltration of the parietal pleura or chest wall by tumor (*black arrows*). A localized chest wall mass with rib destruction also is visible (*white arrows*).

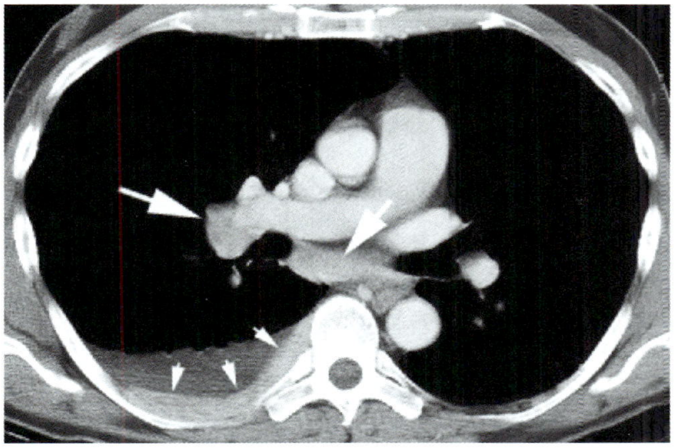

Figure 7.26. Waldenström macroglobulinemia. CT shows hilar and mediastinal lymph node enlargement (*large arrows*), pleura effusion, and pleural or extrapleural tumor (*small arrows*).

Table 7.6 Primary Pulmonary Non-Hodgkin Lymphoma

No evidence of extrathoracic dissemination for at least 3 mo
<1% incidence of pulmonary lymphomas

Low grade (MALToma)
Arises from MALT
Solitary nodule or focal consolidation
Multiple nodules or areas of consolidation
Air bronchograms in 50%
Lymph node enlargement in 5%-30%
Good prognosis

High grade (non-MALT)
Solitary or multiple nodules
Air bronchograms common
Multifocal consolidation

MALT, mucosa-associated lymphoid tissue.

with a 5-year survival of 85% to 95% and a 10-year survival of about 70%.

The most common radiologic manifestation of primary B-cell lymphoma of MALT is a solitary nodule or a focal area of consolidation, ranging in size from a few centimeters to an entire lobe. Multiple nodules or multifocal areas of consolidation also may be present and may appear similar to lung adenocarcinoma. Air bronchograms are visible in 50% of cases. The parenchymal abnormalities typically show an indolent course with slow growth over months or years. On CT, the single or multiple masses or areas of consolidation may appear primarily peribronchial in location. Pleural effusion is present in approximately 10% of cases, usually in association with evidence of parenchymal involvement. Lymphadenopathy is evident radiographically in 5% to 30% of cases at presentation.

Diffuse Large B-Cell Lymphoma

DLBCL accounts for 5% to 20% of primary pulmonary lymphomas. It is not a single disease but may be associated with various morphologies and causes. Some tumors occur in patients who have collagen vascular disease, AIDS, organ transplants (PTLD), EBV infection, or associated with other causes of immunosuppression. The most common radiographic presentation consists of solitary or multiple nodules (Fig. 7.27). As with MALToma, air bronchograms may be visible. Lymph node enlargement may be present. Other manifestations include bilateral consolidation or a diffuse reticulonodular pattern. Treatment often involves immunochemotherapy similar to that used with DLBCL arising in other sites, but patients with lung involvement have a poorer prognosis.

Lymphomatoid Granulomatosis

LG is a rare disease, characterized by an angiocentric, angiodestructive polymorphous lymphoid infiltrate characterized by neoplastic EBV-positive B cells, varying in atypical features,

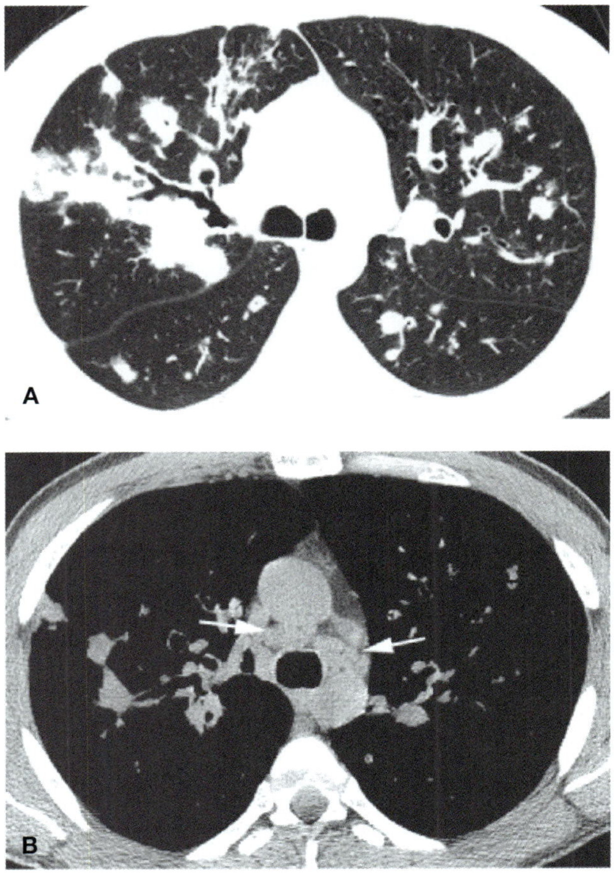

Figure 7.27. High-grade primary pulmonary non-Hodgkin lymphoma. **A:** HRCT shows multiple lung nodules and masses, some containing air bronchograms or arising in relation to bronchi. **B:** HRCT with a tissue window shows mildly enlarged mediastinal lymph nodes (*arrows*).

and a large number of reactive T cells. The median age at presentation is in the 50s; it is most common in men. LG is considered to be an EBV-associated B-cell lymphoproliferative disease. It occurs most commonly in immunodeficient patients, and it may be a manifestation of PTLD (Table 7.7).

Three grades are thought to exist, based on the degree of cytologic atypia: the proportion of EBV-positive cells, presence of necrosis, and their response to treatment. In advanced grades, LG resembles DLBCL, and its prognosis is similar. The lung is the primary site of disease, although other organs, including the skin, brain, kidneys, and heart, may be involved; patients with involvement of other organs have a poorer prognosis. Up to 25% resolve without treatment, but as many as 60% die with a median survival of 14 months. Radiographic and CT findings consist primarily of bilateral, poorly defined nodular lesions, ranging from 0.5 to 8 cm in diameter, with a basal predominance. Lesions may progress rapidly and cavitate, mimicking granulomatosis with polyangiitis. Pleural effusion may be present.

Plasmacytoma

Plasmacytoma is a focal neoplastic proliferation of plasma cells unassociated with a generalized plasma cell disorder, such as multiple myeloma. Plasmacytoma usually originates in bone, resulting in an expansile osteolytic lesion; extraosseous plasmacytoma, which arises in soft tissues, is much less common. Radiologic manifestations of extraosseous plasmacytoma include a tracheal or endobronchial mass or pulmonary nodules or mass lesions. Plasma cell tumor associated with myeloma can show similar findings. Plasmacytoma is a rare form of primary pulmonary lymphoma.

Primary Mediastinal NHL

NHL may occur primarily in the mediastinum. The most common cell types presenting in this fashion are T-cell lymphoblastic lymphoma/leukemia and primary mediastinal (thymic) large B-cell lymphoma (Table 7.8). These resemble mediastinal HL and occur in a similar population.

Table 7.7 Lymphomatoid Granulomatosis

Angiocentric, angiodestructive polymorphous lymphoid lesions
Neoplastic EBV + B cells
Reactive T cells
Associated with immunodeficiency, PTLD
Lung commonly involved
Mimics granulomatosis with polyangiitis (Wegener granulomatosis)
Bilateral, poorly defined nodules or masses
Basal predominance
Cavitation

EBV, Epstein-Barr virus; PTLD, posttransplant lymphoproliferative disorder.

T-Cell Lymphoblastic Lymphoma/Leukemia

T-cell lymphoblastic lymphoma accounts for about 60% of primary mediastinal NHL. If bone marrow and hematologic involvement are predominant features of this disease, it is termed *T-cell lymphoblastic leukemia*. Most patients are children or young adults. A large mediastinal mass representing thymic or lymph node enlargement typically is present; anterior mediastinal lymph nodes are commonly involved (Fig. 7.28). Presenting symptoms usually are related to compression of mediastinal structures. Lymph nodes in other sites suggest leukemia (Fig. 7.29C).

Table 7.8 Primary Mediastinal Non-Hodgkin Lymphoma (NHL)

Lymphoblastic lymphoma
60% of primary mediastinal NHL
Termed *lymphoblastic leukemia* if bone marrow and hematologic abnormalities predominate
Children or young adults
Large anterior mediastinal mass
Primary mediastinal large cell lymphoma
Resembles HL
Median age 35 y
Large anterior mediastinal mass

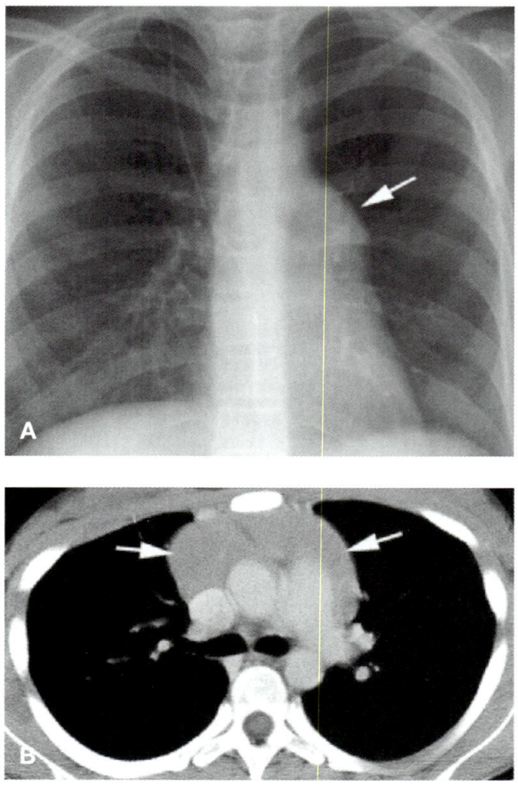

Figure 7.28. T-cell lymphoblastic lymphoma in a 14-year-old patient. **A:** Chest radiograph shows a left mediastinal mass (*arrow*). **B:** CT shows an anterior mediastinal mass (*arrows*) that probably represents thymic enlargement. This appearance in a young patient is typical.

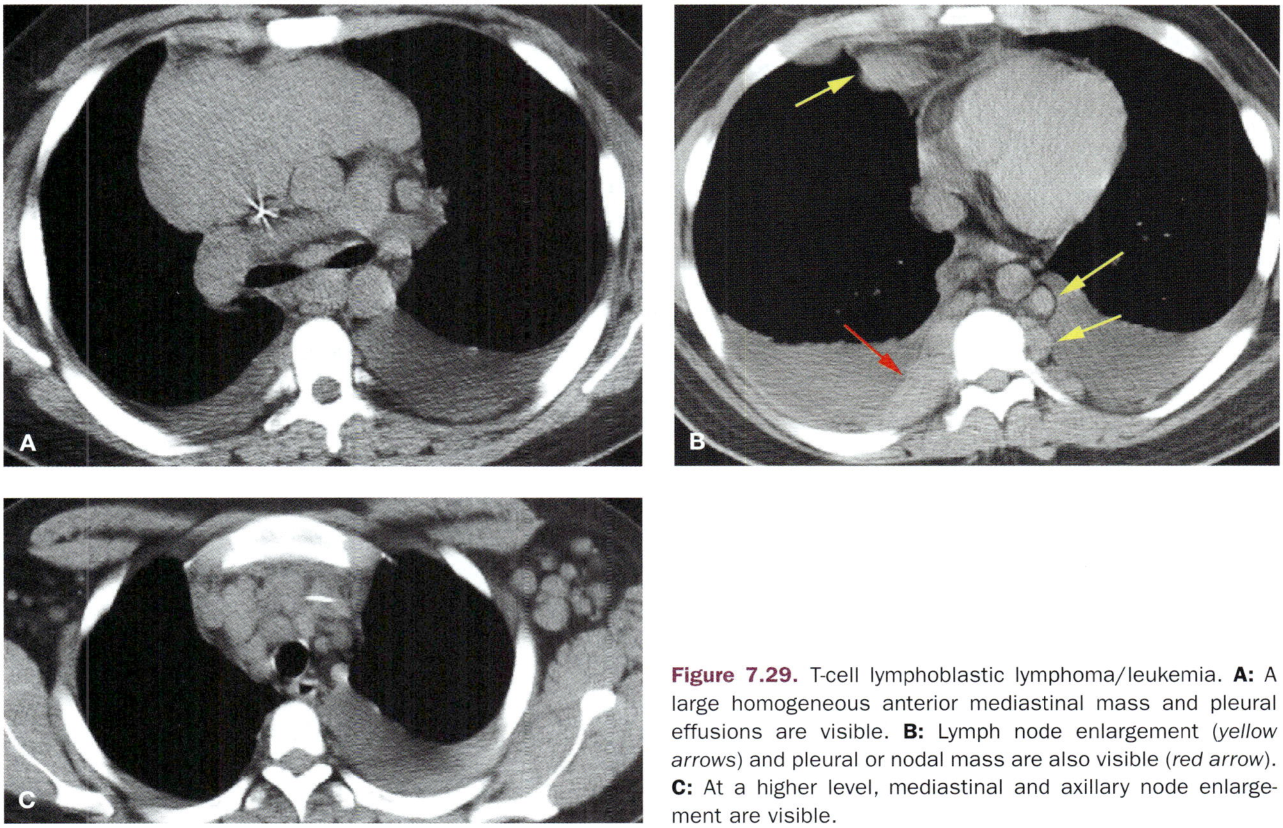

Figure 7.29. T-cell lymphoblastic lymphoma/leukemia. **A:** A large homogeneous anterior mediastinal mass and pleural effusions are visible. **B:** Lymph node enlargement (*yellow arrows*) and pleural or nodal mass are also visible (*red arrow*). **C:** At a higher level, mediastinal and axillary node enlargement are visible.

Primary Mediastinal (Thymic) Large B-Cell Lymphoma

Primary mediastinal B-cell lymphoma is a subtype of DLBCL that accounts for about 2% of all lymphomas. Two-thirds of cases occur in women, and most are in their 30s. It is usually localized to the mediastinum. It is fast growing, but it usually responds well to treatment.

Primary mediastinal large B-cell lymphoma is thought to arise from thymic medullary B cells. This entity is difficult to distinguish from HL, both clinically and radiographically. Affected patients usually are younger than other patients with NHL, with a median age of 35 years. A large, lobulated, anterior mediastinal mass averaging 10 cm in diameter is the predominant finding in nearly all patients (Figs. 7.30 and 7.31). Lymph node enlargement also may be seen in the subcarinal space and posterior mediastinum but is less common. Low-attenuation areas of necrosis within the mass are seen in almost half of cases; calcification is uncommon. Pleural and pericardial effusions are present in about one-third of cases. Cure can be achieved in the majority of patients with combination chemotherapy-immunotherapy or combined-modality therapy.

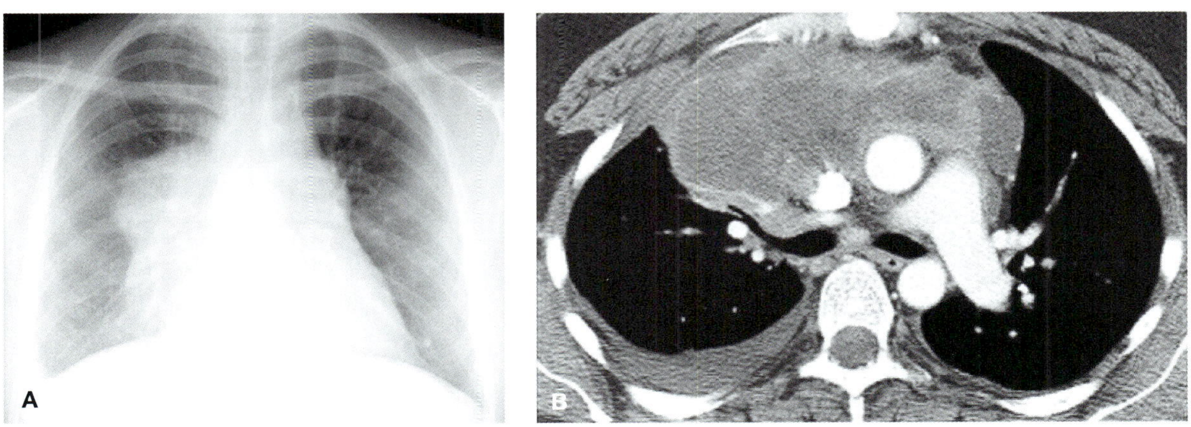

Figure 7.30. Primary mediastinal large B-cell lymphoma in a 36-year-old man. **A:** Chest radiograph shows mediastinal widening. **B:** CT shows a large inhomogeneous anterior mediastinal mass with regions of low attenuation that probably are due to necrosis. A pleural effusion is also visible.

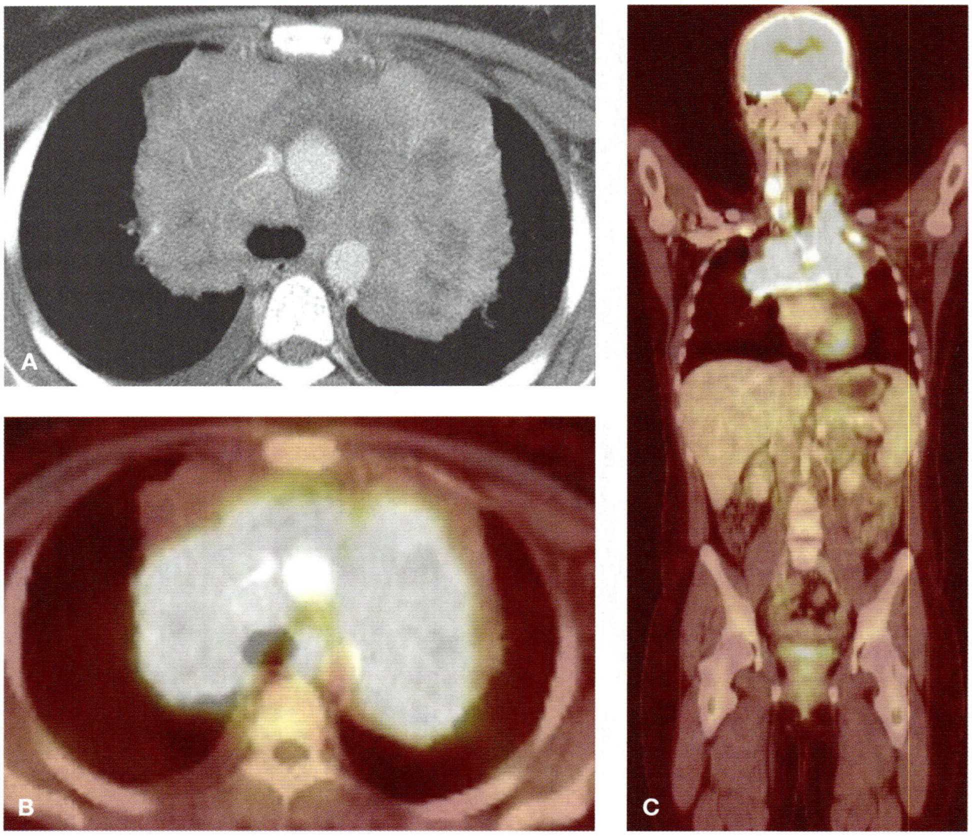

Figure 7.31. CT/FDG-PET in mediastinal large B-cell lymphoma. **A–C:** A large mass limited to the anterior mediastinum is visible on CT and PET.

Primary Effusion Lymphoma

Primary effusion lymphoma (PEL) is a rare and aggressive B-cell NHL that usually presents with malignant pleural, pericardial, or peritoneal effusions, without tumor masses. PEL is universally associated with human herpesvirus 8 (HHV-8, also known as Kaposi sarcoma [KS]-associated herpesvirus). Patients are in immunosuppressed states (HIV infection, post–organ transplantation), and 70% of cases occur with concurrent EBV infection.

Even with combination chemotherapy, prognosis is poor, with median survival only about 6 months.

AIDS-Related Lymphoma

Lymphoma has an incidence of about 2% to 5% in patients with AIDS. In 90% of these patients, it is a B-cell NHL. AIDS-related lymphoma (ARL) typically is characterized by advanced clinical stage, high histologic grade, frequent post-treatment relapse, and poor survival. It originates predominantly in extranodal locations and often involves multiple sites including bone marrow, central nervous system, lung, liver, and bowel. ARL is associated with advanced AIDS and low CD4 counts. HL in AIDS patients is almost always associated with EBV infection.

Thoracic involvement is present in 20% to 40% of patients with ARL (Table 7.9). Primary pulmonary ARL accounts for only 10% to 15% of cases.

Multiple pulmonary nodules and masses, ranging in size from 1 to 5 cm, are seen most commonly on radiographs or CT (Fig. 7.32). The nodules are usually well defined. Cavitation may be present but is not common. Localized consolidation, mass lesions, or reticular opacities also may be seen. Mediastinal lymph node enlargement (30%-50% of cases) is more common in patients with lung involvement associated with disseminated ARL than it is in patients with

Table 7.9 AIDS-Related Lymphoma (ARL)
High histologic grade and poor survival
Thoracic involvement in 20%-40%
Multiple nodules or masses most common, usually well defined
Cavitation in some
Consolidation or reticular opacities
Lymph node enlargement in 30%-50%, usually in those with dissemination
Pulmonary ARL often unassociated with lymph node enlargement

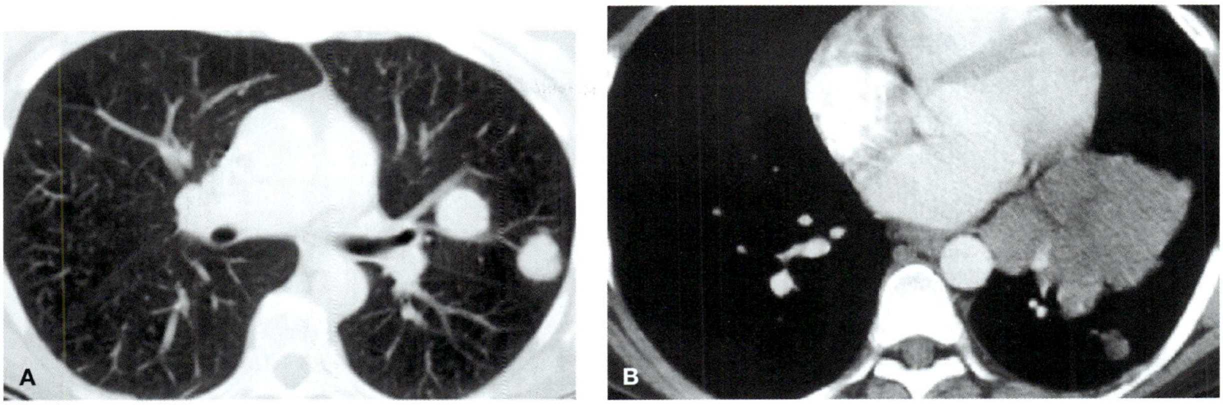

Figure 7.32. AIDS-related ymphoma (ARL). **A:** A typical appearance of an ARL is that of multiple well-defined nodules, without visible lymph node enlargement. **B:** In another patient with AIDS, a large mass represents pulmonary lymphoma.

primary or localized pulmonary ARL. Pleural effusion is common, usually in combination with multiple nodules.

Primary effusion lymphoma accounts for 4% of ARL. As described previously, PEL is a subgroup of B-cell lymphoma that occurs in advanced HIV disease and AIDS and with other causes of immunosuppression. It results in malignant pleural, peritoneal, or pericardial effusion, in the absence of nodal disease or tumor nodules.

Multicentric Castleman disease (MCD), along with KS, and PEL is associated with HHV-8 infection in AIDS patients. Unlike KS, HIV-related MCD has become more common since the development of antiretroviral therapy. Castleman disease is a lymphoproliferative disorder with two main histologic types (hyaline-vascular and plasma cell; the latter either idiopathic or associated with KSHV/HHV8), a unicentric or multicentric distribution, and involvement of multiple nodal stations and organs (see Chapter 8). It may progress to B lymphoma in AIDS patients.

LEUKEMIA

Leukemia may result in lymph node enlargement, lung infiltration, or pleural abnormalities. Imaging findings overlap those of lymphoma (Table 7.10).

Mediastinal Abnormalities

Mediastinal lymph nodes commonly are involved in patients with CLL/SLL and acute T-cell lymphoblastic leukemia (ALL). CLL typically occurs in adults older than 60 years; ALL is more common in children than in adults.

In the WHO classification, requirements for a diagnosis of CLL include an absolute count of greater than 5.0×10^9/L monoclonal B cells with a CLL immunophenotype in the peripheral blood. A diagnosis of SLL is made when lymphadenopathy or splenomegaly is associated with less than 5.0×10^9/L CLL-type cells in the blood.

Mediastinal lymph node enlargement is visible radiographically in about 25% of patients with CLL (Fig. 7.33) and 10% to 20% of patients with ALL, although it is more common at autopsy, being present in more than half of cases. Hilar lymph node enlargement also may be seen but is less common. CLL typically presents with painless lymph node enlargement or hepatosplenomegaly; these abnormalities may be chronic and slowly progressive over a period of years. ALL may present with a large, symptomatic anterior mediastinal mass.

In patients with acute or chronic myelogenous leukemia, masses of malignant myeloid precursor cells may be found in an extramedullary location, including lymph nodes; these masses are termed *granulocytic sarcoma* or *chloroma* (because of their green color). Granulocytic sarcoma occurs in about 5% of adults and 15% of children with myelogenous leukemia; the thorax is involved uncommonly. In about 50%

Table 7.10 Leukemia

Mediastinal lymph node enlargement
25% of CLL
Chronic, slowly progressive
10%-20% of ALL
Large symptomatic anterior mediastinal mass
Acute lymphoblastic lymphoma
5% of acute or chronic myelogenous leukemia
Granulocytic sarcoma (chloroma)
Lung abnormalities
20%-40% lung infiltration at autopsy
Radiographic and CT abnormalities seldom due to leukemia alone
Pneumonia, hemorrhage, drug reactions, edema
Pulmonary leukostasis
Acute myelogenous leukemia
WBC count usually >200,000/mm^3
Pulmonary edema

ALL, acute T-cell lymphoblastic leukemia; CLL, chronic lymphocytic leukemia; WBC, white blood cell.

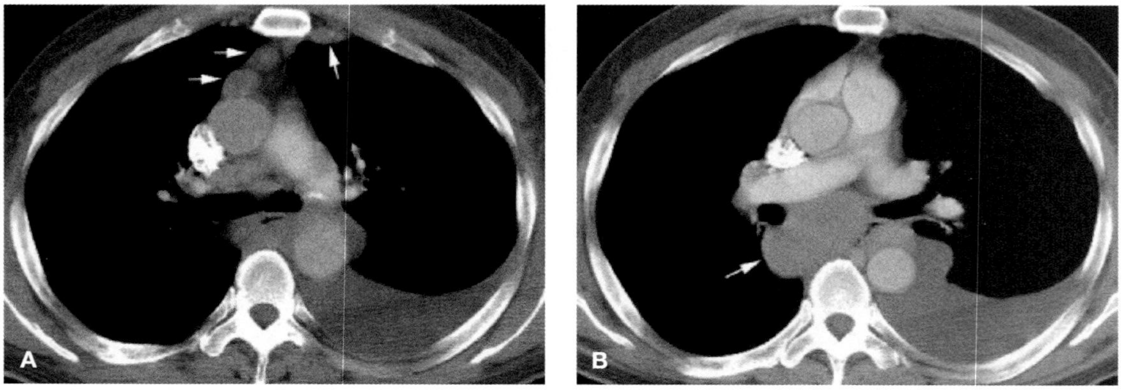

Figure 7.33. Mediastinal lymph node enlargement in chronic lymphocytic leukemia. Enlarged lymph nodes are visible in the prevascular space and internal mammary chain (*arrows* in **A**) and subcarinal space (*arrow* in **B**). A left pleural effusion, which may reflect lymphatic obstruction, also is present.

of cases with thoracic involvement, it involves the mediastinum, as a focal mass, lymph node enlargement, or generalized widening (Fig. 7.34). Less common sites of involvement include the lungs, the pleura, the pericardium, and the hila.

Lung Abnormalities

Pulmonary infiltration is evident at autopsy in 20% to 40% of patients with leukemia. Radiographic findings of pulmonary leukemic infiltration consist of bilateral reticulation that resembles interstitial edema or lymphangitic carcinomatosis. High-resolution CT (HRCT) abnormalities consist of interlobular septal thickening and thickening of the peribronchovascular interstitium.

However, pulmonary abnormalities seen on radiographs or CT in patients with leukemia seldom are due to leukemic infiltration alone. In almost all patients, lung abnormalities are due to pneumonia, hemorrhage, drug-induced lung damage, or pulmonary edema.

Dyspnea in patients with leukemia is sometimes related to *pulmonary leukostasis*. Leukostasis is most common in acute myelogenous leukemia, and it occurs in patients with very high white blood cell counts (usually over 200,000/mm^3). Symptoms result from vascular obstruction (in the lungs and other organs) by leukemic cells. Little, if any, invasion of the pulmonary interstitium occurs in patients with pulmonary leukostasis, and chest radiographs are often normal. In some cases, however, air-space consolidation is visible radiographically due to pulmonary edema (Fig. 7.35). Edema may be due to increased capillary permeability related to the presence of numerous white cells or cardiac failure related to coronary artery leukostasis. Leukostasis is considered an oncologic emergency.

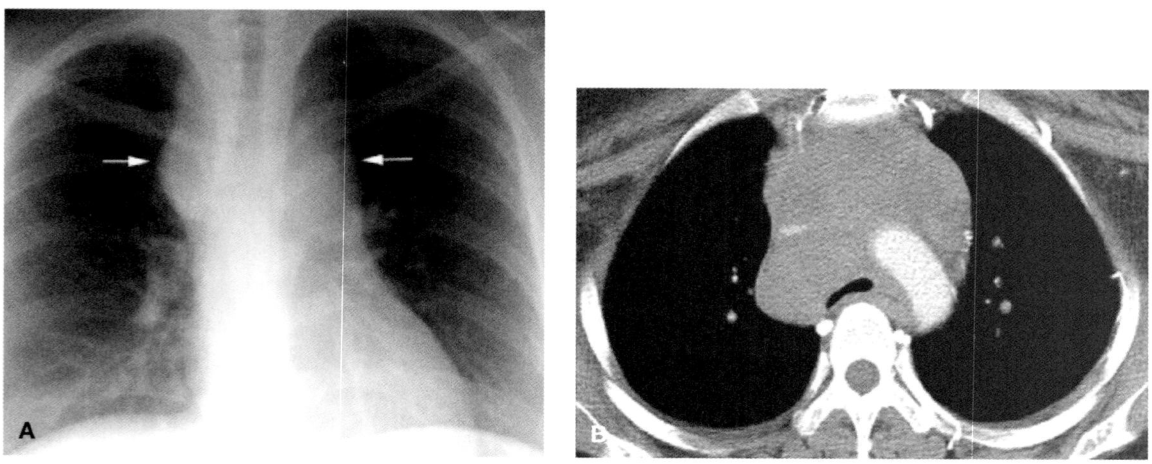

Figure 7.34. Chronic granulocytic leukemia with the involvement of mediastinal lymph nodes, so-called granulocytic sarcoma or "chloroma." **A:** Chest radiograph shows a lobulated mediastinal mass (*arrows*). **B:** CT shows extensive lymph node enlargement in the paratracheal and prevascular mediastinum.

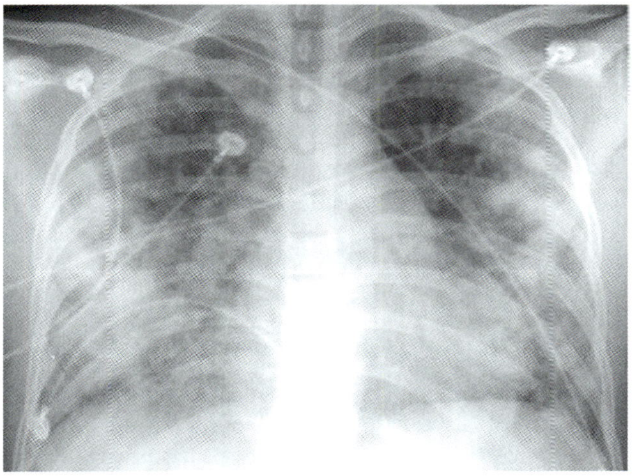

Figure 7.35. Pulmonary leukostasis. A patient with acute leukemia, high white cell count, and leukostasis shows patchy areas of consolidation in the peripheral lung. These usually represent pulmonary edema.

Pleural Disease

As with lymphoma, pleural effusion may reflect lymphatic obstruction (see Fig. 7.33) or pleural involvement by tumor (Fig. 7.36).

LYMPHOPROLIFERATIVE DISEASES

In addition to HL and NHL, pulmonary lymphoproliferative diseases represent a spectrum of focal and diffuse lung abnormalities associated with either a benign or malignant course (Table 7.11). As with MALToma, described earlier, many of these diseases are related to abnormal proliferation of submucosal lymphoid follicles distributed along distal bronchi and bronchioles, termed MALT. Proliferations of MALT may be either hyperplastic or neoplastic. Polyclonal cellular proliferations usually are hyperplastic and benign, whereas most monoclonal cellular proliferations are malignant. However, in some cases, both hyperplasia and neoplasia may be present, and many lymphoproliferative diseases at least have malignant potential.

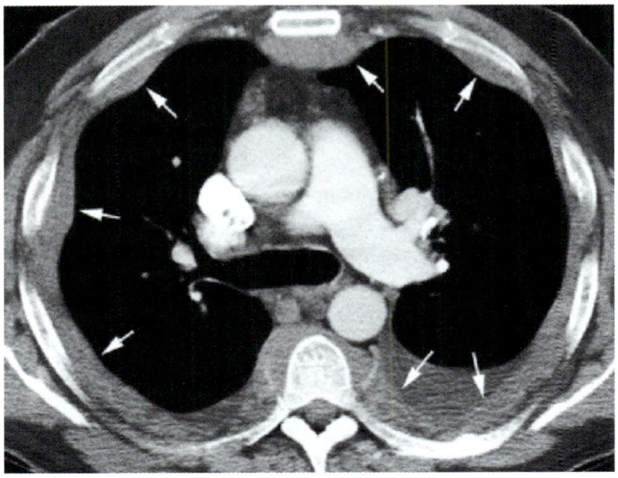

Figure 7.36. Chronic lymphocytic leukemia with extrapleural involvement and pleural effusion. A number of masses (*arrows*) appear to be associated with the sternum and ribs. A left pleural effusion also is present. This appearance is similar to that in Figures 7.25 and 7.26.

Table 7.11 Pulmonary Lymphoproliferative Diseases

Focal lymphoid hyperplasia
Benign focal lesion
Formerly termed pseudolymphoma
Solitary nodule or a focal consolidation
Multiple nodules less common
Air bronchograms
No lymph node enlargement
Follicular bronchiolitis
Hyperplasia of bronchiolar MALT
Peribronchiolar lymphoid follicles
Associations
Collagen diseases, for example, rheumatoid arthritis
Immunodeficiency
Hypersensitivity
Centrilobular nodules
Tree-in-bud
Ground-glass opacity
Lymphocytic interstitial pneumonia
Benign
Diffuse interstitial infiltrate
Collagen diseases, eg, Sjögren syndrome
AIDS or immunosuppression
Ground-glass opacity
Consolidation
Poorly defined centrilobular nodules
Small well-defined nodules
Interlobular septal thickening
Cystic airspaces
Fever and weight loss
Hepatomegaly and splenomegaly
Polyclonal hypergammopathy
Posttransplantation lymphoproliferative disorder
Bone marrow or solid organ transplantation
Occurs in the first year after transplantation
Ranges from benign to HL or NHL
Associated with Epstein-Barr virus infection
85% show single or multiple lung nodules
5%-25% lymph node enlargement

MALT, mucosa-associated lymphoid tissue.

Focal (Nodular) Lymphoid Hyperplasia

Focal or nodular lymphoid hyperplasia is a rare benign condition characterized histologically by localized proliferation of benign mononuclear cells consisting of a mixture of polyclonal lymphocytes, plasma cells, and histiocytes. It has also been referred to as a "pseudolymphoma." The most frequently seen radiologic manifestation of focal lymphoid hyperplasia is a solitary nodule or a focal area of consolidation, but multiple nodules may be seen. The nodules or nodular areas of consolidation usually measure several centimeters in diameter and contain air bronchograms (Fig. 7.37). There is no associated lymphadenopathy. It may occur in association with Sjögren syndrome.

There is a significant overlap between the presentation and appearance of lymphoid hyperplasia and MALT lymphoma, which may also present as a focal lesion, and in a similar clinical setting. The presence of multiple or bilateral nodules suggests that MALToma is more likely.

Follicular Bronchiolitis

Follicular bronchiolitis (FB) is also known as hyperplasia of the BALT or hyperplasia of the MALT. FB results from antigenic stimulation of the BALT and polyclonal lymphoid hyperplasia. Histologically, FB is characterized by abundant peribronchiolar lymphoid follicles, with the lymphoid infiltrate extending into adjacent alveolar interstitium. Although FB lacks the extensive alveolar infiltration of lymphocytic interstitial pneumonia (LIP), a distinction between them is somewhat arbitrary.

FB occurs in several clinical settings including collagen vascular disease (particularly rheumatoid arthritis), immunodeficiency, hypersensitivity disorders, and as a secondary condition associated with a variety of nonspecific airway-centered inflammatory conditions such as bronchiectasis, airway obstruction, and infection. It may occur in adults or children, and typical presenting symptoms include dyspnea and cough.

HRCT typically shows bilateral centrilobular nodules, tree-in-bud opacities, small or large nodules, or ground-glass opacities (Fig. 7.38). Patients with FB typically have a good prognosis, and treatment is aimed at the underlying disease or involves anti-inflammatory drugs.

Lymphoid Interstitial Pneumonia

Lymphoid (lymphocytic) LIP may be classified as a benign lymphoproliferative disorder or an interstitial pneumonia (see Chapter 14). It is characterized histologically by a diffuse interstitial infiltrate of mononuclear cells consisting predominantly of lymphocytes and plasma cells. LIP often occurs in association with Sjögren syndrome, other collagen vascular diseases, immunosuppression, or AIDS. In patients with AIDS, LIP usually occurs in children (Fig. 7.39); most other patients with LIP are adults (mean age, 50 years). The main clinical symptoms are cough and dyspnea.

The radiographic findings vary and may consist of a reticular or reticulonodular pattern involving mainly the lower lung zones. Less common abnormalities include a nodular pattern or air-space consolidation. On HRCT, typical findings include diffuse or patchy areas of ground-glass opacity or consolidation; poorly defined centrilobular nodules; small, well-defined nodules (see Fig. 7.39); and cystic airspaces (typical in Sjögren syndrome; see Chapter 25). The appearance also may mimic lymphangitic spread of carcinoma, with interlobular septal thickening and nodules. FB may be considered a localized form of LIP.

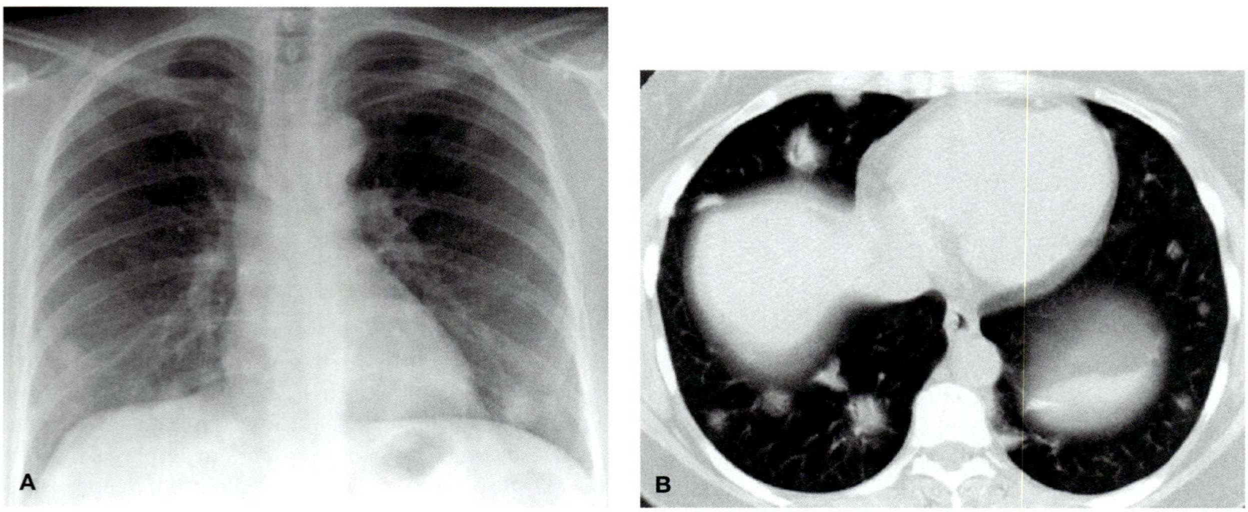

Figure 7.37. Focal lymphoid hyperplasia in a patient with Sjögren syndrome. **A:** Chest radiograph shows multiple nodular opacities. **B:** CT shows multiple ill-defined nodules, many of which contain air bronchograms.

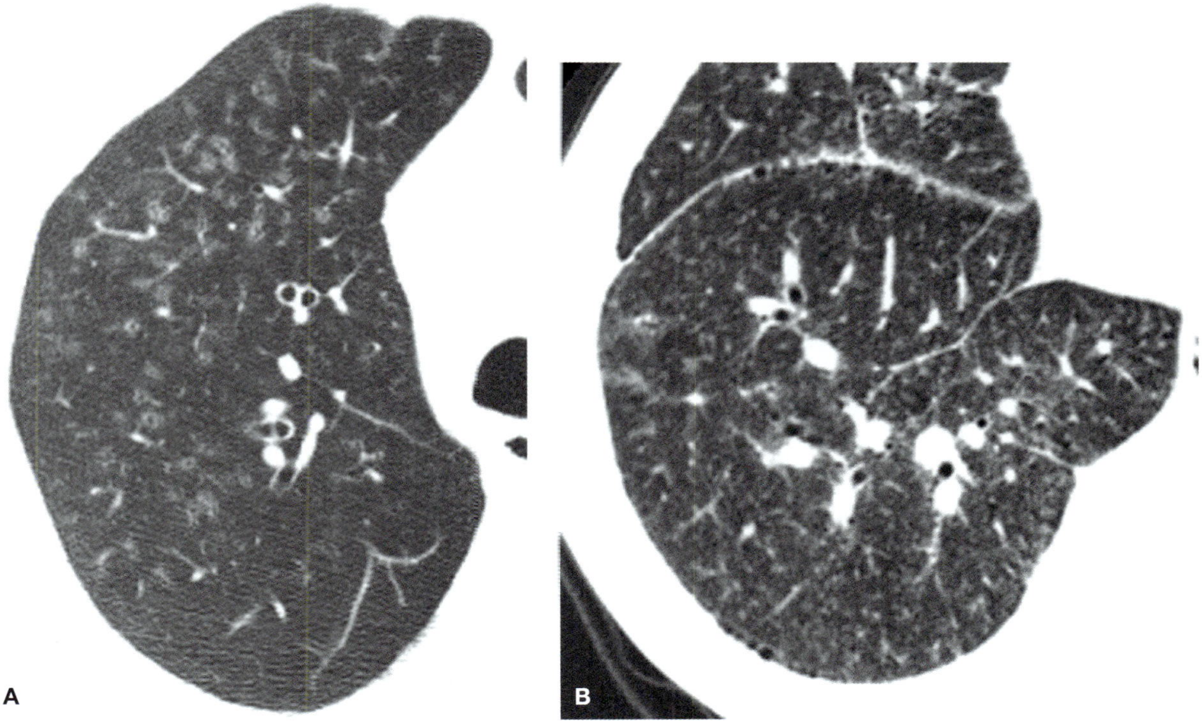

Figure 7.38. Follicular bronchiolitis with centrilobular nodules. **A:** Centrilobular nodules, biopsy-proven follicular bronchiolitis. **B:** Biopsy-proven follicular bronchiolitis in a patient with rheumatoid arthritis. Ground-glass centrilobular nodules are visible.

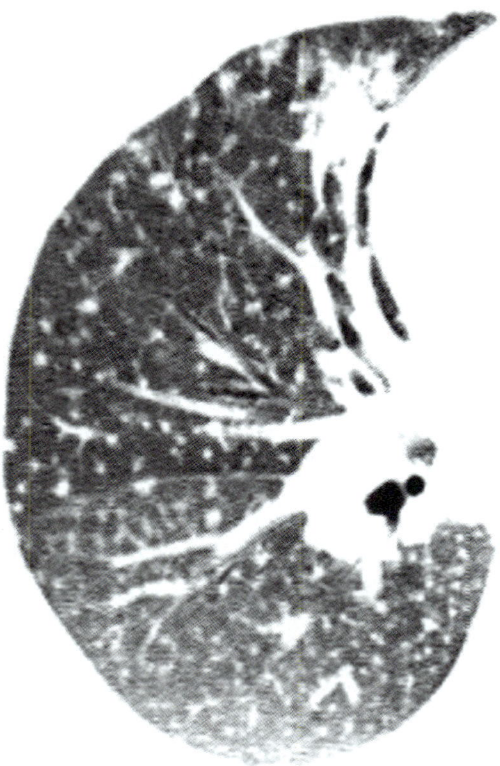

Figure 7.39. Lymphoid (lymphocytic) interstitial pneumonia. An 11-year-old child with AIDS shows multiple small nodules and a focal area of consolidation.

Posttransplantation Lymphoproliferative Disorder

Several histologic patterns of lymphocyte proliferation, known collectively as PTLD, can occur after bone marrow or solid organ transplantation. The histologic patterns range from benign hyperplastic proliferation of lymphocytes to malignant lymphoma, either HL or NHL.

Most cases of PTLD have been associated with EBV infection. PTLD affects up to 10% of transplant recipients. Most patients present in the first year after transplantation. PTLD can manifest as localized or disseminated disease and has a predilection for extranodal involvement. Lung involvement may occur as part of multiorgan disease or in isolation.

In 85% of cases, radiographs and CT show single or multiple pulmonary nodules, which may be small or large (0.3-5 cm) and well or ill defined (Fig. 7.40). Other findings include patchy or focal consolidation or ground-glass opacity, a predominantly peribronchial and subpleural or diffuse distribution of parenchymal abnormalities, and hilar or mediastinal lymphadenopathy (5%-25%). Pleural effusion may be present.

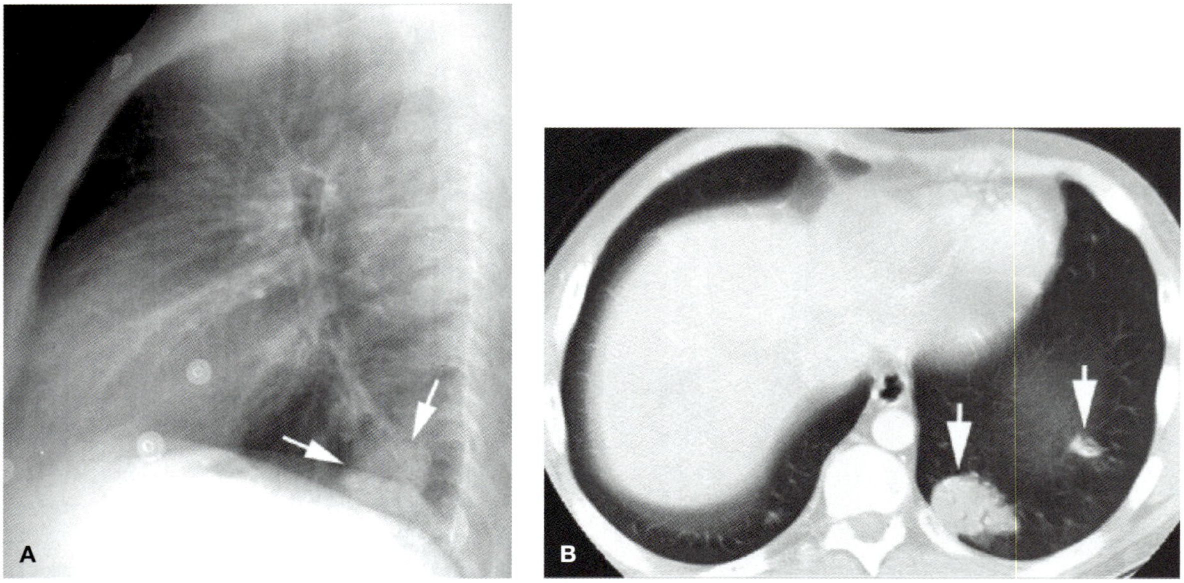

Figure 7.40. Posttransplantation lymphoproliferative disorder. **A:** Lateral radiograph shows a nodule (*arrows*) in the posterior lower lobe. **B:** CT shows two irregular and poorly marginated nodules (*arrows*).

SELECTED READINGS

Alaggio R, Amador C, Anagnostopoulos I, et al. The 5th edition of the World Health Organization classification of haematolymphoid tumours: lymphoid neoplasms. *Leukemia*. 2022;36(7):1720-1748. doi:10.1038/s41375-022-01620-2

Aquino SL, Chen MY, Kuo WT, Chiles C. The CT appearance of pleural and extrapleural disease in lymphoma. *Clin Radiol*. 1999;54(10):647-650.

Au V, Leung AN. Radiologic manifestations of lymphoma in the thorax. *AJR Am J Roentgenol*. 1997;168(1):93-98.

Bae YA, Lee KS. Cross-sectional evaluation of thoracic lymphoma. *Radiol Clin North Am*. 2008;46(2):253-264, viii.

Blunt DM, Padley SP. Radiographic manifestations of AIDS related lymphoma in the thorax. *Clin Radiol*. 1995;50(9):607-612.

Borhani AA, Hosseinzadeh K, Almusa O, Furlan A, Nalesnik M. Imaging of posttransplantation lymphoproliferative disorder after solid organ transplantation. *Radiographics*. 2009;29(4):981-1000; discussion 1000-1002.

Bragg DG, Colby TV, Ward JH. New concepts in the non-Hodgkin lymphomas: radiologic implications. *Radiology*. 1986;159(2):291-304.

Bragg DG, Chor PJ, Murray KA, Kjeldsberg CR. Lymphoproliferative disorders of the lung: histopathology, clinical manifestations, and imaging features. *AJR Am J Roentgenol*. 1994;163(2):273-281.

Camacho JC, Moreno CC, Harri PA, Aguirre DA, Torres WE, Mittal PK. Posttransplantation lymphoproliferative disease: proposed imaging classification. *Radiographics*. 2014;34(7):2025-2038.

Campo E, Swerdlow SH, Harris NL, Pileri S, Stein H, Jaffe ES. The 2008 WHO classification of lymphoid neoplasms and beyond: evolving concepts and practical applications. *Blood*. 2011;117(19):5019-5032.

Carignan S, Staples CA, Müller NL. Intrathoracic lymphoproliferative disorders in the immunocompromised patient: CT findings. *Radiology*. 1995;197(1):53-58.

Castellino RA, Blank N, Hoppe RT, Cho C. Hodgkin disease: contributions of chest CT in the initial staging evaluation. *Radiology*. 1986;160(3):603-605.

Castellino RA, Hilton S, O'Brien JP, Portlock CS. Non-Hodgkin lymphoma: contribution of chest CT in the initial staging evaluation. *Radiology*. 1996;199(1):129-132.

Castellino RA. Hodgkin disease: practical concepts for the diagnostic radiologist. *Radiology*. 1986;159(2):305-310.

Castellino RA. The non-Hodgkin lymphomas: practical concepts for the diagnostic radiologist. *Radiology*. 1991;178(2):315-321.

Cheson BD, Fisher RI, Barrington SF, et al. Recommendations for initial evaluation, staging, and response assessment of Hodgkin and non-Hodgkin lymphoma: the Lugano classification. *J Clin Oncol*. 2014;32(27):3059-3068.

Chou SHS, Prabhu SJ, Crothers K, Stern EJ, Godwin JD, Pipavath SN. Thoracic diseases associated with HIV infection in the era of antiretroviral therapy: clinical and imaging findings. *Radiographics*. 2014;34(4):895-911.

Cobby M, Whipp E, Bullimore J, Goodman S, Davies ER, Goddard P. CT appearances of relapse of lymphoma in the lung. *Clin Radiol*. 1990;41(4):232-238.

Collins J, Müller NL, Leung AN, et al. Epstein-Barr virus–associated lymphoproliferative disease of the lung: CT and histologic findings. *Radiology*. 1998;208(3):749-759.

Costello P, Mauch P. Radiographic features of recurrent intrathoracic Hodgkin's disease following radiation therapy. *AJR Am J Roentgenol*. 1979;133(2):201-206.

Do KH, Lee JS, Seo JB, et al. Pulmonary parenchymal involvement of low-grade lymphoproliferative disorders. *J Comput Assist Tomogr*. 2005;29(6):825-830.

Dodd G, Ledesma-Medina J, Baron RL, Fuhrman CR. Posttransplant lymphoproliferative disorder: intrathoracic manifestations. *Radiology*. 1992;184(1):65-69.

Eisner MD, Kaplan LD, Herndier B, Stulbarg MS. The pulmonary manifestations of AIDS-related non-Hodgkin's lymphoma. *Chest*. 1996;110(3):729-736.

Filly R, Bland N, Castellino R. Radiographic distribution of intrathoracic disease in previously untreated patients with Hodgkin's disease and non-Hodgkin's lymphoma. *Radiology*. 1976;120(2):277-281.

Gibson M, Hansell DM. Lymphocytic disorders of the chest: pathology and imaging. *Clin Radiol*. 1998;53(7):469-480.

Harris NL, Jaffe ES, Stein H, et al. A revised European-American classification of lymphoid neoplasms: a proposal from the International Lymphoma Study Group. *Blood*. 1994;84(5):1361-1392.

Harris NL, Jaffe ES, Diebold J, et al. The World Health Organization classification of neoplastic diseases of the hematopoietic and lymphoid tissues. Report of the Clinical Advisory Committee meeting, Airlie House, Virginia, November, 1997. *Ann Oncol*. 1999;10(12):1419-1432.

Heyneman LE, Johkoh T, Ward S, Honda O, Yoshida S, Müller NL. Pulmonary leukemic infiltrates: high-resolution CT findings in 10 patients. *AJR Am J Roentgenol*. 2000;174(2):517-521.

Jochelson M, Mauch P, Balikian J, Rosenthal D, Canellos G. The significance of the residual mediastinal mass in treated Hodgkin's disease. *J Clin Oncol*. 1985;3(5):637-640.

Johkoh T, Müller NL, Pickford HA, et al. Lymphocytic interstitial pneumonia: thin-section CT findings in 22 patients. *Radiology*. 1999;212(2):567-572.

Johnson SA, Kumar A, Matasar MJ, Schöder H, Rademaker J. Imaging for staging and response assessment in lymphoma. *Radiology*. 2015;276(2):323-338.

Khoury JD, Solary E, Abla O, et al. The 5th edition of the World Health Organization classification of haematolymphoid tumours: myeloid and histiocytic/dendritic neoplasms. *Leukemia.* 2022;36(7):1703-1719. doi:10.1038/s41375-022-01613-1

Kim HJ, Lee S-H, Park J, et al. Primary pulmonary non-Hodgkin lymphoma. *Jpn J Clin Oncol.* 2004;34:510-514.

Kinsely BL, Mastey LA, Mergo PJ, et al. Pulmonary mucosa-associated lymphoid tissue lymphoma: CT and pathologic findings. *AJR Am J Roentgenol.* 1999;172(5):1321-1326.

Koss MN. Pulmonary lymphoid disorders. *Semin Diagn Pathol.* 1995;12(2):158-171.

Lee KS, Kim Y, Primack SL. Imaging of pulmonary lymphomas. *AJR Am J Roentgenol.* 1997;168(2):339-345.

Lee DK, Im JG, Lee KS, et al. B-cell lymphoma of bronchus-associated lymphoid tissue (BALT): CT features in 10 patients. *J Comput Assist Tomogr.* 2000;24(1):30-34.

Lee WK, Duddalwar VA, Rouse HC, Lau EWF, Bekhit E, Hennessy OF. Extranodal lymphoma in the thorax: cross-sectional imaging findings. *Clin Radiol.* 2009;64(5):542-549.

Limpert J, MacMahon H, Variakojis D. Angioimmunoblastic lymphadenopathy: clinical and radiological features. *Radiology.* 1984;152(1):27-30.

Lu P. Staging and classification of lymphoma. *Semin Nucl Med.* 2005;35(3):150-164.

O'Donnell PG, Jackson SA, Tung KT, Hassan B, Wilkins B, Mead GM. Radiological appearances of lymphomas arising from mucosa-associated lymphoid tissue (MALT) in the lung. *Clin Radiol.* 1998;53(4):258-263.

Okada F, Ando Y, Kondo Y, Matsumoto S, Maeda T, Mori H. Thoracic CT findings of adult T-cell leukemia or lymphoma. *AJR Am J Roentgenol.* 2004;182(3):761-767.

Rappaport DC, Chamberlain DW, Shepherd FA, Hutcheon MA. Lymphoproliferative disorders after lung transplantation: imaging features. *Radiology.* 1998;206(2):519-524.

Shaffer K, Smith D, Kirn D, et al. Primary mediastinal large–B-cell lymphoma: radiologic findings at presentation. *AJR Am J Roentgenol.* 1996;167(2):425-430.

Sider L, Weiss AJ, Smith MD, VonRoenn JH, Glassroth J. Varied appearance of AIDS-related lymphoma in the chest. *Radiology.* 1989;171(3):629-632.

Sirajuddin A, Raparia K, Lewis VA, et al. Primary pulmonary lymphoid lesions: radiologic and pathologic findings. *Radiographics.* 2016;36(1):53-70.

Takasugi JE, Godwin JD, Marglin SI, Petersdorf SH. Intrathoracic granulocytic sarcomas. *J Thorac Imag.* 1996;11(3):223-230.

Tateishi U, Muller NL, Johkoh T, et al. Primary mediastinal lymphoma: characteristic features of the various histological subtypes on CT. *J Comput Assist Tomogr.* 2004;28(6):782-789.

Thompson GP, Utz JP, Rosenow EC, Myers JL, Swensen SJ. Pulmonary lymphoproliferative disorders. *Mayo Clin Proc.* 1993;68(8):804-817.

Travis WD, Galvin JR. Non-neoplastic pulmonary lymphoid lesions. *Thorax.* 2001;56(12):964-971.

Travis WD, Brambilla E, Burke AP, et al, eds. *WHO Classification of Tumours of the Lung, Pleura, Thymus and Heart.* WHO Press; 2015.

Zinzani PL. Lymphoma: diagnosis, staging, natural history, and treatment strategies. *Semin Oncol.* 2005;32(1 suppl 1):4-10.

Chapter 8

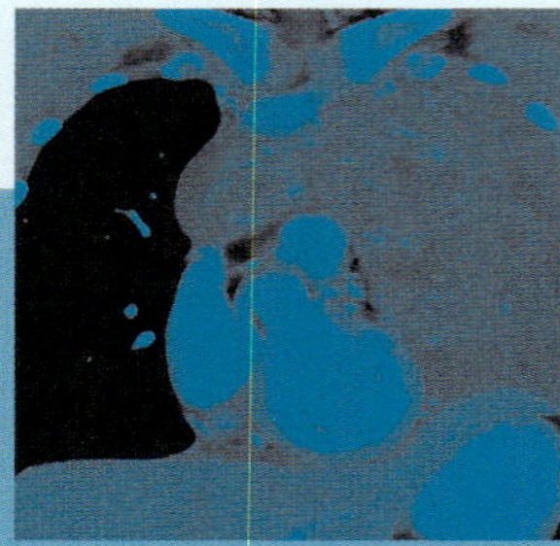

Travis S. Henry

The Mediastinum: Mediastinal Masses

DIAGNOSIS OF MEDIASTINAL MASS

Although radiographs can show recognizable abnormalities in many patients with mediastinal pathology, they are limited in their sensitivity and ability to delineate the extent of mediastinal abnormalities and their relationship to specific mediastinal structures. Computed tomography (CT) is indispensable in the radiographic assessment of the mediastinum, and contrast infusion is typically used.

The differential diagnosis of a mediastinal mass on CT is usually based on several findings:

1. Location (anterior, middle, or posterior mediastinum), or specific mediastinal compartments, such as aortopulmonary window or subcarinal space) or the identification of the specific structure from which it is arising
2. Nature
   a. Solitary lesion
   b. Multifocal (ie, lymph nodes)
   c. Diffuse mediastinal involvement
3. Attenuation
   a. Fat
   b. Fluid
   c. Soft tissue
   d. Calcification
   e. Enhancement following infusion of contrast

MEDIASTINAL COMPARTMENTS

Anatomically, the mediastinum is divided into three compartments. Historically, these were referred to as anterior, middle, and posterior. However, the International Thymic Malignancy Interest Group (ITMIG) recently renamed the compartments as prevascular, visceral, and paravertebral, respectively. The ITMIG classification will primarily be used in this text although the older terms will still be referenced because of their ubiquity in the literature.

Anatomic Divisions

Prevascular (Anterior)

Extent: anterior to the pericardium and posterior to the sternum

Contents: thymus, lymph nodes, left brachiocephalic vein, fat

Visceral (Middle)

Extent: posterior to the prevascular compartment and anterior to the paravertebral compartment (1 cm posterior to the anterior margin of the vertebral bodies); defined by its contents

Contents: heart, pericardium, aorta, superior vena cava, azygos arch, intrapericardial pulmonary arteries, thoracic duct, trachea, carina, esophagus, lymph nodes

Paravertebral (Posterior)

Extent: posterior boundary of the visceral compartment (1 cm from the anterior margin of the vertebral bodies), posterior margin of the chest wall at the transverse process of the thoracic spine

Contents: thoracic spine, paravertebral soft tissues

Plain Radiographic Divisions

The ITMIG compartments allow for localization of mediastinal abnormalities on plain radiographs, and differ only slightly from the traditional Felson classification (the heart, ascending aorta, and portions of the hila are considered part of the anterior mediastinum by Felson) (Fig. 8.1).

A more detailed analysis of the plain film, and localization of mediastinal abnormalities, may be based on identification of specific mediastinal lines, stripes, interfaces, and spaces, listed below and described in Chapter 2.

Prevascular

Extent: posterior to the sternum and anterior to the heart and ascending aorta

Contents: thymus, fat, lymph nodes

Corresponding plain film features: anterior junction line, cardiophrenic angles, retrosternal stripe, and retrosternal space

Visceral

Extent: between the prevascular compartment in front and the paravertebral compartment behind

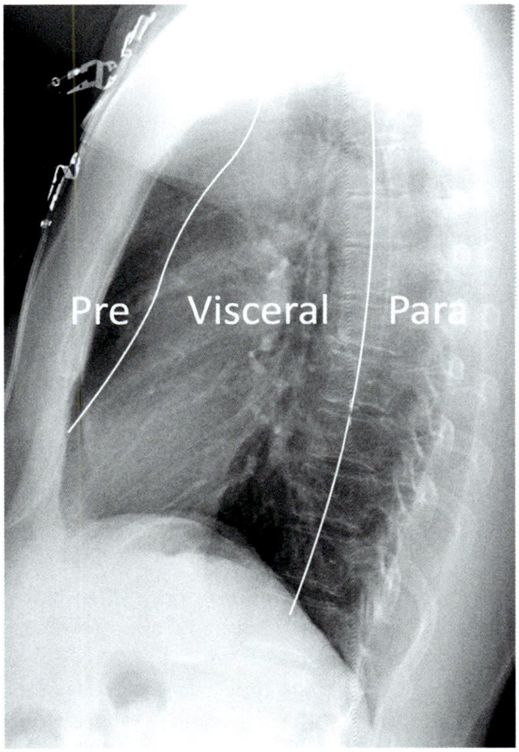

Figure 8.1. Lateral chest radiograph showing the International Thymic Malignancy Interest Group mediastinal divisions. The prevascular compartment (*Pre*) lies posterior to the sternum and anterior to the heart and ascending aorta. The paravertebral compartment (*Para*) lies posterior to a line 1 cm behind the anterior margin of the vertebral column and anterior to the chest wall. The visceral compartment (*Visceral*) lies between these. The major difference between this classification and Felson's classification is the inclusion of the heart and ascending aorta within the visceral compartment rather than the anterior mediastinum.

Contents: heart, pericardium, aorta, pulmonary arteries, trachea and main bronchi, superior vena cava, azygos arch, lymph nodes, esophagus

Corresponding plain film features: right and left paratracheal stripes, superior vena cava interface, aortopulmonary window, left subclavian artery interface, azygoesophageal recess, and preaortic interface

Paravertebral

Extent: posterior to a line 1 cm behind the anterior margin of the vertebral column and anterior to the chest wall

Contents: vertebral bodies, paravertebral tissues, posterior azygos vein, hemiazygos vein, and lymph nodes

Corresponding plain film features: paravertebral stripes

CT Divisions

On CT, it is most appropriate to base the differential diagnosis of a mediastinal mass on a direct observation of the tissue or structure from which the mass is arising (eg, lymph nodes, veins and arteries, thymus, thyroid, trachea, esophagus, vertebral column). If this is not possible, then localizing the mass to specific regions of the mediastinum (eg, prevascular space, paratracheal space, subcarinal space, aortopulmonary window, anterior cardiophrenic angle, paraspinal region) is valuable in differential diagnosis and more specific than considering only the anterior, middle, and posterior divisions (Table 8.1). The normal appearances of these regions are described in Chapter 2.

THE NORMAL THYMUS

The thymus has two lobes, the right and the left, which are fused superiorly near the thyroid gland and smoothly molded to the anterior aspect of the great vessels and anterior heart. It occupies the *thyropericardic space*. The thymus is rarely found in an ectopic location, usually the neck. The left thymic lobe usually is larger than the right.

The thymus weighs an average of about 25 g at birth and increases progressively to reach a maximum weight of approximately 35 to 50 g at puberty. The thymus begins to involute after puberty, and this process continues for a period of 5 to 15 years. During thymic involution, thymic follicles atrophy and are progressively replaced by fat. The relative proportion of fat to thymic tissue increases progressively until after age 60. At this age, little thymic tissue remains.

Plain Radiographs

In adults, the thymus is usually invisible on chest radiographs. In children, the thymus may be quite prominent, mimicking a mass (Fig. 8.2). However, radiographic findings may help in the correct identification of the thymus in children.

Table 8.1 Differential Diagnosis of Mediastinal Masses Based on Common Sites of Origin

Prevascular Compartment
- Thymic masses
  - Hyperplasia
  - Thymoma
  - Thymic carcinoma
  - Thymic neuroendocrine tumor
  - Thymolipoma
  - Thymic cyst
  - Thymic lymphoma and metastases
- Germ cell tumors
  - Teratoma
  - Seminoma
  - Nonseminomatous germ cell tumors
- Thyroid abnormalities (goiter and neoplasm)
- Parathyroid tumor or hyperplasia
- Lymph node masses (particularly Hodgkin lymphoma)
- Vascular abnormalities (aorta and great vessels)
- Mesenchymal abnormalities (eg, lipomatosis, lipoma)
- Foregut cyst
- Lymphangioma and hemangioma

Cardiophrenic Angle
- Pericardial cyst
- Morgagni hernia
- Exuberant epicardial fat
- Mass from prevascular space (eg, thymus, germ cell, lymphoma, metastasis)

Visceral Compartment (paratracheal space)
- Lymph node masses
  - Lung carcinoma
  - Sarcoidosis
  - Lymphoma (Hodgkin lymphoma, non-Hodgkin lymphoma) and leukemia
  - Castleman disease
  - Metastases
  - Infections (eg, tuberculosis)
- Fibrosing mediastinitis
- Foregut cyst
- Tracheal tumor
- Mesenchymal masses
  - Lipomatosis, lipoma, liposarcoma
  - Mediastinal fibromatosis
  - Inflammatory myofibroblastic tumor
  - Solitary fibrous tumor
- Thyroid abnormalities
- Vascular abnormalities (aorta and great vessels)
- Lymphangioma and hemangioma

Visceral Compartment (aortopulmonary window)
- Lymph node masses
  - Lung carcinoma
  - Sarcoidosis
  - Lymphoma
  - Metastases
  - Infections (eg, tuberculosis)
- Mesenchymal masses (see above)
- Vascular abnormalities (aorta or pulmonary artery)
- Chemodectoma
- Foregut cyst

Visceral Compartment (subcarinal space and azygoesophageal recess)
- Lymph node masses
  - Lung carcinoma
  - Sarcoidosis
  - Lymphoma
  - Metastases
  - Infections (eg, tuberculosis)
- Foregut cyst
- Dilated azygos vein
- Esophageal masses
- Varices
- Hernia

Paravertebral Compartment
- Neurogenic tumor
  - Nerve sheath tumors
  - Sympathetic ganglia tumors
  - Paraganglioma
- Foregut cyst
- Meningocele
- Extramedullary hematopoiesis
- Pseudocyst
- Thoracic spine abnormalities
- Hernias
- Esophageal masses
- Varices
- Mesenchymal masses (see above)
- Lymph node masses
  - Lymphoma (particularly non-Hodgkin)
  - Metastases
- Dilated azygos or hemiazygos vein
- Hernia
- Lymphangioma and hemangioma
- Thymic mass or germ cell tumor

The thymus may project to one or both sides of the mediastinum, showing a sharply marginated undersurface, having the appearance of a sail (the "thymic sail" sign). The edge of the thymus may have a wavy appearance because of indentation by the anterior ribs or costal cartilage (the *"thymic wave" sign*).

Computed Tomography

In children, the normal thymus fills the prevascular space, draping itself over the great vessels and cardiac margins (see Fig. 8.2B and C). Cephalad, the thymus extends above the innominate vein (see Fig. 8.2D). In infancy, the thymus is commonly seen to the level of the pulmonary arteries or below, but its inferior extent decreases with age.

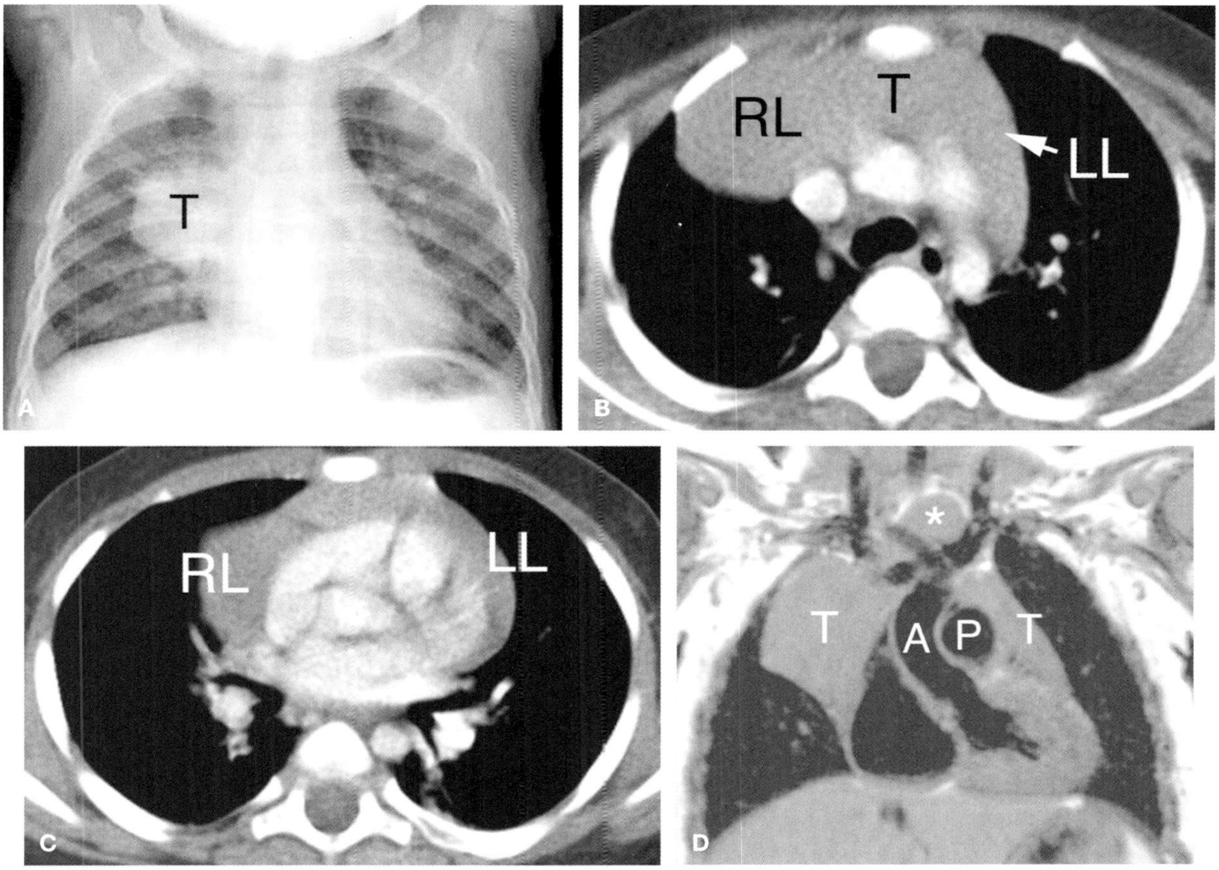

Figure 8.2. Prominent normal thymus-mimicking mass in a 1-year-old infant. **A:** PA chest radiograph shows an apparent right mediastinal mass representing the thymus (*T*). A slight wavy contour laterally is an example of the thymic wave sign. **B:** CT shows a prominent normal thymus (*T*) in the prevascular space. Both the right lobe (*RL*) and left lobe (*LL*) are visible. **C:** The right (*RL*) and left lobes (*LL*) lie lateral to the heart. **D:** T1-weighted coronal MRI showing intermediate-intensity thymus (*T*), with some tissue extending above the innominate vein into the base of the neck (*). Inferiorly, the thymus extends below the pulmonary artery (*P*). *A*, aortic arch.

In infants and young children, the thymus appears quadrilateral on CT. As the child grows, the thymus assumes a more triangular shape, often appearing arrowhead shaped or bilobed, with each of the two thymic lobes contacting the mediastinal pleura. Its margins are sharp, smooth, and convex in infants (see Fig. 8.2B) and often become straight in older children. Each lobe usually measures 1 to 2 cm in thickness (perpendicular to the pleura), but this is variable. On unenhanced CT, the thymus has approximately the same attenuation as muscle. In young subjects, the mean attenuation of the thymus is 36 HU; the thymus shows homogeneous enhancement of 20 to 30 HU after bolus contrast injection.

From puberty to the age of about 25 years, the thymus appears triangular or bilobed, usually outlined by mediastinal fat (Fig. 8.3). The left lobe is usually larger, being seen lateral to the aortic arch; the right lobe may be inconspicuous. Typically, the lateral borders of the thymus are flat or concave where they contact the pleura; uncommonly, they are slightly convex. Its attenuation is usually less than that of muscle because of fatty replacement.

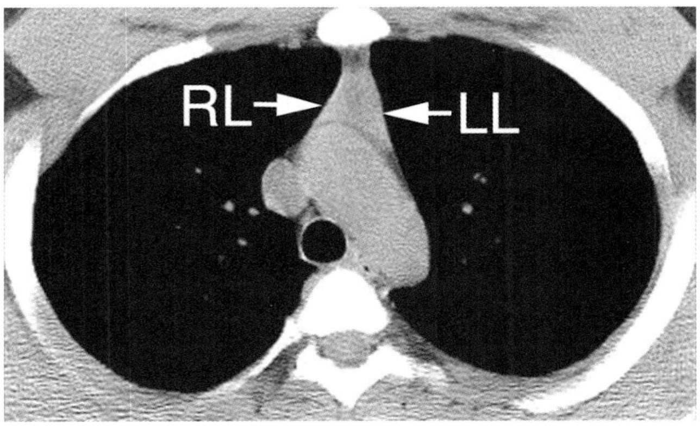

Figure 8.3. Normal thymus in a 21-year-old patient. The thymus occupies the prevascular space and appears triangular and of soft-tissue attenuation, the left lobe (*LL*) being larger than the right (*RL*).

Over the age of 25 years, the thymus is no longer recognizable as a soft-tissue structure on CT because of progressive fatty involution. The thymus appears to be composed primarily of fat, containing islands or wisps of soft tissue (Fig. 8.4). The rapidity and degree of thymic involution are variable, and occasionally, the thymus is still recognized as a discrete structure at the age of 40. With complete thymic involution, the anterior mediastinum appears to be entirely filled with fat; this fat represents the thymic remnant and may have a CT density slightly higher than that of subcutaneous fat.

Thymic Measurement

Thymic size can be quantitated using its length (measured in the cephalocaudal dimension), width (measured in the transverse dimension), and thickness (usually measured perpendicular to the pleura). On CT, the average thickness of the thymus is 1.4 cm in children aged 5 years or less. The maximum normal thickness is 1.8 cm in patients under 20 and 1.3 cm in older adults.

Magnetic Resonance Imaging

On magnetic resonance imaging (MRI), the normal thymus characteristically appears homogeneous and of intermediate signal intensity on T1-weighted images, being less intense than surrounding mediastinal fat but of greater intensity than muscle (see Fig. 8.2D). However, because of progressive involution, the appearance of the thymus is dependent on the age of the patient. In patients over 30 years of age, differentiation between the thymus and adjacent mediastinal fat may be difficult because of thymic involution. The T2 relaxation times of the thymus are similar to fat at all ages. MRI evaluation of the thymus and mediastinum is discussed in Chapter 4.

THYMIC LYMPHOID FOLLICULAR HYPERPLASIA

The term thymic lymphoid follicular hyperplasia (LFH) is used to describe a condition characterized by the presence of hyperplastic lymphoid germinal centers in the thymic medulla, associated with a lymphocytic and plasma cell infiltrate. The presence of LFH is commonly associated with myasthenia gravis (MG), connective tissue disease, pure red blood cell hypoplasia, and infection with HIV; it may also be seen in some normal young subjects.

Plain radiographs are usually normal. On CT, patients with LFH can have a normal-appearing thymus (45%), an enlarged thymus with a normal shape (35%), a focal thymic mass, multiple small soft-tissue nodules, or multilocular thymic cysts (Fig. 8.5).

THYMIC HYPERPLASIA AND REBOUND

Thymic hyperplasia, as distinguished from LFH, is defined by an increase in size of the thymus associated with an otherwise normal gross and histologic appearance. It may be associated with hyperthyroidism (Graves disease; Fig. 8.6), sarcoidosis, red blood cell aplasia, and other entities. It most

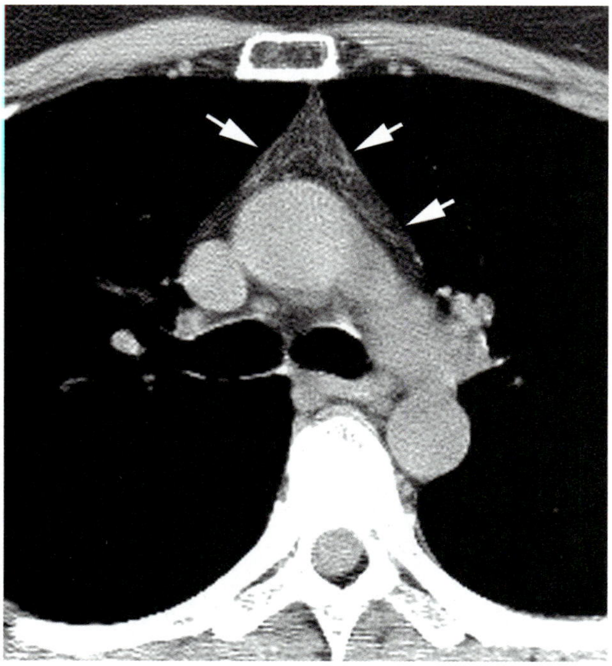

Figure 8.4. Normal thymus in a 51-year-old patient. The thymus (*arrows*) appears to be composed primarily of fat, containing islands or wisps of soft tissue. The left thymic lobe extends more posteriorly than the right.

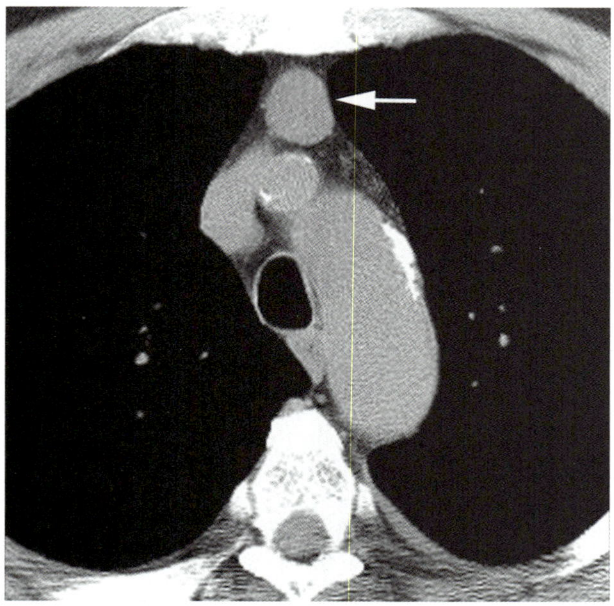

Figure 8.5. Thymic lymphoid follicular hyperplasia. A focal mass (*arrow*) in the prevascular space represented follicular hyperplasia. Its appearance cannot be distinguished from thymoma.

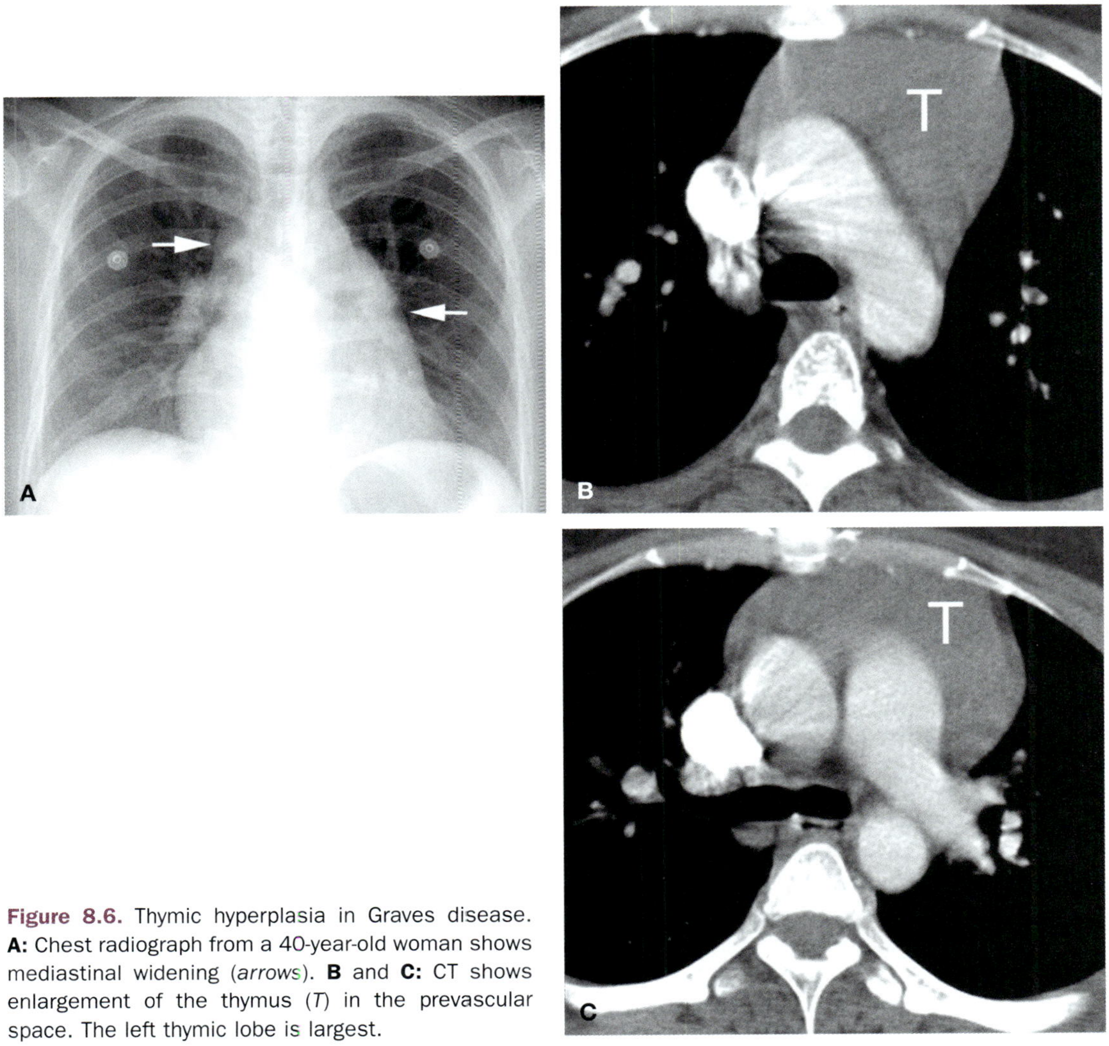

Figure 8.6. Thymic hyperplasia in Graves disease. **A:** Chest radiograph from a 40-year-old woman shows mediastinal widening (*arrows*). **B** and **C:** CT shows enlargement of the thymus (*T*) in the prevascular space. The left thymic lobe is largest.

commonly is seen in association with recovery from chemotherapy, stress, or burns, a phenomenon known as thymic rebound (described below).

Chest radiographs in adults are usually normal. In children, thymic enlargement may be seen. CT demonstrates increased thickness of the thymic lobes but an otherwise normal-appearing thymus.

Thymic Rebound

The thymus involutes during periods of stress (eg, illness, burns, chemotherapy) and may decrease significantly in size, depending on the age of the patient and the severity and duration of the stress. This is most marked in children, but it has also been observed in young adults (Fig. 8.7). A decrease in thymic volume of more than 40% may be seen. The thymus generally regrows to its original size within several months of the stressful episode. It may also exhibit "rebound" or growth to a size significantly larger than its

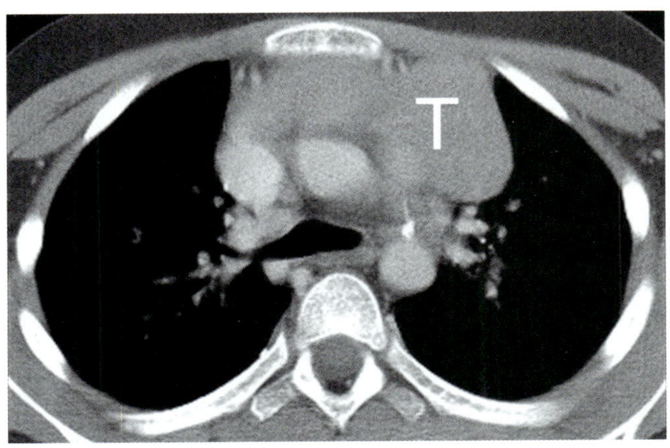

Figure 8.7. Thymic rebound in a 10-year-old patient following chemotherapy for lymphoma. The thymus (*T*) is enlarged.

original size; an increase in thymic volume of 50% in comparison to baseline may be seen. Thymic enlargement may be observed shortly after the stressful episode or from 1 to 9 months afterward. In children and young adults, the incidence of thymic rebound following chemotherapy is 10% to 25%.

Increased thymic size may be seen on plain radiographs, particularly in children, but thymic rebound is detected with greater frequency when CT is used. In patients being treated for an extrathoracic malignancy, the appearance of thymic rebound should not pose a diagnostic problem; however, in patients with lymphoma, distinction from recurrent mediastinal tumor may be difficult. The presence of lymph node enlargement in association with thymic enlargement should suggest recurrent tumor, while isolated thymic enlargement should suggest thymic rebound. On MRI, patients with thymic hyperplasia or thymic rebound may show enlargement of the thymus, but its signal intensity is the same as for normal thymus.

THYMIC MASSES

A number of masses and tumors arise in relation to, or involve, the thymus. The 2021 World Health Organization (WHO) classification of thymic tumors lists more than 50 different lesions. Only the most common are reviewed in this chapter. These include thymic epithelial tumors (thymoma and thymic carcinoma), thymic neuroendocrine tumors, thymic cyst, soft-tissue tumors including thymolipoma, thymic germ cell tumors, and lymphomas. Overall, they account for 20% to 25% of primary mediastinal tumors.

Thymoma

The term *thymoma* should only be used to describe neoplasms originating from thymic epithelium, although these tumors also contain a variable number of lymphocytes. Thymoma is the most common primary thymic tumor. It accounts for about 15% to 20% of primary mediastinal masses (Table 8.2).

Thymomas are rare before age 20 and are most common in patients aged 40 to 60 years. No distinct sex predominance is present. Patients may be asymptomatic, but 20% to 30% have symptoms related to compression of mediastinal structures. MG develops in 30% to 50% of patients with a thymoma, and 10% to 15% of patients with MG have a thymoma. Hematologic abnormalities are also associated with thymoma and include hypogammaglobulinemia and pure red cell aplasia, which occur in 10% and 5% of thymomas, respectively. Autoimmune and connective tissue diseases such as systemic lupus erythematosus, rheumatoid arthritis, Graves disease, and inflammatory bowel disease may also be associated with thymoma.

Thymomas are usually encapsulated and round or lobular in shape. They may contain areas of calcification, necrosis, cysts, or hemorrhage. Most thymomas are slow growing and behave in an indolent fashion. However, about 30% are locally aggressive and invasive or recur following excision. Invasive thymomas infiltrate the tumor capsule and adjacent structures, including the pericardium, pleura, superior vena cava, great vessels, airways, and heart, and may cross the diaphragm to involve the retroperitoneum. Spread to involve one pleural cavity can result in a typical appearance of multiple lenticular pleural implants occurring in the absence of pleural effusion. Thymoma rarely (3%-5%) metastasizes outside the thorax.

Table 8.2 Thymoma
Originates from thymic epithelium
Most common thymic tumor
15%-20% of mediastinal masses
Most common in patients 50-60 years old
Myasthenia gravis in 30%-50%
10%-30% of patients with myasthenia have thymoma
Classified based on behavior as invasive (30%) or noninvasive (70%)
Classified histologically (WHO) as thymic epithelial tumor types A, AB, B1-3
WHO classifications associated with likelihood of invasion and survival (A best, B3 worst)
Metastases outside thorax in 3%-5%
Radiographic findings
Sharply marginated, smooth or lobulated
Usually project to one side of the mediastinum
Retrosternal clear space or costophrenic angles
CT findings
Focal or lobulated mass
Homogeneous or cystic, may calcify
Invasion difficult to diagnose with certainty

Whereas thymomas are generally indolent, thymic carcinoma represents an aggressive tumor that accounts for approximately 20% of thymic epithelial tumors. More than half of patients with thymic carcinoma present with distant metastases at diagnosis. Paraneoplastic syndromes are rare with thymic carcinoma.

Although various systems for the classification of thymic epithelial tumors have been proposed, the simplest consists of three groups based on a combination of histologic features and behavior. These are *noninvasive thymoma* (benign histology and without invasion), *invasive thymoma* (benign histology with invasion), and *thymic carcinoma* (malignant histology).

In 2004, the WHO proposed a detailed histologic classification of thymomas, which remains in use. In the WHO system, thymomas are divided into two groups (type A and B) depending on whether the neoplastic epithelial cells and their nuclei are spindle or oval shaped (type A) or have a dendritic or epithelioid appearance (type B); type AB tumors have mixed features. Type B tumors are further divided into three subtypes (B1 to B3) according to the proportional increase in their epithelial component and the presence of atypical cells. All types of thymic carcinoma are classified as

Table 8.3 WHO Classification of Thymoma Associated With Likelihood of Invasion and Survival

WHO Type	Percent With Invasion (%)	20-year Survival (%)
A	11	100
AB	42	87
B1	47	91
B2	69	59
B3	85	36

Modified from Okumura M, Ohta M, Tateyama H, et al. The World Health Organization histologic classification system reflects the oncologic behavior of thymoma: a clinical study of 273 patients. Cancer. 2002;94:624-632.

type C. The WHO classification of thymic epithelial tumors has been shown to correlate significantly with tumor stage at diagnosis and prognosis. Type A, AB, and B1 thymomas are less likely to be invasive or recur after surgery and are associated with a greater likelihood of complete resection and a better survival than types B2 and B3 (Table 8.3). A detailed knowledge of this classification system is not necessary, but pathology reports in patients with thymoma often use this classification.

A number of immunohistochemical markers and genetic abnormalities have been found in thymic epithelial tumors, but these vary with cell type and are least common in patients with type A thymoma.

Thymomas can be staged at the time of surgery. A simple system (Masaoka-Koga) has long been the most widely used system and is shown below:

Stage I: Tumor capsule is intact
Stage II: Invasion of the tumor capsule, surrounding fat, or mediastinal pleura
Stage III: Invasion of surrounding organs
Stage IVa: Pleural or pericardial implants
Stage IVb: Hematogenous or lymphatic metastases

A TNM system (TNM-8) has also been developed in staging thymic epithelial tumors and is gradually replacing the Masaoka-Koga system. The T and N designations are based on the presence and extent of invasion by the primary tumor and the presence and location of lymph node metastases. M0 and M1 indicate absence or presence of distant metastases. T and N designations are as follows:

T1: Tumor encapsulated or extending into the mediastinal fat
T1a: No mediastinal pleural involvement
T1b: Mediastinal pleural involvement
T2: Tumor with direct invasion of the pericardium
T3: Tumor invasion into: Lung, brachiocephalic vein, superior vena cava, phrenic nerve, chest wall, or extrapericardial pulmonary artery or veins
T4: Tumor invasion into: Aorta, arch vessels, intrapericardial pulmonary artery, myocardium, trachea, esophagus
N0: No regional lymph node metastases
N1: Involvement of anterior (perithymic) lymph nodes
N2: Involvement of deep intrathoracic or cervical lymph nodes
M0: No metastases
M1a: Pleural or pericardial metastasis (separate nodules)
M1b: Pulmonary or distant organ metastasis

Stage grouping is as follows:

Stage I	T1(a,b)	N0	M0
Stage II	T2	N0	M0
Stage IIIA	T3	N0	M0
Stage IIIB	T4	N0	M0
Stage IVA	Any T	N1	M0
	Any T	N0, N1	M1a
Stage IVB	Any T	N2	M0, M1a
	Any T	Any N	M1b

Resection is usually indicated, sometimes in association with radiation, or radiation and chemotherapy. Although invasive thymomas may recur, they tend to grow slowly, and prolonged survival is usually possible. Prognosis for noninvasive thymoma is excellent. Even for invasive thymoma, 10-year survival has been reported as high as 83% for Masaoka stage III disease and 47% for Masaoka stage IV disease.

Plain Radiographs

Most thymomas arise near the junction of the heart and great vessels, although they may be seen superiorly to the level of the clavicles and inferiorly to the level of the costophrenic angles. Their distribution on the frontal radiograph may be likened to an upside-down horseshoe embracing the heart. They may be subtle or invisible on chest radiographs.

In most cases, thymomas appear sharply marginated and smooth or lobulated in contour and usually project to one side of the mediastinum (Figs. 8.8A and 8.9A). They typically range in size from 5 to 10 cm in diameter when visible on radiographs and may obscure the right or left heart border, depending on their location and size. Dense calcification may be seen throughout the mass or in its periphery.

On lateral radiographs, a thymoma may result in a distinct opacity in the inferior aspect of the retrosternal clear space, the relatively lucent triangular region posterior to the sternum and anterior to the aortic arch, main pulmonary

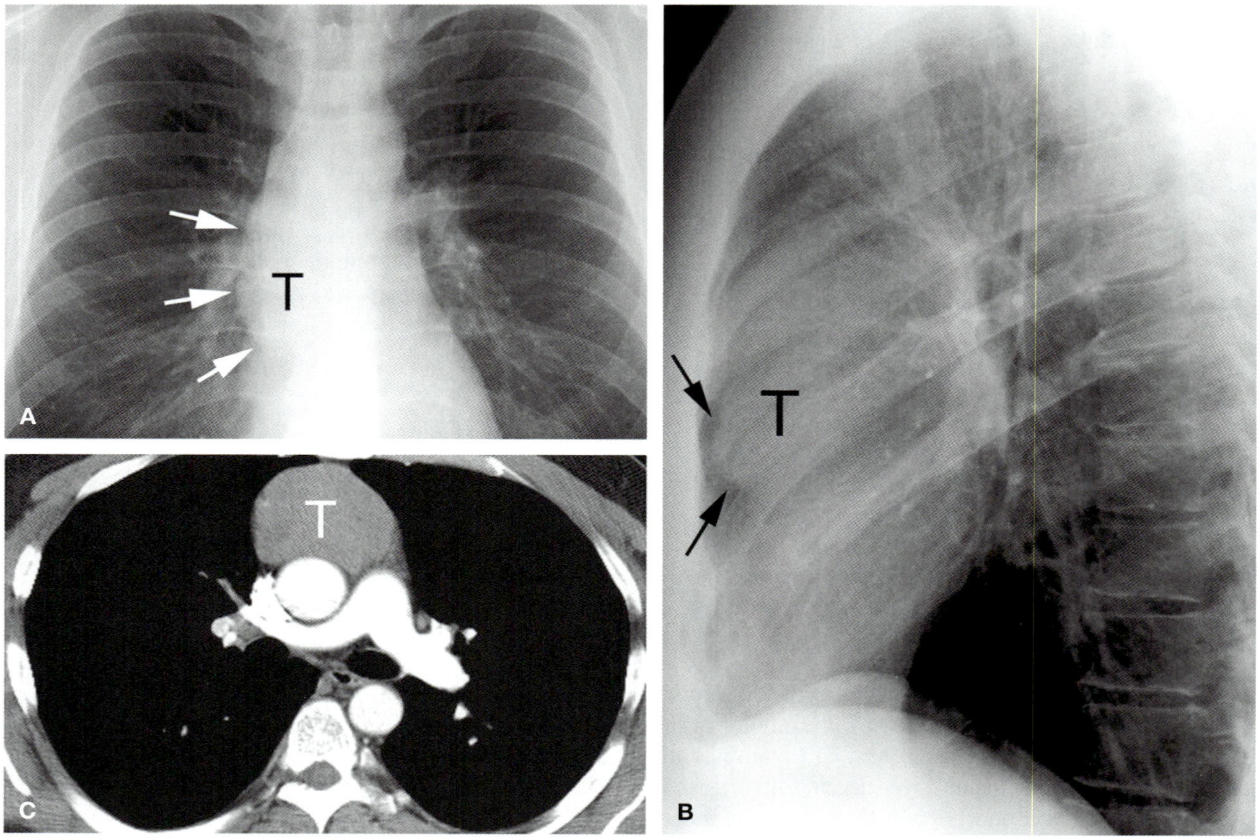

Figure 8.8. Thymoma, invasive. **A:** PA chest radiograph shows prominence of the right mediastinum (*arrows*) due to a thymoma (*T*). **B:** On the lateral radiograph, an opacity (*T*) is visible in the inferior aspect of the retrosternal clear space, with a well-defined edge inferiorly (*arrows*). **C:** CT shows a homogeneous soft-tissue mass in the prevascular space. No fat plane is seen separating the thymoma (*T*) from the ascending aorta. Pericardial invasion was found at surgery. This was WHO type B1.

artery, and heart (see Figs. 8.8B and 8.9B). However, lack of lucency in this space or poor definition or obscuration of the anterior margin of the ascending aorta or pulmonary artery may be normal findings. A mass overlying the heart and region of the cardiophrenic angle may be seen, although this can be mimicked by fat pads and the normal cardiac incisura of the left lung.

Invasive and noninvasive thymomas cannot usually be distinguished on plain radiographs; however, pleural involvement with invasive thymoma occasionally results in pleural thickening, nodularity, or pleural effusion.

Computed Tomography

In nearly all cases, thymomas occur in the prevascular space and displace the great vessels (aorta and its branches, superior vena cava and its branches, and main pulmonary artery) posteriorly (see Figs. 8.8C and 8.9C).

Thymoma or other thymic neoplasm may be distinguished from thymic hyperplasia if enlargement of the thymus is grossly asymmetric, if the thymus has a lobular contour, or if a focal rounded lesion is visible (Fig. 8.10). However, follicular thymic hyperplasia can result in a focal thymic mass up to 5 cm in diameter (see Fig. 8.5).

Approximately 80% of thymomas occur at the base of the heart, as shown on CT (see Fig. 8.9C). They usually appear as masses that are sharply demarcated and oval, round, or lobulated and do not conform to the normal shape of the thymus (see Figs. 8.8C, 8.9C, 8.10). Most often, the tumor grows asymmetrically to one side of the mediastinum. Because ectopic thymic tissue in the neck is found in up to 20% of subjects, thymoma can occur in the neck or at the thoracic inlet, thus mimicking a thyroid mass (Fig. 8.11). Thymoma rarely occurs in the posterior mediastinum.

Thymomas usually appear (paravertebral) homogeneous in attenuation with or without contrast injection (see Figs. 8.8C and 8.11). However, some large thymomas appear cystic (see Fig. 8.9C) or contain areas of necrosis. Calcification may occur in the capsule (see Fig. 8.9C) or within the tumor (see Figs. 8.10B and 8.12).

It is often difficult to distinguish invasive and noninvasive thymomas on CT. The presence of clearly defined fat planes between the tumor and adjacent mediastinal structures suggests the absence of extensive local invasion (Fig. 8.13), but

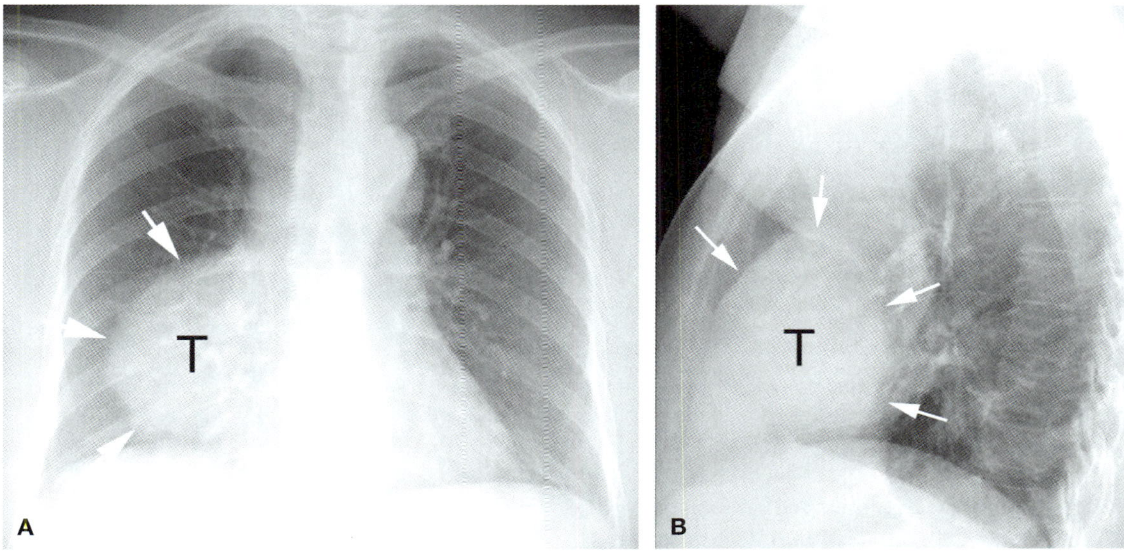

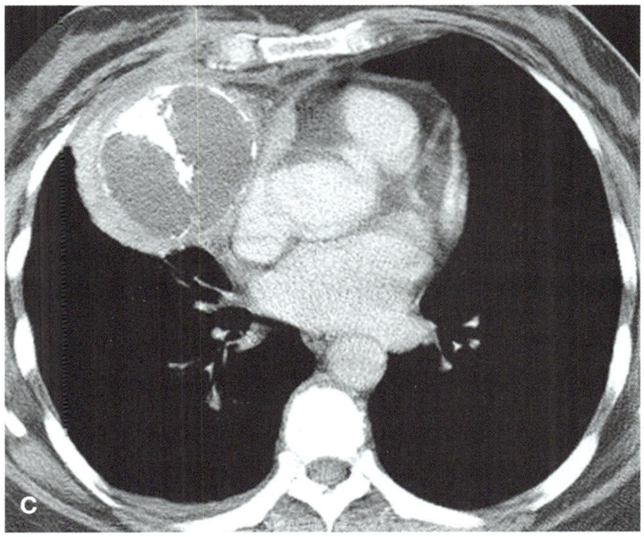

Figure 8.9. Cystic thymoma, noninvasive. **A:** PA chest radiograph shows a large thymoma (*T, arrows*), obscuring the right heart border, extending into the right cardiophrenic angle. **B:** On the lateral radiograph, the thymoma (*T*) is visible overlying the heart shadow (*arrows*). **C:** CT shows a cystic (fluid attenuation) mass in the right cardiophrenic angle. The mass shows dense calcification, including calcification of its capsule. A noninvasive cystic thymoma was found at surgery.

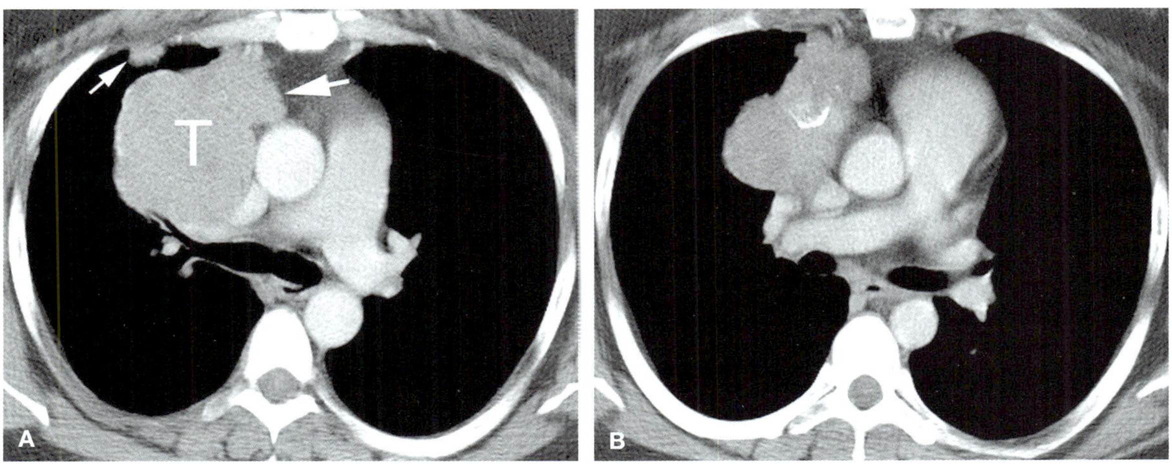

Figure 8.10. Invasive thymoma with calcification in a patient with myasthenia gravis. **A:** CT shows a lobulated mass (*T*) in the prevascular space, typical of thymoma. Medially, the mass invades mediastinal fat (*large arrow*). A small pleural nodule (*small arrow*) is also seen, resulting from pleural invasion. Compression of the superior vena cava is also present. **B:** At a lower level, calcification is visible.

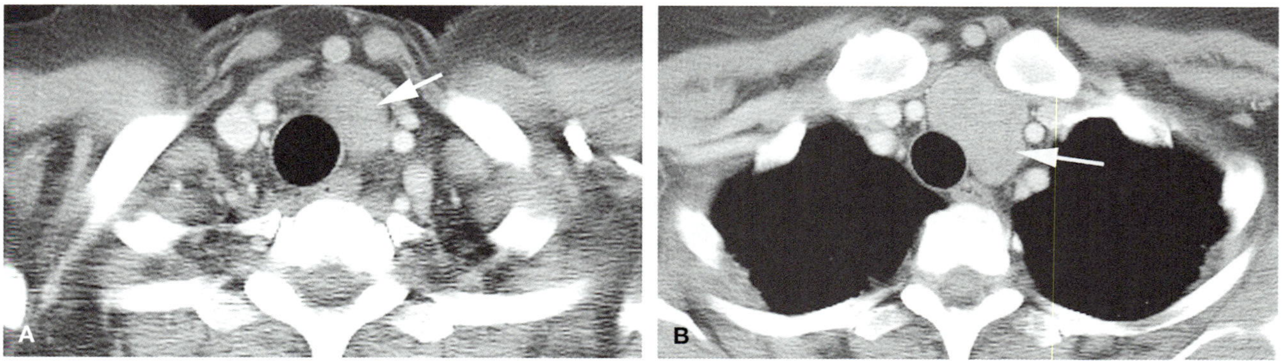

Figure 8.11. Cervical thymoma. **A:** CT through the neck shows a left neck mass (*arrow*), mimicking thyroid enlargement. **B:** The mass (*arrow*) extends into the upper mediastinum. This was a noninvasive thymoma, WHO type A.

limited invasion cannot be determined in many cases. Also, obliteration of fat planes between the tumor and mediastinal structures suggests the possibility of invasion, but this finding cannot be relied upon (see Fig. 8.8C). Findings highly suggestive of invasion include pericardial thickening contiguous with the tumor, pleural thickening, pleural nodules, pleural or pericardial effusion (see Figs. 8.10A, 8.12, 8.14), encasement of mediastinal structures, fat infiltration (see Fig. 8.10A), and an irregular interface between the tumor and lung. Invasive thymomas may extend to involve the posterior mediastinum and, by contiguity, the retroperitoneum. Consequently, it has been recommended that CT staging of thymoma includes the upper abdomen.

MG is commonly associated with thymic pathology (see Fig. 8.10). Sixty-five percent of patients with MG have thymic hyperplasia, and 10% to 30% have thymoma. In patients with myasthenia, a normal-appearing thymus on CT may be associated with normal histology or focal lymphoid hyperplasia; an enlarged but otherwise normal-appearing thymus indicates focal lymphoid hyperplasia; and a focal nodule or mass may represent focal lymphoid hyperplasia or thymoma.

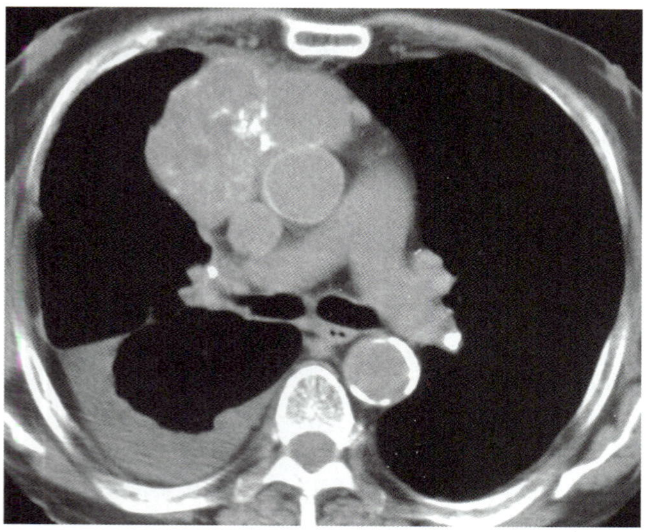

Figure 8.12. Invasive thymoma with calcification. CT shows a lobulated thymoma with multiple calcifications. The presence of pleural effusion strongly suggests invasion.

Magnetic Resonance

On MRI, thymomas typically have a low signal intensity on T1-weighted images, which increases with T2 weighting; they may appear homogeneous in intensity or inhomogeneous with or without cystic components or may show nodules or lobules of tumor separated by relatively low-intensity septations. MRI has proven valuable in identifying the presence or absence of vascular invasion in patients with thymoma, especially in patients to whom intravenous contrast cannot be administered (see Chapter 4).

Fluorodeoxyglucose–positron emission tomography

At present, the role of fluorodeoxyglucose (FDG)-positron emission tomography (PET) in the evaluation of thymic neoplasms is unclear. Thymic hyperplasia may appear similar to thymoma in activity, and high-grade and low-grade thymomas are not easy to distinguish. However, PET may be valuable in detecting metastases in some patients with aggressive tumors.

Thymic Carcinoma

Thymic carcinoma, like thymoma, arises from thymic epithelial cells, but it is much less common. Thymic carcinoma accounts for about 20% of thymic epithelial tumors (Table 8.4). Unlike thymoma, thymic carcinoma can be diagnosed as malignant on the basis of histologic criteria. The list of cell types is long, and the specific histologic pattern and the immunohistochemical and genetic profiles parallel those of lung carcinomas (eg, squamous cell carcinoma, basaloid carcinoma, adenocarcinoma, mucoepidermoid carcinoma, etc). In the WHO classification of thymic epithelial tumors, thymic carcinoma is type C.

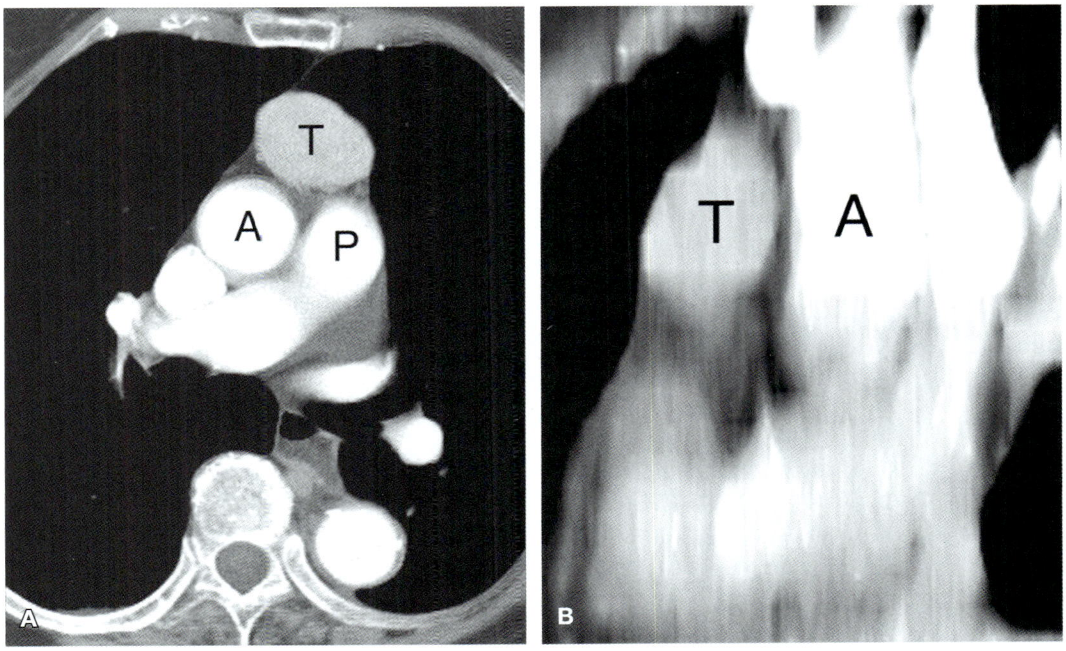

Figure 8.13. Noninvasive thymoma. **A:** CT shows a homogeneous thymoma (*T*) separated from the aorta (*A*) and pulmonary artery (*P*) by a layer of fat. **B:** Oblique sagittal reconstruction shows separation of the thymoma (*T*) from the ascending aorta (*A*).

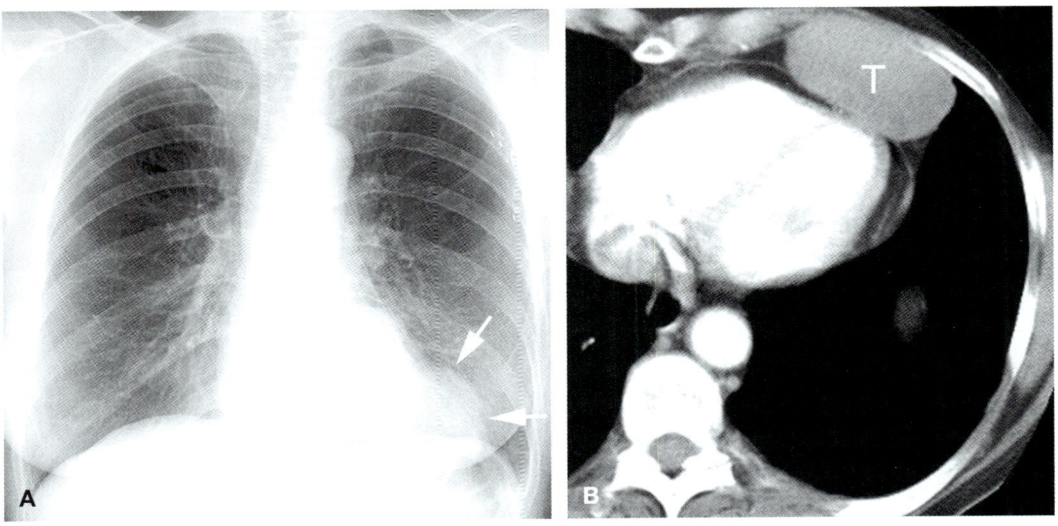

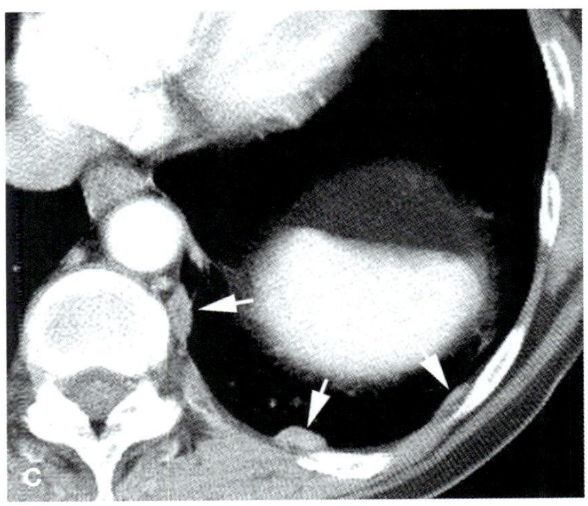

Figure 8.14. Invasive thymoma with pleural metastases. **A:** PA chest radiograph shows a mass at the left cardiophrenic angle (*arrows*). **B:** CT shows a homogeneous rounded mass (*T*) representing thymoma. **C:** At a lower level, CT shows focal pleural thickening or nodules (*arrows*), typical of pleural metastases. Pleural nodules are usually unassociated with pleural effusion. This finding indicates invasion. This thymoma was WHO type B3.

Table 8.4 Thymic Carcinoma

Originates from thymic epithelium
20% of thymic epithelial tumors
Average age 50
Unlike thymoma, appears malignant histologically
Classified histologically (WHO) as thymic epithelial tumor type C
Invasion common, distant metastases in 50%-65%
Myasthenia rare
Appearance indistinguishable from thymoma unless metastases are visible

Thymic carcinomas are aggressive and more likely to result in distant metastases than invasive thymoma. Although distant metastases are found in only about 5% of patients with invasive thymoma, they are present at diagnosis in 50% to 65% of patients with thymic carcinoma. Frequent sites of metastasis include the lungs, liver, brain, and bone. It has a poor prognosis, with a 5-year survival rate of 30%. Average age at presentation is 50 years.

Symptoms are usually attributable to the mediastinal mass. Invasion of mediastinal structures is common, and superior vena cava syndrome may be present. Although paraneoplastic syndromes such as MG, pure red cell aplasia, and hypogammaglobulinemia are common with thymoma, they are rare with thymic carcinoma.

Thymic carcinoma usually results in a mass 5 to 15 cm in diameter, with or without areas of low attenuation (Fig. 8.15). Calcification may be present (see Fig. 8.15) but is uncommon. Thymic carcinoma cannot be distinguished from thymoma on CT, although the presence of enlarged lymph nodes distinct from the primary tumor, distant metastases, and irregular tumor margins are all more common with carcinoma. Thymic carcinoma is less likely than thymoma to result in pleural implants.

On MRI, thymic carcinoma appears higher in signal intensity than muscle on T1-weighted MRI, with an increase in signal on T2-weighted images. Heterogeneous signal may reflect the presence of necrosis, cystic regions within the tumor, or hemorrhage. Thymoma appears to have a greater tendency to show a multinodular appearance on MRI than does thymic carcinoma.

Thymic Neuroendocrine Tumor

Thymic neuroendocrine tumors are rare, accounting for only 2% to 5% of thymic neoplasms. They are believed to arise from thymic cells of neural crest origin (amine precursor uptake and decarboxylase cells). Thymic neuroendocrine tumors are classified in the same manner as pulmonary neuroendocrine tumors, as low-grade carcinoid tumor, intermediate-grade atypical carcinoid tumor, and high-grade large cell neuroendocrine carcinoma or small cell neuroendocrine carcinoma. Most cases represent atypical carcinoid tumor. Diagnostic criteria and markers are the same as for their lung counterparts (see Chapter 5).

The biologic behavior of these tumors shows a direct relation to their cell type and degree of differentiation, with

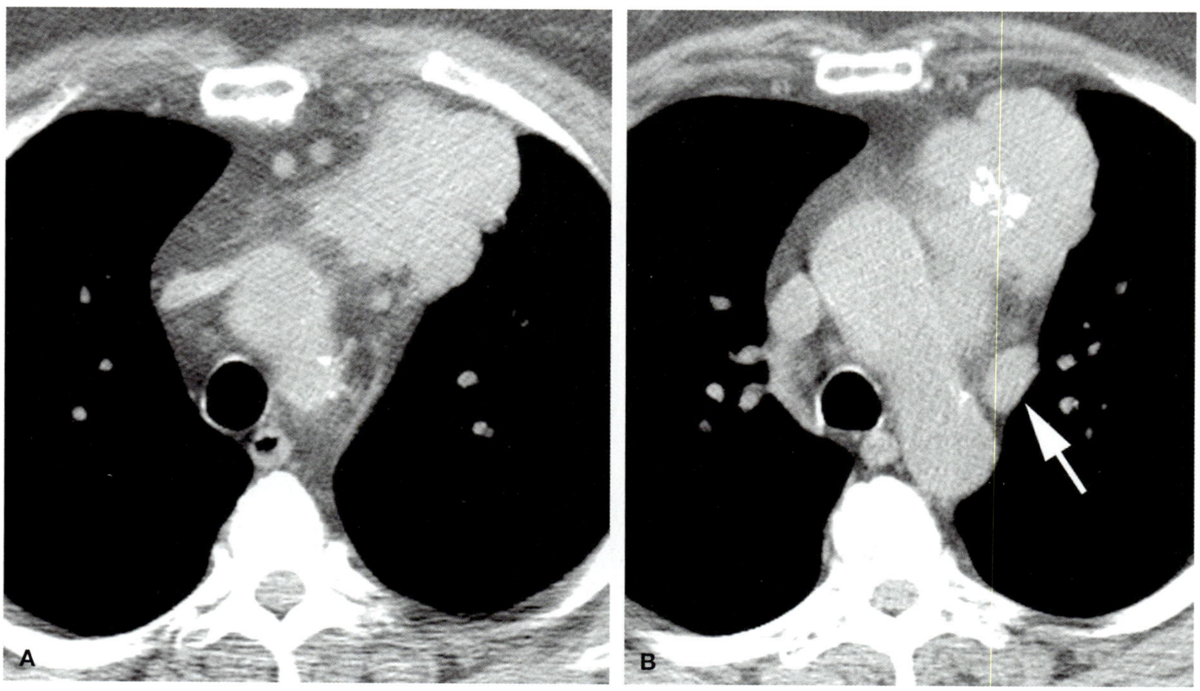

Figure 8.15. Thymic carcinoma. **A:** A large mass is visible in the prevascular space. It is lobulated and poorly marginated. **B:** At a lower level, calcifications are visible within the mass. An enlarged lymph node (*arrow*) adjacent to the mass suggests thymic carcinoma or invasive thymoma as the diagnosis.

Table 8.5 Thymic Neuroendocrine Tumor

Classified as carcinoid, atypical carcinoid, large cell or small cell neuroendocrine carcinoma in order of increasing malignancy
Originates from neural crest cells (APUDoma)
Average age 45
Usually malignant
Cushing syndrome in 25%-40%
Multiple endocrine neoplasia in 20%
Mimics thymoma radiographically
Dense enhancement possibly seen on CT

typical carcinoid having the best prognosis and 5-year survival rates of 50% to 70%. Other cell types tend to behave in a more aggressive and malignant fashion with a tendency for local recurrence or distant metastases following resection; generally speaking, survival rates are similar to those reported for lung tumors of the same cell type (Table 8.5). Average age at presentation is 45 years; men are more commonly involved. Unlike their lung counterparts, there is no association with smoking.

Most patients present with symptoms related to compression of mediastinal structures. Approximately 25% to 40% of patients have Cushing syndrome as a result of tumor secretion of adrenocorticotropic hormone. Nearly 20% of cases have been associated with multiple endocrine neoplasia syndromes I (more common) and II.

Although dense contrast enhancement may be seen on CT in some cases, neuroendocrine tumor does not differ significantly from thymoma in its radiographic or CT appearance (Fig. 8.16). In some patients, a mediastinal mass is not visible on CT despite the presence of endocrine abnormalities. MRI findings are nonspecific and identical to those of thymoma.

This tumor is more aggressive than thymoma, and superior vena cava obstruction is much more common with thymic neuroendocrine tumor than with thymoma. The 5-year survival rate is about 65%. Mediastinal lymph node or distant metastases may be present.

Thymolipoma

Thymolipoma is a rare, benign, well-encapsulated thymic tumor consisting primarily of fat but also containing variable amounts of thymic tissue; it can arise within the thymus or be connected to the thymus by a pedicle. Eighty percent of patients present in the first 4 decades. It accounts for less than 5% of thymic tumors (Table 8.6).

In most cases, thymolipoma is unaccompanied by symptoms and is detected incidentally on chest radiographs. It is often large, averaging nearly 20 cm in diameter at diagnosis, and it may project into both hemithoraces. Because of its fatty content and pliability, thymolipoma tends to drape over the heart, extending inferiorly into the cardiophrenic angles, but may not obscure the cardiac margin (Fig. 8.17A). It can simulate cardiac enlargement, lower lobe collapse, or elevation of a hemidiaphragm. There is no known association with MG.

On CT, thymolipoma may appear to be predominantly fat but usually appears to contain wisps, whorls, or small

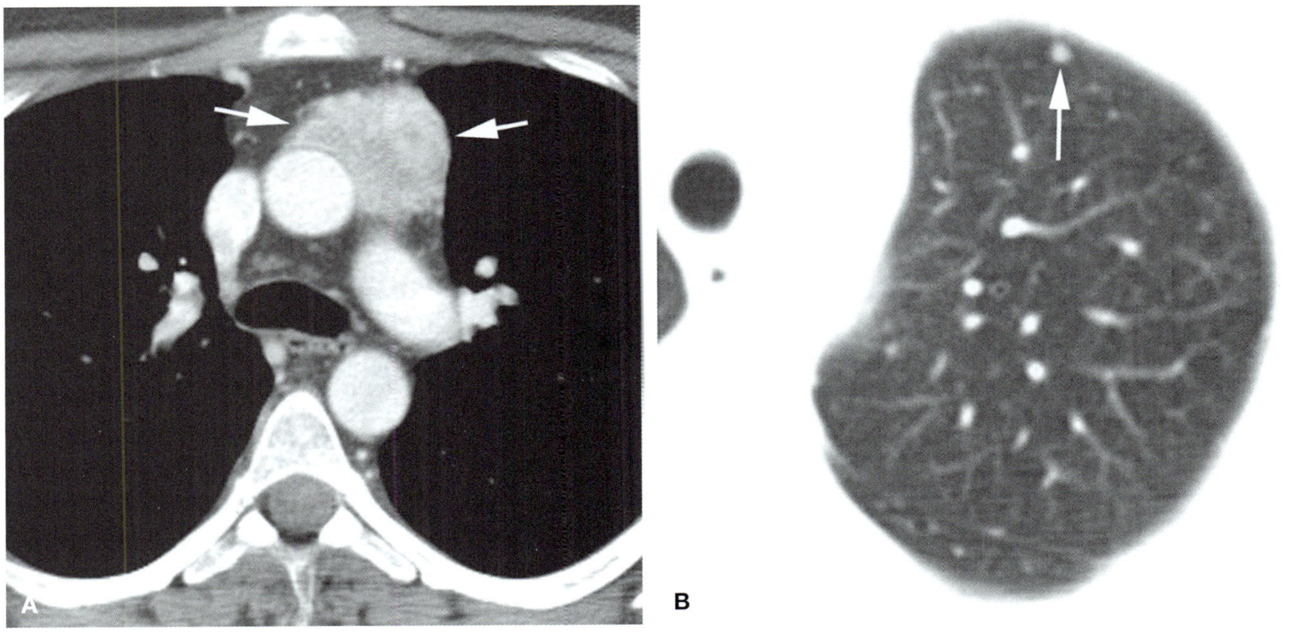

Figure 8.16. Thymic carcinoid tumor in a patient with Cushing syndrome. **A:** A prevascular space mass (*arrows*) shows significant enhancement following contrast infusion. This may be seen in carcinoid tumor. **B:** Lung window scans showed pulmonary metastases (*arrow*).

Table 8.6	Thymolipoma
Consists of fat and thymic tissue	
5% of thymic tumors	
Benign	
Often young patients	
Usually asymptomatic	
Large droopy mediastinal mass containing fat and strands of tissue	

nodules of soft tissue in combination with fat (see Fig. 8.17B). Uncommonly, it appears to be primarily of soft-tissue attenuation. In all cases, CT shows a connection between the mass and the thymic bed.

As would be expected from its fat content, MRI shows areas of high signal intensity on T1-weighted spin-echo images, similar to the intensity of subcutaneous fat, with areas of intermediate signal intensity reflecting the presence of soft tissue. Despite attaining a large size, thymolipomas do not invade surrounding structures. However, some compression of mediastinal structures is visible in half of the cases. They do not recur following resection. Liposarcoma is the primary differential diagnosis (discussed later).

Thymic Cyst

Thymic cysts are uncommon. They can be either congenital or acquired. Congenital thymic cysts are rare; acquired thymic cysts have been reported following radiation therapy, in association with thymic tumors, and following thoracotomy. Their attenuation is usually that of water but can be higher or lower depending on the presence of hemorrhage or fat.

One should be cautious in making the diagnosis of thymic cyst; cystic regions can be seen in a variety of thymic tumors, including thymoma and lymphoma. CT can suggest the diagnosis of thymic cyst if the lesion (a) appears thin walled, (b) is unassociated with a mass lesion, (c) contains fluid with a density close to that of water, and (d) remains unopacified following contrast infusion. Calcification of the cyst wall can also be seen. MRI characteristics are similar to those of other cystic lesions.

Thymic Lymphoma

Hodgkin lymphoma (HL) has a predilection for the involvement of the thymus in conjunction with the involvement of mediastinal lymph nodes. Thymic enlargement may be seen in 30% of patients with intrathoracic HL. Non-Hodgkin lymphoma (NHL) less commonly involves the thymus, but large B-cell lymphoma, extranodal marginal zone lymphoma of mucosa-associated lymphoid tissue, and T-cell lymphoblastic lymphoma/leukemia may arise in the thymus. Lymphomas involving the thymus and mediastinum are reviewed in Chapter 7.

Thymic lymphoma usually results in homogeneous thymic enlargement (Fig. 8.18). However, lobulation or a nodular appearance is seen in some patients, and cystic areas of necrosis are visible on CT in 20% of adults. Calcification uncommonly occurs in the absence of radiation or chemotherapy. Although its appearance is nonspecific, the combination of a thymic mass with mass or lymph node enlargement in other areas of the mediastinum is suggestive of this diagnosis. On MRI, thymic lymphoma shows low intensity on T1-weighted images, with a variable change on T2-weighted images.

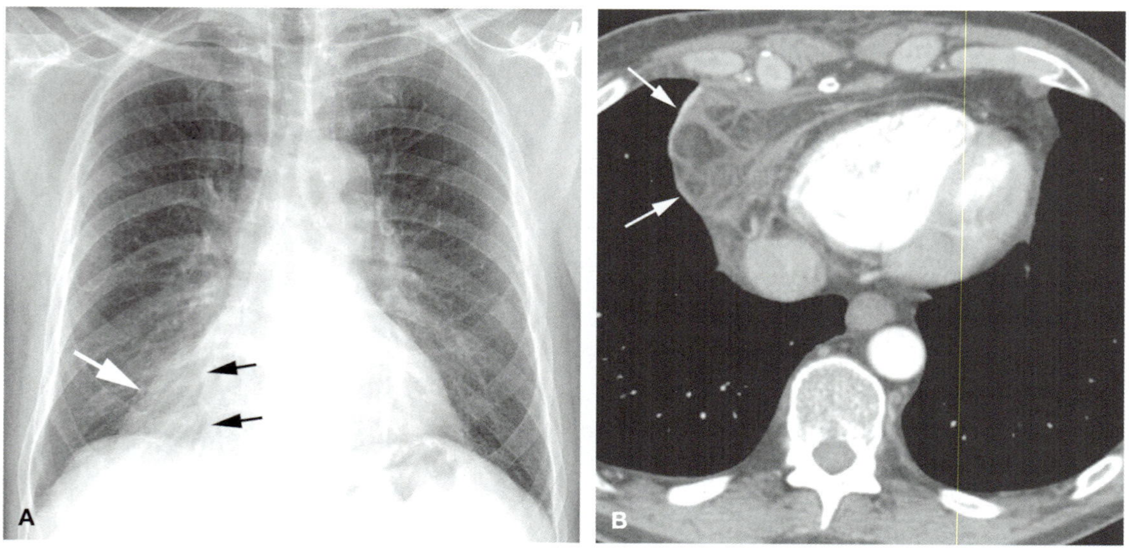

Figure 8.17. Thymolipoma. **A:** PA chest radiograph shows a mass (*white arrow*) in the right cardiophrenic angle. The right heart border remains faintly visible (*black arrows*), a finding that reflects the fatty nature of the mass. **B:** CT shows the mass (*arrows*) to be in the anterior mediastinum. It is composed of fat and strands of soft tissue.

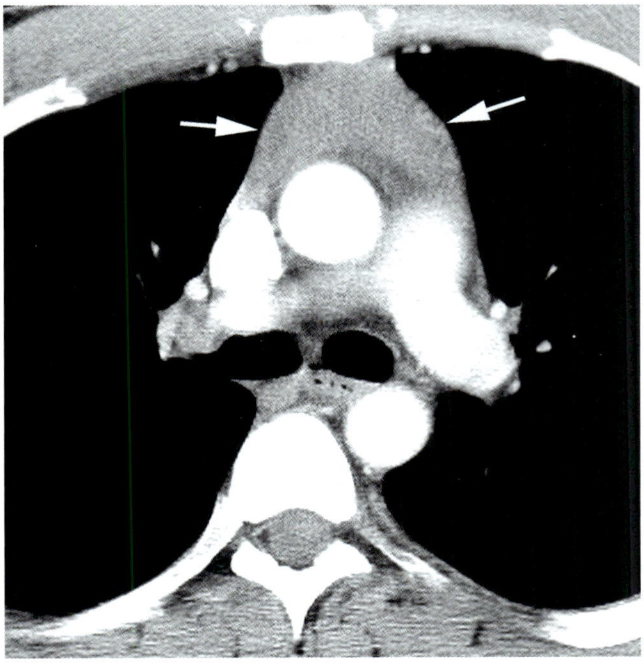

Figure 8.18. Thymic enlargement in Hodgkin disease. The thymus (*arrows*) is homogeneously enlarged.

Thymic Metastases

Metastatic tumors, particularly lung and breast carcinomas, can also involve the thymus. Involvement of mediastinal lymph nodes is also typically present. CT and MRI appearances of thymic metastases are nonspecific.

GERM CELL TUMORS

Germ cell tumors account for about 10% of primary mediastinal masses and arise from primitive germ cells that have arrested their embryologic migration in the mediastinum, frequently within the thymus. They are most common in the anterior mediastinum; only about 5% originate in the posterior mediastinum. Most germ cell tumors present during the second to fourth decades of life.

Germ cell tumors include benign and malignant teratoma, seminoma, embryonal carcinoma, endodermal sinus (yolk sac) tumor, choriocarcinoma, and mixed cell types.

Overall, more than 80% of germ cell tumors are benign, with the large majority of these being teratomas. Although the sex distribution of benign germ cell tumors is about equal, there is a strong preponderance of males among patients with malignant germ cell tumors. Among patients with malignant tumors, seminoma is most common, representing about 30% of cases, with embryonal carcinoma and malignant teratoma each responsible for about 10%, and choriocarcinoma and endodermal sinus tumor responsible for about 5% each; the remainder of malignancies, approximately 40% of cases, represent mixed tumors.

Benign tumors are often asymptomatic, while malignant tumors are more likely to cause symptoms. Confirmation that these lesions are primary to the mediastinum requires that there be no evidence of a testicular or retroperitoneal tumor.

Teratoma

Teratomas contain elements of all germinal layers. They are classified as mature, cystic (dermoid cyst), immature, and malignant (Table 8.7).

Mature teratomas are most common and are composed of well-differentiated tissues, with ectodermal elements such as skin and hair predominating, but they also contain cartilage, fat, and muscle. They are benign. They constitute 60% to 75% of mediastinal germ cell tumors. Sex incidence is equal, and they most commonly occur in children and young adults. They do not usually result in symptoms unless large.

Dermoid cysts are said to contain elements of only the ectodermal layer of germ cells, specifically skin and its appendages, but small rests of endodermal and mesodermal cells are often present; they are benign. Dermoid cysts are also referred to as *mature cystic teratoma*.

Immature teratomas contain less well-developed tissues more typical of those present during fetal development; in infancy or early childhood, these tumors often have a benign course, while in adults, they usually behave in an aggressive and malignant fashion.

Malignant teratomas contain frankly malignant tissues in addition to immature or mature tissues and have a very poor prognosis; they are seen almost exclusively in men.

Table 8.7 Teratoma

- Contains elements of all germinal layers
- Mature teratomas (contain mature tissues)
  - Benign
  - 60%-75% of mediastinal germ cell tumors
  - Occur in children and young adults
  - Dermoid cyst
- Immature teratomas (contain immature tissue)
  - Often have benign course in infants or young children
  - Often aggressive and malignant in adults
- Malignant teratoma (contains frankly malignant tissues)
  - Poor prognosis
  - Usually in men
- Anterior mediastinal mass; posterior in 5%
- Smooth, rounded, or lobulated mass
- Mature teratoma
  - Well defined, smooth, cystic
  - Teeth and bone rare
  - Fluid in 90%; fat in 75%; calcification in 50%
- Immature or malignant teratoma
  - Nodular or poorly defined
  - Fat in 40%
  - Compression or invasion of mediastinal structures
  - Enhancing capsule

Plain Radiographs

Plain radiographs usually show an anterior mediastinal mass projecting to one side of the mediastinum (Fig. 8.19). Their distribution is similar to that of thymoma. Middle mediastinal or posterior masses are occasionally seen. Teratoma appears as a smooth, rounded, or lobulated mass. Mature teratoma is typically well defined and often large at diagnosis, averaging 8 to 10 cm in diameter. Calcification is visible in about 20% of mature teratomas. Teeth and bone are diagnostic but rarely seen.

Computed Tomography

Teratomas are usually found in the prevascular space, although 5% occur in the posterior mediastinum. Regardless of their histology, CT often shows a combination of fluid-filled cysts, fat, soft tissue, and areas of calcification (Fig. 8.20). Calcification is visible in about 50% of cases, being focal or rim like or rarely representing teeth or bone. In patients with mature teratoma, 90% contain fluid and 75% contain fat. Common combinations include fluid, soft tissue, fat, and calcium (40% of cases); fluid, soft tissue, and fat (25% of cases); and fluid and soft tissue (15% of cases). A fat-fluid level within the mass is diagnostic and is present in about 10% of cases. The fluid within cystic parts of the tumors may vary in attenuation. Teratomas are typically encapsulated and well demarcated. Rim enhancement can be seen.

Various CT findings can help in differentiating benign and malignant lesions. Benign lesions are typically well defined, smooth, and cystic, and 90% contain fat. Malignant teratomas are nodular or poorly defined, they are more likely to appear solid, and a smaller proportion (40%) contains fat. Malignant teratoma has a greater tendency to compress surrounding structures. Following contrast infusion, malignant teratoma can show a thick enhancing capsule.

MRI can show various appearances, depending on the composition of the tumor. They commonly contain fat, which is intense on T1-weighted images, and cystic areas, which are low in intensity on T1-weighted images but increase with T2 weighting.

Seminoma

Seminoma occurs almost entirely in males, with a mean age at presentation of 29 years. It is the most common malignant mediastinal germ cell tumor, accounting for up to 30% of cases (Table 8.8). Genetic abnormalities mirror those found in testicular seminoma.

Plain radiographs typically show a large, lobulated, anterior mediastinal mass projecting to one or both sides of the mediastinum and often obscuring a portion of the heart border (Fig. 8.21). On CT, primary mediastinal seminomas present as large, smooth or lobulated, homogeneous soft-tissue masses, although small areas of low attenuation can be seen. Obliteration of fat planes is common, and pleural or pericardial effusion may be present. Seminomas are very radiosensitive and respond well to cisplatin-based chemotherapy, with a 5-year survival rate of 90%.

Germ cell tumors and metastases are typically characterized by a high FDG uptake on PET scans. Pure seminomas are more FDG avid than nonseminomatous lesions.

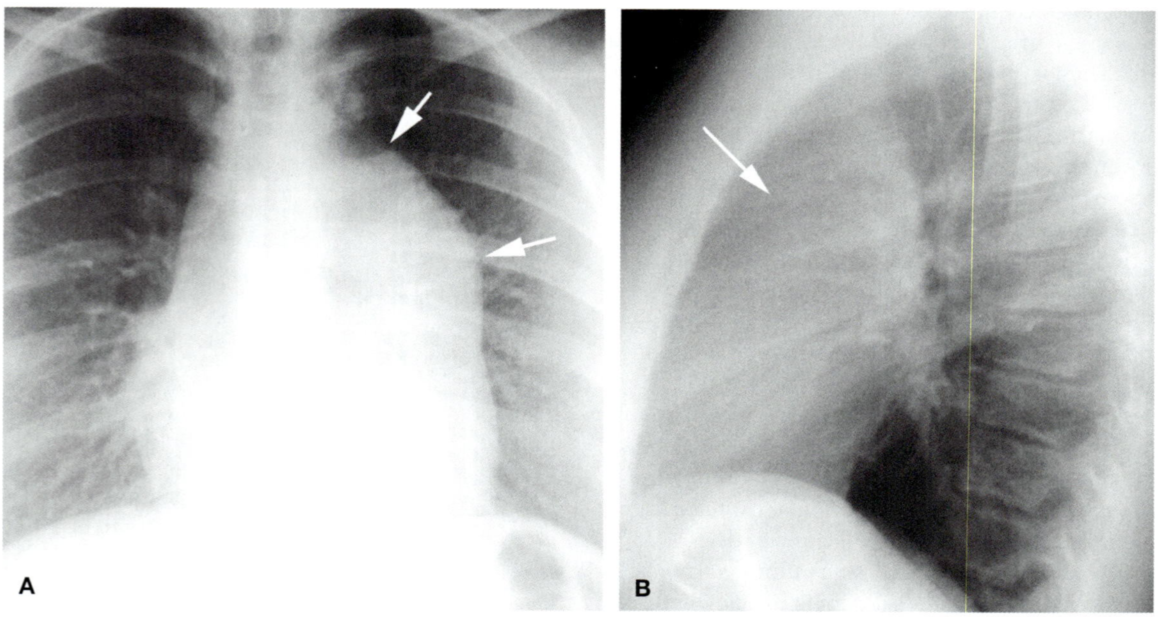

Figure 8.19. Mature mediastinal teratoma. **A:** PA chest radiograph shows a smooth, sharply marginated left mediastinal mass (*arrows*). It obscures the left heart border, indicating its anterior location. **B:** Lateral view shows increased density of the retrosternal clear space (*arrow*), but a discrete mass is not visible.

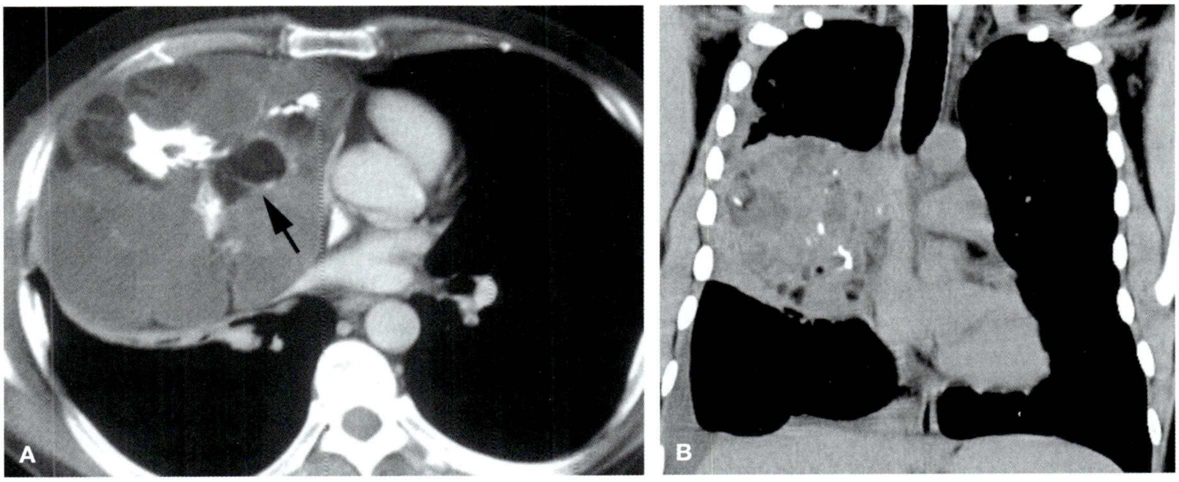

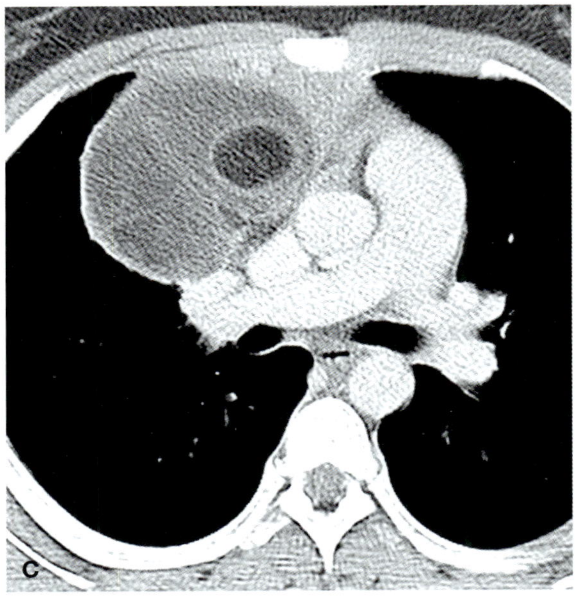

Figure 8.20. Appearance of mediastinal teratoma. **A:** Mature teratoma in an adult appears as a large mass compressing right cardiac structures. It contains calcifications, areas of fat (*arrow*), and cystic or soft-tissue regions. **B:** Mixed mature and immature teratoma in a young man with Klinefelter syndrome appears heterogeneous in attenuation, with areas of fat, calcification, soft tissue, and fluid-filled cysts. **C:** Cystic teratoma in a 12-year-old boy shows fluid attenuation with a localized collection of fat.

Nonseminomatous Germ Cell Tumors

Nonseminomatous germ cell tumors, namely, embryonal carcinoma, endodermal sinus (yolk sac) tumor, choriocarcinoma, and mixed types, are often grouped together because of their relative rarity, similar appearance, and more aggressive behavior (Table 8.9). Their histology and genetics are the same as for testicular tumors. In recent years, there have been significant advances in the treatment of nonseminomatous germ cell tumors. With the introduction of cisplatin-based chemotherapeutic regimens, the likelihood of long-term survival has risen from 10% or less to 45% to 80% and is best for children. Surgery is reserved for those patients with radiologic evidence of persistent masses and may improve survival.

Table 8.8 Seminoma

30% of germ cell tumors
Mean age 29
Large, lobulated, anterior mediastinal mass
Homogeneous in attenuation
Good prognosis; 5-year survival rate 50%-75%

Plain radiographs show large, lobulated, anterior mediastinal masses. They may be ill defined or associated with pleural effusion because of local invasion of lung and pleura.

On CT, these tumors often show heterogeneous opacity, including ill-defined areas of low attenuation secondary to necrosis and hemorrhage or cystic areas (Fig. 8.22). They often appear infiltrative, with obliteration of fat planes, and may be spiculated. Calcification may be seen. MRI findings also reflect the heterogeneous nature of these lesions.

THYROID GLAND AND THYROID ENLARGEMENT

The thyroid gland is in close approximation to the thoracic inlet, and thyroid enlargement is commonly associated with extension into the mediastinum. Multinodular goiter is the

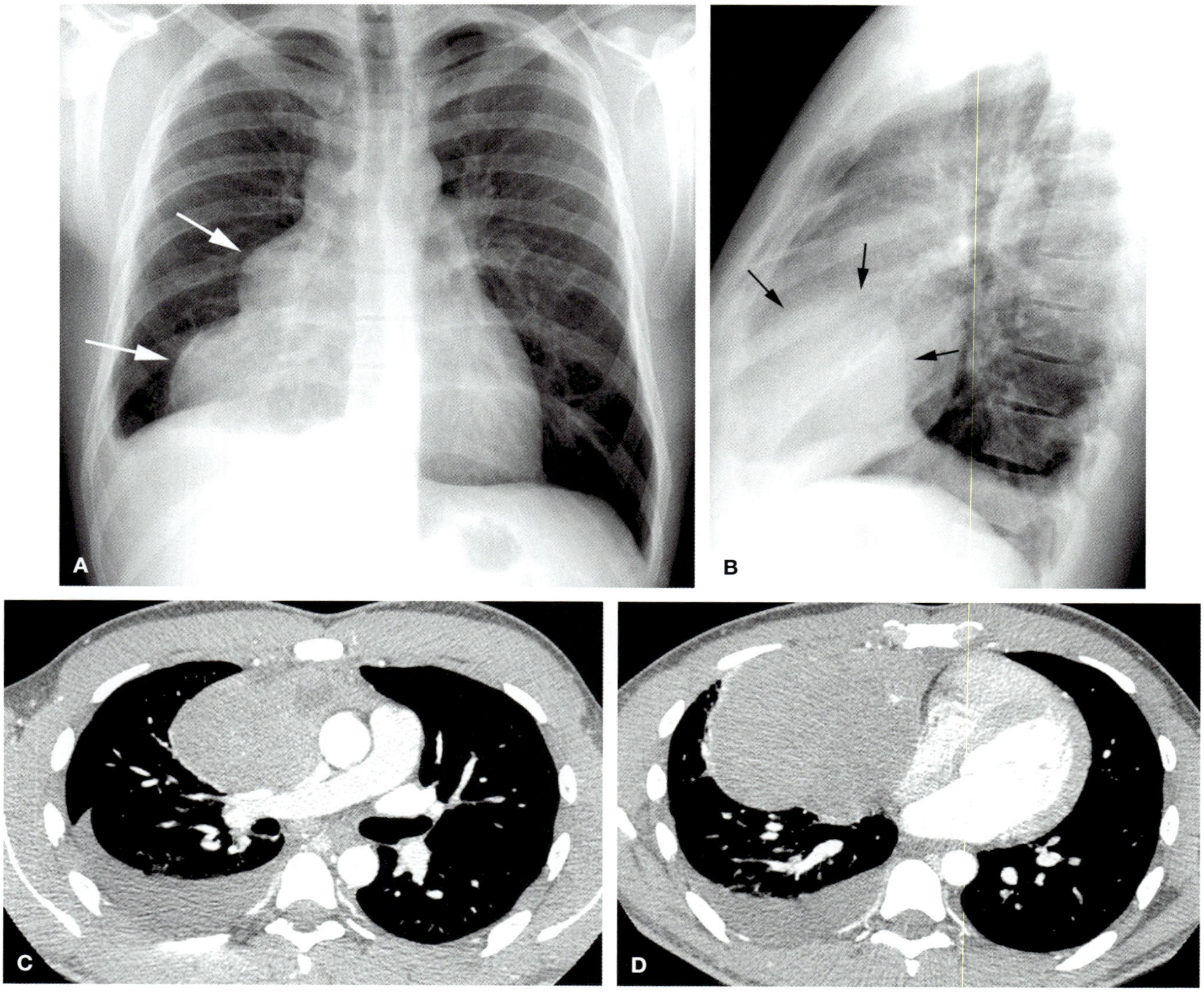

Figure 8.21. Mediastinal seminoma. **A:** PA radiograph shows a large, lobulated mediastinal mass (*arrows*) obscuring the right heart border. A right pleural effusion is also visible. **B:** Lateral view shows a large anterior mediastinal mass (*arrows*). **C** and **D:** CT shows a large, relatively homogeneous mass in the prevascular space, displacing mediastinal structures to the left. A pleural effusion is associated.

most common condition in which a mediastinal thyroid abnormality is detected; carcinoma and thyroiditis are relatively rare causes.

Table 8.9 Nonseminomatous Germ Cell Tumor
Cell types
Embryonal carcinoma
Endodermal sinus (yolk sac) tumor
Choriocarcinoma
Mixed types
Large, lobulated, anterior mediastinal mass
Inhomogeneous in attenuation
Long-term survival 45%-80%

Intrathoracic extension of thyroid lesions is common, representing nearly 10% of mediastinal masses resected at thoracotomy (Table 8.10). Such lesions are almost always connected to the thyroid at the thoracic inlet. Truly ectopic mediastinal thyroid tissue, not showing a connection to the thyroid gland, is uncommon.

Thyroid masses most commonly extend inferiorly into either the prevascular or visceral compartments. Those in the prevascular space are anterior to the subclavian and innominate vessels. Visceral space extension presumably arises from the posterolateral portion of the gland and descends behind the brachiocephalic vessels and are most commonly found on the right side, in proximity to the trachea. Less often, thyroid tissue extends between the esophagus and trachea or posterior to the esophagus.

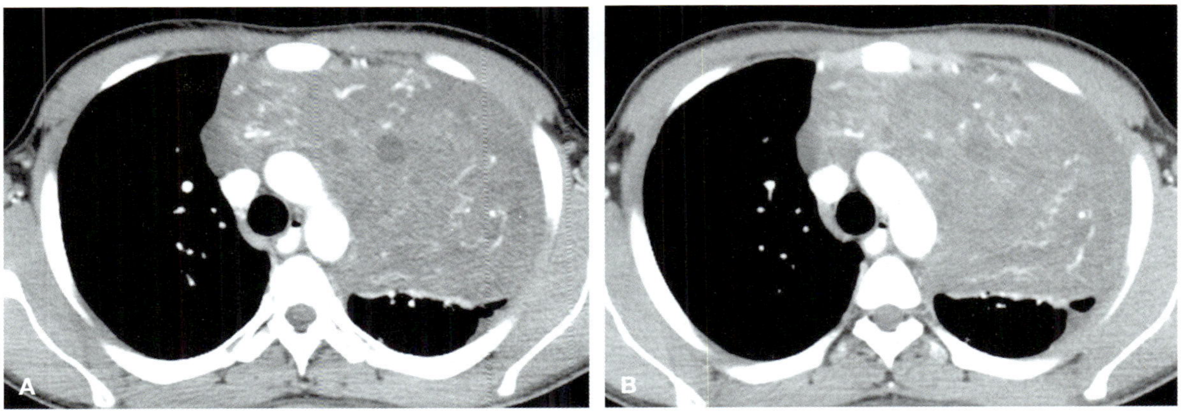

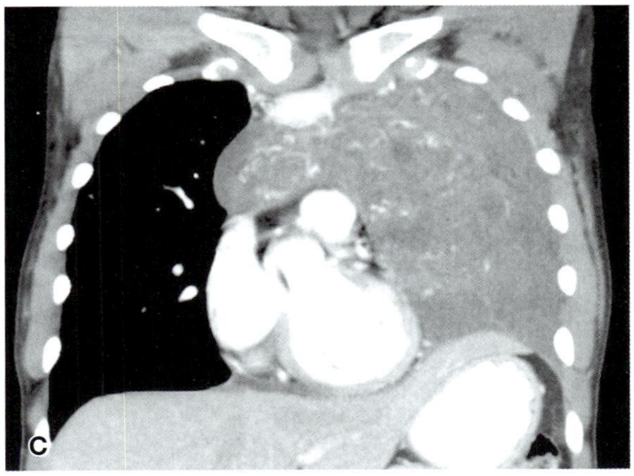

Figure 8.22. Nonseminomatous (mixed) germ cell tumor in a 23-year-old man. **A** and **B:** CT shows a large, heterogeneous mass in the prevascular space, with densely enhancing vessels within it. Cystic areas are visible within the tumor. **C:** Coronal reconstruction shows the large heterogeneous anterior mediastinal mass.

Plain Radiographs

Mediastinal thyroid abnormalities typically present as a sharply marginated, upper mediastinal mass, causing tracheal narrowing or displacement of the trachea to the contralateral side. The mass usually appears poorly marginated above the level of the clavicles (Fig. 8.23A).

Computed Tomography

The appearance of normal thyroid tissue is characteristic. On noncontrast scans, thyroid tissue is high in attenuation relative to adjacent soft tissues because of its high iodine content. Normal thyroid tissue measures around 100 HU, although in hypothyroid patients, thyroid attenuation is only slightly greater than that of soft tissue. Following the administration of contrast, thyroid tissue significantly enhances (see Figs. 8.23B and 8.24).

Table 8.10 Mediastinal Thyroid Mass

10% of mediastinal masses
Almost always connected to cervical thyroid
Anterior in 75%-90%; posterior in 10%-25%
Masses high in attenuation on CT; densely enhance with contrast
Cystic or inhomogeneous
Punctate calcifications
Distinguishing goiter and carcinoma difficult

Recognizing that a mediastinal mass originates from the thyroid gland depends on (a) demonstration of a communication with the cervical portion of the thyroid gland on contiguous slices (see Fig. 8.24), (b) high attenuation of at least a portion of the mass, (c) marked enhancement after contrast injection (see Figs. 8.24 and 8.25), and (d) prolonged enhancement (more than 2 minutes). Mediastinal thyroid masses commonly appear heterogeneous and cystic (see Figs. 8.23B and 8.25) on CT. Curvilinear, punctate, or ring-like calcifications can also be seen. The appearance of thyroid masses is usually nonspecific. Differentiation of goiter and thyroid carcinoma is difficult unless associated lymph node metastases are seen.

Magnetic Resonance

Characteristically, on T1-weighted images, the signal intensity of the normal thyroid is equal to or slightly greater than that seen in the adjacent sternocleidomastoid muscle; on T2-weighted scans, the signal intensity of the thyroid gland is significantly greater (Fig. 8.26). Most focal pathologic processes, including adenomas, cysts, and cancer, are easily identified on T2-weighted sequences because of their

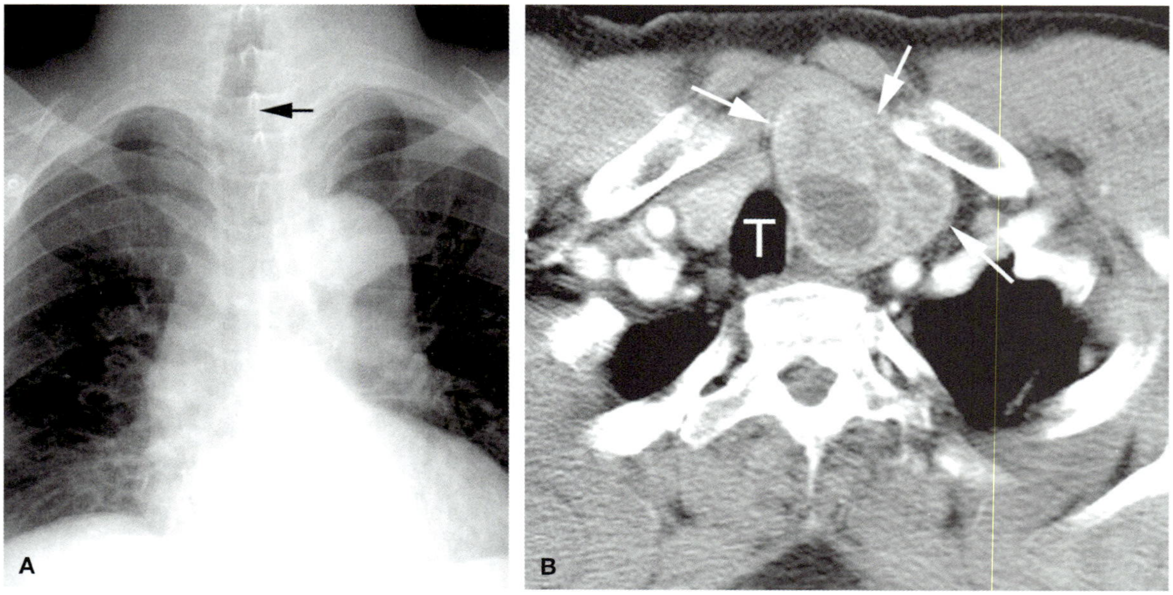

Figure 8.23. Cystic cervical and mediastinal goiter. **A:** Chest radiograph shows displacement of the trachea to the right (*arrow*) and poorly defined superior mediastinal widening at the level of the thoracic inlet. **B:** CT shows an enhancing multicystic mass (*arrows*) at the level of the thoracic inlet. The trachea (*T*) is displaced to the right and slightly narrowed.

markedly prolonged T2 values. Multinodular goiter has heterogeneous signal characteristics.

PARATHYROID ADENOMA

Four parathyroid glands are usually present. The upper pair is typically located dorsal to the superior poles of the thyroid gland, while the lower pair lies just below the lower thyroid poles. However, the precise location of glands may vary, and the lower pair is most variable in location. Most parathyroid adenomas are found in the lower group of parathyroid glands.

Approximately 10% of parathyroid glands are ectopic (Table 8.11). About 60% of these are located in the prevascular (anterior) mediastinum; 30% are embedded within the thyroid tissue; and 10% are found in the visceral (middle) mediastinum, in the region of the tracheoesophageal groove. Prevascular mediastinal parathyroid glands are thought to result from islands of parathyroid tissue that are carried into the mediastinum by the descending thymus during embryologic development. Prevascular mediastinal parathyroid adenomas are intimately associated with the thymus.

Primary hyperparathyroidism results from a solitary adenoma in approximately 85% of cases. Other causes include

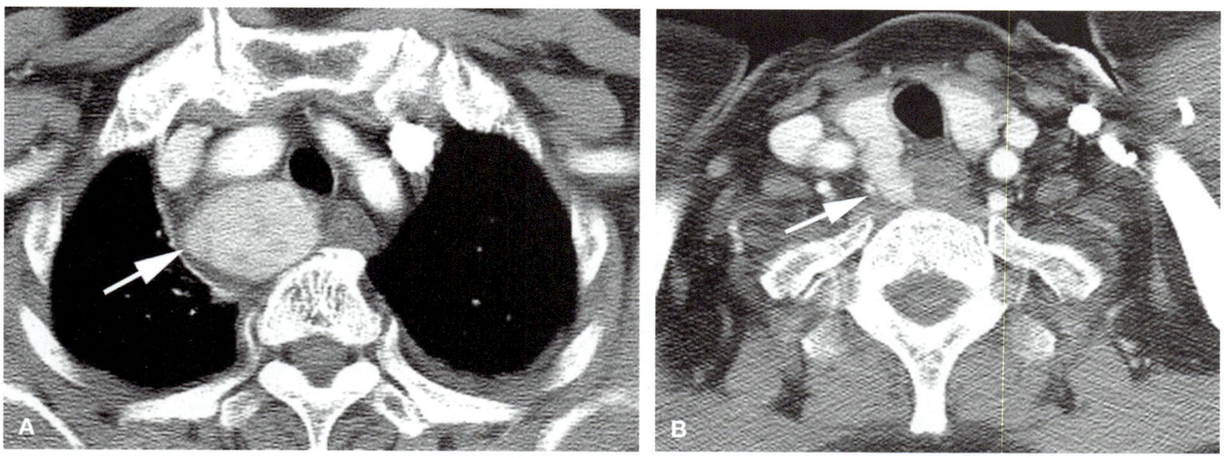

Figure 8.24. Mediastinal goiter. **A:** An enhancing mass is visible in the right paratracheal mediastinum (*arrow*). **B:** At a higher level, this mass is seen to arise from the inferior pole of the right thyroid lobe (*arrow*). The thyroid also densely enhances.

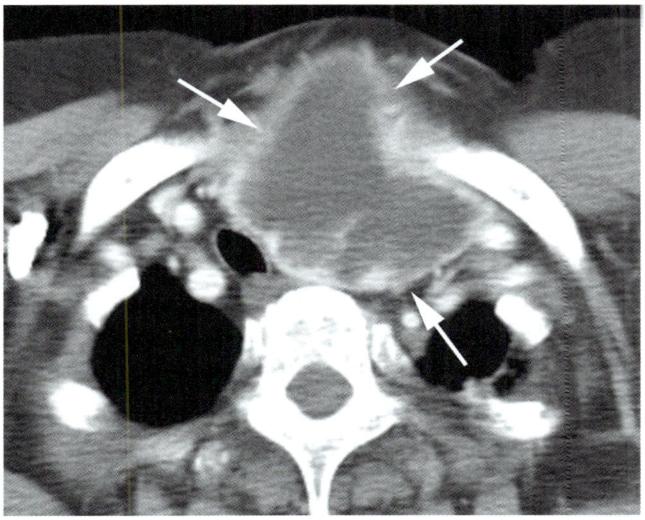

Figure 8.25. Large cystic goiter. A large mass (*arrows*) at the thoracic inlet has a densely enhancing rim and a cystic center. The trachea is displaced to the right and narrowed. The mass protrudes anteriorly into the suprasternal notch.

diffuse hyperplasia (10%), multiple adenomas (5%), and rarely carcinoma (1%). Various studies are available for detecting parathyroid abnormalities. These include high-resolution ultrasonography, radionuclide imaging using thallium or sestamibi, high-resolution contrast-enhanced CT, MRI, and selective venous catheterization.

Normal parathyroid glands cannot be identified on CT. Parathyroid adenomas and hyperplastic glands are usually small but vary in size from 0.3 to 3 cm; rarely, they are large enough to be detected on plain radiographs. When visible on CT, they usually appear homogeneous in density. Rarely, parathyroid adenomas appear calcified. No CT criteria reliably differentiate an adenoma from hyperplasia or carcinoma.

In patients with primary hyperparathyroidism, surgical neck exploration with resection of parathyroid tissues is curative in about 90% to 95% of cases. As a consequence, imaging is not generally performed prior to surgery. However, the persistence of hyperparathyroidism following surgical resection of the cervical glands suggests the presence of an ectopic parathyroid adenoma or ectopic hyperfunctioning gland. Forty to fifty percent of these patients will have mediastinal parathyroid glands. In the prevascular mediastinum, ectopic adenoma is usually found in the expected location of the thymus and may be indistinguishable from a small thymic remnant, small thymoma, or small lymph node (Fig. 8.27). Parathyroid adenomas are rarely found in the aortopulmonary window.

Similar to thyroid adenomas, most parathyroid adenomas, hyperplastic glands, and carcinomas appear intense on T2-weighted images, increasing significantly in intensity compared to T1-weighted images. Enhancement following gadolinium infusion is typical, and fat suppression images can be valuable.

MEDIASTINAL LYMPH NODES AND LYMPH NODE MASSES

On average, more than 60 mediastinal lymph nodes are found at autopsy. Almost 80% of mediastinal lymph nodes are located in relation to the trachea and main bronchi and serve to drain the lungs.

Mediastinal lymph node abnormalities can be seen in any part of the mediastinum, although they most commonly involve visceral (middle) mediastinum regions such as the paratracheal space, aortopulmonary window, and subcarinal space. Their detection and diagnosis is important in the

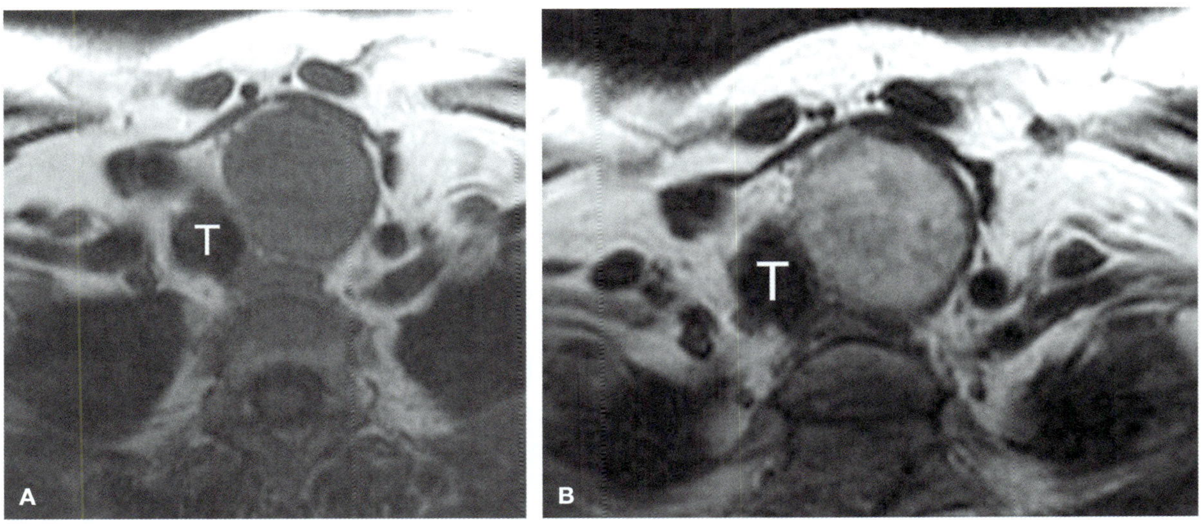

Figure 8.26. MRI of goiter. **A:** T1-weighted image shows a left thyroid mass to be slightly more intense than strap muscles. The trachea (*T*) is displaced to the right. **B:** With T2 weighting, the mass is more intense than muscle. *T*, trachea.

Table 8.11 Mediastinal Parathyroid Mass

10% of parathyroid glands are ectopic
60% in the visceral (anterior) mediastinum
10% in the superior mediastinum
Adenoma and hyperplastic gland usually small
Mediastinal parathyroid gland or adenoma present in 40%-50% of patients with persistent hyperparathyroidism after surgery

evaluation of a number of thoracic diseases, including bronchogenic carcinoma, lymphoma, and granulomatous diseases. The assessment of mediastinal lymph nodes in patients with bronchogenic carcinoma is discussed in detail in Chapter 5.

Mediastinal lymph nodes are generally classified by location, and most descriptive systems are based on Rouvière classification of lymph node groups. Thoracic lymph nodes are usually grouped into parietal and visceral, depending on their location and drainage. The parietal lymph nodes lie outside the parietal pleura, primarily drain structures of the chest wall, and are classified as internal mammary, diaphragmatic, paracardiac, and intercostal. Visceral node groups are located within the mediastinum or are related to the lung hila and include intrapulmonary, bronchopulmonary, tracheobronchial, paratracheal, paraesophageal, and anterior mediastinal lymph nodes.

Lymph Node Groups

The following classification is based on a modification of well-recognized anatomic descriptions of lymphatic anatomy, although some terms have been modified to be consistent with current usage and emphasize the localization of lymph nodes on imaging studies.

Lymph nodes are considered in anterior, tracheobronchial, and posterior node groups, generally corresponding to the plain radiographic divisions of the mediastinum.

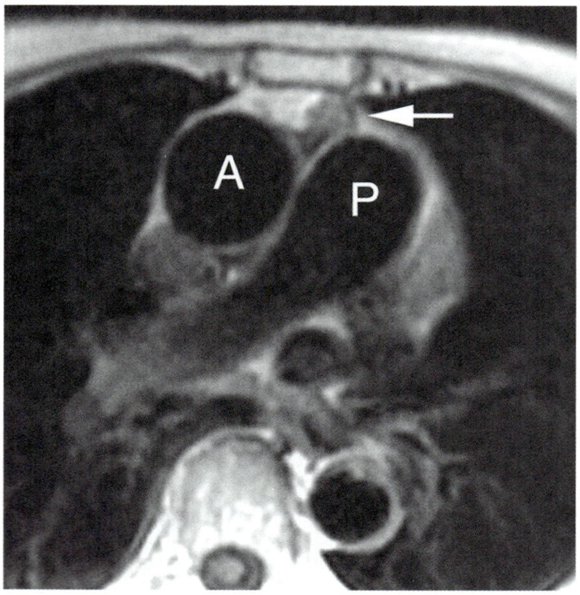

Figure 8.27. Anterior mediastinal parathyroid adenoma on T1-weighted MRI in a patient with persistent hyperparathyroidism after parathyroid surgery. A small mass (*arrow*) is visible anterior to the ascending aorta (*A*) and main pulmonary artery (*P*), in the region of the thymus.

Anterior Lymph Nodes

Internal mammary lymph nodes are located in a retrosternal position, in the anterior intercostal spaces, and near the internal mammary artery and veins; they are considered to be part of the parietal lymph node group. They drain the anterior chest wall, anterior diaphragm, and medial breasts and freely communicate with prevascular lymph nodes and paracardiac or diaphragmatic lymph nodes. They are most often enlarged as a result of lymphoma or metastatic breast cancer (Figs. 8.28A and B, 8.29A and B).

Prevascular lymph nodes lie anterior to the aorta and in relation to the great vessels. These nodes drain most anterior mediastinal structures, including the pericardium, thymus, thyroid, pleura, and the anterior hila. They represent visceral nodes. They communicate with the internal mammary chain of nodes anteriorly and paratracheal and aortopulmonary lymph nodes posteriorly. They may be involved in a variety of diseases, notably lymphoma and granulomatous diseases, and their involvement in lung cancer is less common.

Paracardiac, cardiophrenic angle, or epiphrenic lymph nodes lie anterior to or lateral to the heart and pericardium, on the surface of the diaphragm. They communicate with the lower internal mammary chain and drain the lower intercostal spaces, pericardium, diaphragm, and liver. As with internal mammary nodes, paracardiac nodes are most commonly enlarged in patients with lymphoma (see Fig. 8.28C) and metastatic carcinoma, particularly breast cancer. Paracardiac lymph nodes may also be enlarged in patients with abdominal malignancies and represent a route of spread from the peritoneum.

Paracardiac lymph nodes correspond to the anterior (prepericardiac) and middle (juxtaphrenic) subgroups of the diaphragmatic parietal lymph node group. Prepericardiac nodes are located posterior to the xiphoid process and slightly lateral to it. Juxtaphrenic lymph nodes are situated adjacent to the pericardium, where the phrenic nerves meet the diaphragm. From a clinical standpoint, there is little reason to distinguish between them.

Tracheobronchial Lymph Nodes

Tracheobronchial lymph nodes generally serve to drain the lungs. Lung diseases (eg, lung cancer, sarcoidosis, tuberculosis, fungal infections) that secondarily involve lymph nodes typically involve the tracheobronchial lymph nodes. Tracheobronchial lymph nodes are subdivided into a number of important node groups, which are all closely related.

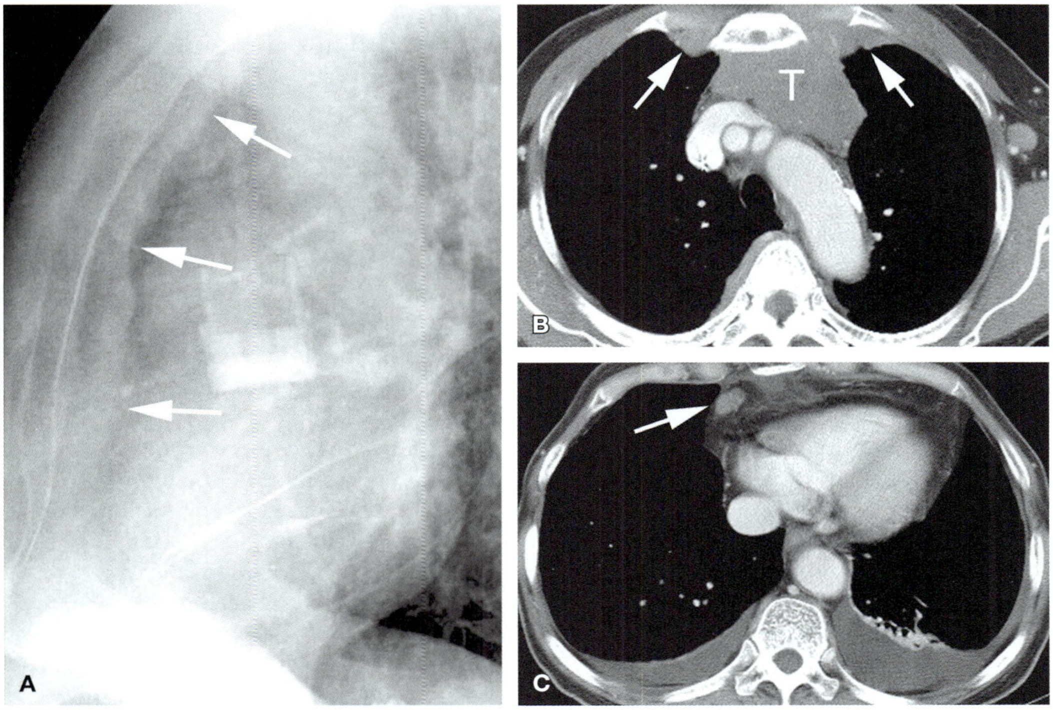

Figure 8.28. Internal mammary and paracardiac lymph node enlargement. **A:** Lateral plain radiograph in a patient with non-Hodgkin lymphoma shows thickening of the retrosternal stripe (*arrows*). **B:** CT shows enlargement of internal mammary lymph nodes (*arrows*) bilaterally, in association with involvement of the thymus (*T*) in the anterior mediastinum, left axillary lymph node enlargement, and pleural effusions. **C:** At a lower level, a right paracardiac lymph node (*arrow*) is also enlarged.

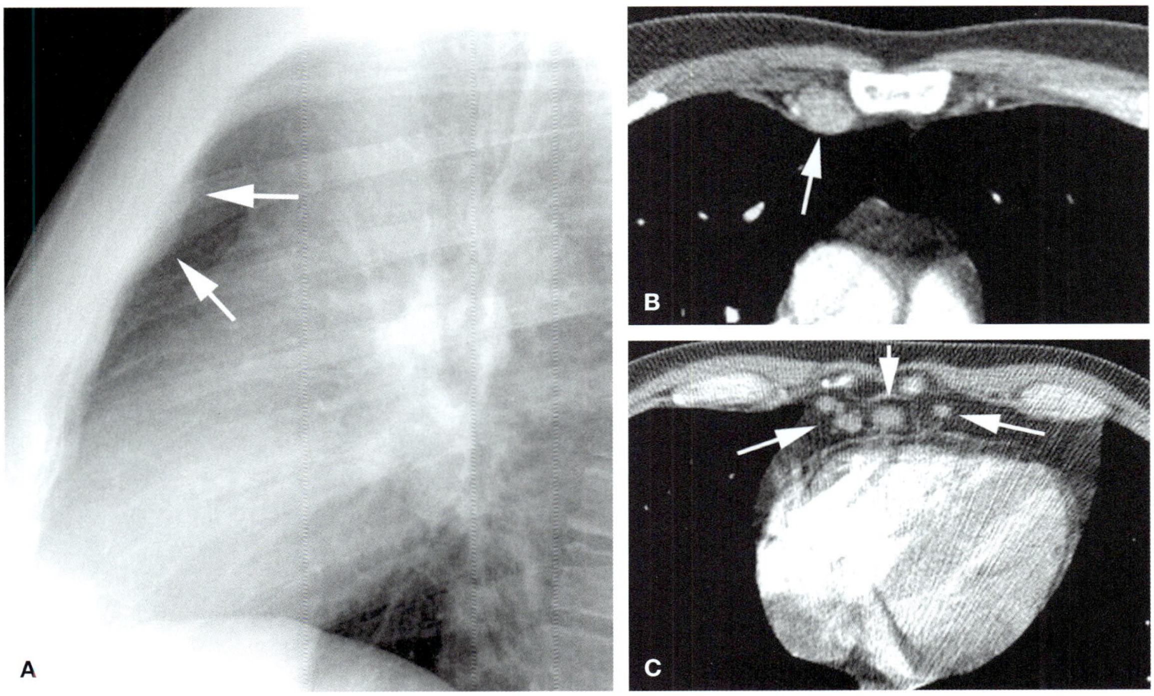

Figure 8.29. Internal mammary and paracardiac lymph node enlargement. **A:** Lateral plain radiograph in a patient with non-Hodgkin lymphoma shows lobulation of the retrosternal stripe (*arrows*). **B:** CT shows enlargement of an internal mammary lymph node (*arrow*), in association with the internal mammary vessels. **C:** At a lower level, a group of enlarged paracardiac lymph nodes (*arrows*) is also visible.

Paratracheal nodes lie anterior to, and on either side of, the trachea, thus occupying the paratracheal space (Figs. 8.30 and 8.31). The left lateral border of the trachea separates right from left paratracheal nodes for purposes of lung cancer staging. Retrotracheal nodes may also be seen. The most inferior node in this region is the so-called azygos node, medial to the azygos arch. These nodes form the final pathway of lymphatic drainage from most of both lungs, excepting the left upper lobe. Because of this, they are commonly abnormal regardless of the location of lung disease.

Aortopulmonary nodes are grouped by Rouvière with prevascular nodes, but because they serve the same function on the left as paratracheal nodes on the right and freely communicate with paratracheal nodes, it is most appropriate to group them together. They lie in the aortopulmonary window, lateral to the left main bronchus and between the aorta and pulmonary artery. The left upper lobe drains via this node group.

Peribronchial nodes surround the main bronchi on each side and lie between the main bronchi in the subcarinal space. These drain the lungs. *Bronchopulmonary nodes* are located distal to the main bronchi and are usually considered to be hilar.

Subcarinal nodes represent peribronchial nodes lying between the main bronchi in the subcarinal space (Fig. 8.32). These nodes drain the inferior hila and lower lobes on both the right and left and communicate in turn with the right paratracheal chain.

Posterior Lymph Nodes

Paraesophageal and inferior pulmonary ligament nodes are associated with the esophagus and descending aorta and lie medial to the inferior pulmonary ligament (Fig. 8.33A and B). They represent visceral nodes and drain the medial lower lobes, esophagus, pericardium, and posterior diaphragm. On the right, they are impossible to distinguish from subcarinal nodes unless they are near the diaphragm.

Intercostal and paravertebral lymph nodes are found in the posterior intercostal spaces and adjacent to thoracic vertebral bodies (see Fig. 8.33B and C). These drain the posterior pleura, chest wall, and spine and communicate with other posterior mediastinal lymph nodes.

Retrocrural lymph nodes lie posterior to the diaphragmatic crura (Fig. 8.34). They communicate with lumbar nodes and posterior mediastinal lymph nodes, drain the diaphragm and liver, and represent the posterior group of diaphragmatic parietal lymph nodes.

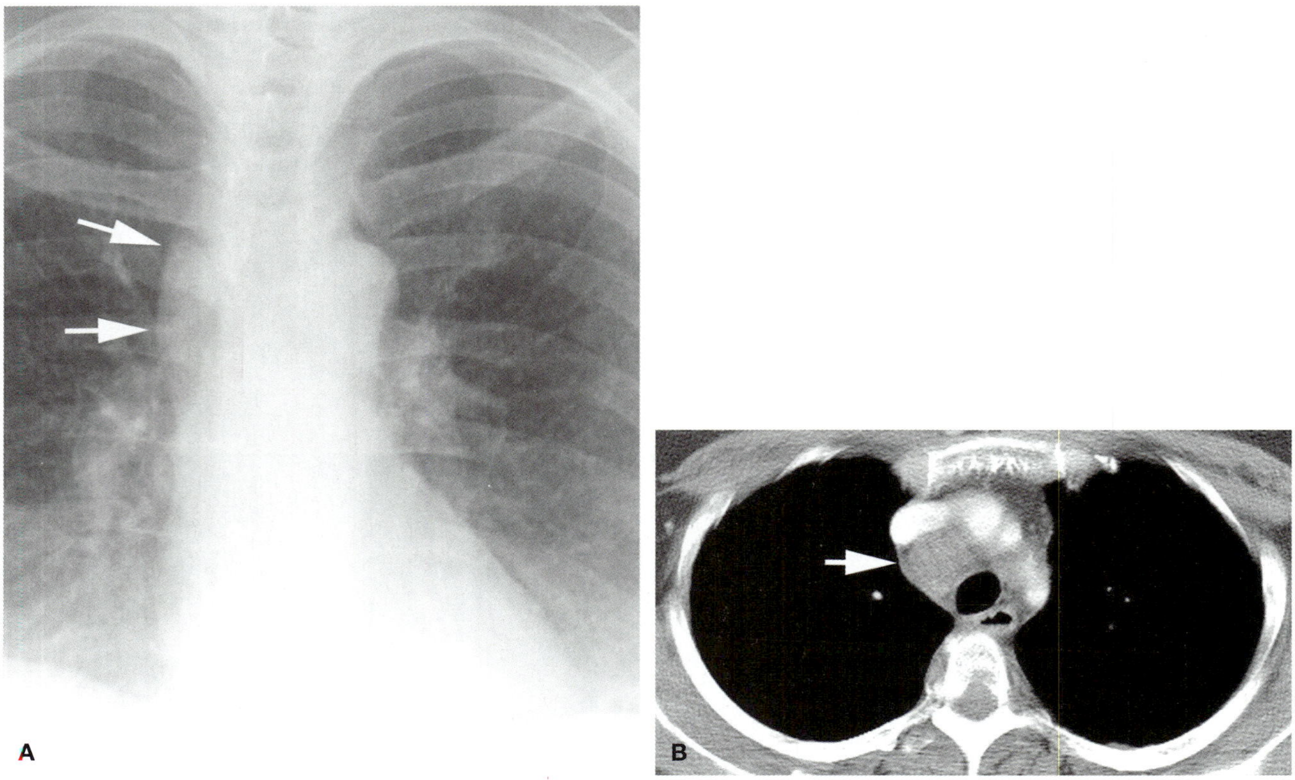

Figure 8.30. Paratracheal lymph node enlargement in metastatic carcinoma. **A:** Chest radiographs show abnormal convexity of the right superior mediastinum (*arrows*). The right paratracheal stripe and the normal contour of the superior vena cava are not visible. **B:** CT shows lymph node enlargement in the right paratracheal space (*arrow*), corresponding to paratracheal lymph nodes. The superior vena cava is displaced laterally and anteriorly, and the normal right paratracheal stripe is obscured by the large nodes.

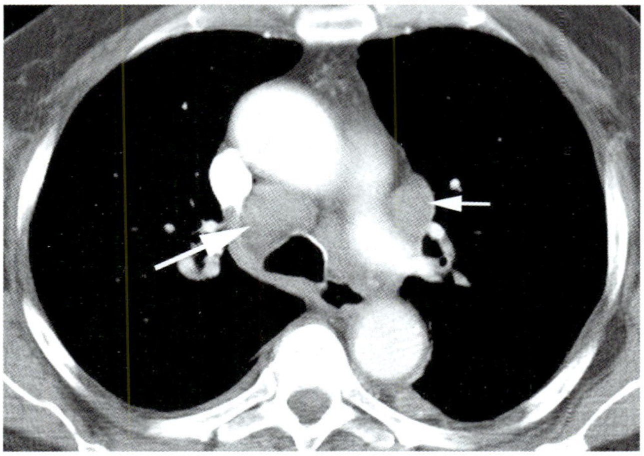

Figure 8.31. Paratracheal and aortopulmonary window lymph node enlargement in non-Hodgkin lymphoma. Enlarged nodes in the right paratracheal space (*large arrow*) and aortopulmonary window (*small arrow*) are visible.

Lymph Node Stations

Numerous lymph node classification schemes have been used since the American Joint Committee on Cancer (AJCC) and the Union for International Cancer Control (UICC) first introduced a numeric system for localization of intrathoracic lymph nodes for the purpose of lung cancer staging in the 1970s. The lymph node map devised by the International Association for the Study of Lung Cancer (IASLC) International Staging Committee is the currently accepted standard and is used in the TNM-8 lung cancer staging system (Table 8.12; Fig. 8.35). The IASLC map supersedes all prior maps, and while a detailed knowledge of lymph node station numbers is not necessary, a basic understanding of nodal groups and zones that alter staging is important as this ensures one can be conversant in appropriate N category designations with lung cancer staging.

The IASLC map groups the lymph nodes into four mediastinal zones (upper zone, aortopulmonary zone, subcarinal zone, lower zone), two pulmonary/hilar zones (hilar/interlobar and peripheral zones), and a supraclavicular zone (Table 8.12). In an analysis of the survival of lung cancer patients with nodal metastases, a consideration of specific lymph node stations within different zones was found to be of little value.

Diagnosis of Lymph Node Enlargement

Radiographs

Normal lymph nodes are not visible on chest radiographs. Abnormally enlarged nodes may be recognized because of distortion of normal mediastinal contours or abnormalities of mediastinal lines, interfaces, or spaces (Table 8.13).

Enlarged right paratracheal lymph nodes usually result in an abnormal convexity of the superior vena cava

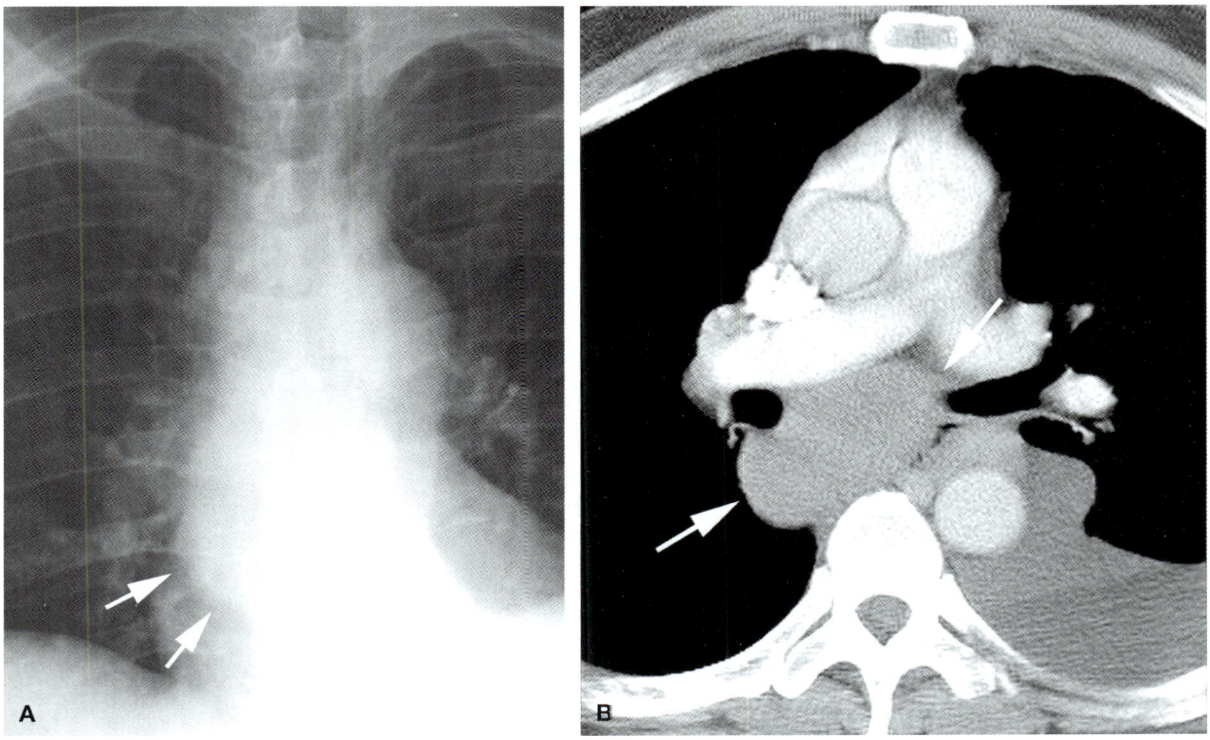

Figure 8.32. Subcarinal lymph node enlargement in chronic lymphocytic leukemia. **A:** Chest radiographs show an abnormal convexity in the region of the azygoesophageal recess (*arrows*), corresponding to subcarinal lymph node enlargement. **B:** CT shows abnormally enlarged subcarinal lymph nodes (*arrows*).

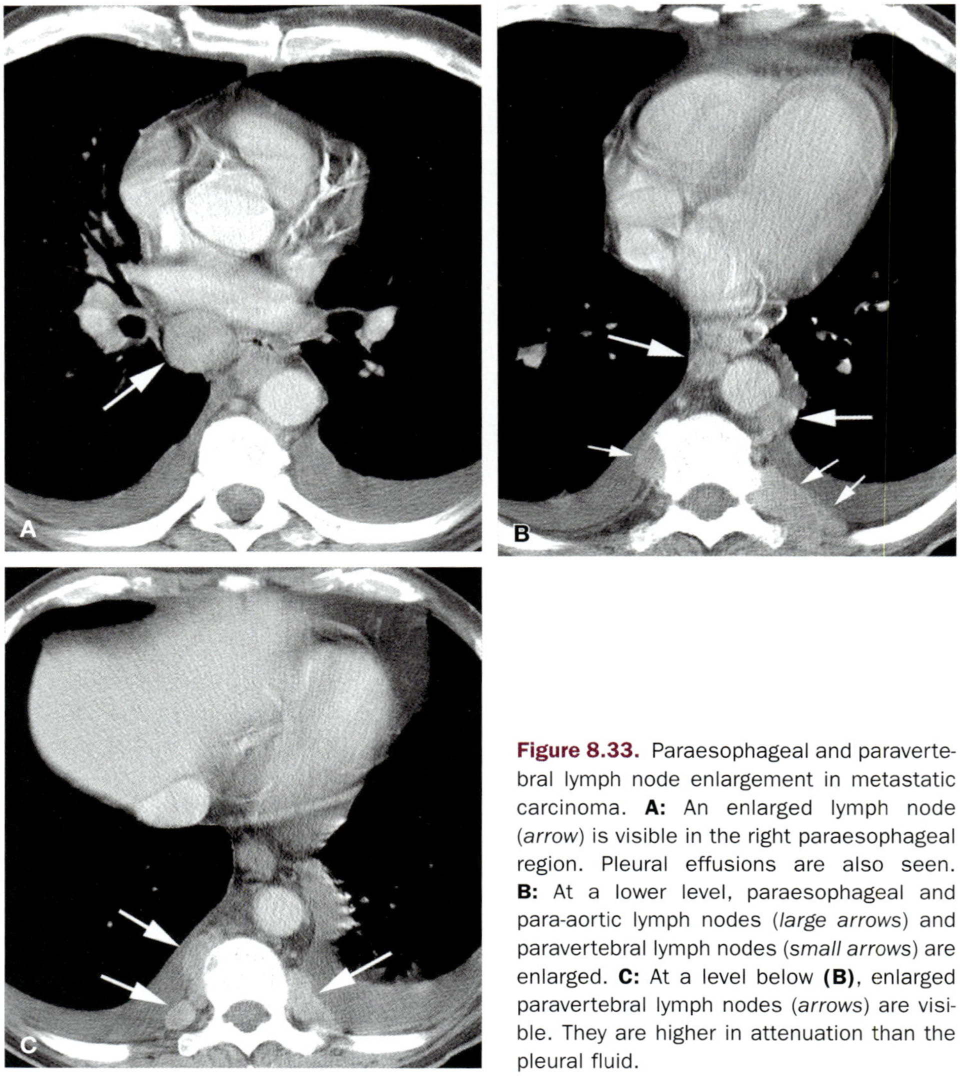

Figure 8.33. Paraesophageal and paravertebral lymph node enlargement in metastatic carcinoma. **A:** An enlarged lymph node (*arrow*) is visible in the right paraesophageal region. Pleural effusions are also seen. **B:** At a lower level, paraesophageal and para-aortic lymph nodes (*large arrows*) and paravertebral lymph nodes (*small arrows*) are enlarged. **C:** At a level below **(B)**, enlarged paravertebral lymph nodes (*arrows*) are visible. They are higher in attenuation than the pleural fluid.

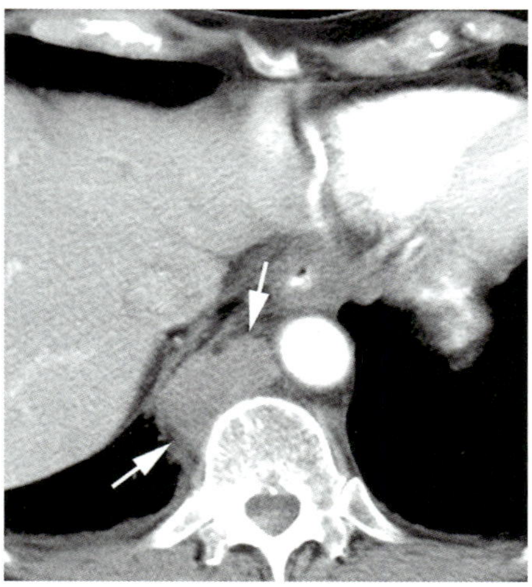

Figure 8.34. Retrocrural lymph node enlargement in lymphoma. Enlarged nodes (*arrows*) are visible in a retrocrural, para-aortic location.

interface or thickening of the right paratracheal stripe (see Fig. 8.30A). Inferiorly, right paratracheal nodes are contiguous with the right tracheobronchial nodes, recognizable when enlarged as a convexity in the region of the azygos arch.

Enlarged left paratracheal lymph nodes are not commonly visible on chest radiographs but may result in a convexity in the region of the left paratracheal stripe or in relation to the left subclavian artery interface, above the aortic arch.

Enlargement of aortopulmonary nodes results in a convexity of the aortopulmonary window.

Enlarged subcarinal lymph nodes result in a convexity in the region of the superior aspect of the azygoesophageal recess (see Fig. 8.32A). Paraesophageal lymph node enlargement also may result in an abnormal convexity in the azygoesophageal recess or an abnormality of the retrotracheal band on the lateral film.

Table 8.12 The International Association for the Study of Lung Cancer Lymph Node Stations

Supraclavicular Zone		
Station 1 (R and L)	Low cervical, supraclavicular, and sternal notch	Lower margin of cricoid cartilage to clavicles/upper border of the manubrium Midline of the trachea serves as the border between 1R and 1L
Upper Zone (visceral compartment)		
Station 2 (R and L)	Upper paratracheal[a]	Apex of the lung/upper border of manubrium at midline to caudal margin of innominate vein (R) or superior margin of aortic arch (L)
Station 3A	Prevascular	Apex of chest to carina Posterior to the sternum and anterior to SVC (right) or carotid artery (left)
Station 3P	Retrotracheal	Apex of chest to carina Posterior to trachea
Station 4 (R and L)	Lower paratracheal[a]	Caudal margin of innominate vein to lower border of azygos vein (4R) Upper margin of aortic arch to upper margin of left PA, medial to ligamentum arteriosum (4L)
Aortopulmonary Zone (visceral compartment)		
Station 5	Subaortic	Upper margin of aortic arch to upper margin of left PA Lateral to ligamentum arteriosum
Station 6	Paraaortic	Upper margin of aortic arch to lower margin of aortic arch Anterior and lateral to the ascending aorta and aortic arch
Subcarinal Zone (visceral compartment)		
Station 7	Subcarinal	Inferior margin of carina to lower border of bronchus intermedius (right) or upper border of left lower lobe bronchus (left)
Lower Zone (visceral compartment)		
Station 8	Paraesophageal	Adjacent to the esophagus below subcarinal space Lower border of the bronchus intermedius on the right or upper border of the lower lobe bronchus on the left to the diaphragm
Station 9	Inferior pulmonary ligament	Nodes within the inferior pulmonary ligament Inferior pulmonary veins to the diaphragm
Hilar and Interlobar Zone (pulmonary nodes)		
Station 10	Hilar	Nodes adjacent to mainstem bronchus and hilar vessels including the proximal portions of the pulmonary veins and main pulmonary artery
Station 11	Interlobar	Between origins of lobar bronchi
Peripheral Zone (pulmonary nodes)		
Station 12	Lobar	Adjacent to lobar bronchi
Station 13	Segmental	Adjacent to segmental bronchi
Station 14	Subsegmental	Adjacent to subsegmental bronchi

[a]Left lateral border of trachea separates R from L (not anatomic midline).

Reprinted from Rusch VW, Asamura H, Watanabe H, et al. The IASLC lung cancer staging project a proposal for a new international lymph node map in the forthcoming seventh edition of the TNM classification for lung cancer. J Thorac Oncol. 2009;4:568-577. Figure 2.

[a]Left lateral border of trachea separates R from L (not anatomic midline).

AJCC, American Joint Committee on Cancer; ATS, American Thoracic Society; L, left; LPA, left pulmonary artery; LUL, left upper lobe; R, right; RUL, right upper lobe, UICC, Union for International Cancer Control.

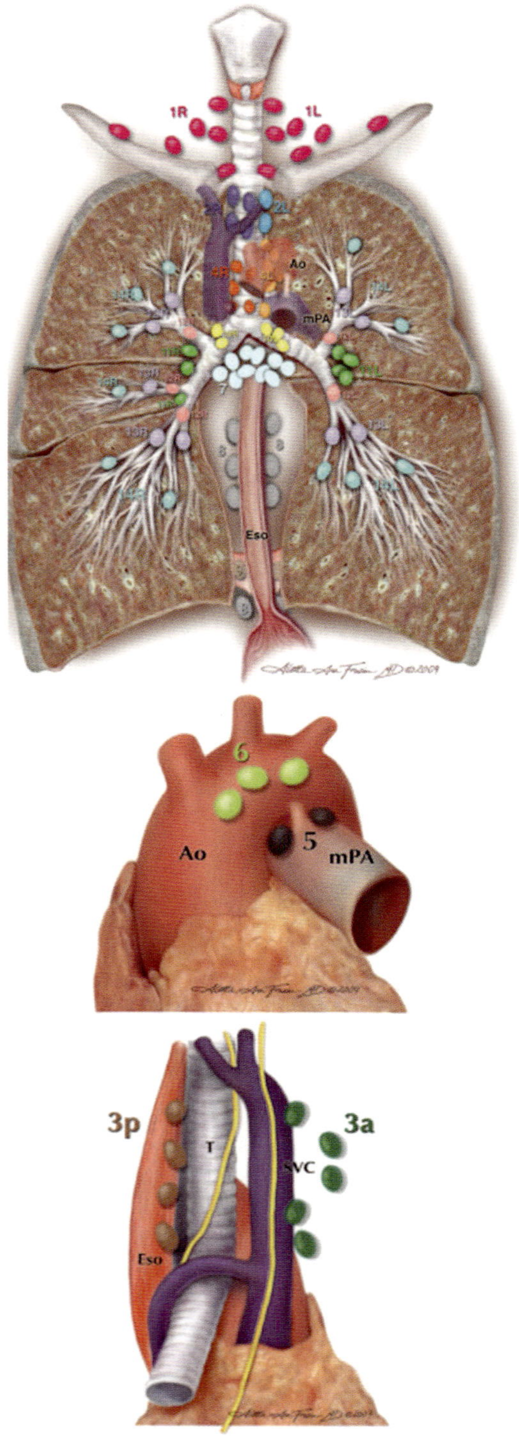

Supraclavicular zone
1 Low cervical, supraclavicular, and sternal notch nodes

Superior mediastinal nodes

Upper zone
2R Upper paratracheal (right)
2L Upper paratracheal (left)
3a Prevascular
3p Retrotracheal
4R Lower paratracheal (right)
4L Lower paratracheal (left)

Aortic nodes

AP zone
5 Subaortic
6 Para-aortic (ascending aorta or phrenic)

Inferior mediastinal nodes

Subcarinal zone
7 Subcarinal

Lower zone
8 Paraesophageal (below carina)
9 Pulmonary ligament

N1 nodes

Hilar/interlobar zone
10 Hilar
11 Interlobar

Peripheral zone
12 Lobar
13 Segmental
14 Subsegmental

Figure 8.35. The International Association for the Study of Lung Cancer (IASLC) lymph node map for staging lung cancer. (From Rusch VW, Asamura H, Watanabe H, et al. The IASLC lung cancer staging project a proposal for a new international lymph node map in the forthcoming seventh edition of the TNM classification for lung cancer. *J Thorac Oncol*. 2009;4: 568-577).

Table 8.13 Plain Film Findings of Lymph Node Enlargement

Node Group	ATS Node Station(s)	Plain Film Finding When Nodes Are Enlarged
Right paratracheal	2R and 4R	1. Convexity of the superior vena cava interface
		2. Thickening of the right paratracheal stripe
Left paratracheal	2L and 4L	1. Convexity of the left subclavian artery interface
		2. Thickening of the left paratracheal stripe (uncommon)
Aortopulmonary	5	Convexity of the aortopulmonary window interface
Prevascular	6	1. Anterior mediastinal mass
		2. Filling in of the retrosternal clear space (lateral film)
Subcarinal	7	Convexity in the superior aspect of the azygoesophageal recess
Paraesophageal	8	1. Thickening of the posterior tracheal band
		2. Convexity of the azygoesophageal recess
Inferior pulmonary ligament	9	Convexity in the inferior aspect of the azygoesophageal recess
Peribronchial (hilar)	10R and L	Hilar enlargement and lobulation (see Chapter 3)
Bronchopulmonary (hilar)	11	Hilar enlargement and lobulation (see Chapter 3)
Paracardiac	14R and L	Convexity in the cardiophrenic angles
Internal mammary	—	Lobulation of the retrosternal stripe
Retrocrural	8R and L	Convexity of the paravertebral stripes
Intercostal or paravertebral	—	Convexity of the paravertebral stripes

ATS, American Thoracic Society.

Computed Tomography

On CT, lymph nodes are generally visible as round, elliptical, or triangular, discrete and surrounded by mediastinal fat, and of soft-tissue attenuation (see Figs. 8.28-8.34). The node hilum is sometimes seen to contain a small quantity of fat.

Lymph nodes can usually be distinguished from vessels by their location. However, the ability to recognize and correctly identify lymph nodes is directly related to the amount of mediastinal fat surrounding them; in patients having little mediastinal fat, lymph nodes can be difficult to distinguish from vessels without contrast infusion. In many parts of the mediastinum, lymph nodes often occur in clusters of a few nodes of similar size.

The short axis or least diameter (ie, the smallest diameter seen in cross section) of a lymph node should generally be used when measuring its size. This measurement more closely reflects the actual node diameter when nodes are obliquely oriented relative to the scan plane and shows less variation among normal subjects than does the long axis or greatest diameter.

There are significant variations in normal node size, depending on the location of the node. However, by convention, the upper limit of normal for mediastinal lymph nodes should generally be considered between 1.0 and 1.5 cm, as measured in its short axis. This measurement should also take into account the morphology as even at the largest end of this range nonpathologic lymph nodes should have an ovoid configuration with a fatty hilum. Internal mammary nodes, paracardiac nodes, and paravertebral nodes are not commonly seen on CT in normals.

The accuracy of lymph node size in the diagnosis of a lymph node abnormality is limited. Significant abnormalities (eg, micrometastases) can be present in the absence of lymph node enlargement. Also, the significance given to the presence of a minimally enlarged lymph node must be tempered by a knowledge of the patient's clinical history. For example, if the patient is known to have lung cancer, an enlarged lymph node has a significant likelihood of being involved by tumor. However, the same node in a patient without neoplasm is much less likely to be of clinical significance. In the absence of a known disease, a mildly enlarged node must be regarded as likely to be hyperplastic or postinflammatory.

Very large lymph nodes, having a short axis of 2 cm or more, often reflect the presence of neoplasm, such as metastatic tumor or lymphoma, granulomatous disease, or infection, and should be regarded as significant. Although mediastinal lymph nodes can become enlarged in a variety of noninfectious and nongranulomatous inflammatory diseases, they are often smaller than 2 cm.

With progression of disease, a pathologic process involving several contiguous nodes may also involve surrounding mediastinal fat, and several adjacent nodes may fuse to form a single larger mass. Poor definition of node margins or poor definition of the margins of the coalescent node mass can indicate extension of the disease process through the node capsule or an associated fibrotic or inflammatory reaction. This appearance is most typical of infection, granulomatous disease, and neoplasm. Diffuse infiltration of mediastinal fat may also occur, with individual nodes or node groups becoming unrecognizable (Fig. 8.36). Typically, mediastinal fat appears to be replaced by soft-tissue density. This pattern suggests lymphoma, undifferentiated carcinoma, generalized infection, or granulomatous mediastinitis.

Lymph Node Calcification

Lymph node calcification may be recognized on chest radiographs or CT. CT, of course, is more sensitive. Typically, calcified lymph nodes indicate prior granulomatous disease, including tuberculosis, histoplasmosis and other fungal infections, and sarcoidosis, although a variety of diseases may be associated with this finding.

Calcification can be dense, involving the node in a homogeneous fashion, stippled, "eggshell" in appearance, or faint and hazy. The abnormal nodes are often enlarged but can also be of normal size. Multiple calcified lymph nodes are often visible, usually in contiguity, and hilar lymph node calcifications are often associated. Dense

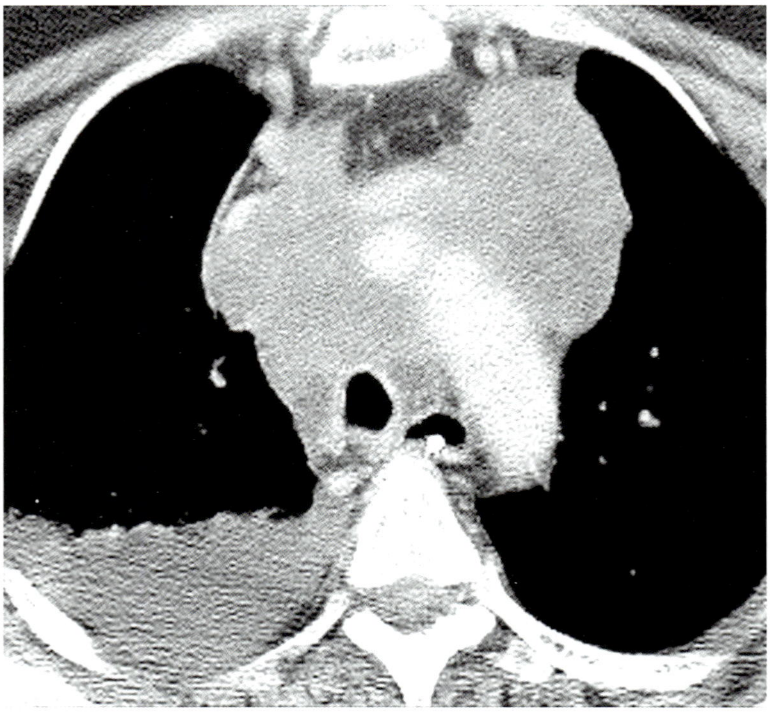

Figure 8.36. Confluent lymph node mass in a patient with metastatic squamous cell carcinoma involving the right and left paratracheal and prevascular spaces. Individual lymph nodes are not visible.

calcification involving all or most of an abnormal node is typical of previous granulomatous infection or sarcoidosis (Fig. 8.37A).

Eggshell calcification is defined by the presence of calcium in the node periphery, which is often ringlike. Eggshell calcification is most often seen in patients with silicosis (see Fig. 8.37B) or in coal workers with pneumoconiosis, sarcoidosis, and tuberculosis, but it also occurs in patients with HL, usually following radiation, and occasionally occurs in patients with other causes of node calcification.

Rarely, lymph node calcification is seen in untreated lymphoma or as a result of metastatic carcinoma, typically mucinous adenocarcinoma or thyroid carcinoma (see Fig. 8.37C). Usually, calcification of adenocarcinomas is stippled or faint and difficult to see on plain radiographs. Lymph node calcification may also be seen in patients with metastatic osteogenic

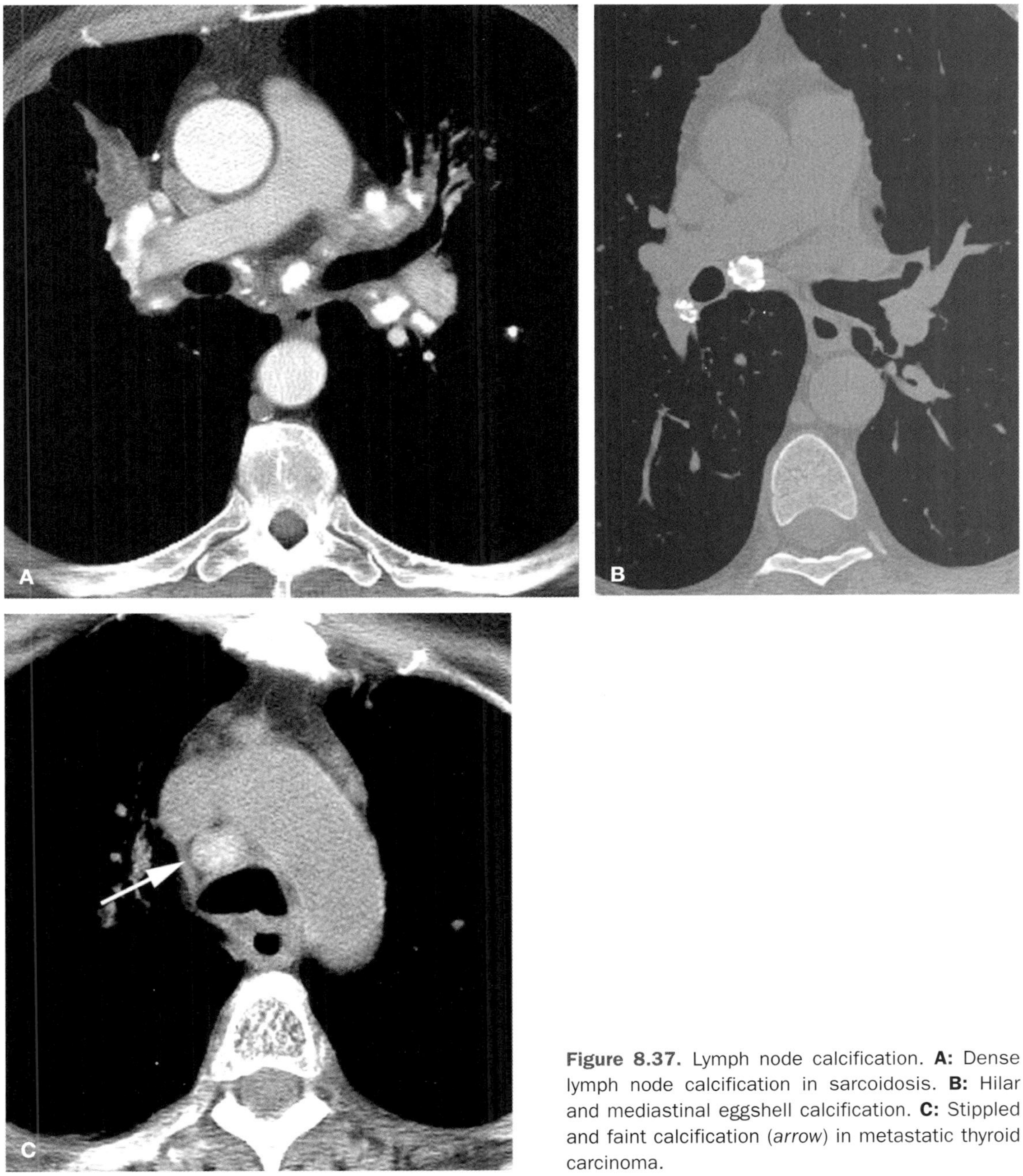

Figure 8.37. Lymph node calcification. **A:** Dense lymph node calcification in sarcoidosis. **B:** Hilar and mediastinal eggshell calcification. **C:** Stippled and faint calcification (*arrow*) in metastatic thyroid carcinoma.

Table 8.14 Calcified Lymph Nodes

Common
Infectious granulomatous diseases
Tuberculosis
Fungal infections (histoplasmosis)
Sarcoidosis
Silicosis
Hodgkin disease (usually following treatment)
Rare
Pneumocystis jiroveci (*Pneumocystis carinii*) pneumonia
Metastases (mucinous adenocarcinoma)
Amyloidosis
Scleroderma
Castleman disease

sarcoma. Calcified hilar and mediastinal lymph nodes have been observed in AIDS patients with *Pneumocystis jiroveci* (*Pneumocystis carinii*) infection (Table 8.14).

Although calcified lymph nodes generally indicate the presence of old disease, densely calcified nodes can remain functional and can become involved by other processes such as metastatic neoplasm.

Calcified lymph nodes in the mediastinum or hila may erode into adjacent bronchi, resulting in *broncholithiasis*. This is most common in histoplasmosis and tuberculosis. The calcified node, or broncholith, may be expectorated or result in atelectasis, postobstructive pneumonia, or hemoptysis (Fig. 8.38A and B).

Low-Attenuation or Necrotic Lymph Nodes

After administration of intravenous contrast agent, enlarged lymph nodes may appear to be low in attenuation, often with an enhancing rim (Fig. 8.39). Typically, low-attenuation nodes reflect the presence of necrosis. They are commonly seen in patients with tuberculosis, fungal infections, and neoplasms such as metastatic carcinoma and lymphoma.

Necrotic lymph nodes are common in patients with active tuberculosis. After injection of intravenous contrast agent, nodes larger than 2 cm in diameter almost always show central areas of low attenuation with peripheral enhancement and an irregular wall. Smaller lymph nodes may also show this finding.

Low-attenuation nodes also occur in patients with metastatic lung cancer (often when the primary tumor also appears necrotic), metastatic seminoma, and metastatic ovarian, thyroid, and gastric neoplasia (Table 8.15). Low-attenuation or necrotic lymph nodes are seen in 10% to 20% of patients with lymphoma, either before or after treatment. Low-attenuation lymph nodes have been described but are rare in sarcoidosis.

Lymph Node Enhancement on CT

Normal lymph nodes may show some increase in attenuation following intravenous contrast infusion. Pathologic lymph nodes with an increased vascular supply may increase significantly in attenuation. The differential diagnosis of densely enhancing mediastinal nodes is limited and includes Castleman disease (CD) (Fig. 8.40A), angioimmunoblastic lymphadenopathy, vascular metastases (eg, renal cell carcinoma, papillary thyroid carcinoma, lung carcinoma, sarcoma, and melanoma; see Fig. 8.40B), tuberculosis, and sometimes sarcoidosis (Table 8.16).

Differentiation between enhancing lymph nodes and enhancing mediastinal mass should be attempted. Enhancing masses include substernal thyroid and parathyroid lesions, neuroendocrine tumor, lymphangioma, hemangioma, and paraganglioma.

MRI Evaluation of Mediastinal Lymph Nodes

MRI is comparable to CT in identifying mediastinal and hilar lymph nodes, even though its spatial resolution is inferior. Although there are some differences in the MRI characteristics of benign and malignant lymph nodes, their differentiation in individual cases is not possible. Furthermore, MRI is unable to detect calcification, rendering identification of granulomatous nodes difficult. Low signal intensity has been noted in calcified nodes on T2-weighted images in patients with fibrosing mediastinitis (FM); however, this appearance is nonspecific.

FDG-PET Evaluation of Mediastinal Lymph Nodes

FDG-PET or PET/CT is commonly used in the diagnosis of mediastinal lymph node abnormalities, particularly when associated with lung tumors, an extrathoracic primary tumor or lymphoma, or a primary mediastinal tumor. FDG-PET is sensitive in the diagnosis of neoplastic involvement of lymph nodes; most neoplasms show increased metabolic activity. However, inflammatory diseases, such as sarcoidosis, may show similar activity in mediastinal lymph nodes.

LYMPHOMA

Lymphomas are primary neoplasms of the lymphoreticular system and are classified in two primary types: HL and NHL. Lymphomas have been recently reclassified and are discussed in detail in Chapter 7. HL is the less common of the two types, representing about 25% to 30% of cases, but it is more common as a cause of mediastinal disease.

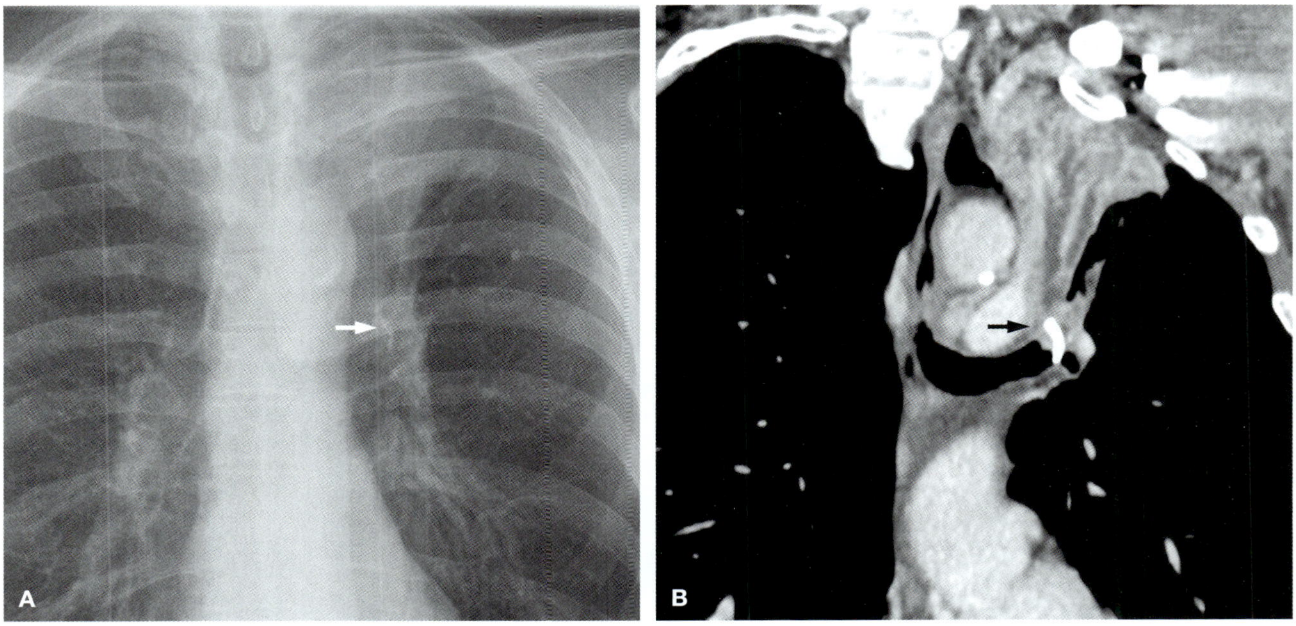

Figure 8.38. Broncholithiasis resulting in lobar collapse mimicking lung cancer. **A:** Frontal chest radiograph showing left upper lobe atelectasis suggestive of an obstructing endobronchial lesion. Calcification is visible within the proximal left upper lobe bronchus (*arrow*). Additional calcified right hilar nodes and small calcified nodules in the aerated left lung are also visible. **B:** Oblique coronal CT shows that the endobronchial lesion is almost entirely calcified (*arrow*) and most suggestive of a broncholith, which was confirmed at bronchoscopy.

Hodgkin Lymphoma

HL has a predilection for thoracic involvement, and up to 85% of patients with HL present with mediastinal adenopathy. HL most often involves the superior mediastinal (prevascular, paratracheal, aortopulmonary) lymph nodes (Figs. 8.41 and 8.42; see also Figs. 7.1-7.7 in Chapter 7); if these nodes appear normal on CT, intrathoracic adenopathy is unlikely to represent HL.

Multiple node groups are commonly involved in patients with HL (see Fig. 8.42). In addition to superior mediastinal node groups, sites of lymph node enlargement, in order of decreasing frequency, include hilar nodes, subcarinal nodes, cardiophrenic angle (paracardiac) lymph nodes, internal mammary nodes, and posterior mediastinal nodes. Enlargement of lymph nodes in a single node group can be seen in some patients with HL, most commonly in the anterior (prevascular) mediastinum. This often indicates the presence of nodular sclerosing HL, which accounts for 50% to 80% of adult HL cases.

In patients with HL, enlarged lymph nodes are variable in appearance. Nodes are usually of homogeneous soft-tissue attenuation, but low attenuation or necrosis may be seen with contrast enhancement. Rarely, nodes show fine flecks of calcification in untreated patients. Multiple enlarged lymph nodes are often seen, and they can be well defined and discrete, matted, or associated with diffuse mediastinal infiltration. HL also has a predilection for involvement of the thymus in association with mediastinal lymph node enlargement.

Non-Hodgkin Lymphoma

The term *non-Hodgkin lymphoma* refers to a large and diverse group of neoplasms, varying in radiologic findings, clinical presentation, course, and prognosis (see Chapter 7). In comparison to HL, these tumors are less common as causes of thoracic disease.

Thoracic involvement is about half as common with NHL (40%-50%) as with HL (85%). As with HL, the most common thoracic abnormality in patients with NHL is mediastinal lymph node involvement, although the pattern of lymph node disease is different (see Figs. 7.15-7.19 in Chapter 7).

Involvement of one node group is much more common in patients with NHL; 40% of patients with thoracic NHL have involvement of only one node group. Enlargement of anterior mediastinal, internal mammary, paratracheal, and hilar nodes is much less common with NHL than with HL. Nonetheless, upper mediastinal node involvement is the most common abnormality seen; 35% of patients have prevascular and/or paratracheal node involvement. Subcarinal lymph nodes, hilar nodes, and cardiophrenic nodes are less often abnormal. Involvement of posterior mediastinal nodal groups is much more common with NHL (10% of cases) than with HL. Rarely, calcification of node masses is seen.

NHL may occur primarily in the mediastinum. The most common cell types presenting in this fashion are T-cell lymphoblastic lymphoma and large B-cell lymphoma. These resemble the appearance of mediastinal HL and are described further in Chapter 7.

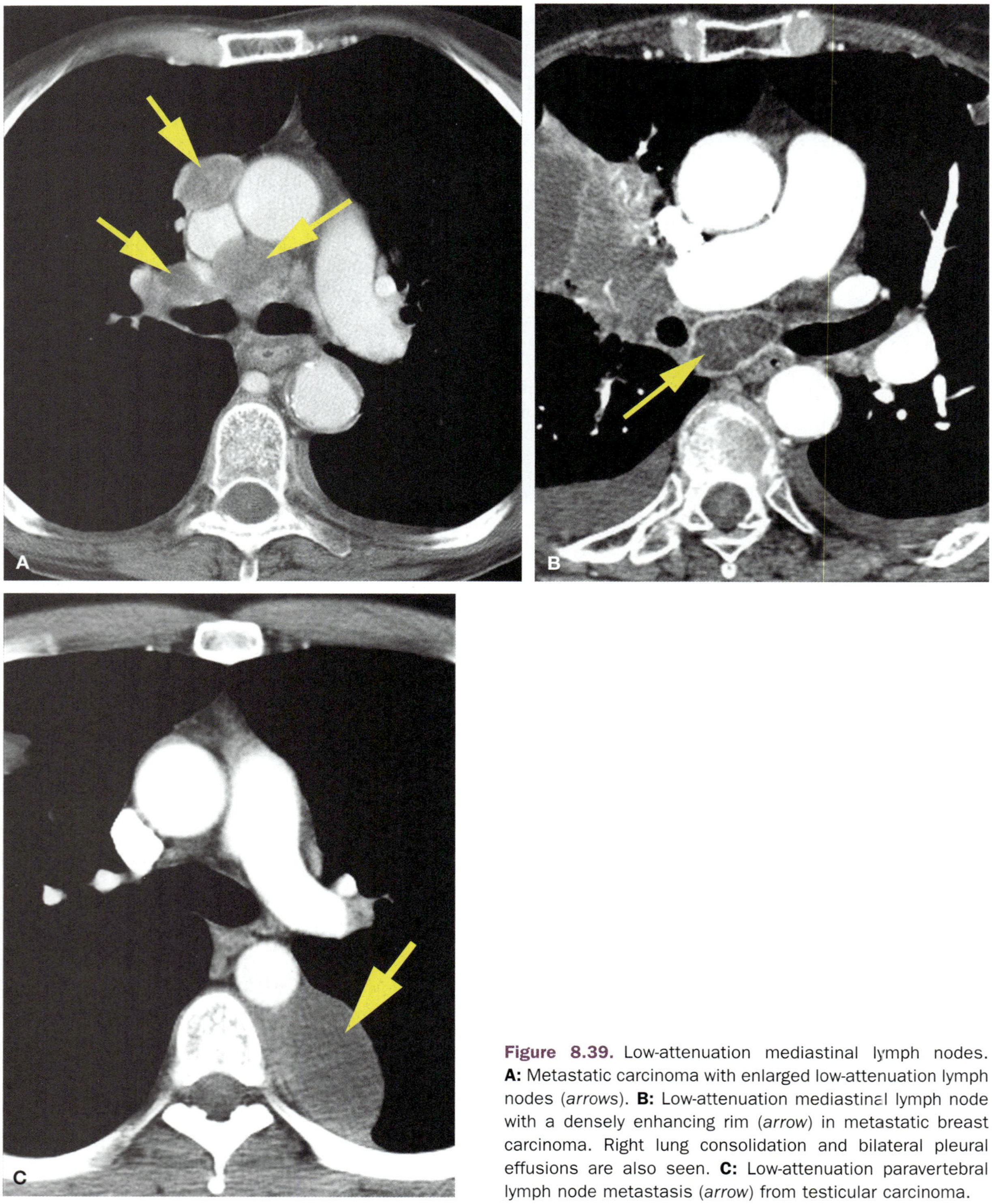

Figure 8.39. Low-attenuation mediastinal lymph nodes. **A:** Metastatic carcinoma with enlarged low-attenuation lymph nodes (*arrows*). **B:** Low-attenuation mediastinal lymph node with a densely enhancing rim (*arrow*) in metastatic breast carcinoma. Right lung consolidation and bilateral pleural effusions are also seen. **C:** Low-attenuation paravertebral lymph node metastasis (*arrow*) from testicular carcinoma.

LEUKEMIA

Mediastinal lymph nodes can be involved in patients with leukemia, particularly lymphocytic leukemia. Mediastinal lymph node enlargement is more common than hilar node enlargement. On chest radiographs, enlarged mediastinal lymph nodes are visible in less than 20% of cases.

In patients with acute or chronic myelogenous leukemia, masses of malignant myeloid precursor cells may be found in an extramedullary location; these masses are termed *granulocytic sarcoma* or *chloroma*. They most commonly are present at the time of first diagnosis of leukemia. In about 50% of cases, masses involve the mediastinum, as either a focal mass

Table 8.15 Low-density/Necrotic Lymph Nodes

Common
Infectious granulomatous diseases
Tuberculosis
Fungal infections (histoplasmosis)
Metastases
Lung cancer
Extrathoracic malignancy
Lymphoma
Rare
Sarcoidosis

or generalized widening (see Figs. 7.33 and 7.34 in Chapter 7). Lymph node enlargement or mediastinal infiltration can be seen. Any portion of the mediastinum can be affected.

CASTLEMAN DISEASE

CD (also referred to by a number of other terms, including angiofollicular mediastinal lymph node hyperplasia, angiomatous lymphoid hamartoma, and giant mediastinal lymph node hyperplasia) is a lymphoproliferative disease. Histologically, three forms of the disease are now recognized: the unicentric or hyaline vascular type, idiopathic multicentric, and the Kaposi sarcoma–associated herpesvirus/human herpesvirus 8 (KSHV/HHV-8)-associated multicentric type (Table 8.17). From a clinical standpoint, these types of CD are also classified as localized or multicentric, respectively.

Unicentric or localized Castleman disease, associated with the hyaline vascular type, involves "Castleman-like" lymph node abnormalities in a single site. It usually is associated with few or no symptoms, other than those resulting from lymph node enlargement. In at least 90% of cases, removal of the enlarged node or nodes is curative with no further complications. Patients are usually children or young adults and are usually asymptomatic; their disease behaves in a benign fashion with cure following complete surgical resection. Typical imaging findings include a localized, mediastinal mass that is hyperenhancing on contrast studies (Fig. 8.43A and B).

Multicentric Castleman disease (MCD) involves "Castleman-like" lymph node abnormalities at multiple sites, and patients often demonstrate intense episodes of systemic inflammation, polyclonal/reactive lymphocyte and plasma cell proliferation, autoimmune symptoms, and multiple organ system impairment. Unlike the hyaline vascular type of CD, the plasma cell variety often presents as a multicentric process, associated with generalized lymphadenopathy and hepatosplenomegaly (see Figs. 8.40A and 8.43C). MCD likely results from hyperactivation of the immune system, excessive release of proinflammatory chemicals (cytokines), proliferation of immune cells (B cells and T cells), and multiple organ system dysfunction. Approximately 50% of MCD are associated

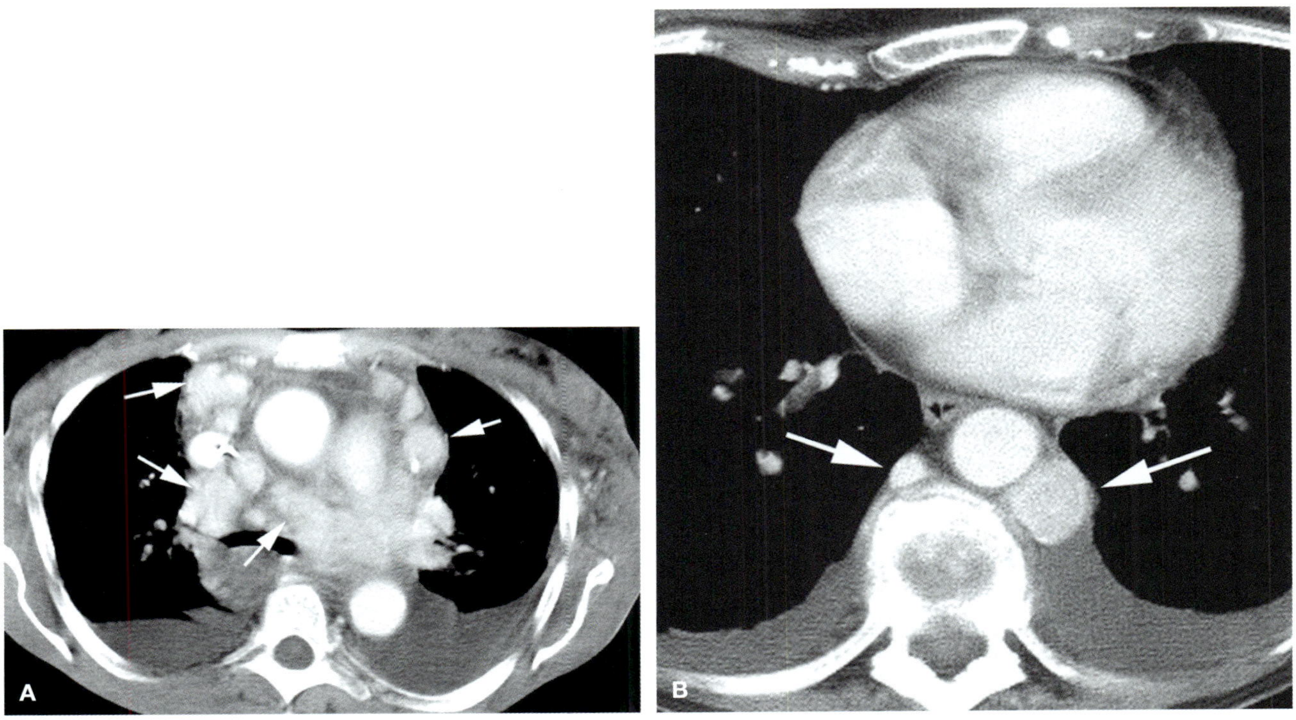

Figure 8.40. Enhancing lymph nodes. **A:** Multiple enlarged lymph nodes (*arrows*) in multicentric plasma cell–type Castleman disease show dense enhancement. **B:** Enhancing paravertebral (para-aortic) lymph node metastases (*arrows*) from a paraganglioma.

Table 8.16 Enhancing Lymph Nodes
Common
Metastases (vascular tumors)
Tuberculosis
Rare
Castleman disease
Sarcoidosis
Angioimmunoblastic lymphadenopathy

with HHV-8, also termed KSHV, which is now considered a specific subtype as described above. Such cases demonstrate "plasmablastic" lymph node abnormalities. Most patients with HHV-8–associated MCD are also HIV positive.

Clinically, multicentric disease occurs in an older population than localized CD, with most patients being in their fifth or sixth decade. It often results in a systemic illness, associated with fever, anemia, infections, and malignancies such as lymphoma or Kaposi's sarcoma. When associated with localized node involvement, such systemic findings usually disappear following total resection; however, the multicentric form of disease is difficult to treat and usually progressive, even with the use of steroids and chemotherapeutic agents.

Plain radiographs may show a well-defined focal mass (localized CD), involving any part of the mediastinum (see Fig. 8.43A and B), or findings of lymph node enlargement (multicentric CD) (see Figs. 8.40A and 8.43C).

On contrast-enhanced CT, localized CD typically shows dense contrast enhancement; any mediastinal compartment can be involved. Central, dense, or flocculent lymph node calcifications are occasionally seen. Patients with multicentric CD evaluated using contrast-enhanced CT have shown early, dense, uniform enhancement of enlarged mediastinal lymph nodes. Axillary, abdominal, and other lymph node groups may also be involved.

OTHER LYMPHOPROLIFERATIVE DISORDERS

In addition to those diseases listed above, a variety of uncommon lymphoproliferative diseases affecting the lung can be associated with hilar or mediastinal lymph node enlargement. These include posttransplantation lymphoproliferative disorders, lymphoid interstitial pneumonia, and lymphomatoid granulomatosis. These are described in Chapter 7.

METASTATIC TUMOR

Metastases to mediastinal or hilar lymph nodes from extrathoracic malignancies are uncommon, occurring in less than 3% of cases. The extrathoracic tumors most likely to metastasize to the mediastinum are carcinomas of the head and

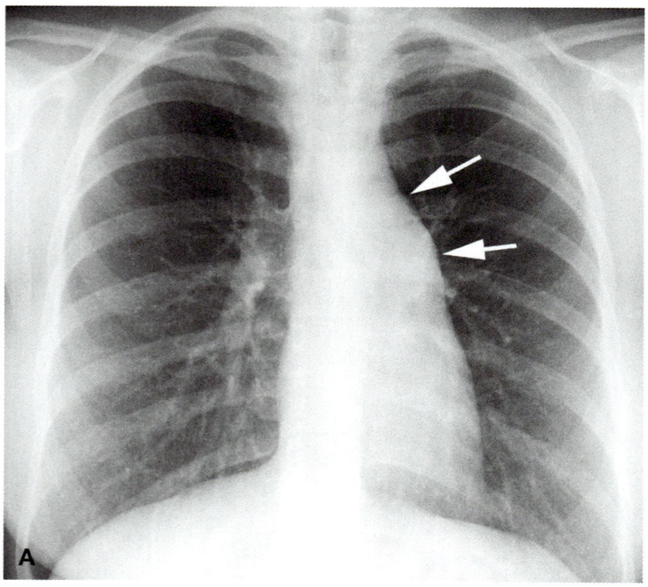

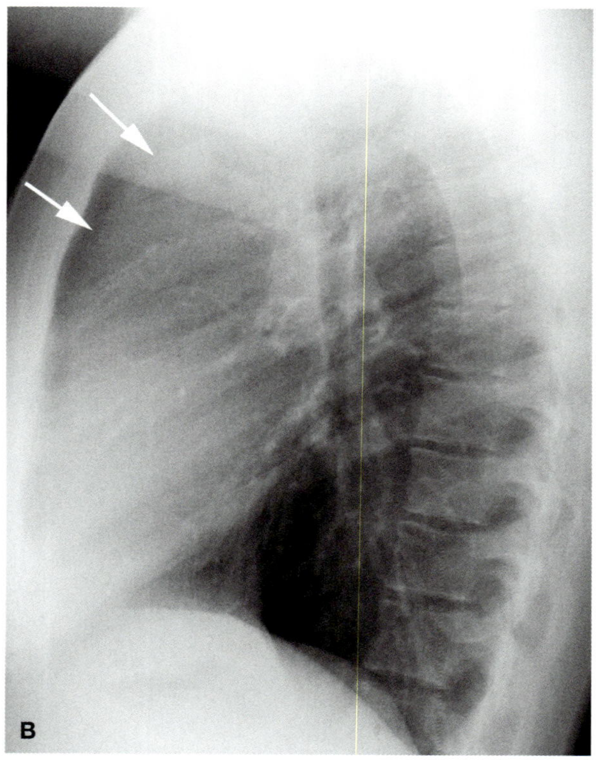

Figure 8.41. Superior mediastinal lymph nodes in Hodgkin disease. **A:** PA radiograph shows a mass (*arrows*) in the region of the aortopulmonary window. **B:** An anterior mediastinal mass (*arrows*) is visible on lateral chest radiograph.

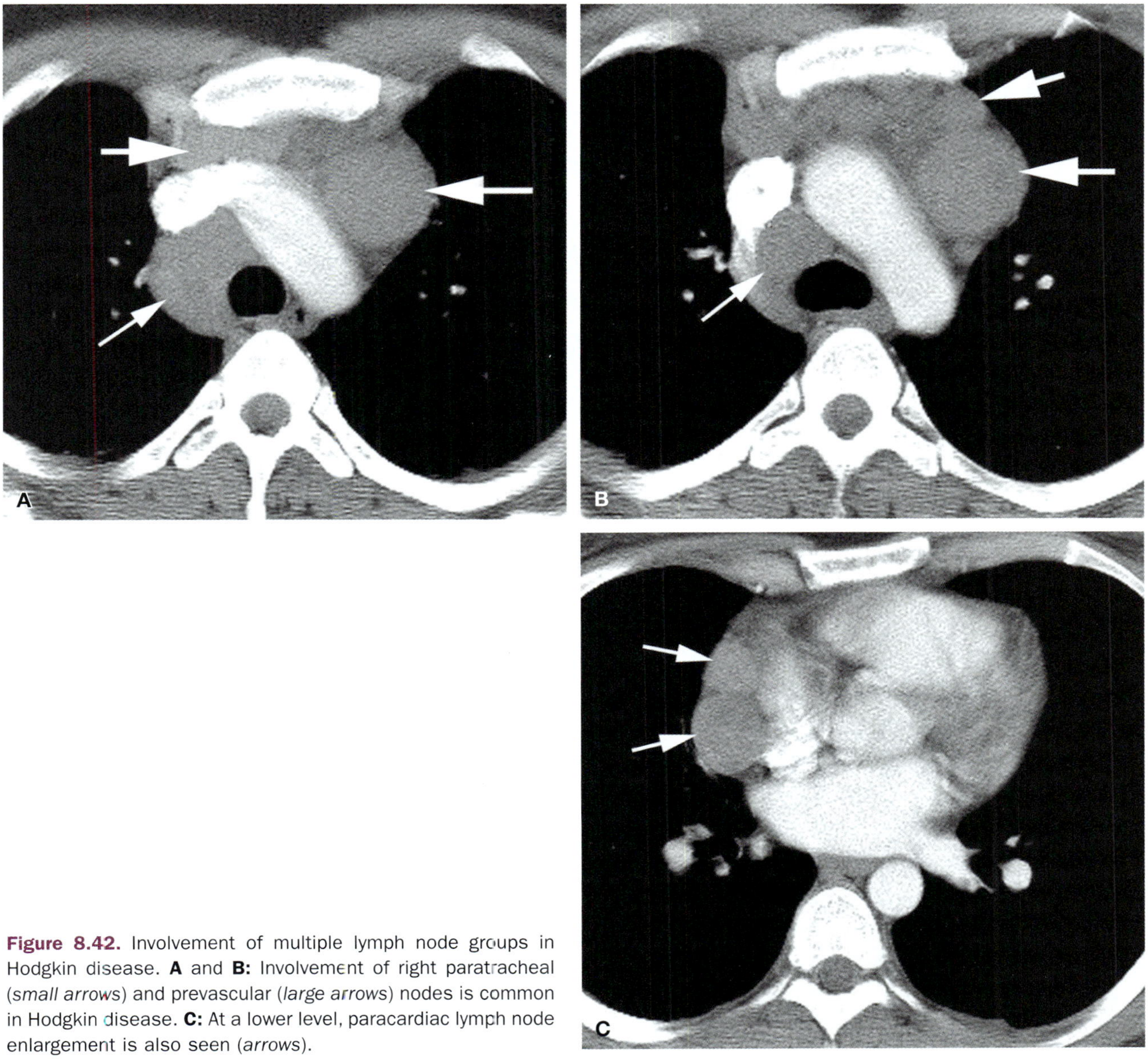

Figure 8.42. Involvement of multiple lymph node groups in Hodgkin disease. **A** and **B:** Involvement of right paratracheal (*small arrows*) and prevascular (*large arrows*) nodes is common in Hodgkin disease. **C:** At a lower level, paracardiac lymph node enlargement is also seen (*arrows*).

neck, genitourinary tract, and breast and malignant melanoma. Metastases are discussed in detail in Chapter 5.

Most metastatic tumors cause lymph node enlargement without distinguishing characteristics. However, enhancing nodes may be seen secondary to metastatic renal cell carcinoma, papillary thyroid carcinoma, lung cancer, sarcomas, and melanoma. Lymph node metastases can also appear cystic, necrotic, or calcified. Calcified lymph node metastases are most typical of thyroid carcinoma or mucinous adenocarcinoma.

The location of enlarged nodes is sometimes suggestive of the primary tumor site. Lymph node enlargement involving posterior mediastinal and paravertebral lymph nodes suggests an abdominal location for the primary tumor, and superior mediastinal lymph node involvement suggests a head and neck tumor. Internal mammary lymph node metastases are most likely due to breast carcinoma. Paracardiac lymph node enlargement can occur as a result of metastasis from abdominal or thoracic tumors in approximately equal numbers. In studies reviewing the causes of paracardiac lymph node enlargement, although a variety of metastatic tumors were responsible, the most common were colon carcinoma, lung carcinoma, ovarian carcinoma, and breast carcinoma.

SARCOIDOSIS

Mediastinal lymph node enlargement is very common with sarcoidosis, occurring in 60% to 90% of patients at some stage in their disease. About half of these will also show findings of lung disease on plain radiographs. A greater percentage

Table 8.17 Castleman Disease

Angiofollicular lymph node hyperplasia
Hyaline vascular (unicentric) and plasma cell (multicentric) types (50% idiopathic; 50% KSHV/HHV-8)
Dense enhancement on CT is typical
Hyaline vascular type
- 90% of cases
- Children or young adults
- Often asymptomatic
- Localized mediastinal or hilar mass
- Behaves in a benign fashion

Plasma cell type (multicentric)
- 10% of cases
- Patients 40-50 years old
- Usually multicentric, multiple node groups involved
- Systemic illness
- Progressive

KSHV/HHV-8, Kaposi sarcoma–associated herpesvirus/human herpesvirus-8.

of patients with lymph node enlargement due to sarcoidosis show evidence of lung disease on CT.

Typically, node enlargement involves the hilar as well as mediastinal node groups, and lymph node masses appear bilateral and symmetrical on chest radiographs (Fig. 8.44A); the combination of bilateral hilar and paratracheal node enlargement usually allows the differentiation of sarcoidosis from lymphoma. The combination of (1) right paratracheal, (2) right hilar, and (3) left hilar node enlargement is termed the 1-2-3 pattern and is typical of sarcoidosis. In patients also having aortopulmonary node enlargement, a 1-2-3-4 pattern is said to be present (see Figs. 8.44A and 8.45A). The presence of hilar lymph node enlargement is so typical of sarcoidosis that the absence of this finding in a patient with mediastinal lymphadenopathy should lead one to question the diagnosis.

On chest radiographs, lymph node enlargement is seen, in order of decreasing frequency, in the hilar (85%-95% of those with lymph node enlargement), right paratracheal (75%), aortopulmonary (50%-75%), subcarinal (20%), and anterior mediastinal (10%-15%) regions; internal mammary, paravertebral, and retrocrural lymph node

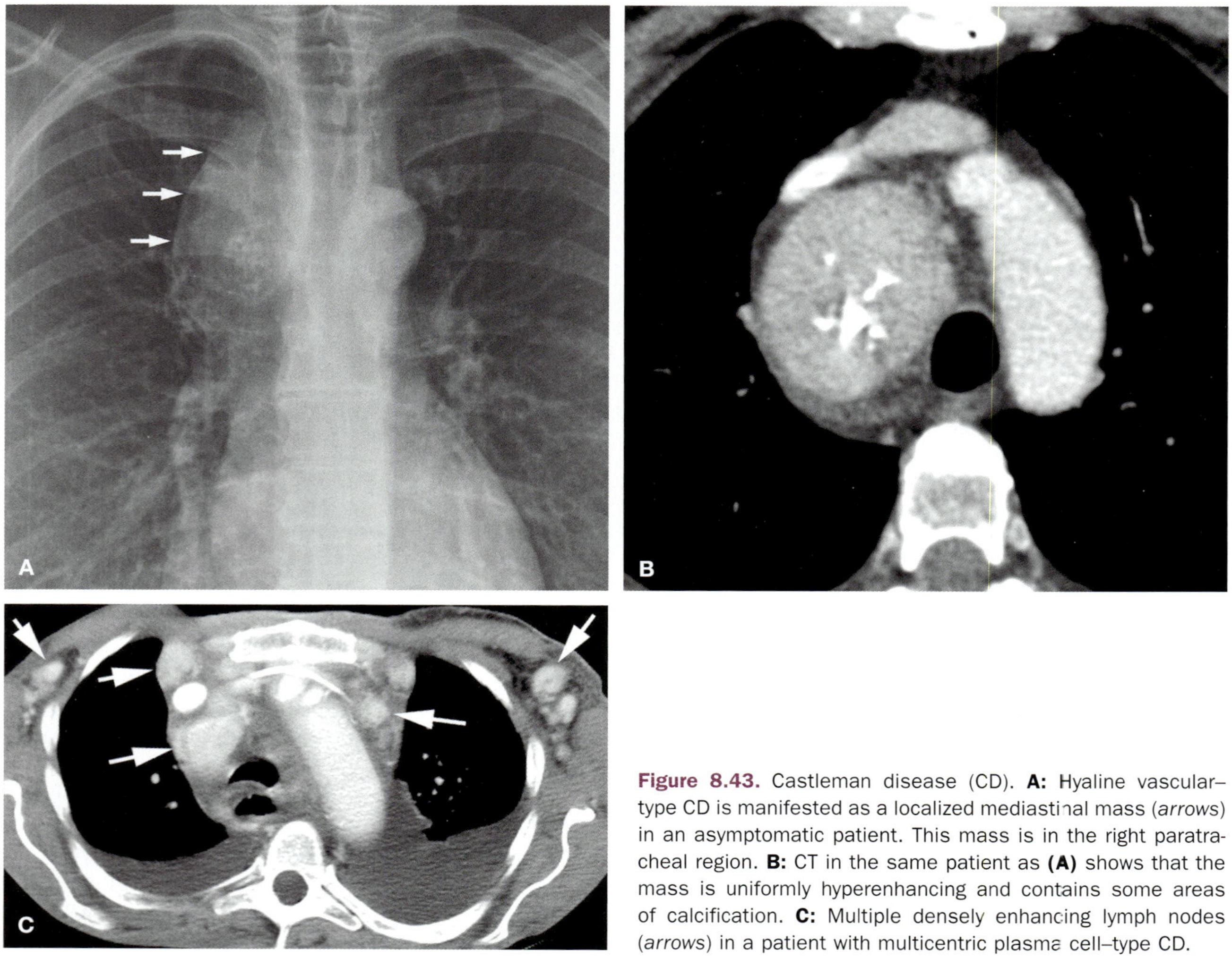

Figure 8.43. Castleman disease (CD). **A:** Hyaline vascular–type CD is manifested as a localized mediastinal mass (*arrows*) in an asymptomatic patient. This mass is in the right paratracheal region. **B:** CT in the same patient as **(A)** shows that the mass is uniformly hyperenhancing and contains some areas of calcification. **C:** Multiple densely enhancing lymph nodes (*arrows*) in a patient with multicentric plasma cell–type CD.

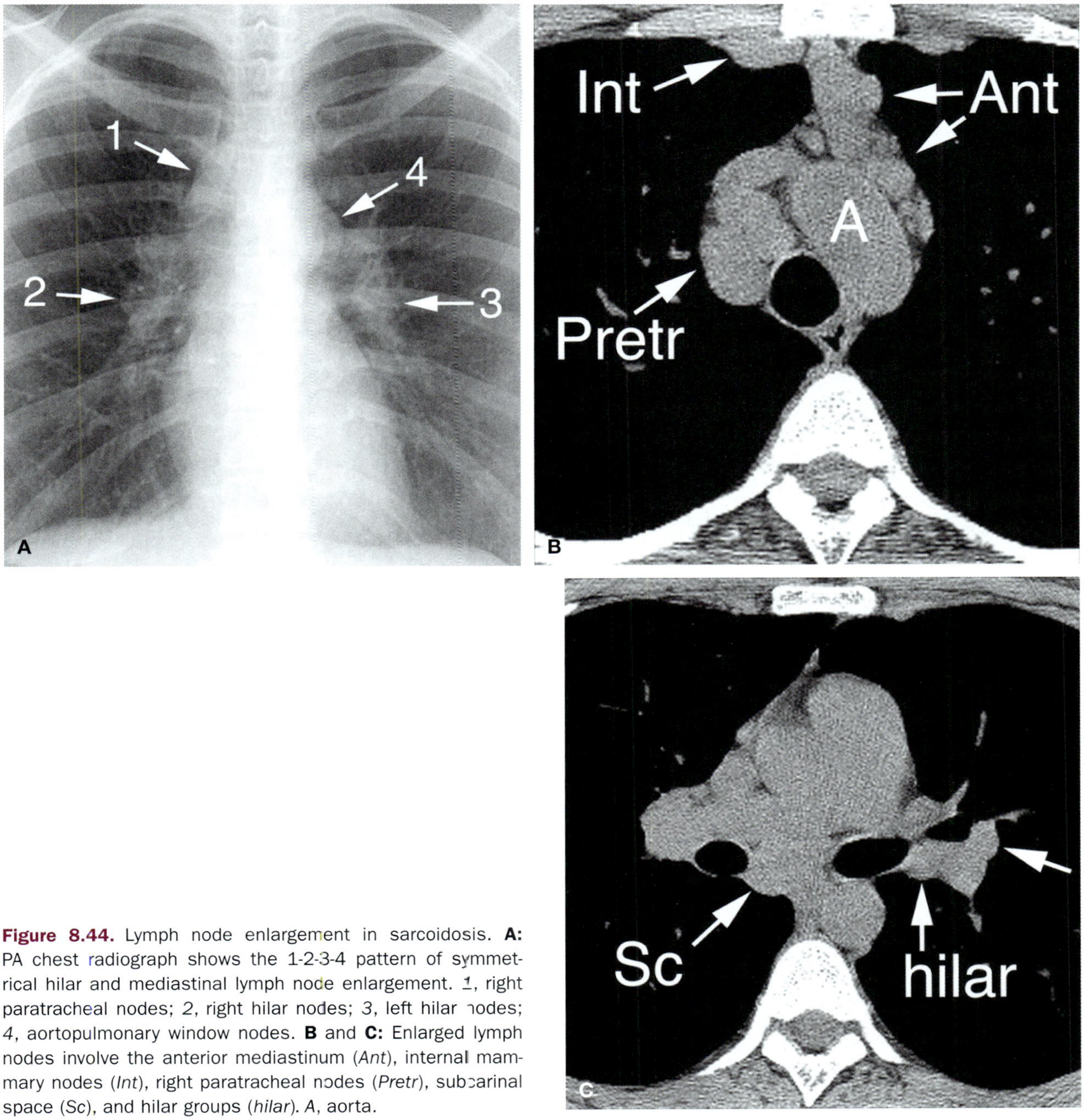

Figure 8.44. Lymph node enlargement in sarcoidosis. **A:** PA chest radiograph shows the 1-2-3-4 pattern of symmetrical hilar and mediastinal lymph node enlargement. *1*, right paratracheal nodes; *2*, right hilar nodes; *3*, left hilar nodes; *4*, aortopulmonary window nodes. **B** and **C:** Enlarged lymph nodes involve the anterior mediastinum (*Ant*), internal mammary nodes (*Int*), right paratracheal nodes (*Pretr*), subcarinal space (Sc), and hilar groups (*hilar*). *A*, aorta.

enlargement can also be seen, but these locations are much less common (Table 8.18; see Figs. 8.44 and 8.45). Unilateral hilar lymph node enlargement shown on plain radiographs is seen in less than 5% of cases. Lymph node calcification may be seen on chest films, appearing dense, stippled, or eggshell in appearance.

On CT, lymph node enlargement is visible in more than 80% to 95% of cases of sarcoidosis, with the great majority showing both hilar and mediastinal lymph node enlargement. A greater frequency of node enlargement is seen on CT than on chest radiographs, and symmetrical adenopathy is more often visible than on chest films. Enlarged lymph nodes may be seen in any part of the mediastinum but are most frequent in the right or left paratracheal or tracheobronchial regions, the aortopulmonary window, subcarinal space, and hila.

In patients with sarcoidosis, lymph nodes can be several centimeters in diameter, but sarcoid is not generally associated with large localized masses as is lymphoma. Lymph node calcification is visible on CT in 25% to 50% of cases (see Fig. 8.45). As on chest radiographs, it may appear hazy or dense or have a stippled or eggshell appearance. Rarely, nodes appear necrotic or low in attenuation or enhancing on contrast-enhanced scans.

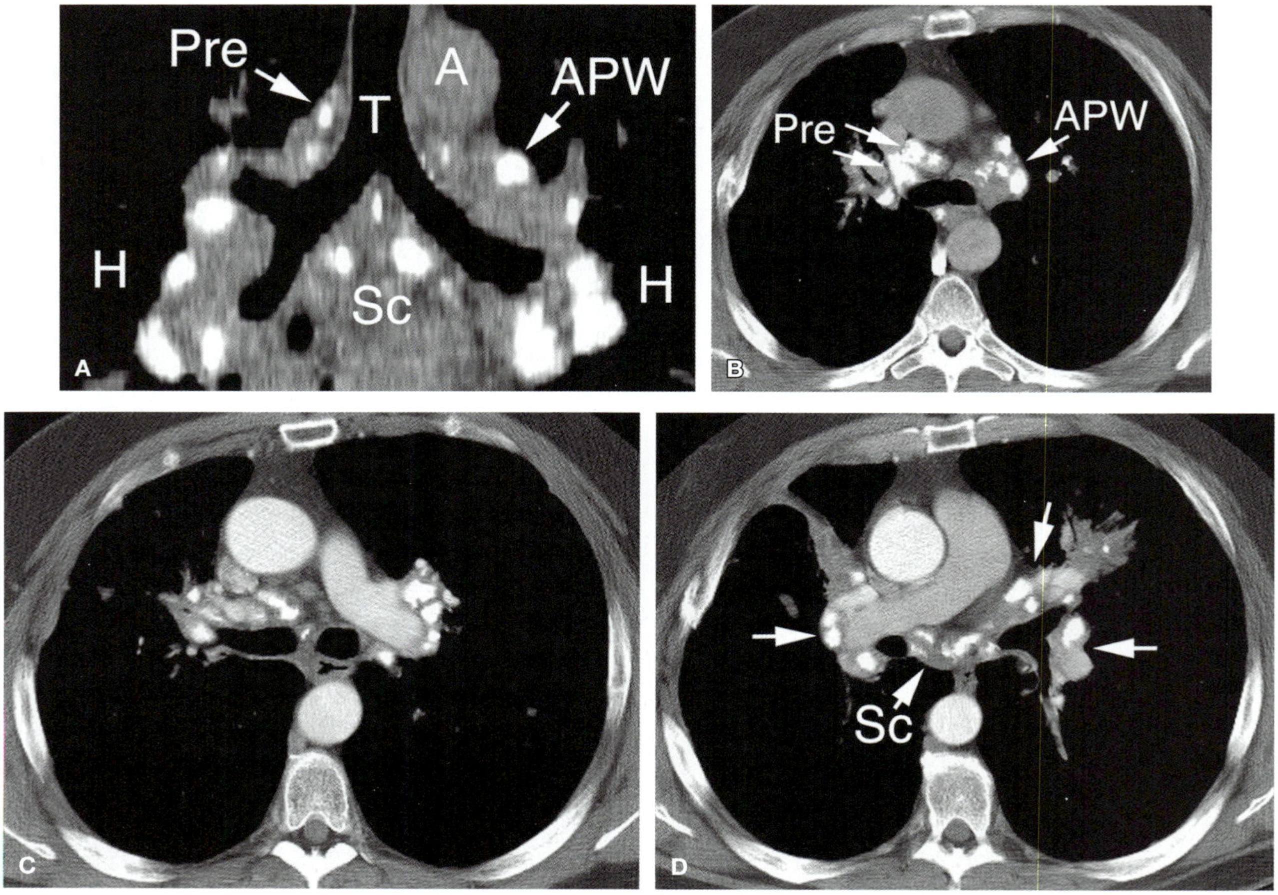

Figure 8.45. Lymph node enlargement and calcification in sarcoidosis. **A:** Coronal reconstruction shows symmetric mediastinal and hilar involvement with sarcoidosis (ie, the 1-2-3-4 pattern). The lymph nodes are densely calcified. *Pre*, right paratracheal; *APW*, aortopulmonary window; *H*, hilar; *Sc*, subcarinal; *A*, aorta; *T*, trachea. **B:** Calcified right paratracheal (*Pre*) and aortopulmonary window (*APW*) nodes in the same patient. **C:** Calcified precarinal and hilar nodes. **D:** Calcified subcarinal (*Sc*) and hilar nodes (*arrows*). Areas of consolidation represent atelectasis due to bronchial narrowing by nodes.

Table 8.18 Sarcoidosis: Frequency of Enlarged Nodes Seen on Chest Radiograph and CT by Lymph Node Group in Patients With Enlarged Nodes

Node Group	Radiograph (%)	CT (%)
Hilar	85-95	90
Right paratracheal	75	100
Aortopulmonary window	50-75	90
Subcarinal	20	65
Anterior mediastinal	10-15	50
Posterior mediastinal	<5	15

A variety of patterns of pulmonary involvement, from small nodules to large ill-defined masses or pulmonary fibrosis, can also be seen in patients with sarcoidosis (see Chapter 16). It is common to see typical features of sarcoid lung involvement on high-resolution CT without lymph node enlargement being visible.

INFECTIONS

A variety of infectious agents can cause mediastinal lymph node enlargement during the acute phase of disease. These include tuberculosis, a number of fungal infections including histoplasmosis and coccidioidomycosis, bacterial infections, and viral infections. Typically, there are symptoms and signs of acute infection and chest radiographs show evidence of lung disease, although this is not always the case. In patients with prior granulomatous infection, lymph node calcification is common, with such nodes appearing normal in size or enlarged.

Tuberculosis

Hilar and mediastinal lymph node enlargement is commonly seen on plain radiographs and CT in patients with active tuberculosis (Table 8.19), although it is more frequently seen in children than adults.

Lymph node enlargement is usually present on the side of lung disease (Fig. 8.46A), but involvement of contralateral nodes is sometimes present. Although the presence of lymphadenopathy on chest radiographs in the absence of visible lung disease is unusual in tuberculosis, this is not always the case (see Fig. 8.46B).

Right-sided adenopathy usually predominates, and specifically, right paratracheal lymph node enlargement is most common (see Fig. 8.46A and B). Bilateral hilar lymph node enlargement is much less common than in sarcoidosis.

In patients with active tuberculosis, nodes larger than 2 cm in diameter commonly show central areas of low attenuation on contrast-enhanced CT, with peripheral rim enhancement (see Fig. 8.46C). The areas of relative low attenuation are not of water density but range from about 40 to 60 HU; they are usually visible only on contrast-enhanced scans. Areas of low attenuation involving the mediastinum with obliteration of mediastinal fat represent tuberculous mediastinitis or a cold abscess. Rim-enhancing lymph nodes have also been reported in nearly 85% of AIDS patients with tuberculosis.

Three patterns of lymph node enlargement have been reported on MRI in patients with tuberculosis, correlating with clinical symptoms and pathologic findings and paralleling the expected CT findings in such patients. In patients

Table 8.19 Lymph Node Enlargement in Patients With Active Tuberculosis Shown on CT

Site	ATS Designation	% Abnormal
Right paratracheal	2R	80
Left paratracheal	2L	5
Right paratracheal	4R	85
Left paratracheal	4L	10
Right tracheobronchial	10R	65
Subcarinal	7	50
Aortopulmonary	5	35
Right hilar	11R	30
Left hilar	11L	10

ATS, American Thoracic Society.

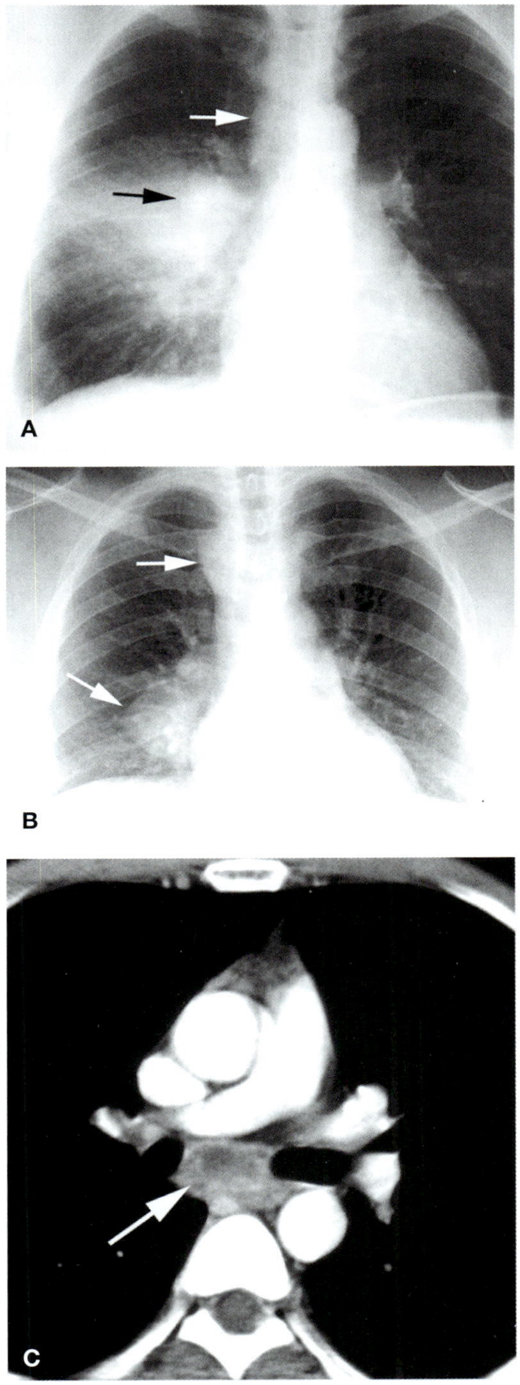

Figure 8.46. Lymph node enlargement in tuberculosis. **A:** Primary tuberculosis with right lung consolidation, right hilar lymph node enlargement (*black arrow*), and right paratracheal lymph node enlargement manifested by widening of the right paratracheal stripe (*white arrow*). **B:** Tuberculosis in AIDS with right hilar and right paratracheal lymph node enlargement (*arrows*). **C:** Tuberculosis with a low-attenuation, rim-enhancing subcarinal lymph node mass (*arrow*).

with necrosis and active TB, nodes are heterogeneous with marked peripheral enhancement after injection of contrast material. Nodes with granulomatous inflammation, but without necrosis, appear relatively homogeneous and hyperintense to muscle on both T1-weighted and T2-weighted images and enhance homogeneously after contrast infusion. Inactive fibrocalcific nodes are homogeneous and hypointense on both T1-weighted and T2-weighted images, without enhancement after contrast infusion.

Histoplasmosis

Infection with *Histoplasma capsulatum* is a well-recognized cause of hilar and mediastinal lymph node enlargement. In patients with acute or subacute histoplasmosis, radiographs and CT may show paratracheal, subcarinal, and hilar lymph node enlargement. On CT, irregular enhancement, rim enhancement, and low-attenuation necrosis may be seen, as in patients with tuberculosis. Masses range up to several centimeters in diameter.

FM AND IGG4-RELATED DISEASE

In some patients with granulomatous disease involving mediastinal lymph nodes, extension of the disease process to involve surrounding mediastinal tissues results in extensive fibrosis (Table 8.20). This is termed *fibrosing mediastinitis* or *granulomatous mediastinitis*. Symptomatic encasement and/or compression of a number of mediastinal structures, particularly vessels, and the trachea or esophagus can result. The most common causes are histoplasmosis, tuberculosis, and sarcoidosis, but FM has also been associated with autoimmune disease, retroperitoneal fibrosis, sclerosing cholangitis, Behçet disease, Riedel thyroiditis, pseudotumor of the orbit, or drugs (ie, methysergide), or may be idiopathic.

Table 8.20 Fibrosing Mediastinitis

Causes
Histoplasmosis
Tuberculosis
Sarcoidosis
Autoimmune diseases
IgG4-related disease (IgG4-RD)
Drugs
Retroperitoneal fibrosis
Idiopathic
Results in narrowing or obstruction of mediastinal or hilar structures, including superior vena cava, trachea, left main bronchus, right pulmonary artery, pulmonary veins, esophagus
Two patterns
Focal: 80% of cases
Localized masses of soft tissue
Calcifications common
Often due to histoplasmosis or IgG4-dRD
Diffuse: 20% of cases
Diffuse infiltration of mediastinum
Calcification less common
Idiopathic or related to causes other than histoplasmosis

It has recently been found that FM, with features identical to those of histoplasmosis-related FM, may be a manifestation of *IgG4-related disease (IgG4-RD),* a relapsing immune-mediated fibroinflammatory condition characterized by tissue-destructive and fibrotic lesions, including many features previously associated with idiopathic FM, including retroperitoneal fibrosis, Riedel thyroiditis, sclerosing cholangitis, pseudotumor of the orbit, and large vessel vasculitis (eg, aortitis or periaortitis). It is likely that up to one-third of patients with either serological or radiological evidence of prior histoplasmosis and typical features of FM, in fact, have IgG4-RD. It is unclear whether typical histologic features of IgG4-RD in these patients occur as an immune response to *Histoplasma* or represent a manifestation of primary IgG4-RD.

Two distinct patterns of mediastinal involvement may be seen in patients with FM. A focal pattern, seen in about 80% of cases, is associated with a localized mass or masses of soft-tissue attenuation, usually in the right paratracheal, subcarinal regions, or hila. Masses often show stippled or diffuse calcification. This localized form of FM is most likely caused by histoplasmosis.

A diffuse pattern of involvement, seen in 20% of cases, results in an infiltrating mass of fibrous tissue, affecting multiple mediastinal compartments. Calcification is less common. The diffuse pattern may be related to causes other than histoplasmosis, such as IgG4-RD. CT shows replacement of low-density mediastinal fat by higher-density fibrous tissue. FDG-PET typically shows increased activity.

Compression and/or encasement of the trachea, main bronchi, or mediastinal vessels is commonly present (Fig. 8.47). Structures most often involved are those that have the thinnest walls (eg, superior vena cava) or the longest mediastinal course (eg, trachea and left main bronchus and right pulmonary artery). In patients with FM, the most common complications are narrowing or obstruction of the superior vena cava (40%), bronchi (35%), pulmonary artery (20%), and esophagus (10%). Rarely, these findings primarily affect the posterior mediastinum, with esophageal encasement and dysphagia predominating.

FAT ATTENUATION LESIONS

Fat is specifically recognized on CT by its low CT numbers, which vary from −40 to −130 HU. Fat is normally present in the mediastinum, and its amount often increases with age.

Normal fat is unencapsulated and equally distributed throughout the connective tissue matrix of the mediastinum.

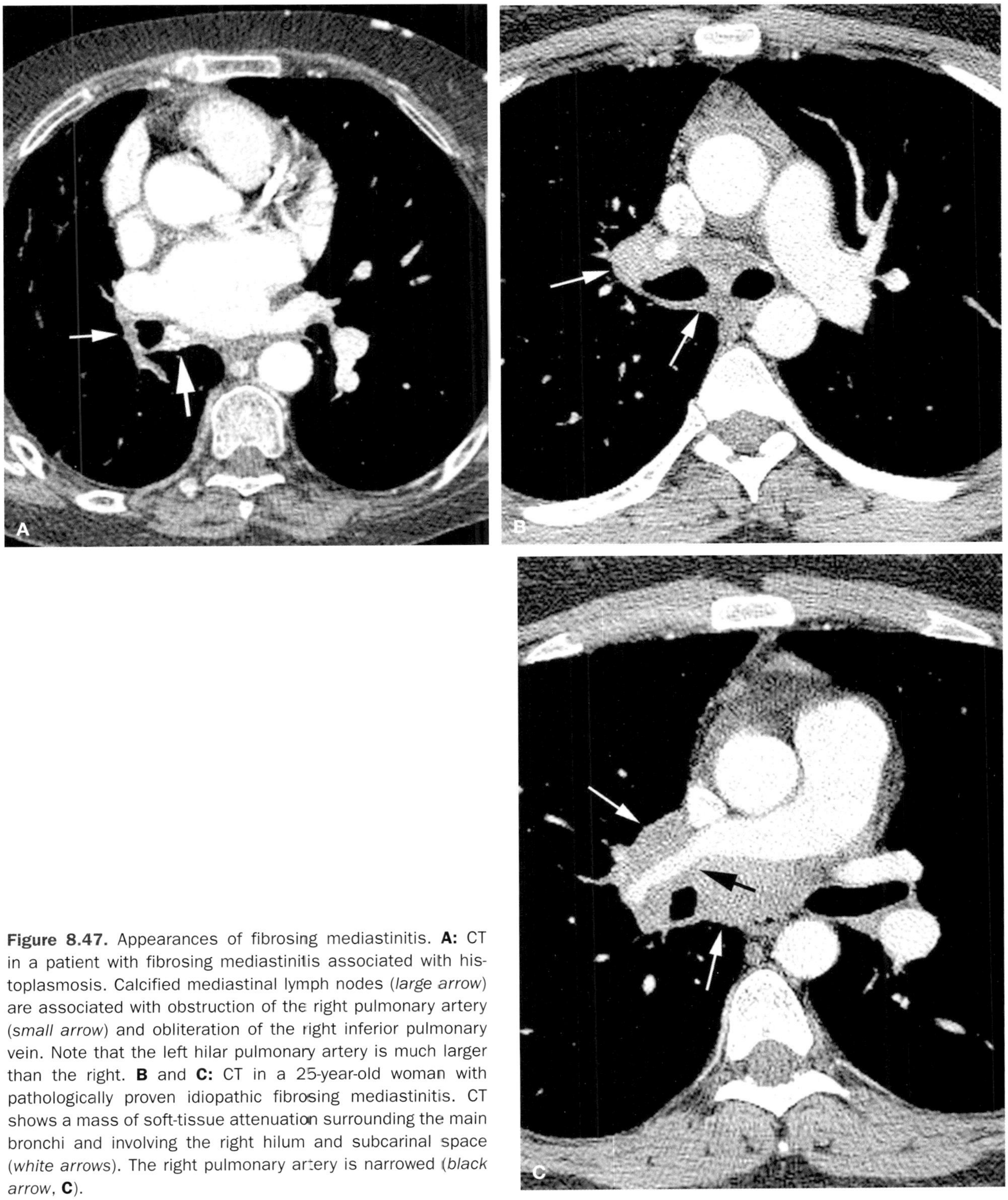

Figure 8.47. Appearances of fibrosing mediastinitis. **A:** CT in a patient with fibrosing mediastinitis associated with histoplasmosis. Calcified mediastinal lymph nodes (*large arrow*) are associated with obstruction of the right pulmonary artery (*small arrow*) and obliteration of the right inferior pulmonary vein. Note that the left hilar pulmonary artery is much larger than the right. **B** and **C:** CT in a 25-year-old woman with pathologically proven idiopathic fibrosing mediastinitis. CT shows a mass of soft-tissue attenuation surrounding the main bronchi and involving the right hilum and subcarinal space (*white arrows*). The right pulmonary artery is narrowed (*black arrow*, **C**).

The contours of the mediastinum are not generally affected by normal amounts of fat. However, accumulations of fat in the anterior cardiophrenic angles, or epicardiac fat pads, can be asymmetric and can suggest the presence of a mass on chest radiographs.

Abnormalities of fat distribution can be diffuse (ie, mediastinal lipomatosis) or focal (eg, lipoma or fat-containing diaphragmatic hernias; Table 8.21). In the large majority of cases, discovery of the fatty nature of a mass indicates its benign nature.

Table 8.21 Masses Containing Fat
Lipomatosis and fat pads
Lipoma or liposarcoma
Thymolipoma
Teratoma
Lymphangioma and hemangioma
Hibernoma
Hernias containing fat
Extramedullary hematopoiesis

Mediastinal Lipomatosis

Lipomatosis is a benign condition in which excessive amounts of histologically normal, unencapsulated fat accumulate in the mediastinum. Lipomatosis may be associated with Cushing syndrome, steroid treatment, or obesity, but these factors are absent in up to half of cases. It is unassociated with symptoms. Lipomatosis is relatively common and is often detected incidentally in patients having chest radiographs or CT.

The excess fat deposition is most prominent in the upper mediastinum, resulting in smooth symmetrical mediastinal widening as shown on chest radiographs (Fig. 8.48A) and convex or bulging mediastinal pleural surfaces on CT. The appearance of smooth mediastinal widening on a plain radiograph is characteristic of mediastinal lipomatosis and, in patients with a suitable clinical history, usually requires no further evaluation. Tracheal compression or displacement is absent. Less commonly, fat also accumulates in the cardiophrenic angles and paraspinal areas. In patients with lipomatosis, the fat should appear homogeneously low in attenuation, sharply outlining mediastinal vessels and lymph nodes (see Figs. 8.48B and 8.49). If the fat appears inhomogeneous or the margins of mediastinal structures are ill defined, superimposed processes such as mediastinitis, hemorrhage, tumor infiltration, and fibrosis may be present.

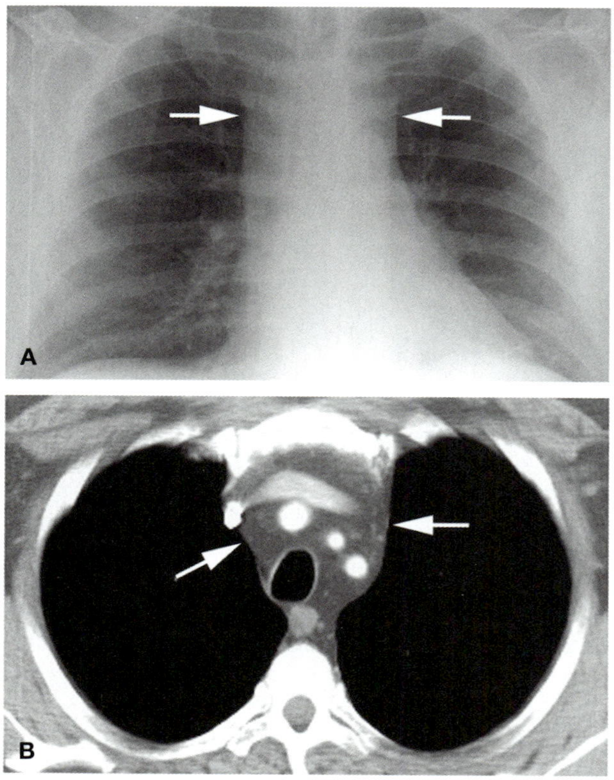

Figure 8.48. Lipomatosis. **A:** Chest radiograph shows smooth symmetrical widening of the upper mediastinum (*arrows*). **B:** CT shows homogeneous fat filling the mediastinum (*arrows*).

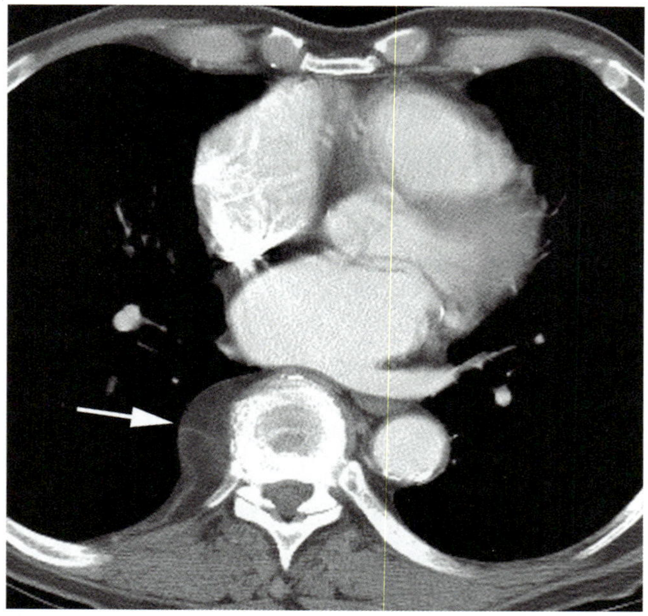

Figure 8.49. Paravertebral lipomatosis. Fat is visible in the posterior mediastinum (*arrow*).

Lipoma and Liposarcoma

Mediastinal *lipoma* is uncommon, constituting approximately 2% of all mediastinal tumors. As with other mesenchymal tumors, lipomas can occur in any part of the mediastinum but are most common in the prevascular space. Lipomas are soft and pliable and do not result in symptomatic compression of adjacent structures unless they are very large. They may or may not be encapsulated. Lipomas appear homogeneously low in attenuation. Their boundaries are typically smooth and sharply defined, and adjacent mediastinal structures appear well defined and sharply marginated.

Mediastinal *liposarcoma* and *lipoblastoma* are rare malignant tumors composed largely of fat. Histologic differentiation between a lipoma and well-differentiated liposarcoma depends on the presence of mitotic activity, cellular atypia, fibrosis, neovascularization, and tumor infiltration. CT findings suggesting liposarcoma or lipoblastoma include (1) heterogeneous attenuation with evidence of significant amounts of soft tissue within the fatty mass (Fig. 8.50), (2) poor definition of adjacent mediastinal structures, or (3)

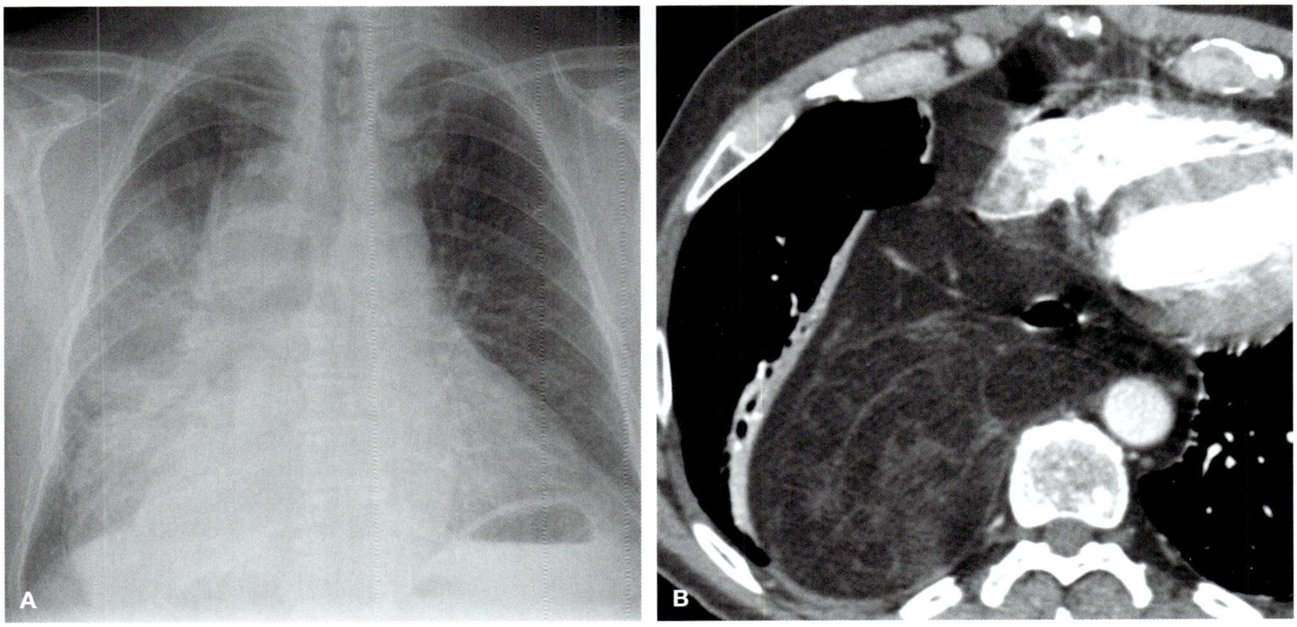

Figure 8.50. Liposarcoma. **A:** Chest radiograph shows a large mass involving much of the right mediastinal borders and the right hemithorax. **B:** The mass is infiltrative in multiple mediastinal compartments, exerting mass effect on the heart and compressing/encasing other mediastinal structures. The mass is predominantly fat attenuation but has central whorls and strands of soft-tissue attenuation.

evidence of infiltration or invasion of mediastinal structures. The diagnosis of a liposarcoma is often difficult using CT but tumors may be large and extend/infiltrate many mediastinal compartments.

Hibernoma and Brown Fat

Hibernoma represents a neoplasm derived from brown adipose tissue. It is usually seen in locations where normal brown fat is found in infants, such as the periscapular or interscapular region, the neck, the axilla, or within the thorax and mediastinum. It appears as a fatty mass, which can be large. There is no known malignant potential, and resection is curative.

Focal collections of brown fat may be present in normal subjects and generally go unrecognized. However, because brown fat is metabolically active, it may show uptake on FDG-PET, mimicking neoplasm. Hypermetabolic mediastinal deposits of fat are more often seen in children than in adults and more common in women than in men. Hypermetabolic brown fat may be seen in the paratracheal, paraesophageal, prevascular, and pericardial regions.

Hernias Containing Fat

There are several direct connections between the abdomen and mediastinum that permit passage of intra-abdominal fat into the thorax. Acquired diaphragmatic hernias may also occur in the setting of trauma or from surgery (see Chapter 27).

Omental fat is freely mobile and can herniate through the foramen of Morgagni to create the appearance of a cardiophrenic angle mass, almost always on the right side (Fig. 8.51A). The transverse colon may accompany the omentum in patients with a Morgagni hernia. Fine linear densities are sometimes seen within herniated omental fat and probably represent omental vessels. When seen within a fatty mass, these linear densities should suggest fat herniation rather than a lipoma.

Fat herniation through the foramen of Bochdalek occurs most frequently on the left side, since the presence of the liver limits its occurrence on the right. Although said to be most often located in the posterolateral diaphragm, they can occur anywhere along the posterior costodiaphragmatic margin and are often seen medially (see Fig. 8.51B). Bochdalek hernias in adults usually contain retroperitoneal fat, although kidney is occasionally present. CT has shown that small Bochdalek hernias occur in as many as 5% of normal individuals. Characteristically, a thinning or defect in the diaphragm is visible on CT, marginating the collection of fat. Lateral chest radiographs usually show a rounded mass in the posterior costophrenic angle.

Herniation of perigastric fat through the phrenicoesophageal membrane surrounding and fixating the esophagus to the diaphragm is the first step in the pathogenesis of hiatus hernias. The herniated fat can extend along the aorta and widen the paraspinal line, or it can appear as a retrocardiac mass.

Other Fatty Masses

Other rare, fatty lesions have been reported to involve the mediastinum. Thymolipoma usually appears on CT as a large

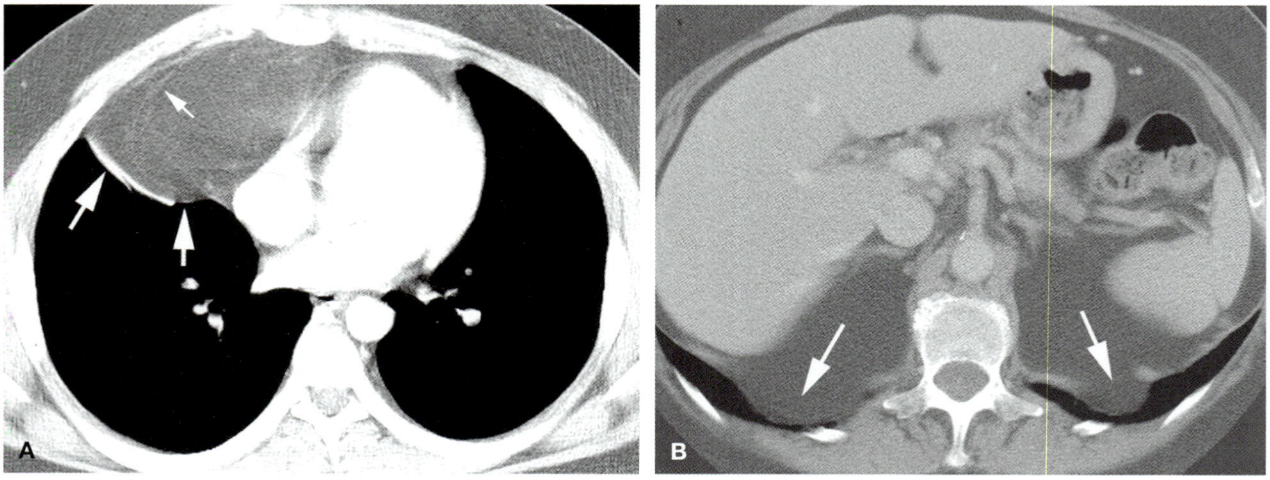

Figure 8.51. Fatty hernias. **A:** Morgagni hernia (*large arrows*) projecting into the right cardiophrenic angle. The hernia consists of omentum. Omental vessels (*small arrow*) are visible within the fatty mass. **B:** Bochdalek hernias (*arrows*) containing fat.

fatty mass in the anterior mediastinum, containing wisps or strands of fibrous tissue. Fat is also commonly identifiable as a component of mediastinal germ cell tumors. In the posterior mediastinum, spinal lipomas rarely present as primary mediastinal masses. Fatty transformation of thoracic extramedullary hematopoiesis may be seen in the posterior mediastinum.

MESENCHYMAL TUMORS AND MASSES NOT COMPOSED OF FAT

Mediastinal Fibromatosis (Desmoid Type)

Mediastinal fibromatosis is a rare entity that affects patients at all ages. It consists of dense and unencapsulated collagenous tissue and highly differentiated fibroblasts. Despite its benign nature, it infiltrates surrounding tissues and may surround or compress mediastinal structures, such as the aorta, trachea, esophagus, or heart. Treatment using surgery may be difficult but is directed at relieving the compression or obstruction of vital mediastinal structures. Although fibromatosis tends to recur locally, metastases do not occur. Imaging features are nonspecific, and biopsy is necessary for diagnosis. Fibromatosis usually appears on CT as a large, slowly growing, infiltrative, soft-tissue mass. It is most frequent in the middle or posterior mediastinum but may occur in any location.

Patients with esophageal involvement may present with dysphagia; a barium swallow may show a regular or eccentric stenosis without dilatation of the proximal esophagus. In such patients, CT typically demonstrates a periesophageal mass and allows evaluation of the extent of the lesion. In some patients, invasion of the chest wall, spinal canal, or abdomen is present.

On T1-weighted MRI, fibromatosis may appear isointense or slightly hyperintense relative to muscle. On T2-weighted images, it appears hyperintense relative to muscle. Enhancement occurs after intravenous administration of gadolinium.

Solitary Fibrous Tumor

Solitary fibrous tumor of the mediastinum is similar to solitary or localized fibrous tumor of the pleura but is much less common. A localized well-circumscribed mass is typically seen. Surgical resection is curative for benign lesions, but aggressive lesions may recur locally or metastasize.

Inflammatory Myofibroblastic Tumor

Inflammatory myofibroblastic tumor (IMT) is a tumor that most frequently arises in the lung; it may involve the mediastinum by direct extension from a pulmonary site of origin. It had been thought to be inflammatory but is now considered neoplastic. CT generally shows a sharply marginated, lobulated mass, ranging up to 13 cm or more in diameter. The mass may be seen to surround mediastinal structures if invasion occurs. IMT may appear homogeneous or heterogeneous in attenuation on CT and may or may not enhance with contrast infusion. It is described in Chapter 5.

Other Mesenchymal Tumors

Fibrosarcoma, malignant fibrous histiocytoma, leiomyoma, leiomyosarcoma, rhabdomyosarcoma, and malignant tumors of bone and cartilage are rare mediastinal tumors. These may occur anywhere in the mediastinum.

MEDIASTINAL CYSTS

Most mediastinal cysts are of congenital origin. Bronchogenic cyst, esophageal duplication cyst, and neurenteric cyst result from abnormalities in foregut development and are termed

Table 8.22 Bronchogenic Cyst

60% of foregut duplication cysts
Wall contains respiratory epithelium, smooth muscle, mucous glands, or cartilage
50% subcarinal; 20% paratracheal; 10% retrocardiac
Round, smooth, sharply defined
Wall thin or invisible on CT; wall may calcify
Fluid contents variable in attenuation on CT (0-40 HU)

"foregut duplication cysts". Pericardial cysts are mesothelial in origin. Thymic cyst, described above, may be congenital or acquired. Cysts account for about 10% of primary mediastinal masses in both adults and children.

Bronchogenic Cyst

Bronchogenic cysts are most common, representing about 60% of foregut duplication cysts (Table 8.22). They probably result from defective growth of the lung bud during fetal development. Bronchogenic cysts are lined by pseudostratified ciliated columnar epithelium, typical of the respiratory system, and frequently are associated with smooth muscle, mucous glands, or cartilage in the cyst wall. Bronchogenic cysts contain fluid, which ranges in color from clear to milky white to brown; the fluid can contain variable amounts of protein and can be serous, hemorrhagic, or highly viscous and gelatinous. Cyst fluid rarely contains milk of calcium.

Bronchogenic cysts can be present in any part of the mediastinum but are most commonly located in the middle or posterior mediastinum, near the carina (50%), in the paratracheal region (20%), adjacent to the esophagus (15%), or in a retrocardiac location (10%). Most occur in contact with the tracheobronchial tree and within 5 cm of the carina. A subcarinal location is most frequently seen. They rarely occur in the prevascular mediastinum or the inferior aspect of the paravertebral mediastinum.

On plain radiographs, bronchogenic cysts appear as smooth, sharply marginated, round or elliptical masses (Fig. 8.52A). They may be large and displace the trachea or bronchi. Subcarinal cysts may result in convexity in the superior aspect of the azygoesophageal recess.

On CT, bronchogenic cysts usually appear rounded or elliptical and smooth in contour; as on chest radiographs, they are sharply marginated (see Figs. 8.52B, 8.53A and B). The wall of a bronchogenic cyst appears thin or is imperceptible (see Fig. 8.52B). Rarely, calcification of the cyst wall is present. Because of the variable composition of the fluid contained within bronchogenic cysts, their attenuation on CT is highly variable. Half of bronchogenic cysts are of water attenuation; in the other half, the CT density ranges from being higher than water to higher than muscle. When dense, bronchogenic cysts may be difficult to distinguish from solid lesions. An important clue to the diagnosis can be their lack of enhancement on scans obtained following intravenous contrast infusion. Mediastinal bronchogenic cysts rarely contain air or become infected, although this is common in patients with a pulmonary bronchogenic cyst.

MRI is valuable in assessing cysts that do not appear fluid filled on CT. High signal intensity is characteristically seen within cysts on T2-weighted sequences regardless of the nature of the cyst contents, but a variable pattern of signal intensity may be seen on T1-weighted sequences, presumably because of variable cyst contents and the presence of protein or mucoid material and/or hemorrhage (see Fig. 8.53C and D). A high intensity on T1-weighted images reflects high protein content and is common with bronchogenic cysts.

Large bronchogenic cysts may be associated with symptoms because of compression of adjacent structures such as

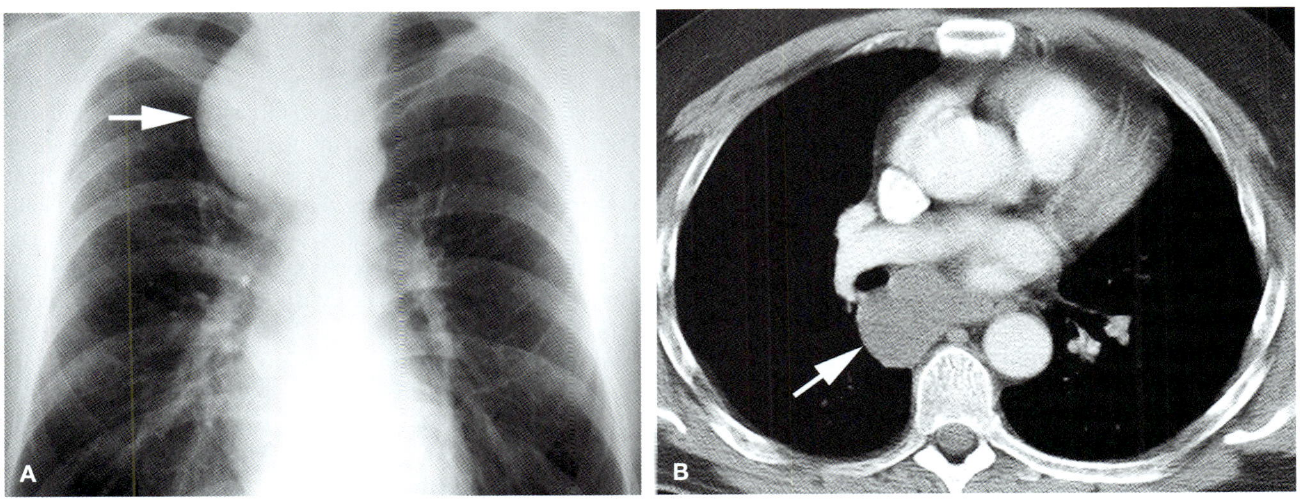

Figure 8.52. Bronchogenic cysts. **A:** A large smooth round right mediastinal mass (*arrow*) is visible on chest radiograph. **B:** In another patient, a low-attenuation subcarinal bronchogenic cyst (*arrow*) is visible. The cyst wall is invisible.

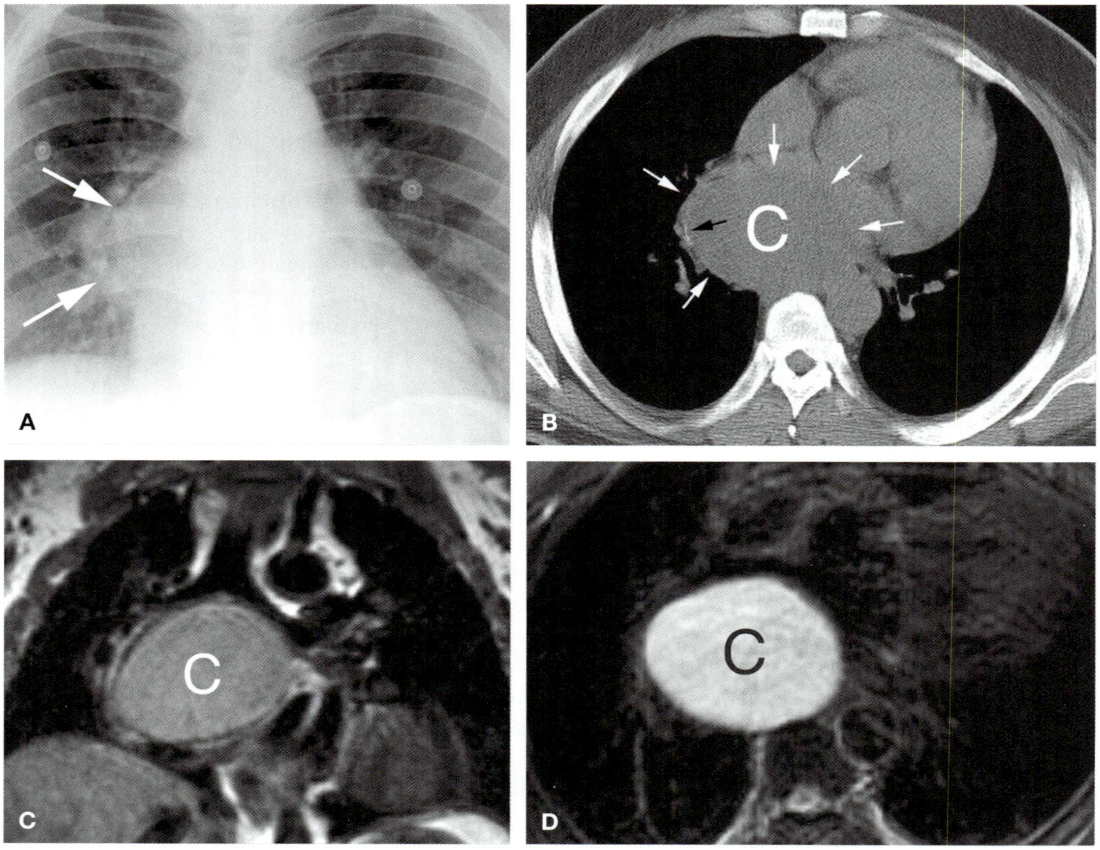

Figure 8.53. Bronchogenic cyst. **A:** A large subcarinal mass (*arrows*) is visible on chest radiograph. **B:** Unenhanced CT shows a large subcarinal bronchogenic cyst (*C, white arrows*), appearing slightly less dense than soft tissue. Focal calcification of the cyst wall is visible (*black arrow*). **C:** Coronal T1-weighted MRI shows a large subcarinal cyst. Signal from the cyst (*C*) is due to its protein content. **D:** Transaxial T2-weighted, fat-saturated image shows high signal intensity. This is typical. *C*, cyst.

the trachea and carina, mediastinal vessels, and left atrium. Small, asymptomatic cysts can be followed. However, enlargement over years is typical, and rapid enlargement associated with pain can indicate hemorrhage or infection. Because of their tendency to enlarge, surgical management has been traditional. Recently, percutaneous and transbronchial needle aspiration has also been used for the diagnosis and treatment of bronchogenic and esophageal duplication cysts.

Esophageal Duplication Cyst

Esophageal duplication cysts are lined by gastrointestinal tract mucosa and are often connected to the esophagus; unlike bronchogenic cysts, they do not contain cartilage. Sixty percent are found in the lower visceral compartment, adjacent to the esophagus, and are sometimes found within its wall. Their appearance on plain radiographs, CT, and MRI is indistinguishable from that of bronchogenic cysts, except for their paraesophageal location (Fig. 8.54). Rarely, the cyst wall calcifies.

Neurenteric Cyst

Neurenteric cyst is rare. It occurs in the paravertebral compartment and is connected to the meninges within the spinal canal through a midline defect in one or more vertebral bodies. They are composed of both neural and gastrointestinal elements, including gastric, salivary gland, adrenal, pancreatic, and intestinal tissues. A connection with the esophagus is often present. The appearance of neurenteric cyst on CT is the same as that of other duplication cysts, but the presence of a vertebral abnormality can point to the diagnosis (Fig. 8.55); vertebral anomalies (eg, hemivertebrae or butterfly vertebrae) or scoliosis is present in about half of cases. The cysts rarely contain air, because of communication with the esophagus. They frequently cause pain and are generally diagnosed at a young age.

Pericardial Cyst

Pericardial cyst reflects a defect in the embryogenesis of the coelomic cavity. The wall of a pericardial cyst is composed of connective tissue and a single layer of mesothelial cells. Most patients are asymptomatic.

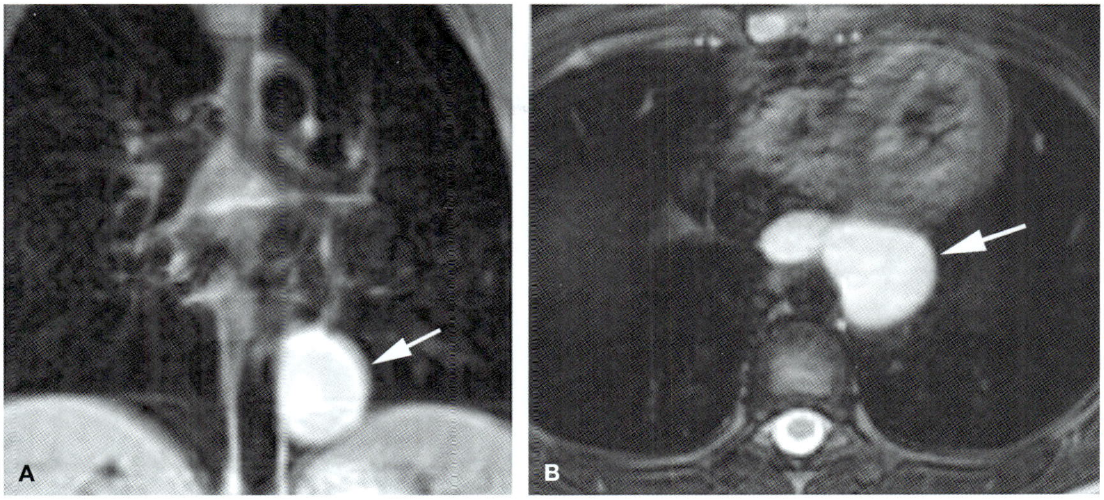

Figure 8.54. Esophageal duplication cyst. **A:** Coronal MRI shows a paraesophageal cyst (*arrow*). **B:** Transaxial T2-weighted, fat-saturated image shows high signal intensity typical of cyst (*arrow*). The cyst is paraesophageal in location.

On plain radiographs, pericardial cysts are smooth and sharply marginated (Fig. 8.56A). Approximately 90% of pericardial cysts contact the diaphragm, with 65% occurring in the right cardiophrenic angle and 25% in the left cardiophrenic angle. In this location, they sometimes are seen to extend into the major fissure, having a lenticular shape on lateral chest films. Ten percent of pericardial cysts do not touch the diaphragm and are seen at higher levels, contiguous with the proximal aorta or pulmonary arteries.

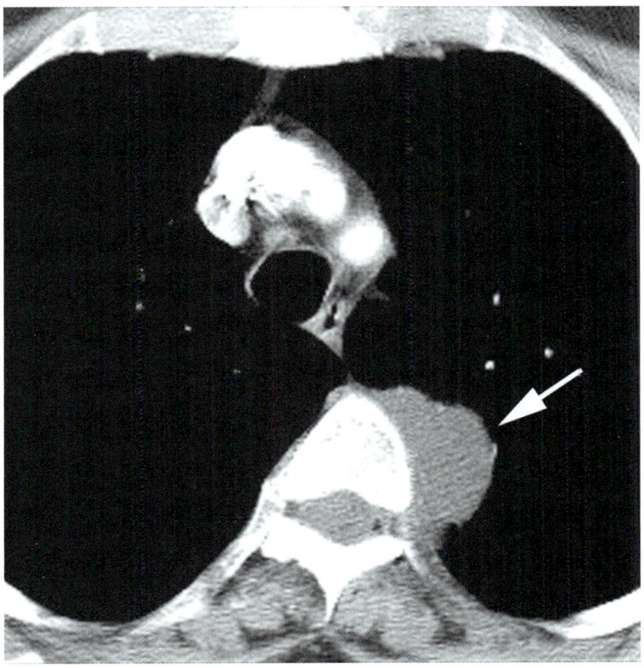

Figure 8.55. Neurenteric cyst. A low-attenuation paravertebral cystic lesion (*arrow*) is associated with scoliosis.

On CT, they appear sharply marginated and their attenuation is usually similar to that of water (see Fig. 8.56B); however, pericardial cysts with high CT numbers are occasionally seen. When occurring within the upper mediastinum, they may be seen to have a relationship to the superior pericardial recesses. Pericardial cysts are not always round; they may assume different shapes when studied at different times. On MRI, pericardial cysts containing serous fluid appear less intense than muscle on T1-weighted images.

Mediastinal Pseudocyst

Pancreatic pseudocyst represents an encapsulated collection of pancreatic secretions, blood, and necrotic material. Mediastinal extension of a pancreatic pseudocyst is rare but can occur via the aortic hiatus or esophageal hiatus or through a defect in the diaphragm. Symptoms are generally those of pancreatitis.

Plain radiographs may show a retrocardiac mediastinal mass. CT shows a cystic and low-attenuation mass in the visceral compartment, associated with compression or displacement of the esophagus or splaying of the diaphragmatic crura. Mediastinal pseudocysts are commonly located under and posterior to the heart, anterior to the aorta and esophagus, and medial to the inferior vena cava. The fluid can be of water attenuation or greater, depending on the presence of blood or infection. An abdominal fluid collection is common but not invariably present.

Other Cystic Lesions

Cystic or fluid-filled mediastinal lesions may represent congenital cysts or cystic masses (Table 8.23). Differentiation of an uncomplicated congenital cyst from other cystic encapsulated lesions, such as abscess, chronic hematoma, cystic lymphangioma or hemangioma, cystic teratoma, or other

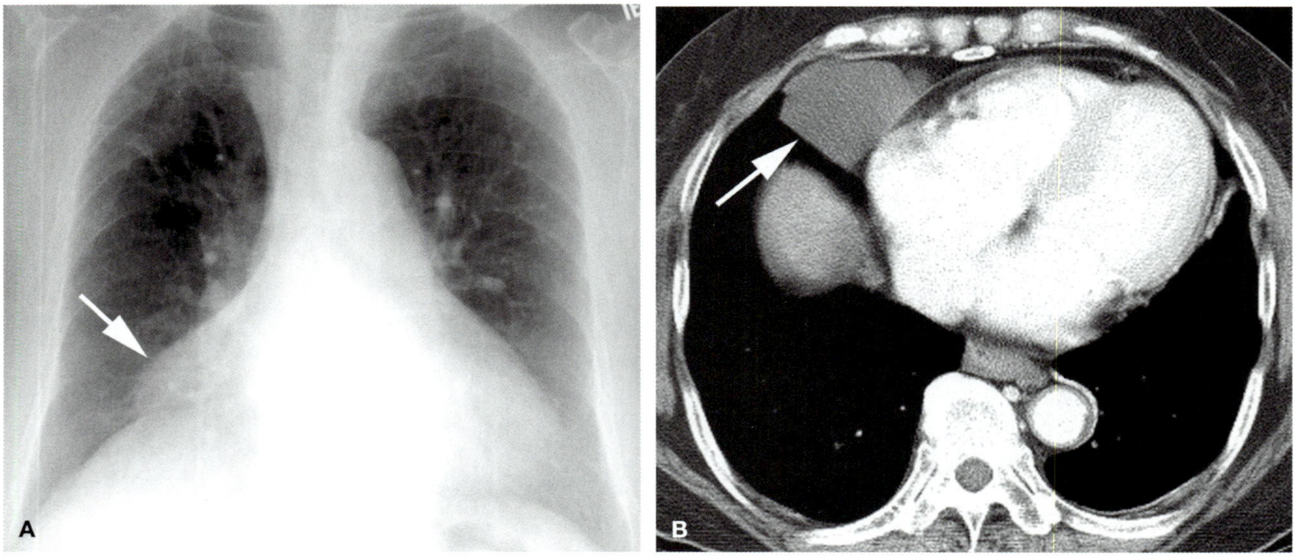

Figure 8.56. Pericardial cyst. **A:** Chest radiograph shows a mass in the right cardiophrenic angle (*arrow*). **B:** CT shows a low-attenuation cyst (*arrow*) contacting the pericardium.

cystic tumor, relies on the clinical presentation, findings on correlative radiographic studies, and the location and CT appearance of the cyst. Abscess, hematoma, and cystic tumors commonly demonstrate thick or irregular walls, septations, and mixed-density fluids. Cystic masses in the prevascular compartment rarely represent a congenital cyst and are more likely related to the presence of a cystic tumor or a thymic cyst. Anterior or lateral meningocele may closely resemble a congenital cyst, but careful examination of adjacent sections should demonstrate the intraspinal connection of the mass through the neural foramen.

VASCULAR TUMORS

Lymphangioma and Cystic Hygroma

Lymphangiomas are rare benign lesions of lymphatic origin and represent 1% to 5% of mediastinal tumors; most are present at birth and are detected in the first 2 years of life (Table 8.24). Patients may be asymptomatic, but compression of mediastinal structures can result in chest pain, cough, or dyspnea. Because of a tendency for local growth, surgery is recommended. Lymphangioma can be seen in adults, with or without a history of incomplete resection as a child.

Lymphangiomas are most common in the neck (75%) and axilla (20%). Although 10% of cervical lymphangiomas extend into the mediastinum, less than 5% of lymphangiomas are limited to the mediastinum. In adults, it is more common for lymphangioma to be localized to the mediastinum.

Lymphangiomas are classified as capillary, cavernous, or cystic (hygroma), depending on the size of the lymph channels they contain. Cystic lymphangioma is most common, accounting for more than 60% cases of lymphangioma in adults (Fig. 8.57). Cystic lymphangioma may be either unilocular or multilocular and can contain either serous or chylous fluid; thin septations within the mass are sometimes seen. In adults, lymphangiomas can be seen in any mediastinal compartment and can be quite large, ranging up to 30 cm in diameter.

Table 8.23 Cystic, Low-Attenuation, or Fluid-Filled Masses
Congenital or acquired cysts (bronchogenic, esophageal, neurenteric, pericardial, and thymic)
Necrotic or cystic neoplasms (germ cell tumors, cystic thymoma, lymphoma)
Necrotic lymph nodes
Cystic lymphangioma (hygroma)
Thoracic meningocele
Mediastinal abscess
Mediastinal hematoma
Mediastinal pseudocyst
Cystic goiter
Dilated, fluid-filled esophagus
Pericardial fluid collections

Table 8.24 Lymphangioma
1%-5% of mediastinal tumors
Usually present in childhood
Compression of mediastinal structures
Most common in neck (75%) and axilla (20%)
10% of cervical masses extend into mediastinum
5% limited to mediastinum
Classified as capillary, cavernous, or cystic (hygroma)
Unilocular or multilocular cystic masses
Contain serous or chylous fluid
May contain fat and enhancing vessels

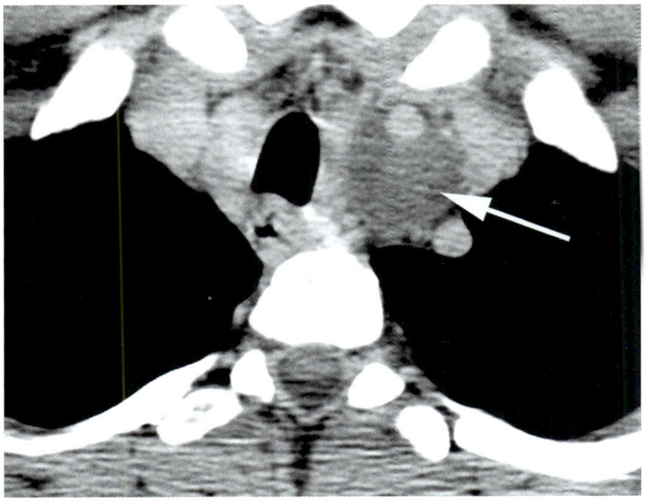

Figure 8.57. Cystic lymphangioma (hygroma). A low-attenuation lesion (*arrow*) is visible in the superior mediastinum.

On plain radiographs, a focal mass in the upper mediastinum may be visible or diffuse mediastinal widening may be seen (Fig. 8.58). An increase in cervical soft tissues may be associated.

On CT, the attenuation of lymphangiomas is usually homogeneous and near to that of water (see Fig. 8.57), but they can be of higher attenuation or variably composed of a combination of fluid, solid tissue, and fat (see Fig. 8.58); calcification is rare. Although they are usually well circumscribed and localized, they may appear to envelop mediastinal structures. Lymphangioma may be associated with vascular malformations that are easily identifiable following the administration of intravenous contrast. Simple lymphangiomas and hemangiomas composed of capillary-sized, thin-walled channels may appear as solid masses. On MRI, heterogeneous signal intensity is typical, with increased signal on T2-weighted images reflecting their fluid content (see Fig. 8.58).

Hemangioma

Hemangiomas are rare benign vascular tumors, accounting for less than 0.5% of mediastinal masses. They are composed of large interconnecting vascular channels with regions of thrombosis and varying amounts of interposed stroma, such as fat and fibrous tissue. Tumors are categorized according to the size and nature of their vascular spaces as capillary, cavernous, or venous; cavernous hemangiomas make up about 75% of cases. They are well defined and rarely are invasive.

Mediastinal hemangiomas are most common in young patients; about 75% present before the age of 35. One-third to one half of cases are asymptomatic, but some patients present with symptoms of compression of mediastinal structures. Occasional cases are associated with peripheral hemangiomas or Osler-Weber-Rendu syndrome.

Hemangiomas most commonly arise in the visceral compartment (45%-70% of cases) and paravertebral compartment (20%-35% of cases). Extension into the neck may occur (7%). Masses may appear well marginated on CT (70%), inseparable from adjacent mediastinal structures (21%), or diffusely infiltrative (7%). Apparent infiltration may or may not predict unresectability.

On CT, tumors are often heterogeneous in attenuation on unenhanced scans, and fat is occasionally seen within them. Heterogeneous enhancement is typical following contrast infusion but is not always present. Enhancement may be dense, multifocal, or diffuse and central or peripheral. Opacified vascular channels can be seen within the mass, with rapid enhancement similar to that of normal mediastinal vessels. Phleboliths, thought to be pathognomonic, are visible in up to 10% of cases on plain radiographs. On CT, punctate calcifications or phleboliths are visible in 10% to 20% (Fig. 8.59). Dilated mediastinal vessels may be associated with the mass (Fig. 8.59).

Other Vascular Lesions

Other mediastinal lesions may be associated with significant enhancement following contrast infusion (Table 8.25).

ESOPHAGUS

At successive levels in the mediastinum, the esophagus is in intimate contact anteriorly with the posterior or posterolateral trachea, the left mainstem bronchus, and the left atrium. The esophagus lies between the aorta on the left and the azygos vein on the right. Intraluminal air or a small amount of fluid is common and a normal finding with CT. Evaluation of esophageal disease is limited if the esophagus is incompletely distended.

CT has several distinct indications in patients with suspected esophageal disease. It is indicated (1) to evaluate and stage patients with esophageal carcinoma and to provide a means for assessing response to therapy and resultant complications, (2) to evaluate and characterize esophageal contour abnormalities detected at esophagography and their relationship to intrinsic or extrinsic masses, and (3) to evaluate patients with suspected esophageal perforation and to assess the extent of pleural and mediastinal fluid collections.

Esophageal Carcinoma

Esophageal carcinoma represents approximately 10% of all cancers of the gastrointestinal tract. Excluding adenocarcinomas of gastric origin with secondary esophageal involvement, 90% to 95% of esophageal tumors are squamous cell carcinoma. These tumors usually present in an advanced stage, with 5-year survival rates varying between 3% and 20%. This poor prognosis results from rapid submucosal extension of the tumor and early transmural invasion. This leads to early spread to regional and distal lymphatics as

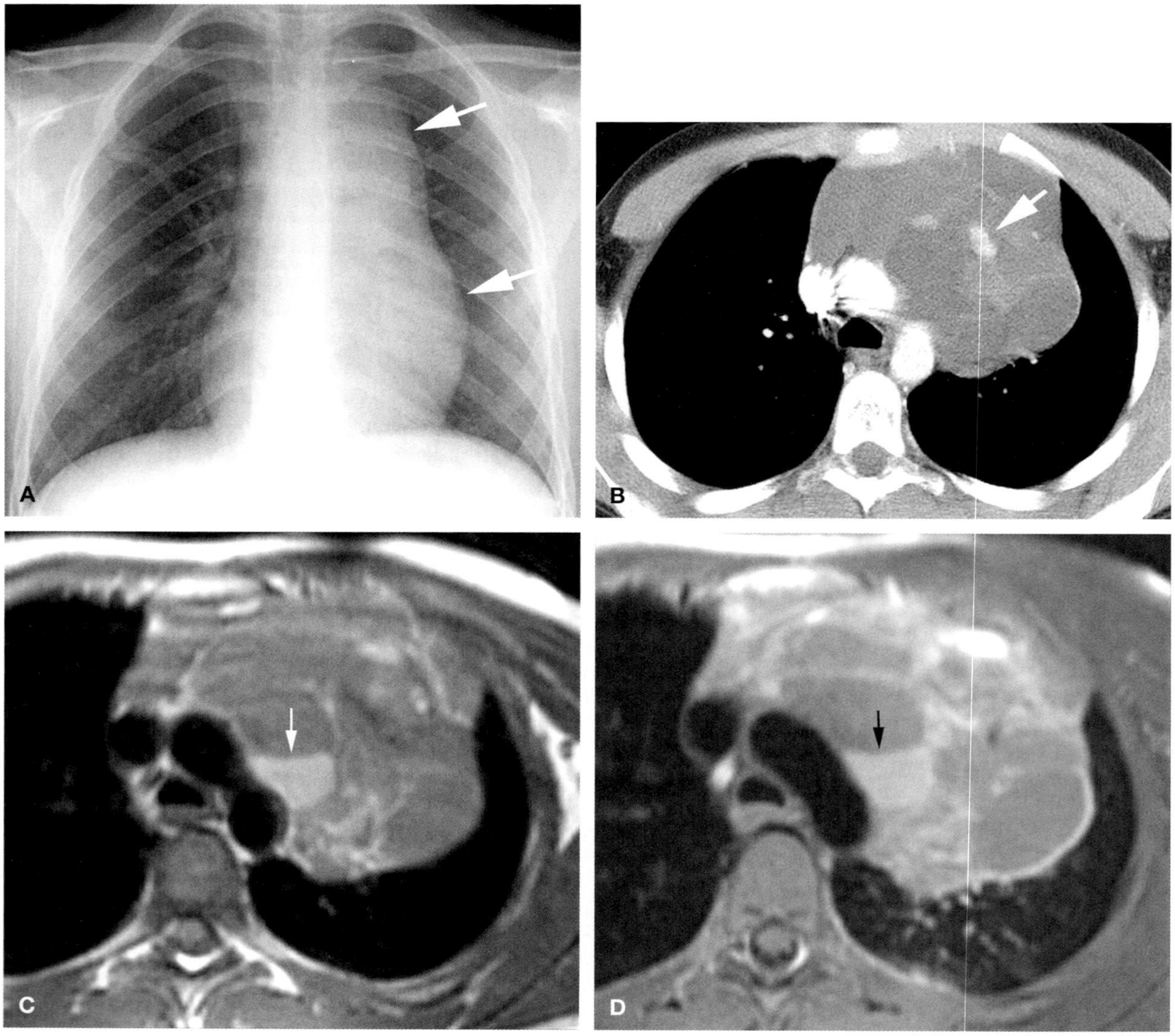

Figure 8.58. Lymphangioma in a young boy. **A:** Chest radiograph shows a mass (*arrows*) involving the left superior mediastinum, obscuring the left heart border. **B:** Contrast-enhanced CT shows a multicystic mass containing enhancing vessels (*arrow*). **C:** Transaxial T1-weighted image shows a large cystic mass with a fluid-fluid level (*arrow*). **D:** Transaxial T2-weighted image shows a complex cystic mass. The fluid-fluid level is visible (*arrow*).

well as the liver, adrenals, and lung. Esophageal carcinoma often presents with symptoms of obstruction, and incidental detection with plain radiographs or CT is unusual.

Plain radiographs show some abnormality in about half of patients with esophageal carcinoma, including an abnormal convexity of the azygoesophageal recess (25%), mediastinal widening (20%), a retrotracheal mass (15%) or thickening of the posterior tracheal band (10%), and tracheal displacement (10%).

The CT manifestations of esophageal carcinoma include (1) narrowing of the esophageal lumen or dilatation due to obstruction; (2) thickening of the esophageal wall, either symmetrical or asymmetrical; (3) loss of periesophageal fat planes, with or without evidence of invasion of surrounding organs; and (4) periesophageal adenopathy. Wall thickening must be distinguished from idiopathic muscular hypertrophy of the esophagus.

Esophageal Mesenchymal Tumors

Mesenchymal tumors of the esophagus, arising from components of the esophageal wall, include gastrointestinal stromal tumor, leiomyoma, fibroma, and lipoma. Unlike esophageal carcinoma, these tumors may be detected incidentally as a mediastinal mass in asymptomatic patients, but symptoms of dysphagia may be present. Leiomyoma is most common and predominates in the middle and lower esophagus. An abnormality in the subcarinal space or involving the

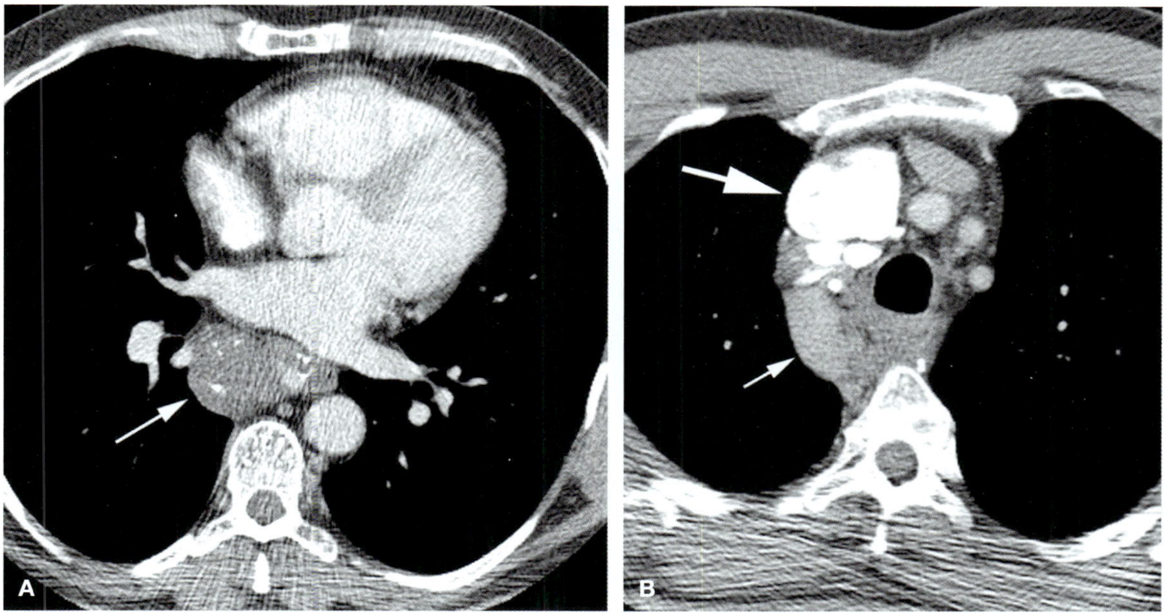

Figure 8.59. Mediastinal hemangioma. **A:** A large mass (*arrow*) in the subcarinal space contains phleboliths. **B:** At a higher level, the superior vena cava (*large arrow*) and azygos vein (*small arrow*) are dilated. Dilated veins are visible in the mediastinum, posterior to the superior vena cava.

azygoesophageal recess may be seen (Fig. 8.60). On lateral radiographs, an abnormality of the posterior tracheal band may be seen.

Esophageal Dilatation

Esophageal dilatation may result from obstructing tumors, stricture, or achalasia. Achalasia or strictures secondary to scleroderma are usually associated with the greatest degree of esophageal dilatation. An increase in air or fluid in the esophageal lumen and retained ingested material are common findings.

With marked esophageal dilatation, or megaesophagus, the esophagus usually projects to the right of the mediastinum, with a marked abnormality of the azygoesophageal recess seen on the chest radiograph (Fig. 8.61A). The left wall of the dilated distal esophagus is often visible in a left retrocardiac location. The trachea may be displaced forward if the upper esophagus is dilated, and there may be thickening of the posterior tracheal band or filling of the retrotracheal triangle. An air-fluid level may be seen (see Fig. 8.61A and B); this is most common with achalasia. CT shows dilatation of the esophageal lumen with air, air and fluid, and sometimes air-fluid or fat-fluid levels (see Fig. 8.61C and D).

Table 8.25 Enhancing Masses

Mediastinal thyroid glands or masses
Ectopic parathyroid glands or masses
Carcinoid tumors
Lymphangioma
Hemangioma
Paraganglioma
Unicentric
Castleman disease
Hypervascular metastases (eg, renal cell carcinoma)

Esophageal Varices

Esophageal or paraesophageal varices occur because of portal hypertension or, less often, systemic venous obstruction. They occasionally result in a chest film abnormality. Findings include convexity of the inferior aspect of the azygoesophageal interface, paravertebral widening (Fig. 8.62A), and dilatation of the azygos arch. Typically, plain film findings are nonspecific, necessitating differentiation from enlarged periesophageal lymph nodes or other posterior mediastinal masses.

CT is able to detect both esophageal and paraesophageal varices. Soft-tissue opacities may be seen on unenhanced scans, sometimes indenting the wall of the air-filled esophagus (see Fig. 8.62B). Using CT with intravenous contrast, esophageal and paraesophageal varices are easily diagnosed.

Hiatal Hernia

Hiatal hernia represents a protrusion of a portion of the stomach through the esophageal hiatus. The esophageal hiatus is an elliptical opening just to the left of the midline, corresponding superiorly to the level of the 10th thoracic vertebral body. It is margined on each side by the diaphragmatic crura. Variation in the normal appearance of the crura is common.

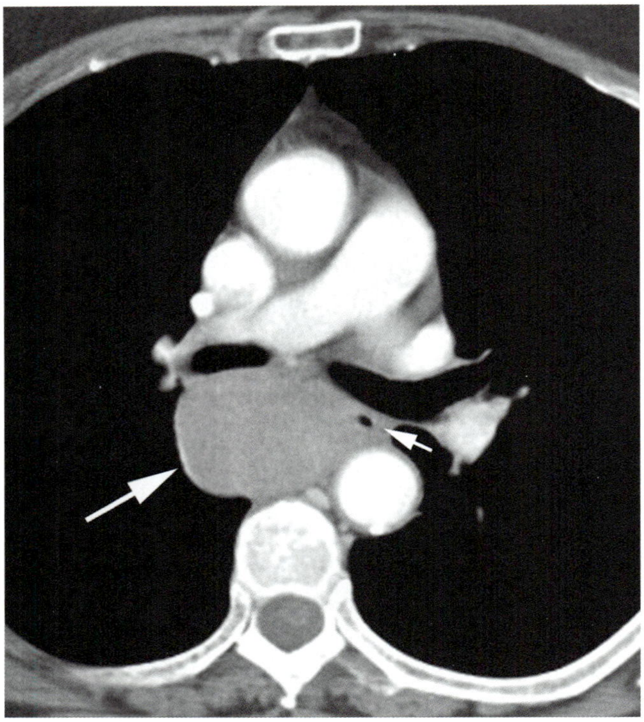

Figure 8.60. Esophageal leiomyoma. An enhancing mass (*large arrow*) is present in the subcarinal space, contiguous with the esophagus (*small arrow*).

In patients with hiatal hernia, chest radiographs show characteristic findings of convexity of the lower aspect of the azygoesophageal interface, sometimes with a similar convexity of the preaortic recess in a retrocardiac location. Air or air and fluid may be seen in association with this convexity. On the lateral view, a retrocardiac opacity may be seen but is usually less conspicuous.

In a patient with sliding hiatal hernia, the most common CT abnormality identified is dehiscence of the diaphragmatic crura, visible as widening of the esophageal hiatus on cross section, with projection of a portion of the stomach into the mediastinum. The width of the esophageal hiatus, defined as the distance between the medial margins of the crura, has a maximum normal value of 15 mm. Sliding hiatal hernias are frequently associated with an increase in the amount of fat surrounding the distal esophagus, secondary to herniation of omentum.

MEDIASTINITIS AND MEDIASTINAL ABSCESS

Acute mediastinal infections are uncommon and usually related to surgery, esophageal perforation, or spread of infection from adjacent regions. Infections may be classified as diffuse mediastinitis or mediastinal abscess, depending on their extent. Diffuse mediastinitis has a relatively poor prognosis.

Plain radiographs generally show diffuse mediastinal widening, most commonly involving the upper mediastinum (Fig. 8.63A). Pneumomediastinum and subcutaneous emphysema may be seen in the neck (see Fig. 8.63A); pneumothorax and pleural effusion may also be associated, depending on the cause of the infection. These are common with esophageal perforation, spontaneous (Boerhaave syndrome), posttraumatic, or iatrogenic, complicating endoscopy, esophageal dilatation, attempted intubation, or surgery. Distal esophageal perforation usually results in left-sided pleural abnormalities, while upper or mid-esophageal perforation usually results in right-sided abnormalities.

CT findings in mediastinitis include diffuse or streaky edema and increased attenuation of mediastinal fat; mediastinal widening; localized fluid collections, sometimes with a thick or enhancing wall; pleural or pericardial effusion; lymph node enlargement; and compression of mediastinal structures (see Fig. 8.63B). Gas bubbles in the mediastinum, with or without associated fluid collections, are seen in up to half of cases and are an important finding in diagnosis. In patients with an abscess, a localized fluid-filled space is visible, often containing air.

Many cases of mediastinitis occur after median sternotomy. In subjects having CT after an uncomplicated sternotomy, findings can closely mimic the appearance of mediastinitis. More than 75% of patients having median sternotomy show retrosternal fluid collections, air, hematoma, or a combination of these in the early postoperative period. After 2 weeks, these abnormalities should largely resolve, although some abnormal findings may persist for up to 3 weeks.

PARAVERTEBRAL ABNORMALITIES

A wide variety of pathologic processes may involve the paravertebral regions. Most frequently, paravertebral masses are neural in origin, including neurogenic tumors, neurenteric cyst, and anterior or lateral thoracic meningocele, or are related to the spine. Infections involving the spine may lead to the development of paraspinal abscess. In addition, lymphoma and other causes of lymph node enlargement may result in abnormalities in this region; paraspinal lymph nodes freely communicate with lymph nodes in the upper abdomen, and contiguous involvement is common. Since the mediastinum communicates with the retroperitoneal space via the esophageal hiatus, aortic hiatus, and other defects in the diaphragm, diseases can spread between the abdomen and thorax by direct extension; inflammatory masses such as pancreatic pseudocysts can involve the paraspinal mediastinal regions. Rare entities such as extramedullary hematopoiesis, primary myelolipomas of the mediastinum, benign hemangioendotheliomas, aggressive fibromatosis, and FM have been reported in the paravertebral regions.

NEUROGENIC TUMORS

Neurogenic tumors account for about 10% to 20% of primary mediastinal masses in adults and 30% to 35% of mediastinal tumors in children. Seventy-five percent of posterior mediastinal masses are neurogenic tumors. Tumors may arise

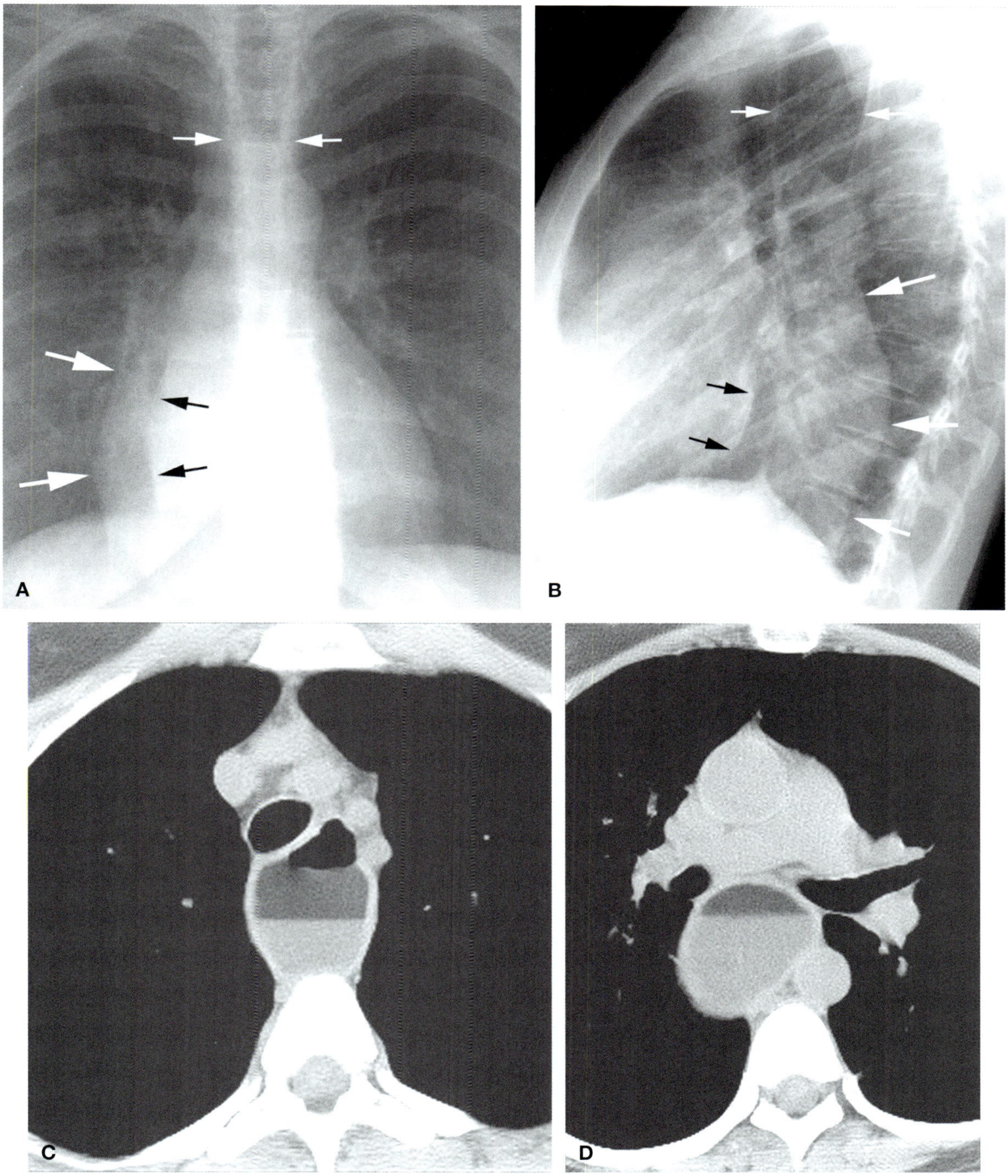

Figure 8.61. Achalasia. **A:** PA chest radiograph shows the dilated esophagus (*large white arrows*) projecting to the right of the right heart border (*black arrows*). An air-fluid level is visible in the esophagus (*small white arrows*). **B:** Lateral chest radiograph shows the dilated esophagus (*large white arrows*) projecting posterior to the heart border (*black arrows*). The air-fluid level is also visible (*small white arrows*) on the lateral view. **C** and **D:** The dilated esophagus shows air-fluid and fat-fluid levels.

from peripheral nerves and nerve sheath (neurofibroma, schwannoma, malignant peripheral nerve sheath tumors) or sympathetic ganglia (ganglioneuroma, ganglioneuroblastoma, neuroblastoma). The most common cell types are schwannoma (35%), ganglioneuroma (25%), neuroblastoma (15%-20%), ganglioneuroblastomas (7%-15%), and neurofibroma (5%-10%), but the incidence varies with the patient's age. Eighty percent are benign.

Nearly 85% of neurogenic tumors in children are of ganglionic origin, while in adults, more than 75% are nerve

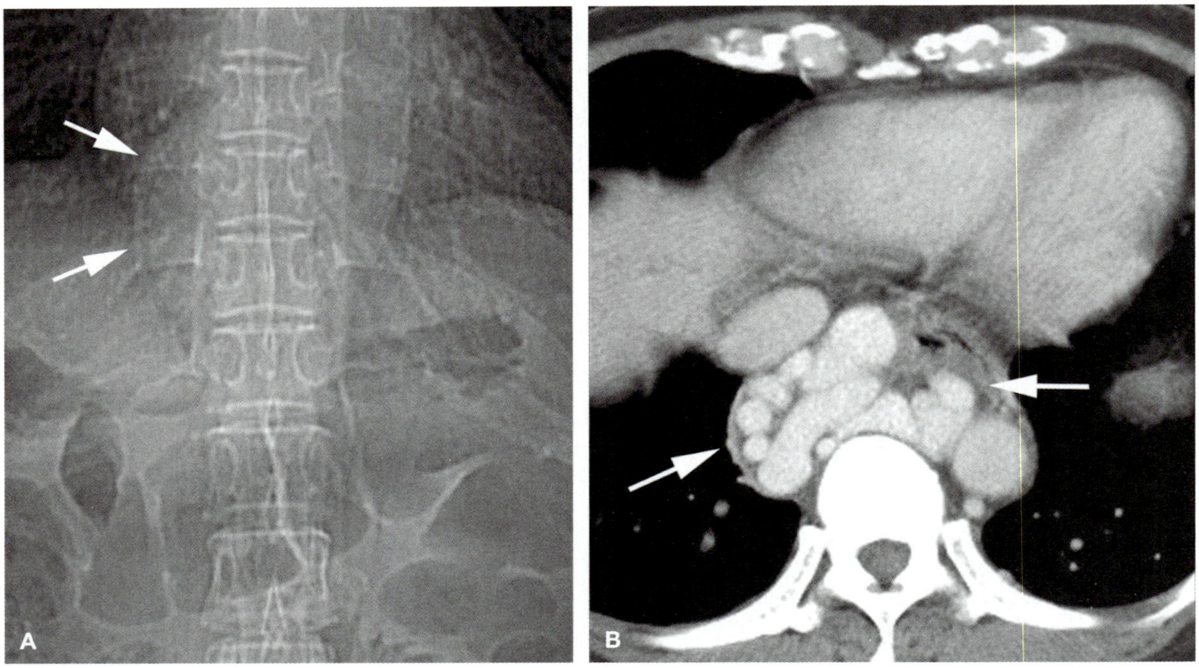

Figure 8.62. Paraesophageal varices appearing as a mediastinal mass in a patient with hepatitis B and portal hypertension. **A:** Scout view shows a convex right posterior mediastinal mass (*arrows*). **B:** CT shows very large paraesophageal varices (*arrows*). The air-filled esophagus is also visible.

sheath tumors. Specifically, schwannoma and neurofibroma are more common in adults, while ganglioneuroblastoma and neuroblastoma are more common in children. The mean age at diagnosis is about 5 years for neuroblastoma, 10 years for ganglioneuroblastoma, 20 years for ganglioneuroma, 30 years for neurofibroma, and 40 years for schwannoma.

Neurogenic tumors occurring in the upper mediastinum commonly show a finding termed the "cervicothoracic sign" on plain radiographs. The sign is said to be present if a mediastinal mass shows a sharply marginated border, outlined by lung, above the level of the clavicles. Only paravertebral mediastinal masses show this finding. Above the level of the clavicles, prevascular and visceral mediastinal masses enter the neck and are no longer outlined by the lung (ie, they no longer have a sharply marginated border).

Peripheral Nerve Sheath Tumors

Nerve sheath tumors include neurilemoma (schwannoma), neurofibroma, and neurogenic sarcoma (malignant schwannoma) (Table 8.26). Schwannomas are composed of spindle cells densely packed together (Antoni A pattern) or organized

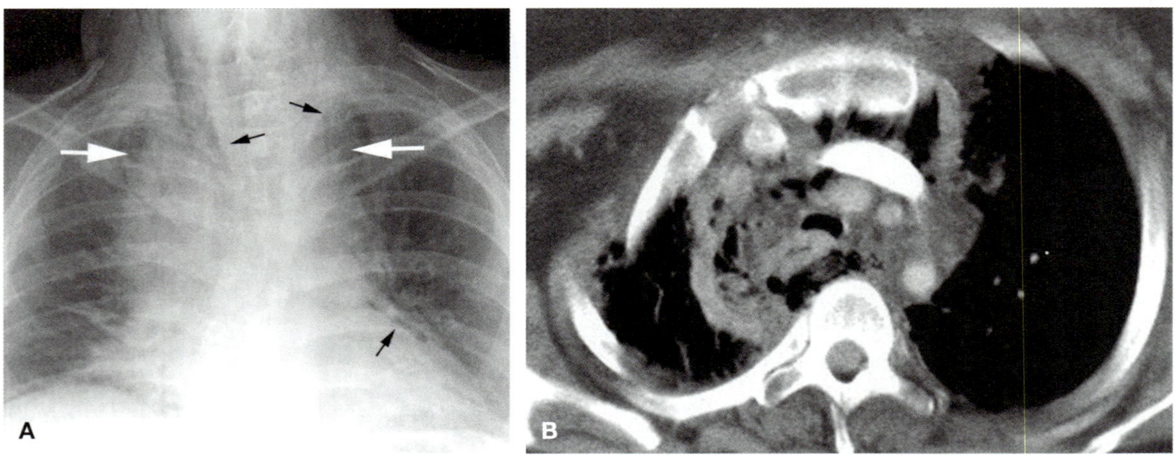

Figure 8.63. Mediastinitis secondary to esophageal perforation. **A:** The mediastinum is widened (*white arrows*) and streaky pneumomediastinum is visible (*black arrows*). Air extends into the neck. **B:** CT shows mediastinal widening, increased attenuation of mediastinal fat, and pneumomediastinum.

Table 8.26 Peripheral Nerve Sheath Tumors

Neurilemoma (schwannoma), neurofibroma, and neurogenic sarcoma
Most common in adults
Round, elliptical, or lobulated paravertebral mass
Often one or two interspaces in length
Rib or vertebral abnormalities in 50%
Lower attenuation than muscle in 70%
One-third of patients with neurofibromas have neurofibromatosis
Plexiform neurofibroma: extensive fusiform or infiltrating mass

more loosely in association with a myxoid stroma (Antoni B pattern); areas of infarction are common. Neurofibromas are also variable in appearance, consisting of spindle cells, a loose myxoid matrix, neurofibrils, and collagen.

On plain radiographs, nerve sheath tumors typically appear as sharply marginated round, elliptical, or lobulated paravertebral masses, although they may be well seen only on the frontal radiograph (Figs. 8.64, 8.65A and B, 8.66A and B, 8.67A). They tend to be limited to one or two interspaces in length but in some patients can be large. Associated rib or vertebral deformity or enlargement of a neural foramen is visible in about 50% of cases (see Fig. 8.64). Nerve sheath tumors may also be seen in the middle or anterior mediastinum, occurring in relation to the vagus, phrenic, or recurrent laryngeal nerves or along the courses of intercostal nerves (Figs. 8.68-8.71).

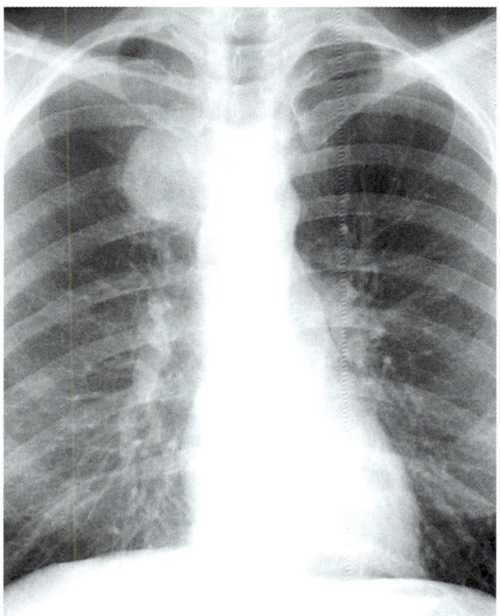

Figure 8.64. Schwannoma. PA chest radiograph shows a well-defined right mediastinal mass associated with deformity of right-sided ribs.

On CT, nerve sheath tumors typically appear as well-marginated, smooth, rounded, or elliptical masses (see Figs. 8.65C, 8.66C and D, 8.67B). Enlargement of neural foramina is better shown on CT than on plain films (see Fig. 8.67B). In over 70% of cases, peripheral nerve or nerve sheath tumors appear to be lower in attenuation than chest wall muscle (see Figs. 8.66C and 8.68A); in the remainder, they are of soft-tissue attenuation. Low-density areas within nerve sheath tumors can be due to the presence of (1) lipid-rich Schwann cells, (2) adipocytes, (3) perineural adipose tissue entrapped by plexiform neurofibromas, or (4) cystic spaces in the tumor. Variable enhancement of the tumor may be seen following contrast infusion; peripheral enhancement is common (Figs. 8.66D and 8.67B). Small areas of calcification are seen in 5% to 10% of cases. Extension into the spinal canal is present in 10% and is best demonstrated with MRI (Fig. 8.67B-D).

Neurofibromas may be associated with neurofibromatosis type 1 (NF1), which can result in vertebral abnormalities including kyphoscoliosis, scalloped vertebrae, and lateral meningocele. More than one-third of patients with neurofibromas have neurofibromatosis, and the neurofibromas are often multiple (Figs. 8.68, 8.70, 8.71).

On MRI, neurogenic tumors typically have slightly greater signal intensity than muscle on T1-weighted images and markedly increased signal intensity on T2-weighted or contrast-enhanced images, although often in an inhomogeneous fashion. On T2-weighted or contrast-enhanced images, the center of the lesion may have a higher or lower intensity than its periphery (see Figs. 8.67D and 8.68C).

Plexiform neurofibroma represents an extensive fusiform or infiltrating mass along the course of the sympathetic chains or mediastinal or intercostal nerves (see Figs. 8.68 and 8.70). It is considered pathognomonic of NF1. As with localized nerve sheath tumors, plexiform neurofibromas often appear low in attenuation compared to muscle, with CT numbers ranging from 15 to 20 HU on unenhanced scans. They are often multiple and lobulated, have ill-defined margins, and tend to surround mediastinal vessels with loss of normally visible fat planes. They can closely mimic the appearance of extensive mediastinal lymph node enlargement. Calcification and contrast enhancement can be seen.

Malignant nerve sheath tumors, termed malignant schwannoma, neurogenic sarcoma, or neurofibrosarcoma, are relatively uncommon but represent up to 15% of nerve sheath tumors. Malignant nerve sheath tumors tend to be large, infiltrating, irregular in contour, and inhomogeneous in attenuation, although these findings are not sufficiently reliable for diagnosis. Both benign and malignant lesions may be symptomatic, rendering attempts at clinical differentiation of limited utility. Calcification and some degree of contrast opacification may be present with either benign or malignant tumors.

Tumors Originating From Sympathetic Ganglia

In children, 80% of paravertebral mediastinal masses are derived from sympathetic ganglia. Included in this group are

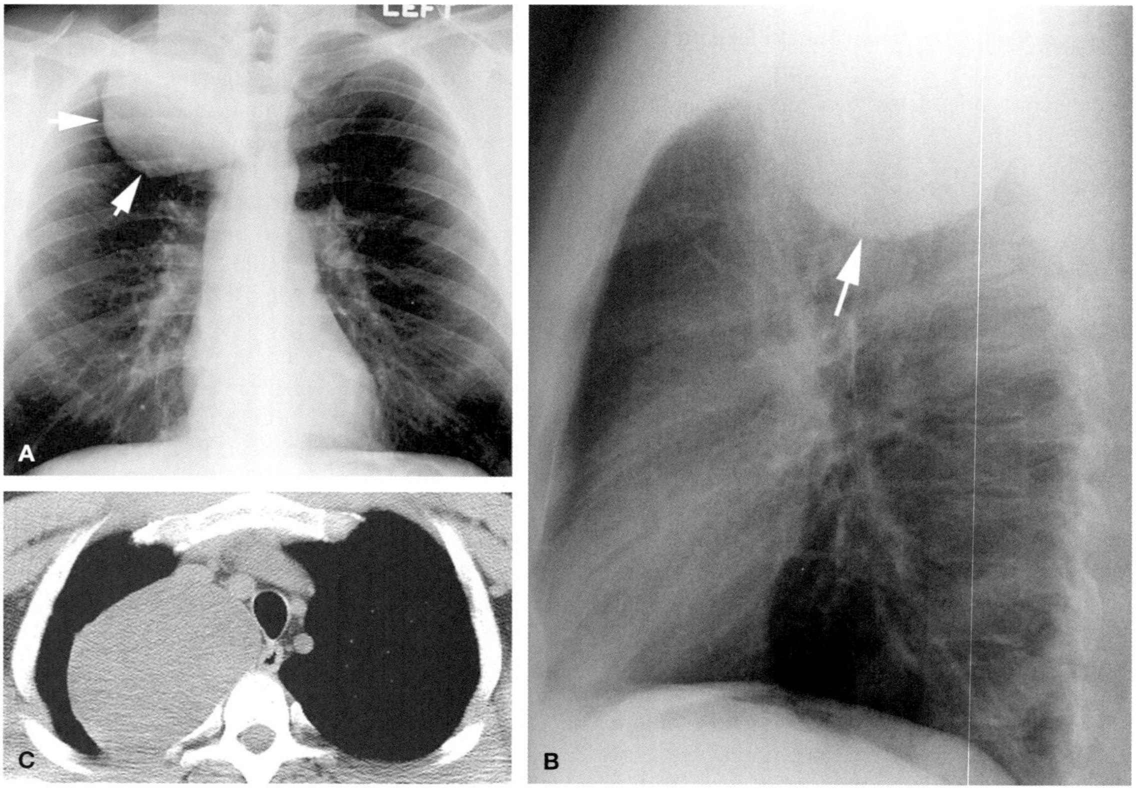

Figure 8.65. Schwannoma. **A:** PA chest radiograph shows a well-defined mass in the superior mediastinum (*arrows*). **B:** On the lateral view, the mass is relatively posterior in location (*arrow*). **C:** A well-defined homogeneous mass is visible on CT.

ganglioneuroma, ganglioneuroblastoma, and neuroblastoma (Table 8.27).

Ganglioneuroma, a benign tumor made up of Schwann cells, collagen, and ganglion cells, is a common neoplasm in teenagers and young adults. On plain radiographs, this tumor often appears as an oblong or sausage-shaped mass in a paravertebral location; it tends to be longer than nerve sheath tumors occurring in a similar location. Ganglioneuroma cannot be distinguished from schwannoma or neurofibroma on the basis of its CT appearance. Calcification is seen in about 20% of cases, and vertebral abnormalities may be seen. On MRI, ganglioneuroma may appear homogeneous in intensity on T1-weighted and T2-weighted images or may show a unique whorled appearance of layers of varying intensity.

Approximately 15% of *neuroblastomas* arise in the mediastinum, and almost all are located posteriorly (Fig. 8.72). Mediastinal neuroblastoma is seen almost exclusively in young children under the age of 5 years. It is malignant and may present with a wide variety of signs and symptoms including chest pain, fever, malaise, anemia, Horner syndrome, and extremity weakness. On CT, neuroblastomas appear as soft-tissue attenuation masses, but up to 40% contain speckled or curvilinear calcifications (see Fig. 8.72C). They are most common in the paravertebral regions and may extend superiorly and inferiorly for several centimeters. Neuroblastoma often shows heterogeneous enhancement following contrast injection. CT and MRI may be used to help determine the presence and extent of mediastinal or vertebral column invasion (see Fig. 8.72D). Invasion of the extradural spinal canal is common, even in the absence of neurologic signs and symptoms. On T2-weighted images, neuroblastoma appears intense (see Fig. 8.72D). MRI has the advantage of allowing tumor and surrounding soft tissues to be distinguished more readily than on CT and is more accurate in the recognition of bone marrow involvement. Neuroblastoma may extend from a primary site in the abdomen into the thorax. Most commonly, this occurs by direct invasion through the retrocrural space and into the lower paravertebral regions, often on both sides. In the rare instance of adult neuroblastoma, differentiation from lymphoma may be difficult.

Ganglioneuroblastoma is found in somewhat older children than neuroblastoma and is less common. Ganglioneuroblastomas are regarded by some as partially matured malignant neuroblastomas and are somewhat intermediate in histology between neuroblastoma and ganglioneuroma. Their imaging characteristics are indistinguishable from neuroblastoma. They can present as either a large, smooth spherical mass or a small, elongated sausage-shaped mass.

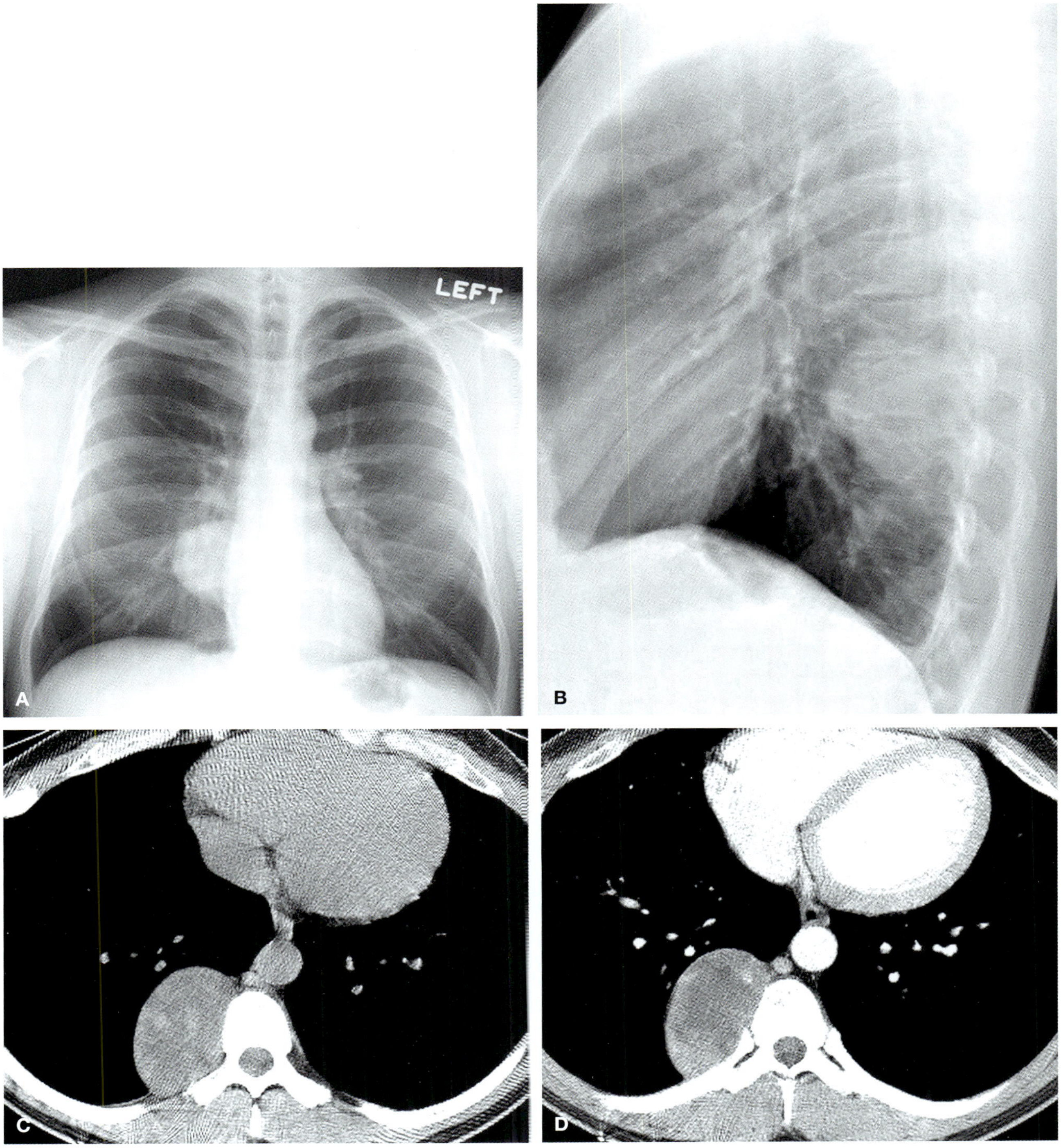

Figure 8.66. Schwannoma. **A:** PA chest radiograph shows a well-defined, rounded right mediastinal mass. **B:** Lateral view shows the mass to be posterior in location. **C:** Unenhanced CT shows a right paravertebral mass of heterogeneous attenuation. Parts of the tumor are of lower attenuation than muscle. **D:** CT following contrast injection shows enhancement of the peripheral portion of the mass.

Paraganglioma

Paraganglioma (chemodectoma) is a rare tumor originating from neuroectodermal cells located in relation to the autonomic nervous system, especially in the region of the aortopulmonary window (Fig. 8.73) and the paravertebral mediastinum; it has also been identified within or adjacent to the atria. It accounts for less than 5% of thoracic neurogenic tumors.

Radiographs usually show a well-defined, round or elliptical mass indistinguishable from other neurogenic tumors.

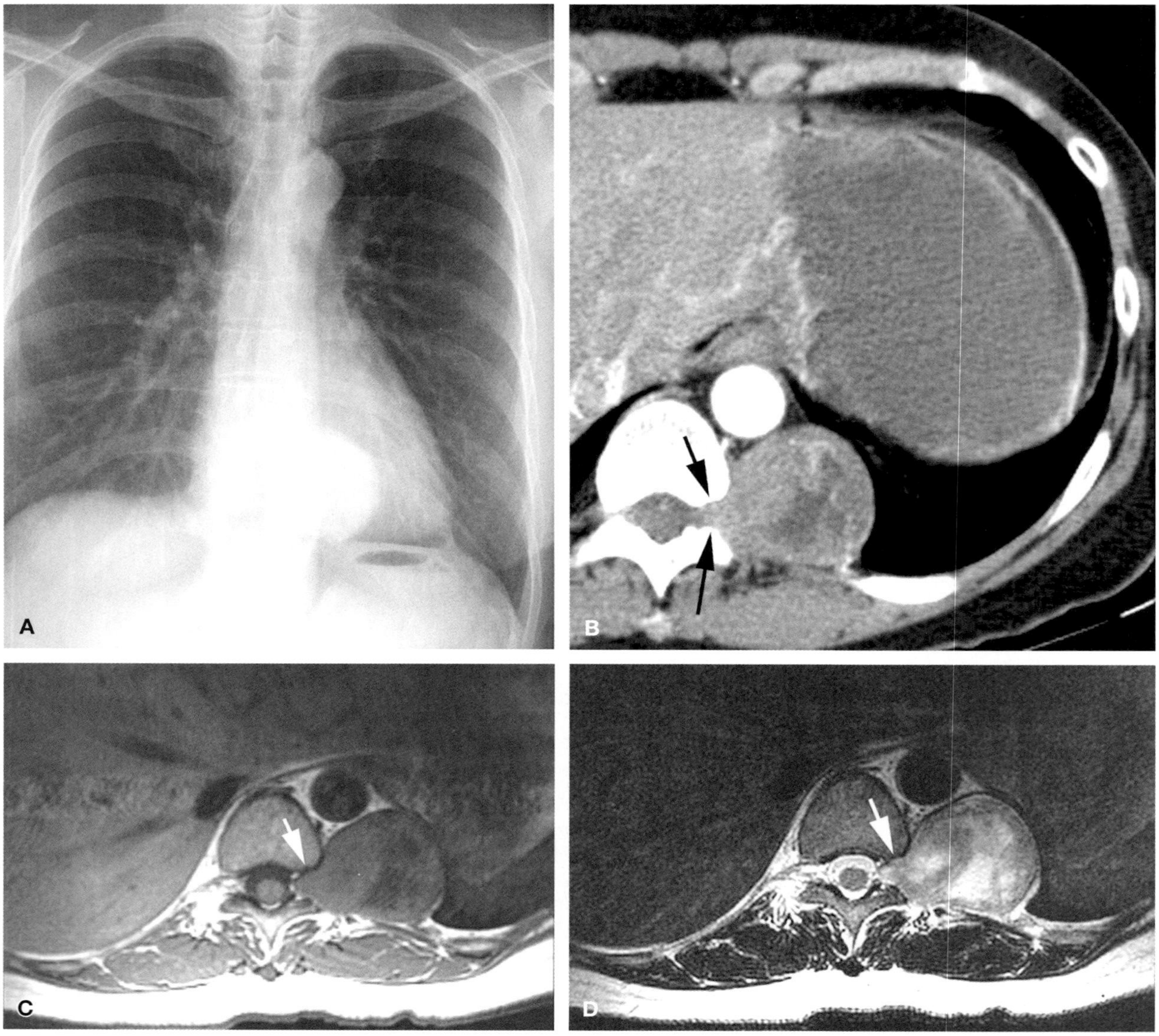

Figure 8.67. Schwannoma. **A:** PA chest radiograph shows a well-defined, rounded retrocardiac mediastinal mass. **B:** CT shows a left paravertebral mass with heterogeneous peripheral enhancement. The mass extends into the left neural foramen (*arrows*), which is enlarged in comparison to the right. **C:** T1-weighted MRI shows extension into the neural foramen (*arrow*) to better advantage. **D:** T2-weighted MRI also shows extension into the neural foramen (*arrow*). The mass has heterogeneous signal intensity.

It has a predilection for the midthoracic region. On unenhanced CT, paraganglioma has no characteristic features. However, scanning with contrast infusion shows dense enhancement (see Fig. 8.40B).

Patients may be asymptomatic, with the tumor being detected incidentally. About half of patients with paravertebral paraganglioma have symptoms of catecholamine secretion by the tumor or associated tumors in other locations, but catecholamine secretion is rare in patients with aortopulmonary window tumors. Compression of mediastinal structures may also result in symptoms.

Identification of hormonally active lesions has been greatly aided recently by use of 131-I metaiodobenzylguanidine scintigraphy, which localizes catecholamine-producing tumors, including neuroblastoma and neuroendocrine tumor. Octreotide scintigraphy is also useful in localization of these lesions.

Approximately 10% of paragangliomas are malignant or invasive. Paravertebral paragangliomas are more easily resectable than those in the visceral compartment and have a better prognosis. Local recurrence is common following surgery in patients with aortopulmonary paraganglioma.

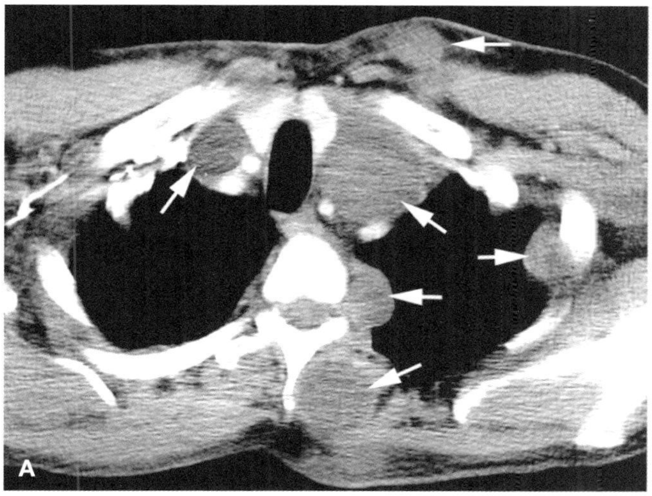
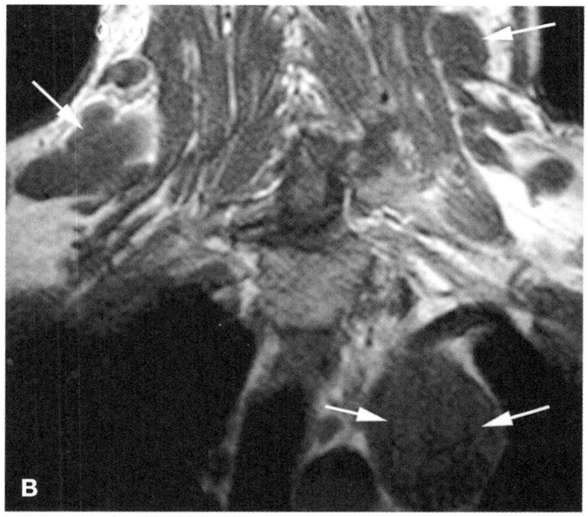
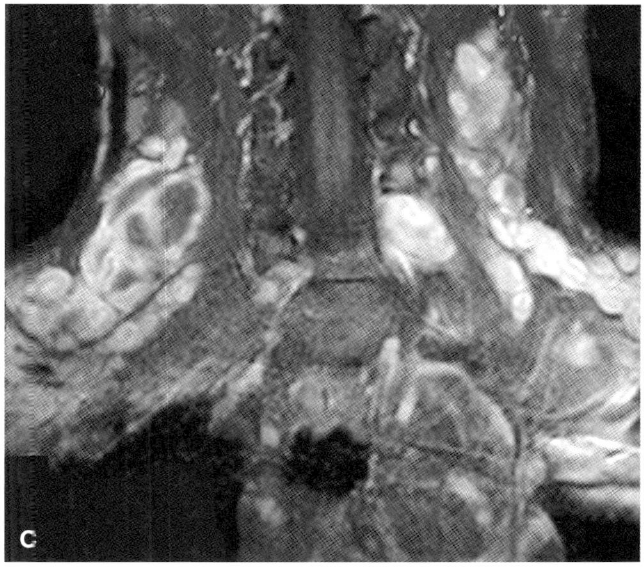

Figure 8.68. Extensive (plexiform) neurofibromas in neurofibromatosis. **A:** CT shows multiple neurofibromas (*arrows*) in the subcutaneous tissues, along the courses of mediastinal and intercostal nerves, and in a paravertebral location. The masses appear low in attenuation on CT, measuring 15 HU. Enlargement of the left neural foramen is visible, contiguous with a left paravertebral neurofibroma. **B:** T1-weighted MRI of the lower neck and upper mediastinum shows numerous neurofibromas along the courses of cervical and mediastinal (*arrows*) nerves. **C:** Contrast-enhanced MRI shows irregular enhancement. The centers of some lesions appear low in intensity.

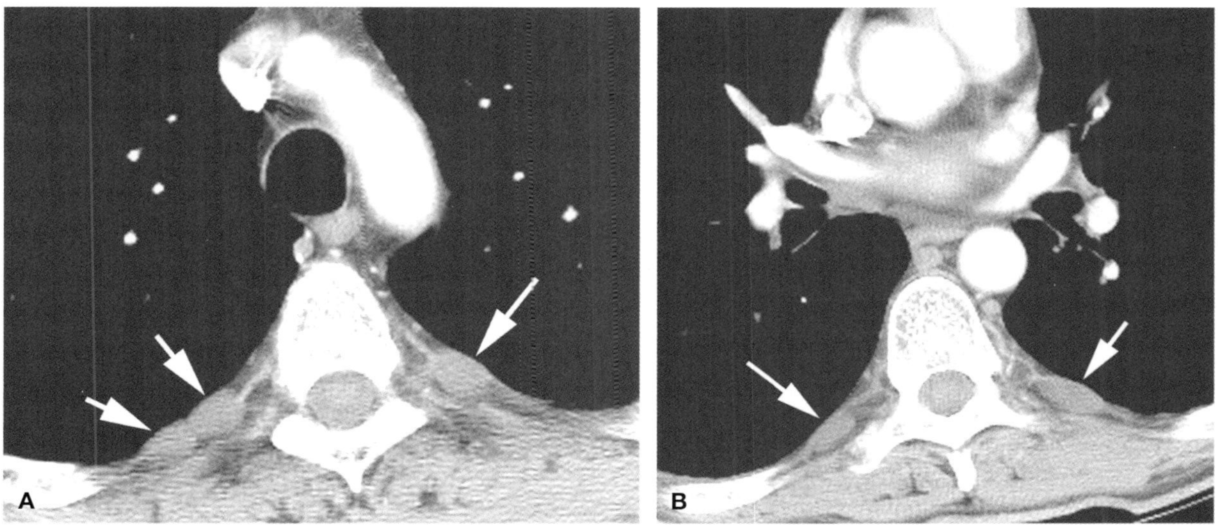

Figure 8.69. Neurofibromatosis with paravertebral and intercostal neurofibromas. **A** and **B:** Multiple paravertebral and intercostal neurofibromas are visible (*arrows*). They appear slightly lower in attenuation than muscle.

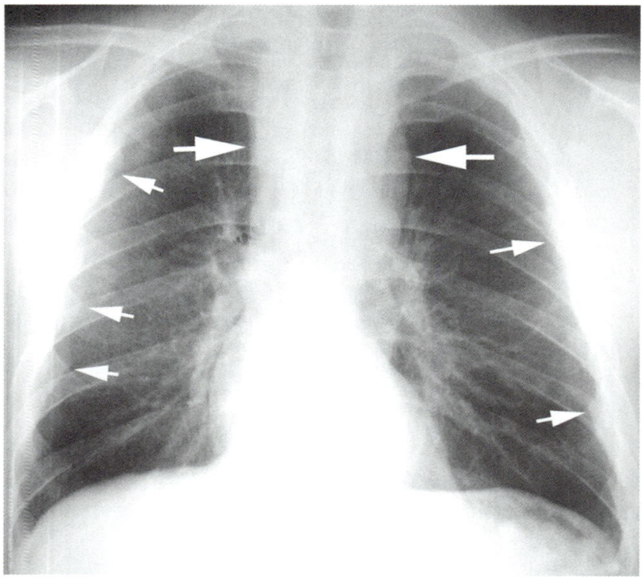

Figure 8.70. Plexiform neurofibromas in neurofibromatosis. Mediastinal widening (*large arrows*) reflects the presence of multiple, infiltrative neurofibromas along the courses of mediastinal nerves. Extensive intercostal neurofibromas (*small arrows*) mimic the appearance of pleural thickening.

ANTERIOR OR LATERAL THORACIC MENINGOCELE

This entity represents anomalous herniation of the spinal meninges through an intervertebral foramen or a defect in the vertebral body. In many patients, this abnormality is associated with neurofibromatosis; most are detected in adults. Meningoceles are described as lateral or anterior, depending on their relationship to the spine. They are slightly more common on the right side.

On chest radiographs, meningoceles commonly result in a sharply marginated paravertebral soft-tissue mass associated with scoliosis or rib and vertebral anomalies at the same level (Fig. 8.74A). When scoliosis is present, meningoceles typically occur at the apex of a convex curve. On CT, they appear low in attenuation, as they contain cerebrospinal fluid (see Fig. 8.74B). MRI is diagnostic (see Fig. 8.74C-E), as is filling of the meningocele with contrast on CT myelography.

EXTRAMEDULLARY HEMATOPOIESIS

Extramedullary hematopoiesis can result in paravertebral masses in patients with severe anemia caused by inadequate production or excessive destruction of blood cells. It can be seen in the presence of thalassemia, hereditary spherocytosis, and sickle cell anemia. These masses are of unknown origin but may arise from herniations of vertebral or rib marrow through small cortical defects or may arise from lymph nodes or elements of the reticuloendothelial system.

Lobulated paravertebral masses, usually multiple and bilateral and caudad to the sixth thoracic vertebra, are typically seen (Fig. 8.75). They appear well marginated. On CT, the paravertebral masses are of homogeneous soft-tissue attenuation (30-65 HU) or may show areas of fat attenuation (−50 HU), which may increase in extent after treatment.

The diagnosis can be suggested by the presence of paravertebral masses in a patient with chronic anemia and skeletal abnormalities visible on radiographs or CT findings suggesting a bone marrow abnormality. Coarsening of the trabecular pattern, rib expansion, and periosteal new bone may be seen. Although not always present, splenomegaly may also be visible.

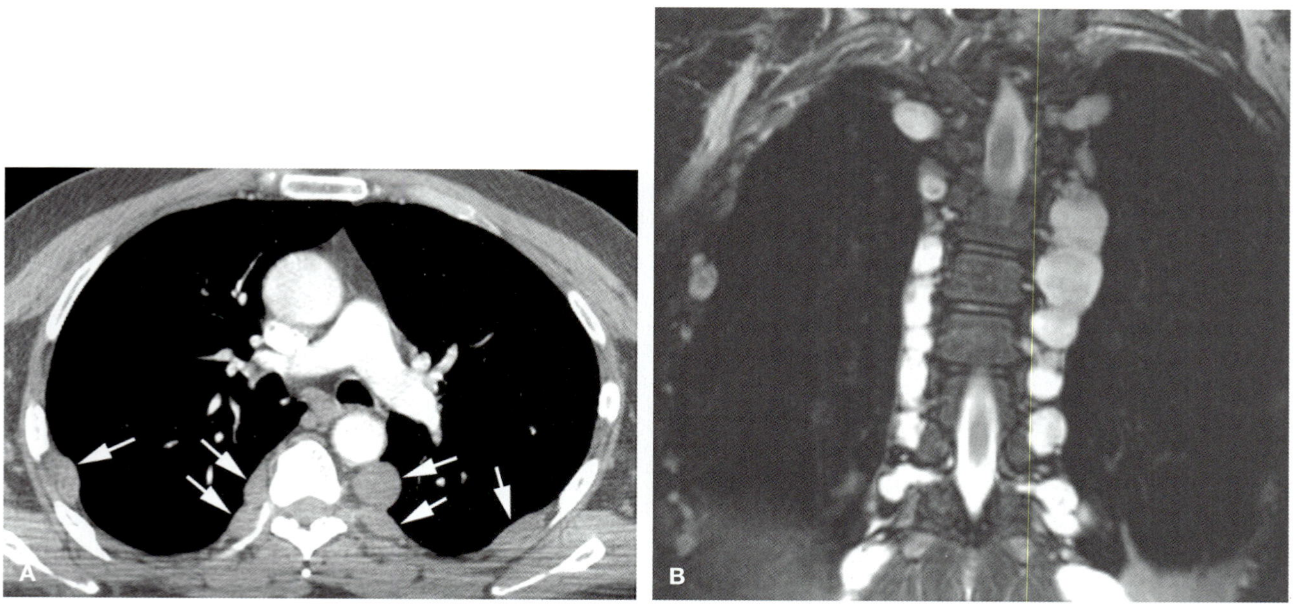

Figure 8.71. Multiple neurofibromas in neurofibromatosis. **A:** CT shows multiple mediastinal and intercostal neurofibromas (*arrows*). **B:** Coronal MRI shows multiple paravertebral neurofibromas.

Table 8.27 Tumors Derived From Sympathetic Ganglia

Ganglioneuroma, ganglioneuroblastoma, and neuroblastoma
20% of posterior masses in children
Oblong or sausage-shaped paravertebral mass
Calcification in 20%

ABNORMALITIES OF THE THORACIC SPINE

Tumors either primary or malignant, infectious spondylitis, or vertebral fracture with associated hemorrhage can produce a paravertebral mass. Frequently, the abnormality is bilateral and fusiform, allowing it to be distinguished from solitary masses such as a neurogenic tumor. Associated abnormalities of the vertebral bodies or discs assist in diagnosis and should be sought.

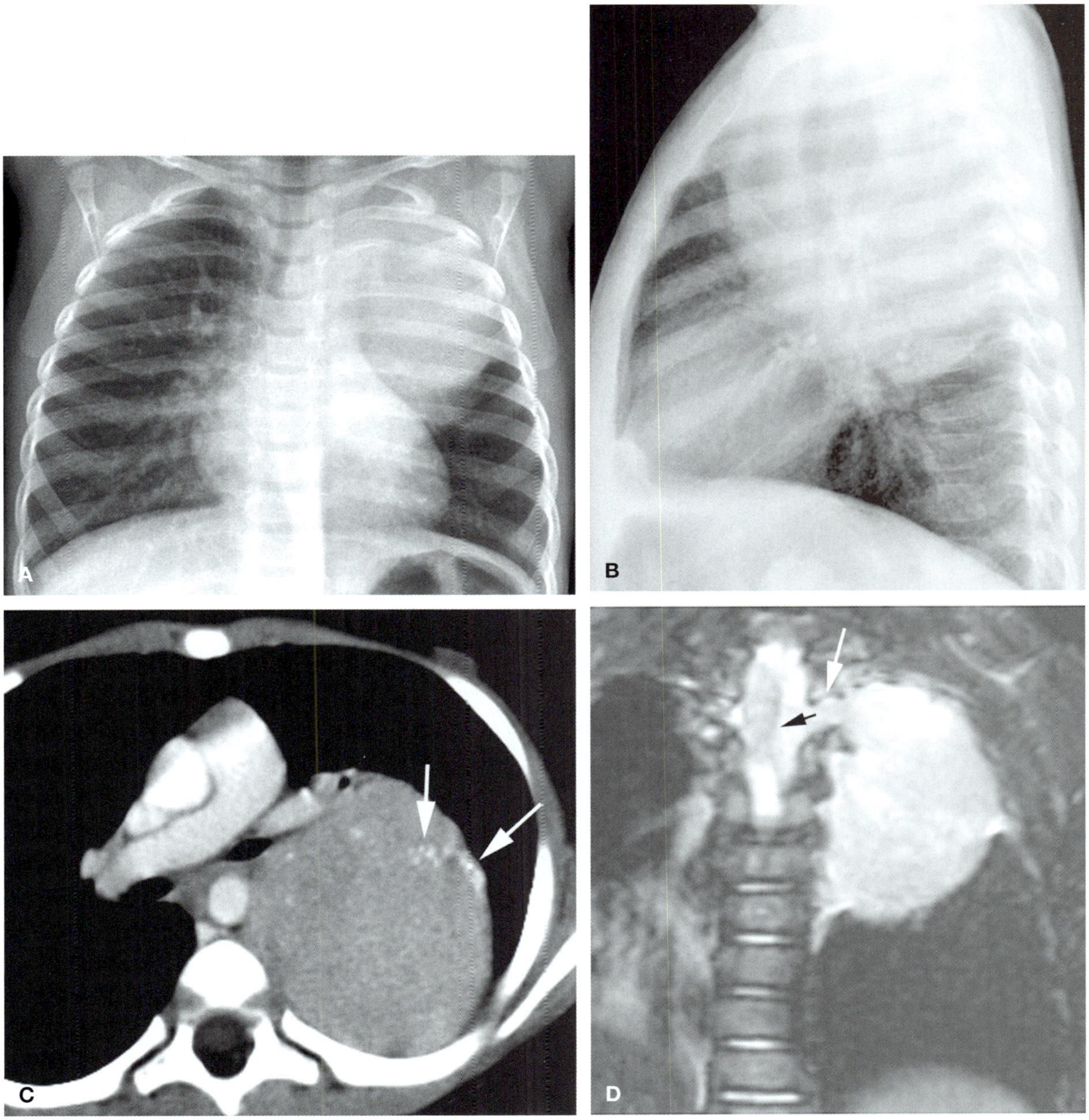

Figure 8.72. Mediastinal neuroblastoma in a 16-month-old child. PA **(A)** and lateral **(B)** chest radiographs show a large superior, posterior mediastinal mass. **C:** CT shows a large paravertebral, posterior mediastinal mass containing small areas of calcification (*arrows*). **D:** T2-weighted MRI shows a large mass in the posterior mediastinum. The tumor extends into the spinal canal through a neural foramen (*white arrow*), displacing the spinal cord to the right (*black arrow*).

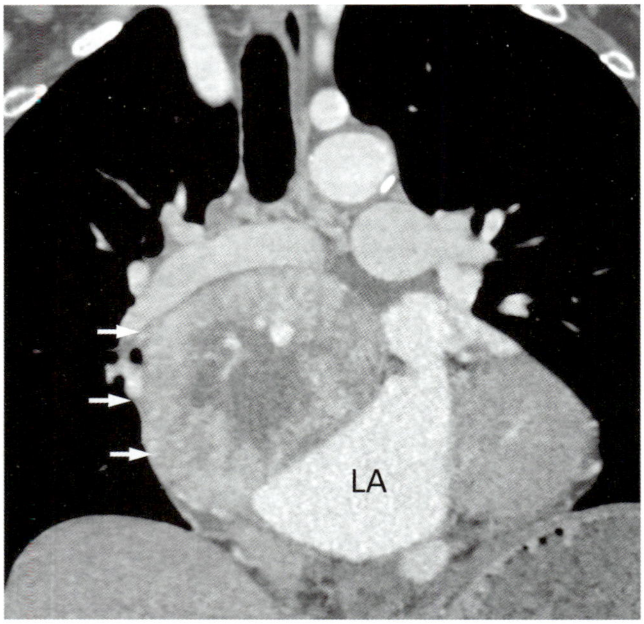

Figure 8.73. Paraganglioma (chemodectoma). Coronal CT shows a hypervascular mass (*arrows*) in the visceral compartment just superior to the left atrium (*LA*). Location and appearance are typical of paraganglioma.

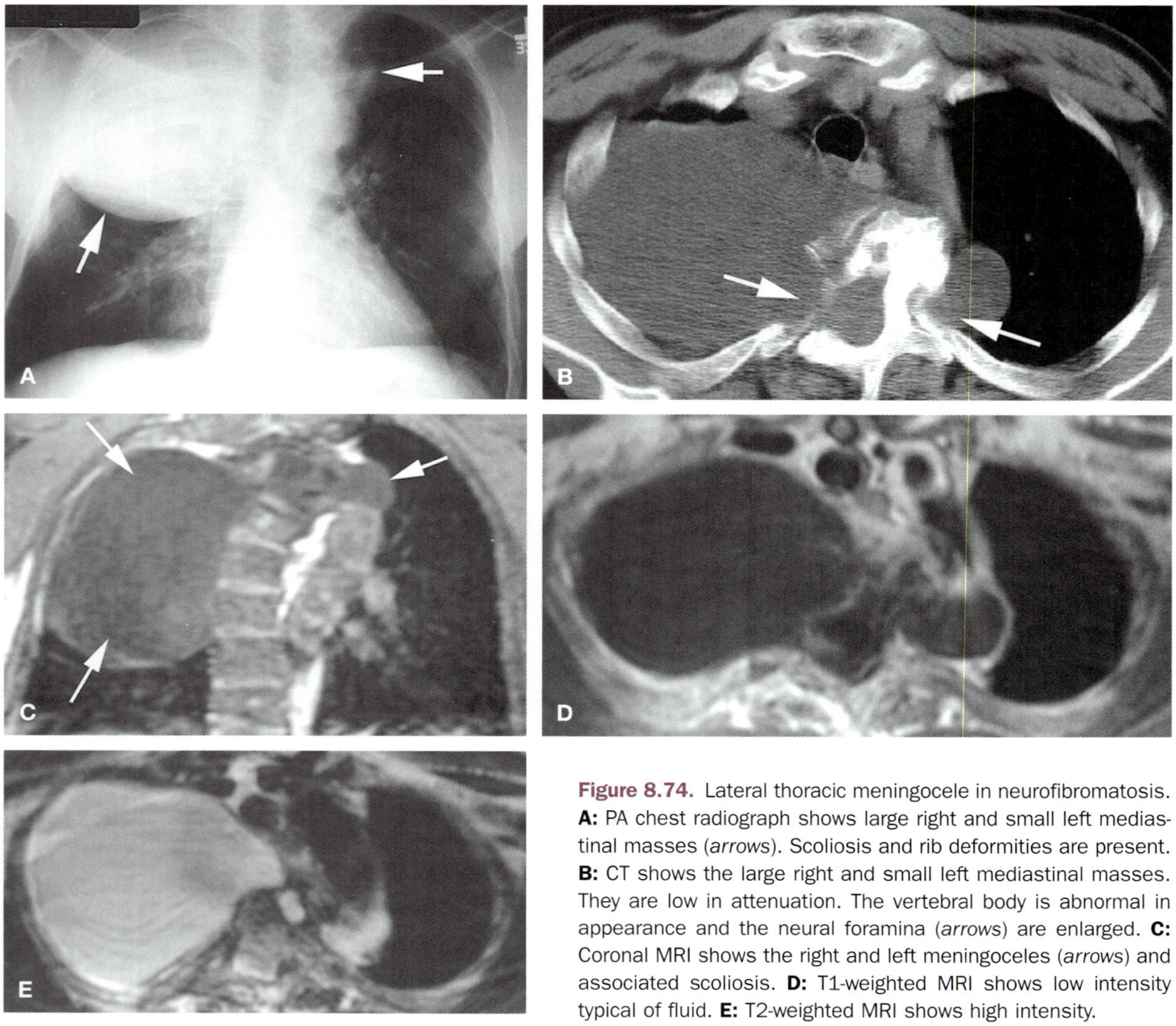

Figure 8.74. Lateral thoracic meningocele in neurofibromatosis. **A:** PA chest radiograph shows large right and small left mediastinal masses (*arrows*). Scoliosis and rib deformities are present. **B:** CT shows the large right and small left mediastinal masses. They are low in attenuation. The vertebral body is abnormal in appearance and the neural foramina (*arrows*) are enlarged. **C:** Coronal MRI shows the right and left meningoceles (*arrows*) and associated scoliosis. **D:** T1-weighted MRI shows low intensity typical of fluid. **E:** T2-weighted MRI shows high intensity.

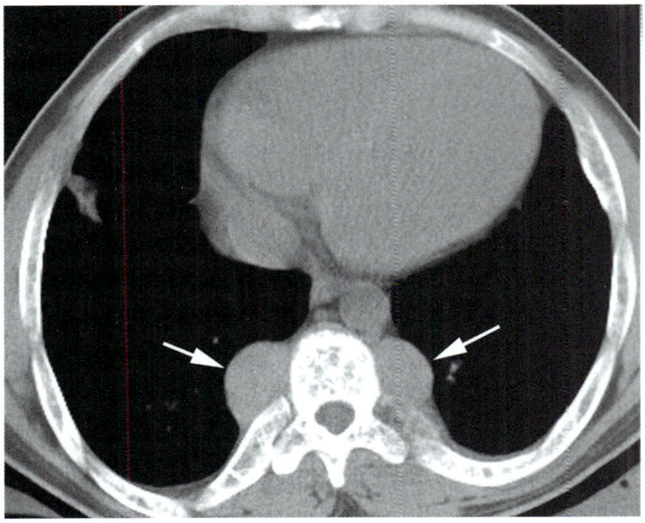

Figure 8.75. Extrathoracic hematopoiesis. CT in a patient with thalassemia major. Paravertebral masses (*arrows*) reflect hematopoietic tissue. Ribs and vertebral bodies are expanded and show an abnormal trabecular pattern, typical of severe anemia.

SUGGESTED READINGS

Agrons GA, Rosado-de-Christenson ML, Kirejczyk WM, Conran RM, Stocker JT. Pulmonary inflammatory pseudotumor: radiologic features. *Radiology*. 1998;206(2):511-518.

Ahn JM, Lee KS, Goo JM, Song KS, Kim SJ, Im JG. Predicting the histology of anterior mediastinal masses: comparison of chest radiography and CT. *J Thorac Imaging*. 1996;11(4):265-271.

Armstrong EA, Harwood-Nash DCF, Ritz CR, Chuang SH, Pettersson H, Martin DJ. CT of neuroblastomas and ganglioneuromas in children. *AJR Am J Roentgenol*. 1982;139(3):571-576.

Balthazar EJ, Naidich DP, Megibow AJ, Lefleur RS. CT evaluation of esophageal varices. *AJR Am J Roentgenol*. 1987;148(1):131-135.

Bashist B, Ellis K, Gold RP. Computed tomography of intrathoracic goiters. *AJR Am J Roentgenol*. 1983;140(3):455-460.

Benveniste MFK, Rosado-de-Christenson ML, Sabloff BS, Moran CA, Swisher SG, Marom EM. Role of imaging in the diagnosis, staging, and treatment of thymoma. *RadioGraphics*. 2011;31(7):1847-1863.

Bourgouin PM, Shepard JO, Moore EH, McLoud TC. Plexiform neurofibromatosis of the mediastinum: CT appearance. *AJR Am J Roentgenol*. 1988;151(3):461-463.

Bragg DG, Chor PJ, Murray KA, Kjeldsberg CR. Lymphoproliferative disorders of the lung: histopathology, clinical manifestations, and imaging features. *AJR Am J Roentgenol*. 1994;163(2):273-281.

Brown LR, Aughenbaugh GL. Masses of the anterior mediastinum: CT and MR imaging. *AJR Am J Roentgenol*. 1991;157(6):1171-1180.

Cakir O, Topal U, Bayram AS, Tolunay S. Sarcomas: rare primary malignant tumors of the thorax. *Diagn Interv Radiol*. 2005;11(1):23-27.

Carter BW, Benveniste MF, Madan R, et al. IASLC/ITMIG staging system and lymph node map for thymic epithelial neoplasms. *RadioGraphics*. 2017;37(3):758-776.

Carter BW, Benveniste MF, Madan R, et al. ITMIG classification of mediastinal compartments and multidisciplinary approach to mediastinal masses. *RadioGraphics*. 2017;37(2):413-436.

Castellino RA, Blank N, Hoppe RT, Cho C. Hodgkin disease: contributions of chest CT in the initial staging evaluation. *Radiology*. 1986;160(3):603-605.

Castellino RA, Hilton S, O'Brien JP, Portlock CS. Non-Hodgkin lymphoma: contribution of chest CT in the initial staging evaluation. *Radiology*. 1996;199(1):129-132.

Cohen LM, Schwartz AM, Rockoff SD. Benign schwannomas: pathologic basis for CT inhomogeneities. *AJR Am J Roentgenol*. 1986;147(1):141-143.

de Geer G, Webb WR, Gamsu G. Normal thymus: assessment with MR and CT. *Radiology*. 1986;158(2):313-317.

Detterbeck FC, Boffa DJ, Tanoue LT. The new lung cancer staging system. *Chest*. 2009;136(1):260-271.

Do YS, Im JG, Lee BH, et al. CT findings in malignant tumors of thymic epithelium. *J Comput Assist Tomogr*. 1995;19(2):192-197.

Drucker EA, McLoud TC, Dedrick CG, Hilgenberg AD, Geller SC, Shepard JA. Mediastinal paraganglioma: radiologic evaluation of an unusual vascular tumor. *AJR Am J Roentgenol*. 1987;148(3):521-522.

Filly R, Bland N, Castellino R. Radiographic distribution of intrathoracic disease in previously untreated patients with Hodgkin's disease and non-Hodgkin's lymphoma. *Radiology*. 1976;120(2):277-281.

Fitch SJ, Tonkin ILD, Tonkin AK. Imaging of foregut duplication cysts. *RadioGraphics*. 1986;6(2):189-201.

Freundlich IM, McGavran MH. Abnormalities of the thymus. *J Thorac Imaging*. 1996;11(1):58-65.

Gal AA, Kornstein MJ, Cohen C, Duarte IG, Miller JI, Mansour KA. Neuroendocrine tumors of the thymus: a clinicopathological and prognostic study. *Ann Thorac Surg*. 2001;72(4):1179-1182.

Glazer GM, Gross BH, Quint LE, Francis IR, Bookstein FL, Orringer MB. Normal mediastinal lymph nodes: number and size according to American Thoracic Society mapping. *AJR Am J Roentgenol*. 1985;144(2):261-265.

Glazer HS, Molina PL, Siegel MJ, Sagel SS. High-attenuation mediastinal masses on unenhanced CT. *AJR Am J Roentgenol*. 1991;156(1):45-50.

Glazer HS, Siegel MJ, Sagel SS, Sagel SS. Low-attenuation mediastinal masses on CT. *AJR Am J Roentgenol*. 1989;152(6):1173-1177.

Glazer HS, Wick MR, Anderson DJ, et al. CT of fatty thoracic masses. *AJR Am J Roentgenol*. 1992;159(6):1181-1187.

Hoeffel C, Floquet J, Regent D, Chen YB, Hoeffel JC. Periesophageal mediastinal fibromatosis. *Abdom Imaging*. 2000;25(3):235-238.

Hoffman OA, Gillespie DJ, Aughenbaugh GL, Brown LR. Primary mediastinal neoplasms (other than thymoma). *Mayo Clin Proc*. 1993;68(9):880-891.

Horger M, Lamprecht HG, Bares R, et al. Systemic IgG4-related sclerosing disease: spectrum of imaging findings and differential diagnosis. *AJR Am J Roentgenol*. 2012;199(3):W276-W282.

Jolles H, Henry DA, Roberson JP, Cole TJ, Spratt JA. Mediastinitis following median sternotomy: CT findings. *Radiology*. 1996;201(2):463-466.

Kang YS, Rosen K, Clark OH, Higgins CB. Localization of abnormal parathyroid glands of the mediastinum with MR imaging. *Radiology*. 1993;189(1):137-141.

Kawashima A, Fishman EK, Kuhlman JE, Nixon MS. CT of posterior mediastinal masses. *RadioGraphics*. 1991;11(6):1045-1067.

Kim DJ, Yang WI, Choi SS, Kim KD, Chung KY. Prognostic and clinical relevance of the world health organization schema for the classification of thymic epithelial tumors: a clinicopathologic study of 108 patients and literature review. *Chest*. 2005;127(3):755-761.

Kirchner SG, Heller RM, Smith CW. Pancreatic pseudocyst of the mediastinum. *Radiology*. 1977;123(1):37-42.

Kirks DR, McCormick VD, Greenspan RH. Pulmonary sarcoidosis: roentgenographic analysis of 150 patients. *AJR Am J Roentgenol*. 1973;117(4):777-786.

Kirsch CFE, Webb EM, Webb WR. Multicentric Castleman's disease and POEMS syndrome: CT findings. *J Thorac Imaging*. 1997;12(1):75-77.

Kiyono K, Sone S, Sakai F, et al. The number and size of normal mediastinal lymph nodes: a postmortem study. *AJR Am J Roentgenol*. 1988;150(4):771-776.

Kushihashi T, Munechika H, Motoya H, et al. CT and MR findings in tuberculous mediastinitis. *J Comput Assist Tomogr*. 1995;19(3):379-382.

Lee KS, Im JG, Han CH, Han MC, Kim CW, Kim WS. Malignant primary germ cell tumors of the mediastinum: CT features. *AJR Am J Roentgenol*. 1989;153(5):947-951.

Long JA, Doppman JL, Nienhuis AW. Computed tomographic studies of thoracic extramedullary hematopoiesis. *J Comput Assist Tomogr*. 1980;4(1):67-70.

Marx A, Chan JKC, Chalabreysse L, et al. The 2021 WHO classification of tumors of the thymus and mediastinum: what is new in thymic epithelial, germ cell, and mesenchymal tumors? *J Thorac Oncol*. 2022;17(2):200-213.

McAdams HP, Rosado de Christenson ML, Moran CA. Mediastinal hemangioma: radiographic and CT features in 14 patients. *Radiology*. 1994;193(2):399-402.

McLoud TC, Kalisher L, Stark P, Greene R. Intrathoracic lymph node metastases from extrathoracic neoplasms. *AJR Am J Roentgenol*. 1978;131(3):403-407.

Miyake H, Shiga M, Takaki H, Hata H, Onishi R, Mori H. Mediastinal lymphangiomas in adults: CT findings. *J Thorac Imaging*. 1996;11(1):83-85.

Moeller KH, Rosado-de-Christenson ML, Templeton PA. Mediastinal mature teratoma: imaging features. *AJR Am J Roentgenol*. 1997;169(4):985-990.

Moon WK, Im JG, Kim JS, et al. Mediastinal Castleman disease: CT findings. *J Comput Assist Tomogr*. 1994;18(1):43-46.

Moon WK, Im JG, Yu IK, Lee SK, Yeon KM, Han MC. Mediastinal tuberculous lymphadenitis: MR imaging appearance with clinicopathologic correlation. *AJR Am J Roentgenol.* 1996;166(1):21-25.

Mountain CF, Dresler CM. Regional lymph node classification for lung cancer staging. *Chest.* 1997;111(6):1718-1723.

Müller NL, Webb WR, Gamsu G. Paratracheal lymphadenopathy: radiographic findings and correlation with CT. *Radiology.* 1985;156(3):761-765.

Müller NL, Webb WR, Gamsu G. Subcarinal lymph node enlargement: radiographic findings and CT correlation. *AJR Am J Roentgenol.* 1985;145(1):15-19.

Nicolaou S, Müller NL, Li DK, Oger JJ. Thymus in myasthenia gravis: comparison of CT and pathologic findings and clinical outcome after thymectomy. *Radiology.* 1996;201(2):471-474.

Okumura M, Ohta M, Tateyama H, et al. The World Health Organization histologic classification system reflects the oncologic behavior of thymoma: a clinical study of 273 patients. *Cancer.* 2002;94(3):624-632.

Patel SN, Levin DL. Distribution of thoracic lymphadenopathy in sarcoidosis using computed tomography. *J Thorac Imaging.* 1999;14(2):114-117.

Rami-Porta R, Crowley JJ, Goldstraw P. The revised TNM staging system for lung cancer. *Ann Thorac Cardiovasc Surg.* 2009;15(1):4-9.

Reed JC, Hallet KK, Feigin DS. Neural tumors of the thorax: subject review from the AFIP. *Radiology.* 1978;126(1):9-17.

Reed JC, Sobonya RE. Morphologic analysis of foregut cysts in the thorax. *AJR Am J Roentgenol.* 1974;120(4):851-860.

Rosado de Christenson ML, Pugatch RD, Moran CA, Galobardes J. Thymolipoma: analysis of 27 cases. *Radiology.* 1994;193(1):121-126.

Rosado de Christenson ML, Templeton PA, Moran CA. From the archives of the AFIP. Mediastinal germ cell tumors: radiologic and pathologic correlation. *RadioGraphics.* 1992;12(5):1013-1030.

Rossi SE, McAdams HP, Rosado-de-Christenson ML, Franks TJ, Galvin JR. Fibrosing mediastinitis. *RadioGraphics.* 2001;21(3):737-757.

Sakai F, Sone S, Kiyono K, et al. Intrathoracic neurogenic tumors: MR–pathologic correlation. *AJR Am J Roentgenol.* 1992;159(2):279-283.

Sherrick AD, Brown LR, Harms GF, Myers JL. The radiographic findings of fibrosing mediastinitis. *Chest.* 1994;106(2):484-489.

Spector JA, Willis DN, Ginsburg HB. Paraganglioma (pheochromocytoma) of the posterior mediastinum: a case report and review of the literature. *J Pediatr Surg.* 2003;38(7):1114-1116.

Strollo DC, Rosado-de-Christenson ML. Primary mediastinal malignant germ cell neoplasms: imaging features. *Chest Surg Clin N Am.* 2002;12(4):645-658.

Tomiyama N, Johkoh T, Mihara N, et al. Using the World Health Organization Classification of thymic epithelial neoplasms to describe CT findings. *AJR Am J Roentgenol.* 2002;179(4):881-886.

Travis WD, Brambilla E, Burke AP, et al. *WHO Classification of Tumours of the Lung, Pleura, Thymus and Heart.* WHO Press; 2015.

Chapter 9

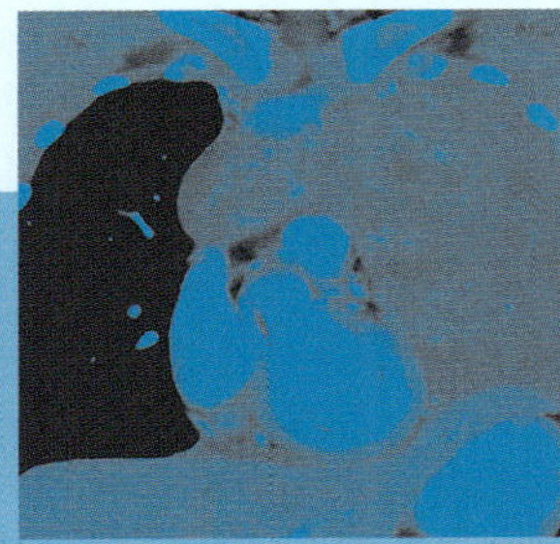

Travis S. Henry

Congenital Lung Abnormalities and Pulmonary Vascular Malformations

INTRODUCTION

A variety of congenital abnormalities may involve the bronchi, lung, and/or its vascular supply. They often have characteristic plain film and computed tomography (CT) findings. Congenital pulmonary malformations can be classified in several ways. A simple classification considers two groups: (1) those usually unassociated with abnormal vessels and (2) those associated with or consisting of abnormal vessels (Table 9.1). Congenital abnormalities of the aorta and great vessels are reviewed in a later chapter.

Table 9.1 Congenital Lung Malformations

Usually Unassociated with Vascular Abnormalities
Bronchial anomalies
Congenital lobar overinflation (congenital lobar emphysema)
Pulmonary bronchogenic cyst
Congenital pulmonary airway malformation
Associated with or Consisting of Vascular Abnormalities
Pulmonary arteriovenous malformation (fistula)
Pulmonary agenesis, aplasia, and hypoplasia
Hypogenetic lung syndrome (scimitar or venolobar syndrome)
Proximal interruption of the pulmonary artery
Unilateral pulmonary vein atresia
Pulmonary vein varix
Anomalous pulmonary vein drainage
Bronchopulmonary sequestration
Systemic artery malformation

BRONCHIAL ANOMALIES

Bronchial anomalies include displaced origins, absent branches, supernumerary branches, and congenital diverticula (Table 9.2). Minor variation in subsegmental bronchial anatomy is common and clinically insignificant; a detailed knowledge of subsegmental bronchial anatomy is not necessary for clinical practice. Variation in segmental bronchial anatomy is less frequent.

Table 9.2 Bronchial Anomalies

Variations in subsegmental branching
Common but insignificant
Tracheal bronchus
Incidence 0.1%
Arises from right tracheal wall; rare on left
Usually supplies apical segment of right upper lobe
Rarely supplies entire right upper lobe
Increased incidence of infection or bronchiectasis
Accessory cardiac bronchus
Incidence 0.1%
Arises from medial wall of bronchus intermedius
Usually blind ending or supplies rudimentary lung
May terminate in the mediastinum
Increased incidence of infection or hemoptysis
Bronchial isomerism
Symmetrical bronchial anatomy
Bilateral right- or left-sided bronchial anatomy
Associated with congenital heart disease, other anomalies

Tracheal Bronchus

A tracheal bronchus is present in about 0.1% of the population. It usually arises from the right tracheal wall, at or within 2 cm of the tracheal bifurcation. It supplies a variable portion of the medial or apical right upper lobe, most often the apical segment (Fig. 9.1). The term "tracheal bronchus" is sometimes used to refer to a displaced bronchus, supplying a part of the upper lobe, even if it does not arise from the trachea; origin from the right main bronchus is most frequent in this case.

Rarely, the entire right upper lobe bronchus arises from the trachea (Fig. 9.2). When a right-sided tracheal bronchus is present, the azygos arch is seen above the tracheal bronchus. Tracheal bronchus is sometimes referred to as a "pig bronchus" or "bronchus suis" as it is common in pigs and other cloven-hoofed animals.

In most cases, this anomaly is insignificant. However, recurrent infection or bronchiectasis may result, since the tracheal bronchus is often slightly narrowed at its origin. A left tracheal bronchus and its variants, supplying the apical posterior segment of the left upper lobe, are rare; it is much less common than a right-sided tracheal bronchus.

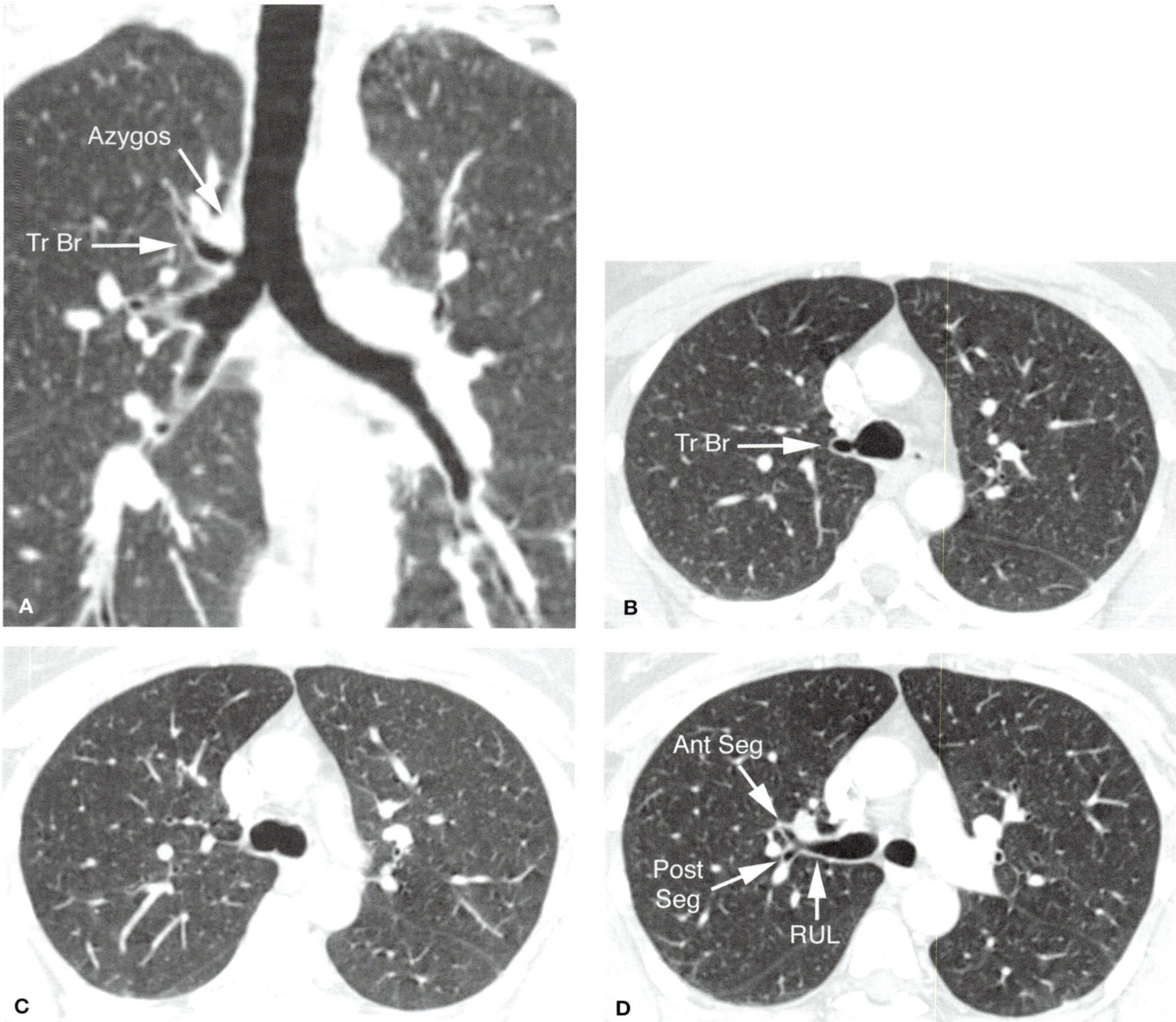

Figure 9.1. Tracheal bronchus. **A:** Coronal CT reconstruction shows a tracheal bronchus (*Tr Br*) arising from the right tracheal wall just above the carina. The azygos arch (*Azygos*) is visible above the bronchus. **B:** CT (1.25-mm slice thickness) shows the origin of the tracheal bronchus (*Tr Br*). As in this case, slight narrowing at the origin of the bronchus is common. The bronchus supplies the apical segment of the right upper lobe. **C:** The tracheal carina is seen slightly below (**B**). **D:** Below (**C**), the main right upper lobe bronchus (*RUL*) gives rise to the anterior (*Ant Seg*) and posterior (*Post Seg*) segmental bronchi.

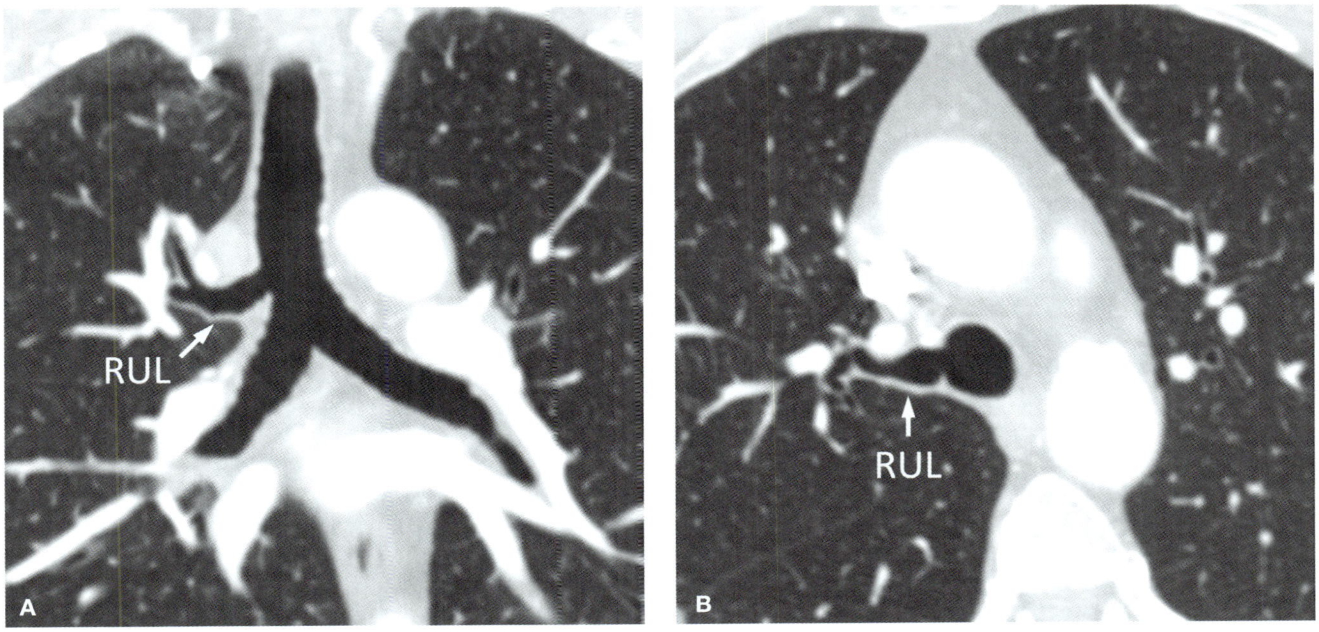

Figure 9.2. Tracheal bronchus. **A:** Coronal reconstruction shows the entire right upper lobe bronchus (*RUL*) arising from the right tracheal wall above the carina. The apical segmental bronchus extends superiorly. **B:** Axial CT shows the right upper lobe bronchus (*RUL*) giving rise to anterior and posterior segments.

Accessory Cardiac Bronchus

Accessory cardiac bronchus is a supernumerary bronchus with an incidence of about 0.1%. It arises from the medial wall of the bronchus intermedius or right lower lobe bronchus and extends inferiorly and medially toward the mediastinum or heart. In some cases, the cardiac bronchus is a short, blind-ending bronchial stump without associated alveolar tissue, and it may terminate in the mediastinum. In others, a longer branching bronchus is present, associated with rudimentary lung tissue (Fig. 9.3). In most cases, this anomaly is an incidental finding; occasionally, chronic infection or hemoptysis is associated.

Bronchial Isomerism

Bronchial isomerism refers to bilateral symmetry of the bronchi and associated pulmonary lobes. It may be isolated or associated with a variety of anomalies, particularly congenital heart disease. Bronchial anatomy may be bilaterally right sided (associated with asplenia) or left sided (associated with polysplenia).

BRONCHIAL ATRESIA

Bronchial atresia is a developmental defect characterized by local narrowing or obliteration of a lobar, segmental, or subsegmental bronchus (Table 9.3). It is most common in the left upper lobe, followed by the right upper and right middle lobes; it is less common in the lower lobes. This entity is usually detected incidentally in adults and is undoubtedly related to some cases of congenital lobar overinflation (CLO). Patients usually have no symptoms, but the lung distal to the obstruction may occasionally become infected. In patients with chronic infection, resection may be necessary.

The lobe or segment distal to the bronchial obstruction usually remains aerated because of collateral ventilation (Figs. 9.4 and 9.5). In 90% of cases, air trapping in the distal lung results in decreased perfusion; radiographs and CT show the affected lung to be hyperlucent and hypovascular. Affected lung is often increased in volume, resulting in mediastinal shift or shift of a fissure. In 80% of cases, mucus accumulates within dilated bronchi distal to the obstruction, resulting in a tubular, branching, or ovoid density (mucous plug or *mucocele*). Mucus within dilated bronchi usually appears low in attenuation. Expiratory radiographs or CT scans show air trapping (see Fig. 9.5B).

The combination of these typical radiographic or CT findings in a young patient is strongly suggestive of the diagnosis. Bronchoscopy may be warranted to rule out another cause of bronchial obstruction, such as tumor.

CONGENITAL LOBAR OVERINFLATION

CLO, formerly known as congenital lobar emphysema, is characterized by marked overinflation of a lobe (Table 9.4). Most cases present within the first month of life; symptoms of respiratory distress are typical, because the overinflated lobe compresses the normal lung. Presentation after the first month may occur.

Most cases of CLO are associated with partial or complete bronchial obstruction occurring as a result of (a) deficient

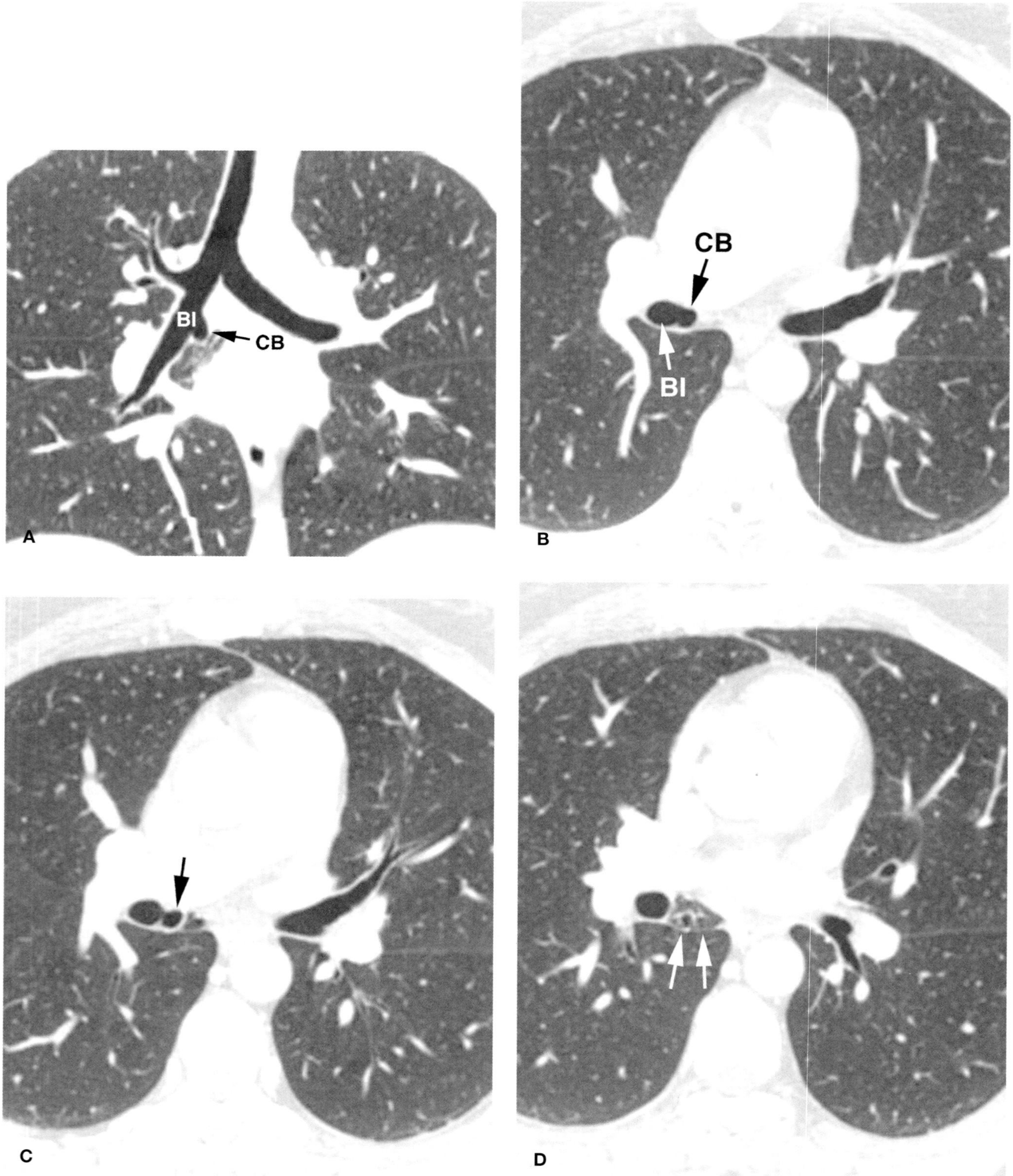

Figure 9.3. Accessory cardiac bronchus. **A:** Coronal CT reconstruction shows an accessory cardiac bronchus (*CB*) arising from the medial aspect of the bronchus intermedius (*BI*), to supply a small region of lung. **B:** Transaxial image shows the cardiac bronchus (*CB*) arising from the medial wall of the bronchus intermedius (*BI*). **C:** Slightly below (**B**), the cardiac bronchus (*arrow*) is seen medial to the bronchus intermedius. **D:** Below (**C**), the bronchus supplies a small segment of lung separated from the lower lobe by an accessory fissure (*arrows*).

Table 9.3 Bronchial Atresia

Bronchial Atresia
Narrowing or obliteration of a lobar, segmental, or subsegmental bronchus
Left upper lobe > right upper lobe > right middle lobe > lower lobes
Detected incidentally in adults
Infection may occur
Mucous plug distal to obstructed bronchial segment
Distal lung
Lucent
Increased in volume
Decreased vessel size
Air trapping on expiration
Rule out obstructing tumor

cartilage; (b) external compression, usually by an anomalous vessel or bronchogenic cyst; or (c) luminal abnormalities such as mucosal folds. Some cases are unassociated with bronchial obstruction.

CLO is most common in the left upper lobe (40%), followed by the right middle lobe (35%) and right upper lobe (20%) (note the similarity of this distribution to that of bronchial atresia). Only a few percent occur in the lower lobes. Radiographs typically show marked overinflation and air trapping in the affected lobe. However, in neonates, the affected lobe may sometimes appear opaque because of retained fetal lung fluid. Mediastinal shift away from the abnormal lobe often occurs, and normal lobes are reduced in volume. Resection is often necessary.

It is reasonable to assume that cases of CLO that go unrecognized at birth may be diagnosed years later as bronchial atresia.

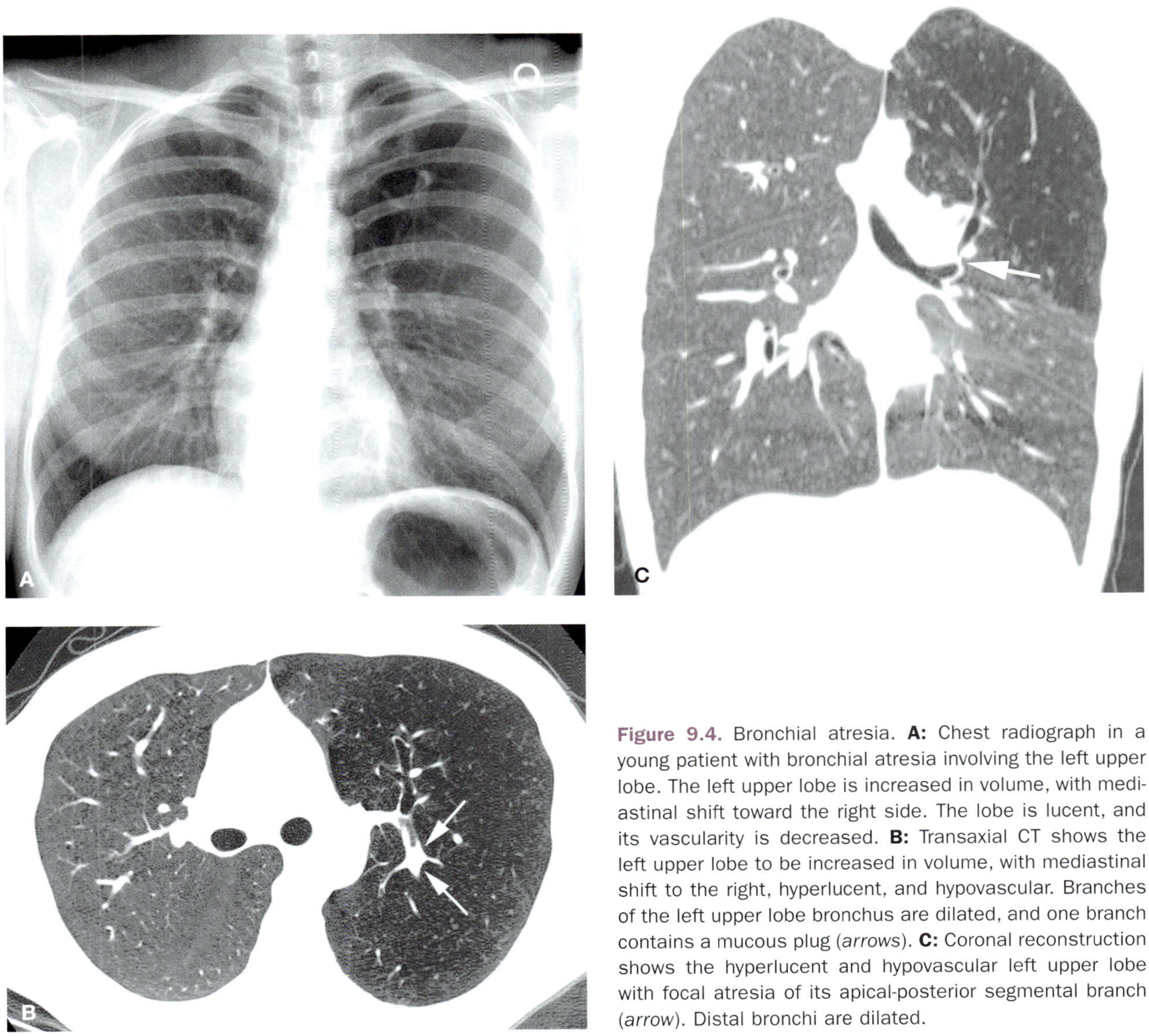

Figure 9.4. Bronchial atresia. **A:** Chest radiograph in a young patient with bronchial atresia involving the left upper lobe. The left upper lobe is increased in volume, with mediastinal shift toward the right side. The lobe is lucent, and its vascularity is decreased. **B:** Transaxial CT shows the left upper lobe to be increased in volume, with mediastinal shift to the right, hyperlucent, and hypovascular. Branches of the left upper lobe bronchus are dilated, and one branch contains a mucous plug (*arrows*). **C:** Coronal reconstruction shows the hyperlucent and hypovascular left upper lobe with focal atresia of its apical-posterior segmental branch (*arrow*). Distal bronchi are dilated.

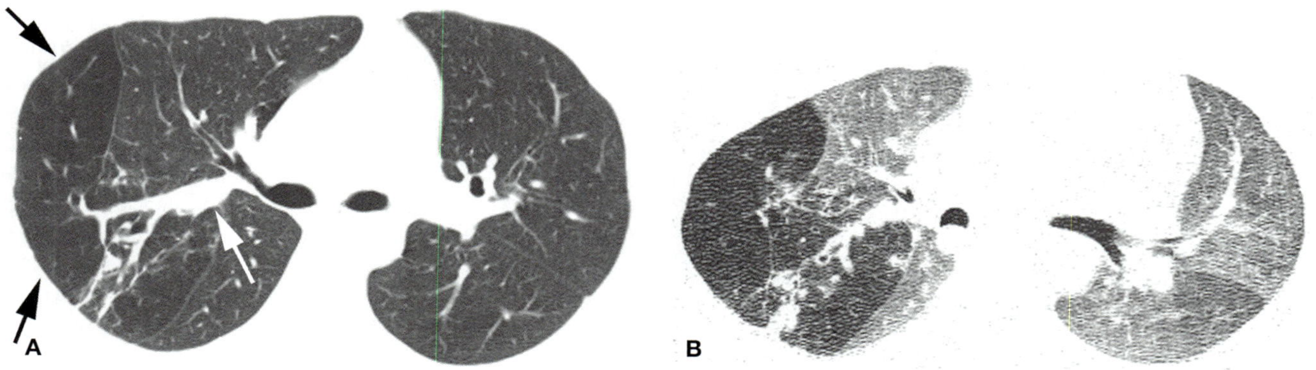

Figure 9.5. Bronchial atresia. **A:** CT shows a branching mucous plug (*white arrow*) in the location of the posterior segmental bronchus of the right upper lobe. Lung distal to the bronchus (*black arrows*) is hyperlucent and hypovascular. Mediastinal shift to the left side is present. **B:** Expiratory CT shows air trapping in the lung distal to the obstructed bronchus. Normal lung increases significantly in attenuation relative to (**A**).

PULMONARY BRONCHOGENIC CYST

Bronchogenic cysts are foregut duplication cysts and result from abnormal development of the lung bud. They are lined by pseudostratified ciliated columnar epithelium, typical of bronchi. The cyst wall may also contain smooth muscle, mucous glands, or cartilage. Bronchogenic cysts are filled with fluid, which can be serous, hemorrhagic, or highly viscous and gelatinous because of its high protein content.

Bronchogenic cysts may be mediastinal or pulmonary. Mediastinal bronchogenic cysts are much more common than pulmonary cysts. They are discussed along with mediastinal masses in Chapter 8.

Pulmonary bronchogenic cysts are most common in the medial lung and the lower lobes (Table 9.5). They are sharply circumscribed and round or oval. The cyst wall may calcify. Rarely, the cyst may contain milk of calcium and appear dense. Cysts may slowly increase in size; a rapid increase in size is unusual unless infection occurs.

About half of fluid-filled bronchogenic cysts appear to be low in attenuation on CT (0-20 HU) (Fig. 9.6). However, as with mediastinal bronchogenic cysts, the CT attenuation of a pulmonary bronchogenic cyst is variable. High CT numbers (40-80 HU), suggesting a solid mass, can be seen. Such cysts contain bloody or thick, proteinaceous fluid. Typically, the cyst wall appears very thin on CT or is invisible. A bronchogenic cyst may sometimes appear to be related to a small bronchus.

Infection eventually occurs in 75% of cases. In the presence of acute infection, a rapid increase in size of the cyst may be seen. Also, the outer cyst wall may become less well defined because of surrounding lung inflammation. During or after infection, a cyst may contain air (Fig. 9.7; see also Figure 10.29 in Chapter 10) or a combination of air and fluid (with an air-fluid level). When the cyst contains air, its wall appears very thin.

CONGENITAL PULMONARY AIRWAY MALFORMATION (CONGENITAL CYSTIC ADENOMATOID MALFORMATION)

Congenital pulmonary airway malformations (CPAM), also known as congenital cystic adenomatoid malformation (CCAM; both terms are used in the literature, although

Table 9.4 Congenital Lobar Overinflation
Partial or complete bronchial obstruction caused by:
Deficient cartilage
External compression
Luminal abnormalities
Some cases unassociated with bronchial obstruction
Left upper lobe > right middle lobe > right upper lobe > lower lobes
Respiratory distress in neonates
Presentation after first month uncommon
Marked overinflation of lobe
Air trapping
Sometimes the abnormal lobe retains fetal lung fluid
Resection often necessary

Table 9.5 Pulmonary Bronchogenic Cyst
Foregut duplication cyst
Lined by bronchial epithelium
Fluid contents can be serous, hemorrhagic, or viscous
Less common than mediastinal bronchogenic cyst
Most common in medial lung and lower lobes
Sharply circumscribed and round or oval
Thin wall; occasionally calcifies
Contents 0-20 HU in half; often 40-80 HU; milk of calcium rare
Infection occurs in 75%
Rapid increase in size
Blurring of outer edge
Air-fluid level
Air in cyst may remain after infection

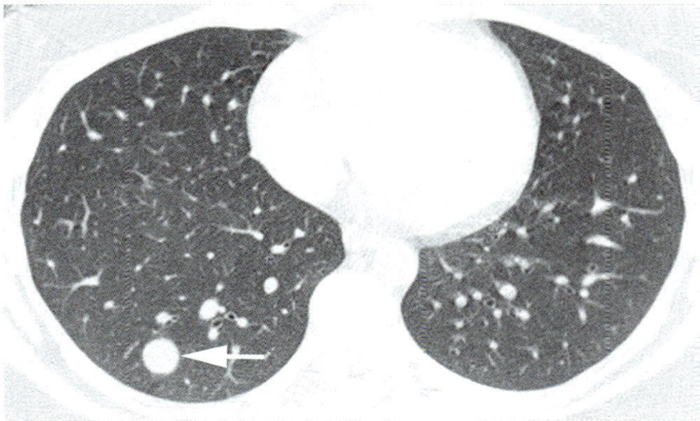

Figure 9.6. Pulmonary bronchogenic cyst. A sharply marginated round nodular opacity (*arrow*) is visible in the right lower lobe. This measured 0 HU in attenuation. This appearance is typical of a fluid-filled bronchogenic cyst.

CPAM is the newer term for this entity), consist of an intralobar mass of disorganized lung tissue, derived primarily from bronchioles, and often cystic or multicystic. About 70% present during the first week of life, but 10% are diagnosed after the first year, and rare cases in adults have been reported.

Lower lobes are most often involved, but any lobe can be affected. CPAM/CCAM can occupy an entire lobe. The CPAM/CCAM communicates with the bronchial tree and is supplied by the pulmonary artery; systemic arterial supply is rarely present.

Understanding these terms requires a little knowledge of history. Initially, the term CCAM was used, because these lesions are typically cystic. CCAMs were classified into three primary types (types 1-3), with different histology, gross pathologic findings, radiographic appearance, and prognosis (Table 9.6). These three types are those most commonly encountered in practice.

Subsequently, types 0 and 4 were proposed by Stocker, based on histopathologic findings and the type of airway epithelium involved in the malformation (Table 9.6). Also, the term CPAM was proposed to encompass this expanded classification, as it was thought that CPAM more accurately described the histology of these lesions. The types of CCAM/CPAM are described below.

Type 1 CCAM (CPAM) (65% of cases) contains one or more cysts more than 2 cm in diameter (Fig. 9.8). They usually appear radiographically as a large, air-filled multicystic lesion, sometimes with air-fluid levels, which may occupy the entire hemithorax.

Type 2 CCAM (CPAM) (20%-25% of cases) contains multiple cysts less than 2 cm in diameter. They present radiographically as an air-filled multicystic mass or a solid mass or area of consolidation (see Fig. 9.9). This type may be associated with a poor prognosis because of associated renal and cardiac abnormalities.

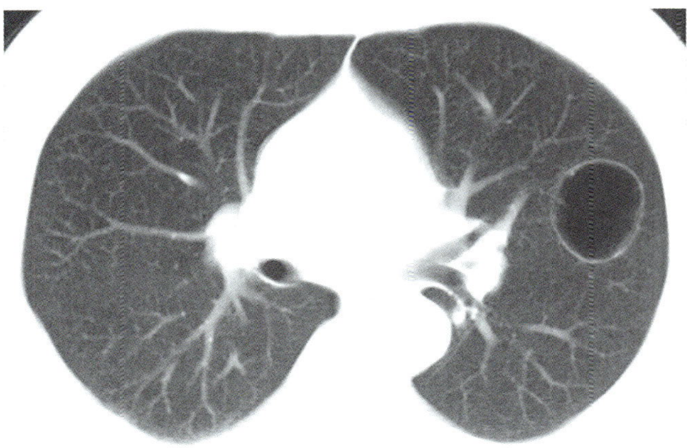

Figure 9.7. Pulmonary bronchogenic cyst. A thin-walled, sharply marginated, air-filled bronchogenic cyst is visible in the left lung. The presence of air within the cyst indicates prior infection.

Table 9.6 Congenital Pulmonary Airway Malformation (Also Known as Congenital Cystic Adenomatoid Malformation)

Multicystic, intralobar mass of disorganized lung tissue
70% present in first week; 10% after first year
Respiratory distress in neonates; recurrent infection in adults
Most common in lower lobe
Three primary types (1-3)
Two additional types (0 and 4) proposed by Stocker, based on histology
Type 1 (65%)
One or more cysts, >2 cm in diameter
May appear initially as solid mass
Large air-filled multicystic lesion
Sometimes with air-fluid levels
May occupy the entire hemithorax
Type 2 (20%-25%)
Multiple cysts <2 cm in diameter
May appear initially as solid mass
Air-filled multicystic mass or focal consolidation
Associated renal and cardiac abnormalities
Often a poor prognosis
Type 3 (10%)
Microscopic (<3-5 mm) cysts
Appears as solid mass
Type 0 (a few %)
Small cysts
Similar to type 3 in appearance
Type 4 (a few %)
Large cysts
Similar to types 1 and 2 in appearance

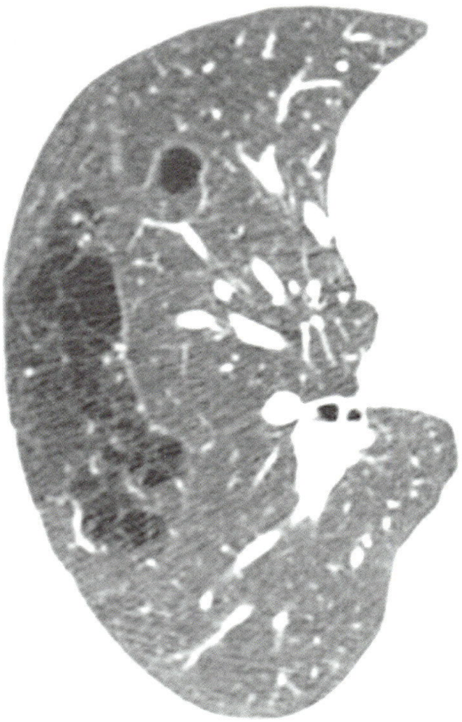

Figure 9.8. Type 1 congenital pulmonary airway malformation (CPAM)/congenital cystic adenomatoid malformation (CCAM). A multicystic lesion is visible in the right lower lobe. This is a typical appearance of type 1 CPAM/CCAM in an adult.

Type 3 CCAM (CPAM) (10% of cases) contains microscopic (less than 3-5 mm) cysts and present radiographically as a solid mass.

Types 0 and 4 CPAM (CCAM) each account for a few percent of cases. Type 0 CCAM/CPAM is associated with small cysts, as in type 3. Type 4 CCAM/CPAM is associated with large cysts, as is type 1; its radiographic and CT appearance is the same as for type 1 or 2. The terms CCAM and CPAM are largely interchangeable and are the same regardless of the acronym used; currently, CPAM tends to be favored, although reports of CCAM still appear in the literature.

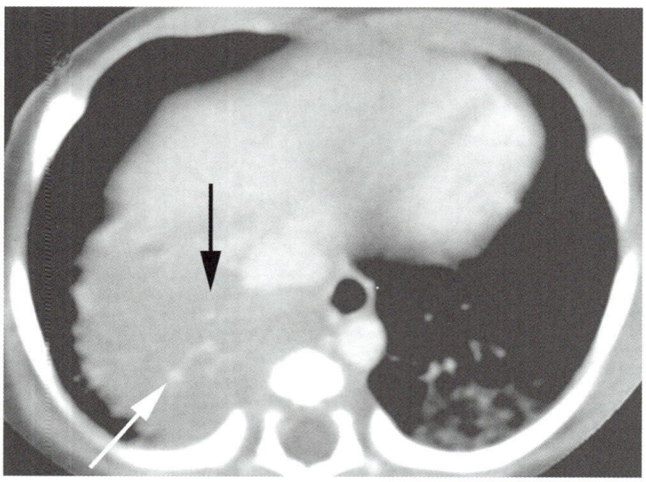

Figure 9.9. Type II congenital pulmonary airway malformation (CPAM)/ congenital cystic adenomatoid malformation (CCAM). A solid mass (*black arrow*) is visible in the right lower lobe of a neonate An opacified vessel is visible within the mass (*white arrow*). Type II CPAM/CCAM may present as an air-filled or fluid-filled mass.

Sonography can be used for prenatal diagnosis. Findings include polyhydramnios, fetal hydrops, and a solid or cystic mass in the fetal thorax. Fetal surgery may be attempted.

In infancy, CCAM/CPAM presents as a space-occupying lesion. Symptoms of respiratory distress are common. In neonates, CCAM/CPAM usually presents as a solid mass regardless of its type. Types 1 and 2 may become air-filled over a period of days to weeks. They are often associated with progressive air trapping and mediastinal shift to the opposite side.

The treatment of choice is excision of the affected lobe. The prognosis of neonates with CCAM/CPAM is adversely affected by large size, underdevelopment of uninvolved lung (ie, the presence of associated lung hypoplasia), and the presence of associated fetal hydrops or other congenital anomalies.

In adults, CCAM/CPAM usually presents as an air-filled or air- and fluid-filled cystic or multicystic mass. Most adults present with recurrent pneumonia, although recurrent pneumothorax has also been associated. Occasionally, adenocarcinoma may arise in relation to a CCAM/CPAM.

PULMONARY ARTERIOVENOUS MALFORMATION

Congenital arteriovenous malformation (AVM), also known as arteriovenous fistula, likely results from deficient formation or abnormal dilation of pulmonary capillaries due to a developmental defect in the capillary wall. From 35% to 67% of cases are associated with Osler-Weber-Rendu syndrome (*hereditary hemorrhagic telangiectasia*), in which AVMs are found in the skin, mucous membranes, and viscera (Table 9.7). Also, AVMs may rarely occur in patients with hepatopulmonary syndrome or as a result of trauma.

Table 9.7 Pulmonary Arteriovenous Malformation (AVM)

35%-67% associated with Osler-Weber-Rendu syndrome
Multiple in 35%
Bilateral in 10%
Single AVM less often symptomatic than multiple AVM (35% vs 60%)
Symptoms: Cyanosis, dyspnea, and hemoptysis
Complications: Rupture and paradoxical embolization
Simple AVM: One feeding artery and one draining vein
Complex AVM: Multiple feeding vessels
Most common in lower lobes, peripheral
Diagnosis by morphology at CT
Treatment by embolization

Pulmonary arteriovenous fistulas slowly enlarge over time and are usually first diagnosed in adulthood. More than two-thirds of AVMs are found in the lower lobes, and they are typically peripheral in location. Fistulas are multiple in 35% of patients and bilateral in 10%.

Simple and Complex AVMs

A *simple AVM* is a single, dilated vascular sac connecting one artery and one vein (Figs. 9.10 and 9.11). It is most frequent and accounts for the bulk of cases of AVM. *Complex AVMs*, which have more than one feeding artery, are rare.

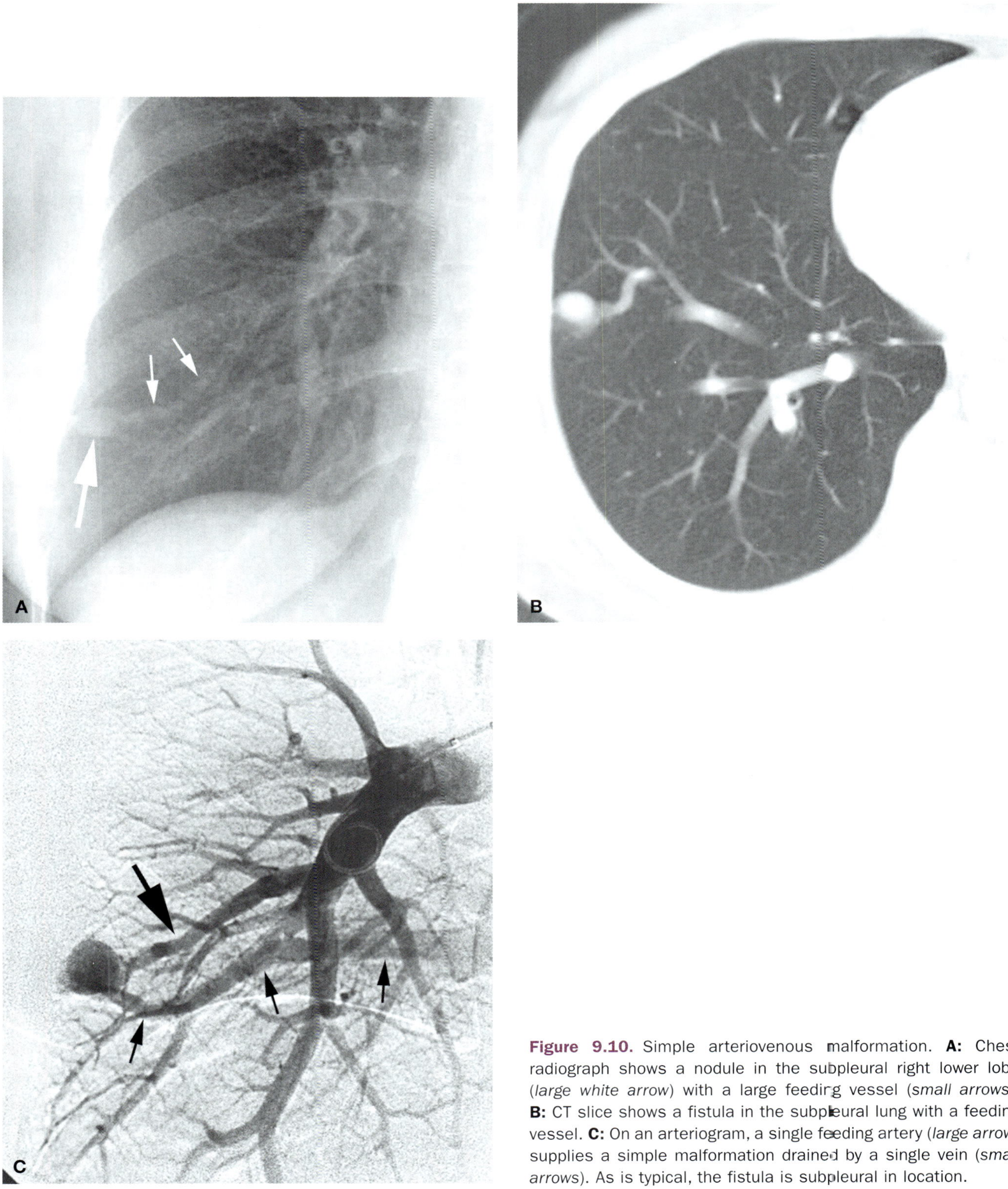

Figure 9.10. Simple arteriovenous malformation. **A:** Chest radiograph shows a nodule in the subpleural right lower lobe (*large white arrow*) with a large feeding vessel (*small arrows*). **B:** CT slice shows a fistula in the subpleural lung with a feeding vessel. **C:** On an arteriogram, a single feeding artery (*large arrow*) supplies a simple malformation drained by a single vein (*small arrows*). As is typical, the fistula is subpleural in location.

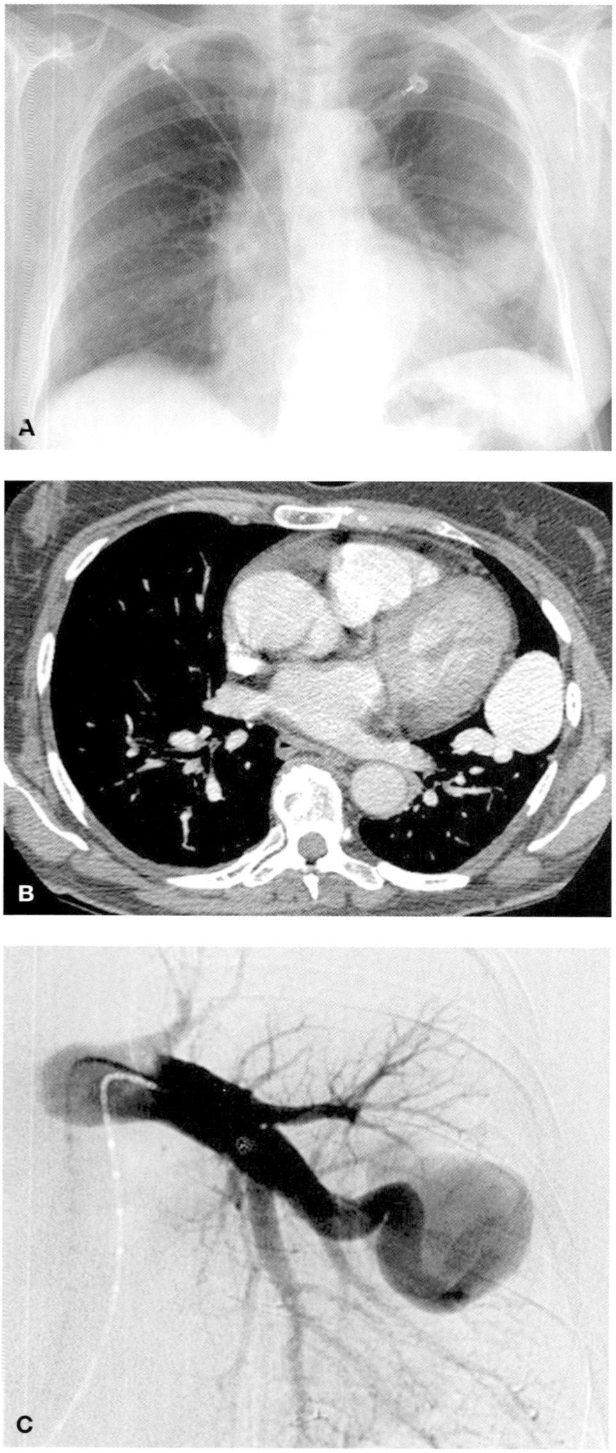

Figure 9.11. Simple arteriovenous malformation (AVM). **A:** A well-defined, smooth, round, 3-cm nodule is visible on chest radiograph in the left lower lobe. **B:** Contrast-enhanced CT shows a densely opacified fistula in the subpleural lung. Its feeding artery is also visible on this slice. **C:** Pulmonary arteriogram shows an AVM and a single feeding artery.

Radiographically, a simple fistula appears as a peripheral, well-defined round, oval, lobulated, or serpentine opacity. Large vessels (feeders) extending centrally toward the hilum are often visible (see Figs. 9.10-9.12). Enlargement of fistulas over a period of months or years is common, and a rapid increase in size can occur.

On CT, a simple AVM is visible as a smooth, sharply defined, round, or elliptical nodule, almost always in a subpleural location (see Figs. 9.12 and 9.13). Arteriovenous fistulas characterized by a tangle of tortuous, dilated vessels are seen as lobulated, serpiginous masses and can often be suspected as being vascular simply by their morphology. In both instances, the feeding pulmonary artery branch and draining pulmonary vein are dilated, and with fistulas of significant size (larger than 1-2 cm), the feeders are easily recognizable. In general, the feeders are about half the diameter of the fistula.

CT is highly accurate in demonstrating AVMs and their architecture (see Figs. 9.10-9.12). In most cases, morphologic findings are sufficient for diagnosis of AVM (see Fig. 9.12B and E), but contrast infusion may be used for confirmation (see Fig. 9.12C). Following the bolus injection of contrast, pulmonary AVMs show rapid contrast opacification and washout, occurring in phase with opacification and washout of the main pulmonary artery and right ventricle.

In general, AVMs less than 2 cm in diameter are asymptomatic. Single fistulas are less commonly symptomatic (35%) or associated with positive physical findings (70%) than are multiple fistulas (60% and 85%, respectively). It is important to trace both the feeding artery and draining vein as, occasionally, a venovenous malformation or pulmonary vein varix can mimic an AVM.

An AVM results in a right-to-left shunt, and cyanosis may be present, depending on the size of the shunt. The most frequent symptoms occurring in patients with AVMs are dyspnea, palpitation, hemoptysis, and chest pain. Stroke (see Fig. 9.12H) may be associated with polycythemia, and paradoxical embolization through the AVM from systemic veins is a serious and potentially fatal complication. Rupture can result in pulmonary hemorrhage (Fig. 9.14) or hemothorax (Fig. 9.15). Without treatment, approximately 25% of patients with AVMs experience worsening of symptoms, and 50% of them will eventually die as a result of complications.

The use of pulmonary arteriography is generally limited to patients having embolization of the fistula (see Fig. 9.12F and G). Historically, transcatheter occlusion of fistulas using wire coils has been the treatment of choice for simple AVMs and is generally reserved for fistulas having an arterial feeder greater than 3 mm in diameter. More recently, microvascular plugs have been employed as an alternative treatment and can be used on feeding vessels 2 mm (or sometimes smaller).

Recanalization of an AVM may occasionally occur after embolization.

Complex AVMs (Fig. 9.16) are more often symptomatic than simple fistulas, because of a larger shunt. They are more difficult to treat because many feeders may be present, but wire coil embolization may be successful.

Pulmonary Telangiectasia

Pulmonary telangiectasia is an uncommon form of AVM characterized by innumerable very small fistulas scattered throughout both lungs. Symptoms are common and progressive, and cyanosis is present in all patients. Unlike simple AVMs, pulmonary telangiectasia is typically discovered

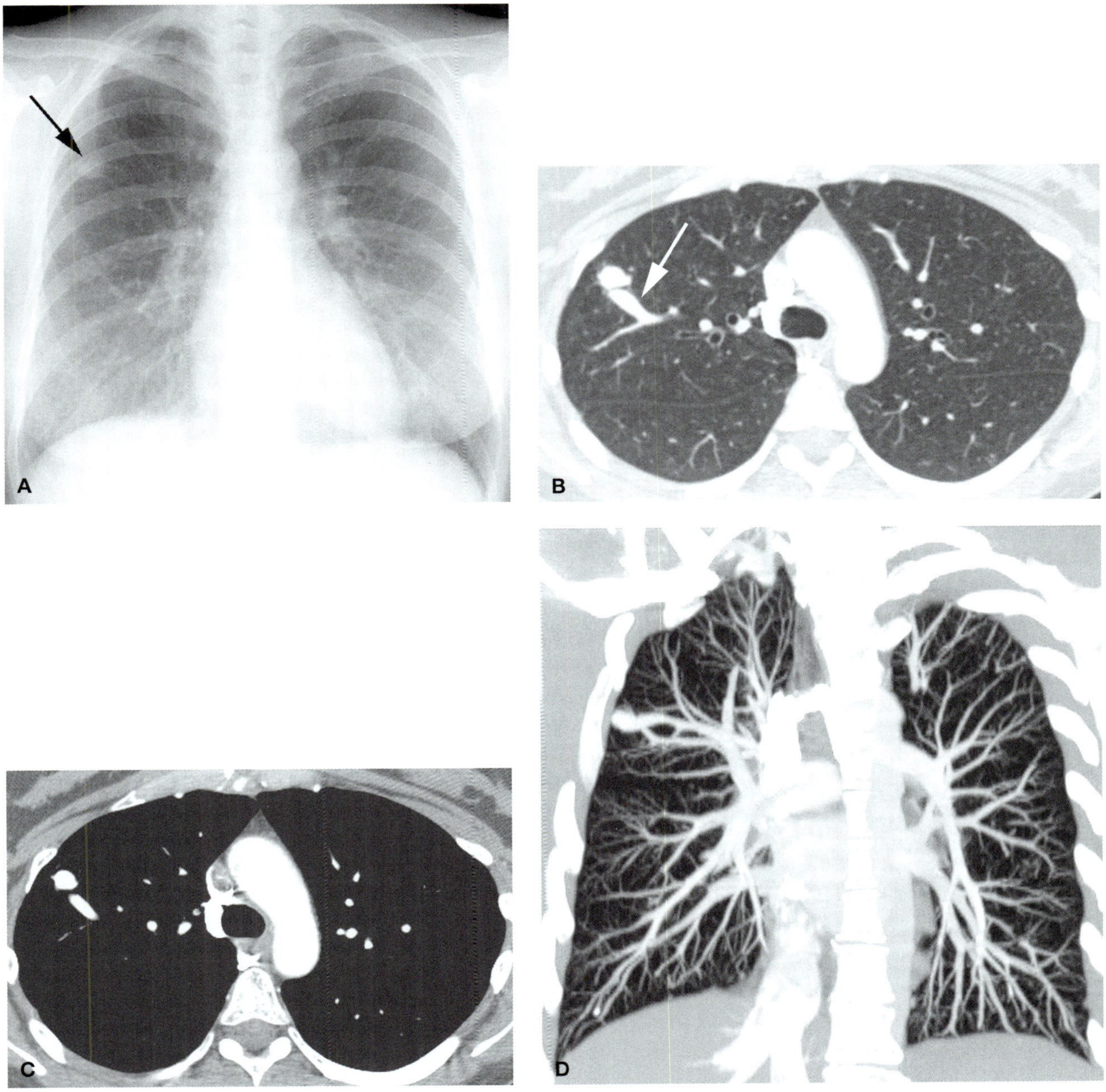

Figure 9.12. Multiple arteriovenous malformations (AVMs) in a 30-year-old woman with Osler-Weber-Rendu syndrome. **A:** Chest radiograph shows a nodule in the right upper lobe (*arrow*). **B:** Spiral CT with 1.25-mm slices shows a well-defined subpleural nodule with a feeding vessel (*arrow*), representing a vein. This appearance is typical of an AVM. **C:** With contrast injection, dense opacification of the fistula and feeding vein is seen. **D:** Coronal reconstruction shows the subpleural fistula, feeding artery, and draining vein.

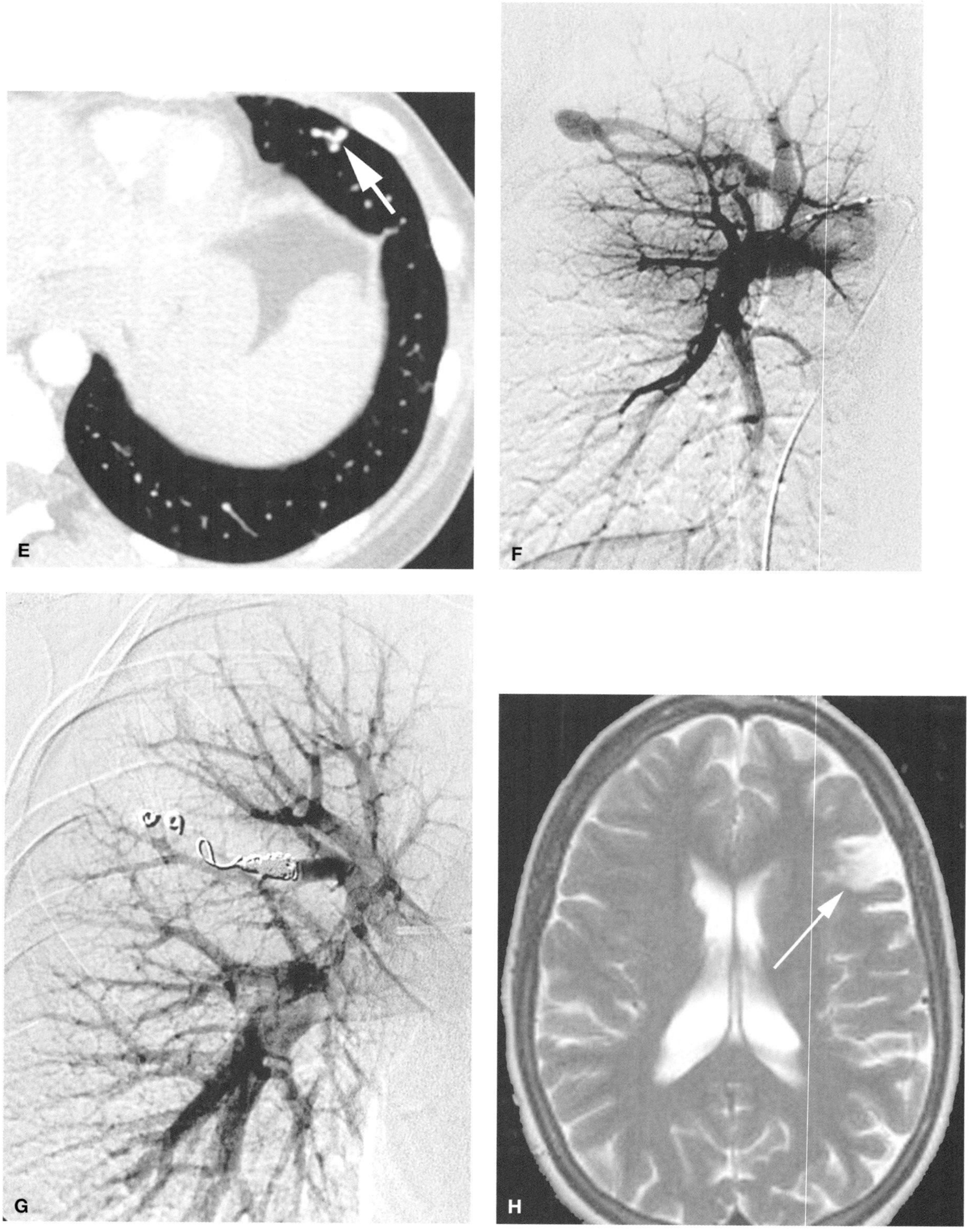

Figure 9.12. *(Continued)* **E:** Multiple other fistulas were visible. A small fistula (*arrow*) in the lower lobe may be diagnosed based on its morphology. **F:** Arteriogram performed at the time of embolization shows the fistula in (**C**) to opacify (**G**). The fistula shown in (**F**) has been occluded by wire coils. **H:** T2-weighted MRI of the brain shows findings of infarction (*arrow*). This is a common complication of AVMs.

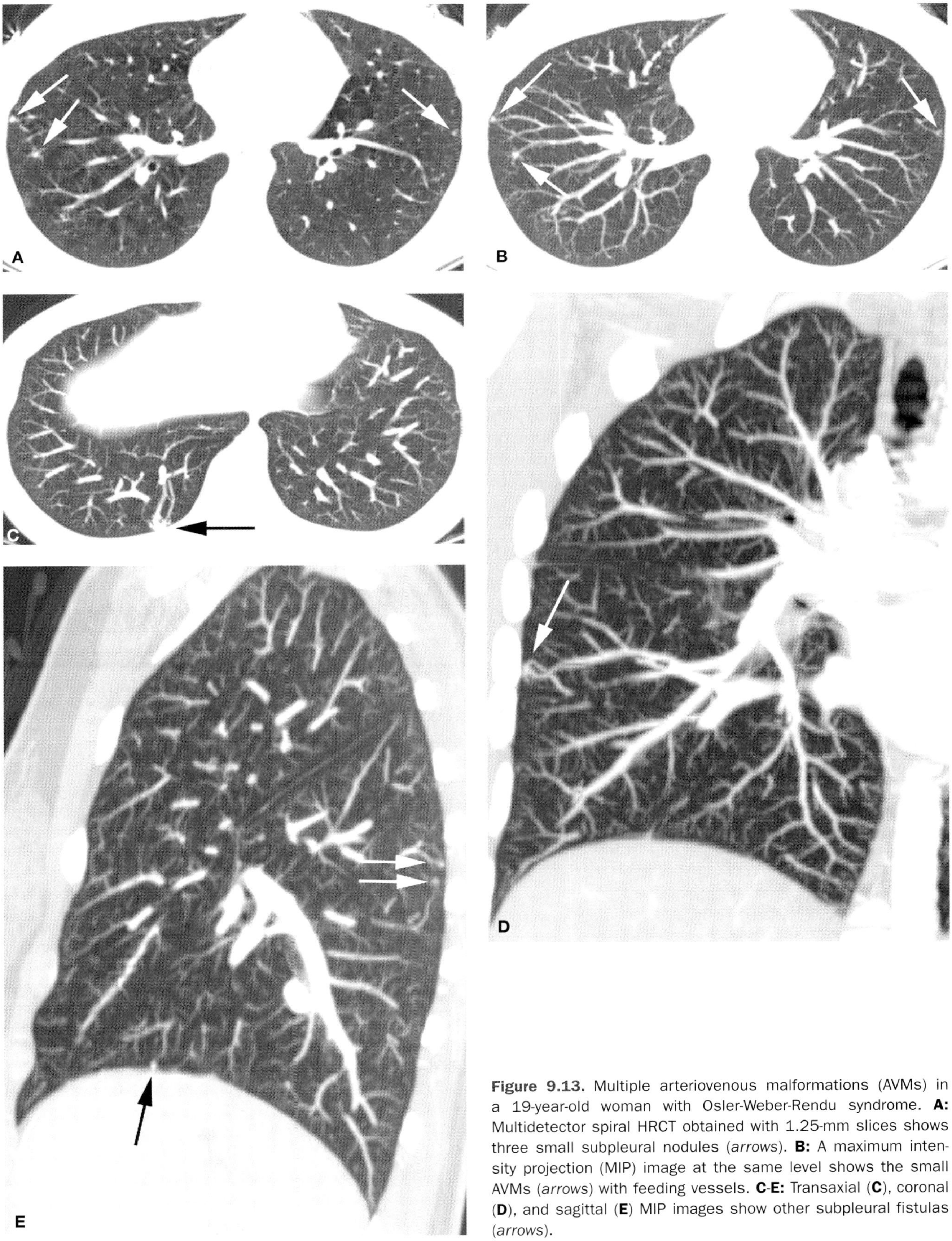

Figure 9.13. Multiple arteriovenous malformations (AVMs) in a 19-year-old woman with Osler-Weber-Rendu syndrome. **A:** Multidetector spiral HRCT obtained with 1.25-mm slices shows three small subpleural nodules (*arrows*). **B:** A maximum intensity projection (MIP) image at the same level shows the small AVMs (*arrows*) with feeding vessels. **C-E:** Transaxial (**C**), coronal (**D**), and sagittal (**E**) MIP images show other subpleural fistulas (*arrows*).

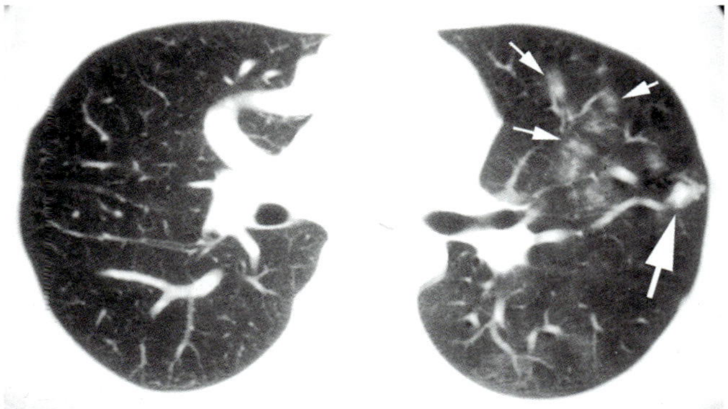

Figure 9.14. Osler-Weber-Rendu syndrome with multiple arteriovenous malformations (AVM) is shown on CT and pulmonary hemorrhage. Patchy areas of ground-glass opacity (*arrows*) in the left lung represent blood due to rupture of an AVM.

by 10 years of age. Radiographs can be normal. If abnormal, radiographic findings are often limited to an abnormal pattern of pulmonary vessels, including (a) a coarse spidery appearance of pulmonary vessels, (b) vascular tortuosity, and (c) areas of hypervascularity. On angiograms, beaded or tortuous vessels, small aneurysmal sacs, or multiple ill-defined areas of vascular blush are visible. Treatment of this condition is difficult, and prognosis is poor. Surgery is not possible because of the multiplicity of lesions.

PULMONARY AGENESIS, APLASIA, AND HYPOPLASIA

These three abnormalities are sometimes classified as types of *pulmonary underdevelopment*.

Pulmonary Agenesis and Aplasia

Pulmonary agenesis and aplasia are nearly the same, and a distinction is not usually necessary. *Pulmonary agenesis* represents complete absence of a lung, its bronchi, and its vascular supply. *Pulmonary aplasia* is characterized by complete absence of a lung and its vascular supply, but a rudimentary bronchus is present (Fig. 9.17), ending in a blind pouch (Table 9.8). Either side may be affected. Associated congenital anomalies are often present. Pulmonary agenesis and aplasia are usually associated with a poor prognosis, with few patients surviving to adulthood.

Radiographically, pulmonary agenesis and aplasia result in opacification of a hemithorax and marked ipsilateral mediastinal shift (see Fig. 9.17). The heart is displaced into the posterior hemithorax on the side of agenesis or aplasia, along with other mediastinal structures. On lateral radiographs, the anterior chest appears abnormally lucent because of herniation of the remaining lung into the opposite hemithorax.

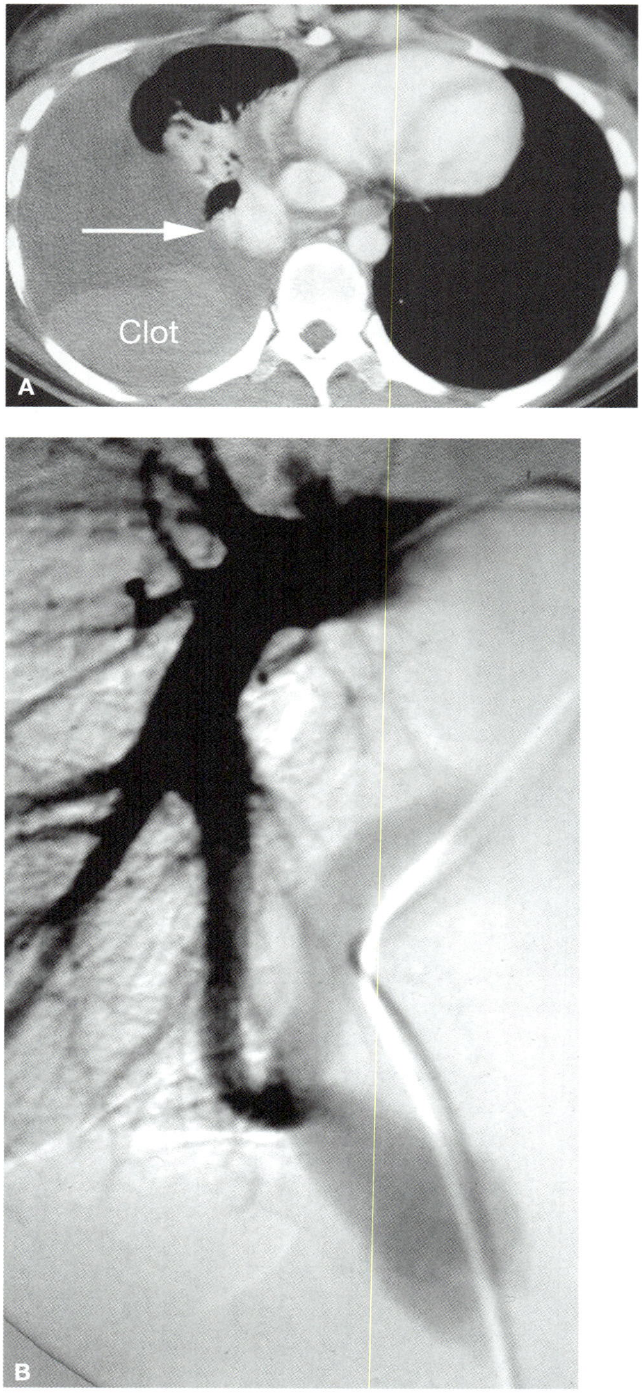

Figure 9.15. Arteriovenous malformation (AVM) and hemothorax in a young woman with acute chest pain and shortness of breath. **A:** CT shows a right pleural effusion with a region of high attenuation indicating clot. A rounded lesion opacified by contrast is visible in the lung periphery (*arrow*). This appearance suggests AVM. **B:** Arteriogram shows a simple AVM in the lung periphery. Wire coil embolization was performed, with resolution of the symptoms.

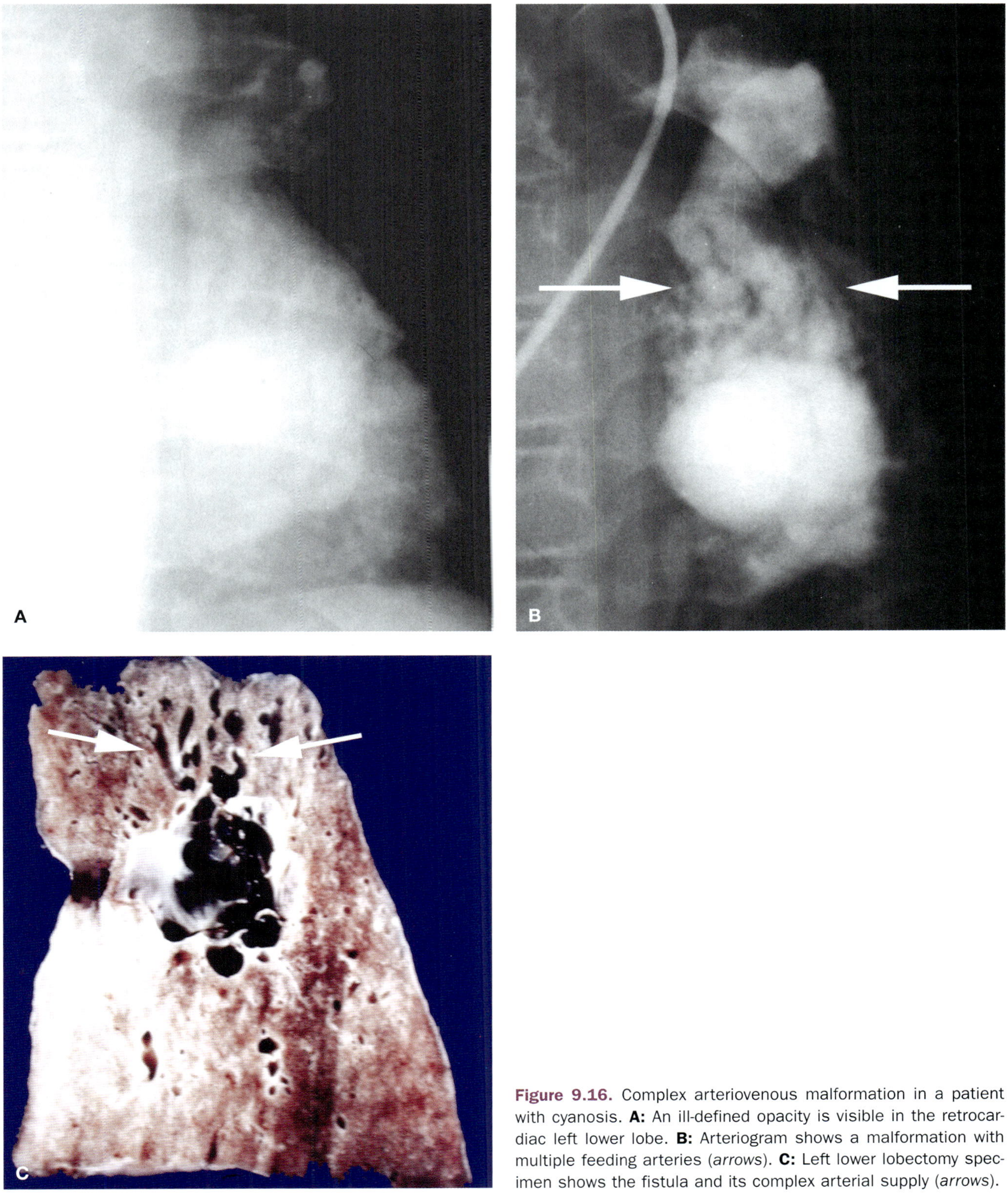

Figure 9.16. Complex arteriovenous malformation in a patient with cyanosis. **A:** An ill-defined opacity is visible in the retrocardiac left lower lobe. **B:** Arteriogram shows a malformation with multiple feeding arteries (*arrows*). **C:** Left lower lobectomy specimen shows the fistula and its complex arterial supply (*arrows*).

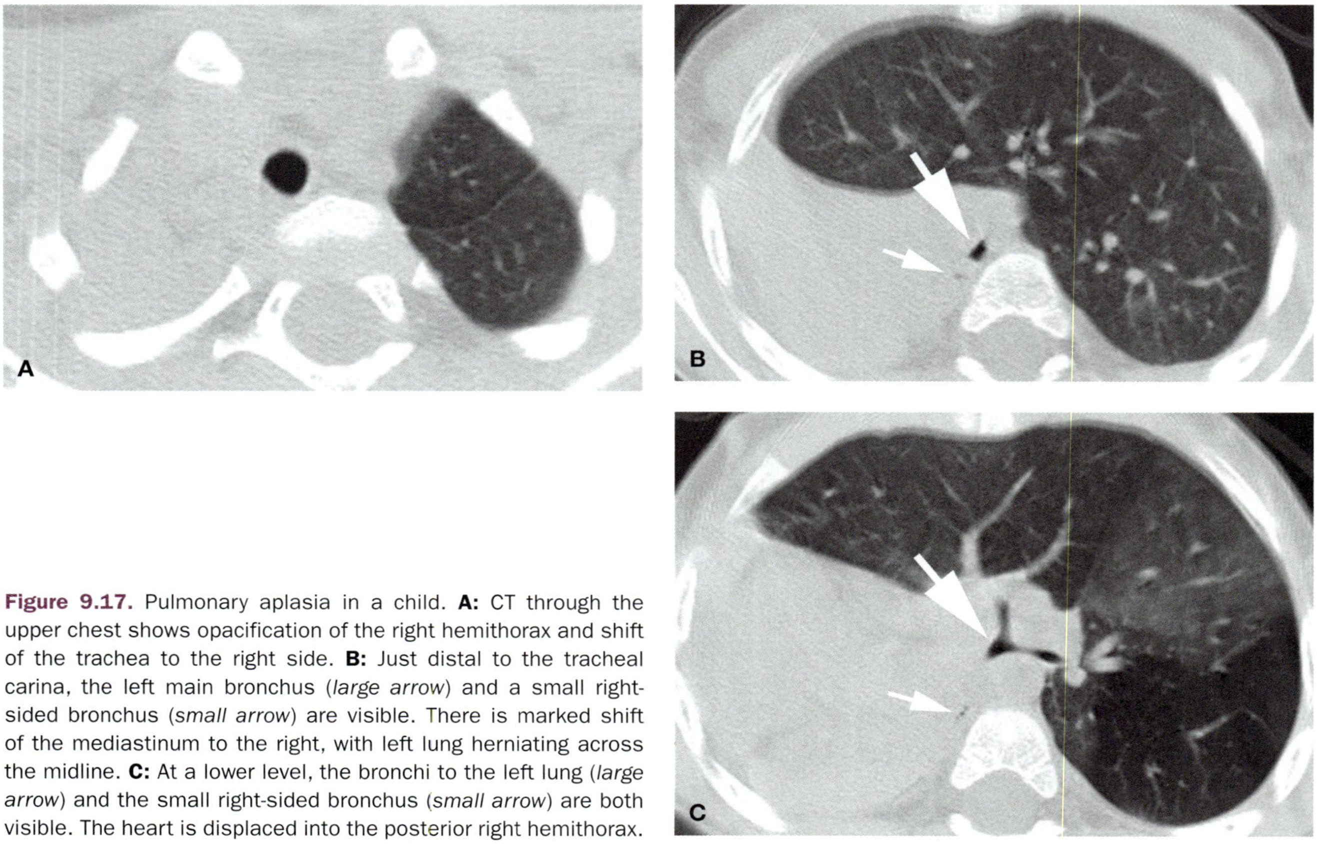

Figure 9.17. Pulmonary aplasia in a child. **A:** CT through the upper chest shows opacification of the right hemithorax and shift of the trachea to the right side. **B:** Just distal to the tracheal carina, the left main bronchus (*large arrow*) and a small right-sided bronchus (*small arrow*) are visible. There is marked shift of the mediastinum to the right, with left lung herniating across the midline. **C:** At a lower level, the bronchi to the left lung (*large arrow*) and the small right-sided bronchus (*small arrow*) are both visible. The heart is displaced into the posterior right hemithorax.

Table 9.8 Pulmonary Agenesis, Aplasia, and Hypoplasia

Agenesis and Aplasia Occur on either side Mediastinal herniation into affected hemithorax Congenital anomalies associated Poor Prognosis
Agenesis: Absence of a lung and its bronchi and vascular supply
Aplasia: Absence of a lung and its vascular supply; a rudimentary bronchus is present
Hypoplasia Abnormal lung development Decreased alveoli and bronchial divisions Deficient lobes or segments may be present Causes: Hypogenetic lung (scimitar) syndrome Proximal interruption of pulmonary artery Lung compression during development

CT demonstrates absence of the lung and pulmonary artery with marked mediastinal shift. In patients with agenesis, bronchi are also absent.

Pulmonary Hypoplasia

Pulmonary hypoplasia represents abnormal lung development associated with a reduction in lung volume and often a decrease in the number of alveoli and bronchial divisions (see Table 9.8). There may also be anomalous lobes or segments, or they may be reduced in number. Hypoplasia is associated with other anomalies in *hypogenetic lung (scimitar) syndrome*. It may also result from abnormal lung development due to deficient vascular supply (eg, *proximal interruption of the pulmonary artery* and *unilateral pulmonary vein atresia*) or lung compression during gestation (eg, congenital diaphragmatic hernia [Fig. 9.18], space-occupying lesions, CPAM, sequestration, thoracic deformity, or oligohydramnios). In patients with lung hypoplasia, the prognosis depends on the degree of abnormality and associated anomalies.

The pulmonary artery supplying the hypoplastic lung is reduced in size or absent (see Fig. 9.18E). On radiographs

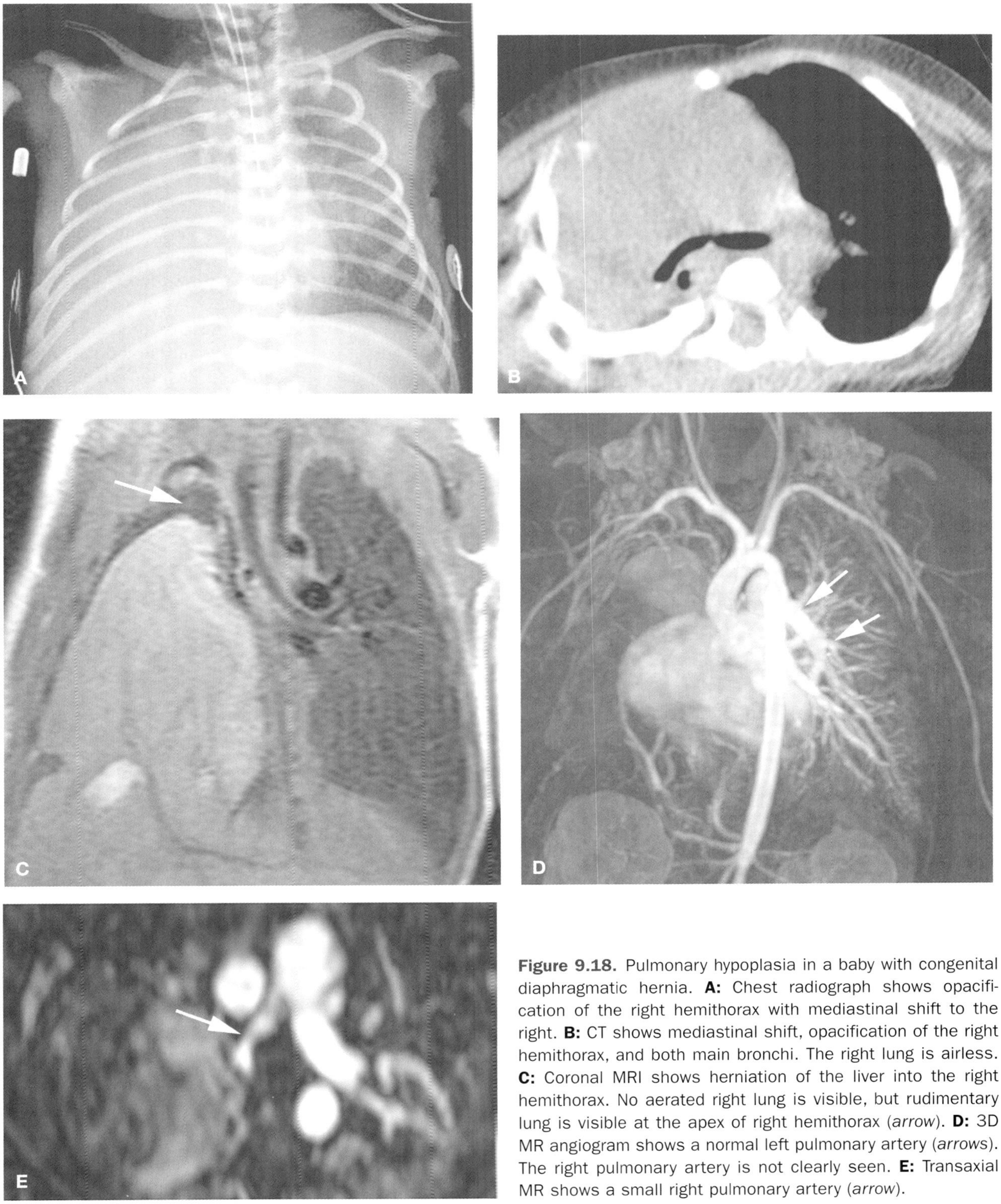

Figure 9.18. Pulmonary hypoplasia in a baby with congenital diaphragmatic hernia. **A:** Chest radiograph shows opacification of the right hemithorax with mediastinal shift to the right. **B:** CT shows mediastinal shift, opacification of the right hemithorax, and both main bronchi. The right lung is airless. **C:** Coronal MRI shows herniation of the liver into the right hemithorax. No aerated right lung is visible, but rudimentary lung is visible at the apex of right hemithorax (*arrow*). **D:** 3D MR angiogram shows a normal left pulmonary artery (*arrows*). The right pulmonary artery is not clearly seen. **E:** Transaxial MR shows a small right pulmonary artery (*arrow*).

or CT, the size of pulmonary vessels may appear reduced on the affected side. Mediastinal shift toward the hypoplastic lung occurs with hypogenetic lung syndrome and proximal interruption of the pulmonary artery. Mediastinal shift may or may not be present when hypoplasia results from an ipsilateral space-occupying lesion.

HYPOGENETIC LUNG (SCIMITAR OR VENOLOBAR) SYNDROME

A rare anomaly, almost always occurring on the right side, hypogenetic lung syndrome is characterized by (a) hypoplasia of the lung with abnormal segmental or lobar anatomy, (b) hypoplasia of the ipsilateral pulmonary artery, (c) anomalous pulmonary venous return to the inferior vena cava (or right atrium, hepatic veins, etc.), and (d) anomalous systemic arterial supply to a portion of the hypoplastic lung, usually the lower lobe (Table 9.9). Although these four features often coexist, hypogenetic lung syndrome shows considerable variation in the degree to which each feature is expressed. Patients may exhibit some features of this syndrome but not others.

This anomaly is usually diagnosed in patients less than 30 years of age, and more than half have symptoms. Recurrent respiratory infections and dyspnea on exertion are most common. Congenital heart lesions, most commonly septal defects and patent ductus arteriosus, are associated in 25%. Surgical treatment involves implantation of the anomalous vein into the left atrium.

The hypogenetic lung syndrome has also been described as the "scimitar syndrome" (because of the resemblance of the anomalous vein to a Turkish scimitar) or the "venolobar syndrome," because of the presence of an anomalous vein and, in some cases, lobar abnormalities. Scimitar syndrome is a commonly used term, and is generally accepted and recognized, in describing this anomaly. The term "venolobar syndrome," proposed by Felson, is used to refer to a variety of anomalies, including sequestration, anomalous pulmonary venous return, hypogenetic lung syndrome, and their variants. Although still used, it is nonspecific and not preferred in describing individual cases.

Radiographically, the appearance of the hypogenetic (scimitar) syndrome is often characteristic (Fig. 9.19). The hypoplastic lung is recognizable because of dextroposition of the heart, mediastinal shift to the right side, and right diaphragmatic elevation. CT may show abnormal bronchial anatomy on the side of the hypoplastic lung.

Hypoplasia of the pulmonary artery may be recognizable by the decreased size of vessels within the hypoplastic lung. Because most of the pulmonary blood flow must traverse the normal artery on the side opposite the hypoplastic lung, the opposite pulmonary artery appears enlarged, further increasing the contrast between the right and left vasculature.

When the anomalous vein is visible radiographically, it appears as a broad arcuate band at the right lung base, paralleling the right heart border and extending to the diaphragmatic surface (see Figs. 9.19 and 9.20). This venous shadow often resembles a scimitar, hence the nickname of this syndrome. In nearly two-thirds of patients, the scimitar vein drains the entire right lung. On CT, the scimitar vein is located in close relation to the major fissure. Left-sided scimitar syndrome, with the anomalous vein entering the coronary sinus, is rarely seen.

Systemic arteries, usually multiple and arising below the diaphragm, typically supply the lower lobe. These may be visible using CT (see Fig. 9.19D and E).

In some patients, findings of the scimitar syndrome may be associated with "horseshoe lung." Horseshoe lung is a rare congenital malformation in which an isthmus of pulmonary parenchyma extends from the right lung base across the midline behind the pericardium and fuses with the base of the left lung. Horseshoe lung may occur in the absence of scimitar syndrome.

Table 9.9 Hypogenetic Lung (Scimitar) Syndrome

Four features typical (although each not always present):
- Hypoplasia of the lung with abnormal segmental or lobar Anatomy
- Hypoplasia of the ipsilateral pulmonary artery
- Anomalous pulmonary venous return (scimitar vein)
- Anomalous systemic arterial supply to lower lobe

Almost always on the right side
Mediastinal shift toward the hypoplastic lung
Reduced size of ipsilateral pulmonary artery
Anomalous (scimitar) vein usually paralleling right heart border
Congenital heart disease in 25% (eg, atrial septal defect and patent ductus arteriosus)
Symptoms: Recurrent infection and dyspnea

PROXIMAL INTERRUPTION OF THE PULMONARY ARTERY

This anomaly can closely resemble hypogenetic lung syndrome. In proximal interruption of the pulmonary artery, the proximal portion of a main pulmonary artery, usually the right, fails to develop (Table 9.10). The ipsilateral lung is hypoplastic because of deficient growth but has a normal number of lobes and segments, and bronchial anatomy is normal. Vessels within the lung appear small (Fig. 9.21), whereas those on the opposite side are much larger. The lung vascular supply is derived from hypertrophied bronchial, intercostal, and other systemic arteries (see Fig. 9.21B).

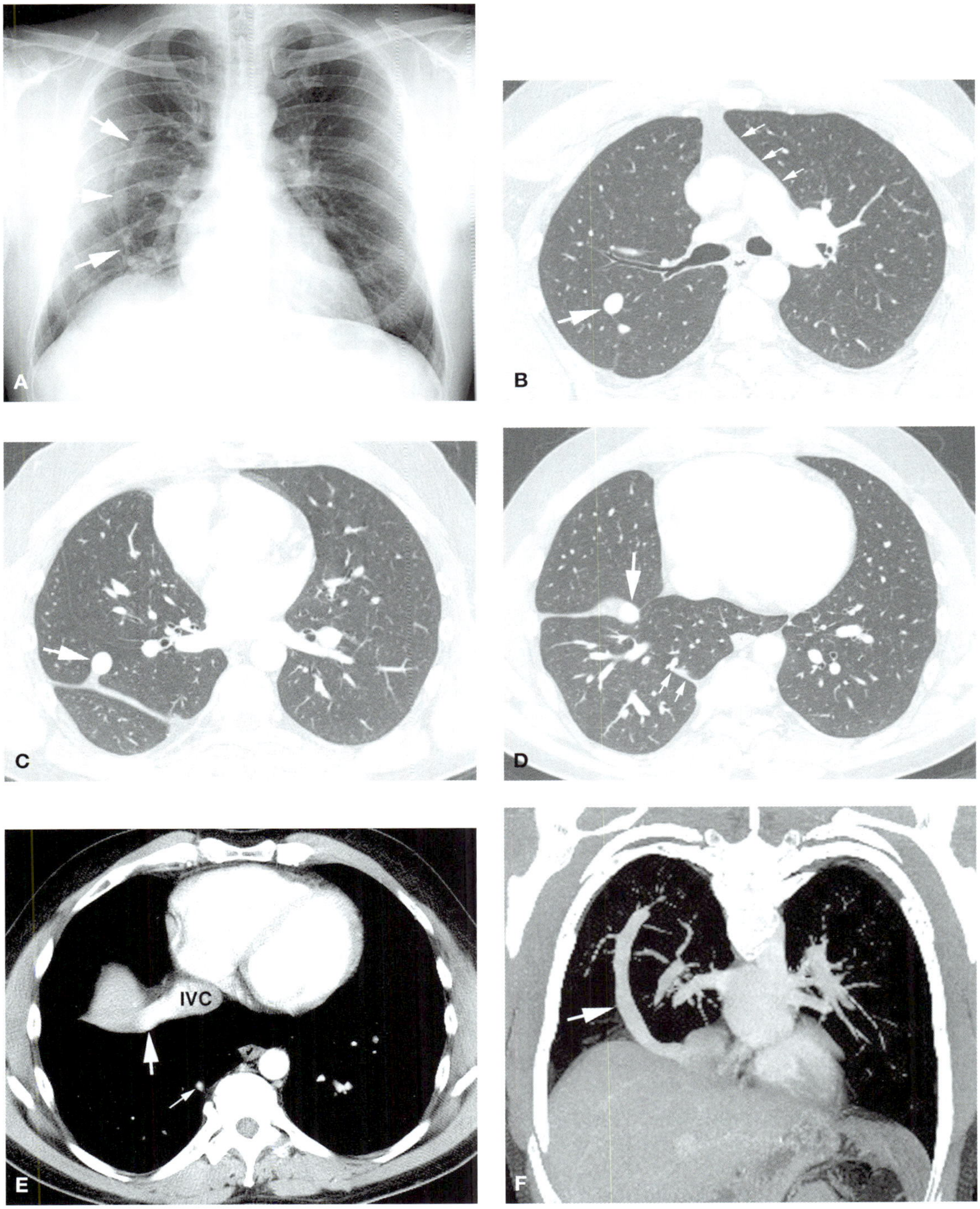

Figure 9.19. Scimitar syndrome. **A:** Plain radiograph shows displacement of the heart toward the right side and elevation of the right hemidiaphragm, because of right lung hypoplasia, and the anomalous pulmonary vein paralleling the right heart border (*arrows*). **B:** CT at the level of the right upper lobe bronchus shows the anomalous pulmonary vein (*large arrow*). Shift of the anterior mediastinum toward the right is visible (*small arrows*). The right pulmonary artery is smaller than the left. **C:** At the lower level, the scimitar vein (*arrow*) is visible in relation to the major fissure, which appears thickened. Mediastinal shift is also visible. **D:** Near the right diaphragm, the scimitar vein (*large arrow*) is within the major fissure. A septum in the posteromedial right lung (*small arrows*) is at the site of systemic arterial supply to the lower lobe. **E:** Soft-tissue window scan at the level of the right hemidiaphragm shows the scimitar vein (*large arrow*) entering the inferior vena cava (*IVC*). A systemic artery (*small arrow*) supplies the lower lobe. **F:** Coronal reconstruction shows the scimitar vein (*arrow*) to best advantage.

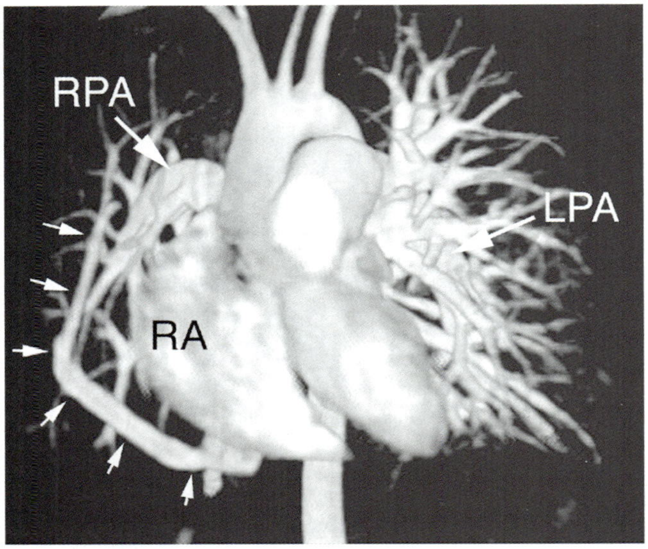

Figure 9.20. 3D MR angiogram in scimitar syndrome. The right pulmonary artery (*RPA*) is smaller than the left (*LPA*). The scimitar vein (*small arrows*) parallels the border of the right atrium (*RA*) and drains into the inferior vena cava.

This entity is often associated with congenital heart disease, most typically tetralogy of Fallot and septal defects. The aortic arch is almost always contralateral to the side of the interrupted pulmonary artery (Fig. 9.22). When the interrupted pulmonary artery and aorta are ipsilateral, the incidence of congenital heart disease is higher than when they are not.

UNILATERAL PULMONARY VEIN ATRESIA

In unilateral pulmonary vein atresia, another rare entity, long segments of the pulmonary veins of one lung are congenitally atretic (Table 9.11). The involved lung can be normal in size or hypoplastic, and it often shows increased interstitial densities and interlobular septal thickening because of venous stasis, edema, and fibrosis (Fig. 9.23). The ipsilateral pulmonary artery may appear small (Fig. 9.23B). Radionuclide imaging shows decreased perfusion. Angiography shows decreased size of the ipsilateral pulmonary artery, peripheral pruning, contrast stasis, and nonvisualization of the pulmonary veins. Symptoms include hemoptysis and infection.

Table 9.10 Proximal Interruption of the Pulmonary Artery

Congenital absence of a main pulmonary artery
Almost always on the side opposite the aortic arch (ie, usually the right)
Hypoplastic ipsilateral lung
Reduced size of ipsilateral pulmonary vessels
Lung vascular supply derived from bronchial arteries
Mediastinal shift toward the hypoplastic lung
Congenital heart disease common (tetralogy of Fallot and septal defects)

PULMONARY VEIN VARIX

Dilation of a pulmonary vein branch (pulmonary vein varix) can be congenital or acquired (Table 9.12). One or more veins appear dilated or tortuous near the point they enter the left atrium. With congenital varices, symptoms are usually absent, although rupture rarely occurs.

Acquired varices are associated with chronically elevated left atrial pressure, as in mitral stenosis. These most commonly involve the right inferior pulmonary vein. On plain radiographs, these are visible through the right part of the heart shadow and often appear rounded and sharply defined (Figure 10.47). They may mimic the appearance of a lung nodule, leading to further evaluation. CT is diagnostic.

ANOMALOUS PULMONARY VEIN DRAINAGE

Anomalous pulmonary vein drainage involves drainage of a pulmonary vein branch into the right atrium, coronary sinus, or systemic vein, producing a left-to-right shunt (Table 9.13).

Partial anomalous pulmonary venous drainage is present in about 0.5% of the population and is usually asymptomatic. The anomalous vein may drain into various vascular structures. On the right, the most common are the superior vena cava (Fig. 9.24), azygos vein, inferior vena cava, and right atrium. On the left, drainage may be through the left brachiocephalic vein, persistent left superior vena cava (vertical vein; Fig. 9.25), or coronary sinus. Drainage may also be below the diaphragm.

Total anomalous pulmonary venous drainage must be associated with a septal defect and is best considered to be a type of congenital heart disease.

BRONCHOPULMONARY SEQUESTRATION

Bronchopulmonary sequestration is a congenital malformation resulting from abnormal budding of the foregut and its associated structures during the period that lung, bronchi, pulmonary vessels, and the pleura are developing. Pathologically, sequestration represents an area of disorganized pulmonary parenchyma without normal pulmonary arterial or bronchial communications (ie, it is sequestered from bronchi and pulmonary arteries). Sequestration usually receives its blood supply from branches of the thoracic or abdominal aorta, and aortography is usually necessary before surgical excision in order to visualize these arterial branches. Fatal hemorrhage can occur if these systemic arteries are accidentally cut during surgery. There are two forms of sequestration: intralobar and extralobar. Although they share some features, they differ significantly in several

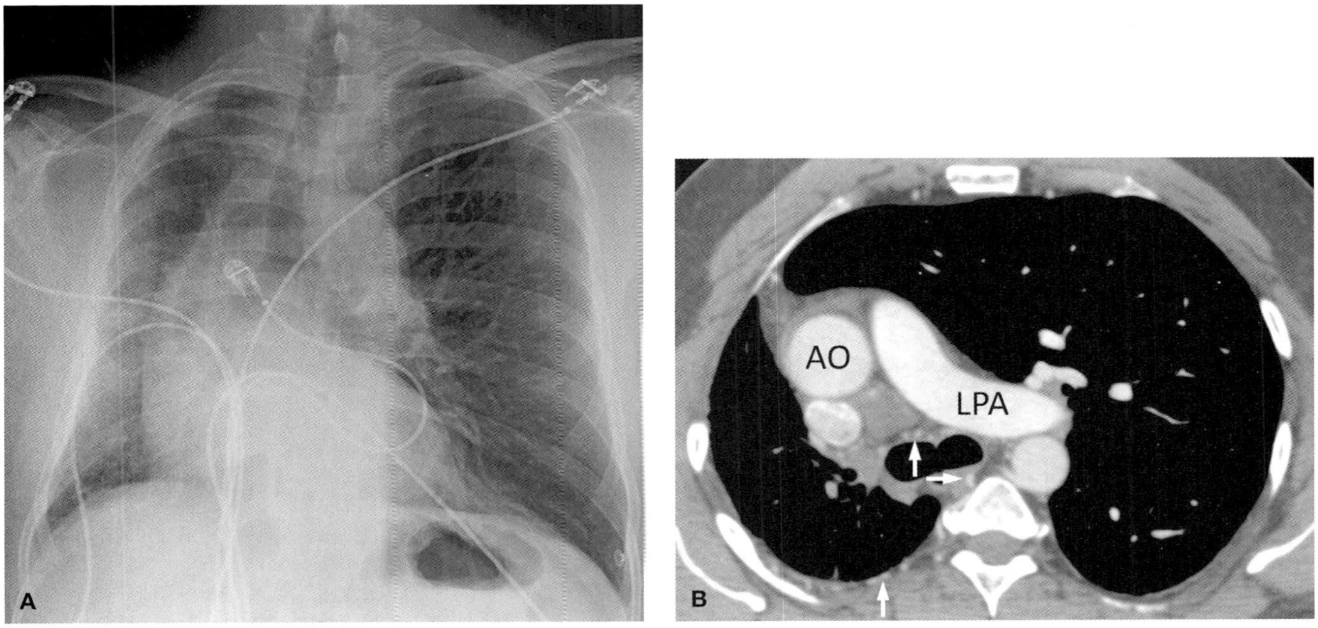

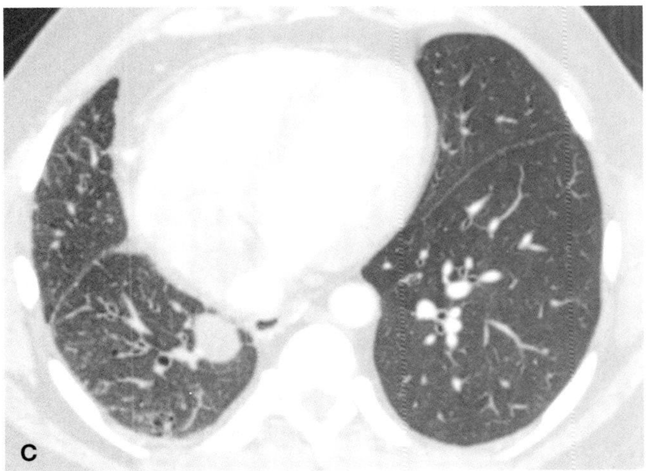

Figure 9.21. Proximal interruption of the right pulmonary artery. **A:** Chest radiograph shows mediastinal shift to the right with a small right lung and diminutive vessels. **B:** Contrast-enhanced CT shows the ascending aorta (*Ao*) and a large left pulmonary artery (*LPA*), but the right pulmonary artery is absent. Large bronchial and intercostal arteries (*arrows*) supply the right lung. **C:** Lung window scan shows hypoplasia of the right lung with chronic septal thickening and small right lung vessels.

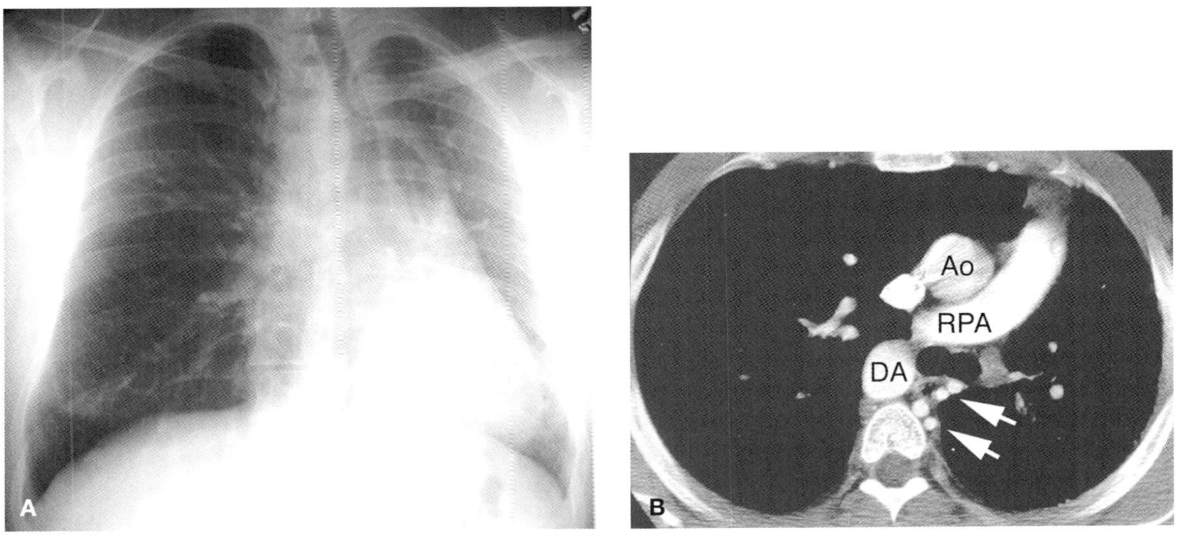

Figure 9.22. Proximal interruption of the left pulmonary artery in a patient with right aortic arch. **A:** Chest radiograph shows mediastinal shift to the left. **B:** Contrast-enhanced CT shows the ascending aorta (*Ao*), a right-sided descending aorta (*DA*), and a large right pulmonary artery (*RPA*), but the left pulmonary artery is absent. Large bronchial arteries (*arrows*) supply the hypoplastic left lung.

Table 9.11 Pulmonary Vein Atresia

Pulmonary veins of one lung atretic
Lung hypoplastic or normal in volume
Reduced size of ipsilateral pulmonary artery
Increased interstitial opacities in affected lung

important clinical and radiographic characteristics. "Hybrid" lesions are well recognized on resected specimens, where a lesion may include features of sequestration, bronchial atresia, and/or CPAM.

Intralobar Sequestration

Intralobar sequestration is the more common of these two malformations. In this anomaly, sequestered lung lies within the visceral pleura of one of the lobes. It occurs most often

Table 9.12 Pulmonary Vein Varix

Congenital
Usually asymptomatic
Acquired
Associated with elevated left atrial pressure (eg, mitral stenosis)
Usually on the right
Mimics a lung nodule

Table 9.13 Anomalous Pulmonary Venous Drainage

Pulmonary vein drainage into the right atrium, coronary sinus, or systemic vein
Left-to-right shunt
Partial: 0.5%, usually asymptomatic
Total: Septal defect present

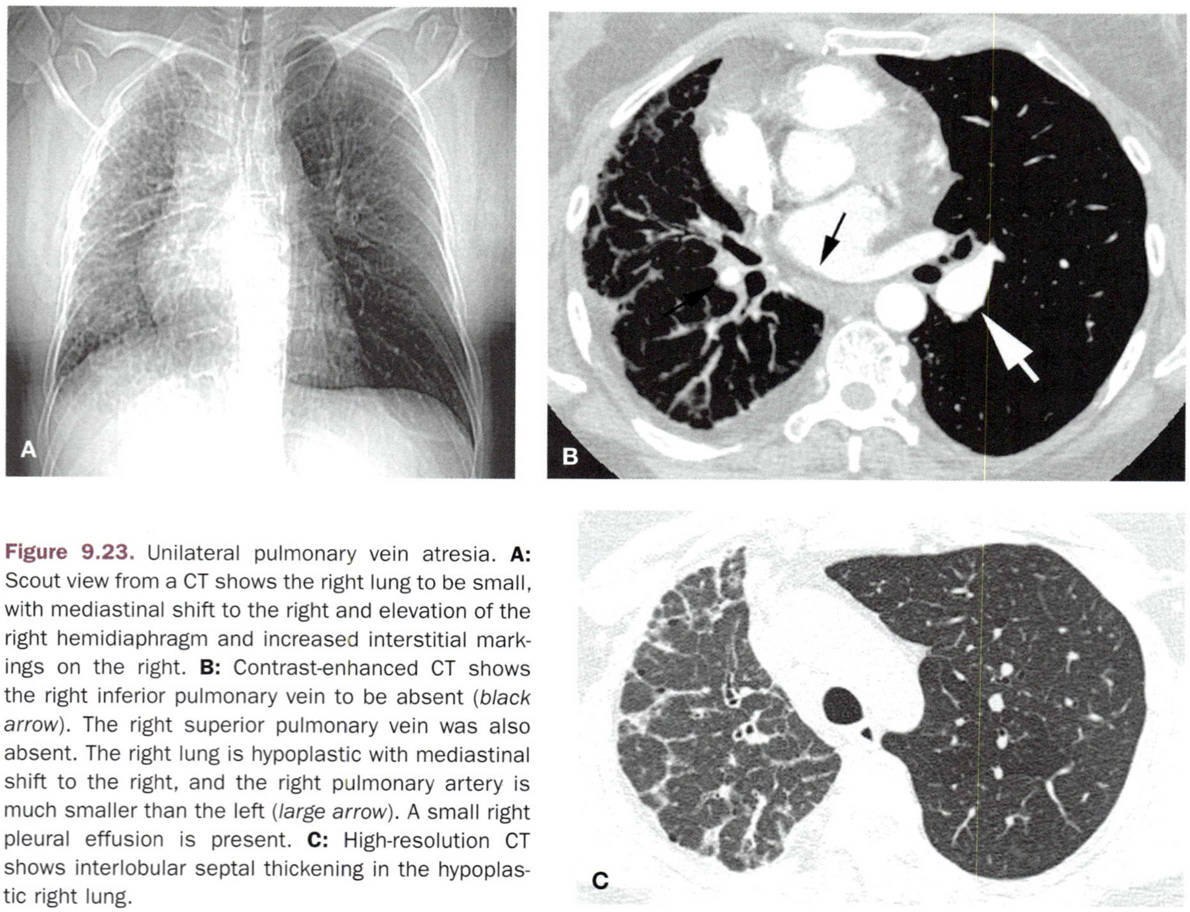

Figure 9.23. Unilateral pulmonary vein atresia. **A:** Scout view from a CT shows the right lung to be small, with mediastinal shift to the right and elevation of the right hemidiaphragm and increased interstitial markings on the right. **B:** Contrast-enhanced CT shows the right inferior pulmonary vein to be absent (*black arrow*). The right superior pulmonary vein was also absent. The right lung is hypoplastic with mediastinal shift to the right, and the right pulmonary artery is much smaller than the left (*large arrow*). A small right pleural effusion is present. **C:** High-resolution CT shows interlobular septal thickening in the hypoplastic right lung.

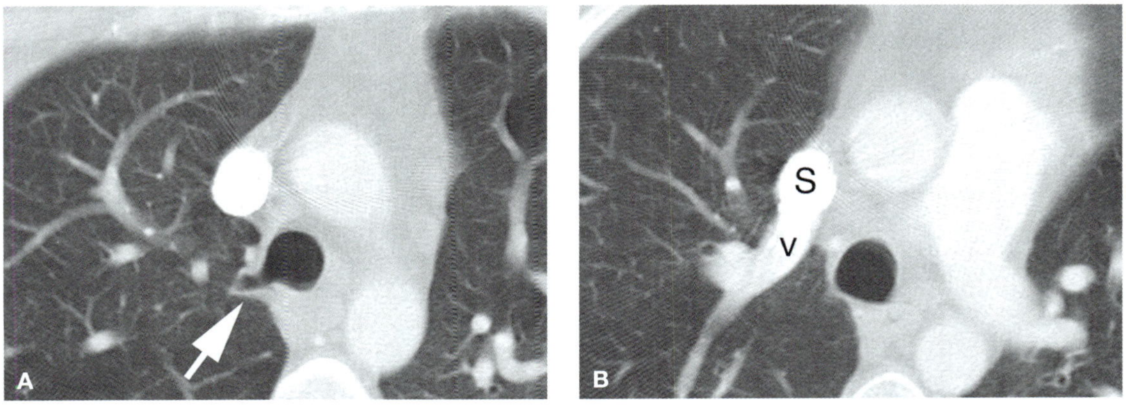

Figure 9.24. Partial anomalous pulmonary vein drainage in a patient with a tracheal bronchus. **A:** The tracheal bronchus is visible arising from the right tracheal wall (*arrow*). **B:** At a lower level, a right superior pulmonary vein (*v*) branch enters the superior vena cava (*S*).

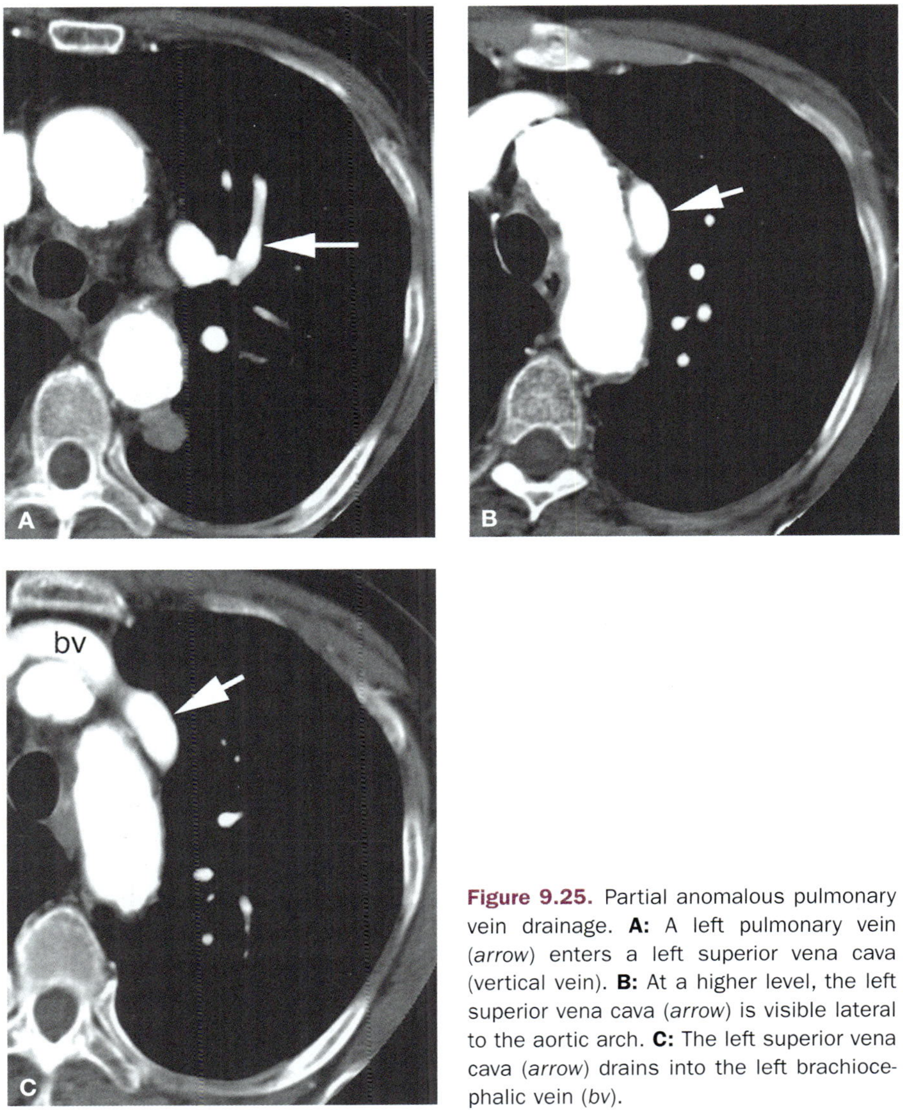

Figure 9.25. Partial anomalous pulmonary vein drainage. **A:** A left pulmonary vein (*arrow*) enters a left superior vena cava (vertical vein). **B:** At a higher level, the left superior vena cava (*arrow*) is visible lateral to the aortic arch. **C:** The left superior vena cava (*arrow*) drains into the left brachiocephalic vein (*bv*).

Table 9.14 Intralobar Sequestration

More common than extralobar sequestration
Within visceral pleura of lobe
65% at left base
No pulmonary artery or bronchial supply
Arterial supply from thoracic aorta in 75%
Drainage via pulmonary veins in most
Presentation in older children or adults
Recurrent infection
Imaging appearances:
- Homogeneous and well-defined mass lesion
- Cystic or multicystic air- and fluid-filled lesion
- Hyperlucent and hypovascular region of lung
- Combination of these

on the left side, and approximately two-thirds are found adjacent to the diaphragm in relation to the posterior basal segment of the left lower lobe (Table 9.14). In almost 75% of cases, the arterial supply of an intralobar sequestration is from the descending thoracic aorta; other cases receive supply from branches of the abdominal aorta or from intercostal arteries. These systemic arteries often enter the lung via the inferior pulmonary ligament. Usually, venous drainage is by pulmonary veins, but drainage into the azygos or hemiazygos system is not uncommon.

Intralobar sequestration usually presents in adults or older children. Acute or recurrent infection is most common as a presenting complaint (Fig. 9.26). Hemoptysis may occur. The systemic arterial to pulmonary venous shunt produced by interlobar sequestration is usually small and clinically insignificant. However, cases resulting in congestive heart failure have been reported. Bilateral sequestrations may occur. Connection to the esophagus is rarely seen. Association with other anomalies is uncommon.

Uncomplicated intralobar sequestration can have a variety of appearances. It may appear as (a) a homogeneous and well-defined mass lesion (Fig. 9.27), (b) a cystic or multicystic air and fluid-filled lesion, (c) a lucent (ie, normal) or hyperlucent and hypovascular region of the lung (Fig. 9.28), or (d) a combination of these. Hyperlucency is common in uncomplicated sequestration due to air trapping; this may be difficult to recognize on chest radiographs but is commonly seen at CT (see Fig. 9.28). The presence of mucous or fluid-filled cysts with air-fluid levels can be seen with or without infection. In such cases, a sequestration can closely mimic lung abscess. Rarely, bilateral sequestrations may be seen. These often are supplied by a single artery (Fig. 9.29).

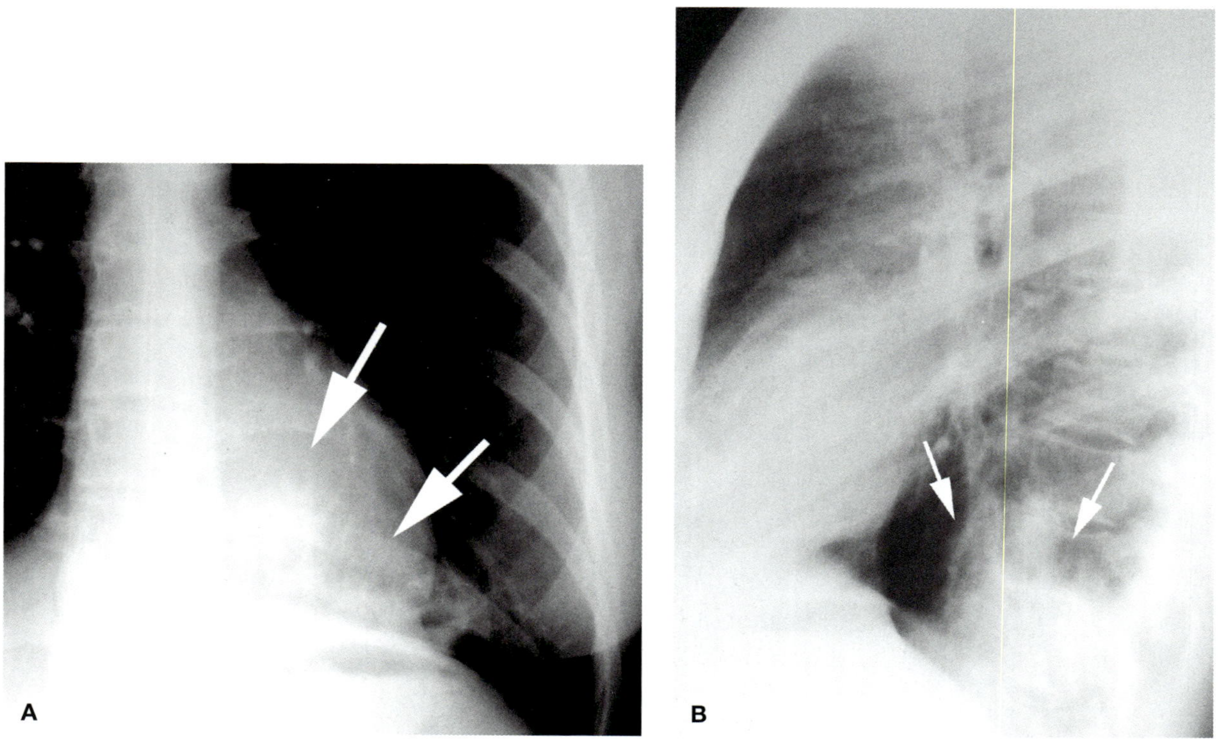

Figure 9.26. Intralobar sequestration in a young woman with recurrent left lower lobe pneumonia. **A, B:** Patchy consolidation is visible in the left lower lobe (*arrows*).

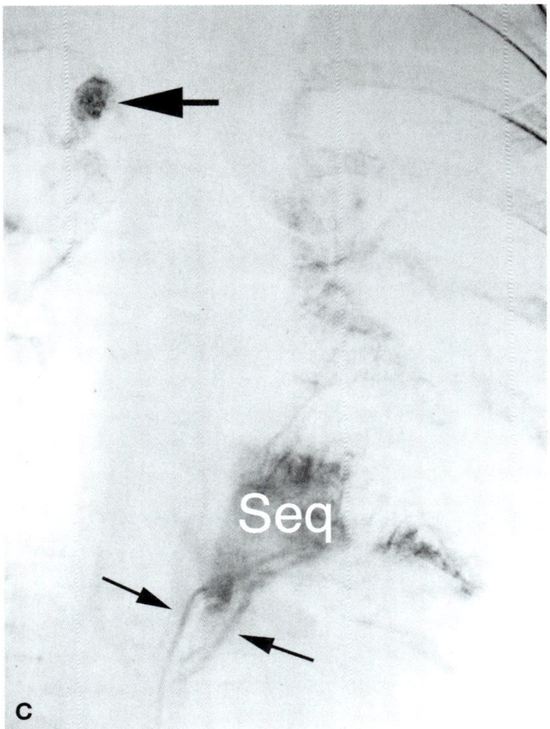

Figure 9.26. *(Continued)* **C:** Angiogram shows several branches (*small arrows*) of the descending aorta resulting in opacification of the sequestration (*Seq*). Drainage is into the azygos vein (*large arrow*).

On CT, bronchi and normal pulmonary arteries can be shown draped over the lesion (see Fig. 9.28) but do not enter a sequestration. With contrast-enhanced spiral CT, the supplying systemic arteries are often visible (see Figs. 9.27 and 9.28). If not, aortography can be used to confirm the diagnosis. The draining veins can also be identified following contrast infusion.

Although it is suggested that intralobar sequestration may be acquired, this is not the case. Chronic lung infection may mimic the appearance of sequestration, with bronchiectasis or lung abscess associated with dilatation of systemic arteries. However, such cases have a different radiographic appearance, abnormalities are unassociated with anomalous vessels, and bronchi may be shown to supply the abnormal lung on CT.

Extralobar Sequestration

Extralobar sequestration represents an anomaly in which the sequestered tissue is enclosed within its only pleural envelope; it is less common than intralobar sequestration. Approximately 90% of cases are present at the left lung base, contiguous with the left hemidiaphragm (Table 9.15). Arterial supply is usually from the abdominal aorta, and drainage is almost always by means of systemic veins (inferior vena cava, azygos, hemiazygos, or portal veins), producing a left-to-right shunt. Rarely, they may be located within

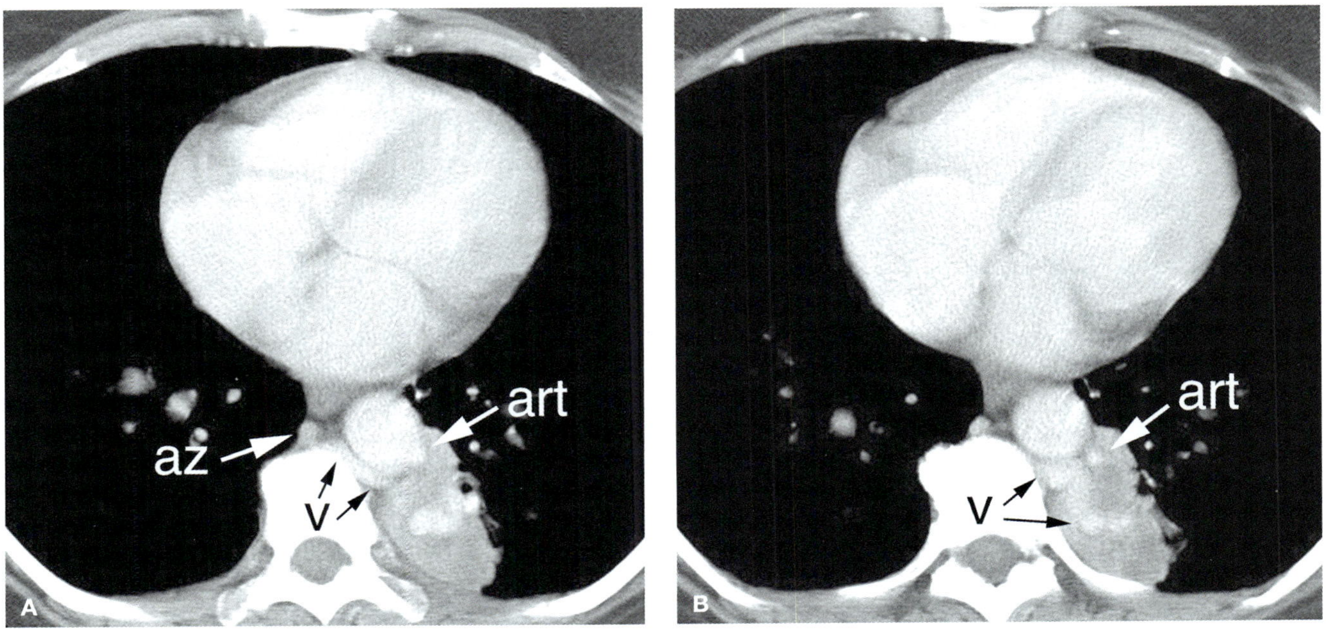

Figure 9.27. Intralobar sequestration presenting as a mass. **A, B:** Contrast-enhanced CTs show a mass lesion posterior to the descending aorta. Large vessels are visible within the mass. An artery (*art*) can be seen arising from the aorta, supplying the sequestration. Venous drainage (*v*) is into the azygos vein (*az*).

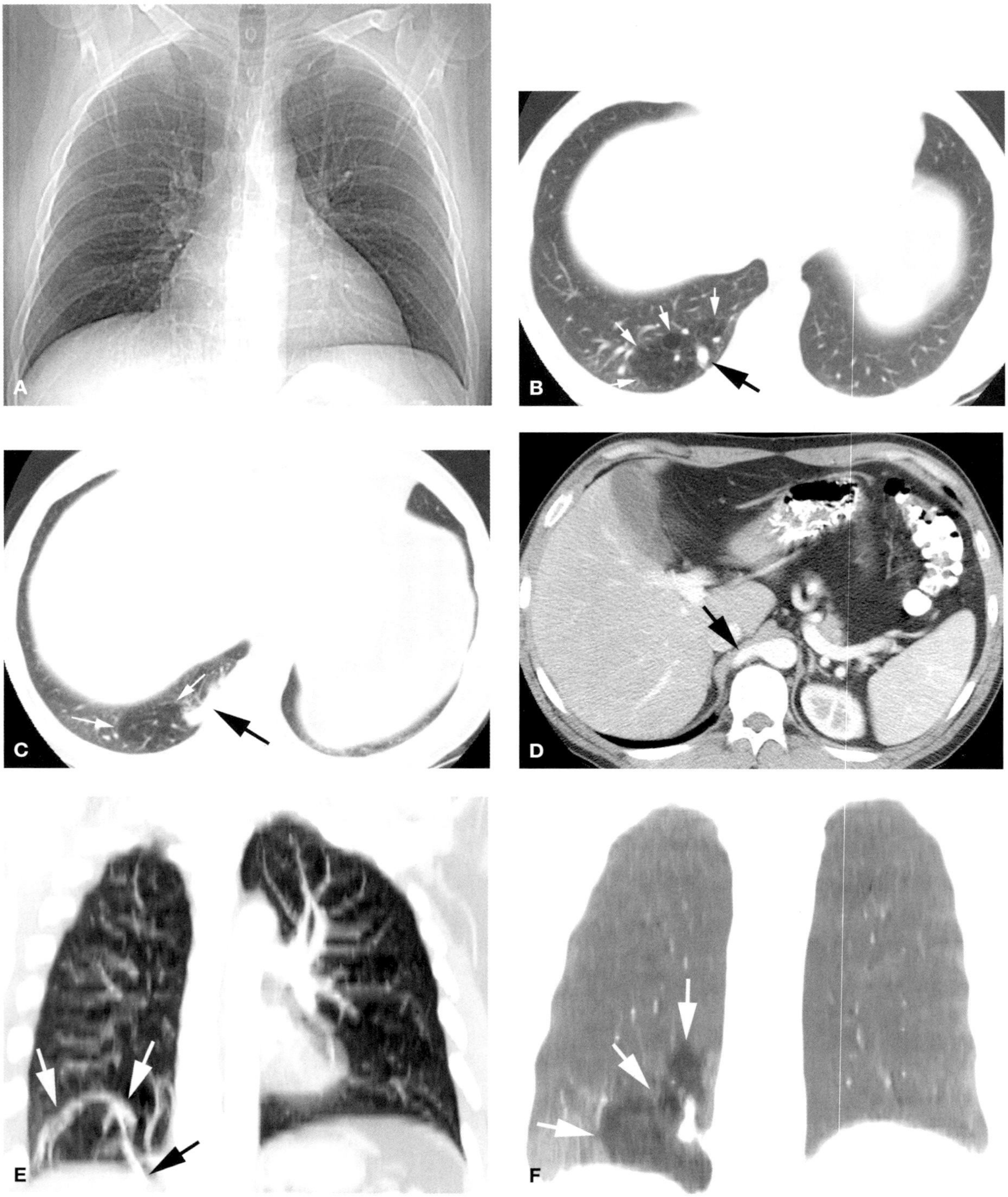

Figure 9.28. Intralobar sequestration presenting as a hyperlucent lesion. **A:** Digital radiograph shows normal-appearing lungs. **B:** CT shows a lucent lesion (*white arrows*) at the right lung base. Pulmonary artery branches are draped over the surface of the lucency. A large, abnormal vessel (*black arrow*) is visible with the region of lucency, but fewer vessels are seen in the lesion than the surrounding lower lobe. **C:** At a lower level, the lucent lesion (*white arrows*) and abnormal vessel (*black arrow*) are visible. **D:** Contrast-enhanced scan at a lower level shows the abnormal vessel (*arrow*) arising from the descending aorta. **E:** Maximum intensity coronal reconstruction shows the abnormal aortic branch (*arrows*) supplying the right lung base. **F:** Minimum intensity coronal reconstruction shows the hyperlucency intralobar sequestration (*arrows*) and its supplying vessel.

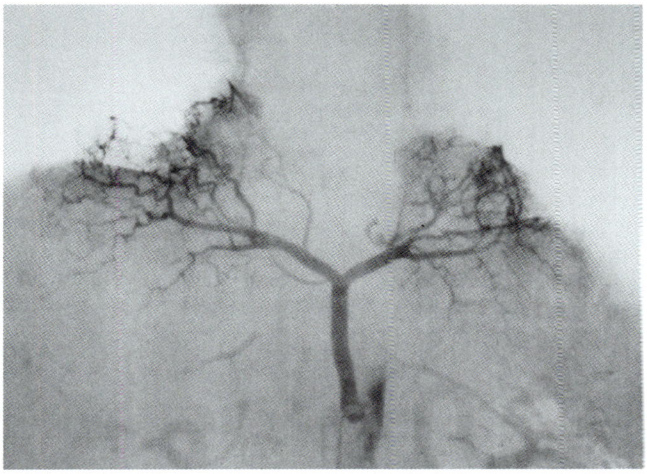

Figure 9.29. Bilateral intralobar sequestrations supplied by a single anomalous branch of the descending aorta (subtracted arteriogram).

the diaphragm or immediately below the diaphragm in the upper abdomen.

Extralobar sequestration is often diagnosed in infancy (unlike intralobar sequestration) (Table 9.16). It is detected incidentally or presents as a mass lesion (Fig. 9.30). Unlike intralobar sequestration, infection is rare. Associated congenital anomalies, particularly diaphragmatic abnormalities and ipsilateral lung hypoplasia, are common. Because of its complete pleural envelope, extralobar sequestration rarely becomes infected.

Radiographically and on CT, extralobar sequestration appears as a sharply marginated mass lesion, which does not contain air (unlike intralobar sequestration) (see Figs. 9.30 and 9.31). It is usually homogeneous in appearance but may contain cystic areas. Its supplying artery may be seen on CT. If not, aortography may be needed for diagnosis.

Table 9.15 Extralobar Sequestration

Within its own pleural envelope
90% at left base
No pulmonary artery or bronchial supply
Arterial supply from abdominal aorta in most
Drainage via systemic (eg, azygos or hemiazygos) veins in most
Presentation in infancy in most
Presents as mass lesion; infection is rare
Imaging appearances:
- Homogeneous and well-defined mass lesion
- May contain fluid-filled cystic areas
- Rarely contains air

Table 9.16 Comparison of Intralobar and Extralobar Sequestration

	Intralobar Sequestration	Extralobar Sequestration
Patient age	Adult or older child	Infant or child
Symptoms	Infection common	Infection rare
Morphology	Within a lobe	Within its own pleural envelope
Location	65% at left base	90% at left base
Arterial supply	Thoracic or abdominal aorta	Usually abdominal aorta
Venous drainage	Usually pulmonary veins	Usually systemic veins
Appearance	Commonly contains air	Rarely contains air

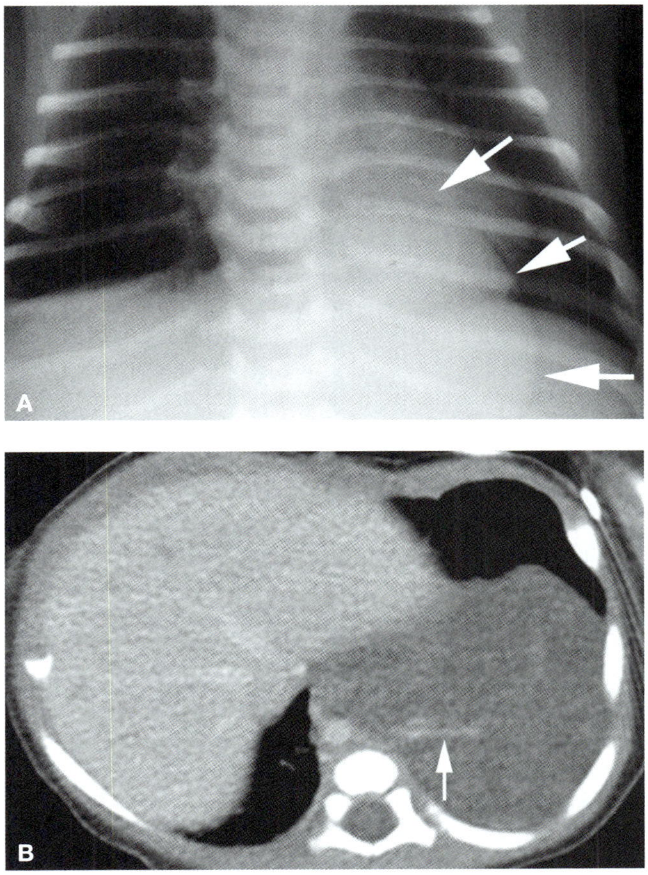

Figure 9.30. Extralobar sequestration in a neonate. **A:** Chest radiograph shows a soft-tissue mass at the left base (*arrows*). **B.**

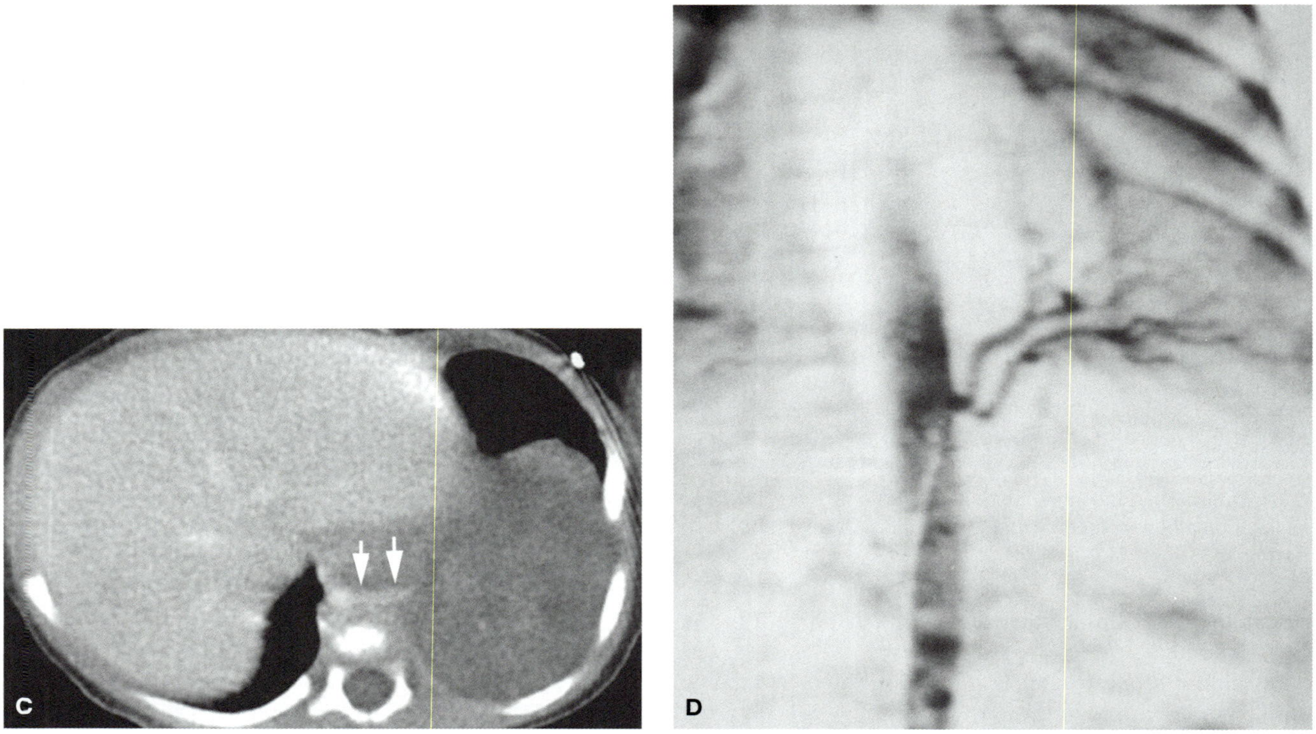

Figure 9.30. *(Continued)* **C:** Contrast-enhanced CTs show a soft-tissue mass with arterial supply (*arrows*) from the aorta. **D:** Aortogram performed via umbilical artery catheter shows anomalous arteries supplying the left base.

ANOMALOUS SYSTEMIC ARTERIES WITHOUT SEQUESTRATION (SYSTEMIC ARTERIAL MALFORMATION)

Systemic arteries may supply normal basal segments of the lung (Table 9.17). Although these lesions can be thought of as representing systemic AVMs, they are unassociated with the large, dilated vascular sac typically seen with pulmonary AVMs. Rather, the arteriovenous communications in patients with systemic arterial malformations usually represent normal capillaries.

This lesion is probably best thought of as anomalous systemic arterial supply to an area of lung due to persistence of an embryonic aortic branch. The pulmonary parenchyma in the region supplied by the anomalous artery is normal, as are bronchial communications (Fig. 9.32). The pulmonary artery supply to these areas can be normal or absent.

A relationship may exist between systemic arterial malformations and pulmonary sequestration, and both these lesions represent different points on the spectrum of anomalies affecting the pulmonary artery, systemic arteries, and bronchial development. Some cases have been reported in which intralobar sequestration on one side coexists with systemic arterial malformation on the other. In such cases, both lesions are typically supplied by the same aortic branch.

Because systemic arterial malformation results in a left-to-left arterial shunt, left ventricular enlargement and congestive heart failure can occur. Hemoptysis may also occur. However, most patients have no symptoms. If the anomalous vessel supplies an area of lung also supplied by the pulmonary artery, treatment involves ligation or embolization of the anomalous vessel.

Table 9.17 Systemic Artery Malformation

Arterial supply to lung from thoracic or abdominal aorta
Lung normal
Bronchi normal
Pulmonary artery normal or absent in affected region
Pulmonary vein drainage normal
Symptoms: Congestive heart failure or hemoptysis

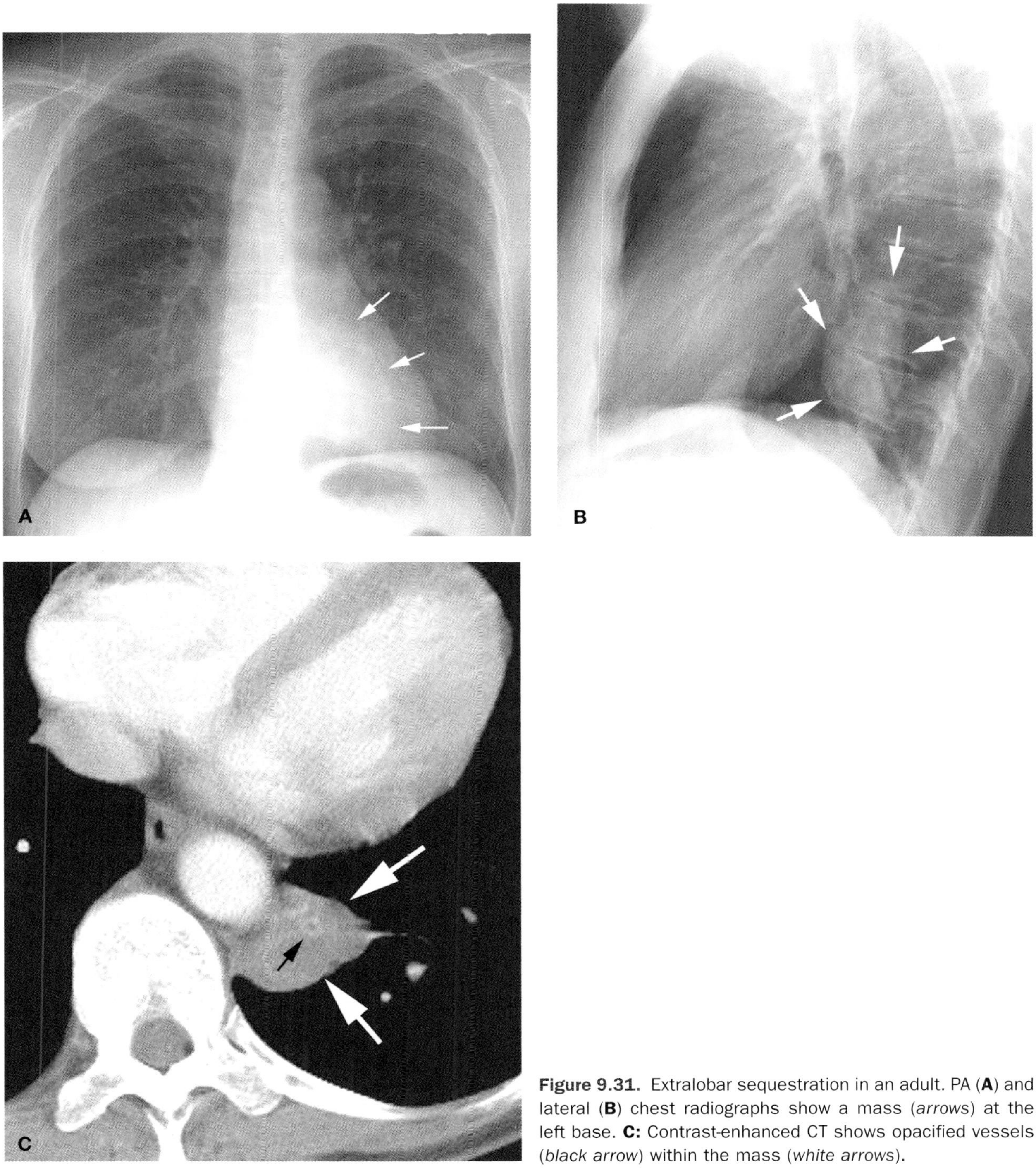

Figure 9.31. Extralobar sequestration in an adult. PA (**A**) and lateral (**B**) chest radiographs show a mass (*arrows*) at the left base. **C:** Contrast-enhanced CT shows opacified vessels (*black arrow*) within the mass (*white arrows*).

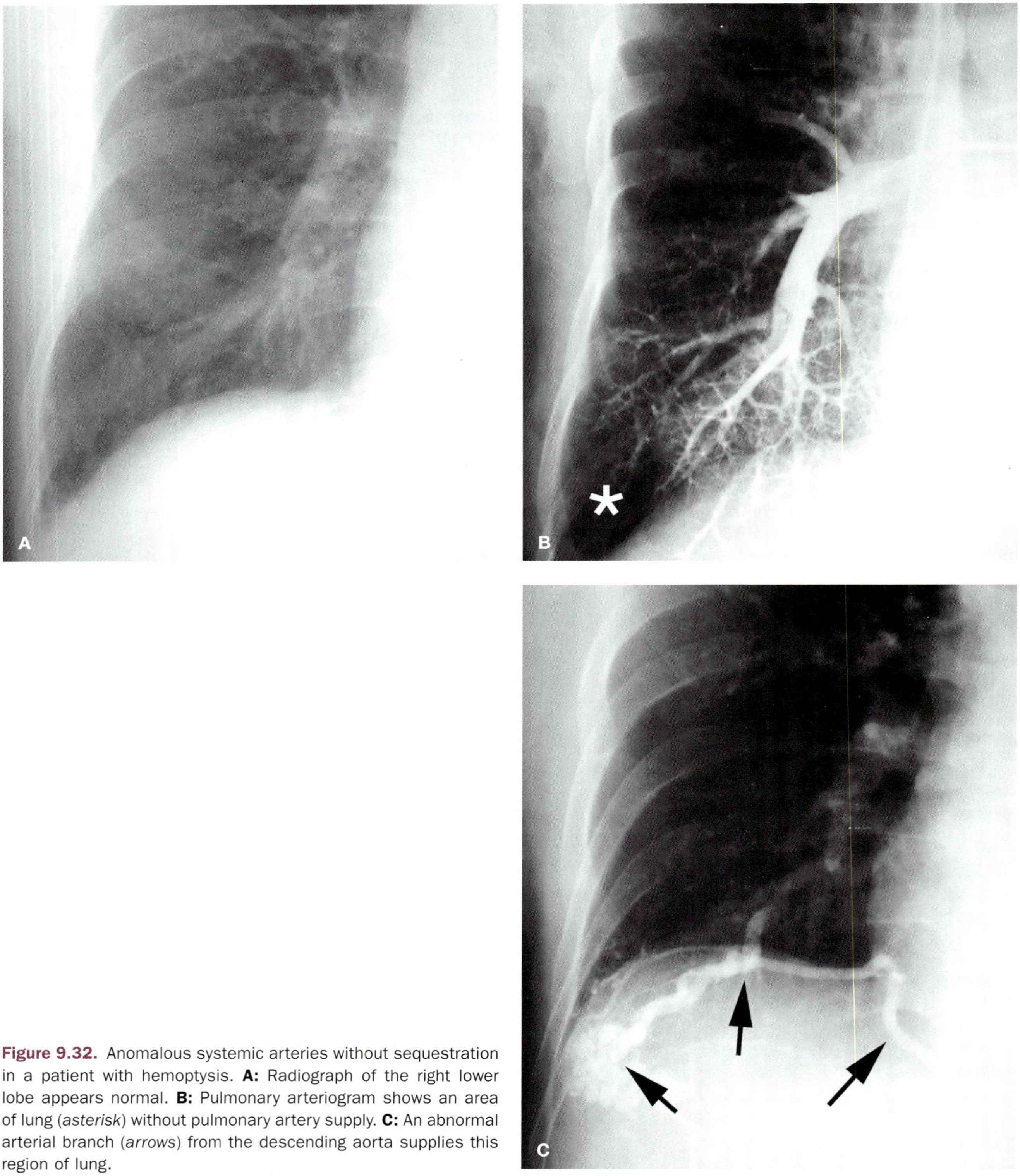

Figure 9.32. Anomalous systemic arteries without sequestration in a patient with hemoptysis. **A:** Radiograph of the right lower lobe appears normal. **B:** Pulmonary arteriogram shows an area of lung (*asterisk*) without pulmonary artery supply. **C:** An abnormal arterial branch (*arrows*) from the descending aorta supplies this region of lung.

SUGGESTED READINGS

Biyyam DR, Chapman T, Ferguson MR Deutsch G, Dighe MK. Congenital lung abnormalities: embryologic features, prenatal diagnosis, and postnatal radiologic-pathologic correlation. *Radiographics*. 2010;30(6):1721-1738.

Chassagnon G, Morel B, Carpentier E, Ducou Le Pointe H, Sirinelli D. Tracheobronchial branching abnormalities: lobe-based classification scheme. *Radiographics*. 2016;36(2):358-373.

Desir A, Ghaye B. Congenital abnormalities of intrathoracic airways. *Radiol Clin North Am*. 2009;47(2):203-225.

Dines DE, Arms RA, Bernatz PE, Gomes MR. Pulmonary arteriovenous fistulas. *Mayo Clin Proc*. 1974;49(7):460-465.

Do KH, Goo JM, Im JG, Kim KW, Chung JW, Park JH. Systemic arterial supply to the lungs in adults: spiral CT findings. *Radiographics*. 2001;21(2) 387-402.

Fitch SJ, Tonkin ILD, Tonkin AK. Imaging of foregut duplication cysts. *Radiographics*. 1986;6(2):189-201.

Fowler DJ, Gould SJ. The pathology of congenital lung lesions. *Semin Pediatr Surg*. 2015;24(4):176-182. https://doi.org/10.1053/j.sempedsurg.2015.02.002

Ghaye B, Szapiro D, Fanchamps JM, Dondelinger RF. Congenital bronchial abnormalities revisited. *Radiographics*. 2001;21(1):105-119.

Griffin N, Devaraj A, Goldstraw P, Bush A, Nicholson AG, Padley S. CT and histopathological correlation of congenital cystic pulmonary lesions: a common pathogenesis? *Clin Radiol*. 2008;63(9):995-1005.

Ikezoe J, Murayama S, Godwin JD, Done SL, Verschakelen JA. Bronchopulmonary sequestration: CT assessment. *Radiology*. 1990;176(2):375-379.

Konen E, Raviv-Zilka L, Cohen RA, et al.. Congenital pulmonary venolobar syndrome: spectrum of helical CT findings with emphasis on computerized reformatting. *Radiographics*. 2003;23(5):1175-1184.

Lee EY, Boiselle PM, Cleveland RH. Multidetector CT evaluation of congenital lung anomalies. *Radiology*. 2008;247(3):632-648.

Mata JM, Caceres J, Lucaya J, Garcia-Conesa JA. CT of congenital malformations of the lung. *Radiographics*. 1990;10(4):651-674.

McAdams HP, Kirejczyk WM, Rosado-de-Christenson ML, Matsumoto S. Bronchogenic cyst: imaging features with clinical and histopathologic correlation. *Radiology*. 2000;217(2):441-446.

Patz EF Jr, Müller NL, Swensen SJ, Dodd LG. Congenital cystic adenomatoid malformation in adults: CT findings. *J Comput Assist Tomogr*. 1995;19(3):361-364.

Porres DV, Morenza OP, Pallisa E, Roque A, Andreu J, Martínez M. Learning from the pulmonary veins. *Radiographics*. 2013;33(4):999-1022.

Rappaport DC, Herman SJ, Weisbrod GL. Congenital bronchopulmonary diseases in adults: CT findings. *AJR Am J Roentgenol*. 1994;162(6):1295-1299.

Raptis DA, Short R, Robb C, et al. CT appearance of pulmonary arteriovenous malformations and mimics. *Radiographics*. 2022;42(1):56-68. https://doi.org/10.1148/rg.210076

Remy J, Remy-Jardin M, Wattinne L, Deffontaines C. Pulmonary arteriovenous malformations: evaluation with CT of the chest before and after treatment. *Radiology*. 1992;182(3):809-816.

Roehm JOF, Jue KL, Amplatz K. Radiographic features of the scimitar syndrome. *Radiology*. 1966;86(5):856-859.

Rosado-de-Christenson ML, Stocker JT. Congenital cystic adenomatoid malformation. *Radiographics*. 1991;11(5):865-886.

Sener RN, Tugran C, Savas R, Alper H. CT findings in scimitar syndrome. *AJR Am J Roentgenol*. 1993;160(6):1361.

Shenoy SS, Culver GJ, Pirson HS. Agenesis of lung in an adult. *AJR Am J Roentgenol*. 1979;133(4):755-757.

Shimohira M, Hara M, Kitase M, et al. Congenital pulmonary airway malformation: CT-pathologic correlation. *J Thorac Imaging*. 2007;22(2):149-153.

Stocker JT. Congenital pulmonary airway malformation: a new name for an expanded classification of congenital cystic adenomatoid malformation of the lung. *Histopathology*. 2002;41(suppl 2):424-430.

Yamanaka A, Hirai T, Fujimoto T, Hase M, Noguchi M, Konishi F. Anomalous systemic arterial supply to normal basal segments of the left lower lobe. *Ann Thorac Surg*. 1999;68(2):332-338.

Chapter 10

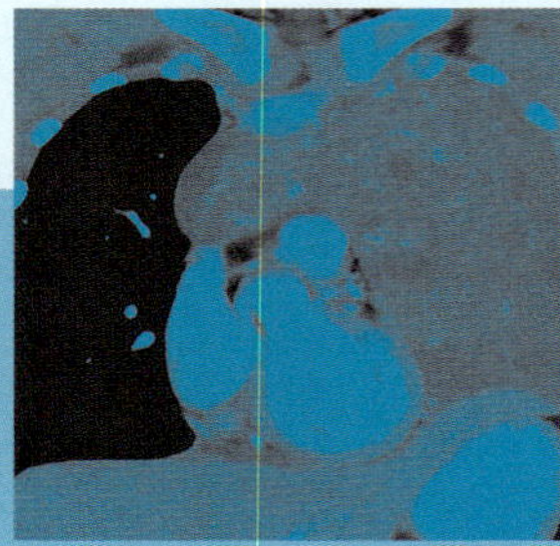

Travis S. Henry

Solitary and Multiple Nodules, Masses, Cavities, and Cysts

INTRODUCTION

The radiographic assessment of patients with solitary or multiple lung nodules, masses, or cavities is a common clinical problem. Lung nodules are incredibly common and are seen in up to a third of patients who undergo MDCT, and the vast majority less than 1 cm are benign. A primary or metastatic tumor usually is the first (and most worrisome) consideration especially for large or growing nodules. However, many other diseases or abnormalities may present with focal lung abnormalities. Some have specific appearances that may suggest the correct diagnosis or limit the differential diagnosis.

THE SOLITARY PULMONARY NODULE

A solitary pulmonary nodule (SPN) usually is defined as a focal opacity, visible on chest radiographs or computed tomography (CT), which fits the following criteria:

1. It is relatively well defined.
2. It is surrounded, at least partially, by lungs.
3. It is roughly spherical in shape.
4. It is 3 cm or less in diameter (Fig. 10.1).

Lesions larger than 3 cm in diameter usually are referred to using the term *mass*. This cutoff also is used to distinguish a T1 lung carcinoma (3 cm or less in diameter) from a T2 carcinoma (more than 3 cm) in the lung cancer TNM staging system.

Clinical Evaluation

Clinical and historical information is helpful in the differential diagnosis of a solitary lung nodule. Important considerations that increase the likelihood of lung cancer include a history of smoking, age over 40, occupational exposures (eg, asbestos), lung fibrosis, coexisting chronic obstructive pulmonary disease (COPD) and emphysema, nodule location in the upper lobe, and a family history of lung cancer. Risk factors for cancer are reviewed in Chapter 5.

Recent travel history, a positive skin test for tuberculosis (TB) or fungus, or the presence of other diseases (eg, rheumatoid arthritis) increases the likelihood of a benign SPN. In a patient younger than 30 years of age, cancer is very uncommon as a cause of SPN.

An SPN found in a patient with a history of extrathoracic malignancy may be a metastasis, a primary lung carcinoma, or an insignificant benign lesion. Certain tumors have a propensity to metastasize as a solitary nodule. Among patients with an SPN, those with a history of melanoma, sarcoma, or testicular carcinoma are more than twice as likely to have a solitary metastasis than a bronchogenic carcinoma. On the other hand, patients with an SPN who have a history of carcinoma of the head and neck, bladder, breast, cervix, bile ducts, esophagus, ovary, prostate, or stomach are more than three times as likely to have primary bronchogenic carcinoma than lung metastasis. In patients with other types of tumors, the relative likelihood of metastasis and lung cancer is about equal.

Radiographic Evaluation

The differential diagnosis of an SPN is extensive (Table 10.1). In patients with an SPN, plain radiographs and CT are used to determine the nodule's (1) size (ie, diameter), (2) morphologic characteristics, (3) density or attenuation (ie, calcium, fat, or contrast enhancement), (4) growth rate, and (5) location (some lesions have a propensity for specific sites).

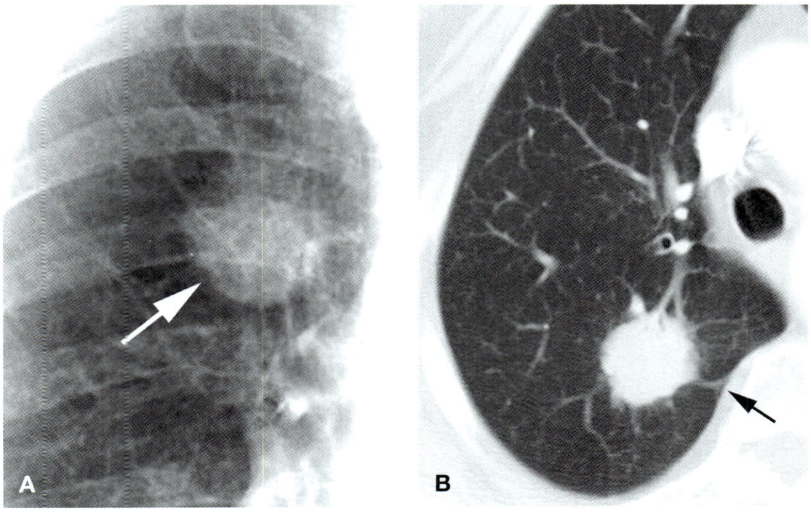

Figure 10.1. Right upper lobe nodule representing an adenocarcinoma. **A:** Chest radiograph shows a right upper lobe nodule (*arrow*). This lesion is classified as a nodule because it is relatively well defined, at least partially surrounded by the lung, roughly spherical in shape, and 3 cm or less in diameter. Because the nodule exceeds 2 cm in diameter, it is very likely malignant. **B:** CT shows the edge of the nodule to be ill defined and lobulated, and a pleural tail (*arrow*) extends to the pleural surface.

Table 10.1 Differential Diagnosis of a Solitary Pulmonary Nodule or Mass (In Alphabetical Order)

Congenital Lesions and Normal Variants
- Arteriovenous fistula
- Bronchogenic cyst
- Congenital cystic adenomatoid malformation (congenital pulmonary airway malformation)
- Intrapulmonary lymph node
- Mucoid impaction (bronchial atresia)
- Pulmonary vein varix
- Sequestration

Malignant Neoplasms
- Lung carcinoma
- Lymphoma
- Lymphoproliferative disease
- Metastatic neoplasm
- Sarcoma (eg, chondrosarcoma, liposarcoma, fibrosarcoma)

Benign Neoplasms and Neoplasm-like Conditions
- Endometrioma
- Hamartoma
- Lymphoproliferative disease
- Miscellaneous benign tumors
  - Mesenchymal tumors (eg, chondroma, lipoma, fibroma)
  - Epithelial tumors (eg, atypical adenomatous hyperplasia, mucous gland adenoma)
  - Vascular tumors

Infection and Parasites
- Aspergillosis, angioinvasive
- *Dirofilaria immitis* (dog heartworm)
- *Echinococcus*
- Focal (round) pneumonia
- Granulomatous infection or granuloma
  - Tuberculosis
  - Nontuberculous mycobacteria (eg, *Mycobacterium avium-intracellulare* complex)
  - Coccidioidomycosis
  - Histoplasmosis
  - *Cryptococcus*
  - Lung abscess
- Mycetoma (aspergilloma)
- Pulmonary gangrene
- Septic embolism

Inflammatory (Noninfectious)
- Churg-Strauss syndrome
- Focal organizing pneumonia
- Rheumatoid nodule
- Sarcoidosis
- Granulomatosis with polyangiitis

Airways and Inhalational Disease
- Mucoid impaction (mucous plug)
  - Asthma
  - Allergic bronchopulmonary aspergillosis
  - Bronchial atresia
  - Bronchiectasis
  - Cystic fibrosis
- Conglomerate mass or progressive massive fibrosis (eg, silicosis)
- Lipoid pneumonia

Vascular Lesions
- Arteriovenous fistula
- Hematoma
- Infarction
- Pulmonary artery aneurysm
- Pulmonary vein varix
- Septic embolism

Idiopathic and Miscellaneous
- Amyloidosis
- Fluid-filled bulla
- Round atelectasis

Table 10.2 Likelihood of Malignancy Related to Nodule Diameter in Patients at Risk (Being Screened Because of Age and Smoking History)

Diameter	Malignancy
<4 mm	<1%
4-7 mm	3%-7%
7-10 mm	15%
10-30 mm	20%-40%

Nodule assessment may also involve 2-(fluorine-18)-fluoro-2-deoxy-D-glucose (FDG)-positron emission tomography (PET) and other nuclear imaging techniques and image-guided biopsy.

Size

Lung nodule size is sometimes measured by using its largest diameter, smallest diameter, or an average of both. The Fleischner Society recommends that a small nodule (<10 mm) be reported as the average of maximal long-axis and perpendicular maximal short-axis longest axial measurement in the same plane. This is consistent with the ACR Lung-RADS 2022 guidelines. Nodules larger than 1 cm should be reported as both long- and short-axis measurements. While some modern software systems allow for 3D nodule volume reporting, this is still not in general practice.

The likelihood of malignancy for a solid nodule seen on CT depends on many nodule and patient characteristics, most notably the size of the nodule (Table 10.2). Based on data from screening trials including the National Lung Screening Trial and Nelson Trial, the likelihood of lung cancer is well under 1% for a nodule less than 6 mm. This risk increases for larger nodules and those with suspicious morphology, ranging from 0.5% to 2% for nodules 6 to 8 mm and higher for larger nodules (see Fig. 10.1). In the general population, the likelihood of cancer is less than reported in screening populations.

In nodules of ground-glass opacity (GGO) less than 6 mm in diameter, fewer than 1% are diagnosed as cancer, while this figure is about 3% for GGO nodules ranging from 6 to 9 mm and 11% for GGO nodules 10 to 30 mm in diameter.

One or more small lung nodules are exceedingly common as an incidental finding on CT scans, and the large majority represent benign lesions such as granuloma or intrapulmonary lymph node (IPLN). IPLNs may show characteristic morphology (see below). Follow-up CT is the only practical method of evaluating the significance of a small nodule.

Morphologic Characteristics of an SPN

Using plain radiographs or CT, an SPN may sometimes be diagnosed as a specific lesion based on its appearance. Some such lesions include mucous plug, arteriovenous malformation (AVM), rounded atelectasis, mycetoma, and focal pleural lesions. These are described later in this chapter.

Much more often, radiographic studies are used to assess less specific morphologic characteristics that suggest that an SPN is more likely malignant or benign.

Edge Appearance

Although plain radiographs do not allow the edge of a lung nodule or mass to be assessed with the precision of CT, cancers often appear to be ill defined, irregular in contour, spiculated, or lobulated on plain films (see Fig. 10.1).

On CT, malignant nodules are much more likely to have an ill-defined, irregular, lobulated, or spiculated margin (see Figs. 10.1B and 10.2). Benign lesions tend to have a smooth, sharply defined edge (Figs. 10.3 and 10.4; Table 10.3). Nearly 90% of nodules with an irregular or spiculated edge are malignant; only 20% of nodules with a smooth, sharp margin are malignant. Malignancies that tend to have a sharp and smooth edge include metastases (Fig. 10.5) and carcinoid tumors (see Fig. 4.18 in Chapter 4). However, despite these differences, such findings should be considered nonspecific in any particular case.

The terms *corona radiata* and *corona maligna* have been used to describe the appearance of spiculation associated with a nodule or mass (see Figs. 10.2 and 10.6). Particularly

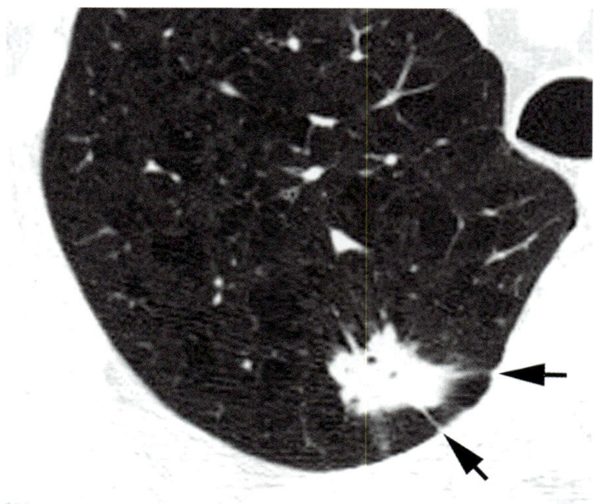

Figure 10.2. Adenocarcinoma with a spiculated margin seen on CT. Two pleural tails (*arrows*) extend to the pleural surface. This appearance has been termed *corona radiata* or *corona maligna*. The surface of the nodule is lobulated and shows notches, both of which are findings indicating malignancy. Several lucencies within the nodule represent air bronchograms of areas of pseudocavitation, typical findings in adenocarcinoma and bronchioloalveolar carcinoma.

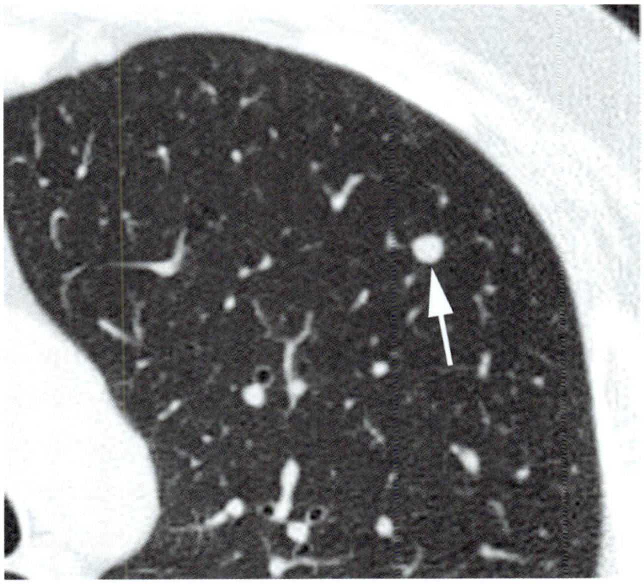

Figure 10.3. Smooth, sharply marginated, rounded nodule representing a granuloma. Its appearance (*arrow*) is typical of a benign lesion. Its small size also makes malignancy less likely.

Table 10.3 Edge Appearances and Common Diagnoses

Sharply marginated
Granuloma
Intrapulmonary lymph node
Hamartoma or benign tumor
Carcinoid tumor
Metastasis
Spiculated (corona radiata) or pleural tail
Adenocarcinoma
Carcinoma
Granuloma or focal scarring

in patients with adenocarcinoma, this appearance reflects the presence of fibrosis surrounding the tumor, although tumor invasion of the adjacent lung also may be present. The fibrosis usually reflects a desmoplastic reaction rather than preexisting lung fibrosis. Spiculation is less common with large cell carcinoma than other cell types that present as a solitary nodule or mass.

In addition, carcinomas can show the presence of a *pleural tail sign*, in which a thin linear opacity is seen extending from the edge of a lung nodule to the pleural surface (see Figs. 10.1B, 10.2, and 10.6). This tail, which can be from a few millimeters to a few centimeters in length, often is seen in association with spiculation. As with spiculation, it reflects the presence of fibrosis and often is associated with a dimpling of the visceral pleura. In patients with lung cancer, a pleural tail sign most often is associated with adenocarcinoma; it uncommonly indicates the presence of a large cell carcinoma. The pleural tail sign also can be seen in association with benign

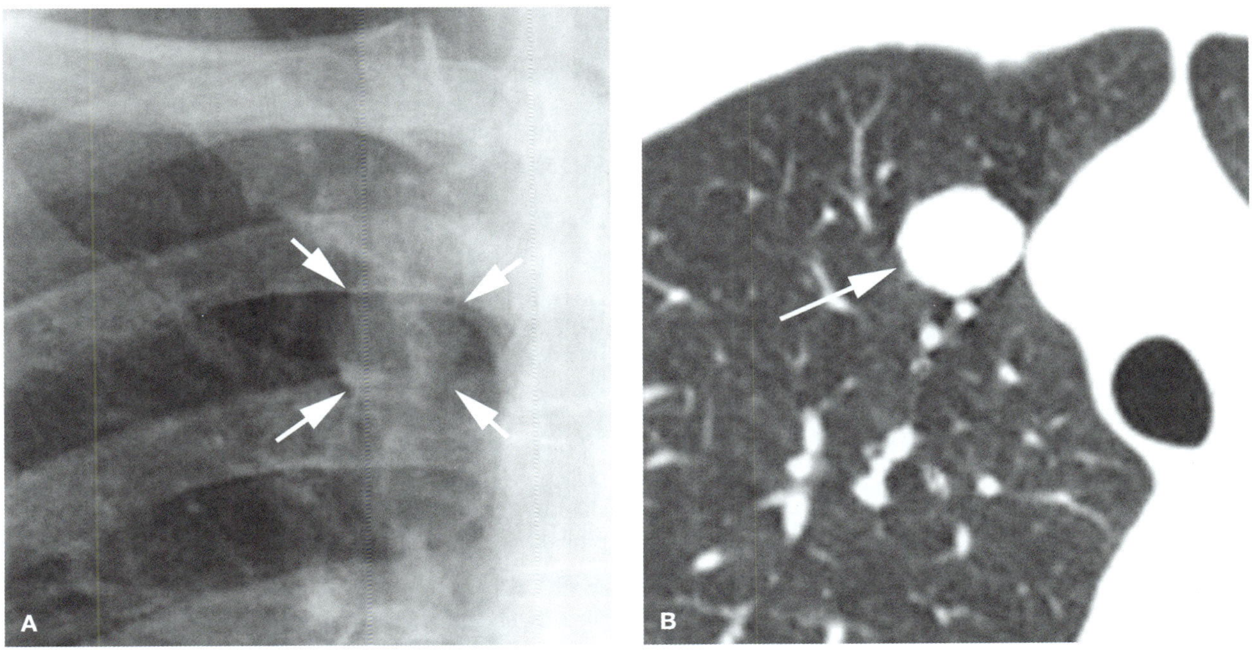

Figure 10.4. Hamartoma presenting as a sharply defined, round nodule. **A:** Chest radiograph shows a round nodule (*arrows*) in the right upper lobe. **B:** CT shows the nodule (*arrow*) to be rounded in shape and sharply marginated. Slight lobulation may be seen with hamartomas.

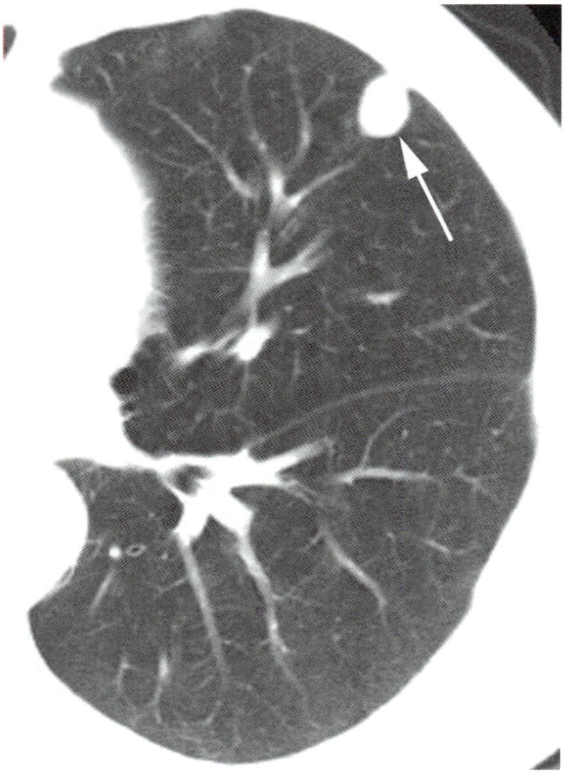

Figure 10.5. Solitary metastasis from a head and neck carcinoma. A left upper lobe nodule (*arrow*) is smooth and sharply defined on CT. This appearance is common with metastases.

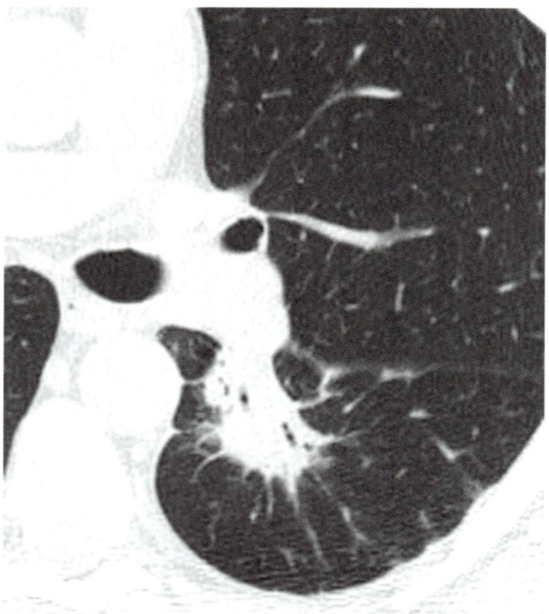

Figure 10.6. Adenocarcinoma. HRCT shows an irregular, spiculated nodule with multiple pleural tails. Air bronchograms are visible within the nodule.

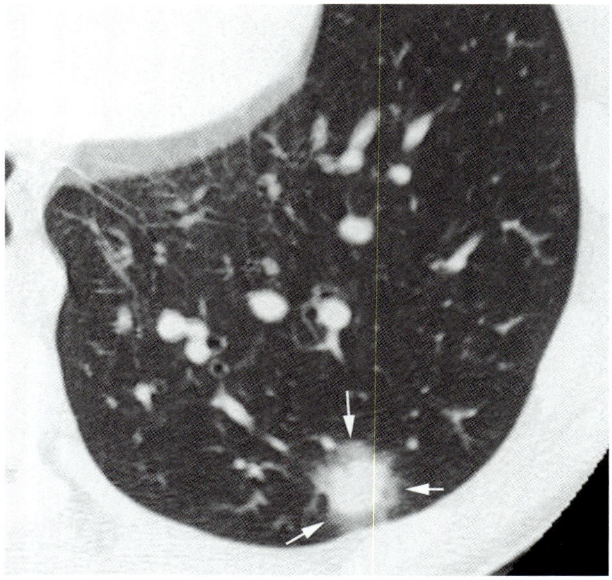

Figure 10.7. Halo sign in invasive aspergillosis. HRCT in a young patient with leukemia and granulocytopenia shows a dense left lower lobe nodule surrounded by a halo (*arrows*) of ground-glass opacity. In patients with invasive aspergillosis, the halo represents hemorrhage surrounding a septic infarction.

lung nodules, which are associated with fibrosis, including various granulomatous diseases. The presence of a spiculated contour is more suggestive of malignancy than a pleural tail.

The *halo sign*, defined by a halo of GGO surrounding a soft-tissue density lung nodule, may be seen in some patients with an SPN. It is commonly present in leukemic patients with angioinvasive aspergillosis (Fig. 10.7) but also can be seen in patients with other infections (see Fig. 10.35C), inflammatory and vascular abnormalities, and in some tumors, particularly adenocarcinoma (Fig. 10.8; Figs. 5.7 and 5.8 in Chapter 5; Table 10.4). The histologic nature of the halo varies with the disease. In patients with invasive aspergillosis, the halo sign represents hemorrhage; in patients with carcinoma, it reflects the presence of lepidic spread of tumor (see Fig. 5.3C in Chapter 5).

Shape

Lung carcinomas tend to be irregular in shape, lobulated, or notched (see Figs. 10.1, 10.2, and 10.6) but uncommonly have concave margins. Granulomas often are round (see Fig. 10.3). Hamartomas and metastases may be round, oval, or lobulated (see Figs. 10.4 and 10.5). Scars or areas of atelectasis or scarring may appear linear or angular or elliptical in shape. A number of other benign lesions (eg, AVM, mucous plugs) may be identified by their characteristic shapes.

Air Bronchograms and Pseudocavitation

On CT, air bronchograms commonly are seen in cancers presenting as an SPN (25% to 65% of cases; see Figs. 10.2 and 10.6). This finding is most typical of adenocarcinoma but

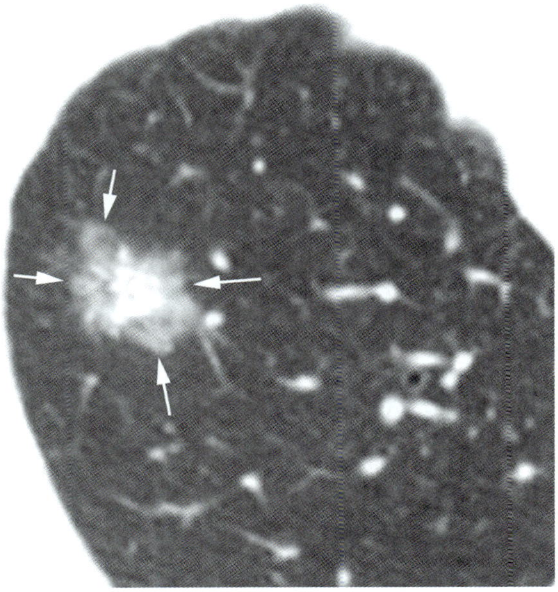

Figure 10.8. Halo sign in adenocarcinoma. HRCT shows a dense central nodule surrounded by a halo (*arrows*). In adenocarcinoma, the dense center usually represents invasive growth, while the halo represents the presence of lepidic tumor growth.

may be seen in other cell types of lung cancer. Air bronchograms are less common in benign lesions but have a variety of causes, such as focal pneumonia, infarction, round atelectasis, or conglomerate masses in patients with silicosis or sarcoidosis (Table 10.5). An appearance mimicking the presence of air bronchograms may be seen in patients with developing mycetoma; the apparent air bronchograms represent air-filled spaces between fronds of fungus. Small bronchi seen in relation to lung cancers often appear abnormal, being narrowed, obstructed, or irregular in contour.

Small rounded lucencies, not representing air bronchograms or cavitation, may be seen in patients with lung cancer, particularly adenocarcinoma (see Fig. 10.2); this appearance is termed *pseudocavitation*. On occasion, an adenocarcinoma may appear as "bubbly" cystic or multicystic lesion with little

Table 10.4 Causes of the Halo Sign

- Fungi: invasive aspergillosis, candidiasis, coccidioidomycosis
- Bacteria: tuberculosis, *Nocardia*, *Legionella*
- Viruses: cytomegalovirus, herpes
- *Pneumocystis jiroveci* (*Pneumocystis carinii*)
- Organizing pneumonia
- Granulomatosis with polyangiitis (Wegener granulomatosis)
- Infarct
- Metastatic tumor
- Kaposi sarcoma
- Adenocarcinoma with lepidic growth

Table 10.5 Causes of Air Bronchograms in Solitary Pulmonary Nodules

- Adenocarcinoma
- Conglomerate mass (eg, silicosis, sarcoidosis)
- Focal pneumonia
- Infarction
- Rounded atelectasis
- Organizing pneumonia
- Lymphoma
- Lymphoproliferative diseases
- Mycetoma (may mimic an air bronchogram)

associated soft tissue or GGO. Although this appearance may suggest a benign lesion, a high degree of suspicion should be maintained.

Cavitation

By general agreement, a *cyst* is an air-filled lesion that has a smooth and uniform wall 3 mm or less in thickness. The term *cavity* usually is used to describe a lesion with a thicker or more irregular wall or a lesion that has *cavitated* (ie, evolved by developing an air-filled space, regardless of how thick the wall is). Thus, a thin-walled lesion may be either a cyst or a cavity, whereas a thick-walled or irregular lesion is a cavity. An exception to this rule is an infected cyst; surrounding lung inflammation may result in a thick "wall."

Cavitation occurs in about 10% of cancers, most commonly in patients with adenocarcinoma and squamous cell carcinoma (Fig. 10.9; see also Figs. 5.13 and 5.44 in Chapter 5). Cavitation of large cell carcinoma also occurs; small cell carcinoma rarely cavitates.

Although a long list of abnormalities may be associated with cysts or cavities, described in Table 10.6 and in detail later, for practical purposes, radiographic evaluation is directed at determining the likelihood of malignancy. Cavitary malignant lesions tend to have a thick, nodular wall (see Fig. 10.9B and C; see also Figs. 5.13 and 5.44 in Chapter 5); benign lesions often have a thin, smooth wall (Fig. 10.10).

The thickness of the wall of a cavity serves as an indicator of its likelihood of being malignant. Nearly 85% of cavities with a wall measuring more than 15 mm in its thickest portion are malignant (see Fig. 10.9B). If the thickest part of the wall is less than 5 mm, 95% are benign (see Fig. 10.10). Seventy-five percent of cavities with a wall 5 to 15 mm in thickness are benign. If the thickest part of the cavity wall measures 1 mm or less, malignancy is rare. However, thin-walled cystic lesions (see pseudocavitation above) may be seen with pulmonary adenocarcinoma, with primary squamous cell carcinoma, or with metastases.

Lung cancer resulting in bronchial obstruction also can be associated with an abscess in the distal lung, mimicking a cavitary carcinoma. In addition, lung cancer sometimes can arise in a bulla or cyst or be associated with a preexisting

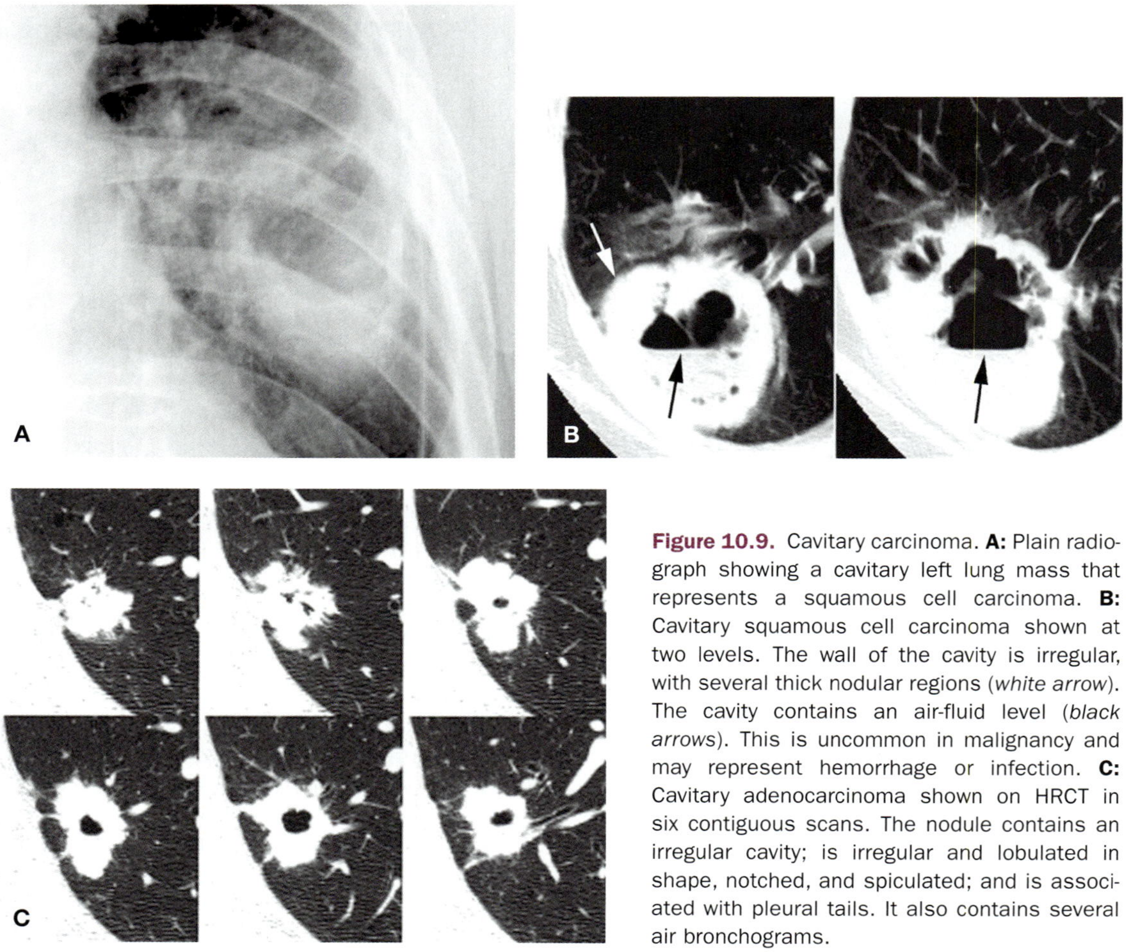

Figure 10.9. Cavitary carcinoma. **A:** Plain radiograph showing a cavitary left lung mass that represents a squamous cell carcinoma. **B:** Cavitary squamous cell carcinoma shown at two levels. The wall of the cavity is irregular, with several thick nodular regions (*white arrow*). The cavity contains an air-fluid level (*black arrows*). This is uncommon in malignancy and may represent hemorrhage or infection. **C:** Cavitary adenocarcinoma shown on HRCT in six contiguous scans. The nodule contains an irregular cavity; is irregular and lobulated in shape, notched, and spiculated; and is associated with pleural tails. It also contains several air bronchograms.

Table 10.6 Causes of a Cyst or Cavity (Solitary or Multiple)

Amyloidosis—solitary or multiple
Aspergillosis, angioinvasive—usually multiple
Aspergillosis, semi-invasive—usually solitary
Bronchogenic cyst—usually single
Bulla—solitary or multiple
Congenital pulmonary airway malformation (CPAM)—solitary, but often multiloculated
Conglomerate mass or progressive massive fibrosis—often bilateral
Cystic bronchiectasis—usually multiple
Cystic lung disease (eg, histiocytosis, lymphangiomyomatosis)—multiple
Echinococcus—solitary or multiple
Endometrioma
Granulomatous infection
- Tuberculosis
- Nontuberculous mycobacteria (eg, *Mycobacterium avium-intracellulare* complex)
- Coccidioidomycosis
- Histoplasmosis
- *Cryptococcus*

Hematoma—solitary or multiple
Intralobar sequestration—may be lucent, cystic, or multicystic
Lung abscess—solitary or multiple
Lung carcinoma, most commonly adenocarcinoma or squamous cell
Lymphoma—solitary or multiple
Metastatic neoplasm—usually multiple
Mycetoma—aspergilloma
Papillomatosis—usually multiple
Paragonimiasis—usually multiple
Pneumatocele—solitary or multiple
Pulmonary gangrene—usually solitary
Pulmonary laceration—traumatic
Rheumatoid nodule—usually multiple
Sarcoidosis—usually multiple
Sarcoma—solitary
Septic embolism—usually multiple
Granulomatosis with polyangiitis—usually multiple

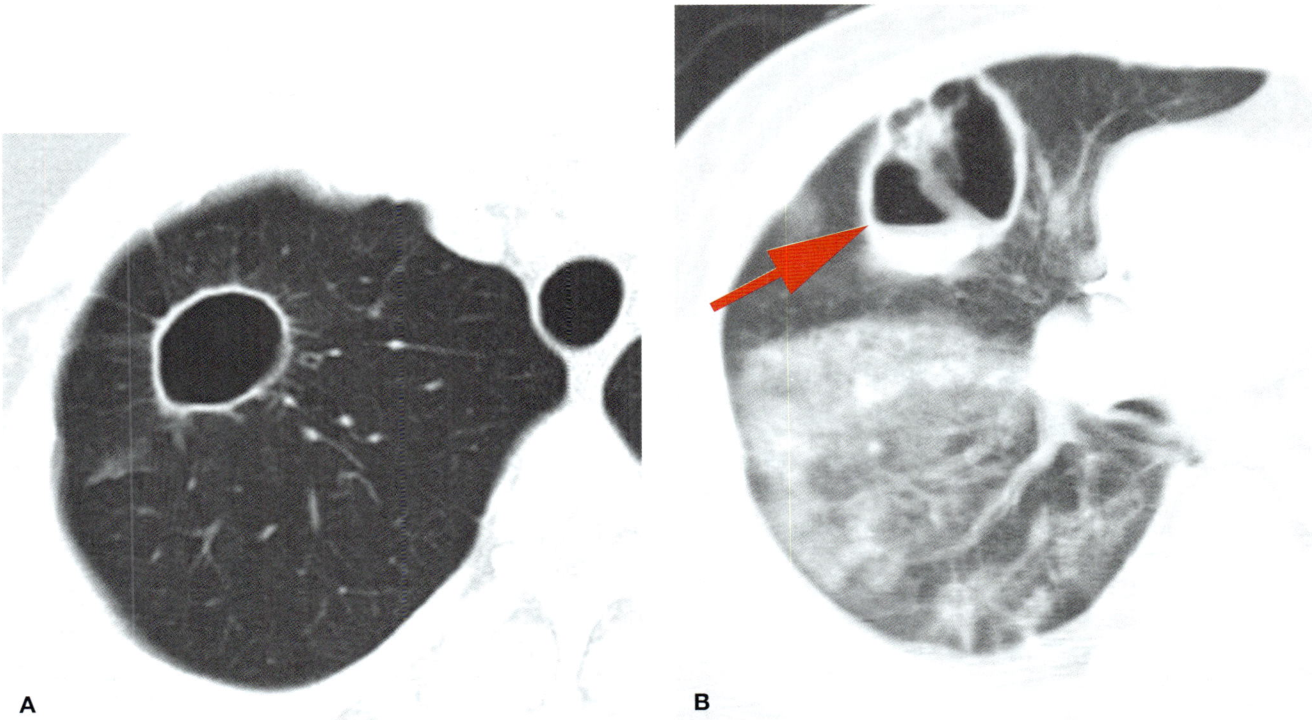

Figure 10.10. Thin-walled lung cavities. **A:** In a patient with a persisting lung cavity from *Coccidioides immitis* infection, the wall is thin and smooth, measuring less than 5 mm in thickness. **B:** In a patient with a bacterial lung abscess, the cavity wall is thin and uniform in thickness. An air-fluid level is visible (*arrow*), typical of abscess. Septations within the abscess may be seen. Ground-glass opacity in the right lower lobe is due to aspiration of abscess fluid.

cavity. In such a case, focal thickening of the cyst or cavity wall or fluid within the cyst may be the only findings suggesting this diagnosis.

Air-Crescent Sign

In some patients with a cavitary nodule or lung cyst, a mass or nodule may be present within the cavity. Air outlining or capping the superior aspect of the mass results in a crescent-shaped collection of air, termed the *air-crescent* sign. The most likely cause of this appearance is aspergilloma (mycetoma), but the differential diagnosis includes other entities as well (Table 10.7). Gravitational shift of the intracavitary mass strongly suggests mycetoma and excludes carcinoma.

Air-Fluid Level

The presence of an air-fluid level in a patient with a cavitary SPN tends to indicate a benign lesion, particularly a bacterial lung abscess (see Fig. 10.10B). However, any infected cystic or cavitary lesion may be associated with an air-fluid level. An air-fluid level is uncommon in a cavitary carcinoma but may be seen in the presence of hemorrhage or superinfection (see Fig. 10.9B). Air-fluid level is also uncommon with cavitary TB or fungal infections (Fig. 10.10A).

Satellite Nodules

Satellite nodules are small nodules seen adjacent to a larger nodule or mass. They tend to predict a benign lesion (Fig. 10.11). Satellites are most common with granulomatous diseases and infections such as TB (Table 10.8). Only a small percentage of carcinomas are associated with satellite nodules. In patients with sarcoidosis, the presence of satellite nodules has been termed the *galaxy sign*.

Table 10.7 Causes of the Air-Crescent Sign

Causes of the Air-Crescent Sign
Aspergilloma (mycetoma)
Angioinvasive aspergillosis
Carcinoma arising in a cyst
Cavitary carcinoma
Clot in a cyst or cavity
Echinococcus
Mucous plug in cystic bronchiectasis
Papillomatosis
Pulmonary gangrene
Rasmussen aneurysm (mycotic pulmonary artery aneurysm in a tubercular cavity)

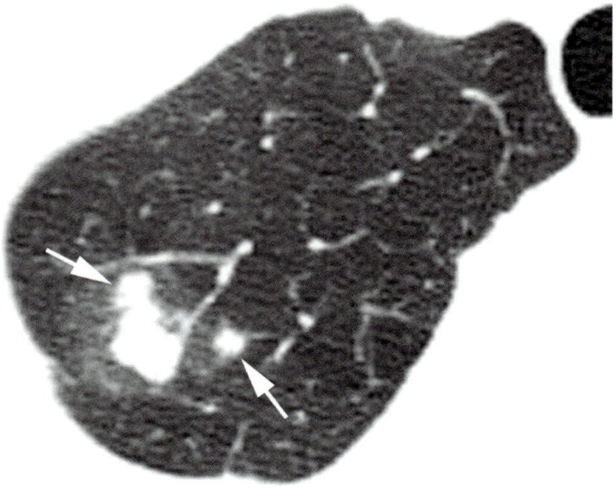

Figure 10.11. Tuberculosis. A right upper lobe nodule is associated with satellites (*arrows*). This appearance is most typical of a benign process but sometimes is seen with carcinoma.

Feeding Vessel Sign

The "*feeding vessel sign*" is present if a small pulmonary artery is seen leading directly to a nodule (Fig. 10.12). This appearance is most common with metastasis, infarct, and AVM. It is less common with primary lung carcinomas or benign lesions such as granuloma. If present, it should suggest the possibility of a vascular abnormality, but is nonspecific.

Nodule Attenuation

CT with thin slices is usually used to determine the attenuation of a lung nodule. This is best assessed without contrast injection. Because of volume averaging, unless an SPN is grossly calcified, CT with thick slices (5 mm) usually cannot be used to accurately determine its attenuation. Most cancers appear to be of soft-tissue attenuation.

Ground-Glass Opacity

With thin slices, some nodules appear to be of GGO. Many focal opacities of GGO are inflammatory and resolve on follow-up. However, *atypical adenomatous hyperplasia, adenocarcinoma* in situ, and *minimally invasive adenocarcinoma* may present as a nodule entirely of GGO (see Fig. 10.13; Figs. 5.3B, 5.5, and 5.6 in Chapter 5). Nodules primarily of GGO, but containing a solid component, may represent *adenocarcinoma* in situ, *minimally invasive adenocarcinoma*, *lepidic adenocarcinoma*, or *invasive adenocarcinoma* (Figs. 10.8; 5.7 and 5.8 in Chapter 5).

Table 10.8 Causes of Satellite Nodules

Causes of Satellite Nodules
Tuberculosis
Nontuberculous mycobacterial infection
Bacterial infections with endobronchial spread
Fungal infections
Sarcoid
Conglomerate masses (silicosis, coal worker's pneumoconiosis, talcosis)
Bronchioloalveolar carcinoma
Adenocarcinoma

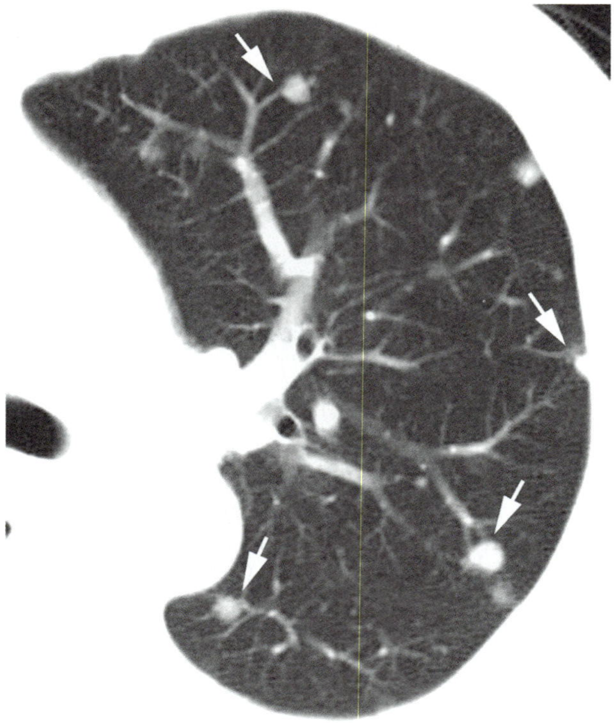

Figure 10.12. Metastatic nasopharyngeal carcinoma. Multiple nodules (*arrows*) are associated with a feeding vessel.

The larger the solid component within a GGO nodule, the more likely that invasion is present; on CT, a solid component larger than 5 mm in diameter is currently used to suggest that a lepidic predominant adenocarcinoma or invasive adenocarcinoma is present (5-year survival of 67%-90%), rather than minimally invasive adenocarcinoma or adenocarcinoma in situ, which have a better prognosis (5-year survival of 100%). Although 5 mm of invasion is the cutoff used pathologically to distinguish these tumors, it has been suggested that 3 mm is a more accurate threshold to use when interpreting CT. Adenocarcinomas presenting as a GGO SPN or a nodule containing both GGO and a solid component are reviewed in detail in Chapter 5. The assessment of such nodules is further discussed later.

Calcification or High Attenuation

The presence of calcium in an SPN increases its chances of being benign (Table 10.9). Diagnosing a small nodule as calcified on chest radiographs is somewhat subjective and subject to error. However, if a nodule a few millimeters in diameter is easily seen on radiographs, it is likely calcified.

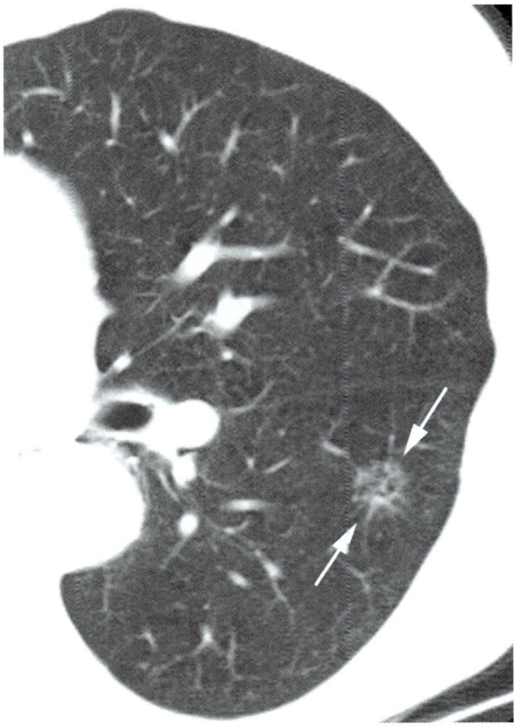

Figure 10.13. Adenocarcinoma in situ. A spiculated nodule (*arrows*) is visible on CT with 3-mm slice thickness. The nodule is of ground-glass opacity.

CT is more sensitive and accurate in diagnosing calcification. Volumetric thin-slice images usually should be obtained through a lung nodule to look for calcium. The pattern of calcification is important in suggesting the diagnosis. Generally, the following four patterns of calcification can be used to predict the presence of a benign lesion with sufficient accuracy to allow appropriate management (Fig. 10.14):

1. Homogeneous calcification (Fig. 10.15)
2. Dense central (bull's-eye) calcification (Fig. 10.16)

Table 10.9 Causes of Calcification or High Attenuation in a Solitary Pulmonary Nodule

Amyloidosis—dense or stippled
Carcinoid tumor—punctuate, eccentric
Carcinoma—punctate, eccentric, chunky
Conglomerate mass—multiple foci
Dirofilaria immitis
Granuloma—diffuse, central, concentric
Hamartoma or chondroma—popcorn, central
Mucoid impaction in allergic bronchopulmonary aspergillosis or bronchial atresia
Metastases—diffuse, punctuate
Talcosis—secondary to talc not calcium
Amiodarone toxicity—due to iodine content

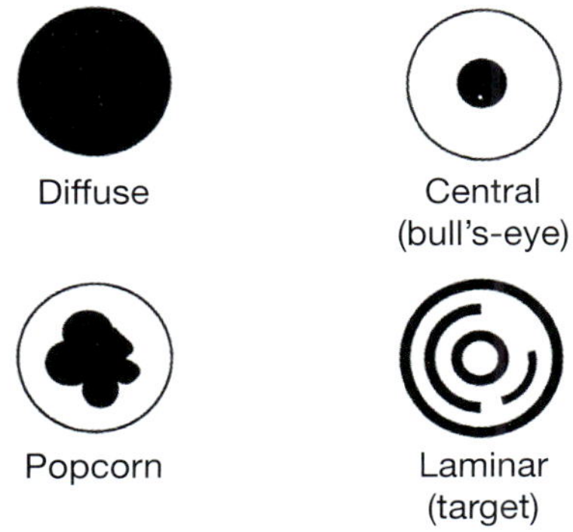

Figure 10.14. Benign patterns of calcification. With rare exceptions, these indicate the presence of a benign lesion.

3. Concentric rings of calcium ("target" calcification; Fig. 10.17)
4. Conglomerate foci of calcification involving a large part of the nodule ("popcorn" calcification; Fig. 10.18)

The first three of these patterns are most typical of granulomas; the last is more typical of hamartoma. In many cases, a calcified nodule thought to be benign should be followed for a year of two, unless the calcification is diffuse.

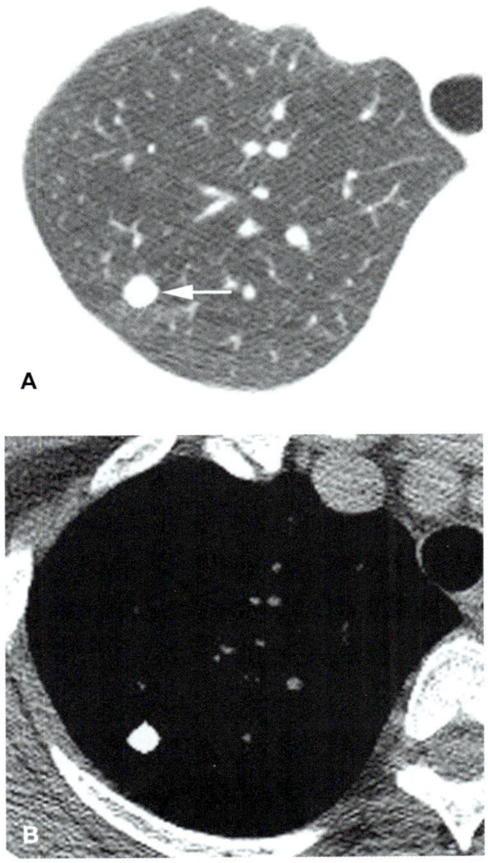

Figure 10.15. Homogeneous calcification. Dense and uniform calcification **(B)** of a small right upper lobe nodule (*arrow*, **A**) is typical of a benign lesion, usually a tuberculoma.

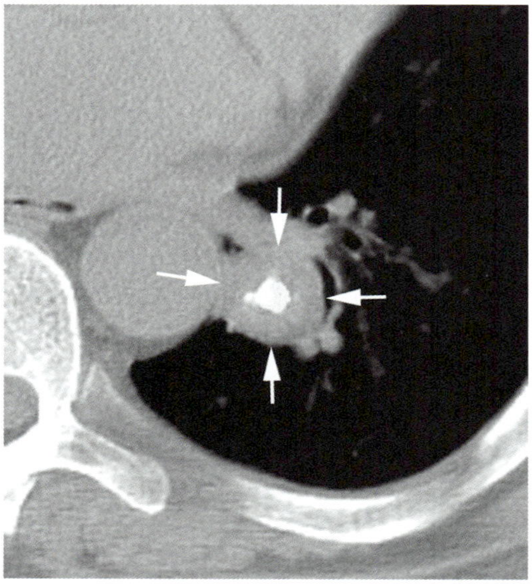

Figure 10.16. Dense central or "bull's-eye" calcification in a hamartoma. A round lung nodule (*arrows*) adjacent to the descending aorta shows dense central calcification. This is typical of histoplasmoma or hamartoma.

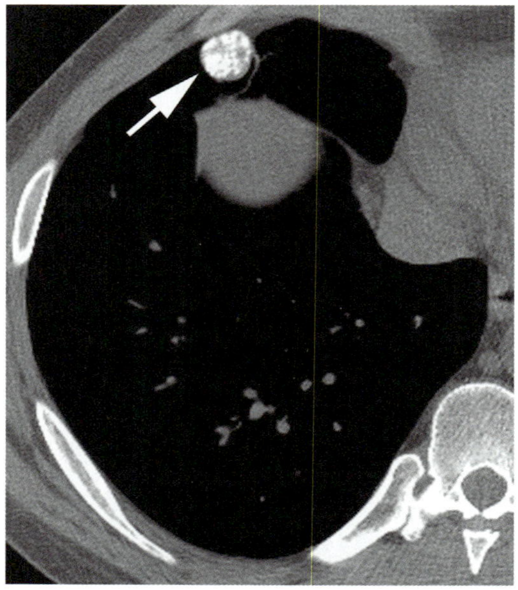

Figure 10.18. Multiple confluent nodular foci of calcification ("popcorn" calcification; *arrow*) in a hamartoma. This appearance is typical of hamartoma and corresponds to the calcification of cartilage nodules.

Stippled calcification or eccentric foci of calcification (Figs. 10.19 and 10.20) may be seen in benign SPNs but are visible in as many as 10% to 15% of cancers; these patterns must be considered indeterminate (see Fig. 10.19).

Calcium in a tumor may reflect dystrophic calcification (occurring in areas of tumor necrosis), engulfing of a preexisting granuloma, or calcification of the tumor itself (as in mucinous adenocarcinoma, carcinoid tumor, or osteogenic sarcoma). A "benign" pattern of calcification occasionally is seen in patients with neoplasm.

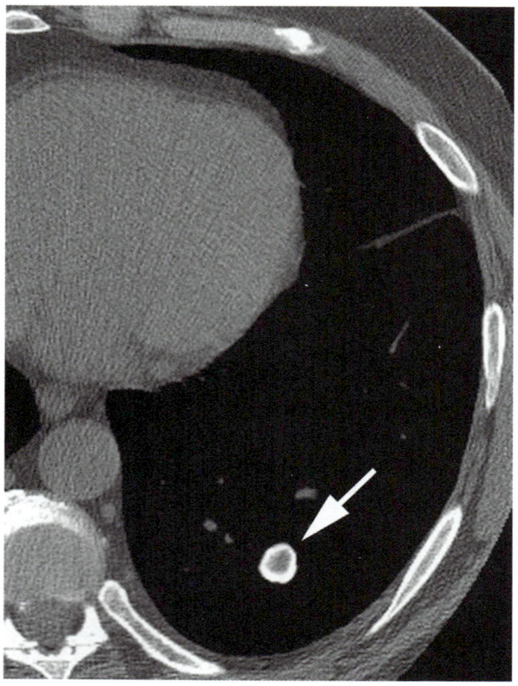

Figure 10.17. Concentric or "target" calcification (*arrow*). One or more rings of calcium may be seen. This pattern is typical of a histoplasmoma.

Carcinoid tumor can show stippled or dense central ("chunky") calcification (Figs. 10.21 and 10.22). Metastases from mucinous adenocarcinoma, osteogenic sarcoma, or chondrosarcoma can show homogenous calcification, but a history of the primary tumor allows a correct diagnosis.

Because of the high likelihood of cancer in patients with spiculated nodules or nodules exceeding 2 cm in diameter, it is inadvisable to call such a nodule benign on the basis of visible calcification, unless the calcification is diffuse and dense. A small central calcification is insufficient for determining whether such a nodule is benign.

Usually, a visible inspection of CT is sufficient for diagnosing calcification. However, the measurement of CT numbers can allow the detection of calcification, which is not clearly seen on the scans. This technique is termed *CT nodule densitometry*. Pixels denser than 100 HU indicate the presence of calcification.

High attenuation of a nodule or mass sometimes is seen using CT in patients who do not have calcification. This may

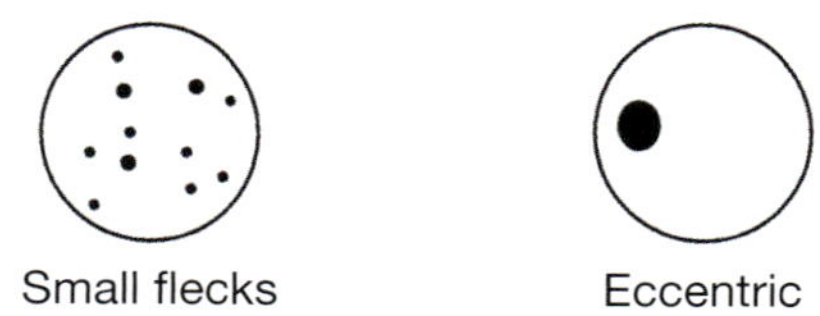

Figure 10.19. Indeterminate patterns of calcification. These may be seen in benign or malignant lesions.

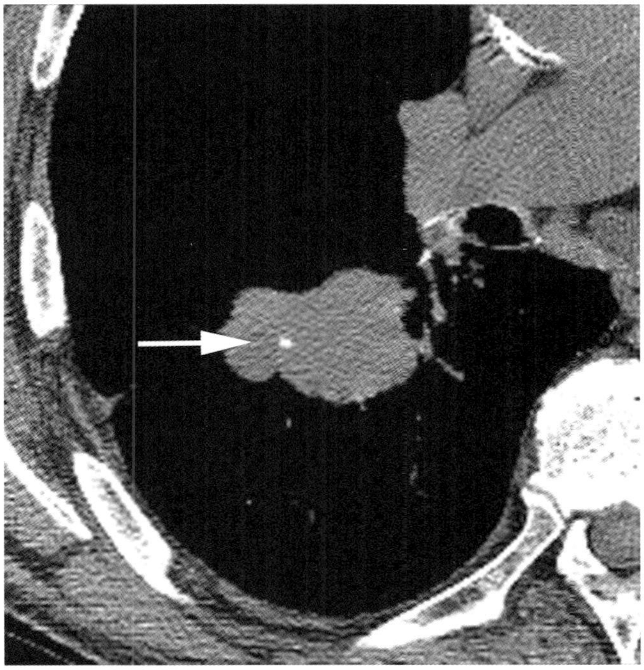

Figure 10.20. Eccentric calcification in an adenocarcinoma. A lobulated mass shows a small focus of eccentric calcification (*arrow*).

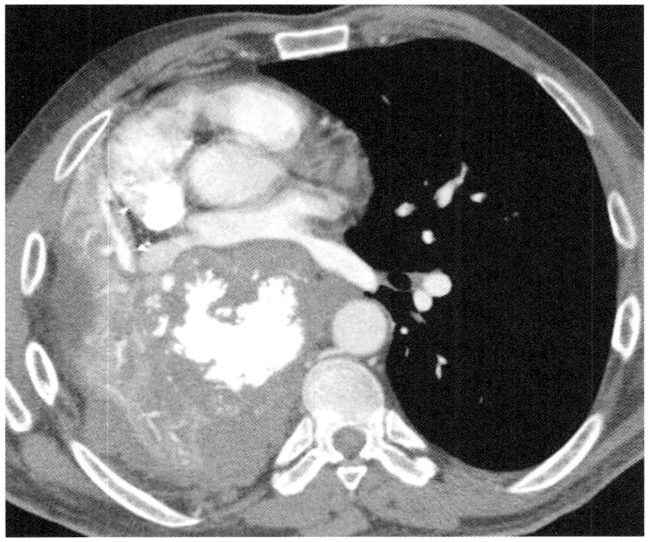

Figure 10.22. Carcinoid tumor with dense calcification and bronchial obstruction. CT shows a large mass with a dense area of "chunky" calcification. The mass is resulting in right lung collapse and impresses the posterior left atrium.

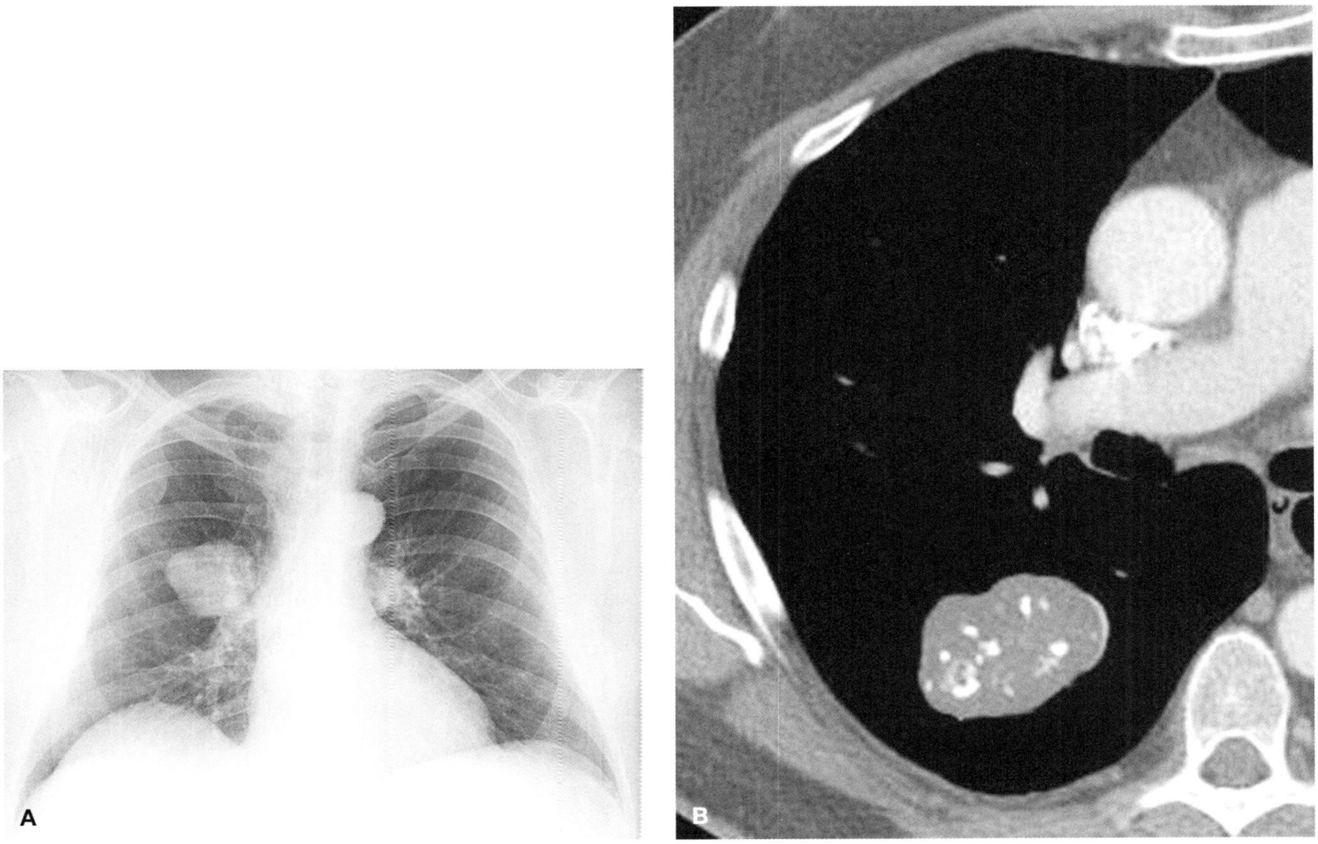

Figure 10.21. Carcinoid tumor with stippled calcifications. **A:** A sharply marginated lung mass is visible. **B:** CT shows a sharply marginated, lobulated mass with multiple small foci of calcification.

Table 10.10 Causes of Solitary Pulmonary Nodules Containing Fat
Pulmonary hamartoma
Lipoma
Liposarcoma (primary or metastatic)
Lipoid pneumonia
Histoplasmoma
Teratoma

be seen in patients with amiodarone toxicity resulting in focal organizing pneumonia (OP): the drug contains iodine, which appears dense. Patients with conglomerate masses from talcosis may show high attenuation due to the talc.

Fat

The presence of fat in an SPN may be diagnosed accurately only on thin-slice HRCT. On HRCT, fat can be accurately diagnosed if low CT numbers are seen (−40 to −120 HU). This most likely indicates the presence of hamartoma (see Figs. 5.27 and 5.29 in Chapter 5), lipoma, or lipoid pneumonia (see Figs. 20.1 and 20.2 in Chapter 20). On occasion, histoplasmoma may show fat deposition with growth (Table 10.10). Nearly 65% of hamartomas show fat on thin-slice CT, sometimes in association with dense popcorn calcification or flecks of calcium. The presence of fat within a lung nodule is sufficient for calling it benign, although follow-up is appropriate.

Low (Water or Fluid) Attenuation

Benign cystic lesions, such as pulmonary bronchogenic cyst, sequestration, congenital pulmonary airway malformations (CPAM, or congenital cystic adenomatoid malformation [CCAM]), or a fluid-filled cyst or bulla (Table 10.11), occasionally may be diagnosed on CT by their low attenuation (0-20 HU) and very thin or invisible walls (see Fig. 9.6 in Chapter 9). Mucoid impaction of a bronchus also may appear to be of low attenuation. On the other hand, bronchogenic

Table 10.11 Causes of Fluid Density Solitary Pulmonary Nodules
Bronchogenic cyst
Carcinoma (necrotic or infected)
Congenital cystic adenomatoid malformation
Conglomerate mass (necrotic)
Fluid-filled or infected cyst, cavity, or bulla
Hematoma
Lung abscess (bacterial and fungal)
Lymphoma (necrotic)
Metastatic neoplasm (necrotic)
Mucoid impaction
Sequestration

Table 10.12 Causes of a Solitary Pulmonary Nodule With Contrast Enhancement
Carcinoma
Carcinoid tumor
Granuloma (active)
Hamartoma or other benign tumor
Hemangioma
Focal pneumonia
Round atelectasis
Vascular metastases

cysts or other fluid-filled cystic lesions may have a higher attenuation because of their protein content. A hematoma may have the attenuation of blood (50 HU) or may have low attenuation, depending on its age.

A necrotic neoplasm, conglomerate mass, or lung abscess or infarction may have a low attenuation center on CT, but these lesions have a thick and perceptible wall.

Contrast Enhancement of an SPN

Cancers have a greater tendency to opacify following contrast infusion than do some types of benign nodules. Specific contrast enhancement techniques have been suggested to help diagnose malignancy, but these are uncommonly used in clinical practice (Table 10.12). Round atelectasis tends to enhance densely, as does any area of atelectasis.

Contrast Opacification

Some solitary (or multiple) lesions densely opacify following contrast injection, thus representing vascular structures (Table 10.13). These have a limited differential diagnosis and specific morphology, described in the following sections.

Nodule Growth and Doubling Time

Carcinomas grow (Fig. 10.23). The growth rate of an SPN has been used to determine its likelihood of being malignant. *Doubling time*, the time required for a lesion to double in volume, is used to measure the growth rate. For easy reference, a 26% increase in nodule diameter is one doubling, and a doubling of diameter means that three volume doublings have occurred. However, not all carcinomas grow in a concentric fashion, and estimating their volume may be difficult, even using current computer algorithms.

Table 10.13 Solitary Pulmonary Nodules Associated With Contrast Opacification
Arteriovenous fistula
Pulmonary vein varix
Pulmonary artery aneurysm

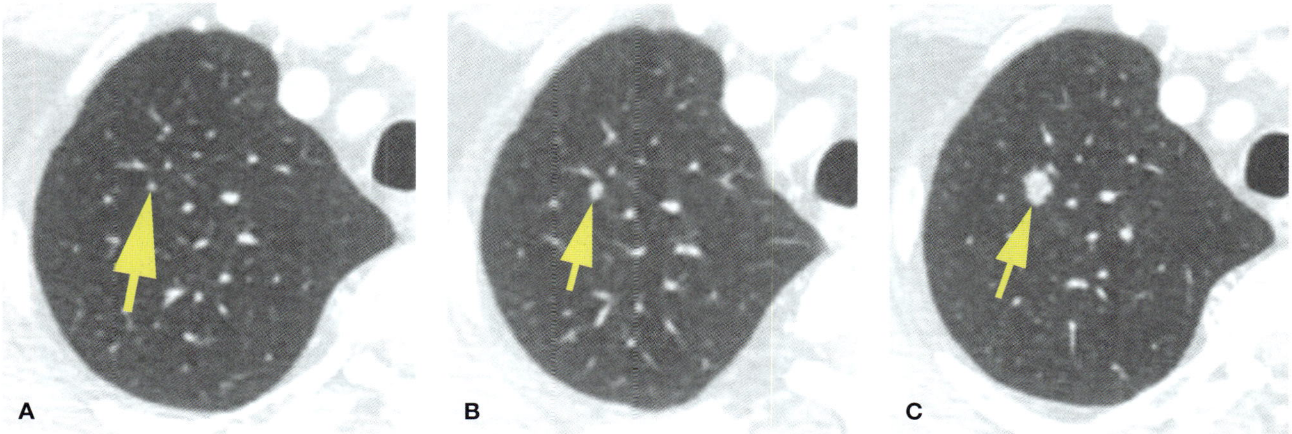

Figure 10.23. Adenocarcinoma with growth. **A:** CT shows very small nodule (*arrow*) in the anterior lung, similar in size to vessels and seen only in retrospect. **B:** Follow-up CT a year later shows an increase in nodule size (*arrow*). **C:** A second follow-up CT scan obtained 1 year after that shown in (**B**) shows further increase in size (*arrow*).

The range of doubling times associated with carcinoma has been reported to be 1 month to 16 months, although reported values vary. Doubling times ranging from 1 month to 200 days encompass most cancers.

Average doubling times vary for different cell types of lung cancer. The average doubling time is estimated as 30 days for small cell carcinoma, 100 days for squamous cell and large cell carcinomas, and 180 days for invasive adenocarcinoma. The doubling of slow-growing adenocarcinomas, characterized by lepidic growth, may be more than 1000 days. Nearly all carcinomas will show some growth over a follow-up period of 2 years, although with lepidic adenocarcinomas appearing as nonsolid nodules (GGO or GGO with a solid component), growth over a 2-year period may be difficult to detect with CT, because of their slow growth and poorly defined margins.

Doubling time of cancers varies with CT nodule attenuation. Nodules appearing solid on CT have an average doubling time of 150 days, while for those appearing part solid and part GGO, doubling time is 500 days, and for those nodules that are entirely GGO, doubling time is more than 800 days.

It has been suggested that a typical lung cancer has doubled approximately 30 times by the time it reaches a diameter of 1 cm and becomes visible radiographically. Metastasis occurring before the primary tumor is recognized radiographically probably accounts for the poor prognosis of many lung cancer patients.

Determining nodule growth rate is relatively easy if prior studies are available. In their absence, for nodules not evaluated using other means such as biopsy or FDG-PET, or not considered appropriate for resection, follow-up CT is often recommended. Follow-up schedules are discussed later.

Nodule Location

About two-thirds of lung cancers occur in the upper lobes, and the right upper lobe is most commonly involved (see Fig. 10.1). Sixty percent of cancers presenting as an SPN on chest radiographs are seen in the lung periphery; only 10% are visible in the medial third of the lung.

A metastatic tumor presenting as an SPN tends to be located in the subpleural or outer third of the lung. Two-thirds of metastatic lesions occur in the lower lobes. TB appearing as a nodule or cavity favors the apical or posterior upper lobes or the superior segment of the lower lobes.

PET and SPECT Imaging

PET obtained following an injection of FDG may be used to characterize pulmonary nodules. FDG is a D-glucose analog labeled with a positron emitter (^{18}F) that is transported through the cell membrane and phosphorylated using normal glycolytic pathways. Increased uptake and accumulation of FDG have been shown to occur in tumor cells, although the effect is nonspecific and may be seen with inflammation.

The degree of FDG accumulation is measured using the standardized uptake value (SUV); the SUV of lung cancers usually is more than 2.5. FDG-PET has a sensitivity of about 95% in detecting malignant SPNs 1 cm or more in diameter, with a specificity of about 80% (Fig. 10.24). False-positive studies occur with inflammatory lesions. False-negative scans may occur with carcinoid tumors, tumors appearing on CT as GGO, and lesions smaller than 1 cm.

Radionuclide single-photon emission computed tomography (SPECT) employing depreotide (a somatostatin analog), thallium, or FDG also may be used to diagnose malignancy in a large lung nodule but is less sensitive than PET for nodules smaller than 2 cm.

Biopsy of Lung Nodules

Methods for biopsy of an SPN include fiberoptic bronchoscopy (FOB), transthoracic needle biopsy (TNB), and surgery, including video-assisted thoracoscopic surgery (VATS).

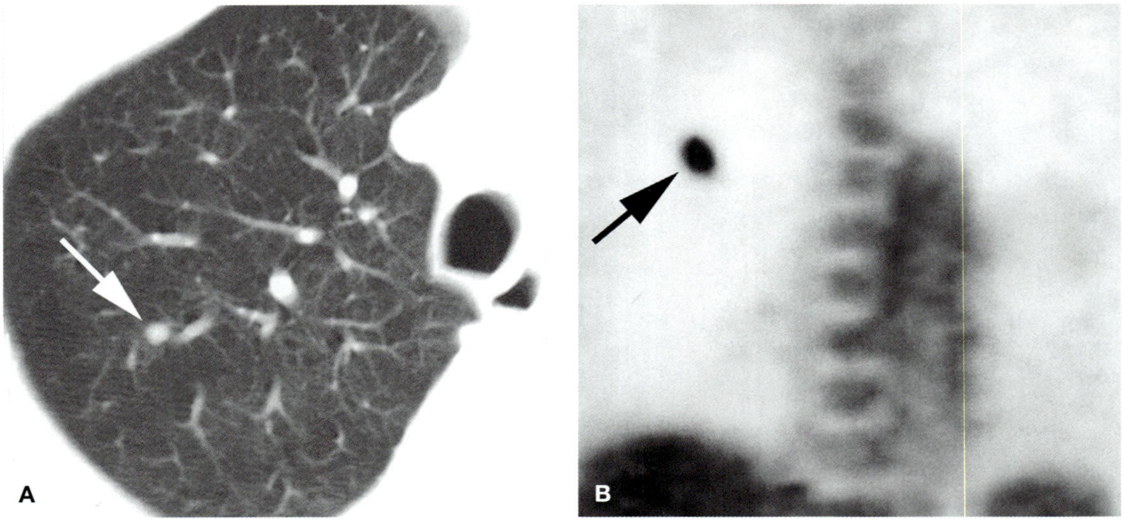

Figure 10.24. FDG-PET in a patient with adenocarcinoma. **A:** HRCT shows a small right upper lobe nodule (*arrow*). **B:** PET (coronal plane) shows the nodule to have a very high activity (*arrow*). The size of the nodule on PET exceeds its real size. PET is poor at showing the specific location of abnormalities.

Bronchoscopy

Conventional FOB with transbronchial biopsy and bronchial washing has a limited role in evaluating an SPN. Although transbronchial biopsy is accurate for assessing endobronchial lesions, the yield of FOB for peripheral nodules is less than 60% and is only 25% to 30% for an SPN smaller than 2 cm. The sensitivity of FOB is best when a bronchus leads directly to or is seen within the SPN (the "positive bronchus" sign; Fig. 10.25). Navigational bronchoscopy is an advanced bronchoscopic technique that allows physicians to access and biopsy peripheral lung nodules that are typically beyond the reach of conventional bronchoscopy. Navigational bronchoscopy uses preprocedure volumetric CT to produce a "virtual 3D roadmap" of the lungs that guides the bronchoscope to the lesion.

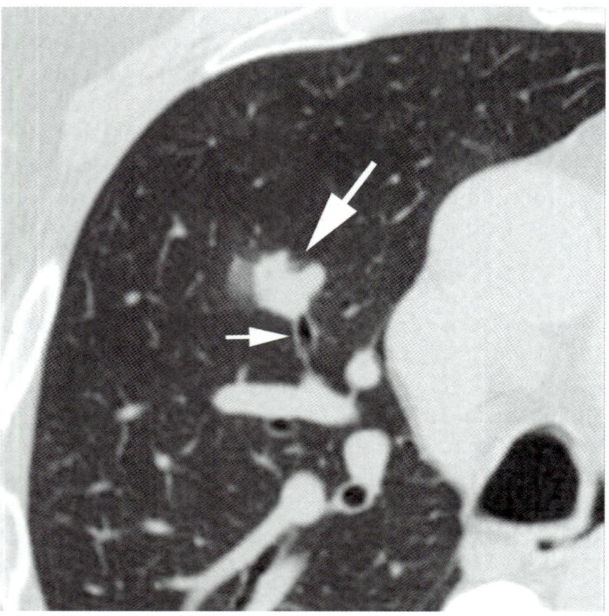

Figure 10.25. The positive bronchus sign. A small right upper lobe nodule (*large arrow*) with a bronchus (*small arrow*) leading to it. This sign predicts a higher likelihood of a diagnosis being made at bronchoscopy.

Transthoracic Needle Biopsy

TNB is often used for assessing an SPN. The sensitivity of TNB in diagnosing cancer is over 90%. Unfortunately, the accuracy of TNB for diagnosing benign disease other than active infections is limited. Malignancy cannot be ruled out if a biopsy is "negative" but no specific benign diagnosis is made; 30% of such cases later prove to represent cancer. Biopsy of nodules smaller than 1 cm in diameter is associated with an increased false-negative rate. Complications include pneumothorax, hemorrhage, and air embolism.

Video-Assisted Thoracic Surgery

VATS also is used to assess indeterminate pulmonary nodules. Wedge resections and, less commonly, lobar resections may be performed using either an endoscopic stapler or a laser. CT nodule localization before surgery may be accomplished using methylene blue or a hooked wire.

Strategies for CT Nodule Follow-Up

Patients with an acute process, such as pulmonary embolism, focal pneumonia, or other inflammatory process, can present with an SPN on chest radiographs or CT. Short-term follow-up may be indicated, particularly in patients with acute symptoms. A decrease in the size of a nodule suggests it is benign, although lung cancers sometimes show a transient decrease in size because of necrosis. A single follow-up study showing a decrease in the size of a lung nodule should not be considered proof of a benign process. Further follow-up showing continued resolution or stability is a good idea.

If a nodule is definitely benign, based on lack of growth on sequential examinations or because of CT findings (ie, it has specific morphologic characteristics of a benign lesion, contains fat, or benign calcification), further evaluation should be limited to plain film or occasional CT follow-up.

For an indeterminate nodule (ie, one that is not definitely benign), CT is often used for follow-up, to determine if the nodule is stable in size, and likely benign, or is growing and likely malignant. The patient's risk for cancer, the size of the nodule detected, the nodule's attenuation characteristics, and whether or not the nodule is found as a result of lung cancer screening are all used to determine the appropriate interval for CT follow-up, or whether a more aggressive approach should be taken.

Solid Nodules

For solid nodules that are detected incidentally (ie, not as a result of lung cancer screening), the Fleischner Society (and other societies) has published recommendations for evaluation and CT follow-up, which are generally accepted and are summarized in Table 10.14.

For nodules less than 6 mm in diameter, follow-up CT in a year is adequate for a high-risk patient (eg, a smoker), while a nodule of this size requires no follow-up in a low-risk patient. A high proportion of small nodules are IPLNs and can be comfortably ignored (see discussion in IPLNs later). For larger nodules or nodules with suspicious features, recommended follow-up intervals are shorter, again stratified on the basis of risk.

The management of a solid SPN larger than 8 mm is often based on an assessment of risk factors and the patient's likelihood of having lung cancer. The likelihood of lung cancer may be determined using published algorithms (see McWilliams et al in Selected Reading for an example), which consider various aspects of the patient's history and the size and appearance of the nodule. For patients with a low likelihood of lung cancer based on the absence of risk factors, age, small nodule size or appearance, and other factors, CT follow-up at 3 to 6 and 12 to 24 months is often appropriate with the goal of establishing at least 2 years of stability. In patients with an intermediate probability of lung cancer, additional testing (ie, PET, contrast-enhanced CT, needle biopsy, bronchoscopy) is appropriate. In patients with a high probability of cancer, VATS or resection is most appropriate.

For example, if an SPN larger than 8 mm has benign characteristics on CT (eg, it is smooth, round, and sharply defined) but is not definitely benign and risk factors for cancer (eg, history of malignancy, smoking history) are absent, follow-up using CT would be appropriate. However, depending on the clinician's or patient's wishes, needle biopsy or PET may be performed. If the patient is a smoker or has a history of malignancy or the nodule has malignant characteristics on CT (eg, it is uncalcified, irregular in shape or spiculated, or contains air bronchograms), a surgeon should generally be consulted. The surgeon may request a needle biopsy or PET scanning for further evaluation, or VATS or resection may be performed.

Table 10.14 Fleischner Society 2017 Guidelines for Management of Incidentally Detected Pulmonary Nodules in Adults—Solid Nodules

Nodule Size[a]	Low-Risk Patient	High-Risk Patient
Single Solid Nodule		
<6 mm	No routine follow-up	Optional CT at 12 mo
6-8 mm	CT at 6-12 mo, then consider CT at 18-24 mo	CT at 6-12 mo, then CT at 18-24 mo
>8 mm	CT at 3 mo, PET-CT, or tissue sampling	Same as low risk
Multiple Solid Nodules		
≤6 mm	No routine follow-up	Optional CT at 12 mo
6-8 mm	CT at 3-6 mo, then consider CT at 18-24 mo	CT at 3-6 mo, then CT at 18-24 mo
>8 mm	CT at 3-6 mo, then consider CT at 18-24 mo	CT at 3-6 mo, then at 18-24 mo

Low-risk patient, minimal or absent history of smoking or other known risk factors.

High-risk patient, history of smoking or other known risk factors.

Modified from MacMahon H, Naidich DP, Goo JM, et al. Guidelines for Management of incidental pulmonary nodules detected on ct images: from the Fleischner Society 2017. Radiology. *2017;284(1):228-243. https://doi.org/10.1148/radiol.2017161659*

[a]*Average of long and short axis rounded to nearest mm. Multiple nodules management based on most suspicious nodule.*

Nonsolid Nodules

Recommendations for CT follow-up of incidental nodules that are entirely of GGO, or GGO with a solid component, have also been reported by the Fleischner Society (Table 10.15). Since persistent nonsolid nodules usually represent an adenocarcinoma with lepidic growth and have relatively slow growth rates, longer-term follow-up is recommended.

Table 10.15 Fleischner Society 2017 Guidelines for Management of Incidentally Detected Pulmonary Nodules in Adults—Subsolid Nodules

Nodule Size[a]	Recommendation
Solitary Ground-Glass Nodule	
<6 mm	No routine follow-up
≥6 mm	CT at 6-12 mo to confirm persistence, then CT every 2 y until 5 y
Solitary Part-Solid Nodule	
<6 mm	No routine follow-up
≥6 mm	CT at 3-6 mo to confirm persistence. If unchanged and solid component remains <6 mm, annual CT should be performed for 5 y
Multiple	
<6 mm	CT at 3-6 mo. If stable, consider CT at 2 and 4 y
≥6 mm	CT at 3-6 mo. Subsequent management based on the most suspicious nodule(s)

[a]Average of long and short axis rounded to nearest mm. Multiple nodules management based on most suspicious nodule.

At present, a GGO nodule measuring less than 6 mm in diameter requires no follow-up using these criteria, because of the likelihood that such nodules represent atypical adenomatous hyperplasia or a small adenocarcinoma in situ. However, some studies indicate that a small percentage (less than 1%) of such nodules represent or may progress to invasive carcinoma, and future recommendations may include follow-up of such nodules at an extended interval (eg, every 2 years). For a GGO nodule 6 mm or larger, follow-up in 3 months (to exclude an acute process) and then every 1 to 2 year follow-up for a minimum of 5 years is recommended. About 10% of GGO nodules that are 1 to 3 cm in size represent a carcinoma.

For a part-solid nodule (a GGO nodule with a smaller solid component), initial follow-up at 3 to 6 months is recommended. If the nodule persists and the solid component is less than 6 mm, then yearly follow-up for a minimum of 5 years is indicated. If the nodule persists and the solid component is ≥6 mm, then biopsy or surgical resection is recommended. In each of these instances, progression is considered present if the nodule or its solid component increase in size.

As a general rule, if multiple nonsolid nodules are present, the largest nodule, or the nodule with the largest solid component, determines the evaluation or follow-up interval. Multiple primary adenocarcinomas having these characteristics are not uncommon.

Screening-Detected Nodules

Lung nodules detected as a result of CT lung cancer screening are reported and followed using a different system, such as that developed by the American College of Radiology, termed *Lung-RADS* (Lung Imaging Reporting and Data System) (Table 10.16). This system is designed to reduce false positives, reduce confusion in lung cancer screening CT interpretations, provide reporting and management recommendations, and facilitate outcome monitoring and development of a nationwide database. It is likely that Fleischner criteria will continue to be revised to be closer to Lung-RADS, or some common ground will be sought to avoid confusion in interpreting and reporting CT in a patient with a nodule or nodules.

Lung-RADS includes criteria for follow-up of solid and nonsolid nodules, but follow-up intervals and size criteria differ from those recommended by the Fleischner Society (Tables 10.14 and 10.15) and are difficult to remember. Having a copy of the Lung-RADS criteria on hand is essential when reading lung cancer screening studies. Since patients reported using this system are being screened with yearly CT, nodules with a low likelihood of being a cancer only require yearly rescreening. Some modifiers used in scoring, including a history of lung cancer (C) or clinically significant findings suggesting a diagnosis of a disease other than lung cancer (S), are also used.

MULTIPLE NODULES AND MASSES

This section reviews the differential diagnosis of multiple large nodules (ie, 1 cm or larger) and masses (Table 10.17). A nodular pattern of diffuse lung disease (ie, innumerable nodules 1 cm or less in diameter) is discussed in Chapter 11. Obviously, there is some overlap in their differential diagnosis.

Metastases should be considered most likely when multiple nodules or masses are visible (see Chapter 6). The initial evaluation of multiple nodules usually is based on history, clinical studies, and assessment of radiographic findings. Bronchoscopy or percutaneous biopsy may be needed for eventual diagnosis. An organized radiographic approach to the evaluation of multiple nodules and masses is more difficult to summarize than that for the SPN, but it is based on many of the same principles.

Size

Benign and malignant lesions may be either small or large. A clear-cut relation of size to malignancy does not exist as it does with SPN. There is a tendency for multiple nodular metastases to vary in size (see Fig. 6.8 in Chapter 6), whereas benign processes result in nodules of similar size.

Table 10.16 The Lung-RADS v2022 System for Lung Cancer Screening (ACR.org)

Lung-RADS	Category Descriptor	Findings	Management
0	**Incomplete** Estimated Population Prevalence: ~1%	Prior chest CT examination being located for comparison (see note 9)	Comparison to prior chest CT;
		Part or all of lungs cannot be evaluated	Additional lung cancer screening CT imaging needed;
		Findings suggestive of an inflammatory or infectious process (see note 10)	1-3 month LDCT
1	**Negative** Estimated Population Prevalence: 39%	**No lung nodules OR** **Nodule with benign features:** • Complete, central, popcorn, or concentric ring calcifications **OR** • Fat-containing	12-month screening LDCT
2	**Benign -** Based on imaging features or indolent behavior Estimated Population Prevalence: 45%	**Juxtapleural nodule:** • <10 mm (<524 mm^3) mean diameter at baseline or new **AND** • Solid; smooth margins; and oval, lentiform, or triangular shape **Solid nodule:** • <6 mm (<113 mm^3) at baseline **OR** • New <4 mm (<34 mm^3) **Part solid nodule:** • <6 mm total mean diameter (<113 mm^3) at baseline **Non solid nodule (GGN):** • <30 mm (<14,137 mm^3) at baseline, new, or growing **OR** • ≥30 mm (≥14,137 mm^3) stable or slowly growing (see note 7) **Airway nodule,** subsegmental - at baseline, new, or stable (see note 11) Category 3 lesion that is stable or decreased in size at 6-month follow-up CT **OR** Category 4B lesion proven to be benign in etiology following appropriate diagnostic workup	

Table 10.16 The Lung-RADS v2022 System for Lung Cancer Screening (ACR.org) (Continued)

Lung-RADS	Category Descriptor	Findings	Management
3	**Probably Benign** Based on imaging features or behavior Estimated Population Prevalence: 9%	**Solid nodule:** • ≥6 to <8 mm (≥113 to <268 mm^3) at baseline **OR** • New 4 mm to <6 mm (34 to <113 mm^3)	6-month LDCT
		Part solid nodule: • ≥6 mm total mean diameter (≥113 mm^3) with solid component <6 mm (<113 mm^3) at baseline **OR** • New <6 mm total mean diameter (<113 mm^3)	
		Non solid nodule (GGN): • ≥30 mm (≥14,137 mm^3) at baseline or new	
		Atypical pulmonary cyst: (see note 12) • Growing cystic component (mean diameter) of a thick-walled cyst	
		Category 4A lesion that is stable or decreased in size at 3-month follow-up CT (excluding airway nodules)	
4A	**Suspicious** Estimated Population Prevalence: 4%	**Solid nodule:** • ≥8 to <15 mm (≥268 to <1,767 mm^3) at baseline **OR** • Growing <8 mm (< 268 mm^3) **OR** • New 6 to <8 mm (113 to <268 mm^3)	3-month LDCT; PET/CT may be considered if there is a ≥ 8 mm (≥268 mm^3) solid nodule or solid component
		Part solid nodule: • ≥ 6 mm total mean diameter (≥113 mm^3) with solid component ≥6 to <8 mm (≥113 to <268 mm^3) at baseline **OR** • New or growing <4 mm (<34 mm^3) solid component	
		Airway nodule, segmental or more proximal - at baseline (see note 11)	
		Atypical pulmonary cyst: (see note 12) • Thick-walled cyst **OR** • Multilocular cyst at baseline **OR** • Thin- or thick-walled cyst that becomes multilocular	

(continued)

Table 10.16 The Lung-RADS v2022 System for Lung Cancer Screening (ACR.org) (Continued)

Lung-RADS	Category Descriptor	Findings	Management
4B	**Very Suspicious** Estimated Population Prevalence: 2%	**Airway nodule,** segmental or more proximal - stable or growing (see note 11)	Referral for further clinical evaluation
		Solid nodule: • ≥15 mm (≥1767 mm³) at baseline **OR** • New or growing ≥8 mm (≥268 mm³)	Diagnostic chest CT with or without contrast; PET/CT may be considered if there is a ≥8 mm (≥268 mm³) solid nodule or solid component; tissue sampling; and/or referral for further clinical evaluation Management depends on clinical evaluation, patient preference, and the probability of malignancy (see note 13)
		Part solid nodule: • Solid component ≥8 mm (≥268 mm³) at baseline **OR** • New or growing ≥4 mm (≥34 mm³) solid component	
		Atypical pulmonary cyst: (see note 12) • Thick-walled cyst with growing wall thickness/nodularity **OR** • Growing multilocular cyst (mean diameter) **OR** • Multilocular cyst with increased loculation or new/increased opacity (nodular,ground glass, or consolidation)	
		Slow growing solid or part solid nodule that demonstrates growth over multiple screening exams (see note 8)	
4X	Estimated Population Prevalence: <1%	Category 3 or 4 nodules with additional features or imaging findings that increase suspicion for lung cancer (see note 14)	
S	**Significant or Potentially Significant** Estimated Population Prevalence: 10%	**Modifier:** May add to category 0-4 for clinically significant or potentially clinically significant findings unrelated to lung cancer (see note 15)	As appropriate to the specific finding

See https://www.acr.org/-/media/ACR/Files/RADS/Lung-RADS/Lung-RADS-2022.pdf for additional footnotes and details.

Number

Multinodular metastases may be few in number or innumerable, but a large number of nodules suggest this diagnosis (see Figs. 6.6-6.9 in Chapter 6). Most infectious and inflammatory diseases result in less than a dozen nodules.

Location

Metastases, infarction, and septic emboli have a predilection for the lung periphery and the lung bases. Abscesses related to aspiration often are posterior or basal in distribution. Metastases tend to have a peripheral and basal predominance.

Edge Appearance

Metastases are usually sharply marginated (see Figs. 6.8-6.11 in Chapter 6), as are nodules in amyloidosis, rheumatoid nodules, AVMs, hematomas, and Caplan syndrome. Infectious lesions, invasive mucinous adenocarcinoma (see Figs. 5.9 and 5.10 in Chapter 5), lymphoma (see Figs. 7.10-7.12 in Chapter 7), conglomerate masses and progressive massive fibrosis, and granulomatosis with polyangiitis (GPA) are often ill defined.

An increase in sharpness of the edge of a lesion with time suggests the resolution of a benign inflammatory process. For example, septic emboli, lung abscesses, infections, and GPA result in masses that are ill defined early in their course and become sharply defined as they heal.

Table 10.17 Multiple Pulmonary Nodules or Masses
Congenital lesions and normal variants
Arteriovenous malformations
Intrapulmonary lymph nodes
Malignant neoplasm
Invasive mucinous adenocarcinoma
Carcinoma
Lymphoma
Lymphoproliferative disease
Metastatic neoplasm
Benign neoplasms and neoplasm-like conditions
Endometriomas
Lymphoproliferative disease
Multiple chondromas (Carney triad)
Papillomas (papillomatosis)
Infection and parasites
Aspergillosis, angioinvasive
Bronchopneumonia
Echinococcus
Granulomatous infection or granulomas
Tuberculosis
Nontuberculous mycobacteria (eg, *Mycobacterium avium-intracellulare* complex)
Coccidioidomycosis
Histoplasmosis
Cryptococcus
Lung abscesses
Mycetomas (aspergillomas)
Paragonimiasis
Septic embolism
Inflammatory (noninfectious)
Churg-Strauss syndrome
Focal organizing pneumonia
Rheumatoid nodules
Sarcoidosis
Granulomatosis with polyangiitis
Airways and inhalational disease
Mucoid impaction (mucous plug)
Asthma
Allergic bronchopulmonary aspergillosis
Bronchiectasis
Cystic fibrosis
Conglomerate masses or progressive massive fibrosis (eg, silicosis)
Lipoid pneumonia
Vascular lesions
Arteriovenous malformations
Hematomas
Infarctions
Pulmonary artery aneurysms
Septic embolism
Miscellaneous
Amyloidosis
Fluid-filled bullae
Round atelectasis

The halo sign may be seen in patients with multiple nodules; its differential diagnosis is described in Table 10.4.

Attenuation

Metastases are usually of soft-tissue attenuation, but invasive mucinous adenocarcinoma may result in multiple nodules of GGO. About 10% of patients with pulmonary adenocarcinoma show multiple lung nodules representing multiple primary tumors. These may be solid or of GGO or may have mixed attenuation.

Infection and diffuse inflammatory lung diseases such as hypersensitivity pneumonitis may result in multiple GGO nodules; these may be diffuse and centrilobular in location. OP may result in multiple nodules, either solid or of GGO. Some diseases, particularly granulomatous infections, sarcoidosis, and amyloidosis, result in multiple nodules, which may be calcified.

Cavitation

As with SPNs, thick-walled cavities are consistent with malignancy, but thick walls may be seen with inflammatory, nonmalignant lesions as well. Very thin-walled cavities usually are benign, although metastatic tumors, particularly squamous cell carcinoma of the head and neck or sarcomas and tracheobronchial papillomatosis, may be associated with thin-walled lesions. As with SPNs, an air-fluid level tends to predict benign disease. The differential diagnosis of multiple cystic or cavitary lesions is reviewed in Table 10.6.

Growth

Rapid growth with an increase in size over a period of a few days suggests infection (eg, bacterial infection or fungus or TB in an immunosuppressed patient). Progression over a period of a few weeks is typical of indolent infections (eg, TB or fungus in an immunocompetent patient), noninfectious inflammatory disease, or rapidly progressing malignancy (Fig. 10.26). Nodules that appear stable over a period of weeks or show slow growth during a few months are likely to be either malignant or due to indolent inflammatory conditions (eg, rheumatoid nodules). Masses that show little change over a period of months are typical of amyloidosis, AVMs, benign tumors, and conglomerate masses. Some metastatic tumors (eg, thyroid carcinoma or benign metastasizing leiomyoma) may show very slow growth.

Resolution of lesions with or without treatment suggests benign disease. Slow resolution is typical of hematoma and infarction. Rapid resolution is typical of treated infections.

DIFFERENTIAL DIAGNOSIS OF LUNG NODULES, MASSES, AND CAVITIES

A large number of diseases and abnormalities associated with solitary or multiple nodules, masses, or cysts are reviewed in the following sections in alphabetical order. Many of these are discussed in more detail elsewhere in this book.

Amyloidosis

Patients with localized nodular amyloidosis usually are asymptomatic. Nodular amyloidosis may manifest as single or multiple lung nodules or masses, usually well defined and round (see Fig. 21.5 in Chapter 21). Bilateral lung nodules are most typical, and they tend to be peripheral or subpleural in location. Nodules range from 0.5 to 5 cm in diameter in most cases but may be as large as 10 cm. Calcification is visible in 30% to 50% of cases and may be stippled or dense. Cavitation may be seen in approximately 5%. Nodules may grow slowly or remain stable over a number of years. Needle biopsy may be diagnostic.

Arteriovenous Malformation

Congenital AVM, also known as arteriovenous fistula (AVF), is associated with Osler-Weber-Rendu syndrome in 35% to 67% of cases. *Simple AVM* represents a single, dilated vascular sac connecting one artery and one vein (see Figs. 9.10-9.15 in Chapter 9). It is the most common type and accounts for almost all cases of AVM. *Complex AVM* has multiple feeding arteries or draining veins.

Radiographically, a simple fistula appears as a peripheral, well-defined, round, oval, lobulated, or serpentine opacity. Large vessels (feeders) extending centrally toward the hilum are easily seen on CT. AVFs typically are subpleural in location, and more than two-thirds are found in the lower lobes. Fistulas are multiple in 35% of patients and bilateral in 10%. Multiple AVMs are most common in patients with Osler-Weber-Rendu syndrome. Enlargement of fistulas over a period of months or years is common, and a rapid increase in size can occur. Opacification occurs following contrast enhancement.

Aspergillosis

Invasive aspergillosis almost always occurs in immunosuppressed patients and is particularly common in association with (1) neutropenia in patients with acute leukemia, (2) treatment using corticosteroids or other immunosuppressive agents, (3) organ transplantation, and (4) malignancy. Angioinvasive aspergillosis accounts for about 80% of cases of invasive aspergillosis, while airway-invasive aspergillosis accounts for 15%. Chronic necrotizing aspergillosis and mycetoma are other manifestations of *Aspergillus* infection.

Angioinvasive Aspergillosis

Angioinvasive aspergillosis is characterized by the involvement of normal lung tissue by *Aspergillus* organisms, usually resulting in significant tissue damage and necrosis. Pathologic examination shows infiltration of lung tissue by fungus, with invasion of small arteries, vascular occlusion, and, often, infarction of the involved lung.

Early in the course of disease, ill-defined nodules up to several centimeters in diameter or focal areas of consolidation typically are seen on chest radiographs. At this stage, CT typically shows the *halo sign*, in which a halo of GGO surrounds a central nodule (see Figs. 10.7 and 10.27). The halo and central nodule reflect, respectively, a rim of hemorrhage surrounding a central fungal nodule or infarct. In an immunosuppressed patient, the CT appearance of early invasive aspergillosis with a visible halo sign is sufficiently characteristic to justify a presumptive diagnosis and treatment.

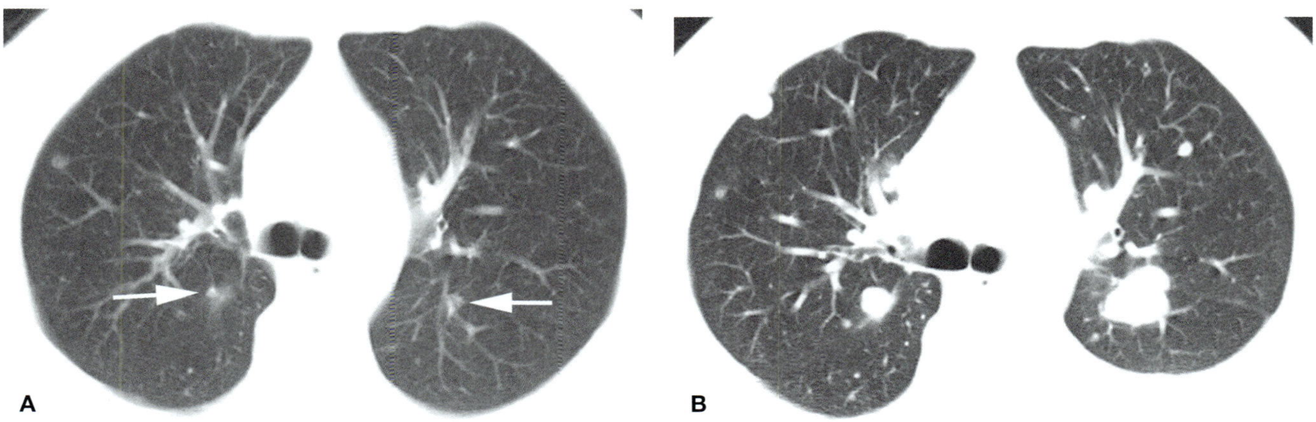

Figure 10.26. Metastases from a spindle cell sarcoma with rapid growth. **A:** CT scan shows multiple small nodules (*arrows*). **B:** A follow-up scan 6 wk later shows marked increase in size. Such rapid growth suggests an infectious or inflammatory process but may be seen with very rapidly growing neoplasms.

However, as described previously, the *halo sign* can be associated with a variety of infectious and noninfectious processes.

If patients with angioinvasive aspergillosis survive their acute infection, nodules often cavitate, showing the *air-crescent sign* (see Fig. 10.27). The presence of an air crescent in angioinvasive aspergillosis reflects lung necrosis with the presence of a sequestrum or ball of devitalized and necrotic lung occupying part of the cavity. Although this appearance mimics that of a mycetoma, the two conditions are unrelated.

Cavitation, when present, generally occurs about 2 weeks after the appearance of nodular opacities and is associated with a white blood cell count of more than 1000. Thus, the presence of cavitation is generally considered to be a good prognostic sign.

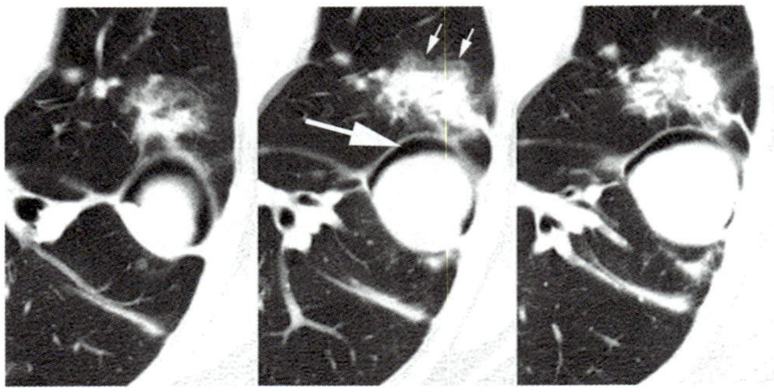

Figure 10.27. Angioinvasive aspergillosis with halo sign and air-crescent sign. CT scans at three adjacent levels in a patient with leukemia show an air-crescent sign (*large arrow*) outlining a "lung ball" within a cavity. Anterior to it is an ill-defined nodule with a halo sign (*small arrows*).

Airway-Invasive Aspergillosis

In some immunosuppressed patients, aspergillus infection centers on small airways, resulting in multiple small nodules or the finding of tree-in-bud. The CT findings are those of a bronchopneumonia.

Chronic (Necrotizing) or Semi-Invasive Aspergillosis

Chronic (necrotizing) aspergillosis, also described as semi-invasive aspergillosis, is typically associated with slowly progressive upper lobe consolidation, cavitation, or cysts. Most patients have an underlying chronic lung disease such as TB, COPD, fibrosis, or pneumoconiosis. Patients may be mildly immunocompromised (eg, chronic disease, advanced age, diabetes, poor nutrition, alcoholism, low-dose corticosteroid treatment) but lack the severe immune deficiencies typical of patients with invasive aspergillosis. Pathology reveals a combination of granulomatous inflammation, necrosis, and fibrosis similar to that seen in TB. Symptoms are nonspecific, consisting of cough, sputum production, weight loss, fever, and hemoptysis.

Radiographs and CT typically show upper lobe consolidation, with progressive cavitation over a period of weeks to months, often indistinguishable from active TB. It is common to see an irregular or thick-walled cavity, and frondlike intracavitary opacities may be present, representing masses of fungus and associated material. Obvious aspergillomas, with an air-crescent sign, may develop over time. With progressive disease, pleural and chest wall involvement may be present. *Aspergillus* infection is discussed in detail in Chapter 12.

Bronchiectasis

Bronchiectasis may result in the presence of multiple cystic lung lesions (ie, cystic bronchiectasis). These often have thin but easily recognizable walls and may be focal or diffuse in distribution. Air-fluid levels are common, representing secretions or pus, and help to distinguish cystic bronchiectasis from cystic lung diseases such as lymphangioleiomyomatosis, histiocytosis, and lymphoid interstitial pneumonia, in which the cysts do not typically contain fluid. Because the cystic areas communicate with each other (via the bronchial tree), the amount of fluid in each "cyst" is similar or more fluid tends to be seen in cysts located at the lung bases (Fig. 10.28).

Bronchogenic Cyst

Pulmonary bronchogenic cysts are most common in the medial lung and the lower lobes. Uninfected cysts are sharply circumscribed and round or oval in shape; their wall is invisible on CT or appears very thin. Fluid-filled bronchogenic cysts may appear low in attenuation on CT (0-20 HU; see Fig. 9.6 in Chapter 9) or may have high CT numbers (40-80 HU). Rarely, the cyst wall may calcify or the cyst may contain milk of calcium and appear dense. Infection eventually occurs in 75% of cases. In the presence of acute infection, a rapid increase in size of the cyst may be seen. In addition, the outer cyst wall may become less well defined because of surrounding lung inflammation (Fig. 10.29A). A previously infected cyst may contain air, showing a thin and well-defined wall, and may contain an air-fluid level (see Fig. 10.29B and Fig. 9.7 in Chapter 9).

Bullae

By definition, a bulla is a sharply demarcated area of emphysema, measuring 1 cm or more in diameter and possessing a wall less than 1 mm thick. Bullae usually are a manifestation of paraseptal emphysema but also may be seen in patients with centrilobular emphysema. Bullae usually are subpleural in location, largest at the lung apices, and very thin walled (Fig. 10.30A); these findings often allow their accurate diagnosis on chest radiographs or CT. On HRCT, other areas of emphysema usually are visible.

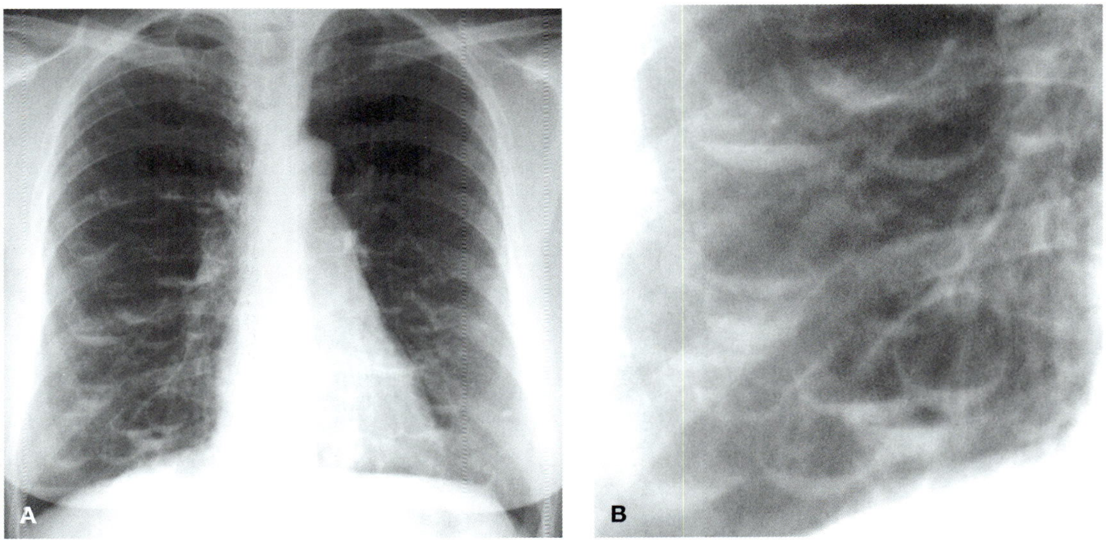

Figure 10.28. Cystic bronchiectasis. **A:** Multiple thin-walled cysts represent cystic bronchiectasis. **B:** Detail view of the right lower lobe. Air-fluid levels are visible, with the largest amount of fluid being in cysts at the lung bases. This implies communication between the cysts and is diagnostic of bronchiectasis.

A bulla may contain fluid, showing an air-fluid level or appearing as a focal mass. This may result from infection, hemorrhage, tumor arising in a bulla, or bland fluid accumulation (see Fig. 10.30B and C). The identification of other bullae may be helpful in diagnosis. CT may show the fluid nature of the opacity or associated wall thickening in patients with tumor.

Carcinoma

Adenocarcinoma accounts for 50% to 70% of lung cancers presenting as an SPN or lung mass. As currently defined by WHO, other cell types presenting as a lung nodule are squamous cell carcinoma (15%-20%), large cell carcinoma (5%), small cell carcinoma (5%), and unspecified non–small cell carcinoma or other cell types (15%). Nearly two-thirds of lung cancers presenting as a lung nodule occur in the upper

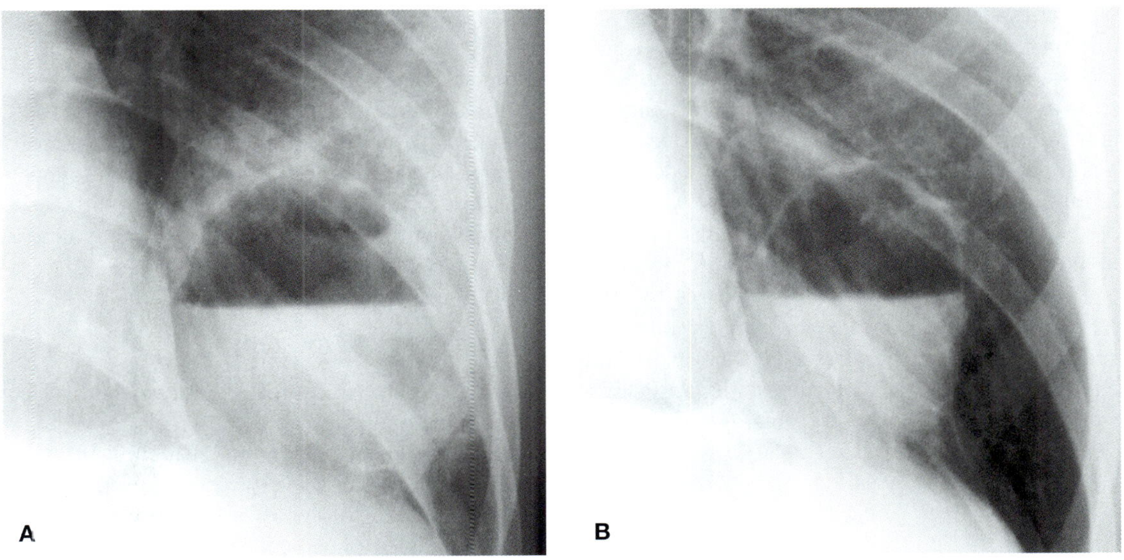

Figure 10.29. Bronchogenic cyst. **A:** When it is acutely infected, the air- and fluid-filled cyst is very ill defined, resembling a lung abscess. **B:** After treatment, a thin-walled cystic lesion is visible in the left lung. This was found to represent a bronchogenic cyst. The presence of an air-fluid level indicates prior infection.

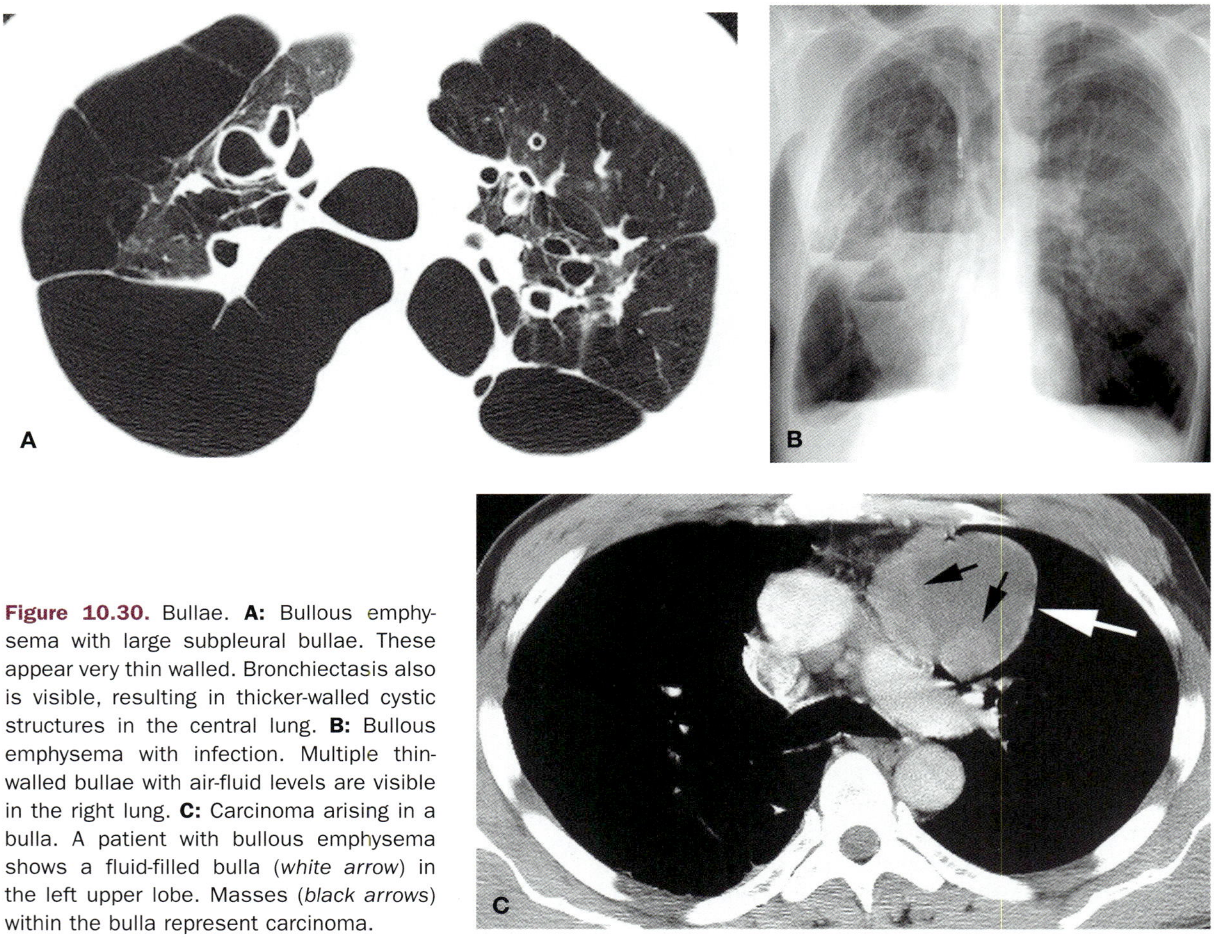

Figure 10.30. Bullae. **A:** Bullous emphysema with large subpleural bullae. These appear very thin walled. Bronchiectasis also is visible, resulting in thicker-walled cystic structures in the central lung. **B:** Bullous emphysema with infection. Multiple thin-walled bullae with air-fluid levels are visible in the right lung. **C:** Carcinoma arising in a bulla. A patient with bullous emphysema shows a fluid-filled bulla (*white arrow*) in the left upper lobe. Masses (*black arrows*) within the bulla represent carcinoma.

lobes. Because they are not usually associated with symptoms, lung cancers presenting as an SPN often are large when first detected; it has been reported that nearly 60% of lung cancers are larger than 2 cm when first detected, but this has changed with lung cancer screening and wider use of CT, and smaller lung cancers are now commonly found. The appearances of lung carcinoma are described earlier in this chapter and in Chapter 5. Primary carcinomas may contain air bronchograms and may be cystic or cavitary.

Multiple lung nodules may occur in patients with lung cancer in the presence of multiple synchronous primary tumors, satellite nodules associated with the primary tumor due to local spread, or hematogenous metastases to lung from the primary lung cancer or may occur in patients with invasive mucinous adenocarcinoma (see Figs. 5.9, 5.10, and 5.40 in Chapter 5). In patients with metastatic lung carcinoma, the primary lesion usually is visible as a dominant mass (Fig. 10.31).

Carcinoid Tumor

Carcinoid tumors account for 1% to 2% of tracheobronchial neoplasms. Approximately 20% of carcinoid tumors present as a peripheral nodule or mass. They often are well defined, round or oval, and slightly lobulated in contour (see Fig. 5.18 in Chapter 5). Calcification is uncommonly seen on radiographs but is visible on CT in nearly 40% (Figs. 10.21 and 10.22). Approximately 10% to 25% of carcinoid tumors can be classified as *atypical carcinoid tumor* because of histologic features suggesting a more aggressive behavior. Atypical carcinoid tumors tend to present as a lung nodule or mass somewhat larger than seen with carcinoid tumor. Cavitation is rare. Dense enhancement may be seen following contrast infusion. Small cell carcinoma is part of the spectrum of pulmonary neuroendocrine carcinomas that included carcinoid and atypical carcinoid tumors.

Churg-Strauss Syndrome

Churg-Strauss syndrome is characterized by a combination of necrotizing vasculitis, extravascular granulomas, and tissue infiltration by eosinophils. Patients with this syndrome usually are middle-aged (average onset, 40-50 years) and often have a history of allergic diseases including asthma, nasal polyps, or sinusitis. One or more ill-defined pulmonary nodules, up to 3.5 cm, are seen in 20% of cases. Cavitation is uncommon, a finding that is helpful in distinguishing Churg-Strauss syndrome from GPA, which may have a similar

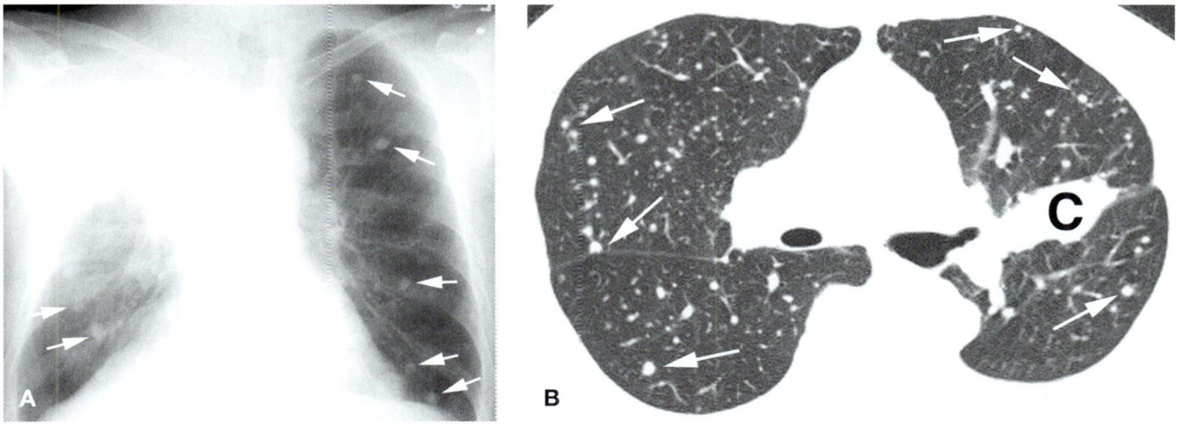

Figure 10.31. Lung cancer with multiple nodules representing metastases. **A:** A patient with right upper lobe collapse due to right hilar carcinoma shows multiple small nodules (*arrows*) representing metastases. **B:** CT in a patient with left-sided carcinoma (*C*) who shows diffuse nodular metastases (*arrows*).

presentation. Other common radiographic abnormalities, which may be seen in combination, consist of transient multifocal areas of consolidation indistinguishable from simple pulmonary eosinophilia or chronic eosinophilic pneumonia. Pulmonary hemorrhage may be associated. Churg-Strauss syndrome is described in detail in Chapter 17.

CPAM and CCAM

CPAM, also known as CCAM, consists of an intralobar mass of disorganized lung tissue, derived primarily from bronchioles, and often is cystic or multicystic. About 70% of cases present during the first week of life, but 10% are diagnosed after the first year. Lower lobes are involved most often, but any lobe can be affected. CCAM often is classified into three types that have different histology, gross pathologic findings, and radiographic appearances.

Type 1 CPAM (65% of cases) contains one or more cysts, which are larger than 2 cm in diameter (see Fig. 9.8 in Chapter 9). Type 1 CPAM usually presents as a large, air-filled, multicystic lesion, sometimes with air-fluid levels, which may occupy the entire hemithorax.

Type 2 CPAM (20% to 25% of cases) contains multiple cysts less than 2 cm in diameter. It presents as an air-filled multicystic mass or a solid mass or area of consolidation (see Fig. 9.9 in Chapter 9).

Type 3 CPAM (10% of cases) contains microscopic (less than 3-5 mm) cysts and presents radiographically as a solid mass.

Types 0 and 4 CPAM each account for a few percent of cases. Type 0 CPAM/CCAM is associated with small cysts, as in type 3. Type 4 CPAM/CCAM is associated with large cysts, as is type 1; its radiographic and CT appearance is the same as for type 1 or 2. The terms *CCAM* and *CPAM* are largely interchangeable and are the same regardless of the acronym used; currently, CPAM tends to be favored, although reports of CCAM still appear in the literature.

Type 1 and 2 CPAM may become air filled over a period of days to weeks after birth. They often are associated with progressive air trapping and mediastinal shift to the opposite side. In adults, CPAM usually presents as an air-filled or air- and fluid-filled cystic or multicystic mass.

Conglomerate Masses

Large conglomerate masses may develop in patients with sarcoidosis, long-standing silicosis or coal worker's pneumoconiosis, and talcosis and in association with some granulomatous infections. Their appearances are similar. In silicosis, conglomerate masses reflect the presence of progressive massive fibrosis (see Chapter 16).

These masses represent a conglomeration of small interstitial nodules in combination with a variable degree of fibrosis. A background pattern of multiple small lung nodules often is visible (*satellite nodules*). Conglomerate masses are typically, but not always, seen in the upper lobes or midlung, are usually oval or lenticular in shape, are distinct from the hila, and are separated from peripheral pleural surface (Fig. 10.32). Nearly all have irregular borders. They often are bilateral and symmetrical.

Distortion of lung architecture usually is evident due to fibrosis and volume loss. Traction bronchiectasis with air bronchograms may be seen within the masses, and surrounding bullae may be present. Calcification in association with conglomerate masses is common. Central necrosis or cavitation may be present and may indicate superinfection by TB or bacteria. Cavities usually are thick walled. Talcosis, secondary to intravenous injection of talc, is seen almost exclusively in drug users who inject medications intended for oral use; the masses may appear high in attenuation on CT because of the talc they contain.

Cysts and Cystic Lung Disease

Cyst is a nonspecific term describing the presence of a thin-walled (usually less than 3 mm), well-defined, and

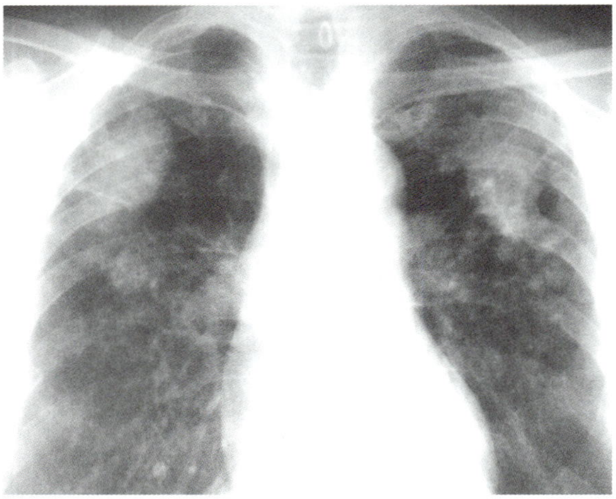

Figure 10.32. Conglomerate masses (progressive massive fibrosis) in silicosis. Conglomerate masses typically—but not always—are seen in the upper lobes or midlung and usually are oval or lenticular in shape. They often are bilateral and symmetrical.

circumscribed, air- or fluid-containing lesion, 1 cm or more in diameter, and having an epithelial or fibrous wall. The term usually is used to describe the presence of a thin-walled lesion when a more specific diagnosis cannot be made. Cysts may be congenital (eg, bronchogenic cyst) or acquired (eg, honeycombing, bullae, pneumatocele). It is not uncommon to see one or more (ie, up to a few) lung cysts in an asymptomatic patient without known disease. These are usually undiagnosed and are rarely of significance.

Multiple lung cysts as a manifestation of diffuse lung disease are seen in patients with Langerhans cell histiocytosis, lymphangioleiomyomatosis, sarcoidosis, lymphoid interstitial pneumonia, Birt-Hogg-Dube syndrome, and other causes (see Chapter 25).

Lung cysts may contain fluid as a result of accumulated secretions or in the presence of infection, hemorrhage, or tumor. Thickening of the wall of a cyst suggests infection or tumor. Fluid filling cysts is uncommon in patients with cystic lung diseases such as lymphangiomyomatosis, histiocytosis, and lymphoid interstitial pneumonia.

Dirofilaria immitis

Dirofilaria immitis is the dog heartworm. Humans may become infected by a mosquito bite. Larvae travel to right-sided cardiac chambers, but cannot live in humans, and eventually embolize to the pulmonary vascular bed, where they result in an infarct and granulomatous response. A small lung nodule may result, usually less than 2 cm in diameter, rounded, sharply marginated, and subpleural in location (Fig. 10.33). Calcification may be visible on CT. Eosinophilia usually is absent. It is most common in eastern and southern states.

Echinococcosis

Echinococcus granulosus and *Echinococcus multilocularis* are intestinal tapeworms of canine carnivores such as the dog and wolf. Ova are dispersed in feces and ingested by an intermediate host. Larvae develop in the intestine of the intermediate host and migrate via the circulation to organs such as the liver and lungs, where they develop and encyst. When the larva is consumed by the carnivore (at the same time the intermediate host is consumed), the adult tapeworm develops in the carnivore.

The development of parasites in the intermediate host results in one or more hydatid cysts, usually in the liver or

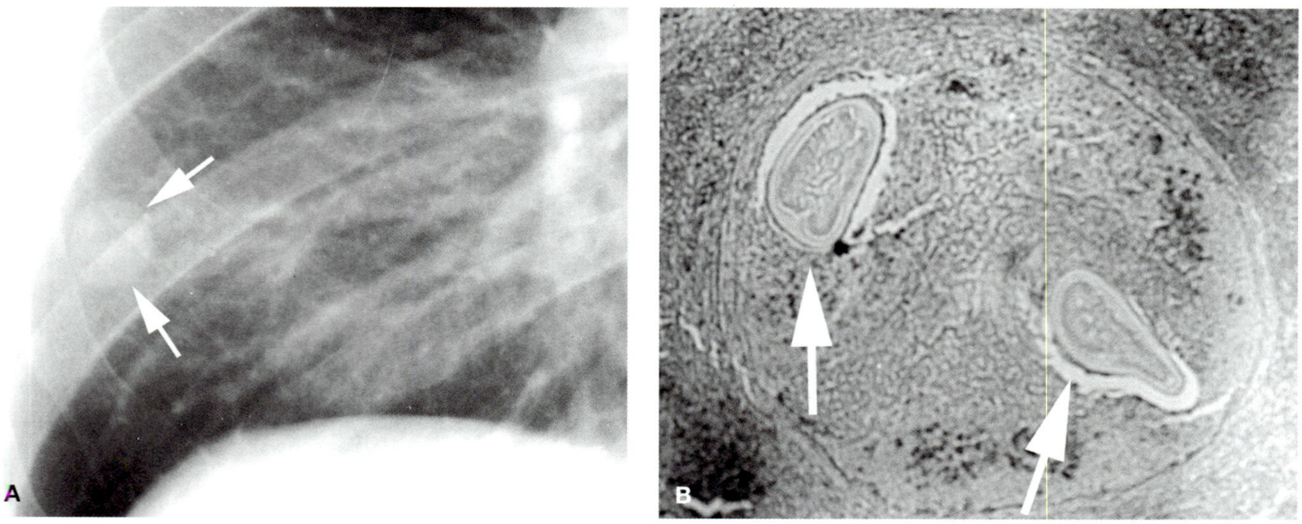

Figure 10.33. Lung nodule secondary to *Dirofilaria immitis* infection. **A:** A sharply marginated, rounded nodule (*arrows*) is visible in the peripheral right lung. **B:** The histologic specimen following resection shows an intravascular worm (*arrows*) within the nodule.

lungs, an occurrence termed *hydatid disease*. Hydatid disease occurs in two forms. In the *pastoral* form, a dog is the primary host and sheep are the intermediate host; it occurs in sheep-raising countries and is most common in the Mediterranean regions of Europe and North Africa, in South America, and in Australia. In the *sylvatic* or *sylvian* form, the wolf is the primary host, and wild animals such as deer, moose, and caribou are intermediate hosts; it is endemic in Arctic regions such as Alaska or Siberia. Humans may serve as an intermediate host of either form.

Pulmonary lesions have three components, knowledge of which is important in understanding the radiographic appearance of pulmonary hydatid cysts. The outermost part is termed the *pericyst*. It consists of compressed lung tissue and fibrosis adjacent to the parasite. The parasite itself is composed of two layers, an outer layer or *ectocyst* and an inner layer or *endocyst*, from which daughter cysts bud.

Uncomplicated pulmonary hydatid cysts are fluid filled and rounded and may be quite large (over 10 cm; Fig. 10.34). Pulmonary cysts are solitary in more than half of cases. They occur most commonly in the lower lobes. Rapid growth may be seen. CT may show a wall ranging up to 1 cm in thickness, largely depending on the thickness of the pericyst. Cyst contents are of fluid attenuation on CT, but septations may be visible, representing the walls of daughter cysts. Although common in the liver, calcification of the walls of cysts is rare in the lung. Liver cysts may or may not be present in a patient with lung cysts.

Rupture of the pericyst leads to dissection of air between the pericyst and the ectocyst, resulting in an air-crescent sign. Rupture of the exocyst, with the expulsion of some fluid contents, produces an air-fluid level and allows the endocyst to collapse. The presence of the endocyst floating on the fluid may be visible as the "water lily" or *camalote* sign. Rupture of the cyst into the pleural space may result in effusion or seeding of the pleural space with cysts. Rupture of the cyst into a bronchus may be associated with an allergic reaction or infection. Mediastinal cysts may be seen. Diagnosis usually is based on serologic tests. Biopsy should be avoided because of the risk of rupture. Echinococcosis is discussed in detail in Chapter 13.

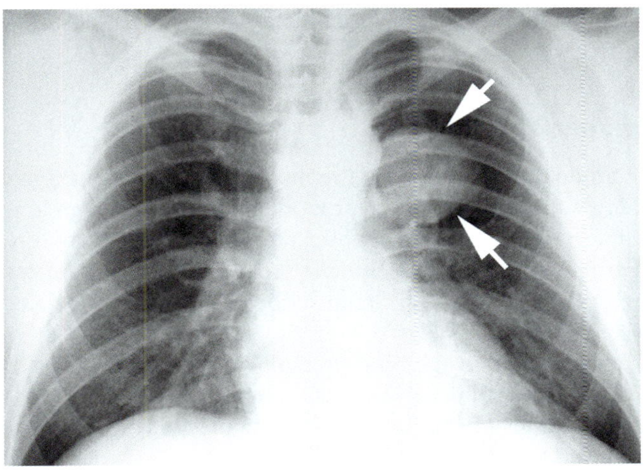

Figure 10.34. Pulmonary hydatid cyst (*arrows*) resulting from the sylvatic form of disease. A fisherman from Alaska shows a focal rounded opacity.

Endometrioma

Nodules of the endometrium may rarely involve the lung parenchyma. They typically occur in women who have previously given birth or have had uterine surgery and probably reflect embolism and implantation of endometrial tissue. Pelvic endometriosis need not be present. Pulmonary endometrioma may result in catamenial hemoptysis or pulmonary hemorrhage, symptoms that strongly suggest the diagnosis. Pneumothorax may result if the implants involve the pleural surface. Pulmonary endometrioma usually is solitary, appearing in most cases as a well-defined, rounded nodule up to a few centimeters in diameter. Cavitation may occur, with the cavity often appearing thin walled. Treatment is hormonal or by excision.

Focal OP

OP, previously known as bronchiolitis obliterans organizing pneumonia, is characterized pathologically by the presence of granulation tissue polyps within bronchioles and alveolar ducts and patchy areas of inflammation in the surrounding lung (OP). Many cases are idiopathic, but OP also may be seen in patients with pulmonary infection, drug reactions, collagen vascular diseases, GPA, and after inhalation of toxic fumes.

Most often, OP presents with patchy, unilateral or bilateral areas of air-space consolidation, which may be peripheral or peribronchial. Small or large nodules are seen in up to 50%, with or without associated consolidation (see Figs. 14.18 and 14.19 in Chapter 14 and Fig. 18.3 in Chapter 18). Large nodules or masses usually are multiple and may appear very irregular in shape, mimicking carcinoma. A finding termed the *reversed halo sign* or *atoll sign*, in which ring-shaped or crescentic opacities are seen, often with GGO in the center of the ring (resembling a coral atoll or the opposite of the halo sign), may be seen with OP. This finding strongly suggests the diagnosis. High-attenuation nodules or masses may be seen in patients with OP related to amiodarone toxicity due to its iodine content. Cavitation and calcification do not occur.

Focal (Round) Pneumonia

Pneumonias may be focal, mimicking the appearance of carcinoma. This configuration has been termed *round pneumonia*. Findings suggestive of focal pneumonia include satellite nodules (Fig. 10.35A), tree-in-bud, centrilobular nodules, or a lobular or multilobular pattern, but these do not need to be seen to establish the diagnosis. Focal infections are common with bacterial bronchopneumonia (see Fig. 10.35A),

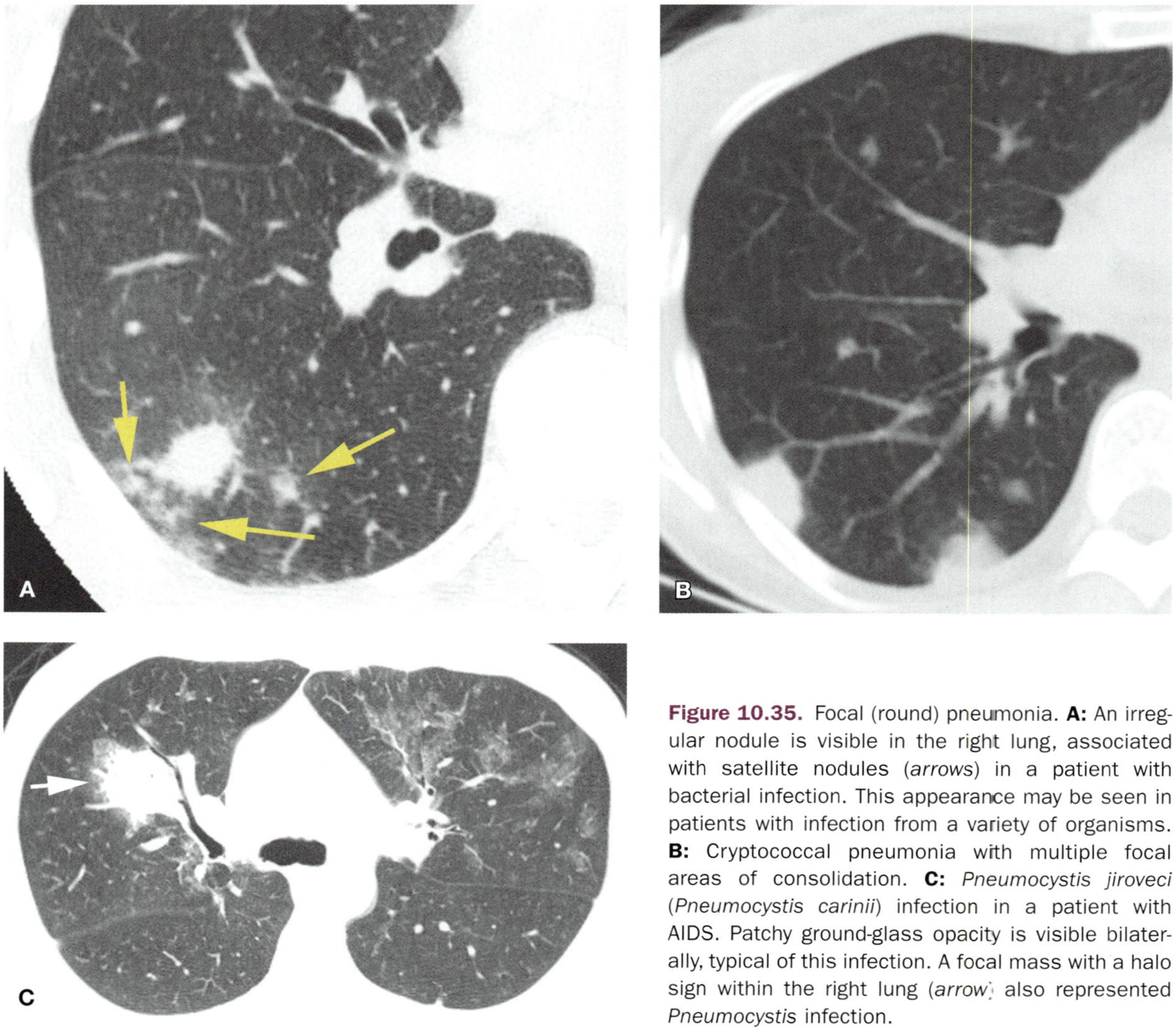

Figure 10.35. Focal (round) pneumonia. **A:** An irregular nodule is visible in the right lung, associated with satellite nodules (*arrows*) in a patient with bacterial infection. This appearance may be seen in patients with infection from a variety of organisms. **B:** Cryptococcal pneumonia with multiple focal areas of consolidation. **C:** *Pneumocystis jiroveci* (*Pneumocystis carinii*) infection in a patient with AIDS. Patchy ground-glass opacity is visible bilaterally, typical of this infection. A focal mass with a halo sign within the right lung (*arrow*) also represented *Pneumocystis* infection.

TB, nontuberculous mycobacteria, and fungal infection (see Fig. 10.35B) and occasionally are seen with viral infection or infection with *Pneumocystis jiroveci* (formerly *Pneumocystis carinii*; see Fig. 10.35C). Focal opacities associated with infection may be solitary or multiple. The halo sign is common with angioinvasive aspergillosis (see Figs. 10.7 and 10.27) but may be seen with focal infection of various causes (see Fig. 10.35C).

Granuloma

Granulomas usually result from TB, nontuberculous mycobacteria, and fungal infections, most commonly coccidioidomycosis and histoplasmosis. They usually are well defined and rounded (see Fig. 10.3). Granulomas associated with surrounding lung fibrosis (common in TB) may appear very irregular and spiculated in contour, mimicking carcinoma. Granulomas also may be associated with irregular cavitation. Calcification is common but may have a variety of appearances—dense and homogeneous, central, lamellar, eccentric, or stippled. Granulomas usually are smaller than 2 cm in diameter and often are solitary or few in number. Numerous small granulomas, a few millimeters in diameter, also may be seen.

Hamartoma

Pulmonary hamartoma is the most common mesenchymal lung tumor and accounts for more than 75% of benign lung tumors. More than 85% appear radiographically as an SPN. Peripheral hamartomas usually are 1 to 4 cm in diameter, well defined, sharply circumscribed, and often lobulated (see Fig. 10.4 and Figs. 5.27, 5.28, 5.29, 5.30 in Chapter 5). Calcification is visible on plain radiographs in approximately 30% of hamartomas and is seen more commonly on CT. The calcification of hamartomas can be stippled or conglomerate, referred to as "popcorn" calcification. Nearly 65% of hamartomas may be diagnosed using HRCT because of visible fat (−40 to −120 HU), either focal or diffuse or a combination of fat and calcification. Cavitation is rare.

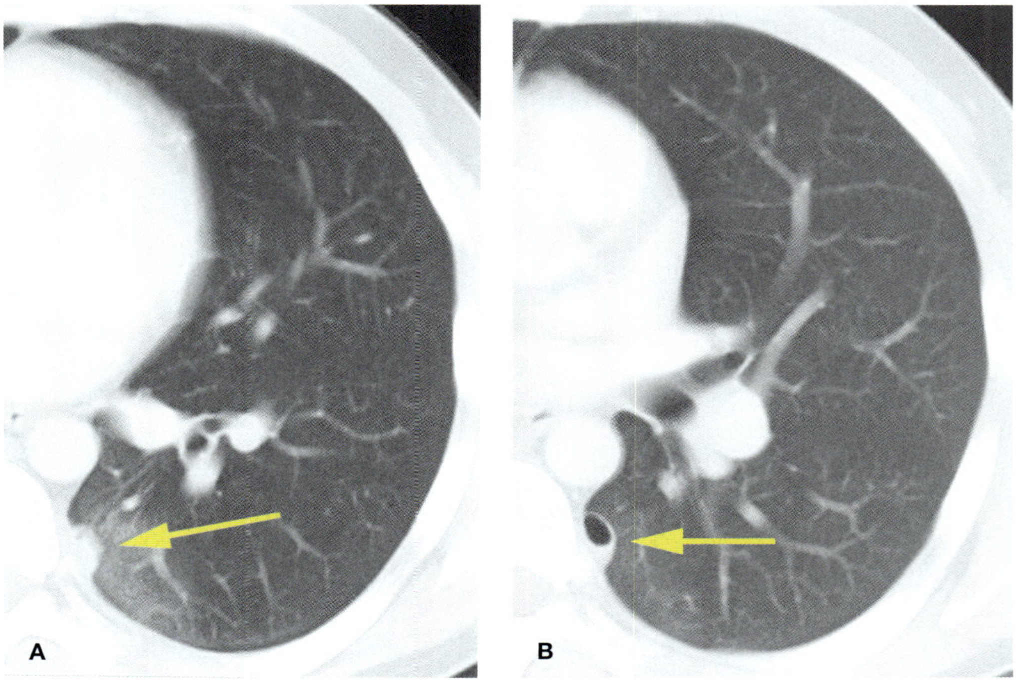

Figure 10.36. Pulmonary laceration with hematoma in a hockey player with hemoptysis after a "bad body check." **A:** A focal lung opacity (*arrow*) represents a focal hematoma. Some surrounding ground-glass opacity is due to hemorrhage. **B:** At a different level, an air-fluid level (*arrow*) is visible within a focal cystic lesion.

Other benign tumors may arise from mesenchymal tissues. They are usually solitary, well defined, and rounded in shape. Benign tumors usually are solitary. Multiple chondromas may be associated with *Carney triad* (ie, multiple pulmonary chondromas, gastric epithelioid leiomyosarcoma, and extra-adrenal paraganglioma).

Hematoma and Laceration

Hematomas are often the result of trauma (blunt or penetrating), representing focal lung contusion or pulmonary laceration containing blood. *Contusion* represents focal bleeding without disruption of lung architecture. *Traumatic laceration* is associated with tearing of the lung; a laceration contains blood or air (or both), with air-fluid levels sometimes visible (Figs. 10.36 and 10.37). These lesions usually are thin walled. They may be solitary or multiple. High-attenuation clot may be detectable using CT. Focal hematoma also may result from other causes of bleeding.

Infarction

Focal consolidation distal to a pulmonary embolus may be due to ischemia with focal pulmonary hemorrhage or frank infarction. Because the lung is supplied by both pulmonary and bronchial arteries, pulmonary infarction occurs in the minority (10%-15%) of patients with pulmonary embolism and often is associated with underlying cardiovascular disease, the presence of peripheral emboli, or multiple emboli.

Hemorrhage or infarction in the peripheral lung may result in a wedge-shaped or rounded, pleural-based opacity, the classic *Hampton hump*. Subpleural opacities are seen more often in the lower lobes, where most emboli occur. On plain films, these opacities usually are unassociated with air bronchograms; the absence of air bronchograms is likely due to blood filling the bronchi. Pulmonary opacities due to hemorrhage usually resolve within a week, but pulmonary infarctions may require months to heal. They typically resolve by maintaining the same shape while decreasing in size, an occurrence called the "melting sign" because of its resemblance to a melting ice cube. Infarctions often leave linear scars.

On CT (Fig. 10.38), a pulmonary infarction may be characterized by the following features:

1. A wedge-shaped opacity (sometimes with a truncated apex)
2. Contact with the pleural surface
3. Convex borders
4. A linear opacity directed from the apex of the density toward the hilum (ie, its feeding vessel)
5. Scattered areas of low attenuation (necrosis) within the lesion
6. A halo sign due to adjacent hemorrhage

Some or all of these findings are seen on CT in about half of patients with pulmonary embolism.

Following the administration of a bolus of intravenous contrast medium, the perimeter of an infarct

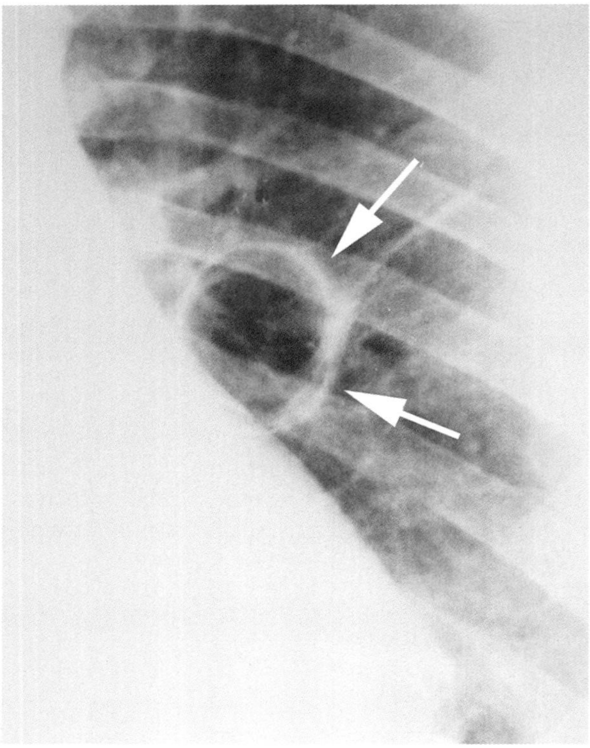

Figure 10.37. Pulmonary laceration. A cystic air-filled lesion in the left lung (*arrows*) represents a laceration from a stab wound.

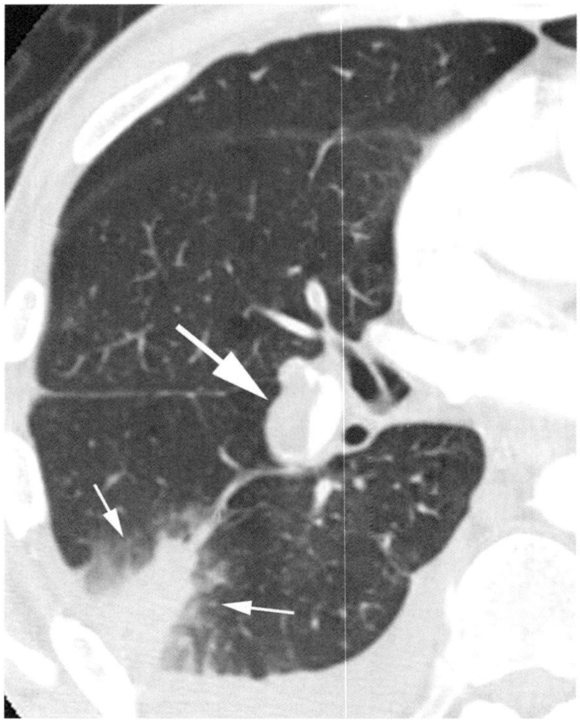

Figure 10.38. Pulmonary infarction in a patient with pulmonary embolism. CT shows a pulmonary embolus in the right interlobar pulmonary artery (*large arrow*). A wedge-shaped opacity (*small arrows*) is visible in the peripheral lung, contacting the pleural surface, and associated with surrounding ground-glass opacity (halo sign). A vessel is noted at the apex of the opacity. A pleural effusion is associated.

characteristically enhances, possibly because of collateral blood flow from adjacent bronchial arteries, while the center of the lesion remains lucent. Cavitation of an infarction suggests septic embolism or infection of a bland infarct.

Intrapulmonary Lymph Nodes

IPLNs (also referred to as juxtapleural nodules, perifissural nodules or PFNs) are very common on thin-section CT and, while estimates vary, likely make up 20% to 40% of subcentimeter noncalcified nodules in adults. Analyses of lung cancer screening cohorts have shown that for typical IPLNs found in the lower lobes or middle lobes, the chance of a primary lung cancer is close to zero. The Fleischner Society and Lung-RADS both consider these lesions to be benign in their most recent publications.

Different authors have used slightly different criteria for PFNs (see review by Schruder et al at the end of this chapter), but familiarity with these general principles will allow a confident diagnosis of these benign nodules in most cases. Typical IPLNs are solid, noncalcified nodules with sharp margins; triangular, oval, or polygonal in shape; abutting a fissure/pleural surface or within 15 mm of pleura/fissure in the middle or lower lobes (Fig. 10.39). Analysis in multiple planes may be helpful to confirm morphology. IPLNs may fluctuate in size on follow-up studies.

Nodules not meeting these criteria may represent atypical IPLNs but could also represent small lung cancers and thus should be treated with caution. If the nodule is not completely solid or has even a hint of an irregular margin, it should be managed like other incidental nodules. Nodules in the upper lobes are also less likely to be IPLNs although precise data are lacking.

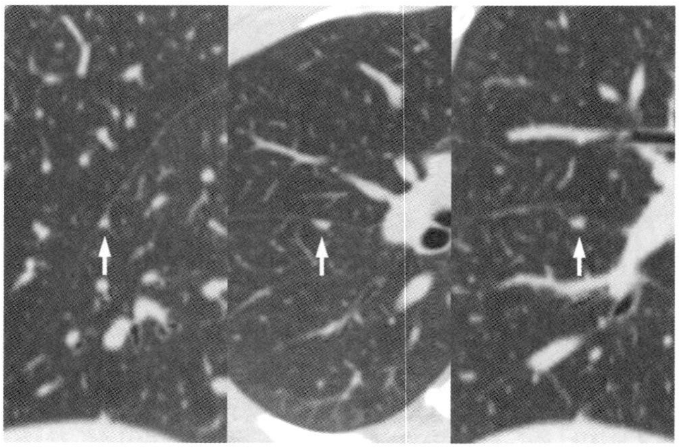

Figure 10.39. Typical intrapulmonary lymph node. Sagittal, axial, and coronal images show a sharply defined, triangular, solid nodule along the major fissure in the right lung (arrows) that measures 7 × 3 mm in the axial plane. This intrapulmonary lymph node is benign and does not warrant additional follow-up.

Lipoid Pneumonia

Lipoid pneumonia (lung consolidation containing lipid) may be endogenous or exogenous.

Endogenous lipoid pneumonia may occur due to bronchial obstruction with accumulation of lipid-rich cellular debris distal to the obstructing lesion.

Exogenous lipoid pneumonia results from the chronic aspiration of animal-, vegetable-, or petroleum-based oils or fats. Consolidation, ill-defined masses, or (sometimes) findings of fibrosis are seen on chest radiographs. A posterior or lower lobe distribution is typical. Opacities may be bilateral or unilateral. If a large amount of lipid has been aspirated, CT can show rounded or irregular areas of low-attenuation consolidation (−35 to −75 HU); this appearance is most common in patients with chronic mineral oil aspiration (see Figs. 20.1 and 20.2 in Chapter 20). Because inflammation or fibrosis may accompany the presence of the lipid material, the CT attenuation of the consolidation need not be low, but in many cases, small areas of low-attenuation oil are visible within larger masses. In some patients, necrosis and cavitation may be present.

Lung Abscess

Lung abscess represents an infected, necrotic, pus-filled cavity. If communication with a bronchus occurs, partial drainage of the abscess contents may occur. With a chronic abscess, the wall of the cavity may be surrounded by granulation tissue or fibrosis.

Lung abscess may result from pyogenic bacteria, mycobacteria, fungal organisms, parasites, and, rarely, viral infections. Many cases are caused by anaerobic organisms in association with poor oral hygiene and periodontal disease, conditions predisposing to aspiration, and old age. Lung abscess may also be associated with infection by *Klebsiella pneumoniae, Staphylococcus aureus, Pseudomonas aeruginosa, Nocardia* spp., *Actinomyces* spp., and TB. They may occur as complications of infarction, cavitary neoplasm, and cavitary conglomerate mass.

In patients with an anaerobic abscess, symptoms include low-grade fever, cough, and sputum production, often of several weeks' duration. In patients with other causes of bacterial abscess, symptoms usually are acute and resemble those of pneumonia.

On plain radiographs, acute lung abscesses usually appear as irregular masses. The outer aspect of an abscess may be very ill defined because of surrounding inflammation and lung consolidation. An air-fluid level may be seen if communication with a bronchus and partial drainage has occurred.

On CT, when contrast medium is infused, lung abscesses typically show a densely enhancing wall that is variable in thickness and irregular in contour (Fig. 10.40A). The internal wall of the abscess cavity often is shaggy (Fig. 10 40C). The outer wall may be sharply marginated and smooth, irregular, or obscured by surrounding consolidation. The contents of a lung abscess appear low in attenuation (ie, fluid attenuation) compared to the density of the enhancing wall or surrounding consolidated lung. An air-fluid level may be seen (see Fig. 10.10). Bronchi may be seen entering the abscess, an appearance that helps to distinguish lung abscess from empyema.

With healing, the wall of an abscess becomes thinner and more sharply defined (see Fig. 10.40B). The abscess tends to decrease in size, and the amount of fluid in the abscess decreases. Complete resolution or focal scarring is typical.

In patients with clinical symptoms of infection, the diagnosis of lung abscess usually is not difficult. However, the appearance of a peripheral abscess may overlap that of an empyema. This distinction is important to make because an empyema is often treated by tube drainage, whereas an abscess is not. Several findings usually assist in distinguishing these two entities.

Lung abscesses typically are round or oval in shape and form acute angles where they touch the pleural surface. Abscesses tend to have an irregularly thick wall in their acute stage. Because an abscess represents necrotic lung, pulmonary vessels or bronchi may be seen entering an abscess wall or may be seen within its center.

Empyemas typically are oval, lenticular, or crescentic in shape and usually show obtuse angles at the pleural surface. The walls of an empyema cavity tend to be smooth and uniform in thickness, although the wall may be partially obscured by adjacent atelectasis. Pulmonary vessels and bronchi are displaced by an empyema.

Lymphoma

Lymphoma may be associated with single or multiple lung nodules, masses, or focal masslike areas of consolidation. Cavitation may occur. The presence of associated lymph node enlargement is variable. Lymphomas are discussed in detail in Chapter 7.

Hodgkin Lymphoma

Hodgkin lymphoma (HL) involves lung in 10% of patients at the time of presentation. It is uncommon in untreated patients in the absence of radiographically visible mediastinal or ipsilateral hilar adenopathy. However, lung recurrence can be seen without node enlargement in patients with prior mediastinal and hilar radiation. Discrete, single or multiple, well-defined or ill-defined, large or small nodules or masslike lesions, or localized areas of air-space consolidation associated with air bronchograms may all be seen (see Figs. 7.10-7.12 in Chapter 7). These can cavitate, with either thick or thin walls. Peripheral, subpleural masses are common.

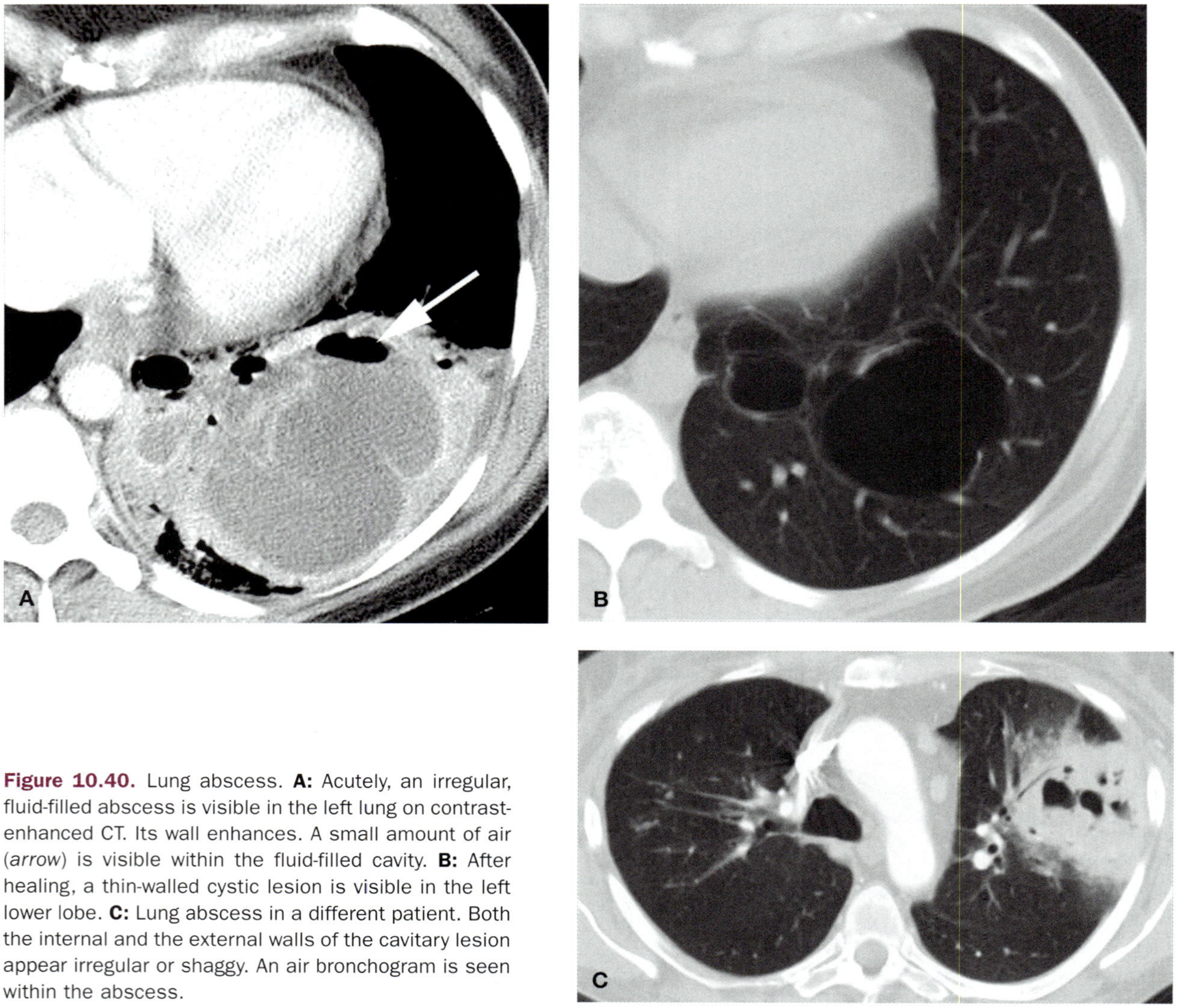

Figure 10.40. Lung abscess. **A:** Acutely, an irregular, fluid-filled abscess is visible in the left lung on contrast-enhanced CT. Its wall enhances. A small amount of air (*arrow*) is visible within the fluid-filled cavity. **B:** After healing, a thin-walled cystic lesion is visible in the left lower lobe. **C:** Lung abscess in a different patient. Both the internal and the external walls of the cavitary lesion appear irregular or shaggy. An air bronchogram is seen within the abscess.

Non-Hodgkin Lymphoma

Non-Hodgkin lymphoma (NHL) usually is a disseminated disease, and the lung is involved in 10% to 15% of cases. Lung involvement may appear as discrete nodules or masses, air-space consolidation, or infiltration contiguous with enlarged lymph nodes (see Figs. 7.21, 7.22, and 7.32 in Chapter 7). Specific types of NHL include primary pulmonary lymphoma, AIDS-related lymphoma, mycosis fungoides, and plasmacytoma.

Primary pulmonary lymphoma is considered to be present if there is no evidence of extrathoracic disease for at least 3 months after the initial diagnosis of lung lymphoma. Primary pulmonary lymphoma may be classified as a low-grade B-cell lymphoma, usually derived from bronchus- or mucosa-associated lymphoid tissue (malt lymphoma or MALToma), or high-grade lymphoma. Both may present as a solitary nodule or mass, multiple nodules or masses, or multifocal areas of consolidation, with or without associated lymph node enlargement.

AIDS-related lymphoma originates primarily in extranodal locations and commonly involves multiple sites, including the lung. Multiple pulmonary nodules and masses, ranging in size from 1 to 5 cm, are seen most commonly on radiographs or CT. The nodules usually are well defined. Cavitation may be present but is not common.

Plasmacytoma usually originates in bone; much less common is extramedullary plasmacytoma. Pulmonary nodules or mass lesions may be seen.

Lymphoproliferative Disease

In addition to HL and NHLs, pulmonary lymphoproliferative diseases represent a spectrum of focal and diffuse lung abnormalities associated with either a benign or a malignant course. As with the lymphomas, these may be associated with single or multiple lung nodules, masses, or focal masslike areas of consolidation, and cavitation may occur.

Focal lymphoid hyperplasia is an uncommon benign condition characterized histologically by localized proliferation of benign mononuclear cells including polyclonal lymphocytes, plasma cells, and histiocytes. Its most common radiologic manifestation is that of a solitary nodule or a focal area of consolidation, often containing air bronchograms (see Fig. 7.37 in Chapter 7). There is no associated lymphadenopathy.

Lymphomatoid granulomatosis encompasses a group of angiocentric, angiodestructive abnormalities characterized by a lymphoid infiltrate and a variable degree of cellular atypia; it is considered to be an NHL. The lung is the primary site of disease. Radiographic and CT findings consist of bilateral, poorly defined nodular lesions, ranging from 0.5 to 8 cm in diameter, with a basal predominance. Lesions may progress rapidly and cavitate, mimicking GPA.

Posttransplantation lymphoproliferative disorder (PTLD). Several histologic patterns of disease, ranging from a benign proliferation of lymphocytes to overtly malignant lymphoma, can occur after bone marrow or solid organ transplantation. These are known collectively as PTLD. PTLD can manifest as localized or disseminated disease and has a predilection for extranodal involvement. Lung involvement may occur as part of multiorgan disease or in isolation. In 85% of cases, radiographs and CT show single or multiple pulmonary nodules, which may be small or large (0.3-5 cm), well defined or ill defined (see Fig. 7.40 in Chapter 7). Other findings include patchy or focal consolidation. Hilar or mediastinal lymphadenopathy is common.

Metastatic Neoplasm

Lung nodules are the most common thoracic manifestation of metastatic tumors, usually due to hematogenous spread (see Chapter 6).

Nodules of metastatic tumor tend to be sharply marginated. Poorly marginated nodules may be seen in the presence of surrounding hemorrhage, local invasion of adjacent lung, or lepidic growth. They tend to predominate in the lung bases because of relatively greater blood flow. Individual metastases may arise from the tips of small arteries, suggesting their hematogenous origin (ie, the feeding vessel sign). Nodules may be of any size.

Cavitation of metastases is not as common as with primary lung carcinoma, but it does occur in 5% of cases. The likelihood of cavitation varies with histology. Cavitation is most common with squamous cell tumors, but it also may be seen in adenocarcinomas and in some sarcomas.

Calcification of metastases occurs most commonly with osteogenic sarcoma, chondrosarcoma, synovial sarcoma, thyroid carcinoma, and mucinous adenocarcinoma.

A subpleural predominance of nodules is common unless the nodules are very numerous. On HRCT, numerous nodules tend to involve the lung in a diffuse fashion without regard for specific anatomic structures, a distribution termed *random*.

Multiple nodules are most common, and often the nodules vary in size. Benign nodular disease most often results in nodules of similar size. The size and number of nodules vary greatly. Nodules may be small and very numerous (ie, miliary); this appearance often is seen with very vascular tumors. Fewer, larger metastases also may be seen; when these are well defined, they are referred to as *cannonball metastases*.

Most patients (80%-90%) with multiple metastases have a history of neoplasm. In some patients, however, a history of a primary tumor is lacking at the time of diagnosis; in others, the primary tumor may never be found.

A metastatic tumor occasionally presents as a solitary nodule. About 5% to 10% of solitary nodules represent a solitary metastasis. Solitary metastases are most common with carcinoma of the colon, sarcomas, melanoma, and carcinomas of the kidney and testicle. Solitary metastases more often have a smooth margin than do the lesions of primary lung carcinoma.

Solitary metastases are least common in patients with carcinomas of the head and neck, bladder, breast, cervix, bile ducts, esophagus, ovary, prostate, and stomach; in patients with these tumors, a solitary nodule more likely represents a primary lung carcinoma.

Multiple pulmonary "leiomyomas" associated with smooth muscle tumors of the uterus in women (*benign metastasizing leiomyoma*) may represent (a) pulmonary dissemination of benign uterine tumors, (b) metastasis from a low-grade uterine leiomyosarcoma, or (c) a primary leiomyomatous process involving multiple sites. The smooth muscle lung tumors have benign histology, are clonal, and are identical to the patient's uterine tumors. Single or multiple lung masses usually are present, but cysts may be present (Figs. 5.31 and 5.32 in Chapter 5). They may be quite large, may calcify, and grow very slowly over a period of years.

Mucoid Impaction (Mucous Plug)

Mucous plugs mimicking the appearance of a lung nodule or nodules may be seen in a variety of conditions, including bronchial atresia (see Figs. 9.4 and 9.5 in Chapter 9), bronchial obstruction by a stricture or tumor, asthma, allergic bronchopulmonary aspergillosis, cystic fibrosis, and other causes of bronchiectasis (Fig. 10.41). In many cases, the characteristic branching appearance of the mucoid impaction allows it to be distinguished from other causes of a lung nodule. Air trapping or atelectasis may be associated. Mucous plugs often appear low in attenuation on CT, being less dense than the bronchial wall. High-attenuation mucous plugs may be seen on CT in patients with allergic bronchopulmonary aspergillosis due to calcification or metal salt deposition associated with the presence of aspergillus. Resolution of the mucous plug, revealing a dilated bronchus, may mimic cavitation of a solid lesion.

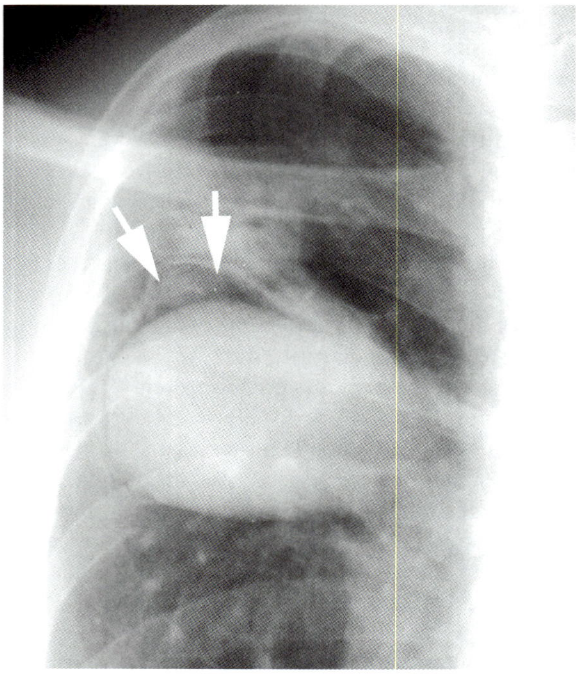

Figure 10.41. Mucoid impaction in bronchial atresia. A large oval mass in the right upper lobe represents a mucous plug distal to the atretic bronchial segment. Air in the dilated bronchial lumen (*arrows*) outlines the bronchial wall and mucous plug, resulting in an air-crescent sign.

Mycetoma (Aspergilloma)

In patients with a preexisting cyst or cavity, a mycetoma or fungus ball can form as a result of saprophytic infection, usually by aspergillus; other fungi occasionally are involved. Patients may be asymptomatic. However, hemoptysis and hemorrhage are common presenting complaints because of inflammation in the wall of the cyst.

Chest radiographs often show a cyst or cavity containing a mass within its dependent portion (Fig. 10.42). Cysts are commonly found in the upper lobe and often result from prior TB or sarcoidosis (see Fig. 16.10 in Chapter 16). However, early in the development of the mycetoma, thickening of the wall of the preexisting cyst or adjacent pleural thickening may be the only recognizable finding and should suggest the diagnosis. Gravitational shift of the intracavitary mass may be seen with change in the patient's position. A rim of air outlining the top of the mycetoma and the inner wall of the cavity is characteristic and is termed the *air-crescent* sign (see Table 10.7).

On CT, a round or oval mass (the fungus ball) can be seen within the cavity, usually in a dependent location. An air-crescent sign may be seen. The wall of the associated cyst or cavity usually is thick. In patients with a developing mycetoma, the fungus ball can contain multiple bubbles of air.

Papillomatosis

In 2% to 5% of patients with a history of laryngeal papillomas, distal spread occurs, with involvement of the tracheobronchial tree, a condition referred to as *tracheobronchial papillomatosis*. The extension of papillomas to the bronchi, bronchioles, and lung parenchyma is rare but may occur. Papillomas may be visible radiographically as nodular mass lesions within the lung, usually multiple, which often cavitate. Eventually, cavitary lesions may progress to large, thick- or thin-walled cysts. Nodules representing papillomas may be seen within cysts (Fig. 10.43; see also Fig. 5.25 in Chapter 5). Squamous cell carcinoma may develop.

Paragonimiasis

Paragonimiasis results from infection by the lung fluke *Paragonimus westermani*. It is common in Southeast Asia

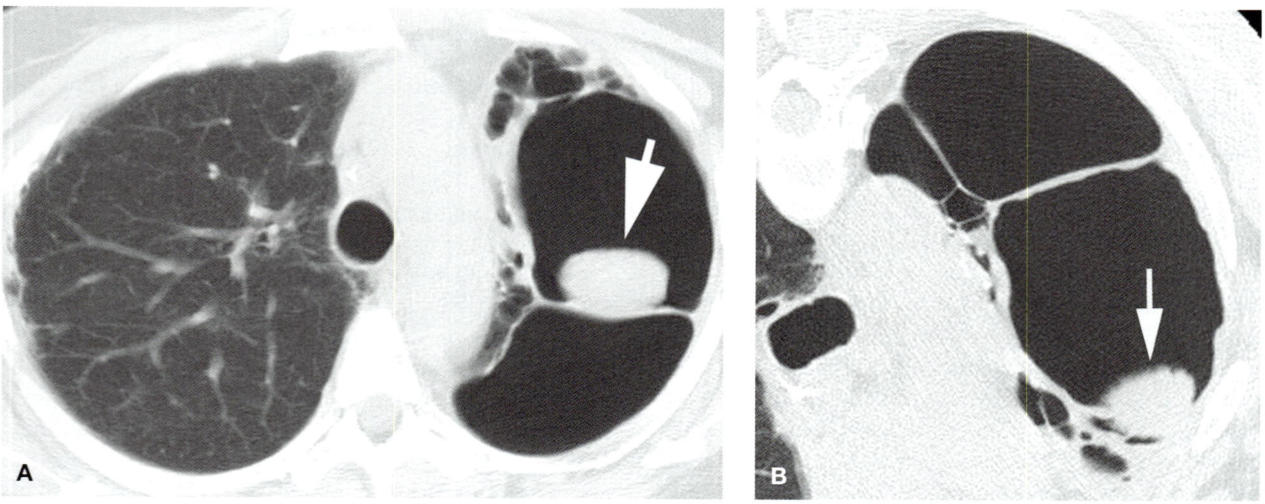

Figure 10.42. Mycetoma (aspergilloma) seen on chest radiograph. **A:** Cystic lung disease in the left upper lobe is associated with an intracavitary mass (*arrow*). **B:** On the prone image, the mass moves anteriorly (*arrow*).

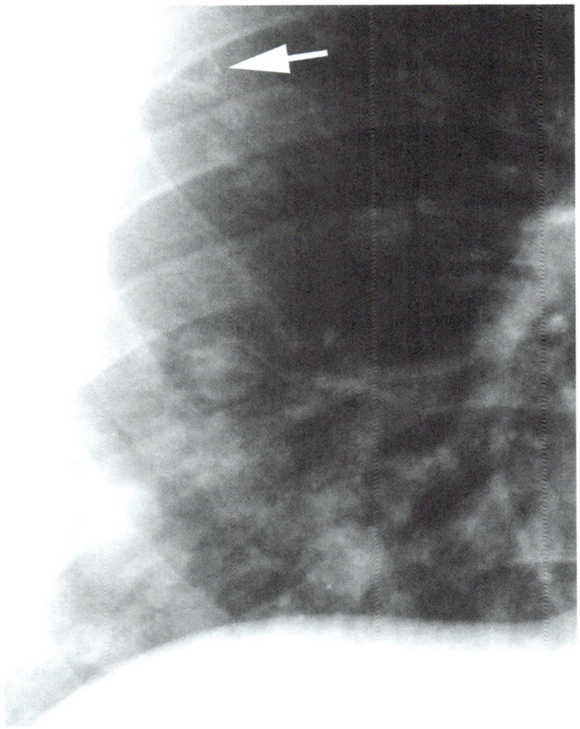

Figure 10.43. Papillomatosis with multiple nodules. Detail view of the right lower lobe. Multiple well-defined nodules are visible, one of which is cavitary (*arrow*).

and thus may be seen in recent immigrants to the United States. It is acquired by eating freshwater crustaceans. Flukes migrate through the bowel wall, peritoneum, diaphragm, and pleura to reach the lungs, where they develop. They may result in the presence of ill-defined nodules or linear opacities, often multiple, with predominance at the lung bases (Fig. 10.44). Cysts or cavities may also be seen; irregular wall thickening may reflect the presence of the adult worm within a lung cyst (see also Fig. 13.58 in Chapter 13).

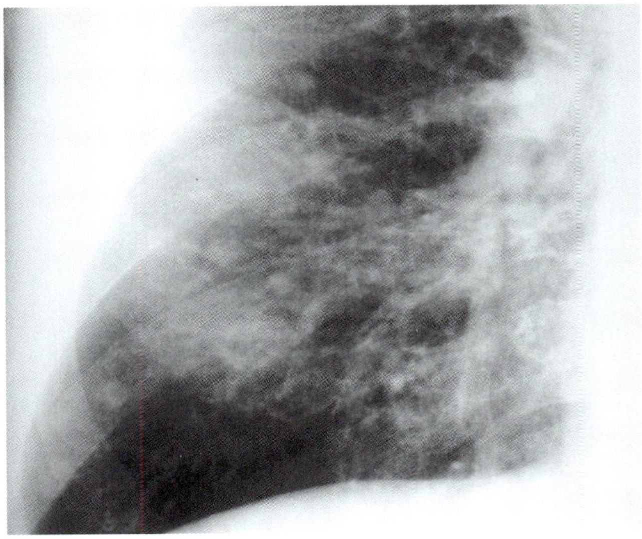

Figure 10.44. Paragonimiasis in a world traveler with hemoptysis. Radiograph coned to the right lung base shows multiple small nodules. Some cystic or cavitary lesions also are visible.

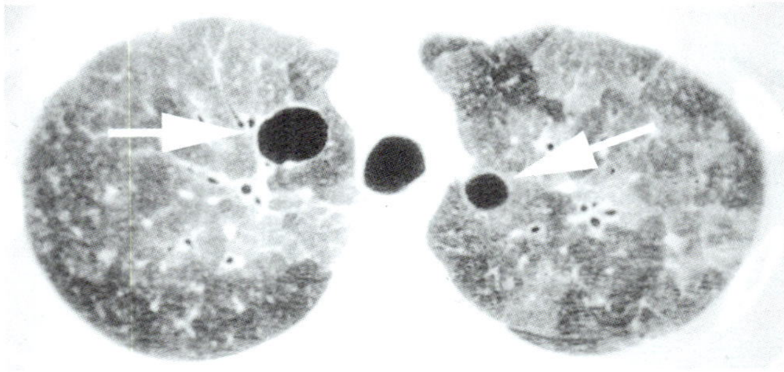

Figure 10.45. Pneumatoceles in *Pneumocystis jiroveci* (*Pneumocystis carinii*) pneumonia. High-resolution CT in a patient with AIDS shows ground-glass opacity consistent with *P. jiroveci* pneumonia. Thin-walled pneumatoceles (*arrows*) are visible bilaterally.

Pneumatocele

Pneumatoceles are thin-walled, air-filled cysts that typically occur in association with infection. They may increase in size due to air trapping. Pneumatoceles are commonly seen in patients with *P. jiroveci* (*P. carinii*) pneumonia in association with AIDS, *S. aureus* pneumonia, and other bacterial infections. In distinction to lung abscess or pulmonary gangrene, the wall of an air-filled pneumatocele tends to be thin and of uniform thickness (Fig. 10.45).

Pulmonary Artery Aneurysm

Pulmonary artery aneurysms are rare. When they occur in relation to lobar, segmental, or smaller arteries, they may present as a lung nodule (Fig. 10.46). CT with contrast infusion is diagnostic, resulting in dense opacification.

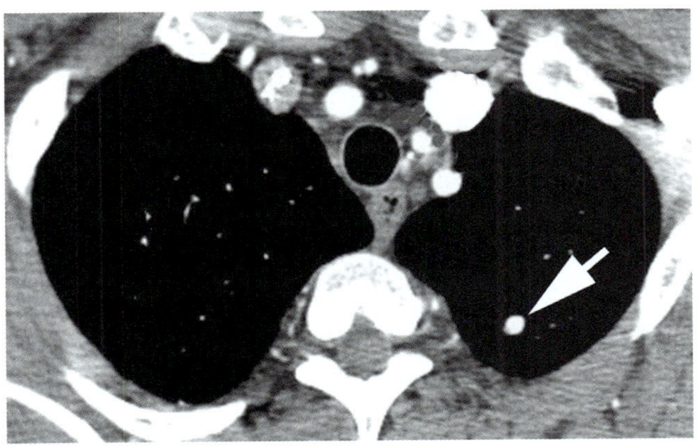

Figure 10.46. Pulmonary artery aneurysm following septic embolism. A small, densely opacified aneurysm (*arrow*) is visible at the left lung apex.

Pulmonary artery aneurysms may be (1) mycotic (see Fig. 10.46), (2) the result of catheter-related complications, or (3) associated with pulmonary hypertension (see Fig. 3.29 in Chapter 3) or diseases such as Takayasu arteritis, Williams syndrome, Behçet syndrome (Fig. 19.2 in Chapter 19), and prenatal varicella. *Rasmussen aneurysm* is a mycotic aneurysm occurring in relation to an infectious cavity and is most typical of TB.

Pulmonary Vein Varix

Pulmonary vein varix represents a segmental dilatation of a pulmonary vein at or near its junction with the left atrium. Although varix may result from a congenital defect of the vein wall, many varices are associated with elevated pulmonary venous pressure and mitral valve disease. They are radiographically visible as round or oval densities in the medial third of either lung, typically adjacent to the left atrial shadow (Fig. 10.47). On the lateral view, they are noted in the typical location of pulmonary veins. They rarely cause symptoms but can enlarge in response to increasing left atrial pressure and may rupture with hemorrhage. A varix can be confused for AVM so it is important to trace the proximal and distal connection, which should both be to the left atrium/pulmonary veins with a varix.

Pulmonary Gangrene

Rarely, patients with a lung infection develop an abscess containing a sequestrum of necrotic lung, identical to what is seen in patients with angioinvasive aspergillosis. This is termed *pulmonary gangrene*. Lung necrosis may be the result of direct action by bacterial toxins or ischemia resulting from thrombosis of small pulmonary arteries. It may occur in patients infected with *Klebsiella, Streptococcus pneumonia, Haemophilus influenzae, S. aureus*, or anaerobic bacteria. The presence of a mass in a cavity or an air-crescent sign is typical on radiographs or CT (Fig. 10.48).

Rheumatoid Nodules and Caplan Syndrome

Rheumatoid (necrobiotic) nodules are an uncommon manifestation of rheumatoid arthritis. They often are asymptomatic but tend to appear and disappear in conjunction with subcutaneous nodules. They range in size from a few millimeters to 5 cm or more and may be solitary or multiple and numerous (Fig. 10.49). Rheumatoid nodules predominate in the lung periphery and typically are well defined. They may cavitate, having thick walls that become thin with healing. Pleural effusion may be associated, and cavitary nodules in the periphery may lead to pneumothorax.

Caplan syndrome is a rare manifestation of rheumatoid arthritis that occurs in coal miners or patients with silicosis. It is characterized by single or multiple lung nodules ranging from a few millimeters to 5 cm in diameter, similar to those seen with rheumatoid nodules. Nodules may have an upper lobe predominance, resembling the appearance of silicosis, but nodules in Caplan syndrome appear rapidly and in "crops," in contrast to the slow progression of pneumoconiosis.

Round Atelectasis

Round atelectasis represents focal rounded lung collapse, usually associated with pleural thickening or effusion. It typically appears as a focal mass lesion and is described in detail in Chapter 1.

Round atelectasis often shows characteristic findings on chest radiographs or CT. It usually is (1) round or oval in shape, (2) peripheral in location and abutting the pleural surface, (3) associated with curving of pulmonary vessels or bronchi into the edge of the lesion (the "comet tail" sign), and

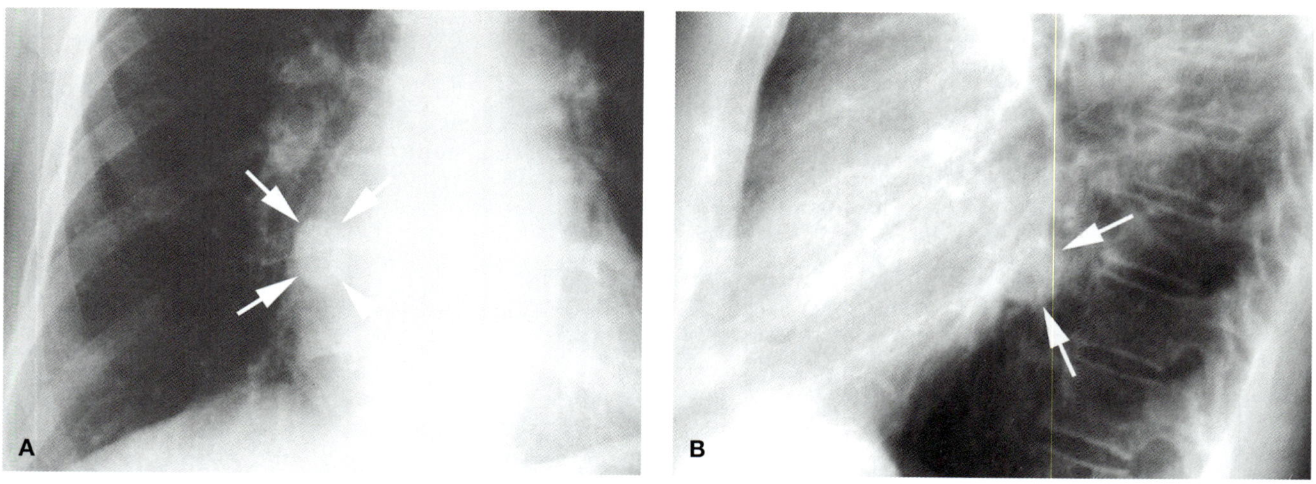

Figure 10.47. Pulmonary vein varix in mitral stenosis. **A:** On the PA radiograph, a well-defined oval opacity (*arrows*) overlies the shadow of the left atrium. **B:** On the lateral view, the opacity is localized to the junction of the pulmonary veins with the left atrium (*arrows*).

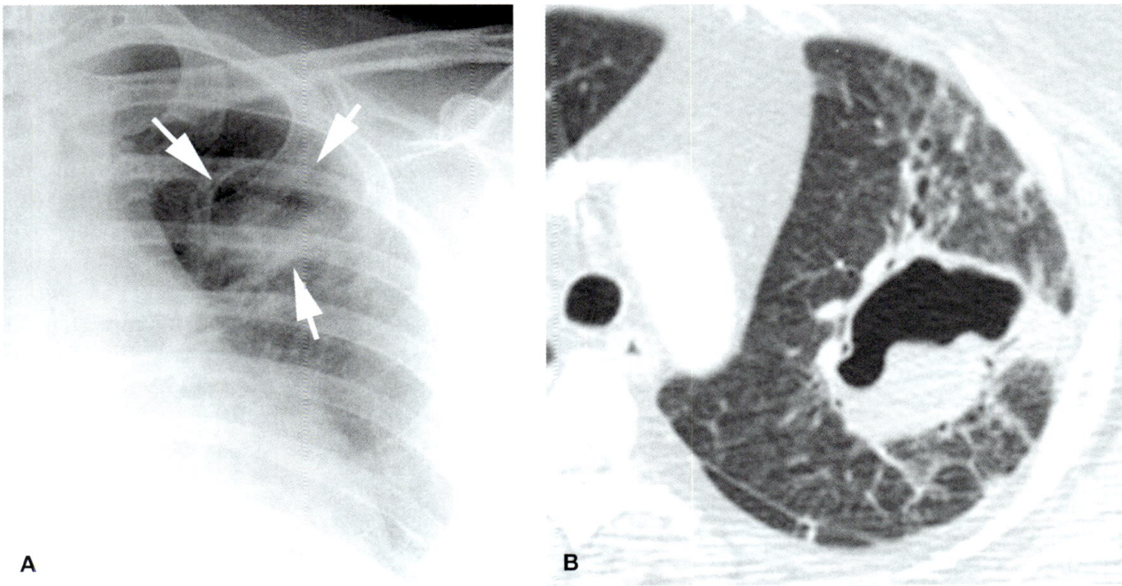

Figure 10.48. Pulmonary gangrene in *Staphylococcus aureus* infection. **A:** Chest radiograph shows a thin-walled cavity (*arrows*) in the left upper lobe. The cavity contains an ill-defined opacity, representing a sequestrum of necrotic lung. **B:** HRCT shows the thin-walled cavity, a sequestrum of necrotic lung, and an air-crescent sign. This appearance is very similar to that seen with angioinvasive aspergillosis.

(4) associated with an ipsilateral pleural abnormality, either effusion or pleural thickening, with the lesion contacting the abnormal pleural surface. If these criteria for rounded atelectasis are met, a confident diagnosis usually can be made, and radiographic follow-up should be sufficient. Rounded atelectasis is most common in the posterior lower lobes and, sometimes, is bilateral or symmetrical (see Figs. 1.44-1.47 in Chapter 1).

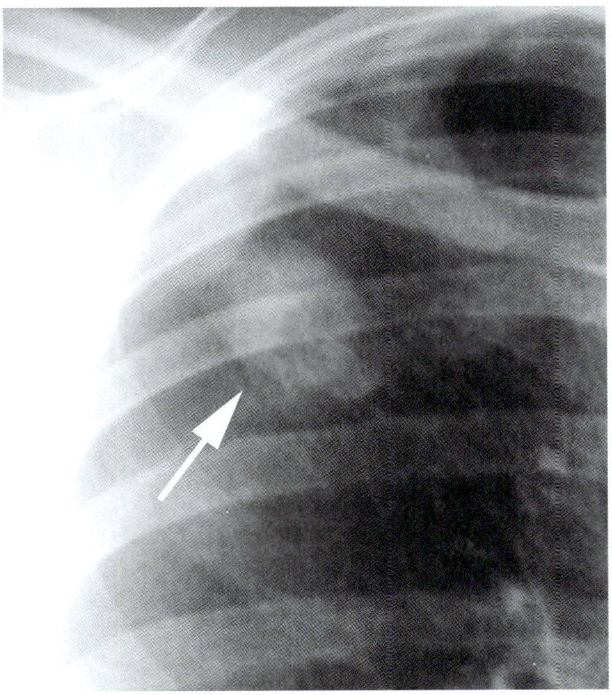

Figure 10.49. Rheumatoid nodule. A well-defined nodule (*arrow*) is visible in the peripheral right upper lobe. A central lucency represents cavitation. Focal pleural thickening is visible adjacent to the nodule.

Sarcoidosis

Large masses or areas of consolidation, measuring 4 cm in diameter or larger, are seen in 15% to 25% of patients with active sarcoidosis (see Chapter 16). Because they may contain air bronchograms, they sometimes are termed *alveolar sarcoid*. These masses are due to the confluence of large numbers of small interstitial granulomas. They may be parahilar or peripheral in location, and they rarely cavitate. On CT, small nodules (*satellite nodules*) often are visible at the periphery of these masses. This occurrence is also termed the *galaxy sign*.

Pulmonary masses also may be seen in patients with end-stage sarcoidosis. Progressive fibrosis may lead to abnormal central conglomeration of parahilar bronchi and vessels, associated with masses of fibrous tissue, typically most marked in the upper lobes. This finding often is associated with bronchial dilatation, a finding referred to as *traction bronchiectasis*. It is similar in appearance to that of progressive massive fibrosis in silicosis.

Septic Embolism With Infarction

Septic pulmonary emboli, with or without infarction, generally result in multiple parenchymal abnormalities; rarely does septic embolism present as a solitary lesion. The correct radiographic diagnosis usually is suggested by the finding of relatively well-defined, bilateral peripheral nodules with or without cavitation, especially in the setting of known intravenous drug abuse, or some other known source of sepsis.

In patients with septic embolism, peripheral nodules in varying stages of cavitation often are present, presumably due to intermittent seeding of the lungs by infected material (Fig. 10.50). The *feeding vessel sign* is visible in 65% of cases (see Fig. 10.50C). CT is helpful in showing the peripheral and subpleural location of the nodules (see Fig. 10.50B and C).

Sequestration

Sequestration represents an area of disorganized pulmonary parenchyma without normal pulmonary arterial or bronchial communications. Sequestration usually receives its blood supply from branches of the thoracic or abdominal aorta. There are two forms of sequestration, intralobar and extralobar.

Intralobar sequestration is more common. Two-thirds of intralobar sequestrations are found adjacent to the diaphragm in relation to the posterior basal segment of the left lower lobe. Intralobar sequestration usually presents in adults or older children. Uncomplicated intralobar sequestration can have a variety of appearances. It may appear as (1) a homogeneous and well-defined mass lesion, (2) a cystic or multicystic air- and fluid-filled lesion, (3) a hyperlucent and hypovascular region of lung, or (4) a combination of these. Bilateral intralobar sequestrations may occur (see Figs. 9.26-9.29 in Chapter 9).

Extralobar sequestration represents an anomaly in which the sequestered tissue is enclosed within its only pleural envelope; it is less common than intralobar sequestration and often is diagnosed in neonates. Approximately 90% of cases are visible at the left lung base, contiguous with the left hemidiaphragm (see Figs. 9.30 and 9.31 in Chapter 9). Extralobar sequestration appears as a sharply marginated mass lesion, which does not contain air (unlike intralobar sequestration). It usually is homogeneous in appearance but may contain cystic areas. Its supplying artery may be seen on CT.

Granulomatosis With Polyangiitis

GPA, formerly termed *Wegener granulomatosis*, is a multisystem disease of unknown cause associated with the involvement of the upper respiratory tract (nasal, oral, or sinus inflammation), lower respiratory tract (airway or lung), and kidney (see Chapter 19). The presence of antineutrophilic cytoplasmic antibody (C-ANCA) is characteristic and is seen in 90% of cases.

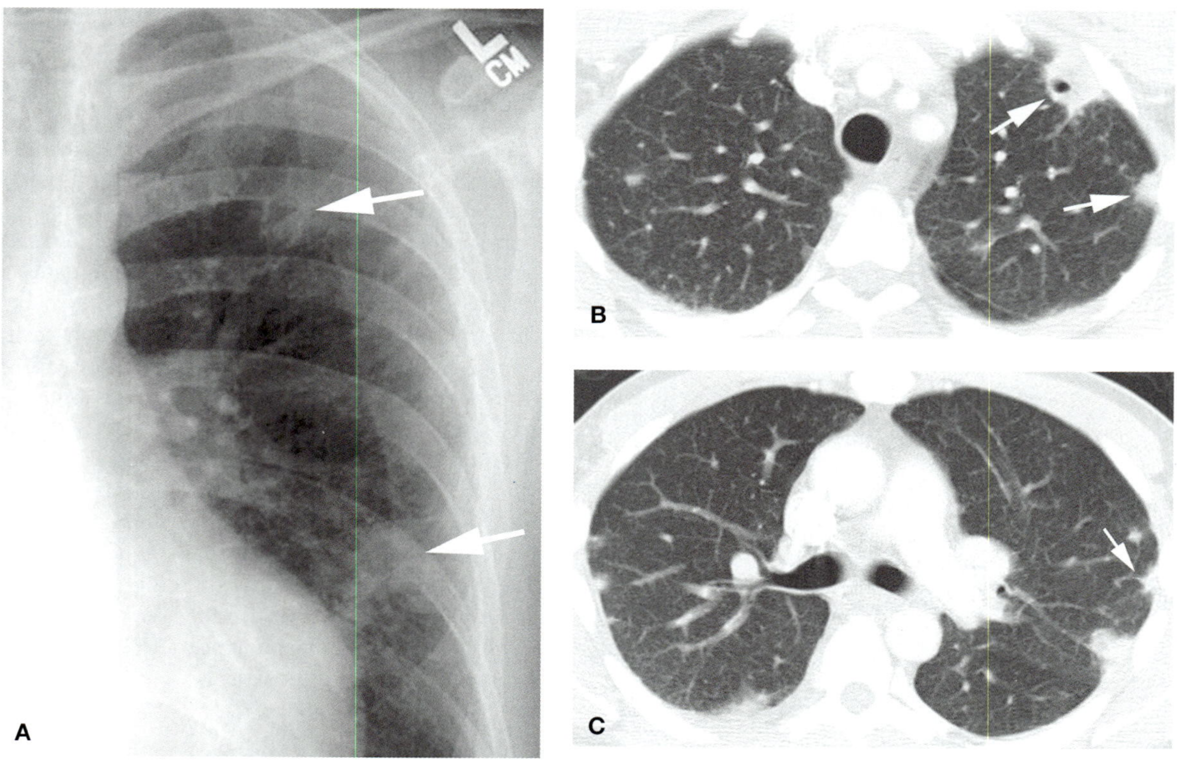

Figure 10.50. Septic embolism in a patient with intravenous drug abuse and endocarditis. **A:** Chest radiograph shows lung nodules, which appear cavitary (*arrows*). **B:** CT shows the peripheral nature of the nodules (*arrows*), relatively well-defined margins, and a variable degree of cavitation. **C:** Several examples of the feeding vessel sign are visible (*arrow*). The nodules are peripheral in location.

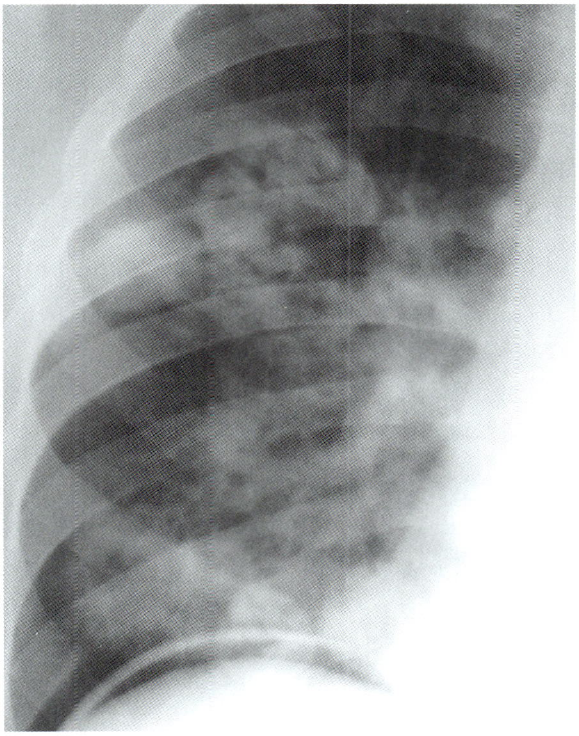

Figure 10.51. Granulomatosis with polyangiitis with multiple nodules. Multiple, poorly marginated nodules are visible in the right lung. Some appear cavitary. Free intraperitoneal air is the result of peritoneal dialysis for associated renal failure.

Patients usually are between the ages of 30 and 60. At presentation, chest radiographic abnormalities are visible in 75% of patients with GPA. The most common radiographic abnormality is multiple lung nodules or masses; these are visible in more than half of patients at presentation. Typically, fewer than a dozen nodules are visible, but they may be more numerous. In most cases, the nodules are bilateral and widely distributed without predominance in any lung region. A solitary nodule or mass may be seen, but this appearance is less common.

Masses usually range from 2 to 4 cm but may be up to 10 cm in diameter (Fig. 10.51; see also Figs. 19.3 and 19.4 in Chapter 19). Masses are round or oval in shape and may be well or poorly defined. Cavitation occurs in approximately 50% of cases. Cavities usually are thick walled with an irregular inner margin. Air-fluid levels may be present. Calcification of the masses does not occur.

With the progression of disease, nodules and masses tend to increase in size and number. With treatment, nodules usually resolve over a period of months. Typically, cavitary nodules and masses become thin walled and decrease in size with treatment. Complete resolution may occur.

SUGGESTED READINGS

Au V, Leung AN. Radiologic manifestations of lymphoma in the thorax. *AJR Am J Roentgenol.* 1997;168(1):93-98.

Balakrishnan J, Meziane MA, Siegelman SS, Fishman EK. Pulmonary infarction: CT appearance with pathologic correlation. *J Comput Assist Tomogr.* 1989;13(6):941-945.

Bankier AA, MacMahon H, Goo JMo, Rubin GD, Schaefer-Prokop CM, Naidich DP. Recommendations for measuring pulmonary nodules at CT: a statement from the Fleischner society. *Radiology.* 2017;285(2):584-600. doi:10.1148/radiol.2017162894

Bankoff MS, McEniff NJ, Bhadelia RA, Garcia-Moliner M, Daly BD. Prevalence of pathologically proven intrapulmonary lymph nodes and their appearance on CT. *AJR Am J Roentgenol.* 1996;167(3):629-630.

Bernard A, Azorin J, Bellenot F, et al. Resection of pulmonary nodules using video-assisted thoracic surgery. *Ann Thorac Surg.* 1996;61:202-204.

Calhoun P, Feldman PS, Armstrong P, et al. The clinical outcome of needle aspirations of the lung when cancer is not diagnosed. *Ann Thorac Surg.* 1986;41(6):592-596.

Davis SD. CT evaluation for pulmonary metastases in patients with extrathoracic malignancy. *Radiology.* 1991;180:1-12.

Dewan NA, Shehan CJ, Reeb SD, Gobar LS, Scott WJ, Ryschon K. Likelihood of malignancy in a solitary pulmonary nodule: comparison of Bayesian analysis and results of FDG-PET scan. *Chest.* 1997;112(2):416-422.

Fintelmann FJ, Bernheim A, Digumarthy SR, et al. The 10 pillars of lung cancer screening: rationale and logistics of a lung cancer screening program. *Radiographics.* 2015;35(7):1893-1908.

MacMahon H, Austin JH, Gamsu G, et al; Fleischner Society. Guidelines for management of small pulmonary nodules detected on CT scans: a statement from the Fleischner Society. *Radiology.* 2005;237(2):395-400.

Gaeta M, Pandolfo I, Volta S, et al. Bronchus sign on CT in peripheral carcinoma of the lung: value in predicting results of transbronchial biopsy. *AJR Am J Roentgenol.* 1991;157(6):1181-1185.

González Maldonado S, Delorme S, Hüsing A, et al. Evaluation of prediction models for identifying malignancy in pulmonary nodules detected via low-dose computed tomography. *JAMA Netw Open.* 2020;3(2):e1921221. doi:10.1001/jamanetworkopen.2019.21221

Gould MK, Fletcher J, Iannettoni MD, et al; American College of Chest Physicians. Evaluation of patients with pulmonary nodules: when is it lung cancer? ACCP evidence-based clinical practice guidelines (2nd ed.). *Chest.* 2007;132(3 suppl l):108S-130S.

Gupta NC, Maloof J, Gunel E. Probability of malignancy in solitary pulmonary nodules using fluorine-18-FDG and PET. *J Nucl Med.* 1996;37(6):943-948.

Gurney JW, Lyddon DM, McKay JA. Determining the likelihood of malignancy in solitary pulmonary nodules with Bayesian analysis. Part II: application. *Radiology.* 1993;186(2):415-422.

Gurney JW. Determining the likelihood of malignancy in solitary pulmonary nodules with Bayesian analysis. Part 1: theory. *Radiology.* 1993;186(2):405-413.

Hasegawa M, Sone S, Takashima S, et al. Growth rate of small lung cancers detected on mass CT screening. *Br J Radiol.* 2000;73(876):1252-1259.

Hirakata K, Nakata H, Haratake J. Appearance of pulmonary metastases on high-resolution CT scans: comparison with histopathologic findings from autopsy specimens. *AJR Am J Roentgenol.* 1993;161(1):37-43.

Huang RM, Naidich DP, Lubat E, Schinella R, Garay SM, McCauley DI. Septic pulmonary emboli: CT-radiographic correlation. *AJR Am J Roentgenol.* 1989;153(1):41-45.

Jang HJ, Lee KS, Kwon OJ, Rhee CH, Shim YM, Han J. Bronchioloalveolar carcinoma: focal area of ground-glass attenuation at thin-section CT as an early sign. *Radiology.* 1996;199(2):485-488.

Kakinuma R, Muramatsu Y, Kusumoto M, et al. Solitary pure ground-glass nodules 5 mm or smaller: frequency of growth. *Radiology.* 2015;276(3):873-882.

Kuhlman JE, Fishman EK, Siegelman SS. Invasive pulmonary aspergillosis in acute leukemia: characteristic findings on CT, the CT halo sign, and the role of CT in early diagnosis. *Radiology.* 1985;157(3):611-614.

Kui M, Templeton PA, White CS, Cai ZL, Bai YX, Cai YQ. Evaluation of the air bronchogram sign on CT in solitary pulmonary lesions. *J Comput Assist Tomogr.* 1996;20(6):983-986.

Kushihashi T, Munechika H, Ri K, et al. Bronchioloalveolar adenoma of the lung: CT-pathologic correlation. *Radiology.* 1994;193(3):789-793.

Larici AR, Farchione A, Franchi P, et al. Lung nodules: size still matters. *Eur Respir Rev.* 2017;26(146):170025. doi:10.1183/16000617.0025-2017

Li HQ, Boiselle PM, Shepard JO, Trotman-Dickenson B, McLoud TC. Diagnostic accuracy and safety of CT-guided percutaneous needle aspiration biopsy of the lung: comparison of small and large pulmonary nodules. *AJR Am J Roentgenol.* 1996;167(1):105-109.

Libby DM, Henschke CI, Yankelevitz DF. The solitary pulmonary nodule: update 1995. *Am J Med.* 1995;99(5):491-496.

MacMahon H, Naidich DP, Goo JM. Guidelines for management of incidental pulmonary nodules detected on CT images: from the Fleischner society 2017. *Radiology*. 2017;284(1):228-243. doi:10.1148/radiol.2017161659

Mahoney MC, Shipley RT, Corcoran HL, Dickson BA. CT demonstration of calcification in carcinoma of the lung. *AJR Am J Roentgenol*. 1990;154(2):255-258.

McWilliams A, Tammemagi MC, Mayo JR, et al. Probability of cancer in pulmonary nodules detected on first screening CT. *N Engl J Med*. 2013;369(10):910-919. doi:10.1056/NEJMoa1214726

Munden RF, Pugatch RD, Liptay MJ, Sugarbaker DJ, Le LU. Small pulmonary lesions detected at CT: clinical importance. *Radiology*. 1997;202(1):105-110.

Naidich DP, Bankier AA, MacMahon H, et al. Recommendations for the management of subsolid pulmonary nodules detected at CT: a statement from the Fleischner Society. *Radiology*. 2013;266(1):304-317.

Nathan MH, Collins VP, Adams RA. Differentiation of benign and malignant pulmonary nodules by growth rate. *Radiology*. 1962;79:221-232.

National Lung Screening Trial Research Team; Church TR, Black WC, Aberle DR, et al. Results of initial low-dose computed tomographic screening for lung cancer. *N Engl J Med*. 2013;368(21):1980-1991.

Patz EF, Lowe VJ, Hoffman JM, et al. Focal pulmonary abnormalities: evaluation with F-18 fluorodeoxyglucose PET scanning. *Radiology*. 1993;188(2):487-490.

Primack SL, Hartman TE, Lee KS, Müller NL. Pulmonary nodules and the CT halo sign. *Radiology*. 1994;190:513-515.

Quint LE, Park CH, Iannettoni MD. Solitary pulmonary nodules in patients with extrapulmonary neoplasms. *Radiology*. 2000;217(1):257-261.

Remy J, Remy-Jardin M, Giraud F, Wattinne L. Angioarchitecture of pulmonary arteriovenous malformations: clinical utility of three-dimensional helical CT. *Radiology*. 1994;191(3):657-664.

Schreuder A, Jacobs C, Scholten ET, Van Ginneken B, Schaefer-Prokop CM, Prokop M. Typical CT features of intrapulmonary lymph nodes: a review. *Radiol Cardiothorac Imaging*. 2020;2(4):e190159. doi:10.1148/ryct.2020190159

Schultz EM, Sanders GD, Trotter PR, et al. Validation of two models to estimate the probability of malignancy in patients with solitary pulmonary nodules. *Thorax*. 2008;63(4):335-341.

Siegelman et al., 1986 Siegelman SS, Khouri NF, Leo FP, Fishman EK, Braverman RM, Zerhouni EA. Solitary pulmonary nodules: CT assessment. *Radiology*. 1986;160(2):307-312.

Siegelman SS, Khouri NF, Scott WW, et al. Pulmonary hamartoma: CT findings. *Radiology*. 1986;160(2):313-317.

Theros EG. 1976 Caldwell Lecture: varying manifestation of peripheral pulmonary neoplasms—a radiologic-pathologic correlative study. *AJR Am J Roentgenol*. 1977;128(6):893-914.

Travis WD, Brambilla E, Noguchi M, et al. International association for the study of lung cancer/American Thoracic Society/European Respiratory Society International multidisciplinary classification of lung adenocarcinoma. *J Thorac Oncol*. 2011;6(2):244-285.

Travis WD, Brambilla E, Nicholson AG, et al. The 2015 World Health Organization classification of lung tumors: impact of genetic, clinical and radiologic advances since the 2004 classification. *J Thorac Oncol*. 2015;10(9):1243-1260.

Truong MT, Ko JP, Rossi SE, et al. Update in the evaluation of the solitary pulmonary nodule. *Radiographics*. 2014;34(6):1658-1679.

Webb WR. The pleural tail sign. *Radiology*. 1978;127(2):309-313.

Webb WR. Radiologic evaluation of the solitary pulmonary nodule. *AJR Am J Roentgenol*. 1990;154(4):701-708.

Weisbrod GL, Towers MJ, Chamberlain DW, Herman SJ, Matzinger FR. Thin-walled cystic lesions in bronchioalveolar carcinoma. *Radiology*. 1992;185(2):401-405.

Yankelevitz DF, Yip R, Smith JP, et al. CT screening for lung cancer: nonsolid nodules in baseline and annual repeat rounds. *Radiology*. 2015;277(2):555-564.

Zwiebel BR, Austin JHM, Grimes MM. Bronchial carcinoid tumors: assessment with CT of location and intratumoral calcification in 31 patients. *Radiology*. 1991;179(2):483-486.

Zwirewich CV, Vedal S, Miller RR, Müller NL. Solitary pulmonary nodule: high-resolution CT and radiologic-pathologic correlation. *Radiology*. 1991;179(2):469-476.

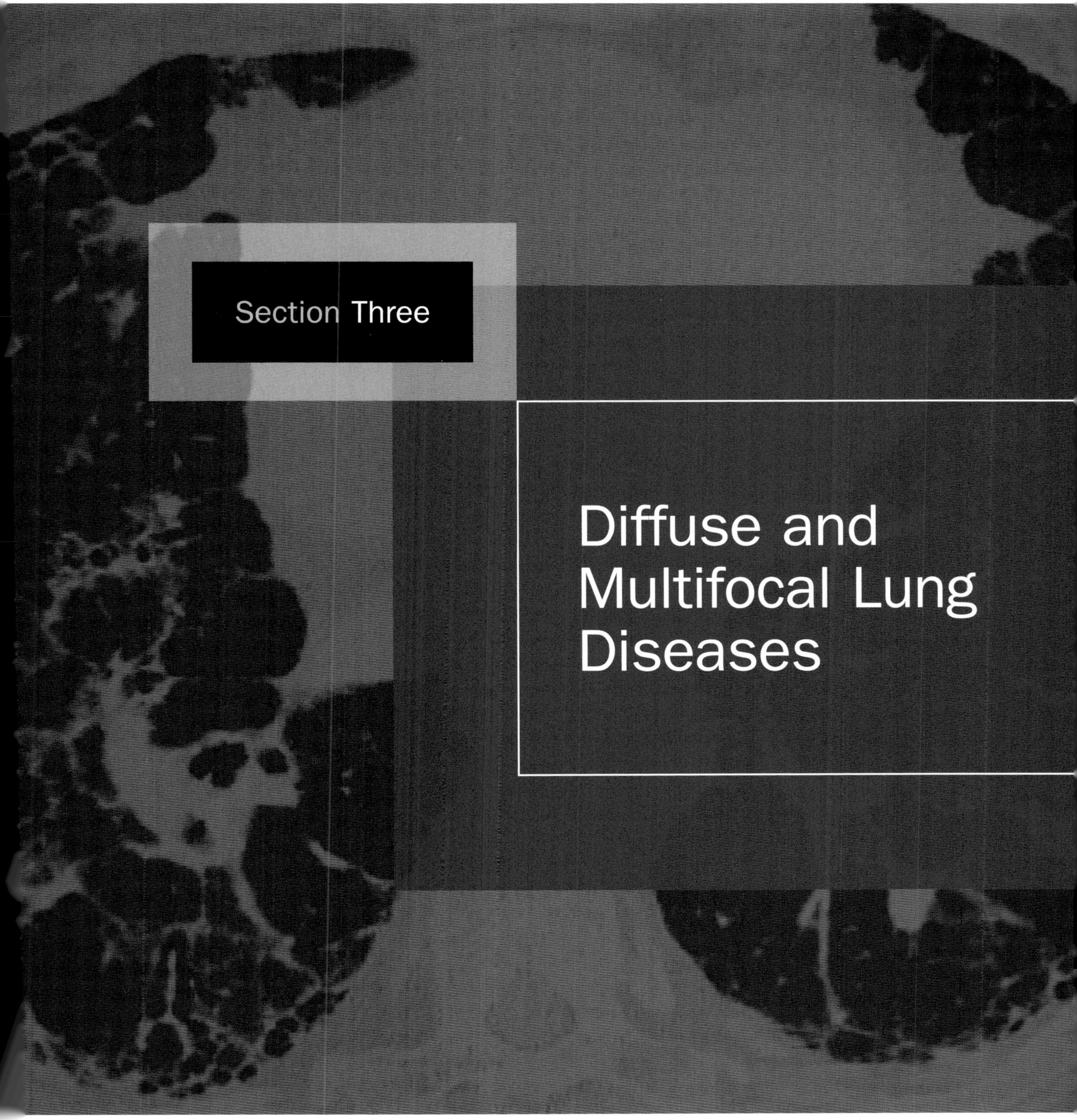

Section Three

Diffuse and Multifocal Lung Diseases

Chapter 11

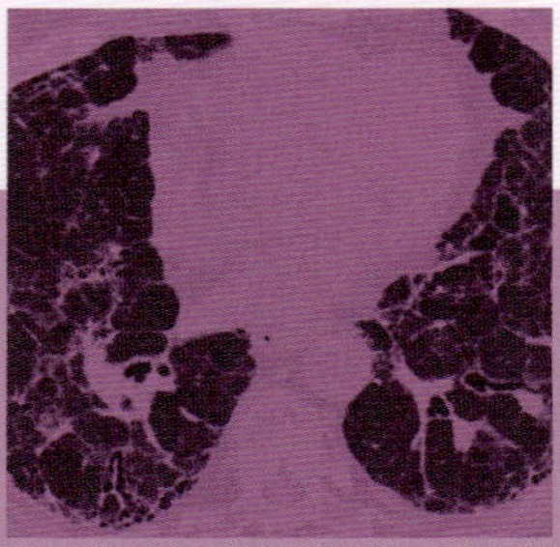

Travis S. Henry

Plain Film and Computed Tomographic Assessment of Diffuse Lung Disease

INTRODUCTION

Diffuse infiltrative lung diseases (DILDs) may be acute or chronic, involving the interstitium, alveolar spaces, or both. Specific DILDs are discussed in other chapters in this book. This chapter reviews the radiographic and high-resolution computed tomography (HRCT) diagnosis of DILDs, including a review of important findings and the differential diagnosis of various patterns of disease. Airways disease and emphysema, although diffuse lung diseases and often diagnosed with HRCT, are not considered DILDs and are discussed in Chapters 23 and 24.

PLAIN RADIOGRAPHIC ASSESSMENT OF DILD

On plain radiographs, infiltrative diseases usually are classified according to the pattern of abnormality they produce. There are six basic patterns:

1. Air-space or alveolar consolidation
2. Linear or septal
3. Reticular
4. Nodular
5. Reticulonodular
6. Ground-glass opacity (GGO)

Air-Space or Alveolar Consolidation

The terms *air-space consolidation* and *alveolar consolidation* refer to diseases associated with pathologic filling of alveoli (ie, replacement of alveolar air) as the predominant abnormality. As discussed in detail in Chapter 1, radiographic abnormalities indicating the presence of air-space or alveolar disease include (1) confluent or homogeneous opacities obscuring vessels, (2) air bronchograms, (3) ill-defined or fluffy opacities, (4) air alveolograms, (5) air-space or "acinar" nodules, (6) preserved lung volume, and (7) a tendency for opacities to extend to pleural surfaces.

The differential diagnosis of diffuse air-space consolidation is reviewed in detail in Chapter 1 and Table 1.1. Simply stated, alveolar filling may be caused by:

1. Water (eg, pulmonary edema)
2. Blood (eg, pulmonary hemorrhage)
3. Pus (eg, pneumonia)
4. Cells (eg, eosinophilic pneumonia, organizing pneumonia [OP])
5. Other substances (eg, lipoprotein in alveolar proteinosis, lipid in lipoid pneumonia, mucin in invasive mucinous adenocarcinoma [IMA])

Linear or Septal Pattern

A linear pattern is defined by the presence of Kerley A or B lines. Kerley A and B lines result from thickening of interlobular septa; this pattern also may be referred to as *septal* (Table 11.1).

Kerley B lines are most common (Fig. 11.1). They are horizontal lines, 1 to 2 cm in length. They are seen in contact with the pleural surface and are best seen laterally at the costophrenic angles. The characteristic appearance of Kerley B lines results from the consistent size and regular organization of pulmonary lobules at the lung bases.

Kerley A lines are seen less often. They are oblique in orientation, several centimeters in length, and located within

Table 11.1 Linear or Septal Pattern: Differential Diagnosis

Pulmonary edema (hydrostatic most common), typically symmetric
Lymphangitic spread of neoplasm, often asymmetric
Chronic or recurrent pulmonary hemorrhage and hemosiderosis
Pulmonary fibrosis (sarcoidosis most common)

the central or parahilar lung. Kerley A lines (Fig. 11.2) also represent thickened septa, but their appearance is different from that of B lines because of the different arrangement of pulmonary lobules in the central lungs.

Kerley C lines are seen at the lung bases and represent interlobular septa en face rather than in profile. They result in a nonspecific, reticular pattern and are unimportant in diagnosis, because B lines invariably are visible as well.

Peribronchial cuffing results from thickening of the peribronchovascular interstitium and also contributes to a linear pattern. This abnormality is seen as thickening of end-on bronchi or as lines radiating outward from the hila. To some extent, peribronchial cuffing contributes to the appearance of Kerley A lines on chest radiographs.

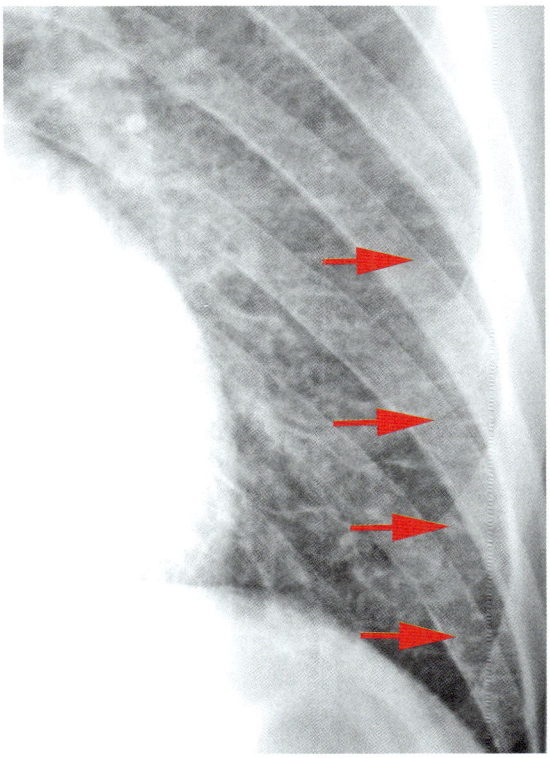

Figure 11.1. Kerley B lines. Coned-down views of the left lateral costophrenic angle in a patient with cardiogenic interstitial pulmonary edema. Thin horizontal lines in the lung periphery, 1 to 2 cm in length, represent Kerley B lines (*arrows*). Kerley B lines result from thickened interlobular septa.

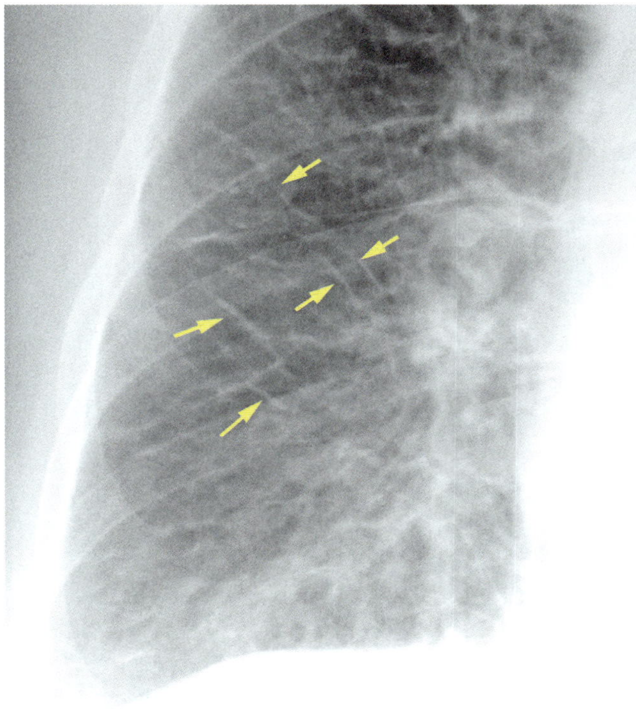

Figure 11.2. Kerley A lines. A patient with pulmonary edema associated with fluid overload shows multiple Kerley A lines. Thin oblique lines in the parahilar lung (*arrows*) represent A lines. Thickening of the minor fissure also is seen.

Well-defined and easily recognized Kerley lines are indicative of interstitial lung disease and have a limited differential diagnosis. They are typical of interstitial pulmonary edema and lymphangitic spread of carcinoma. Edema usually is symmetrical. Lymphangitic spread often is asymmetrical; asymmetrical Kerley lines strongly suggest lymphangitic spread of carcinoma. Other causes are rare.

Although consolidation may be seen with any type of pulmonary edema (eg, hydrostatic, increased permeability with or without diffuse alveolar damage, or mixed), a septal pattern more often represents hydrostatic edema or increased permeability edema occurring in the absence of diffuse alveolar damage (see Chapter 11). A septal pattern also can result from chronic or recurrent pulmonary hemorrhage and hemosiderosis.

Pulmonary fibrosis sometimes can result in well-defined Kerley lines, but a reticular pattern is more typical.

Reticular Pattern

"Reticular" means "netlike," which is an excellent description of the appearance of this pattern. A reticular pattern is characterized by multiple intersecting lines, often irregular in appearance, outlining what appear to be round or irregular "spaces" (Fig. 11.3). Although a few Kerley lines may

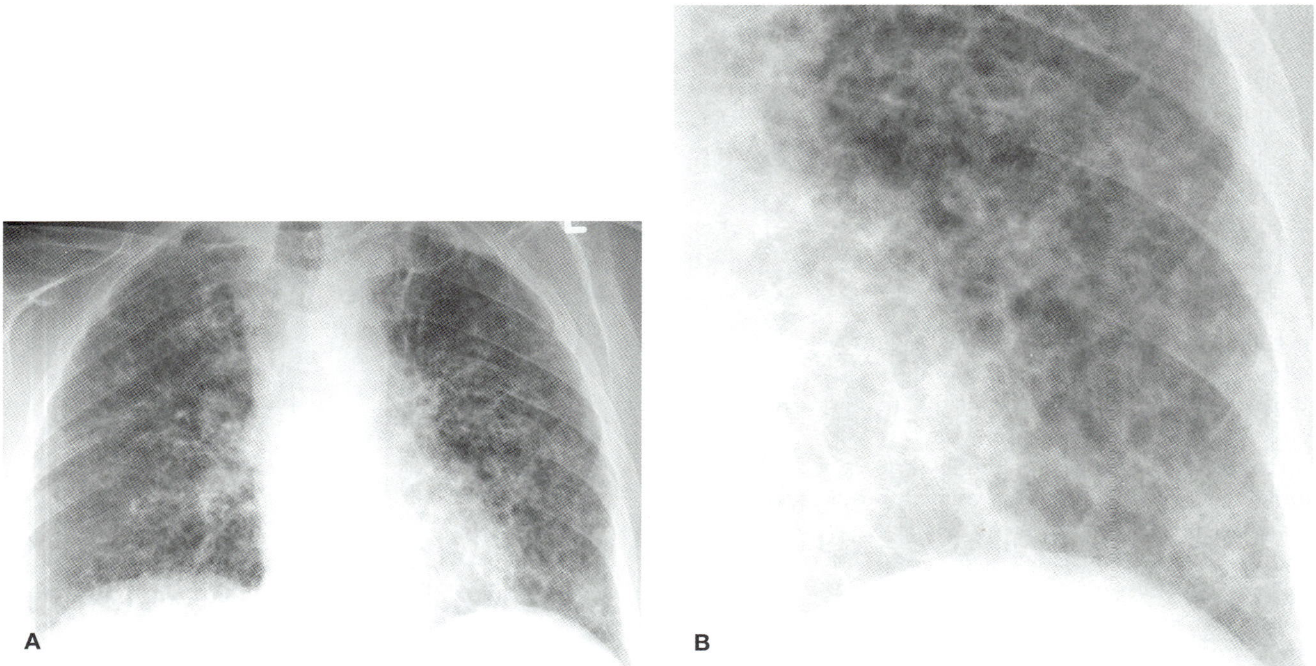

Figure 11.3. Reticular pattern in rheumatoid lung disease. **A:** Chest radiograph shows decreased lung volumes and irregular reticular opacities at the lung bases. Kerley B lines are inconspicuous. The lines appear to outline spaces 1 cm or less in diameter, representing a medium reticular pattern. **B:** Coned-down view of the left lower lobe in the same patient shows the irregular reticular pattern.

be visible, they do not predominate (if they did, the pattern would be linear). A reticular pattern indicates the presence of interstitial lung disease (Table 11.2).

The reticular pattern has been subdivided into three subpatterns, based on the size of the "spaces" surrounded by lines: a fine pattern ("spaces" smaller than 3 mm; Fig. 11.4), a medium pattern ("spaces" 3-10 mm; Fig. 11.5), and coarse pattern ("spaces" larger than 10 mm; Fig. 11.6). It should be kept in mind, however, that the size of the spaces visible on chest radiograph does not necessarily reflect the presence or size of any "spaces" present pathologically. Superimposition of the reticular opacities often confuses the picture; in the presence of extensive reticulation, the outlined spaces usually appear smaller than they really are (see Fig. 11.4). Medium or coarse patterns are the most common and the most easily seen on chest radiographs.

Table 11.2 Reticular Pattern: Differential Diagnosis

Usual Interstitial Pneumonia
Idiopathic pulmonary fibrosis
Collagen vascular disease
Drug-related fibrosis
Asbestosis
End-stage hypersensitivity pneumonitis
End-stage sarcoidosis
Nonspecific interstitial pneumonia
Radiation
End-stage adult respiratory distress syndrome
Cystic Lung Disease
Langerhans cell histiocytosis
Lymphangiomyomatosis
Tuberous sclerosis
Sjögren syndrome with LIP
Lymphoid interstitial pneumonia (LIP)
Birt-Hogg-Dube syndrome
Cystic bronchiectasis
Pneumonia with pneumatoceles (eg, pneumocystis)
Papillomatosis

A medium pattern is typical of patients with pulmonary fibrosis and "honeycombing"; the reticulation often appears to have a peripheral, posterior, and lower lobe predominance. The abnormality usually is best seen on the lateral view, just above the diaphragm, in the posterior costophrenic angles. Because of lung fibrosis, lung volumes usually appear reduced.

Honeycombing with a medium reticular pattern usually indicates the presence of *usual interstitial pneumonia* (UIP). UIP can be seen in a variety of conditions; however, over 90% of cases of honeycombing result from a small group of diseases, including idiopathic pulmonary fibrosis (IPF), collagen vascular disease, drug-related fibrosis, asbestosis, fibrotic hypersensitivity pneumonitis, or end-stage sarcoidosis. *Nonspecific interstitial pneumonia* (NSIP) less commonly results in honeycombing; it often is associated with collagen vascular disease. Honeycombing also may result from radiation lung fibrosis, as an end stage of acute respiratory distress syndrome, and other entities. Lung volumes are characteristically reduced in the presence of honeycombing.

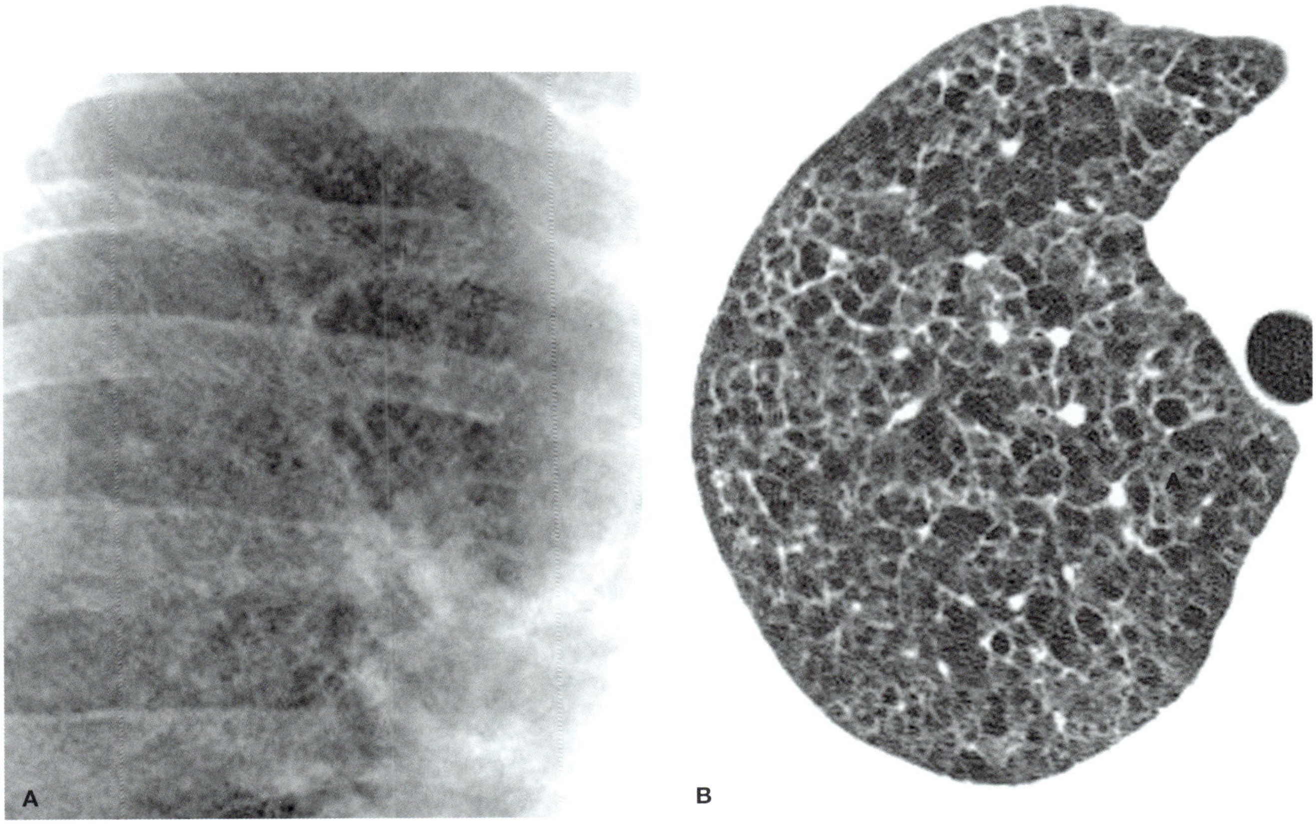

Figure 11.4. Fine reticular pattern in Langerhans cell histiocytosis. **A:** Coned-down view of the right upper lobe shows fine reticular opacities with poor definition of pulmonary arteries. **B:** HRCT shows cystic disease. Superimposition of the cyst walls results in the fine reticular pattern that is visible on chest radiographs.

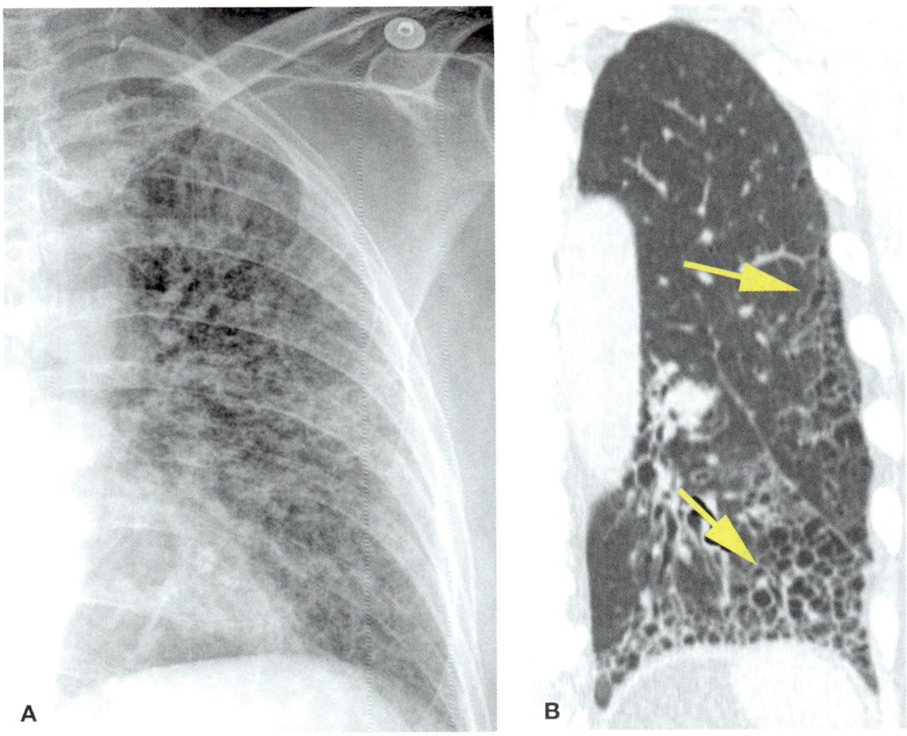

Figure 11.5. Medium reticular pattern in rheumatoid lung disease. **A:** Chest radiograph shows irregular reticular opacities, best classified as a medium pattern. **B:** Coronal HRCT through the left lung in a different patient with rheumatoid lung disease and usual interstitial pneumonia shows honeycombing (*arrows*).

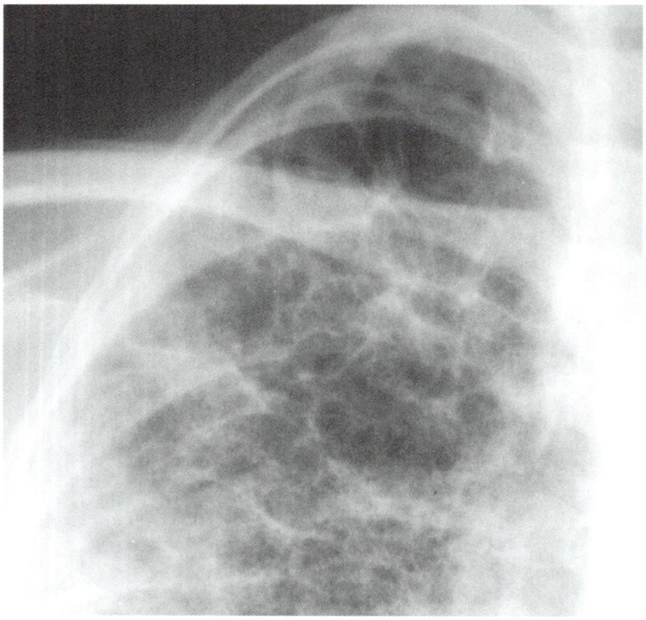

Figure 11.6. Coarse reticular pattern in cystic lung disease. Coned-down view of the right apex shows reticular opacities outlining spaces exceeding 1 cm.

Some cystic lung diseases (eg, Langerhans cell histiocytosis [LCH], lymphangioleiomyomatosis [LAM]) result in a reticular pattern because of superimposition of the walls of cysts ranging in size from several millimeters to several centimeters in diameter (see Fig. 11.6). Depending on the size of the cysts, the pattern may be fine, medium, or coarse. This appearance can mimic honeycombing, but significant lung fibrosis is absent, and lung volumes are not reduced. In fact, in many such patients, lung volumes appear increased. An upper lobe predominance may be seen rather than predominance at the lung bases, depending on the responsible disease.

A fine reticular pattern may indicate fine lung fibrosis or lung infiltration by a variety of processes (see Fig. 11.4). This pattern is less common, more difficult to see, and less specific.

Nodular Pattern

Innumerable small nodules, ranging from a few millimeters to 1 cm in diameter, may indicate interstitial or air-space disease. The differential diagnosis of multiple larger nodules and masses is reviewed in Chapter 9.

Interstitial nodules usually are sharply marginated, despite being very small (Figs. 11.7 and 11.8). Air-space disease also may result in nodules (air-space or acinar nodules), typically 5 to 10 mm in diameter and poorly marginated. The term *miliary pattern* describes the presence of diffuse or widespread, well-defined nodules, 2 to 3 mm or less in diameter (see Figs. 11.7 and 11.8). Miliary nodules usually are interstitial.

Nearly all patients with nodules visible on chest radiographs that are 5 mm or less in size, either well-defined or ill-defined, have a predominant interstitial abnormality; many will have metastases (Fig. 11.9) or a granulomatous disease (see Figs. 11.7 and 11.8; Table 11.3). Granulomatous diseases that may produce this appearance include infections (eg, miliary tuberculosis and fungus), noninfectious granulomatous diseases (eg, sarcoidosis, Langerhans

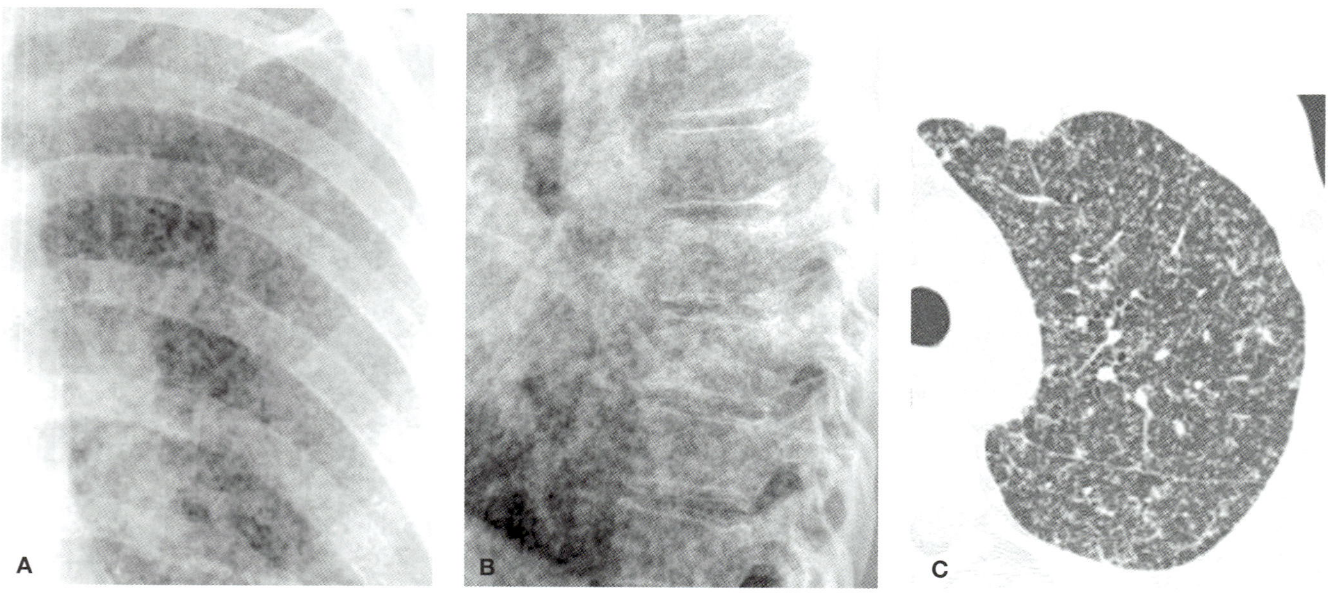

Figure 11.7. Miliary nodules in hematogenous spread of coccidioidomycosis. Coned-down views from PA (**A**) and lateral (**B**) radiographs show innumerable nodules a few millimeters in diameter. **C:** HRCT shows innumerable, very small lung nodules in a random distribution.

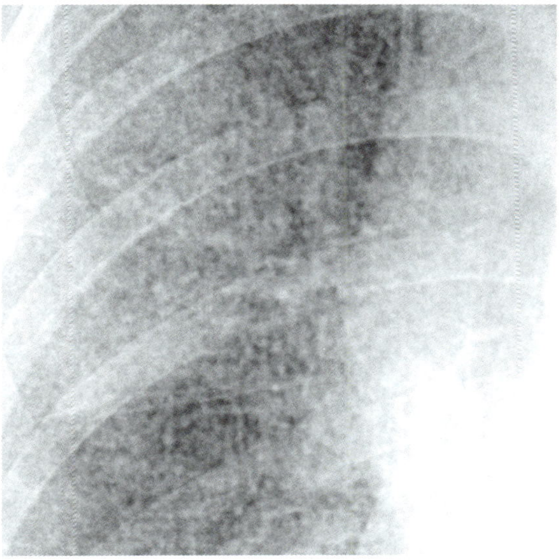

Figure 11.8. Miliary tuberculosis. Coned-down view of the right upper lobe shows innumerable, discrete, very small nodules.

histiocytosis), and some pneumoconioses (primarily silicosis and coal worker's pneumoconiosis [CWP]). Metastases tend to have a basal predominance because of greater blood flow to the bases; the granulomatous diseases and pneumoconioses, for a variety of reasons, often have an upper lobe predominance.

Nodules measuring 5 to 10 mm in diameter may be seen in these same diseases but are more typical of infection, particularly endobronchial spread of infection or bronchopneumonia. Common causes include tuberculosis (Fig. 11.10) and other mycobacterial, bacterial, viral infections such as cytomegalovirus or varicella, and *Pneumocystis* infection in patients with AIDS. Other causes of air-space consolidation also may result in ill-defined nodules. IMA often results in this appearance.

Reticulonodular Pattern

The term *reticulonodular*, indicating a perceived combination of lines and dots, is used commonly by radiologists but

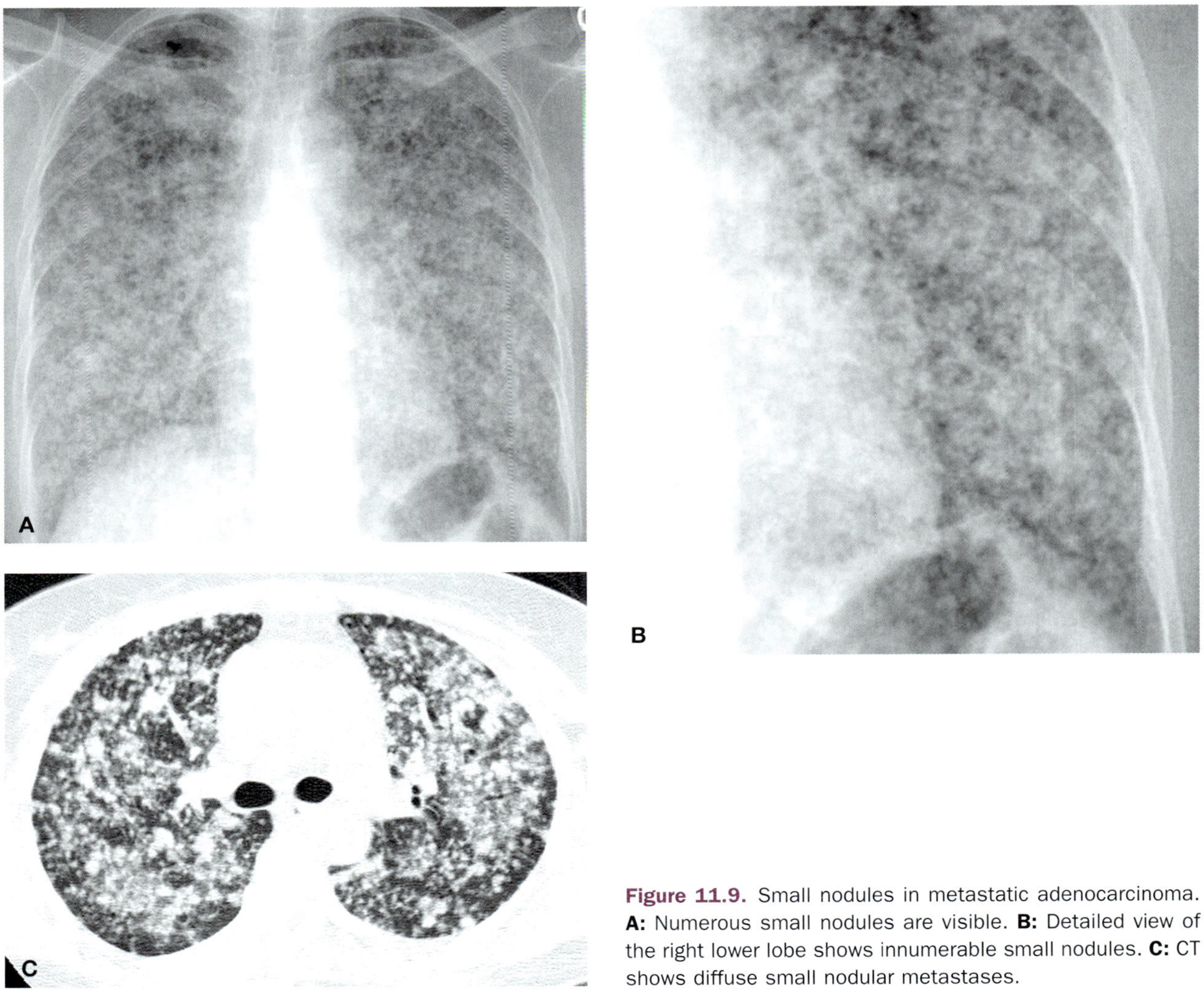

Figure 11.9. Small nodules in metastatic adenocarcinoma. **A:** Numerous small nodules are visible. **B:** Detailed view of the right lower lobe shows innumerable small nodules. **C:** CT shows diffuse small nodular metastases.

Table 11.3 Nodular Pattern: Differential Diagnosis

Metastases: Diffuse or basal, well-defined
Invasive mucinous adenocarcinoma (diffuse or patchy, ill-defined)
Miliary tuberculosis (diffuse, well-defined, may be upper lobe)
Miliary fungus or nontuberculous mycobacterium (diffuse, well-defined)
Sarcoidosis (upper lobe, may be asymmetric, adenopathy)
Silicosis and coal worker's pneumoconiosis (posterior, upper lobe, symmetric, adenopathy with eggshell calcification)
Histiocytosis (upper lobe predominance, cysts)
Hypersensitivity pneumonitis (ill-defined)
Endobronchial infection (diffuse or patchy, ill-defined)

is of limited value in diagnosis. Reticulonodular opacities observed on plain radiographs often are artifactual, resulting from the superimposition of mostly lines or mostly nodules. Thus, it is generally a good idea, if a reticulonodular pattern appears to be present on plain radiographs, to decide whether a reticular or nodular pattern predominates and use that finding for differential diagnosis. Cases actually characterized histologically by a combination of reticular and nodular opacities are relatively uncommon but include sarcoidosis, lymphangitic spread of tumor, and diffuse amyloidosis.

Ground-Glass Opacity

GGO represents an increase in lung density without the presence of frank consolidation (Fig. 11.11A). A slight

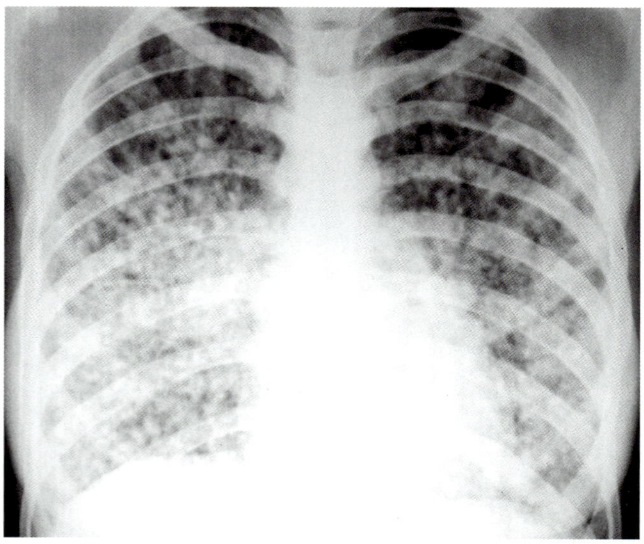

Figure 11.10. Endobronchial spread of tuberculosis. Ill-defined nodules ranging from 5 to 10 mm in diameter are visible.

A

B

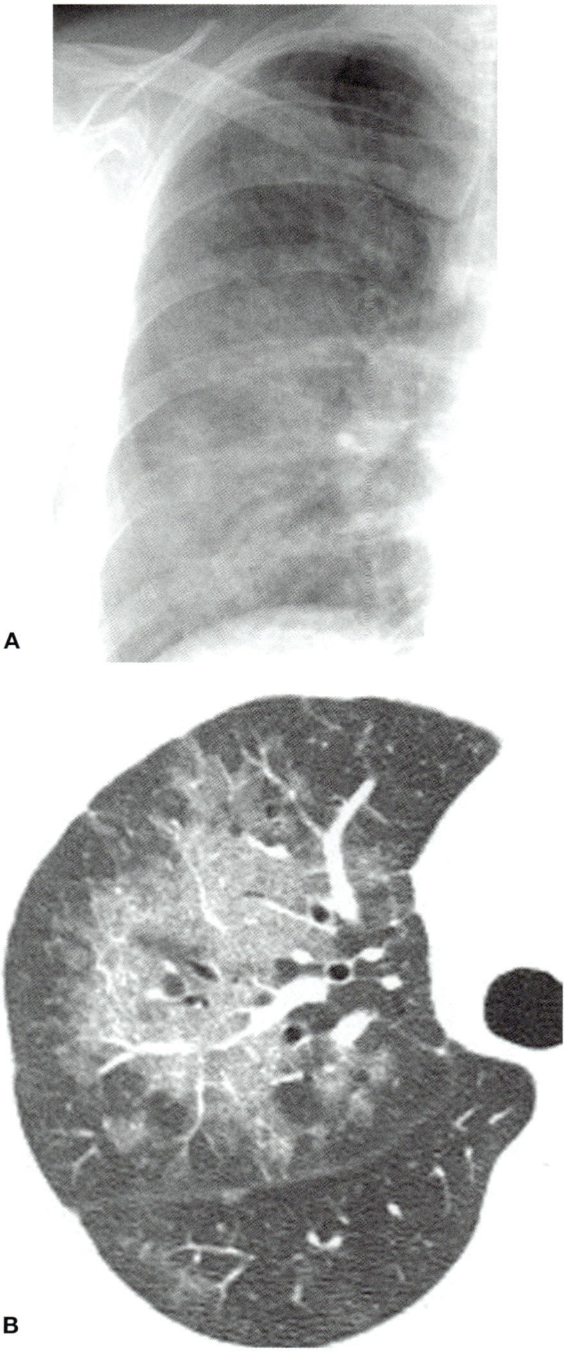

Figure 11.11. Ground-glass opacity in exogenous lipoid pneumonia. **A:** Chest radiograph shows a subtle increase in lung opacity in the right parahilar region. Pulmonary vessels are poorly defined. **B:** HRCT coned down to the right lung shows patchy ground-glass opacity.

fuzziness of pulmonary vessels is usually visible, but this abnormality can be quite subtle and difficult to diagnose with certainty. It is a nonspecific pattern (see the following section on HRCT) and may indicate the presence of either air-space disease or interstitial disease. Because it is nonspecific, its differential diagnosis is very long. It may be seen with edema, hemorrhage, infections, and a wide variety of different DILDs. When visible on a chest film, it is best evaluated by assessment of the history and clinical presentation in patients with acute symptoms or by further imaging (eg, HRCT) in patients with chronic symptoms (see Fig. 11.11B).

HRCT ASSESSMENT OF DILDS

HRCT techniques optimize the radiographic demonstration of lung architecture and are invaluable in the assessment of patients with suspected DILD. The use of thin collimation (1.5 mm or less) and a high-resolution algorithm for image reconstruction are essential.

HRCT may be obtained with volumetric imaging or with spaced axial scans. In current practice, volumetric imaging is most commonly employed. Using a reduced or modulated mA with volumetric imaging results in a significant reduction in radiation dose. Spaced axial images (eg, every 1 cm) are usually sufficient for diagnosis of a diffuse lung disease and this technique is inherently low dose.

Obtaining prone scans in addition to supine imaging is advisable in a patient with suspected DILD, at least for the initial HRCT examination. Some dependent (posterior) lung collapse often is seen on supine scans (Fig. 11.12A). Prone scans are valuable in distinguishing true posterior lung disease from dependent collapse; posterior lung collapse disappears in the prone position (Fig. 11.12B). If spaced axial imaging is employed, scanning at 1-cm intervals in both the supine and the prone positions would be an appropriate protocol. In patients having volumetric HRCT, prone scans may be obtained volumetrically or at spaced intervals. Patients with normal or minimal chest film abnormalities benefit the most from prone scans. Prone scans are not generally needed in patients being imaged for diagnosis of airway disease, chronic obstructive pulmonary disease, infections, tumors, or neoplasm.

Postexpiratory scans at selected levels can demonstrate air trapping and may be valuable in diagnosing airway disease in patients with normal inspiratory scans.

NORMAL ANATOMY: THE SECONDARY PULMONARY LOBULE AND ACINUS

A *secondary pulmonary lobule* (also simply known as a *pulmonary lobule*) ranges from 1 to 2.5 cm in size and is marginated by connective tissue interlobular septa, which contain pulmonary veins and lymphatics (Figs. 11.13 and 11.14). Within the peripheral lung, normal interlobular septa are at the lower limit of HRCT resolution. On clinical HRCT in normal patients, a few interlobular septa often can be seen, but they tend to be inconspicuous.

The central portion of the secondary lobule, referred to as *centrilobular*, contains the pulmonary artery and bronchiole that supply the lobule. The pulmonary artery supplying a secondary lobule measures somewhat less than 1 mm in diameter and can be seen in normal lungs as a dot or branching structure 5 to 10 mm from the pleural surface; the centrilobular bronchiole is normally invisible.

An *acinus* is the largest unit of lung structure in which all airways participate in gas exchange. Anatomically, it is located distal to a terminal bronchiole and is supplied by a first-order respiratory bronchiole (see Fig. 11.13). Acini average 7 to 8 mm in diameter. A pulmonary lobule usually consists of a dozen or fewer acini, although large lobules may contain twice that number. Acini are not visible on HRCT.

HRCT FINDINGS IN DILDS

Chest radiographs are normal in 10% to 15% of patients with interstitial lung disease. HRCT is more sensitive, specific, and accurate. HRCT characterizes morphologic abnormalities

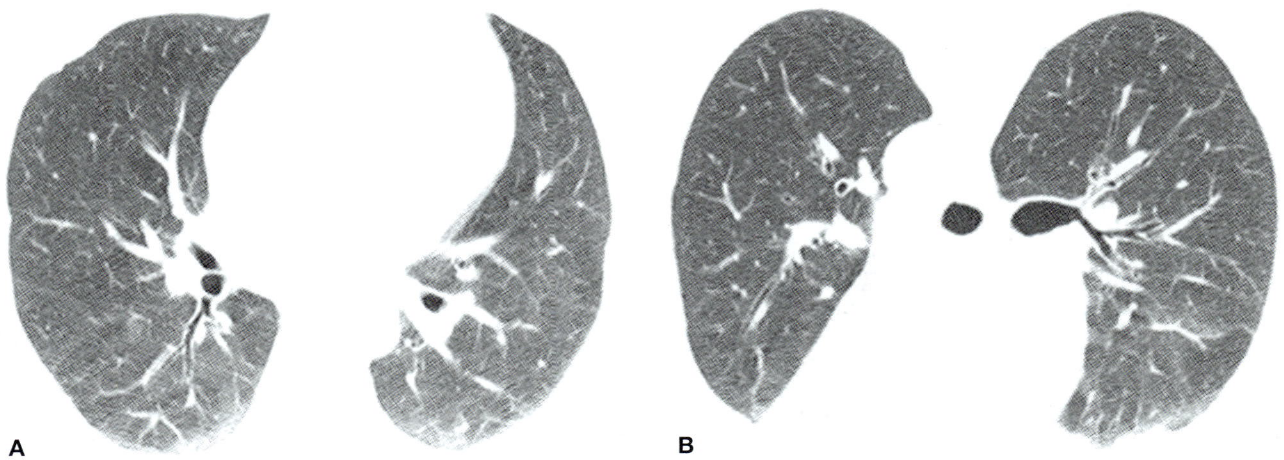

Figure 11.12. Normal dependent lung collapse and the use of prone scans. **A:** Supine HRCT in a normal subject shows increased opacity in the posterior (dependent) lung. This appearance cannot be distinguished from lung disease. **B:** Prone scan shows that the posterior lung is normal.

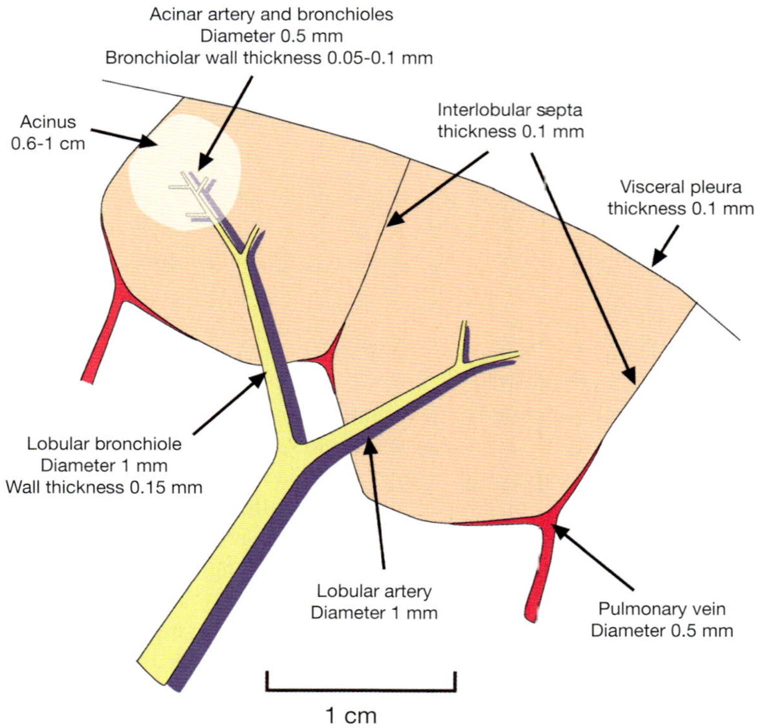

Figure 11.13. Normal anatomy of the pulmonary lobule. Two lobules are shown.

much more precisely and allows a more accurate diagnosis than do chest radiographs.

An approach to the HRCT diagnosis of DILD is fundamentally based on the recognition of specific abnormalities, together with an assessment of their distribution. Generally speaking, HRCT findings of lung disease can be considered in four groups or categories, which reflect the types of histologic abnormalities present. These abnormalities include reticular opacities, nodular opacities, increased lung opacity, and decreased lung opacity and cystic lesions. Within each of these four categories, a relatively short list of findings may be recognized. Although some findings (eg, "tree-in-bud" pattern, emphysema, mosaic perfusion, and air trapping) are features of airways and obstructive lung diseases rather than DILD, they are discussed briefly in this chapter in order to describe an overall approach to HRCT.

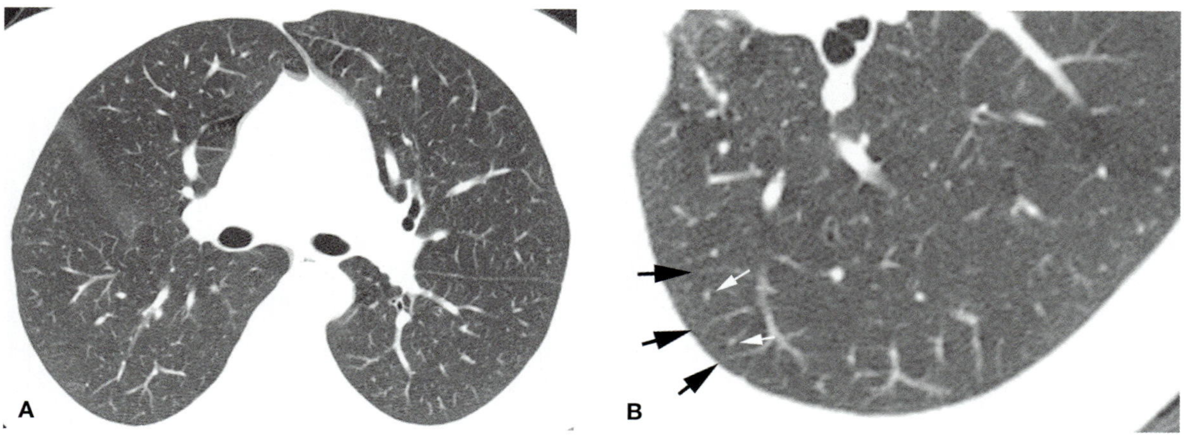

Figure 11.14. Normal HRCT. **A:** The lung appears homogeneous in attenuation, with the posterior lung appearing slightly denser than the anterior lung. Fissures are smooth and uniform in thickness. Vessels are smooth in contour and sharply marginated. The most peripheral vessels visible are 5 to 10 mm from the pleural surface and represent centrilobular arteries or, sometimes, veins in interlobular septa. Centrilobular bronchioles and interlobular septa are not visible. **B:** Coned-down HRCT of the left lower lobe. Two pulmonary lobules are outlined by pulmonary veins within interlobular septa (*black arrows*). Centrilobular arteries are visible as dots (*white arrows*).

Reticular Opacities

Thickening of the interstitial fiber network of the lung by fluid or fibrous tissue, or because of cellular infiltration, results in an increase in reticular lung opacities.

Interlobular Septal Thickening

Thickened interlobular septa can be recognized as such because they outline what can be recognized as pulmonary lobules, because of their characteristic size and shape. In the peripheral lung, thickened septa measure 1 to 2 cm in length and often are seen extending to the pleural surface; in the central lung, the thickened septa can outline lobules that are 1 to 2.5 cm in diameter and appear polygonal in shape (Figs. 11.15 and 11.16). Visible lobules commonly contain a central dotlike or branching centrilobular artery.

Associated findings, regardless of the cause of septal thickening, often include peribronchial interstitial thickening recognized as peribronchial cuffing, thickening of fissures, and abnormal prominence of the centrilobular arteries because of thickening of the interstitium that surrounds them (see Fig. 11.16).

Septal thickening can be smooth, nodular, or irregular in contour in different pathologic processes. *Smooth septal thickening* is most typical of pulmonary edema (see Fig. 11.15), lymphangitic spread of tumor (see Fig. 11.16), or, rarely, deposition of material such as amyloid protein (Table 11.4). *Nodular septal thickening* reflects a perilymphatic distribution of nodules and is typical of sarcoidosis and lymphangitic spread of tumor. Septal thickening is not common in patients with interstitial fibrosis; other reticular patterns usually predominate. When visible, septal thickening due to fibrosis often is irregular in appearance and associated with distortion of lung architecture.

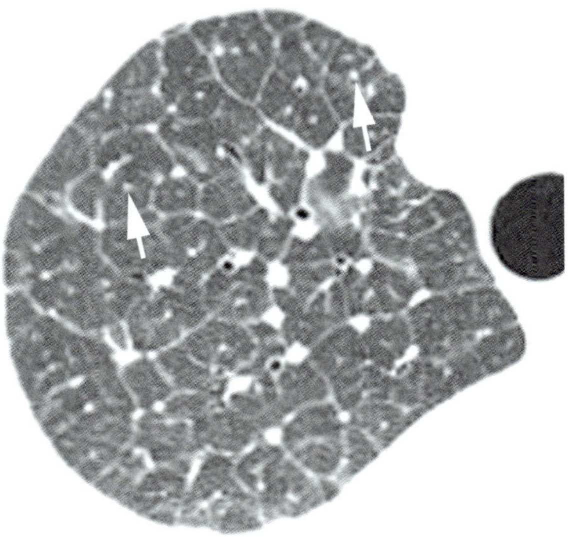

Figure 11.15. Interlobular septal thickening in interstitial pulmonary edema. Smooth thickening of numerous septa is visible in the right lung. The thickened septa outline lobules of characteristic size and shape. Centrilobular arteries (*arrows*) are visible within many of the lobules.

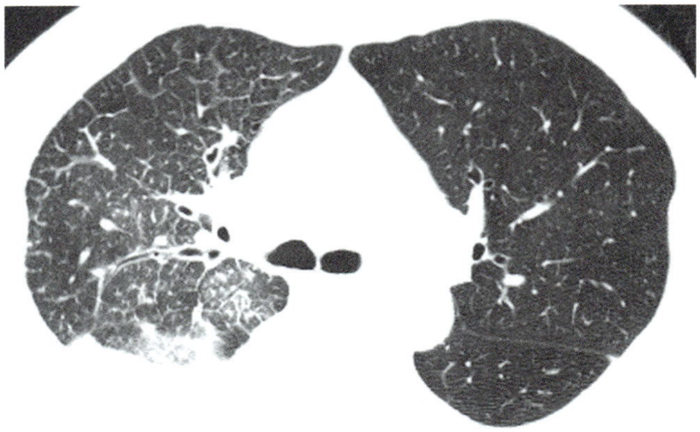

Figure 11.16. Interlobular septal thickening in lymphangitic spread of lung cancer. Smooth thickening of septa is visible within the right lung. The left lung appears normal. Peribronchial interstitial thickening recognized as peribronchial cuffing on the right. The right bronchi appear thicker walled than do those on the left. A right pleural effusion also is present.

Honeycombing

Honeycombing reflects extensive lung fibrosis with alveolar destruction and results in a characteristic reticular appearance. On HRCT, necessary findings for the diagnosis of honeycombing are

1. air-filled (ie, black) cysts
2. the cysts have a thick (ie, easily recognizable) wall
3. the cysts are usually from 3 mm to 1 cm in diameter (although they may be larger or smaller in some cases)
4. cysts are immediately beneath the pleural surface
5. cysts share walls

Three cysts in a row, at the pleural surface, is a minimum for the diagnosis of honeycombing; scattered isolated cysts are not sufficient for this diagnosis (Fig. 11.17). When extensive honeycombing is present, the cysts occur in several layers and characteristically share walls (Fig. 11.17).

Table 11.4 Smooth Interlobular Septal Thickening: Differential Diagnosis

Lymphangitic spread of tumor (asymmetrical or symmetrical)
Pulmonary edema (symmetrical)
Amyloidosis (rare)
Lymphoid interstitial pneumonia
Lymphoma or Leukemia
Lymphangiomatosis
Erdheim-Chester disease

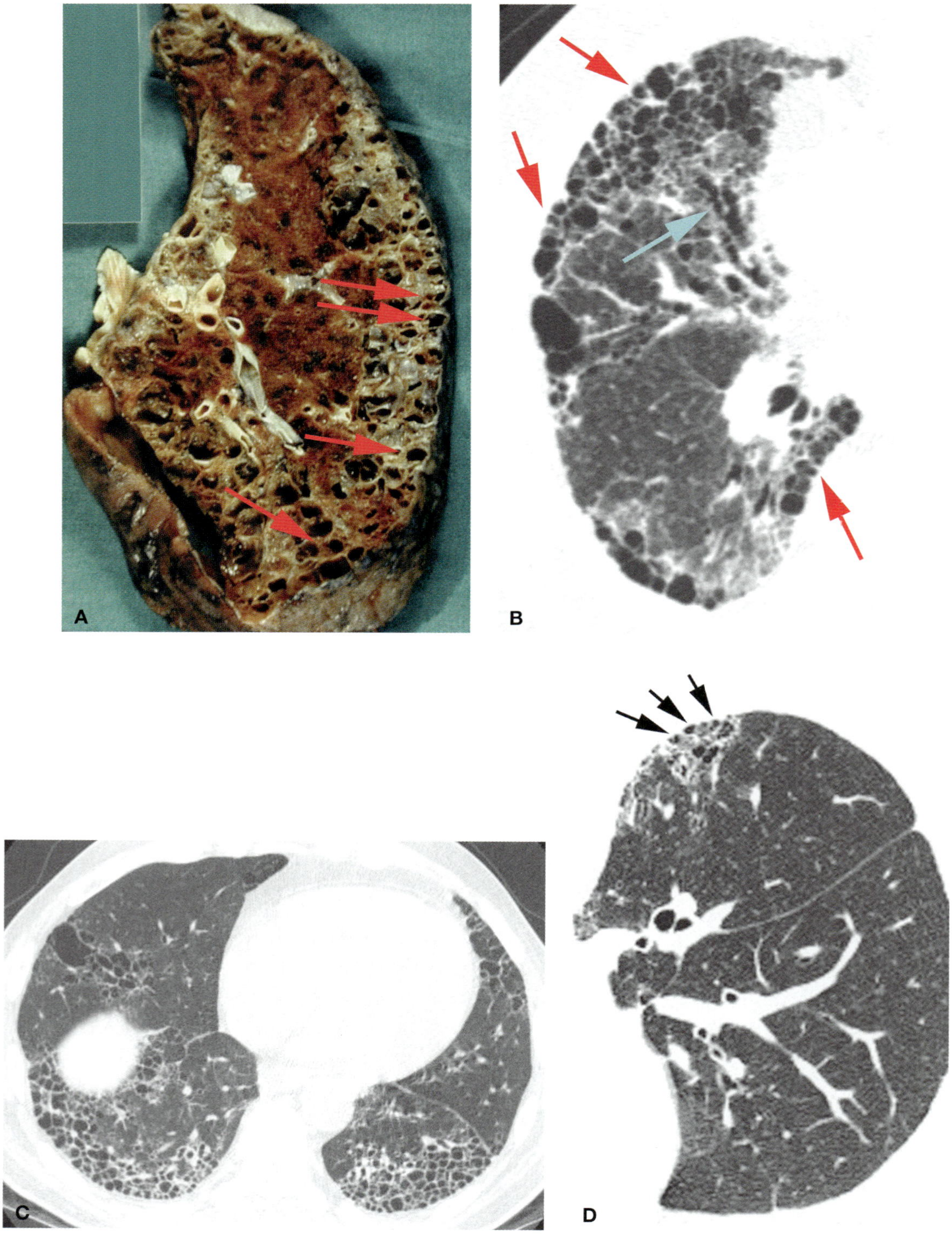

Figure 11.17. Honeycombing. **A:** A lung slice in a patient with usual interstitial pneumonia (UIP) and idiopathic pulmonary fibrosis (IPF). Patchy areas of subpleural honeycombing (*arrows*) are visible. The cysts are air filled, thick walled, and less than 1 cm in diameter. They share walls and occur in multiple layers in the subpleural lung. **B:** Honeycombing in a patient with UIP and IPF. Honeycombing is visible in the peripheral lung (*red arrows*). Cysts tend to be clustered. A reticular pattern and traction bronchiectasis is also present (*blue arrow*). **C:** Honeycombing in a patient with UIP associated with rheumatoid arthritis. **D:** Mild honeycombing in a patient with lupus. Focal fibrosis is visible posteriorly on a prone scan. A cluster of subpleural honeycomb cysts are visible (*arrows*).

Cysts that are not at the pleural surface may or may not represent honeycombing.

When honeycombing is present, normal lung architecture is distorted, and secondary lobules are difficult or impossible to recognize. Associated findings of fibrosis, including reticular opacities, traction bronchiectasis, and traction bronchiolectasis, are usually present.

The presence of honeycombing usually predicts the presence of UIP, although a basal and peripheral predominance is also required for making this diagnosis. The differential diagnosis of honeycombing is that of UIP and includes IPF, which accounts for 60% to 70% of cases of honeycombing; collagen vascular diseases (most often rheumatoid arthritis and scleroderma); fibrotic drug reactions; asbestosis; chronic or end-stage hypersensitivity pneumonitis; and, occasionally, sarcoidosis (Table 11.5). This appearance also may be seen with fibrotic NSIP, but honeycombing in NSIP tends to be inconspicuous and of minimal extent.

The identification of honeycombing on HRCT is of great clinical importance for the following reasons:

1. It indicates fibrotic lung disease, although further progression can be seen in patients with honeycombing.
2. It indicates that a lung biopsy probably will not prove diagnostic (other than showing UIP). Lung biopsy is not often performed in patients with obvious honeycombing on HRCT.
3. In a patient without an associated disease (eg, collagen vascular disease) or exposure (eg, asbestos, drugs, organic antigens), IPF is likely the diagnosis.
4. It points to a poor prognosis in patients with IPF (the 5-year survival rate in patients with IPF is 20% without treatment, although antifibrotic drugs may slow the progression of disease).

Nonspecific Reticular Patterns

Reticular patterns other than interlobular septal thickening and honeycombing are somewhat nonspecific and may indicate lung fibrosis or lung infiltration without fibrosis. The reticular opacities may be very fine or coarse and irregular. Fine reticulation often reflects the presence of intralobular interstitial thickening (ie, *intralobular lines*) or thickening of the lung interstitium at a sublobular level (Fig. 11.18).

Intralobular lines may represent mild fibrosis, and a clue is associated "traction bronchiectasis" (Fig. 11.18A). Intralobular lines may be seen in association with GGO, nodules, or other findings in patients with infiltrative or inflammatory lung disease (see Fig. 11.18B). When this is the case, it is most appropriate to ignore the reticulation and base the differential diagnosis on the other findings present.

Table 11.5 Honeycombing: Differential Diagnosis

Usual Interstitial Pneumonia
- Idiopathic pulmonary fibrosis
- Collagen vascular disease (often rheumatoid arthritis or scleroderma)
- Drug-related fibrosis
- Asbestosis
- Fibrotic hypersensitivity pneumonitis
- End-stage sarcoidosis

Nonspecific interstitial pneumonia
Radiation
End-stage acute respiratory distress syndrome

Traction Bronchiectasis

The term *traction bronchiectasis* refers to bronchial dilatation occurring as a result of lung fibrosis. It typically is associated with a reticular pattern, lung distortion, or honeycombing. Bronchi tend to be irregular or corkscrewed in appearance (Figs. 11.17B, 11.18A, and 11.19). In comparison to garden variety bronchiectasis that is the result of irreversible damage to the airway wall such as with infection, mucous plugging or fluid within the bronchi is absent. The appearance of traction bronchiectasis in the peripheral lung may overlap with that of honeycombing.

Dilatation of small peripheral bronchioles also may be seen in the presence of lung fibrosis and is termed *traction bronchiolectasis*. Normally, bronchi are not visible in the peripheral 1 to 2 cm of lung; if they are visible, bronchiolectasis is present. If this finding is seen in combination with a reticular pattern, fibrosis is the likely cause.

Traction bronchiectasis and traction bronchiolectasis are very helpful in suggesting the presence of fibrosis when honeycombing is absent (Fig. 11.19B and C). Although the differential diagnosis of traction bronchiectasis without honeycombing includes UIP (eg, a probable UIP pattern), other diseases commonly cause traction bronchiectasis, including fibrotic NSIP, hypersensitivity pneumonitis, and sarcoidosis (Table 11.6). Because of this possibility and the greater likelihood that treatment may be effective when this pattern is present, lung biopsy may be performed. However, if the patient has a known collagen vascular disease, treatment is generally instituted without biopsy.

Nodules

Nodules as small as 1 to 2 mm in diameter can be detected on HRCT in patients with DILD. Nodules can be classified by (1) their appearance as well-defined (and thus most likely interstitial) or ill-defined (and most likely "airspace"), (2) their overall distribution, or (3) their specific anatomic distribution relative to lung structures. Although taking account of each of these features is important, recognition of the specific anatomic distribution of nodules is fundamental to their accurate diagnosis. Based on their anatomic distribution, nodules can be classified as *perilymphatic*, *random*, or *centrilobular*.

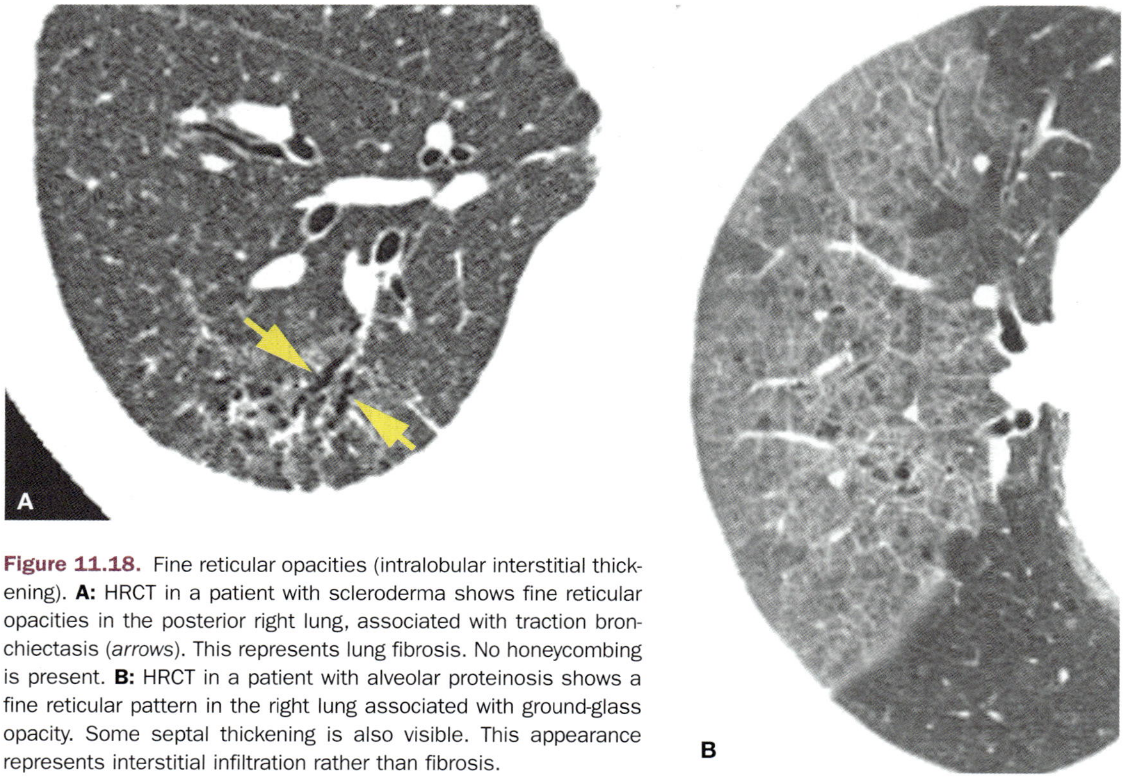

Figure 11.18. Fine reticular opacities (intralobular interstitial thickening). **A:** HRCT in a patient with scleroderma shows fine reticular opacities in the posterior right lung, associated with traction bronchiectasis (*arrows*). This represents lung fibrosis. No honeycombing is present. **B:** HRCT in a patient with alveolar proteinosis shows a fine reticular pattern in the right lung associated with ground-glass opacity. Some septal thickening is also visible. This appearance represents interstitial infiltration rather than fibrosis.

Perilymphatic Nodules

Perilymphatic nodules occur in relation to lung lymphatics. They usually are well-defined. They involve specific lung regions: (1) the subpleural interstitium at the pleural surfaces and fissures, (2) the peribronchovascular interstitium in the parahilar lung, (3) the interlobular septa, and (4) the peribronchovascular interstitium in a centrilobular location (Fig. 11.20).

In clinical practice, perilymphatic nodules usually are the result of sarcoidosis (see Chapter 15), which tends to have a peribronchovascular and subpleural predominance of nodules (Fig. 11.21), or lymphangitic spread of tumor (see Chapter 5), which typically predominates in relation to interlobular septa and the peribronchovascular interstitium (Fig. 11.22; Table 11.7). Sarcoidosis usually shows

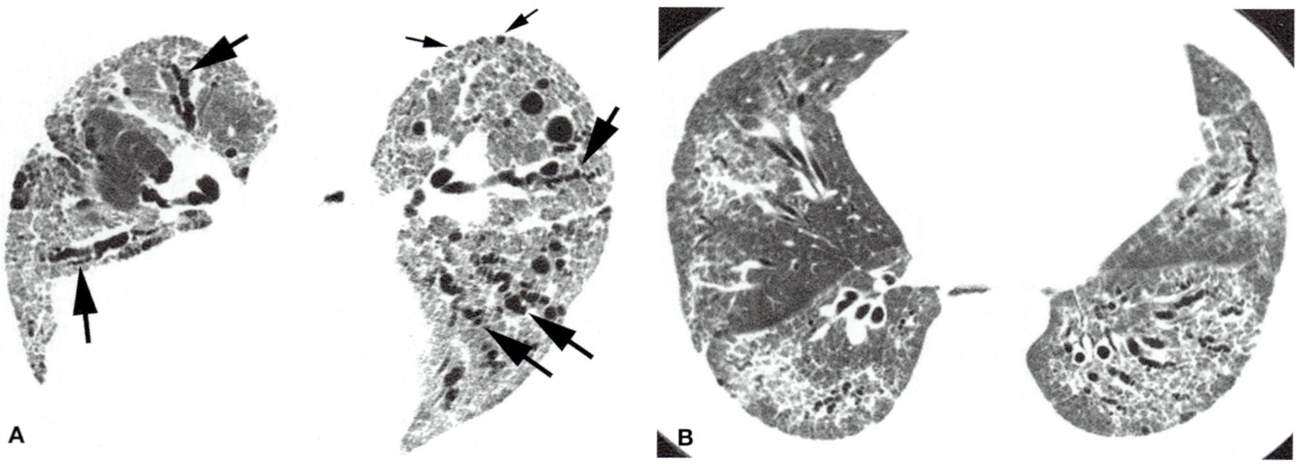

Figure 11.19. Reticular opacities with traction bronchiectasis. **A:** Prone HRCT in a patient with lung fibrosis shows an extensive reticular pattern associated with multiple irregularly dilated (corkscrewed) bronchi (*large arrows*). This is termed *traction bronchiectasis*. A few scattered subpleural cysts also are visible in the posterior subpleural lung (*small arrows*), insufficient for a diagnosis of honeycombing. **B:** A patient with fibrotic nonspecific interstitial pneumonia shows reticular opacities with irregular dilatation of multiple bronchi (ie, traction bronchiectasis). This finding indicates the presence of lung fibrosis. There is no evidence of honeycombing.

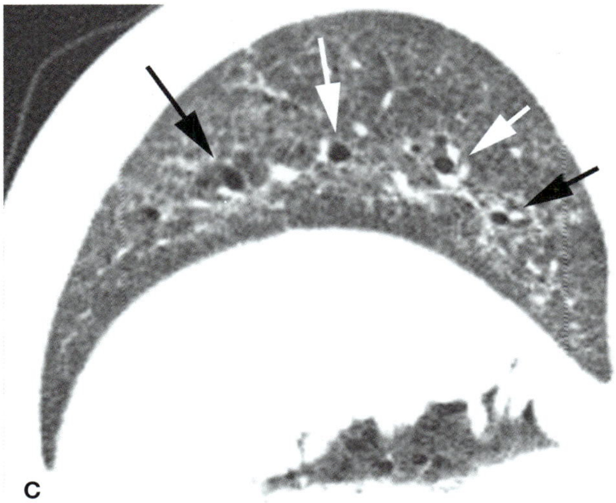

C

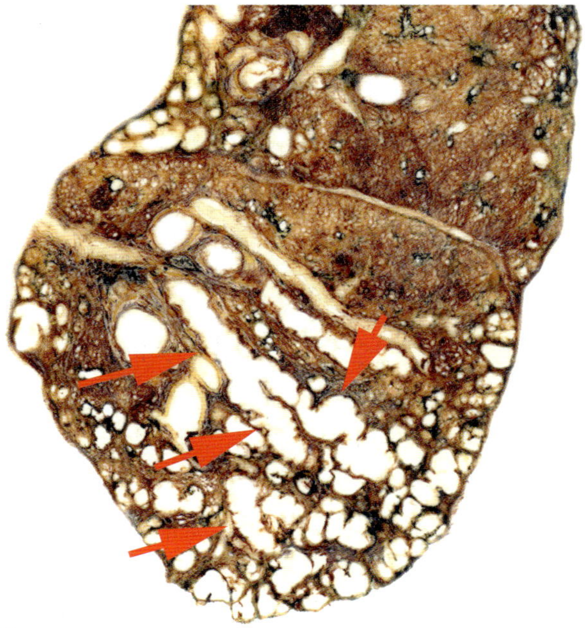

D

Figure 11.19. *(Continued)* **C:** Prone HRCT in a patient with mixed connective tissue disease shows a fine reticular pattern. This appearance is nonspecific, but the presence of multiple dilated bronchi (*arrows*) indicates that lung fibrosis is present. There is no evidence of honeycombing. This appearance probably is due to nonspecific interstitial pneumonia. **D:** Lung slice in a patient with idiopathic pulmonary fibrosis, traction bronchiectasis (*arrows*), and honeycombing in the subpleural lung.

more extensive abnormalities in the upper lobes and may be symmetrical or asymmetrical. Lymphangitic spread of carcinoma usually is most severe at the lung bases and often is asymmetrical.

Silicosis and CWP also may result in this pattern, predominating in the subpleural and centrilobular peribronchovascular regions (see Chapter 18). However, silicosis and CWP are best recognized by a symmetrical, posterior, upper lobe predominance of nodules. Also, an exposure history usually is available. Granulomatous infection and, rarely, amyloidosis (see Chapter 21) or lymphoid interstitial pneumonitis (LIP; see Chapter 13) results in this pattern.

Random Nodules

Random nodules are randomly distributed relative to structures of the secondary lobule and lung and appear diffuse and uniform in distribution (Figs. 11.7C and 11.23). Subpleural nodules are often present. Nodules usually are well-defined.

The random pattern is most typical of hematogenous diseases, such as miliary tuberculosis (Fig. 11.24), miliary fungal infection (see Fig. 11.7C), and hematogenous metastases (Fig. 11.25), but sarcoidosis, when diffuse, also can show this pattern (Table 11.8).

Table 11.6 Traction Bronchiectasis Without Honeycombing: Differential Diagnosis

Nonspecific interstitial pneumonia
Usual interstitial pneumonia and its causes (see above)
Sarcoidosis
Hypersensitivity pneumonitis
Radiation
End-stage acute respiratory distress syndrome

Centrilobular Nodules

Centrilobular nodules often reflect bronchiolar or peribronchiolar abnormalities in a centrilobular location, although abnormalities occurring in relation to small arterioles also may result in this finding. The most peripheral nodules present are usually centered 5 to 10 mm from the pleural surface and do not touch the pleura unless they are large (unlike the other two patterns) (Fig. 11.26). Because lobules are all of similar size, centrilobular nodules tend to be evenly spaced. Nodules may be well-defined or ill-defined, or a centrilobular rosette of small nodules may be seen (Figs. 11.26A and 11.27). Nodules may involve the lung diffusely or be patchy in distribution and may be solid or of GGO.

Centrilobular nodules can be seen in endobronchial spread of tuberculosis or other causes of bronchopneumonia (see Fig. 11.27A); endobronchial spread of tumor (eg, IMA; see Figs. 4.9, 4.10, and 4.40 in Chapter 4); hypersensitivity

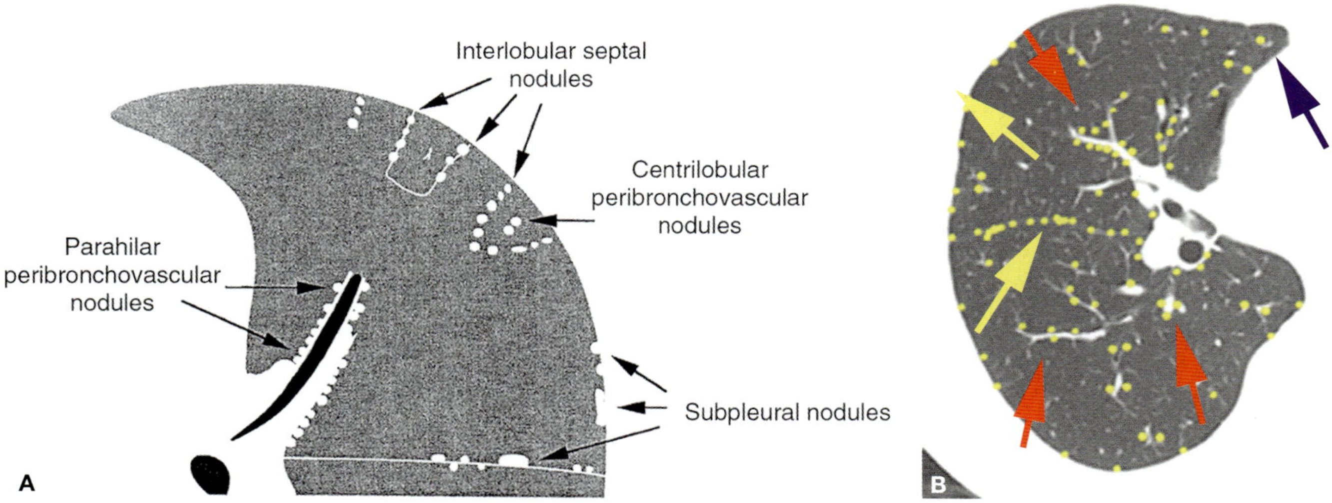

Figure 11.20. Locations of "perilymphatic" nodules. **A:** Nodules are visible in the subpleural regions and adjacent to fissures, the parahilar region adjacent to vessels and bronchi, the interlobular septa, and the peribronchovascular interstitium in a centrilobular location. **B:** Simulated perilymphatic nodules. Nodules are visible in the subpleural regions (*yellow arrows*), peribronchovascular regions (*red arrows*), and in relation to interlobular septa (*blue arrow*).

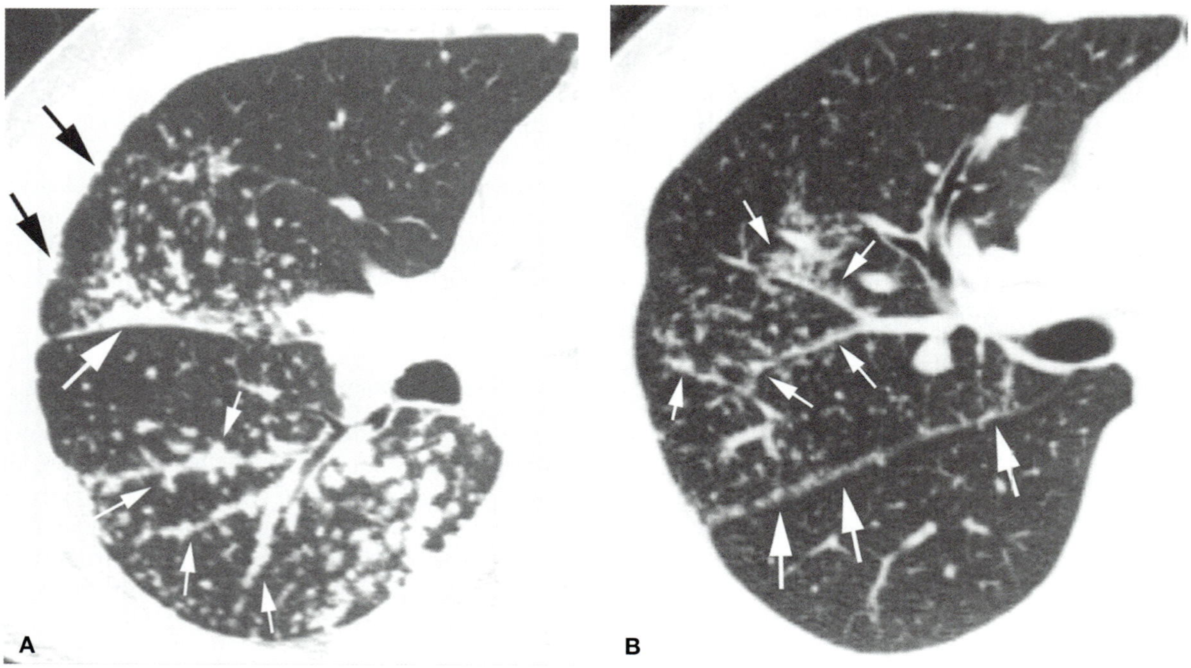

Figure 11.21. A and **B:** Perilymphatic nodules on HRCT in two patients with sarcoidosis. Nodules involve the subpleural interstitium (*large arrows*) in the lung periphery and adjacent to the fissure. Parahilar peribronchovascular nodules (*small arrows*) also are visible. Septal nodules and centrilobular nodules are visible but are less numerous.

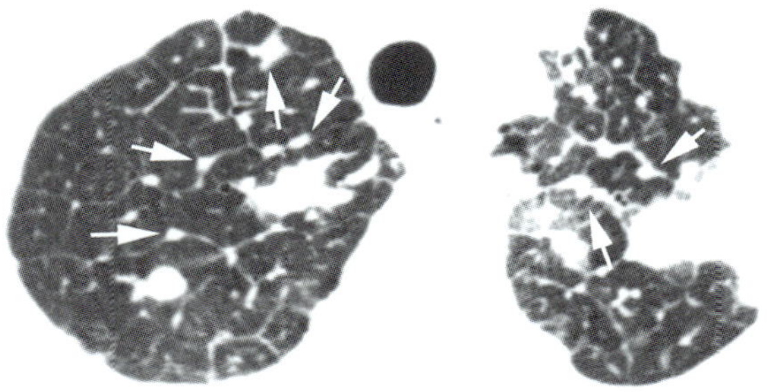

Figure 11.22. Lymphangitic spread of breast carcinoma. Multiple nodules (*arrows*) are visible in relation to interlobular septa.

pneumonitis (see Fig. 11.27B and C); OP, silicosis and CWP, histiocytosis, or vascular diseases such as vasculitis and pulmonary edema (Table 11.9).

When centrilobular nodules are the predominant finding, diseases involving the small airways are most likely. Consider infection, hypersensitivity pneumonitis (which may be diagnosed by history), and remember mucinous adenocarcinoma.

Table 11.7 Perilymphatic Nodules: Differential Diagnosis

Sarcoidosis
Lymphangitic spread of tumor
Silicosis and coal worker's pneumoconiosis
Granulomatous infection
Amyloidosis (rare)
Lymphoid interstitial pneumonitis (rare)

Centrilobular Tree-In-Bud Pattern

The "tree-in-bud" pattern represents a specific subset of centrilobular nodules (see Fig. 11.26A) and nearly always represents the presence of dilated and fluid-filled (with mucus or pus) centrilobular bronchioles (Fig. 11.28). Nodular branching opacities are visible in the lung periphery, and these are considerably larger than normal branching vessels. Trees-in-bud, which are centrilobular, tend to be centered 5 to 10 mm from the pleural surface when they are seen in the peripheral lung. Centrilobular nodules or clusters of nodules (rosettes) also may be seen.

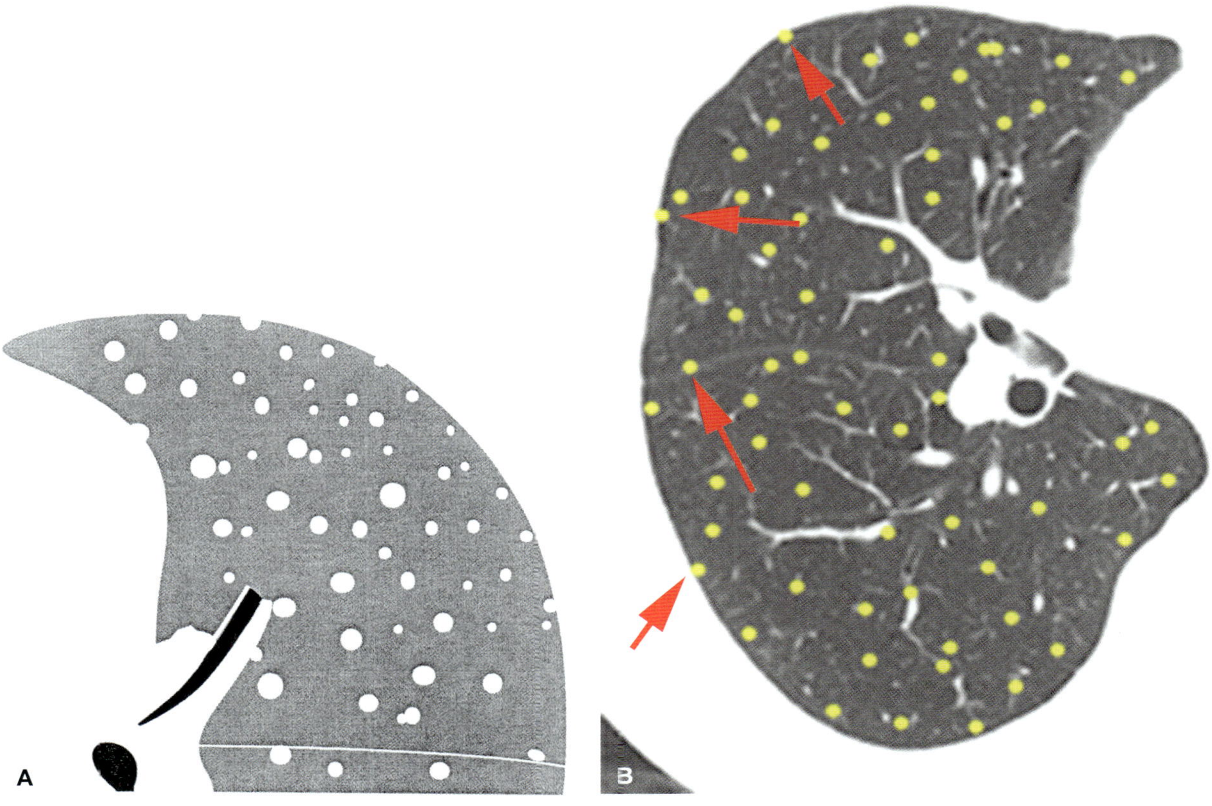

Figure 11.23. Random nodules. **A:** Nodules may involve the pleural surfaces, peribronchovascular interstitium, and interlobular septa but do not show a predominance in relation to these structures as is present with a perilymphatic pattern. The overall distribution appears diffuse and uniform. **B:** Simulated random nodules. Some nodules involve the pleural surfaces (*arrows*), but the overall distribution is uniform. Compare with Figure 11.20B.

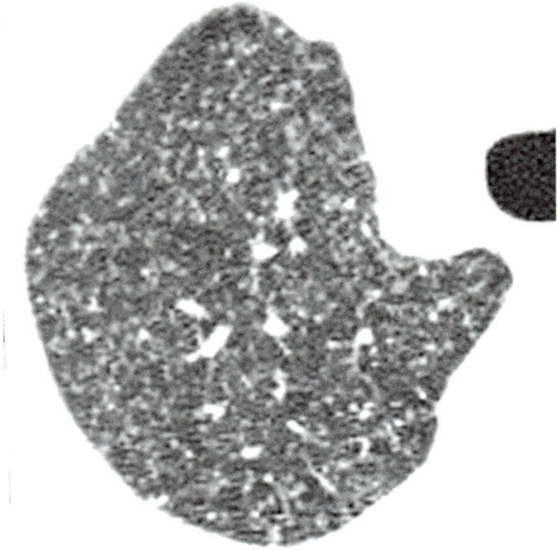

Figure 11.24. Random nodules in a patient with miliary tuberculosis. The nodules are small, sharply defined, and diffuse and uniform in distribution. Some nodules are seen at the pleural surface.

The presence of the tree-in-bud pattern is of great value in differential diagnosis. Because this finding represents dilatation and impaction of small centrilobular bronchioles, it indicates airway disease. Furthermore, the tree-in-bud appearance almost always (90%) indicates the presence of infection (eg, tuberculosis, *Mycobacterium avium* complex, bacteria, fungus), infected airway disease (eg, bronchiectasis, cystic fibrosis; Fig. 11.28), or aspiration. On occasion, it may

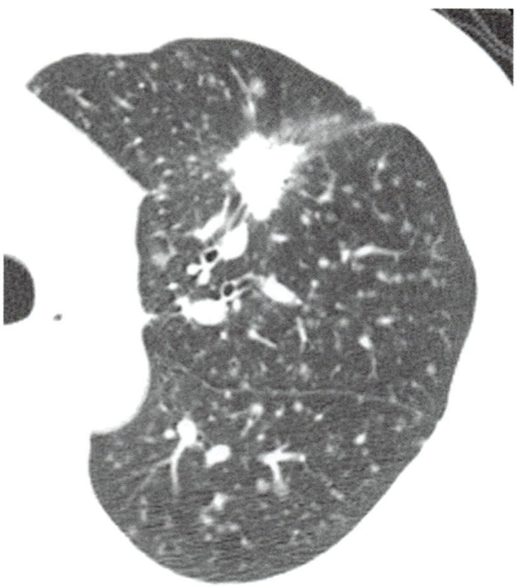

Figure 11.25. Random nodules of metastatic lung carcinoma. The primary carcinoma is visible in the left upper lobe. The nodules are diffuse and uniform in distribution.

Table 11.8 Random Nodules: Differential Diagnosis
Miliary infections
Hematogenous metastases
Sarcoidosis

be due to asthma with mucous plugging, allergic bronchopulmonary aspergillosis, or endobronchial spread of tumor (Table 11.10).

This finding means that the diagnosis should be made by examination or culture of sputum. If not, bronchoalveolar lavage is likely to be diagnostic.

Distribution of Nodules: A Diagnostic Algorithm

On HRCT, it is possible to distinguish these three specific distributions of nodules—perilymphatic, random, and centrilobular nodules—by using a simple algorithm (Fig. 11.29A).

The first step is to look for subpleural nodules and nodules seen in relation to the fissures. If they are absent, the nodules are centrilobular. Once it has been confirmed that the nodules are centrilobular, the presence of tree-in-bud should be sought (Fig. 11.29B).

If pleural or fissural nodules are present, then the pattern is either perilymphatic or random. These two patterns are then distinguished by looking at the distribution of other nodules. If they are patchy in distribution, particularly if a distinct peribronchovascular or septal distribution is present, then the nodules are perilymphatic; if the nodules are diffuse and uniform, the pattern is random. Using this approach, 94% of cases can be accurately classified.

Increased Lung Opacity

Increased lung opacity may be classified as consolidation or GGO.

Air-Space Consolidation

Air-space consolidation is said to be present when alveolar air is replaced by fluid, cells, or other things. On HRCT, consolidation results in an increase in lung opacity associated with obscuration of underlying vessels. Air bronchograms may be present.

If another pattern also is present (eg, small nodules), the consolidation probably represents confluent disease and should be ignored for the purposes of differential diagnosis. Attention should be paid to the areas of less affected lung to try and tease out other features of disease distribution.

The differential diagnosis of consolidation is based primarily on the duration of symptoms. In patients with acute symptoms, pneumonia, pulmonary edema, pulmonary hemorrhage, aspiration, and diffuse alveolar damage (often associated with the acute respiratory distress syndrome) are

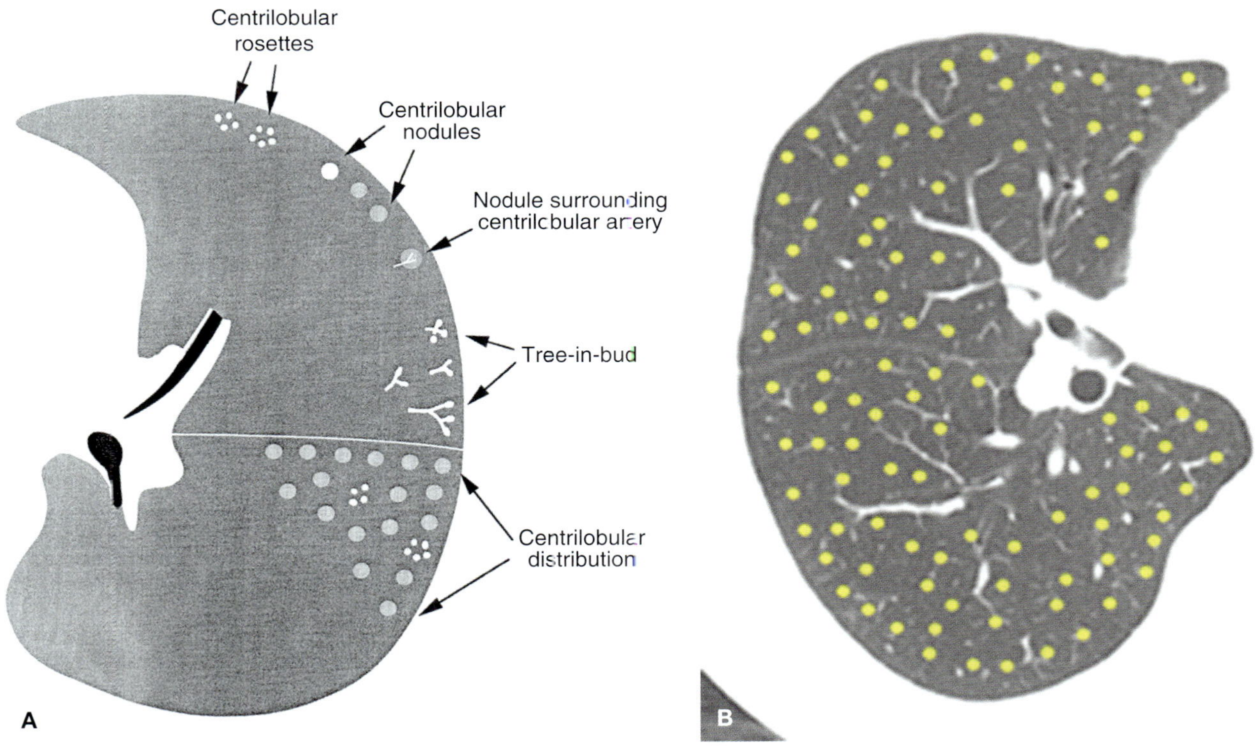

Figure 11.26. Centrilobular nodules. **A:** Nodules spare the pleural surfaces unless they are large and tend to be centered 5 to 10 mm from the pleural surface or fissures. Because lobules are of similar size, nodules appear evenly spaced. Nodules may be well- or ill-defined or may appear as a rosette of smaller nodules. The finding of the tree-in-bud pattern, which almost always represents dilatation and impaction of bronchioles, also is centrilobular in location. **B:** Simulated centrilobular nodules. Compare with Figure 11.20B.

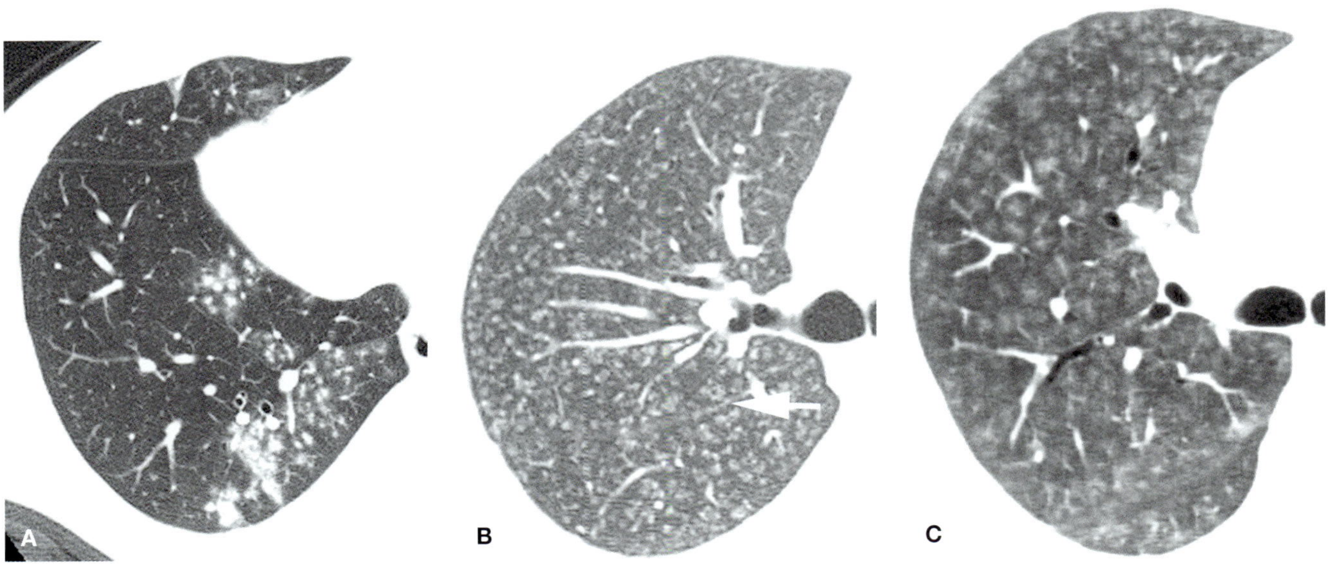

Figure 11.27. Centrilobular nodules. **A:** Bacterial bronchopneumonia with patchy centrilobular nodules in the lower lobe. The most peripheral nodules are centered 5 to 10 mm from the pleural surface and spare the pleura. Small rosettes also are visible. **B:** Centrilobular nodules in hypersensitivity pneumonitis. Note that the nodules spare the fissure (*arrow*) and pleural surface. The nodules are diffuse and appear evenly spaced. **C:** Hypersensitivity pneumonitis with centrilobular nodules of ground-glass opacity.

Table 11.9 Centrilobular Nodules: Differential Diagnosis

Bronchopneumonia or infectious bronchiolitis of any cause
Endobronchial spread of infection (bacteria, virus, tuberculosis, mycobacteria, fungus)
Endobronchial spread of tumor (Invasive mucinous adenocarcinoma)
Hypersensitivity pneumonitis
Respiratory bronchiolitis in a smoker
Follicular bronchiolitis (eg, collagen vascular disease)
Organizing pneumonia
Silicosis and coal worker's pneumoconiosis
Langerhans cell histiocytosis
Aspiration
Pulmonary edema or hemorrhage
Pulmonary hypertension (pulmonary veno-occlusive disease, capillary hemangiomatosis)
Excipient lung disease/IV talcosis (rare)
Vasculitis

most likely (see Table 11.10). Among patients with chronic symptoms, the most common causes of this finding include chronic eosinophilic pneumonia (Fig. 11.30A), OP (Fig. 11.30B), and interstitial pneumonia such as NSIP (Table 11.11). IMA also may result in this pattern.

Ground-Glass Opacity

GGO is a common finding that refers to a hazy increase in lung opacity that is not associated with obscuration of underlying vessels (see Figs. 11.11B, 11.18B, and 11.31). This finding can reflect the presence of a number of diseases and can be seen in patients with either minimal interstitial thickening or air-space disease. Although GGO is a nonspecific finding, its presence is very significant. As with consolidation, the differential diagnosis is based primarily on the duration of symptoms.

In patients with acute symptoms, the presence of GGO reflects active or ongoing disease such as pulmonary edema (Fig. 11.31A) or hemorrhage, aspiration, pneumonia, often

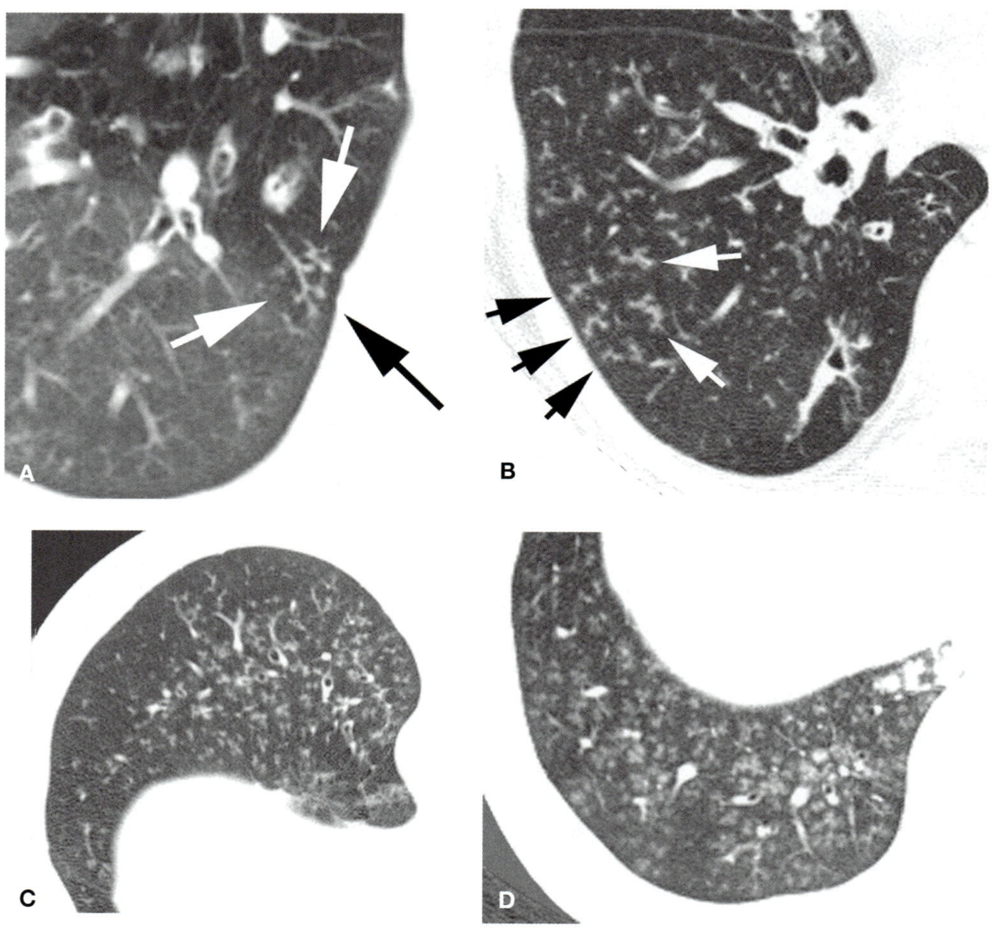

Figure 11.28. Tree-in-bud. **A:** Tree-in-bud (*arrows*) in the right lower lobe in a patient with cystic fibrosis. A branching opacity in the peripheral lung (ie, the tree) represents a dilated centrilobular bronchiole impacted with mucus and pus. Small, rounded opacities at the tips of the branches (ie, the buds) represent peribronchiolar inflammation. Bronchial wall thickening and mosaic perfusion also are visible. **B:** Several examples of tree-in-bud (*arrows*) in another patient with airway infection. These appear larger than normal branching vessels in the peripheral lung, visible posteriorly. **C:** Tree-in-bud in a patient with *Pseudomonas* bronchopneumonia. **D:** Centrilobular nodules and tree-in-bud in a patient with *Haemophilus influenzae* bronchopneumonia.

Table 11.10 Tree-In-Bud: Differential Diagnosis

Endobronchial spread of infection (bacteria, tuberculosis, mycobacteria, fungus)
Airways diseases with infection (eg, cystic fibrosis, bronchiectasis)
Mucous plugging (asthma, allergic bronchopulmonary aspergillosis)
Aspiration
Invasive mucinous adenocarcinoma (rare)
Intravascular metastasis

atypical (eg, *Pneumocystis* or viral pneumonias; Fig. 11.31B and C), diffuse alveolar damage, acute interstitial pneumonia, and acute hypersensitivity pneumonitis (Table 11.12).

In patients with subacute or chronic symptoms, GGO usually (60%-80% of cases) indicates an acute, active, and potentially treatable process, such as NSIP, OP, smoking-related interstitial lung disease, hypersensitivity pneumonitis (Fig. 11.31D), pulmonary alveolar proteinosis (PAP) (see Figs. 11.18B and 11.32), sarcoidosis, lipoid pneumonia (see Fig. 11.11B), and IMA. Because of its association with active lung disease, the clinical diagnosis should be pursued in patients with GGO. The presence of this finding may lead

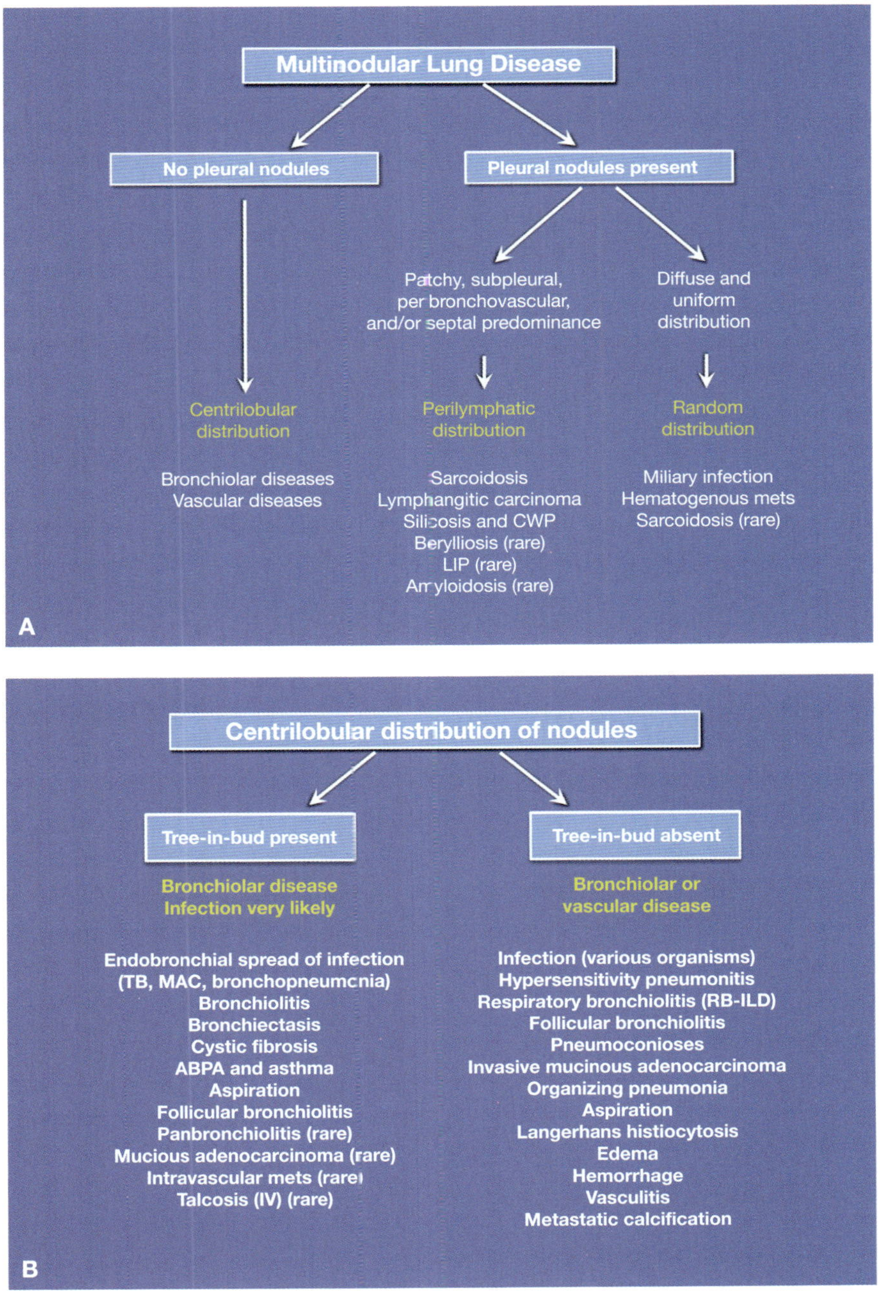

Figure 11.29. Algorithms for classification and diagnosis of multiple small nodules. **A:** Classification of nodules. **B:** Classification of centrilobular nodules. ABPA, allergic bronchopulmonary aspergillosis; CWP, coal worker's pneumoconiosis; IV, intravenous; LIP, lymphoid interstitial pneumonitis; MAC, *Mycobacterium avium* complex; RB-ILD, respiratory bronchiolitis–associated interstitial lung disease; TB, tuberculosis.

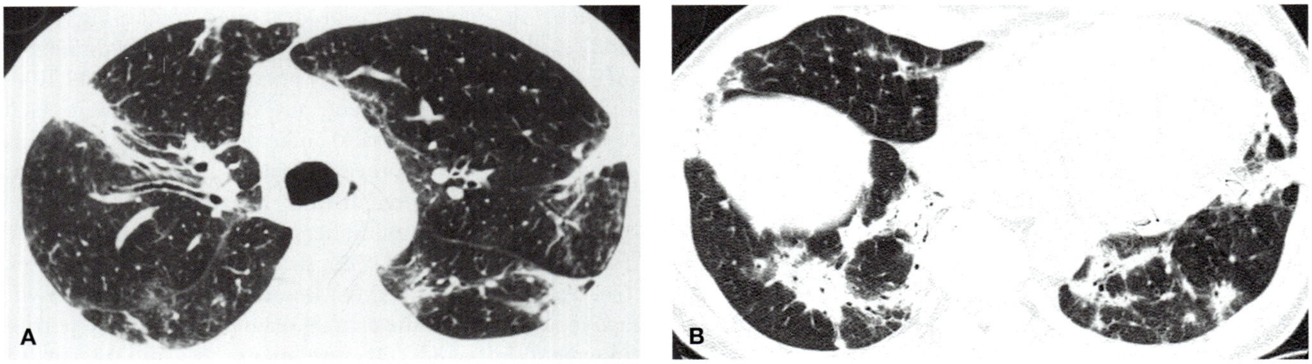

Figure 11.30. Consolidation. **A:** Homogeneous areas of consolidation are visible in the peripheral lung. This represents chronic eosinophilic pneumonia. **B:** Patchy areas of consolidation with air bronchogram in a patient with organizing pneumonia.

to lung biopsy, depending on the history and clinical status of the patient.

The combination of GGO and interlobular septal thickening is termed *crazy paving* (see Fig. 11.32). This appearance is nonspecific and may be seen with a variety of acute lung diseases such as *Pneumocystis* or viral pneumonia, edema, hemorrhage, and acute lung injury. Among patients with chronic lung disease, it is a classic finding for PAP, although it may be seen in any chronic infiltrative lung disease characterized by GGO.

When GGO is associated with reticulation and findings of fibrosis such as traction bronchiectasis (Fig. 11.33), and particularly when they are seen in the same lung regions, the GGO is likely to be due to fibrosis rather than active disease. In this situation, it is necessary to hedge in the interpretation; in most cases, the differential diagnosis is the same as for fibrosis with traction bronchiectasis (Table 11.6). Biopsy may be warranted and can be directed to areas showing the least evidence of fibrosis.

Decreased Lung Opacity and Cystic Lesions

Geographic areas of decreased lung attenuation may represent emphysema, mosaic perfusion, or air trapping (on expiratory scans). Circumscribed areas of decreased lung attenuation may represent emphysema or lung cysts.

Table 11.11 Air-Space Consolidation: Differential Diagnosis

Acute Symptoms
Pneumonia
Pulmonary edema
Pulmonary hemorrhage
Acute respiratory distress syndrome
Aspiration
Chronic Symptoms
Chronic eosinophilic pneumonia or other eosinophilic lung disease
Organizing pneumonia
Interstitial pneumonias
Lipoid pneumonia
Invasive mucinous adenocarcinoma

Emphysema

Emphysema results in areas of very low attenuation, usually less than −950 HU. The appearance of emphysema is characteristic and depends on the type of emphysema present (Fig. 11.34). Typical appearances are as follows:

Centrilobular emphysema: Focal areas of lucency without (or sometimes with) visible walls, usually with an upper lobe predominance (see Fig. 24.6 in Chapter 24).

Panlobular emphysema: Large areas of low attenuation, usually diffuse and associated with decreased vessel size (see Fig. 24.9 in Chapter 24). Focal, sharply marginated areas of emphysema and bullae are typically absent.

Paraseptal emphysema: Subpleural lucencies marginated by interlobular septa, or subpleural bullae, usually with an upper lobe predominance (see Fig. 24.11 in Chapter 24).

Lung Cysts

Lung cyst is used to describe a thin-walled (usually less than 3 mm), well-defined, and circumscribed air-containing lesion 1 cm or more in diameter (as opposed to fluid-filled cysts in other organs). Cysts may be seen in various cystic lung disease or may represent bullae in association with emphysema, honeycombing in patients with fibrosis, pneumatoceles in association with pneumonia, or cystic bronchiectasis (see Table 11.13). Bullae, honeycombing, pneumatoceles, and cystic bronchiectasis usually can be distinguished from cystic lung disease by associated findings. Scattered lung cysts may be seen in some patients with hypersensitivity pneumonitis.

Cystic lung diseases (ie, lung disease characterized by numerous cysts) are rare. LAM and LCH often are associated with multiple lung cysts as a primary manifestation. The cysts have a thin but easily discernible wall, ranging up to a few millimeters in thickness (Fig. 11.35). In these diseases,

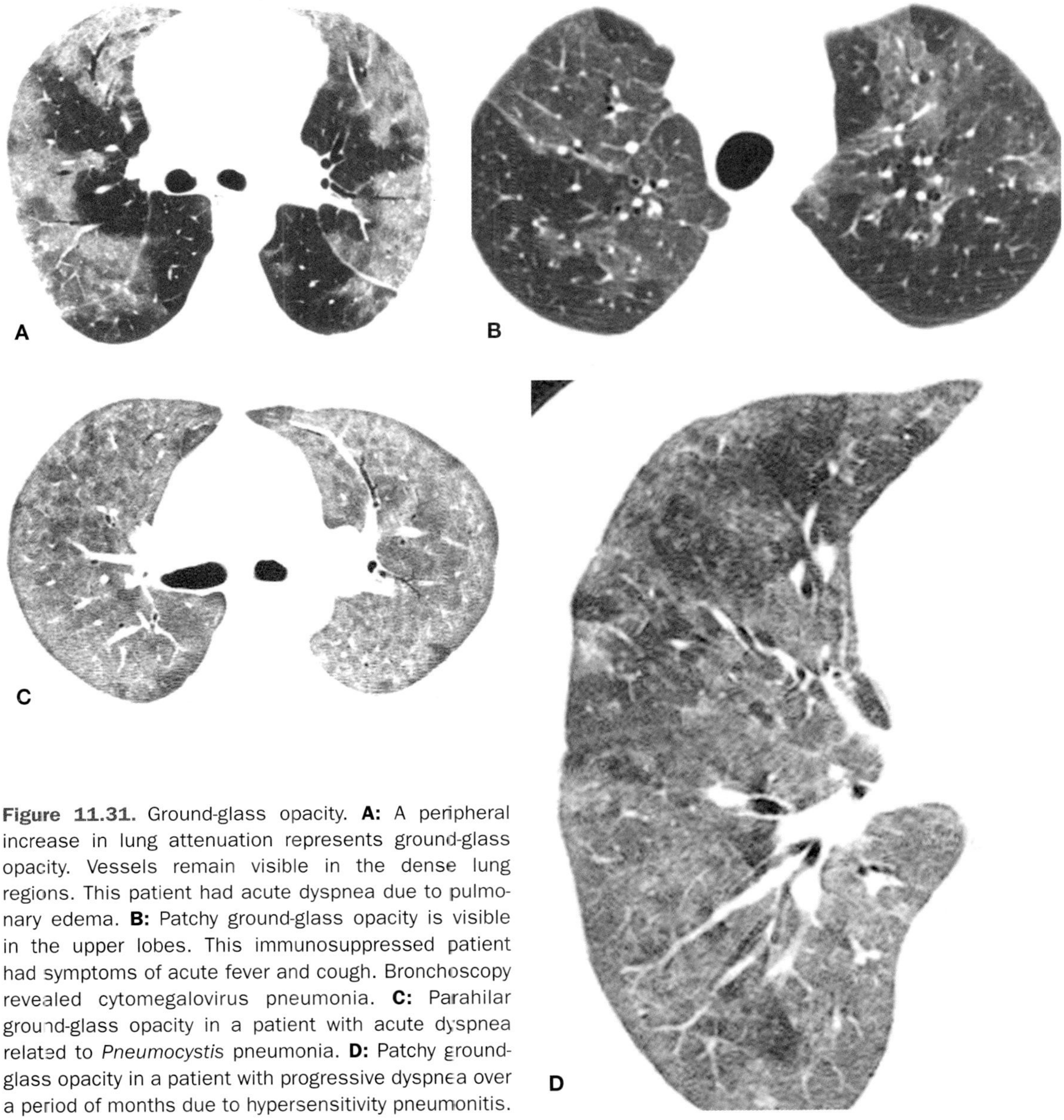

Figure 11.31. Ground-glass opacity. **A:** A peripheral increase in lung attenuation represents ground-glass opacity. Vessels remain visible in the dense lung regions. This patient had acute dyspnea due to pulmonary edema. **B:** Patchy ground-glass opacity is visible in the upper lobes. This immunosuppressed patient had symptoms of acute fever and cough. Bronchoscopy revealed cytomegalovirus pneumonia. **C:** Parahilar ground-glass opacity in a patient with acute dyspnea related to *Pneumocystis* pneumonia. **D:** Patchy ground-glass opacity in a patient with progressive dyspnea over a period of months due to hypersensitivity pneumonitis.

the cysts usually are interspersed with areas of normal-appearing lung.

LAM, related to abnormalities of the so-called tuberous sclerosis genes 1 and 2, almost always occurs in females, usually of childbearing age; typically, the cysts are uniformly distributed, round, and similar in size and shape (see Fig. 11.35A). They represent a PECOMA, a neoplastic proliferation of perivascular epithelioid cells (See Chapter 4). A small percentage of patients with tuberous sclerosis have LAM.

In patients with LCH, the cysts can be irregularly or bizarrely shaped (see Fig. 11.35B), have an upper lobe predominance, may be associated with nodules and cavitary nodules in early stages of the disease, and tend to spare the costophrenic angles. Almost all patients with LCH are smokers.

Multiple cysts also may be seen in LIP, particularly in patients with Sjögren syndrome and other collagen vascular diseases (Table 11.13); cysts are limited in number and are predominant at the lung bases. It is common to see vessels associated with the walls of cysts.

Birt-Hogg-Dube syndrome is another cause of cystic lung disease. Cysts are limited in number and may be large, oddly shaped, and subpleural. In this syndrome, they are associated with fibrofolliculomas of the face, neck, and trunk and oncocytomas or renal cell carcinoma.

Protein deposition including amyloid or light chain deposition disease also causes cysts that may overlap in appearance with LIP. These cysts often have small foci of calcium that represents ossification.

Table 11.12 Ground-Glass Opacity: Differential Diagnosis

Acute Symptoms
- Pulmonary edema
- Hemorrhage
- Pneumonia (eg, *Pneumocystis jirovecii* [*Pneumocystis carinii*] or viral pneumonias)
- Diffuse alveolar damage
- Acute interstitial pneumonia
- Hypersensitivity pneumonitis (acute)

Chronic Symptoms
- Nonspecific interstitial pneumonia
- Smoking-related interstitial lung disease
- Hypersensitivity pneumonitis (subacute or chronic)
- Alveolar proteinosis
- Sarcoidosis
- Lipoid pneumonia
- Invasive mucinous adenocarcinoma

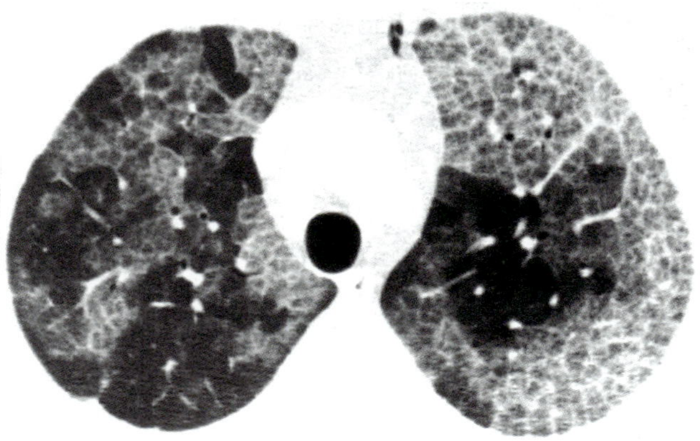

Figure 11.32. Ground-glass opacity with "crazy paving." Patchy ground-glass opacity is associated with interlobular septal thickening in the abnormal regions. This represents alveolar proteinosis.

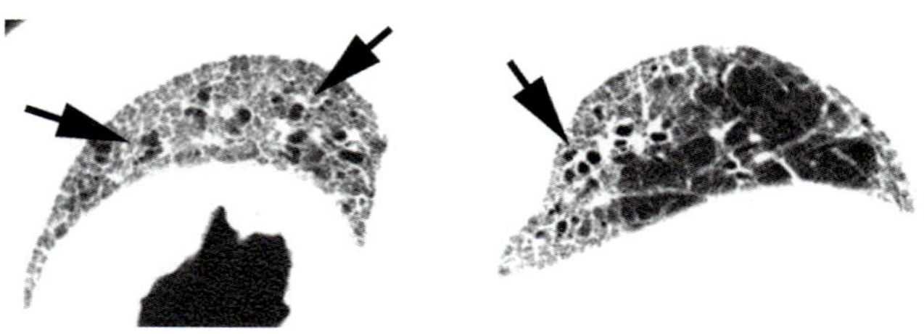

Figure 11.33. Ground-glass opacity associated with traction bronchiectasis. Fibrosis in the posterior lung bases is associated with ground-glass opacity and reticulation. The presence of traction bronchiectasis (*arrows*) indicates that the ground-glass opacity is likely due to fibrosis.

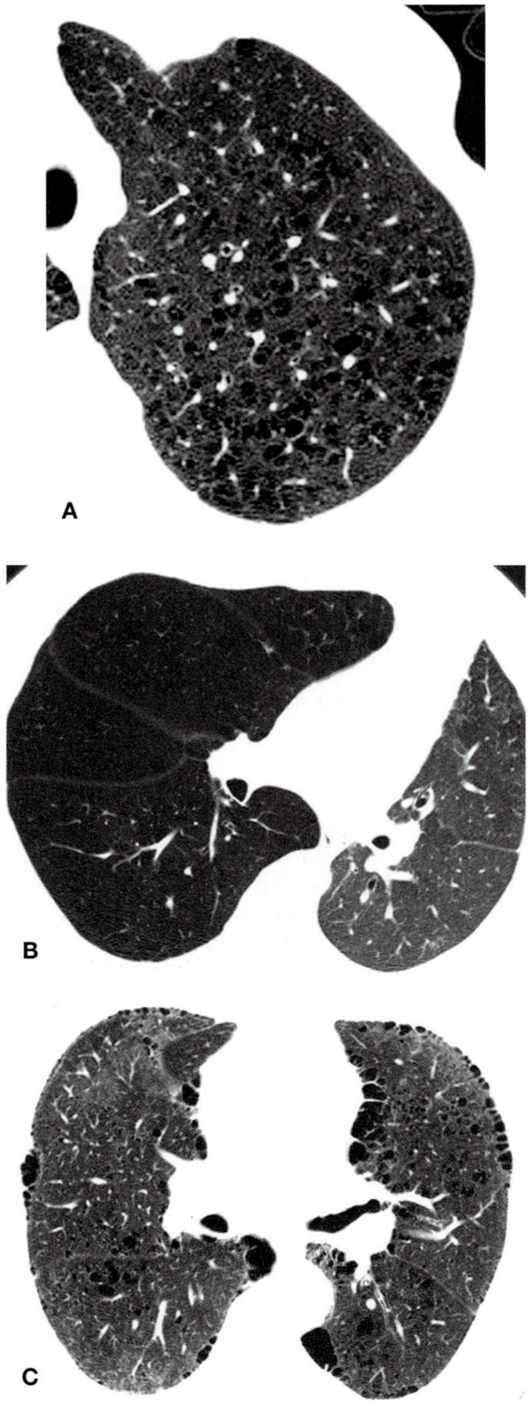

Figure 11.34. Appearances of emphysema. **A:** Centrilobular emphysema. Focal areas of lucency without visible walls are visible in the left upper lobe. **B:** Panlobular emphysema in a patient with a left lung transplant. The right lung is hyperlucent, and vessels are reduced in size and number. **C:** Paraseptal emphysema. Subpleural lucencies marginated by interlobular septa and subpleural bullae are visible.

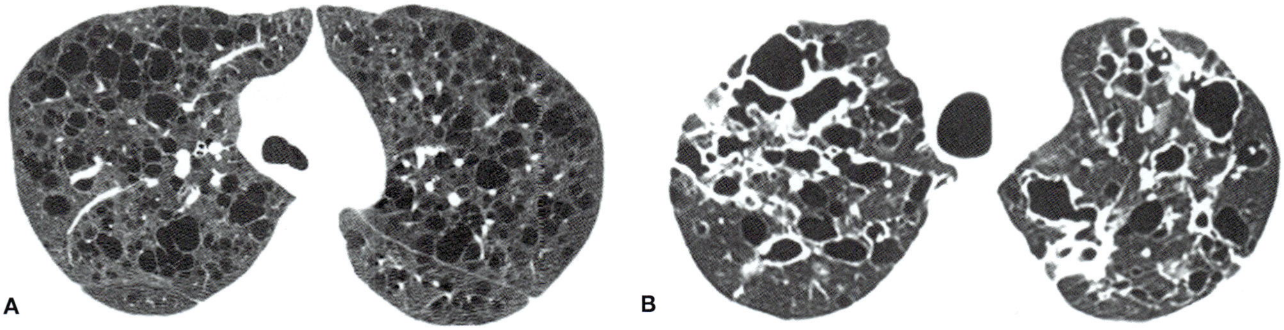

Figure 11.35. Lung cysts. **A:** HRCT in a young woman with lymphangiomyomatosis (LAM). Multiple lung cysts are visible, having thin but easily discernible walls. In this disease, the cysts usually are interspersed within areas of normal-appearing lung and appear rounded. **B:** Lung cysts in histiocytosis. The cysts are more irregular in shape than those in patients with LAM and have an upper lobe predominance. In this patient, the cysts appear thick walled.

Mosaic Perfusion

Patchy areas of decreased lung attenuation sometimes can be recognized on HRCT in patients with abnormal lung perfusion and reduced regional pulmonary blood volume (Fig. 11.36). The term *mosaic perfusion* is used to describe this appearance. Mosaic perfusion most often results from airway diseases such as cystic fibrosis or other causes such as airway infection, asthma, or bronchiolitis obliterans; in this setting, abnormal regional lung ventilation leads to vasoconstriction and decreased perfusion. Mosaic perfusion also can be seen with vascular obstruction (eg, chronic pulmonary embolism; Table 11.14), but this is less common.

The key to diagnosing mosaic perfusion as the cause of heterogeneous lung attenuation on HRCT is recognizing the presence of reduced vessel size in relatively lucent lung regions (see Figs. 11.36A and 11.38A). If abnormal bronchi are visible in lucent lung regions (see Fig. 11.36A), and bronchi appear normal in relatively dense regions, airway disease

Table 11.13 Lung Cysts: Differential Diagnosis

Common Causes of Cysts
- Bullae
- Honeycombing
- Pneumatoceles in association with pneumonia
- Cystic bronchiectasis
- Cysts in hypersensitivity pneumonitis

Cystic Lung Disease (Uncommon)
- Lymphangioleiomyomatosis (LAM)
- Langerhans cell histiocytosis
- Tuberous sclerosis
- Sjögren syndrome
- Lymphoid interstitial pneumonia
- Birt-Hogg-Dube syndrome
- Papillomatosis

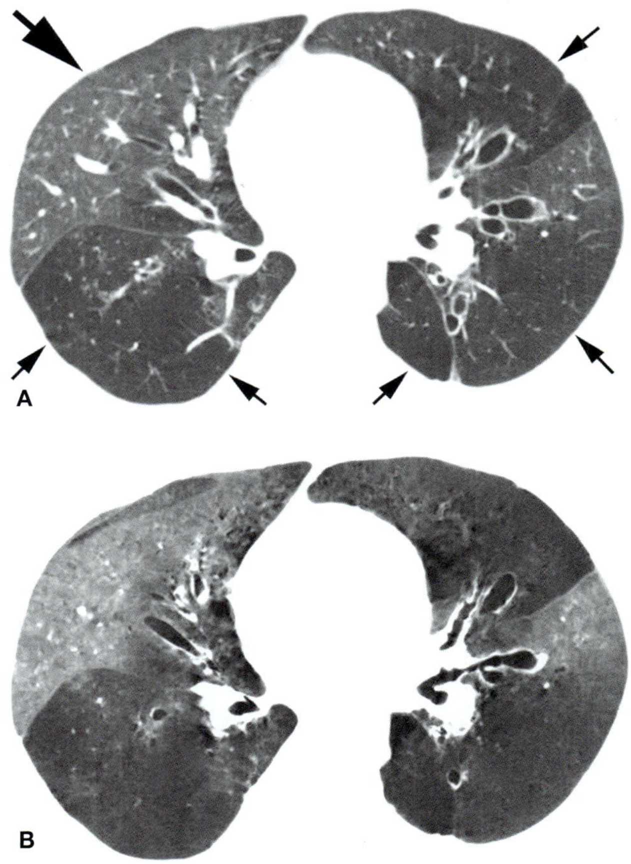

Figure 11.36. Mosaic perfusion due to bronchiolitis obliterans. **A:** HRCT shows decreased lung attenuation in the lower lobes and left upper lobe (*small arrows*). Note that vessels appear smaller in these regions than in the relatively dense right upper lobe (*large arrow*). This is typical of mosaic perfusion. Abnormal bronchi are also seen in the lucent lung regions, suggesting an airway disease as the cause. **B:** Minimum intensity projection from a stack of HRCT images at the same level shows the density differences between lung regions resulting from differences in lung perfusion.

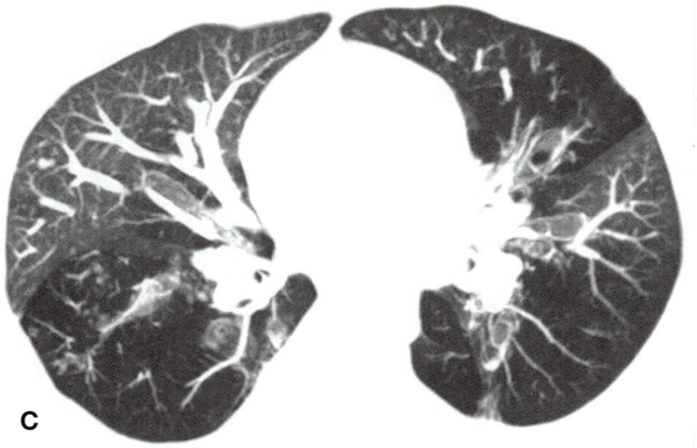

Figure 11.36. *(Continued)* **C:** Maximum intensity projection at the same level shows the difference in vascular size between lucent and dense lung regions.

Table 11.14 Mosaic Perfusion: Differential Diagnosis

Airway Diseases
- Large airway diseases (eg, cystic fibrosis, bronchiectasis)
- Small airway diseases
- Asthma
- Hypersensitivity pneumonitis
- Bronchiolitis obliterans
- Small airway infection
- Mucous plugging

Vascular Diseases
- Chronic pulmonary embolism
- Other causes of vascular obstruction

very likely is the cause. Also, mosaic perfusion related to airway disease often shows lobular regions of low attenuation; mosaic perfusion related to vascular obstruction often shows larger, peripheral regions of low attenuation.

Air Trapping on Expiratory Computed Tomography

In patients with mosaic perfusion resulting from airway disease, air trapping often is visible on expiratory scans in lucent lung regions. Although mosaic perfusion and air trapping look the same, and often are related, they are distinct findings. Mosaic perfusion is an inspiratory scan finding, and air trapping is an expiratory scan finding. Also, in some patients with airway disease, air trapping may be visible on expiratory scans even though inspiratory scans are normal.

A variety of techniques can be used to obtain expiratory scans. Postexpiratory scans may be obtained following exhalation (ie, the patient breathes out and suspends respiration). Dynamic expiratory scans are more sensitive. These are obtained by scanning at the same level, for 5 to 6 seconds, as the patient forcefully exhales, obtaining a series of five or six scans at a single level. This should be done with reduced milliamperage settings so that the entire dynamic series equals the radiation dose of a single HRCT slice.

Normally, lung increases homogeneously in attenuation on expiratory scans (usually by more than 100 HU), although dependent lung increases in attenuation more than nondependent lung (Fig. 11.37). In the presence of air trapping, lung regions remain lucent on expiration with little increase in attenuation and show little change in volume (see Fig. 11.38). Patchy air trapping is characteristic of small airway diseases. Larger areas of air trapping (eg, an entire lobe) suggest a large airway abnormality. Air trapping on HRCT is associated principally with bronchiolitis; its appearance is discussed in detail in Chapter 23.

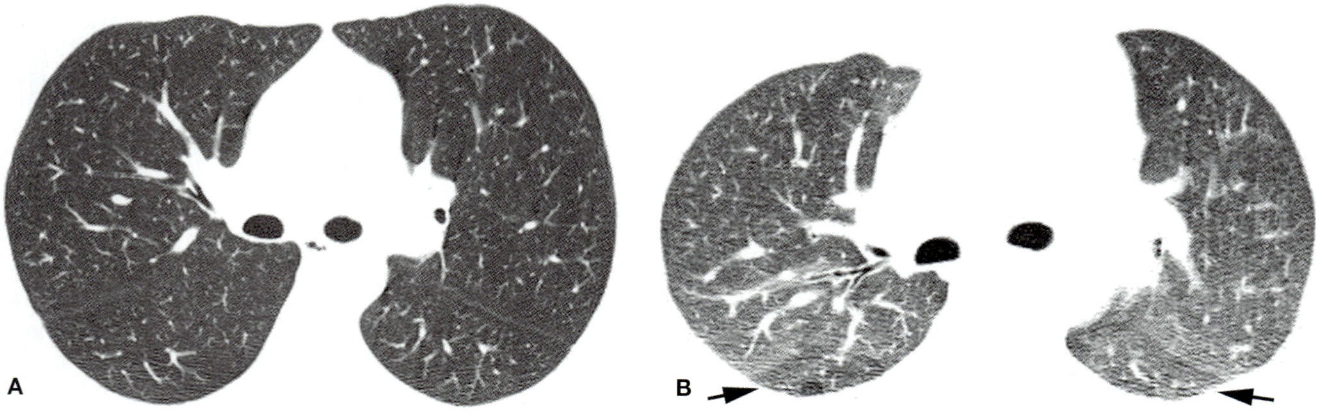

Figure 11.37. Normal expiratory HRCT. **A:** Inspiratory scan shows the lung to be homogeneous in attenuation. **B:** Following expiration, the lung increases in attenuation. Posterior, dependent lung usually increases in density more than nondependent lung. Mild air trapping posterior to the major fissures in the superior segments of the lower lobes (*arrows*) is common in healthy individuals.

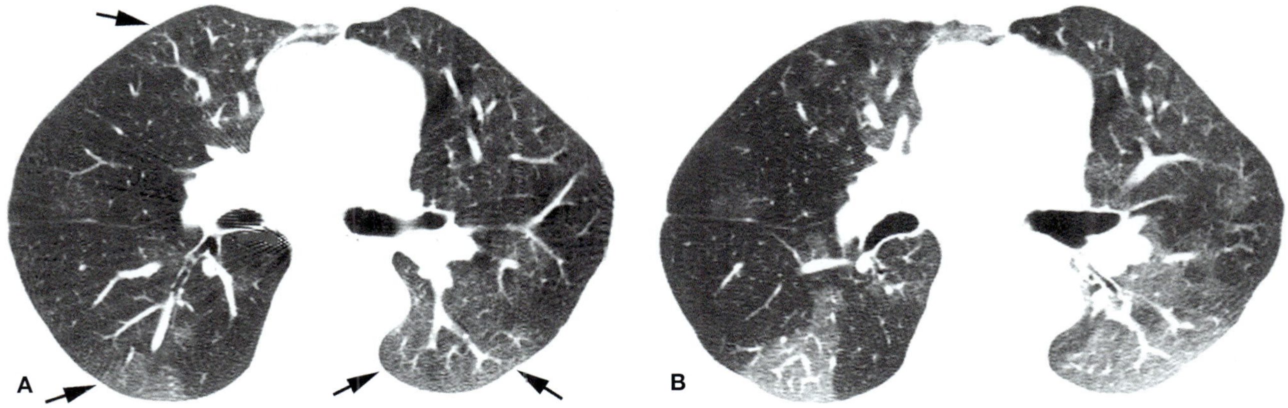

Figure 11.38. Mosaic perfusion and air trapping in a patient with bronchiolitis obliterans secondary to lung transplant rejection. **A:** Inspiratory scan shows inhomogeneous lung attenuation due to mosaic perfusion. Several lung regions (*arrows*) appear relatively dense and contain larger vessels. Other lung regions appear relatively lucent and contain small vessels. **B:** Expiratory scan shows a normal increase in attenuation of the dense regions shown in (**A**). The relatively lucent regions in (**A**) show little change in attenuation on the expiratory scan due to air trapping.

SUGGESTED READINGS

Aquino SL, Gamsu G, Webb WR, Kee ST. Tree-in-bud pattern: frequency and significance on thin section CT. *J Comput Assist Tomogr*. 1996;20(4):594-599.

Arakawa H, Webb WR. Expiratory high-resolution CT scan. *Radiol Clin North Am*. 1998;36(1):189-209.

Austin JH, Müller NL, Friedman PJ, et al. Glossary of terms for CT of the lungs: recommendations of the Nomenclature Committee of the Fleischner Society. *Radiology*. 1996;200(2):327-331.

Colby TV, Swensen SJ. Anatomic distribution and histopathologic patterns in diffuse lung disease: correlation with HRCT. *J Thorac Imaging*. 1996;11:1-26

Felson B. A new look at pattern recognition of diffuse pulmonary disease *AJR Am J Roentgenol*. 1979;133(2):183-189.

Godwin JD, Müller NL, Takasugi JE. Pulmonary alveolar proteinosis: CT findings. *Radiology*. 1988;169(3):609-613.

Gruden JF, Webb WR, Warnock M. Centrilobular opacities in the lung on high-resolution CT: diagnostic considerations and pathologic correlation. *AJR Am J Roentgenol*. 1994;162(3):569-574.

Gruden JF, Webb WR, Naidich DP, McGuinness G. Multinodular disease: anatomic localization at thin-section CT—multireader evaluation of a simple algorithm. *Radiology*. 1999;210(3):711-720.

Hansell DM, Bankier AA, MacMahon H, McLoud TC, Müller NL, Remy J. Fleischner society: glossary of terms for thoracic imaging. *Radiology*. 2008;246(3):697-722.

Hewitt MG, Miller WT Jr, Reilly TJ, Simpson S. The relative frequencies of causes of widespread ground-glass opacity: a retrospective cohort. *Eur J Radiol*. 2014;83:1970-1976.

Johkoh T, Müller NL, Cartier Y, et al. Idiopathic interstitial pneumonias: diagnostic accuracy of thin-section CT in 129 patients. *Radiology*. 1999;211(2):555-560.

Kligerman SJ, Henry T, Lin CT, Franks TJ, Galvin JR. Mosaic attenuation: etiology, methods of differentiation, and pitfalls. *Radiographics*. 2015;35(5):1360-1380. doi:10.1148/rg.2015140308

Lee KS, Kim TS, Han J, et al. Diffuse micronodular lung disease: HRCT and pathologic findings. *J Comput Assist Tomogr*. 1999;23(1):99-106.

Leung AN, Miller RR, Müller NL. Parenchymal opacification in chronic infiltrative lung diseases: CT-pathologic correlation. *Radiology*. 1993;188(1):209-214.

Mayo JR. High resolution computed tomography: technical aspects. *Radiol Clin North Am*. 1991;29(5):1043-1049.

Miller WT Jr. Chest radiographic evaluation of diffuse infiltrative lung disease: review of a dying art. *Eur J Radiol*. 2002;44:182-197.

Miller WT Jr, Chatzkel J, Hewitt MG. Expiratory air trapping on thoracic computed tomography. A diagnostic subclassification. *Ann Am Thorac Soc*. 2014;11(6):874-881.

Müller NL, Miller RR. Computed tomography of chronic diffuse infiltrative lung disease: part 1. *Am Rev Respir Dis*. 1990;142(5):1206-1215.

Müller NL, Miller RR. Computed tomography of chronic diffuse infiltrative lung disease: part 2. *Am Rev Respir Dis*. 1990;142(6 pt 1):1440-1448.

Müller NL, Miller RR. Diseases of the bronchioles: CT and histopathologic findings. *Radiology*. 1995;196(1):3-12.

Okada F, Ando Y, Yoshitake S, et al. Clinical/pathologic correlations in 553 patients with primary centrilobular findings on high-resolution CT scan of the thorax. *Chest*. 2007;132(6):1939-1948.

Primack SL, Hartman TE, Hansell DM, Müller NL. End-stage lung disease: CT findings in 61 patients. *Radiology*. 1993;189(3):681-686.

Webb WR. High resolution lung computed tomography: normal anatomic and pathologic findings. *Radiol Clin North Am*. 1991;29(5):1051-1063.

Webb WR. Thin-section CT of the secondary pulmonary lobule: anatomy and the image—the 2004 Fleischner lecture. *Radiology*. 2006;239(2):322-338.

Chapter 12

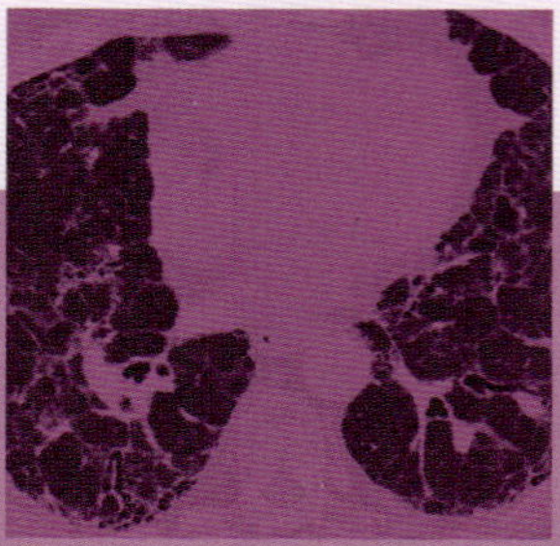

Travis S. Henry

Pulmonary Edema, the Acute Respiratory Distress Syndrome, and Radiology in the Intensive Care Unit

INTRODUCTION

Chest radiographs are routinely obtained in critically ill patients in the intensive care unit. Radiographs are generally used to detect significant changes in cardiopulmonary status; to search for pleural abnormalities; to evaluate the position of the numerous tubes, lines, and catheters used in monitoring and treatment; and to detect complications arising from the use of monitoring and support devices.

In accordance with the American College of Radiology (ACR), Society for Pediatric Radiology (SPR), and Society of Thoracic Radiology (STR) guidelines, the goal of portable chest radiography is to help determine the presence or absence of thoracic disease, to follow known abnormalities, and to evaluate clinical support devices such as endotracheal tubes, chest tubes, vascular catheters, and ventricular assist devices.

In the ICU, some practices still perform routine daily radiographs, although in clinically stable patients this is not supported by data or ACR appropriateness guidelines. On-demand radiograph performance (eg, for patients with clinical deterioration or new support device placement) resulted in change in patient management in 10% to 60% of studies as compared to only 10% to 20% for routine daily radiographs.

The ACR-SPR-STR recommend portable chest radiography for patients:

1. Evaluation of patients with cardiopulmonary signs and/or symptoms following cardiac or thoracic surgery or major trauma, when chest CT has not already been performed, and when PA and lateral examinations cannot be performed
2. Patients with life-support devices
3. Patients who are critically ill or medically unstable
4. Patients who, because of their clinical condition, cannot be transported for standard chest radiography
5. Immediate assessment for pneumothorax following an interventional procedure in the chest or abdomen
6. Intraoperative indications, such as verification of line or device placement or assessment for retained foreign bodies

The ACR-SPR-STR also have published guidelines for (1) qualifications and responsibilities of personnel, (2) technical specifications for the examination, (3) documentation and reporting, (4) equipment specification, (5) quality control and improvement, and (6) radiation safety.

For patients who are pregnant or potentially pregnant, see the ACR–SPR Practice Parameters for Imaging Pregnant or Potentially Pregnant Adolescents and Women.

RADIOGRAPHIC TECHNIQUE

Adequate radiographs are difficult to obtain in the ICU. Portable chest radiographs usually are done using relatively low kilovoltage, long exposure times, no grids, and short source (tube)-to-detector distance. These result in high-contrast films, often with portions of the mediastinum

Table 12.1 ACR-SPR Technical Standards for Bedside Portable Radiographs

1. 72 in source-to-image distance (SID) and upright position in cooperative adults and older pediatric patients (although this is uncommonly possible in ICU patients), or
2. Infants and young children and comatose or uncooperative patients may be imaged supine or semierect with a 40 in or greater SID
3. kVp of 70-100 should be used in radiographs obtained without a grid. In newborns, infants, or small children, lower kVp may be used to optimize contrast and decrease the radiation dose. Grids should be avoided in children less than 10-12 cm thickness
4. kVp of more than 100 may be used for radiographs obtained with a grid
5. Exposure times as short as possible
6. Technical parameters such as mAs, kVp, distance, and patient position should be recorded (to allow consistency in performance)
7. The radiographic beam should be collimated to limit radiation exposure

ACR, American College of Radiology; SPR, Society for Pediatric Radiology.

Adapted from https://www.acr.org/-/media/ACR/Files/Practice-Parameters/Port-Chest-Rad.pdf.

or pulmonary parenchyma poorly seen, motion-related blur, and increased scatter radiation. The ACR-SPR-STR have recommended technical standards for the performance of bedside portable radiographs (Table 12.1).

Even if the technique is optimized, it often is not possible to obtain optimal radiographs because of the patient's inability to cooperate. Patients in the ICU often are too ill to be positioned perfectly for radiographic examinations. Portable radiographs are performed in the anteroposterior (AP) projection, usually supine or semierect rather than upright. Position must be taken into account in interpreting radiographs for the presence of cardiomegaly, pulmonary vascular congestion, and pleural effusion. Furthermore, variation in patient position from day to day also must be considered.

PULMONARY DISEASE IN THE CRITICALLY ILL PATIENT

Common pulmonary complications that occur in critically ill patients include pulmonary edema (hydrostatic and increased capillary permeability), the acute respiratory distress syndrome (ARDS), atelectasis, pneumonia, aspiration, pulmonary embolism, and pulmonary hemorrhage.

The radiographic findings in a patient in the ICU with acute pulmonary disease may be nonspecific, but the distribution of lung disease, the time course of developing radiographic abnormalities, and associated radiographic findings may help in reaching a useful differential diagnosis. Knowledge of the clinical history or physical findings also may be essential in suggesting the appropriate diagnosis.

PULMONARY EDEMA AND THE ARDS

Pulmonary edema often is classified as either hydrostatic (cardiogenic) or due to increased capillary permeability (noncardiogenic). It should be recognized, however, that it is not always possible—or entirely appropriate—to make a simple distinction between hydrostatic edema and permeability edema. Attempting to classify as (1) hydrostatic edema, (2) increased permeability edema associated with diffuse alveolar damage (DAD), (3) increased permeability edema without associated DAD, and (4) mixed edema agrees better with pathology, physiology, and radiology. Although these types of edema cannot always be distinguished on the basis of plain film or CT findings, their appearances do tend to differ.

HYDROSTATIC PULMONARY EDEMA

Hydrostatic pulmonary edema results from alterations in the normal relation between intra- and extravascular hydrostatic and oncotic pressures. In most cases, an increased intravascular pressure due to pulmonary venous hypertension is the predominant cause, resulting in a transudation of fluid into the interstitium. This may result from left heart failure, left atrial or pulmonary venous obstruction, volume overload in renal failure, or overhydration. Hypoalbuminemia, which is associated with peripheral edema, does not contribute as much to pulmonary edema as once thought. Alveolar capillaries have a higher baseline permeability to albumin and thus have greater protection to edema than other tissues. Rapid administration of large volumes of saline, however, can cause acute dilutional hypoalbuminemia and result in hydrostatic pulmonary edema before the levels of albumin equilibrate.

Radiographic abnormalities associated with hydrostatic or cardiogenic pulmonary edema may be difficult to evaluate on portable radiographs. Heart size is difficult to determine accurately on portable AP radiographs, particularly when lung volume is reduced. Pulmonary vascular congestion also may be difficult to identify with certainty because of patient position. Upper lobe vessels appear larger than normal when patients are supine or semierect. Similarly, dilatation of the azygos vein, useful as a sign of increased right atrial pressure, occurs normally in the supine position. The apparent width of the mediastinum (vascular pedicle, see Chapter 2) is increased by supine position, AP projection, and decreased inspiratory level. Associated pleural effusion is common but may be difficult to see on supine radiographs.

In patients with hydrostatic pulmonary edema, chest radiographs and high-resolution CT (HRCT) may show findings of interstitial or airspace edema or both.

Interstitial Edema

Interstitial edema is manifested on chest radiographs by (1) Kerley A or B lines, (2) thickening of the fissures, (3) "peribronchial cuffing," and (4) poor definition of pulmonary vessels or "perihilar haze."

On CT, these findings correspond to the presence of (1) smooth interlobular septal thickening, (2) subpleural edema, (3) thickening of the peribronchovascular interstitium, and (4) ground-glass opacity.

Kerley Lines (Thickening of Interlobular Septa)

Kerley B lines visible on chest radiographs result from thickening of interlobular septa (Fig. 12.1; see also Fig. 11.1 in Chapter 11). They are horizontal, are 1 to 2 cm in length, touch the pleural surface, and are best seen laterally in the costophrenic angles. Their characteristic appearance results from the regular organization of pulmonary lobules at the lung bases.

Kerley A lines (see Fig. 12.1; see also Fig. 11.2 in Chapter 11) are less commonly seen. They are oblique, several centimeters in length, and are seen within the central or perihilar lung. They also represent thickened septa, but their appearance is different from that of B lines because of the different organization of lobules in this location.

In patients with Kerley lines visible on radiographs, HRCT shows smooth interlobular septal thickening (Fig. 12.2; see also Fig. 11.15 in Chapter 11).

Thickening of the Fissures (Subpleural Edema)

The subpleural interstitial space is contiguous with peripheral interlobular septa. If interlobular septal thickening and Kerley lines are present, subpleural interstitial thickening is often visible as well. It is recognized as thickening of the fissures on both chest radiographs and CT (see Figs. 12.1B and 12.2). This finding also may be due to pleural effusion thickening the fissure.

Peribronchial Cuffing (Thickening of the Peribronchovascular Interstitium)

Thickening of the peribronchovascular interstitium often occurs in patients with interstitial edema, resulting in apparent bronchial wall thickening on chest radiographs, or *peribronchial cuffing* (see Fig. 12.2). Peribronchial cuffing is

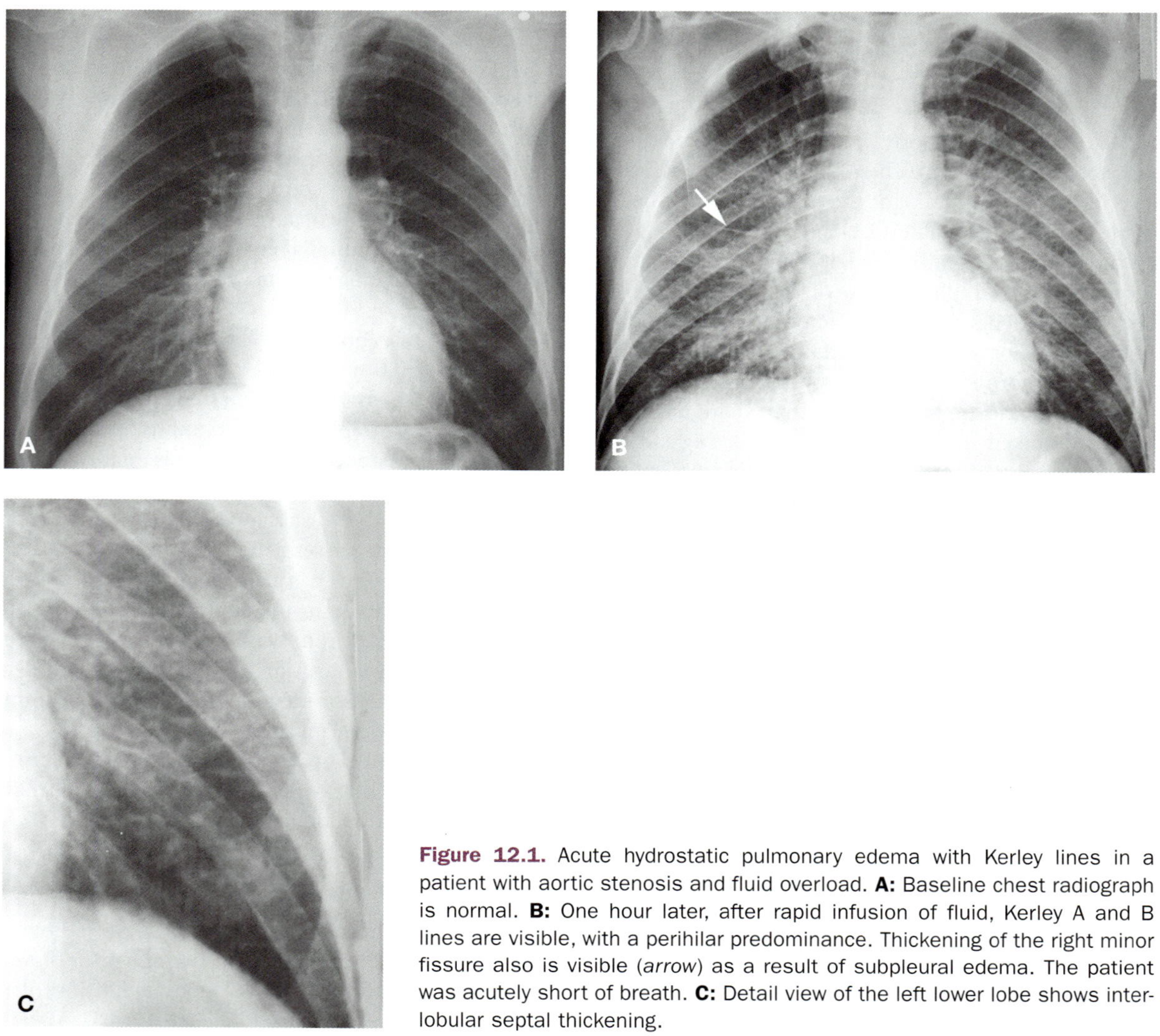

Figure 12.1. Acute hydrostatic pulmonary edema with Kerley lines in a patient with aortic stenosis and fluid overload. **A:** Baseline chest radiograph is normal. **B:** One hour later, after rapid infusion of fluid, Kerley A and B lines are visible, with a perihilar predominance. Thickening of the right minor fissure also is visible (*arrow*) as a result of subpleural edema. The patient was acutely short of breath. **C:** Detail view of the left lower lobe shows interlobular septal thickening.

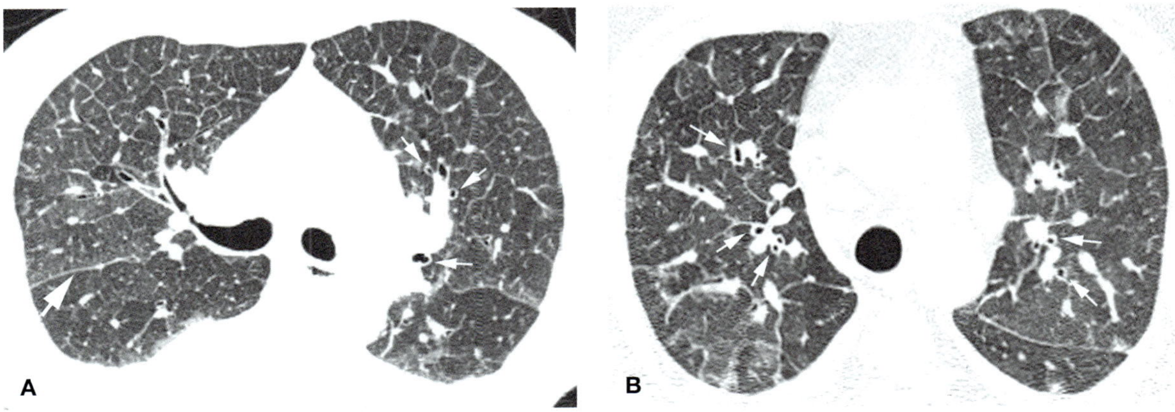

Figure 12.2. Interlobular septal thickening on HRCT in acute hydrostatic pulmonary edema in two different patients. **A:** There is extensive thickening of interlobular septa. Subpleural edema results in thickening of the fissures (*large arrow*). Apparent parahilar bronchial wall thickening ("peribronchial cuffing") results from edema fluid thickening the peribronchovascular interstitium (*small arrows*). Bilateral pleural effusions also are present. **B:** Interlobular septal thickening and thickening of the left major fissure are visible. Peribronchial cuffing (*arrows*) is well seen in this case. Patchy areas of increased lung attenuation represent ground-glass opacity, which may be seen with or without septal thickening in patients with interstitial edema.

easiest to recognize in the perihilar regions where bronchi are seen end on; sometimes lines radiating outward from the hila reflect the thickened peribronchial interstitium. On CT, thickening of the peribronchovascular interstitium resembles bronchial wall thickening; pulmonary arteries adjacent to the bronchi appear increased in diameter because the thickened interstitium surrounds them as well.

Poor Definition of Perihilar Vessels and Perihilar Haze (Ground-Glass Opacity)

On chest radiographs, edema fluid surrounding pulmonary vessels blurs their margins, making them difficult to see or poorly defined on chest radiographs. This finding is easiest to recognize when comparison films are available. Poor definition of lower lobe vessels usually is the first abnormality noted in pulmonary edema and may be seen when Kerley lines are unrecognizable.

Poor definition of hilar or perihilar vessels is a common finding in patients with mild pulmonary edema (Fig. 12.3). On radiographs, this finding, sometimes referred to as *perihilar haze*, is often useful in diagnosing pulmonary edema in bedridden patients with lower lobe atelectasis or pneumonia in whom the lower lobe vessels cannot be assessed. This appearance may progress to a frank "batwing" pattern of pulmonary edema.

An overall increase in lung water or interstitial thickening often is recognizable as a poorly defined, generalized increase in lung density, or ground-glass opacity. It may be difficult to recognize on chest radiographs in the absence of comparison films but is easily seen on HRCT (Fig. 12.4).

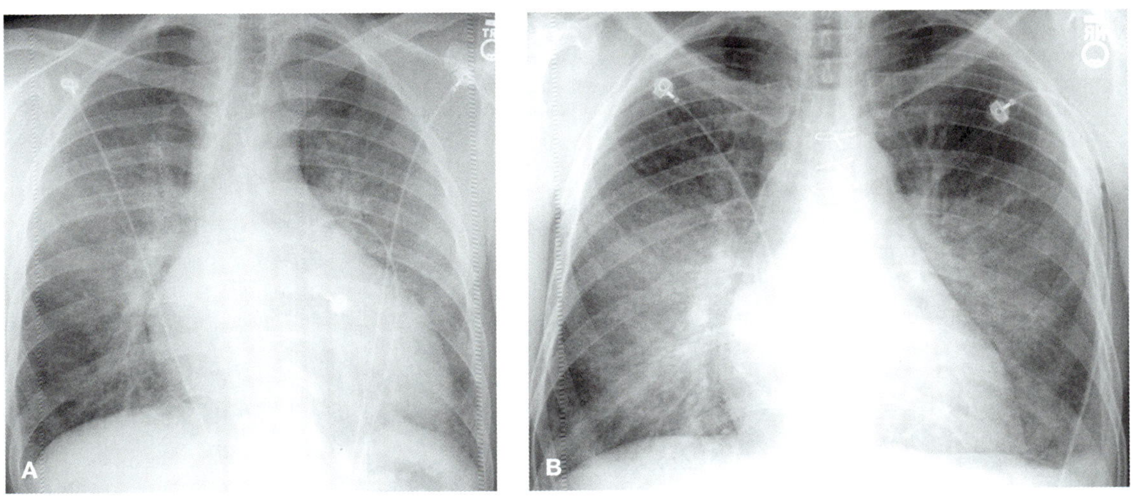

Figure 12.3. Poor definition of perihilar and lower lobe vessels ("perihilar haze") in two patients with hydrostatic edema. **A:** Chest radiograph in a patient with congestive heart failure and cardiomegaly shows poor definition of perihilar and lower lobe vessels as the first sign of pulmonary edema. **B:** In another patient with cardiomegaly and pulmonary edema, hazy opacity obscures perihilar and lower lobe vessels.

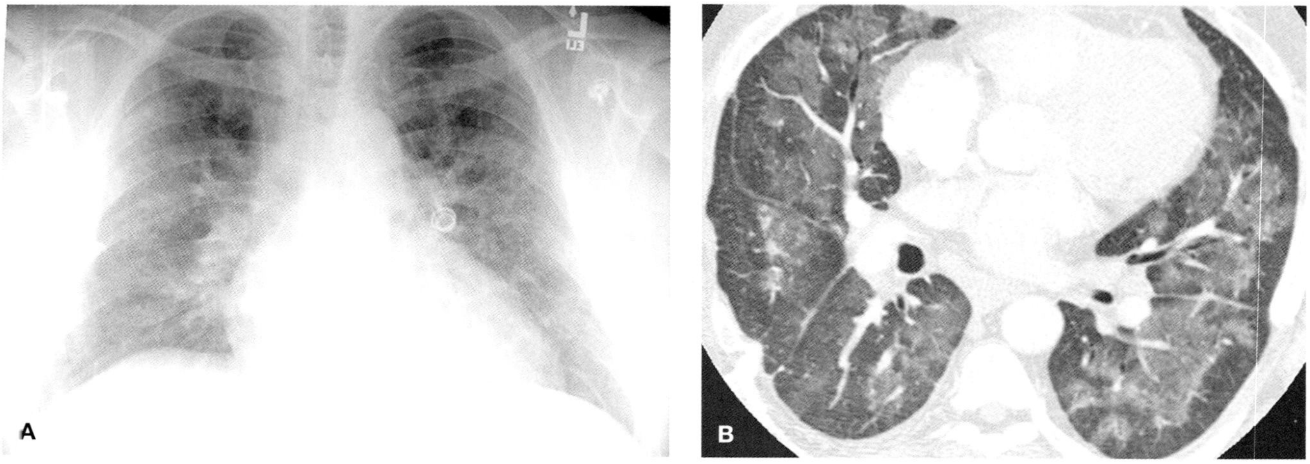

Figure 12.4. Hydrostatic edema with ground-glass opacity. **A:** Chest radiograph in a patient with edema shows poor definition of perihilar vessels and a subtle increase in lung density. **B:** HRCT shows patchy perihilar ground-glass opacity. Thickening of the fissures and small pleural effusions are present, but septal thickening is absent in this patient.

In patients with perihilar haze visible on chest radiographs, ground-glass opacity often is seen on HRCT.

On HRCT, ground-glass opacity due to edema may be perihilar and perivascular (see Fig. 12.4B), peripheral and subpleural (see Fig. 11.31A in Chapter 11), patchy (Fig. 12.5) and lobular, or centrilobular in distribution. It may be seen in isolation or in combination with septal thickening (see Fig. 12.2B).

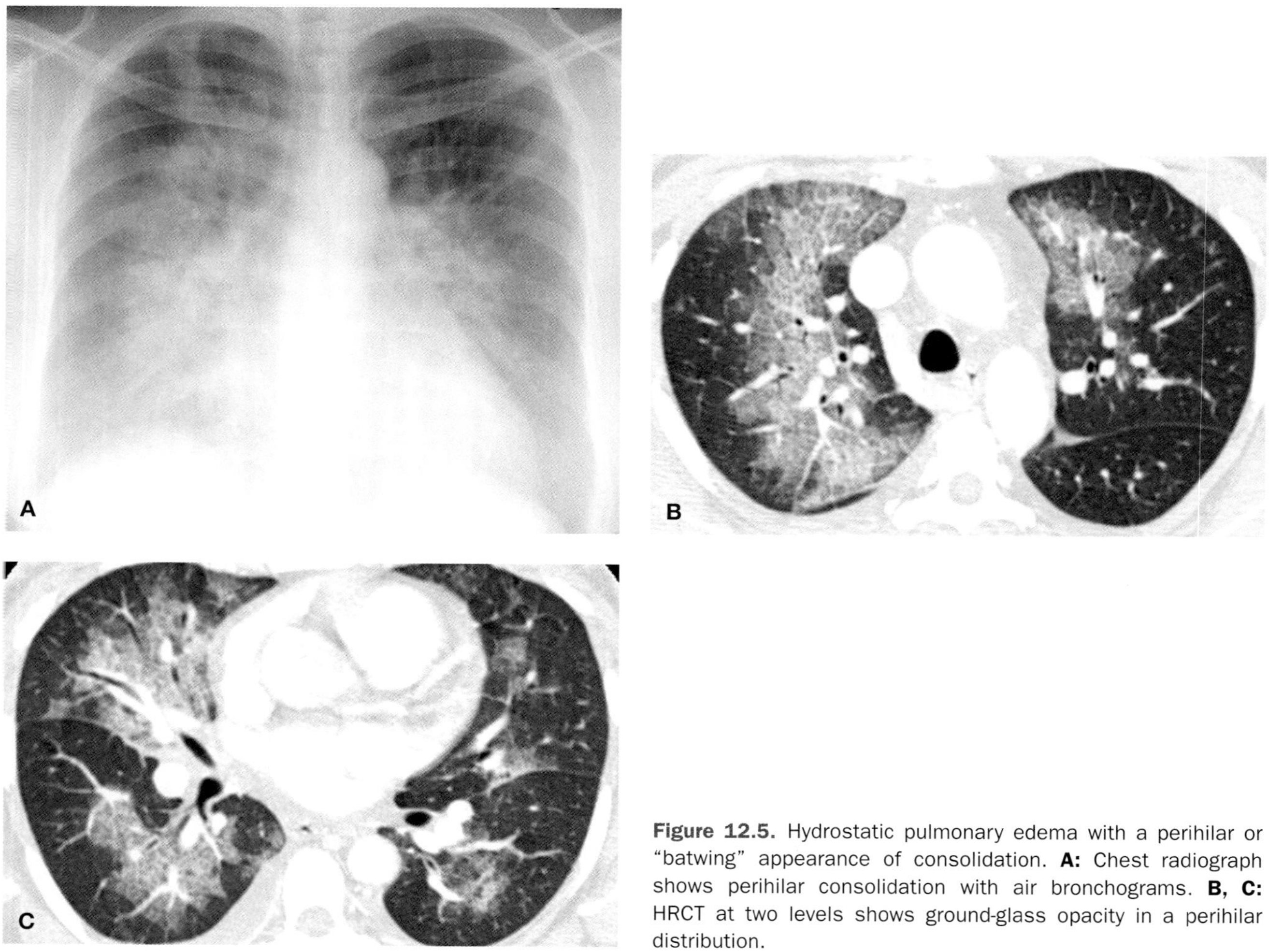

Figure 12.5. Hydrostatic pulmonary edema with a perihilar or "batwing" appearance of consolidation. **A:** Chest radiograph shows perihilar consolidation with air bronchograms. **B, C:** HRCT at two levels shows ground-glass opacity in a perihilar distribution.

Airspace Edema

With an increase in interstitial pressure and a worsening of edema, fluid overflows the interstitium and fills the alveoli. Findings of airspace edema are the same as those of airspace consolidation. They include ill-defined or confluent opacities with obscuration of underlying vessels and "acinar" or airspace nodules. Air bronchograms may be seen in some patients but are not always visible. HRCT may show frank consolidation or dense ground-glass opacity in patients with the appearance of consolidation on plain radiographs. Homogeneous dense consolidation is unusual on HRCT in patients with edema unless atelectasis is associated.

Airspace edema may be patchy, multifocal, or diffuse, but usually it is bilateral and symmetric. In upright patients, a basal distribution often is visible. A perihilar "batwing" or "butterfly" distribution occurs occasionally, often related to rapid accumulation of edema fluid (Fig. 12.5). This pattern also has been attributed to better clearance of edema fluid in the lung periphery because of a richer lymphatic network in this region, but why it is seen in some patients and not in others is unclear.

Unilateral or Asymmetric Edema

Hydrostatic edema usually is bilateral and symmetric. In patients with edema, variations in the distribution of the edema fluid may result from variations in blood flow or hydrostatic pressure (or other mechanisms). Unilateral or asymmetric edema may result (Table 12.2).

The most common cause of unilateral edema is the decubitus position (Fig. 12.6). Right upper lobe edema may be seen in patients with papillary muscle rupture and mitral regurgitation; this is caused by a jet of regurgitant blood directed into the right superior pulmonary vein (Fig. 12.7).

Table 12.2 Unilateral Pulmonary Edema

Unilateral edema associated with ipsilateral abnormalities
Decubitus position
Reexpansion edema
Pulmonary vein occlusion
Congenital or acquired systemic to pulmonary artery shunt (eg, Blalock-Taussig)
Papillary muscle rupture and mitral regurgitation with a jet effect
Unilateral edema associated with contralateral abnormalities
Pulmonary artery occlusion (eg, pulmonary embolism, tumor)
Hypoplastic pulmonary artery or interruption of the pulmonary artery
Swyer-James syndrome
Unilateral emphysema or bullae
Transient atelectasis

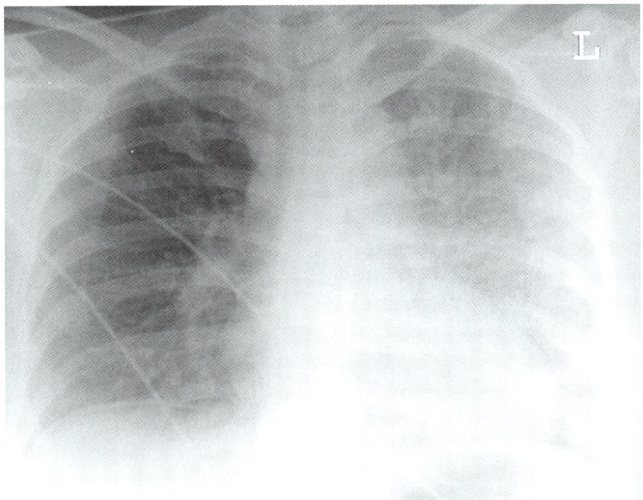

Figure 12.6. Unilateral left-sided pulmonary edema. Postoperative radiograph in a patient who had a right nephrectomy in the left lateral decubitus position. Note free air under the right hemidiaphragm secondary to surgery.

Patients with decreased blood flow to one lung (eg, pulmonary artery occlusion) tend to develop edema on the opposite side. This also may be seen in patients with unilateral lung abnormalities resulting in decreased blood flow, such as pulmonary embolism or Swyer-James syndrome (Fig.12.8).

Course and Clearing of Hydrostatic Edema

Hydrostatic edema may appear rapidly in association with acute heart failure or fluid overload (see Fig. 12.1). Often the radiograph becomes abnormal at the same time that symptoms appear. However, it is important to recognize

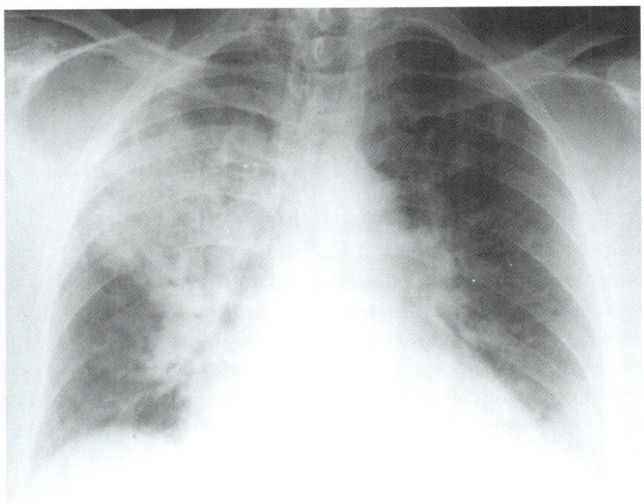

Figure 12.7. Right upper lobe edema due to acute myocardial infarction with papillary muscle rupture, prolapse of the posterior leaflet of the mitral valve, and acute mitral regurgitation. Note cardiomegaly.

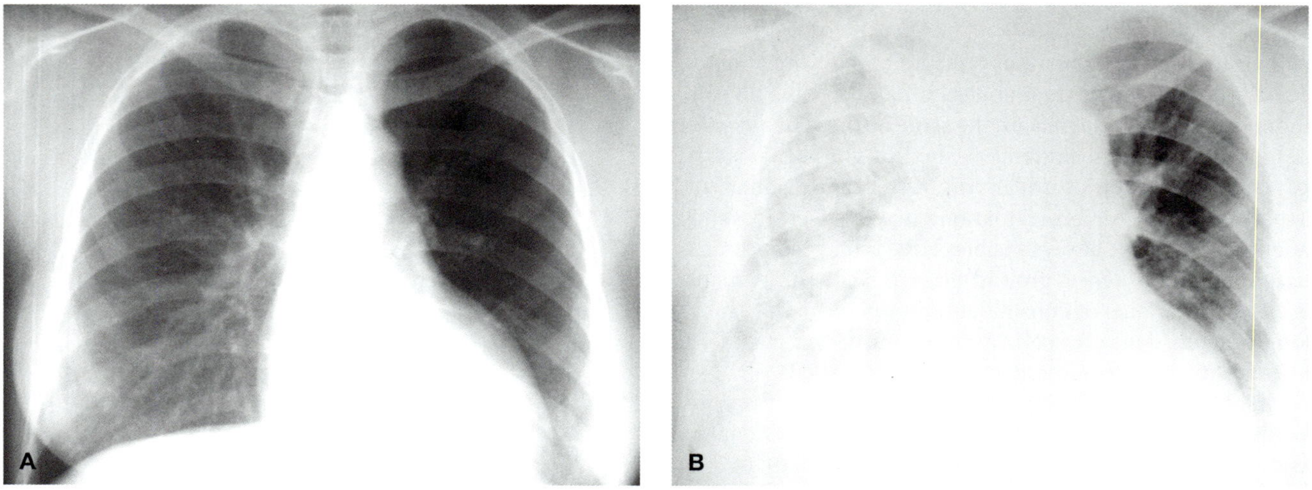

Figure 12.8. Left-sided Swyer-James syndrome with predominant right-sided pulmonary edema. **A:** Baseline chest radiograph shows a hyperlucent and hypovascular left upper lobe. This appearance is typical of Swyer-James syndrome. **B:** Subsequently, congestive heart failure with cardiomegaly is associated with pulmonary edema. The edema spares the left upper lobe.

that hydrostatic edema may be visible on chest radiographs before the symptoms develop (clinical lag) or after pulmonary venous pressure has returned to normal (radiographic lag).

Because hydrostatic edema is relatively low in protein, it may show rapid clearing with improvement in patient status. Similarly, a gravitational shift in the distribution of edema fluid may occur within minutes to hours of a change in patient position. Airspace edema reacts more slowly than does interstitial edema to changes in patient status.

Although a progression of edema from an interstitial to an airspace pattern may be seen with worsening, this is not always the case. Many patients show airspace edema as the initial finding. Similarly, in patients with airspace edema, the edema does not typically assume an interstitial appearance as it clears.

PERMEABILITY EDEMA, DAD, AND THE ARDS

Permeability edema is a manifestation of injury to the alveolar-capillary membrane, with resultant leakage of fluid and protein into the lung interstitium. It results in a high-protein edema and, therefore, is slow to clear. It often, but not always, is associated with a histologic diagnosis of *diffuse alveolar damage* (*DAD*). DAD often results in the clinical syndrome known as *acute respiratory distress syndrome* (*ARDS*), although ARDS may occur in patients without histologic DAD. It is important to note that the two terms are not interchangeable.

In the current international definition and classification of ARDS, termed the Berlin definition, the term *acute lung injury* (*ALI*), previously used to refer to lung injury with less severe hypoxemia than that seen in ARDS, has been dropped.

ARDS is characterized by progressive dyspnea and hypoxemia over a period of hours to days. Specific Berlin criteria for the diagnosis and classification of ARDS include the following:

1. Acute onset of respiratory failure, within a week of a known clinical insult or new or worsening respiratory symptoms
2. Bilateral opacities on chest radiographs or CT, not fully explained by effusions, lobar or lung atelectasis, or nodules
3. Respiratory failure not fully explained by cardiac failure or fluid overload. Need objective assessment (eg, echocardiography) to exclude hydrostatic edema, if no risk factor present
4. Oxygenation (criteria modified if altitude greater than 1000 m), dividing ARDS into three severity categories for intubated patients (PEEP ≥ 5 5 cm H_2O in all categories):
   Mild: 200 mm Hg < PaO_2/FiO_2 ≤ 300 mm Hg
   Moderate: 100 mm Hg < PaO_2/FiO_2 ≤ 200 mm Hg
   Severe: PaO_2/FiO_2 ≤ 100 mm Hg

CPAP, continuous positive airway pressure; FiO_2, fraction of inspired oxygen; PaO_2, partial pressure of arterial oxygen; PEEP, positive end-expiratory pressure.

ARDS can be related to a variety of pathologic processes, not all of which are associated with pulmonary edema or DAD, including the following:

1. Infection (eg, pneumonia, including COVID-19 and sepsis)
2. Inhalation or aspiration of toxic or irritating substances (eg, EVALI)
3. Trauma with lung or extrathoracic injury

Table 12.3 Direct and Indirect Causes of Acute Respiratory Distress Syndrome

Direct injury
Pneumonia (including virus, bacteria, mycoplasma, fungus, tuberculosis, *Pneumocystis jiroveci* [*Pneumocystis carinii*] pneumonia, rickettsia)
Miliary tuberculosis or other disseminated infections
Inhalation (smoke, toxic gases, oxygen in high concentration vaping)
Aspiration (gastric acid, ingested substances, drowning, chemicals, blood)
Thoracic trauma with contusion or crush injury
Thoracic radiation
Cardiopulmonary bypass
Fat embolism
Air embolism
Amniotic fluid embolism
Reexpansion or reperfusion edema
Sickle cell crisis
Acute interstitial pneumonia
Usual interstitial pneumonia with acute exacerbation
Indirect injury
Sepsis (particularly gram-negative organisms)
Shock
Toxic shock syndrome
Disseminated intravascular coagulation
Extrathoracic trauma
Burns
Neurogenic edema
Drugs
Anaphylaxis
Transfusion reactions
Leukoagglutinin reactions
Diabetic ketoacidosis
Pancreatitis
Uremia
High altitude

4. Hemodynamic abnormalities (eg, shock, high altitude, anaphylaxis)
5. Hematologic disorders (eg, disseminated intravascular coagulation, transfusion reaction)
6. Embolic disease (eg, fat embolism, amniotic fluid embolism)
7. Drugs, either therapeutic or nontherapeutic
8. Metabolic disorders (eg, pancreatitis, ketoacidosis)
9. Neurologic disease (eg, head injury, stroke)

An idiopathic form of ARDS is termed acute interstitial pneumonia (AIP). AIP is discussed in Chapter 14.

Most simply, the mechanism of lung injury in ARDS may be considered to be *direct*, in which the lungs themselves are injured (eg, pneumonia, aspiration, and inhalational injury), or *indirect*, in which extrapulmonary abnormalities (eg, sepsis, shock, pancreatitis) lead to lung injury (Table 12.3).

The Stages of ARDS Associated With DAD

ARDS is considered to occur in stages, within the time frame of hours, days, weeks, and months (Table 12.4), which have close pathologic and radiographic correlates.

Pathologic Abnormalities

Pathologic abnormalities in DAD with ARDS are similar regardless of its cause.

Hours. Within hours of the precipitating insult, endothelial cell edema, widening of intracellular junctions, congestion of capillaries, and limited interstitial pulmonary edema and hemorrhage are present. These manifestations represent the early *exudative (injury) stage* of DAD with ARDS.

Days. The period from a day to a week after the initial insult is characterized by progressive capillary endothelial injury, necrosis of alveolar lining cells (type I pneumocytes), proteinaceous interstitial and alveolar edema, and

Table 12.4 The Stages of Acute Respiratory Distress Syndrome

Time Frame	Stage	Pathologic Findings	Radiologic Findings
Hours	Early exudative (injury)	Endothelial edema, early edema	Normal
Days	Late exudative (injury)	Progressive endothelial injury, necrosis of alveolar lining cells, progressive alveolar edema and hemorrhage	GGO/consolidation, often bilateral, progressive confluence, dependent atelectasis
Weeks	Proliferative (reparative)	Proliferation of alveolar lining cells and fibroblasts, organization of alveolar exudates	Slow resolution of GGO/consolidation, development of reticular opacities, airway dilation, organization
Months	Fibrosis	Depending on the degree of injury, resolution or fibrosis	Clearance of GGO/consolidation, progressive fibrosis with reticulation, traction, possibly honeycombing; may be anterior

GGO, ground-glass opacity.

hemorrhage. Hyaline membranes form within the alveoli. This represents the late *exudative (injury) stage*.

Weeks. The *proliferative (organizing) stage* usually occurs from 1 week to 1 month following the onset of DAD. It is characterized by proliferation of type II pneumocytes, which reline the denuded alveolar walls, organization of the alveolar exudates, fibroblast proliferation within the alveolar walls and interstitium, and deposition of collagen.

Months. In many patients, these abnormalities resolve, and little respiratory disability results. In patients with more severe lung injury, interstitial fibrosis develops. This is termed the *fibrotic stage*.

Radiographic Abnormalities

Hours. Radiographs typically are normal for the first 12 to 24 hours after the acute injury, despite the presence of dyspnea (Fig. 12.9A). This latent period is suggestive of ARDS (Table 12.4).

Days. Radiographs typically become abnormal within 24 hours of the inciting insult and the development of symptoms. Radiographs show bilateral patchy areas of airspace consolidation; these tend to have a more peripheral distribution than those seen in patients with hydrostatic edema (see Fig. 12.9B and C). They increase over time and eventually become confluent (see Fig. 12.9D and E). Dependent

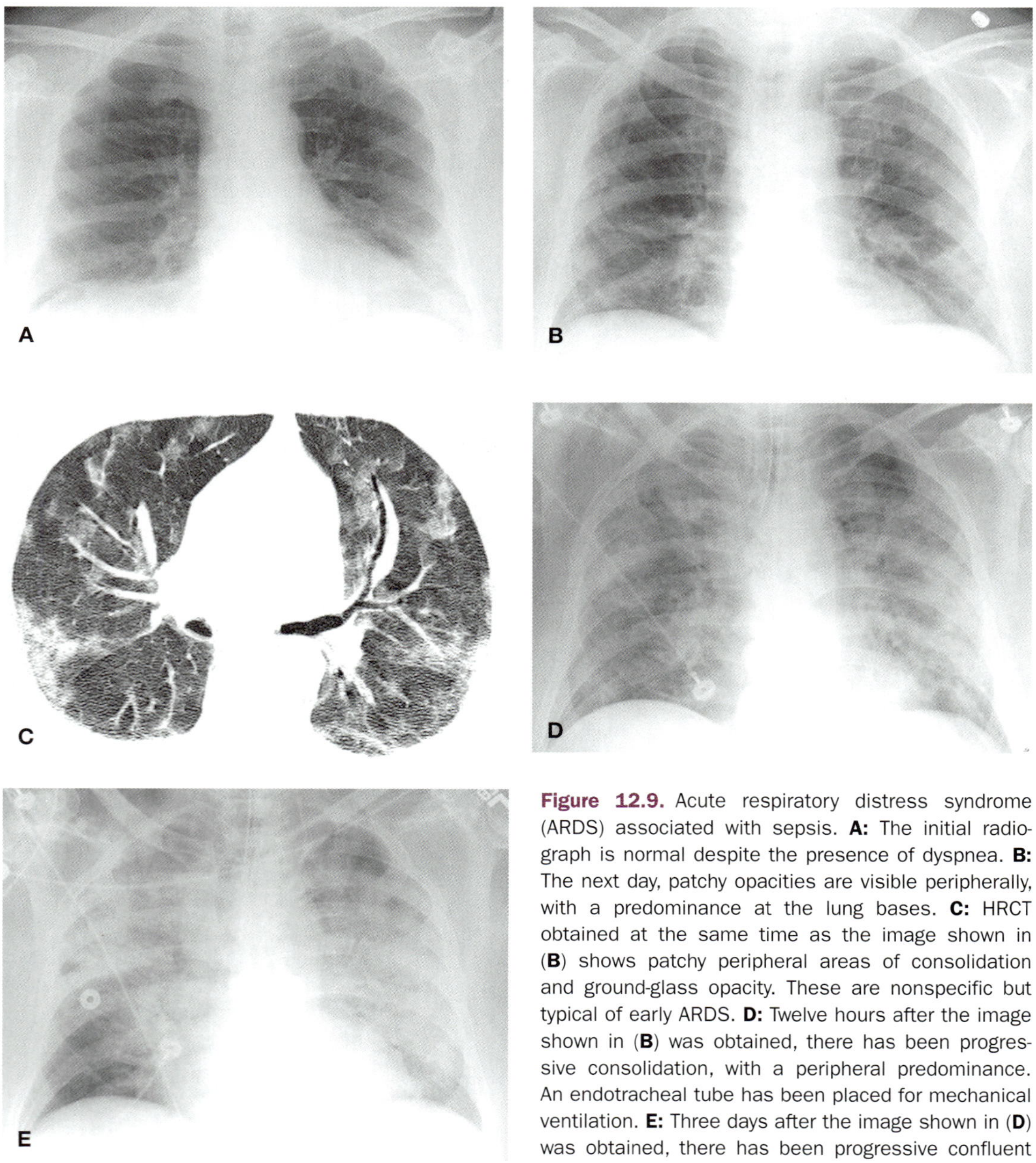

Figure 12.9. Acute respiratory distress syndrome (ARDS) associated with sepsis. **A:** The initial radiograph is normal despite the presence of dyspnea. **B:** The next day, patchy opacities are visible peripherally, with a predominance at the lung bases. **C:** HRCT obtained at the same time as the image shown in (**B**) shows patchy peripheral areas of consolidation and ground-glass opacity. These are nonspecific but typical of early ARDS. **D:** Twelve hours after the image shown in (**B**) was obtained, there has been progressive consolidation, with a peripheral predominance. An endotracheal tube has been placed for mechanical ventilation. **E:** Three days after the image shown in (**D**) was obtained, there has been progressive confluent consolidation, and air bronchograms are visible.

atelectasis often develops. Air bronchograms are more common than with hydrostatic edema. Interstitial abnormalities may be present, but Kerley lines are distinctly uncommon. Pleural effusion is much less common and, when present, is smaller than in patients with hydrostatic edema.

Because of the lung injury occurring with ARDS and the presence of proteinaceous edema fluid, hyaline membranes and hemorrhage, radiographic abnormalities clear much more slowly than with hydrostatic edema. Radiographic improvement, with increased lung volumes and decrease in lung opacity, may occur within the first week, but this often reflects positive pressure ventilation rather than improvement in lung abnormalities.

Mechanical ventilation (see Fig. 12.9D) usually is required to maintain oxygenation. High ventilator pressures often are necessary in patients with ARDS, and barotrauma with pneumothorax and pneumomediastinum often occurs during this stage.

On HRCT, pulmonary edema occurring with ARDS generally is associated with ground-glass opacity or consolidation, with predominance in dependent lung regions (see Fig. 12.9C). Opacities can be diffuse or patchy. Interlobular septal thickening is less commonly seen than in hydrostatic edema. Depending on the etiology of the lung injury, opacities may predominate in the peripheral and subpleural regions or can spare the lung periphery. Unilateral or bilateral pleural effusions may be seen, but they typically are small.

Differences may be seen in the CT appearances of patients with ARDS due to pulmonary disease (eg, pneumonia) and those with ARDS resulting from extrapulmonary causes (eg, sepsis). In patients with ARDS due to pulmonary disease, consolidation and ground-glass opacity are equally prevalent, and lung abnormalities often are asymmetric, reflecting the presence of the predisposing lung disease. In patients with an extrathoracic cause of ARDS, ground-glass opacity is predominant, and symmetric lung involvement is more typical (see Fig. 12.9C).

The CT findings in patients with pulmonary *fat embolism syndrome*, a cause of ARDS, include diffuse ground-glass opacity, focal areas of consolidation or ground-glass opacity, or nodules. Focal abnormalities predominate in the upper lobes. Gravity-dependent opacities predominate in the lower lobes.

Weeks. After 1 week, consolidation may begin to resolve slowly, becoming more patchy or being replaced by reticular opacities and areas that look like organizing pneumonia. New confluent areas of consolidation or new centrilobular nodules after 1 week may indicate superimposed pneumonia. Over time, consolidation clears in patients with DAD, but ground-glass opacity and findings of lung fibrosis may persist.

Months. In patients developing pulmonary fibrosis, chest films show a persisting reticular pattern or findings of honeycombing. Reticulation and honeycombing may be seen on HRCT and tend to have a striking anterior distribution (Fig. 12.10). This unusual distribution probably reflects the fact that patients with ARDS typically develop posterior lung atelectasis and consolidation during the exudative stage of disease; it is thought that this consolidation protects the posterior lung regions from the adverse effects of mechanical ventilation, including high ventilatory pressures and high oxygen tension. This unusual distribution may be offset in some patients when prone positioning is used while on ventilatory support.

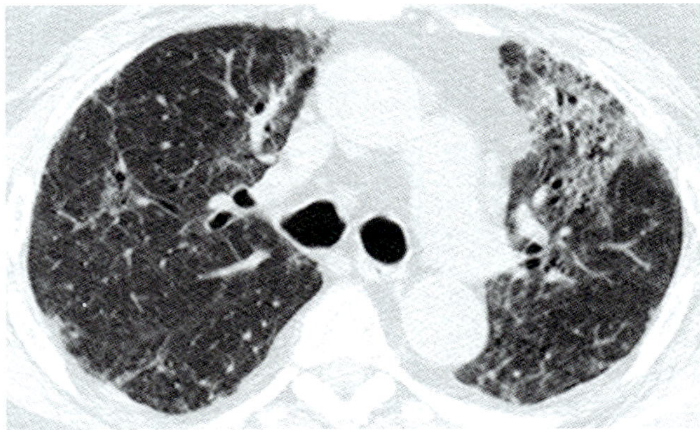

Figure 12.10. Anterior lung fibrosis in a patient recovering from acute respiratory distress syndrome. There is asymmetric reticulation with traction bronchiectasis and mild honeycombing. The posterior lung also is abnormal, but to a lesser degree.

PERMEABILITY EDEMA WITHOUT DAD

Permeability pulmonary edema may occur without accompanying DAD in patients with drug reactions, interleukin-2 treatment, transfusion reaction, or hantavirus pulmonary syndrome, or as a result of a mild insult of a type usually resulting in ARDS, such as air embolism or toxic shock syndrome. It has been suggested that the absence of a pulmonary epithelial injury in such patients reduces the extent of alveolar edema.

In patients with permeability pulmonary edema occurring in the absence of DAD, radiographic abnormalities typically resemble hydrostatic edema, with interlobular septal thickening being a predominant feature in many cases (Fig. 12.11). Edema may clear rapidly, because of the absence of epithelial injury.

MIXED EDEMA

Mixed permeability and hydrostatic edema may be seen in diseases resulting in increased intravascular pressure and capillary endothelial injury. A mixed etiology is thought to exist in patients with neurogenic pulmonary edema, reexpansion edema, high-altitude pulmonary edema, reexpansion or reperfusion edema, edema associated with tocolytic therapy or the postpartum state (Fig. 12.12), posttransplantation edema, postpneumonectomy or post–volume reduction edema, and edema related to air embolism; in some drug reactions (Fig. 12.13); and in patients with ARDS who

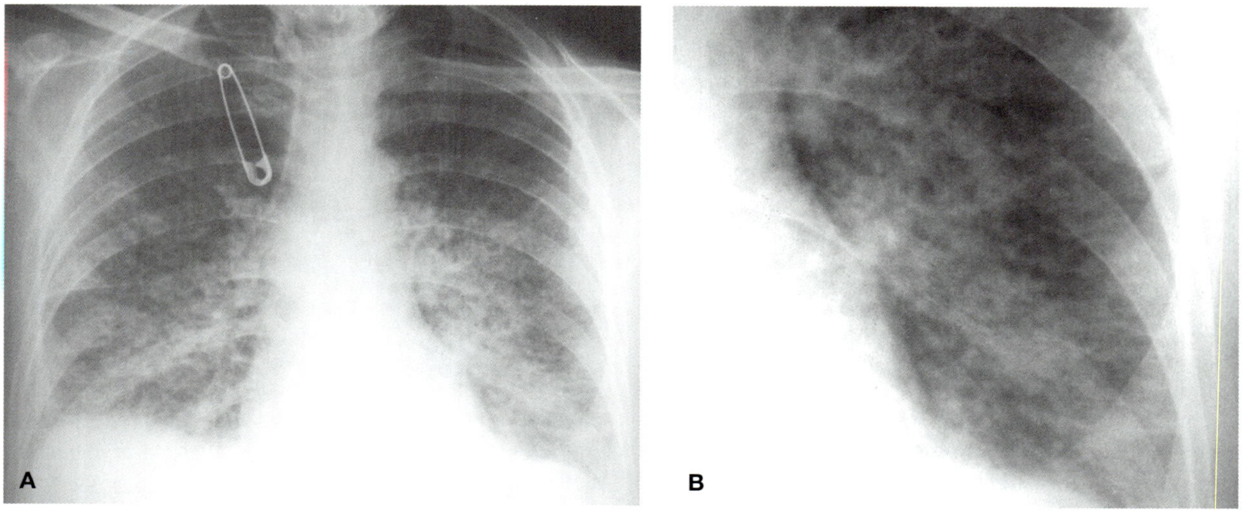

Figure 12.11. Acute drug reaction (to bleomycin) showing permeability pulmonary edema. **A:** Chest radiograph shows increased reticular opacities at the lung bases with Kerley lines. Although this appearance resembles hydrostatic edema, the heart size is normal. **B:** Coned-down view of the left base shows Kerley B lines.

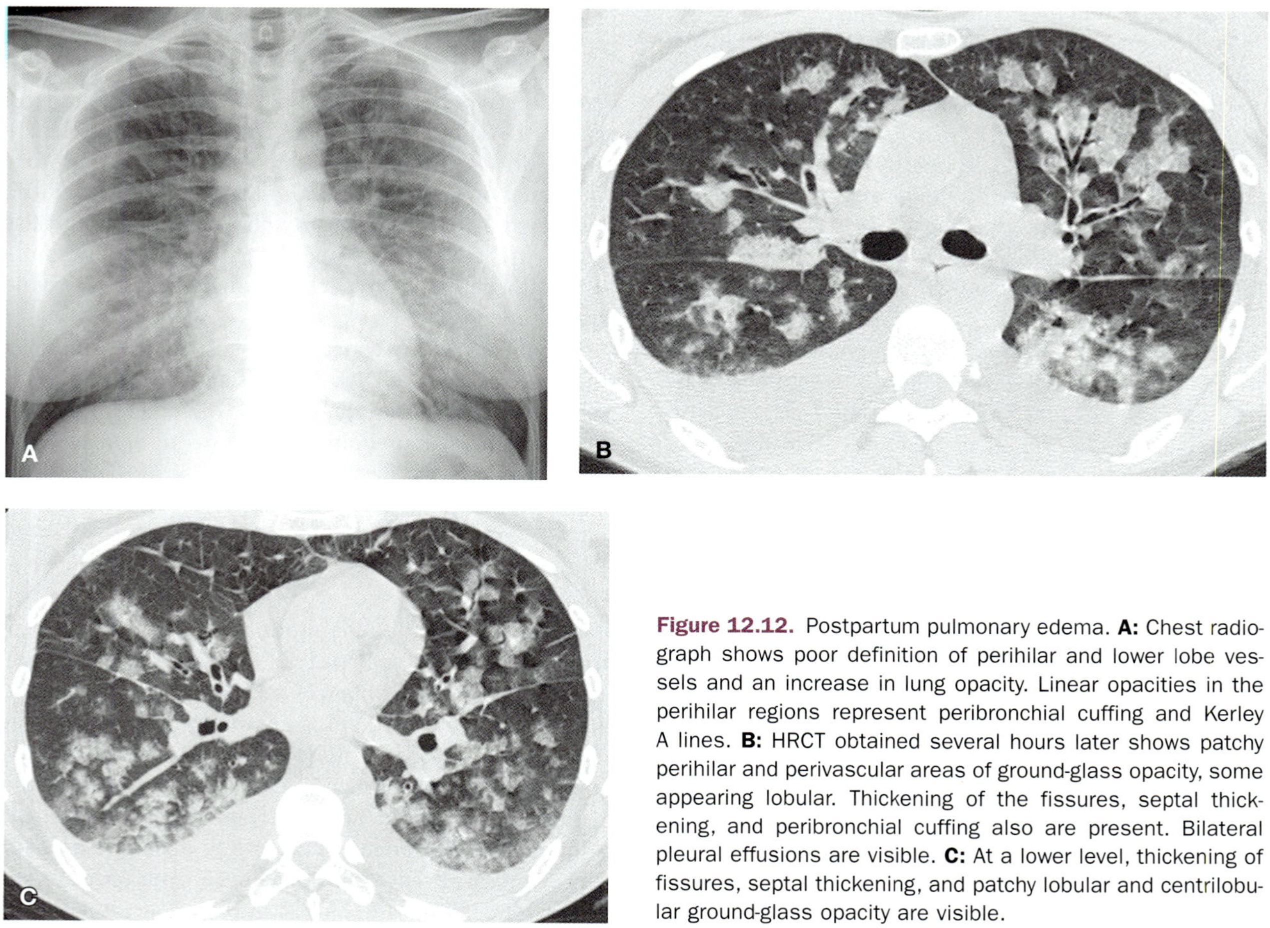

Figure 12.12. Postpartum pulmonary edema. **A:** Chest radiograph shows poor definition of perihilar and lower lobe vessels and an increase in lung opacity. Linear opacities in the perihilar regions represent peribronchial cuffing and Kerley A lines. **B:** HRCT obtained several hours later shows patchy perihilar and perivascular areas of ground-glass opacity, some appearing lobular. Thickening of the fissures, septal thickening, and peribronchial cuffing also are present. Bilateral pleural effusions are visible. **C:** At a lower level, thickening of fissures, septal thickening, and patchy lobular and centrilobular ground-glass opacity are visible.

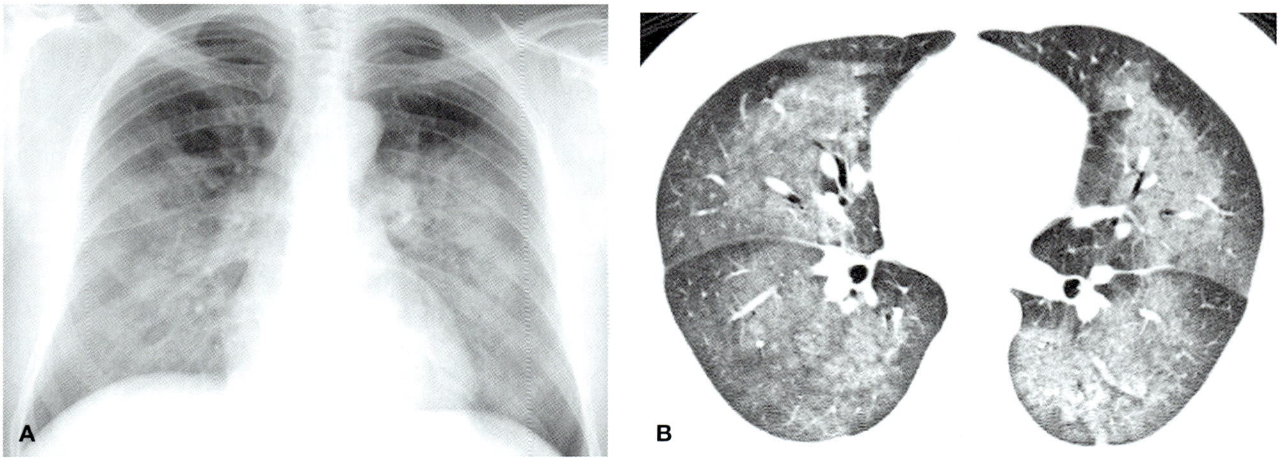

Figure 12.13. Mixed permeability and hydrostatic pulmonary edema in a patient with cocaine abuse. Transient hypertension and capillary leak are thought to be responsible. **A:** Chest radiograph shows a perihilar "batwing" appearance of pulmonary edema. **B:** HRCT shows perihilar ground-glass opacity, with sparing of the lung periphery. This cleared over a period of a few days.

are overhydrated or develop renal or heart failure. As would be expected, the radiographic appearances of these different types of edema are variable.

DISTINGUISHING THE TYPES OF EDEMA

Although it is sometimes impossible to distinguish among these types of edema, attention to specific findings allows more than two-thirds of cases to be classified correctly.

In hydrostatic edema, findings of cardiomegaly and vascular congestion often are valuable in making the diagnosis. Radiographic findings of edema often appear soon after the inciting incident and may change rapidly. The presence of interstitial edema with Kerley lines suggests hydrostatic edema, although they may be seen in patients with permeability edema without DAD and in mixed edema. Pleural effusion is common with hydrostatic edema and may be large.

In patients with ARDS, radiographic abnormalities often are delayed 24 hours after the onset of symptoms, and radiographic abnormalities change slowly. Air bronchograms are more typical of ARDS, and Kerley lines are unusual. Pleural effusions are uncommon and usually small.

SPECIFIC CAUSES OF PULMONARY EDEMA

Neurogenic Pulmonary Edema

Pulmonary edema developing in patients with head trauma, intracranial hemorrhage, increased intracranial pressure, seizures, or other acute neurologic conditions most likely occurs because of both hydrostatic mechanisms and increased permeability (ie, mixed edema). Sympathetic discharge resulting from central nervous system injury results in systemic vasoconstriction, increased systemic blood pressure, and acute left heart failure. The edema fluid may be high in protein, indicating increased permeability. Edema may appear very rapidly, within minutes of the responsible episode (ie, "flash" *pulmonary edema*). The appearance is usually that of airspace edema (Fig. 12.14). Clearing occurs within 1 or 2 days.

Reexpansion Pulmonary Edema

Rapid reexpansion of lung after being collapsed for more than 2 or 3 days may result in focal edema of the reexpanded lung. It typically occurs within 2 to 4 hours of reexpansion but may progress for 1 or 2 days. It typically appears as airspace edema.

Two mechanisms probably are responsible. First, following collapse, lung perfusion decreases, lung becomes

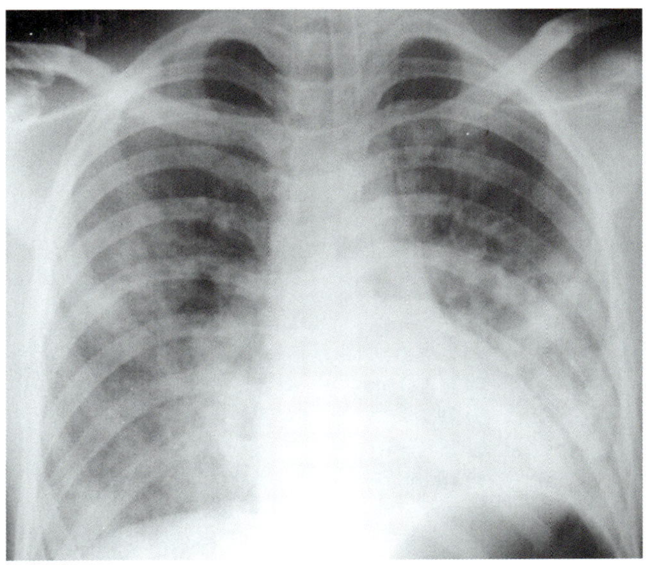

Figure 12.14. Neurogenic pulmonary edema following head trauma. Bilateral consolidation is visible.

hypoxemic, surfactant production decreases, and the lung becomes less compliant. Because of this, a more negative intrapleural pressure is required (during thoracentesis or chest tube drainage) to achieve lung reexpansion. This may contribute to the development of edema by hydrostatic mechanisms. Secondly, prolonged hypoxemia with release of free radicals may result in capillary endothelial injury, with increased permeability edema developing with reperfusion. A transient decrease in pulmonary lymphatic or venous return has also been suggested as a contributing mechanism. Edema usually resolves in less than 1 week.

Although the edema usually is localized to the part of lung that was previously collapsed, it sometimes may be seen in other lobes or in the opposite lung. This occurrence may be due to the release of free radicals and vasoactive substances into the bloodstream following reperfusion of hypoxemic lung. Reexpansion pulmonary edema usually appears as consolidation or ground-glass opacity (Figs. 12.15 and 12.16).

Reexpansion edema usually is not problematic, but in some cases, it may result in a worsening of the patient's symptoms even though lung compression due to the pleural air or fluid collection has been alleviated. In patients with large pleural collections, slow removal over a period of days may be appropriate, reducing the chance that reexpansion edema will occur.

High-Altitude Pulmonary Edema

Pulmonary edema may develop after rapid ascent to high altitude, usually in excess of 10,000 feet. Edema usually develops between 12 hours and 3 days after ascent; most cases occur in the first day. Less commonly, it develops in people with prolonged residence at high altitude.

Reduction in the partial pressure of oxygen in inspired air is responsible for this type of edema. In susceptible people, it results in patchy spasm of some small pulmonary arteries, resulting in high pressure in those arterial branches that remain patent. This high pressure not only results in hydrostatic edema but also injures the capillary endothelium, leading to increased permeability. Patchy airspace edema typically is seen. Administration of oxygen or a return to sea level results in resolution within 1 or 2 days.

ATELECTASIS

Atelectasis often develops in patients in the ICU because of depressed sensorium, pain, endotracheal intubation, mechanical ventilation, and the supine position. Particularly in postsurgical patients, areas of basal atelectasis are common and typically appear in the first 24 to 48 hours. Obstruction

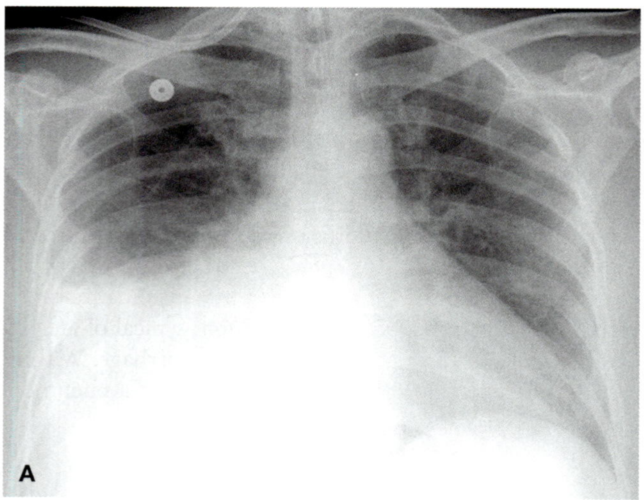

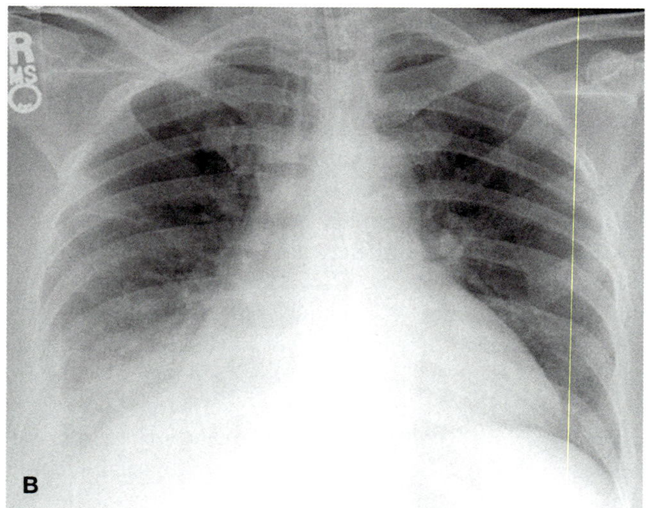

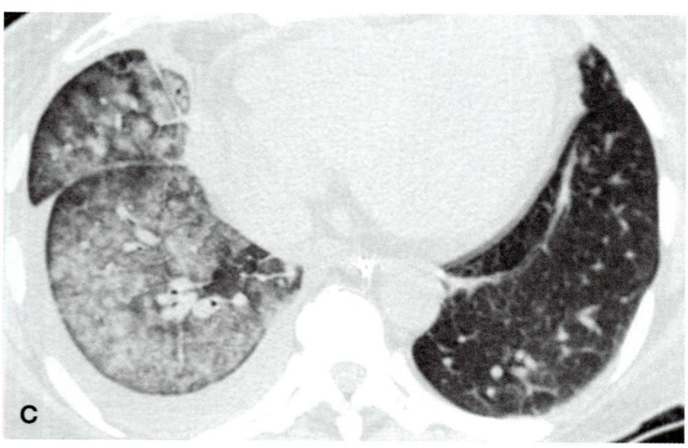

Figure 12.15. Reexpansion pulmonary edema following thoracentesis. **A:** A patient with cardiomegaly shows a right-sided pleural effusion. **B:** Radiograph following thoracentesis shows a small residual effusion and increased opacity in the right lower lobe due to reexpansion edema. **C:** HRCT shows a small residual right-sided effusion and ground-glass opacity involving right middle and lower lobes. The opacities show a centrilobular predominance.

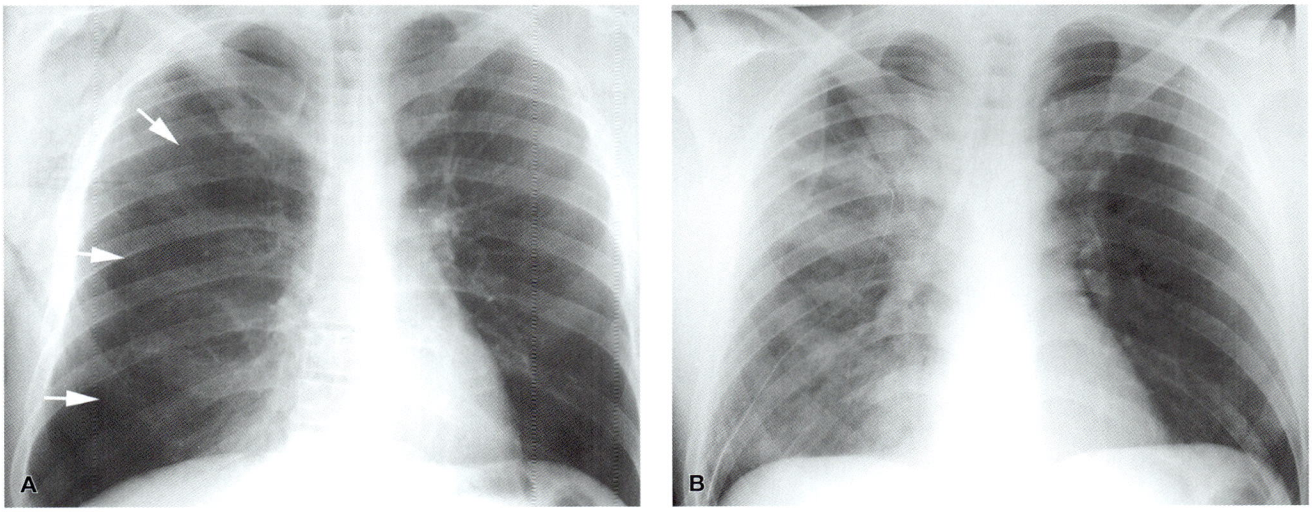

Figure 12.16. Reexpansion pulmonary edema following evacuation of pneumothorax. **A:** Chest radiograph following trauma shows a large right pneumothorax (*arrows*) and subcutaneous emphysema. **B:** Following rapid lung reexpansion using a chest tube, patchy consolidation is visible in the right lung.

of small peripheral airways by retained secretions is the usual cause.

A localized area of consolidation is the most common radiographic finding with atelectasis, and its radiographic appearance is impossible to distinguish from pneumonia or aspiration unless associated findings of volume loss are visible. On AP portable radiographs, signs of lower lobe volume loss include depression of the hilum, a vertical orientation of the main bronchus, crowding of segmental lower lobe bronchi, and a visible and vertically oriented major fissure. Left lower lobe atelectasis is almost universal in patients having open heart surgery with cold cardioplegia.

Because the mucous plugging resulting in atelectasis in these patients usually is peripheral and involves small bronchi, air bronchograms often are visible within collapsed lung. Small pleural effusions can be present.

Areas of consolidation resulting from atelectasis may change rapidly in appearance, a finding that helps to distinguish them from pneumonia. Acute opacification of a hemithorax may represent atelectasis and drowned lung; little volume loss may be seen in this situation.

PNEUMONIA

Pneumonias occur in 10% to 20% of patients in the ICU. They are associated with high mortality because these patients often are debilitated; hospital-acquired infections are notoriously antibiotic resistant and difficult to treat; and normal mechanisms of mucociliary clearance are suppressed or made ineffective by oxygen therapy and mechanical ventilation. Gram-negative organisms such as *Pseudomonas* and *Klebsiella* species and *Staphylococcus aureus* are the most common culprits.

Although the diagnosis of pneumonia usually is based on the association of fever, culture of pathogenic organisms from the sputum, and an abnormal chest radiograph, a patient in the ICU may have each of these findings without having pneumonia. Endotracheal intubation often results in tracheal colonization by pathogenic bacteria without producing pneumonia. Many such patients will also have some sort of pulmonary abnormality on chest radiographs, usually representing atelectasis, aspiration, or pulmonary edema. A misdiagnosis of pneumonia is common, and bacteriologic confirmation of pneumonia may not be obtained.

Radiographically, pneumonias may appear as localized or diffuse areas of airspace consolidation, often patchy and heterogeneous. Depending on the organism responsible and the patient's immunocompetence, pneumonias generally appear and progress over a few days. Uncommonly, pneumonia shows a dramatic worsening in consolidation over a matter of hours; this occurrence is more typical of atelectasis, pulmonary edema, aspiration, or hemorrhage. Within 1 or 2 days of appropriate antibiotic treatment, a pneumonic consolidation should stabilize and begin to clear. Further, progression suggests superinfection with a second organism, a mixed infection, or a superimposed second process such as pulmonary edema.

ASPIRATION

Aspiration of bland substances such as water, blood, or neutralized gastric contents elicits little inflammatory response and does not result in severe lung disease unless the volume of aspirated fluid is large. Radiographs may show areas of consolidation in dependent portions of lung resulting from the aspirated substance, but these areas rapidly clear with ventilatory therapy or coughing.

Aspiration of irritating substances, particularly acid gastric contents with a pH less than 2.5, causes marked inflammation of pulmonary parenchyma and results in pulmonary

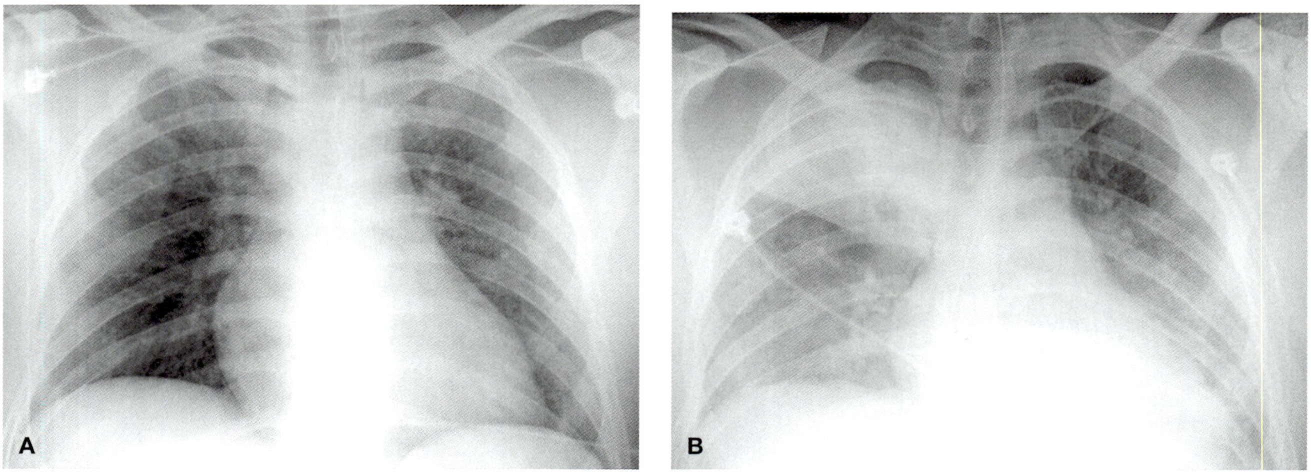

Figure 12.17. Acute aspiration. A: Baseline radiograph appears normal. B: Several hours later, following an acute aspiration, there has been rapid appearance of right upper lobe and left lower lobe consolidation, with lesser consolidation at the right base. The distribution of consolidation varies with the patient's position at the time of aspiration.

edema. Patients in the ICU are predisposed to aspiration of gastric contents because of nasogastric or endotracheal intubation, diminished level of consciousness, and a supine position. Inflation of the cuff of the endotracheal tube does not entirely prevent aspiration.

In general, within several hours of aspiration of acid material, the patient experiences fever, dyspnea, and hypoxemia. Radiographs usually show rapidly appearing and progressing consolidation, homogeneous or patchy, favoring dependent areas of lung (Fig. 12.17). HRCT may show ground-glass opacity (often acute), centrilobular/tree-in-bud nodules, or consolidation (Fig. 12.18). Within the next few days, clinical improvement and at least some clearing of consolidation should occur. If the symptoms progress and the radiograph fails to show clearing or worsens, superimposed infection or ARDS must be suspected. Pleural effusion is not generally associated with aspiration unless pneumonia supervenes (see Fig. 12.18B).

PULMONARY EMBOLISM

Pulmonary embolism may be considered in the differential diagnosis of early ARDS. Both conditions are characterized by progressive respiratory insufficiency in the face of a normal or slightly abnormal radiograph. However, the diffuse consolidation typically occurring with ARDS rarely is seen in patients with pulmonary embolism. Rather, pulmonary embolism usually produces more localized areas of consolidation, and pleural effusion is common. The diagnosis of pulmonary embolism in ICU patients primarily rests with CT pulmonary angiography.

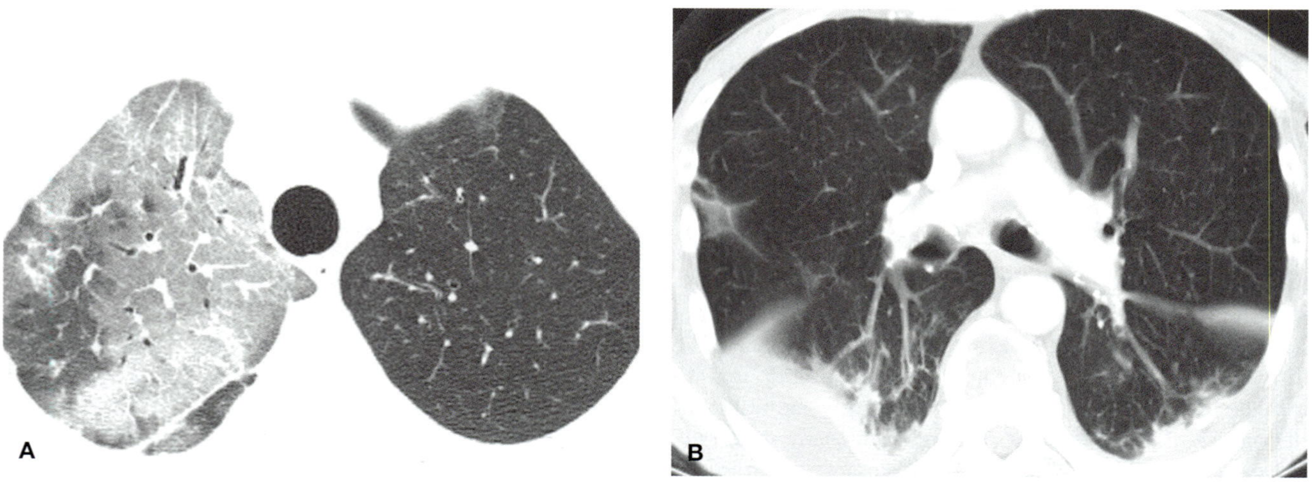

Figure 12.18. Aspiration. A: HRCT in a patient with acute aspiration shows ground-glass opacity in the right upper lobe. B: Aspiration pneumonias in a different patient. Consolidation involves dependent lung regions. Small pleural effusions thickening the fissures suggest superimposed infection.

PULMONARY HEMORRHAGE

Pulmonary parenchymal hemorrhage can occur in anticoagulated patients, patients with a bleeding diathesis, patients with pulmonary vasculitis, and patients with Goodpasture syndrome, among others. Typically, areas of consolidation appear rapidly, are bilateral, and are associated with a drop in hematocrit. Resolution may be slow. Aspiration of blood from the trachea resulting from traumatic intubation can produce a similar appearance. Hemoptysis need not be present in patients with significant pulmonary hemorrhage. Pulmonary hemorrhage syndromes are discussed in Chapter 19.

PLEURAL EFFUSION

Pleural effusion may be extremely difficult—if not impossible—to distinguish from basal areas of consolidation on portable supine or semierect radiographs. Costophrenic angle blunting and a meniscus often are absent, and poor definition of the ipsilateral hemidiaphragm or homogeneous opacity in the inferior hemithorax may be the only findings visible. The presence of air bronchograms indicates that at least some consolidation is present but does not rule out the presence of fluid; in fact, the lung consolidation and air bronchograms may reflect atelectasis secondary to effusion.

Unless diagnostic thoracentesis is being considered, small pleural fluid collections rarely are significant in patients in the ICU, and the differentiation of fluid and consolidation may not be necessary. If a definite diagnosis of effusion is desired in a bedridden patient, decubitus films or bedside ultrasonography may be performed.

In patients in the ICU, the presence or absence of pleural effusion usually does not help in diagnosing the cause of coexisting lung disease. Although pleural effusion is uncommonly associated with ARDS, aspiration, and hemorrhage, patients with these diseases may have pleural effusion resulting from another process, such as congestive heart failure, recent surgery, or abdominal disease.

Large pleural effusions, significantly reducing ventilation and pulmonary function, usually are treated by thoracentesis or pleural drainage tubes.

MECHANICAL VENTILATION AND PULMONARY BAROTRAUMA

Mechanical ventilators commonly are used in the ICU to treat ventilatory or respiratory failure. High peak ventilator pressure and continuous positive airway pressure usually are employed in the treatment of hypoxemia resulting from ARDS, edema, and other respiratory diseases.

Ventilator therapy may alter the appearance of lung disease. Increasing ventilator pressures result in increased lung volume and produce an apparent clearing of lung consolidation, whereas decreasing pressure produces a decrease in lung volume and an apparent worsening of disease. Thus, knowledge of changes in ventilator settings is helpful in allowing the correct interpretation of radiographs.

Barotrauma

The use of mechanical ventilators and high ventilatory pressures can result in barotrauma with alveolar rupture and subsequent development of pneumomediastinum, subcutaneous emphysema, pneumothorax, and air within the retroperitoneum or free within the abdominal cavity. Prompt recognition of extra-alveolar air is important, because pneumothorax may be life threatening in ICU patients.

In a small minority of patients, extra-alveolar air is first recognized in the pulmonary interstitial space as collections of perivascular air (*interstitial emphysema*; Fig. 12.19) or as irregular bubbles within areas of consolidation. Subpleural blebs may develop and threaten impending pneumothorax due to their rupture. Interstitial emphysema visible on plain radiographs is very uncommon in adults.

From the interstitial space, air dissects centrally to produce pneumomediastinum (Fig. 12.20; see also Fig. 12.19). This may be visible as a lucency adjacent to the mediastinum or outlining specific mediastinal structures, such as the aorta

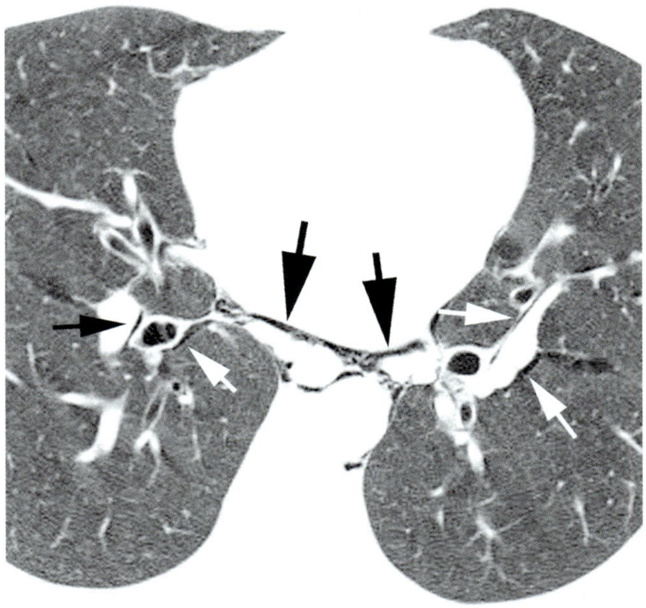

Figure 12.19. Interstitial emphysema and pneumomediastinum. In a postoperative patient, streaks of air (*small arrows*) are seen surrounding the central bronchi and vessels. This appearance represents interstitial emphysema. Although this is thought to be the first manifestation of barotrauma, it is not commonly seen in adults. Interstitial emphysema leads directly to pneumomediastinum. In this patient, mediastinal air is seen surrounding the esophagus and aorta (*large arrows*).

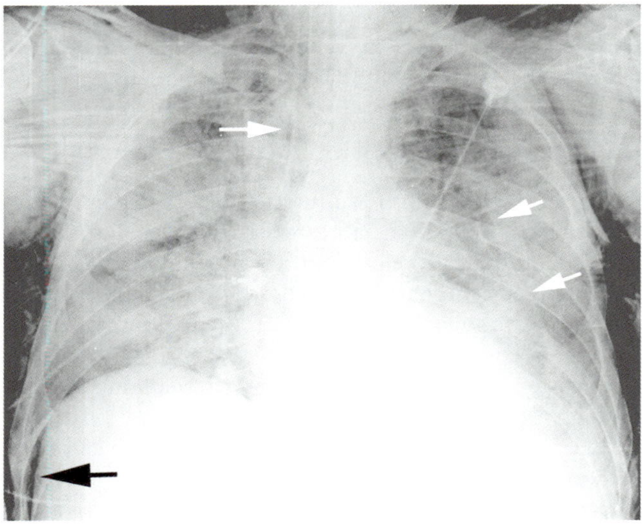

Figure 12.20. Pneumomediastinum, subcutaneous emphysema, and retroperitoneal air. In a patient with barotrauma, pneumomediastinum (*white arrows*) is visible outlining the tracheal wall and displacing the mediastinal pleura laterally. The presence of subcutaneous emphysema, seen outlining the pectoralis major muscles, is presumptive evidence of pneumomediastinum in the absence of penetrating trauma or chest tube placement. A crescent of air lateral to the liver (*black arrow*) is retroperitoneal. Free air in the abdomen is seen above the liver rather than lateral to it.

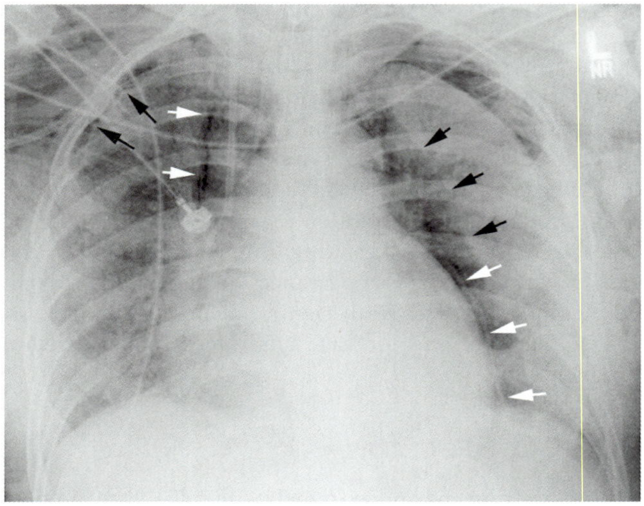

Figure 12.21. Pneumomediastinum, subcutaneous emphysema, and pneumothorax. In a patient with barotrauma, pneumomediastinum (*white arrows*) is visible, outlining and displacing the mediastinal pleura laterally. Bilateral pneumothorax is present (*black arrows*). Little lung collapse had occurred despite the presence of pneumothorax (likely under tension because of mechanical ventilation). This is due to underlying lung consolidation. Subcutaneous emphysema is present.

or trachea. Air outlining the tracheal wall is common with pneumomediastinum.

Pneumopericardium may occur because of interstitial air dissecting along pulmonary vessels. This finding is relatively common in infants but is uncommon in adults, except following cardiac surgery or pericardial intervention.

In the absence of penetrating trauma or chest tube placement, the presence of subcutaneous emphysema is evidence that pneumomediastinum is present, even if it is not visible (see Fig. 12.20).

Pneumothorax may result from rupture of mediastinal air into the pleural space, but the opposite does not occur: pneumothorax does not lead to pneumomediastinum under normal circumstances. In mechanically ventilated patients, pneumothorax should be considered to be under tension; this is commonly the case. With tension pneumothorax, the diaphragm often is depressed, and the mediastinum may be displaced to the opposite side. However, because of underlying lung disease (ie, consolidation), significant lung collapse on the side of the pneumothorax may not occur even in the presence of tension (Fig. 12.21). In supine patients, pneumothorax may be seen in atypical locations, either medial to the lungs or at the lung base (see Chapter 26). Care must be taken to distinguish skin folds from pneumothorax.

Air dissecting inferiorly from the mediastinum can reach the retroperitoneum (Fig. 12.22; see also Fig. 12.20) and may rupture into the peritoneal space, producing free abdominal air (see Fig. 12.22C). Generally, retroperitoneal air is seen lateral to the liver; free air is seen above it. Almost all patients with ventilator-related abdominal air will also have a visible pneumomediastinum.

TUBES AND LINES AND THEIR COMPLICATIONS

The first step in interpreting a radiograph of a patient in the ICU is an evaluation of indwelling catheters and tubes. Misplaced catheters can result in serious complications. Tube or catheter misplacement occurs in up to 10% of cases.

Endotracheal Tubes

Mechanical ventilators require the use of an endotracheal tube. The tube's tip should be positioned several centimeters above the tracheal carina. The tracheal carina is often visible; if it is not visible, it can be located by looking for the main bronchi and following them to the point they meet. Also, the carina may be assumed to be near the level of the undersurface of the aortic arch (Fig. 12.23) or near the level of the T4-T5 vertebral bodies.

The ideal position for an endotracheal tube depends on the degree of extension or flexion of the patient's neck. An endotracheal tube's tip may descend as much as 3 cm when the neck is flexed from a neutral position and may ascend as much as 5 cm with neck extension. With the patient's neck in a neutral position, the tube's tip should lie approximately 4 to 7 cm above the carina (Fig. 12.24). If the neck is extended,

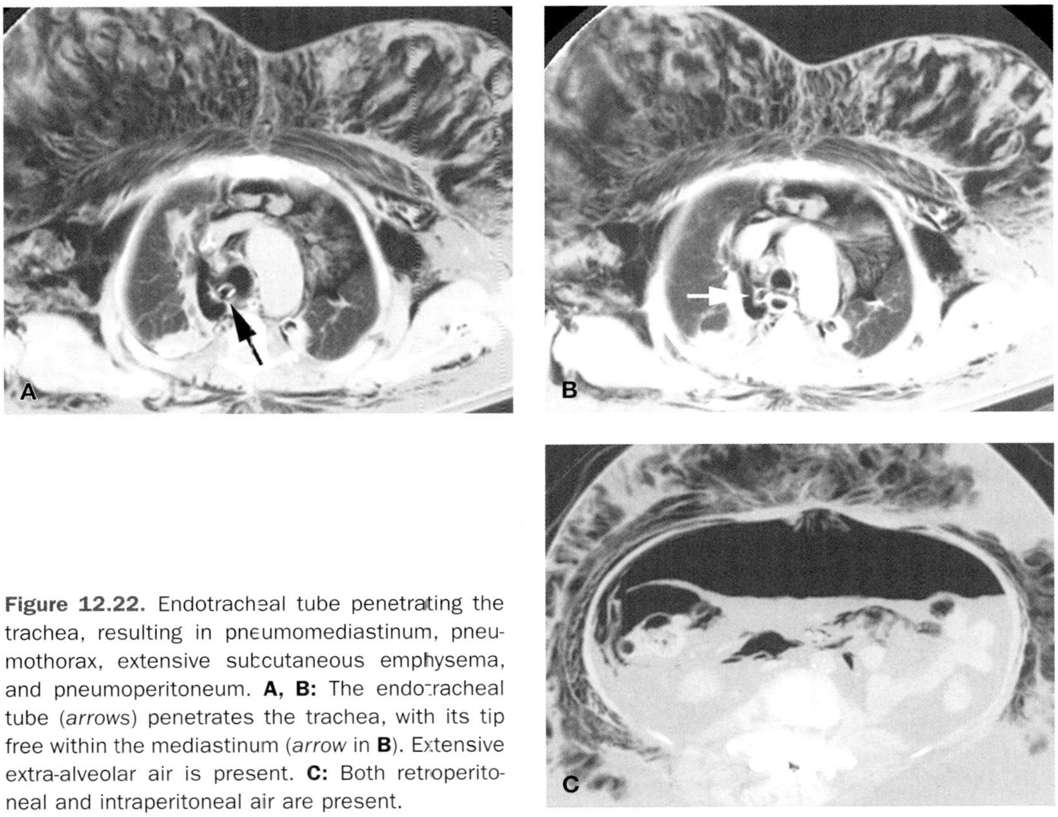

Figure 12.22. Endotracheal tube penetrating the trachea, resulting in pneumomediastinum, pneumothorax, extensive subcutaneous emphysema, and pneumoperitoneum. **A, B:** The endotracheal tube (*arrows*) penetrates the trachea, with its tip free within the mediastinum (*arrow* in **B**). Extensive extra-alveolar air is present. **C:** Both retroperitoneal and intraperitoneal air are present.

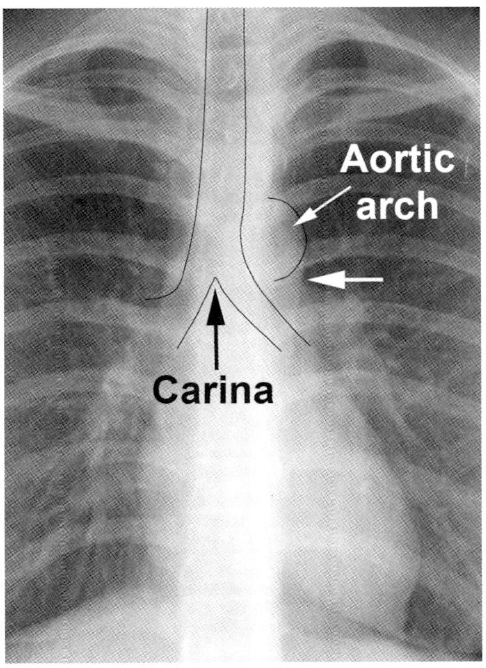

Figure 12.23. Relation of the carina to the aortic arch. If the carina is not clearly visible, it is located near the level of the undersurface of the rounded opacity of the aortic arch (*white arrow*).

the tip should be higher (7-9 cm above the carina) to allow for possible downward migration. If the neck is flexed, the reverse is true, and the tip should be lower (2-4 cm above the carina).

Flexion and extension of the neck can be judged by the position of the patient's mandible on the chest radiograph. In a neutral position, the mandible overlies the lower cervical spine. If the chin or mandible is higher, the neck is extended; if it is lower, the neck is flexed. It is simplest to remember that the tube tip moves in the same direction as the chin with flexion or extension of the neck (Fig. 12.25).

Placing an endotracheal tube too low usually results in its entering the right main bronchus (Fig. 12.26A). This position can produce right lung overinflation, alveolar rupture and pneumothorax, or right upper lobe or left lung collapse because of lack of ventilation of these areas. Intubation of the left main bronchus is less common because of its more horizontal orientation (see Fig. 12.26B).

A tube placed too high may lodge in the hypopharynx or larynx (Fig. 12.27), resulting in poor ventilation or gastric distention. If the tube tip or cuff lies at the level of the vocal cords, ulceration and scarring may result, leading to stricture.

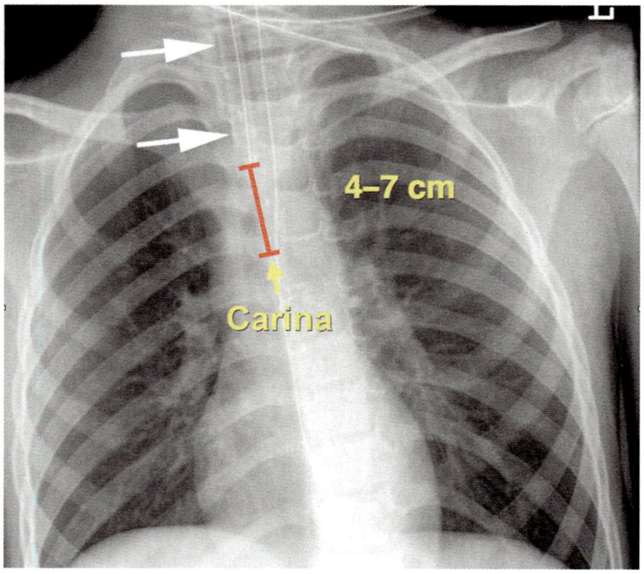

Figure 12.24. A properly placed endotracheal tube (*white arrows*), identified by its radiopaque marker, should be positioned with its tip 4 to 7 cm above the carina, to account for movement of the tube with neck flexion. A nasogastric tube is also in place.

Esophageal intubation may be recognized by an unusual tube course, with the tube not overlying the tracheal air column or because of gastric distention (Fig. 12.28). A lateral view is very helpful in diagnosis; although the trachea and esophagus overlap on the frontal projection, they can be easily distinguished on the lateral view.

Overinflation of the tube cuff or balloon (see Fig. 12.27) may result in ulceration of the tracheal wall, with perforation or scarring and stricture as complications. Overinflation may be recognized if there is a bulge in the tracheal air column at the site of the balloon, several centimeters above the tube tip. Tracheal stenosis or tracheal malacia may occur as a late complication of endotracheal intubation (see Chapter 22). These complications have been minimized by the use of low-pressure balloons, but they still occur.

Rarely, tracheal perforation occurs with intubation (see Fig. 12.22). The endotracheal tube may have an abnormal course, or pneumomediastinum may be present.

Tracheostomy Tubes

A tracheostomy tube is placed if a patient requires chronic mechanical ventilation or for upper airway obstruction. The tube tip position relative to the carina is not critical, because this is determined by the location of the tracheostomy stoma. Tracheostomy tubes that are angled relative to the tracheal lumen may cause erosion of the tracheal wall, with perforation or subsequent tracheal stenosis, or may occasionally fall out. Tracheostomy balloons may be overinflated.

Central Venous Catheters

Central venous catheters used for measuring central venous pressure or for intravenous infusion of fluids often are placed by means of percutaneous puncture of the internal jugular or subclavian veins. Complications of venous puncture include laceration of the subclavian or carotid artery (Fig. 12.29), mediastinal hemorrhage (Fig. 12.30) or infusion of intravenous fluids into the mediastinum or pleural space (Fig. 12.31), pneumomediastinum, and pneumothorax (see Fig. 12.29). Pneumothorax is most common, occurring between 1% and 7% of patients (see Fig. 12.29), with higher incidences

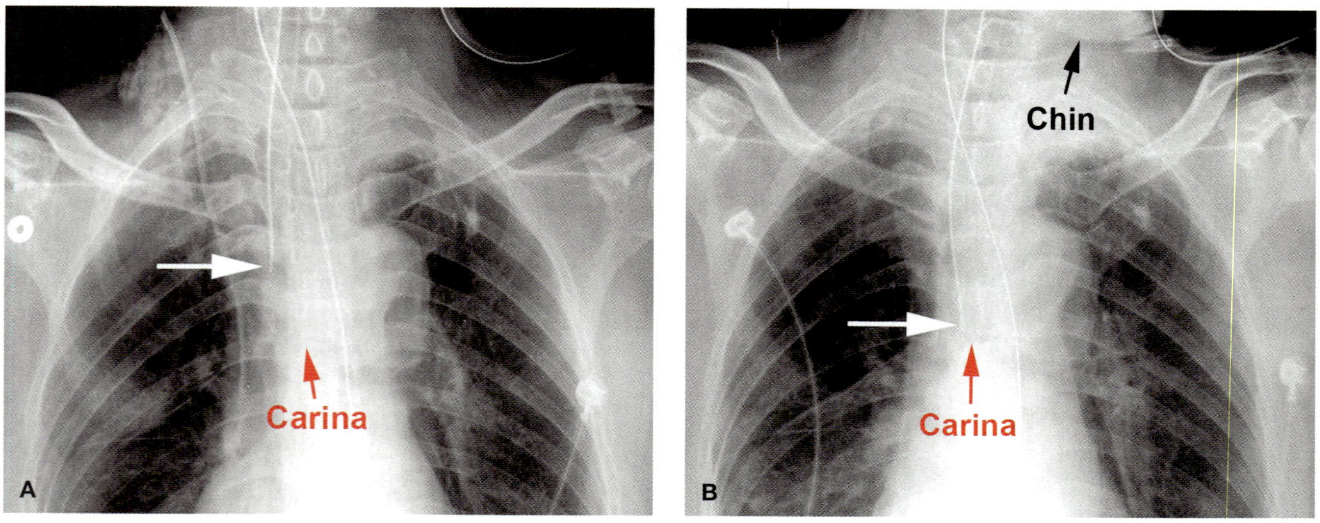

Figure 12.25. Migration of an endotracheal tube with neck flexion. **A:** Chest radiograph shows an endotracheal tube with its tip (*white arrow*) about 3 cm above the carina. Note that the patient's chin is not visible overlying the lower cervical spine. This means the patient's neck is extended. **B:** On a subsequent radiograph, the chin is visible overlying the lower cervical spine, indicating the neck is in a neutral position or slightly flexed. The endotracheal tube tip (*white arrow*) has migrated downward and is a few millimeter above the carina.

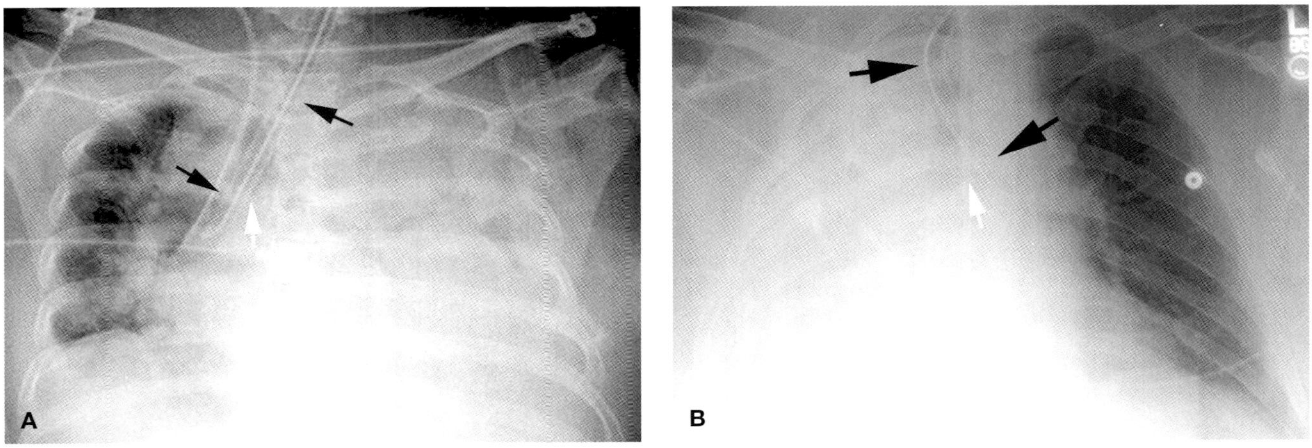

Figure 12.26. Intubation of a main bronchus. **A:** Right main bronchus intubation. The endotracheal tube (*black arrows*) enters the right main bronchus. The tracheal carina is indicated by the *white arrow*. Left lung collapse has resulted. **B:** Left main bronchus intubation. The endotracheal tube (*black arrows*) extends into the proximal left main bronchus. This is less common than is intubation of the right main bronchus. Right lung collapse has resulted. The *white arrow* indicates the location of the carina.

being reported in emergency situations, increased number needle passes, and larger bore catheters. Because of these possible complications, a portable chest radiograph should be obtained after every attempted or successful subclavian or jugular puncture.

A catheter placed properly should be in the superior vena cava (SVC). On chest radiographs, the first anterior intercostal space is the approximate site of the junction of the brachiocephalic veins to form the SVC (Fig. 12.32). Because many catheters have two or three lumens, each with a different orifice, the catheter tip should be as near to the azygos arch as possible. This position allows each orifice, which may be as much as 5 cm proximal to the tip, to be distal to the last venous valve. This valve is located at the junction of the

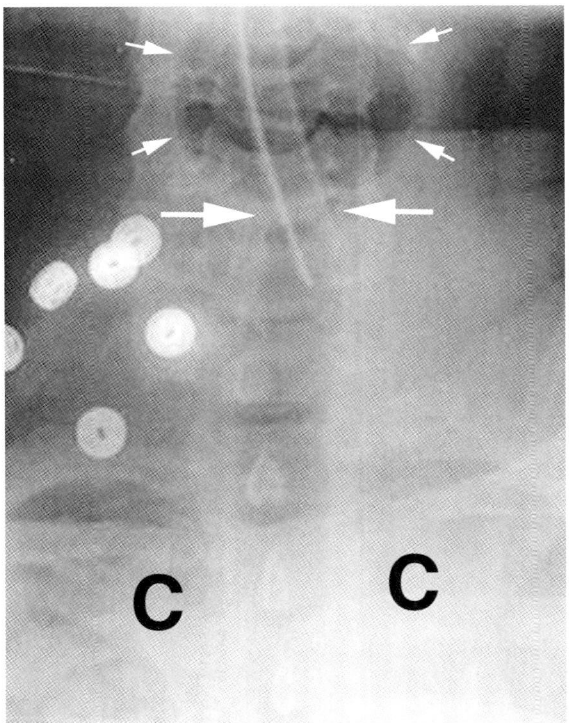

Figure 12.27. Endotracheal tube located too high. The tube tip is just below the vocal cords (*large arrows*) at the level of C6. The tube balloon (*small arrows*) is overinflated and at the level of the piriform sinuses. C, clavicular heads.

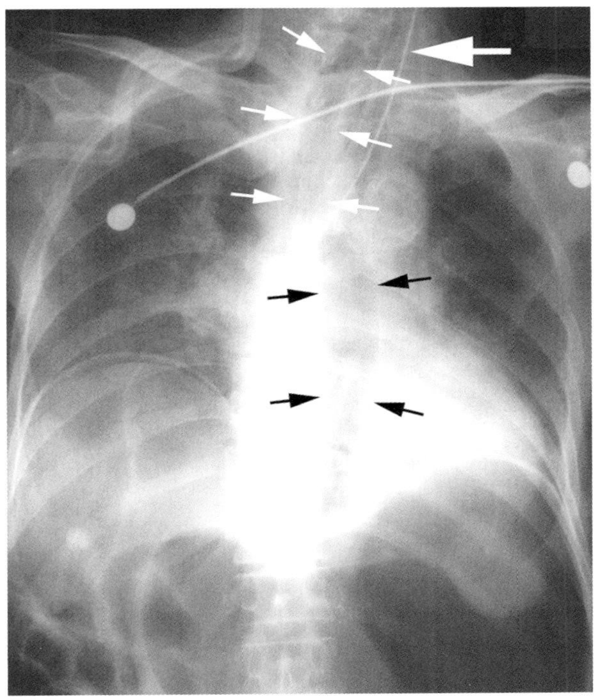

Figure 12.28. Esophageal intubation. The endotracheal tube (*large white arrow*) does not overlie the shadow of the trachea (*small white arrows*). Below the level of the tube tip, the esophagus (*black arrows*) is dilated and air filled. The stomach and bowel are dilated by air.

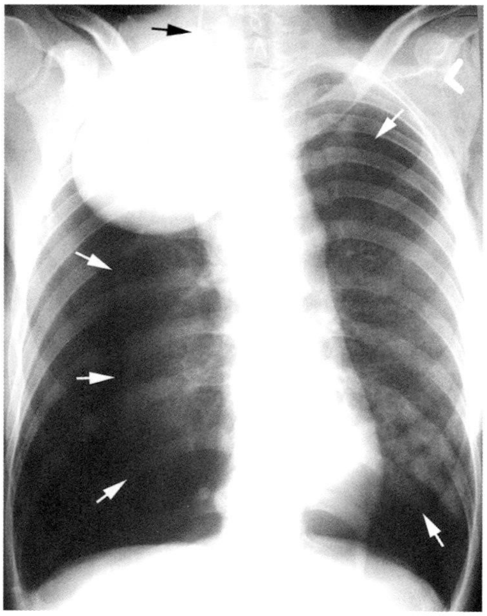

Figure 12.29. Chest radiograph following attempted bilateral subclavian and internal jugular vein catheter placement. A catheter (*black arrow*) overlies the right neck. A large mass at the right apex represents an extrapleural hematoma due to laceration of the right carotid artery. Bilateral pneumothoraces (*white arrows*) also are present, with mediastinal shift to the left. The heart appears small, suggesting tension with decreased venous return. This patient subsequently died.

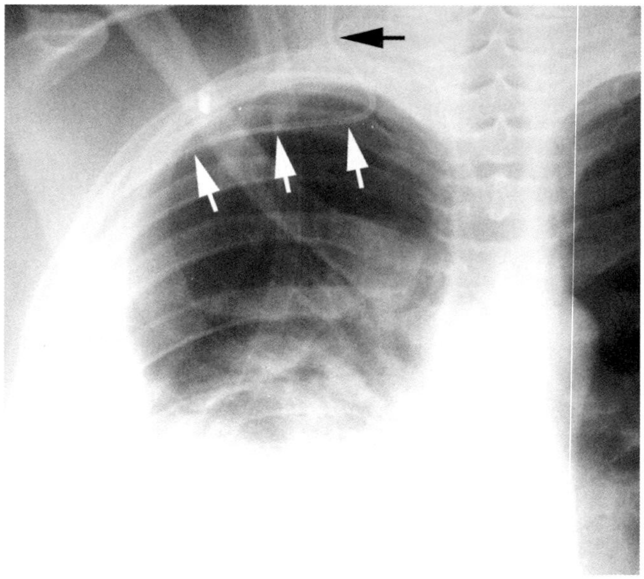

Figure 12.31. Catheter placement in the pleural space. A right internal jugular catheter (*black arrow*) follows an unusual course and is directed laterally (*white arrows*) at a level above the clavicle (and the subclavian vein). This catheter is within the right pleural space. A large right pleural effusion is due to intravenous fluid infusion.

internal jugular and subclavian veins, at the level of the inner aspect of the first rib (Fig. 12.32B).

It usually is not desirable to place a catheter in the right atrium; this may result in dysrhythmia or injection of undiluted toxic drugs into the heart. If the chest radiograph shows the catheter tip to be at the level of the lower aspect of the bronchus intermedius, it generally is considered to be at the junction of the SVC and RA or *cavoatrial junction* (Fig. 12.32B), although this relationship is not precise. A catheter below this level is in the RA. It should be kept in mind that the relative positions of the catheter and RA change with inspiratory level. A catheter positioned at the cavoatrial

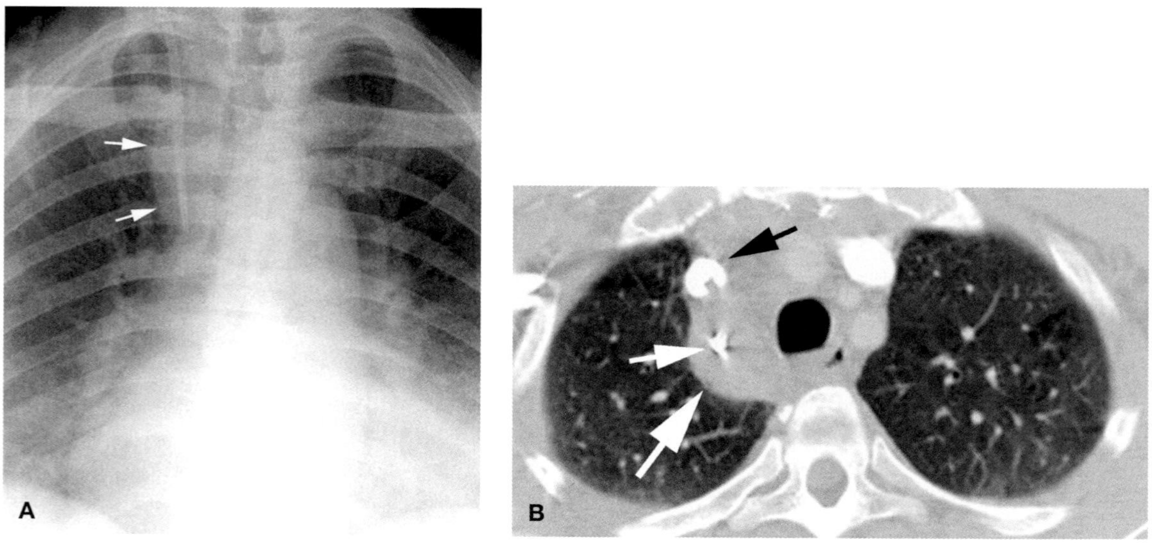

Figure 12.30. Mediastinal hemorrhage following catheter placement. **A:** Chest radiograph shows a catheter overlying the superior vena cava. The mediastinum is widened (*arrows*). Blood return from the catheter was poor. **B:** CT shows the catheter (*small white arrow*) to be extravascular and associated with mediastinal hematoma (*large white arrow*). The catheter should be within the right brachiocephalic vein (*black arrow*).

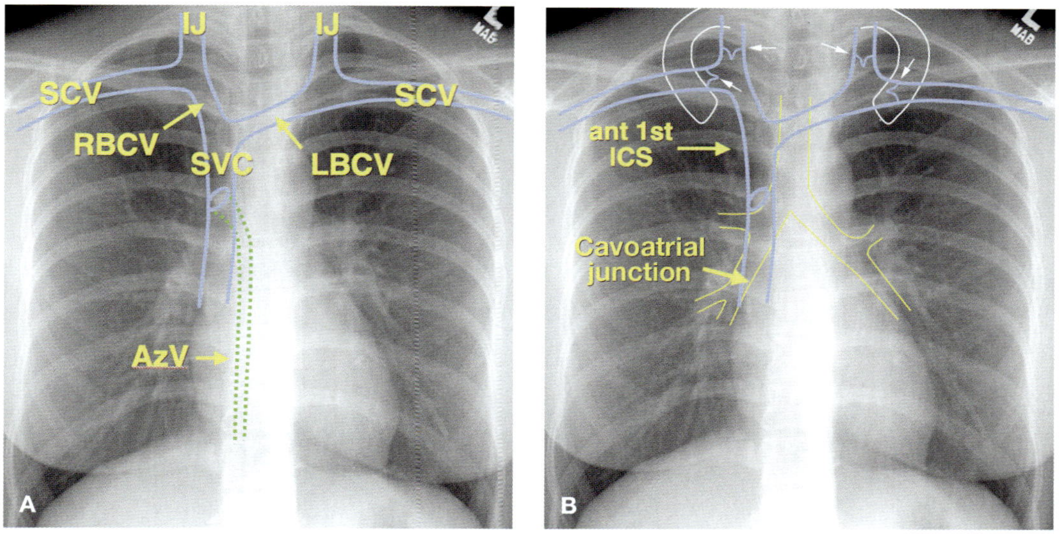

Figure 12.32. Anatomy of major thoracic veins and radiographic landmarks. **A:** The right and left internal jugular (*IJ*) and subclavian veins (*SCV*) join to form the right and left brachiocephalic veins (*RBCV*; *LBCV*), which in turn join to form the superior vena cava (SVC). The azygos vein (*AzV*) is shown as a dashed green line. The azygos arch results in an oval shadow at the point it enters the posterior SVC. The AzV is located anterior to the spine. **B:** The veins shown in (**A**) are localized relative to important landmarks visible on chest radiographs. The trachea and major bronchi are shown in yellow. The last valves in the internal jugular and subclavian veins (*white arrows*) are located near the inner aspects of the first ribs (*outlined in white*). The internal jugular veins and subclavian veins merge medial to the first ribs. The brachiocephalic veins join to form the SVC near the first anterior intercostal space (*ant 1st ICS*). The cavoatrial junction is near the point the vena cava crosses the bronchus intermedius.

junction on inspiration may be located in the RA on an expiratory radiograph. Catheters directed laterally against the wall of the SVC are at risk for perforation. This occurs most often with catheters placed via the left subclavian vein or left internal jugular vein.

Catheters that follow an unusual course may be (1) in a variant vein; (2) in an artery; or (3) extravascular. Catheters may inadvertently extend into smaller veins, increasing the risk of inaccurate pressure measurements, thrombosis, or perforation (Figs. 12.33 and 12.34). A catheter placed in a persistent left SVC (Fig. 12.35) may mimic placement in a small vein.

Occasionally, a catheter may be placed in the subclavian artery or carotid artery rather than in a vein (Fig. 12.36). In the case of a subclavian artery, the catheter may be seen above the clavicle since the artery is superior and posterior to the vein. Arterial catheters tend to have a more medial course than the corresponding veins, and the tip is usually projecting over the aorta.

A catheter taking an unusual course may be free within the mediastinum or pleural space rather than within a vein, and fluids should be administered with care. A good return of blood through the catheter does not ensure proper positioning.

Improperly placed catheters sometimes can be sheared off at the needle tip and embolize to the heart or pulmonary arteries (Fig. 12.37). Perforation, infection, and thrombosis can result.

Improper technique may lead to air embolism, with air visible in the pulmonary artery.

Pulmonary Artery (Swan-Ganz) Catheters

Swan-Ganz catheters are double-lumen, balloon-tipped catheters allowing measurement of pulmonary arterial and wedge pressures when the balloon is inflated. Normally, the tube tip should lie within a large central pulmonary artery; with inflation of the balloon, the tube tip migrates distally to a wedged position. A catheter positioned in a main or interlobar pulmonary artery is usually adequate for pressure measurements (Fig. 12.38). Thus, the catheter tip should overlie the main or hilar arteries (Fig. 12.39). If the catheter lies in a small (lobar or segmental) artery, it may remain wedged with the balloon uninflated, and thrombosis and pulmonary infarction or pulmonary artery aneurysm can result (Fig. 12.40). Care also must be taken that the balloon does not remain inflated between measurements; continued inflation also may result in infarction. Coiling of the catheter within the heart should be avoided. Coiling can result in knotting or sudden peripheral migration of the catheter with wedging.

Transvenous Pacemakers and Implanted Cardiac Defibrillators

Transvenous pacemaker and implanted cardiac defibrillator leads vary in number and location in different patients.

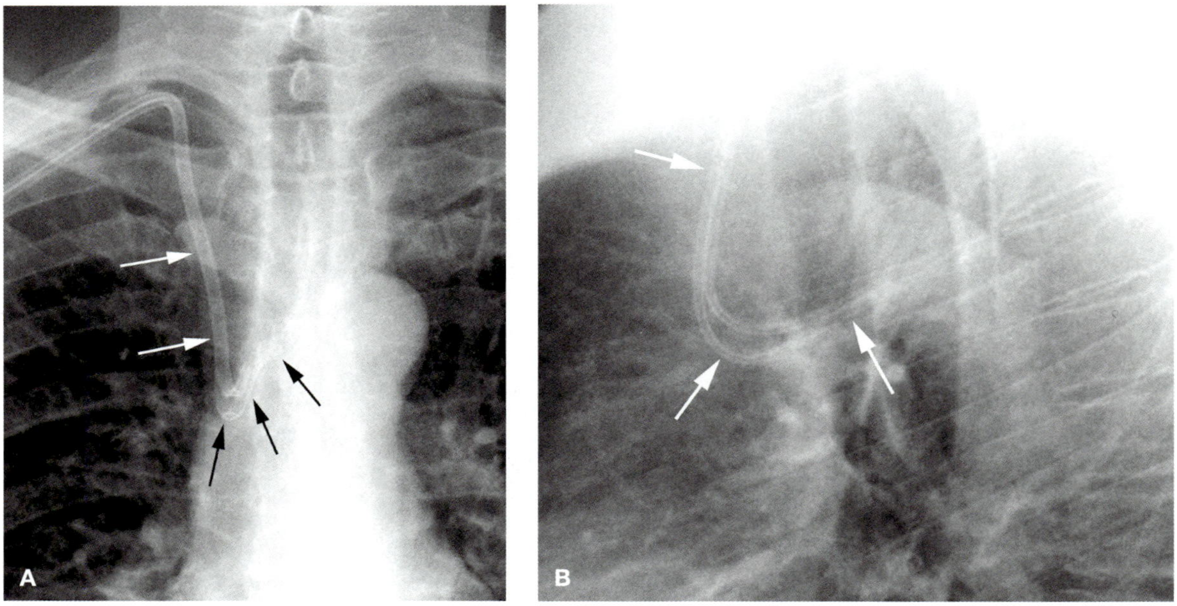

Figure 12.33. Catheter placement into the azygos vein. **A:** A dialysis catheter (*arrows*) enters the azygos arch with it distal tips directed medially and upward. **B:** On a lateral view, the distal catheter tips are directed posteriorly into the azygos arch (*arrows*).

Defibrillator leads are usually indicated by coils of wire overlying the SVC and right ventricle. A right ventricular lead is typically positioned with its tip in the apex of the right ventricle, pointing to the left, anteriorly, and inferiorly (Fig. 12.41A).

A second lead is often present, positioned in the right atrium, with its tip usually directed anteriorly into the atrial appendage (Fig. 12.41B) or laterally against the right atrial wall. In some patients, a third lead is positioned in a coronary vein by means of the coronary sinus, to allow biventricular pacing.

Rarely, pacemaker leads perforate the coronary sinus or myocardium, resulting in pericardial tamponade or diaphragmatic pacing (with hiccoughs). If this occurs, the lead tip may be seen very close to the edge of the heart shadow or may project beyond it.

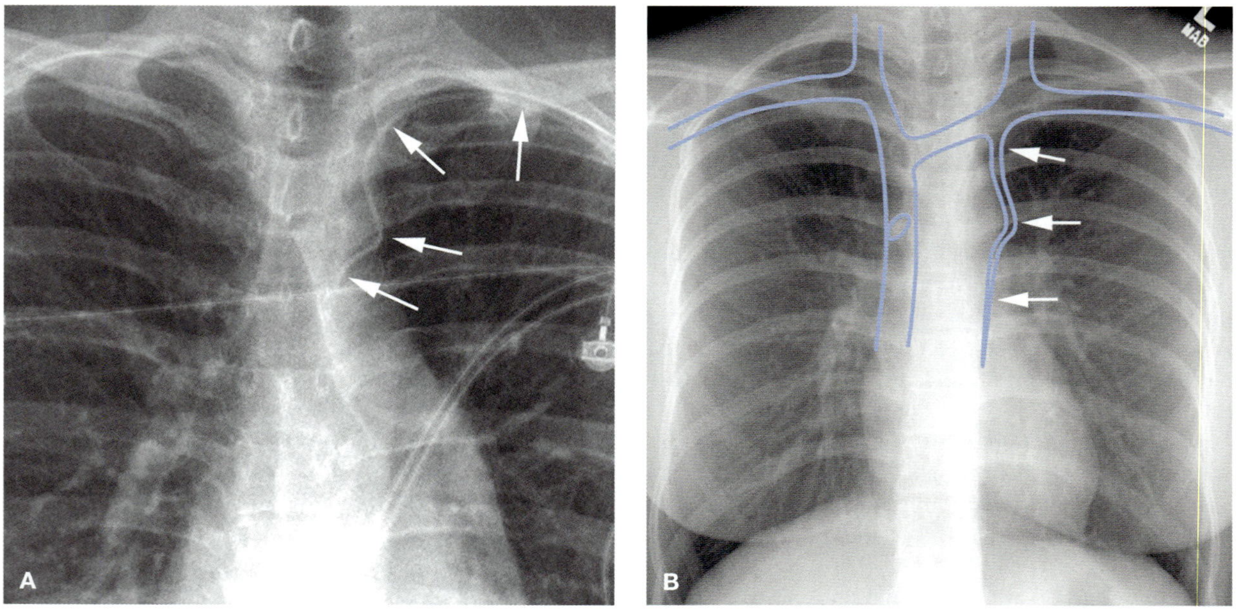

Figure 12.34. Catheter placement into the left superior intercostal vein. **A:** A left venous catheter (*arrows*) is positioned along the left mediastinum. The catheter curves around the aortic arch, a course that is typical. **B:** Typical course of the left superior intercostal vein (*arrows*) relative to other mediastinal veins.

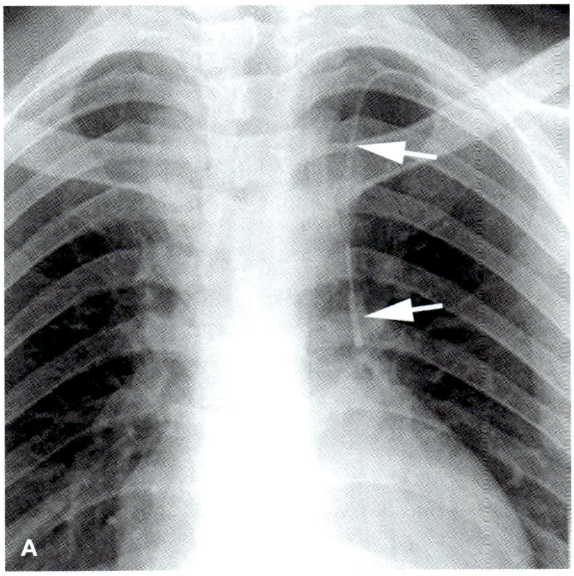

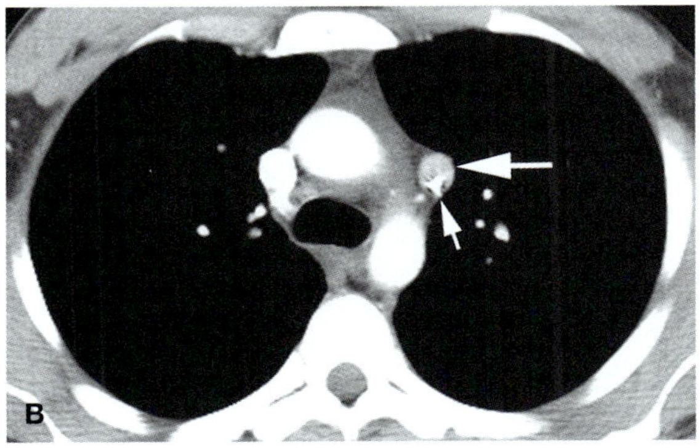

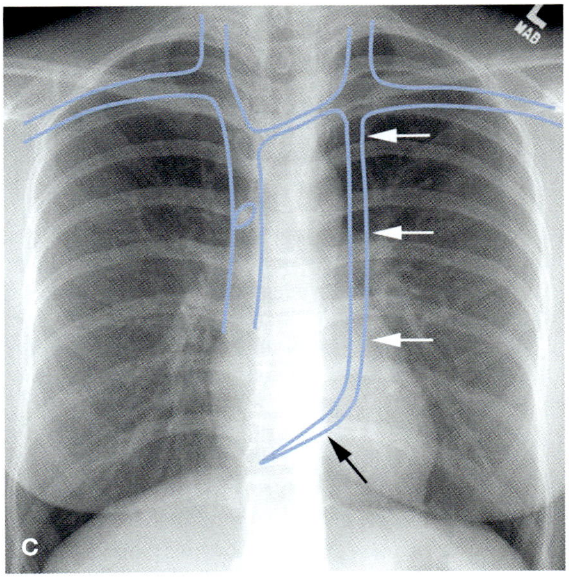

Figure 12.35. Catheter placement in a persistent left superior vena cava (SVC). **A:** A left internal jugular venous catheter (*white arrows*) descends along the left mediastinum. This course is typical of a persistent left SVC. However, this catheter position also may be extravascular or in a small mediastinal vein (eg, internal mammary or left pericardiophrenic vein). **B:** CT shows the catheter (*small arrow*) to be within a persistent left SVC (*large arrow*). **C:** Typical course of a persistent left SVC. The left SVC descends along the left mediastinum (*white arrows*) and enters the coronary sinus (*black arrow*). In patients with a left SVC, the left brachiocephalic vein is small or absent.

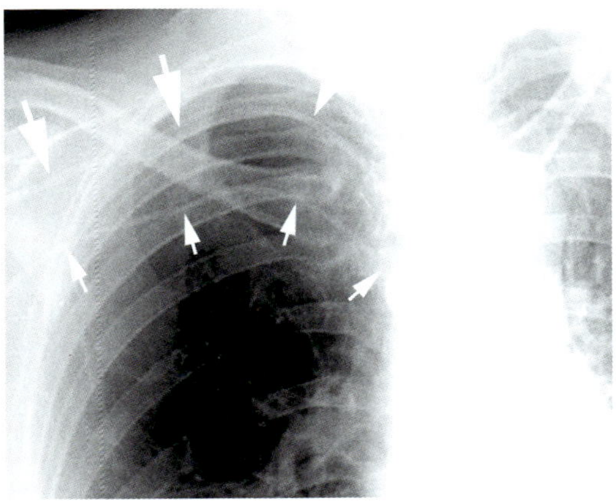

Figure 12.36. Subclavian artery catheter. A peripherally placed right venous catheter (*small arrows*) is visible in the typical location of the subclavian vein, beneath and overlying the clavicle. A second catheter, placed using a subclavian approach (*large arrows*), is too high to be within the subclavian vein, and its tip is medially located, overlying the aortic arch rather than the superior vena cava.

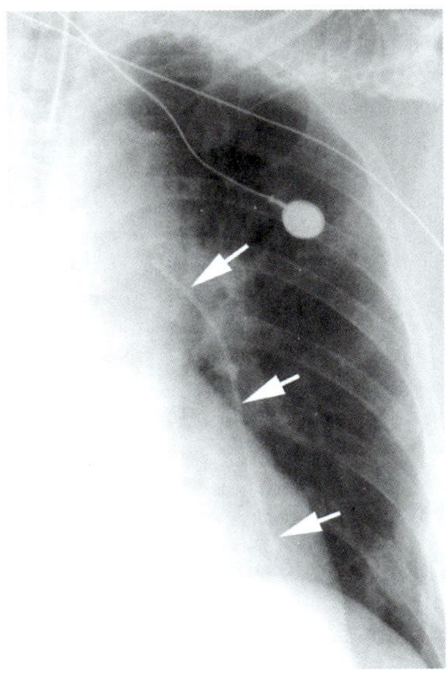

Figure 12.37. Catheter embolization. A venous catheter (*arrows*) was sheared off during insertion and has embolized to the left pulmonary artery.

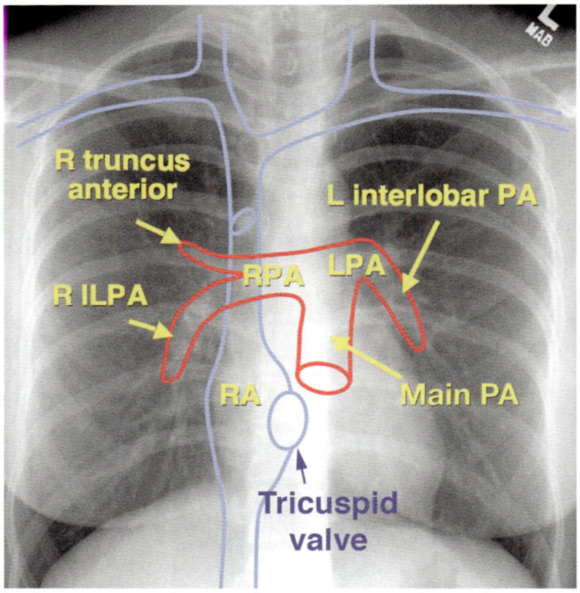

Figure 12.38. Pulmonary artery anatomy on the chest radiograph. A Swan-Ganz catheter tip should overlie the main or hilar arteries. The thoracic systemic veins are shown in blue as in Figure 12.32. The right atrium (*RA*) and location of the tricuspid valve are shown. PA, pulmonary artery; RPA, right pulmonary artery; R ILPA, right interlobar pulmonary artery; LPA, left pulmonary artery.

Pacemaker failure may result from poor lead position, fracture of the pacemaker lead usually near the pacemaker (this often is difficult to see), or failure of the pacemaker itself. Some patients play with their pacemaker device (so-called "twiddler's syndrome"), which may result in coiling of the pacemaker wire around the pacemaker and retraction of the lead tip into the right atrium or vena cava.

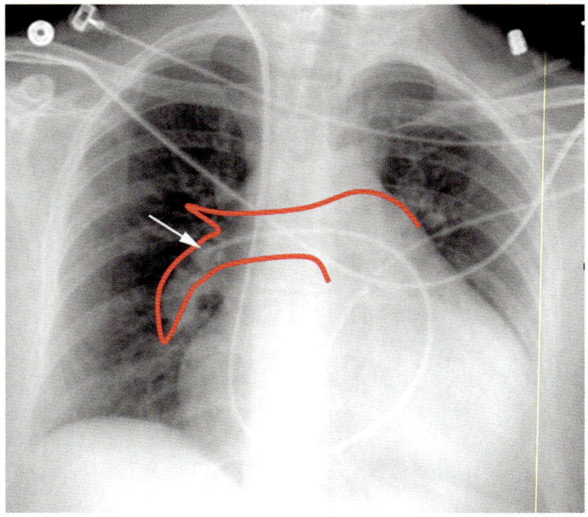

Figure 12.39. Properly positioned Swan-Ganz catheter. The catheter tip (*arrow*) overlies the hilar shadow and is within the right interlobar pulmonary artery.

Pleural Drainage Tubes

Pleural drainage tubes commonly are used to evacuate pneumothorax or pleural effusion. Ideally, tubes placed for pneumothorax should occupy the least dependent portion of the pleural space (anterosuperior in a bedridden patient). For the treatment of pleural fluid, tubes should be placed within the dependent portion of the pleural space (posteroinferior).

If a tube functions poorly, it may be occluded or kinked, it may be positioned in the chest wall or with its side hole (marked by a discontinuity in the radiopaque tube marker) outside the thoracic cavity, or it may be positioned in the major fissure with the two adjacent lobes occluding the tube. A tube located within the major fissure is most easily

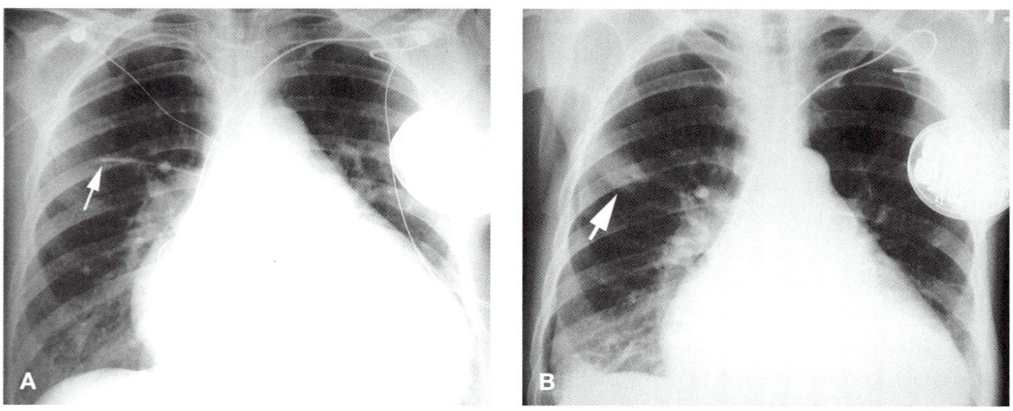

Figure 12.40. Peripheral location of a Swan-Ganz catheter with infarction. **A:** A patient with cardiomegaly shows a peripherally located (segmental or subsegmental) Swan-Ganz catheter (*arrow*). The catheter should overlie the large hilar vessels. **B:** Following withdrawal of the catheter 1 day later, a focal opacity representing a lung infarction is visible in the right lung (*arrow*).

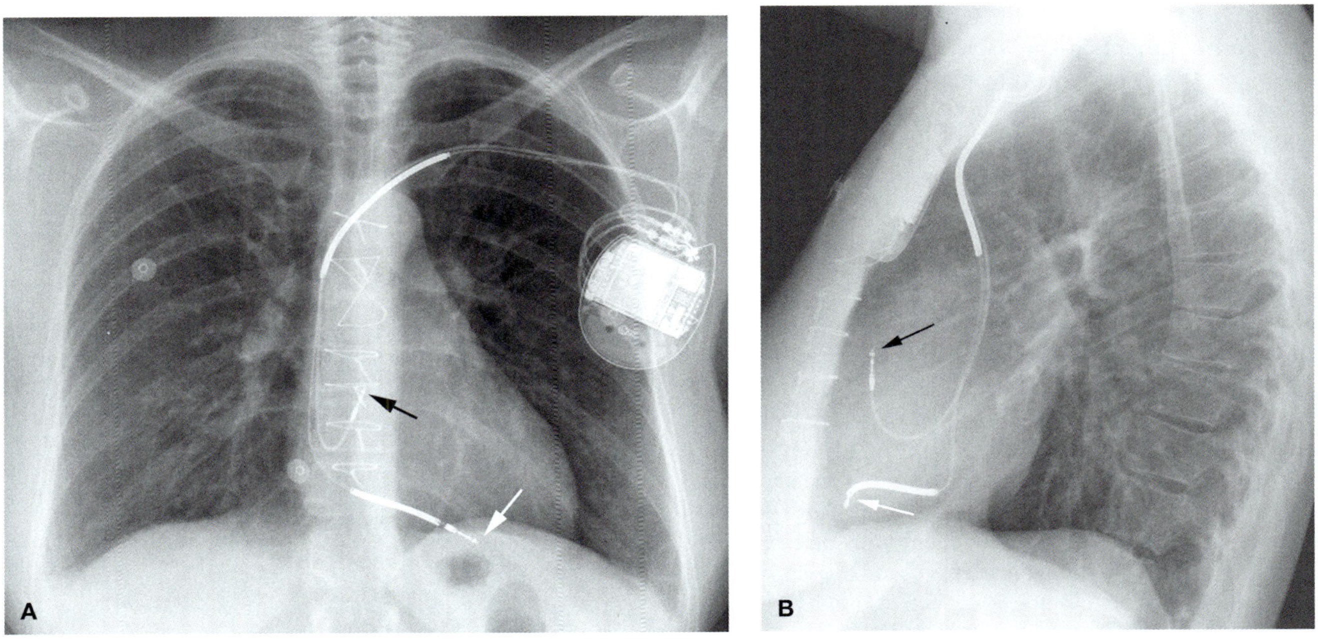

Figure 12.41. Transvenous pacemaker (implanted defibrillator) leads. **A, B:** Pacemaker leads are positioned with tips in right ventricular apex (*white arrows*) and right atrial appendage (*black arrows*). The dense bands along the superior vena cava and right ventricular pacemaker leads indicate this is an implanted defibrillator.

recognized by comparing its position on the frontal and lateral radiographs and localizing this to the plane of the fissure.

Rarely, the lung may be perforated during tube placement with the tube tip lying within lung parenchyma. Obviously, such tubes function poorly and lead to pneumothorax. CT may be needed to confirm this location.

Enteric Tubes

Enteric tubes or feeding tubes occasionally may be placed in the tracheobronchial tree (Fig. 12.42). This placement may result in perforation of the visceral pleura and pneumothorax, bronchial obstruction and atelectasis, or delivery of a tube feeding into the lung, which may result in severe pneumonia. Coiling of a nasogastric tube in the hypopharynx can

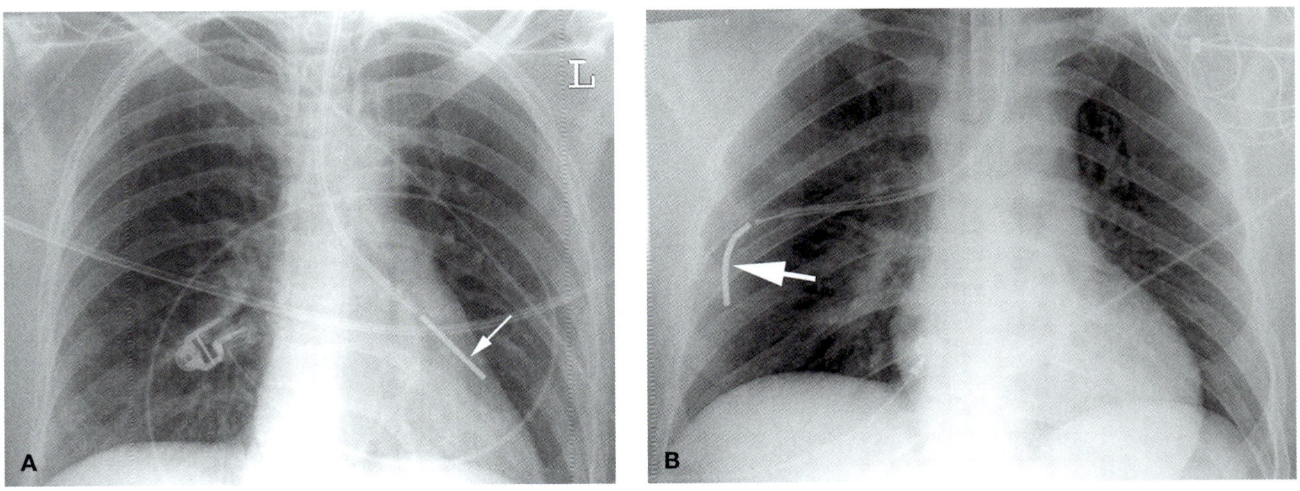

Figure 12.42. Feeding tubes placed in the tracheobronchial tree. **A:** A feeding tube (*arrow*) is placed in the left lower lobe and is oriented along the course of bronchi. **B:** In another patient, the tube follows the course of bronchi in the central lung but curves in a manner inconsistent with an endobronchial location in the periphery (*arrow*). This suggests perforation of the visceral pleura, with the tube tip in the pleural space.

contribute to aspiration. If the tube is coiled in the esophagus, gastric distention and aspiration may result. Feeding tubes characteristically have a dense marker at their tip; nasogastric tubes placed for suction have a dense marker along their length.

Aortic Balloon Pump

A catheter-based, gas-filled intra-aortic balloon pump (IABP) may be used to improve peripheral blood flow in patients with left ventricular failure and low cardiac output. The long (25-30 cm), sausage-shaped balloon may be visible when inflated as a relative lucency within the descending aorta (Fig. 12.43). The catheter itself is difficult to see, although a small radiopaque line usually marks its tip. Ideally, the catheter tip is positioned just below the origin of the left subclavian artery and therefore should overlie the aortic knob on the radiograph (see Fig. 12.43). If a femorally placed IABP is advanced too far, the catheter may occlude the left vertebral artery; if located too low, it is less effective, and its lower portion may partially obstruct the renal arteries.

Extracorporeal Membrane Oxygenation

Extracorporeal membrane oxygenation (ECMO) is used after cardiac surgery or failure to wean from cardiopulmonary bypass and in patients with severe respiratory failure. ECMO cannulae are large and easily recognized on chest radiographs, which are commonly obtained to check appropriate cannula placement (Fig. 12.44).

Numerous ECMO cannula placement sites and ECMO configurations exist and depend on the need for cardiac support, pulmonary support, or both. The most common

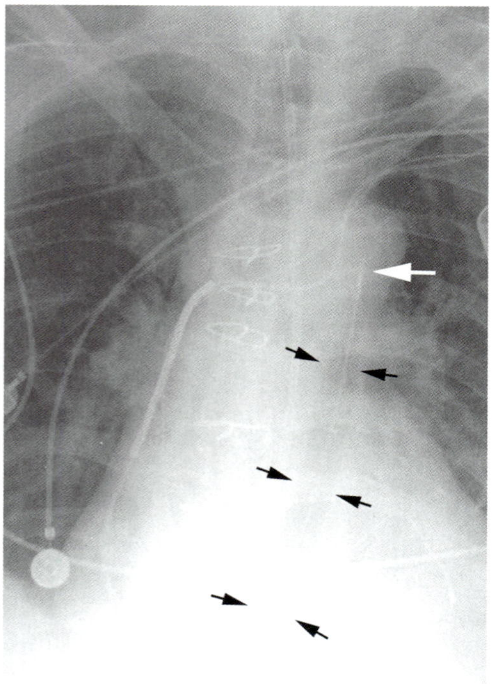

Figure 12.43. Aortic balloon pump. The balloon tip (*white arrow*) is radiopaque and is properly positioned slightly below the superior aspect of the aortic arch. In this patient, the balloon (*black arrows*) was inflated at the time the radiograph was performed and is visible as a long lucency overlying the descending aorta.

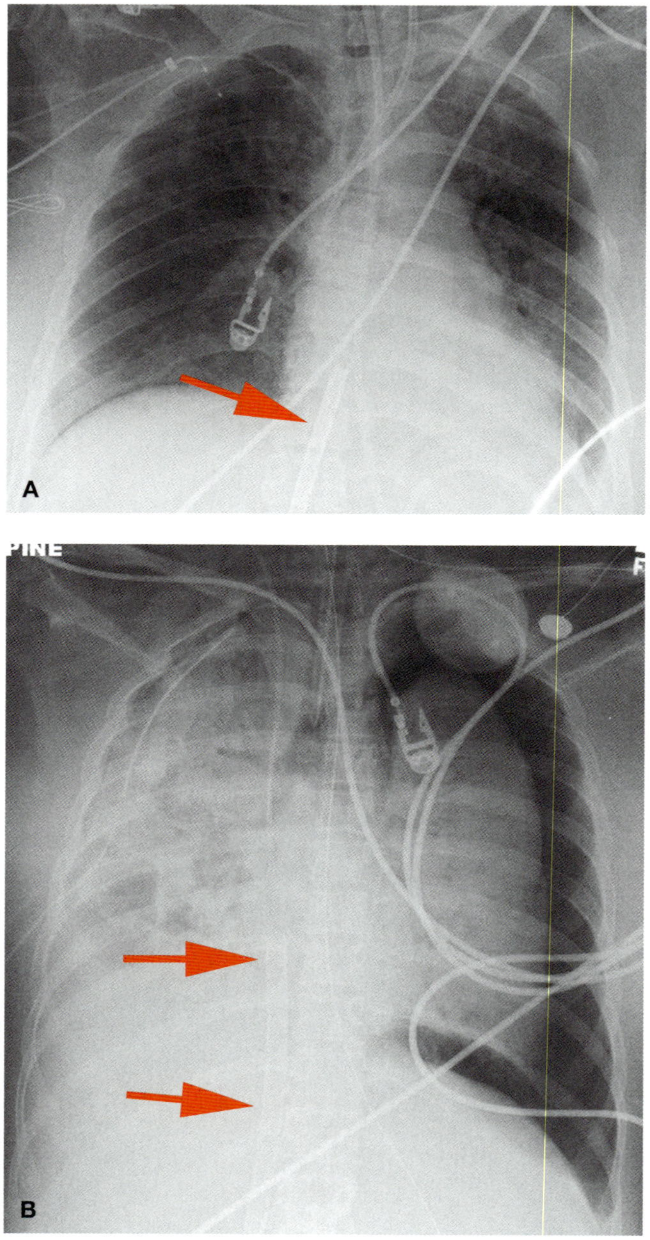

Figure 12.44. Extracorporeal membrane oxygenation (ECMO). **A:** A large ECMO catheter (*arrow*) is positioned with its tip in the right atrium. Side holes in the cannula are in the inferior vena cava (IVC). **B:** A different patient with acute respiratory distress syndrome and tension pneumothorax shows an ECMO catheter (*arrows*) in the right atrium or IVC, at the level of the diaphragm.

Table 12.5 Expected ECMO Cannulae Sites and Possible Complications

ECMO	Drainage Cannula	Blood Return Cannula
Central VA	Right atrium	Aorta
Peripheral VA	Distal IVC or SVC	Femoral, subclavian, or axillary artery
Femoro-atrial VV	IVC at the diaphragm	Distal SVC or right atrium via SVC
Femoro-femoral VV	IVC at the diaphragm	Right atrium via the iliofemoral vein
Dual-lumen cannula VV	IVC below the diaphragm	Right atrium via the SVC

ECMO, extracorporeal membrane oxygenation; IVC, inferior vena cava; SVC, superior vena cava; VA, venoarterial; VV, venovenous.

include double cannulation venoarterial (VA) routes and venovenous (VV) routes:

1. *peripheral VA ECMO:* peripheral venous drainage with peripheral arterial return
2. *central VA ECMO:* right atrial drainage with aortic return
3. *femoro-atrial VV ECMO:* femoral vein drainage with right atrial return
4. *femoro-femoral VV ECMO:* return and drainage placed in femoral veins
5. *dual-lumen single cannula VV ECMO:* drainage using the distal part of a dual-lumen cannula with its tip in the IVC and RA and reintroduction by a second lumen into the right atrium

More sophisticated techniques like VAV, VVA, and VAA exist to help mitigate the downsides of the double cannulation routes but are beyond the scope of this text. Knowledge the particular ECMO circuit being used, and the expected locations of cannulae and possible complications are essential for accurate image interpretation (Table 12.5). Commonly encountered ECMO complications include cannula malposition, adjacent or distal hemorrhage, stasis thrombus in access vessels, and distal emboli.

Left Ventricular Assist Devices

Left ventricular assist devices (LVADs) are increasingly used for patients with end-stage heart failure, prior to transplantation. A wide variety of LVADs are being used, and radiographic appearances vary (Fig. 12.45). Percutaneous VADs are also used at many institutions, and appropriate placement

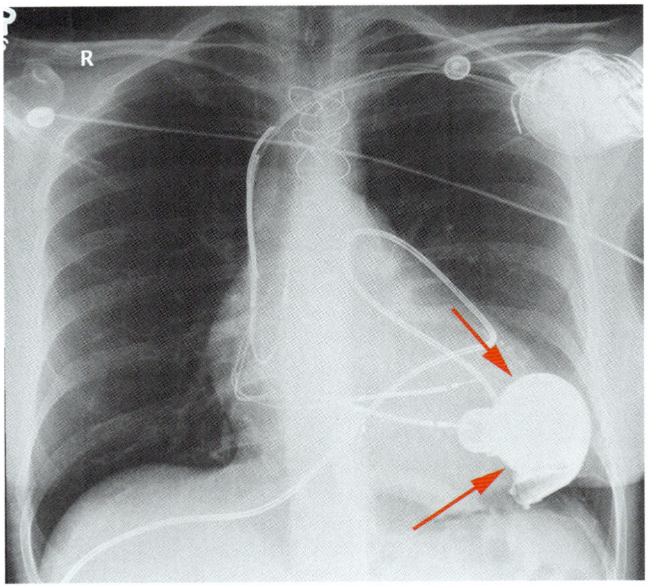

Figure 12.45. Left ventricular assist device (LVAD). An LVAD (*arrows*) overlies the left ventricle. Conduits used with LVADs are not visible on radiographs.

is usually known based on built-in sensors. Several publications listed below review the expected radiographic appearances of commonly used devises. Potential complications include inflow and outflow cannula complications, hemorrhage, pericardial tamponade, thrombus formation, aortic valve stenosis and insufficiency, right-sided heart failure, and infection.

SUGGESTED READINGS

American College of Radiology. *ACR–SPR–STR Practice Parameter for the Performance of Portable (Mobile Unit) Chest Radiography.* Accessed February 6, 2023. https://www.acr.org/-/media/ACR/Files/Practice-Parameters/Port-Chest-Rad.pdf

ARDS Definition Task Force; Ranieri VM, Rubenfeld GD, Thompson BT, et al. Acute respiratory distress syndrome: the Berlin Definition. *JAMA.* 2012;307:2526-2533.

Bartsch P. High altitude pulmonary edema. *Respiration.* 1997;64(6):435-443.

Beasley MB. Acute lung injury—from Cannabis to COVID. *Mod Pathol.* 2022;35(suppl 1):1-7. doi:10.1038/s41379-021-00915-6

Bernard GR, Artigas A, Brigham KL, et al. The American-European Consensus Conference on ARDS. Definitions, mechanisms, relevant outcomes, and clinical trial coordination. *Am J Respir Crit Care Med.* 1994;149(3 pt 1):818-824.

Carr C, Jacob J, Park SJ, Karon BL, Williamson EE, Araoz PA. CT of left ventricular assist devices. *Radiographics.* 2010;30(2):429-444.

Desai SR, Wells AU, Rubens MB, Evans TW, Hansell DM. Acute respiratory distress syndrome: CT abnormalities at long-term follow-up. *Radiology.* 1999;210(1):29-35.

Expert Panel on Thoracic Imaging; Laroia AT, Donnelly EF, Henry TS, et al. ACR appropriateness Criteria® intensive care unit patients. *J Am Coll Radiol.* 2021;18(5S):S62-S72. doi:10.1016/j.jacr.2021.01.017

Gluecker T, Capasso P, Schnyder P, et al. Clinical and radiologic features of pulmonary edema. *Radiographics.* 1999;19(6):1507-1533.

Goodman LR, Fumagalli R, Tagliabue P, et al. Adult respiratory distress syndrome due to pulmonary and extrapulmonary causes: CT, clinical, and functional correlations. *Radiology.* 1999;213(2):545-552.

Hommeyer SH, Godwin JD, Takasugi JE. Computed tomography of air-space disease. *Radiol Clin North Am.* 1991;29(5):1065-1084.

Hunter TB, Taljanovic MS, Tsau PH, Berger WG, Standen JR. Medical devices of the chest. *Radiographics*. 2004;24(6):1725-1746.

Ketai LH, Godwin JD. A new view of pulmonary edema and acute respiratory distress syndrome. *J Thorac Imaging*. 1998;13(3):147-171.

Lee S, Chaturvedi A. Imaging adults on extracorporeal membrane oxygenation (ECMO). *Insights Imaging*. 2014;5:731-742.

Mohamed I, Lau CT, Bolen MA, et al. Building a bridge to save a failing ventricle: radiologic evaluation of short-and long term cardiac assist devices. *Radiographics*. 2015;35(2):327-356.

Müller-Leisse C, Klosterhalfen B, Hauptmann S, et al. Computed tomography and histologic results in the early stages of endotoxin-injured pig lungs as a model for adult respiratory distress syndrome. *Invest Radiol*. 1993;28(1):39-45.

Murata K, Herman PG, Khan A, Todo G, Pipman Y, Luber JM. Intralobular distribution of oleic acid–induced pulmonary edema in the pig: evaluation by high-resolution CT. *Invest Radiol*. 1989;24(9):647-653.

Obadina ET, Torrealba JM, Kanne JP. Acute pulmonary injury: high-resolution CT and histopathological spectrum. *Br J Radiol*. 2013;86(1027):20120614. doi:10.1259/bjr.20120614

Owens CM, Evans TW, Keogh BF, Hansell DM. Computed tomography in established adult respiratory distress syndrome. Correlation with lung injury score. *Chest*. 1994;106(6):1815-1821.

Schuster DP. What is acute lung injury? *Chest*. 1995;107(6):1721-1726.

Storto ML, Kee ST, Golden JA, Webb WR. Hydrostatic pulmonary edema: high-resolution CT findings. *AJR Am J Roentgenol*. 1995;165(4):817-820.

Chapter 13

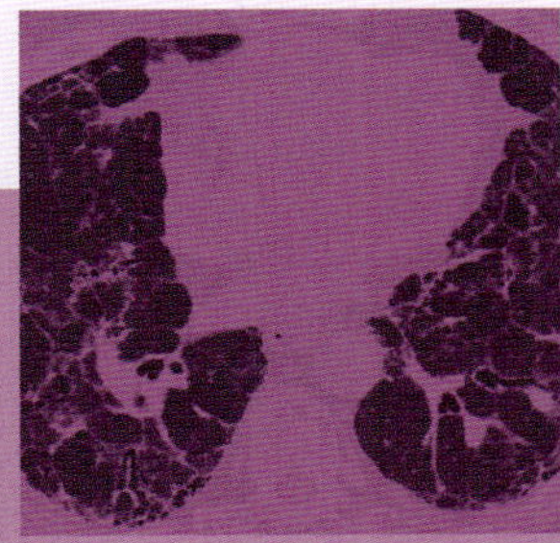

Katherine Cheng • Travis S. Henry

Pulmonary Infections

INTRODUCTION

Pulmonary infections are among the most common causes of morbidity and mortality worldwide and contribute substantially to annual medical expenditures in the United States. The causes of pulmonary infection are numerous, and the clinical presentations of pulmonary infection are frequently nonspecific. Thoracic imaging plays a central role in the evaluation of patients suspected of pulmonary infection. The recent COVID-19 pandemic underscores this point as imaging became central to the diagnosis of these patients.

MECHANISMS

Microorganisms gain access to the respiratory system and cause infection in a variety of ways. The most common route of entry is inoculation via the tracheobronchial tree, usually by the inhalation of aerosolized respiratory droplets or by the microaspiration or gross aspiration of oropharyngeal secretions. Pulmonary infections may also occur through inoculation via the pulmonary vasculature, usually in the presence of a definable extrapulmonary infectious source, such as endocarditis or thrombophlebitis. Finally, pulmonary infections may rarely result from direct extension of organisms into the respiratory system from adjacent sources, such as infected mediastinal or hilar lymph nodes, from an adjacent organ such as transdiaphragmatic spread from a liver abscess or esophageal rupture with esophagopulmonary fistula formation.

Whether or not overt pulmonary infection takes place depends on a variety of factors, including the number of inoculating organisms, the integrity of the host's immune system, and the virulence of the infecting organisms. Many organisms exhibit characteristics that enhance the likelihood of pulmonary infection and promote tissue destruction.

PATTERNS

Pathologically, pulmonary infections may be divided into infections involving the central airways (tracheobronchitis), the small airways (bronchiolitis), and the pulmonary parenchyma (pneumonia).

Pneumonia may be subdivided into several categories: lobar pneumonia, bronchopneumonia, and interstitial pneumonia (not to be confused with "interstitial pneumonia" in the context of ILD). Lung abscess is an additional pattern of pulmonary infection that may be seen with lobar pneumonia or bronchopneumonia.

Imaging manifestations often are sufficiently different to allow the recognition of these patterns of infection. Although it is usually not possible to suggest a specific microbiological diagnosis in individual cases, specific patterns tend to be associated with specific organisms.

Tracheobronchitis

Infection of the central airways may predominantly affect the trachea, the central bronchi, or both. Tracheobronchitis is often the result of viral infection.

Viral tracheobronchitis, also known as croup, is a common infection in children, particularly those under the age of 3 years. Narrowing of the subglottic trachea may be seen on chest radiographs.

In adults, viral tracheobronchitis is usually of little clinical consequence, and patients rarely undergo imaging. Occasionally, viral infections impair host immunity sufficiently to predispose to bacterial superinfection, in which case the radiographic pattern will primarily be that of a bacterial pneumonia.

Bacterial tracheitis is rare. It most often affects children, although adults may be affected as well. It often occurs after an upper respiratory viral infection. The most common etiologic agents are *Staphylococcus aureus* and *Haemophilus influenzae*; anaerobes and *Corynebacterium diphtheriae* are rare causes. Bacterial tracheitis produces inflammatory exudates that may lead to the obstruction of the tracheal lumen.

Bacterial bronchial infections in adults are most common in patients with chronic obstructive pulmonary disease (COPD) or cystic fibrosis. Bacterial bronchitis is usually diagnosed clinically and treated conservatively. Imaging is not necessary in most cases, although airway wall thickening may be visible on chest radiographs. Often, chest radiographs are performed to exclude associated pneumonia. CT, particularly high-resolution CT (HRCT), may show airway wall thickening, and air trapping may be evident on postexpiratory imaging.

Airway inflammation and stenoses may result from tuberculosis or other granulomatous infections. Smooth, tapered narrowing affecting the lobar bronchi and associated with bronchial wall thickening is most typical. The distal trachea may be involved, usually in concert with main stem bronchial involvement.

Acute tracheobronchitis may be seen with *Aspergillus fumigatus* infection. It is an uncommon form of invasive aspergillosis occurring in immunosuppressed patients. Chest radiography and CT are often normal in this form of disease. Focal airway wall thickening or plaques are seen on CT in some cases (Fig. 13.1).

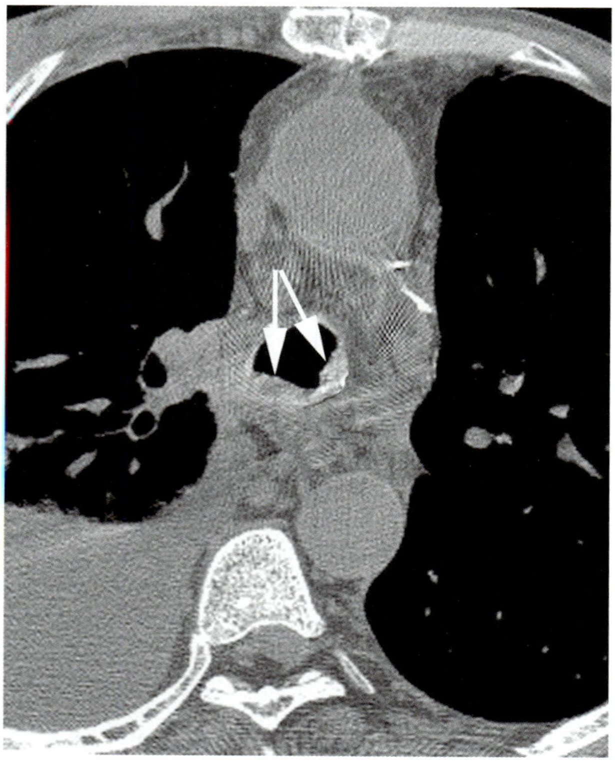

Figure 13.1. *Aspergillus* tracheobronchitis. Axial CT image in an immunosuppressed heart transplant recipient shows irregular, mildly high-attenuation plaques (*arrows*) along the posterior and left lateral tracheal wall, consistent with *Aspergillus* tracheobronchitis.

Bronchiolitis

The term *bronchiolitis* refers to the inflammation of small airways, particularly membranous and respiratory bronchioles.

Acute bronchiolitis consists of predominantly peribronchiolar neutrophilic and lymphocytic inflammation associated with necrosis of the respiratory epithelium. The organisms most commonly associated with acute bronchiolitis are viruses, especially respiratory syncytial virus (RSV) but also human metapneumovirus (hMPV); parainfluenza virus; adenovirus types 3, 7, and 21; and rhinoviruses. *Mycoplasma pneumoniae* and *Chlamydia* spp. may also cause acute bronchiolitis. Bacterial and fungal organisms involving the large airways may also result in infectious bronchiolitis.

Most clinically significant viral bronchiolar infections are encountered in small children. RSV is the most common offending agent and usually afflicts children between the ages of 2 months and 2 years. Infants below the age of 6 weeks may be relatively protected by maternal IgG. hMPV is a viral pathogen that is responsible for infant bronchiolitis in 5% to 15% of cases. Serologic studies suggest that infection with hMPV is nearly ubiquitous by the age of 5.

Chest radiographic findings of acute bronchiolitis may show a combination of peribronchiolar thickening, perihilar linear opacity, and peribronchiolar consolidation, often bilateral (Fig. 13.2A). Air trapping, manifested as areas of increased lucency, is also common in patients with acute bronchiolitis. Air trapping may be effectively demonstrated with postexpiratory imaging. In very young patients who are unable to cooperate with the instructions required for postexpiratory imaging, lateral decubitus imaging may be used to demonstrate air trapping.

CT and HRCT manifestations of acute bronchiolitis include patchy areas of atelectasis, frequently combined with bronchial wall thickening and mosaic perfusion (see Fig. 13.2B), the latter due to air trapping.

Acute bronchiolitis, particularly related to adenovirus infection acquired during early childhood, may result in the Swyer–James syndrome (constrictive bronchiolitis or bronchiolitis obliterans see also Chapter 23). Histopathology in the Swyer–James syndrome shows constrictive bronchiolitis, chronic bronchiolitis, bronchiectasis, and some destruction of the lung parenchyma.

The Swyer–James syndrome is usually encountered incidentally in a patient undergoing radiography for unrelated reasons. Patients occasionally complain of dyspnea on exertion. Many patients provide a history of childhood infection.

Inspiratory chest radiographs in patients with Swyer–James syndrome show increased lucency involving affected parts of the lung(s). While historically described as a unilateral process, many cases do involve both lungs to varying degrees. The inspiratory volume of the affected areas is usually normal or perhaps slightly diminished with attenuated peripheral vasculature. The hilum on the affected side is usually small (Fig. 13.3A). Postexpiratory imaging shows air trapping in the affected areas, with shift of the mediastinum

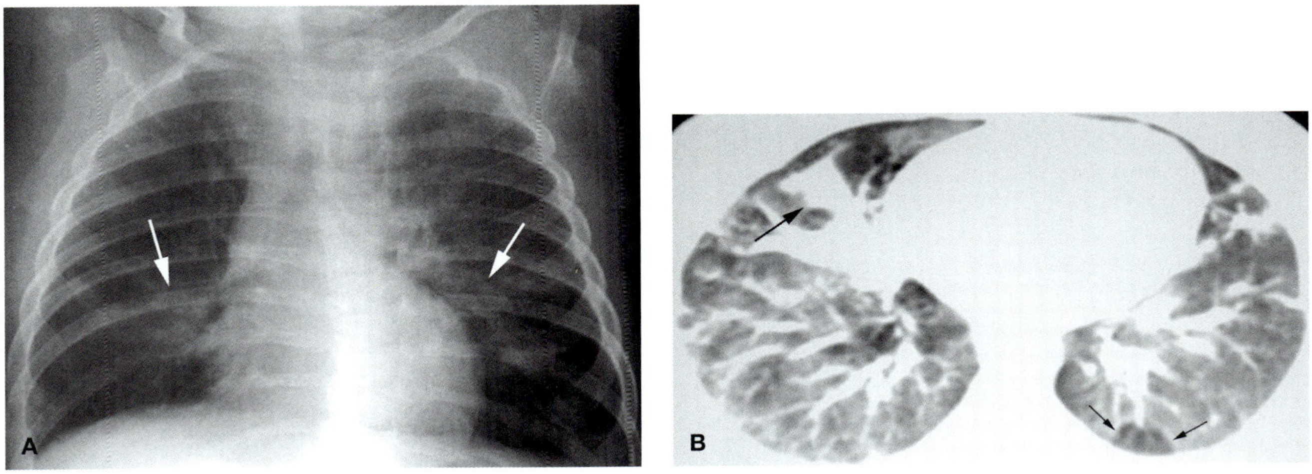

Figure 13.2. Viral bronchiolitis in a 3-year-old boy. **A:** Frontal chest radiograph shows bilateral perihilar linear opacities (*arrows*) consistent with bronchial wall thickening and atelectasis. **B:** Axial CT image shows patchy atelectasis (*large arrow*) and lobular air trapping (*small arrows*).

away from the more severely affected side. CT and HRCT easily demonstrate the findings of Swyer–James syndrome. CT shows increased lucency with diminished vascular size in the affected area in most patients (see Fig. 23.26 in Chapter 23). Bronchiectasis is often seen as well (see Fig. 13.3B). Air trapping, seen as failure of the expected increase in lung attenuation (and decrease in volume) following exhalation or a paradoxical decrease in attenuation following exhalation, is always present.

Lobar Pneumonia

Lobar pneumonia is typically caused by organisms such as *Streptococcus pneumoniae* (*Pneumococcus*) and *Klebsiella pneumoniae*. This pattern is characterized by the initial development of peripheral opacity that rapidly evolves into confluent, homogeneous consolidation (Fig. 13.4 and Fig. 1.15 in Chapter 1), often conforming to anatomic boundaries such as the interlobar fissures. Lobar pneumonia uncommonly affects the entire lobe, and the term *air-space pneumonia* is often used instead. Air bronchograms are common with lobar or air-space pneumonia (Fig. 13.5). Usually, lobar or air-space pneumonia is nonsegmental, meaning that it easily crosses pulmonary segments (bronchopneumonia is usually segmental and patchy—see below). Lobar or air-space pneumonia may produce expansion of a lobe, the "bulging fissure" sign (Fig. 13.6 and Fig. 1.15 in Chapter 1); this sign has been associated with *K. pneumoniae* infection

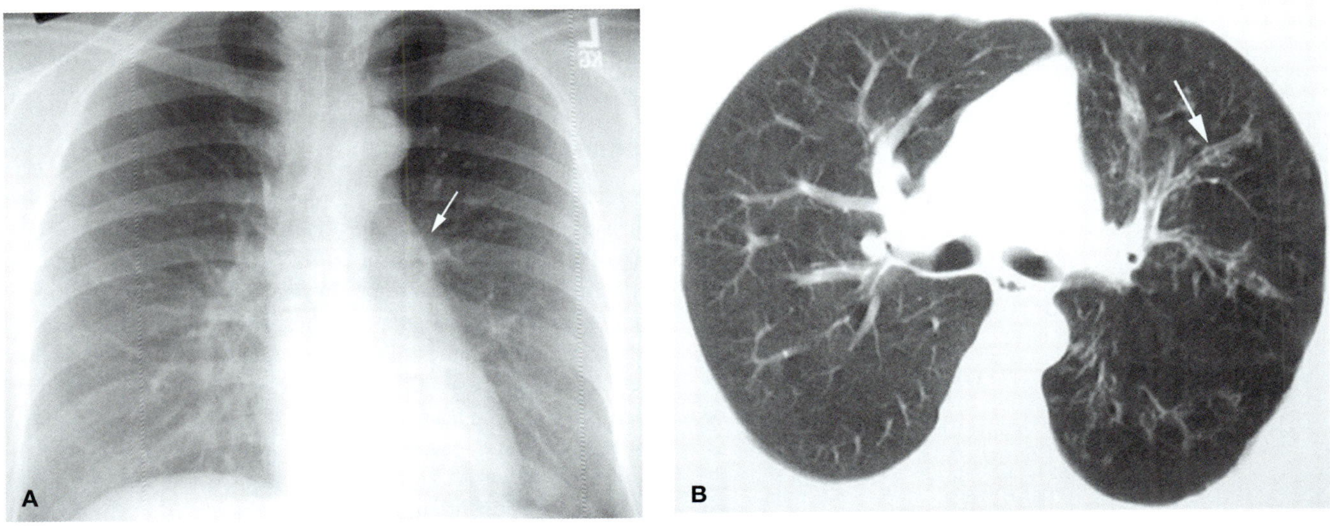

Figure 13.3. Swyer–James syndrome. **A:** Frontal chest radiograph shows a diminutive left hilum (*arrow*) and relatively decreased attenuation throughout the left upper lobe. Note the leftward shift of the trachea, indicating diminished left upper lobe volume. **B:** Axial CT image shows relatively decreased attenuation of the left upper lobe associated with irregular bronchial wall thickening and dilation (*arrow*).

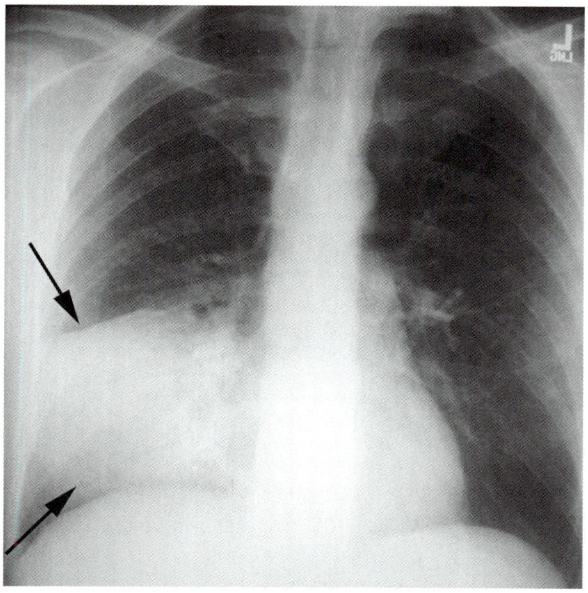

Figure 13.4. Lobar pneumonia. Frontal chest radiograph shows homogeneous right middle lobe consolidation (*arrows*), representing pneumococcal pneumonia.

but probably is more commonly the result of pneumococcal pneumonia owing to the latter's greater prevalence. If the patient survives the infection, air-space pneumonia usually heals without sequelae.

Bronchopneumonia

Bronchopneumonia begins with infection of the airway mucosa and subsequently extends into the adjacent alveoli. The bronchopneumonia pattern consists of patchy areas of consolidation that may be initially limited to one or more pulmonary segments (Fig. 13.7), but it then progresses to multifocal,

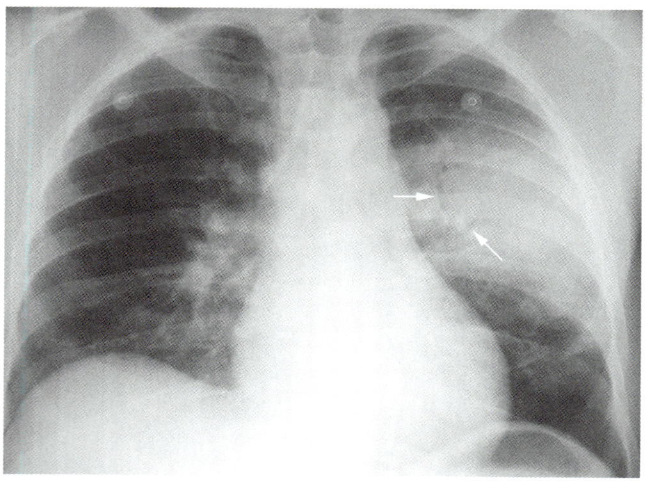

Figure 13.5. Air-space pneumonia: air bronchograms. Frontal chest radiograph in a patient with pneumococcal pneumonia shows homogenous consolidation associated with tubular lucencies (*arrows*), representing air bronchograms.

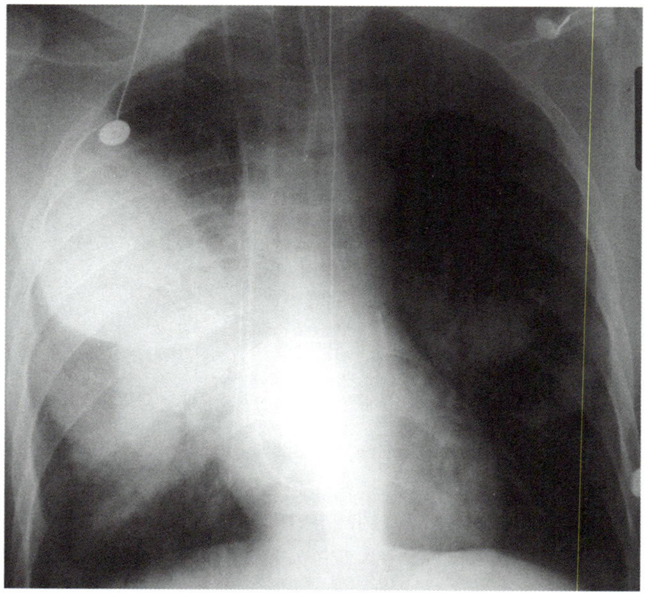

Figure 13.6. Air-space pneumonia: the bulging fissure sign. Frontal chest radiograph shows homogenous right upper lobe consolidation associated with inferior displacement of the major fissure. *Klebsiella pneumoniae* was recovered in both blood and sputum.

often bilateral, consolidation (see Fig. 1.7 in Chapter 1). Less affected areas will show tree-in-bud nodules or more confluent air-space nodules (also known as acinar nodules), which are ill defined and usually range from 5 to 10 mm in size. These nodules represent infection of the terminal and respiratory bronchioles with peribronchiolar consolidation. Because of the prominent airway involvement with bronchopneumonia, some volume loss is common. The bronchopneumonia pattern is often associated with virulent organisms such as *S. aureus* or Gram-negative organisms. Because these organisms are commonly aggressive, tissue destruction is common and complications such as necrosis or abscess may occur. Healing of bronchopneumonia often results in scarring.

Interstitial Pneumonia

Infectious interstitial pneumonias are commonly caused by viruses, *M. pneumoniae*, and *Pneumocystis jirovecii* pneumonia. Pathologically, inflammation in interstitial pneumonia is primarily limited to the pulmonary interstitium, although not exclusively so. The typical chest radiographic appearance of interstitial pneumonia is bilateral, symmetric, linear, or reticular opacities (Fig. 13.8). Interstitial pneumonias, particularly *P. jirovecii* pneumonia, may produce a fine granular or ground-glass pattern on chest radiography that subsequently evolves to consolidation if not treated. Ground-glass opacity or consolidation is usually associated with alveolar filling superimposed on the interstitial abnormality. Treated infectious interstitial pneumonias typically resolve without sequelae, if the patient survives. COVID-19 often presents with ground-glass opacity and is discussed later in the chapter.

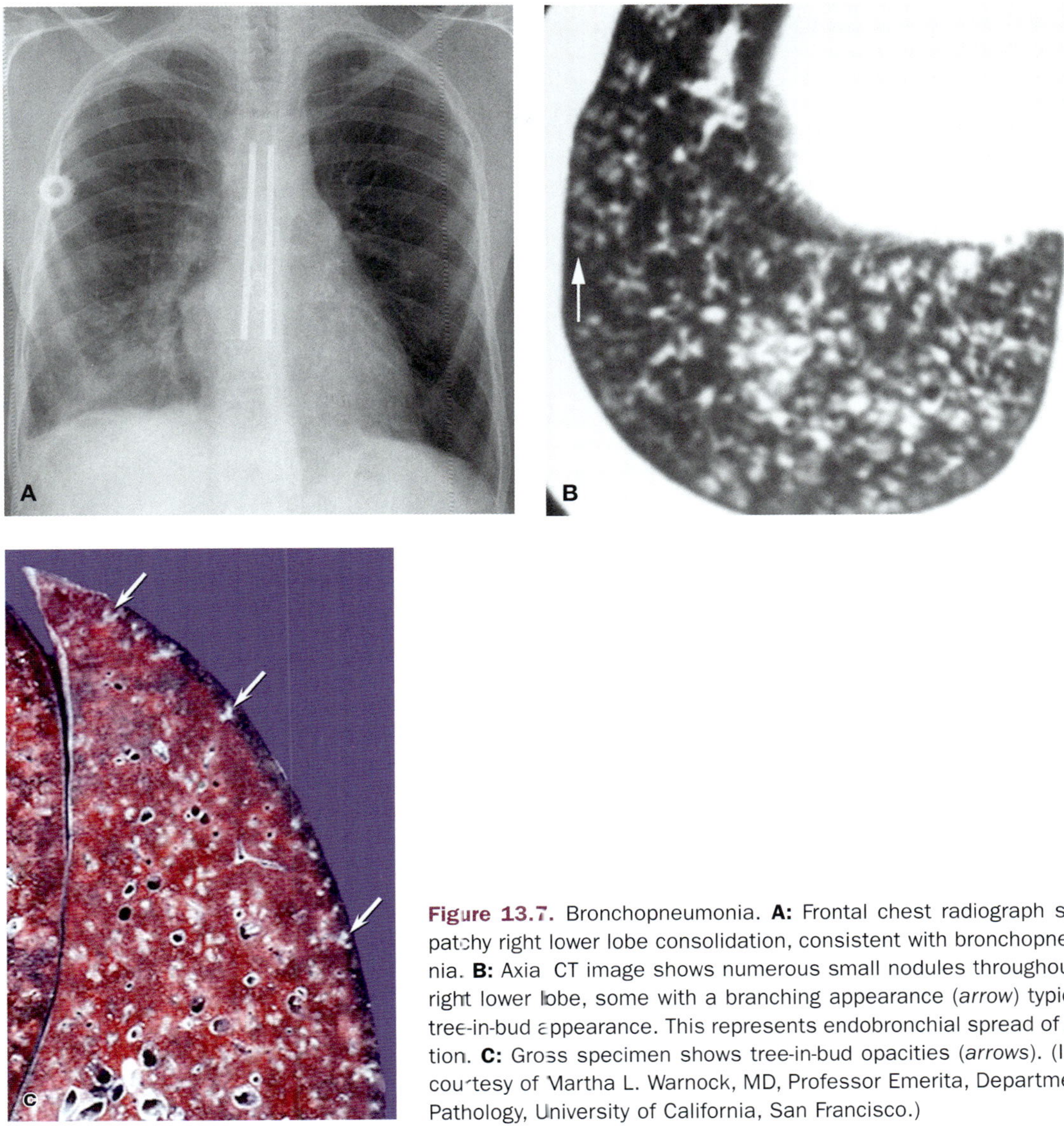

Figure 13.7. Bronchopneumonia. **A:** Frontal chest radiograph shows patchy right lower lobe consolidation, consistent with bronchopneumonia. **B:** Axial CT image shows numerous small nodules throughout the right lower lobe, some with a branching appearance (*arrow*) typical of tree-in-bud appearance. This represents endobronchial spread of infection. **C:** Gross specimen shows tree-in-bud opacities (*arrows*). (Image courtesy of Martha L. Warnock, MD, Professor Emerita, Department of Pathology, University of California, San Francisco.)

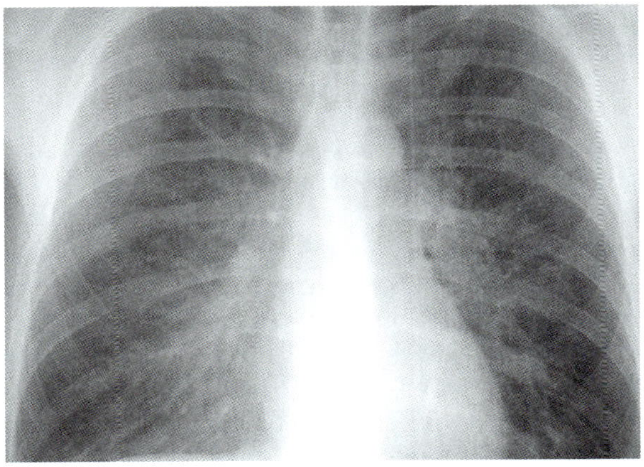

Figure 13.8. Infectious interstitial pneumonia. Frontal chest radiograph shows diffuse, bilateral interstitial prominence. *Pneumocystis jirovecii* was recovered with sputum induction.

Lung Abscess

A lung abscess represents a localized infection that undergoes tissue destruction and necrosis. When a communication with the tracheobronchial tree is present, cavitation and an air-fluid level may be evident (Fig. 13.9 and Figs. 10.10, 10.40 in Chapter 10). The inner wall of an abscess varies from smooth to shaggy and irregular, and maximum wall thickness usually ranges from 5 to 15 mm. Pulmonary abscesses are most commonly caused by mixed anaerobic infections, followed in frequency by *S. aureus* and *Pseudomonas aeruginosa*. Such infections are often the result of aspiration. Consequently, a lung abscess is often encountered in patients at risk for aspiration, such as patients with poor dental hygiene, impaired consciousness, esophageal motility disorders, and neurologic diseases. Multiple abscesses may result from septic embolism.

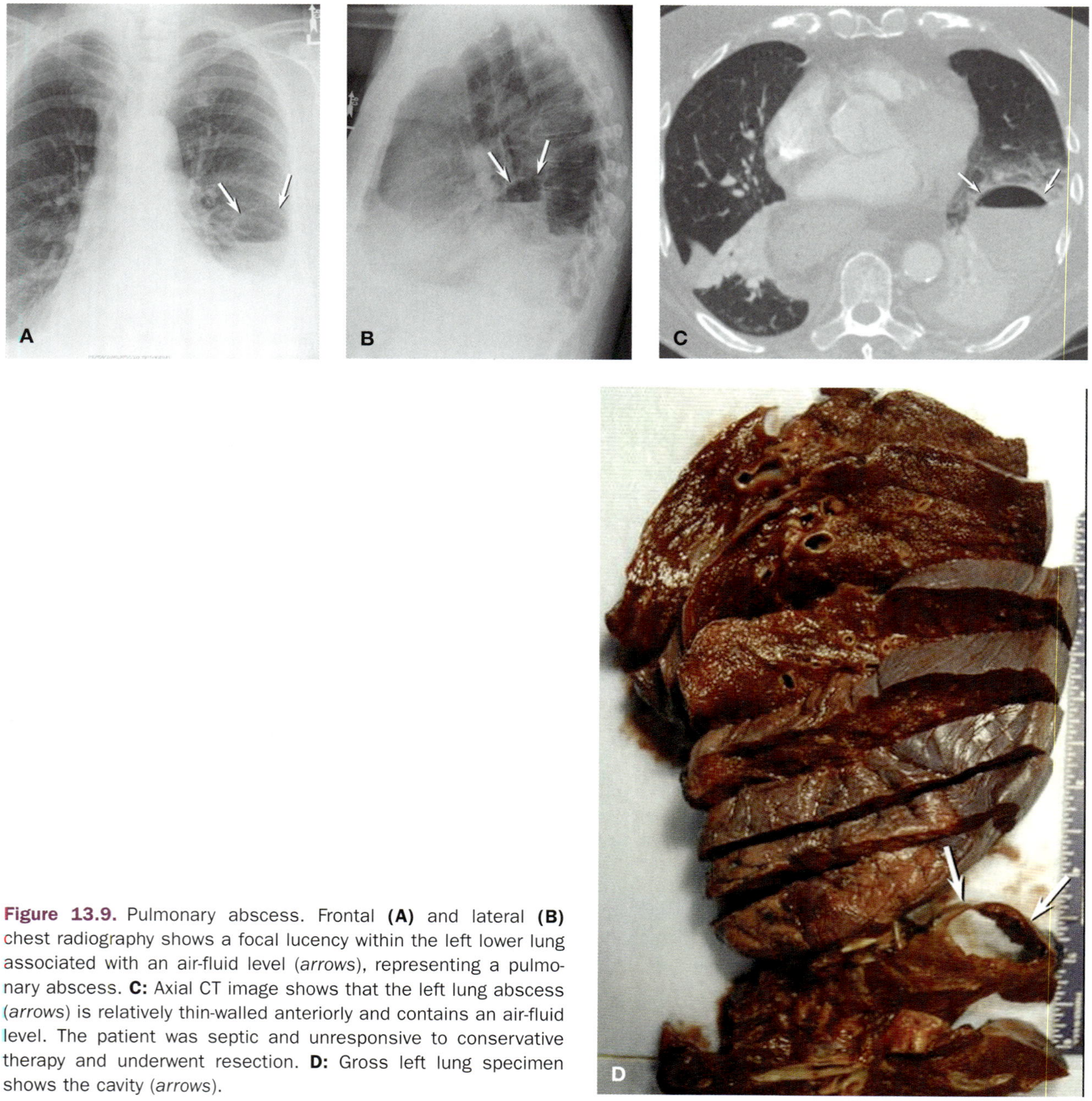

Figure 13.9. Pulmonary abscess. Frontal **(A)** and lateral **(B)** chest radiography shows a focal lucency within the left lower lung associated with an air-fluid level (*arrows*), representing a pulmonary abscess. **C:** Axial CT image shows that the left lung abscess (*arrows*) is relatively thin-walled anteriorly and contains an air-fluid level. The patient was septic and unresponsive to conservative therapy and underwent resection. **D:** Gross left lung specimen shows the cavity (*arrows*).

Approach to Imaging of the Immunocompromised Patient

Imaging of immunocompromised patients, including those with HIV infection, organ transplantation, and patients with hematopoietic stem cell transplantation or bone marrow suppression, requires special consideration. An organized approach to the imaging evaluation of such patients is critical to ensure accurate and timely diagnosis.

It is critical to understand the pathogenesis of the various causes of immunosuppression for such patients and to recognize that the use of any prophylactic medications may alter the interpretation of imaging studies. For example, the pathogenesis of immunosuppression for patients with HIV infection is related to the progressive depletion of T-cell immunity (specifically depletion of CD4 cells). Because opportunistic infections occur with greater frequency as the CD4 cell count falls, awareness of the CD4 cell count is critical for accurate interpretation of imaging studies. Furthermore, because the use of highly active antiretroviral therapy (HAART) has dramatically changed the course of HIV infection, every effort should be made to determine whether a patient is receiving HAART before providing a differential diagnosis for abnormal thoracic imaging findings.

For patients with bone marrow suppression from chemotherapy or hematopoietic stem cell transplantation and for patients with solid organ transplantation, certain infectious and noninfectious complications are more likely to occur at different times following the institution of chemotherapy or transplantation. Awareness of these time courses is important for accurate diagnosis.

Imaging of immunosuppressed patients usually begins with chest radiography. While chest radiographic findings in immunosuppressed patients are often nonspecific, recognizing certain basic radiographic patterns is important. The discussion below details a basic imaging approach to the immunosuppressed patient.

Focal Air-space Opacities

Infected immunosuppressed patients with focal air-space opacities are most likely to have bacterial infection, particularly if such opacities are unilateral, if they show air bronchograms and/or pleural effusions or if either a segmental or a lobar distribution is evident. This is true for patients with HIV infection, regardless of CD4 count, and is generally the case for patients with immunosuppression unrelated to HIV infection. With advancing severity of immunosuppression, infection with *Mycobacterium tuberculosis* (MTB) must be considered as a cause of focal air-space consolidation. Although uncommon in patients with HIV infection, *Nocardia asteroides* infection may present with focal, often mass-like, air-space opacity, particularly in organ transplant recipients (Fig. 13.10). This pattern may reflect lobar pneumonia or bronchopneumonia. In neutropenic patients, about one-third of patients with mucormycosis presents with a solitary area of consolidation that often has a reversed halo appearance (which may resemble a pulmonary infarct) or surrounding perilesional ground-glass halo.

Multifocal Air-space Opacities

When bilateral opacities are present, the differential diagnosis must be expanded, and it becomes very important to integrate information regarding the degree of immunosuppression in the imaging assessment of such patients. Bilateral opacities may represent bacterial pneumonia, but for severely immunosuppressed patients (HIV infection with CD4 cell counts below 200 cells/μL and non-HIV-immunosuppressed patients with neutropenic fever), opportunistic infections, such as *P. jirovecii* pneumonia (still often referred to as *Pneumocystis carinii* pneumonia or PCP), fungal infections (most commonly *Cryptococcus neoformans* and *A. fumigatus*, but also other invasive fungal species, including mucormycosis), and less commonly, viruses and infection with unusual bacterial organisms, such as mycobacteria and *N. asteroides*, must be considered. Fungal, mycobacteria, or *N. asteroides* infections are more likely if the radiographic abnormalities are nodular in appearance, whereas PCP or viral infections are more likely when opacities are appearing interstitial (see Fig. 13.8) or have a ground-glass appearance and are unaccompanied by either pleural effusion or lymphadenopathy.

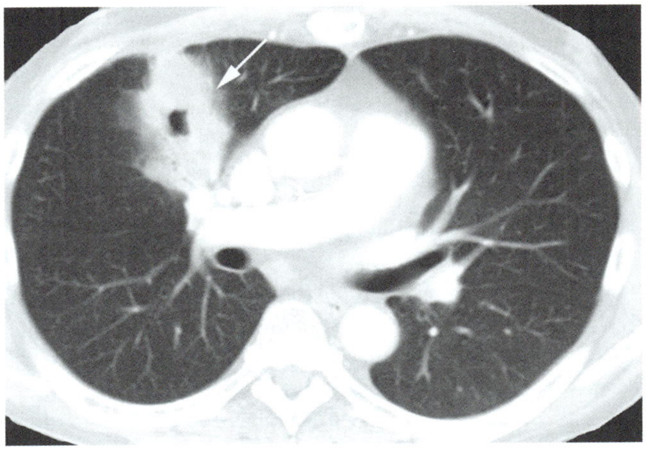

Figure 13.10. *Nocardia asteroides* infection in a heart transplant recipient. Axial CT image shows nodular right lung consolidation with central cavitation (*arrow*). *N. asteroides* was recovered following biopsy of this lesion.

Linear (Interstitial-appearing) Opacities

Linear, or interstitial-appearing, radiographic abnormalities in immunosuppressed patients may reflect atypical pneumonia, such as viral infections or PCP. These infections usually occur in HIV-infected patients with CD4 cell counts below 200 cells/μL and in hematopoietic stem cell transplant patients between 1 and 6 months after transplantation, although viral infections may occur in lung transplant recipients any time after lung transplantation. PCP is, however, very uncommon in patients receiving appropriate prophylactic therapy.

Cavitation

Cavitation within either focal or diffuse lung parenchymal opacities in immunosuppressed patients is usually caused by bacterial infection, including *N. asteroides* (see Fig. 13.10), mycobacterial infections, and fungal infection. In patients with severe bone marrow suppression, such as chemotherapy patients or patients several weeks after hematopoietic stem cell transplantation, bilateral, multifocal, and nodular opacities that quickly undergo cavitation are highly suggestive of invasive aspergillosis.

Cavitation of upper lobe parenchymal opacities may occur in relatively immunocompetent patients with mycobacterial infections. Cavitation in mycobacterial infections in HIV-infected patients with CD4 cell counts below 200 cells/μL is uncommon, however, and the presence of cavitation within focal or diffuse opacities in such patients favors either necrotizing pyogenic pneumonia or fungal infection.

Pleural Effusions

Pleural effusions are commonly present in immunosuppressed patients with pyogenic bacterial infections of any etiology. They may be present in patients with fungal infections, although they are extremely uncommon in patients with PCP.

Lymphadenopathy

Lymphadenopathy is commonly encountered in immunosuppressed patients with pyogenic bacterial infections, although enlarged nodes are usually seen only with CT and not on chest radiographs. Visibly enlarged nodes on chest radiographs in HIV-infected patients with CD4 cell counts below 200 cells/μL should specifically suggest the diagnosis of MTB (Fig. 13.11). The development of lymphadenopathy in patients who have recently been started on HAART therapy has been associated with mycobacterial infection. It has been postulated that HAART allows the reconstituted immune system to react to latent pulmonary infection. It is therefore important to know whether an HIV-infected patient is taking HAART, and when HAART was started, if lymphadenopathy is encountered on chest radiographs in patients with AIDS.

SPECIFIC INFECTIONS

The epidemiology, pathogenesis, clinical presentation, and imaging findings of specific infections (Table 13.1) are reviewed in this section.

Bacteria

Gram-Positive Cocci

Streptococcus pneumoniae

Streptococcus pneumoniae is overwhelmingly the most common cause of pneumonia associated with Gram-positive cocci (Table 13.2). Numerous antigenic types have been identified. Pneumococcus may colonize nearly 20% of the population, and this figure is higher in COPD patients.

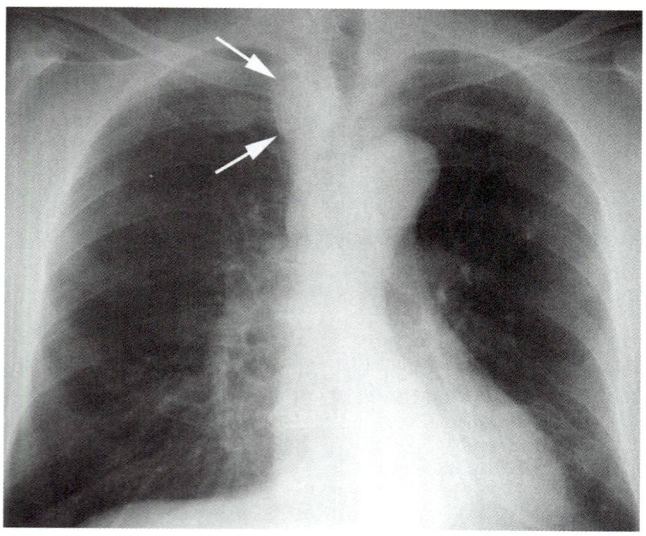

Figure 13.11. *Mycobacterium tuberculosis* infection in an AIDS patient with a low CD4 cell count. Frontal chest radiograph shows right paratracheal lymph node enlargement (*arrows*).

Table 13.1 Classification of Important Pulmonary Infections by Organism

Bacteria

Gram-positive cocci
- *Streptococcus pneumoniae*
- *Staphylococcus aureus*
- *Streptococcus pyogenes*

Gram-positive bacilli
- *Bacillus anthracis*
- *Rhodococcus equi*

Gram-negative cocci
- *Moraxella catarrhalis (Branhamella catarrhalis)*
- *Neisseria meningitidis*

Gram-negative rods
- *Escherichia coli*
- *Klebsiella pneumoniae*
- *Pseudomonas aeruginosa*
- *Yersinia pestis*
- *Serratia* and *Enterobacter* spp.

Gram-negative coccobacilli
- *Haemophilus influenzae*
- *Legionella pneumophila*
- *Bordetella* species
- *Bartonella henselae* and *Quintana*
- *Francisella tularensis*

Anaerobic bacteria

Mycobacteria

Mycobacterium tuberculosis

Mycobacterium bovis

Nontuberculous mycobacteria
- *M. avium* complex
- *M. kansasii*
- *M. abscessus*

Actinomyces

Nocardiosis

Actinomycosis

Fungi

Histoplasmosis

Coccidioidomycosis

North American blastomycosis

South American blastomycosis (paracoccidioidomycosis)

Cryptococcosis

Aspergillosis

Invasive aspergillosis

Chronic necrotizing aspergillosis
- Chronic cavitary pulmonary aspergillosis
- Subacute invasive pulmonary aspergillosis

Aspergilloma

Mucormycosis

Pneumocystis jirovecii (P. carinii) pneumonia

***Mycoplasma*, *Chlamydia*, and Rickettsiae pneumonias**

Mycoplasma pneumoniae

Chlamydia
- *C. trachomatis*
- *C. psittaci*
- *C. pneumoniae*

Rickettsiae

RNA viruses

Influenza virus

Parainfluenza virus

Respiratory syncytial virus

Human metapneumovirus

Measles

Coronaviruses
- COVID-19
- SARS
- MERS-CoV

Hantaviruses

Togaviruses (rubella)

DNA viruses

Herpesviruses
- Herpes simplex
- Varicella-zoster

Cytomegalovirus

Epstein-Barr virus

Adenoviruses

Parasites: protozoans, roundworms (nematodes), and flatworms

Amebiasis

Toxoplasmosis

Ascariasis

Strongyloidiasis

Dirofilariasis

Tropical eosinophilia

Toxocariasis (visceral larva migrans)

Paragonimiasis

Schistosomiasis

Echinococcosis (hydatid disease)

Cysticercosis

Table 13.2 Streptococcus pneumoniae

Most common pneumonia associated with Gram-positive cocci
Most common pneumonia requiring hospitalization or resulting in death
Air-space (lobar) pneumonia often with air bronchograms
Multifocal consolidation consistent with a bronchopneumonia less common
Pleural effusion in <50%

The development of pneumococcal pneumonia has been associated with several risk factors, including advanced age; immunosuppression; chronic heart, lung, and renal diseases; sickle cell disease; cirrhosis; prior splenectomy; and hematologic malignancies. *S. pneumoniae* is the most commonly isolated pathogen in hospitals, and pneumococcal pneumonia is the most common cause of pneumonia requiring hospitalization or resulting in death. In recent years, the emergence of resistant strains of *S. pneumoniae* has caused great concern in the medical community.

Pulmonary infection with *S. pneumoniae* is typically preceded by colonization of the nasopharynx. Once the organism reaches the lower respiratory tract, infection is facilitated by several virulence factors, including the antiphagocytic properties of the organism's capsule as well as the organism's ability to elaborate various proteins that augment the infection.

Pneumococcal pneumonia classically presents with the abrupt onset of high fever, classically preceded by a single rigor, cough that may be productive of rusty brown sputum, shaking chills, and pleuritic chest pain. Manifestations of pneumococcal pneumonia in the elderly may be somewhat atypical and are occasionally overshadowed by other chronic illnesses. Physical examination may reveal crackles, dullness to percussion, decreased breath sounds, and bronchial breathing.

Complications of pneumococcal pneumonia include empyema, meningitis, disseminated intravascular coagulation, hepatocellular damage, renal damage, and acute respiratory distress syndrome (ARDS). Pneumococcal pneumonia may leave the patient vulnerable to superinfection by other bacterial organisms.

Imaging Findings Pneumococcal pneumonia appears on the chest radiograph as classical air-space pneumonia: consolidation extending to pleural surfaces, often with air bronchograms (Fig. 13.12A). Volume loss is minimal. Pneumococcal pneumonia may also present with patchy, multifocal consolidation consistent with bronchopneumonia (Fig. 13.12B and C) or, rarely, as an interstitial-appearing process associated with some air-space consolidation. Occasionally, pneumococcal pneumonia appears as a focal nodule or mass (Fig. 13.13), often referred to as "round pneumonia." Cavitation and abscess formation are uncommon. Pleural disease, either pleural effusion or empyema, is found in 50% or fewer patients. Thoracic CT often shows lobar air-space consolidation, often with areas of ground-glass opacity surrounding the consolidation, lobular opacity, poorly defined centrilobular nodules measuring 3 to 10 mm, bronchial wall thickening, and smooth interlobular septal thickening. Localization of opacity in the middle and outer third of the lung is common. It has been suggested that small (less than 3 mm) centrilobular nodules are less commonly seen in bacterial pneumonias, such as pneumococcus, and may favor another infectious etiology, such as other bacteria, *M. pneumoniae*, or viral pneumonia.

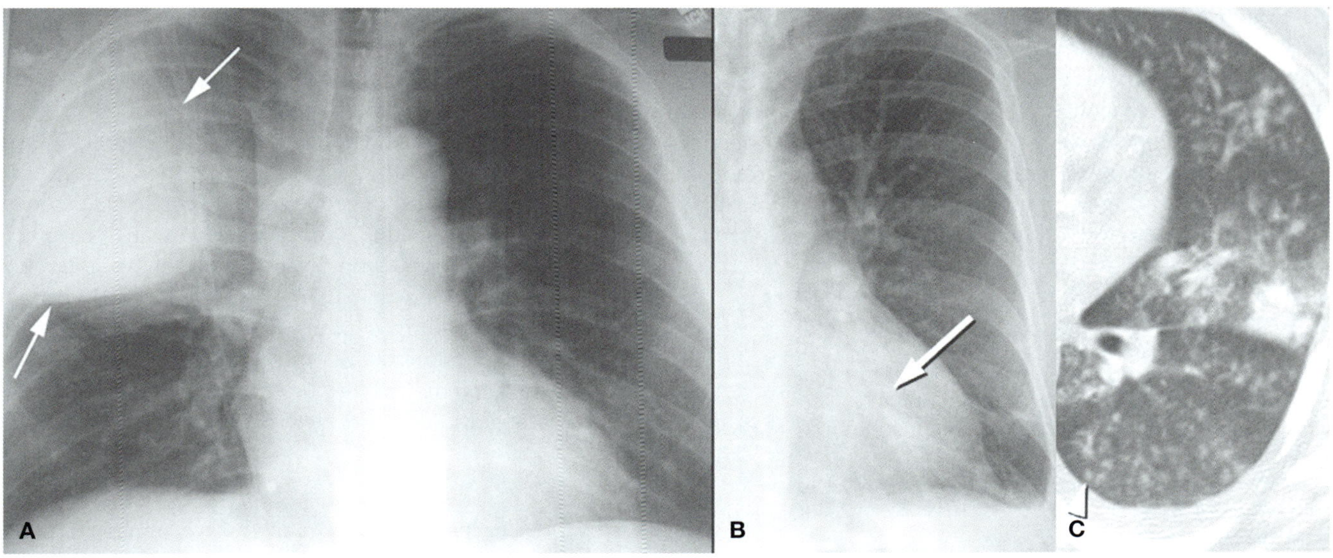

Figure 13.12. Pneumococcal pneumonia: air-space and bronchopneumonia patterns. **A:** Frontal chest radiograph shows homogenous right upper lobe consolidation (*arrows*) associated with air bronchograms, typical of air-space, or lobar, pneumonia. **B:** Frontal chest radiograph shows left lower lobe bronchovascular thickening (*arrow*). **C:** Axial CT shows patchy consolidation in lingula and small centrilobular nodules (*arrowhead*), consistent with the bronchopneumonia pattern.

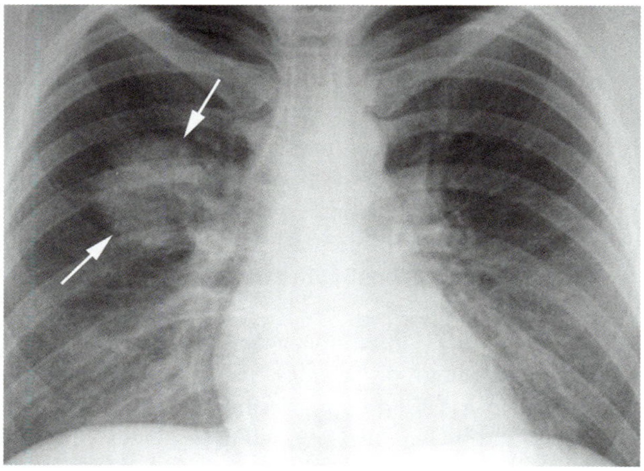

Figure 13.13. Round pneumonia caused by pneumococcus. Frontal chest radiograph shows a round, mass-like opacity within the right upper lobe (*arrows*). Pneumococcus was recovered in the patient's sputum, and the opacity resolved following antibiotic therapy.

With appropriate treatment, pneumococcal pneumonia may completely resolve within 14 days, although complete resolution may take longer in elderly or very ill patients.

Staphylococcus aureus

Staphylococcus aureus is an uncommon cause of community-acquired pneumonia but an important cause of nosocomial pneumonia (Table 13.3). It possesses several virulence factors that allow the organism to infect susceptible hosts. While *S. aureus* infection usually occurs via the tracheobronchial tree, hematogenous spread of organisms to the lungs from staphylococcal endocarditis or cellulitis is another common mode of pulmonary infection.

Staphylococcus aureus pneumonia has a well-recognized propensity for occurring following influenza infection. When pneumonia occurs in these settings, abrupt onset of chest pain, fever, cough, and purulent sputum, occasionally with hemoptysis, is typical. Factors that place patients at risk for pneumonia include COPD and other chronic illnesses, advanced age, immunosuppression, and cystic fibrosis. Most commonly, *S. aureus* pneumonia is encountered in hospitalized patients and presents with fever and cough productive of purulent, occasionally blood-streaked, sputum. The mortality rate associated with *S. aureus* pneumonia in hospitalized patients is often substantial. While *S. aureus* pneumonia has traditionally been considered an uncommon cause of community-acquired pneumonia, *S. aureus* is a common cause of pneumonia severe enough requiring intensive care unit admission. Furthermore, a community-acquired strain of methicillin-resistant *S. aureus* pneumonia is being increasingly encountered.

Table 13.3 *Staphylococcus aureus*
Common cause of nosocomial pneumonia
Associated with influenza and hematogenous pulmonary dissemination from endocarditis
Usually bronchopneumonia with patchy lower lobe consolidation
Cavitation frequent
Pneumatoceles may be seen
Septic emboli
Pleural effusion in nearly 50%; empyema may result

Imaging Findings S. aureus usually causes bronchopneumonia, with homogeneous or patchy, often multifocal, consolidation (Fig. 13.14), often predominating in the lower lobes. Volume loss is common, but air bronchograms are not. Abscess formation with cavitation is frequent (see Fig. 10.48 in Chapter 10). Occasionally, pneumatoceles are seen, especially in children. Pneumatoceles, unlike abscesses, appear as thin-walled cystic structures that may contain air-fluid levels. The inner wall of a pneumatocele is usually thin and regular, unlike that of a pulmonary abscess. Pneumatoceles tend to resolve spontaneously in weeks or a few months following infection.

On CT or HRCT, pneumonia usually appears as segmental consolidation often associated with centrilobular nodules or tree-in-bud opacity.

Pleural effusions occur in nearly 50% of patients with *S. aureus* pneumonia; empyema may complicate such effusions. The latter may be suggested when loculation is present, particularly when extensive pleural thickening (the "split-pleura" sign) is seen on CT.

Hematogenous dissemination (septic embolization) of *S. aureus* to the lungs, as may be encountered with intravenous drug abuse and bacterial tricuspid valve endocarditis, typically presents as multiple, poorly defined nodules that cavitate over a period of several days (Fig. 13.15A). These nodules are usually peripherally located and predominate in the lower lobes. CT may show the presence of cavitation (see Fig. 13.15B) to better advantage than radiography and may also reveal that the nodules are closely associated with pulmonary vessels; this association, termed the "feeding vessel sign," is typical of processes that are hematogenously disseminated to the lung. Wedge-shaped areas of peripheral consolidation, representing septic pulmonary infarction, are commonly seen in patients with septic embolization. Diffuse alveolar damage rarely follows septic embolization. The imaging manifestations of septic embolization are not specific to *S. aureus* and may be encountered with other bacterial pathogens, such as *S. epidermidis*.

Streptococcus pyogenes

Streptococcus pyogenes, a Gram-positive organism that is usually arranged in chains on smear, predominantly causes pneumonia in the very young and the elderly.

Pathologically, a bronchopneumonia pattern is usually observed with *S. pyogenes*. Much like *S. aureus*, *S. pyogenes*

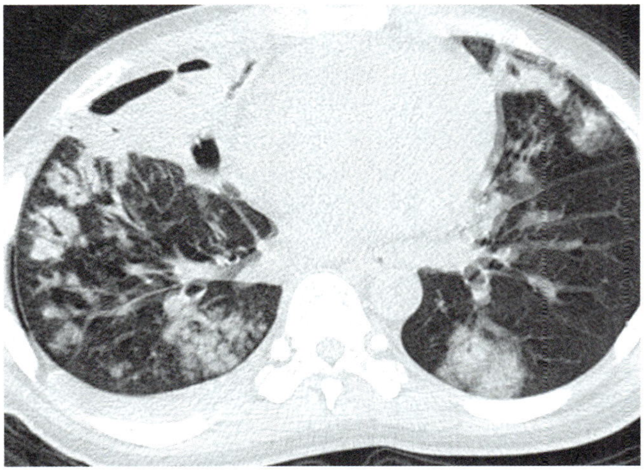

Figure 13.14. Staphylococcal pneumonia. Axial chest CT shows a wide range of findings from bronchopneumonia including consolidation with cavitation in the right middle lobe, patchy bilateral nodular areas of consolidation, and smaller centrilobular nodules in the right lower lobe. A small right pneumothorax is due to bronchopleural fistula from the right middle lobe. Staphylococcal pneumonia was proven by blood and sputum cultures.

pneumonia frequently follows other respiratory infections, especially measles and whooping cough (*Bordetella pertussis*), although the frequency of these two infections has declined and *S. pyogenes* pneumonia is rarely seen.

Streptococcus pyogenes pneumonia usually presents with high fever, cough productive of purulent sputum, pleuritic chest pain, and shaking chills. The sputum may be blood streaked. Rarely, *S. pyogenes* pneumonia is accompanied by other *S. pyogenes* infections, such as scarlet fever and toxic shock syndrome.

Streptococcus pyogenes pulmonary infection typically causes patchy, segmental, multifocal consolidation that is often accompanied by pleural effusion. Unlike *S. aureus* pneumonia, pneumatocele formation is uncommon with *S. pyogenes* pneumonia, although lung abscesses may occur.

Other Gram-Positive Cocci

Other Gram-positive cocci that rarely produce pulmonary infection include *S. viridans*, *S. faecalis* (*Enterococcus—now classified as a separate genus from Streptococcus*), *S. agalactiae*, and *S. intermedius*, among a number of other species. These organisms usually produce a bronchopneumonia pattern that is radiographically indistinguishable from *S. pyogenes* pneumonia or *S. aureus* pneumonia or may result in abscesses or endocarditis.

Gram-Positive Bacilli

Bacillus anthracis

Bacillus anthracis is an encapsulated Gram-positive rod that forms spores (Table 13.4). The organism is most commonly found in agricultural areas, especially in Central and South America, Eastern and Southern Europe, Asia, the Middle East, and Africa. The spores are found in soil. Once they germinate, they are ingested by an animal, usually wild or domestic herbivores such as sheep, cattle, camels, and goats. Individuals who come in contact with these animals or their tissues may be exposed and become infected. Therefore, the highest risk occupations include farmers, individuals who work with animal hides, and butchers.

Anthrax was largely unknown in the United States until October 2001, shortly following the terrorist attacks on the World Trade Center and Pentagon on September 11, 2001. From September 18 to November 20, 2001, 22 cases of anthrax (11 inhalational and 11 cutaneous) occurred following exposure to mail contaminated with anthrax spores. Five of the 11 patients with inhalational anthrax died. In 2008, the Federal Bureau of Investigation identified a single perpetrator—a scientist in the biodefense industry—who committed suicide while awaiting prosecution.

Anthrax infection occurs in three forms: cutaneous (the most common form), gastrointestinal, and inhalational. Humans usually become infected when they inhale spores

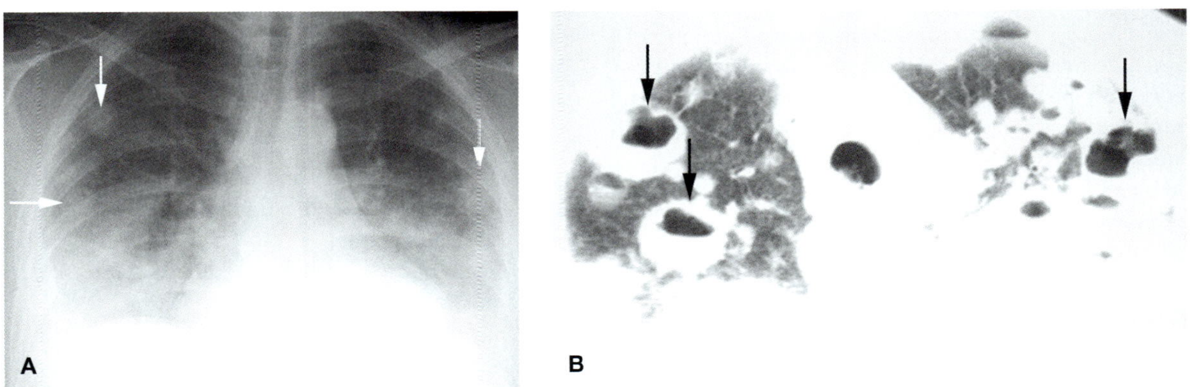

Figure 13.15. Infective endocarditis with septic embolization. **A:** Frontal chest radiograph shows multiple, bilateral, peripheral nodules and cavities (*arrows*) representing septic emboli in a patient with *Staphylococcus aureus* infection of the tricuspid valve. **B:** Axial CT shows multiple, bilateral cavities (*arrows*) representing septic embolization.

Table 13.4 Bacillus Anthracis
Most common in agricultural areas (Central and South America, Eastern and Southern Europe, Asia, the Middle East, and Africa)
Contact with animals or their tissues
Three forms: cutaneous, gastrointestinal, and inhalational
Inhalational anthrax occurs when spore-containing dust is inhaled
Mediastinal widening, due to lymphadenopathy
Progressive pleural effusions

after being exposed to infected animals or animal tissue. Rarely, infection is acquired through the ingestion of undercooked meat from infected animals.

Inhaled anthrax spores are ingested by macrophages and are transported to the pulmonary lymphatics and eventually into the mediastinal and hilar lymph nodes. There the organisms may germinate and produce endotoxin, which results in hemorrhage and edema within the affected nodes. The organisms may then reach the bloodstream and cause sepsis.

Cutaneous anthrax occurs when the organism enters a host through an abrasion or laceration on the skin while an individual is handling infected animal tissue. This may be fatal if not treated, but treatment usually results in complete recovery.

Gastrointestinal anthrax occurs if infected animal tissue is ingested; it results in nausea, anorexia, vomiting, fever, and abdominal pain. Severe diarrhea is often present, and hematemesis is occasionally noted.

Inhalational anthrax occurs when spore-containing dust is inhaled. Symptoms of infection may initially resemble an upper respiratory tract viral infection, although an abrupt onset of high fever and chest pain occurs in some individuals. Inhalational anthrax often progresses to respiratory failure and shock. Inhalational anthrax is often fatal, although early antibiotic treatment may be curative for some patients.

Imaging Findings Chest radiographic manifestations of anthrax include mediastinal widening, due to bulky lymphadenopathy and progressively enlarging pleural effusions. Hilar lymphadenopathy may also be present. Lung opacity is usually minimal in comparison to the lymph node enlargement and pleural effusions. CT often shows high-attenuation lymphadenopathy and may also show peribronchiolar thickening resulting from lymphatic stasis.

Rhodococcus equi

Rhodococcus equi is a weakly acid-fast coccobacillus that has been primarily associated with pulmonary infection in immunocompromised individuals, particularly AIDS patients. The organism lives in soil, and human infection occurs via inhalation. Once a susceptible host inhales the organisms, they enter and replicate within alveolar macrophages. The presence of the organism induces an inflammatory response within the pulmonary parenchyma. Infection with *R. equi* is usually subacute in nature. Patients present with fever, productive cough, and chest pain. Infection with *R. equi* carries a high mortality rate. Imaging findings of *R. equi* pulmonary infection include nodules and rounded areas of consolidation, favoring the upper lobes and may develop cavitation.

Gram-Negative Cocci

Moraxella catarrhalis (Branhamella catarrhalis)

Infection with *M. catarrhalis* usually occurs in patients with chronic illnesses such as COPD or patients on corticosteroid therapy. Other forms of immunocompromise may also place patients at risk for infection. *M. catarrhalis* is frequently found in the oral cavity. Upper and lower respiratory tract infection may occur in susceptible hosts. Patients present with fever and cough, usually mild. Infection with *M. catarrhalis* is usually mild, manifesting as a bronchopneumonia or bronchitis, and radiographic findings are nonspecific. Complications such as pleural effusion and empyema are uncommon.

Neisseria meningitidis

Pulmonary infection with *N. meningitidis* is uncommon and may occur with or without associated meningitis. Either lobar pneumonia or bronchopneumonia patterns may occur, occasionally with pleural effusion.

Gram-Negative Rods

Gram-negative rods are the leading cause of hospital-acquired pneumonia. Most ventilator-associated pneumonias are due to Gram-negative rods, and these infections are associated with high mortality. Gram-negative rod infection is also an increasing cause of community-acquired pneumonia, and these infections are often severe, requiring intensive unit care.

Escherichia coli

Escherichia coli is a normal inhabitant of the small and large bowel and may also be found within the oropharynx and nasopharynx following antibiotic treatment. Pulmonary infection occurs when the organism is aspirated into the lower respiratory tract. Gram-negative rods, including *E. coli*, typically cause a bronchopneumonia pattern.

Patients with *E. coli* pulmonary infection are usually either hospitalized or have chronic illnesses; they usually present with fever, cough productive of yellow sputum, shortness of breath, and pleuritic chest pain. When infection occurs in the outpatient setting, abrupt onset of fever, productive cough, pleuritic chest pain, and shortness of breath are the major presenting features.

The typical radiographic pattern of *E. coli* pulmonary infection is lower lobe bronchopneumonia. Pleural effusion is common.

Klebsiella pneumoniae

Although several *Klebsiella* species are known, *K. pneumoniae* is the most important organism from the point of view of human infection. *K. pneumoniae* classically affects older patients, particularly chronic alcoholics (Table 13.5). Other chronic illnesses, such as diabetes mellitus and COPD, are associated with a higher prevalence of *K. pneumoniae* infection.

Klebsiella pneumoniae is occasionally a normal commensal in the human gastrointestinal tract. The organism may also colonize the upper airway in some patients, particularly those who are hospitalized. Lower respiratory tract infection may occur when oral secretions are aspirated. Bronchopneumonia and air-space pneumonia patterns may be observed, and tissue necrosis and abscess formation are common.

Klebsiella pneumoniae usually presents with rapid onset of fever, painful respiration, and shortness of breath. Cough productive of purulent green sputum is suggestive of *K. pneumoniae* infection, although occasionally the sputum is red and gelatinous ("currant jelly" sputum). Patients are usually quite ill and may even be hypotensive.

Imaging Manifestations When *K. pneumoniae* presents with an air-space pattern, nonsegmental homogeneous consolidation resembling pneumococcal pneumonia is present. Air bronchograms are commonly seen. *K. pneumoniae* is known for its peculiar tendency to produce a large volume of consolidation, which causes expansion of a lobe, resulting in the bulging fissure sign (see Fig. 13.6). Pulmonary abscess formation (Fig. 13.16A-C) is common, as are pleural effusion and empyema. A bronchopneumonia pattern (Fig. 13.16D-G) may be seen with *K. pneumoniae* pulmonary infection, especially when the infection is hospital acquired.

Pseudomonas aeruginosa

Pseudomonas aeruginosa is typically found in soil and water but also in small numbers in the gastrointestinal tract of humans. *P. aeruginosa* is a common cause of nosocomial pneumonia, particularly in patients in the intensive care unit (Table 13.6). The organism typically lives within moist areas, such as showers, sinks, nebulizers, respiratory therapy equipment, and so forth. Infection with *P. aeruginosa* pneumonia is associated with numerous risk factors, including COPD, immunosuppression, mechanical ventilation, and prolonged antibiotic use.

Aspiration of organisms colonizing the upper respiratory tract is the usual cause of respiratory infection with *P. aeruginosa*. The organism elaborates a number of toxins and virulence factors that contribute to the ability to cause infection. The pattern of infection is bronchopneumonia, with peribronchiolar microabscess formation, hemorrhage, and associated inflammation being common.

Patients usually present with fever, shaking chills, cough productive of purulent sputum (occasionally blood streaked), and shortness of breath. Mortality in ventilated patients or patients in the intensive care unit is high.

Imaging Findings Chest radiographs show a pattern typical of bronchopneumonia, including segmental, often multifocal, patchy consolidation that favors the lower lobes. Pleural effusions may occur, as may empyema. Cavitation may also be seen (see Fig. 13.9). Tree-in-bud or centrilobular nodules may be seen on HRCT (see Fig. 11.28C in Chapter 11). The pattern of *P. aeruginosa* infection is insufficiently specific to distinguish it from other causes of bronchopneumonia.

Yersinia pestis

Yersinia pestis is the Gram-negative rod that causes plague. Historically, it has caused great epidemics, one of the largest of which occurred throughout Europe from 1347 to 1367, killing over one quarter of the population. While public health measures have largely controlled this disease, *Y. pestis* is still endemic in several areas of the world, including South America, China, parts of Eastern and Southern Africa, and the Western United States. An outbreak of pneumonic plague occurred as recently as 2014 in Eastern Colorado, related to an infected dog, affecting four people, and sporadic cases have been reported in the United States since then but usually number in the single digits annually. The disease usually occurs in the late spring through early fall. It affects men more commonly than women.

Yersinia pestis is a zoonosis, usually infecting wild rodents (squirrels are the most important disease reservoir in the United States), although dogs, cats, prairie dogs, and rabbits may become infected and serve as reservoirs as well. In urban areas, rats are an important disease reservoir. The disease is transferred from animal to animal or animal to person by the bite of a tick or flea. Rare cases of plague occur following the inhalation of the organism from other infected patients.

Following a bite from an infected flea or tick, a local skin reaction occurs, after which regional lymphadenopathy develops. Infected lymph nodes are usually very enlarged and tender, and the skin overlying these lymph nodes is often discolored, giving rise to the "buboes" of **bubonic plague**. Without treatment, dissemination may then occur,

Table 13.5 *Klebsiella pneumoniae*

Risk factors: old age, chronic alcoholism, chronic illness, and chronic obstructive pulmonary disease (COPD)
Occurs with aspiration
Green sputum
Lobar pneumonia, sometimes bulging fissure sign
Abscesses common
Bronchopneumonia may be seen

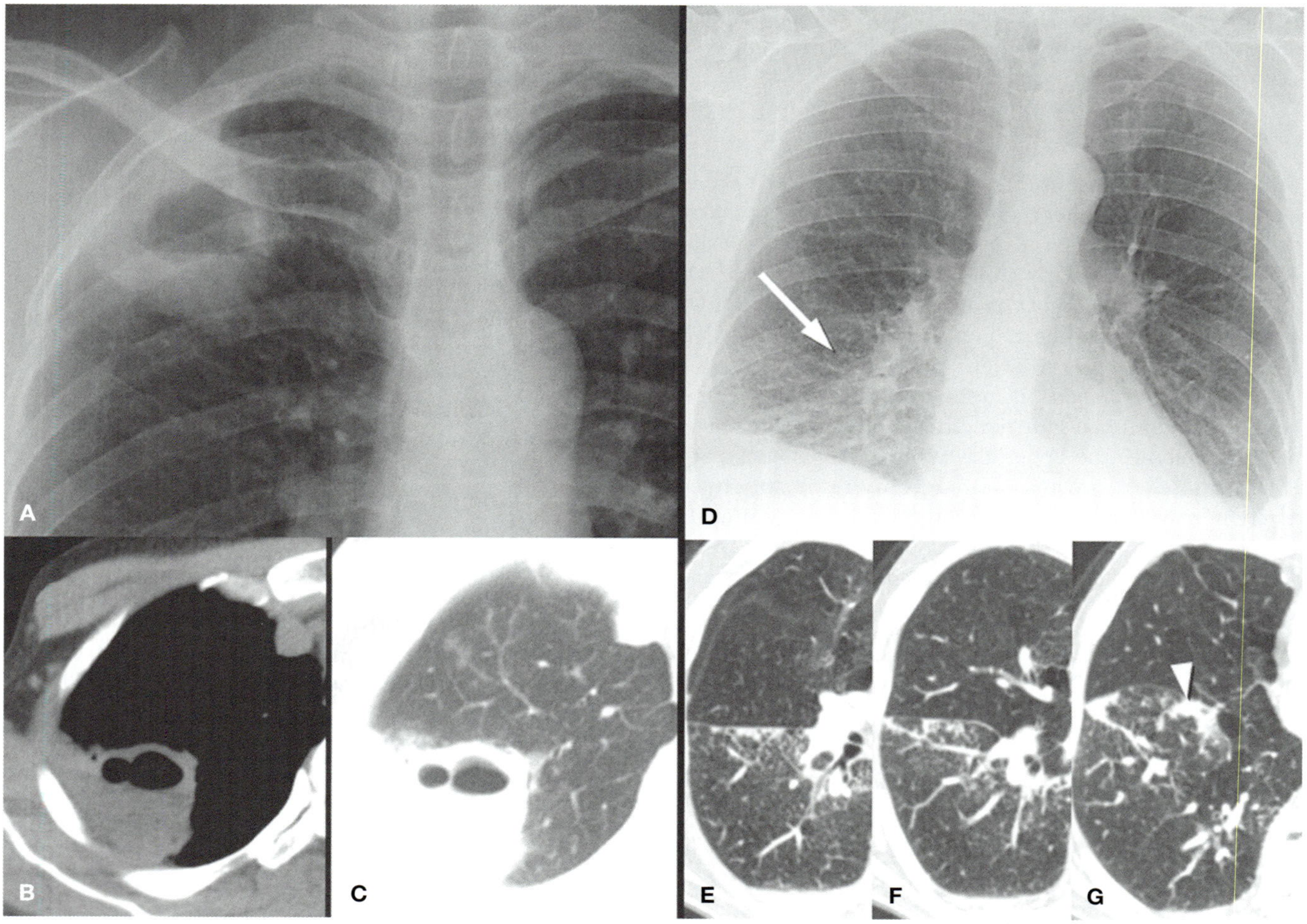

Figure 13.16. *Klebsiella pneumoniae* pulmonary infection: lung abscess (**A-C**) and bronchopneumonia (**D-G**) patterns. **A:** Frontal chest radiograph shows a subpleural right apical cavity with an air-fluid level, consistent with a pulmonary abscess. **B and C:** Axial thoracic shows a nonspecific cavity containing and air-fluid level consistent with a pulmonary abscess. **D:** Frontal chest radiograph shows patchy right lower lobe bronchovascular thickening (*arrow*). **E-G:** Axial CT shows small nodules and patchy areas of consolidation (*arrowhead*), consistent with a bronchopneumonia pattern.

potentially affecting the lungs and producing pneumonic plague. Person-to-person disease transmission may occur during this phase. **Septicemic plaque**, without formation of a bubo, may occur, and **pneumonic plague**, while typically occurring following bubonic or septicemic plague, may develop after exposure to infected humans or animals, or even bioterrorism.

Table 13.6 *Pseudomonas aeruginosa*
Nosocomial pneumonia, particularly in intensive care patients
Risk factors: chronic obstructive pulmonary disease, immunosuppression, mechanical ventilation, and antibiotic use
Bronchopneumonia pattern, lower lobe involvement
Cavitation

Yersinia pestis has several virulence factors that promote infection. The organism has a capsule that resists phagocytosis, and several surface antigens allow the organism to resist destruction and multiply within monocytes even if phagocytosed.

Pathologically, *Y. pestis* produces a severe bronchitis and bronchiolitis that rapidly evolve into severe bronchopneumonia. The airspaces may become filled with hemorrhage, edema, organisms, macrophages, and neutrophils, and alveolar necrosis is common.

Patients with pneumonic plague present with high fever, cough productive of bloody fluid, pleuritic chest pain, dyspnea, and cyanosis. Tender peripheral lymphadenopathy is often present. Prior to antibiotics, plague was uniformly fatal within 1 week of presentation. If antibiotic therapy is instituted in a timely fashion, recovery is the rule.

Pneumonic plague presents as severe, bilateral bronchopneumonia without cavitation, simulating ARDS. Pleural effusions may be present. Occasionally, regional lymph node enlargement is present, and this may be a clue to the diagnosis in endemic areas. Rarely, lymphadenopathy occurs without visible lung parenchymal abnormalities.

Serratia and Enterobacter Species

Both *Serratia* (*Serratia marcescens*) and *Enterobacter* spp. can cause pneumonia in debilitated, chronically ill patients, particularly those in the hospital. Bronchopneumonia patterns are typical. Pleural effusions are common with both organisms.

Gram-Negative Coccobacilli

Haemophilus influenzae

Haemophilus influenzae is by far the most important human pathogen within the *Haemophilus* genus. This infection is particularly common in COPD patients (Table 13.7) and in children between the ages of 2 months and 3 years. Other risk factors include chronic illnesses such as diabetes, alcoholism, anatomic or functional asplenia, and immunodeficiency. *H. influenzae* also commonly afflicts young children and the elderly.

Haemophilus influenzae typically causes bronchitis in adults. In patients with viral respiratory infections, *H. influenzae* may cause a bronchopneumonia pattern; the air-space pneumonia pattern is less commonly observed. *H. influenzae* is a major cause of epiglottitis in both children and adults.

The clinical presentation of *H. influenzae* pneumonia consists of fever, cough productive of purulent sputum, and shortness of breath, usually superimposed on a background of chronic illness.

Imaging Findings Chest radiography usually shows multifocal, bilateral patchy consolidation that favors the lower lobes. An air-space pneumonia pattern is occasionally encountered. Centrilobular nodules or tree-in-bud nodules may be seen on HRCT (see Fig. 11.28D in Chapter 11). Pleural effusions occur in about half of affected patients. Cavitation is uncommon.

Legionella pneumophila

Identified as the etiologic agent causing the pneumonia affecting the attendees of the National Convention of the American Legion in Philadelphia in 1976, *L. pneumophila* is recognized as the pathogen that causes a vast majority of cases of legionellosis. *Legionella* pneumonia is a fairly common cause of lower respiratory tract infection and is a frequent cause of nosocomial infection (Table 13.8). The organism is not part of the normal human flora; rather, *Legionella* resides in natural water sources. The organism is indigenous to freshwater lakes and streams, and human infection may occur when *Legionella* contaminates water systems, such as air conditioners and condensers. The organism may also contaminate showerheads and the like. Despite the frequency of *Legionella* nosocomial infection and the propensity of the organism to reside within sources of moisture, *Legionella* pneumonia is an uncommon cause of pulmonary infection in ventilator patients.

Legionella pneumonia usually affects older men, usually those with underlying chronic illnesses. Risk factors for infection include COPD, corticosteroid use, immunosuppression (including both AIDS and following organ transplantation), and malignancy.

Pathologically, *Legionella* causes a bronchopneumonia pattern of infection more commonly than an air-space pattern.

Legionella pneumonia may present with a wide range of severity, ranging from nearly asymptomatic to fulminant respiratory failure. On the mild end of the spectrum is the flulike illness known as Pontiac fever, and on the severe end is respiratory failure with diffuse alveolar damage. The typical presentation is a middle-aged to elderly man with underlying chronic illness such as COPD, presenting with nonproductive cough, fever, headache, myalgia, mental status changes, and gastrointestinal symptoms, particularly diarrhea. As the disease progresses, shortness of breath and chest pain may occur, and the cough may become productive.

Central nervous system symptoms, gastrointestinal symptoms, and renal insufficiency are more commonly encountered in patients with *Legionella* pneumonia than other bacterial pneumonias. Electrolyte disturbances, such as hyponatremia, are also common.

Legionnaire's disease is a severe form of pneumonia primarily caused by *Legionella* pneumophila. Individuals typically contract the disease by inhaling aerosolized water droplets containing the bacteria, often originating from contaminated sources such as air conditioning systems, cooling towers, and hot tubs.

Imaging Findings *Legionella* pneumonia often causes peripheral focal consolidation that rapidly progresses to

Table 13.7 *Haemophilus influenzae*

Risk factors: chronic obstructive pulmonary disease, chronic illness, alcoholism, and immunodeficiency
Bronchitis and bronchopneumonia pattern
Lobar pneumonia less common

Table 13.8 *Legionella pneumophila*

Resides in natural water sources, contamination of water systems
Risk factors: old age, chronic obstructive pulmonary disease, steroid use, chronic illness, and immunodeficiency
Bronchopneumonia or lobar pneumonia
Cavitation in immunosuppressed patients
Pleural effusion in 30%-60%

involve an entire lobe or perhaps several lobes on the side of initial presentation (see Fig. 1.16 in Chapter 1). Soon after, the consolidation becomes bilateral in majority of patients, and this progression tends to occur even with proper antibiotic therapy. Cavitation is uncommon in immunocompetent patients but occurs frequently in immunocompromised patients. Pleural effusion is encountered in 30% to 60% of patients. Radiographic clearing of *Legionella* pneumonia is slow compared to other bacterial pneumonias.

Bordetella Species

Bordetella pertussis is by far the most important organism in the *Bordetella* genus to cause human disease. *B. pertussis* is the pathogen that causes the majority of cases of whooping cough. *B. pertussis* infection results in extensive mucous production, bronchitis, and bronchiolitis in infected patients. Infection can range from mild to quite serious, and bronchiectasis can result from severe infections.

Whooping cough classically presents in patients under the age of 2. The characteristic component of the infection is paroxysmal coughing that ends with a "whoop." Posttussive emesis may also occur. Adult infection is more common than previously recognized. Infection in adults may not follow the same pattern as in children, although the infection can be severe in some individuals.

Imaging Findings The radiographic manifestations of *B. pertussis* infection include multifocal atelectasis and consolidation, occasionally accompanied by hilar lymphadenopathy. Radiographic abnormalities are most commonly found in the lower lobes, and central opacities obscuring the cardiac borders are common.

Bartonella henselae and Quintana

Bartonella henselae and *quintana* are the causative agents of cat scratch disease and bacillary angiomatosis in patients with AIDS.

Bartonella henselae and *quintana* pulmonary infections occur almost exclusively in patients with AIDS. Cat scratch disease is an infection that primarily affects children and causes local lymphadenopathy. The mode of transmission of thoracic bacillary angiomatosis is unknown, but because cat scratch disease is transmitted by animal–human contact, a similar mechanism may apply for thoracic bacillary angiomatosis.

Bartonella henselae and *quintana* infections produce extensive vascular proliferation, commonly involving the skin, mucous membranes, and internal organs, including the lungs.

Patients infected with *B. henselae* and *quintana* may present with fever, chest pain, weight loss, and night sweats. Hemoptysis has also been reported. Palpable lymphadenopathy may be evident on physical examination. The infection usually responds rapidly to antibiotic therapy.

Imaging Findings Bacillary angiomatosis most commonly causes lung nodules. If large enough, the nodules may show intense enhancement. Large pleural effusions are often evident, and mediastinal lymphadenopathy is common. Enlarged lymph nodes often show extensive enhancement.

Francisella Tularensis

Francisella tularensis is the cause of tularemia. This disease is a zoonosis and usually occurs in small animals, but accidental human infection may occur when individuals come in contact with infected animals or insect vectors.

Infection is usually acquired by contact with infected animals, often through an open cut or skin abrasion while handling animal hides. Infection may also occur by ingesting contaminated meat or being bitten by infected insect vectors, such as ticks or deer flies. Infection is most frequently encountered in rural areas.

Several patterns of *F. tularensis* infection have been described. The most common patterns of pulmonary infection are the **typhoidal** and **ulceroglandular** forms of the disease. The typhoidal form of tularemia results from the ingestion of meat or water contaminated with organisms, whereas the ulceroglandular form of the disease results from direct patient skin inoculation through the handling of contaminated skins or hides. A rare pulmonary form of tularemia acquired by inhalation has been reported in laboratory employees working with *F. tularensis* and would be the pattern expected if the organism were used as a bioweapon.

The ulceroglandular form of tularemia causes ulcerated skin lesions and regional lymphadenopathy. The typhoidal form of the disease causes bacteremia. Clinical pneumonia develops in one third and three quarters of patients with the ulceroglandular and typhoidal forms of the disease, respectively. Patients present with high fever, weakness, and headaches, often with variable pharyngeal symptoms ranging from mild inflammation to ulcerative tonsillitis.

A nonspecific air-space pattern of pneumonia is most often encountered in patients with tularemia. Pleural effusion and hilar or mediastinal lymphadenopathy are also seen in nearly 50% of affected patients.

Anaerobic Bacteria

The major anaerobic bacteria implicated in human disease include organisms of the genus *Bacteroides*, *Fusobacterium*, *Porphyromonas*, and *Prevotella* (all Gram-negative bacilli); *Clostridium*, *Actinomyces*, and *Eubacterium* (Gram-positive bacilli); *Peptostreptococcus* and *Peptococcus* (Gram-positive cocci); and *Veillonella* (Gram-negative coccus).

These organisms are normally found in the oral cavity, and they may result in disease when aspirated (Table 13.9). Therefore, conditions that favor the occurrence of aspiration, such as impaired consciousness, seizure, stroke, drug ingestion, and alcoholism, or conditions that impair the ability to clear aspirated secretions, such as obstructing endobronchial lesions or bronchostenoses, favor the development of anaerobic pulmonary infections. Additionally, factors that favor

Table 13.9 Anaerobic Bacteria

Organisms are normally found in the oral cavity
Risk factors: poor dental hygiene or gingivitis
Pneumonia occurs with aspiration
Few symptoms: foul-smelling sputum, fever, nonproductive cough
Involves gravitationally dependent regions
- Superior segments of lower lobes and posterior segments of upper lobes
- Right lower lobe more common than left lower lobe

Bronchopneumonia or lung abscess most common
Empyema may be associated

overgrowth of these organisms in the oral cavity, particularly poor dental hygiene or gingivitis, also predispose to the development of pulmonary anaerobic infections. Tonsillitis or chronic sinus infections are also associated with pulmonary anaerobic infections.

Pulmonary or pleural anaerobic infection begins with the aspiration of infectious material from the oral cavity. Anaerobic bacterial infection produces several syndromes, including **aspiration pneumonia** (which may be preceded by **chemical pneumonitis**), **anaerobic pleuropneumonia**, and **primary anaerobic empyema**. Typically, anaerobic pneumonia begins as a bronchopneumonia pattern, potentially complicated by tissue necrosis if anaerobic pleuropneumonia develops; the latter produces radiographic evidence of cavitation.

Patients may initially present with fever and nonproductive cough and then develop foul-smelling sputum production once abscess formation occurs. Chest pain and hemoptysis may also occur. Quite often, anaerobic infection presents with few symptoms, making the infection difficult to diagnose.

Imaging Findings

Because anaerobic pulmonary infection is strongly related to aspiration, anaerobic bronchopneumonia most commonly involves the gravitationally dependent regions of the lung: the superior segments of the lower lobes and the posterior segments of the upper lobes in the recumbent patient and the basal segments of the lower lobes in upright patients (Fig. 13.17). As a result of the relatively vertical orientation of the right main stem bronchus, the right lung is more commonly involved by aspiration events than the left lung.

Bronchopneumonia in a basilar and dependent distribution is most common in patients with aspiration-induced anaerobic infection. Pleural effusion commonly accompanies the lung parenchymal abnormalities. Parenchymal cavitation is common and may evolve into a discrete lung abscess (Fig. 13.18). Necrotizing pneumonia, manifesting as areas of consolidation with multiple areas of cavitation, is common. Lymphadenopathy may be present, and when focal, the radiographic appearance occasionally resembles pulmonary carcinoma. With treatment, cavities may close, but residual scarring and bronchiectasis may occur. Occasionally, pleural effusion or empyema, without significant lung parenchymal abnormality, is the primary manifestation of anaerobic infection.

Mycobacteria

Mycobacteria are aerobic, non-spore-forming rods with unusually long doubling times. Numerous species of mycobacteria exist in nature, but the mycobacteria that cause human disease may be divided into two broad groups: the

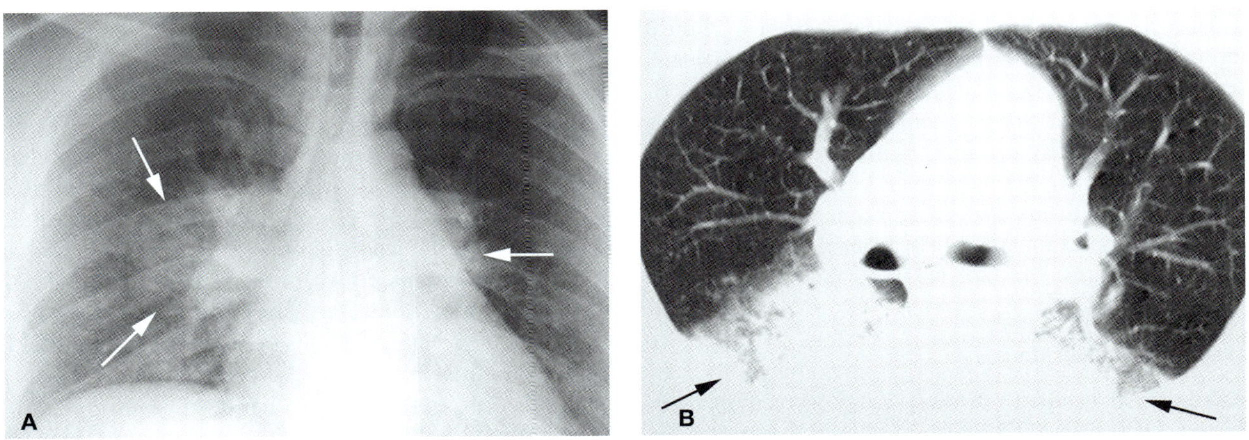

Figure 13.17. Aspiration pneumonia. **A:** Frontal chest radiograph shows bilateral, poorly defined opacities in the superior segments of both lower lobes (*arrows*). **B:** Axial CT image shows an air-space opacity within the superior segments of the lower lobes (*arrows*), associated with volume loss. The right lung is more abnormal than the left. The relatively vertical orientation of the right main stem bronchus predisposes the right lower lobe to aspiration pneumonia.

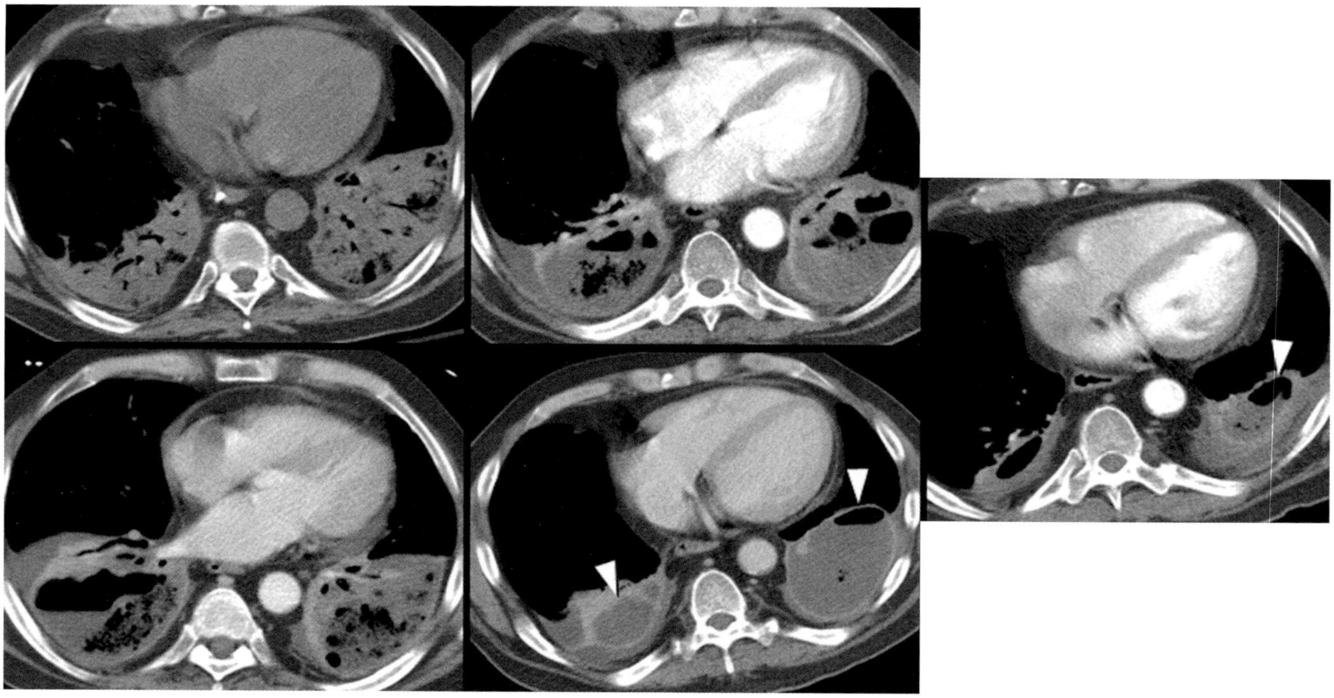

Figure 13.18. Anaerobic pneumonia beginning as aspiration pneumonia, evolving into pleuropneumonia anaerobic pneumonia, and eventually developing into lung abscesses (*arrowheads*) over a period of several weeks.

tuberculosis complex and the **nontuberculous**, or **atypical**, mycobacteria.

Another classification scheme for mycobacteria groups the organisms according to their rate of growth on solid medium: rapid growers usually show visible colonies within 7 days and slow growers require longer than 7 days to form visible colonies. Organisms classified as rapid growers that cause human pulmonary disease include *M. abscessus*, *M. fortuitum*, and *M. chelonae*. Organisms in the slow-growing group that cause pulmonary infection in humans include MTB, *Mycobacterium avium* complex (MAC), and *M. kansasii*. This classification scheme is useful from a clinical standpoint because rapid-growing mycobacteria are usually resistant to first-line antituberculosis drugs. Grouping mycobacteria into the tuberculosis complex and nontuberculous mycobacteria (NTMB) is more useful from an imaging standpoint.

The major organisms that cause human disease in the tuberculosis complex include MTB, *M. bovis*, *M. africanum*, and *M. microti*.

Mycobacterium tuberculosis

Tuberculosis has been an infection of importance throughout history. Although MTB infection rates had been steadily declining in the United States since the middle of the 19th century, worldwide MTB infection rates remain quite high. The World Health Organization estimates that nearly 25% of the global population have been infected with MTB, with 10.6 million new symptomatic cases in 2022.

Numerous factors influence the likelihood of contracting tuberculosis. These include socioeconomic status, immune system integrity, age, general state of health, gender, and ethnicity. Patients with low socioeconomic status are at relatively higher risk for acquiring tuberculosis infection. Such patients often include those living in crowded housing conditions, individuals living in inner city areas, homeless individuals, and drug abusers. Immunosuppressed patients, especially AIDS patients, are clearly at higher risk than the general population for the development of tuberculosis. Patients treated with corticosteroids or those who have undergone organ transplantation are also at increased risk for the development of MTB infection. Chronic illnesses, including diabetes mellitus, silicosis, and alveolar proteinosis, also place patients at increased risk for the development of tuberculosis. Very young and elderly patients are also at relatively increased risk for MTB infection, and men are more commonly affected than women. Finally, African American and Native American patients are at relatively higher risk for tuberculosis compared with other ethnic groups. In North America, immigrants from areas of the world who have a high prevalence of tuberculosis are at high risk for the development of infection.

MTB infection occurs with the inhalation of airborne respiratory droplets containing the organisms. Many factors influence the likelihood of contagion, including the presence of cavitation on imaging examinations, the burden of organisms, and the severity of cough. Person-to-person transmission is also more likely if exposure occurs in a poorly ventilated area or if contact with the infectious person is prolonged, such as occurs in relatively confined situations such as prisons, schools, and nursing homes.

Several different patterns of tuberculous infection have been described, differing in pathologic, clinical, and radiologic manifestations. These include primary MTB, progressive primary MTB, and postprimary MTB. This classification scheme for MTB infection has been challenged in the era of molecular epidemiology as DNA fingerprinting techniques have shown that the radiographic pattern of MTB infection does not correlate well with the time since infection. It is now recognized that the patient's immune status (and to some extent, patient age), but *not* the time since infection, is the primary determinant of the radiographic appearance of MTB infection. Nevertheless, the time-honored classification of MTB infection into *primary* or *postprimary* (*reactivation*) patterns remains a useful organizational approach to imaging of the MTB-infected patient and will be employed here, but the reader should recognize the limitations of this approach.

Primary Tuberculosis Primary tuberculosis is said to occur when clinical infection occurs following the first exposure to the organism, typically within the first year following exposure. Ultimately, the ability of MTB to cause human infection is related to the organism's ability to survive dormant within host macrophages for long periods of time and to incite a T-cell-mediated, delayed hypersensitivity response by the infected host. The host organism, under normal circumstances, will sequester the MTB organism by forming granulomas. Usually, these granulomas show **caseous necrosis**, a pattern characteristically, but not exclusively, associated with tuberculous infection. This initial infection has been termed the **Ghon focus** and usually heals by the development of a fibrous capsule around the focus of infection, which often calcifies. Shortly after the infection occurs, organisms may spread through the lymphatics to hilar and mediastinal lymph nodes, where a similar histopathologic reaction may occur. The combination of the lung parenchymal and lymph node MTB infection has been termed the **Ranke complex**. Organisms within the Ghon focus often gain access to the bloodstream and may disseminate to extrathoracic organs, but usually, host defenses are sufficient to prevent overt infection from developing in extrathoracic sites. Although the pulmonary, lymphatic, and extrathoracic foci of infection are usually inactive at this point, organisms remain viable and may serve as the nidus for reactivation of disease when the circumstances are favorable.

Primary MTB infection in children is usually asymptomatic and may be detected only with the conversion of skin tests. When symptoms occur, cough and fever are most common. By contrast, adults with primary MTB infection are usually symptomatic and may present with weight loss, failure to thrive, fever, cough, and hemoptysis. Night sweats may also occur.

Imaging Findings Patients with primary MTB most often show no radiologic abnormalities. If overt infection occurs, the pattern is usually one of air-space consolidation (Fig. 13.19), often involving an entire lobe. The right lung is more commonly affected than the left, although no definite zonal predominance is seen. Cavitation in primary MTB is unusual, and miliary dissemination is similarly uncommon.

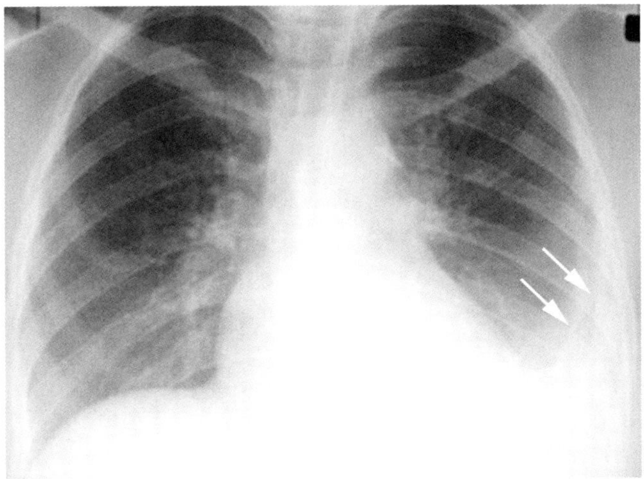

Figure 13.19. Primary *Mycobacterium tuberculosis* infection. Frontal chest radiograph shows left lower lobe consolidation associated with a small left effusion (*arrows*). MTB was recovered in the sputum, and the radiographic abnormalities resolved with antituberculous therapy.

Atelectasis is often encountered in children with primary MTB and may be related to airway compression by enlarged lymph nodes. Less commonly, rupture of an infected lymph node into an adjacent bronchus may cause endobronchial dissemination of infection associated with atelectasis. Adults with primary MTB uncommonly present with pulmonary atelectasis.

Radiographic abnormalities in primary MTB infections are often slow to resolve, even with prompt treatment. Air-space opacities may take more than 6 months to clear, and lymphadenopathy may take even longer to resolve. The pulmonary lesion in primary MTB often heals with calcification, leaving a residual nodule; infected lymph nodes may heal in a similar fashion.

Lymphadenopathy commonly occurs in children with primary MTB infection. Usually hilar lymph nodes are involved (Fig. 13.20), and mediastinal lymph nodes, particularly in the right paratracheal region, may be enlarged as well. Unilateral lymphadenopathy is more often seen than bilateral disease, and occasionally, lymph node enlargement is the only radiographic finding present. Lymphadenopathy is uncommon in adults with primary MTB unless they are immunocompromised (see below; see Fig. 13.11). Lymph nodes actively infected with MTB quite commonly show central low attenuation, representing necrosis, on contrast-enhanced CT (Fig. 13.21).

Pleural effusion may occur in patients with primary MTB infection (see Fig. 13.19). Often when tuberculosis is discovered as the cause of pleural effusion, no parenchymal focus of disease is radiographically evident; this pattern is considered characteristic of primary MTB pleural infection. Usually, such effusions are small and unilateral (Table 13.10).

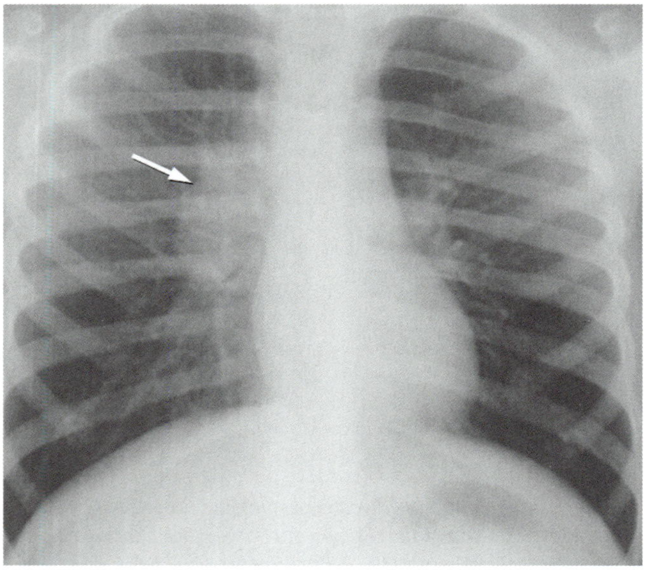

Figure 13.20. Lymphadenopathy associated with primary *Mycobacterium tuberculosis* infection. Frontal chest radiograph in a young patient shows enlargement of right hilar lymph nodes (*arrow*).

Table 13.10 Primary *Mycobacterium tuberculosis*
Clinical infection following first exposure
Ghon focus: local infection
Ranke complex: local infection with lymph node spread
Often asymptomatic in children
Adults: weight loss, fever, cough, and hemoptysis
Radiographs may be normal
Air-space consolidation, may be lobar; often slow to clear
Atelectasis in children
Cavitation and miliary spread uncommon
Lymphadenopathy common in children, uncommon in adults (unless immunocompromised)
Pleural effusion may be seen without lung disease

Progressive Primary Tuberculosis Rarely, a parenchymal focus of primary MTB infection becomes rapidly progressive. Extensive consolidation and cavitation develop, either at the site of the initial pulmonary parenchymal focus of infection or in the apical and posterior segments of the upper lobes. Thus, progressive primary MTB infection may closely resemble postprimary MTB infection.

Postprimary (Reactivation) Tuberculosis. Usually, postprimary MTB occurs as a result of previously latent infection (Table 13.11). During the initial infection, organisms may be transported by the bloodstream to the apical and posterior segments of the upper lobes and to the superior segments of the lower lobes. Later, reactivation of infection in these regions may be favored by the relatively high oxygen tension and relatively decreased lymphatic drainage in these lung segments and tends to occur when host defenses become impaired. The latent organisms then become active, inflammation with necrosis occurs, and overt infection develops. Unlike the healing that commonly occurs with primary MTB infection, postprimary MTB infection is often associated with progressive disease. As the inflammation mounts, tissue destruction occurs, and caseous material liquefies and may acquire communication with the tracheobronchial tree, producing the characteristic pathologic and radiologic finding of postprimary MTB: cavitation. The presence of cavitation tends to promote worsening infection by allowing more oxygen to reach the inflammatory focus and also creates the opportunity for endobronchial spread of infection and communication of infection to others.

If host defenses triumph, cavities in postprimary MTB usually heal by scar formation. Bronchiectasis, volume loss, and areas of emphysema are common sequelae. Chronic cavities, often very thin walled, may persist.

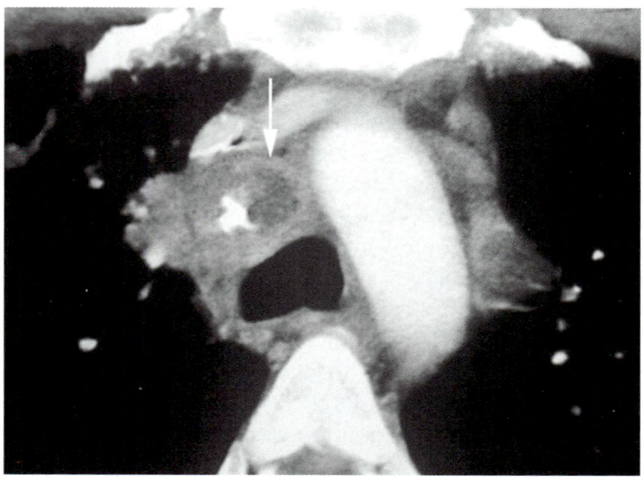

Figure 13.21. Necrotic lymphadenopathy due to *Mycobacterium tuberculosis* infection. Axial contrast-enhanced CT in a patient with AIDS shows low attenuation and calcification within right paratracheal lymph nodes (*arrow*).

Table 13.11 Postprimary *Mycobacterium tuberculosis*
Reactivation of latent infection
Most often involves apical and posterior segments of upper lobes and superior segments of lower lobes
Often associated with progressive disease
Cavitation common; endobronchial spread may occur.
Fatigue, night sweats, weight loss, low-grade fever, hemoptysis
Radiographic findings:
Poorly defined areas of consolidation
Cavitation visible in 20%-45%
Tree-in-bud or centrilobular nodules on HRCT
Lymphadenopathy and effusions uncommon
Miliary spread
Airway stenosis
Tuberculoma

Typical clinical manifestations of postprimary MTB include failure to thrive, fatigue, night sweats, weight loss, and low-grade fever. Hemoptysis may occur and is commonly due to bronchiectasis, although the presence of this symptom has been associated with active disease. The presence of chest pain may indicate spontaneous pneumothorax, and shortness of breath may herald the presence of extensive tuberculous bronchopneumonia or developing ARDS.

Imaging Findings The most typical finding of postprimary MTB is that of poorly defined areas of consolidation favoring the apical and posterior segments of the upper lobes (Fig. 13.22) and, to a lesser extent, the superior segments of the lower lobes. Opacities may also be found in other segments. Often, small, poorly defined opacities, or satellite nodules, are seen on the periphery of the dominant foci of consolidation (see Fig. 10.11 in Chapter 10). On HRCT, such nodules characteristically show centrilobular branching linear patterns or so-called tree-in-bud opacities (Fig. 13.23). These opacities represent impaction of small airways with pus. Areas of cavitation are seen in 20% to 45% of patients with active postprimary MTB on chest radiographs, but small cavities are more easily appreciated with CT and HRCT. Cavities may be thick or thin walled; air-fluid levels are relatively uncommon.

Lymphadenopathy is uncommon in postprimary MTB, as are pleural effusions. When effusions occur, they are often discovered in elderly patients, and a parenchymal focus of infection is frequently evident.

Occasionally, poorly defined nodules ranging in size from 2 to 10 mm are seen in a patchy distribution, spatially separated from areas of cavitation. These nodules often represent endobronchial spread of MTB infection (Fig. 13.24). Endobronchial spread of infection usually occurs as a result of spillage of caseous material from cavities, although rarely it occurs following the rupture of an infected lymph node into a bronchus; the latter mechanism may allow an endobronchial spread pattern of infection to occur in primary MTB infection.

MTB infection may result in a miliary pattern. This pattern manifests as numerous, well-defined nodules that measure 1 to 2 mm in size, diffusely distributed throughout the lungs (Fig. 13.25). On HRCT, these small nodules show a random distribution (Fig. 13.26). The miliary pattern represents hematogenous dissemination of infection from a pulmonary nidus and may be seen in both primary and postprimary diseases. Radiographs occasionally appear normal in patients with miliary tuberculosis.

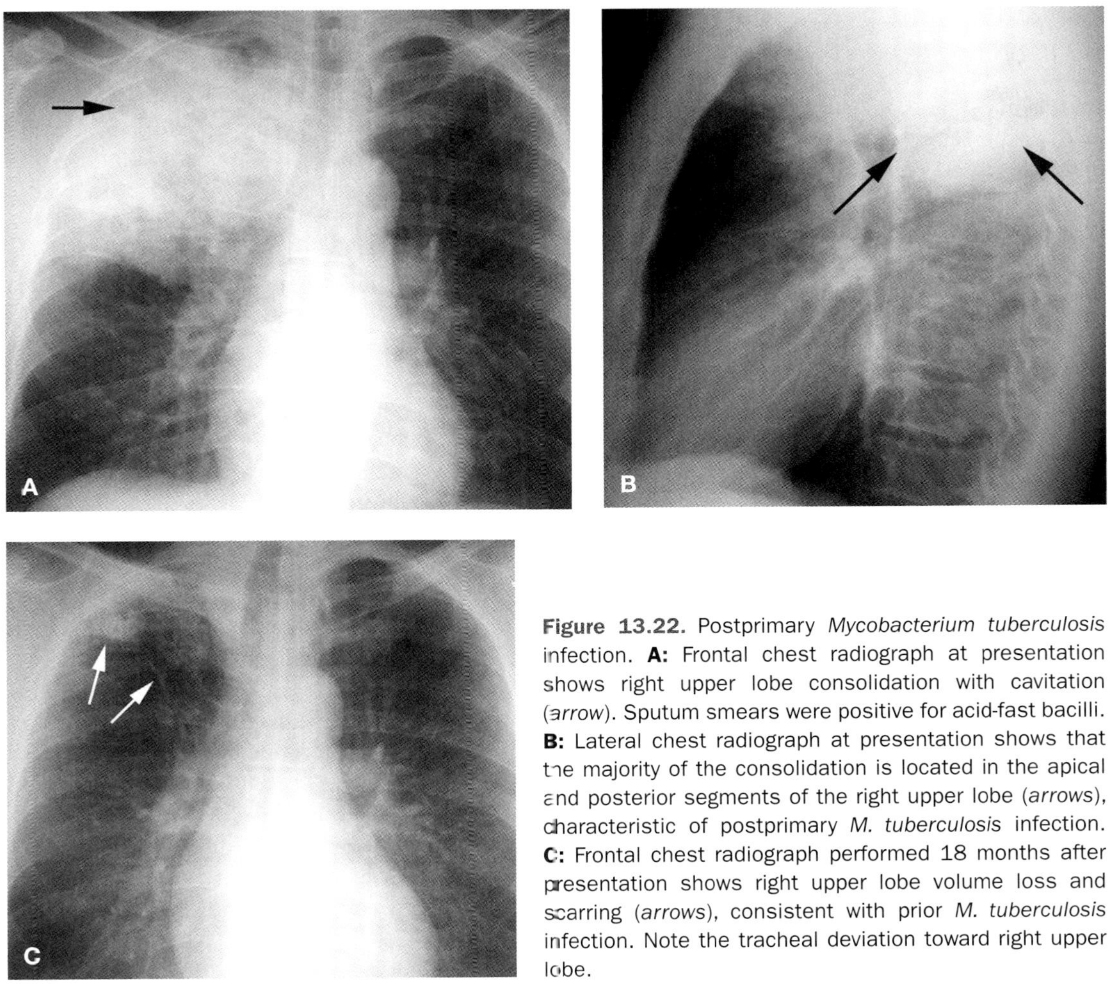

Figure 13.22. Postprimary *Mycobacterium tuberculosis* infection. **A:** Frontal chest radiograph at presentation shows right upper lobe consolidation with cavitation (*arrow*). Sputum smears were positive for acid-fast bacilli. **B:** Lateral chest radiograph at presentation shows that the majority of the consolidation is located in the apical and posterior segments of the right upper lobe (*arrows*), characteristic of postprimary *M. tuberculosis* infection. **C:** Frontal chest radiograph performed 18 months after presentation shows right upper lobe volume loss and scarring (*arrows*), consistent with prior *M. tuberculosis* infection. Note the tracheal deviation toward right upper lobe.

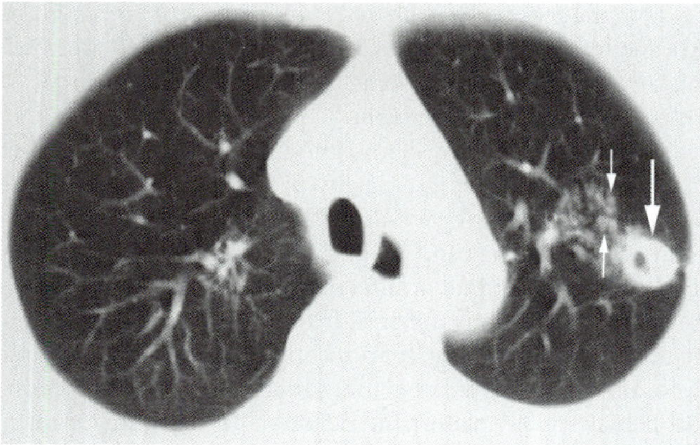

Figure 13.23. Postprimary *Mycobacterium tuberculosis* infection. Axial CT image shows a cavity in the apical-posterior segment of the left upper lobe (*large arrow*), with small surrounding centrilobular nodules (*small arrows*), representing endobronchial dissemination of the infected material.

MTB may affect the main or lobar bronchi, and the pattern is usually one of bronchial obstruction associated with airway wall thickening and inflammation. Airway strictures most commonly involve the left main stem bronchus. Tracheal disease is less common and is usually accompanied by bronchial disease; MTB preferentially affects the distal portion of the trachea. Airway lesions usually result from local extension of infection from affected lymph nodes or lung parenchyma. They are less commonly related to endobronchial or hematogenous dissemination of MTB. Active infection appears as irregular or smooth circumferential airway thickening and narrowing, often accompanied by lymphadenopathy and strand-like densities within the mediastinum. Chronic airway stenoses from MTB are due to fibrosis and are not generally accompanied by other signs of active infection. Chronic stenoses are associated with less wall thickening than with acute infection.

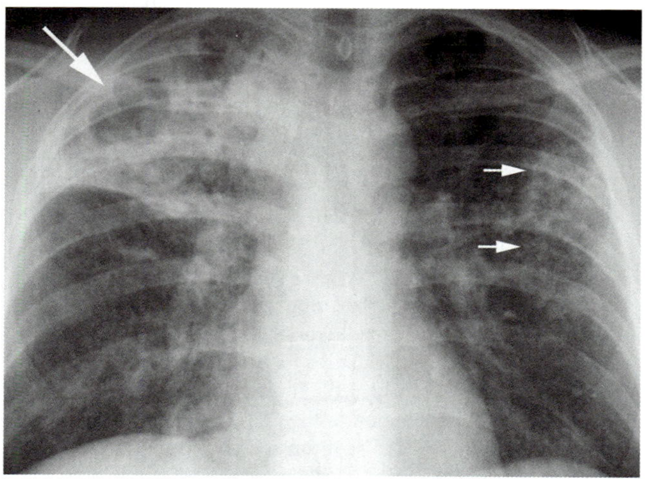

Figure 13.24. Endobronchial spread of *Mycobacterium tuberculosis* infection. Frontal chest radiograph shows right upper lobe cavitation (*large arrow*) associated with numerous small nodules in the left upper lobe (*small arrows*), representing airway spread of infectious material.

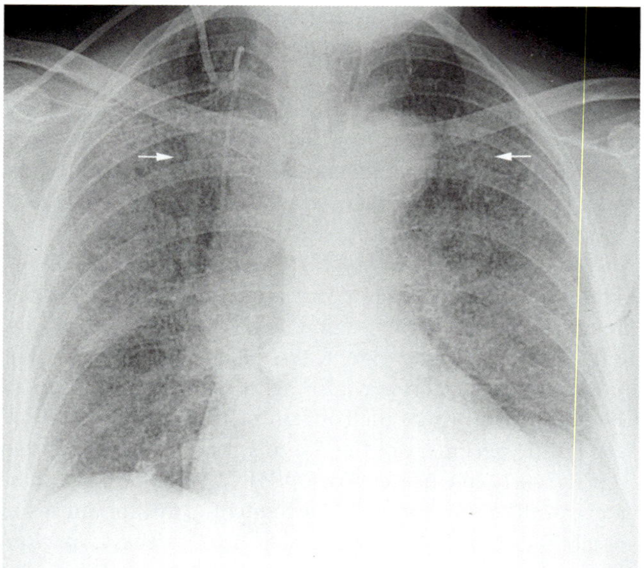

Figure 13.25. Miliary spread of *Mycobacterium tuberculosis* infection. Frontal chest radiograph shows innumerable, bilateral, diffusely distributed small nodules (*arrows*) representing miliary (hematogenous) spread of MTB infection.

Occasionally, MTB infection manifests as a solitary pulmonary nodule or tuberculoma. Tuberculomas may result from either primary or postprimary MTB infection. Tuberculomas appear as rounded nodules, often circumscribed (see Fig. 13.23), but occasionally with a spiculated margin and are usually located in the upper lobes. Small satellite nodules are often present as well. These lesions often do not show enhancement following CT performed with intravenous contrast administration, although peripheral enhancement may occur. Calcification may develop over time.

Active versus Inactive Tuberculosis Radiologists are often asked to determine whether a particular radiographic pattern suggests the presence of active tuberculous infection or more frequently whether active tuberculous infection can be confidently excluded by radiography. In general, one must have prior radiographs for comparison to determine disease activity, and the radiographic pattern should be stable for 6 months or more before suggesting that disease is not active. An exception to this rule is that one may confidently assume that calcified lung nodules represent inactive disease.

Radiographic patterns that usually suggest active disease include consolidation, endobronchial spread patterns (see Fig. 13.24), the miliary pattern (see Figs. 13.25 and 13.26), and cavities (see Fig. 13.24). On HRCT, centrilobular nodules, particularly when tree-in-bud opacities are present (see Fig. 13.23), usually suggest active disease. Such nodules often resolve with treatment. Findings more often associated with inactive disease include bronchiectasis, linear opacities, and calcified nodules.

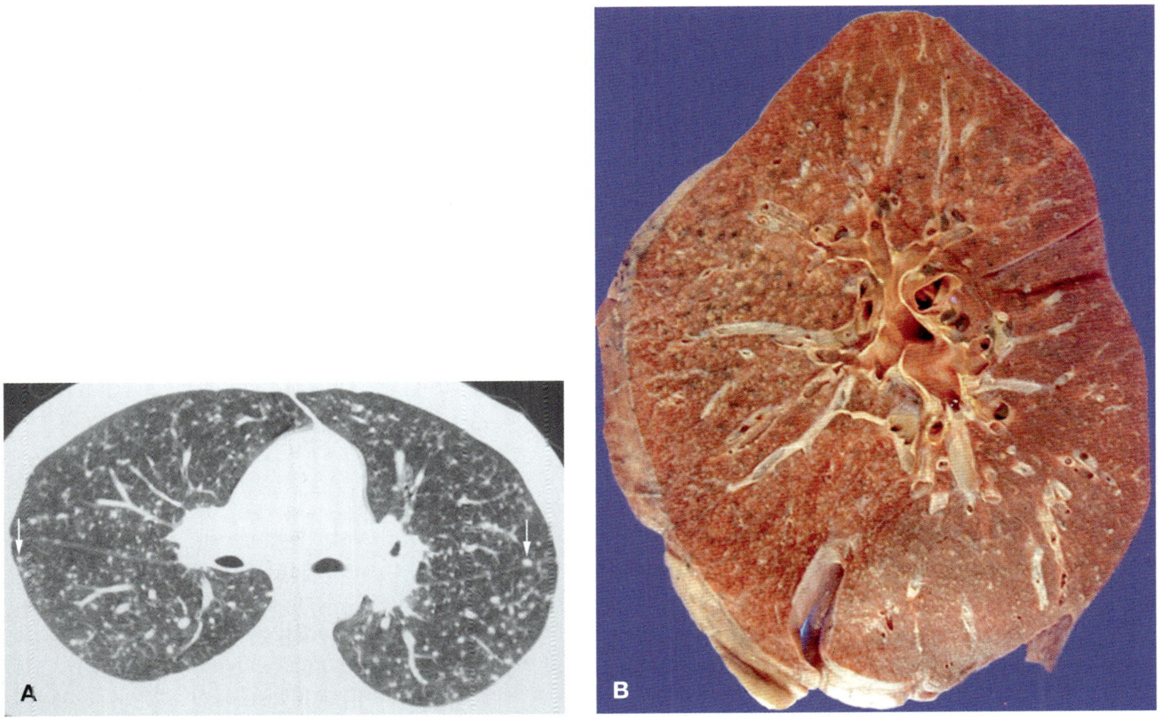

Figure 13.26. Miliary spread of *Mycobacterium tuberculosis* infection. **A:** Axial HRCT image shows numerous, bilateral, randomly distributed small nodules (*arrows*) representing miliary spread of MTB infection. **B:** Gross specimen shows numerous randomly disseminated nodules, correlating with the HRCT study. (Image courtesy of Martha L. Warnock, MD, Professor Emerita, Department of Pathology, University of California, San Francisco.)

AIDS and Tuberculosis AIDS is a major risk factor for the development of tuberculosis. This phenomenon is at least in part related to the fact that HIV adversely affects macrophage function and also destroys CD4 lymphocytes, both of which are part of the normal host defense mechanisms involved in combating MTB.

The radiographic manifestations of MTB in patients with AIDS depend on the CD4 count. Patients with relatively preserved immunity (CD4 counts above 200 cells/μL) usually present with the typical postprimary pattern of MTB infection seen in immunocompetent patients. These findings include upper lobe consolidation, cavitation, and nodules, usually without pleural effusion or lymphadenopathy. Patients who are comparatively immunosuppressed, usually with CD4 counts less than 200 cells/μL, present with a pattern of disease resembling primary MTB infection. Such findings include consolidation associated with lymphadenopathy. Often, lymphadenopathy is the dominant or only finding (see Fig. 13.11), and on CT, affected lymph nodes may show low central attenuation with peripheral enhancement following contrast administration (Fig. 13.27). HRCT commonly shows centrilobular nodules, often with tree-in-bud patterns. Pleural effusions may also occur. Normal radiographs are occasionally encountered in patients with AIDS and MTB, and extrapulmonary dissemination is also more frequent in this setting than in immunocompetent patients.

Mycobacterium bovis

The BCG (bacille Calmette-Guérin) vaccine, composed of an avirulent strain of *M. bovis*, is used to generate immunity against MTB in certain high-risk patients. BCG has also been used as an immune stimulant in the treatment of certain conditions, particularly carcinoma of the bladder. Although the organism used for this vaccine is not usually pathogenic in humans, in certain populations, particularly immunosuppressed patients, disseminated disease may develop, often manifesting as a miliary pattern on chest radiographs and HRCT.

Nontuberculous Mycobacteria

NTMB include at least 20 organisms that potentially cause human disease, although only a fraction of these organisms are important as a cause of thoracic infection. The NTMB have traditionally been subclassified according to Runyon criteria, based on their rate of growth and the presence or absence of pigment production: photochromogens (*M. kansasii*), scotochromogens (*M. szulgai* and *M. gordonae*), the nonphotochromogens (*M. avium* complex), and the rapid growers (*M. fortuitum* and *M. abscessus* among others), but this classification scheme has been supplanted by molecular methods. Furthermore, the use of molecular methods has resulted in the identification of numerous new NTMB

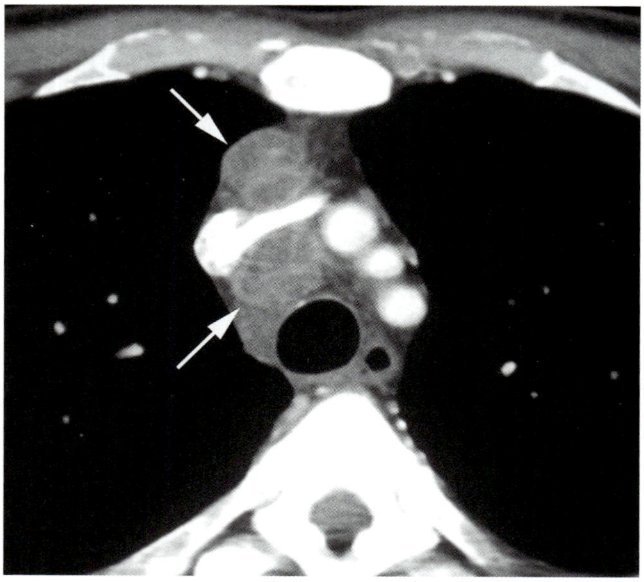

Figure 13.27. Low-attenuation lymph nodes due to *Mycobacterium tuberculosis* infection in AIDS. Axial CT image shows low-attenuation lymphadenopathy anterior and posterior to the left brachiocephalic vein and superior vena cava (*arrows*).

species—currently, more than 160 such species are identified, at least 50 of which are associated with pulmonary disease. Most NTMB are inhabitants of natural water sources, such as lakes, rivers, and ponds, and some species may be found in soil or on animals. Infection may occur by various routes, including inhalation, ingestion, direct inoculation, or iatrogenic infection.

Many patients who develop NTMB infections are chronically ill. Risk factors include COPD, bronchiectasis, silicosis, cystic fibrosis, and AIDS. Other conditions associated with NTMB infection include diabetes mellitus, alcoholism, malignancy, and achalasia.

The pathologic patterns of most NTMB infections are similar to that of MTB infection. Pathologic features of NTMB infection include tissue destruction, necrosis, cavitation, and occasionally, endobronchial spread of infection or miliary disease. Often, these disease patterns are superimposed on underlying chronic pulmonary abnormalities, complicating the pathologic appearance of NTMB infection.

For many patients, the symptoms of NTMB infection are indistinguishable from those of MTB pulmonary infection. One of the most common presenting symptoms is chronic cough.

Mycobacterium avium-intracellulare complex *M. avium-intracellulare* complex (MAC) is one of the most common human NTMB pathogens, and several patterns of infection in immunocompetent patients have been described (Table 13.12).

The first pattern resembles that of postprimary MTB, with upper lobe (often the apical and posterior segments) consolidation, cavities, scar formation, and small nodules suggesting endobronchial spread of infection—often referred to as the *apical fibrocavitary pattern* of NTMB pulmonary infection. Pleural effusions and lymphadenopathy are relatively infrequent. This pattern of MAC infection is most often encountered in older men with some degree of mild underlying immunocompromise, such as COPD.

Table 13.12 *Mycobacterium avium* Complex (MAC): Patterns of Disease

MAC resembling postprimary *Mycobacterium tuberculosis*
Most often in older men with mild immunocompromise or chronic obstructive pulmonary disease (apical fibrocavitary)
MAC infection associated with bronchiectasis and nodules (nodular bronchiectatic)
Usually females >60 y of age
Often involves right middle lobe and lingula
Patchy consolidation, bronchiectasis, nodules, and tree-in-bud
MAC with hypersensitivity pneumonitis
Patchy ground-glass opacity or small nodules
"Hot-tub lung"

The second pattern of MAC infection consists of bronchiectasis and centrilobular nodules and is often referred to as the *nodular/bronchiectatic pattern* of NTM pulmonary infection. The bronchiectasis and nodules may be found in all lobes, but they predominate in the right middle lobe and lingula (Fig. 13.28). Large nodules (more than 1 cm) are seen in some patients (see Fig. 13.28C). Patchy consolidations, representing foci of organizing pneumonia, are also seen. This pattern of infection most often affects older (more than 60 years of age) females.

A third pattern of MAC infection resembles hypersensitivity pneumonitis, with patchy ground-glass opacities and poorly defined ground-glass centrilobular nodules, and air trapping. MAC in this context is usually acquired via exposure to contaminated hot tubs, and the term "hot-tub lung" has been applied to this exposure (see Fig. 17.5 in Chapter 17).

Mycobacterium kansasii The radiographic pattern of *M. kansasii* infection closely resembles that of postprimary MTB (Fig. 13.29). Several studies examining the differences in the radiographic abnormalities between these two infections have found no consistent features that can distinguish the two infections, except that pleural effusions are very uncommon with *M. kansasii* infection.

Mycobacterium abscessus *M. abscessus* pulmonary infection may be more common than previously thought. *M. abscessus* tends to cause bronchiectasis and centrilobular nodules, often with tree-in-bud morphology, predominating in the right middle lobe and lingula.

Nontuberculous Mycobacteria in AIDS NTMB infection, especially MAC, is very common in patients with AIDS, and the incidence of infection rises as the CD4 cell count falls. Most patients with clinically overt MAC infection have CD4 cell counts below 50 cells/μL. Although MAC is often found in the sputum of patients with advanced AIDS, true pulmonary

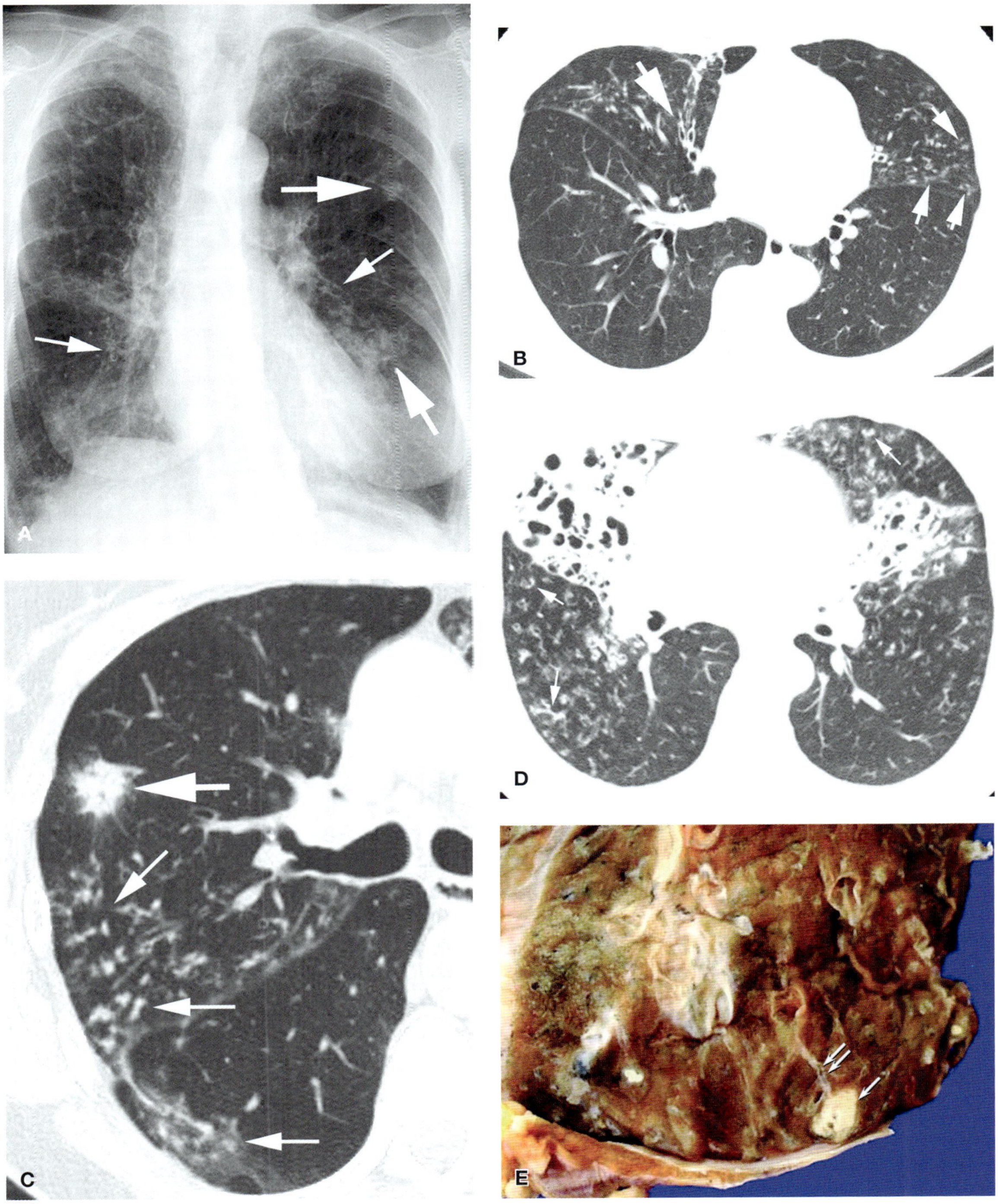

Figure 13.28. Spectrum of *Mycobacterium avium* complex (MAC) infection. **A:** Chest radiograph in a 72-year-old woman with MAC infection. Ill-defined nodular opacities (*large arrows*) are associated with bronchial wall thickening (*small arrows*) in the middle lobe and lingula. **B:** HRCT in a 70-year-old woman with MAC. Right middle lobe bronchiectasis (*large arrow*) is associated with centrilobular nodules (and tree-in-bud) (*small arrows*). **C:** HRCT of the right lung in an elderly woman with MAC. Small nodules and tree-in-bud opacities are visible (*small arrows*). Large nodules (*large arrow*) are also due to MAC. **D:** Axial HRCT image in a 67-year-old woman shows extensive right middle lobe and lingular bronchiectasis with centrilobular nodules and "tree-in-bud" opacities (*arrows*). **E:** Gross specimen shows centrilobular nodule (*arrow*) related to a dilated, irregular centrilobular bronchus (*double arrows*). (Image courtesy of Martha L. Warnock, MD, Professor Emerita, Department of Pathology, University of California, San Francisco.)

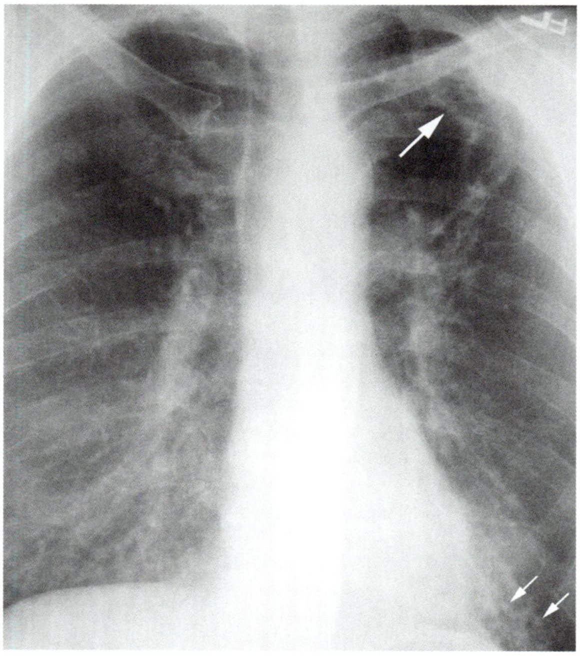

Figure 13.29. *Mycobacterium kansasii* infection. Frontal chest radiograph shows a left upper lobe cavity (*large arrow*) and numerous small nodules in the lower lobes (*small arrows*), representing endobronchial spread of infection.

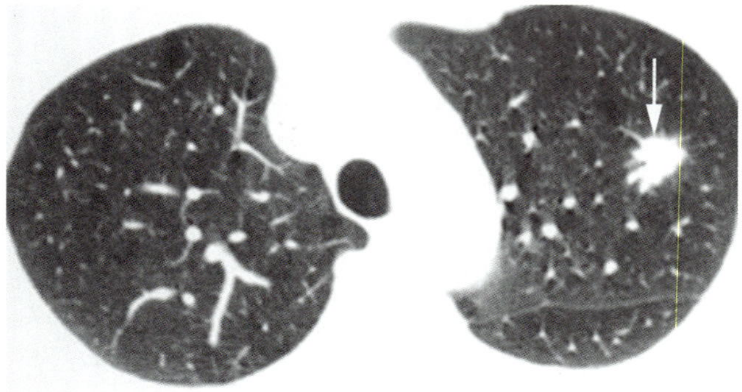

Figure 13.30. *Mycobacterium avium* complex infection in AIDS. Axial CT image shows a spiculated nodule (*arrow*) in the left upper lobe mimicking the appearance of carcinoma. Resection revealed that the nodule was caused by *M. avium* complex infection.

disease due to MAC is relatively uncommon. Clinically overt MAC infection in patients with AIDS often presents with small nodules, usually centrilobular in distribution, combined with air-space consolidation. Mediastinal lymph node enlargement may occur. Enlarged lymph nodes may show low attenuation, although this finding is more predictive of MTB than MAC infection. Occasionally, patients present with solitary pulmonary nodules resembling pulmonary carcinoma (Fig. 13.30). Hepatosplenomegaly is common.

Mycobacterium kansasii infection may also occur in patients with AIDS and most commonly present with consolidation and nodules located in the mid- and lower lung zones; this presentation contrasts with the upper lobe cavitary pattern that often occurs in patients without HIV infection. When cavitation is present in these patients, it portends a worse outcome. Other concurrent infections are common.

Actinomyces

The actinomyces resemble fungi morphologically and are often classified with fungi, but they respond to antibiotics and are more appropriately considered bacteria. Disease is usually caused by *Nocardia* and *Actinomyces*.

Nocardiosis

The most important disease-causing *Nocardia* sp. is *N. asteroides*. Nocardiae are aerobic, Gram-positive, weakly acid-fast organisms that live in soil. Human disease is acquired via inhalation of the organism, although person-to-person transmission can occur (Table 13.13). *Nocardia* infection may occur in otherwise healthy patients but is most common in patients with underlying immunodeficiency, such as transplant recipients on immunosuppressive therapy, patients with connective tissue disease on corticosteroid therapy, patients with malignancy on cytotoxic therapy, or patients with AIDS. *N. asteroides* has a propensity for infecting patients with alveolar proteinosis.

Nocardia asteroides infection usually appears as either bronchopneumonia or multiple nodules, often accompanied by a neutrophilic exudate. Cough, chest pain, and fever are the most common presenting symptoms, and the course of the illness is often protracted. However, the disease course may be quite rapid in severely immunocompromised patients. In such patients, dissemination may occur, often affecting the brain.

Imaging Findings

Chest radiography or CT may show one or more areas of consolidation (ie, bronchopneumonia) or a solitary pulmonary nodule or mass, which may be cavitary (Fig. 13.31; also see Fig. 13.10). Multiple nodules, either large or small, may be seen, particularly in immunosuppressed patients (Fig. 13.32). Nodules are often sharply defined. Areas of decreased attenuation may be seen on CT within nodules or areas of consolidation due to necrosis. Pleural effusion or empyema occurs in nearly 50% of patients. Chest wall invasion is uncommon but may occur.

Table 13.13 Nocardiosis

Organisms live in soil
Acquired via inhalation of the organism; human-to-human spread less common
Immunodeficiency usually present
Bronchopneumonia pattern or multiple nodules
Cavitation may occur.
Pleural effusion in 50%
Chest wall involvement may occur

Actinomycosis

Among the various species within the genus *Actinomyces*, *Actinomyces israelii* is the most important cause of human infection. *A. israelii* is an anaerobic or microaerophilic organism that occasionally stains in a weakly Gram-positive fashion. The organisms uncommonly show minimal acid-fast staining characteristics if a weak decolorizing solution is used. *A. israelii* forms mycelia that, in tissue, may cluster to form sulfur granules. These granules are so named because of their yellow color, although they contain relatively little actual sulfur.

Actinomyces israelii is a normal inhabitant of the oropharynx. The organism causes disease when it is aspirated into the lungs or swallowed into the gastrointestinal tract. The organism is ubiquitous, and no specific factors predisposing to infection are found in many patients, although alcoholics may be relatively predisposed to *A. israelii* infection due to their increased risk of aspiration and poor oral hygiene. The organism usually causes mandibular osteomyelitis following dental extraction, with gastrointestinal and thoracic diseases occurring less commonly.

When the organism reaches the lungs, it has a propensity for causing abscesses and sinus tracts. Acute and chronic inflammation, often with some degree of fibrosis, is present surrounding the sulfur granules.

Actinomyces israelii infection may start as a nonproductive cough that may become purulent over time, occasionally accompanied by hemoptysis. Fever may also be present. Pleuritic chest pain may occur if the infection involves the pleural space. If the infection remains untreated, patients may develop stigmata of chronic pulmonary disease, such as weight loss and digital clubbing. As infection extends into the pleural space and then into the chest wall, bronchopleural-cutaneous fistulas and sinus tracts may develop. *A. israelii* infection may also invade the diaphragm and extend into the abdomen, into the mediastinum, or through the lung apex into the neck. Extrathoracic dissemination may occur.

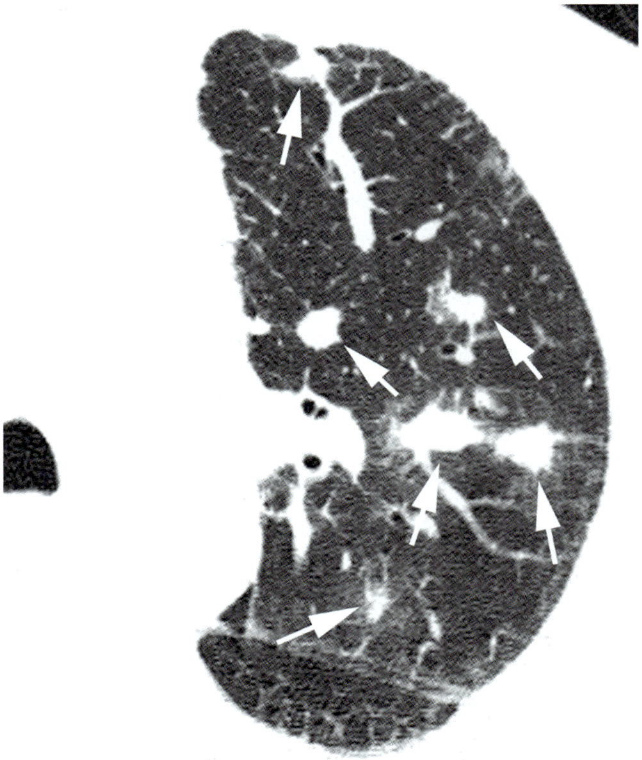

Figure 13.32. *Nocardia* infection in a patient with a heart transplant. CT shows multiple left lung nodules (*arrows*).

Imaging Findings

Actinomyces israelii typically causes lower lobe peripheral air-space consolidation that may progress to abscess formation if proper therapy is not instituted in a timely fashion. On CT, foci of air-space consolidation may show areas of low attenuation, representing microabscess formation. If a frank abscess occurs, pleural effusion and empyema commonly develop, and chest wall invasion may also occur. The latter

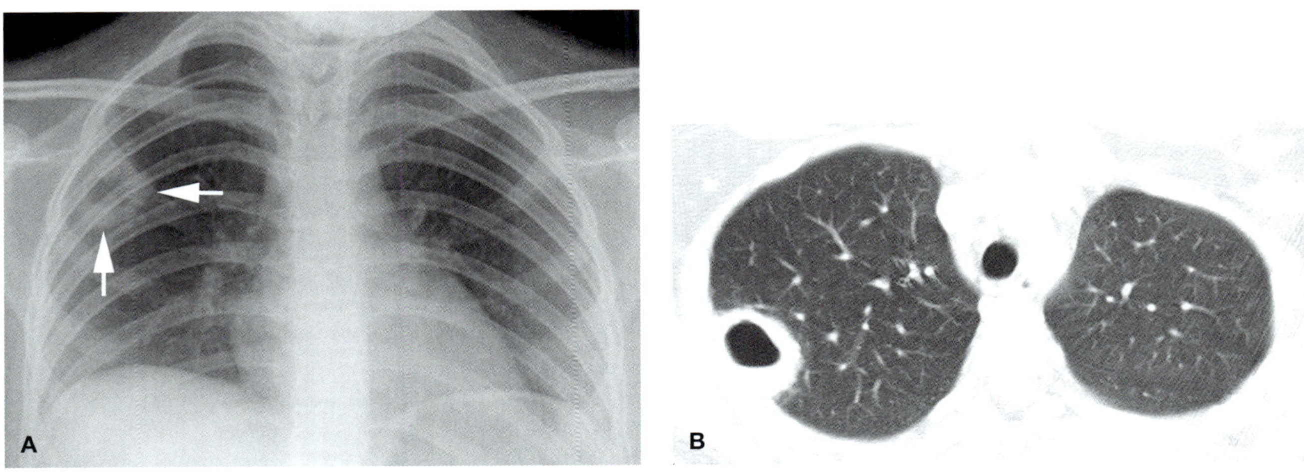

Figure 13.31. *Nocardia* infection. **A:** Chest radiograph in an immunosuppressed patient shows a cavitary mass in the right upper lobe (*arrows*). **B:** CT shows a cavity containing an air-fluid level.

usually appears as a chest wall mass, often with periosteal reaction involving the ribs or frank rib destruction. A pattern particularly suggestive of *A. israelii* chest wall infection is wavy periosteal reaction affecting several contiguous ribs; this pattern may be seen in the absence of associated empyema. Although chest wall invasion has classically been associated with *A. israelii* infection, it is becoming very uncommon due to effective early antibiotic treatment.

Actinomyces israelii may present on chest radiography as a mass, often with cavitation, simulating lung carcinoma. Rare reported manifestations of thoracic *A. israelii* infection include endobronchial lesions, isolated pleural effusions, a miliary pattern, and biapical consolidation resembling pulmonary tuberculosis. For patients who develop chronic *A. israelii* pulmonary infection, extensive lung fibrosis and architectural distortion may occur.

Fungal Infections

Certain fungi—including *Histoplasma capsulatum*, *Coccidioides immitis*, North American blastomycosis, *Paracoccidioides brasiliensis*, and *Blastomyces dermatitidis*—are endemic to particular geographic areas and in these regions tend to affect otherwise healthy persons; these fungi are known as **endemic fungi**. These organisms typically live in soil as saprophytes and infect humans when their spores are inhaled.

Histoplasmosis

Histoplasma capsulatum is by far the most important *Histoplasma* species from a human disease perspective. Infection with *H. capsulatum* is usually asymptomatic, but clinically overt infection may result from overwhelming inoculation or infection in immunocompromised patients.

Histoplasma capsulatum normally lives in soil. The organism thrives in nitrogen-rich environments and is thus often found in soil contaminated with guano from bats or birds. Particularly high-risk environments include caves, pigeon roosts, chicken houses, or other environments where guano becomes concentrated.

Histoplasma capsulatum infection occurs most commonly in individuals living in the Ohio and Mississippi River valleys in the United States and less commonly in South America, Africa, Southeast Asia, and Europe. In these areas, infection is endemic, with 70% or more of the population showing positive histoplasmin skin tests.

Histoplasma capsulatum exists in a mycelial form in soil and may produce microconidia that may be inhaled by humans. The initial polymorphonuclear leukocytic response to the inhaled microconidia is ineffective in killing the organisms, and soon, lymphocytes and macrophages are recruited. These cells are capable of killing the microconidia and the budding yeast into which microconidia transform. The recruitment of lymphocytes is part of the cell-mediated immunity that is important in the pathogenesis of *H. capsulatum* infection, and granulomatous inflammation very similar to tuberculosis is common. Early in the course of infection, spread to lymph nodes is ubiquitous, and extrathoracic dissemination, often to the liver, spleen, bone marrow, and lymph nodes, is also frequent. Healing with the formation of a fibrous capsule around the inflammatory focus usually occurs, often with calcification.

The vast majority of *H. capsulatum* infections are not associated with symptoms. When symptoms are associated with clinical evidence of infection, the term "acute histoplasmosis" is often used. Patients often present with fever, headache, chest pain, and cough, usually mild. Uncommonly, overwhelming exposures may produce severe infection, with hemoptysis, pericarditis, and even ARDS.

Imaging Findings

In the majority of patients with *H. capsulatum* infection, the chest radiograph appears normal. When findings are present, nonspecific multifocal areas of consolidation are often found. If infection is severe, the pattern may resemble bacterial air-space pneumonia. Lymphadenopathy is common, but pleural effusions are not.

In patients with large exposures, diffusely distributed, variably sized but usually small (occasionally small enough to resemble a miliary pattern) nodules may be seen, usually associated with lymphadenopathy. Such nodules may eventually undergo calcification when healing occurs (Fig. 13.33).

The development of a solitary pulmonary nodule from *H. capsulatum* infection, or **histoplasmoma**, is a well-recognized pattern of disease. Such nodules are often circumscribed, measuring up to 3 cm and occasionally more (Fig. 13.34), and often contain central "bull's-eye" or "target" calcification (see Fig. 10.16 in Chapter 10). Adjacent satellite nodules may be present, and calcified lymph nodes are also common. Occasionally, histoplasmomas are multiple but usually not more than five in number.

Uncommonly, lymphadenopathy is the only abnormality seen on chest radiography. Enlarged lymph nodes may compress adjacent bronchi, causing atelectasis.

Chronic pulmonary histoplasmosis may appear as upper lobe fibrocavitary consolidation that closely resembles post-primary MTB. Often, these findings are superimposed on COPD, and air-fluid levels within bullae and increasing wall thickness of bullae may be seen. Over time, linear opacities develop, indicating the presence of fibrosis.

Histoplasma capsulatum infection of mediastinal lymph nodes may result in extensive necrosis and fibrosis of the affected lymph nodes (see Fig. 8.47 in Chapter 8). This pattern of infection may result in granulomatous or fibrosing mediastinitis, with venous obstruction, bronchial stenoses, and narrowing of the pulmonary arteries visible on CT scanning; the former is recognized by the formation of extensive mediastinal venous collateral vessels. Soft tissue masses in the distribution of lymph node stations are present, and *H. capsulatum* may be assumed to be the cause when extensive calcifications of lymph nodes are seen. Esophageal obstruction and esophageal diverticula may occur.

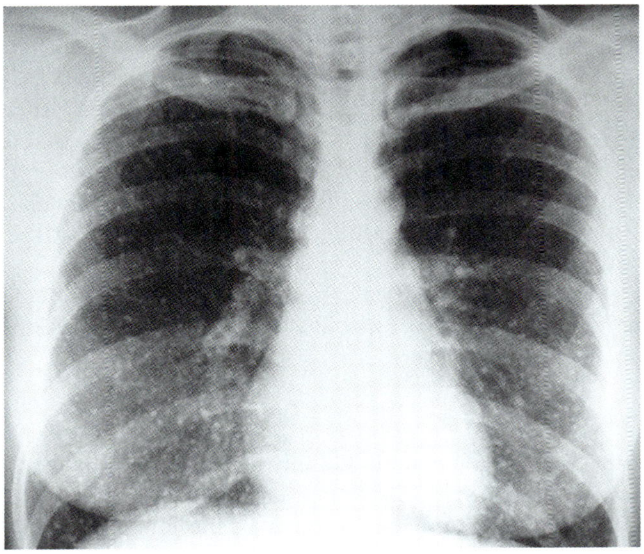

Figure 13.33. Healed histoplasmosis with multiple calcified nodules. This appearance reflects the healing of diffuse nodular histoplasmosis.

Acute disseminated histoplasmosis usually occurs in very young children or in severely immunocompromised individuals, such as AIDS patients or transplant recipients. The typical radiographic appearance is a miliary pattern, and the liver, spleen, lymph nodes, adrenal glands, and bone marrow are often affected. The disease course may be fulminant (Table 13.14).

Coccidioidomycosis

Coccidioides immitis is a dimorphic fungus that exists in soil in a mycelial form. The mycelia produce arthrospores that may cause human infection when inhaled (Table 13.15). Once in tissue, the organisms exist as spherules and may undergo reproduction while in this form.

Coccidioides immitis infection is endemic in the Southwestern United States, Northern Mexico, and areas of Central and South America. Strong winds may carry infection beyond these areas, and travel through endemic areas may account for other cases that are noted outside endemic areas of the country. Within endemic regions, infection rates (often measured by conversion of skin tests) are high. Risk factors associated with *C. immitis* infection include living in endemic areas and immunosuppression. It has been suggested that Filipinos, Native Americans, and African Americans are at relatively higher risk for infection than whites. Miniepidemics have occurred in situations when soil has been disturbed in endemic areas, such as construction projects and earthquakes.

Coccidioides immitis infection has traditionally been divided into primary infection, persistent primary infection, and disseminated infection patterns. The primary infection pattern usually occurs at initial exposure. When inhaled, *C. immitis* arthrospores develop into sporangia, which induce pulmonary inflammation. Initially, the pattern of inflammation resembles bronchopneumonia, but later granulomatous inflammation develops. In most patients, the inflammatory focus resolves without sequelae.

In a few individuals, the initial site of inflammation progresses and necrosis develops. Such progressive disease may occupy an entire lobe or even a whole lung, and hilar and mediastinal lymph node involvement is common in this setting.

Persistent primary infection with *C. immitis* is said to be present when primary infection lasts longer than 6 weeks. This pattern of infection may result in progressive pneumonia or the formation of nodular lesions, often with central necrosis, residing within a fibrous capsule.

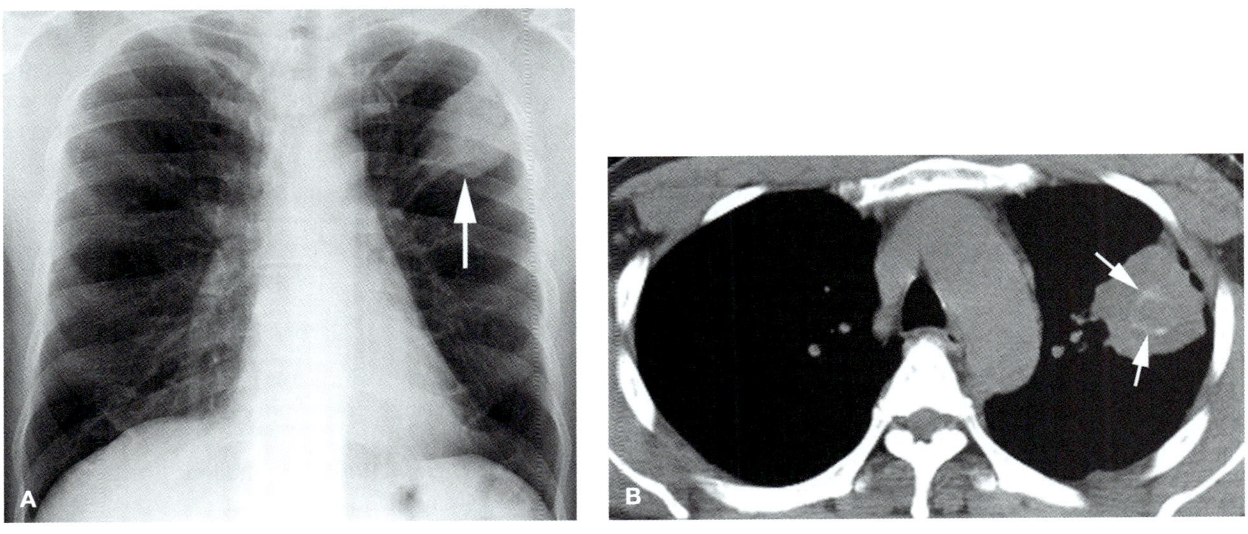

Figure 13.34. Histoplasmoma. **A:** Chest radiograph shows a left upper lobe mass (*arrow*). **B:** CT shows ring-like calcification (*arrows*).

Table 13.14 Histoplasmosis

Organisms live in soil
Thrives in nitrogen-rich environments (soil contaminated with guano); high-risk environments: caves, pigeon roosts, and chicken houses
Ohio and Mississippi River valleys
Infection usually asymptomatic; if not, fever, headache, chest pain, and cough
Radiographs may be normal
Radiographic findings:
- Patchy pneumonia
- Lymphadenopathy common
- Effusion uncommon
- Diffuse small nodules due to large exposure, may calcify
- Histoplasmoma, central "bull's-eye" or "target" calcification
- Chronic disease may mimic postprimary *Mycobacterium tuberculosis.*
- Fibrosing mediastinitis
- Miliary spread, usually in children or immunocompromised patients

Disseminated infection tends to occur in male Filipino, African American, and immunocompromised patients. Using the lungs as an entry portal, *C. immitis* infection may disseminate to the brain and meninges, bones, skin, joints, and kidneys. Radiographic evidence of coincident pulmonary infection is usually present but occasionally is lacking. Miliary disease with *C. immitis* infection may occur and is usually accompanied by the evidence of extrathoracic infection.

Table 13.15 Coccidioidomycosis

Organisms live in soil
Southwestern United States, Northern Mexico, Central and South America
Infection often asymptomatic
Primary infection pattern: usually occurs at initial exposure
- Resembles bronchopneumonia
- Unilateral consolidation
- Hilar lymphadenopathy may be present
- Resolves in most patients

Persistent primary infection: infection lasting >6 wk
- Progressive pneumonia
- Development of nodular lesions, often with cavitation
- Cavities may be thin-walled
- Calcification uncommon

Disseminated infection
- Male Filipino, Native American, African American, and immunocompromised patients
- Miliary pattern often with lymph node enlargement

For most patients, primary *C. immitis* infection is asymptomatic. In some cases, flulike symptoms are present, including fever, cough, headache, and chest pain. An erythematous rash may also be encountered. A syndrome known as "valley fever" has been noted with *C. immitis* infection; it consists of a flu-like constellation of symptoms in addition to erythema nodosum or erythema multiforme and arthralgias. Peripheral blood eosinophilia may be present in patients with valley fever.

Patients with persistent primary *C. immitis* pneumonia are often symptomatic, whereas those with nodular lesions are not.

Imaging Findings

When chest radiographic findings are present, primary *C. immitis* pulmonary infection usually manifests as unilateral air-space consolidation, often in the lower lobe (Fig. 13.35). The consolidation occasionally shows the tendency to resolve in one area and recur in another (phantom infiltrates). Lymphadenopathy is not uncommon, and pleural effusions, usually ipsilateral to the consolidation, are present in a few cases.

Progressive primary infection is associated with increasing multifocal pneumonia or the development of pulmonary nodules, either of which may cavitate. Occasionally, consolidation resolves into a peripheral nodule, which may then undergo progressive cavitation into a thin-walled (grape-skin) cyst, which then spontaneously resolves (Fig. 13.36). Such nodules are more commonly single than multiple, and they calcify in very few patients.

Similar to MTB and histoplasmosis, a progressive form of *C. immitis* infection has been described, variously referred to as chronic progressive coccidioidomycosis or progressive coccidioidal pneumonia. Radiographically, chronic progressive coccidioidomycosis appears as upper lobe consolidation associated with linear opacities and cavitation (Fig. 13.37) and therefore may closely resemble either postprimary MTB or chronic histoplasmosis.

Disseminated coccidioidomycosis occurs most frequently in immunocompromised patients, African Americans, or Filipinos. A miliary pattern is often present on chest radiographs or CT (Fig. 13.38), usually accompanied by hilar or mediastinal lymphadenopathy. Extrathoracic dissemination occurs frequently, often affecting the bones, brain and meninges, and spleen.

North American Blastomycosis

North American blastomycosis is caused by *B. dermatitidis.* This organism resides in soil but may assume a yeast form at body temperature.

Blastomyces dermatitidis is endemic in the central and southeastern United States and Canada (especially the Ohio and Mississippi River valleys, particularly Wisconsin) but may also be found in Central and South America and parts

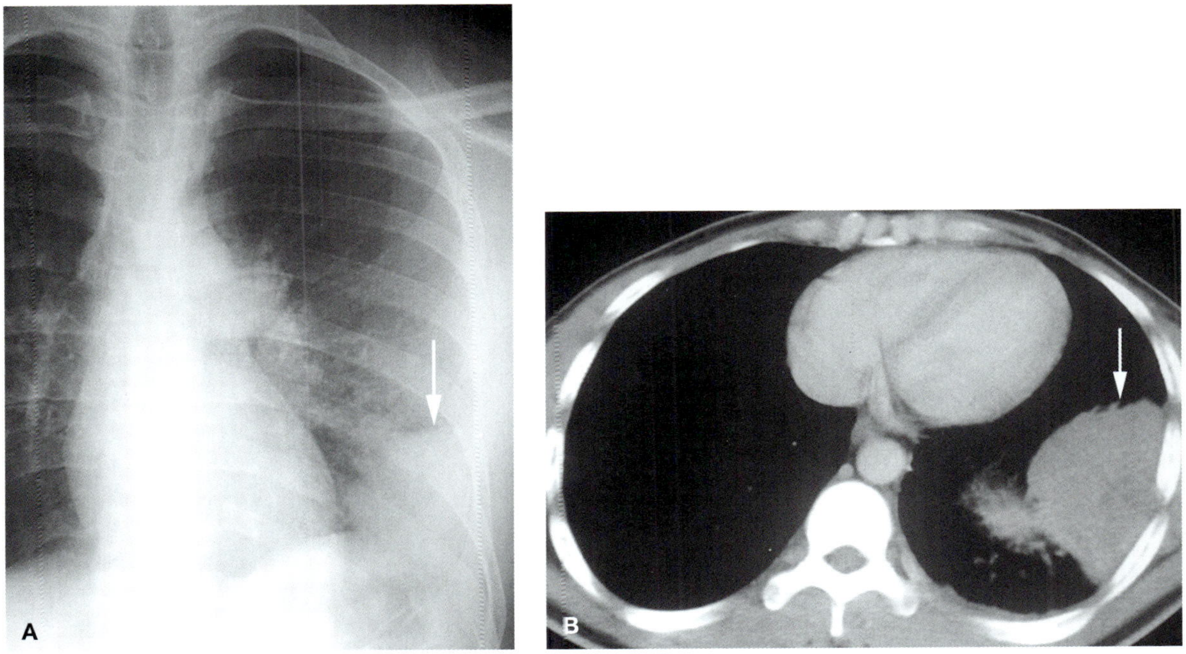

Figure 13.35. Primary coccidioidomycosis pulmonary infection proven by serology and bronchoscopy. **A:** Frontal chest radiograph shows homogenous left lower lobe consolidation (*arrow*). Left hilar enlargement reflects lymphadenopathy. **B:** Axial CT image shows homogenous left lower lobe mass-like opacity (*arrow*) without air bronchograms.

of Africa. Infection occurs by the inhalation of aerosolized fungal spores, often in previously healthy individuals, and has been associated with people living and working in wooded areas, particularly near water. Certain risk factors for *B. dermatitidis* have been identified, including immunosuppression and corticosteroid therapy. Similar to the other endemic fungi, disseminated disease is more likely in immunosuppressed patients.

Following inhalation of the organisms, bronchopneumonia occurs. The initial neutrophilic reaction is subsequently replaced with lymphocytes and macrophages and granulomatous inflammation, although caseous necrosis is uncommon.

Blastomyces dermatitidis infection may be asymptomatic, much like the other endemic fungi, but the frequency of asymptomatic primary infection may be less than the other endemic fungi. Symptomatic infection presents either as a flu-like illness or as an acute bronchopneumonia, with fever, chills, sputum production, and chest pain. Musculoskeletal symptoms and skin findings may be present.

Imaging Findings

Infection with *B. dermatitidis* may present as consolidation resembling other causes of bronchopneumonia. Occasionally, disease is rapidly progressive, with the development of multifocal bilateral air-space opacities or even ARDS. Miliary disease has been reported. Extrathoracic dissemination may occur, especially in immunocompromised patients, usually affecting the skin, musculoskeletal structures, and characteristically the genitourinary tract.

South American Blastomycosis (Paracoccidioidomycosis)

The causative agent of South American blastomycosis is the dimorphic fungus *P. brasiliensis*. Much like *B. dermatitidis*, *P. brasiliensis* exists in soil as a mycelial form but converts to a yeast form at body temperature.

Paracoccidioides brasiliensis is endemic in Central and South America, particularly Brazil. Patients outside these regions with *P. brasiliensis* infection usually have a history of travel to an endemic area. Asymptomatic infection may show no gender predilection, but clinically apparent infection is far more common in men than women. Infection occurs following the inhalation of organisms, and dissemination may then occur. Patients at greatest risk for the development of infection are those who come in contact with soil in endemic regions, such as farmers and manual laborers.

Much like the other endemic fungi, cell-mediated immunity is important in the host response to *P. brasiliensis* infection. Patterns of infection include bronchopneumonia, nodules with or without cavitation, and miliary disease. A combination of granulomatous inflammation and a neutrophilic infiltrate may be seen pathologically.

Patients may be asymptomatic or present with a flu-like illness. Immunocompromised patients are at higher risk for developing disseminated disease and may present with hepatosplenomegaly, lymphadenopathy, and possibly central nervous system or gastrointestinal findings.

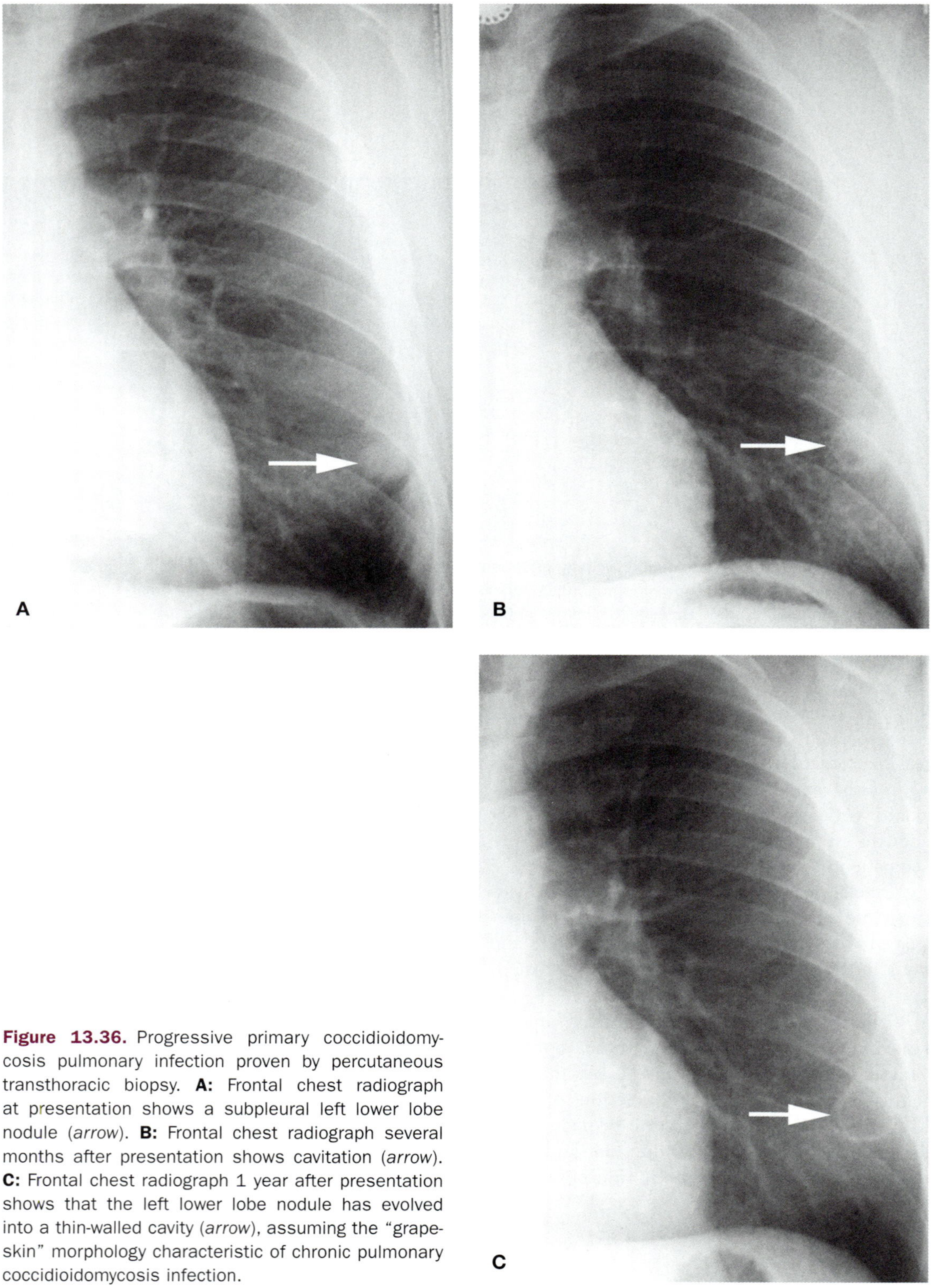

Figure 13.36. Progressive primary coccidioidomycosis pulmonary infection proven by percutaneous transthoracic biopsy. **A:** Frontal chest radiograph at presentation shows a subpleural left lower lobe nodule (*arrow*). **B:** Frontal chest radiograph several months after presentation shows cavitation (*arrow*). **C:** Frontal chest radiograph 1 year after presentation shows that the left lower lobe nodule has evolved into a thin-walled cavity (*arrow*), assuming the "grape-skin" morphology characteristic of chronic pulmonary coccidioidomycosis infection.

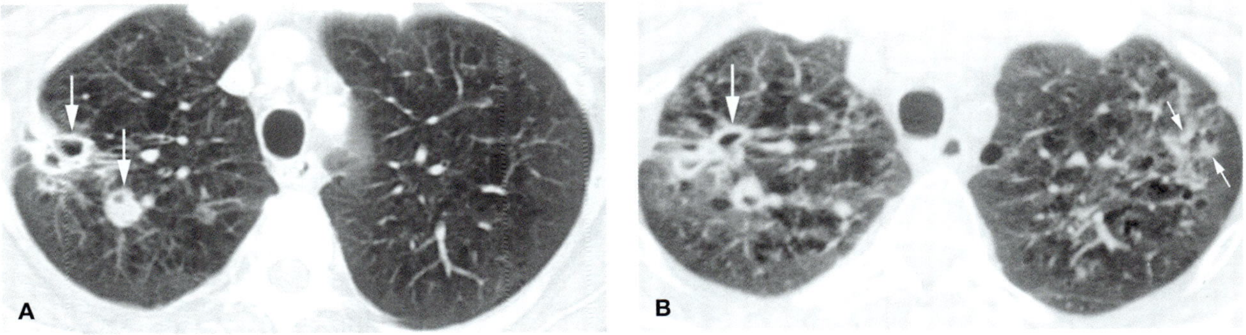

Figure 13.37. Chronic progressive primary coccidioidomycosis pulmonary infection. **A:** Axial CT image shows thin-walled cavities (*arrows*) in the right upper lobe. **B:** Axial CT image obtained several months later, and after the initiation of antifungal therapy, shows persistence of the right upper lobe cavities (*large arrow*) and the development of nodular opacities in the left upper lobe (*small arrows*). Sputum examination was persistently positive for *Coccidioides immitis*.

Imaging Findings

The imaging manifestations of *P. brasiliensis* pulmonary infection are similar to the other endemic fungi and include air-space consolidation and single or multiple nodules (Fig. 13.39) that may cavitate. Lymphadenopathy may occur, either alone or together with pulmonary parenchymal disease. The most commonly visible thoracic CT findings in patients with *P. brasiliensis* include focal, multifocal, or diffuse areas of consolidation and ground-glass opacity with variably sized nodules. Areas of low attenuation and interlobular septal thickening may also be evident. In the minority of patients, a "reversed halo" sign (the "atoll" sign) may be encountered. Over time and following treatment, findings of fibrosis, including architectural distortion, traction bronchiectasis, peribronchovascular thickening, and irregular air-space enlargement, may be seen.

Cryptococcus

Cryptococcus neoformans is the most common etiologic agent resulting in cryptococcosis. Unlike the endemic fungi, *C. neoformans* exists only in a yeast form in both nature and when it infects humans. The organism often has a characteristic capsule that becomes visible with India ink preparations. Two variants of *C. neoformans* cause human disease: *C. neoformans* variant *neoformans* and *C. neoformans* variant *grubii (serotype A)*. Previously classified as a variant of *C. neoformans*, *C. gattii* is now classified as a distinct species.

Cryptococcus neoformans is typically found in pigeon droppings and is distributed globally, although it is unclear if contact with pigeons actually results in a demonstrably increased risk of developing cryptococcosis. *C. neoformans* var. *neoformans* infections primarily occur in immunocompromised patients and are prevalent in Northern Europe, whereas *C. neoformans* var. *grubii* infections may be found worldwide. *C. gattii* infections were previously found mostly in tropical regions, particularly in association with eucalyptus and fir trees, but have been recently encountered in the Pacific Northwest and Canada and may occur in otherwise healthy adults.

Inhalation of the yeast provides the route for infection. It is likely that the capsule of the organism contributes to its ability to cause disease because organisms without a capsule are usually easily destroyed by neutrophils. Infection by

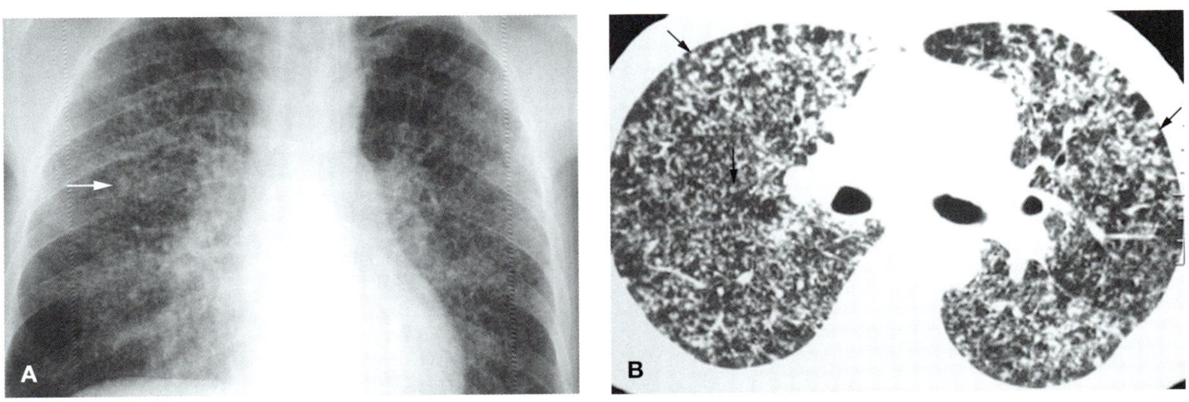

Figure 13.38. Hematogenous dissemination of coccidioidomycosis pulmonary infection in AIDS. **A:** Frontal chest radiograph shows numerous bilateral small nodules, some of which are larger (*arrow*) than is typical for miliary *Mycobacterium tuberculosis* infection. **B:** Axial chest CT shows numerous, variably sized, randomly distributed nodules (*arrows*), consistent with hematogenous dissemination.

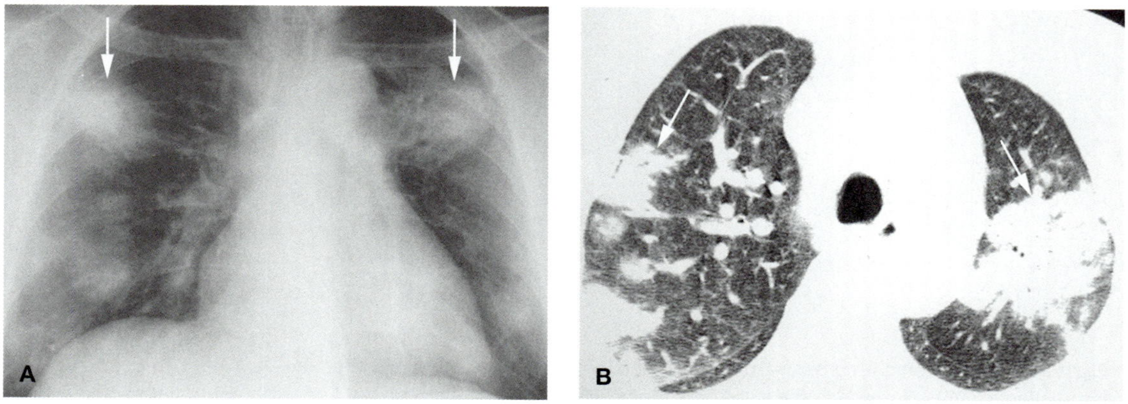

Figure 13.39. Paracoccidioidomycosis proven by transthoracic needle biopsy. **A:** Frontal chest radiograph shows bilateral, poorly defined masses (*arrows*). **B:** Axial CT image shows poorly defined areas of nodular consolidation (*arrows*). Note the presence of air bronchograms within the left upper lobe opacity.

Cryptococcus may take the form of single or multiple nodules, bronchopneumonia, or miliary nodules. The pattern of inflammation is variable, occasionally with elements of a granulomatous response in some and a suppurative response in others. In patients with AIDS, there may be little inflammation associated with the organisms.

Cryptococcus infection in otherwise healthy patients is often asymptomatic. When symptoms occur, a flu-like illness is common. Patients with AIDS and *Cryptococcus* infection may present with a variety of respiratory complaints as well as headache. The latter may indicate the presence of meningitis and may occur in the absence of radiographic evidence of pulmonary disease.

Imaging Findings

In healthy patients, cryptococcal infection usually manifests as one or more peripheral, circumscribed nodules, usually without cavitation. Less commonly, air-space consolidation is seen.

In patients with AIDS, a diffuse interstitial pattern, variously described as reticular or nodular, resembling *P. jirovecii* pneumonia (Fig. 13.40), may be seen. A miliary pattern may occur (Fig. 13.41), as may single (Fig. 13.42) or multiple nodules (see Fig. 10.35B in Chapter 10), occasionally with cavitation (Fig. 13.43). Lymph node enlargement is uncommon as is pleural effusion. Dissemination to extrathoracic structures is common in patients with AIDS, particularly to the brain and meninges.

Candida

Several species of *Candida* are capable of causing human disease, but *Candida albicans* is the most common and most important. *C. albicans* is found in the gastrointestinal tract and on the skin of normal individuals, but clinically overt pulmonary infection almost always occurs in the setting of immunosuppression. Such conditions include cytotoxic therapy for malignancy, AIDS, chronic antibiotic use, organ transplant recipients, chronic granulomatous disease of childhood, and patients with severe burns. As with other fungi, cell-mediated immunity is important for the prevention of *C. albicans* infection.

Candida albicans pulmonary infection usually occurs in the setting of multiorgan involvement in patients with disseminated disease. In this circumstance, the lungs show numerous small nodules with associated inflammation. Very rarely, *C. albicans* infection occurs as a result of aspiration of organisms from the oral cavity into the lungs. Symptoms of infection are nonspecific and include purulent cough and fever. Findings suggesting extrathoracic dissemination are often present.

The most common chest radiographic appearance of *C. albicans* pulmonary infection is focal or multilobar consolidation (Fig. 13.44), occasionally with linear abnormalities suggesting an interstitial component. Cavitation and lymphadenopathy

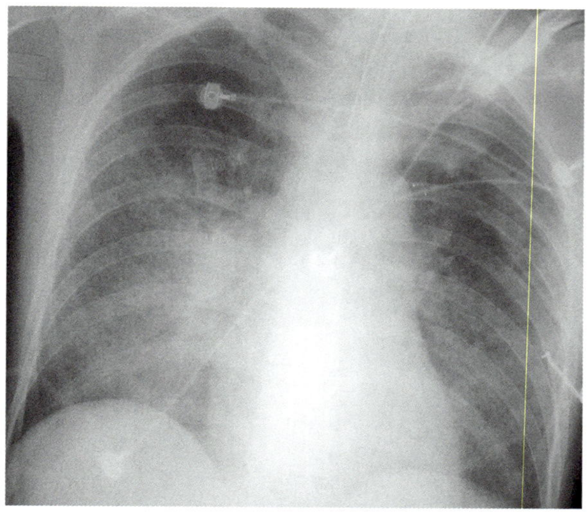

Figure 13.40. Cryptococcosis in AIDS. Frontal chest radiograph shows bilateral linear and ground-glass opacity that resembles *Pneumocystis jirovecii* pneumonia. Bronchoscopy proved cryptococcal pneumonia.

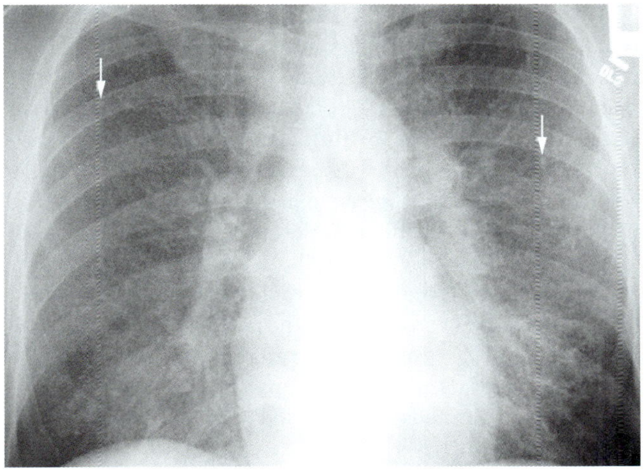

Figure 13.41. Cryptococcosis in AIDS. Frontal chest radiograph shows innumerable, bilateral, very small, and well-defined pulmonary nodules (*arrows*), consistent with a miliary pattern, proven to represent pulmonary cryptococcosis. Note the right paratracheal and bilateral hilar lymphadenopathy.

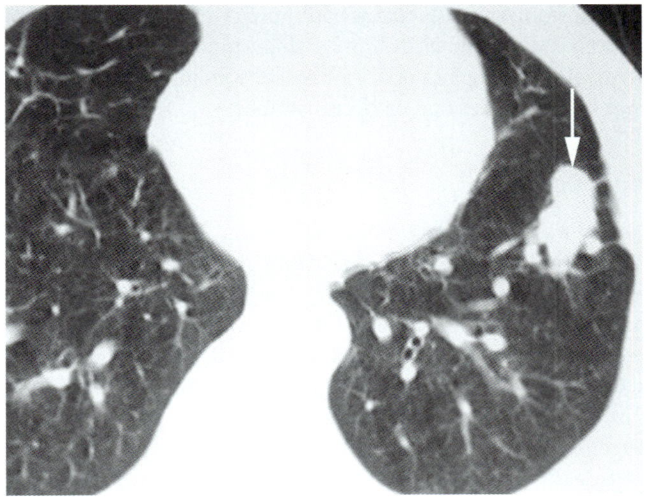

Figure 13.42. Cryptococcosis in AIDS. Axial CT image shows an irregular left lower lobe nodule (*arrow*) with associated pleural reaction. Percutaneous biopsy recovered *Cryptococcus neoformans*.

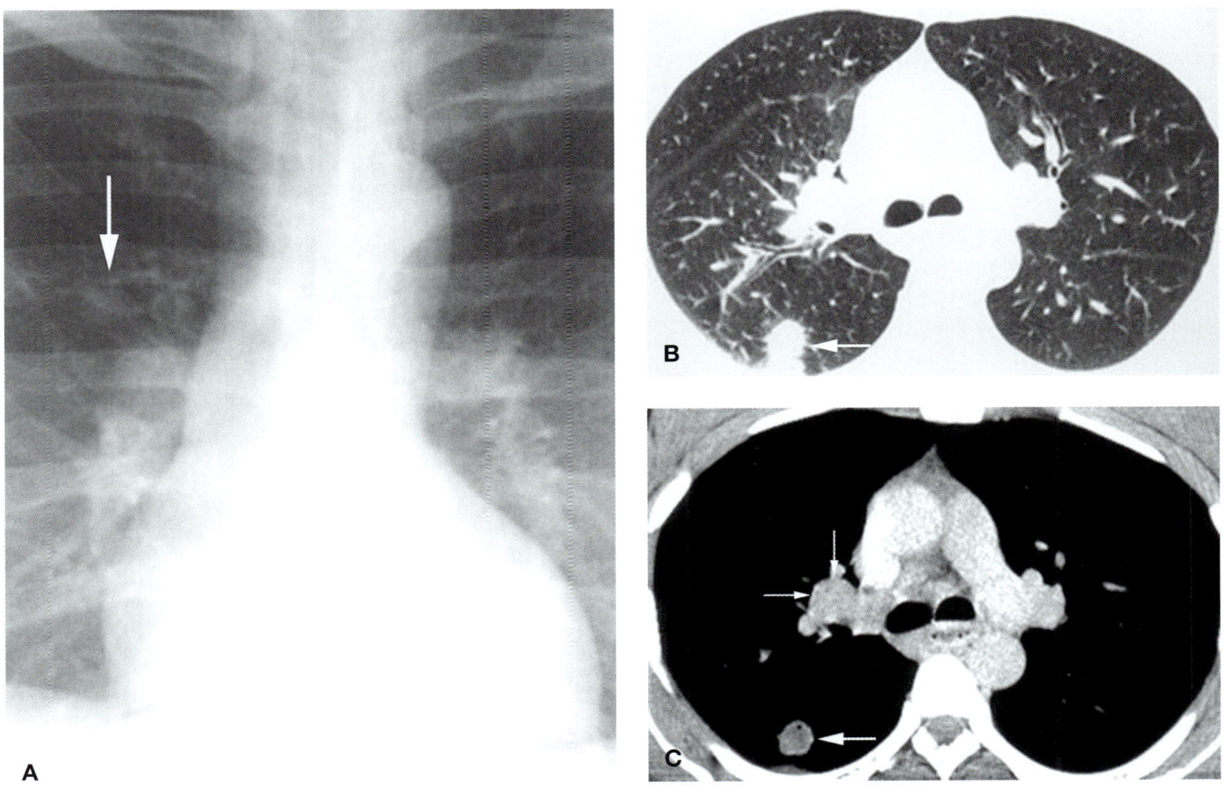

Figure 13.43. Cryptococcosis in AIDS. **A:** Frontal chest radiograph shows a poorly defined nodule in the right lung (*arrow*) associated with right hilar lymphadenopathy. **B:** Axial CT image photographed in lung windows shows a spiculated nodule (*arrow*) within the superior segment of the right lower lobe. **C:** Axial CT image photographed in soft tissue windows shows that the nodule (*larger arrow*) is low in attenuation (necrotic) and contains a small amount of air due to cavitation. Right hilar lymphadenopathy (*smaller arrows*) is also present.

are not features of *C. albicans* pulmonary infection. A miliary pattern may occur. HRCT may show multiple nodules with areas of ground-glass opacity and consolidation; the nodules may be poorly defined or circumscribed.

Aspergillus

Aspergillus species are ubiquitous fungi found throughout nature that may result in disease in susceptible hosts when inhaled. The most important *Aspergillus* species from a human infectious disease point of view is *A. fumigatus*. The organism exists in a mycelial form with hyphae that characteristically branch at 45-degree angle and may be found throughout nature. Other *Aspergillus* species, particularly *A. terreus*, are of growing importance as well.

Infections caused by *A. fumigatus* have traditionally been classified into four different forms: invasive aspergillosis, chronic necrotizing aspergillosis (also known as semi-invasive aspergillosis), allergic aspergillosis (including allergic bronchopulmonary aspergillosis [ABPA] and hypersensitivity pneumonitis; see Chapters 17 and 23), and aspergilloma. An uncommon manifestation of *A. fumigatus* infection that primarily affects AIDS patients, known as obstructing bronchial aspergillosis, also has been described.

Aspergillus infection may occur when a susceptible host inhales the organism. Various risk factors for the development of *A. fumigatus* infection exist, and each is related to a particular pattern of infection.

Invasive Aspergillosis

In normal hosts, inhaled *Aspergillus* organisms are rapidly destroyed by macrophages, with neutrophils providing additional immunity. The presence of granulocytopenia or neutropenia allows *Aspergillus* spores to germinate and develop into hyphae; the latter may invade tissues.

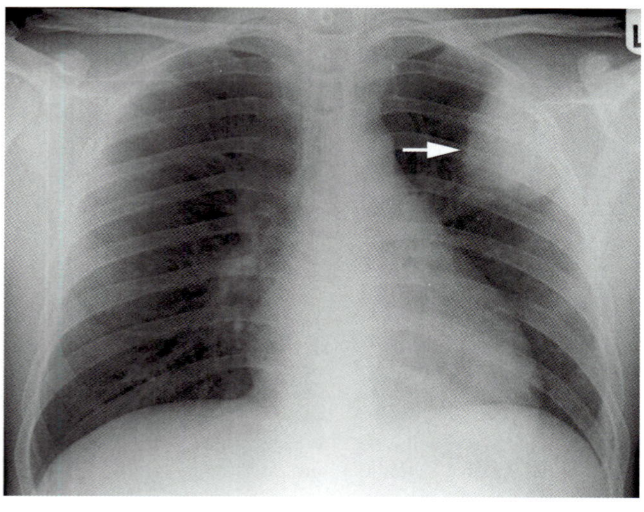

Figure 13.44. Candidal pneumonia in a patient receiving steroids for collagen vascular disease. Chest radiograph shows a focal left upper lobe pneumonia (*arrow*).

Aspergillus hyphae may invade the pulmonary vasculature, causing thrombosis, pulmonary hemorrhage, and infarction. This occurrence, termed **angioinvasive aspergillosis**, accounts for about 80% of cases of invasive aspergillosis (Table 13.16). *Aspergillus* within airways may invade the airway wall and peribronchial or peribronchiolar lung, a condition known as **airway invasive aspergillosis** or *Aspergillus* bronchopneumonia. This manifestation accounts for about 15% of cases of invasive aspergillosis. A third form of invasive aspergillosis, termed **acute tracheobronchitis**, results in more limited invasion of the trachea or bronchi; it accounts for about 5% of cases of invasive aspergillosis. Pathologically, ulcerated mucosa, fungal hyphae, mucus, and sloughed epithelial cells, combined with extensive submucosal inflammation, are present.

Invasive aspergillosis is primarily an infection of severely immunocompromised patients, such as hematopoietic stem cell transplant recipients, solid organ transplant recipients, patients with hematologic malignancy, patients treated with high doses of corticosteroids, and patients with AIDS. Invasive aspergillosis is characterized by tissue invasion and destruction caused by *Aspergillus* organisms. Less commonly, invasive aspergillosis is seen in patients with milder forms of immunocompromise, such as obstructive lung disease and interstitial fibrosis. Rarely, invasive aspergillosis develops in patients with normal immune systems following massive inhalation of spores, a condition known as **primary invasive aspergillosis**.

Usually, the immune defect predisposing to invasive aspergillosis is known. Nonproductive cough, shortness of breath, and chest pain are some of the more common symptoms encountered. Fever may also occur, but often, the febrile response is blunted in patients with severe immunodeficiency, especially those receiving high-dose corticosteroid therapy. The time course of angioinvasive aspergillosis following hematopoietic stem cell transplantation is frequently predictable. Infection is typically encountered at the point of most profound immunosuppression, generally about 15 to 25 days after induction chemotherapy or hematopoietic stem cell transplantation. Risk is maximal while the white blood cell count remains below 500 cells/mm^3.

Imaging Findings The imaging manifestations of invasive aspergillosis depend on the type of invasion present.

Angioinvasive Aspergillosis Chest radiographs are often abnormal but nonspecific, revealing patchy segmental or lobar consolidations or multiple, ill-defined nodular opacities. Nodular opacities may show the "halo" sign on CT (Fig. 13.45; see also Fig. 10.7 in Chapter 10), a halo of ground-glass opacity surrounding a denser central nodule; this finding correlates with the presence of hemorrhage (the halo) surrounding a region of septic infarction (the central nodule). As the patient's immune system recovers, about 2 weeks after the onset of infection, chest radiography or CT may demonstrate the "air-crescent" sign (see Fig. 10.27 in Chapter 10). The air-crescent sign consists of a nodular opacity that represents retracted, infarcted lung associated with crescentic

Table 13.16 Invasive Aspergillosis

Associated with granulocytopenia and neutropenia
Severely immunocompromised patients, transplant recipients, patients with hematologic malignancy, AIDS
Occurs in three forms:
Angioinvasive aspergillosis
- 80% of cases of invasive aspergillosis
- Results in thrombosis, pulmonary hemorrhage, infarction
- Patchy consolidations or multiple, ill-defined nodules
- Halo sign on CT in early disease
- Air-crescent sign after 2 wk

Airway invasive aspergillosis (*Aspergillus* bronchopneumonia)
- 15% of cases of invasive aspergillosis
- Results in thrombosis, pulmonary hemorrhage, infarction
- Patchy air-space opacity
- Centrilobular nodules, centered on airways
- Tree-in-bud on HRCT

Acute tracheobronchitis
- 5% of cases of invasive aspergillosis
- Invasion of the walls of trachea or bronchi
- Radiographs often normal; CT may show plaques in airways.

or circumferential cavitation. Although this finding is not specific for angioinvasive aspergillosis, it is highly characteristic in the proper clinical setting. It is seen in nearly 50% of patients with invasive aspergillosis, particularly those in whom the initial lesion was consolidation or a mass.

Airway Invasive Aspergillosis (Aspergillus Bronchopneumonia) Radiographs usually show as patchy air-space opacity, often accompanied by small nodules. The radiographic appearance is nonspecific, and the differential diagnosis is extensive and includes pyogenic bronchopneumonia, pulmonary hemorrhage, noncardiogenic pulmonary edema, and other acute lung injury patterns. CT shows multifocal areas of air-space consolidation or nodules that may be peribronchiolar in distribution (Fig. 13.46). Small centrilobular nodules, indicative of bronchiolitis, may also be seen.

Acute Tracheobronchitis Chest radiography is unrevealing, but CT may reveal multifocal irregular plaques within the trachea, which are occasionally high in attenuation due to the ability of *Aspergillus* to fix calcium (see Fig. 13.1). Bronchoscopy is the procedure of choice for diagnosis and will reveal raised, white fungal plaques coating the airways.

Chronic Necrotizing Aspergillosis. Chronic necrotizing aspergillosis, previously known as semi-invasive aspergillosis, commonly occurs in patients with low-grade forms of immunocompromise, such as COPD, low-dose corticosteroid use, alcoholism, tuberculosis, diabetes mellitus, and collagen vascular diseases (Table 13.17). Risk is compounded in those with preexisting structural lung disease, such as pneumoconiosis, prior mycobacterial disease, sarcoidosis, obstructive

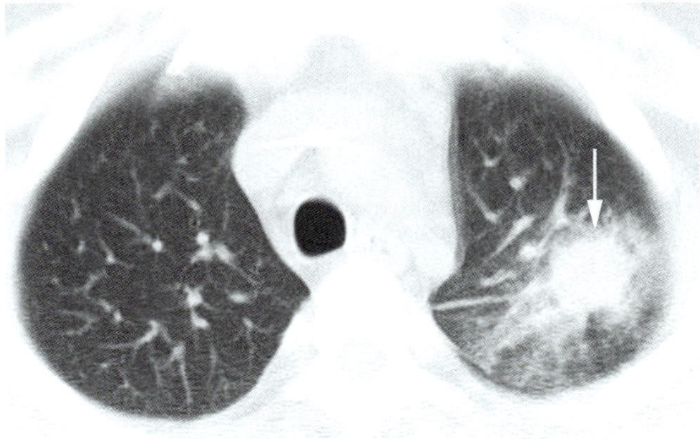

Figure 13.45. Invasive aspergillosis in a bone marrow transplant patient. Axial CT image shows a left upper lobe nodule (*arrow*) with surrounding ground-glass opacity. This combination represents the halo sign.

lung disease, or prior radiation treatment. Chronic necrotizing aspergillosis has recently been subdivided into three forms: (1) *chronic cavitary pulmonary aspergillosis*, a chronic cavitary disease in which new cavity formation may occur, but the *Aspergillus* hyphae do not invade surrounding pulmonary tissues; (2) *subacute invasive pulmonary aspergillosis*, in which hyphal tissue invasion occurs, typically beginning with a thin-walled cavity, but over a slower time course compared with angioinvasive aspergillosis (typically months with the former, compared with days to weeks for the latter); and (3) *chronic fibrosing pulmonary aspergillosis*, which is characterized by extensive cavity wall fibrosis.

Patients with chronic necrotizing aspergillosis present with low-grade fever and productive cough, often over a period of months. Hemoptysis may also occur. These symptoms may be superimposed on a background of chronic illness.

Imaging Findings Chronic necrotizing aspergillosis mimics the appearance of active TB. It often presents with irregular upper lobe consolidation and pleural thickening that slowly progresses to cavitation over weeks or months. The upper lobe disease commonly contacts thickened pleura. The cavity may contain an internal opacity resembling an

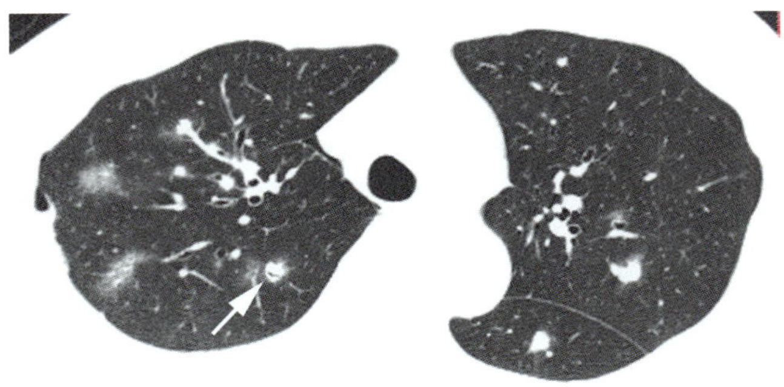

Figure 13.46. Airway invasive aspergillosis in an immunosuppressed patient. Ill-defined nodules are visible bilaterally. A nodule on the right (*arrow*) surrounds a small bronchus.

Table 13.17 Chronic Necrotizing Aspergillosis
Also known as semi-invasive aspergillosis
Subdivided into two types:
Chronic cavitary pulmonary aspergillosis
Subacute invasive pulmonary aspergillosis
Associated with mild immunocompromise (chronic obstructive pulmonary disease, low-dose corticosteroid use, alcoholism, tuberculosis, diabetes, collagen vascular diseases)
Low-grade fever, productive cough, often over a period of months
Mimics active *Mycobacterium tuberculosis* radiographically
Progressive upper lobe consolidation
Cavitation
Pleural thickening
Mass within the cavity due to fungus

aspergilloma, largely consisting of fungus. Irregular strands may be seen extending from the intracavitary mass to the cavity wall (Fig. 13.47). Occasionally, regions of high attenuation are visible within the cavity on CT. This probably represents calcification occurring in relation to the fungus.

Aspergilloma

Aspergilloma, or mycetoma, is a saprophytic infection that occurs in patients with underlying structural lung disease. Patients with mycetoma generally have normal immunity, although coexistent chronic diseases are often present. Pathologically, aspergilloma consists of a combination of fungal hyphae, cellular debris, and mucus within a cavity. The cavity wall commonly consists of fibrous tissue, inflammatory cells, and granulation tissue, the latter derived from the bronchial circulation. The most common cause of underlying structural lung disease in patients with aspergilloma is cavitary disease from prior TB. Structural lung disease due to sarcoidosis is the second most common condition predisposing to aspergilloma formation. Bullae, abscesses, and bronchiectasis are less common predisposing factors. The preexisting lung disease presumably impairs normal clearance of the organisms, allowing infection to occur. Characteristically, the fungus does not usually produce tissue invasion.

Often, patients with aspergilloma are asymptomatic. When symptoms are present, cough, weight loss, and hemoptysis are common. Hemoptysis may range from minor blood streaking to massive, life-threatening hemorrhage. The latter is commonly temporized with bronchial embolization, although pulmonary resection may be required. Although the overall prognosis of patients with aspergilloma is good, death from massive hemoptysis may occur, and rare cases of severe local parenchymal destruction and even dissemination have occurred.

Imaging Findings Aspergilloma usually appears as a round or oval mass partially filling a cavity and with a crescent of air, which may show mobility when the patient is imaged in different positions (Fig. 13.48A).

Aspergillomas are usually located in the upper lobes, adjacent to the pleura, which may be thickened. Aspergillomas rarely calcify, and they may diminish or remain unchanged in size over time. An air-fluid level is usually not present within the cavity. The cavity itself is usually thin walled, although thickening of the cavity walls before a discrete internal opacity is seen may indicate early infection.

CT shows a mobile, intracavitary mass (see Fig. 13.48B and C; see also Fig. 10.42 in Chapter 10) and may also reveal

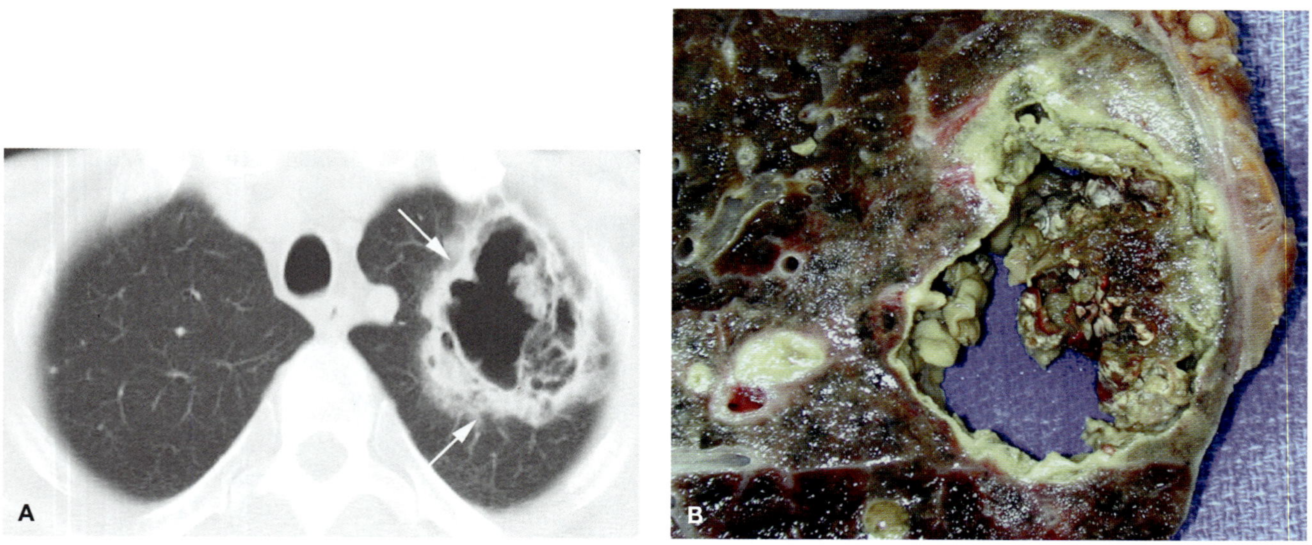

Figure 13.47. Chronic necrotizing aspergillosis in a patient with diabetes mellitus. **A:** Axial CT image through the lung apices shows an irregular left upper lobe cavity (*arrows*). Internal opacities reflect the presence of fungus. **B:** Gross specimen at autopsy shows the internal elements within the cavitary lesion.

small fungal strands bridging the fungus ball and the cavity wall in cases when the air-crescent sign is not visible on chest radiographs. CT may also demonstrate foci of increased attenuation within the fungal ball, presumably reflecting calcium. As with chest radiography, CT may reveal thickening of the wall of a preexisting cavity before the fungus ball is evident.

Zygomycosis

Fungal organisms, formerly of the class *Zygomycetes*, now of the order *Mucorales*, the most important of which are *Rhizopus*, *Rhizomucor*, and *Mucor*, may produce infections referred to as Mucormycosis.

The fungi that cause mucormycosis are found worldwide, usually in decaying matter. These organisms produce spores that may result in disease when inhaled. Disease almost always occurs in patients with impaired immunity, including patients with diabetes mellitus (especially in the context of ketoacidosis), corticosteroid therapy, AIDS (often when corticosteroid therapy is employed concomitantly), hematologic malignancy, lymphoma, and chronic renal failure. In particular, neutropenic patients are at risk for mucormycosis.

The pattern of infection caused by the *Mucorales* fungi is variable, depending on the degree of underlying immunity. An extensive neutrophilic infiltrate may be present, but granulomatous inflammation is rare. Vascular invasion by the fungal organisms is common.

Patients with *Mucorales* infections, especially mucormycosis, present with chest pain, fever, and hemoptysis; the latter can be massive. The organisms can be very destructive, and invasion of the mediastinum, pleura, chest wall, and spine may occur. Bronchopleural-cutaneous fistulas may also result from mucormycosis. Vascular catastrophes, such as pulmonary artery aneurysms, pulmonary vein thrombosis with subsequent pulmonary infarction, and superior vena cava thrombosis, may also occur.

Imaging Findings

Chest radiography in patients with mucormycosis may show multifocal, occasionally bilateral, air-space consolidation, a single nodule or mass, or multiple, ill-defined nodules or masses. CT findings include single or multiple large nodules or consolidations with ground-glass halos or a reverse halo sign (appearing as an infarct) usually in peripheral distribution (Fig. 13.49). In some patients with severe disease, imaging features evolved to show a multifocal pneumonia similar to other organisms. An air-crescent sign may also occur, especially as the patient's immune system recovers following chemotherapy. Pleural effusions and lymphadenopathy may also occur.

Fusariosis

Fusarium spp. are fungal organisms commonly found in soil and water and are second only to *Aspergillus* as the leading cause of fungal infections in immunocompromised patients.

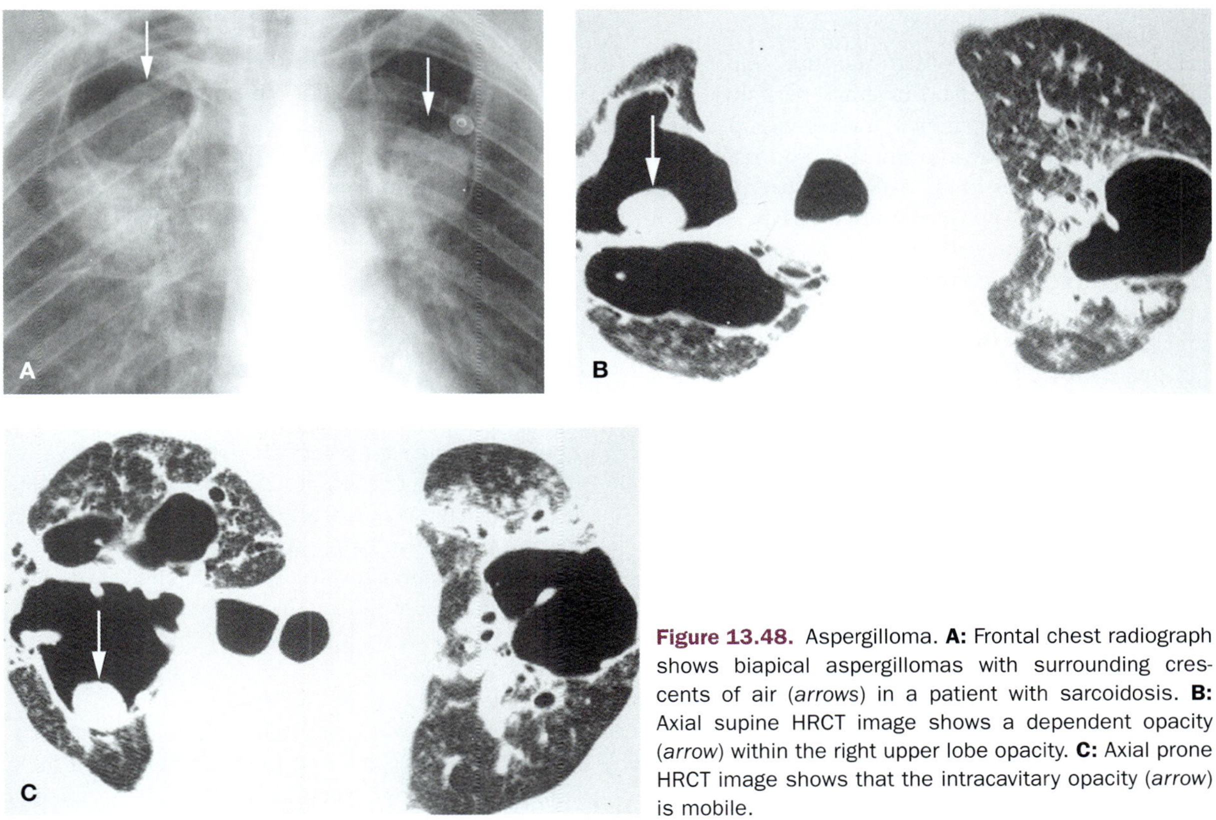

Figure 13.48. Aspergilloma. **A:** Frontal chest radiograph shows biapical aspergillomas with surrounding crescents of air (*arrows*) in a patient with sarcoidosis. **B:** Axial supine HRCT image shows a dependent opacity (*arrow*) within the right upper lobe opacity. **C:** Axial prone HRCT image shows that the intracavitary opacity (*arrow*) is mobile.

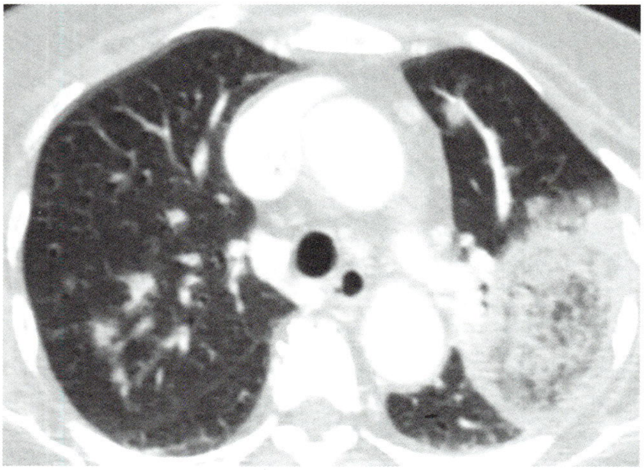

Figure 13.49. Mucormycosis. Axial contrast-enhanced CT image in a neutropenic patient with proven mucormycosis. The rounded area of consolidation in the left upper lobe demonstrates a reverse halo with a rind of consolidation and central ground-glass opacity that has the appearance of an infarct, which is a common appearance in mucor. There is a small surrounding ground-glass halo.

Fusarium spp. may also produce infections in immunocompetent patients with wounds or foreign bodies and rarely in immunocompetent patients with no underlying identifiable risk factors. A number of *Fusarium* species may be responsible for human infection, including *F. solani*, *F. dimerum*, *F. moniliforme*, *F. oxysporum*, *F. proliferatum*, and *F. verticillioides*. Infection is acquired via the inhalation of airborne conidia, which eventually germinate and invade tissues, including blood vessels.

The clinical manifestations of *Fusarium* spp. infection are variable, including pneumonia, fungemia, peritoneal space infection (particularly in patients undergoing peritoneal dialysis), ulcers, septic arthritis, sinusitis, and osteomyelitis. A manifestation resembling ABPA has been reported. Patients with *Fusarium* spp. pneumonia may present with cough, dyspnea, fever, pleuritic chest pain, and hemoptysis. Infection is most commonly encountered in profoundly immunosuppressed patients, such as those with hematologic malignancies and stem cell transplantation. Most patients are neutropenic at the time of diagnosis.

Imaging Findings

The most common imaging finding of pulmonary fusariosis is variably sized pulmonary nodules or masses. Multiple nodules are more commonly seen than solitary nodules, and areas of consolidation may also be present. Mild lymphadenopathy, typically only appreciable at thoracic CT, and pleural effusions may be present in a minority of patients.

Unlike pulmonary aspergillosis, mucormycosis, and *Candida* infections, the ground-glass halo sign is not a typical finding in patients with pulmonary fusariosis. Cavitation may occur but, unlike invasive aspergillosis, is relatively uncommon.

The treatment of fusariosis is difficult, as these organisms are frequently resistant to antifungal medications.

Scedosporium Species and *Pseudallescheria boydii*

Scedosporium spp., including *Scedosporium apiospermum* and *Scedosporium prolificans*, are filamentous fungi with a worldwide distribution that are becoming increasingly important from a human infectious disease perspective. The sexual state of *S. apiospermum*, known as *Pseudallescheria boydii*, is an organism that is known to infect cystic fibrosis patients and has been reported in lung transplant recipients as well. *Scedosporium* infections typically affect severely immunosuppressed patients, such as patients with hematologic malignancies, neutropenic patients with HIV infection, patients on corticosteroid therapy, hematopoietic stem cell transplant recipients, and organ transplant recipients. *S. prolificans* may infect immunocompetent patients also, particularly traumatically injured patients and surgical patients. *Scedosporium* spp./*P. boydii* infections also occur following near-drowning episodes, and it has been suggested that infection with *Scedosporium* spp./*P. boydii* should be specifically sought when pneumonia and brain abscesses occur in such patients.

Although infection with *Scedosporium* spp. is uncommon, in the United States, the largest number of cases is reported from Texas and California.

Scedosporium spp. may produce a wide variety of infections, including sinopulmonary infections, skin and soft tissue infections, septic arthritis, osteomyelitis, endocarditis, CNS infections, and ocular infections. *Scedosporium* spp. may colonize the damaged regions of lung, particularly patients with bronchiectasis (especially cystic fibrosis patients) and patients with previous mycobacterial infection and pulmonary cavities. Such colonization may be transient and may result in localized airway infection, the organisms may invade locally or extend deeply into surrounding tissue, or the infection may widely disseminate to distant regions of the body.

Imaging Findings

Radiologic manifestations of *pulmonary scedosporiosis* are nonspecific and include progressive, multifocal, often bilateral areas of consolidation that may have a nodular character. Cavitation may occur, but the air-crescent sign is less commonly seen with pulmonary scedosporiosis than with aspergillosis. In lung transplant recipients, *P. boydii* pulmonary infection may present with airway thickening, tree-in-bud opacities, patchy areas of ground-glass opacity, and mediastinal lymphadenopathy. These findings may closely resemble infection with more commonly encountered organisms, such as *Aspergillus* spp. *Scedosporium* spp. may produce mycetomas radiologically indistinguishable from mycetomas related to *Aspergillus* infection.

The diagnosis of scedosporiosis may be suggested by serology but usually depends on the identification of the organism by microscopy and culture. Treatment of *Scedosporium* spp. infections is difficult because these organisms are often resistant to the antifungal agents typically employed to treat the more commonly encountered *Aspergillus* infections. In particular, *S. prolificans* infection is associated with high mortality. Reversal of immunosuppression and surgical debridement is favored whenever possible.

Pneumocystis jirovecii (Pneumocystis carinii)

Pneumocystis jirovecii, previously known as *P. carinii*, was initially classified as a protozoan but is now thought to be a fungus. The organism exists as a cyst containing trophozoites, which may then be liberated to develop into cysts themselves.

Pneumocystis jirovecii pneumonia occurs almost exclusively in patients with underlying disease. Patients with AIDS are most vulnerable, with transplant recipients on immunosuppression and patients on low-dose corticosteroid therapy for vasculitis or connective tissue disorders also at risk. Patients with malignancies undergoing cytotoxic therapy are also at relatively increased risk for infection with *P. jirovecii*. *P. jirovecii* infection in the general population, as evidenced by the presence of IgG antibodies against the organism's surface antigens, is common and is usually asymptomatic in immunocompetent individuals.

Infection with *P. jirovecii* probably occurs as a result of the reactivation of a latent infection, occurring because of immunosuppression. Furthermore, the risk of developing infection with *P. jirovecii* increases with worsening immunosuppression. Exogenous sources of *P. jirovecii*, such as animal reservoirs, have been postulated but are considered unlikely, although documented outbreaks suggest that the infection can be transferred among susceptible individuals.

The development of clinically overt *P. jirovecii* infection is strongly related to CD4 lymphocyte function. In patients with AIDS, the risk of infection with *P. jirovecii* is low in patients with CD4 cell counts greater than 200 cells/μL, but the risk of infection increases substantially with CD4 counts below this level. Neutrophil and macrophage activity, as well as humoral immunity, also play some role in the pathogenesis of *P. jirovecii* infection.

Pneumocystis jirovecii infection causes alveolar inflammation with an eosinophilic exudate containing cysts and trophozoites as well as other material. Lymphocytes and plasma cells may also be present. The organisms are identifiable within the exudate when a sputum sample is obtained, either by sputum induction or with bronchial lavage. Hyaline membrane formation, interstitial edema, and type II pneumocyte hyperplasia are often present to a variable degree. *P. jirovecii* infection less commonly is associated with granulomatous inflammation, cyst formation, calcification, and interstitial fibrosis.

Infection usually presents with a variable duration of dyspnea on exertion, shortness of breath, a dry, nonproductive cough, and high fever; the duration of symptoms prior to diagnosis is typically longer with *P. jirovecii* pneumonia than bacterial pneumonia. Patients with AIDS who are infected with *P. jirovecii* are usually severely immunocompromised (CD4 cell count less than 200 cells/μL) and are usually not on trimethoprim-sulfamethoxazole prophylaxis. In the current era of combination antiretroviral therapy (ART), the risk of *P. jirovecii* pneumonia is low in HIV-infected individuals with CD4 cell counts between 100 and 200 cells/μL but with suppressed HIV RNA levels. Hypoxia is common in patients with *P. jirovecii* pneumonia, and serum levels of lactate dehydrogenase are often elevated.

Diagnosis is usually established with the demonstration of organisms on sputum induction. In patients at risk for infection with *P. jirovecii* but with negative sputum induction results, bronchoscopy with bronchial lavage usually establishes the diagnosis.

Imaging Findings

The earliest chest radiographic manifestation of *P. jirovecii* infection is bilateral perihilar ground-glass opacity or interstitial thickening (see Fig. 13.8) or poor definition of pulmonary vessels (Fig. 13.50A and C). Later, multifocal air-space consolidation may be present, particularly if the patient has been ill for some time. Pleural effusions are characteristically absent.

Some patients with AIDS and *P. jirovecii* infection develop cystic areas, termed pneumatoceles. Such pneumatoceles are characteristically thin walled and are usually found in the upper lobes. The presence of these lesions may predispose to the development of pneumothorax.

Atypical chest radiographic manifestations of *P. jirovecii* infection include an upper lobe distribution, focal consolidation, single or multiple nodules, cavitation of a nodule, lymphadenopathy, and pleural effusions. A normal chest radiograph occurs uncommonly in patients with AIDS and *P. jirovecii* infection.

CT, in particular HRCT, shows multifocal ground-glass opacity predominantly in a perihilar distribution (see Fig. 13.50B and D); HRCT shows this finding in all AIDS patients with this infection. Smooth interlobular septal thickening may be present, and foci of consolidation are often encountered. Pneumatoceles and pneumothorax may also be evident (Fig. 13.51). Patients with a granulomatous response to *P. jirovecii* infection may show small nodules in addition to ground-glass opacities. Rarely, evidence of fibrosis may be seen in patients who have recovered from *P. jirovecii* infection. Larger nodules or masses are occasionally seen (Table 13.18; see Fig. 10.35C in Chapter 10).

Mycoplasma, Chlamydia, and Rickettsiae Pneumonias

Mycoplasma pneumoniae

Mycoplasmas are the smallest free-living culturable organisms. They share some similarities with bacteria, but their lack of a cell wall and certain genetic features make them

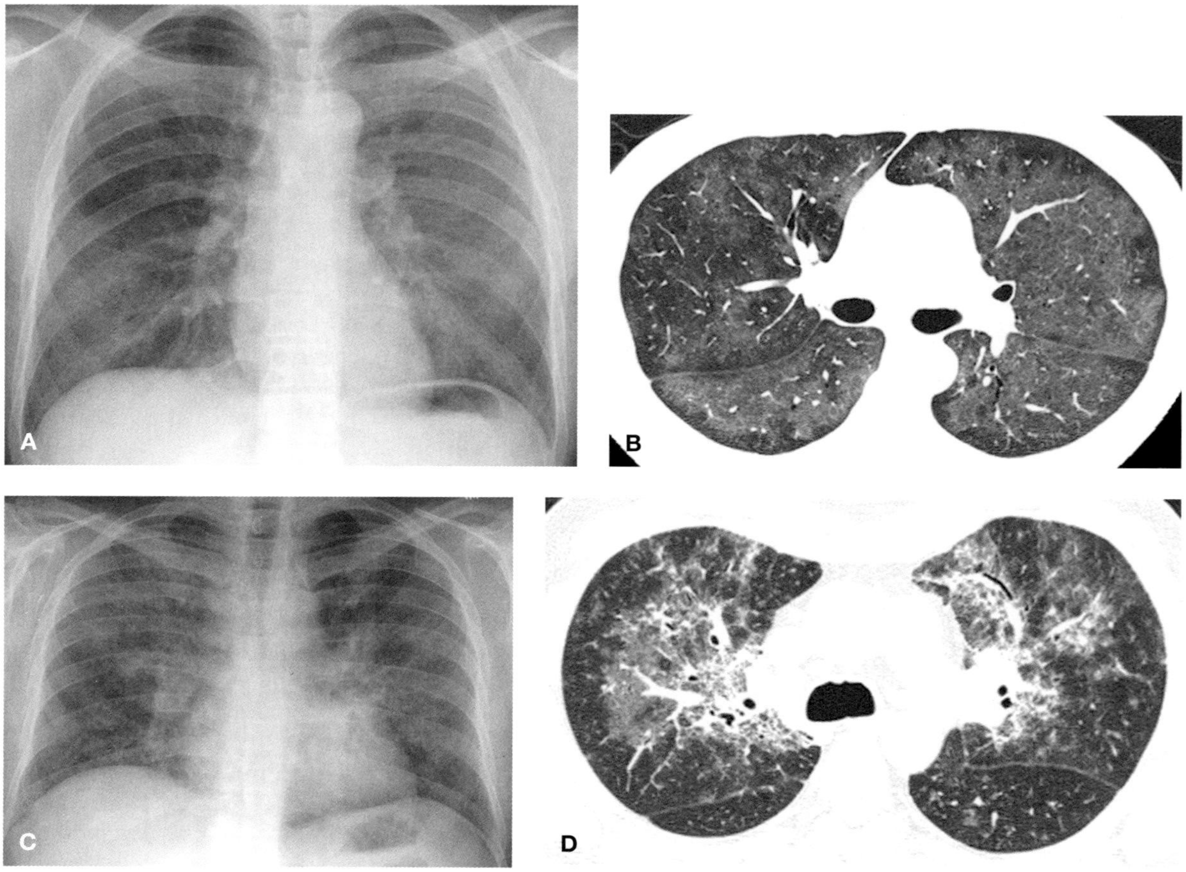

Figure 13.50. *Pneumocystis jirovecii* pneumonia in two patients. **A:** Chest radiograph shows subtle perihilar ground-glass opacity with poor definition of pulmonary vessels. **B:** HRCT shows diffuse, patchy ground-glass opacity typical of *Pneumocystis* pneumonia. The lung periphery is spared. This patient was being treated with immunosuppression for connective tissue disease and was not on appropriate prophylaxis. **C:** Chest radiograph shows perihilar ground-glass opacity, interstitial opacities, and poor definition of pulmonary vessels. **D:** HRCT shows perihilar ground-glass opacity and reticular opacities. The lung periphery is spared. This patient had AIDS with a CD-4 count of less than 200.

distinctly different than most bacteria. There are several distinct *Mycoplasma* spp., but *M. pneumoniae* is the most important from the human infectious disease standpoint.

Mycoplasma pneumoniae is a common cause of community-acquired pneumonia. *M. pneumoniae* pulmonary infection occurs mostly in younger patients, and infection is particularly common among families, military recruits, and other closed populations. Infection is transmitted by person-to-person contact and respiratory droplets; infection rates peak in the fall and winter.

Mycoplasma pneumoniae causes infection by both direct cytotoxicity and damage incurred from the host inflammatory response. A peribronchiolar mononuclear cell infiltrate is one of the more common pathologic findings, although neutrophilic infiltration, chronic inflammatory cell infiltration, fibrosis, diffuse alveolar damage, organizing pneumonia, and pulmonary hemorrhage are additional reported pathologic features.

Upper respiratory tract infectious symptoms may precede overt *M. pneumoniae* infection. Patients develop nonproductive cough, headache, malaise, and fever, somewhat resembling a viral infection, although unlike viral infections, arthralgias and myalgias are usually absent. Rarely, infection is severe, resulting in hypoxemic respiratory failure, particularly in patients with sickle cell disease. Superimposed bacterial infection occurs rarely.

Patients with *M. pneumoniae* may develop extrathoracic disease manifestations, including aseptic meningitis, encephalitis, and transverse myelitis (among other neurologic syndromes); hemolysis, venous thrombosis, pericarditis, and myocarditis; and skin rashes.

Imaging Findings

The earliest chest radiographic findings are commonly interstitial in appearance, consisting of fine linear opacities followed by segmental air-space consolidation. Occasionally,

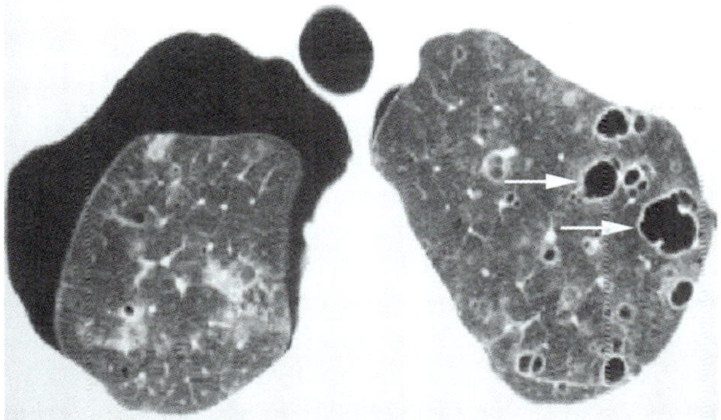

Figure 13.51. *Pneumocystis jirovecii* pneumonia with pneumatoceles and pneumothorax in an AIDS patient with a low CD4 cell count. Axial HRCT image shows numerous thin-walled cysts (*arrows*), representing pneumatoceles, surrounded by ground-glass opacity. Pneumothorax is present on the right side, likely due to rupture of a pneumatocele.

these patterns are seen separately rather than sequentially. Pleural effusion occurs in fewer than 20% of patients, and lymphadenopathy is uncommon.

CT scanning typically shows patchy, segmental, and lobular consolidation or ground-glass opacity (Fig. 13.52), sometimes associated with thickening of the perihilar interstitium. Mosaic perfusion may be seen due to small airway obstruction. Air trapping may be present on expiratory scans.

Chlamydia

Chlamydia spp. are obligate intracellular organisms that possess their own cell walls and share some other characteristics with other bacteria. They exist in an extracellular form known as elementary bodies and then change to reticular bodies once they enter a cell. Three *Chlamydia* spp. are important in the pathogenesis of human disease: *Chlamydia trachomatis*, *C. psittaci*, and *C. pneumoniae*.

Table 13.18 *Pneumocystis jirovecii* (*Pneumocystis carinii*)

- Associated with AIDS, with transplant recipients on immunosuppression, low-dose corticosteroid therapy, cytotoxic therapy for malignancy
- Associated with low CD4 count (<200)
- Shortness of breath; dry, nonproductive cough; and high fever
- Hypoxia, elevated lactate dehydrogenase level
- Radiographs and HRCT
  - Perihilar ground-glass opacity
  - Air-space consolidation may be present
  - Effusion rare
  - Pneumatoceles may develop
  - May present with pneumothorax
- HRCT is highly sensitive in AIDS patients
  - Ground-glass opacity visible in all patients

Chlamydia trachomatis

Chlamydia trachomatis infection usually causes a sexually transmitted disease, but an infant born through the birth canal of an infected patient may acquire pulmonary infection. Pathologically, *C. trachomatis* causes peribronchiolar inflammation, but few data regarding the pathologic appearance of *C. trachomatis* infection are available. Infants born to mothers infected with *C. trachomatis* may acquire pneumonia; such patients manifest disease shortly after birth, usually between 2 days and 2 weeks, and always by 6 months of age. Cough and tachypnea, often in the absence of significant fever, are common. Radiographs of infants infected with *C. trachomatis* often show multifocal air-space consolidation combined with interstitial opacities and areas of air trapping. Patchy areas of atelectasis are often seen.

Chlamydia psittaci

Chlamydia psittaci primarily infects birds. Humans usually acquire the disease from pigeons, parakeets, or poultry following the inhalation of dried bird excrement containing the organisms. Peribronchiolar mononuclear inflammatory cell infiltration that eventually extends into the alveoli is one of the most common pathologic findings of *C. psittaci* pneumonia. Hyaline membrane formation may occur. Patients with *C. psittaci* pneumonia usually present with fever, nonproductive cough, headache, fever, and chills. The illness is usually mild, with cases of overwhelming infection with hypoxemic respiratory failure occurring rarely.

Chest radiographs in patients with *C. psittaci* pneumonia may show perihilar linear opacities, air-space consolidation, and multifocal or diffuse ground-glass opacities. Hilar lymph node enlargement has been reported as a common finding on the radiographs of patients infected with *C. psittaci*.

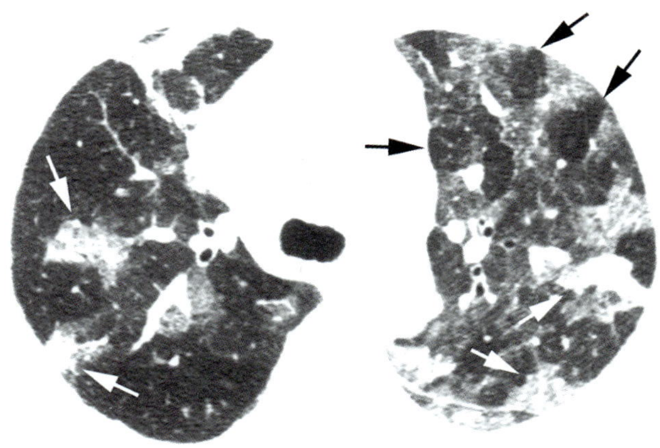

Figure 13.52. Mycoplasmal pneumonia. HRCT shows patchy, lobular areas of ground-glass opacity and consolidation (*white arrows*). Lobular lucencies (*black arrows*) reflect mosaic perfusion due to small airway abnormalities.

Chlamydia pneumoniae

Chlamydia pneumoniae is a fairly common cause of community-acquired pneumonia. The disease is rarely severe or fatal. Patients with *C. pneumoniae* pulmonary infection usually present with pharyngitis, fever, and nonproductive cough. The disease is usually self-limited.

The imaging appearances of *C. pneumoniae* pulmonary infection are nonspecific and include air-space consolidation, linear opacities simulating interstitial disease, or a combination of these findings. Pleural effusions occur in about one fifth of patients and may be moderate in size. The radiographic pattern of *C. pneumoniae* infection tends to progress to multilobar opacities over time.

Rickettsiae

Rickettsiae are small obligate intracellular organisms that cause disease when humans are bitten by the arthropods, often ticks, in which the organisms live. The *Rickettsia* that most commonly causes human pulmonary disease is *Coxiella burnetii*.

Coxiella burnetii causes Q fever. The organism usually lives in a variety of wild and domestic animals and insects, most notably ticks. Humans may acquire disease when bitten by the arthropod vector, although disease can be transmitted to humans by inhalation when humans come into contact with animals infected by the bacteria.

Few data regarding the pathologic appearance of Q fever are available. Interstitial and alveolar inflammation associated with hemorrhage, edema, and necrosis may occur.

Patients with Q fever present with fever, myalgia, malaise, headache, chills, nonproductive cough, and occasionally shortness of breath and chest pain. Extrathoracic disease manifestations, such as meningoencephalitis, myocarditis, venous thrombosis, and hepatitis, often occur.

Chest radiographs in patients with Q fever often show multifocal, bilateral, basilar predominant areas of consolidation that may be somewhat rounded. Segmental or lobar consolidation may also occur. Pleural effusions are uncommon. Areas of linear atelectasis may also be seen.

Viruses

The viruses that cause thoracic infection are usually transmitted from person to person by hand-to-hand contact, contact with infected surfaces, or aerosol transmission. Viral organisms may be deposited in the nasopharynx and cause upper respiratory infection only, although smaller organisms may be carried into the lungs, causing lower respiratory tract infections such as bronchitis, bronchiolitis, and pneumonia.

Viruses infect cells by interaction with various receptors on cell membranes. Once the virus enters the cell, the virus undergoes replication. This replication may kill the host cell, releasing more viruses to infect other cells. Alternatively, the viral replication may not kill the cell, but the virus continues to replicate within the cell and releases virions. In this situation, the infected cells may express viral antigens that may provoke a reaction from the host immune system. Last, viral infection may result in the virus incorporating itself into the DNA of the host cell, only to cause disease later upon reactivation of this latent infection.

Viral infections may be classified into the RNA virus group and the DNA virus group. RNA viruses that produce human infection include influenza virus, parainfluenza virus, hMPV, RSV, measles virus, coronaviruses, hantaviruses, togaviruses, reoviruses, picornaviruses, arenaviruses, and retroviruses. The DNA viruses that may result in human infection include herpesviruses, adenoviruses, papovaviruses, and poxviruses.

RNA Viruses

Influenza Virus

Worldwide, influenza is responsible for nearly 3 to 5 million severe respiratory illnesses and results in 250,000 to 500,000 deaths per year. Each year, according to the Centers for Disease Control, approximately more than 200,000 hospitalizations in the United States result from influenza and estimates of deaths related to influenza-related complications range from a low of 3000 to as many as 49,000 patients per year. Influenza occurs sporadically, in epidemics and in worldwide pandemics. Transmission of influenza virus occurs by respiratory aerosols and droplets. Although direct transmission from animals to humans may occur, it is generally not sustained.

Influenza outbreaks tend to occur in the winter. Patients at greatest risk for contracting disease include those with diabetes mellitus, COPD, chronic renal disease, cystic fibrosis or heart disease, the elderly, immunocompromised patients, and cigarette smokers.

Influenza viruses are divided into types A, B, and C. Type A is most often responsible for serious illnesses, and both epidemics and pandemics are almost exclusively caused by influenza A. Influenza A virus includes several subtypes, the most important of which, from the human disease perspective, are H1N1, the virus that was responsible for the 1918 flu pandemic and the pandemic H1N1/09 virus (also known as the novel H1N1 virus, antigenically distinct from human H1N1 influenza viruses circulating since 1977) responsible for the 2009 "swine flu" pandemic, first recognized in April of 2009; H2N2, the "Asian flu" virus (pandemic in 1957); H1N2, endemic in human and pig populations; H3N2, the cause of Hong Kong flu and seasonal flu (and pandemic in 1968); and the recently described H5N1 (emerged in Hong Kong in 1997) and H7N9 (emerged in Shanghai in March 2013) avian influenza viruses, so-called bird flu. Type B influenza tends to cause upper respiratory tract infections, and type C influenza causes sporadic, mild, lower respiratory tract infections. Influenza pulmonary infection causes hemorrhagic and edematous consolidation with diffuse alveolar damage and an associated mononuclear cell inflammatory infiltrate. Infection with influenza renders the host more susceptible to superinfection, usually with bacteria such as pneumococci and staphylococci. Such superinfection may prove fatal.

Influenza A H1N1 infection presents with dry cough, headache, myalgia, low-grade fever, and conjunctivitis. Young children may present with croup or otitis media. When overt pulmonary infection occurs, symptoms of bronchitis occur, followed shortly by signs of severe illness, including cyanosis, hypoxemia, shortness of breath, and chest pain. Bacterial superinfection may be heralded by the onset of purulent cough and worsening fever and chest pain, often in a patient who was improving.

The clinical features of influenza A H1N1/09 infection are similar to influenza A H1N1 infection, although vomiting and diarrhea may be more common among swine flu patients. Fever and cough are the most common symptoms, with shortness of breath, fatigue, weakness, chills, and myalgias occurring less commonly, in descending frequency. In contrast to seasonal flu (influenza A H1N1), in which the greatest fatality rate is seen in patients older than 65 years, the risk of death from swine flu is highest in younger patients, particularly those aged 25 to 49 years.

Chest radiography in patients with influenza A H1N1 often shows multifocal patchy consolidation that may be unilateral or bilateral. When unilateral, the pulmonary opacities may rapidly progress to bilateral disease. Pleural effusion is relatively uncommon. CT and HRCT may show multifocal, patchy air-space consolidation and ground-glass opacities. Imaging findings are usually nonspecific and resemble noncardiogenic pulmonary edema.

Patients infected with influenza A H1N1/09 (swine flu) may have normal chest radiographs, although some patients will show multifocal, commonly bilateral, central, and lower lung predominant areas of consolidation; pleural effusion is uncommon and lymphadenopathy is typically not seen. Thoracic CT studies in patients infected with influenza A H1N1/09 have been reported to show patchy areas of rounded ground-glass opacity, even in patients with normal chest radiographs; consolidation may be present as well. A peribronchovascular and peripheral distribution of parenchymal infiltration may be encountered. Severely ill patients infected with influenza H1N1/09, particularly those admitted to the intensive care unit, may have an elevated prevalence of pulmonary embolism, and radiographic abnormalities in these patients are typically extensive. Thoracic CT images from four patients with swine flu infection are shown in Figure 13.53. The images show a variable appearance for influenza A H1N1/09 respiratory infection, including patchy areas of ground-glass opacity, small poorly defined centrilobular nodules and bronchial wall thickening resembling other causes of bronchopneumonia, and areas of dense consolidation. It is possible that the thoracic imaging appearances of swine flu will be influenced by the presence or absence of other underlying medical conditions as well as the duration of infection prior to imaging.

Parainfluenza Virus

Parainfluenza viruses are classified into types 1 through 4. Types 1, 2, and 3 are responsible for the majority of human disease. Parainfluenza virus types 1 and 2 usually cause outbreaks of croup or acute bronchiolitis in young children, usually in the fall and winter. Parainfluenza type 3 may cause pneumonia and acute bronchiolitis in infants and children, often in the spring. Parainfluenza viral infections are usually self-limited.

Because parainfluenza viral infection is usually self-limited, little information regarding the pathologic characteristics of infection is available. Infection with parainfluenza virus does render the host more susceptible to bacterial superinfection.

In children, parainfluenza viral infection usually results in croup or, less commonly, acute bronchiolitis. Symptoms of parainfluenza viral acute bronchiolitis include coughing, dyspnea, and wheezing; physical examination may disclose crackles. Parainfluenza viral infection in adults usually causes tonsillitis and pharyngitis. Lower respiratory tract infection by a parainfluenza viral infection is rare in adults.

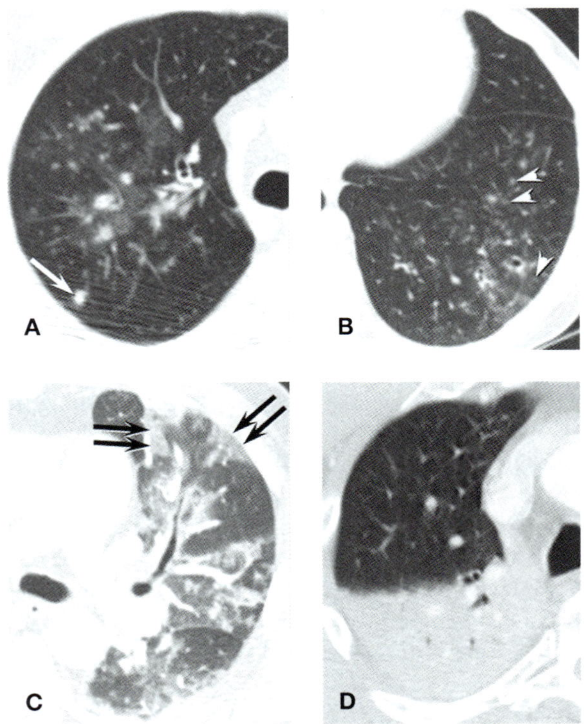

Figure 13.53. Thoracic CT findings of influenza A H1N1/09 (swine flu) respiratory infection in four patients. **A:** Patchy, faintly lobular ground-glass opacity and small solid nodules (*arrow*). **B:** Small, poorly defined ground-glass opacity centrilobular nodules (*arrowheads*) associated with airway thickening and peribronchial opacity, resembling other causes of community-acquired bronchopneumonia. **C:** More extensive disease, including areas of lobular and peribronchial ground-glass opacity (*double arrows*). **D:** Posterior dependent dense consolidation. (Images courtesy of Brett M. Elicker MD, Department of Radiology and Biomedical Imaging, University of California, San Francisco.)

Radiographs in children with croup may show smooth subglottic tracheal narrowing, the so-called "steeple" sign. Acute bronchiolitis may manifest as a combination of multifocal atelectasis and areas of air trapping. HRCT may more effectively demonstrate these findings but is rarely indicated unless the patient is immunocompromised and the diagnosis is not straightforward. When parainfluenza virus pneumonia occurs, radiographs are often normal or may show only vague ground-glass opacity or interstitial prominence. HRCT reveals multifocal ground-glass opacity in many patients.

Respiratory Syncytial Virus

RSV is an important cause of both upper and lower respiratory tract diseases in infants and young children. Sporadic infection may occur, but outbreaks often occur in schools or nurseries. Infection is transmitted by respiratory droplets or hand-to-hand contact, often in the winter. Infants with congenital heart disease, immunodeficiency, or pulmonary bronchodysplasia are at particularly high risk.

RSV may cause direct bronchiolar and pulmonary parenchymal damage, although hypersensitivity may also contribute to the pathogenesis of infection. The size of the viral inoculum may also play a role in the pathogenesis of RSV bronchiolar and pulmonary parenchymal infection. In children, RSV typically causes upper respiratory tract symptoms such as pharyngitis, rhinitis, and otitis media. Lower respiratory tract infection produces coughing, dyspnea, wheezing, and intercostal retractions. Physical examination may reveal crackles.

In adults, RSV usually causes symptoms of common cold, and lower respiratory tract infection is rare. When the latter occurs, it usually affects chronically ill, debilitated, elderly, or immunocompromised patients (especially hematopoietic stem cell transplant recipients) and produces symptoms suggestive of pneumonia. Respiratory failure resulting from ARDS may occur.

Chest radiographs in patients with RSV infection commonly show perihilar linear opacities, bronchial wall thickening, patchy areas of consolidation, and areas of air trapping (see Fig. 13.2). Often, the radiographic findings seem unimpressive in comparison to the patient's clinical presentation. Hilar lymphadenopathy may occur in a few patients. HRCT may show patchy areas of ground-glass opacity and interstitial thickening (Fig. 13.54).

Human Metapneumovirus

hMPV is a negative-sense nonsegmented RNA virus of the pneumovirus subfamily, family Paramyxoviridae. hMPV is a recently recognized respiratory pathogen of the paramyxovirus family, although the virus has probably been responsible for human infection for at least 50 years. Initially described in infants in the Netherlands, hMPV is now recognized as a common cause of upper and lower respiratory tract infections worldwide, primarily in infants and young children and those greater than 65 years of age, but the virus may affect patients of practically any age. Patients with malignancy, COPD, and immunocompromised patients are at greater risk for hMPV respiratory infection. In children, additional risk factors for hMPV include congenital heart disease, chronic lung disease, organ or stem cell transplantation, and prematurity. hMPV infection is the second leading identifiable cause of lower respiratory tract infection in children of all age groups, second only to RSV.

The pathophysiology of respiratory infection with hMPV resembles RSV infection. The rate of infection with hMPV peaks in late winter and early spring in the United States, whereas peak infection rates in tropical regions occur during the spring and summer months.

The clinical features of hMPV infection range from asymptomatic to severe pneumonia. The clinical presentation of most symptomatic patients resembles RSV infection, with typical symptoms including rhinorrhea, cough, dyspnea, tachypnea, myalgia, fever, and wheezing. In severe cases, particularly immunosuppressed patients, hypoxemic respiratory failure may occur. Coinfection with other respiratory pathogens may occur, but it is unclear if disease severity is related to such coinfection.

The chest radiographic appearance of hMPV respiratory tract infection is indistinguishable from other forms of viral bronchitis or community-acquired pneumonia. Thoracic CT and HRCT may show multifocal, patchy, bilateral, ground-glass opacity, and small nodular opacities. Air-space consolidation is present in less than half of patients.

hMPV infection can be difficult to identify during routine virologic procedures performed on nasal washes, swabs, endotracheal tube aspirates, or bronchoalveolar lavage fluid. Commercial tests to identify the presence of hMPV are available, including reverse transcriptase polymerase chain reaction, enzyme-linked immunosorbent assays, and shell vial amplification.

Treatment of hMPV infection is supportive, including hydration, supplemental oxygen, and mechanical ventilation

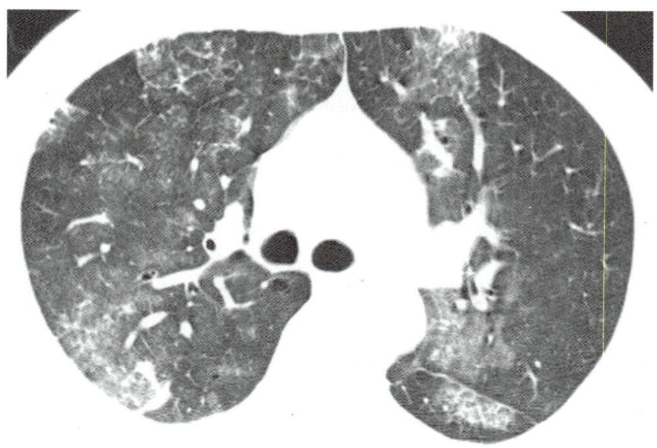

Figure 13.54. Respiratory syncytial virus pneumonia in an adult. HRCT shows patchy ground-glass opacity associated with interstitial thickening. Interlobular septal thickening is visible.

as necessary. Clinical trials of anti-hMPV monoclonal antibodies for the prevention of hMPV infection in high-risk infants are underway.

Measles (Rubeola) Virus

The incidence of measles infection has been dramatically reduced in recent years due to the introduction of immunization programs. Epidemics, particularly in underdeveloped countries, are still a problem. Adults may rarely contract the disease, possibly from lack of exposure to the infection during childhood.

Measles classically produces giant cell pneumonia, manifest as multinucleated giant cells containing viral inclusions infiltrating the alveoli and bronchial epithelium. Giant cell pneumonia is characteristic of measles but may also be seen with parainfluenza and RSV infections.

Patients with measles viral infection initially usually present with fever, myalgia, headache, conjunctivitis, cough, and rhinorrhea followed by the characteristic skin rash. Measles pneumonia develops either before or at the onset of the skin rash and presents with worsening cough and dyspnea. Bacterial superinfection may occur with measles infection, usually after the patient has begun to improve clinically, and presents with worsening purulent cough, fever, and chest pain.

Measles pneumonia usually manifests on chest radiography as bilateral patchy air-space consolidation associated with perihilar linear opacities, bronchial wall thickening, and small nodules. Radiographs in children may show lymph node enlargement, but radiographs in adults usually do not. CT of measles pneumonia may show multifocal ground-glass opacity and consolidation, often with small nodular opacities.

Coronaviruses

Until 2002, coronaviruses were considered relatively unimportant respiratory pathogens, causing primarily mild upper respiratory tract ailments such as coryza and pharyngitis. However, in the fall of 2002, a new respiratory illness, known as Severe Acute Respiratory Syndrome (SARS), emerged in southern China. The disease rapidly spread worldwide, eventually affecting 29 countries. By the end of the outbreak in 2003, 8098 cases of SARS had been reported, with 774 deaths, equating to a case fatality rate of just under 10%. The outbreak was declared contained by late 2003. The source of the SARS outbreak is thought to have been from the civet cat.

In 2012, another coronavirus named Middle East Respiratory Syndrome (MERS) emerged, mainly in the Arabian Peninsula and caused severe respiratory illness with a high fatality rate.

Then, in late 2019, a novel coronavirus, SARS-CoV-2, emerged and led to the global pandemic of coronavirus disease 2019 (COVID-19). This virus has caused an unprecedented impact on global health and economies. As of the end of 2022, COVID-19 has affected millions of people worldwide, with a significantly higher number of cases and deaths compared to the SARS and MERS outbreaks. The disease presents with a range of symptoms, from mild respiratory illness to severe pneumonia and death, with older adults and those with underlying health conditions at higher risk for severe disease.

The World Health Organization (WHO) and other health agencies have set criteria for defining and diagnosing COVID-19 cases. Similar to SARS, COVID-19 cases can be categorized based on clinical symptoms, exposure history, and laboratory testing. Radiographic evidence, particularly from chest CT scans, has been an essential tool for assessing the severity of respiratory involvement in COVID-19. Patients affected by COVID-19 span all age groups, with no definite gender predilection, and include both individuals with underlying chronic illnesses and those who were previously healthy. The rapid development and distribution of vaccines have been critical in the fight against COVID-19.

Imaging Findings

Radiographic abnormalities in patients with SARS typically begin to appear about 12 days after viral exposure (range, 4-26 days) or about 5 days after the onset of fever. The abnormalities observed in SARS consist of poorly marginated consolidation which may start focally and remain unilateral or become multifocal and bilateral. The abnormalities tend to have a lower lobe predominant location and peripheral distribution. Lymphadenopathy is not a feature, and pleural effusions are rare. Radiographic resolution may lag behind clinical improvement. Volume loss and scarring have been reported in a few patients.

The HRCT findings of SARS include lower lobe predominant ground-glass opacity associated with thickening of the interlobular septa, occasionally with consolidation. A peripheral distribution of the opacities is common. Nearly half of patients undergoing HRCT for SARS show fibrosis, including architectural distortion, traction bronchiectasis, and coarse linear opacities.

Middle East Respiratory Syndrome Coronavirus (MERS-CoV) was identified in 2012 and has since caused several outbreaks, primarily in the Middle East. Chest radiographic findings in MERS-CoV infection include patchy, peripheral ground-glass opacity and consolidation, favoring the lower lungs. Thoracic CT findings in MERS-CoV infection are also nonspecific and resemble organizing pneumonia.

Imaging features of COVID-19 center on an inflammatory reaction to the virus, often stimulating a response of organizing pneumonia and sequela of acute lung injury. Therefore, the imaging findings in COVID-19 overlap with other coronaviruses and viruses such as influenza as well as other pathologies including drug reaction (Fig. 13.55). The Radiological Society of North America (RSNA) published a consensus to categorize the imaging appearance of COVID-19: (1) typical appearance including peripheral and bilateral ground glass opacities, crazy paving,

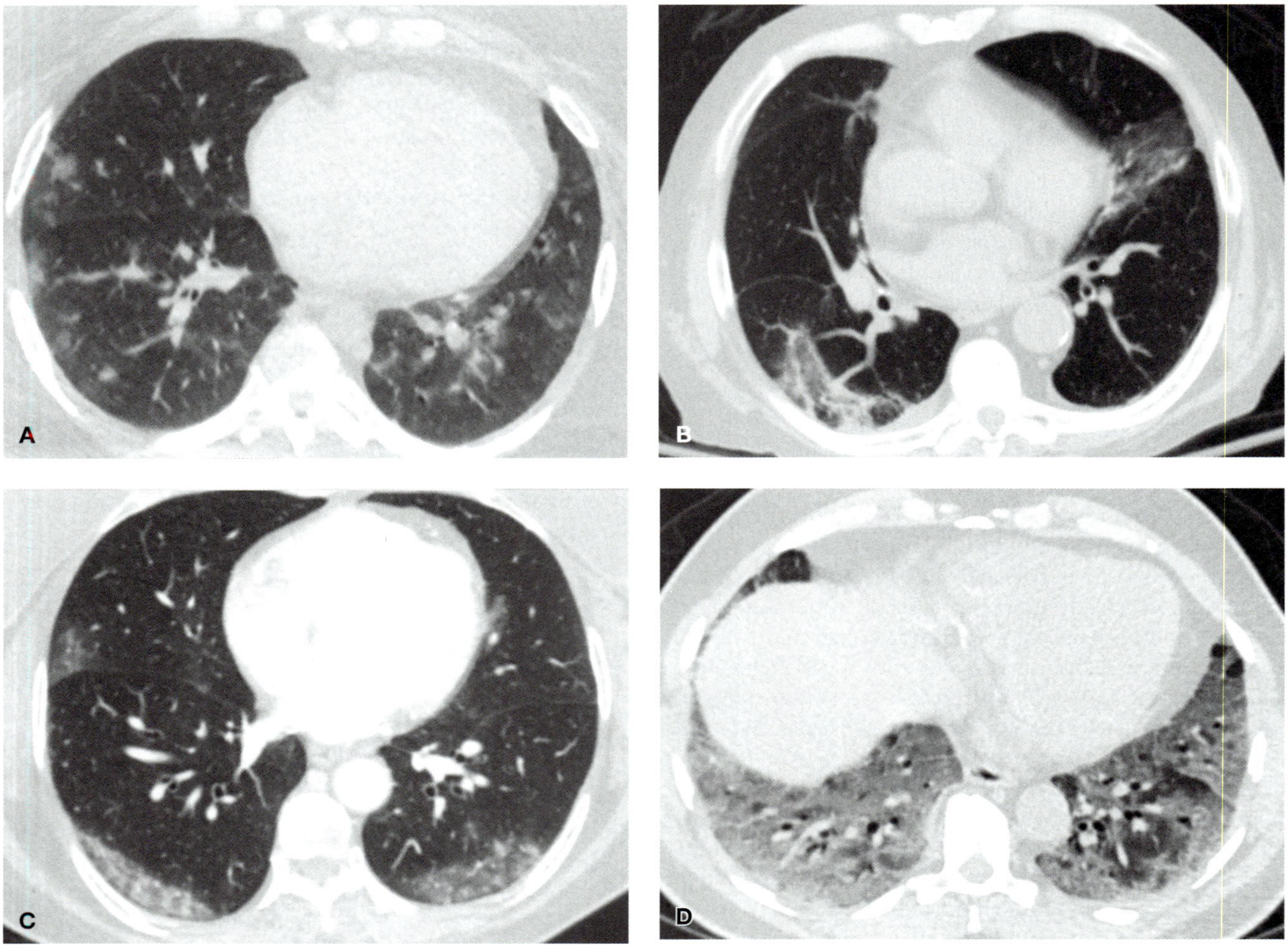

Figure 13.55. CT findings of COVID-19 pneumonia in four patients. **A:** Bilateral ground-glass nodules. **B:** Bilateral peripheral and peribronchovascular ground-glass opacities. **C:** Peripheral ground-glass opacities. **D:** Confluent ground-glass opacities and traction bronchiectasis indicative of more severe disease.

and organizing pneumonia; (2) indeterminate appearance including absence of typical features and presence of diffuse, unilateral, or multifocal ground glass opacities without consolidation, (3) atypical appearance including isolated consolidation, discrete micronodules, smooth interlobular septal thickening with pleural effusions, and lung cavitation, (4) negative for pneumonia without CT features to suggest pneumonia.

In addition, imaging features of COVID-19 evolve over the progression of the virus. Over time, ground-glass opacities will become more extensive and areas of consolidation will develop, peaking around days 9 to 13 after symptoms present. Gradually, the consolidation will decrease, and crazy paving may be more prevalent. Depending on the degree of acute lung injury and severity of the inflammatory response, the opacities can become more reticular, and features of fibrosis may evolve with traction bronchiectasis and architectural distortion. Besides demonstrating the progression of disease and prognosis, radiology has been utilized to detect other thoracic complications of COVID-19 including ARDS, superimposed pneumonia, pulmonary embolism, and myocarditis.

Hantaviruses

There are several antigenically different hantaviruses known to cause human disease, such as hemorrhagic fever with renal syndrome and the hantavirus pulmonary syndrome. The natural reservoir of hantaviruses is rodents, in particular the deer mouse. Hantavirus pulmonary syndrome is most commonly encountered in rural areas, especially in the Southwestern United States. Human disease is acquired by the inhalation of dried rodent excrement containing the virus.

Hantavirus infection causes both interstitial and air-space edema accompanied by lymphocytic infiltration, but with little evidence of vascular thrombosis or hyaline membrane formation.

Patients with hantavirus pulmonary syndrome present with fever, myalgia, and headache that progress to worsening cough, shortness of breath, and then hypotension

Hypoxemic respiratory failure may occur. The death rate approaches 50%.

Chest radiographic findings of hantavirus pulmonary syndrome include peribronchiolar thickening, perihilar indistinctness, and interlobular septal thickening. Air-space consolidation may also be encountered. For patients who do not present with air-space consolidation on the initial chest radiograph, subsequent films may show developing consolidation. Pleural effusions occur in more than half of patients and may be large.

Togaviruses (Rubella)

Rubella is the only significant togavirus from a human respiratory infection viewpoint. Infants born to mothers infected with rubella during the first trimester may develop congenital anomalies. The teratogenic effects of congenital rubella infection include pulmonary abnormalities such as pulmonary artery stenoses and interstitial pneumonitis.

Infants born with pulmonary arterial stenoses from congenital rubella infection may be largely asymptomatic or they may develop pulmonary hypertension and right heart failure. Interstitial pneumonitis related to congenital rubella infection may be mild or may produce fulminant respiratory failure.

DNA Viruses

Herpesviruses

Numerous antigenically different types of herpesviruses are known to exist, but herpesvirus types 1, 2, 6, 8, varicella-zoster virus, cytomegalovirus (CMV), and Epstein–Barr virus (EBV) are the most important from the standpoint of human diseases.

Herpesviruses infect patients and incorporate themselves into the cell of the host, and there they may remain latent for the lifetime of the individual. On occasion, particularly when the host becomes immunocompromised, the herpes infection reactivates and causes clinically overt disease. While reactivation episodes are usually minor, they may become quite significant in immunocompromised patients.

Herpes Simplex Herpes simplex virus type 1 (HSV-1) and herpes simplex virus type 2 (HSV-2) infections usually cause mucosal ulcerations following the reactivation of latent infection.

HSV-1 infection is often acquired during childhood and usually affects the oral cavity. Following the reactivation of latent disease, lower respiratory tract infection may occur if the organisms are transported into the trachea and bronchi, as could occur with aspiration or endotracheal intubation. However, overt oral cavity infection is not always present, implying that other mechanisms are operative. Patients with HSV-1 infection of the trachea and bronchi are often severely immunocompromised. Tracheobronchial involvement is suggested by the presence of fever and productive cough, occasionally in the presence of the oral ulcerative lesions. Symptoms of HSV-1 pneumonia are nonspecific. Chest radiographs may show multifocal consolidation due to bronchopneumonia. CT and HRCT also show patchy, multifocal ground-glass opacity and consolidation, often associated with small nodules.

HSV-2 pulmonary infection is acquired during birth as the fetus passes through the infected maternal birth canal. The newborn may present with fever, jaundice, seizure, and signs of pneumonia. Radiographs may show patchy air-space consolidation, usually without effusions.

HSV-6 causes roseola (a childhood skin infection). Pulmonary disease is exceedingly rare, usually occurring in immunocompromised patients.

HSV-8 (also called Kaposi's sarcoma-associated herpesvirus) has been implicated in the pathogenesis of both Kaposi's sarcoma and primary effusion lymphoma (previously known as body cavity-based lymphoma). Primary effusion lymphoma presents with fluid accumulation in body cavities, especially the pleural space and peritoneal cavity. Primary effusion lymphoma tends to present in patients with AIDS and a low CD4 cell count; shortness of breath is commonly present, and the pleural effusions may be quite large. Kaposi's sarcoma is discussed in Chapter 6.

Varicella-Zoster Virus Hematogenous dissemination of the varicella virus develops soon after the organism is inhaled, and the organism subsequently invades the respiratory epithelium. Viral replication eventually results in a second viremic episode, which causes skin eruption. If pneumonia occurs, the virus will induce diffuse alveolar damage and produce giant cell pneumonia.

Varicella represents the initial varicella-zoster infection in previously uninfected patients, also called chickenpox. Varicella is a very contagious skin infection that usually affects children. About one in six patients with skin infection caused by varicella develops coincident pulmonary infection; this figure is higher for patients ill enough to be admitted to the hospital or for immunocompromised patients. Zoster, also known as shingles, represents the reactivation of a latent herpes varicella-zoster infection. Pulmonary infection may occur with either form of herpes varicella-zoster, although it is more commonly seen with varicella. Varicella pneumonia presents as high fever that is usually rapidly followed by a painful skin rash. Chest pain, nonproductive cough, and shortness of breath are common. Radiographic abnormalities often persist after clinical improvement.

Varicella pneumonia appears on chest radiography as diffuse small nodules in the range of 5 to 10 mm that progress to air-space consolidation rather rapidly. Hilar lymphadenopathy is common, but pleural effusion is rare. Radiographic clearing of pulmonary opacities may take weeks or months. Some patients develop multiple, bilateral small calcified pulmonary nodules measuring 2 to 3 mm without hilar lymph node calcification.

Cytomegalovirus

Congenital CMV infection may occur by transplacental spread of the organism, or neonatal infection may occur when the fetus passes through an infected birth canal.

Acquired infection with CMV is very common; infection is usually asymptomatic. Pulmonary infection with CMV is usually significant only in patients with impaired immunity. Cell-mediated immunity is particularly important in defense against CMV infection. Clinically overt CMV infection usually occurs as a result of reactivation of latent disease, although reinfection from an endogenous source can occur.

CMV infection may cause direct cellular damage, although the host reaction to infection also contributes to the infectious process. Nevertheless, it is clear that in most patients from whom CMV is isolated, the organism is not a primary pulmonary pathogen. When CMV infects cells, it often produces a characteristic pattern of intranuclear inclusions that fill most of the nucleus and are separated from the remaining nuclear membrane by a characteristic halo, resulting in the so-called owl-eye appearance.

Congenital CMV infection presents with hepatosplenomegaly, jaundice, chorioretinitis, microcephaly, seizures, and thrombocytopenic purpura; mental retardation often results. Neonatal CMV infection, acquired through maternal transmission from an infected birth canal, is often asymptomatic.

CMV infection acquired in childhood or adulthood is often asymptomatic or presents with low-grade fever, lymphadenopathy, and organomegaly.

In immunocompromised patients, CMV infection presents with nonproductive cough, fever, and shortness of breath. CMV pneumonia is a very common cause of infectious pneumonia in hematopoietic stem cell transplant patients and has a high mortality if untreated. In this context, the risk of infection is highest between 30 and 90 days following transplant, although late-onset (>180 days) CMV infections are encountered with increasing frequency. Diagnosis rests on demonstrating the presence of the organism and viral inclusions, usually with associated tissue damage, to prove that CMV is the culprit organism, or by quantitative polymerase chain reaction detection in serum or bronchoalveolar lavage fluid.

Imaging Findings CMV infection usually occurs in the setting of impaired immunity. Chest radiographic findings associated with CMV infection include bilateral reticulation or interstitial opacities, diffuse ground-glass opacities, or multifocal consolidation; chest radiographs may be normal (Fig. 13.56). Diffuse, small nodules are a less common pattern of infection with CMV, and lobar consolidation in CMV infection is uncommon. Bilateral opacities are more commonly encountered than unilateral disease.

CT may reveal multifocal, bilateral areas of ground-glass opacity and foci of air-space consolidation, occasionally accompanied by small centrilobular nodules (see Fig. 13.56; see also Fig. 11.31B in Chapter 11). Small pleural effusions are encountered in less than half of the patients, and lymphadenopathy is infrequent.

Epstein–Barr Virus

EBV infects B lymphocytes and cells lining the pharynx. Direct person-to-person transmission is most common, although spread via blood transfusions may also occur.

EBV causes infectious mononucleosis, which presents as hepatosplenomegaly, lymphadenopathy, pharyngitis, and fever. When intrathoracic involvement occurs, lymphadenopathy is the most common manifestation; interstitial pneumonia may occur but is rare.

Patients with infectious mononucleosis present with fever, malaise, weakness, a minimally productive cough, and pharyngitis. One of the most compelling physical examination findings of infectious mononucleosis is splenomegaly.

EBV is an important pathogen in the pathogenesis of lymphoproliferative disorders, especially Burkitt's lymphoma, lymphomas in patients with AIDS, and posttransplant lymphoproliferative disease.

Adenoviruses

Sporadic adenoviral infection is not an uncommon cause of respiratory infection in childhood. Epidemic outbreaks of adenoviral infection have been reported in military recruits and other situations in which the living quarters are close.

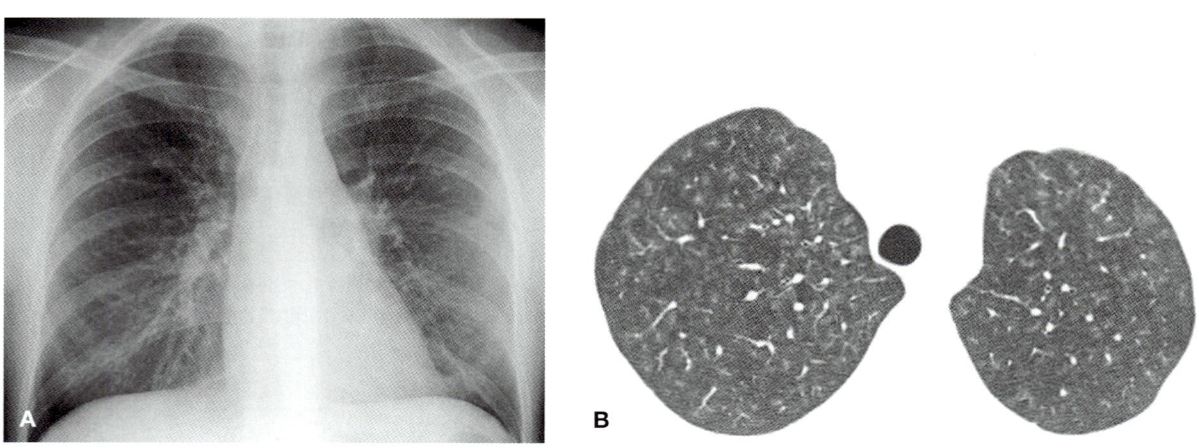

Figure 13.56. Cytomegalovirus infection in an immunosuppressed patient. **A:** Chest radiograph is normal. **B:** Axial CT image shows multiple small centrilobular areas of ground-glass opacity.

Adenoviral infection causes bronchitis and bronchiolitis that, in severe cases, progresses to hemorrhagic bronchopneumonia with edema and hyaline membranes.

Adenoviral infection usually presents with pharyngoconjunctival fever, myalgia, malaise, and cough; tracheitis and bronchitis may be present as well. Disease is usually mild, but rare cases of hypoxemic respiratory failure occur. As discussed previously, adenoviral infection may result in bronchiectasis and bronchiolitis obliterans, including Swyer–James syndrome.

Adenoviral pneumonia may present on chest radiography with multifocal, bilateral bronchopneumonia associated with air trapping. In one of the largest series detailing the chest radiographic appearance of adenoviral infection, lobar collapse was a common event; the right upper lobe was particularly commonly involved. Resolution of infection may be complete but occasionally results in pulmonary scarring, especially when infection occurs in patients under the age of 2 years.

Parasites: Protozoans, Roundworms (Nematodes), and Flatworms

Amebiasis

Amebiasis is caused by the protozoan *Entamoeba histolytica*. The organism usually causes amebic dysentery, with pulmonary disease occurring as a complication of colon or liver disease.

Amebic dysentery is most prevalent in underdeveloped countries, where transmission of the organism from person to person occurs by the fecal–oral route. In the United States, many cases of amebic dysentery occur in immigrants who have been in the United States for only a short time. Pulmonary amebiasis is far more common in men and usually occurs in young to middle-aged adults.

The life cycle of *E. histolytica* begins with the host-ingesting cysts in contaminated food or water. The cyst form of the organism is acid-resistant, so it is capable of passing through the stomach and into the small intestine unharmed. Once in the small intestine, *E. histolytica* excysts and forms trophozoites, which then migrate to the colon. From there, organisms may be passed in feces to complete the life cycle of the organism.

The organisms may be transported to the liver, where an amebic abscess may form; such abscesses are almost always located in the cranial portion of the liver, usually in the right lobe. From there, direct transdiaphragmatic spread of infection may cause pleural effusion or lung abscess formation. Very rarely, pulmonary or pleural infection forms in the absence of a liver abscess by the extension of the organisms through the hemorrhoidal veins, the transdiaphragmatic lymphatics or the thoracic duct, or the hepatic veins.

Patients with pulmonary or pleural amebic abscesses usually present with right upper quadrant pain, fever, and cough. Chest pain may also be present. Patients may also expectorate the characteristic "anchovy paste" or "chocolate sauce" material that usually represents amebic abscesses. Rarely, biloptysis occurs. Gastrointestinal symptoms are often, but not invariably, present.

Amebic pulmonary infection usually presents as lower lobe air-space consolidation, usually on the right, often accompanied by a pleural effusion (Fig. 13.57). The latter may be quite large. Cavitation within the consolidation may occur. Amebic abscesses in the liver, uncomplicated by pulmonary abscesses, often cause elevation of the right diaphragm with basilar atelectasis; a small pleural effusion may be present.

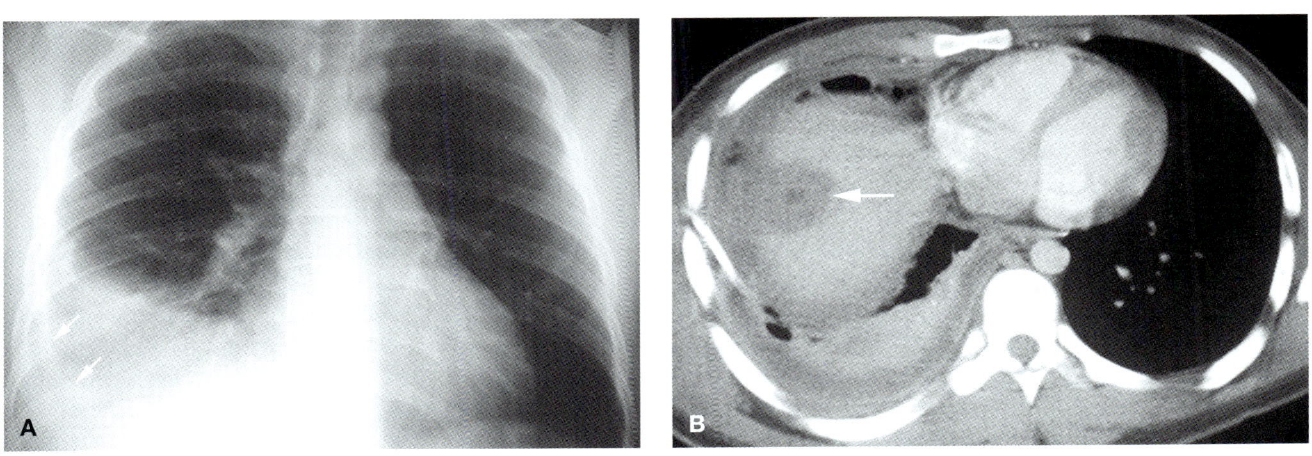

Figure 13.57. Amebic pneumonia and liver abscess. **A:** Frontal chest radiograph shows right lower lobe pneumonia and right pleural effusion (*arrows*), initially interpreted as community-acquired pneumonia and parapneumonic effusion. The patient's symptoms and the radiographic abnormalities failed to resolve with therapy directed toward community-acquired pneumonia. **B:** Axial CT image through the cranial aspect of the liver shows right lower lobe consolidation and a low-attenuation lesion within the liver (*arrow*).

Toxoplasmosis

Toxoplasmosis is caused by the protozoan *Toxoplasma gondii*. *T. gondii* is an intracellular protozoan that commonly causes human infection, although such infections are often not clinically apparent. *T. gondii* is distributed worldwide. Human infection is extremely common but usually asymptomatic.

The organism's definitive host is the cat, and mice or rats may serve as an intermediate host. Humans acquire disease when they ingest the oocyte form of the parasite in contaminated water or food or in undercooked meat. Once ingested, the oocyte excysts and forms trophozoites, which may cross the intestine and disseminate through the bloodstream. The trophozoites usually travel to the heart, skeletal muscle, and brain most commonly, where they may remain viable and cause infection when the host becomes immunocompromised. *T. gondii* can also be transmitted from women to their fetuses by the transplacental route.

Most infections caused by *T. gondii* are asymptomatic. When symptoms are present, they most often include low-grade fever and lymphadenopathy; the presentation somewhat resembles mononucleosis. Immunocompromised patients may develop disseminated disease; when *T. gondii* pneumonia occurs in this setting, fever, dry cough, and shortness of breath may be encountered. Neurologic symptoms, due to *T. gondii* brain infection, may occur.

Overt pulmonary infection in patients without impaired immunity is uncommon. Chest radiographs may show bilateral linear opacities suggesting an interstitial process, perhaps accompanied by hilar lymphadenopathy. HRCT will reveal patchy areas of ground-glass opacity, possibly with some foci of consolidation.

Ascariasis

Ascaris lumbricoides is a nematode (roundworm) that causes the majority of cases of the infection known as ascariasis. *A. suum* may also cause this infection.

Ascaris lumbricoides infection is acquired by the ingestion of food or water contaminated by the worm's ova. The larval forms of the worm develop within the ovum inside the small intestine of the host. Once the larval forms hatch, they may burrow through the wall of the small intestine to reach the portal venous circulation. The larvae may then migrate to the pulmonary capillary circulation and then into the alveoli. From there, the larvae may migrate into the proximal airways and into the larynx, where they are swallowed. Eventually, they reach the small intestine and develop into adult worms, where they may produce eggs that are passed in the feces to complete the worm's life cycle. *A. lumbricoides* infection is most commonly encountered in Southeast Asia, Africa, and Central and South America. However, infection does occur in the United States, especially in the southeastern region.

Although the worms can be comparatively large (often over 30 cm in length), *A. lumbricoides* infection is usually asymptomatic. Most patients who experience symptoms develop gastrointestinal complaints. As the worms migrate through the lungs, they can cause bronchopneumonia, producing symptoms of chest pain, shortness of breath, cough, and hemoptysis.

When pulmonary infection is present, air-space consolidation is usually encountered. Pneumonia may be caused by the migration of the larvae or by vomiting with aspiration. Often, the air-space opacities are transient.

Strongyloidiasis

Strongyloides stercoralis is the nematode (roundworm) that causes most cases of strongyloidiasis. *S. stercoralis* infection is endemic in tropical areas, although infection does occur in the United States. Immunocompromised patients, particularly those with AIDS, are at increased risk.

Human infection with *S. stercoralis* begins with larvae penetrating the skin of the human host, after which they travel to the lungs via the bloodstream. Once the larvae reach the lungs, they migrate through the airways into the larynx, then into the esophagus, and finally into the small intestine. There, the larvae develop into adult worms and lay eggs. The eggs may be passed in feces to perpetuate the life cycle, although eggs also have the ability to develop into larval forms while still in the intestine. Once larvae form in the intestine, they may directly penetrate the intestinal wall and migrate to the lungs and back to the gut. This ability is termed **autoinfection** and allows the organism to perpetuate infection within the host.

Most patients with *S. stercoralis* infection are asymptomatic. When symptoms occur, cough, shortness of breath, and hemoptysis may be seen.

Chest radiography in patients with *S. stercoralis* infection may show patchy areas of air-space consolidation. Other patterns, such as nodular consolidation, small nodules, or reticulation, have been reported. Pleural effusions occur in a few patients.

Dirofilariasis

Dirofilaria are nematodes. Several species of *Dirofilaria* may cause dirofilariasis, but the most common species is *Dirofilaria immitis*.

Dirofilaria immitis infection is primarily encountered in the Eastern United States, although the infection has been seen in Europe, Canada, and South America. Adults are far more commonly affected than children. Dogs are the most common definitive hosts for *D. immitis*; the organism is the cause of dog heartworm. The infection is transmitted by mosquito bites, and humans become intermediate hosts when they are bitten by an infected mosquito. Because the filarial organisms cannot complete their life cycles in humans, the organisms die and are transported to the pulmonary arterial circulation where they may incite an inflammatory reaction

Patients with *D. immitis* infection are usually asymptomatic. Cough, hemoptysis, and chest pain may occur. The diagnosis is usually discovered upon biopsy of a pulmonary nodule. Serum eosinophilia may occur but is not marked.

The typical chest radiographic appearance of *D. immitis* infection is a peripheral, circumscribed solitary pulmonary nodule (see Fig. 10.33 in Chapter 10). Less commonly, multiple nodules or air-space consolidation is seen.

Tropical Eosinophilia

Tropical eosinophilia refers to an asthma-like condition caused primarily by two nematodes: *Wuchereria bancrofti* and *Brugia malayi*. As the name implies, tropical eosinophilia is most commonly seen in the tropics, particularly Southeast Asia, India, and the West Indies.

Tropical eosinophilia is acquired when an infected mosquito bites a person and injects the larvae into the lymphatics. Larvae mature into adult worms in the lymphatics and produce microfilariae; the latter reach the bloodstream and are ingested by an uninfected mosquito, thus completing the life cycle. As the microfilariae travel the bloodstream, they may become trapped within pulmonary capillaries and induce a hypersensitivity reaction.

Patients often present with a mildly productive cough, occasionally with hemoptysis. Low-grade fever, weight loss, and other constitutional symptoms may occur. Blood eosinophilia is common.

Chest radiographs in patients with tropical eosinophilia usually show a basilar predominant, symmetric, small nodular or reticular and nodular pattern. Lymphadenopathy may occur. Pleural effusions are uncommon.

Toxocariasis (Visceral Larval Migrans)

Toxocara canis and *Toxocara cati* are the two organisms that cause the roundworm infection toxocariasis. The former organism generally infects dogs and the latter cats. Toxocariasis occurs in tropical and temperate regions alike, with symptomatic human disease occurring more commonly in the former.

Dogs and cats normally serve as the definitive hosts for *Toxocara* sp. The parasite eggs reach the soil when the definitive hosts pass them, through feces, into soil. Toxocariasis may occur when humans, often children, ingest soil containing the eggs of the organism. Once ingested, the eggs develop into larvae in the intestine of the human host and are then carried in the bloodstream to various organs, including the brain, liver, eyes, lungs, and heart. The larvae cannot develop properly in these organs and instead migrate into the surrounding tissues, where they often eventually die, evoking a host granulomatous inflammatory reaction.

Patients are often asymptomatic. When clinically overt pulmonary infection occurs, cough, shortness of breath, and symptoms referable to other involved organs (such as the brain) may be present.

Patchy, poorly defined areas of air-space consolidation may be encountered on chest radiographs during the course of pulmonary infection. Recent CT descriptions of thoracic toxocariasis suggest that peripheral and lower lobe predominant nodular opacities, which may show completely subsolid, or solid, or part-solid attenuation, as well as linear opacities, may be encountered.

Paragonimiasis

Paragonimiasis is caused by worms of the flatworm genus *Paragonimus*. Most human disease is caused by infestation by *Paragonimus westermani*. Paragonimiasis occurs most frequently in Southeast Asia and less commonly in South and Central America and Africa. The infection is particularly common in the Philippines. North American disease occurs in immigrants from these regions or from comparatively rare infections by a related organism found in North America, *P. kellicotti*.

Humans acquire paragonimiasis by ingesting the organism when they eat infected shellfish. The ingested organisms, called *metacercariae*, develop in the small intestine of the human host and then migrate through the intestinal wall into the peritoneum. From there, the organisms burrow through the diaphragm into the lungs where they develop into adult worms. In the lungs, adult worms lay eggs that are either coughed up or swallowed and excreted in feces where they reach the soil. In the soil, the eggs develop into miracidia, which can then infect freshwater snails. Within the snails, the miracidia develop further and form cercariae, which then infect shellfish (crab and crayfish) to complete the life cycle.

The typical symptoms of fever, cough, and chest pain occur when the organisms are migrating through the lung parenchyma. Hemoptysis becomes a common symptom in patients with chronic disease.

Imaging Findings

Chest radiographs in patients infected with *P. westermani* often show basilar predominant small, thin-walled cystic lesions or ring shadows, with or without nodules with surrounding ground-glass opacity or poorly defined areas of nodular consolidation (see Fig. 10.44 in Chapter 10). The cystic areas are usually small, often less than 1 cm, but may be as large as 5 cm. Patchy areas of nonsegmental consolidation may also be seen, and the ring shadows, nodules, and consolidation may be seen together or separate from one another. On CT, there may be crescentic thickening of a portion of the cystic lesions, perhaps representing the worm itself. Pleural effusions are common and lymphadenopathy may be present. A linear "track" between a nodule and the visceral pleural surface has been reported as a distinguishing finding of North American paragonimiasis (*P. kellicotti*) infection (Fig. 13.58).

Pleural effusions occur in more than half of patients. The pulmonary parenchymal lesions may calcify in chronic cases.

In patients immigrating to the United States from endemic regions, a pattern resembling postprimary TB has been described.

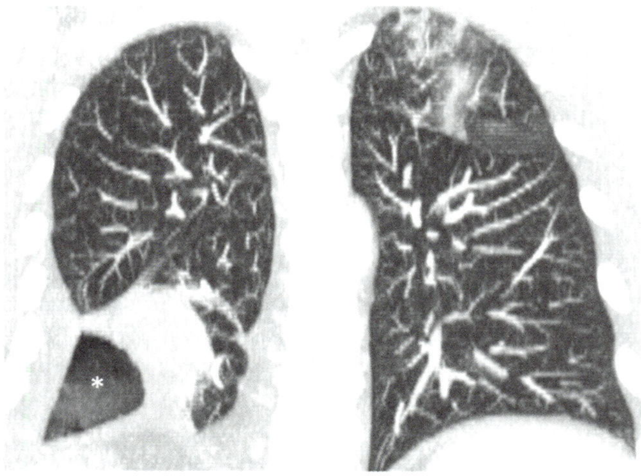

Figure 13.58. Coronal maximum intensity projection (MIP) image in a patient with paragonimiasis. Linear areas of consolidation in the left upper lobe that are contiguous with the pleura represent presumed worm tracks. A chronic right hydropneumothorax (asterisk) is due to chronic untreated paragonimiasis of several years duration. Diagnosis was finally confirmed with PCR and patient responded to anti-parasitic therapy.

Schistosomiasis

Schistosomiasis is caused by flatworms of the genus *Schistosoma*; the species *Schistosoma mansoni*, *S. japonicum*, *S. mekongi*, and *S. haematobium* are the most important etiologic agents of this infection.

Schistosomiasis is a very important parasitic infection worldwide. *S. mansoni* and *S. haematobium* are endemic in the Middle East and Africa, whereas *S. japonicum* is endemic in Japan, China, and the Philippines. *S. mekongi* infection occurs in Southeast Asia. *S. mansoni* may also be found in South America and the West Indies. Schistosomiasis infection in North America is most often encountered in individuals emigrating from endemic regions.

Cercariae living in water in endemic regions may infect humans when they drink infected water, or the organisms may burrow into skin when humans work in infected waters. Once the cercariae penetrate human integument, they change into a form known as a schistosomules and migrate into the pulmonary venous circulation. From here, the organisms migrate to the hepatic portal circulation and develop further. The worms then migrate to the mesenteric venous circulation (*S. mansoni*, *S. japonicum*, and *S. mekongi*) or the perivesicular veins (*S. haematobium*), and then adult worms reproduce in these venules. Laden with eggs, the adult female worm burrows into the submucosa of either the bowel or the bladder and lays eggs, which then may be passed into water via feces or urine. In the water, the eggs develop into miracidia, which then infect snails. Within the snail, cercariae develop, eventually to leave the snail to infect humans and complete the organism's life cycle.

The release of eggs into human tissue by the adult female worm precipitates a host inflammatory response and is usually the cause of clinically overt disease. These eggs may produce inflammation within the wall of the organ in question (either bladder or bowel), or they may be released into the associated venous circulation and embolize downstream organs. In the case of *S. japonicum*, *S. mansoni*, and *S. mekongi*, the eggs may travel from the mesenteric venous system to the liver; eggs released by *S. haematobium* may reach the inferior vena cava and travel to the lungs. If cirrhosis develops, eggs from the organisms that typically inhabit the mesenteric vasculature may also reach the lungs through portosystemic shunts. Once these eggs reach the lungs, they may extend through the capillaries into the surrounding tissue and induce a fibrotic reaction that obliterates small vessels, inducing pulmonary hypertension.

A transitory febrile reaction, associated with gastrointestinal symptoms, cough, and constitutional findings, may occur with initial infection. As eggs embolize to the lungs, patients may develop cough, shortness of breath, and hypoxemia. Chronically, pulmonary hypertension, which develops in a minority of patients and usually after repeated infection, presents with right heart failure. *S. haematobium* may cause hematuria.

Imaging Findings

Transient opacities (a Loeffler-like syndrome) may occur on chest radiography as the schistosomules enter the pulmonary circulation shortly after infection. The migration of the organism from the pulmonary vessels into the surrounding tissues, and the host inflammatory reaction that results, may produce radiographically evident abnormalities, commonly focal or multifocal consolidation. Pulmonary hypertension caused by schistosomiasis has the same appearance as other causes of pulmonary hypertension: dilation of the main and central pulmonary arteries with peripheral tapering. Cirrhosis may be caused by the organisms that inhabit the mesenteric venous circulation.

Echinococcosis (Hydatid Disease)

Echinococcosis is primarily caused by the tapeworms (Cestodes) *Echinococcus granulosus* and *E. multilocularis*. *E. granulosus* is responsible for most cases of hydatid disease.

Epidemiology

Echinococcus granulosus causes infection in two basic varieties, the pastoral and the sylvatic forms, that differ in terms of their definitive and intermediate hosts and the geographic disease distribution. The clinical and imaging appearances are also slightly different between these two disease forms.

The intermediate hosts for the more common pastoral variety of echinococcosis are domestic farm animals, such as sheep, cows, pigs, and horses; dogs are the usual definitive hosts. This form of the disease is endemic in southeastern Europe, North Africa, the Middle East, and Russia.

The definitive hosts for the sylvatic form of echinococcosis are canines such as foxes, wolves, and coyotes. The intermediate hosts for the sylvatic disease form are moose, deer, and the like. This form of echinococcosis is found primarily in Alaska and Canada.

The definitive hosts for *E. multilocularis* are also canines, including dogs, foxes, and wolves. The intermediate hosts include various rodents. *E. multilocularis* is endemic in southern Europe (especially Switzerland and Germany), Alaska, Russia, and Canada.

The normal life cycle begins with the usual intermediate hosts ingesting the eggs, passed from definitive hosts, in contaminated food, water, or soil. The eggs develop into larvae in the gut of the intermediate host and eventually penetrate through the intestinal wall and migrate into the portal venous system and then to the liver. Many larvae are trapped in the liver, but some escape the liver and come to rest in the pulmonary circulation. Most larvae are killed, but some develop into cysts containing immature worms. The life cycle is completed when the definitive host feeds on the remains of the intermediate host, and the cysts develop into adult worms in the gut of the definitive hosts.

Humans acquire disease by the ingestion of food, water, or soil contaminated by intermediate-host feces containing the organisms (which usually live in the small intestine of the intermediate host). In this fashion, humans become an inadvertent intermediate host.

About 60% to 70% of cases of *E. granulosus* occur in the liver, and 15% to 30% occur in the lung parenchyma. The few remaining cases occur in a variety of other organs, including the brain, heart, and kidneys. Lung abnormalities are more common than liver findings in the sylvatic form of the disease.

The hydatid cysts that occur in intermediate hosts consist of an outer fibrotic capsule called the **pericyst**, an outer **exocyst**, and an inner **endocyst**. The endocyst produces fluid and gives rise to immature forms called **brood capsules**. Larval forms develop within these brood capsules. Daughter cysts may develop directly from the larval forms within the brood capsules or directly from the exocyst, creating the overall appearance of a multilocular cystic lesion on imaging studies.

Echinococcus multilocularis has a life cycle similar to *E. granulosus*. However, the structure of the cyst that forms in *E. multilocularis* is different than that of *E. granulosus*. In contrast to *E. granulosus*, the exocyst is rather poorly formed and the pericyst does not form at all.

Hydatid disease causes symptoms by the compression of adjacent structures or by rupture of a cyst with an ensuing host inflammatory response, although most patients remain asymptomatic. Cyst rupture may be heralded by the sudden onset of cough, hemoptysis, chest pain, fever, and systemic hypersensitivity. Purulent sputum production may occur with bacterial superinfection of hydatid cysts.

Imaging Findings

Chest radiographs in patients with echinococcosis often show a single, lower lobe, circumscribed nodule or mass of variable size, ranging from 1 cm to more than 15 cm (see Fig. 10.34 in Chapter 10). Multiple lesions are seen in 20% to 30% of patients. Pulmonary hydatid cysts grow slowly and, unlike their liver counterparts, usually do not calcify.

Pulmonary hydatid cysts may change shape with respiration and are often irregularly deformed by adjacent anatomy, such as vessels or mediastinal structures.

If the cyst acquires a communication with the tracheobronchial tree, several radiographic patterns may occur. If the pericyst ruptures, allowing air to gain access to the potential space between the pericyst and the exocyst, a meniscus or crescent sign may be observed. This sign is not very common overall and is practically seen only with the pastoral form of echinococcosis. If a communication develops between the tracheobronchial tree and the endocyst, an air-fluid level may form within the cyst, accompanied by surrounding pulmonary parenchymal consolidation that represents expelled cyst fluid. Additionally, once tracheobronchial communication with the cyst occurs, the cyst membrane may collapse and float on the resulting air-fluid level, creating an irregular contour to the air-fluid level, representing the characteristic "water lily (camalote)" sign.

CT often shows that the rounded or oval lesions in patients with pulmonary echinococcosis have fluid attenuation. CT may also effectively show the collapsed cyst membranes as well as the configuration of daughter cysts. CT also effectively shows chest wall invasion or pleural extension by the cysts. In the uncommon patient in whom hydatid pulmonary disease results from extension of an infectious focus from the liver across the diaphragm, CT may show the cystic liver lesion in continuity with pulmonary and pleural disease.

Cysticercosis

The larval form of the tapeworm *Taenia solium* is the cause of cysticercosis. The adult *T. solium* tapeworms usually live asymptomatically in the intestine of the human definitive host. Cysticercosis is endemic in parts of Africa, Europe (especially Spain and Portugal), and Central America.

Humans acquire infection by ingesting undercooked meat containing cysticerci from an intermediate host, usually a pig. The ingested immature forms develop into adult worms within the human gut, shedding eggs in the feces, which are in turn eaten by the intermediate host, completing the organism's life cycle. Humans may also serve as both intermediate and definitive hosts, creating a pattern known as **autoinfection**. This occurs when humans ingest the eggs of the tapeworm directly or if the eggs are regurgitated back into the stomach. With autoinfection, the ingested eggs hatch into immature forms that migrate through the intestinal wall into the mesenteric veins and are then carried to various organs, such as the brain, eyes, and skeletal muscle, where they develop into cysticerci. Cysticercosis is often asymptomatic. Neurologic involvement may cause seizures, and respiratory muscle involvement may cause chest pain.

Cysticercosis may present as small calcified nodules, which may be oval or cigar-shaped and are often seen in the musculature of the thorax on chest radiographs.

SUGGESTED READINGS

Ajlan AM, Ahyad RA, Jamjoom LG, Alharthy A, Madani TA. Middle East respiratory syndrome coronavirus (MERS-CoV) infection: chest CT findings. *AJR Am J Roentgenol*. 2014;203(4):782-787.

Antonio GE, Wong KT, Hui DS, et al. Thin-section CT in patients with severe acute respiratory syndrome following hospital discharge: preliminary experience. *Radiology*. 2003;228(3):810-815.

Brecher CW, Aviram G, Boiselle PM. CT and radiography of bacterial respiratory infections in AIDS patients. *AJR Am J Roentgenol*. 2003;180(5):1203-1209.

Cattamanchi A, Nahid P, Marras TK, et al. Detailed analysis of the radiographic presentation of Mycobacterium kansasii lung disease in patients with HIV infection. *Chest*. 2008;133(4):875-880.

Erasmus JJ, McAdams HP, Farrell MA, Patz EF Jr. Pulmonary nontuberculous mycobacterial infection: radiologic manifestations. *Radiographics*. 1999;19(6):1487-1505.

Franquet T, Müller NL, Gimenez A, Guembe P, de La Torre J, Bagué S. Spectrum of pulmonary aspergillosis: histologic, clinical, and radiologic findings. *Radiographics*. 2001;21(4):825-837.

Franquet T. Imaging of pulmonary viral pneumonia. *Radiology*. 2011;260(1):18-39.

Gotway MB, Dawn SK, Caoili EM, Reddy GP, Araoz PA, Webb WR. The radiologic spectrum of pulmonary Aspergillus infections. *J Comput Assist Tomogr*. 2002;26(2):159-173.

Grinblat L, Shulman H, Glickman A, Matukas L, Paul N. Severe acute respiratory syndrome: radiographic review of 40 probable cases in Toronto, Canada. *Radiology*. 2003;228(3):802-809.

Gruden JF, Huang L, Turner J, et al. High-resolution CT in the evaluation of clinically suspected Pneumocystis carinii pneumonia in AIDS patients with normal, equivocal, or nonspecific radiographic findings. *AJR Am J Roentgenol*. 1997;169(4):967-975.

Hammer MM, Madan R, Hatabu H Pulmonary mucormycosis: radiologic features at presentation and over time. *AJR Am J Roentgenol*. 2018;210(4):742-747.

Henry TS, Cummings KW. Role of imaging in the diagnosis and management of parasitic infections. *Curr Opin Pulm Med*. 2013;19(3):310-317.

Kim EA, Lee KS, Primack SL, et al. Viral pneumonias in adults: radiologic and pathologic findings. *Radiographics*. 2002;22 Spec No:S137-S149.

Leung AN. Pulmonary tuberculosis: the essentials. *Radiology*. 1999;210(2):307-322.

Lieberman D, Ben-Yaakov M, Lazarovich Z, et al. Chlamydia pneumoniae community-acquired pneumonia: a review of 62 hospitalized adult patients. *Infection*. 1996a;24(2):109-114.

Lieberman D, Porath A, Schlaeffer F, Lieberman D, Boldur I. Legionella species community-acquired pneumonia. A review of 56 hospitalized adult patients. *Chest*. 1996b;109(5):1243-1249.

Marom EM, Holmes AM, Bruzzi JF, Truong MT, O'Sullivan PJ, Kontoyiannis DP. Imaging of pulmonary fusariosis in patients with hematologic malignancies. *AJR Am J Roentgenol*. 2008;190(6):1605-1609.

McAdams HP, Rosado de Christenson ML, Lesar M, Templeton PA, Moran CA. Thoracic mycoses from endemic fungi: radiologic-pathologic correlation. *Radiographics*. 1995a;15(2):255-270.

McAdams HP, Rosado de Christenson ML, Templeton PA, Lesar M, Moran CA. Thoracic mycoses from opportunistic fungi: radiologic-pathologic correlation. *Radiographics*. 1995b;15(2):271-286.

Miller WT Jr, Barbosa E Jr, Mickus TJ, Mullin C, Van Deerlin VM, Shiley KT. Chest computed tomographic imaging characteristics of viral acute lower respiratory tract illnesses: a case–control study. *J Comput Assist Tomogr*. 2011;35(4):524-530.

Reittner P, Muller NL, Heyneman L, et al. Mycoplasma pneumoniae pneumonia: radiographic and high-resolution CT features in 28 patients. *AJR Am J Roentgenol*. 2000;174(1):37-41.

Saurborn DP, Fishman JE, Boiselle PM. The imaging spectrum of pulmonary tuberculosis in AIDS. *J Thorac Imaging*. 2002;17(1):28-33.

Simpson S, Kay FU, Abbara S, et al. Radiological Society of North America expert consensus document on reporting chest CT findings related to COVID-19: endorsed by the Society of Thoracic Radiology, the American College of Radiology, and RSNA. *J Thorac Imaging*. 2020;35(4):219-227.

Chapter 14

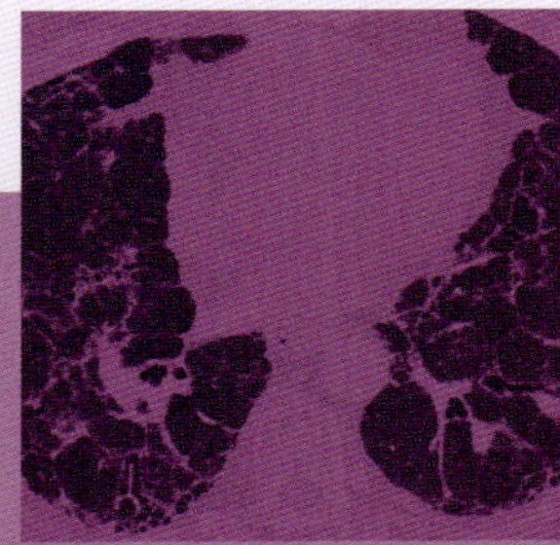

Travis S. Henry

The Idiopathic Interstitial Pneumonias

INTRODUCTION

The idiopathic interstitial pneumonias (IIPs) are a heterogeneous group of diffuse parenchymal lung diseases associated with varying degrees of interstitial lung inflammation and fibrosis. The IIPs are classified by a consensus committee of the American Thoracic Society and the European Respiratory Society into eight types, based on their histologic pattern, clinical features, and radiographic appearances (Table 14.1). Each of the IIPs is referred to using an acronym. Knowing these acronyms is appropriate, as they are in common usage.

In this classification, a distinction is made between the histologic pattern of the interstitial pneumonia and the IIP associated with it. In several cases, these have different names (see Table 14.1).

The IIPs are as follows:

1. Usual interstitial pneumonia (UIP) and idiopathic pulmonary fibrosis (IPF)
2. Nonspecific interstitial pneumonia (NSIP)
3. Respiratory bronchiolitis-interstitial lung disease (RB-ILD)
4. Desquamative interstitial pneumonia (DIP)
5. Cryptogenic organizing pneumonia (COP)
6. Acute interstitial pneumonia (AIP)
7. Lymphoid interstitial pneumonia (LIP)
8. Pleuropulmonary fibroelastosis (PPFE)

The first six are considered *major IIPs*, while the last two are classified as *rare IIPs*. The major IIPs are further subclassified as *chronic fibrosing IIPs* (UIP/IPF and NSIP), smoking-related IIPs (RB-ILD and DIP), and *acute/subacute IIPs* (COP and AIP). An additional category of unclassifiable IIP is also included for atypical cases. Interstitial lung abnormality or ILA is a recently introduced term for very early or mild cases of fibrosis in asymptomatic individuals and is discussed at the end of the chapter.

Although the IIPs are defined as idiopathic, identical histologic patterns, radiographic and high-resolution CT (HRCT) appearances, and clinical symptoms occur in association with specific diseases or exposures, including autoimmune or connective tissue diseases (CTD), drug reactions, smoking, environmental exposures, and infection. It is helpful to think of the histologic patterns (the IPs) as having a differential diagnosis, with one of the possible causes being an idiopathic syndrome (an IIP) (see Table 14.1).

Since the radiographic appearances of the IIP parallel their histologic patterns, this approach allows the appropriate radiographic or HRCT differential diagnosis to be suggested.

UIP AND IPF

UIP is a histologic pattern. It is the most common interstitial pneumonia, accounting for about 40% of cases. *IPF* is the idiopathic disease associated with the histologic pattern termed UIP.

Histologically, UIP is characterized by a heterogeneous pattern with different parts of the biopsy showing normal lung, interstitial fibrosis, fibroblastic proliferation, and honeycombing; in other words, the biopsy shows *spatial heterogeneity*. Histologic abnormalities appear to represent different stages in the temporal evolution of fibrosis, a combination of end-stage and more active lesions. This is termed *temporal heterogeneity*. Spatial and temporal heterogeneity

Table 14.1 Idiopathic Interstitial Pneumonias: Classification and Differential Diagnosis

Category		Histologic Pattern (IP)	Idiopathic Syndrome (IIP)	Associated Diseases and Exposures
Major IIPs	Chronic fibrosing IIPs	Usual IP (UIP)	Idiopathic pulmonary fibrosis (IPF)	CTD, drugs, asbestosis, hypersensitivity pneumonitis, radiation, familial
		Nonspecific IP (NSIP)	Idiopathic NSIP	CTD, drugs, hypersensitivity pneumonitis, immunodeficiency
	Smoking-related IIPs	Desquamative IP (DIP)	DIP	Smoking, toxic fumes
		Respiratory bronchiolitis (RB)	Respiratory bronchiolitis-interstitial lung disease (RB-ILD)	Smoking, toxic fumes
	Acute/subacute IIPs	Organizing pneumonia (OP)	Cryptogenic organizing pneumonia	CTD, drugs, infection, aspiration, bronchial obstruction
		Diffuse alveolar damage (DAD)	Acute interstitial pneumonia (AIP)	Causes of ARDS (eg, sepsis, shock, infection, drug toxicity, toxic inhalations, trauma)
Rare IIPs		Lymphoid IP (LIP)	Idiopathic LIP	CTD (Sjögren's syndrome) immunosuppression
		Pleuropulmonary fibroelastosis (PPFE)	Idiopathic PPFE	Infection, autoantibodies, familial, posttransplantation

ARDS, acute respiratory distress syndrome; CTD, connective tissue disease; IIP, idiopathic interstitial pneumonia; IP, interstitial pneumonia; LIP, lymphoid interstitial pneumonia.

is characteristic of UIP and is not seen in other IIPs. Lung involvement is patchy, although there is a predominance in the subpleural and basal lung regions (Table 14.2).

UIP may be associated with CTDs, asbestosis, drug toxicity, radiation, fibrotic hypersensitivity pneumonitis, or familial pulmonary fibrosis. Idiopathic UIP is termed idiopathic pulmonary fibrosis. IPF accounts for about 70% of cases of UIP.

IPF occurs most frequently in patients older than 50 years (see Table 14.2). Symptoms include progressive dyspnea, cough, weight loss, and finger clubbing; symptoms usually precede presentation by 6 months. Pulmonary function tests (PFTs) show restriction with a reduced diffusing capacity. IPF has a poor prognosis, with a mean survival of 3 to 4 years from the onset of symptoms. The 5-year survival rate is 25% to 40%.

Since 2014, two antifibrotic agents – Ofev (nintedanib) and Esbriet (pirfenidone) – have been approved in the United States and other countries for the treatment of IPF. Although the mechanism of action of the drugs is unclear, they appear to inhibit fibrosis, and although they do not cure IPF, they slow progression of the disease measured using PFTs. Before these drugs were available, treatments other than lung transplantation were ineffective.

The diagnosis of IPF is limited to patients with histologic findings of UIP; in other words, if it is not UIP, it is not IPF. Histologic diagnosis traditionally relies on surgical open lung biopsy; in 2022 conditional recommendation was made to consider transbronchial lung cryobiopsy as an acceptable alternative to surgical lung biopsy.

Radiographic Findings in UIP/IPF

In 80% of patients with UIP/IPF, radiographs show a bilateral reticular pattern predominantly involving the lower lung zones and subpleural lung regions (Figs. 14.1 and 14.2). In its earliest stages, a fine reticular pattern may be visible in the posterior costophrenic angles on the lateral radiograph (see Figs. 14.1C and 14.2B), and the lateral radiograph is often more sensitive than the PA view in making this diagnosis. As fibrosis progresses, the reticular pattern becomes coarse, and cystic areas of honeycombing are visible in about half of cases (see Fig. 14.2). Pleural thickening or effusion is very uncommon.

Table 14.2 Usual Interstitial Pneumonia and Idiopathic Pulmonary Fibrosis: Histologic, Clinical, and HRCT Features

UIP: Histologic Pattern

Characteristics
- Spatial and temporal inhomogeneity
- Dense fibrosis, often with honeycombing
- Fibroblastic foci
- Patchy lung involvement
- Subpleural and basal predominance

Differential diagnosis
- Idiopathic (IPF)
- Connective tissue disease
- Asbestosis
- Drug toxicity
- Radiation
- Chronic hypersensitivity pneumonitis
- Familial pulmonary fibrosis

IPF: idiopathic clinical syndrome

Age >50 y

Progressive dyspnea; duration of symptoms 3 months or more

Pulmonary function tests: restriction and impaired gas exchange

Historical 5-year survival rate 25%-40%

Two drugs now approved that slow progression

HRCT findings highly accurate in diagnosis
- Honeycombing
- Reticulation
- Subpleural and basal predominance

Little ground-glass opacity

HRCT, high-resolution CT; IPF, idiopathic pulmonary fibrosis.

Because of lung fibrosis, decreased lung volume is typical (see Fig. 14.1A), and serial chest radiographs are often used to monitor progressive reduction in lung volume with time. Because of greater fibrosis and volume loss in the lower lobes, the major fissures may be seen to bow posteriorly (see Fig. 14.1C).

A combination of clinical and radiographic findings is sufficient to make an accurate diagnosis of IPF in about 70% of cases. In 10% of cases, the radiograph appears normal.

HRCT Findings of UIP/IPF

On HRCT, UIP/IPF is characterized by traction bronchiectasis/bronchiolectasis and/or honeycombing, usually with a subpleural and lower lobe predominance (see Figs. 14.1 and 14.2; Table 14.2).

In its earliest stages, the only HRCT abnormality may be fine reticulation in the subpleural lung, at the lung bases (Fig. 14.3); as the disease progresses, the reticular opacities become more pronounced, involving more of the lung, and traction bronchiectasis/bronchiolectasis and/or honeycombing may be seen.

Honeycomb cysts, identified in the immediate subpleural lung, usually range from 3 mm to 2 cm in diameter, but may occasionally be larger. Honeycomb cysts must be visible in the immediate subpleural lung, and seeing three cysts in a row, with thick and recognizable walls, is considered to be a minimum finding in making this diagnosis. Seeing stacked honeycomb cysts is preferable, as a single row of cysts may be difficult to distinguish from paraseptal emphysema. An isolated subpleural cyst should not be considered sufficient to call honeycombing (Figs. 14.1D, 14.2C and D, 14.4, 14.5).

Recent radiologic-pathologic correlation has shown that honeycombing exists along a spectrum with traction bronchiolectasis. Honeycombing cysts develop as a result of alveolar collapse and dilation of terminal airways; in some cases, the cysts are seen to be connected with each other and in continuity with the bronchiolar tree. Thus, in IPF, there appears to be a continuum from traction bronchiolectasis to honeycombing, and the conceptual separation of the two processes may be misleading. Nonetheless, the current ATS/ERS/JRS/ALAT guidelines discussed below still distinguish the two, but the differences are less important than in the past, as either a UIP or Probable UIP pattern can confer a confident diagnosis of IPF without surgical lung biopsy.

On HRCT, a basal and peripheral predominance of fibrosis is characteristic of UIP/IPF. A subpleural predominance is evident on HRCT in 80% to 95% of cases, either concentric (Fig. 14.5) or patchy and clustered (Fig. 14.6). In approximately 80% of patients, the fibrosis is most severe in the lower lung zones; in about 20%, all zones are involved to a similar degree. The upper lobes will be affected in almost all cases, but the extent and severity of abnormalities are typically less than at the lung bases. Subpleural, basal honeycombing associated with irregular reticular opacities in the upper lobes is characteristic of IPF. Findings of fibrosis and honeycombing may be asymmetrical (Fig. 14.6).

Ground-glass opacity may be seen in patients with UIP/IPF, but this finding typically reflects the presence of fine lung fibrosis. Thus, ground-glass opacity is almost always seen in the same lung regions where reticulation and traction bronchiectasis are also present (Fig. 14.7); it is rare as an isolated finding. Ground-glass opacities seen in regions that do not show findings of lung fibrosis suggest a diagnosis other than UIP/IPF.

In some patients, IPF may be associated with emphysema. This has been termed *combined pulmonary fibrosis and emphysema* (*CPFE*). CPFE is most common in patients with IPF but can occur in patients with smoking-related fibrosis. It is characterized by dyspnea, upper lobe emphysema, and lower lobe fibrosis. This syndrome frequently is complicated by pulmonary hypertension, acute lung injury, and lung cancer. The CPFE syndrome typically occurs in male smokers, and the mortality associated with this syndrome is significant particularly if associated with IPF and

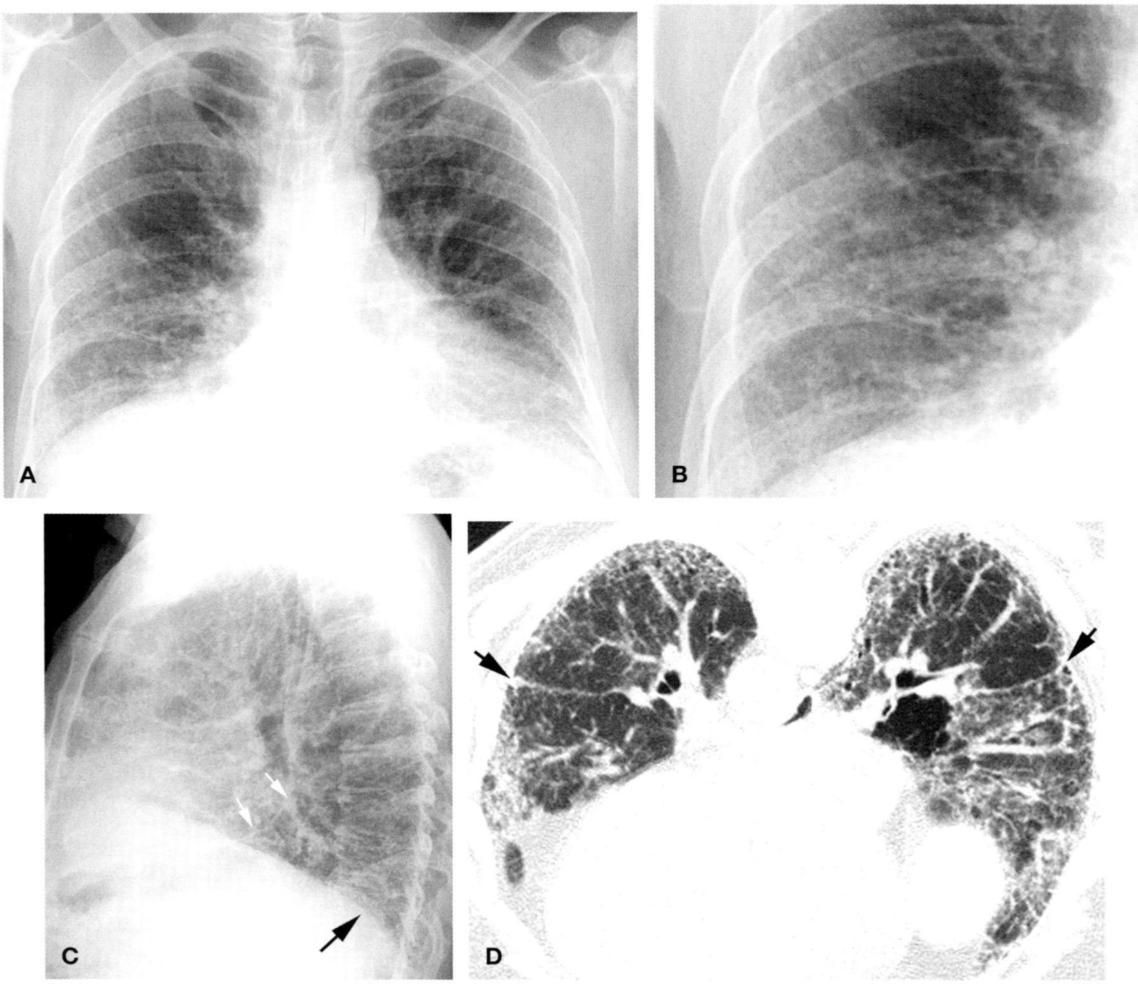

Figure 14.1. Chest radiograph and HRCT in a patient with histologically proven idiopathic pulmonary fibrosis. **A:** PA radiograph shows reduced lung volumes. There is an increase in reticular opacities in the lung periphery and at the lung bases. The appearance and distribution are typical of idiopathic pulmonary fibrosis. **B:** Detailed view of the right lower lobe shows increased reticular opacities. **C:** Lateral view shows increased reticular opacities in the posterior costophrenic angles (*black arrow*). A major fissure (*white arrows*) is bowed posteriorly because of more severe fibrosis in the lower lobe. **D:** Prone HRCT shows extensive subpleural reticular opacities with mild honeycombing. The major fissures (*arrows*) are displaced posteriorly because of lower lobe fibrosis. HRCT, high-resolution CT.

pulmonary hypertension. HRCT typically shows upper lobe emphysema and lower lobe honeycombing, with a gradual transition from one to the other (Fig. 14.8). While the combination of emphysema and pulmonary fibrosis is relatively common, CPFE is still an incompletely understood clinical syndrome.

Mediastinal lymph node enlargement is visible on CT in more than 70% of cases. The enlarged nodes typically measure less than 15 mm.

In the vast majority of patients with IPF, serial HRCT scans show an increase in the extent of reticulation and honeycombing. This progression usually occurs gradually over several months or years. Occasionally, a patient develops a fulminant and sometimes fatal *acute exacerbation* characterized by consolidation or ground-glass opacity (Fig. 14.9); biopsy typically shows diffuse alveolar damage (DAD). When such exacerbations occur, pulmonary function decreases in a series of acute stair-step increments coincident with the exacerbations.

Clinical Diagnosis of IPF

Diagnostic criteria for the multidisciplinary diagnosis of UIP/IPF have been revised multiple times over the past 2 decades. In 2018 both a Fleischner Society White Paper and a multispecialty committee of the American Thoracic Society, European Respiratory Society, Japanese Respiratory Society, and Latin American Thoracic Society Clinical Practice Guideline were published. The ATS/ERS/JRS/ALAT guidelines were updated in 2022 and serve as the most up-to-date reference.

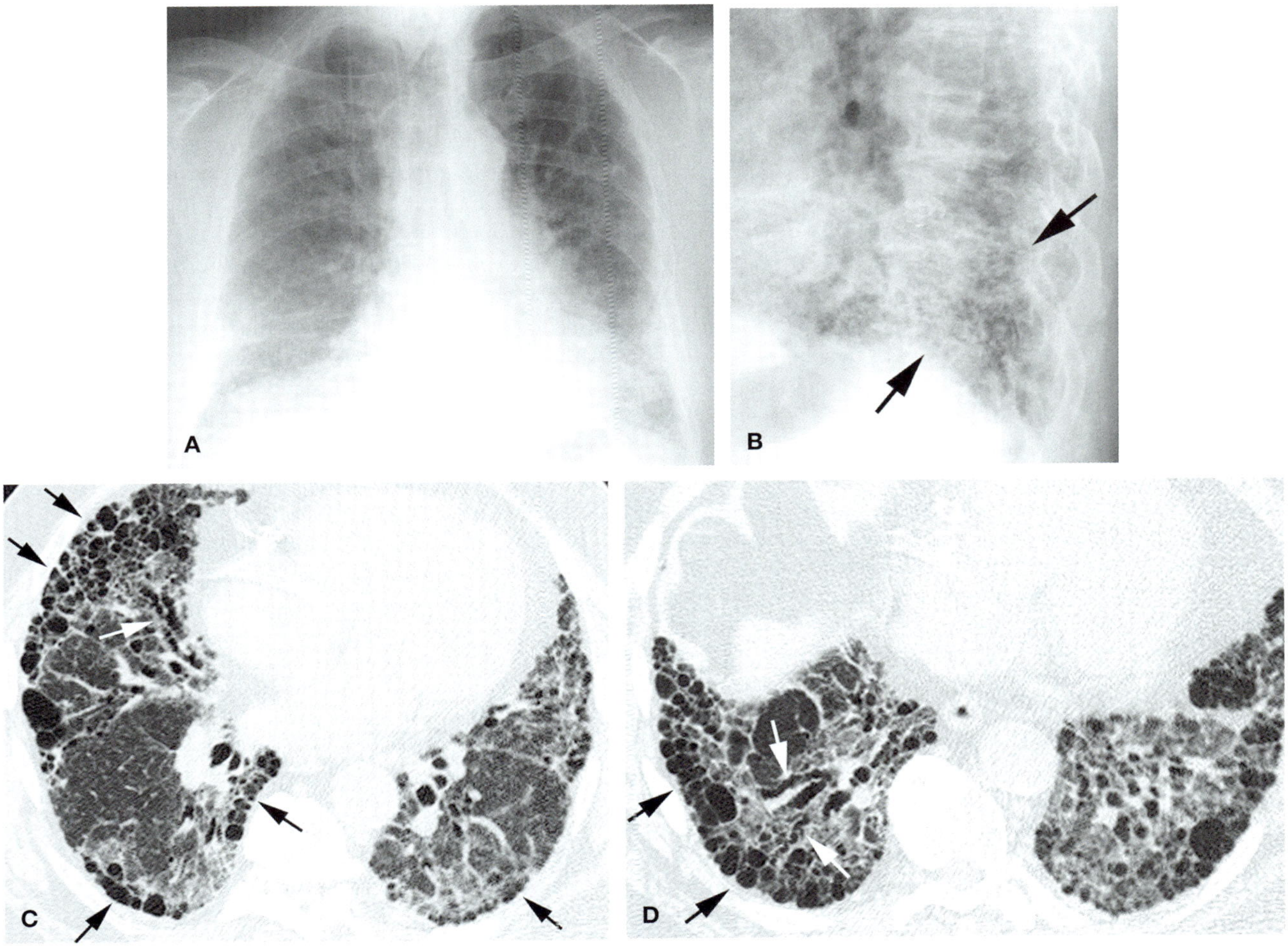

Figure 14.2. Chest radiograph and HRCT in a patient with idiopathic pulmonary fibrosis. **A:** PA radiograph shows ill-defined reticular opacities at the lung bases. **B:** Coned-down lateral view shows a coarse reticular pattern (*arrows*) in the posterior costophrenic angles. **C and D:** HRCT shows extensive subpleural honeycombing (*black arrows*), reticular opacities, and traction bronchiectasis (*white arrows*). The honeycomb cysts range from a few millimeters to 2 cm in diameter. This is a "usual interstitial pneumonia pattern" of fibrosis. HRCT, high-resolution CT.

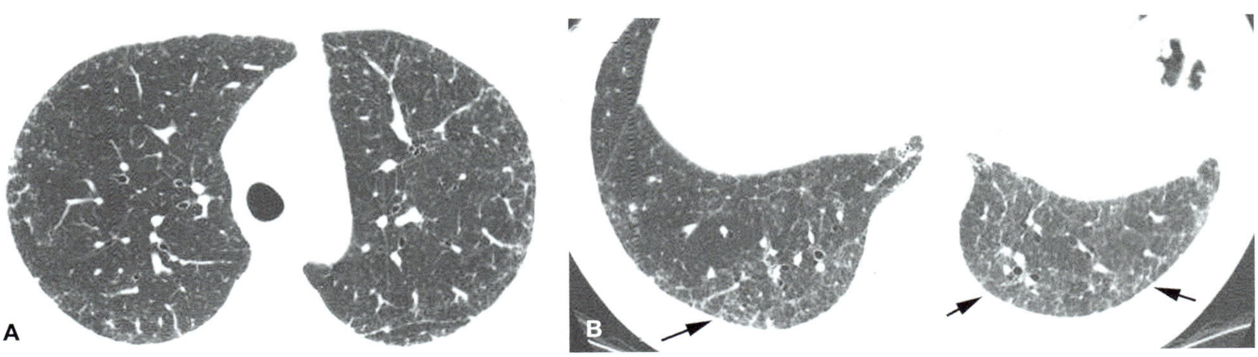

Figure 14.3. Reticulation in early/mild usual interstitial pneumonia/idiopathic pulmonary fibrosis. **A and B:** Concentric subpleural reticulation is the only abnormality. It is most severe in the lung bases (*arrows*, **B**). Reticulation is the earliest abnormality seen on HRCT in patients with IPF. Because no honeycombing is visible in this patient, the HRCT would be read as "Probable UIP pattern" using current criteria. Biopsy confirmed a diagnosis of UIP/IPF as this case predated the update in guidelines. HRCT, high-resolution CT; IPF, idiopathic pulmonary fibrosis; UIP, usual interstitial pneumonia.

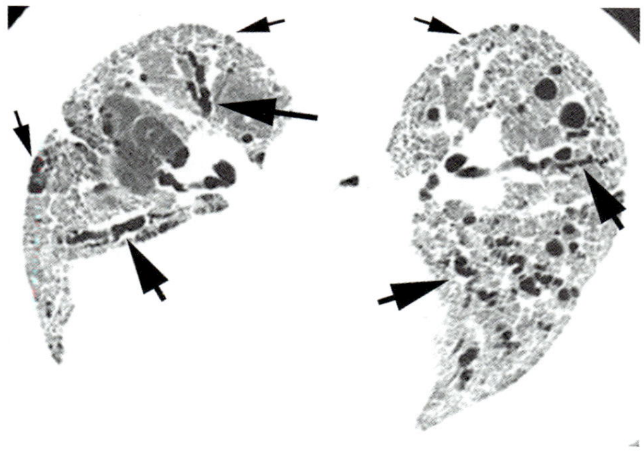

Figure 14.4. Reticular opacities, traction bronchiectasis, and honeycombing in idiopathic pulmonary fibrosis. Prone HRCT shows a diffuse, coarse, reticular pattern at the lung bases, with traction bronchiectasis (*large arrows*) and mild subpleural honeycombing (*small arrows*). While the fibrosis is severe, there are still some areas of normal lung interspersed (spatial heterogeneity) best seen in the right lower lobe on this image. This is a "usual interstitial pneumonia pattern" of fibrosis. UIP, usual interstitial pneumonia.

The purpose of the guidelines is to provide a framework to simplify and standardize the diagnosis of IPF emphasizing a multidisciplinary approach including clinical, serologic, imaging, and histologic data. The guidelines put forth criteria for four categories of imaging: *UIP Pattern*, *Probable UIP Pattern*, *Indeterminate for UIP*, and *Alternative Diagnosis*. In patients with a UIP pattern on HRCT, lung biopsy is rarely performed as the positive predictive value of the HRCT for IPF is between 90% and 100% (in the appropriate clinical context). Patients with Probable UIP pattern have a similar disease course to UIP pattern, and the likelihood of pathologic UIP in these patients is 80% to 85%. Thus, many patients in the Probable UIP category may also forego lung biopsy and be diagnosed with IPF after careful multidisciplinary discussion. As mentioned above, this has lessened the necessity of relying on honeycombing to make a confident diagnosis and obviate the need for surgical lung biopsy.

Applying the ATS guidelines requires an approach to the HRCT that incorporates both the distribution of fibrosis and the specific CT features of fibrosis that are present. These are presented in detail in Table 14.3, and summarized below for

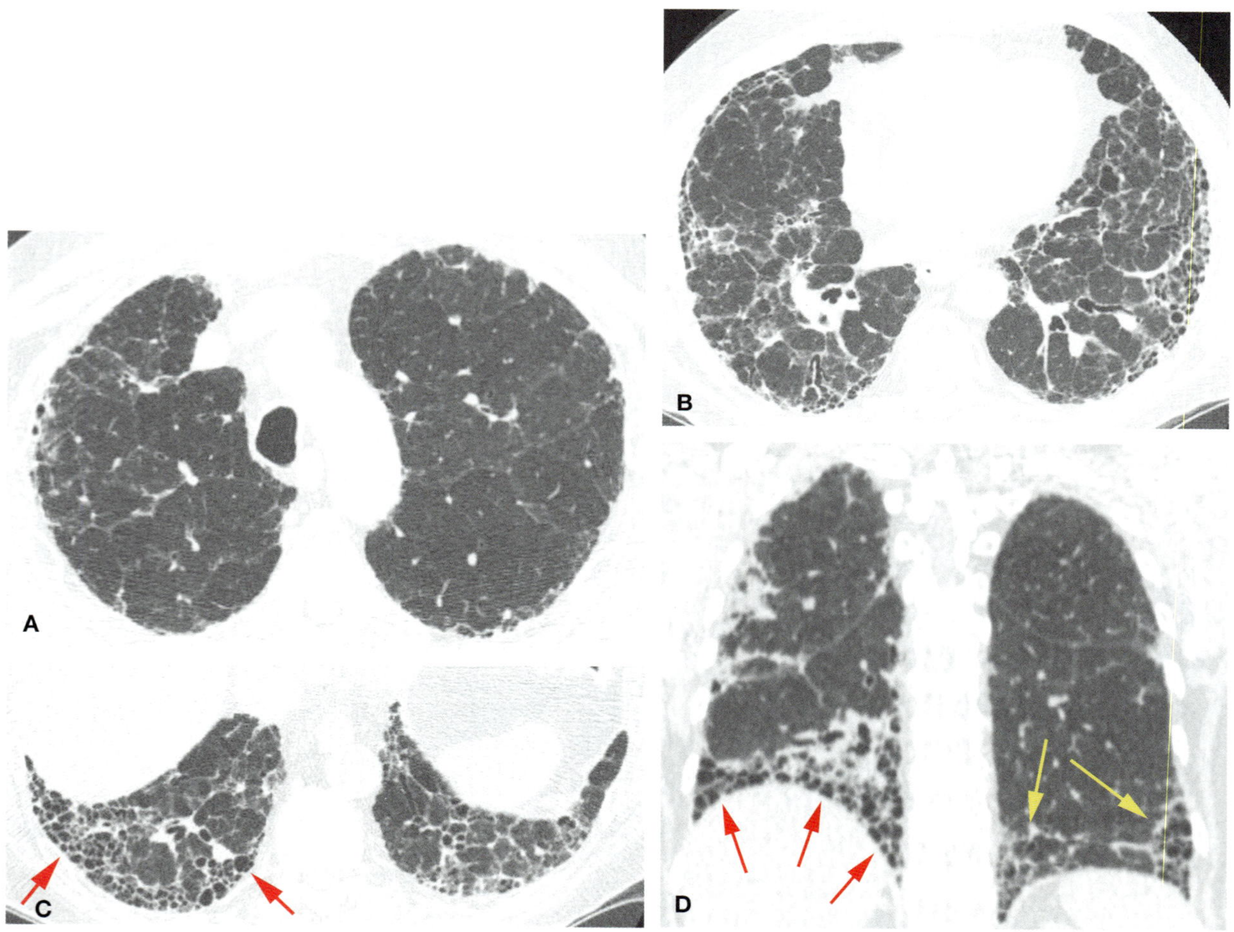

Figure 14.5. Honeycombing and a "usual interstitial pneumonia pattern" on high-resolution CT in a patient with idiopathic pulmonary fibrosis. **A:** Mild peripheral reticulation is visible in the upper lobes. **B and C:** Concentric subpleural honeycombing is visible in the lung periphery and at the lung bases (*arrows*). Most cysts are less than 1 cm in size. Reticulation and traction bronchiectasis are also present. **D:** Coronal reconstruction shows the predominance of honeycombing (*arrows*) at the bases.

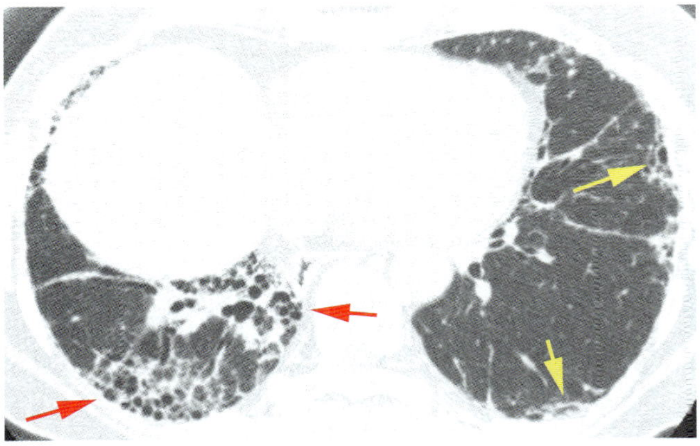

Figure 14.6. Patchy, asymmetric subpleural reticular opacities and honeycombing in idiopathic pulmonary fibrosis. Areas of fibrosis and honeycombing (*arrows*) involve the peripheral lung in a patchy fashion. Although the findings are mild this is still sufficient for a "usual interstitial pneumonia pattern".

each category. It is important to note that the presence of features suggesting an alternative diagnosis to UIP supersede the diagnosis of either a UIP Pattern or Probable UIP Pattern.

For an HRCT diagnosis of a *UIP pattern*, the required findings (see Figs. 14.2, 14.3, 14.5) are as follows:

Distribution – subpleural and basal; spatially heterogeneous with areas of normal lung and areas of fibrosis on the same image; may be asymmetric in some cases and may be diffuse in craniocaudal plane.

CT features – reticulation; honeycombing with or without traction bronchiectasis; absence of features suggesting an alternative diagnosis

For an HRCT diagnosis of a *Probable UIP*, findings are essentially the same as the UIP pattern minus the

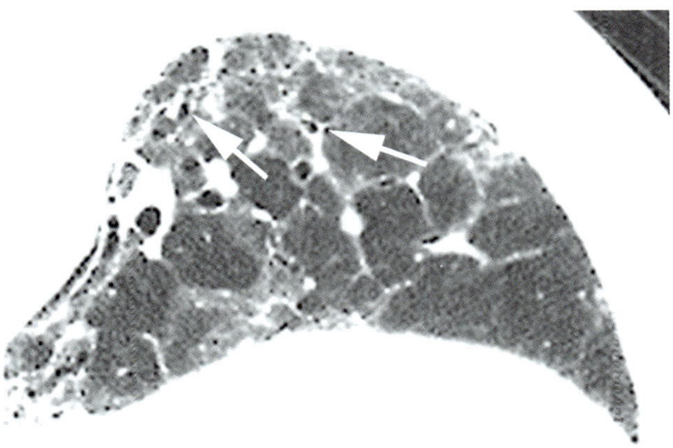

Figure 14.7. Ground-glass opacity (GGO) in idiopathic pulmonary fibrosis. Detail of the left lower lobe on a prone HRCT shows patchy ground-glass opacity. Note that the GGO is confined to areas that also have irregular reticular opacities and traction bronchiectasis (*arrows*) and bronchiolectasis, indicating the presence of fibrosis. Also note the areas of normal lung (ie, spatial heterogeneity). This amount of GGO and distribution is insufficient for the "suggestive of an alternative diagnosis" designation. HRCT, high-resolution CT.

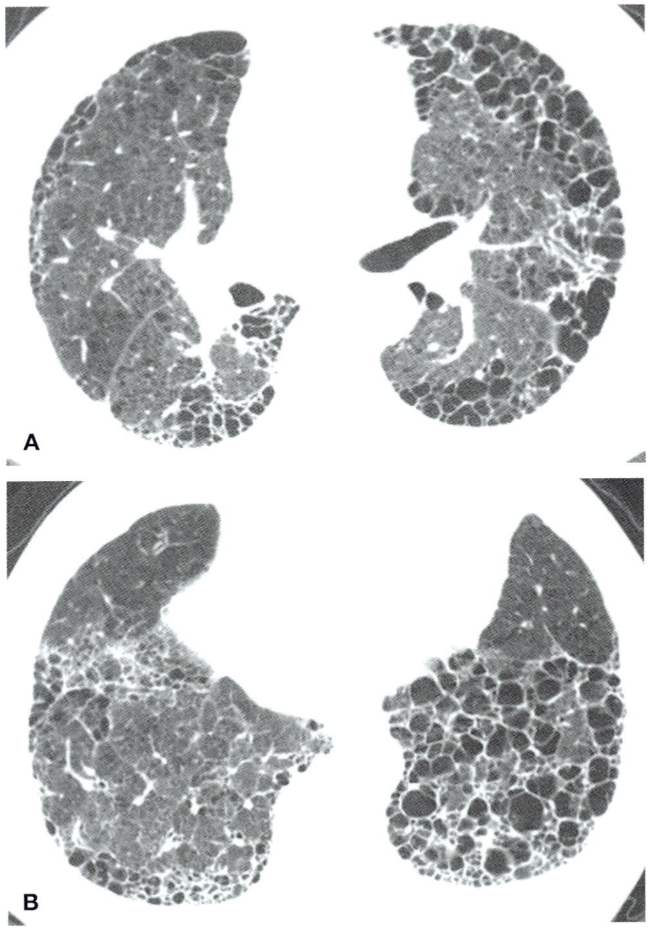

Figure 14.8. Combined pulmonary fibrosis and emphysema. **A:** High-resolution CT through the upper lobes shows centrilobular and paraseptal emphysema. **B:** Honeycombing is more conspicuous at the lung bases. The fibrosis, in this case, is a "usual interstitial pneumonia pattern".

honeycombing (see Fig. 14.3). As discussed previously these patients may forego surgical lung biopsy and be diagnosed with IPF after multidisciplinary discussion.

Distribution – subpleural and basal; spatially heterogeneous with areas of normal lung and areas of fibrosis on the same image.

CT features – reticulation, traction bronchiectasis without honeycombing; Absence of features suggesting an alternative diagnosis.

The *Indeterminate for UIP* pattern was added in the 2018 ATS guidelines and is used when fibrosis is present on CT but "does not meet UIP or probable UIP criteria and does not explicitly suggest an alternative diagnosis." Sometimes the findings are extremely mild and some authors have classified this as "interstitial lung abnormality" or ILA (see section at the end of this chapter):

Distribution – diffuse distribution without subpleural predominance

CT Features – findings of fibrosis that do not suggest a specific diagnosis

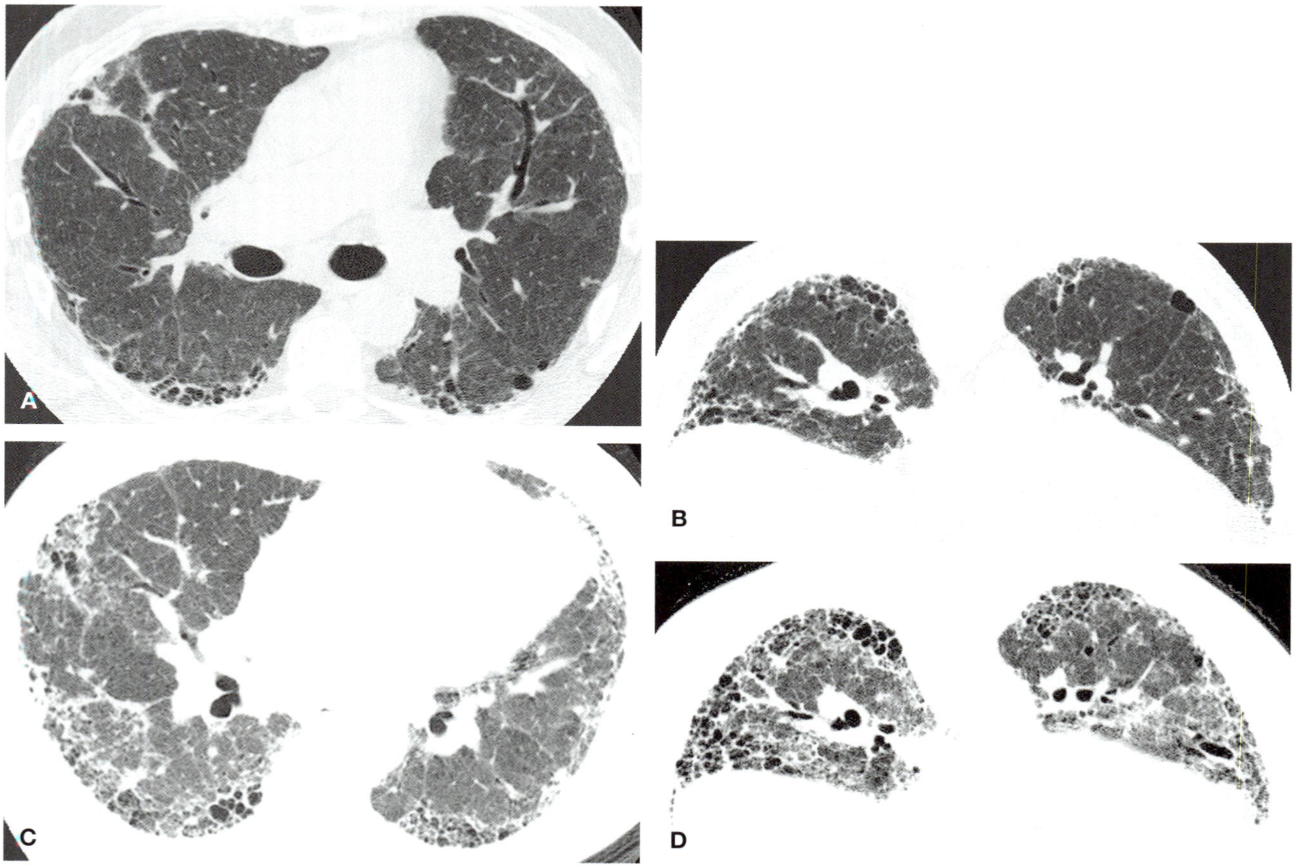

Figure 14.9. Acute exacerbation of idiopathic pulmonary fibrosis. Supine **(A)** and prone **(B)** HRCTs show subpleural reticulation and honeycombing in the lower lobes, typical of idiopathic pulmonary fibrosis. Supine **(C)** and prone **(D)** HRCTs at the time of an acute exacerbation show progression of honeycombing and an increase in ground-glass opacity. This reflects diffuse alveolar damage. HRCT, high-resolution CT.

HRCT findings suggestive of an *Alternative Diagnosis to UIP* are features typical of other interstitial pneumonia or other forms of lung disease. The presence of these findings supersedes a UIP pattern and are as follows:

Distribution – peribronchovascular with subpleural sparing (think NSIP); perilymphatic (think sarcoid); upper or mid-lung predominant (think HP, sarcoid, or CTD)

CT Features – cystic lung disease; mosaic attenuation or three-density sign (think HP); profuse nodules; consolidation (think OP); pleural plaques (think asbestos); dilated esophagus (think CTD)

Note that in all cases the final diagnosis should be made by multidisciplinary discussion. Being conversant in the UIP/IPF guidelines and HRCT classification is essential (Table 14.3).

NONSPECIFIC INTERSTITIAL PNEUMONIA

NSIP is less common than UIP. The histologic pattern is termed NSIP; it accounts for 20% of IPs. The idiopathic form of NSIP is termed *idiopathic NSIP*.

Despite its name, it is best to think of NSIP as a specific pathologic entity, not a "nonspecific" diagnosis. NSIP is characterized histologically by alveolar wall thickening or fibrosis. Abnormalities are described as showing spatial and temporal homogeneity. In other words, all parts of the biopsy look the same and represent the same stage of the disease; in UIP/IPF, the biopsy appears heterogeneous. NSIP may demonstrate cellular (ie, *cellular NSIP*) or fibrotic (ie, *fibrotic NSIP*) patterns (Table 14.4).

NSIP is often associated with CTDs, drug toxicity, hypersensitivity pneumonitis, infection, or immunodeficiency; it is uncommonly idiopathic. An association with CTDs is particularly common, and NSIP is the most common histologic abnormality present in patients with CTD and lung disease.

Clinically, patients with NSIP present with symptoms similar to those of IPF, including dyspnea and cough. The average duration of symptoms is 18 to 30 months at diagnosis (see Table 14.4). The average age at diagnosis is 40 to 50 years. Patients typically respond to treatment with steroids, and the prognosis is good, although this varies with the degree of fibrosis present. Overall, 5-year survival rate is 80% to 90%. Patients with cellular NSIP have a 5-year survival rate exceeding 90%; in patients with fibrotic NSIP, 5-year survival rate is 65% to 90%. Patients with NSIP may suffer an acute

Table 14.3 HRCT Pattern for Diagnosis of UIP/IPF

	UIP Pattern	Probable UIP Pattern	Indeterminate for UIP	CT Findings Suggestive of an Alternative Diagnosis
Level of Confidence for Histologic UIP	Confident (>90%)	Provisional high confidence (70%-89%)	Provisional low confidence (51%-69%)	Low to very low confidence (≤50%)
Distribution	Subpleural and basal predominant Spatial heterogeneity (normal lung and fibrosis interspersed) Occasionally diffuse in craniocaudal plane May be asymmetric	Subpleural and basal predominant Spatial heterogeneity	Diffuse distribution without subpleural predominance	Peribronchovascular with subpleural sparing (NSIP) Perilymphatic (sarcoidosis) Upper or mid-lung (fibrotic HP, CTD, sarcoidosis)
CT Features	Honeycombing with or without traction bronchiectasis/ bronchiolectasis Reticular pattern, irregular thickening of interlobular septa May have mild GGO May have pulmonary ossification	Reticular pattern with traction bronchiectasis/ bronchiolectasis May have mild GGO Absence of subpleural sparing	CT features that do not suggest a specific etiology	Cysts (LAM, PLCH, LIP, DIP) Mosaic attenuation or three-density sign (HP) Predominant GGO (HP, smoking-related disease, drug toxicity, acute exacerbation) Centrilobular nodules (HP or smoking-related) Nodules (sarcoid) Consolidation (OP) Pleural plaques (asbestosis) Dilated esophagus (CTD)

HRCT, high-resolution CT; IPF, idiopathic pulmonary fibrosis; UIP, usual interstitial pneumonia.

 Raghu G, Remy-Jardin M, Richeldi L, et al. Idiopathic pulmonary fibrosis (an update) and progressive pulmonary fibrosis in adults: an official ATS/ERS/JRS/ALAT clinical practice guideline. Am J Respir Crit Care Med. *2022;205(9):e18-e47.The American Journal of Respiratory and Critical Care Medicine is an official Journal of the American Thoracic Society.*

exacerbation similar to that occurring in UIP/IPF. Clinical trials are ongoing for the use of antifibrotic agents in NSIP.

Radiographic Findings

The radiographic findings consist mainly of ill-defined opacity, ground-glass opacity, or consolidation predominantly involving the lower lung zones (Figs. 14.10A and 14.11A). Other manifestations include a reticular pattern or a combination of reticular and air-space patterns. In 10% or more of cases, the chest radiograph is normal.

HRCT Findings

Because the histology associated with NSIP is variable, HRCT may show a variable combination of ground-glass opacity, patchy consolidation, reticular opacities, and traction bronchiectasis, usually with a concentric and symmetrical, peribronchovascular or peripheral, and basal predominance. Although honeycombing may be present in patients with NSIP, it is uncommon, being seen in a few percent of cases, and when present, tends to be inconspicuous and limited in extent, particularly in comparison to patients with UIP and IPF.

In most cases, patchy or concentric subpleural ground-glass opacity with a lower lobe predominance is seen on HRCT; superimposed fine reticulation is common, being seen in 50% of cases (see Figs. 14.10-14.13). Although it usually predominates in the peripheral lung, NSIP commonly shows sparing of the immediate subpleural lung region (20%-60% of cases). This finding, termed *subpleural sparing*, strongly suggests the diagnosis of NSIP and helps distinguish NSIP from UIP and IPF (see Figs. 14.12-14.16).

Ground-glass opacity suggests cellular NSIP (Fig. 14.12). GGO may be quite subtle in early or mild cases, being visible with certainty only on prone scans. Ground-glass opacity may resolve with treatment (Fig. 14.17). Reticulation and traction bronchiectasis occurring in the absence of ground-glass opacity correlate with the fibrotic pattern of NSIP (Figs. 14.15 and 14.16); traction bronchiectasis also may be seen in some patients with cellular NSIP.

The diagnosis of NSIP should be considered if HRCT shows ground-glass opacity or reticulation, without honeycombing,

Table 14.4 Nonspecific Interstitial Pneumonia: Histologic, Clinical, and HRCT Features

Histologic Pattern
Spatially and temporally homogeneous
Cellular pattern
  Mild to moderate interstitial inflammation
  Alveolar wall thickening
  Type II pneumocyte hyperplasia
  Dense fibrosis absent
Fibrotic pattern
  Mild to moderate chronic interstitial inflammation
  Fibrosis lacking the temporal heterogeneity and/or patchy distribution of usual interstitial pneumonia (UIP)
  Fibroblastic foci absent or inconspicuous
Differential diagnosis
  Idiopathic (nonspecific interstitial pneumonia)
  Connective tissue disease
  Hypersensitivity pneumonitis
  Drug toxicity
  Infection
  Immunodeficiency

Idiopathic clinical syndrome
Age 40-50 (younger than UIP)
Progressive dyspnea, for 18 mo or more (longer than UIP)
Pulmonary function tests: restriction and impaired gas exchange (less severe than UIP)
Treatment (steroids) usually effective
Prognosis good
HRCT findings
  Ground-glass opacity
  Irregular reticulation
  Patchy consolidation
  Honeycombing absent, inconspicuous, or minimal
  Concentric subpleural and basal predominance
  Subpleural sparing

HRCT, high-resolution CT.

in the subpleural and basal lung, particularly if subpleural sparing is present. These features are "Suggestive of an alternative diagnosis to UIP" when ATS criteria are applied. A lung biopsy may be necessary for diagnosis because fibrotic NSIP may resemble early UIP/IPF (Fig. 14.3). In patients with known CTD, treatment is often undertaken without biopsy if the HRCT suggests or is consistent with either cellular or fibrotic NSIP.

ORGANIZING PNEUMONIA (CRYPTOGENIC ORGANIZING PNEUMONIA)

Organizing pneumonia (*OP*) is a histologic pattern of lung injury characterized by the presence of patchy areas of organizing pneumonia, consisting largely of mononuclear cells, foamy macrophages, and organizing fibrosis in peripheral airspaces, including bronchioles, alveolar ducts, and alveoli (Table 14.5). It is common, accounting for 10% to 20% of IP. Formerly, OP was termed bronchiolitis obliterans organizing pneumonia (BOOP), a term which is still sometimes used.

Idiopathic OP is termed *COP*. However, OP is more often seen in association with a variety of diseases, including connective tissue diseases (particularly myositis syndromes), pulmonary infection (most recently COVID-19), drug reactions, bronchial obstruction, aspiration, and after toxic fume inhalation. It may also accompany radiation pneumonitis, hypersensitivity pneumonitis, UIP, NSIP, and other patterns.

Patients with OP typically present with a subacute history of nonproductive cough, low-grade fever, malaise, and shortness of breath. Mean age at presentation is 55. PFTs characteristically show a restrictive pattern. Clinically and functionally, the findings may be similar to IPF, although the duration of symptoms in patients with OP is shorter, and systemic symptoms are more common. Patients usually respond well to corticosteroid therapy and have a good prognosis.

Radiographic Findings

The characteristic radiologic features of OP/COP consist of patchy, unilateral, or bilateral areas of air-space consolidation. Small nodular opacities or larger nodules may be seen as the only finding or, more commonly, are seen in association with areas of air-space consolidation. In some patients, consolidation is peripheral, a pattern similar to that seen in chronic eosinophilic pneumonia.

HRCT Findings

HRCT findings in patients with OP/COP vary and may include the following:

1. Patchy consolidation (80% of cases) or ground-glass opacity (60%), often with a subpleural and/or peribronchial distribution (Figs. 14.18-14.20).
2. Small, ill-defined nodules (30%-50% of cases), which may be peribronchial or peribronchiolar (ie, centrilobular; Fig. 14.21).
3. Large nodules or masses, which may be irregular in shape (see Figs. 14.19 and 14.21).
4. Focal or lobar consolidation (Fig. 14.22).
5. The "reversed halo sign" or "atoll sign," in which ring-shaped or crescentic consolidation is seen, with ground-glass opacity in the center of the ring (thus resembling a coral atoll or the reverse of the halo sign; see Figs. 14.19A and 14.23). It is most common with drug reactions.
6. A "perilobular pattern," with opacities in the periphery of pulmonary lobules, mimicking the appearance of interlobular septal thickening (Fig. 14.24). However, what appear to be thickened septa are thicker than is usually seen. This pattern is often associated with peripheral

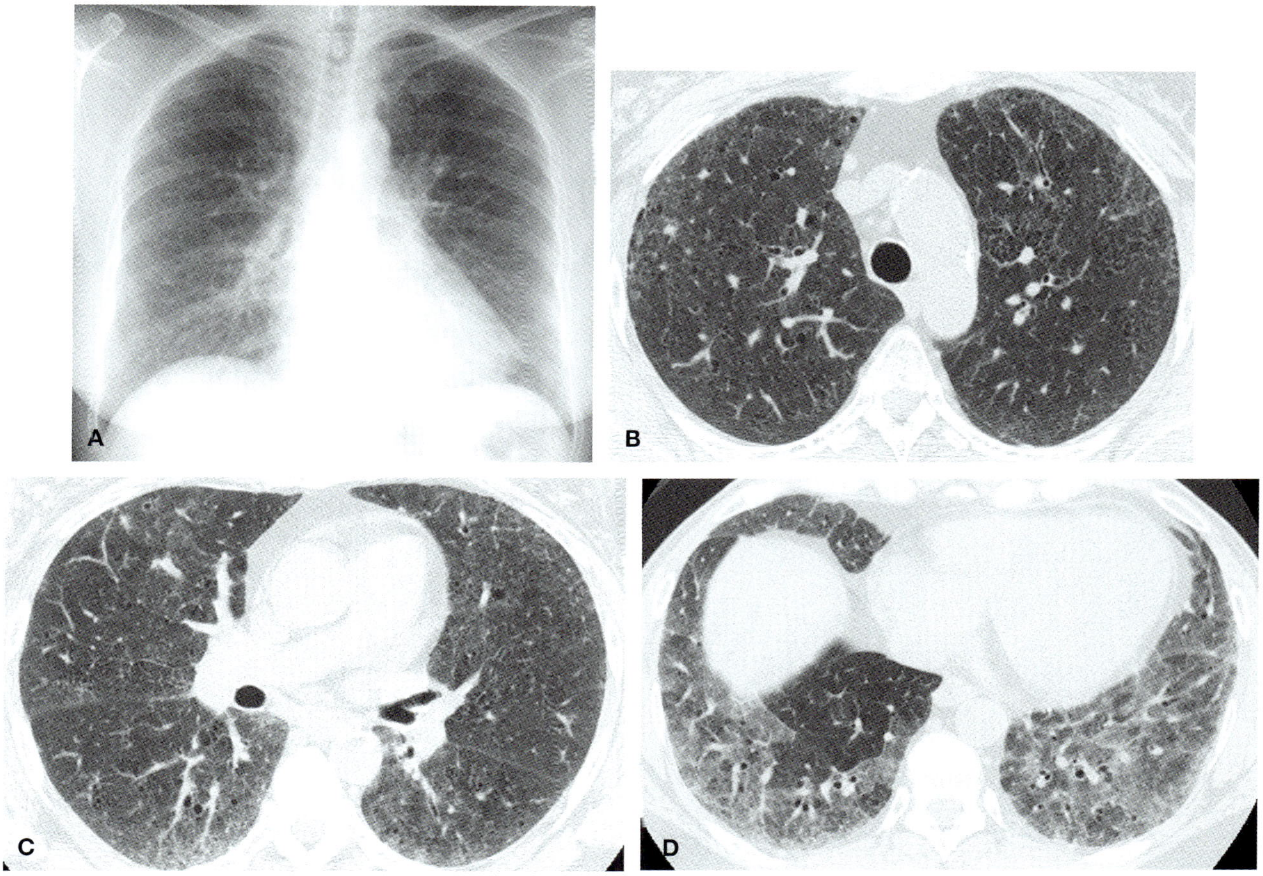

Figure 14.10. Cellular nonspecific interstitial pneumonia. **A:** Chest radiograph shows a subtle increase in opacity at the lung bases. **B-D:** High-resolution CTs at three levels shows an increase in ground-glass opacity and reticular opacities, which is predominant at the lung bases and in the lung periphery.

ground-glass opacity, typical of NSIP, or consolidation, typical of OP. It is common in myositis syndromes.

OP/COP often involves the lower lung zones to a greater degree than the upper lung zones. A pattern of patchy peripheral or peribronchial consolidation is common, seen in more than 70% of cases, and should be sufficient to suggest the diagnosis in a patient with a typical history of progressive dyspnea and low-grade fever. There is considerable overlap between the presentation, CT appearance, treatment, and prognosis of OP and chronic eosinophilic pneumonia, differing only in the presence of eosinophilia in the latter.

Other findings in patients with OP/COP include small pleural effusions, present in 30% to 35% of cases, irregular linear opacities, mild honeycombing, and "crazy paving," with a superimposition of ground-glass opacity and interlobular septal thickening.

ACUTE INTERSTITIAL PNEUMONIA

AIP is a fulminant disease of unknown cause, usually occurring in a previously healthy person. It is associated with the histologic pattern of *DAD* with alveolar hyaline membranes and diffuse, active interstitial fibrosis (Table 14.6); it accounts for about 5% of IIPs. The appearance of DAD in AIP is indistinguishable from DAD in patients with acute respiratory distress syndrome (ARDS) caused by sepsis, shock, infection, drug toxicity, toxic inhalations, trauma, or other insults; DAD in the setting of one of these conditions is relatively common.

The mean age at presentation is 50. A prodromal illness associated with symptoms of a viral upper respiratory infection is often present, followed by rapidly increasing dyspnea and respiratory failure. Patients with AIP usually require mechanical ventilation within 1 to 2 weeks of the onset of symptoms. Fifty percent or more die within 6 months of presentation.

Because of its acute presentation and histologic pattern identical to that of ARDS, AIP has been referred to as idiopathic ARDS. It was formerly known as *Hamman-Rich syndrome* (see Chapter 12).

Radiographic Findings

Chest radiographs show bilateral air-space consolidation or ground-glass opacity that is diffuse (50%) or may predominate in the upper (25%) or lower (25%) lung zones

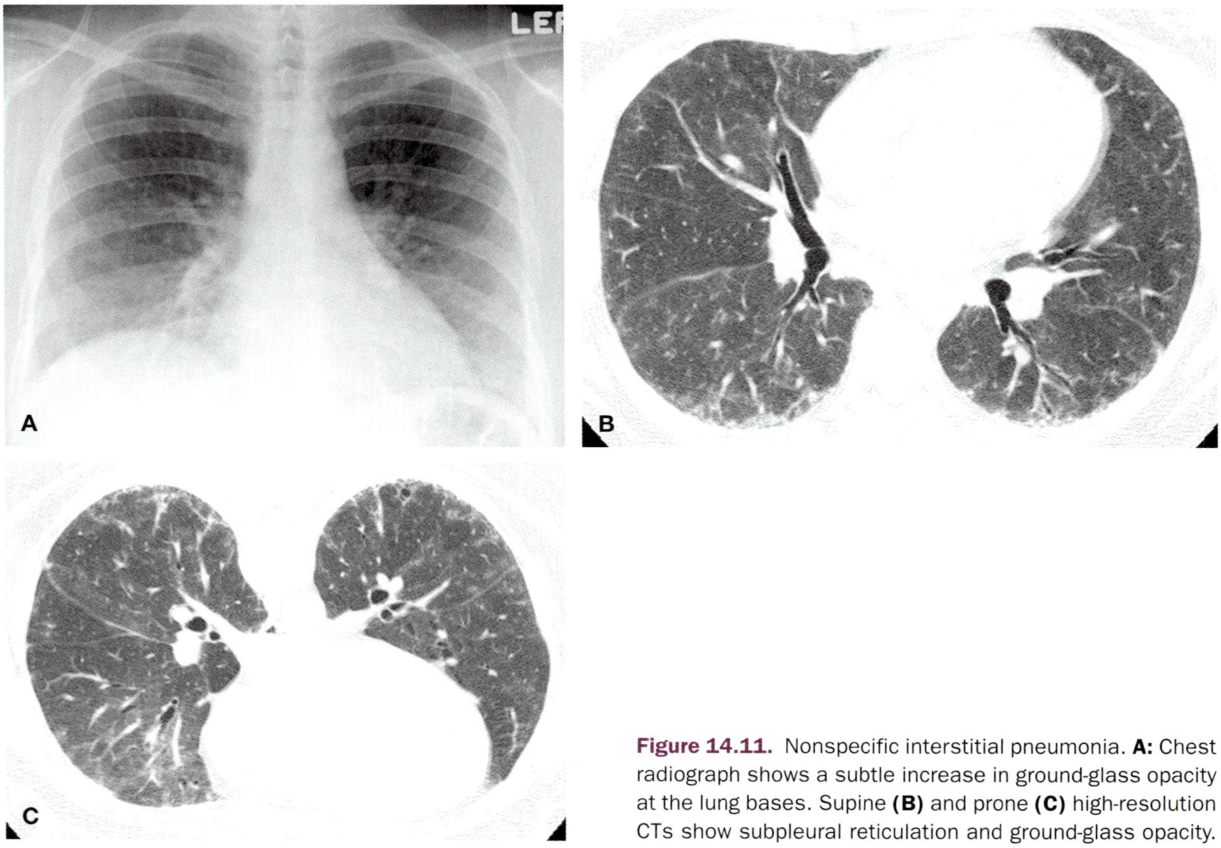

Figure 14.11. Nonspecific interstitial pneumonia. **A:** Chest radiograph shows a subtle increase in ground-glass opacity at the lung bases. Supine **(B)** and prone **(C)** high-resolution CTs show subpleural reticulation and ground-glass opacity.

(Figs. 14.25-14.27). Honeycombing may be seen late in the disease. Findings are similar to other causes of ARDS.

HRCT Findings

There is little reason to obtain HRCT in a patient with AIP. Findings are similar to those of any patient with ARDS.

In the early stages of AIP, HRCT shows patchy bilateral ground-glass opacity and consolidation, which tend to be diffuse or patchy, indistinguishable from other causes of ARDS. Abnormalities are most severe in the posterior lungs (see Figs. 14.26C and 14.27C). Architectural distortion, traction bronchiectasis, and honeycombing may be seen as the disease progresses.

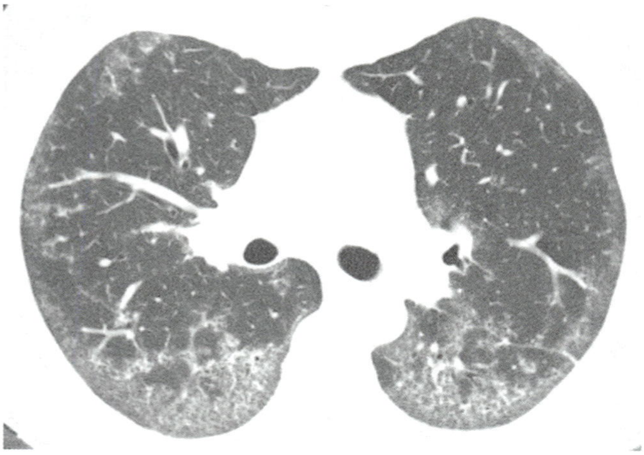

Figure 14.12. Cellular nonspecific interstitial pneumonia with ground-glass opacity. Supine high-resolution CT shows ground-glass opacity with superimposed fine reticulation. Abnormalities predominate at the lung bases. There is subpleural sparing.

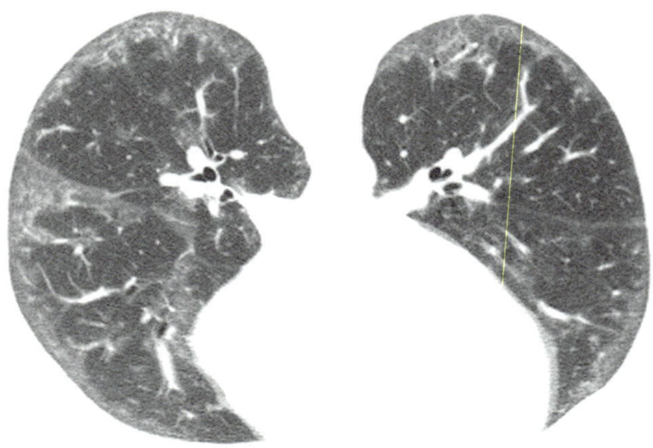

Figure 14.13. Nonspecific interstitial pneumonia with ground-glass opacity. Ground-glass opacities are concentric and predominate in the lung periphery but spare the immediate subpleural lung.

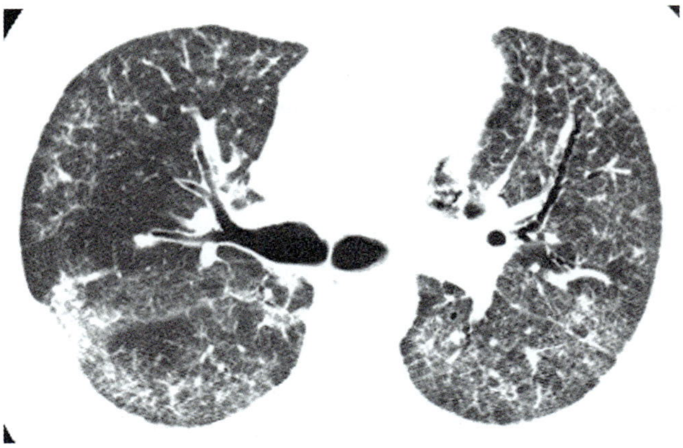

Figure 14.14. Nonspecific interstitial pneumonia with ground-glass opacity and reticulation. Supine high-resolution CTs show a combination of ground-glass opacity and reticulation. There is sparing of the immediate subpleural lung. This finding helps to distinguish nonspecific interstitial pneumonia from usual interstitial pneumonia.

DIP, RB, AND RB-ILD

DIP is a rare condition characterized histologically by the presence of numerous macrophages filling alveoli, mild inflammation of alveolar walls, and minimal fibrosis. DIP is typically diffuse in distribution (Table 14.7).

Although DIP is classified as an IIP, more than 90% of patients with DIP are cigarette smokers. In most cases, DIP is considered to be a smoking-related disease. It also can be seen in association with toxic inhalation, drug reactions, Langerhans cell histiocytosis, leukemia, asbestosis, and hard-metal pneumoconiosis.

If the alveolar macrophage infiltrate is localized, having a peribronchiolar predominance, it is usually referred to using the term *RB* rather than DIP (see Table 14.7). RB is a common

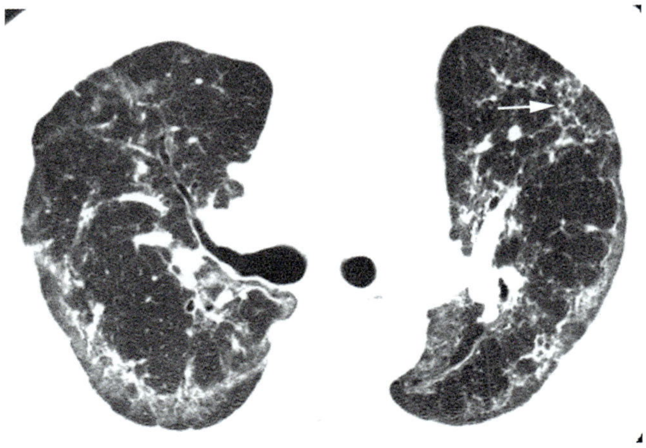

Figure 14.15. Fibrotic nonspecific interstitial pneumonia. Supine high-resolution CTs show reticular opacities and ground-glass opacity. The presence of traction bronchiectasis (*arrow*) suggests that fibrosis is likely present. There is sparing of the immediate subpleural lung. Honeycombing is absent.

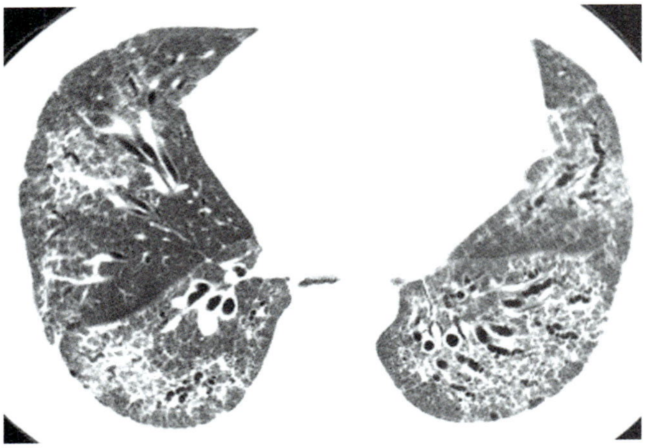

Figure 14.16. Fibrotic nonspecific interstitial pneumonia. Supine high-resolution CTs show coarse reticular opacities and extensive traction bronchiectasis. There is sparing of the immediate subpleural lung. Honeycombing is absent despite the findings of fibrosis.

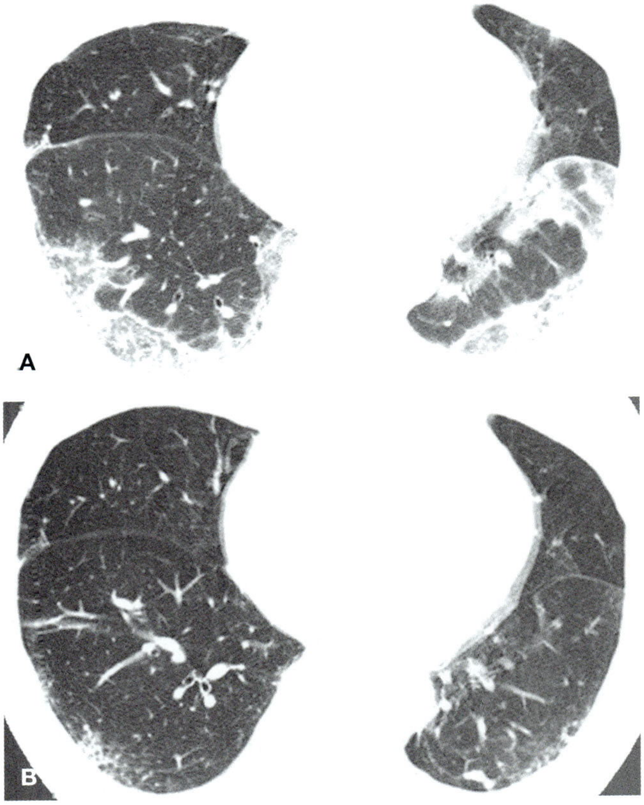

Figure 14.17. Clearing of nonspecific interstitial pneumonia with treatment. **A:** Baseline high-resolution CT shows subpleural ground-glass opacity with superimposed reticulation and focal areas of consolidation. **B:** After treatment with steroids, there has been a significant reduction in ground-glass opacity and consolidation. Some reticulation persists, due to fibrosis.

Table 14.5 Organizing Pneumonia and Cryptogenic Organizing Pneumonia: Histologic, Clinical, and HRCT Features

OP: histologic pattern
Characteristics
- Organizing fibrosis in distal airspaces
- Lack of interstitial fibrosis
- Patchy distribution
- Mild chronic interstitial inflammation

Differential diagnosis
- Idiopathic (COP)
- Pulmonary infection
- Bronchial obstruction
- Aspiration
- Drug reactions
- Connective tissue diseases
- Toxic fume inhalation
- Radiation pneumonitis
- Hypersensitivity pneumonitis

COP: idiopathic clinical syndrome
Mean age 55 y
Several months of cough, fever, and dyspnea
PFT: restriction and impaired gas exchange (less severe than usual interstitial pneumonia)
Treatment (steroids) effective
Prognosis very good
HRCT findings
- Patchy consolidation or ground-glass opacity
- Subpleural or peribronchial distribution
- Air bronchograms
- Small, ill-defined nodules, centrilobular
- Large irregular nodules or masses
- Focal consolidation
- "Atoll" or "reversed halo" sign
- "Perilobular" pattern

COP, cryptogenic organizing pneumonia; HRCT, high-resolution CT; OP, organizing pneumonia.

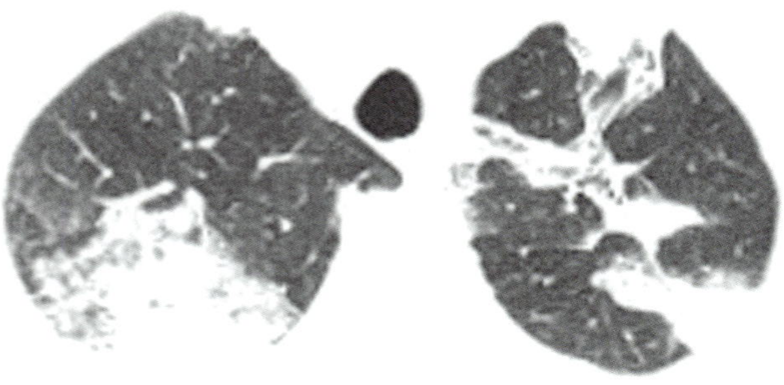

Figure 14.18. HRCT in organizing pneumonia. The classic appearance of cryptogenic organizing pneumonia is patchy subpleural and peribronchial consolidation. In this patient, subpleural consolidation predominates.

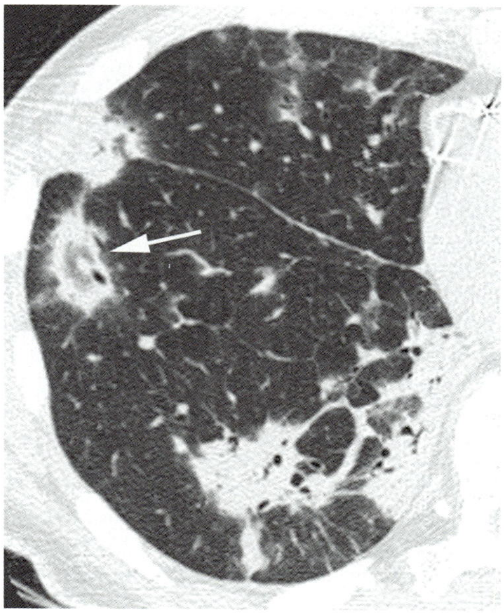

Figure 14.19. Subpleural and peribronchial consolidation in organizing pneumonia. High-resolution CT shows irregular nodular areas of consolidation, many occurring in relation to bronchi. Air bronchograms are visible within the opacities. An example of the "atoll" or "reversed halo" sign is visible in the midlung (*arrow*). The opacities have irregular margins.

incidental finding in the lungs of asymptomatic smokers. If the histologic finding of RB is associated with pulmonary symptoms, the resulting syndrome is called RB-ILD. The association of smoking with RB and RB-ILD is even stronger than with DIP.

DIP, RB, and RB-ILD represent different degrees of lung involvement by the same process, with RB being the mildest and most localized and DIP being the most extensive. RB and RB-ILD are more common than DIP (see Table 14.7).

DIP and RB-ILD occur most commonly in patients between 30 and 50 years of age. The clinical symptoms usually consist of slowly progressive dyspnea and dry cough. They account for about 10% of IPs.

The prognosis of patients with DIP and RB-ILD is very good. Smoking cessation leads to an improvement in symptoms. Patients who continue to smoke may improve clinically, but those with persistent complaints may benefit from oral steroid therapy. It has been suggested that RB may be the precursor to chronic airway abnormalities or centrilobular emphysema in susceptible smokers.

Radiographic Findings

The most common abnormality on chest radiographs in patients with DIP is ground-glass opacities seen in the lower lung zones (Fig. 14.28A). However, in up to 25% of patients with DIP, the chest radiographs are normal. Chest radiographs in patients with RB-ILD can be normal or can show nonspecific bilateral, ill-defined opacities, usually with a lower zonal predominance.

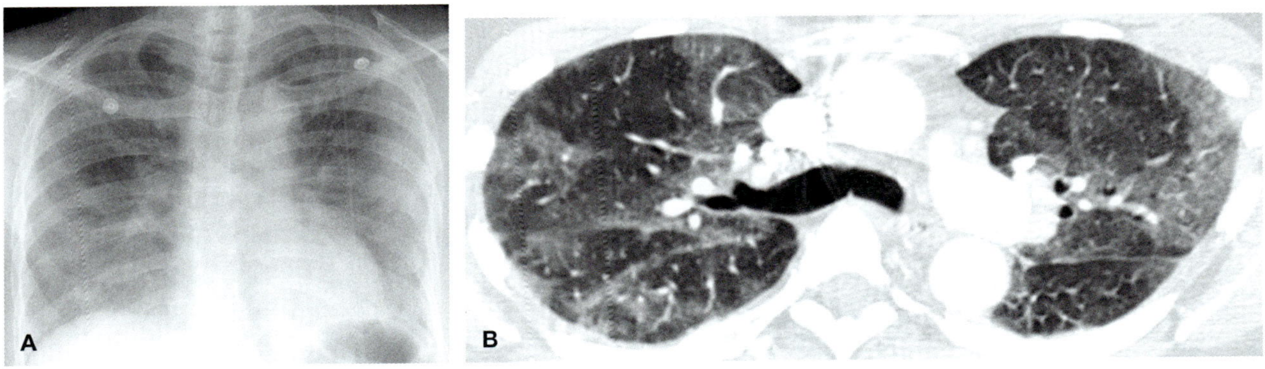

Figure 14.20. Patchy ground-glass opacity in organizing pneumonia. **A:** Chest radiograph shows an increase in lung opacity. **B:** High-resolution CT shows patchy areas of ground-glass opacity.

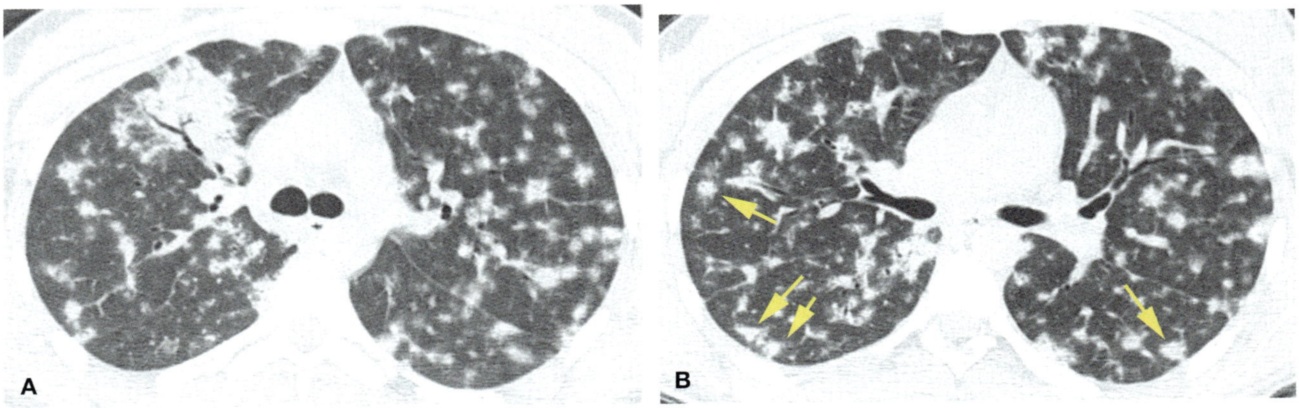

Figure 14.21. Irregular nodular opacities in organizing pneumonia. **A:** CT shows irregular nodular opacities. Focal consolidation is visible in the right upper lobe. **B:** At a lower level, multiple nodular opacities are visible, many occurring in relation to bronchi. Some of the nodules (*arrows*) appear centrilobular in location.

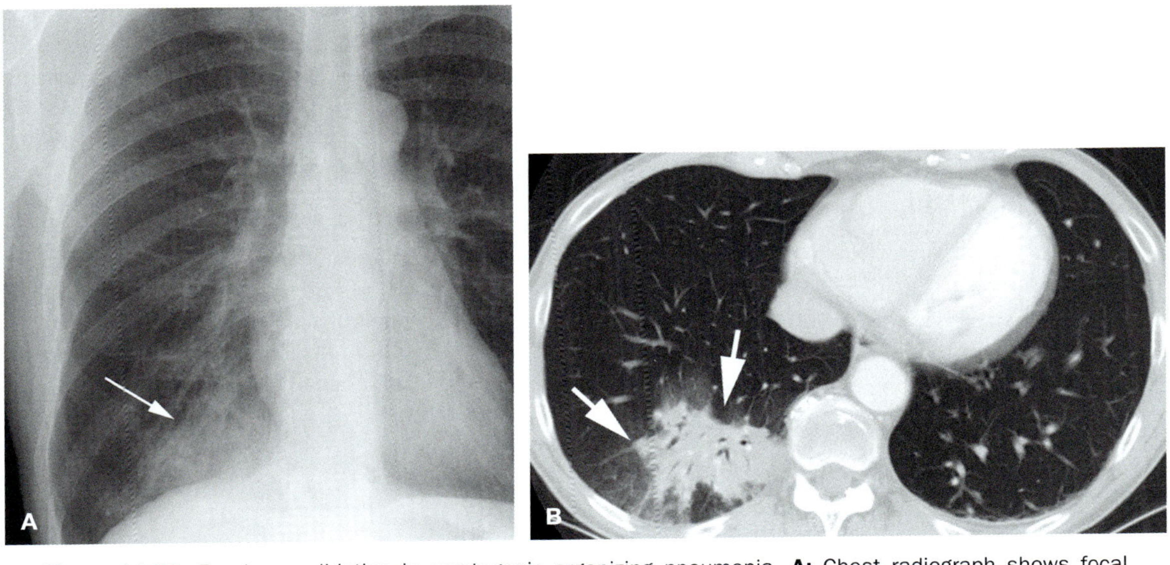

Figure 14.22. Focal consolidation in cryptogenic organizing pneumonia. **A:** Chest radiograph shows focal consolidation in the right lower lobe (*arrow*) **B:** High-resolution CT shows an irregular peripheral area of consolidation in the right lower lobe (*arrows*), containing air bronchograms.

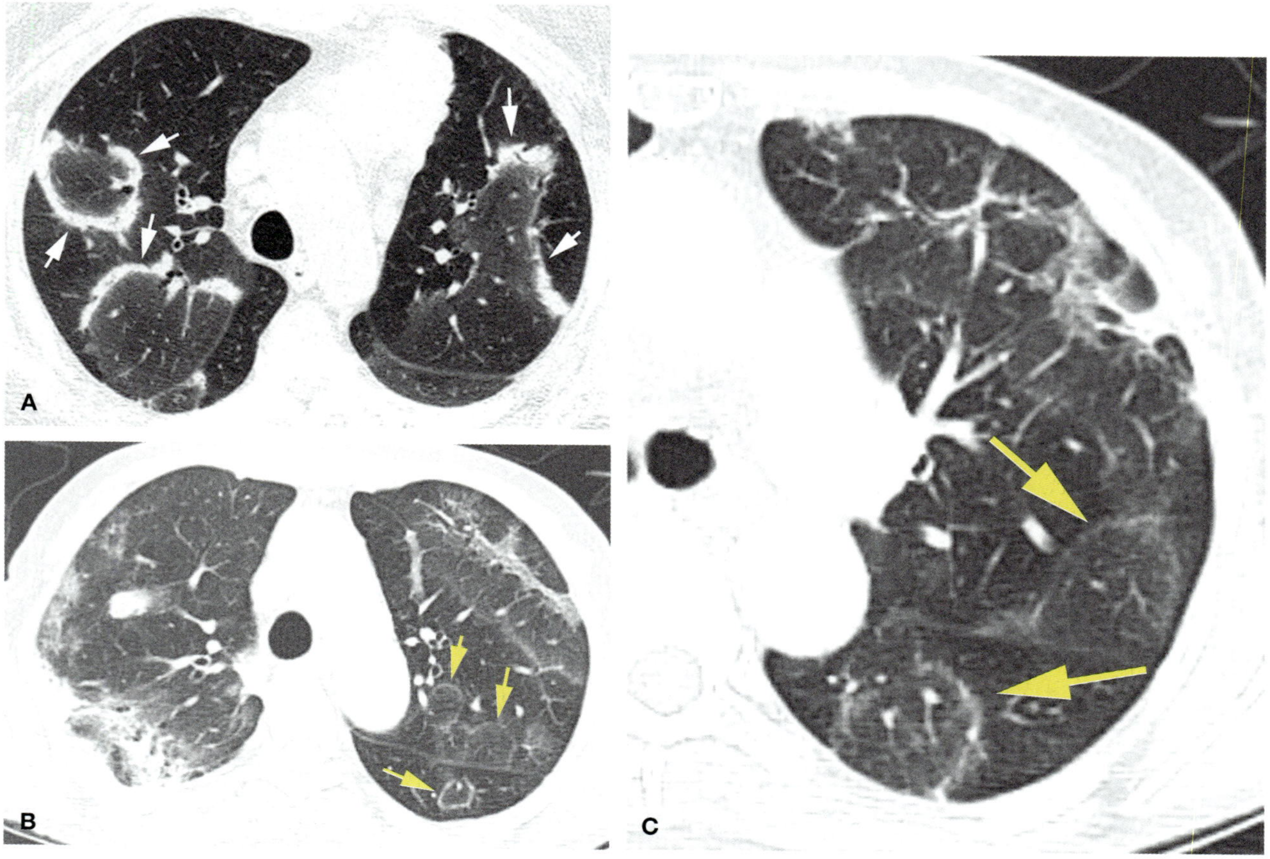

Figure 14.23. **A:** The "reversed halo" or "atoll" sign in organizing pneumonia. Crescentic regions of consolidation (*arrows*) surround or outline areas of ground-glass opacity. **B and C:** In another patient with organizing pneumonia, patchy peripheral and peribronchial consolidation is associated with thin-walled "atolls" (*arrows*).

HRCT Findings

In patients with DIP, the predominant abnormality on HRCT consists of areas of ground-glass opacity (see Figs. 14.28 and 14.29). A subpleural and lower lobe predominance is seen in 60% to 75%; a diffuse distribution may also be seen. Although reticular opacities are commonly associated with ground-glass opacity, honeycombing or obvious fibrosis is rare.

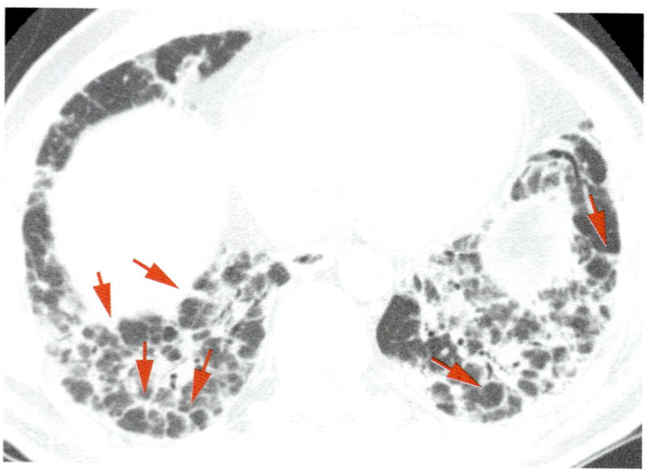

Figure 14.24. The "perilobular" pattern in organizing pneumonia . Opacities at the lung bases mimic the appearance of interlobular septal thickening (*arrows*).

Because of its association with smoking, centrilobular emphysema may be visible. Small cystic lucencies, not representing emphysema, may also be seen in patients with DIP (see Fig. 14.29A). Patchy air trapping may be seen on expiratory scans, presumably associated with smoking-related small airway disease (see Fig. 14.29B).

Not all patients with RB-ILD show abnormalities on HRCT. When abnormal, HRCT findings include centrilobular ground-glass opacity nodules (40% of cases), patchy ground-glass opacities (50%), and thickening of bronchial walls, probably related to smoking and bronchitis (Fig. 14.30).

Unlike patients with DIP, an upper lobe predominance is typical of RB-ILD. A small percentage of patients (25%) show some reticular opacities due to fibrosis. The fibrosis in RB-ILD is mild and tends to involve mainly the lower lung zones.

LYMPHOID INTERSTITIAL PNEUMONIA

LIP is characterized histologically by a dense lymphoid interstitial infiltrate consisting predominantly of lymphocytes, plasma cells, and histiocytes (Table 14.8). Alveolar

Table 14.6 Diffuse Alveolar Damage and Acute Interstitial Pneumonia: Histologic, Clinical, and HRCT Features

DAD: histologic pattern
Characteristics
Diffuse distribution
Uniform temporal appearance
Hyaline membranes
Alveolar wall thickening due to organizing fibrosis
No evidence of infection
Differential diagnosis
Any cause of acute respiratory distress syndrome (ARDS)
AIP: idiopathic clinical syndrome
Idiopathic ARDS or Hamman-Rich syndrome
Mean age 50 y
Prodromal illness suggesting viral infection
1-2 wk of progressive dyspnea
Pulmonary function tests: restriction and impaired gas exchange
Severe hypoxemia
Prognosis poor (50% die)
Radiographic features of ARDS
HRCT findings
Diffuse or patchy consolidation
Diffuse or patchy ground-glass opacity
Posterior, lower lobe predominance

AIP, acute interstitial pneumonia; DAD, diffuse alveolar damage; HRCT, high-resolution CT.

walls are extensively involved. Lymphoid follicles may be present. If the interstitial infiltrate occurs primarily in relation to small airways, in association with lymphoid follicles, the abnormality may be termed *follicular bronchiolitis.* LIP is considered by some to be a lymphoproliferative disease rather than an IIP.

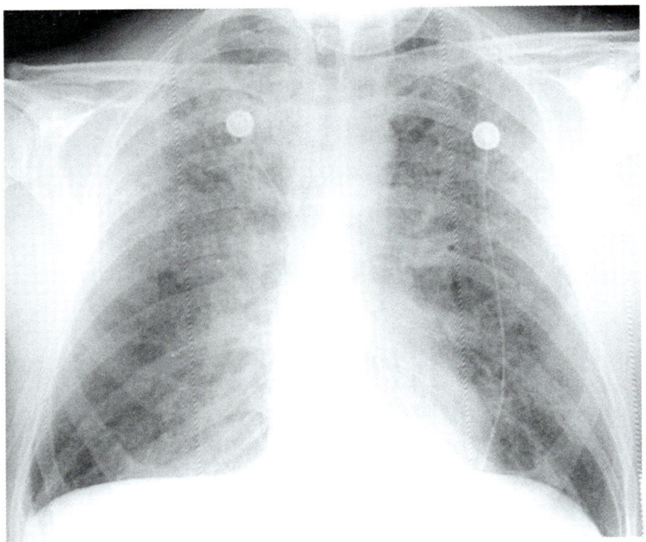

Figure 14.25. Acute interstitial pneumonia. Chest radiograph at presentation shows diffuse, ill-defined areas of ground-glass opacity and consolidation.

LIP is rarely idiopathic and frequently occurs in association with CTD (particularly Sjögren's syndrome, rheumatoid arthritis, and lupus), immunologic disorders (eg, Hashimoto's thyroiditis, autoimmune hemolytic anemia, myasthenia gravis, pernicious anemia, chronic active hepatitis), infection, immunodeficiency (eg, AIDS), and drug toxicity. LIP occurring in AIDS patients usually occurs in children; otherwise, most patients with LIP are adults (mean age, 50 years). LIP is more common in women.

The presentation of LIP is often that of the underlying disease (if present). The main clinical symptoms are cough and dyspnea, progressing over a period of a few years. Steroids are helpful in treatment, but about one-third of patients progress to lung fibrosis.

Radiographic Findings

The radiographic appearance of LIP is variable and nonspecific. Most often, radiographs show a reticular pattern predominantly involving the lower lung zones. Less common abnormalities include a nodular pattern or air-space consolidation.

HRCT Findings

HRCT findings reflect the predominant sites of lymphocytic infiltration and tend to vary with the underlying disease. The HRCT findings of LIP include the following:

1. Diffuse or patchy areas of ground-glass opacity (Figs. 14.31 and 14.32A) or consolidation (see Fig. 7.37 in Chapter 7). This appearance reflects the presence of alveolar infiltration and is most frequent in patients with immune deficiency.
2. Poorly defined centrilobular nodules (see Figs. 14.31 and 14.32A). This appearance correlates with the presence of lymphocytic infiltration predominantly involving bronchioles (follicular bronchiolitis) and is most frequent in connective tissue disease or acquired immunodeficiency syndrome (AIDS).
3. Small, well-defined nodules with a perilymphatic distribution or septal thickening (Fig. 14.33) mimicking lymphangitic spread of carcinoma. This is due to interstitial infiltration and most common in AIDS.
4. Isolated cystic airspaces, which may appear perivascular and are usually limited in number (see Figs. 14.33 and 14.34), or diffuse cystic disease that may resemble honeycombing (see Figs. 14.32B and 14.35). This is most often associated with Sjögren's syndrome and CTD. The cysts may be due to bronchiolar obstruction or represent protein deposition (see Chapters 15 and 25).

PLEUROPARENCHYMAL FIBROELASTOSIS

PPFE is a recently described, very rare condition characterized by an upper lobe predominance of elastotic fibrosis of the pleura and adjacent parenchyma. The characteristic

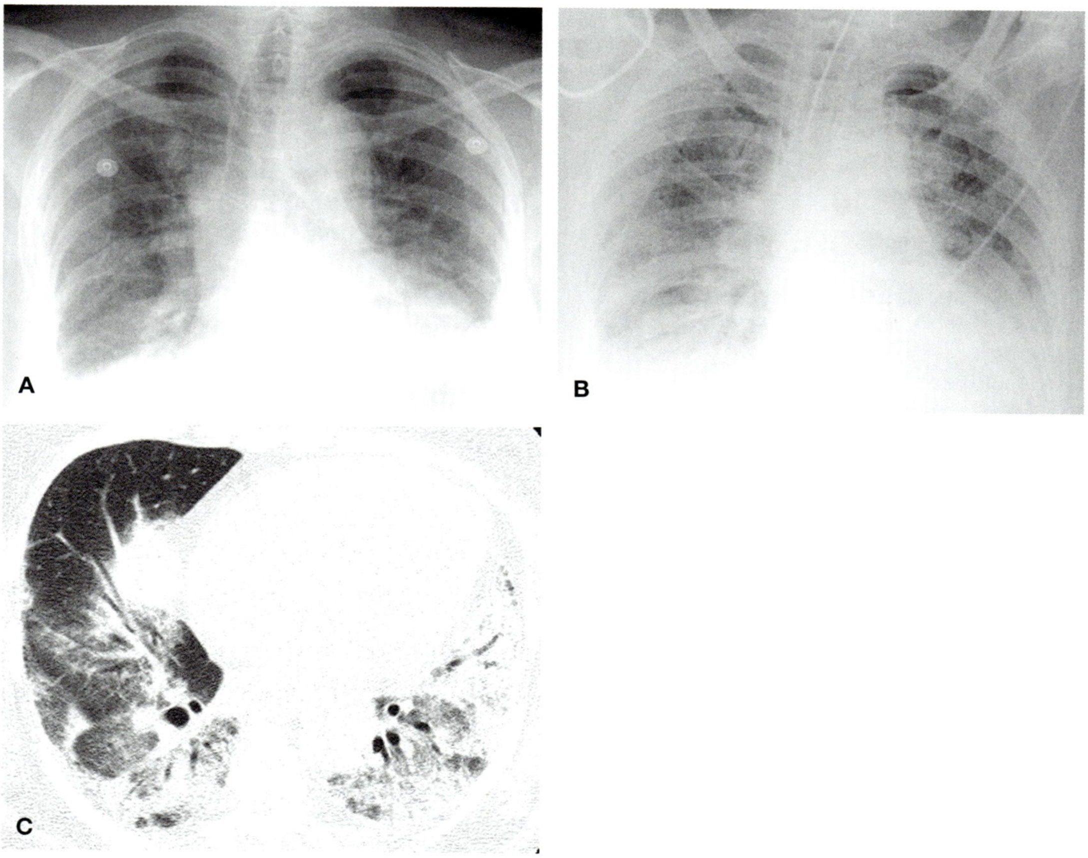

Figure 14.26. Acute interstitial pneumonia proved at autopsy. **A:** At presentation, chest radiograph shows ill-defined consolidation at the lung bases. **B:** After 1 week, the patient is intubated and consolidation has progressed. The appearance is similar to other causes of acute respiratory distress syndrome. **C:** High-resolution CT shows ground-glass opacity and consolidation consistent with DAD.

histologic findings consist of marked thickening of the visceral pleura due to a homogeneous mixture of elastic tissue and dense collagen associated with parenchymal fibrosis and septal elastosis. The histologic findings tend to be temporally homogeneous as opposed to the temporally heterogeneous pattern seen in UIP. The majority of cases are idiopathic, although some patients may have nonspecific autoantibodies, a familial history, bone marrow transplantation, lung transplantation with restrictive allograft syndrome, or infection. Mean age is 50 to 60 years; there is no sex predilection.

The most common symptoms are dry cough and shortness of breath present for several months or years prior to diagnosis. Approximately 50% of patients have a history of recurrent lower respiratory tract infections. In approximately 60% of patients, the clinical course is progressive despite treatment with corticosteroids and immunosuppressants, and death from the disease occurs in approximately 40% of patients.

Radiographic Findings

Chest radiographs are nonspecific and typically show marked pleural thickening mainly in the peripheral upper lungs, associated with upward hilar retraction.

HRCT Findings

The characteristic HRCT features of PPFE consist of predominantly upper lung zone pleural thickening and subpleural reticulation, associated with upper lobe volume loss and upward retraction of the hila (Figs. 14.36 and 14.37). Architectural distortion, traction bronchiectasis, reticulation, and honeycombing may be seen. The abnormalities involved mainly the upper lobes, lower lobe involvement being less marked or absent. Evidence of interstitial fibrosis in lung regions remote from the upper lobe pleuroparenchymal abnormalities, and involving the mid or lower lungs, may be seen, with an HRCT pattern suggestive of NSIP or UIP.

INTERSTITIAL LUNG ABNORMALITY

ILAs are incidental findings of fibrosis at HRCT in asymptomatic patients without a known diagnosis of ILD and are reported in up to 9% of smokers and 7% of nonsmokers on CT. Understanding of ILAs is evolving, and recent publications have subclassified ILA into non-subpleural (which do not progress), and subpleural (which can progress) subtypes. Subpleural ILAs are important as they may represent the earliest manifestation of UIP/IPF. Estimates for progression of subpleural ILAs are 20% and >70% at 2 and 5 years,

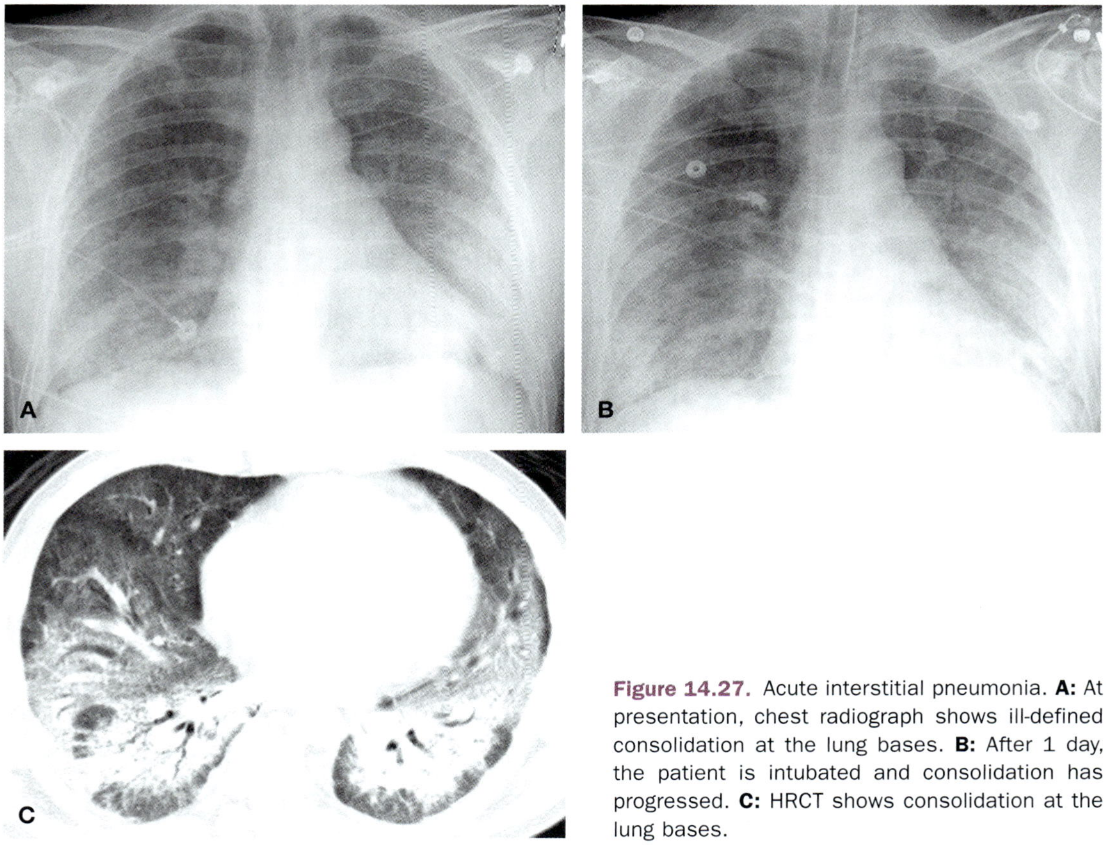

Figure 14.27. Acute interstitial pneumonia. **A:** At presentation, chest radiograph shows ill-defined consolidation at the lung bases. **B:** After 1 day, the patient is intubated and consolidation has progressed. **C:** HRCT shows consolidation at the lung bases.

respectively, with some of these patients becoming clinically symptomatic.

HRCT imaging findings of subpleural ILAs include mild ground-glass opacity and/or mild reticulation (Fig. 14.38). The distribution is basal and peripheral predominant just like UIP. Prone imaging may be helpful to differentiate mild fibrosis from dependent atelectasis. If traction bronchiolectasis or honeycombing are present, or if the patient is symptomatic, then it is better to classify the imaging as either a UIP or Probable UIP pattern depending on the specific findings. See the 2022 review article by Hata et al in the references for more information on ILAs.

A HRCT APPROACH TO THE DIAGNOSIS OF THE INTERSTITIAL PNEUMONIAS: THE HRCT "PATTERN"

The radiologist is often asked to suggest a diagnosis based on HRCT in a patient with chronic and progressive respiratory symptoms. In these patients, the diagnosis is most often sarcoidosis, hypersensitivity pneumonitis, or an interstitial pneumonia. Fortunately, the HRCT appearances of these entities are usually sufficiently different from provide guidance.

The HRCT appearances seen in the interstitial pneumonias are very helpful in suggesting the diagnosis. HRCT findings and the key findings in diagnosis are listed in Table 14.9. Familiarity with diagnostic guidelines (either ATS or Fleischner Society as mentioned above and referenced at the end of this chapter) provides a framework for your approach to interstitial pneumonia on HRCT. A few important rules should be remembered:

1. Honeycombing with a basal and subpleural predominance, in the absence of a known disease or exposure, is highly suggestive of UIP/IPF. Lung biopsy is uncommonly performed when HRCT shows these findings.
2. Uniform lower lobe ground-glass opacity without honeycombing suggests NSIP. In a patient with CTD, biopsy is uncommonly performed.
3. Subpleural sparing of abnormalities (reticulation or ground-glass opacity) strongly suggests NSIP.
4. Patchy or nodular subpleural or peribronchial consolidation is typical of OP or COP. The atoll or reversed halo sign suggests this diagnosis.
5. ARDS with typical plain film or CT findings of lung injury, without known cause, may be AIP.
6. Diffuse or centrilobular ground-glass opacity in a smoker is typical of DIP or RB-ILD.
7. Cystic airspaces or ground-glass opacity may represent LIP. LIP is usually associated with other diseases.

When interpreting HRCT, typical findings of an interstitial pneumonia should lead to the diagnosis of the *pattern* considered to be present. Although a definite diagnosis

Table 14.7 Desquamative Interstitial Pneumonia, Respiratory Bronchiolitis, and Respiratory Bronchiolitis-Interstitial Lung Disease: Histologic, Clinical, and HRCT Features

DIP and RB: histologic patterns
DIP characteristics
Diffuse distribution
Intra-alveolar macrophages
Minimal fibrosis
RB characteristics
Bronchiolocentric (peribronchiolar) distribution
Intra-alveolar macrophages
Minimal fibrosis
Differential diagnosis
90% cigarette smokers (DIP), RB higher incidence
Idiopathic
Inhalations
Drug reactions
Langerhans cell histiocytosis
Leukemia
Asbestosis
Hard-metal pneumoconiosis
DIP and RB-ILD: idiopathic clinical syndromes
Age 30-50
Progressive cough and dyspnea
Pulmonary function tests: restriction and impaired gas exchange
Prognosis very good with smoking cessation or steroids
DIP HRCT findings
Diffuse or patchy ground-glass opacity
Posterior, lower lobe predominance in 60%-75%
Fibrosis rare
Cystic lucencies or emphysema
Air trapping on expiratory scans
Progression to fibrosis in a few
RB-ILD HRCT findings
Normal
Centrilobular or patchy ground-glass opacity
Upper lobe predominance in 60%-75%
Bronchial wall thickening

AIP, acute interstitial pneumonia; DAD, diffuse alveolar damage; DIP, desquamative interstitial pneumonia; HRCT, high-resolution CT; RB, respiratory bronchiolitis; RB-ILD, respiratory bronchiolitis-interstitial lung disease.

usually cannot be made, HRCT is used to predict the histology likely to be present. For example, the HRCT appearance of subpleural honeycombing indicates a "UIP pattern," subpleural sparing of ground-glass opacity is typical of a "NSIP pattern," and patchy consolidation or the atoll sign indicates an "OP pattern."

Recognize that a minimum clinical workup for a new suspected UIP/IPF includes family history, exposure and drug history, and a basic CTD serology panel. So even if a patient has a UIP pattern on imaging, the final diagnosis may not be IPF, but at least the radiologist can help accurately classify the imaging.

Table 14.8 Lymphoid Interstitial Pneumonia: Histologic, Clinical, and HRCT Features

Histologic pattern
Characteristics
Diffuse interstitial and alveolar wall involvement
Infiltration by lymphocytes, plasma cells, and histiocytes
Lymphoid hyperplasia
Differential diagnosis
Idiopathic (rare)
Connective tissue diseases
Sjögren's syndrome
Rheumatoid arthritis
Systemic lupus erythematosus
Immunologic disorders
Hashimoto's thyroiditis
Autoimmune hemolytic anemia
Myasthenia gravis
Pernicious anemia
Chronic active hepatitis
Primary biliary cirrhosis
Infection
Immunodeficiency (eg, AIDS)
Drug toxicity
Idiopathic clinical syndrome
Age 40-50
Progressive cough and dyspnea
Dysproteinemia in 75%
Pulmonary function tests: restriction and impaired gas exchange
Steroids helpful in treatment
HRCT findings variable
Diffuse or patchy areas of ground-glass opacity
Poorly defined centrilobular nodules
Small well-defined nodules or septal thickening
Isolated cystic airspaces (suggestive of LIP)
Diffuse cystic disease

HRCT, high-resolution CT; LIP, lymphoid interstitial pneumonia.

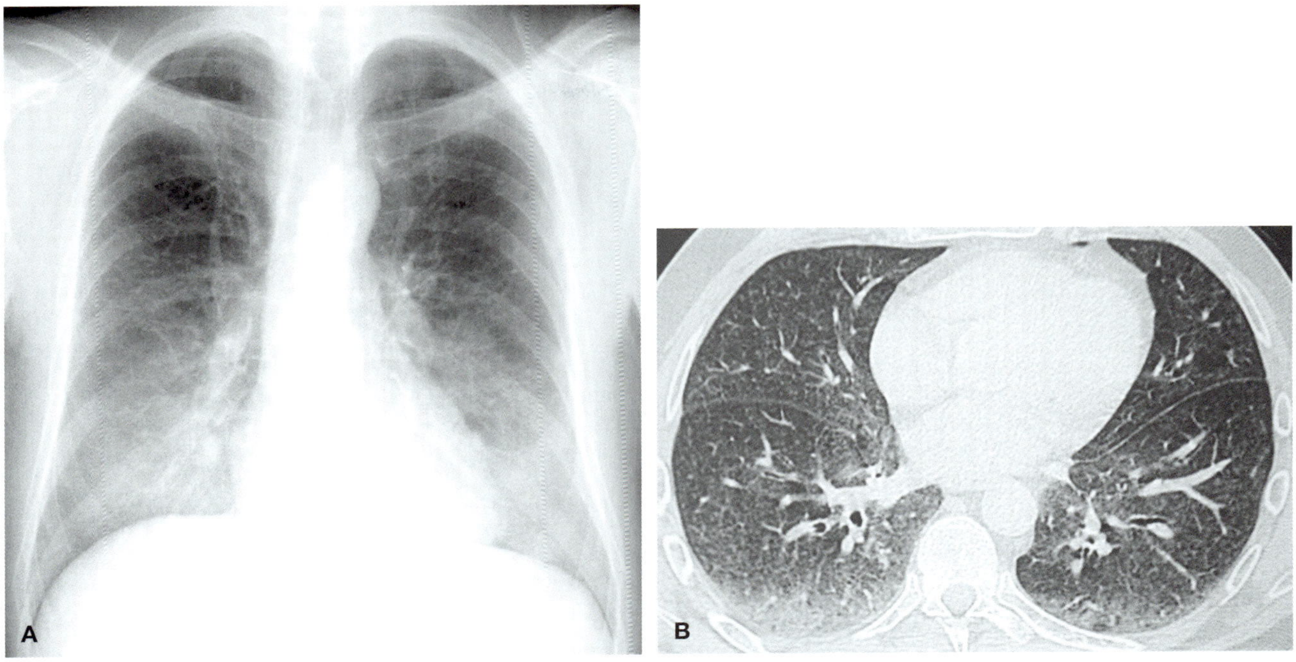

Figure 14.28. Desquamative interstitial pneumonia. **A:** Chest radiograph shows reduced lung volume and hazy ground-glass opacity in the peripheral lung. **B:** High-resolution CT shows ground-glass opacity in the peripheral lung.

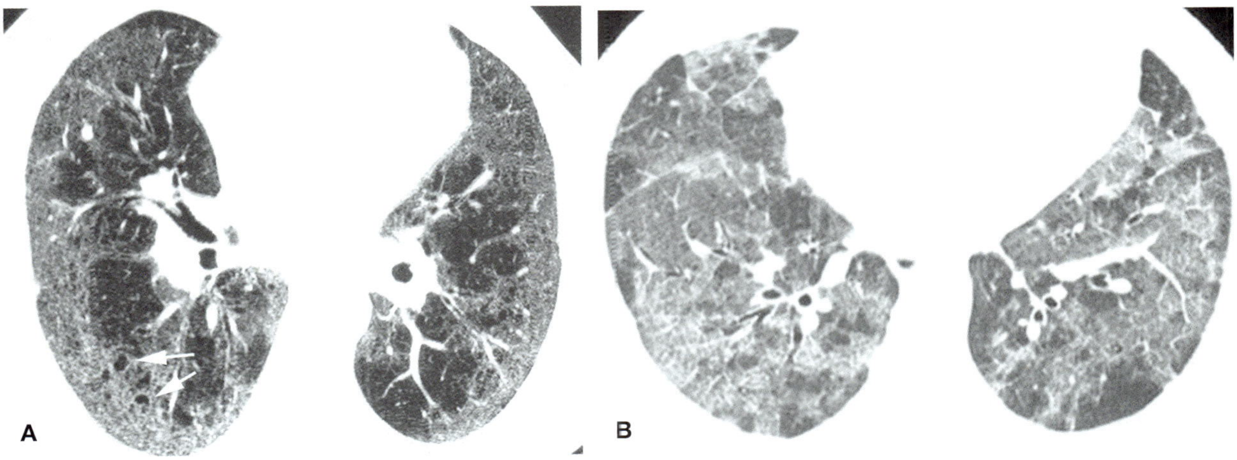

Figure 14.29. Desquamative interstitial pneumonia in two different patients. **A:** Peripheral ground-glass opacity associated with small cystic lesions (*arrows*). These may resolve with treatment. **B:** Patchy ground-glass opacity associated with fine reticulation. Areas of lucency likely reflect air trapping.

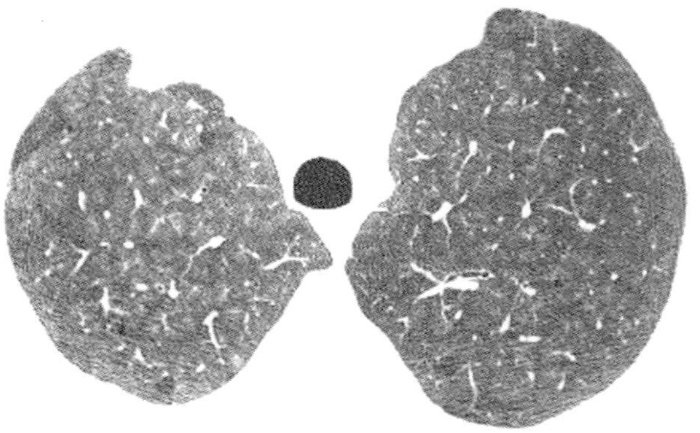

Figure 14.30. Biopsy-proven respiratory bronchiolitis-interstitial lung disease. High-resolution CT shows patchy areas of ground-glass opacity. Many of the opacities are centrilobular.

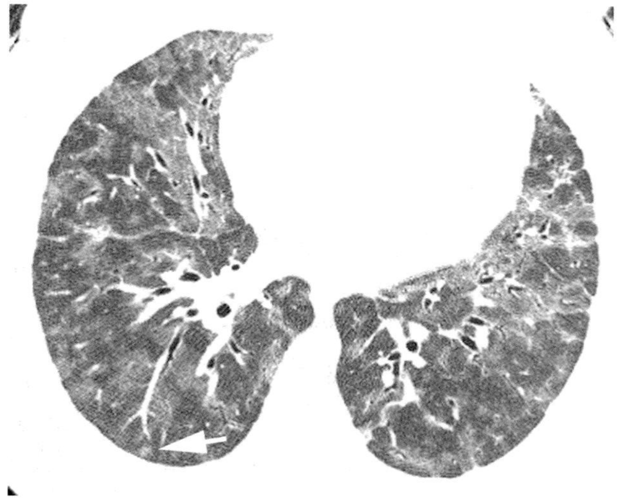

Figure 14.31. Biopsy-proven lymphoid interstitial pneumonia in a patient with common variable immunodeficiency. High-resolution CT shows patchy areas of ground-glass opacity. Some of the opacities appear centrilobular.

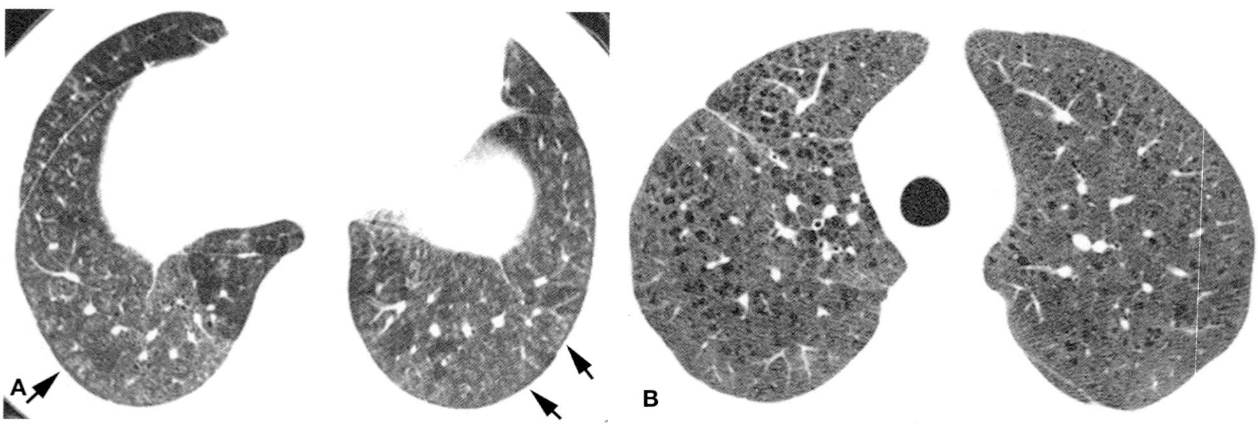

Figure 14.32. Biopsy-proven lymphoid interstitial pneumonia in a 20-year-old woman with a history of juvenile rheumatoid arthritis. **A:** High-resolution CT shows patchy areas of ground-glass opacity at the lung bases. In some areas (*arrows*), the ground-glass opacities appear predominantly centrilobular. **B:** High-resolution CT through the upper lobes shows thin-walled cysts also typical of lymphoid interstitial pneumonia.

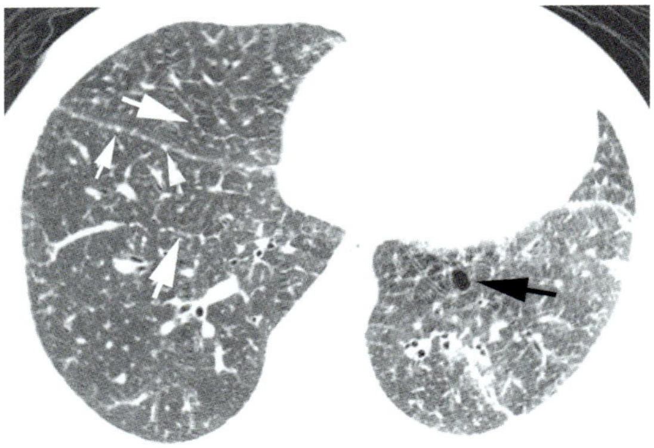

Figure 14.33. Biopsy-proven lymphoid interstitial pneumonia in a woman with AIDS. Small, sharply defined nodules are visible, particularly along the right major fissure (*small white arrows*). Interlobular septal thickening and nodules are visible (*large white arrows*). Ground-glass opacity is also present on the left side, and a single cyst is visible in the left lower lobe (*black arrow*).

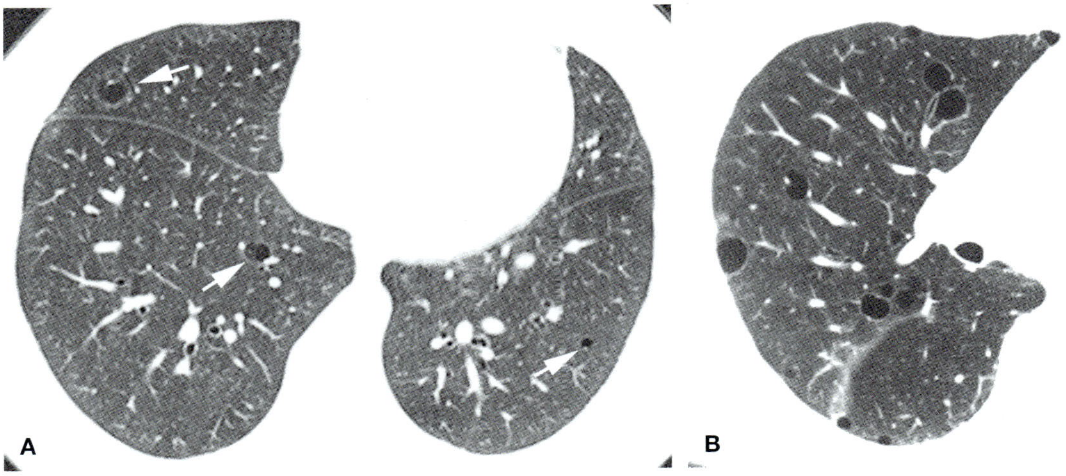

Figure 14.34. Lung cysts in two patients with Sjögren's syndrome and lymphoid interstitial pneumonia. **A:** Several isolated lung cysts are visible (*arrows*). **B**: Detailed view of the right lung. Multiple scattered thin-walled cysts are present. This appearance is typical of lymphoid interstitial pneumonia in Sjögren's syndrome. The cysts are usually limited in number.

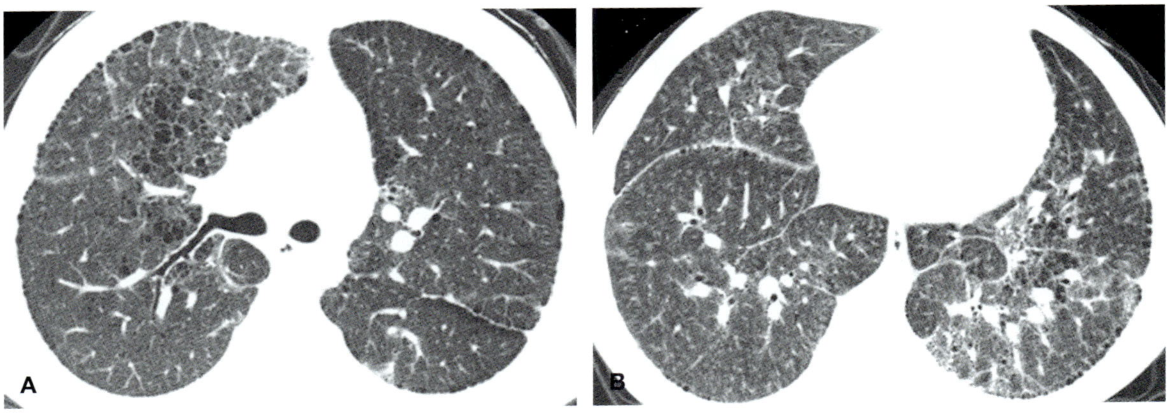

Figure 14.35. Cystic disease mimicking honeycombing in lymphoid interstitial pneumonia associated with juvenile rheumatoid arthritis. **A:** Scattered and clustered cysts, many subpleural in location, are visible in the upper lobes. **B:** High-resolution CT at the lung bases shows ground-glass opacity, interlobular septal thickening, and subpleural cysts. The predominance of cysts in the upper lobes is unusual in honeycombing.

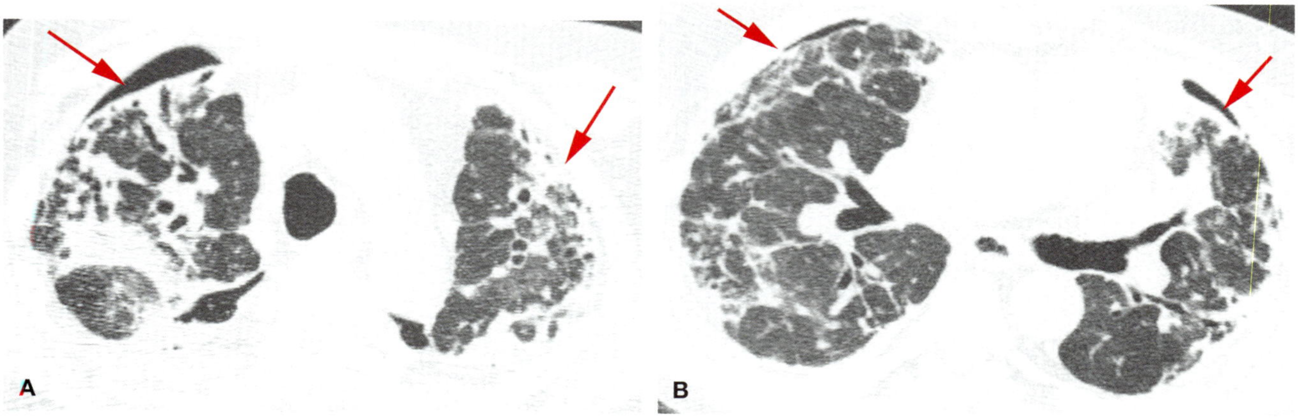

Figure 14.36. Pleuroparenchymal fibroelastosis in a patient with lung transplantation. **A and B:** High-resolution CT shows peripheral lung fibrosis in the upper lobes, with reticulation and traction bronchiectasis (*arrows*). Pneumothoraces are present, and visceral pleural thickening is visible.

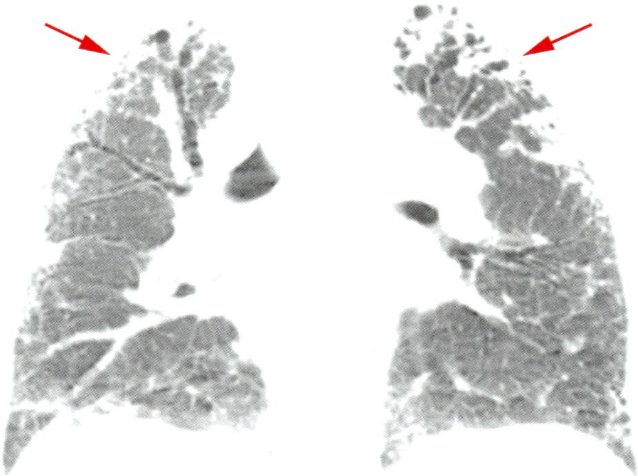

Figure 14.37. Pleuroparenchymal fibroelastosis. A coronal high-resolution CT reconstruction shows peripheral upper lobe fibrosis with traction bronchiectasis (*arrows*).

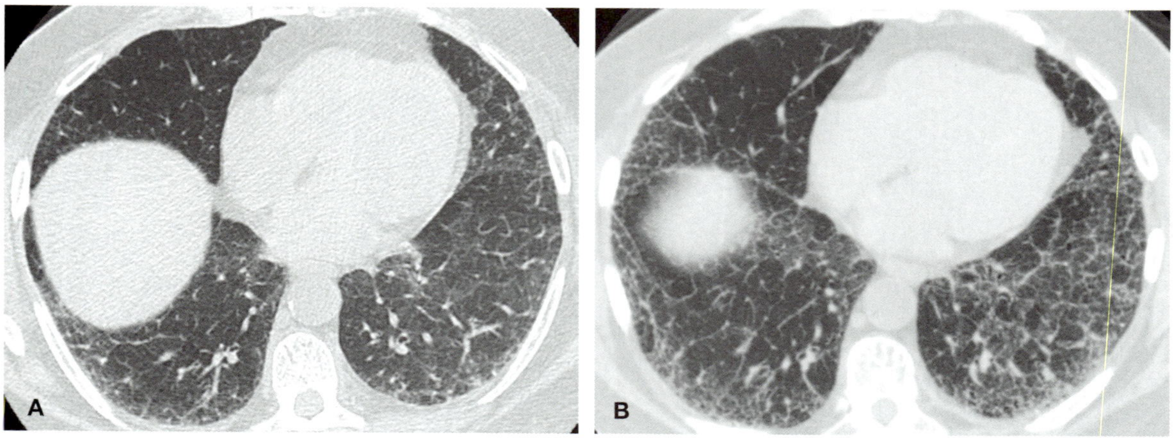

Figure 14.38. Interstitial lung abnormality with progression to probable usual interstitial pneumonia pattern. **A:** Axial HRCT in an asymptomatic 70-year-old man shows very mild subpleural reticulation and GGO. There is no significant traction bronchiolectasis or honeycombing. This patient was categorized as having interstitial lung abnormality as he was asymptomatic. **B:** Follow-up HRCT at age 76 shows progression to a Probable usual interstitial pneumonia pattern with worsening reticulation, and traction bronchiolectasis now visible. Patient had a notable decline in PFTs and was symptomatic at the later time point. HRCT, high-resolution CT.

Table 14.9 HRCT Findings in the Interstitial Pneumonias

Histologic Pattern	Idiopathic Clinical Syndrome	HRCT Findings	Distribution	Key HRCT Findings
UIP	IPF	Reticulation Honeycombing Traction bronchiectasis Ground-glass opacity rare	Peripheral, basal, subpleural, patchy	Subpleural, basal traction bronchiolectasis, honeycombing
NSIP	NSIP	Ground-glass opacity Reticulation Consolidation Honeycombing uncommon	Peripheral, basal, concentric, subpleural sparing	Concentric peripheral ground-glass opacity without honeycombing, subpleural sparing
OP	COP	Patchy consolidation or GGO Centrilobular nodules Large nodules Focal consolidation Reversed halo sign Perilobular pattern	Basal, subpleural, peribronchovascular	Patchy irregular subpleural and peribronchial consolidation or nodules, reversed halo sign, perilobular pattern
DAD	AIP	Consolidation Ground-glass opacity	Diffuse, lower lobe predominance	Typical findings of ARDS
RB	RB-ILD	Centrilobular nodules Patchy ground-glass opacity	Diffuse, upper lobe predominance	Centrilobular nodules of ground-glass opacity
DIP	DIP	Ground-glass opacity Reticulation Cysts	Peripheral, lower lobe predominance	Diffuse ground-glass opacity, cysts
LIP	LIP	Ground-glass opacity Centrilobular nodules Septal thickening or nodules Cysts	Diffuse	Ground-glass opacity or air-filled cysts
PPFE	PPFE	Reticulation, traction bronchiectasis, honeycombing, and visceral pleural thickening	Upper lobes	Upper lobe distribution

AIP, acute interstitial pneumonia; COP, cryptogenic organizing pneumonia; DAD, diffuse alveolar damage; DIP, desquamative interstitial pneumonia; HRCT, high-resolution CT; ILD, interstitial lung disease; IPF, idiopathic pulmonary fibrosis; LIP, lymphoid interstitial pneumonia; NSIP, nonspecific interstitial pneumonia; OP, organizing pneumonia; RB, respiratory bronchiolitis; UIP, usual interstitial pneumonia.

SUGGESTED READINGS

Akira M, Yamamoto S, Sakatani M. Bronchiolitis obliterans organizing pneumonia manifesting as multiple large nodules or masses. *AJR Am J Roentgenol.* 1998;170(2):291-295.

American Thoracic SocietyEuropean Respiratory Society. American Thoracic Society/European Respiratory Society International Multidisciplinary Consensus Classification of the Idiopathic Interstitial Pneumonias. This joint statement of the American Thoracic Society (ATS), and the European Respiratory Society (ERS) was adopted by the ATS board of directors, June 2001 and by the ERS Executive Committee, June 2001. *Am J Respir Crit Care Med.* 2002;165(2):277-304.

Colby TV, Myers JL. The clinical and histologic spectrum of bronchiolitis obliterans including bronchiolitis obliterans organizing pneumonia (BOOP). *Semin Respir Dis.* 1992;13:119-133.

Gruden JF, Green DB, Girvin FG, Naidich DP. Current imaging of idiopathic pulmonary fibrosis. *Radiol Clin North Am.* 2022;60(6):873-888.

Hartman TE, Primack SL, Swensen SJ, Hansell D, McGuinness G, Müller NL. Desquamative interstitial pneumonia: thin-section CT findings in 22 patients. *Radiology.* 1993;187(3):787-790.

Hartman TE, Swensen SJ, Hansell DM, et al. Nonspecific interstitial pneumonia: variable appearance at high-resolution chest CT. *Radiology.* 2000;217(3):701-705.

Hata A, Hino T, Yanagawa M, et al. Interstitial lung abnormalities at CT: subtypes, clinical significance, and associations with lung cancer. *Radiographics.* 2022;42(7):1925-1939.

Heyneman LE, Ward S, Lynch DA, Remy-Jardin M, Johkoh T, Müller NL. Respiratory bronchiolitis, respiratory bronchiolitis-associated interstitial lung disease, and desquamative interstitial pneumonia: different entities or part of the spectrum of the same disease process?. *AJR Am J Roentgenol.* 1999;173(6):1617-1622.

Johkoh T, Müller NL, Cartier Y, et al. Idiopathic interstitial pneumonias: diagnostic accuracy of thin-section CT in 129 patients. *Radiology*. 1999;211(2):555-560.

Johkoh T, Müller NL, Colby TV, et al. Nonspecific interstitial pneumonia: correlation between thin-section CT findings and pathologic subgroups in 55 patients. *Radiology*. 2002;225(1):199-204.

Johkoh T, Müller NL, Pickford HA, et al. Lymphocytic interstitial pneumonia: thin-section CT findings in 22 patients. *Radiology*. 1999;212(2):567-572.

Johkoh T, Müller NL, Taniguchi H, et al. Acute interstitial pneumonia: thin-section CT findings in 36 patients. *Radiology*. 1999;211(3):859-863.

Katzenstein AL, Myers JL. Idiopathic pulmonary fibrosis: clinical relevance of pathologic classification. *Am J Respir Crit Care Med*. 1998;157(4 Pt 1):1301-1315.

Kim SJ, Lee KS, Ryu YH, et al. Reversed halo sign on high-resolution CT of cryptogenic organizing pneumonia: diagnostic implications. *AJR Am J Roentgenol*. 2003;180(5):1251-1254.

Lee KS, Kullnig P, Hartman TE, Müller NL. Cryptogenic organizing pneumonia: CT findings in 43 patients. *AJR Am J Roentgenol*. 1994;162(3):543-546.

Lynch DA, Sverzellati N, Travis WD, et al. Diagnostic criteria for idiopathic pulmonary fibrosis: a Fleischner Society White Paper. *Lancet Respir Med*. February 2018;6(2):138-153.

Lynch DA, Travis WD, Müller NL, et al. Idiopathic interstitial pneumonias: CT features. *Radiology*. 2005;236(1):10-21.

Müller NL, Coiby TV. Idiopathic interstitial pneumonias: high-resolution CT and histologic findings. *Radiographics*. 1997;17(4):1016-1022.

Park JS, Lee KS, Kim JS, et al. Nonspecific interstitial pneumonia with fibrosis: radiographic and CT findings in seven patients. *Radiology*. 1995;195(3):645-648.

Primack SL, Hartman TE, Ikezoe J, Akira M, Sakatani M, Müller NL. Acute interstitial pneumonia: radiographic and CT findings in nine patients. *Radiology*. 1993;188(3):817-820.

Raghu G, Collard HR, Egan JJ, et al. An official ATS/ERS/JRS/ALAT statement: idiopathic pulmonary fibrosis–evidence-based guidelines for diagnosis and management. *Am J Respir Crit Care Med*. 2011;183(6):788-824.

Raghu G, Remy-Jardin M, Myers JL, et al, American Thoracic Society, European Respiratory Society, Japanese Respiratory Society, and Latin American Thoracic Society. Diagnosis of idiopathic pulmonary fibrosis. An official ATS/ERS/JRS/ALAT clinical Practice guideline. *Am J Respir Crit Care Med*. 2018;198(5):e44-e68.

Raghu G, Remy-Jardin M, Richeldi L, et al. Idiopathic pulmonary fibrosis (an update) and progressive pulmonary fibrosis in adults: an official ATS/ERS/JRS/ALAT clinical practice guideline. *Am J Respir Crit Care Med*. 2022;205(9):e18-e47.

Travis WD, Costabel U, Hansell DM, et al. An official American Thoracic Society/European Respiratory Society statement: update of the international multidisciplinary classification of the idiopathic interstitial pneumonias. *Am J Respir Crit Care Med*. 2013;188(6):733-748.

Travis WD, Hunninghake G, King TE, et al. Idiopathic nonspecific interstitial pneumonia. Report of an American Thoracic Society Project. *Am J Respir Crit Care Med*. 2008;177(12):1338-1347.

Connective Tissue Diseases

INTRODUCTION

Connective tissue diseases (CTDs; also referred to as collagen vascular diseases) and autoimmune syndromes may be associated with focal or diffuse pulmonary abnormalities. The type and frequency of lung abnormalities vary with the specific disease. The two most common conditions associated with lung disease are rheumatoid arthritis (RA) and scleroderma (progressive systemic sclerosis [PSS]).

Most CTDs can cause chronic interstitial pneumonia with clinical, radiographic, high-resolution CT (HRCT) and pathologic features indistinguishable from those of the idiopathic interstitial pneumonias (Table 15.1; see Chapter 14). CTDs may result in usual interstitial pneumonia (UIP), nonspecific interstitial pneumonia (NSIP), lymphoid interstitial pneumonia (LIP), organizing pneumonia (OP), and diffuse alveolar damage (DAD). Individual CTDs may also be associated with specific thoracic manifestations of lung disease. It is important to remember that a minority of patients present with lung disease as the initial manifestation of their CTD.

The diagnosis of a specific CTD in patients with a lung abnormality of interstitial lung disease (ILD) is based on a consideration of both clinical features and the presence or absence of various autoantibodies (Table 15.2).

Table 15.1 Pulmonary Abnormalities in Collagen Vascular Diseases (CTDs)

	Pulmonary Abnormality								
CTD	**UIP**	**NSIP**	**OP**	**LIP**	**DAD**	**Hemorrhage**	**Airways Disease**	**Pericardial or Pleural Disease**	**Pulmonary Hypertension**
RA	+++	++	++	+	+		+++	+++	+
PSS	+	+++	+		+			+	+ (CREST ++)
SLE	+	+	+	+	+	+++	+	+++	
PM-DM	+	++	+++	+	+		+		
MCTD	+	+	+					+	+
SS	+	++	+	++	+		+		

DAD, diffuse alveolar damage; LIP, lymphoid interstitial pneumonia; MCTD, mixed connective tissue disease; NSIP, nonspecific interstitial pneumonia; OP, organizing pneumonia; PM-DM, polymyositis-dermatomyositis; PSS, progressive systemic sclerosis; RA, rheumatoid arthritis; SLE, systemic lupus erythematosus; SS, Sjögren syndrome; UIP, usual interstitial pneumonia.

Table 15.2 **Common Autoantibodies in Collagen Vascular Disease**

	RA	PSS	CREST	SLE	PM-DM	MCTD	SS
RF	+	+		+	Rare	+	+
ANA	+	+		+	+	+ speckled	+
Anti-dsDNA				+			
Anticentromere		+ limited	+		Rare		Rare
Scl-70		+ diffuse	+		Rare		
Anti-Jo-1					+		Rare
ANCA	Rare			Rare			
Anti-Smith				+			
Anti-Ro/SSA Anti-La/SSB							+
Anti-U1-RNP Anti-UN-70 kd						+	
Anti-CCP	+						

ANA, antinuclear antibody; ANCA, antineutrophilic cytoplasmic antibody; CCP, cyclic citrullinated peptide; dsDNA, double-stranded DNA antibody; MCTD, mixed connective tissue disease; PM-DM, polymyositis-dermatomyositis; PSS, scleroderma; RA, rheumatoid arthritis; RF, rheumatoid factor; RNP, ribonucleoprotein; SLE, systemic lupus erythematosus; SS, Sjögren syndrome.

RHEUMATOID ARTHRITIS

RA is commonly associated with thoracic abnormalities, including interstitial pneumonia and fibrosis (UIP, NSIP, and OP are most common), pleural effusion or pleural thickening, necrobiotic nodules, bronchiectasis, and bronchiolitis obliterans (Tables 15.1 and 15.3).

Clinical evidence of arthritis precedes the development of pulmonary or pleural disease in about 90% of patients, and 90% have a positive serum rheumatoid factor. Although RA is twice as common in females, extra-articular manifestations of RA, including lung disease, are more common in males. Radiographic findings vary with the manifestation of RA present (see Table 15.3).

Table 15.3 **Rheumatoid Arthritis**

- Arthritis precedes lung disease in 90%
- Lung disease more common in males
- Pleural effusion or pleural thickening in 5%-20%
- Interstitial pneumonia 10%-25%
  - Histologic pattern may be UIP, NSIP, OP, or LIP
  - Ground-glass, reticulation, honeycombing
  - Reticulation usually finer than IPF
  - Basal and peripheral predominance
  - Immediate subpleural sparing may be present in NSIP
  - Consolidation with OP
  - Cystic lucencies with LIP may mimic honeycombing.
- Rheumatoid nodules
  - Peripheral, well defined
  - Caplan syndrome
- Bronchiectasis in 20%
- Bronchiolitis obliterans rare
- LIP with follicular bronchiolitis
  - Centrilobular nodules or tree-in-bud
- Pulmonary hypertension

IPF, idiopathic pulmonary fibrosis; LIP, lymphoid interstitial pneumonia; NSIP, nonspecific interstitial pneumonia; OP, organizing pneumonia; UIP, usual interstitial pneumonia.

Pleural Disease

Pleural disease, either pleural effusion or pleural thickening, is common in patients with RA being seen in up to 40% of patients at autopsy. However, radiographic evidence of pleural thickening or pleural effusion is present in only 5% to 20% of patients, and it often is asymptomatic. Pleural effusions are usually small and unilateral, being more common on the right. Generally, effusion is not associated with radiographic evidence of lung disease. On HRCT, pleural effusion is visible more often than on radiographs and is seen in more than 40% of patients with findings of interstitial pneumonia.

Interstitial Pneumonia and Fibrosis

Interstitial pneumonia and fibrosis, the most common pulmonary manifestation of RA, is most common in middle-aged males, occurring in 20% to 30% of cases. Dyspnea is common. Histologically, it may represent UIP, NIP, OP, or LIP.

Although pulmonary function abnormalities are present in up to 40% of patients with RA, only about 5% to 10% of patients with RA have radiologically detectable interstitial disease.

On HRCT, interstitial pneumonia may be associated with a spectrum of abnormalities ranging from ground-glass opacity to fine reticulation or coarse reticulation with honeycombing. Findings of pulmonary fibrosis (irregular reticulation, traction bronchiectasis, honeycombing) are seen on HRCT in about 10% of patients; ground-glass opacity is seen in 15%.

The appearance of RA with interstitial fibrosis may be indistinguishable from that of idiopathic pulmonary fibrosis (IPF) (Figs. 15.1 and 15.2). A UIP pattern in RA tends to be associated with a poor prognosis.

Some patients with RA have lung disease associated with the histologic pattern of NSIP (see Chapter 14); in these patients, reticular opacities visible tend to be finer than those seen with IPF (Figs. 15.3 and 15.4), and honeycombing is less common and minimal in extent.

Also, anterior upper lobe honeycombing appears to be more common in the CTDs than in IPF (see Fig. 15.2B). In some patients, this may be a manifestation of LIP with lung cysts, rather than UIP with fibrosis.

Predominance in the posterior and subpleural lung and at the lung bases is typical of reticular opacities and ground-glass opacity in patients with RA (Fig. 15.5). Relative sparing of the immediate subpleural lung may be seen, a finding associated with the histologic pattern of NSIP (see Fig. 15.4).

OP may also occur in patients with RA, having typical radiographic and CT features of patchy consolidation, nodules, or the "reversed halo or atoll sign" (see Chapter 14).

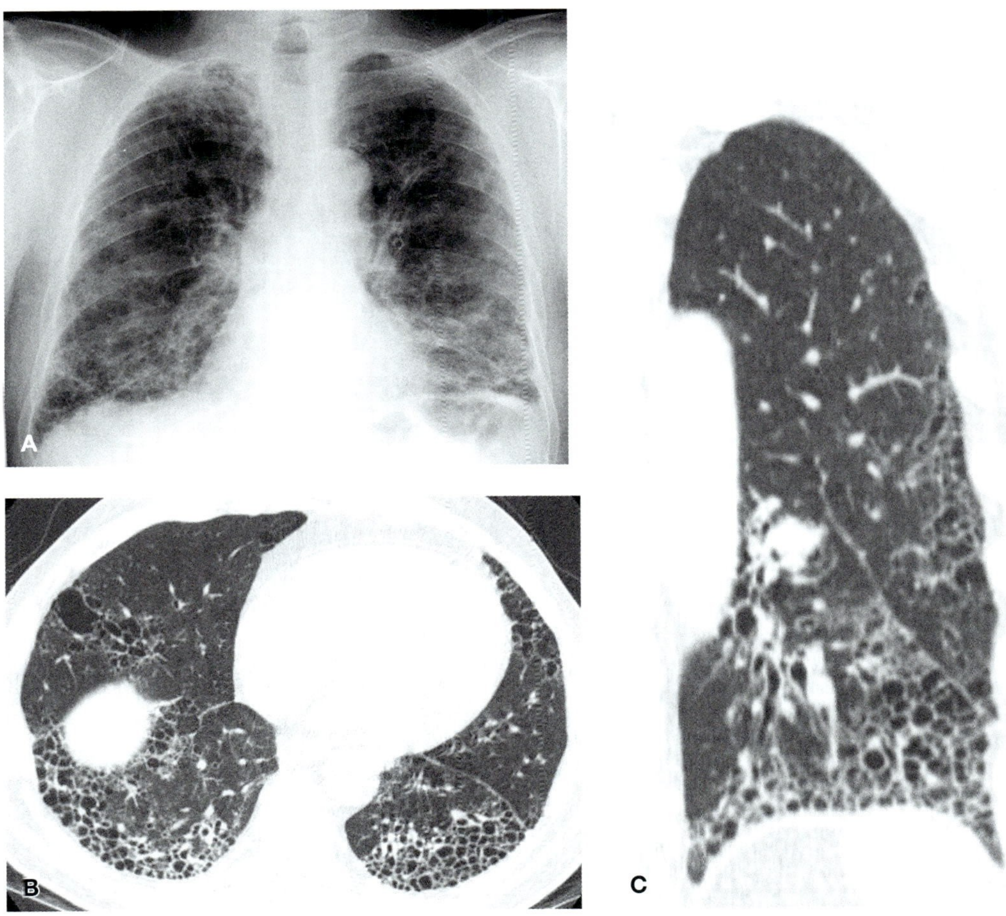

Figure 15.1. Pulmonary fibrosis with honeycombing in a male with rheumatoid arthritis (RA). **A:** Chest radiograph shows a coarse reticular pattern typical of honeycombing. Lung volume is reduced. Axial **(B)** and coronal **(C)** HRCT in a different patient with RA show subpleural and basal predominant honeycombing, consistent with a usual interstitial pneumonia pattern.

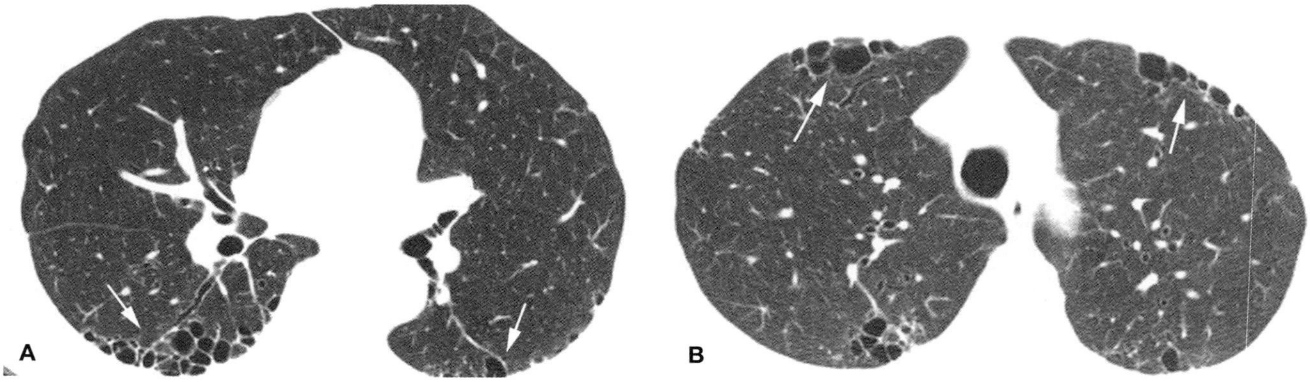

Figure 15.2. Honeycombing in a female with rheumatoid arthritis. **A:** Patchy subpleural honeycombing (*arrows*) is visible in the posterior lung. **B:** Patchy cystic disease (*arrows*) is also present in the upper lobes. This abnormality may represent usual interstitial pneumonia or lymphoid interstitial pneumonia.

In patients with CTD, lung disease may reflect an overlap of various interstitial pneumonia patterns, with features of NSIP, OP, and LIP superimposed. Findings include peripheral reticulation and fibrosis; ground-glass opacity; OP, particularly with a perilobular pattern; and cystic abnormalities due to LIP. DAD is sometimes seen with acute exacerbation.

Rheumatoid Nodules

Rheumatoid (necrobiotic) nodules are an uncommon manifestation of RA. Their histology is identical to that of subcutaneous rheumatoid nodules. They are often asymptomatic but tend to appear and disappear in conjunction with subcutaneous nodules. They range in size from a few millimeters

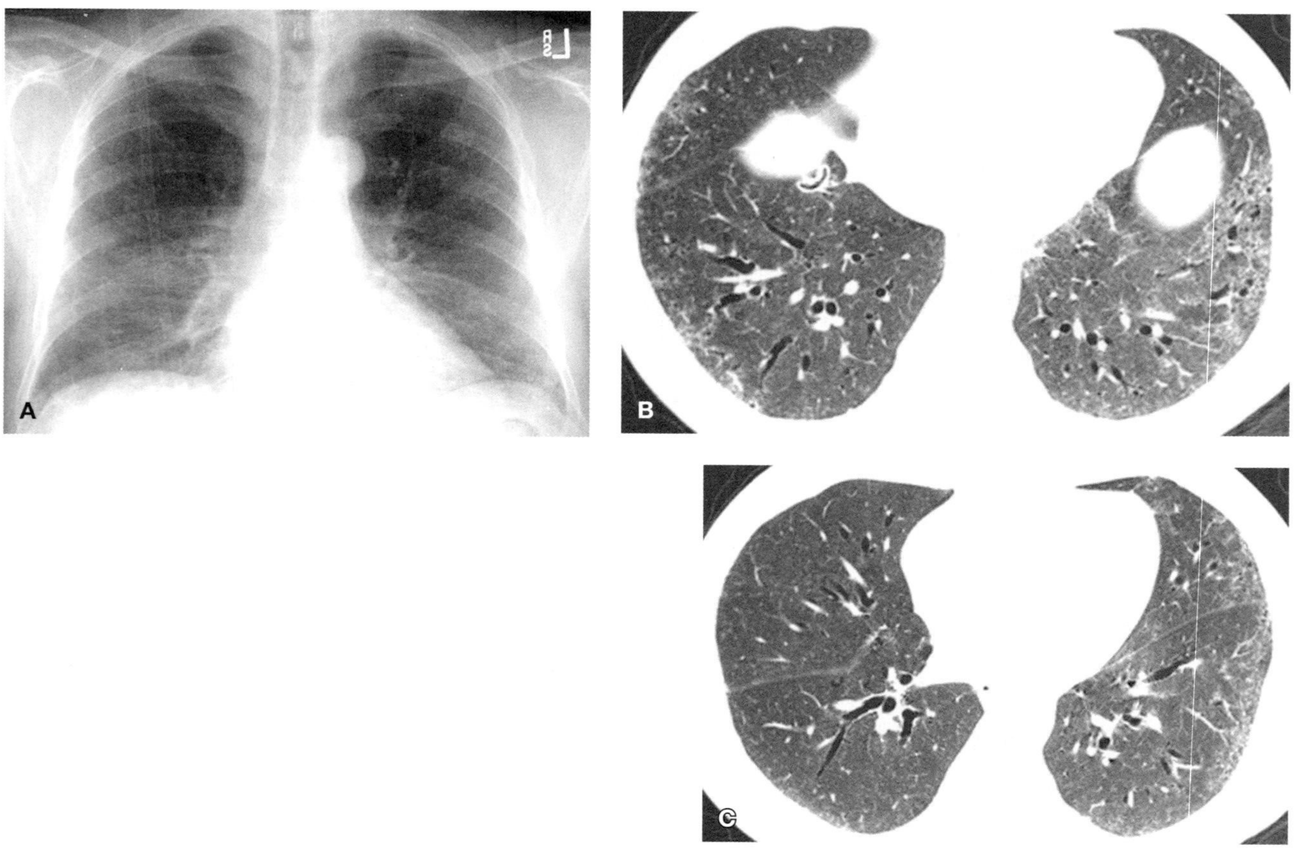

Figure 15.3. Pulmonary fibrosis in rheumatoid arthritis with reticular opacities. **A:** Chest radiograph shows some reduction in lung volume and a mild nonspecific reticular abnormality at the lung bases. **B:** Fine reticular opacities are visible at the lung bases with evidence of traction bronchiectasis. There is no evidence of honeycombing. **C:** At a higher level, reticular opacities are less severe and predominate on the left. A distinct subpleural and lower lobe predominance is visible. This abnormality may represent nonspecific interstitial pneumonia or usual interstitial pneumonia.

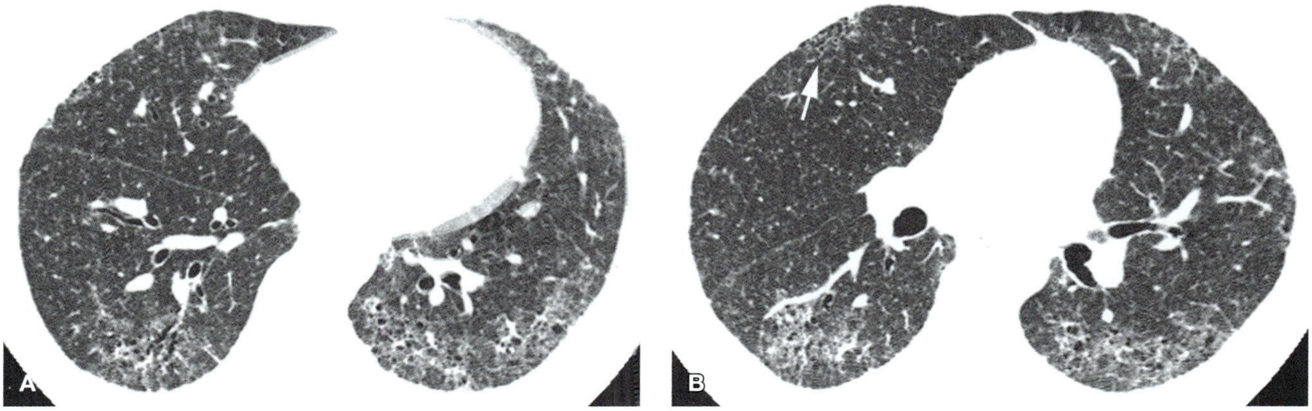

Figure 15.4. Rheumatoid arthritis with reticular opacities and subpleural sparing. **A:** Fine reticular opacities are visible at the lung bases with evidence of traction bronchiectasis. Although there is a predominance in the subpleural lung, the immediate subpleural lung is less severely involved. This appearance is typical of fibrotic nonspecific interstitial pneumonia. **B:** At a higher level, subpleural sparing is also visible. A cluster of lung cysts in the anterior upper lobe (*arrow*) may represent honeycombing or cystic lymphoid interstitial pneumonia.

to 5 cm or more and may be solitary or multiple and numerous. Rheumatoid nodules predominate in the lung periphery and are typically well defined (Fig. 15.6; see also Fig. 10.49 in Chapter 10). They may cavitate, having thick walls that become thin with healing. Pleural effusion may be associated, and cavitary nodules in the periphery may lead to pneumothorax.

Caplan Syndrome

Caplan syndrome is a very rare manifestation of RA occurring in coal miners or patients with occupational exposures to silicates. Nodules are present, which resemble necrobiotic nodules histologically but are characterized by concentric layers of light collagen and black dust-laden cells. Caplan syndrome is characterized by single or multiple lung nodules ranging from a few millimeters to 5 cm in diameter, similar to rheumatoid nodules. The nodules may cavitate. An upper lobe predominance may be seen, resembling silicosis or coal worker's pneumoconiosis, but nodules in Caplan syndrome appear rapidly in "crops" in contrary to the slow progression of silicosis.

Bronchiectasis

Bronchiectasis is associated with RA, particularly in smokers. It may reflect chronic infection, which has an increased incidence in rheumatoid patients, or, associated with infection, it may be a factor in the development of RA. Also, bronchiectasis is commonly present in patients with bronchiolitis obliterans (Fig. 15.7). On CT, it is present in 20% of patients.

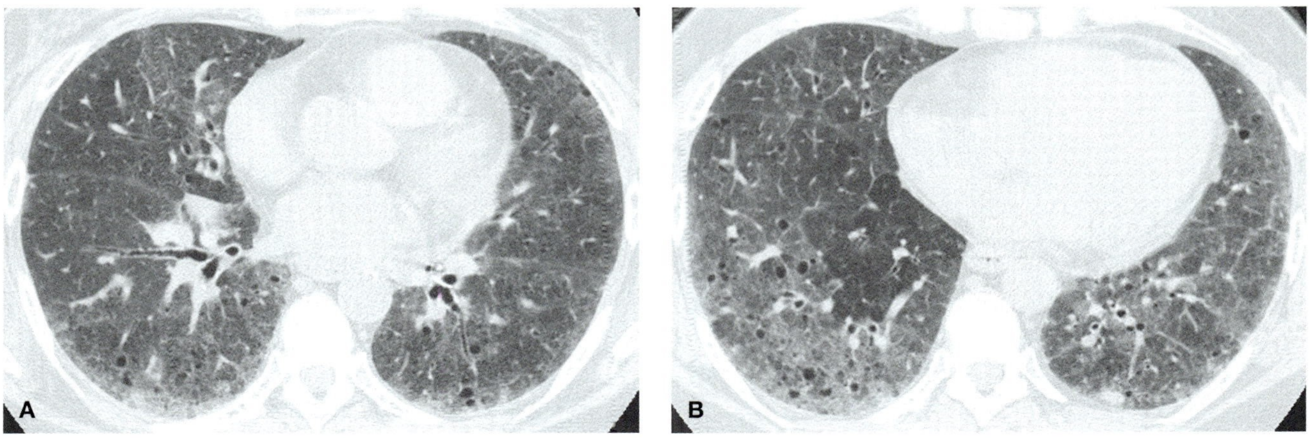

Figure 15.5. Ground-glass opacity in a female with rheumatoid arthritis. **A:** HRCT shows patchy ground-glass opacity with a subpleural predominance. **B:** The abnormality is more extensive at the lung bases. This appearance may reflect nonspecific or lymphoid interstitial pneumonia (LIP). Small cystic lucencies are visible within the abnormal lung. These may represent traction bronchiectasis associated with lung fibrosis or cysts associated with LIP.

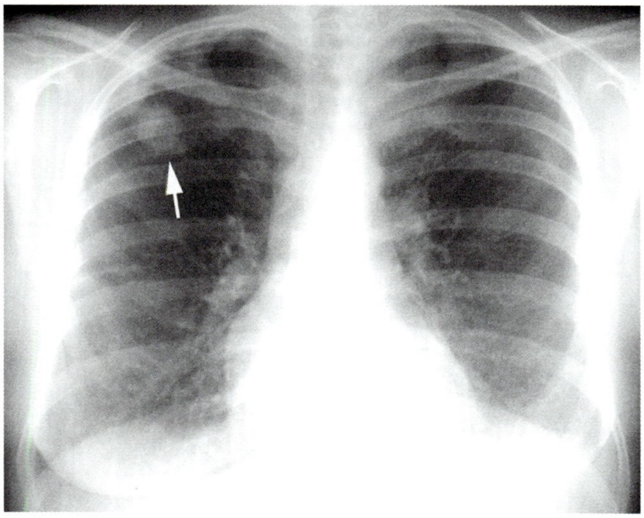

Figure 15.6. Rheumatoid nodule. A young male with rheumatoid arthritis shows a well-defined nodule in the peripheral right upper lobe. Small pleural effusions are also present (*arrow*).

Constrictive Bronchiolitis (Bronchiolitis Obliterans)

Bronchiolitis obliterans (see Chapter 23) is a rare manifestation of RA. It has been associated with penicillamine treatment, but this is not always the case and may be a result of the disease rather than the treatment. Radiographs are normal or show increased lung volumes. HRCT may show bronchiectasis, mosaic perfusion, and air trapping (see Fig. 15.7).

Follicular Bronchiolitis and LIP

Follicular bronchiolitis is also a rare airway manifestation of RA; it is associated with dyspnea. A lymphocytic infiltrate in the walls of small airways is present histologically. Radiographs may show a reticular or reticulonodular pattern. HRCT shows small centrilobular nodules or tree-in-bud. More extensive lymphocytic infiltrations may be associated with findings of LIP such as ground-glass opacity or lung cysts (see Fig. 15.5; see also Figs. 14.32 and 14.35 in Chapter 14).

Pulmonary Hypertension

Pulmonary hypertension usually occurs secondary to pulmonary fibrosis. Rarely, it develops in the absence of lung disease, perhaps related to vasculitis.

PROGRESSIVE SYSTEMIC SCLEROSIS (SCLERODERMA)

PSS (or systemic sclerosis), also known as scleroderma, is a generalized disease of connective tissue often associated with vasculitis. Females outnumber males by three to one. Only 1% present with pulmonary symptoms but up

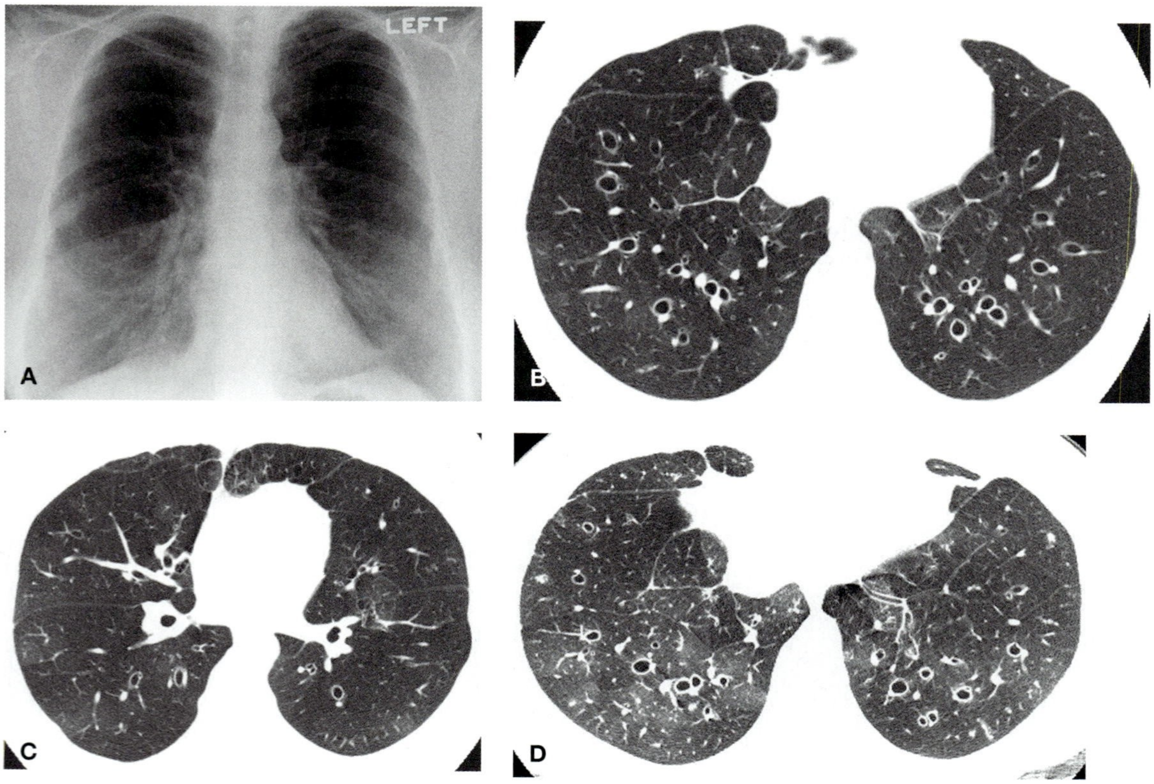

Figure 15.7. Bronchiectasis and bronchiolitis obliterans in a young female with rheumatoid arthritis. **A:** Chest radiograph shows large lung volume. **B, C:** HRCT scans at two levels show extensive bronchiectasis and regional differences in lung attenuation due to mosaic perfusion. **D:** Postexpiratory HRCT at the same level as (**B**) shows patchy air trapping typical of bronchiolitis obliterans.

to 75% have evidence of pulmonary disease at some point in their disease course.

PSS is most commonly associated with NSIP, UIP, OP, and DAD. Pulmonary vasculitis, pericardial and pleural disease, and pulmonary hypertension also may be seen (Tables 15.1 and 15.4). There is an increased incidence of lung cancer in patients with PSS and pulmonary fibrosis. NSIP is the most common pattern.

Table 15.4 Progressive Systemic Sclerosis (Scleroderma)

Lung disease in 75%
More common in females
Interstitial pneumonia
Histologic pattern may be NSIP, UIP, or OP
Ground-glass, reticulation, honeycombing
HRCT appearances similar to RA
Pleural effusion or thickening in 35%
Esophageal dilatation in 40%-80%
Mediastinal lymph node enlargement in 60%

NSIP, nonspecific interstitial pneumonia; OP, organizing pneumonia; RA, rheumatoid arthritis; UIP, usual interstitial pneumonia.

Interstitial Pneumonia and Fibrosis

As with RA, chest radiographs may appear normal despite abnormal pulmonary function tests. The incidence of radiographically recognizable interstitial disease is about 25%. Chest radiographs may show a reticular abnormality with lower lobe predominance indistinguishable from that of IPF. In early cases, ill-defined ground-glass opacity may be seen in the bases (Fig. 15.8A). With progression, reticulation may progress from fine to coarse, associated with progressive loss of lung volume.

HRCT findings of interstitial pneumonia in PSS include (1) ground-glass opacity (see Fig. 15.8), (2) consolidation (Fig. 15.9), (3) fine reticular opacities (Fig. 15.10), (4) coarse or irregular reticulation (Fig. 15.11), (5) traction bronchiectasis (see Figs. 15.11 and 15.12), and, less commonly, (6) honeycombing. Abnormalities typically show a subpleural and lower lobe predominance and often involve the lung periphery in a concentric fashion. As with other collagen diseases, there is a tendency for PSS to show a finer reticular pattern than is typical of IPF, and honeycombing is less frequent.

The HRCT appearance reflects the histologic pattern of the interstitial pneumonia present. Ground-glass opacity

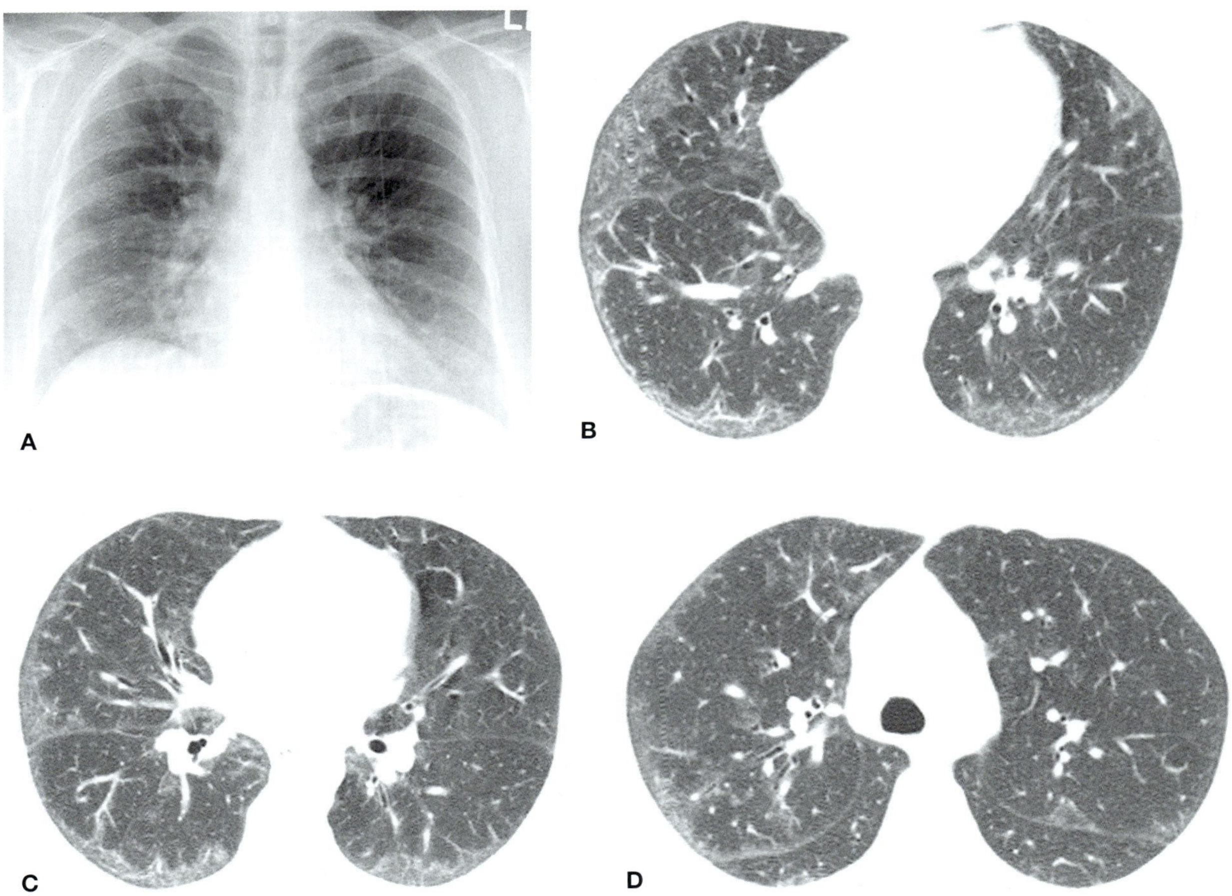

Figure 15.8. Scleroderma with ground-glass opacity. **A:** Chest radiograph shows a very subtle increase in opacity at the lung bases. **B-D:** HRCT scans at three levels show ground-glass opacity and minimal reticulation with a subpleural and lower lobe predominance. There is subpleural sparing. This appearance usually reflects the presence of cellular nonspecific interstitial pneumonia and is typical of scleroderma.

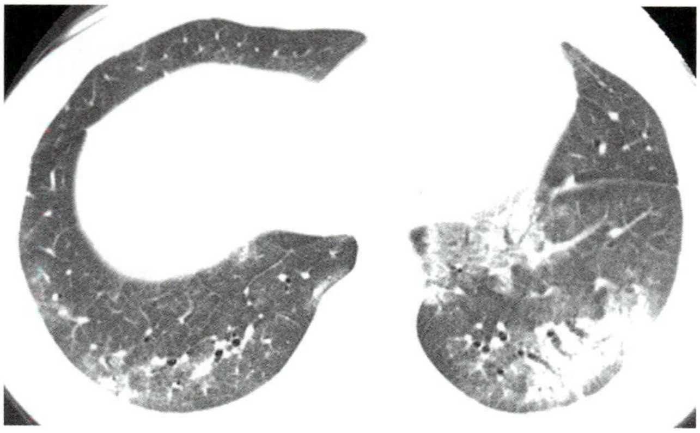

Figure 15.9. Scleroderma with consolidation. HRCT shows peripheral consolidation and ground-glass opacity in the lower lobes. Subpleural sparing is visible on the left. This may represent organizing pneumonia, nonspecific interstitial pneumonia, or a mixed abnormality.

with fine reticulation is often due to cellular NSIP, which is the most frequent histologic pattern seen in PSS (see Fig. 15.8). Subpleural sparing strongly suggests NSIP (see Figs. 15.8 and 15.9). Consolidation may indicate NSIP or OP (see Fig. 15.9). Reticulation and traction bronchiectasis usually indicate fibrotic NSIP. UIP with honeycombing is much less frequent.

Interstitial pneumonia associated with PSS follows a less progressive course and has a better long-term prognosis than does IPF. Improvement following treatment is more common in patients with a prominent ground-glass component than in those with predominant reticular abnormalities.

Pleural Disease

Pleural effusion or thickening is less common than with other collagen diseases and is visible on radiographs in 10% to 15%. On CT, diffuse pleural thickening is seen in one-third of cases.

Other Findings

Asymptomatic esophageal dilatation is present in 40% to 80% of cases (see Figs. 15.10B and 15.11C). Pulmonary hypertension may occur due to lung disease or vasculitis (Fig. 15.13), but this is more typical of CREST syndrome (see below). Enlarged mediastinal nodes are seen on CT in approximately 60% of cases. Pulmonary hypertension may also develop and portends a poor prognosis.

CREST SYNDROME

CREST syndrome (limited systemic sclerosis) is a variant of PSS (Table 15.5). It is defined by the presence of **C**alcification (subcutaneous), **R**aynaud phenomenon, **E**sophageal dysmotility, **S**clerodactyly, and **T**elangiectasia. Pulmonary hypertension is more common than in PSS, occurring in nearly 10% of patients. Otherwise, pleural and pulmonary manifestations of CREST syndrome are similar to those of PSS (Fig. 15.14) but tend to be less severe and are associated with a better prognosis.

SYSTEMIC LUPUS ERYTHEMATOSUS

Systemic lupus erythematosus (SLE) is a multisystem autoimmune disease that is associated with increased circulating serum antinuclear antibodies (ANAs) in 95% of cases. Clinical diagnosis is based on the presence of at least four of the following 11 features: malar rash, discoid rash, photosensitivity, oral ulcers, arthritis, serositis, renal disorders, neurologic disorders, hematologic disorders, immunologic disorders (anti-DNA, anti-Sm, or positive antiphospholipid antibodies), or positive ANA. SLE is much more common in females than in men. Over 50% of patients with SLE develop pleural or pulmonary disease (Tables 15.1 and 15.6).

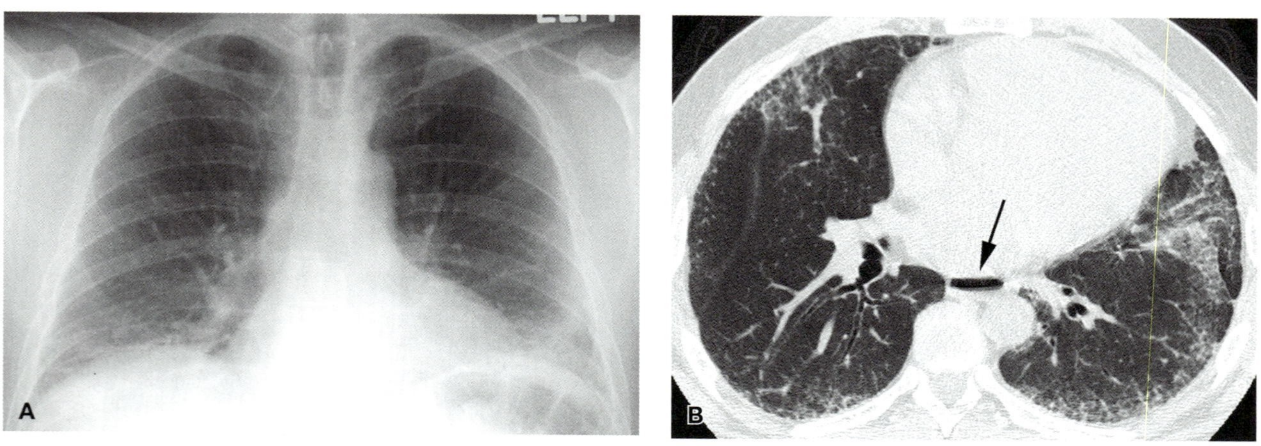

Figure 15.10. Scleroderma with fine reticular opacities and esophageal dilatation. **A:** Chest radiograph shows reduced lung volume and ill-defined reticular opacities at the lung bases. **B:** HRCT at the lung bases shows a fine reticular pattern without definite honeycombing. The esophagus (*arrow*) is dilated and filled with air and fluid.

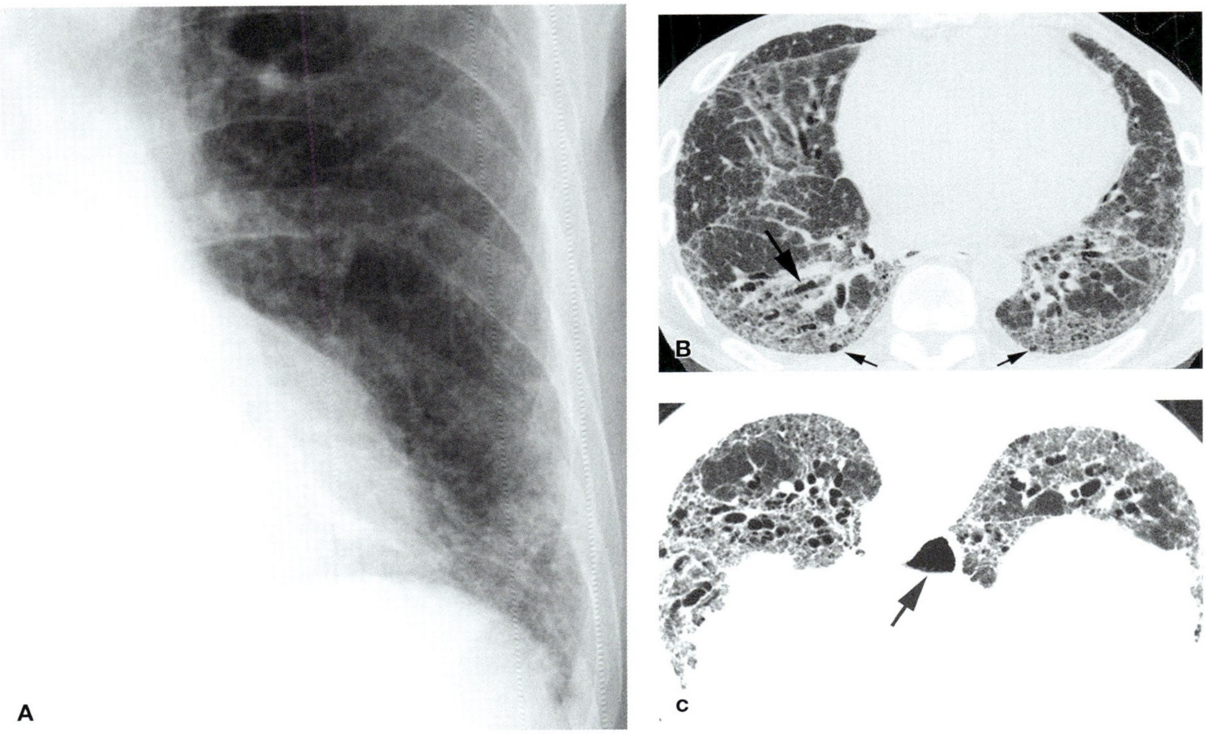

Figure 15.11. Scleroderma with coarse reticulation and traction bronchiectasis. **A:** Detail radiographic view of the left lower lobe shows reticular opacities in the subpleural region. **B:** HRCT at the lung base shows coarse reticulation with traction bronchiectasis (*large arrow*). Very early honeycombing (*small arrows*) may be present. **C:** Prone HRCT at the lung base shows the reticular pattern and traction bronchiectasis. The esophagus (*arrow*) is dilated and air filled. Except for the presence of esophageal dilatation, this appearance is indistinguishable from idiopathic pulmonary fibrosis.

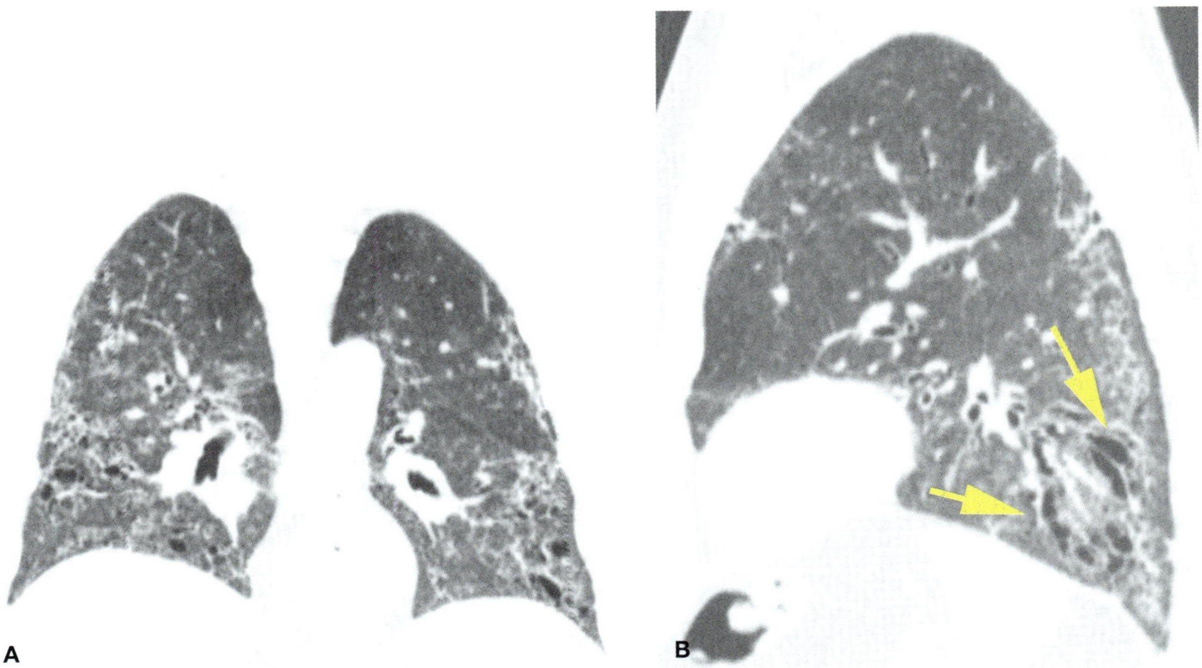

Figure 15.12. Scleroderma with traction bronchiectasis. **A:** Coronal HRCT shows reticulation and traction bronchiectasis representing fibrotic nonspecific interstitial pneumonia. **B:** Sagittal HRCT shows traction bronchiectasis (*arrows*). Note that the dilated bronchi do not reach the pleural surface and subpleural sparing is visible posteriorly.

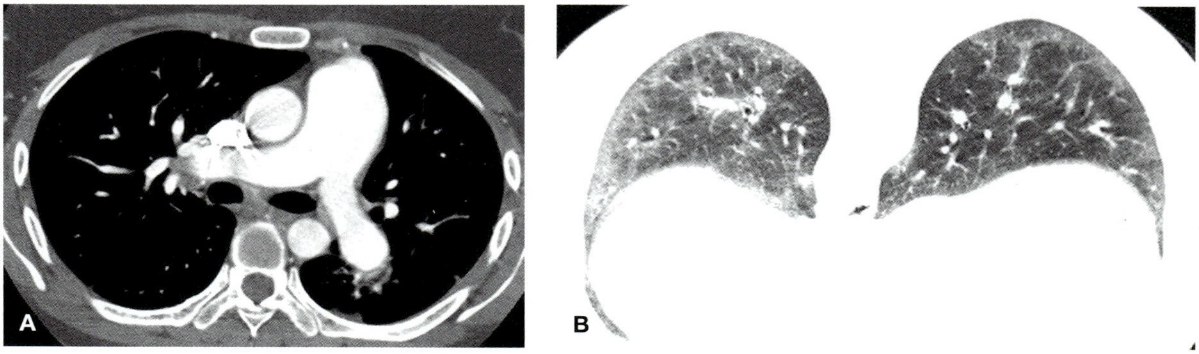

Figure 15.13. Scleroderma with pulmonary hypertension. A: Contrast-enhanced CT shows dilatation of the main pulmonary artery due to pulmonary hypertension. B: Prone HRCT shows ground-glass opacity with subpleural sparing consistent with a nonspecific interstitial pneumonia pattern.

Pleural and Pericardial Disease

Pleural disease is the most common abnormality present. Pleural effusion or pleural thickening occurs in 70% of cases, and pleural effusion is visible on chest radiographs in 35% of patients presenting with SLE. Effusions are usually bilateral and small.

Pericardial effusion or cardiomegaly is present in 35% of cases on chest radiographs. Pericardial effusion is seen much more commonly on CT than on chest radiographs. Cardiomegaly may also reflect lupus cardiomyopathy.

Pulmonary Disease

A variety of pulmonary abnormalities may be seen in SLE. These often appear nonspecific on chest radiographs, resulting in focal or patchy opacities predominantly at the lung bases.

Pneumonia

Pneumonia, usually bacterial, is the most common cause of pulmonary abnormality in SLE, accounting for two-thirds of cases of lung disease. It may be related to immunosuppression due to SLE or to drug treatment.

Table 15.5 CREST Syndrome

Variant of scleroderma
Findings
Calcification (subcutaneous)
Raynaud phenomenon
Esophageal dysmotility
Sclerodactyly
Telangiectasia
Pulmonary hypertension in 10%
Pleural and pulmonary disease similar to PSS but less severe

PSS, progressive systemic sclerosis.

Lupus Pneumonitis

Lupus pneumonitis occurs in about 5% of cases and is characterized by fever, dyspnea, cough, and sometimes hemoptysis. It tends to be associated with concurrent multisystem involvement. Chest radiographs and CT show patchy unilateral or bilateral areas of consolidation or ground-glass opacity (Fig. 15.15), with or without pleural effusion. A lower lobe predominance may be seen. Histology may show DAD, capillaritis, or hemorrhage often associated with immune complexes visible on immunofluorescent staining. The diagnosis is usually made by exclusion of other manifestations, such as pneumonia.

Diffuse Pulmonary Hemorrhage

Diffuse pulmonary hemorrhage occurs in a few patients with SLE and is likely a manifestation of lupus pneumonitis. It typically presents with worsening anemia and progressive lung consolidation on radiographs (Fig. 15.16). Hemoptysis is variably present. Lupus nephritis is commonly associated, making this a pulmonary-renal syndrome. Radiographic improvement may be rapid, occurring within several days.

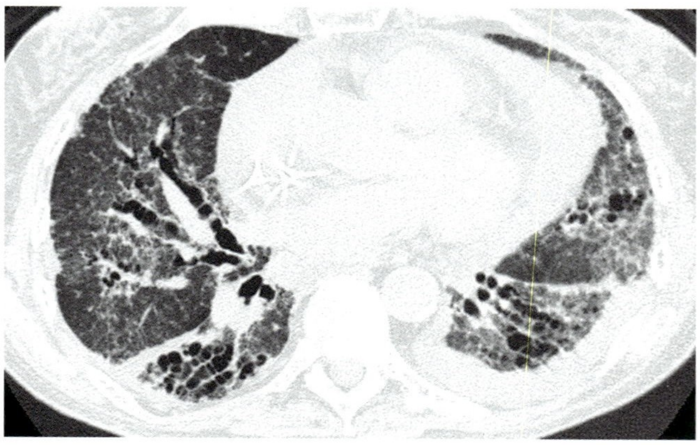

Figure 15.14. CREST syndrome. HRCT shows reticulation and traction bronchiectasis indicating lung fibrosis. Pericardial and pleural effusions are present.

Table 15.6 Systemic Lupus Erythematosus

Pleural effusion or pleural thickening in 70%
Pericardial effusion or cardiomegaly in 35%
Lung disease
Pneumonia most common
Lupus pneumonitis in 5%
Pulmonary hemorrhage
"Shrinking lung syndrome"
OP, NSIP, UIP, or LIP
Pulmonary fibrosis in 30%-35% on HRCT
Findings similar to other CTDs
Bronchiectasis
Pulmonary hypertension
Antiphospholipid syndrome (thrombosis) in 20%

CTDs, connective tissue diseases; LIP, lymphoid interstitial pneumonia; NSIP, nonspecific interstitial pneumonia; OP, organizing pneumonia; UIP, usual interstitial pneumonia.

Consolidation is typically replaced by an interstitial abnormality during resolution.

"Shrinking Lung" Syndrome

Progressive loss of lung volume, the so-called shrinking lung syndrome, is a common manifestation of SLE. The etiology is unclear, but it is thought to be due to diaphragmatic dysfunction or pleuritic chest pain with restriction of respiration. Patients present with dyspnea. Radiographs show progressive loss of volume in the lower lobes, sometimes associated with linear or focal areas of atelectasis, but obvious parenchymal abnormalities are usually absent. In some patients, this appearance on chest radiographs correlates with mild lung fibrosis.

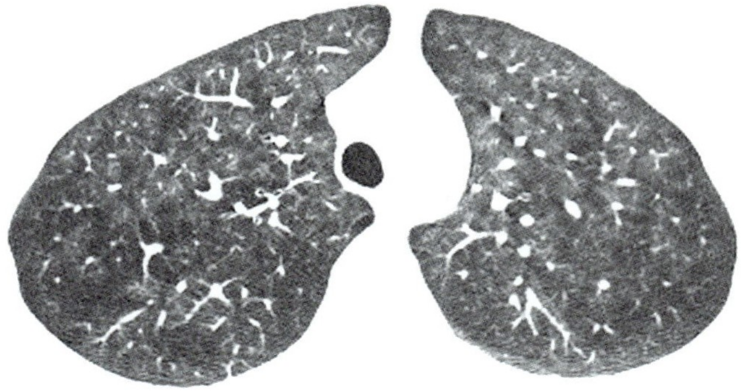

Figure 15.15. Lupus pneumonitis proven by biopsy. HRCT shows patching ground-glass opacities. Some opacities are lobular or centrilobular in distribution.

Interstitial Pneumonia and Pulmonary Fibrosis

Pulmonary fibrosis is uncommon in SLE, compared with other CTDs. Biopsy may show NSIP or less likely UIP. Pulmonary fibrosis is evident on radiographs in approximately 3% to 5% of patients, showing a basal predominance of reticular opacities. The incidence of HRCT abnormalities consistent with fibrosis is higher. OP occurring in SLE shows typical findings of patchy lower lobe consolidation, ground-glass opacity, or ill-defined nodular opacities (Fig. 15.17) with a peripheral or peribronchial distribution. Symptoms include low-grade fever and dyspnea. Its appearance closely mimics that of pneumonia.

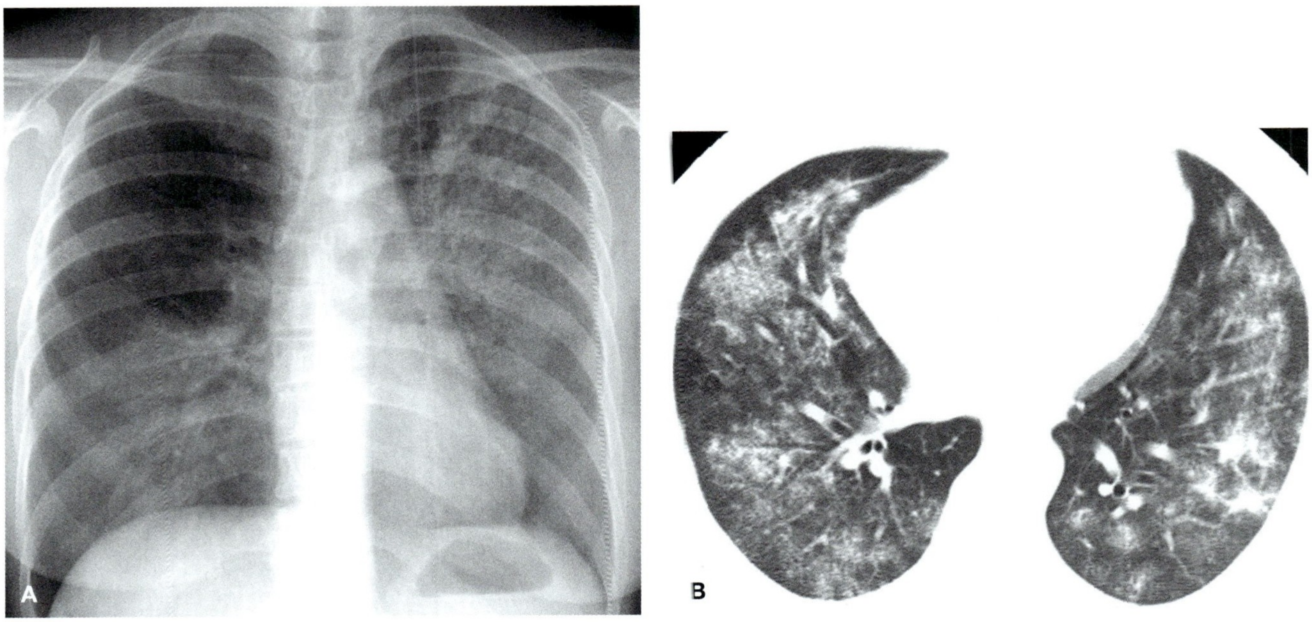

Figure 15.16. Systemic lupus erythematosus with pulmonary hemorrhage. **A:** Chest radiograph shows areas of consolidation and ground-glass opacity involving the left lung and right lower lobe. Hemoptysis was present. **B:** CT in a different patient shows patchy consolidation and ground-glass opacity with subpleural sparing.

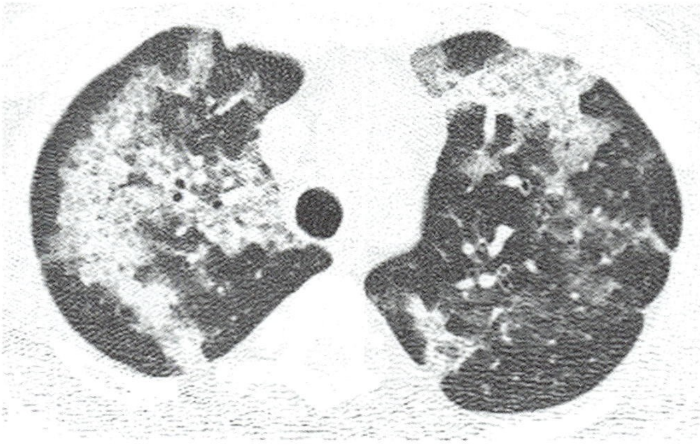

Figure 15.17. Systemic lupus erythematosus (SLE) with organizing pneumonia (OP). CT in a patient with SLE and low-grade fever shows ill-defined areas of ground-glass opacity in the upper lobes. The appearance is nonspecific. Lung biopsy showed OP.

HRCT findings of interstitial pneumonia and fibrosis include ground-glass opacity, fine reticulation, traction bronchiectasis, and honeycombing in advanced cases (Fig. 15.18). Ground-glass opacity is seen in 10% to 15% of patients with SLE, and consolidation is seen in 5% to 10%. These may be associated with pneumonia, lupus pneumonitis, pulmonary hemorrhage, NSIP, or OP. There is a tendency for fibrosis in patients with SLE to be finer than in patients with IPF, and honeycombing is very uncommon. Lung fibrosis predominates in the periphery and at the lung bases, although anterior upper lobe involvement is common. Fibrosis tends to be patchy rather than concentric.

LIP may be associated with cystic lung disease (Fig. 15.19) that is unassociated with obvious fibrosis. It may occur in association with OP or NSIP.

Airway Disease

Bronchial wall thickening and bronchiectasis are seen on HRCT in about 20% of patients but are uncommonly visible on chest radiographs.

Pulmonary Hypertension

Pulmonary hypertension is rare in SLE. It may be secondary to lung disease or pulmonary emboli or may be similar to primary pulmonary hypertension.

Antiphospholipid Syndrome

About 20% of patients with SLE have the antiphospholipid syndrome, associated with venous and arterial thrombosis, and complications such as pulmonary embolism, stroke, or coronary occlusion.

POLYMYOSITIS-DERMATOMYOSITIS AND THE ANTISYNTHETASE SYNDROME

Polymyositis-dermatomyositis (PM-DM) is a group of disorders characterized by weakness in the proximal limb muscles. About 50% of patients show a characteristic rash diagnostic of dermatomyositis. Autoantibodies are detectable in the sera of 50% of PM-DM patients and consist of myositis-associated and myositis-specific antibodies. Females are involved twice as often as are males. Carcinoma, which may originate from a number of different sites, is associated in 5% to 15% of cases (Table 15.7).

PM-DM is less commonly associated with pulmonary involvement than are other CTDs. The reported incidence of pulmonary function abnormalities is about 30%, and approximately 5% of patients show chest radiographic abnormalities. Pharyngeal muscle weakness may be also associated with recurrent aspiration.

In some reviews, however, up to 75% of PM-DM patients have some evidence of ILD. The pattern of involvement is typically that of OP, NSIP, or UIP (Table 15.1). Involvement of the diaphragm can lead to diaphragmatic elevation and decreased lung volumes. OP is particularly common with myositis syndromes and may be associated with NSIP and LIP. Basal and peripheral ground-glass opacity, consolidation, and a perilobular pattern (see OP in Chapter 14) are common.

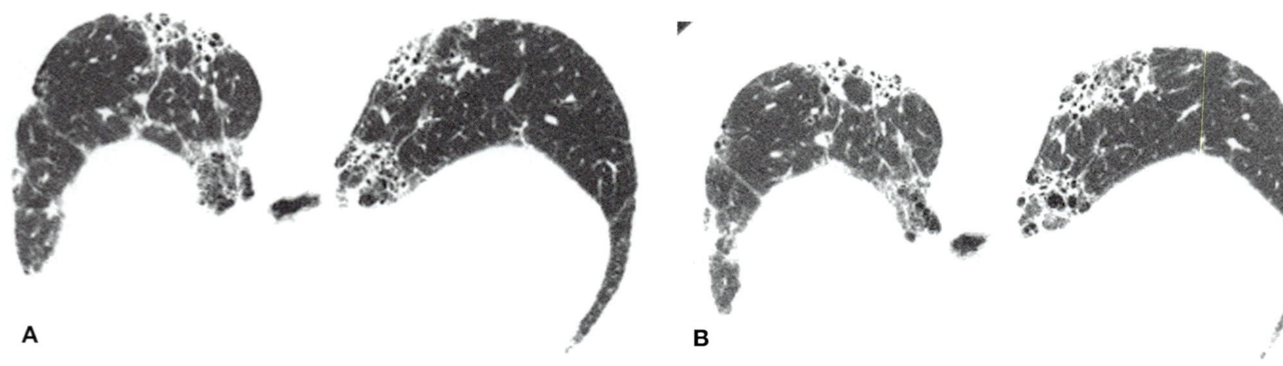

Figure 15.18. Systemic lupus erythematosus with reticular opacities and traction bronchiectasis. **A, B:** Prone HRCT scans at two levels show patchy reticular opacities with traction bronchiectasis.

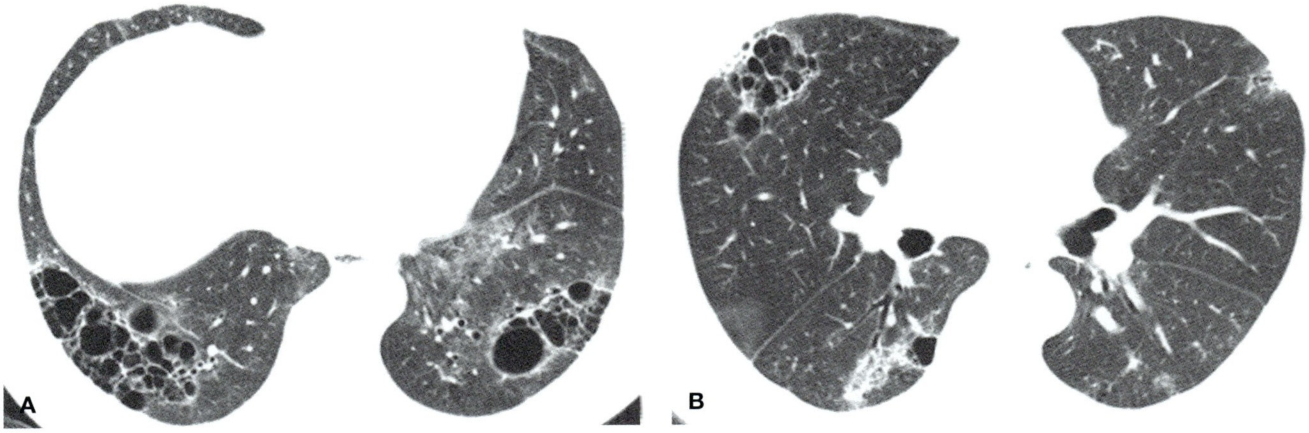

Figure 15.19. Systemic lupus erythematosus with lung cysts. HRCT scans at the lung base (**A**) and through the midlung (**B**) show patchy areas of consolidation and lung cysts. This appearance most likely represents lymphoid interstitial pneumonia.

HRCT findings in PM-DM include (1) ground-glass opacity (90% of abnormal cases; Fig. 15.20), which resembles NSIP or OP; (2) fine reticular opacities indicating fibrosis (90% of abnormal cases; Fig. 15.21); (3) patchy consolidation typical of OP and sometimes showing the "reversed halo" or "atoll sign" (50%) (Fig. 15.22); (4) a perilobular pattern of opacities typical of OP, often associated with NSIP (Fig. 15.23); and (5) honeycombing (15%) with a basal and subpleural predominance. The pattern of lung fibrosis is similar to that of other collagen diseases.

After treatment with corticosteroids and immunosuppressants, abnormal findings typically improve (with the exception of fibrosis and honeycombing).

PM-DM may present with acute symptoms and DAD, leading to lung fibrosis.

Antisynthetase Syndrome

About 20% to 30% of PM-DM patients have the antisynthetase syndrome (AS), characterized by (1) the presence of one or more antisynthetase antibodies, such as anti-Jo-1, which target tRNA synthetase enzymes, important in protein synthesis, (2) ILD, (3) inflammatory myopathy, and/or (4) inflammatory polyarthritis affecting small joints. Lung disease is present in about 70% of PM-DM patients with a positive anti-Jo-1 and 10% of those who do not have a positive anti-Jo-1. Antisynthetase antibodies are more commonly associated with PM (20%-40%) than DM (5%).

Other features of AS include fever, Raynaud phenomenon, and the so-called mechanics hands characterized by the presence of thick, cracked skin, usually on the palms and radial surfaces of the digits. Lung disease is common, may be an isolated abnormality in the absence of myositis, and is similar to that seen in patients with PM-DM. Lung abnormalities are typically basal predominant and represent OP and/or NSIP (Fig. 15.23). Mixed OP/NSIP patterns are common.

Table 15.7 Polymyositis-Dermatomyositis

More common in females
Carcinoma in 5%-15%
Lung involvement less common than with other collagen diseases
Pattern may be OP (most common), NSIP, UIP, or LIP
HRCT findings similar to other collagen diseases
Antisynthetase syndrome in 20%-30%

LIP, lymphoid interstitial pneumonia; NSIP, nonspecific interstitial pneumonia; OP, organizing pneumonia; UIP, usual interstitial pneumonia.

MIXED CONNECTIVE TISSUE DISEASE

Mixed connective tissue disease (MCTD) is associated with clinical and laboratory findings overlapping those of PSS, SLE, and PM-DM. High titers of circulating antibodies

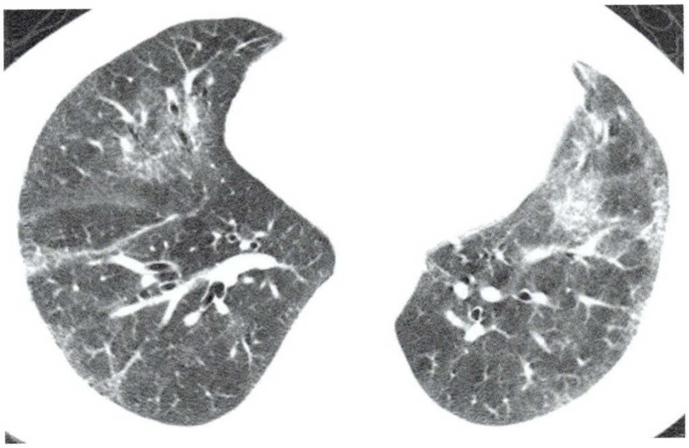

Figure 15.20. Dermatomyositis with ground-glass opacity. Patchy and subpleural ground-glass opacity is visible on HRCT at the lung bases.

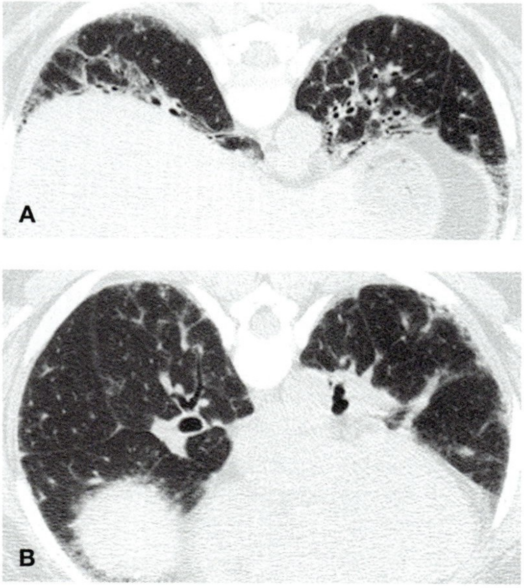

Figure 15.21. Dermatomyositis with reticular opacities. **A, B:** Prone HRCT scans at two levels show reticulation in the posterior lung bases. Traction bronchiectasis is present (**A**), indicative of fibrosis.

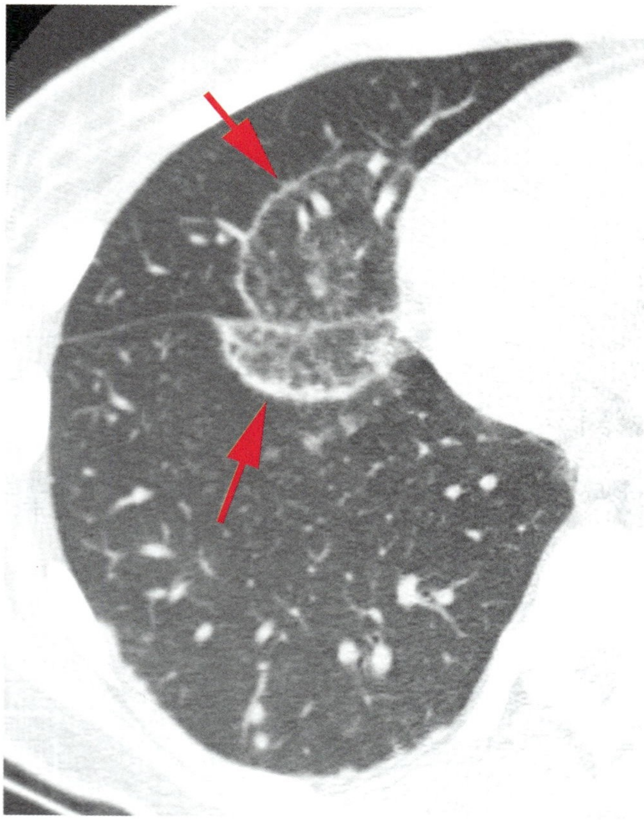

Figure 15.22. Polymyositis-dermatomyositis with organizing pneumonia (OP). HRCT shows examples of the "reversed halo" or "atoll sign" (*arrows*) typical of OP.

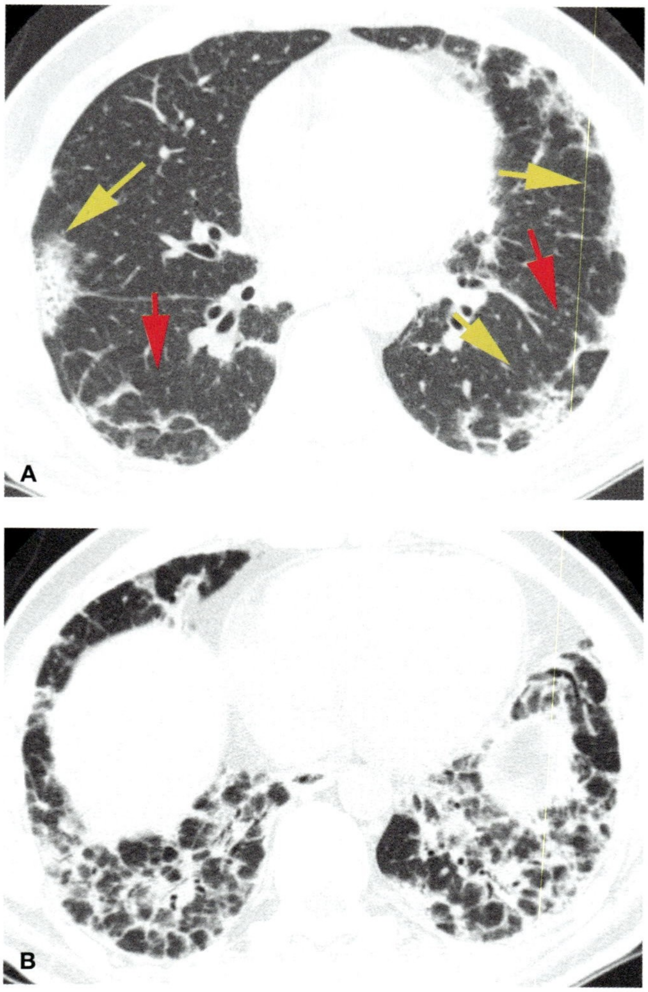

Figure 15.23. Antisynthetase syndrome associated with polymyositis-dermatomyositis. **A:** Patchy consolidation (*yellow arrows*) and a perilobular pattern (*red arrows*) are typical of organizing pneumonia (OP). **B:** More extensive abnormalities are visible at the lung bases. This appearance may represent an overlap of interstitial pneumonia and OP in this syndrome.

against small nuclear ribonucleoprotein are required for diagnosis (Table 15.8).

MCTD is commonly associated with radiologic and functional evidence of ILD or pleural effusion, with a prevalence of up to 80%. Pulmonary vasculitis with pulmonary hypertension and pulmonary hemorrhage is also associated with MCTD.

More than two-thirds of patients with MCTD have abnormal pulmonary function tests, but chest radiographic abnormalities are visible in only about 20%. The ILD of MCTD appears identical to that of other CTDs on histologic examination, radiographs, and HRCT (Table 15.1; Fig. 15.24). Pleural effusion or pleural thickening is present in less than 10% of cases of MCTD.

Table 15.8 Mixed Connective Tissue Disease

Findings of PSS, SLE, and PM-DM
Pleural effusion or thickening in 10%
Lung involvement in 80%
Pattern may be NSIP, UIP, or OP
HRCT findings similar to other collagen diseases
Pulmonary hemorrhage
Pulmonary hypertension

NSIP, nonspecific interstitial pneumonia; OP, organizing pneumonia; PM-DM, polymyositis-dermatomyositis; PSS, progressive systemic sclerosis; SLE, systemic lupus erythematosus; UIP, usual interstitial pneumonia.

SJÖGREN SYNDROME

Sjögren syndrome (SS) consists of the clinical triad of keratoconjunctivitis sicca (dryness of the cornea and conjunctiva), xerostomia (dryness of the mouth and lips), and recurrent swelling of the parotid gland (Table 15.9). Although SS can occur in isolation (primary SS), most patients have coexistent collagen vascular disease (secondary SS), most commonly RA (less often SLE and PSS). Primary SS is associated with nuclear and cytoplasmic antibodies. SS occurs in patients ranging from 40 to 70 years of age and is much more common in females.

Pleuropulmonary manifestations are relatively common and include LIP, follicular bronchiolitis, NSIP, OP, UIP, tracheobronchial gland inflammation, and pleuritis with or without effusion (Table 15.1). Focal lymphoid hyperplasia and lymphoma have an increased incidence in SS.

The frequency of reported radiographic abnormalities ranges from 2% to 30%. The most common radiographic finding consists of a reticular or reticulonodular pattern, usually with a basal predominance. This pattern may be caused by LIP, interstitial fibrosis, or occasionally lymphoma.

HRCT findings are largely nonspecific, including ground-glass opacity, fibrosis, and bronchiectasis, typically present in the lower lobes. However, a characteristic appearance in SS is that of multiple lung cysts occurring as an isolated abnormality (Fig. 15.25; see Fig. 14.34 in Chapter 14) or in association with ground-glass opacity. These reflect the presence of LIP, which is common in this disease. The HRCT manifestations of LIP in SS are similar to those seen in LIP associated with other conditions, although multiple lung cysts are most typical (see Chapter 14).

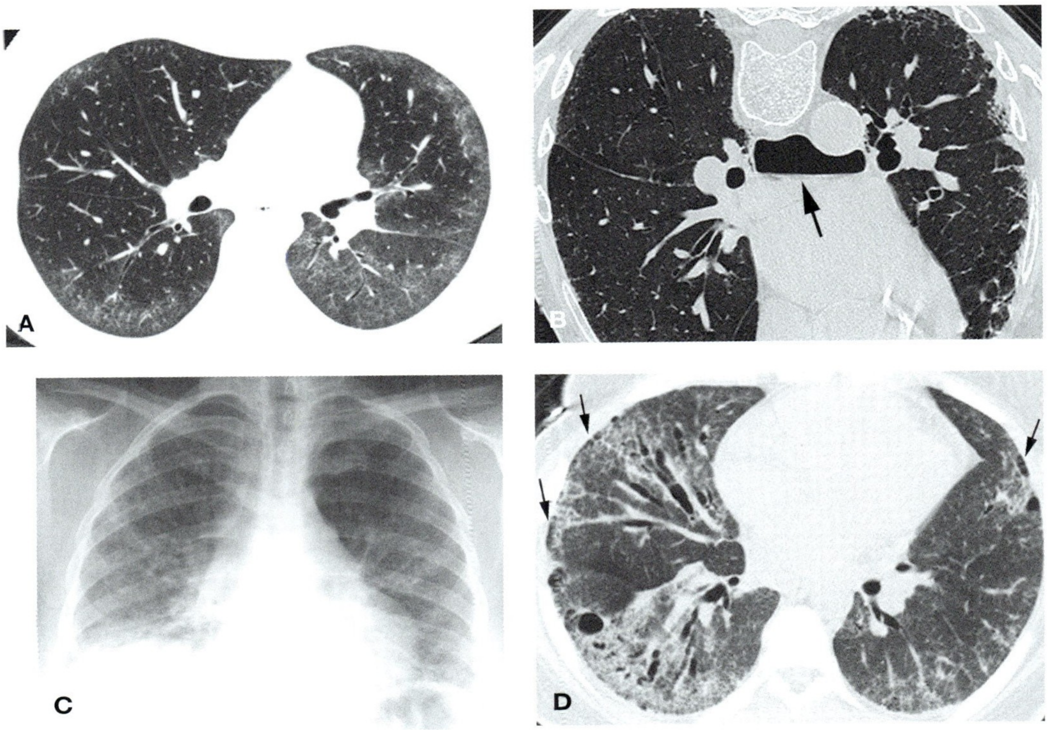

Figure 15.24. Manifestations of mixed connective tissue disease with ground-glass opacity in three different patients. **A:** Concentric peripheral ground-glass opacity and fine reticulation are visible with sparing of the immediate subpleural lung. This appearance is typical of nonspecific interstitial pneumonia. **B:** Prone HRCT shows reticular opacities in the lung periphery. The esophagus is dilated and filled with air and fluid (*arrow*). **C:** Chest radiograph shows decreased lung volumes with reticular opacities at the lung bases. **D:** HRCT in the same patient as (**C**) shows reticular opacities in the lung periphery with traction bronchiectasis and early honeycombing (*arrows*).

Table 15.9 Sjögren Syndrome

Primary or secondary (associated collagen disease)
Triad of
- Keratoconjunctivitis sicca
- Xerostomia
- Parotid swelling

More common in females
LIP and follicular bronchiolitis
- Lung cysts characteristic

Lung disease with pattern of NSIP, OP, or UIP
- HRCT similar to other collagen diseases

Tracheobronchial gland inflammation
Pleuritis with or without effusion
Focal lymphoid hyperplasia and lymphoma
- Lung nodules or masses

LIP, lymphoid interstitial pneumonia; NSIP, nonspecific interstitial pneumonia; OP, organizing pneumonia; UIP, usual interstitial pneumonia.

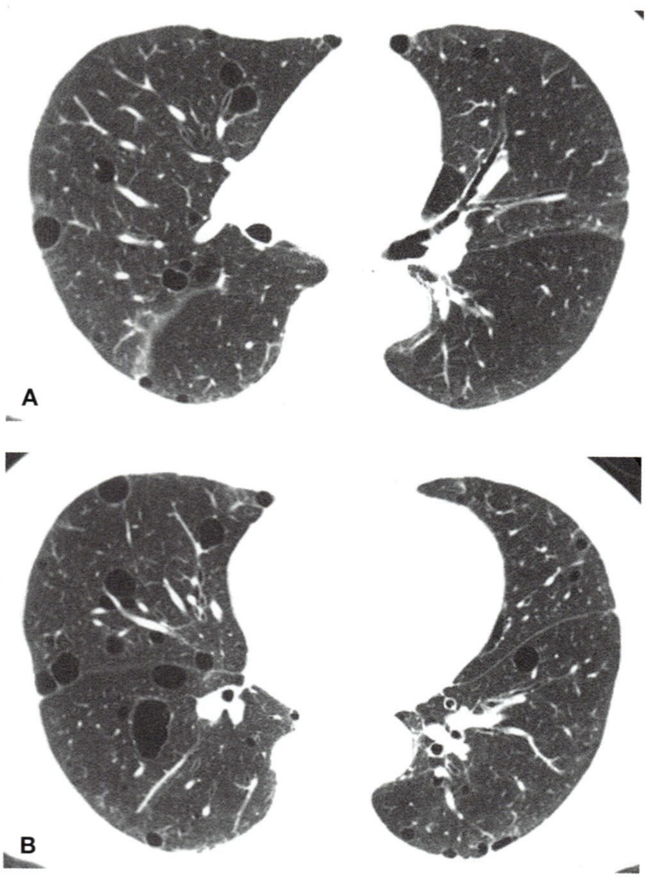

Figure 15.25. Sjögren syndrome (SS) with lung cysts. **A, B:** Multiple thin-walled cysts are visible. These are characteristic of SS and represent lymphoid interstitial pneumonia.

Table 15.10 Ankylosing Spondylitis

Upper lobe fibrosis in 1%
Apical pleural thickening
Cystic lung destruction, bronchiectasis, and paraseptal emphysema
Associated aspergilloma

Lymphoma in patients with SS may result in diffuse interstitial infiltration or multiple nodules. Focal lymphoid hyperplasia may present as solitary or multiple lung nodules (Fig. 7.37 in Chapter 7).

ANKYLOSING SPONDYLITIS

Upper lobe and apical lung fibroses are seen in less than 1% of patients with ankylosing spondylitis, usually 10 years or more after the onset of the disease. Histologic abnormalities include nonspecific inflammation, fibrosis, and sometimes bronchiolitis obliterans or lipoid pneumonia (Table 15.10). Autoantibodies are typically lacking.

Radiologically, the process begins as apical pleural thickening; an apical infiltrate characteristically develops and progresses to cystic lung destruction. It may be unilateral or bilateral. The chest radiographic findings may closely mimic those of tuberculosis (Fig. 15.26). Symptoms are usually

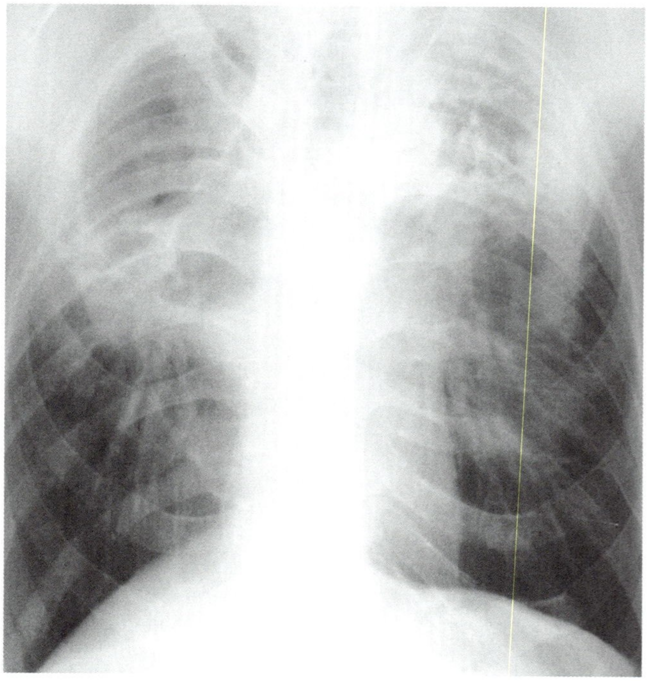

Figure 15.26. Upper lobe fibrosis in ankylosing spondylitis. There is upward retraction of the hila with fibrosis in both apices.

absent, but the cavities become secondarily infected, most commonly by *Aspergillus fumigatus*. HRCT more commonly shows abnormalities than do chest radiographs. The most common findings are apical fibrosis, bronchiectasis, paraseptal emphysema, and pleural thickening.

INTERSTITIAL PNEUMONIA WITH AUTOIMMUNE FEATURES

It is not uncommon for a patient with ILD to present with clinical, imaging, and/or serologic findings that are suggestive of CTD but do not meet criteria for a specific diagnosis (such as RA, scleroderma, etc.). These patients were historically described with varying terms including "undifferentiated CTD-ILD," "lung-dominant CTD," "forme frustes" of CTD, "autoimmune-featured ILD," and others. In 2015, a task force of the European Respiratory Society and American Thoracic Society proposed the term "interstitial pneumonia with autoimmune features" (IPAF) to help provide consensus definition and terminology. The term IPAF represents more of a category of disease for research purposes rather than a true diagnosis, but at least 20% of patients initially diagnosed with IPAF will later develop a definable CTD. Differentiating ILD related to a potential autoimmune disease from idiopathic counterparts can have significant prognostic and treatment implications.

A diagnosis of IPAF requires the following: (1) the presence of ILD (either HRCT or surgical lung biopsy); (2) exclusion of known causes of ILD; and (3) not meeting criteria for a defined CTD. Furthermore, patients must meet criteria from two of the three "domains"—clinical, serologic, and morphologic. Imaging findings are part of the morphologic domain and include patterns described earlier in this chapter that are seen in CTD including NSIP, OP, NSIP and OP overlap, or LIP. Note that a UIP pattern is not part of the criteria for the morphologic domain, but it does not exclude IPAF either (patients must still meet other criteria). A full list of the current IPAF criteria is included in Table 15.11.

Table 15.11 Diagnostic Criteria for IPAF

Presence of an interstitial pneumonia (by HRCT or surgical lung biopsy) *and*
Exclusion of alternative etiologies *and*
Does not meet criteria of a defined connective tissue disease *and*
At least one feature from at least two of these domains:
a. clinical domain
b. serological domain
c. morphological domain

Clinical domain
- Distal digital fissuring (ie, "mechanic hands")
- Distal digital tip ulceration
- Inflammatory arthritis *or* polyarticular morning joint stiffness ≥60 min
- Palmar telangiectasia
- Raynaud phenomenon
- Unexplained digital edema
- Unexplained fixed rash on the digital extensor surfaces (Gottron sign)

Serological domain
- ANA ≥1:320 titer, diffuse, speckled, homogeneous patterns *or*
  1. ANA nucleolar pattern (any titer) *or*
  2. ANA centromere pattern (any titer)
- Rheumatoid factor ≥2× upper limit of normal
  - Anti-CCP
  - Anti-dsDNA
  - Anti-Ro (SS-A)
  - Anti-La (SS-B)
  - Anti-ribonucleoprotein
  - Anti-Smith
  - Anti-topoisomerase (Scl-70)
  - Anti-tRNA synthetase (Jo-1, PL-7, PL-12, EJ, OJ, KS, Zo, tRS)
  - Anti-PM-Scl
  - Anti-MDA-5

Morphological domain
- Suggestive radiology patterns by HRCT (see text for descriptions):
  - NSIP
  - OP
  - NSIP with OP overlap
  - LIP
- Histopathology patterns or features by surgical lung biopsy:
  - NSIP
  - OP
  - NSIP with OP overlap
  - LIP
- Multicompartment involvement (in addition to interstitial pneumonia):
  - Unexplained pleural effusion or thickening
  - Unexplained pericardial effusion or thickening
  - Unexplained intrinsic airways disease (by PFT, imaging or pathology)
  - Unexplained pulmonary vasculopathy

ANA, antinuclear antibody; CCP, cyclic citrullinated peptide; dsDNA, double-stranded DNA antibody; IPAF, interstitial pneumonia with autoimmune features; LIP, lymphoid interstitial pneumonia; NSIP, nonspecific interstitial pneumonia; OP, organizing pneumonia; PFT, pulmonary function test; UPI, usual interstitial pneumonia.

Reproduced with permission of the © ERS 2024: Fischer A, Antoniou KM, Brown KK, An official European Respiratory Society/American Thoracic Society research statement: interstitial pneumonia with autoimmune features. Eur Respir J. *2015;46(4):976-987.*

SUGGESTED READINGS

Aquino SL, Webb WR, Golden J. Bronchiolitis obliterans associated with rheumatoid arthritis: findings on HRCT and dynamic expiratory CT. *J Comput Assist Tomogr*. 1994;18(4):555-558.

Arroliga AC, Podell DN, Matthay RA. Pulmonary manifestations of scleroderma. *J Thorac Imaging*. 1992;7(2):30-45.

Bankier AA, Kiener HP, Wiesmayr MN, et al. Discrete lung involvement in systemic lupus erythematosus: CT assessment. *Radiology*. 1995;196(3):835-840.

Bhalla M, Silver RM, Shepard JA, McLoud TC. Chest CT in patients with scleroderma: prevalence of asymptomatic esophageal dilatation and mediastinal lymphadenopathy. *AJR Am J Roentgenol*. 1993;161(2):269-272.

Capobianco J, Grimberg A, Thompson BM, Antunes VB, Jasinowodolinski D, Meirelles GSP. Thoracic manifestations of collagen vascular diseases. *Radiographics*. 2012;32(1):33-50.

Corte TJ, Copley SJ, Desai SR, et al. Significance of connective tissue disease features in idiopathic interstitial pneumonia. *Eur Respir J*. 2012;39(3):661-668.

Cottin V. Idiopathic interstitial pneumonias with connective tissue diseases features: a review. *Respirology*. 2016;21(2):245-258.

Fenlon HM, Doran M, Sant SM, Breatnach E. High-resolution chest CT in systemic lupus erythematosus. *AJR Am J Roentgenol*. 1996;166(2):301-307.

Fenlon HM, Casserly I, Sant SM, Breatnach E. Plain radiographs and thoracic high-resolution CT in patients with ankylosing spondylitis. *AJR Am J Roentgenol*. 1997;168(4):1067-1072.

Fischer A, Antoniou KM, Brown KK, et al; ERS/ATS Task Force on Undifferentiated Forms of CTD-ILD. An official European Respiratory Society/American Thoracic Society research statement: interstitial pneumonia with autoimmune features. *Eur Respir J*. 2015;46(4):976-987. doi:10.1183/13993003.00150-2015

Franquet T, Giménez A, Monill JM, Díaz C, Geli C. Primary Sjögren's syndrome and associated lung disease: CT findings in 50 patients. *AJR Am J Roentgenol*. 1997;169(3):655-658.

Fujii M, Adachi S, Shimizu T, Hirota S, Sako M, Kono M. Interstitial lung disease in rheumatoid arthritis: assessment with high-resolution computed tomography. *J Thorac Imaging*. 1993;8(1):54-62.

Gamsu G. Radiographic manifestations of thoracic involvement by collagen vascular diseases. *J Thorac Imaging*. 1992;7(3):1-12.

Henry TS, Little BP, Veeraraghavan S, Bhalla S, Elicker BM. The spectrum of interstitial lung disease in connective tissue disease. *J Thorac Imaging*. 2016;31(2):65-77. doi:10.1097/RTI.0000000000000191

Kim JS, Lee KS, Koh EM, Kim SY, Chung MP, Han J. Thoracic involvement of systemic lupus erythematosus: clinical, pathologic, and radiologic findings. *J Comput Assist Tomogr*. 2000;24(1):9-18.

Kim HC, Ji W, Kim MY, et al. Interstitial pneumonia related to undifferentiated connective tissue disease: pathologic pattern and prognosis. *Chest*. 2015;147(1):165-172.

Kinder BW, Collard HR, Koth L, et al. Idiopathic nonspecific interstitial pneumonia lung manifestation of undifferentiated connective tissue disease? *Am J Respir Crit Care Med*. 2007;176(7):691-697.

Lee HK, Kim DS, Yoo B, et al. Histopathologic pattern and clinical features of rheumatoid arthritis-associated interstitial lung disease. *Chest*. 2005;127(6):2019-2027.

Mackintosh JA, Wells AU, Cottin V, Nicholson AG, Renzoni EA. Interstitial pneumonia with autoimmune features: challenges and controversies. *Eur Respir Rev*. 2021;30(162):210177. doi:10.1183/16000617.0177-2021

Mino M, Noma S, Taguchi Y, Tomii K, Kohri Y, Oida K. Pulmonary involvement in polymyositis and dermatomyositis: sequential evaluation with CT. *AJR Am J Roentgenol*. 1997;169(1):83-87.

Prakash UB. Respiratory complications in mixed connective tissue disease. *Clin Chest Med*. 1998;19(4):733-746.

Primack SL, Müller NL. Radiologic manifestations of the systemic autoimmune diseases. *Clin Chest Med*. 1998;19(4):573-586.

Remy-Jardin M, Remy J, Wallaert B, Bataille D, Hatron PY. Pulmonary involvement in progressive systemic sclerosis: sequential evaluation with CT, pulmonary function tests, and bronchoalveolar lavage. *Radiology*. 1993;188(2):499-506.

Remy-Jardin M, Remy J, Cortet B, Mauri F, Delcambre B. Lung changes in rheumatoid arthritis: CT findings. *Radiology*. 1994;193(2):375-382.

Schurawitzki H, Stiglbauer R, Graninger W, et al. Interstitial lung disease in progressive systemic sclerosis: high-resolution CT versus radiography. *Radiology*. 1990;176(3):755-759.

Schwarz MI. Pulmonary and cardiac manifestations of polymyositis-dermatomyositis. *J Thorac Imaging*. 1992;7(2):46-54.

Solomon J, Swigris JJ, Brown KK. Myositis-related interstitial lung disease and antisynthetase syndrome. *J Bras Pneumol*. 2011;37(1):100-109.

Souza AS Jr, Müller NL, Marchiori E, Soares-Souza LV, de Souza Rocha M. Pulmonary abnormalities in ankylosing spondylitis: inspiratory and expiratory high-resolution CT findings in 17 patients. *J Thorac Imaging*. 2004;19(4):259-263.

Tanaka N, Kim JS, Newell JD, et al. Rheumatoid arthritis-related lung diseases: CT findings. *Radiology*. 2004;232(1):81-91.

Tanaka N, Newell JD, Brown KK, Cool CD, Lynch DA. Collagen vascular disease-related lung disease: high-resolution computed tomography findings based on the pathologic classification. *J Comput Assist Tomogr*. 2004;28(3):351-360.

Tanoue LT. Pulmonary involvement in collagen vascular disease: a review of the pulmonary manifestations of the Marfan syndrome, ankylosing spondylitis, Sjögren's syndrome, and relapsing polychondritis. *J Thorac Imaging*. 1992;7(2):62-77.

Taormina VJ, Miller WT, Gefter WB, Epstein DM. Progressive systemic sclerosis subgroups: variable pulmonary features. *AJR Am J Roentgenol*. 1981;137(2):277-285.

Tazelaar HD, Viggiano RW, Pickersgill J, Colby TV. Interstitial lung disease in polymyositis and dermatomyositis: clinical features and prognosis as correlated with histologic findings. *Am Rev Respir Dis*. 1990;141(3):727-733.

Wiedemann HP, Matthay RA. Pulmonary manifestations of systemic lupus erythematosus. *J Thorac Imaging*. 1992;7(2):1-18.

Chapter 16

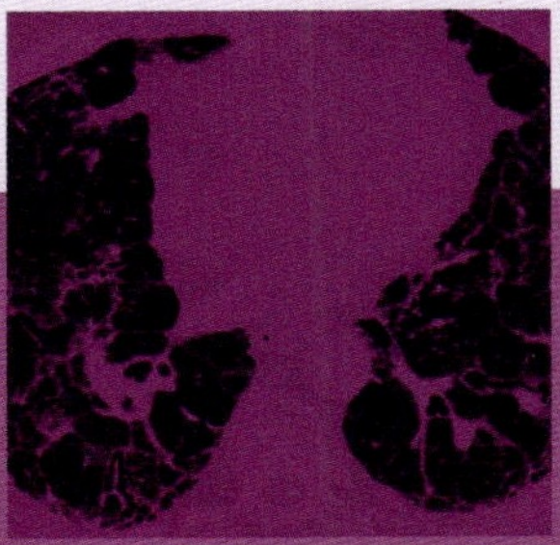

Jeff Kanne

Sarcoidosis and Occupational Lung Diseases

SARCOIDOSIS

Sarcoidosis is a systemic disease characterized by the accumulation of nonnecrotizing granulomata in tissues. While the exact causes of sarcoidosis are unclear, an inhalational etiology is suspected in many cases. Occasionally, medications such as tumor necrosis factor alpha inhibitors can cause a sarcoid-like reaction in the lungs. The lungs and intrathoracic lymph nodes are most commonly affected. Patients with pulmonary sarcoidosis can be asymptomatic or develop cough or shortness of breath.

The Scadding system of chest radiographic staging for sarcoidosis (Table 16.1) was in common use for many decades until the widespread use of CT, which is more sensitive for both lung and lymph node abnormalities. While patients with earlier stages of disease are more likely to have radiographic resolution of abnormalities, sarcoidosis does not necessarily progress from one stage to the next. On chest radiographs, lung disease is apparent in about 40% of patients with sarcoidosis, usually in combination with lymphadenopathy, in contrast to over 80% of patients on CT (Table 16.2).

LYMPH NODE ABNORMALITIES

Lymph node enlargement develops in up to 90% of patients with sarcoidosis, most commonly in the central mediastinum and pulmonary hila. Lymphadenopathy is typically bilateral and often symmetric (Fig. 16.1). Enlargement of lymph nodes elsewhere in the chest such as cardiophrenic, internal mammary (thoracic), and posterior mediastinum occurs in fewer than 5% of patients.

Lymph node calcification is apparent in up to 50% of patients on CT and ranges from faint central ("icing sugar") or stippled to eggshell or dense. The faint central pattern is highly suggestive of sarcoidosis (Fig. 16.2), whereas eggshell calcification also occurs in silicosis and coal worker's pneumoconiosis (CWP). Although lymph node calcification suggests subacute or chronic disease, fluorodeoxyglucose (FDG)-positron emission tomography (PET)/CT is superior to CT in determining disease activity (Fig. 16.3). Central low attenuation or lack of contrast enhancement, which can indicate the presence of necrotizing granulomata, occurs in fewer than 5% of patients.

Table 16.1 Scadding System for Radiographic Staging of Sarcoidosis

Stage	Radiographic Abnormalities	Patients at Presentation	Resolution of Radiographic Abnormalities
0	None	10%	N/A
1	Mediastinal or hilar lymphadenopathy	50%	65%
2	Mediastinal or hilar lymphadenopathy and lung abnormalities	30%	50%
3	Lung abnormalities without lymphadenopathy	10%	20%
4	End-stage or fibrosis	N/A	0%

Table 16.2 CT Findings of Sarcoidosis

Small sharply defined nodules Typical of active lung disease Perilymphatic distribution of nodules most common Patchy upper lobe predominance typical Calcification may occur
Large nodules and masses 15%-25% of patients Due to confluence of small granulomas ± Air bronchograms Commonly parahilar (peribronchovascular) Associated with satellite nodules (galaxy sign)
Ground-glass opacity Uncommon Due to numerous very small granulomas Small nodules may be associated
Reticular opacities and fibrosis Develops in 15% of patients Peribronchovascular fibrosis with traction bronchiectasis Upper lobe volume loss Air-filled cysts Honeycombing in some Aspergilloma may develop
Bronchial or bronchiolar abnormalities Endobronchial granulomas Atelectasis in some Mosaic perfusion and expiratory air trapping

Lung Nodules and Masses

A perilymphatic distribution of lung nodules is the imaging hallmark of sarcoidosis and usually is bilateral and upper lung predominant (Fig. 16.4). Perilymphatic nodules are located along the costal pleura, interlobar fissures, interlobular septa, bronchovascular bundles, and pulmonary veins (see Chapter 11 for further description of perilymphatic nodules). Unlike centrilobular and randomly distributed nodules, perilymphatic nodules often cluster or clump together. The small nodules of sarcoidosis usually have irregular shapes in contrast to the more rounded nodules of some pneumoconioses.

Larger nodules and masses ranging from 10 to 40 mm occur in 15% to 20% of patients with sarcoidosis and are more readily apparent on chest radiography than small nodules (Fig. 16.5). Cavitation and necrosis are rare in contrast to many neoplasms and infections. The presence of small satellite nodules, which create the "galaxy sign," strongly favors a diagnosis of sarcoidosis over infection or neoplasm (Fig. 16.6). Cavitation of large nodule and masses associated with sarcoidosis is rare.

Sometimes, the large masses of sarcoidosis have irregular margins and mimic the appearance of consolidation. This pattern has been referred to "alveolar sarcoidosis," although this term has fallen out of favor presumably because it is a misnomer. These large opacities are the result of numerous granulomata coalescing in the pulmonary interstitium and not in the alveolar spaces.

Ground-Glass Opacity

Pure ground-glass opacity (GGO) is not a characteristic finding of sarcoidosis on CT. However, areas of GGO can be associated with small perilymphatic nodules and reflect the presence of tiny granulomata in the interstitium. On close inspection, especially on thin-section CT, the apparent GGO sometimes has a subtle nodular texture (Fig. 16.7).

Fibrosis

Lung fibrosis develops in up to 15% of patients with sarcoidosis. The fibrosis is usually patchy, has a mid and upper zone predominance, and is concentrated along the bronchovascular bundles (Fig. 16.8). Upper lobe volume loss and upward hilar retraction of the hila are indirect signs of fibrosis. Reticulation or soft-tissue thickening along the bronchovascular bundles is characteristic, and paracicatricial emphysema or cystic spaces can form adjacent to areas of fibrosis. Honeycombing and a lower lobe predominant distribution of fibrosis similar to usual interstitial pneumonia are rare.

Airway Involvement

The airways are commonly involved in sarcoidosis with nodular bronchial wall thickening and endobronchial granulomata reported in up to two-thirds of patients. Extrinsic narrowing of bronchi results in distal atelectasis, and small airway narrowing can lead to inspiratory mosaic attenuation with expiratory air trapping (Fig. 16.9).

Pleural Involvement

Pleural involvement by sarcoidosis is rare and can manifest as pleural thickening or effusion.

Complications

Patients with sarcoidosis can develop aspergillomas in cystic spaces or cavities (Fig. 16.10). Patients with aspergillomas sometimes present with hemoptysis, which can be life threatening. Embolization therapy or resection may be required to prevent further hemorrhage. Compression of pulmonary veins leading to pulmonary hypertension can result from lymphadenopathy and rarely mediastinal fibrosis.

OCCUPATIONAL LUNG DISEASES

Despite increased regulations and improved personal safety equipment and monitoring, occupational exposures to chemicals, dusts, and other compounds continue to cause a range of acute and chronic lung diseases in exposed workers. Occupational asthma is the most common work-related

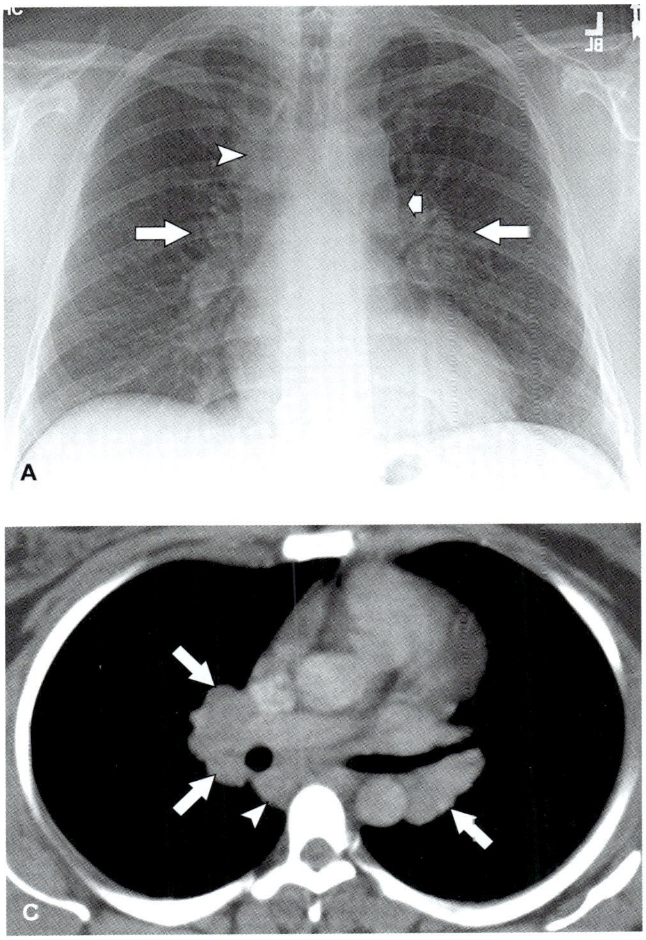

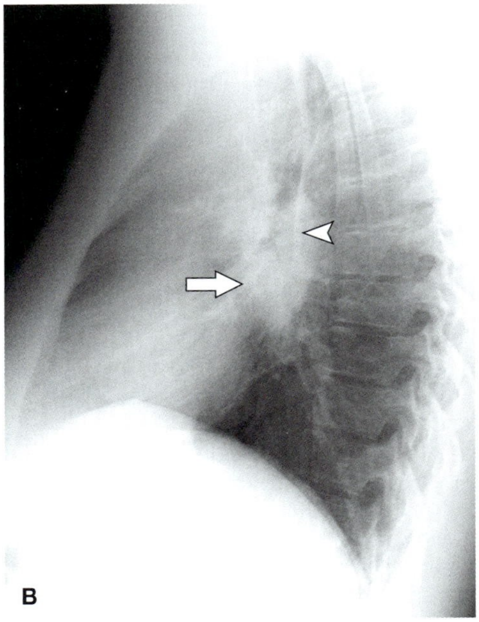

Figure 16.1. Sarcoidosis with lymphadenopathy. **A:** PA radiograph shows enlargement of bilateral hilar (*thin arrows*), right paratracheal (*arrowhead*), and subaortic (*wide arrow*) lymph nodes. **B:** Lateral radiograph shows filling in of the infrahilar window (*arrow*) and thickening of the posterior wall of the bronchus intermedius or intermediate stem line (*arrowhead*). **C:** Contrast-enhanced CT image shows bilateral hilar (*arrows*) and subcarinal (*arrowhead*) lymphadenopathy.

respiratory illness. Other common occupational lung diseases include acute lung injuries from toxic gas exposures, chronic pneumoconiosis related to dust exposure, and hypersensitivity pneumonitis from organic and inorganic antigen exposures.

Establishing a diagnosis of occupational lung disease requires a full clinical evaluation including detailed

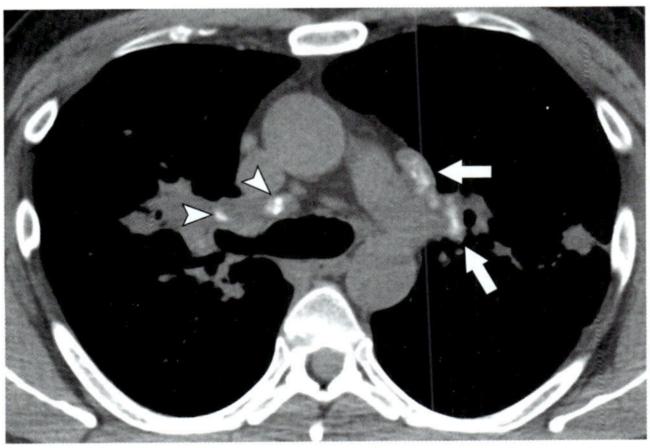

Figure 16.2. Sarcoidosis with lymph node calcifications. Unenhanced CT image shows a mix of dense (*arrowheads*) and "icing sugar" (*arrows*) calcifications.

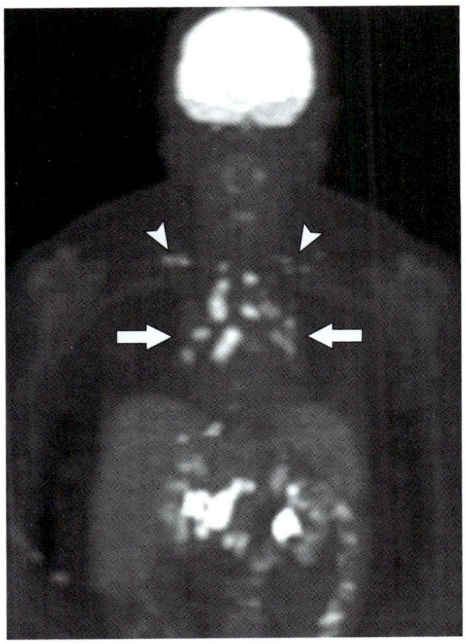

Figure 16.3. Sarcoidosis with extensive lymphadenopathy and metabolic activity. Maximum intensity projection FDG-PET image shows metabolically active mediastinal and bilateral hilar (*arrows*) lymph nodes. Extrathoracic lymph node hypermetabolism is also present in the upper abdomen and supraclavicular fossae (*arrowheads*).

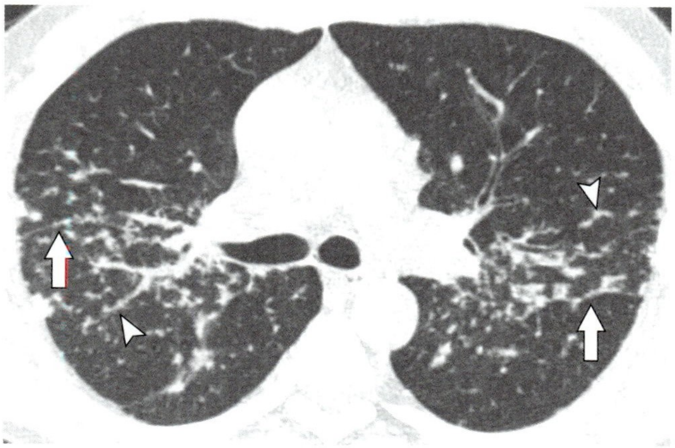

Figure 16.4. Sarcoidosis with typical perilymphatic distribution of small lung nodules. Unenhanced CT image shows numerous tiny nodules along the interlobar fissures (arrows), costal pleura, pulmonary veins (arrowheads), and bronchovascular bundles. Coalescence and clustering of small nodules is typical of a perilymphatic pattern.

occupational and exposure history, physical examination, laboratory and physiologic testing, and imaging. Because some inhaled substances can cause a variety of clinical and radiologic manifestations and because some industries are associated with a variety of exposures, establishing a confident diagnosis of a specific occupational lung disease, even with a thorough clinical evaluation, can be challenging.

This section will focus primarily on the three most common pneumoconiosis: CWP, silicosis, and asbestos-related lung disease. Less common occupational lung diseases will be briefly discussed.

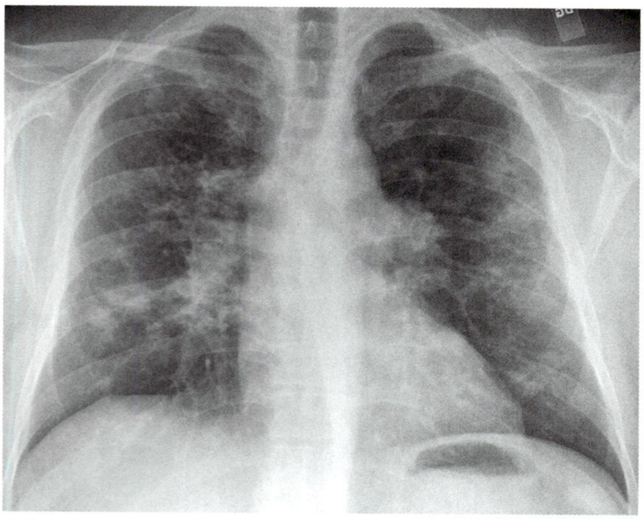

Figure 16.5. Sarcoidosis with large nodule. PA chest radiograph shows bilateral large nodules with irregular margins. The nodules can result from coalescence of smaller nodules or larger areas of granulomatous inflammation. Hilar and mediastinal lymph nodes are also enlarged.

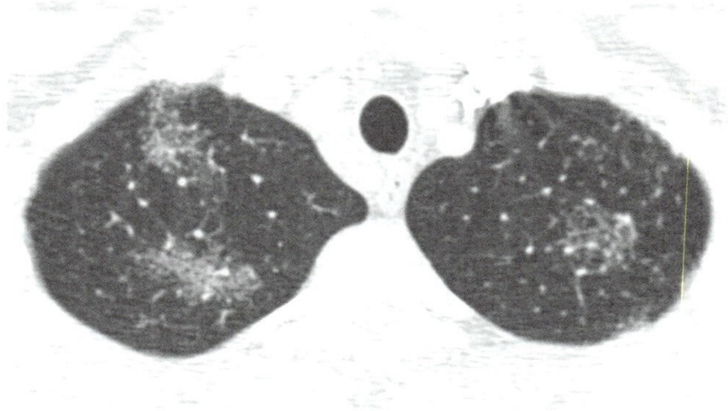

Figure 16.6. Sarcoidosis with galaxy signs. Unenhanced CT image shows bilateral rounded clusters of tiny lung nodules. In contrast to large nodules and masses, the individual tiny nodules are still readily apparent.

COAL WORKER'S PNEUMOCONIOSIS

CWP is a chronic disease almost exclusively of miners who are exposed to dust containing coal, silica, kaolin, and mica. Typically, at least 20 years of dust exposure is required to develop CWP, and factors such as type and concentration of coal dust, mining methods and environment, and use of personal protective equipment affect development and severity of disease.

CWP can be simple or complicated, the latter characterized by development of progressive massive fibrosis (PMF). The coal macule is the characteristic histopathologic lesion of CWP and consists of a microscopic aggregate of coal dust-laden macrophages surrounding a dilated respiratory bronchiole. Pathologically, complicated CWP is characterized by irregularly arranged collagen fibers surrounded by fibers associated with numerous pigment-laden macrophages and free coal dust.

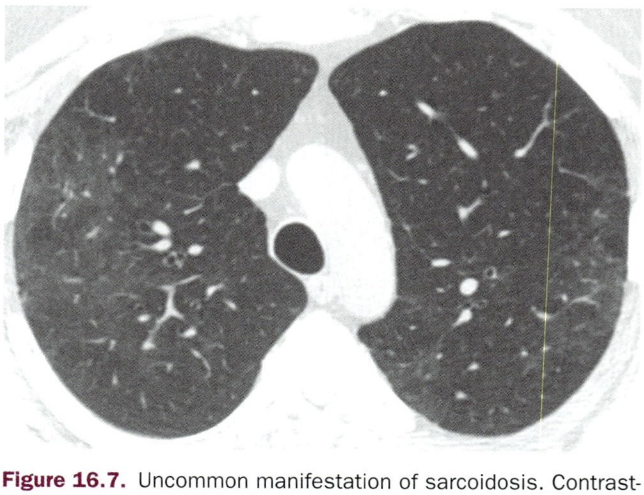

Figure 16.7. Uncommon manifestation of sarcoidosis. Contrast-enhanced CT image shows bilateral patchy, peripheral predominant ground-glass opacity. Histopathologically, this reflects extensive granulomata in the pulmonary interstitium.

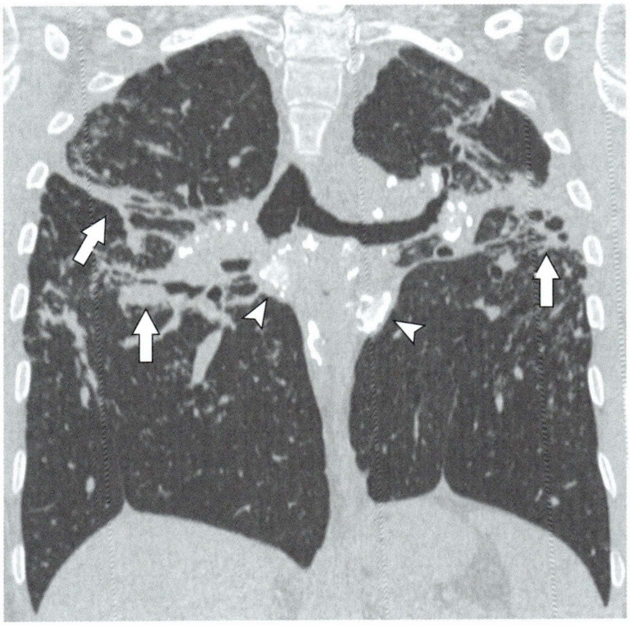

Figure 16.8. Lung fibrosis resulting from sarcoidosis. Coronal reformatted unenhanced CT image shows thickening along the upper lobe bronchovascular bundles (*arrows*) with upper lobe volume loss and upward retraction of the hila. Note the background of small perilymphatic nodules and "eggshell" calcification of enlarged mediastinal and hilar lymph nodes (*arrowheads*).

Radiographically, CWP is characterized by round, well-defined small lung nodules predominating in the upper zones (Table 16.3). Small nodules typically are 2 to 5 mm in diameter but can be as large as 10 mm (Fig. 16.11). The presence of a nodule or nodules larger than 10 mm (large opacity) is the radiographic criterion for PMF. Large opacities form from coalescence of smaller nodules, most commonly in the mid and upper zones resulting in volume loss and hilar retraction. The margins of large opacities are typically smooth and parallel the curvature of the costal pleura (Fig. 16.12). Mediastinal and hilar lymphadenopathy occurs in up to one-third of patients.

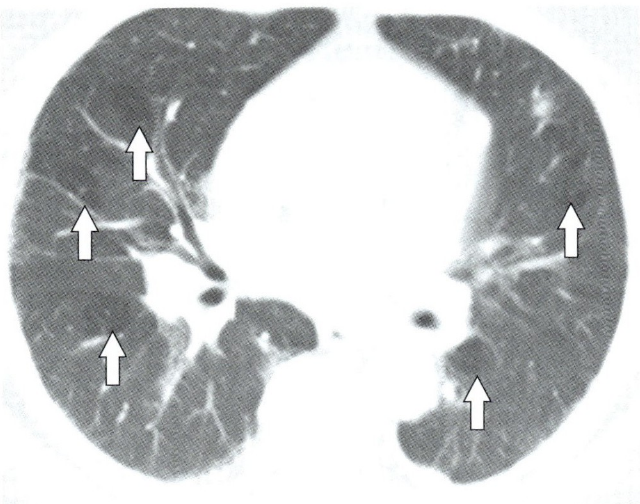

Figure 16.9. Sarcoidosis with small airways involvement. Contrast-enhanced CT image shows bilateral lobular areas of air trapping (*arrows*).

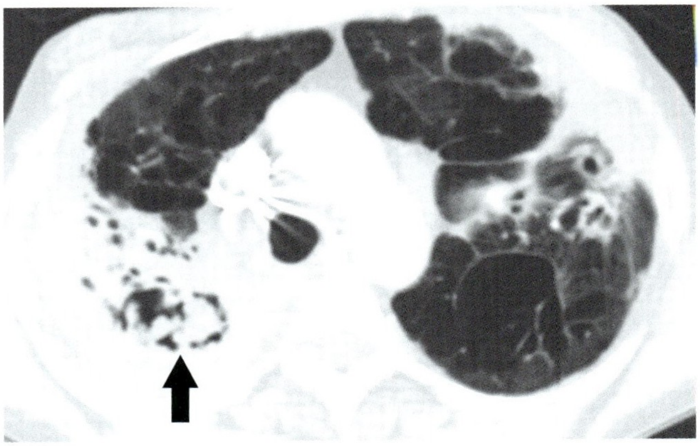

Figure 16.10. Aspergilloma complicating chronic sarcoidosis. Contrast-enhanced CT image shows a thick-walled cavity in the right upper lobe containing a fungus ball layering dependently (*arrow*). Note the background of scaring, bronchiectasis, and emphysema.

CT is more sensitive than radiographs for low profusion small nodules in CWP. In addition to the upper zone predominance, a perilymphatic and slightly posterior distribution is evident. In up to 20% of patients, small pneumoconiotic

Table 16.3 Radiographic and CT Findings of CWP and Silicosis

Simple silicosis and CWP
Well-circumscribed nodules usually measuring 2-5 mm, sometimes larger in silicosis
Predominate in the posterior upper lungs and superior lower lobes
Centrilobular and subpleural distribution on HRCT
Calcification especially with silicosis (10%-20%)
Complicated silicosis and CWP
Large opacities and conglomerate masses (>10 mm diameter)
Termed progressive massive fibrosis
Lenticular masses in upper lobes
Upper lobe nodules decrease in number
Calcification common
Architectural distortion and adjacent paracicatricial emphysema
Masses may cavitate (ischemia, tuberculosis, bacterial infection)
Lymph node enlargement
Hilar and mediastinal node enlargement in 30%-40%
Calcification common (especially eggshell calcification with silicosis)

CWP, coal worker's pneumoconiosis.

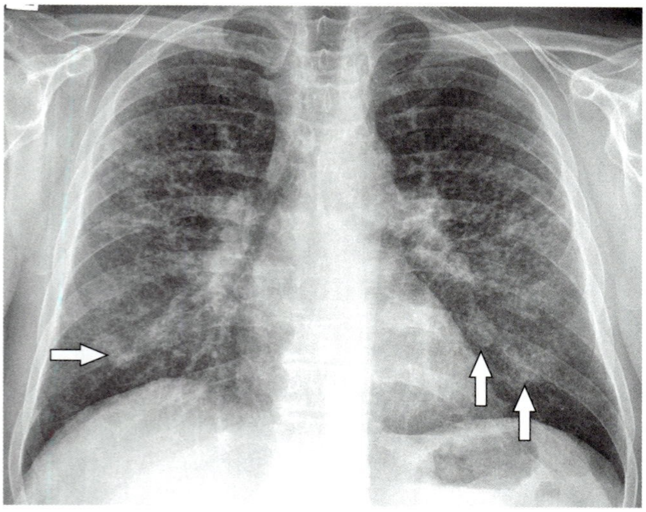

Figure 16.11. Coal worker's pneumoconiosis. PA radiograph shows numerous small (3-5 mm) nodules throughout both lungs with a mid and upper lung predominance. A few larger opacities (≥10 mm) are in the lower lung zones (*arrows*), indicative of progressive massive fibrosis or complicated pneumoconiosis. Mild mediastinal and hilar lymph node enlargement is also present.

nodules calcify. On CT, the coalescence of small nodules into large opacities is more apparent, as are internal calcifications and background small nodules. Paracicatricial emphysema can develop adjacent to the large opacities as the affected lung loses volume.

SILICOSIS

Silicosis results from inhalation of crystalline silicone dioxide (silica) and usually develops after 20 years of exposure. Occupations associated with silicosis include sandblasting, mining, quarrying, tunneling, foundry work, drilling, polishing, and ceramics manufacturing in the lungs and results in tissue reaction and injury. As with CWP, silicosis can be simple or complicated. Additionally, acute and accelerated forms of silicosis can occur.

The silicotic nodules are the pathologic hallmark of silicosis. Alveolar macrophages ingest silica particles, and resultant cell injury leads to release of inflammatory cytokines. Fibroblasts migrate to the lung and form the silicotic nodules, which consist of mature collagen centrally and silica-laden macrophages peripherally.

Radiographically, silicosis is for the most part indistinguishable from CWP with simple silicosis consisting of round, small nodules predominating in the upper lung zones (Table 16.3). In some patients, the nodules of silicosis are slightly larger and better defined than those of CWP, and calcification is more common, occurring in 10% to 15%. Lymphadenopathy develops in up to 75% of patients, and lymph nodes can have punctate or peripheral "eggshell" calcifications (Fig. 16.13). In patients with lower levels of exposure, lymphadenopathy or increased lymph node attenuation can precede development of lung findings. PMF is defined as the presence of one or more large opacities greater than 10 mm (Fig. 16.14).

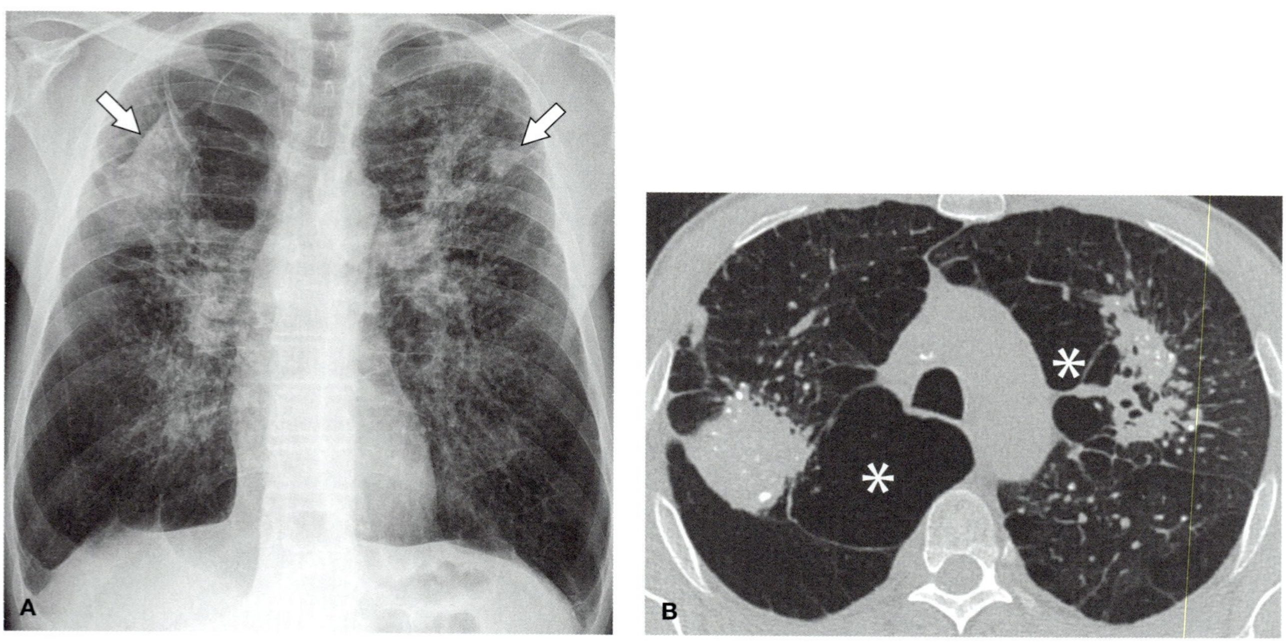

Figure 16.12. Progressive massive fibrosis in a coal miner. **A:** PA radiograph shows bilateral upper lung large opacities (*arrows*) on a background of small nodules. Note how the lateral margin of the large opacity in the right upper lung parallels the contours of the chest wall. The lungs are hyperinflated despite upward hilar retraction and upper lobe volume loss. **B:** Unenhanced CT shows scattered calcifications in the small nodule and large opacities. Note paracicatricial emphysema (*) adjacent to the large opacities.

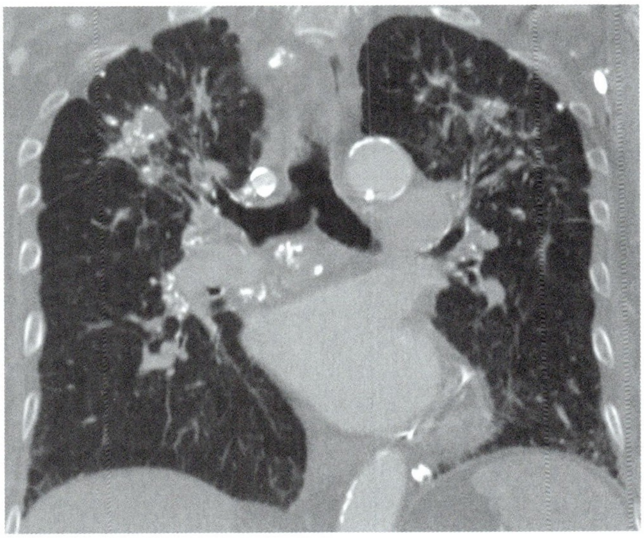

Figure 16.13. Complicated silicosis in a sand blaster. Coronal reformatted contrast-enhanced CT image shows bilateral larger opacities with background small nodules. As small nodules coalesce into large opacities, the profusion of small nodules decreases. Note "eggshell" calcification in enlarged mediastinal and hilar lymph nodes.

As with CWP, CT is more sensitive than radiography for small and large opacities and shows a similar upper lung and perilymphatic distribution. Coalescence of small subpleural nodules along the costal pleura into pseudoplaques can mimic asbestos-related pleural plaques (Fig. 16.15).

Accelerated silicosis occurs with prolonged high-level silica dust exposure resulting in disease development in under 10 years. Recent clusters of accelerated silicosis cases have been attributed to workers exposed to dust of countertops made from artificial or engineered stone, which has a very high concentration of silica content. The clinical and radiographic manifestations are like those of complicated silicosis.

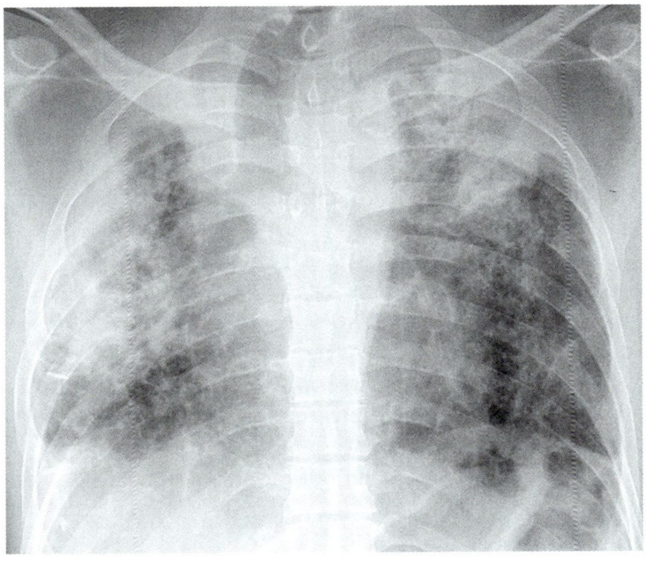

Figure 16.14. Advanced complicated silicosis. PA radiograph shows extensive bilateral large opacities with architectural distortion and volume loss. Even with this extent of disease, a background of small nodules can still be recognized.

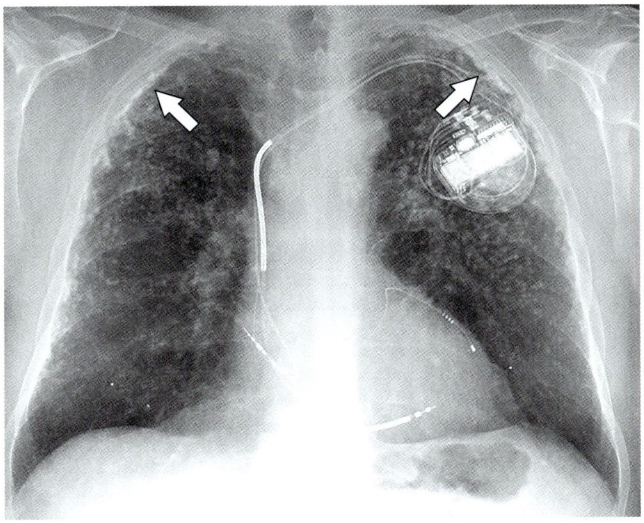

Figure 16.15. Silicosis in a sandblaster. PA radiograph shows upper lung predominant, mostly calcified small round nodules. Coalescence of subpleural nodules forms pseudoplaques (*arrows*), which can mimic asbestos-related pleural plaques.

Acute silicosis or silicoproteinosis is a rare manifestation of silicosis resulting from exposure to very high concentrations of silica dust in an enclosed environment and is most often associated with sandblasting. Acute lung injury results and leads to proliferation of type 2 pneumocytes and surfactant production overfilling the air spaces. Histopathologic and imaging findings are similar to pulmonary alveolar proteinosis. On CT, patchy GGO, consolidation, and poorly defined centrilobular nodules are seen (Fig. 16.16). A "crazy-paving" pattern consisting of GGO with superimposed lines has also been reported. Silicoproteinosis is usually progressive and leads to fatal respiratory failure.

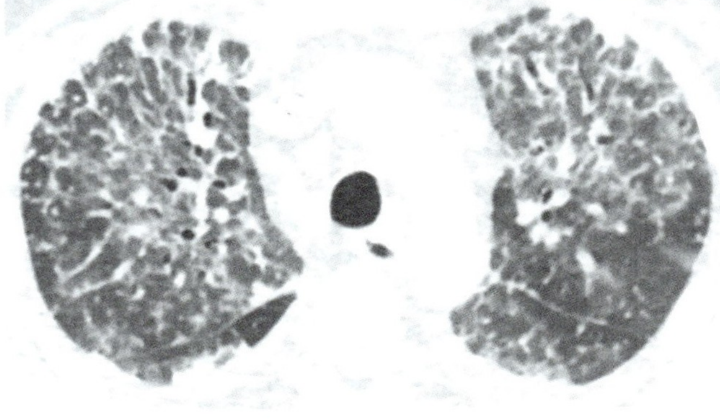

Figure 16.16. Silicoproteinosis. Unenhanced CT image shows patchy ground-glass opacity, scattered perilymphatic nodules, and reticular opacities. (Courtesy of Seth Kligerman, MD, Denver, CO.)

PMF Versus Lung Carcinoma

Patients with CWP and silicosis are at increased risk of developing lung cancer regardless of smoking history, and distinguishing PMF from lung carcinoma is important. A developing nodule or mass without associated fibrosis or architectural distortion or one in a location atypical for large opacities should be further investigated for the possibility of lung cancer (Fig. 16.17). On CT, spiculated or lobulated margins or the absence of background small nodules are findings suggestive of lung carcinoma. For equivocal cases, MRI might help guide further management. On T2-weighted images, lung carcinomas usually have increased signal intensity, whereas large opacities of PMF have low signal intensity because of fibrosis within the lesion. The role of FDG-PET/CT remains unclear because both lung carcinomas and large pneumoconiotic opacities can have increased metabolic activity.

Other Complications

Besides malignancy, patients with silicosis and CWP are at increased risk of acute and chronic infections including tuberculosis (Fig. 16.18). Cavitation in large opacities can result from ischemia or infection. Silicosis and CWP have also been linked to autoimmune diseases including systemic sclerosis and rheumatoid arthritis. Caplan syndrome is a very rare condition consisting of CWP, rheumatoid arthritis, and rheumatoid arthritis–associated necrobiotic lung nodules.

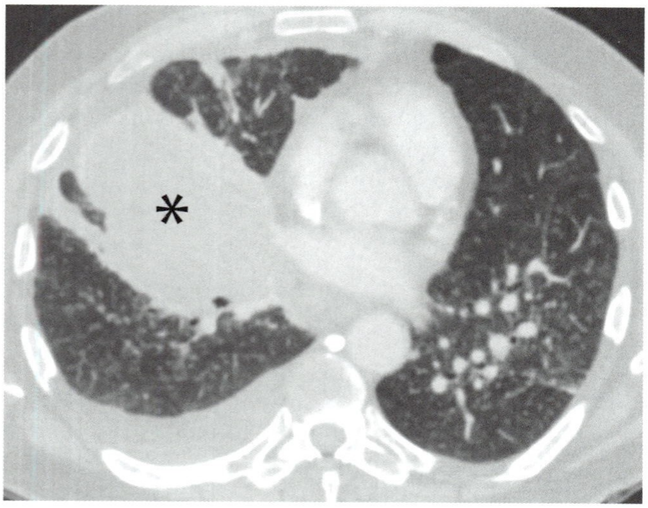

Figure 16.17. Lung carcinoma in the setting of silicosis. Contrast-enhanced chest CT image shows a large mass in the right upper and middle lobes (*). Note the background of small nodules. In contrast to large opacities, there is no volume loss from coalescence. A small right pleural effusion is present, which is not typical of pneumoconiosis and should suggest an alternative or other diagnosis.

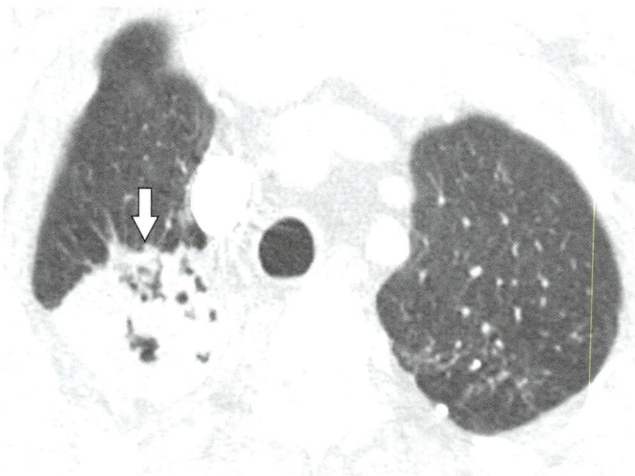

Figure 16.18. Tuberculosis in the setting of silicosis. Contrast-enhanced CT image shows a large cavitary right apical mass (*arrow*). Low profusion small pneumoconiotic nodules, some of which are calcified, are located posteriorly in the left lung apex.

ASBESTOS-RELATED LUNG DISEASE

Asbestos fibers have at least a 3:1 aspect ratio and consist of a variety of silicate minerals. Two morphologic types of asbestos fibers exist. Serpentine fibers are curly, flexible, and smooth, whereas amphibole fibers are straight, rigid, and needlelike. Chrysotile, a serpentine fiber, accounts for 90% of the asbestos found in the United States. Crocidolite and amosite are the most common amphibole fibers.

Asbestos was used extensively in construction and manufacturing because of its heat resistance and tensile strength. However, with the recognition of carcinogenic and fibrotic effects of asbestosis, asbestos use has been discontinued in much of the world. Nevertheless, asbestos-related disease is still encountered because of the decades of latency between exposure and clinical presentation as well as exposure from preexisting asbestos especially in older buildings. In contrast to silicosis and CWP, identifying exposure to asbestos can be quite challenging.

Inhaled asbestos fibers first accumulate in the alveoli and respiratory bronchioles and then penetrate the interstitium and pleura. Because of their morphology and lower clearance rate in the lungs, amphiboles more readily reach the pleural surface as compared to serpentines. Peribronchial fibrosis can lead to airway narrowing and subsequent air trapping, causing obstructive lung disease.

Thoracic manifestations of asbestos-related disease include benign pleural processes, lung fibrosis, and lung and pleural malignancies (Table 16.4). Asbestos exposure has also been linked to extrathoracic malignancies including peritoneal mesothelioma, leukemia, gastrointestinal carcinoma, and head and neck carcinoma.

Table 16.4 Asbestos-Related Pleuropulmonary Findings

Pleural plaques
10-20 y after the onset of exposure
Nearly always parietal pleural
Overlie ribs
Most often posterolateral and along domes of hemidiaphragms
Spare apices and costophrenic sulci
Radiographs
Calcified in 10%-15%
Irregular with discrete margins
CT
Mesa shaped
Often high attenuation
Calcified in up to 50%
Parietal pleural thickening may occur without plaques
Visceral pleural thickening
Lateral lower lobes
May be associated with rounded atelectasis
Benign exudative pleural effusion
Early finding
First 10 y after exposure
Up to 7% of exposed individuals
Small, unilateral, or bilateral
Diffuse pleural thickening
5% of patients
Related to prior benign pleural effusion
Radiographs and CT
Often involves costophrenic sulci
Asbestosis (pulmonary fibrosis)
Almost always associated with pleural plaque
Similar to usual interstitial pneumonia
Reticulation
Traction bronchiectasis
Subpleural honeycombing
Subpleural and basal predominant distribution
Other findings
Peripheral centrilobular nodules
Subpleural curvilinear opacities
Parenchymal bands

Pleural Effusion

Pleural effusion is the earliest thoracic manifestation of asbestos exposure, usually developing in the first 5 to 10 years after exposure and sometimes as late as 20 years. Asbestos-related pleural effusion, however, is uncommon, reported in only up to 7% of exposed workers. The pleural fluid is exudative and often blood tinged and typically resolves without treatment. Most patients are asymptomatic. Signs and symptoms include mild chest pain, fever, or leukocytosis. Significant chest pain, pleural effusion developing more than 20 years after exposure or in the setting of pleural plaques, and persistent or recurrent effusion should raise concern for mesothelioma or other malignancy.

Pleural Plaque

Pleural plaques are the most common manifestation of asbestos exposure, occurring in up to 80% of exposed workers. Plaques usually develop 20 to 30 years after exposure and calcify over time in up to 50%. Plaques consist of discrete bundles of acellular collagen in an undulating basketweave pattern. Asbestos fibers can be identified in plaques with electron microscopy. Most plaques form on the parietal pleura. Plaques are considered biomarkers of asbestos exposure and, as a rule, do not produce symptoms or clinically significant functional impairment.

On radiographs and CT, plaques can be seen along the anterolateral and posterolateral chest wall between the sixth and tenth ribs and along the dome of the diaphragm (Fig. 16.19). Sparing of the costophrenic sulci and lung apices is characteristic, and the mediastinal pleura is only occasionally involved. Plaques are bilateral in nearly 75% of patients.

Diffuse Pleural Thickening

In contrast to pleural plaque, diffuse pleural thickening (DPT) can result from other causes besides asbestosis including trauma, surgery, infection, and autoimmune disease such as rheumatoid arthritis (see Chapter 26). Asbestos-related DPT (Fig. 16.20) is usually the result of asbestos-related pleural effusion and occurs in up to 25% of exposed individuals. Chronic pleural inflammation can lead to fusion of the parietal and visceral layers and, in contrast to plaque, can lead to respiratory impairment.

Pleural Mesothelioma

Asbestos exposure is the leading cause of pleural mesothelioma, a pleural malignancy which is discussed in detail in Chapter 26.

Asbestosis

Pulmonary fibrosis resulting from asbestos exposure is termed asbestosis and normally develops 20 years or more after initial exposure. The extent of asbestos dust exposure correlates with the risk of asbestosis. Asbestos bodies are often detected in bronchoalveolar lavage fluid or biopsy tissue samples.

Chest radiographic findings of asbestos include basal predominant coarse reticular opacities and are indistinguishable from other causes of pulmonary fibrosis. However, on radiographs and CT, the presence of pleural plaques can help establish a diagnosis of asbestosis.

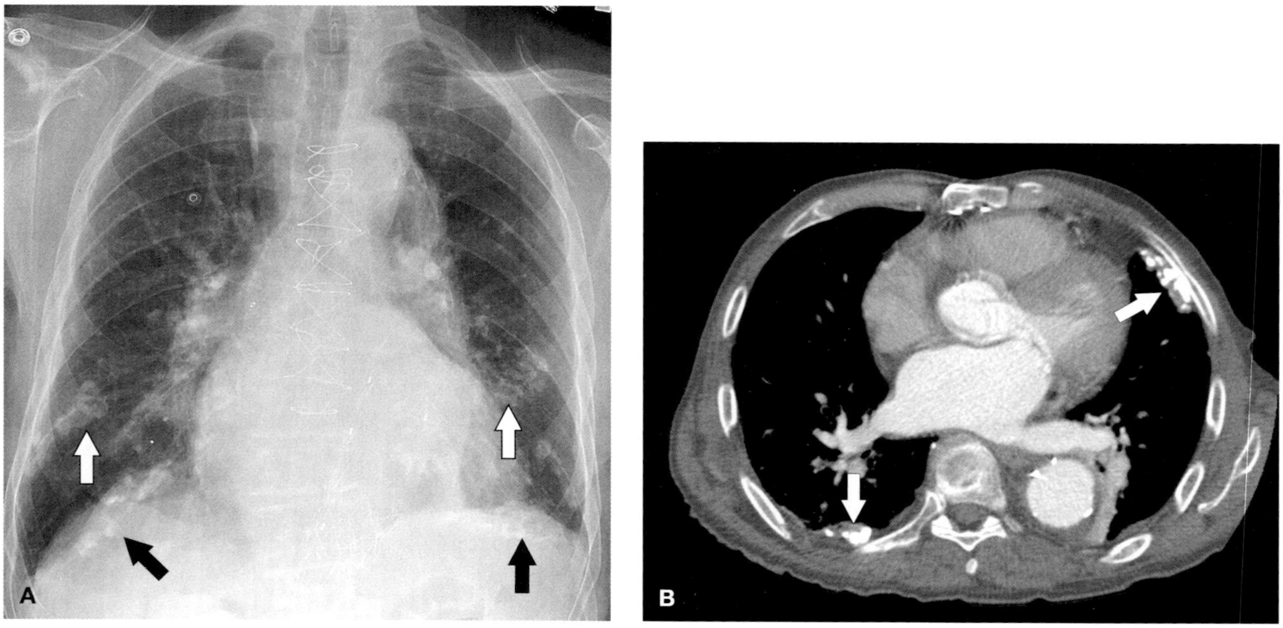

Figure 16.19. Asbestos-related pleural plaques. **A:** PA radiograph shows calcified pleural plaques face on (*white arrows*) and along the hemidiaphragms (*black arrows*). **B:** Contrast-enhanced CT image shows the relatively smooth margins of the pleural plaques (*arrows*).

On CT, findings are similar to those of usual interstitial pneumonia, which include subpleural and basal predominant reticulation with traction bronchiectasis and subpleural honeycombing developing in more advanced disease (Fig. 16.21). Other CT findings associated with asbestosis include poorly defined centrilobular nodules in the lung periphery, subpleural curvilinear opacities, and parenchymal bands. Peribronchial fibrosis can lead to expiratory air trapping. In select cases, prone imaging can be used to distinguish mild posterior fibrosis from dependent atelectasis.

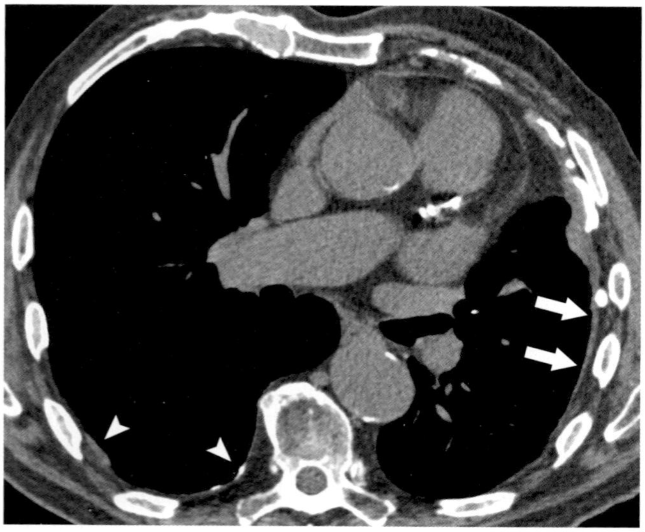

Figure 16.20. Asbestos-related pleural disease. Contrast-enhanced CT image shows calcified and noncalcified pleural plaques (*arrowheads*) and left diffuse pleural thickening (*arrows*).

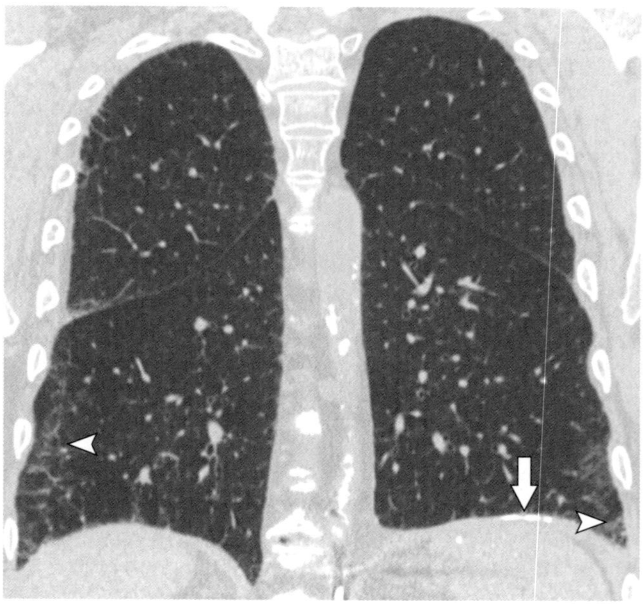

Figure 16.21. Asbestosis. Coronal reformatted unenhanced CT image shows subpleural and basal predominant reticulation (*arrowheads*). With the presence of pleural plaque (*arrow*), the presumption is the fibrosis reflects asbestosis.

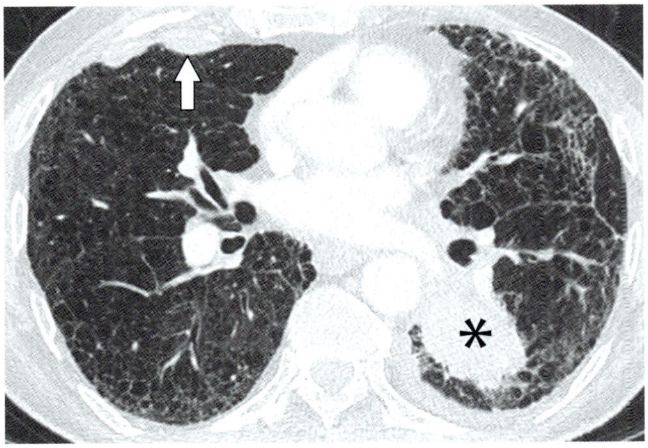

Figure 16.22. Asbestosis and lung carcinoma. Contrast-enhanced CT image shows a mass (*) in the left lower lobe. There is background emphysema and fibrosis. Note the small left pleural effusion and right anterior pleural plaque (*arrow*).

Lung Cancer

Asbestos exposure is a risk factor for lung cancer independent of cigarette smoking (Fig. 16.22). Lung cancer is discussed in detail in Chapter 5.

HARD METAL LUNG DISEASE

Hard metal lung disease results from exposure to alloys containing tungsten carbide and cobalt, the latter of which is believed to be the main contributor to lung toxicity. Occupational asthma, constrictive bronchiolitis, and giant cell interstitial pneumonia (GIP) comprise hard metal lung disease. Associated occupational exposures include cutting, polishing, and drilling where hard metals are routinely used because of their strength and heat resistance. Criteria for establishing a diagnosis of hard metal lung disease have been proposed and include history of exposure to hard metal dust, prolonged dyspnea or dyspnea on exertion with or without chronic cough, diffuse lung disease on imaging studies, histopathologic findings of GIP, and documentation of metal in lung tissue.

Radiographic and CT findings of hard metal lung disease vary (Fig. 16.23). Constrictive bronchiolitis is one of the earliest manifestations and presents with mosaic attenuation on inspiratory CT and associated expiratory air trapping. Other CT findings include GGO, consolidation, small nodules, reticulation, and traction bronchiectasis. Honeycombing is a manifestation of more advanced fibrosis.

CHRONIC BERYLLIUM DISEASE

Beryllium is a low-molecular-weight metal used in manufacturing, nuclear power plants and weaponry, and industrial ceramics. Chronic beryllium disease is a systemic disease resulting from long-term exposure to beryllium. It is characterized by granulomatous inflammation and is clinically and

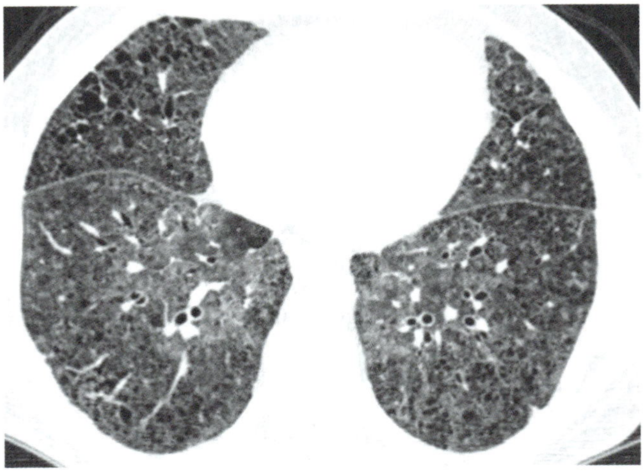

Figure 16.23. Giant cell interstitial pneumonia in a dental laboratory technician exposed to hard metals while polishing and finishing dental crowns. Axial unenhanced CT image shows relatively diffuse axial distribution of fibrosis including ground-glass opacity, reticulation, traction bronchiolectasis, and peripheral cystic spaces. This pattern of fibrosis is difficult to classify and was proven to represent giant cell interstitial pneumonia at surgical lung biopsy.

radiographically identical to sarcoidosis. Differentiation of the two entities requires special laboratory testing.

ALUMINUM-RELATED LUNG DISEASE

Inhalation of aluminum or aluminum oxide dust has been associated with a variety of lung diseases including fibrosis, alveolar proteinosis (Fig. 16.24), and granulomatous inflation. Imaging findings include dense or enlarged mediastinal and hilar lymph nodes, varying degrees of pulmonary fibrosis, and small predominantly centrilobular nodules.

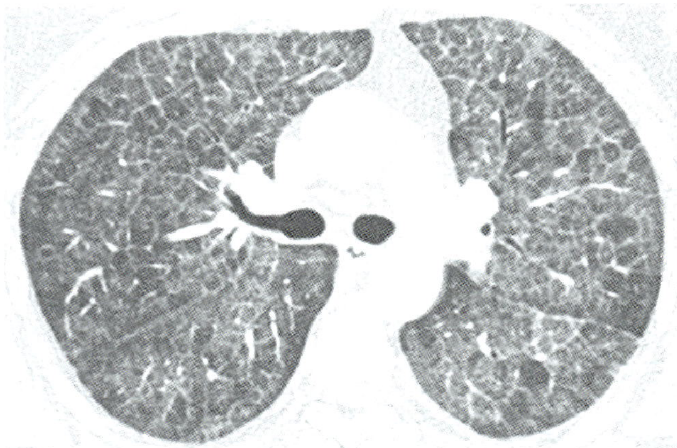

Figure 16.24. Alveolar proteinosis resulting from chronic aluminum exposure. Unenhanced CT image shows a "crazy-paving" pattern consisting of ground-glass opacity with superimposed septal lines and reticular opacities.

SUGGESTED READINGS

Ahuja J, Kanne JP, Meyer CA. Occupational lung disease. *Semin Roentgenol.* 2015;50(1):40-51.

Akira M, Yamamoto S, Yokoyama K, et al. Asbestosis: high-resolution CT-pathologic correlation. *Radiology.* 1990;176(2):389-394.

Akira M, Yokoyama K, Yamamoto S, et al. Early asbestosis: evaluation with high-resolution CT. *Radiology.* 1991;178(2):409-416.

Akira M. High-resolution CT in the evaluation of occupational and environmental disease. *Radiol Clin North Am.* 2002;40(1):43-59.

Antao VC, Pinheiro GA, Terra-Filho M, Kavakama J, Müller NL. High-resolution CT in silicosis: correlation with radiographic findings and functional impairment. *J Comput Assist Tomogr.* 2005;29(3):350-356.

Carroll MB, Kanne JP. Imaging of occupational and environmental lung disease. *Semin Respir Crit Care Med.* 2022;43(6):874-886.

Chong S, Lee KS, Chung MJ, Han J, Kwon OJ, Kim TS. Pneumoconiosis: comparison of imaging and pathologic findings. *Radiographics.* 2006;26(1):59-77.

Copley SJ, Wells AU, Sivakumaran P, et al. Asbestosis and idiopathic pulmonary fibrosis: comparison of thin-section CT features. *Radiology.* 2003;229(3):731-736.

Criado E, Sánchez M, Ramírez J, et al. Pulmonary sarcoidosis: typical and atypical manifestations at high-resolution CT with pathologic correlation. *Radiographics.* 2010;30(6):1567-1586.

Flors L, Domingo ML, Leiva-Salinas C, Mazon M, Roselló-Sastre E, Vilar J. Uncommon occupational lung diseases: high-resolution CT findings. *AJR Am J Roentgenol.* 2010;194(1):20-26.

Gevenois PA, de Maertelaer V, Madani A, Winant C, Sergent G, De Vuyst P. Asbestosis, pleural plaques and diffuse pleural thickening: three distinct benign responses to asbestos exposure. *Eur Respir J.* 1998;11(5):1021-1027.

Greco FG, Spagnolo P, Muri M, et al. The value of chest radiograph and computed tomography in pulmonary sarcoidosis. *Sarcoidosis Vasc Diffuse Lung Dis.* 2014;31(2):108-116.

Gupta R, Baughman RP. Advanced pulmonary sarcoidosis. *Semin Respir Crit Care Med.* 2020;41(5):700-715.

Hansell DM, Milne DG, Wilsher ML, Wells AU. Pulmonary sarcoidosis: morphologic associations of airflow obstruction at thin-section CT. *Radiology.* 1998;209(3):697-704.

Jun JS, Jung JI, Kim HR, et al. Complications of pneumoconiosis: radiologic overview. *Eur J Radiol.* 2013;82(10):1819-1830.

Kalshetty A, Basu S. PET/computed tomography in pulmonary and thoracic inflammatory diseases (including cardiac sarcoidosis): the current role and future promises. *PET Clin.* 2020;15(2):163-173.

Laney AS, Weissman DN. Respiratory diseases caused by coal mine dust. *J Occup Environ Med.* 2014;56(suppl 10):S18-S22.

Llanos O, Hamzeh N. Sarcoidosis. *Med Clin North Am.* 2019;103(3):527-534.

Lynch DA, Webb WR, Gamsu G, Stulbarg M, Golden J. Computed tomography in pulmonary sarcoidosis. *J Comput Assist Tomogr.* 1989;13(3):405-410.

Mossman BT, Churg A. Mechanisms in the pathogenesis of asbestosis and silicosis. *Am J Respir Crit Care Med.* 1998;157(5 pt 1):1666-1680.

Müller NL, Mawson JB, Mathieson JR, Abboud R, Ostrow DN, Champion P. Sarcoidosis: correlation of extent of disease at CT with clinical, functional, and radiographic findings. *Radiology.* 1989;171(3):613-618.

Nakatsu M, Hatabu H, Morikawa K, et al. Large coalescent parenchymal nodules in pulmonary sarcoidosis: "sarcoid galaxy" sign. *AJR Am J Roentgenol.* 2002;178(6):1389-1393.

Newman LS, Buschman DL, Newell JD, Lynch DA. Beryllium disease: assessment with CT. *Radiology.* 1994;190(3):835-840.

Nishimura K, Itoh H, Kitaichi M, Nagai S, Izumi T. Pulmonary sarcoidosis: correlation of CT and histopathologic findings. *Radiology.* 1993;189(1):105-109.

Remy-Jardin M, Degreef JM, Beuscart R, Voisin C, Remy J. Coal worker's pneumoconiosis: CT assessment in exposed workers and correlation with radiographic findings. *Radiology.* 1990;177(2):363-371.

Savranlar A, Altin R, Mahmutyazicioglu K, et al. Comparison of chest radiography and high-resolution computed tomography findings in early and low-grade coal worker's pneumoconiosis. *Eur J Radiol.* 2004;51(2):175-180.

Seaman DM, Meyer CA, Kanne JP. Occupational and environmental lung disease. *Clin Chest Med.* 2015;36(2):249-268.

Sette A, Neder JA, Nery LE, et al. Thin-section CT abnormalities and pulmonary gas exchange impairment in workers exposed to asbestos. *Radiology.* 2004;232(1):66-74.

Spagnolo P, Rossi G, Trisolini R, Sverzellati N, Baughman RP, Wells AU. Pulmonary sarcoidosis. *Lancet Respir Med.* 2018;6(5):389-402.

Traill ZC, Maskell GF, Gleeson FV. High-resolution CT findings of pulmonary sarcoidosis. *AJR Am J Roentgenol.* 1997;168(6):1557-1560.

Chapter 17

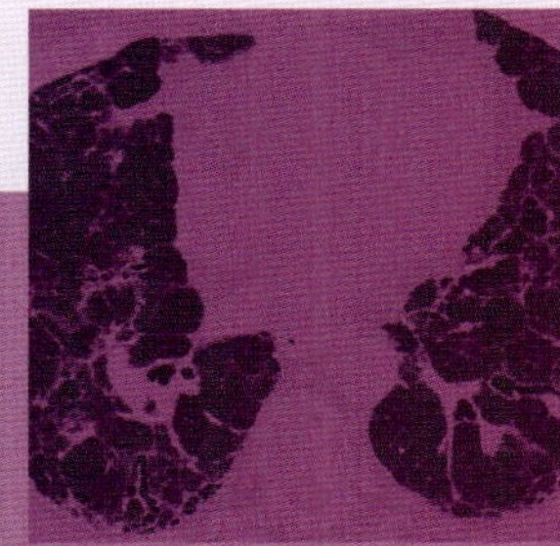

Travis S. Henry

Allergic Lung Diseases: Hypersensitivity Pneumonitis and Eosinophilic Lung Disease

HYPERSENSITIVITY PNEUMONITIS

Hypersensitivity pneumonitis (HP), formerly known as extrinsic allergic alveolitis, is an allergic lung disease caused by the inhalation of various antigens, including microbes, animal and plant proteins, and low-molecular-weight chemicals that combine with host proteins to form haptens. Farmer's lung, the best-known HP syndrome, results from the inhalation of fungal organisms (thermophilic actinomycetes) growing in moist hay. Many other HP syndromes have been reported, and the list continues to grow. As with farmer's lung, HP syndromes are usually named after the setting in which exposure occurs or the substance involved. HP syndromes include bird fancier's lung (bird proteins), mushroom worker's lung (thermophilic actinomycetes), malt worker's lung (*Aspergillus* species), maple bark disease (*Cryptostroma* species), bagassosis (thermophilic actinomycetes in sugarcane fibers), building-associated HP, and hot tub lung (mycobacteria). Hundreds of causes of HP exist and in about 50% of cases, the responsible antigen cannot be determined despite a careful history and environmental assessment.

The exact mechanisms of developing HP are unclear. Variants in genes associated with both innate and adaptive immunity may promote sensitivity to inciting agents, a phenomenon evidenced in polymorphisms present in major histocompatibility complex class II, proteasomes, transporter proteins, and tissue inhibitors of matrix metalloproteinases, all linked with HP. In particular, among patients with fibrotic HP, the MUC5B promoter polymorphism is more common than in the general population and is linked to decreased survival rates. Furthermore, HP has been reported in familial pulmonary fibrosis probands, including those with mutations in telomere-related genes.

Other potential sensitizing factors for HP include preceding respiratory viral infection, which is suggested to enhance susceptibility to the condition. Additionally, exposure to pesticides seems to amplify the risk of HP in farmers. This variety of influencing factors suggests that HP is a complex condition with various contributing genetic and environmental factors.

Clinical Presentation and Natural History of HP

Despite the complex pathogenesis, the clinical, radiographic, and pathologic abnormalities occurring in patients with HP are similar regardless of the antigen responsible. Historically, HP was classified into three forms based on the duration of symptoms at presentation: acute, subacute, and chronic. However, these classifications were loosely defined and inconsistently associated with outcomes. More recent work has focused on distinguishing between the inflammatory and fibrotic manifestations of HP. This culminated in a 2020 multidisciplinary expert panel of the American Thoracic Society, Japanese Respiratory Society, and Asociación Latinoamericana de Tórax (ATS/JRS/ALAT) clinical practice guideline revising the classification of HP into two forms—nonfibrotic (purely inflammatory) and fibrotic (fibrosis with or without an inflammatory component)—determined by the presence or absence of significant fibrosis on imaging and/or pathology. This new classification is intended to be more objective, and better reflect disease presentation, clinical course, and outcomes. Similar classification schemes have more recently been adopted by other organizations.

The 2020 ATS/JRS/ALAT classification does not distinguish the symptoms between the two phenotypes as presentations of nonfibrotic HP and fibrotic HP overlap. Any patient with HP may present with acute-onset symptoms (days to weeks), or the presentation may be insidious (months to years). Episodes may be recurrent based on repeated exposures to antigens.

Presenting symptoms of both nonfibrotic and fibrotic types of HP include dyspnea, cough, and midinspiratory squeaks. Less common symptoms include weight loss, flulike symptoms, chest tightness, wheezing, and physical examination findings of rales and cyanosis. The onset of symptoms can be acute, developing rapidly over days to weeks, sometimes with pleural effusion, or insidious, with the disease developing and worsening over months to years. Despite an acute presentation often being more consistent with nonfibrotic HP and the insidious presentation more likely with fibrotic HP, a precise characterization of symptoms with respect to fibrosis status has not been conclusively established.

The prevalence of HP is highest among older individuals, specifically those aged 65 years and older, with the average diagnosis occurring in the fifth or sixth decade of life. Nonetheless, the condition can also be diagnosed in younger adults and, rarely, children. Patients with fibrotic HP are more likely to be older and exhibit a lower vital capacity, diffusion capacity, and percentage of lymphocytes in their bronchoalveolar lavage (BAL) fluid compared to patients with nonfibrotic HP. Furthermore, these patients often have an unidentified inciting agent, indicating the complex nature of HP's underlying causes.

The natural history of HP is variable and can range from improvement to progressive decline and eventual death due to respiratory failure. Nonfibrotic HP patients who successfully avoid further exposure to the causative agent may have a favorable prognosis, with possibilities of stabilization or full recovery. However, patients with fibrotic HP, especially those with a usual interstitial pneumonia (UIP)-like pattern, tend to have reduced survival.

The prevalence of HP demonstrates regional variations, depending on disparities in climate, occupational exposures, and environmental exposures. Incidence rates range from 0.3 to 0.9 per 100,000 individuals in general populations, but may be increased in certain occupational groups. For example, one study found an incidence of 4.9 per 100,000 bird breeders per year over a decade. Additionally, insurance claim–based analyses conducted from 2004 to 2013 estimated a 1-year prevalence of HP between 1.67 and 2.71 per 100,000 in the U.S. population.

HP's proportion among all interstitial lung disease (ILD) cases significantly varies, ranging from 2% to 47% in various studies and registries. Although HP in children is rare, it could account for up to 50% of all childhood ILDs. There have been reports of sporadic HP outbreaks in groups exposed to certain conditions, including lifeguards at swimming pools, automobile workers exposed to polyurethane, and office workers exposed to contaminated humidifiers or forced-air climate control systems.

As with all ILD, a clinical diagnosis of HP (either fibrotic or nonfibrotic) is best made by a multidisciplinary team that includes pulmonologists, radiologists, and pathologists.

Imaging Findings of Nonfibrotic HP

Radiographs may show ill-defined air-space consolidation, predominantly in the middle and lower lung zones, but may be normal even in the face of marked symptoms (Fig. 17.1). Ill-defined air-space nodules can also be seen. HRCT is the mainstay for diagnosis of nonfibrotic HP with diagnostic criteria put forth by the 2020 ATS/JRS/ALAT guidelines (Table 17.1).

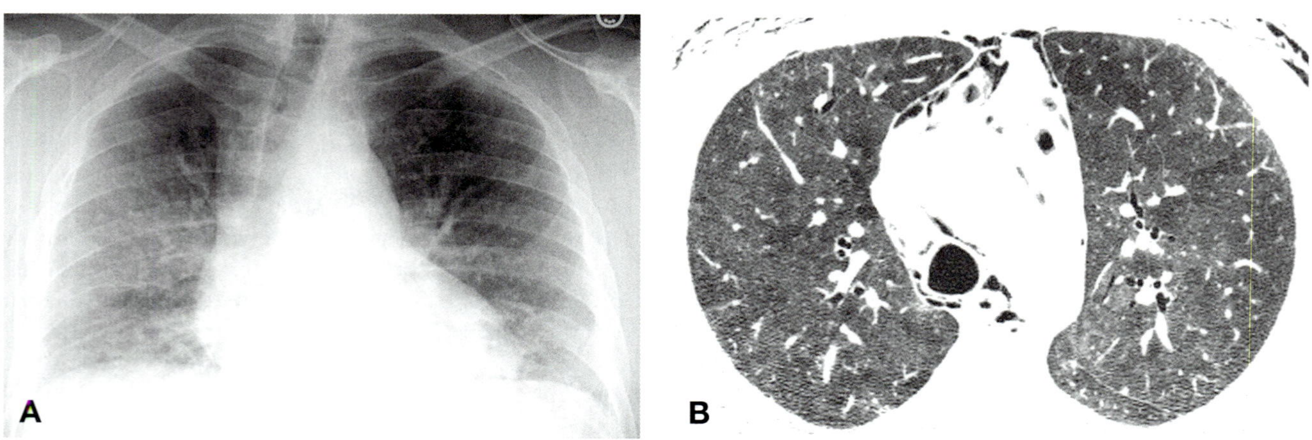

Figure 17.1. Nonfibrotic hypersensitivity pneumonitis (HP). **A:** Chest radiograph shows reduced lung volumes and ill-defined increased lung opacity at the lung bases. **B:** HRCT shows mosaic attenuation from bilateral ground-glass opacity subacute from nonfibrotic HP. Pneumomediastinum and subcutaneous emphysema are also present.

Table 17.1 Nonfibrotic Hypersensitivity Pneumonitis (HP)

Typical Nonfibrotic HP
Requires findings of both parenchymal infiltration and small airways disease in a diffuse distribution
Parenchymal infiltration—GGO and/or mosaic attenuation
Small airways disease—ill defined centrilobular nodules and/or air trapping

Findings Compatible With Nonfibrotic HP
Isolated air trapping
Uniform, subtle GGO
Consolidation
Lung cysts

GGO, ground-glass opacity.

On CT, nonfibrotic HP can be separated into findings of parenchymal infiltration, and findings of small airways disease. Findings of parenchymal infiltration include ground-glass opacity (GGO, which reflects the presence of alveolitis) and mosaic attenuation. Findings of small airways disease include ill-defined centrilobular ground-glass nodules (which correlates with peribronchiolar inflammation) and air trapping (Figs. 17.2-17.5). The distribution of findings is usually diffuse in the axial and craniocaudal planes, but there may be some relative basal sparing in the craniocaudal direction (Fig. 17.6). This distribution is unlike that of some other diseases, particularly nonspecific interstitial pneumonia (NSIP) and UIP/idiopathic pulmonary fibrosis (IPF), with which it may be confused clinically.

Mosaic attenuation represents a patchwork of differing lung densities (see Chapter 11), and in the case of HP is usually due to the presence of areas of decreased attenuation on inspiratory HRCT (see Figs. 17.2B, 17.7, and 17.8) or air trapping on expiratory HRCT (see Figs. 17.8 and 17.9). These areas usually have sharply defined margins and a configuration consistent with involvement of single lobule or multiple adjacent pulmonary lobules. The areas of decreased attenuation and air trapping result from the cellular bronchiolitis seen in patients with HP. In some patients with HP, evidence of expiratory air trapping is seen in the absence of inspiratory scan abnormalities. The three-density sign, formerly the headcheese sign, is inconsistently seen in nonfibrotic HP and is discussed later in this chapter with fibrotic HP.

When both parenchymal infiltration and small airways disease are present in a diffuse distribution, it is highly suggestive of nonfibrotic HP (Figs. 17.2-17.7 and 17.9). Additional imaging manifestations that are suggestive of nonfibrotic HP but nonspecific include isolated air trapping, uniform and subtle GGO, consolidation, or thin-walled lung cysts. In most patients, fewer than five cysts are visible and may range from millimeters in size to 2 cm. The cysts are randomly distributed and often associated with GGO or mosaic perfusion. They likely result from bronchiolitis and bronchiolar obstruction.

Imaging findings in nonfibrotic HP may be reversible with removal of the antigen or medical treatment.

Imaging Findings of Fibrotic HP

On chest radiographs, findings of fibrosis include irregular reticular opacities that predominate in the upper, mid, or lower lung zones and may be parahilar, peribronchovascular, or peripheral in distribution (Fig. 17.10A). Lung volumes are usually reduced. In some cases, fibrosis in HP can mimic the appearance of IPF with honeycombing. A confident

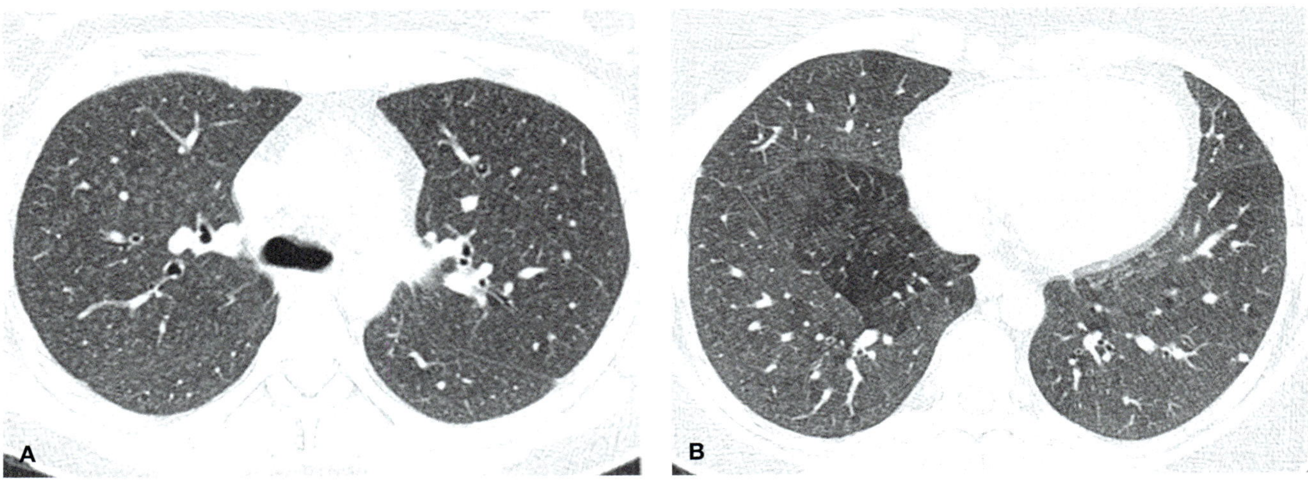

Figure 17.2. Nonfibrotic hypersensitivity pneumonitis (HP) in a bird fancier. **A:** HRCT through the upper lobes shows patchy areas of ground-glass opacity and ill-defined nodular opacities with a centrilobular predominance. **B:** HRCT at the lung base shows patchy ground-glass opacities. Focal areas of relatively lucency represent mosaic attenuation. The distribution of abnormalities is relatively diffuse in both the axial and craniocaudal planes, typical of nonfibrotic HP.

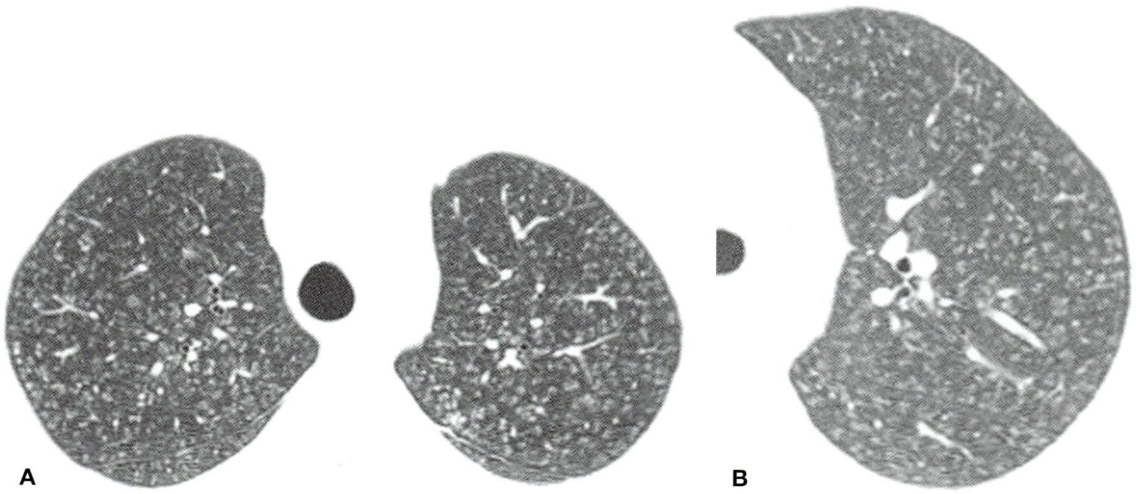

Figure 17.3. Nonfibrotic hypersensitivity pneumonitis with diffuse centrilobular nodules. **A:** Scan through the upper lobes show diffuse centrilobular nodules. **B:** Detail view of the left upper lobe. The nodules do not involve the fissures or peripheral pleural surface. This appearance correlates with the presence of peribronchiolar infiltrates and ill-defined granulomas.

diagnosis of fibrotic HP is generally not possible on a radiograph alone.

On HRCT, fibrosis is seen with or without superimposed findings of parenchymal infiltration and small airways disease (Figs. 17.10-17.12). The degree of fibrosis may vary from mild reticulation and architectural distortion to more severe traction bronchiectasis and/or honeycombing.

A typical task of the radiologist is to differentiate fibrotic HP from more common causes of fibrosis such as UIP and NSIP. Once it is determined that fibrosis is present, assessing the distribution of fibrosis and the presence of small airways disease/bronchiolar obstruction can help to categorize the CT findings. Based on the 2020 ATS/JRS/ALAT guidelines, CT findings can be considered as "typical," "compatible with," or "indeterminate for" fibrotic HP (Table 17.2).

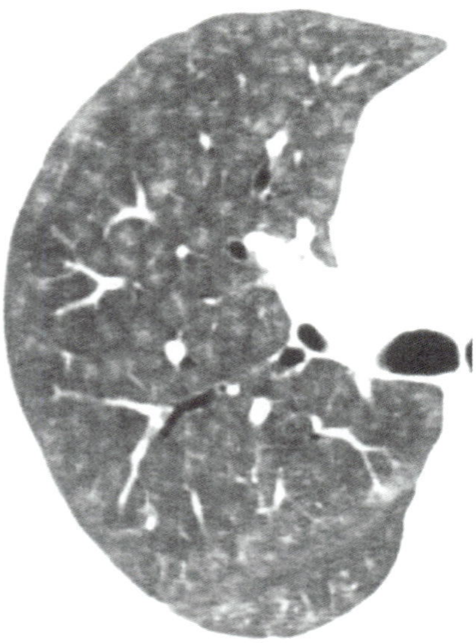

Figure 17.4. Nonfibrotic hypersensitivity pneumonitis in a bird fancier, with ill-defined centrilobular nodules of ground-glass opacity. The nodules surround small vessels and spare the pleural surfaces. The chest radiograph in this patient was normal.

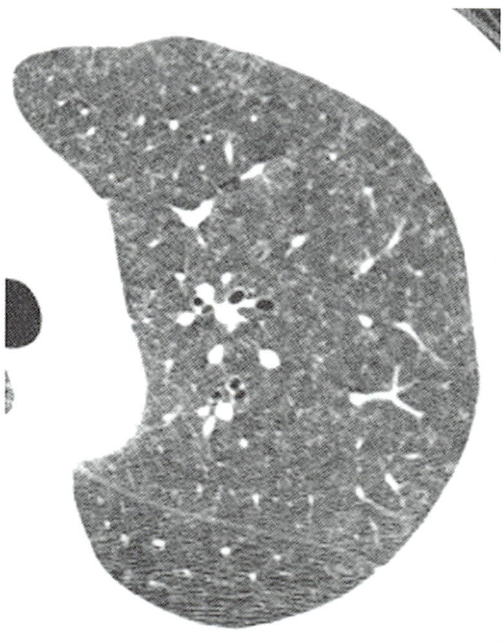

Figure 17.5. Nonfibrotic hypersensitivity pneumonitis with diffuse ground-glass opacity (GGO) and centrilobular nodules, representing "hot tub lung." Small, ill-defined nodules are visible with other areas of more confluent GGO.

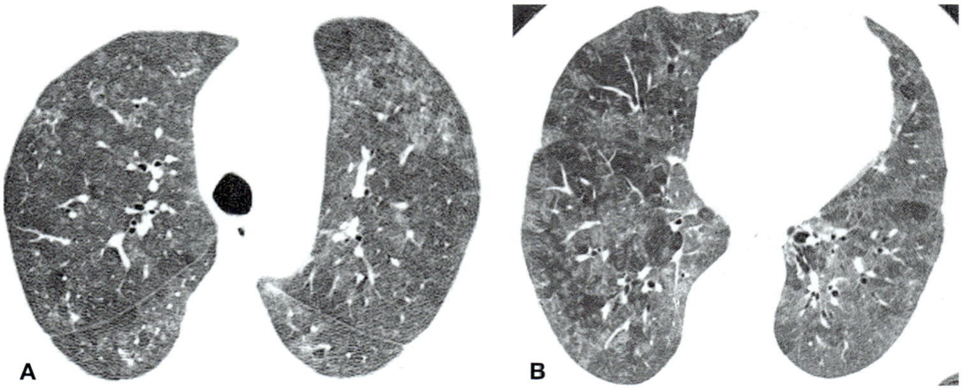

Figure 17.6. Nonfibrotic hypersensitivity pneumonitis in a bird fancier. **A, B:** CT scans through the upper and lower lobes show diffuse ground-glass opacity with more discrete centrilobular ground-glass nodules in the upper lobes. Some basal sparing is evident, a common finding in nonfibrotic hypersensitivity pneumonitis.

In typical cases, a confident diagnosis may be made at multidisciplinary discussion based on imaging and history alone, but less classic cases may involve surgical lung biopsy.

The "typical" pattern for fibrotic HP has the highest diagnostic confidence. This is based on the combination of small airways disease and fibrosis in a pattern that would be atypical for other causes of fibrosis such as UIP or NSIP. The findings of small airways disease include those discussed above in the nonfibrotic HP section, and the three-density sign (discussed below). The distribution in typical fibrotic HP may be random (both axial and craniocaudal), mid-lung predominant, or relatively spared at the lung bases (Figs. 17.10-17.13).

A "compatible with" fibrotic HP pattern is present when small airways disease and fibrosis are both present, but the distribution of fibrosis varies from the typical pattern. In this category, fibrosis may be in a UIP pattern with basal/peripheral reticulation, traction, and/or honeycombing or when the fibrosis is predominantly in the upper lobes (Fig. 17.14).

When fibrosis is present without findings of small airways disease, the CT is considered "indeterminate for" fibrotic HP pattern and is better characterized according to UIP/IPF guidelines discussed in Chapter 14 (Fig. 17.15).

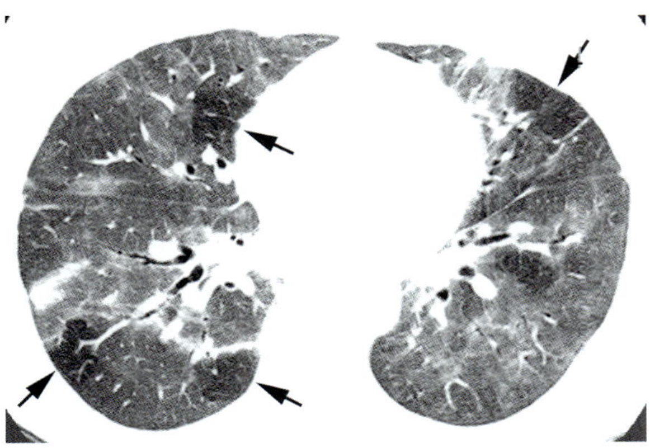

Figure 17.7. Nonfibrotic hypersensitivity pneumonitis with ground-glass opacity (GGO) and air trapping. HRCT shows patchy GGO and consolidation. Also, areas of lucency (*arrows*) containing small vessels represent mosaic perfusion.

The Three-Density Sign and Mosaic Attenuation

The "three-density sign" or "three-density pattern" is now the accepted term in place of the "headcheese sign," which was used in previous editions of this book and other radiology texts as many people are unfamiliar with the previous term. The three-density sign is defined as a combination of three different densities that are sharply demarcated on inspiratory imaging—normal appearing lung, GGO, and lobules of decreased attenuation/vascularity (Table 17.3). This sign indicates the presence of severe bronchiolar obstruction and has been shown to be a highly specific finding of fibrotic HP, especially when combined with expiratory air trapping (Figs. 17.11 and 17.13).

Mosaic attenuation, when applied to fibrotic HP, has been defined by subjective terms including "extensive" or "marked" that did not quantify the finding. For fibrotic HP, using a threshold of five or more lobules in three or more lobes bilaterally has a reasonably high specificity (Figs. 17.10, 17.12, and 17.14). It is important to note that up to half of patients with IPF may have some low attenuation lobules, and patients with other fibrotic lung diseases may have air trapping as an isolated finding.

Imaging findings in fibrotic HP are generally irreversible and may progress.

EOSINOPHILIC LUNG DISEASE

The term *eosinophilic lung disease* describes a group of entities characterized by an abundant accumulation of eosinophils in the pulmonary interstitium and airspaces. Peripheral blood eosinophilia is commonly present. Diagnostic criteria include (1) radiographic or CT findings of lung disease in association with peripheral eosinophilia, (2) biopsy-confirmed lung eosinophilia, and (3) increased eosinophils at BAL.

Eosinophilic lung disorders can be classified into those of unknown cause and those with a known cause (Table 17.4). Some overlap exists between these categories.

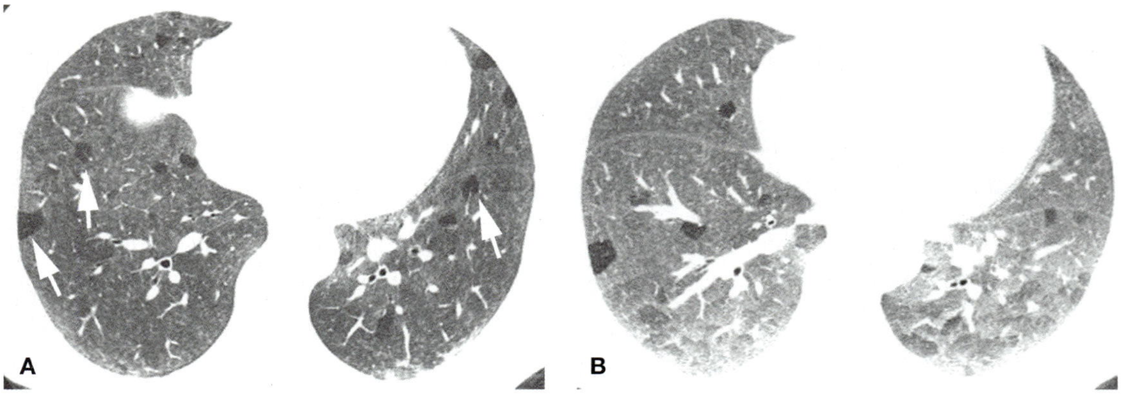

A B

Figure 17.8. Nonfibrotic hypersensitivity pneumonitis with air trapping. **A:** Inspiratory scan shows diffuse ground-glass opacity and centrilobular nodules, with numerous focal, lobular areas of lucency (*arrows*) due to mosaic perfusion. **B:** Expiratory scan at the same level shows air trapping in the lucent lung regions.

IDIOPATHIC EOSINOPHILIC LUNG DISEASE

Common idiopathic eosinophilic lung diseases include (1) simple pulmonary eosinophilia, (2) chronic eosinophilic pneumonia (CEP), (3) acute eosinophilic pneumonia (AEP), (4) idiopathic hypereosinophilic syndrome, and (5) eosinophilic granulomatosis with polyangiitis (EGPA) (formerly Churg-Strauss syndrome). These conditions reflect a spectrum, being associated with symptoms ranging from mild to severe and radiographic abnormalities ranging from focal to diffuse.

Other idiopathic diseases also may be associated with blood or tissue eosinophilia and may be considered in the differential diagnosis of eosinophilic lung disease; vasculitis is typically present. These diseases include granulomatosis with polyangiitis (GPA; see Chapter 19), polyarteritis, and collagen vascular diseases such as rheumatoid arthritis, scleroderma, CREST syndrome, polymyositis-dermatomyositis, and Sjögren syndrome (see Chapter 15). They are sometimes included in a category of eosinophilic lung disease with angiitis.

Simple Pulmonary Eosinophilia (Loeffler Syndrome)

Simple pulmonary eosinophilia, also known as Loeffler syndrome, is characterized by blood eosinophilia and radiographic findings of focal areas of consolidation, which are usually transient (Table 17.5). Although similar findings can be seen in association with a number of etiologic agents, particularly parasites and drugs, use of the term *simple pulmonary eosinophilia* should be limited to cases in which the cause is unknown. Approximately one-third of patients with this pattern have idiopathic disease. The disease may be self-limited, resolving within a month.

Patients typically have cough and mild shortness of breath; often, a history of asthma or atopic disease is present. Pathologically, eosinophils and histiocytes accumulate in the alveolar walls and alveoli.

The radiographic manifestations are characteristic and consist of patchy transient (fleeting) and migratory areas of consolidation that usually clear spontaneously within 1 month. These may be single or multiple and usually have

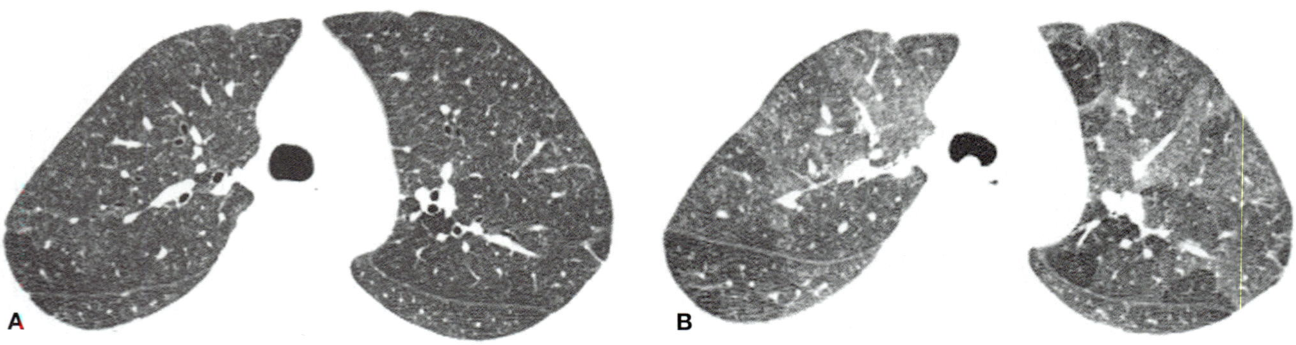

A B

Figure 17.9. Nonfibrotic hypersensitivity pneumonitis with air trapping and very subtle ground-glass opacity. **A:** Inspiratory scan shows a fine nodular appearance and subtle mosaic perfusion from ground-glass opacity. **B:** Expiratory scan shows patchy air trapping with geographic areas of lucency. Anterior bowing of the posterior tracheal membrane indicates a good expiration.

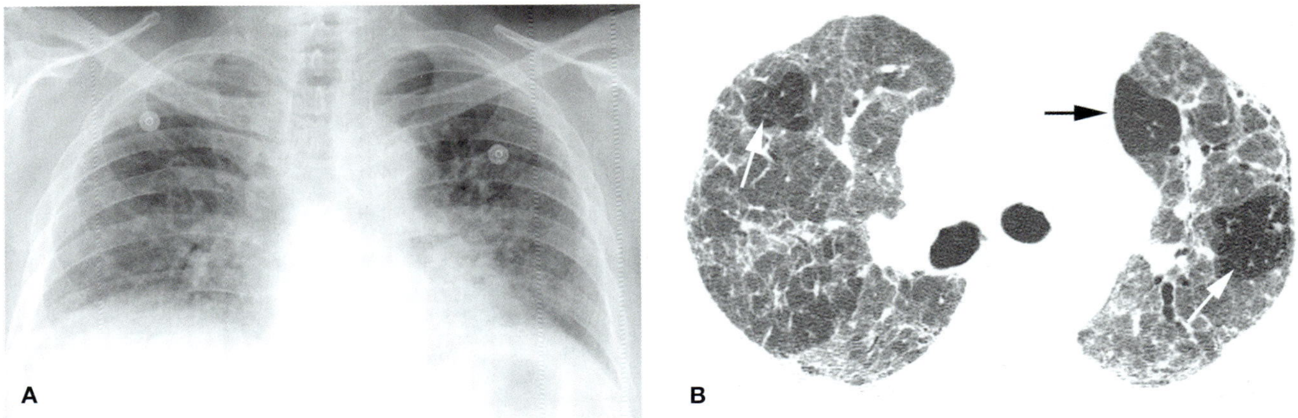

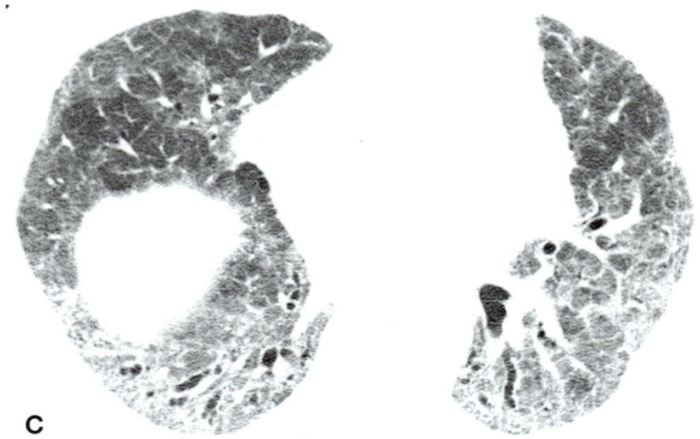

Figure 17.10. Fibrotic hypersensitivity pneumonitis (HP). **A:** Chest radiograph shows marked reduction in lung volume with poorly defined reticular opacities at the lung bases. **B:** HRCT through the upper lobes shows typical findings of fibrotic HP with diffuse fibrosis including irregular reticular opacities and traction bronchiectasis. Evidence of small airways disease is also present with ground-glass opacity and mosaic attenuation (arrows). **C:** HRCT at the lung bases shows similar findings. Traction bronchiectasis is visible in both lower lobes. This is a "typical fibrotic HP" appearance.

ill-defined margins. On radiographs and HRCT, the areas of consolidation often have a predominantly peripheral distribution. On HRCT, areas of GGO, focal areas of consolidation, or large nodules may be seen.

Chronic Eosinophilic Pneumonia

CEP is an idiopathic condition characterized by extensive infiltration of the alveoli and interstitium by a mixed inflammatory infiltrate consisting primarily of eosinophils and lymphocytes (Table 17.6); histologic findings may resemble organizing pneumonia (OP). CEP is usually associated with increased eosinophils in the peripheral blood. Clinically, patients present with fever, cough, weight loss, malaise, and shortness of breath. Symptoms may be insidious, being present for months before diagnosis, but in some patients are severe. Life-threatening respiratory compromise may occur, but this is unusual.

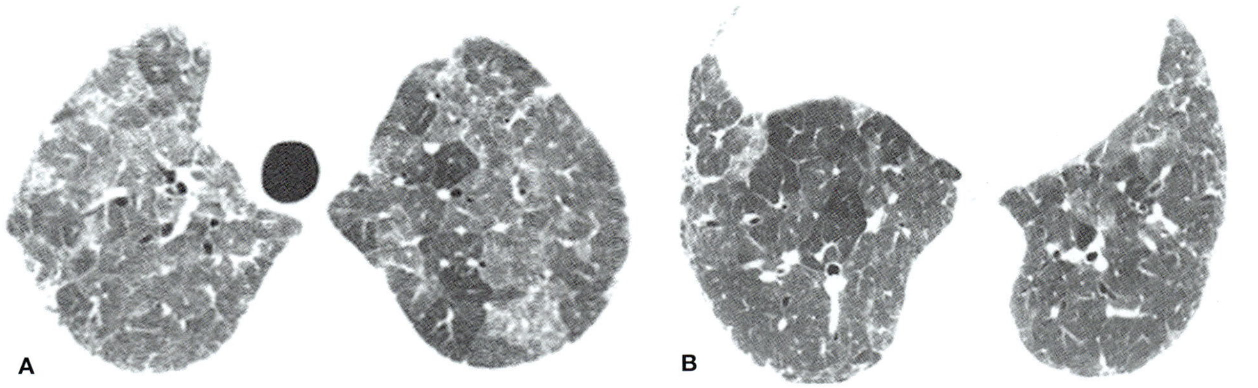

Figure 17.11. Fibrotic hypersensitivity pneumonitis (HP) with three-density sign. **A:** Inspiratory HRCT through the upper lobes shows sharply demarcated lobules ground-glass opacity, normal lung, and slightly lucent lung as well as irregular reticular opacities indicating early fibrosis. **B:** At the lung bases, irregular reticular opacities indicative of fibrosis and the three-density sign predominate. This is a "typical fibrotic HP" appearance.

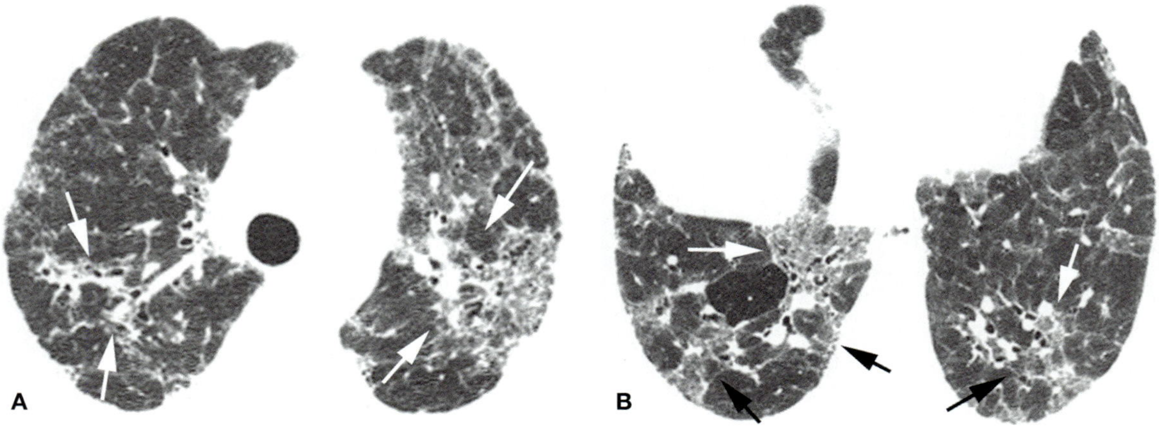

Figure 17.12. Fibrotic hypersensitivity pneumonitis (HP). **A:** HRCT through the upper lobes shows patchy irregular reticular opacities. Traction bronchiectasis is visible bilaterally, with a patchy and parahilar predominance (*arrows*). **B:** At the lung bases, areas of fibrosis (*arrows*) are patchy and lack the subpleural predominance of idiopathic pulmonary fibrosis. Lobular lucencies are also visible in all lobes indicative of mosaic attenuation. This is a "typical fibrotic HP" appearance.

Radiographically, CEP is characterized by the presence of homogeneous peripheral air-space consolidation, "the photographic negative of pulmonary edema" (Figs. 17.16 and 17.17; see also Fig. 1.12A in Chapter 1). Consolidation may be patchy. This pattern can remain unchanged for weeks or months unless steroid therapy is given; CEP responds promptly to the administration of steroids. An upper lobe predominance is common (see Fig. 17.17).

Table 17.2 Fibrotic Hypersensitivity Pneumonitis (HP)

Typical Fibrotic HP Fibrosis and Small Airways Disease Fibrosis—random; mid-lung predominant; or craniocaudal with some basal sparing Small Airways Disease—centrilobular nodules and/or GGO; or mosaic attenuation, three-density pattern, and/or air trapping
Compatible With Nonfibrotic HP Variant Fibrosis AND Small Airways Disease Fibrosis—UIP pattern; extensive GGO with subtle fibrosis; peribronchovascular or upper lung Small Airways Disease—same as typical
Indeterminate for Fibrotic HP Fibrosis without additional findings of small airways disease Fibrosis—UIP; Probable UIP; Indeterminate for UIP; Fibrotic NSIP; OP

GGO, ground-glass opacity; NSIP, nonspecific interstitial pneumonia; OP, organizing pneumonia; UIP, usual interstitial pneumonia.

The combination of blood eosinophilia, peripheral consolidation visible on radiographs, and rapid response to steroid therapy is often sufficiently characteristic to obviate the need for lung biopsy. However, this classic radiologic picture is seen in only about 50% of cases. The diagnosis may be difficult in patients with minimal blood eosinophilia or those in whom the peripheral distribution of infiltrates is not apparent.

On CT, CEP is characterized by (1) consolidation, often peripheral and patchy in distribution (90%; Figs. 17.16, 17.18, and 17.19); (2) patchy or peripheral GGO (80%), sometimes associated with "crazy paving"; (3) linear or bandlike opacities (Fig. 17.20), usually seen during resolution (5%); (4) the "reversed halo" or "atoll sign" (Fig. 17.16); and (5) an upper lobe predominance of abnormalities.

An appearance identical to that of CEP can be seen in patients with simple pulmonary eosinophilia or Loeffler syndrome, but CEP has a more protracted course, and areas of consolidation remain unchanged over weeks or months.

The presence of peripheral air-space consolidation should be considered suggestive of CEP in the appropriate clinical setting (ie, in patients with eosinophilia). However, an identical appearance of peripheral air-space consolidation can be seen in OP, although OP often involves the lower lung zones to a greater degree. CEP and OP are similar in presentation, symptoms, course, treatment, and response. Generally, if one diagnosis is considered, the other should be in the differential diagnosis.

Acute Eosinophilic Pneumonia

AEP is an acute febrile illness associated with rapidly increasing shortness of breath and hypoxemic respiratory failure

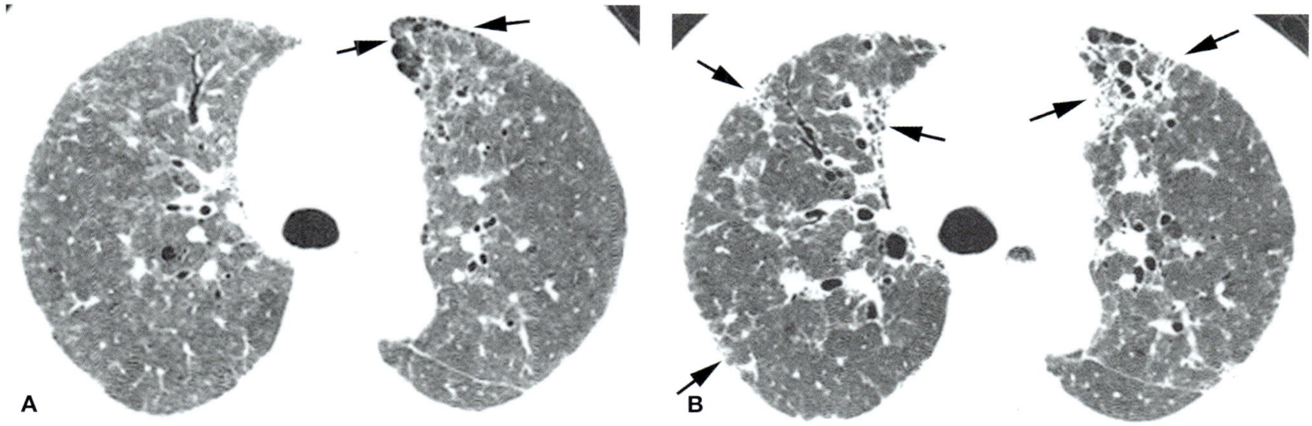

Figure 17.13. Progression of fibrotic hypersensitivity pneumonitis in a bird fancier. **A:** HRCT shows diffuse ground-glass opacity, ill-defined ground-glass opacity nodules, and lobular mosaic attenuation. Mild fibrosis is present in the left upper lobe (*arrows*). **B:** HRCT 15 months later shows progression of fibrosis with reticulation and traction bronchiectasis (*arrows*). Ground-glass opacity has diminished.

(Table 17.7). The diagnosis is based on clinical findings of acute respiratory failure and the presence of markedly elevated numbers of eosinophils in BAL fluid. Blood eosinophilia is usually absent. Histology shows diffuse alveolar damage with alveolar and interstitial eosinophilia. Response to steroids is prompt, and the prognosis is good, with no residual disability.

The etiology of AEP remains unknown, but several studies have proposed a close relationship between cigarette smoking and AEP. Nearly all patients are smokers, either new smokers or former smokers who resumed smoking after a year or two, or are smokers who increased the number of cigarettes smoked, all within a month of onset.

The radiographic manifestations are similar to those of pulmonary edema. The earliest radiographic manifestation is reticular opacities, frequently with Kerley B lines. This progresses over a few hours or days to bilateral interstitial opacities and air-space consolidation involving mainly the lower lung zones. Small bilateral pleural effusions are present in most patients.

The HRCT findings of acute eosinophilic pneumonia include bilateral areas of GGO, smooth interlobular septal thickening, small pleural effusions, and occasionally areas of consolidation (Fig. 17.21). The combination of GGO and septal thickening may result in the appearance of "crazy paving."

Idiopathic Hypereosinophilic Syndrome

Hypereosinophilic syndrome is characterized by blood eosinophilia persisting for at least 6 months, associated with multiorgan tissue infiltration by mature eosinophils (Table 17.8). An underlying cause may or may not be evident. The main causes of morbidity and mortality are cardiac and central nervous system involvement. Pulmonary and

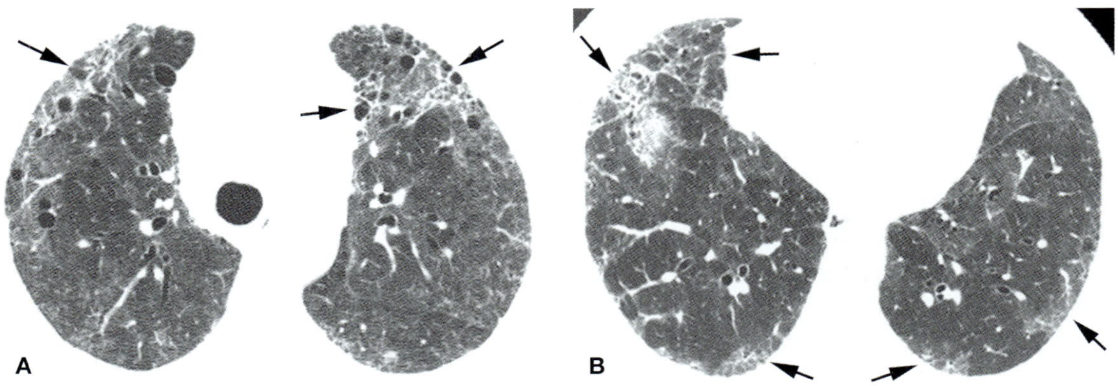

Figure 17.14. Fibrotic hypersensitivity pneumonitis (HP). **A:** HRCT through the upper lobes shows irregular reticular opacities, traction bronchiectasis, and honeycombing (*arrows*) predominantly anteriorly. **B:** At the lung bases, patchy areas of fibrosis (*arrows*) are visible. Superimposed ground-glass opacities are also visible in the upper lobes. This imaging is considered "compatible with fibrotic HP."

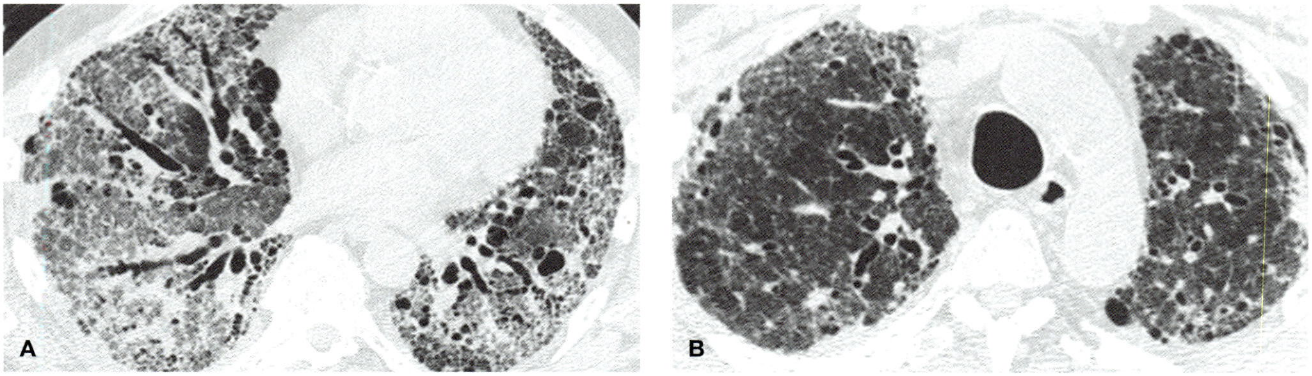

Figure 17.15. End-stage fibrotic hypersensitivity pneumonitis (HP) with honeycombing. **A:** HRCT at the lung bases shows extensive lung fibrosis with mild subpleural honeycombing, traction bronchiectasis, and irregular reticulation. **B:** Similar findings are noted in the upper lobes. While based on imaging alone, this would be indeterminate for fibrotic HP; because of the absence of small airways disease, final diagnosis was made based on exposure history and surgical lung biopsy.

pleural abnormalities are present in approximately 40% of cases, often related to heart failure and pulmonary edema. Pulmonary symptoms include cough, wheezing, and shortness of breath.

The radiographic manifestations are nonspecific and consist of transient hazy GGO or areas of consolidation. Cardiac involvement eventually leads to cardiomegaly, pulmonary edema, and pleural effusion. The prognosis is poor.

The predominant HRCT findings reflect pulmonary edema and pleural effusion. Bilateral pulmonary nodules, 1 cm or less in diameter, mainly involving the peripheral lung regions, are likely related to eosinophilic infiltration and perhaps necrosis. Nodules may show the halo sign.

EGPA (Churg-Strauss Syndrome)

EGPA (formerly known as Churg-Strauss syndrome or Churg-Strauss granulomatosis) is a multisystem disorder characterized by the presence of (1) necrotizing vasculitis, (2) extravascular granuloma formation, and (3) eosinophilic infiltration of various organs, particularly the lungs, skin, heart, nerves, gastrointestinal tract, and kidneys. Not all of these three findings need be present (Table 17.9).

Patients with this syndrome are usually middle aged (average onset 40-50 years) and often have a history of allergic diseases, including asthma, nasal polyps, or sinusitis. Criteria for diagnosis include (1) asthma, (2) blood eosinophilia greater than 10%, (3) neuropathy, (4) migratory or transient pulmonary opacities visible radiographically, (5) paranasal sinus abnormalities, and (6) extravascular eosinophilia on biopsy. The presence of four or more of these criteria is 85% sensitive and nearly 100% specific for EGPA. EGPA may be associated with antineutrophil cytoplasmic antibody (ANCA), usually p-ANCA (perinuclear pattern).

Table 17.3 Three-Density Sign

Formerly known as "headcheese sign"
Combination of three attenuations sharply demarcated on *inspiratory imaging*: 1. Normal Lung 2. GGO 3. Lucent Lung
Indicates parenchymal infiltration + obstruction
Highly specific for fibrotic HP (not shown to be specific for nonfibrotic HP)

GGO, ground-glass opacity; HP, hypersensitivity pneumonitis.

Table 17.4 Classification of Eosinophilic Lung Disease

Idiopathic eosinophilic lung disease Simple pulmonary eosinophilia Chronic eosinophilic pneumonia Acute eosinophilic pneumonia Idiopathic hypereosinophilic syndrome Eosinophilic granulomatosis with polyangiitis (Churg-Strauss syndrome)
Eosinophilic lung disease with angiitis Granulomatosis with polyangiitis Polyarteritis Collagen vascular diseases
Eosinophilic lung disease with a known cause Drugs Parasitic disease and tropical pulmonary eosinophilia Fungi Bronchocentric granulomatosis

Table 17.5 Simple Pulmonary Eosinophilia (Loeffler Syndrome)

Idiopathic
Blood eosinophilia
Mild dyspnea
History of asthma or atopy often present
Focal consolidation, usually transient or fleeting
May be self-limited

Cough and hemoptysis are common, but symptoms may reflect the involvement of various organs; these include skin rash, diarrhea, neuropathy, and congestive heart failure. Patients usually respond well to treatment with steroids, but without treatment, patients may die within months. With treatment, the 5-year survival rate is good, up to 80%. Associated renal failure is associated with a poor prognosis.

Churg-Strauss syndrome may evolve in three phases:

1. An *allergic phase* with rhinitis, sinusitis, and asthma as the primary features.
2. A *eosinophilic phase* associated with blood and tissue eosinophilia, usually involving the lung and gastrointestinal tract. Lung abnormalities usually resemble simple pulmonary eosinophilia or CEP.
3. A *systemic or small vessel vasculitis phase* in which other organs (heart, skin, musculoskeletal system, nervous system, and kidney) are also involved. This may occur years after the development of eosinophilia.

Table 17.6 Chronic Eosinophilic Pneumonia

Idiopathic
Blood eosinophilia
Fever, weight loss, dyspnea, often severe
Patchy peripheral consolidation, often persistent
Patchy ground-glass opacity
Mimics organizing pneumonia, but usually shows an upper lobe predominance
Rapid resolution with steroids

Radiographic abnormalities are common. Pulmonary opacities have been identified in 50% to 70% of patients in the eosinophilic or vasculitic phases of the disease, often consisting of transient multifocal areas of consolidation

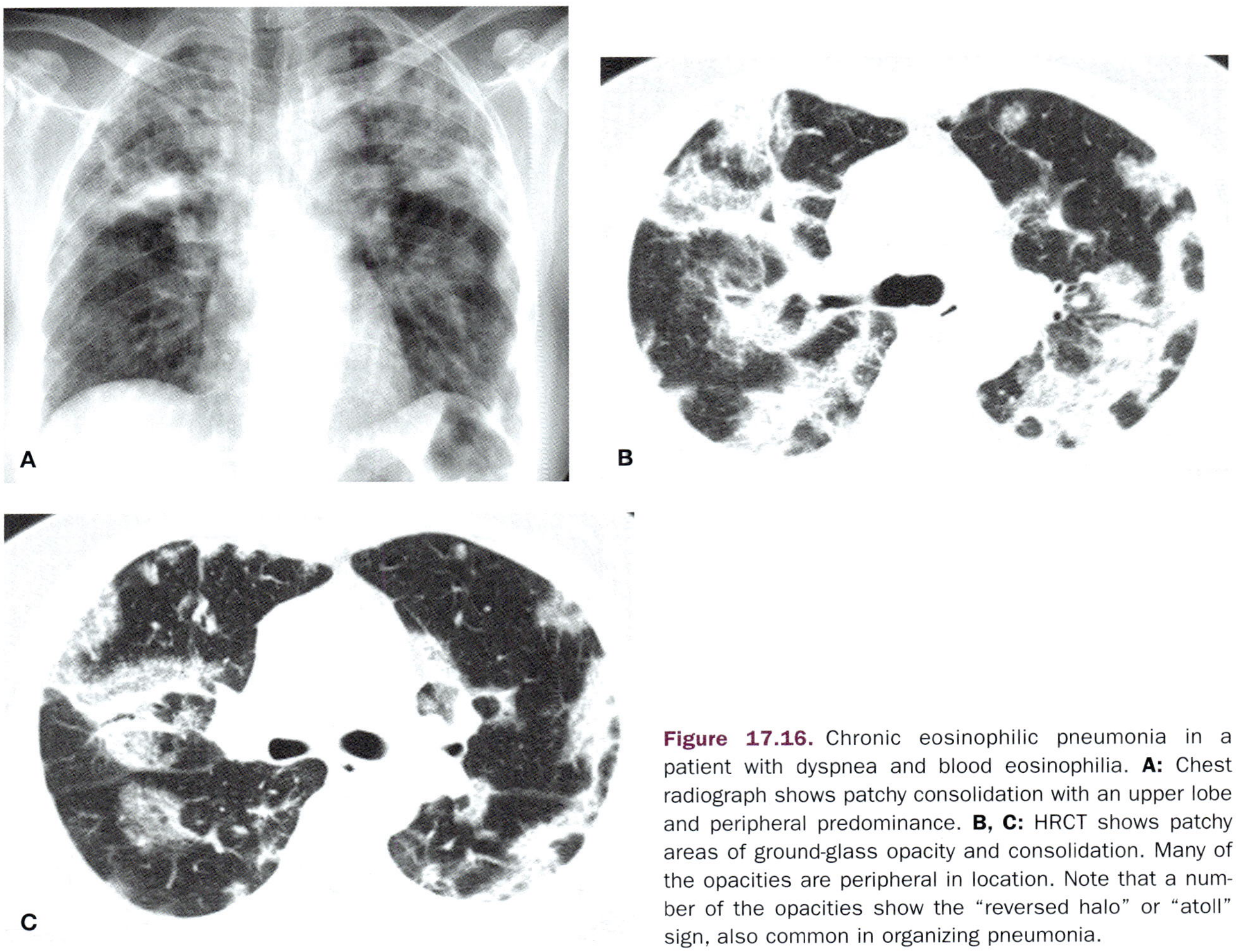

Figure 17.16. Chronic eosinophilic pneumonia in a patient with dyspnea and blood eosinophilia. **A:** Chest radiograph shows patchy consolidation with an upper lobe and peripheral predominance. **B, C:** HRCT shows patchy areas of ground-glass opacity and consolidation. Many of the opacities are peripheral in location. Note that a number of the opacities show the "reversed halo" or "atoll" sign, also common in organizing pneumonia.

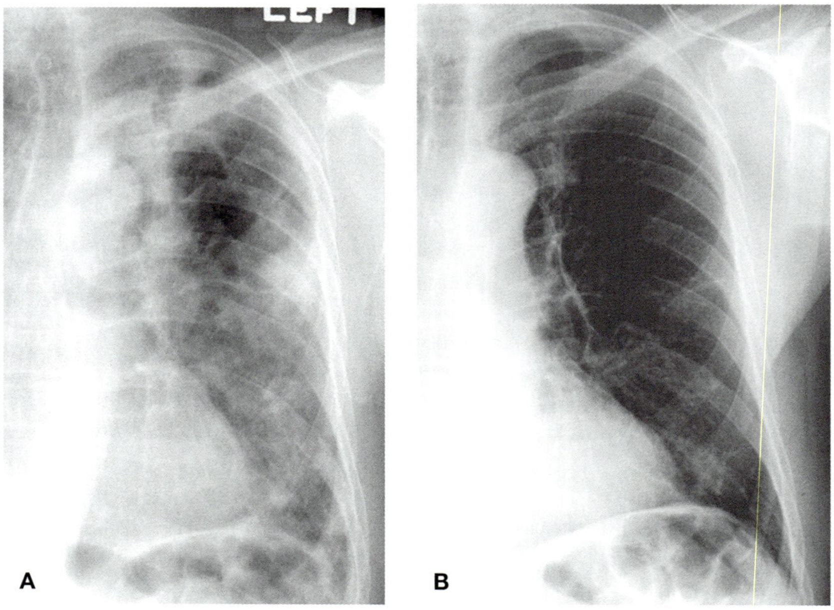

Figure 17.17. Chronic eosinophilic pneumonia. **A:** Chest radiograph shows patchy peripheral consolidation. **B:** Following steroid treatment, the abnormalities have resolved.

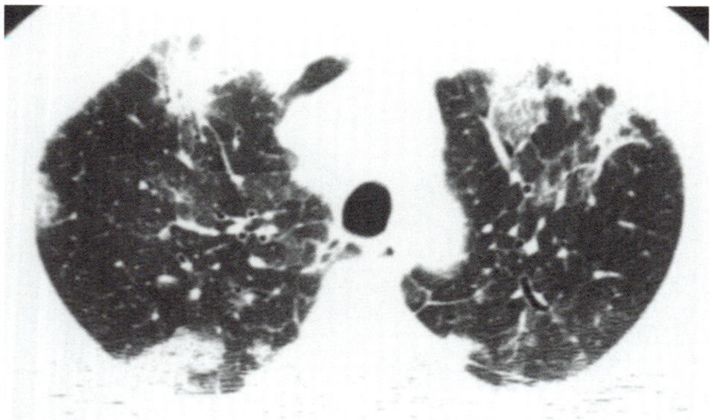

Figure 17.18. Chronic eosinophilic pneumonia. HRCT shows patchy areas of consolidation involving the peripheral lung.

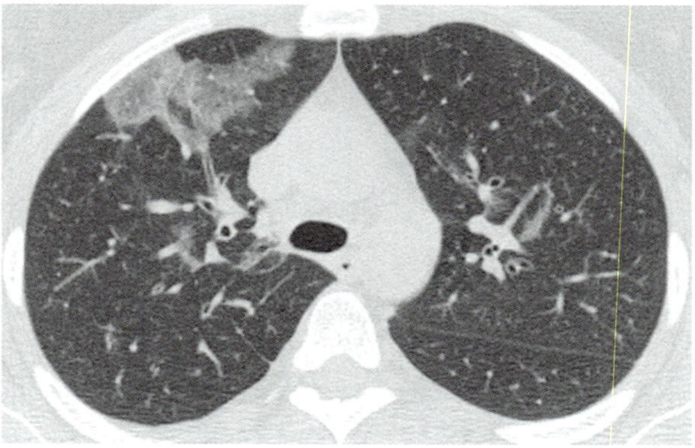

Figure 17.19. Chronic eosinophilic pneumonia. HRCT shows patchy ground-glass opacity in the peripheral right upper lobe. Similar abnormalities were visible at other levels.

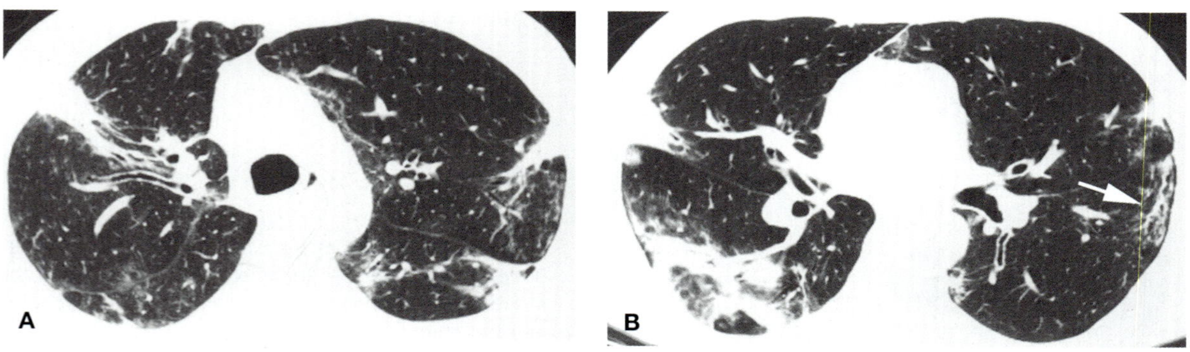

Figure 17.20. Chronic eosinophilic pneumonia. HRCTs at two levels (**A, B**) show patchy consolidation in the peripheral lung. A bandlike opacity is visible (*arrow* in **B**), paralleling the pleural surface. This appearance mimics that of organizing pneumonia/bronchiolitis obliterans organizing pneumonia.

Table 17.7 Acute Eosinophilic Pneumonia

Close association with onset or increase in smoking
Eosinophilia on bronchoalveolar lavage
Rapidly progressing respiratory failure
Radiographic and CT findings resemble pulmonary edema

indistinguishable from simple pulmonary eosinophilia or CEP. Pulmonary nodules or masses, hemorrhage, pulmonary edema, and pleural effusions may be present. In 40% of cases, pulmonary radiographic abnormalities precede the development of systemic vasculitis. Involvement of the heart may result in cardiomegaly with findings of congestive heart failure; otherwise, pleural effusion is uncommon.

HRCT findings are variable and nonspecific, reflecting the different pulmonary manifestations of this disease. Findings include (1) consolidation or GGO (60%), which may have a peripheral distribution or be patchy and geographic; (2) pulmonary nodules or masses (20%) ranging from 0.5 to 3.5 cm in diameter, which may appear centrilobular or may contain air bronchograms (Fig. 17.22); (3) bronchial wall thickening or bronchiectasis (35%); and (4) interlobular septal thickening due to pulmonary edema (5%). Although cavitation of nodules or masses may occur, it is much less common than with GPA, which it may resemble clinically and radiographically. The absence of cavitation is helpful in distinguishing Churg-Strauss syndrome from GPA.

EOSINOPHILIC LUNG DISEASE HAVING A SPECIFIC ETIOLOGY

Known causes of eosinophilic lung disease include drugs, parasites, and fungi.

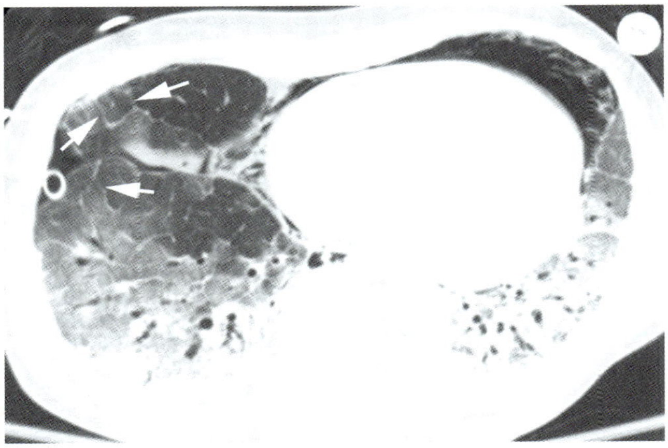

Figure 17.21. Acute eosinophilic pneumonia. HRCT shows extensive ground-glass opacity and consolidation with a lower lobe predominance. Interlobular septal thickening is also seen (*arrows*). Pneumomediastinum and right pneumothorax are present and a right chest tube is in place. The patient had rapidly progressive respiratory failure and was intubated. Bronchoalveolar lavage revealed numerous eosinophils.

Table 17.8 Idiopathic Hypereosinophilic Syndrome

Idiopathic
Blood eosinophilia
Multiorgan infiltration by eosinophils
Pulmonary and pleural involvement in 40%
Ground-glass opacity or areas of consolidation
Small nodules in some
Cardiac involvement: cardiomegaly, pulmonary edema, pleural effusion
Poor prognosis

Drug-Related Disease

Drugs are an important cause of eosinophilic lung disease. Many drugs have been reported to be associated with eosinophilic lung disease; implicated drugs include antibiotics, nonsteroidal anti-inflammatory agents, and cytotoxic drugs. Reactions range from those similar to simple pulmonary eosinophilia to those imitating acute eosinophilic pneumonia (see Table 17.7).

Parasitic Infestations

Parasites most commonly result in findings similar to simple pulmonary eosinophilia. Most cases are due to roundworms such as *Ascaris lumbricoides*, *Toxocara*, *Ancylostoma*, and *Strongyloides stercoralis*.

Tropical pulmonary eosinophilia is caused by the worms *Wuchereria bancrofti* and *Brugia malayi*, with most cases being reported in India, Africa, South America, and Southeast Asia. In the Far East, the lung fluke *Paragonimus*

Table 17.9 Eosinophilic Granulomatosis With Polyangiitis (Churg-Strauss Syndrome)

Idiopathic
Multisystem disorder
- Necrotizing vasculitis
- Extravascular granulomas
- Eosinophilic infiltration

History of atopy
Neuropathy
Sinus disorders
Renal involvement
Perinuclear antineutrophil cytoplasmic antibodies
Three phases
- *Allergic phase with rhinitis, sinusitis, and asthma*
- *Eosinophilic phase*
  - Blood and tissue eosinophilia
  - Findings of simple pulmonary eosinophilia or chronic eosinophilic pneumonia
- *Systemic or small vessel vasculitis phase*

Heart, kidney, musculoskeletal, and nervous systems involved
- Nodules or masses; may cavitate

Responds well to steroids

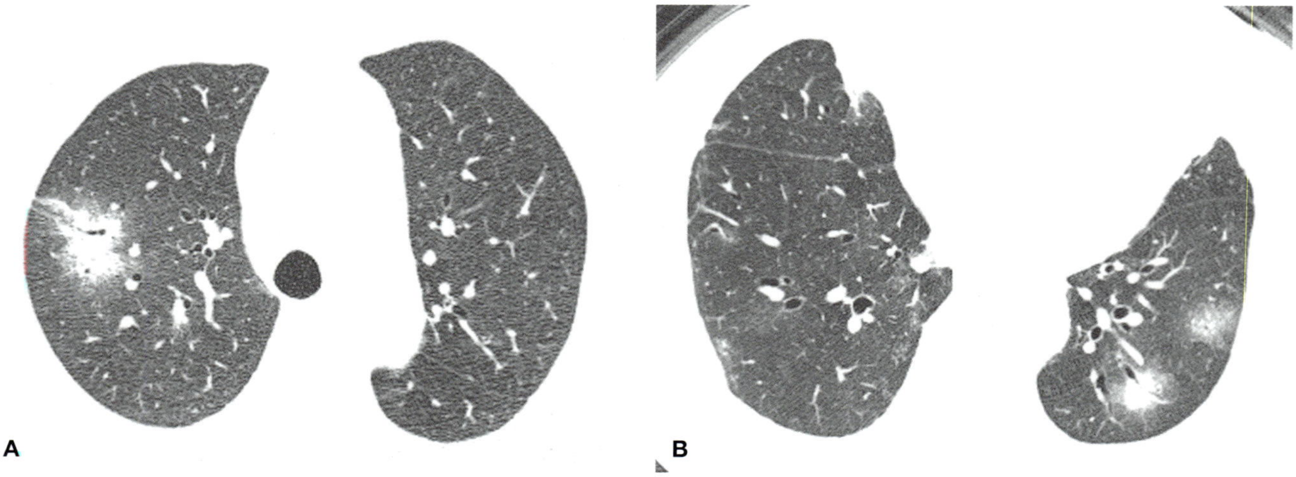

Figure 17.22. Eosinophilic granulomatosis with polyangiitis (Churg-Strauss syndrome). **A, B:** HRCT shows ill-defined focal regions of consolidation and ground-glass opacity. The nodular opacities contain air bronchograms.

westermani is typically responsible. Symptoms are nonspecific but include fever, weight loss, dyspnea, cough, and hemoptysis. CT findings reported in paragonimiasis include patchy lung consolidation, cystic lesions filled with air or fluid, pneumothorax, and pleural effusion (see Chapter 13).

Fungal Disease

The primary fungal disease associated with pulmonary eosinophilia is allergic bronchopulmonary aspergillosis (ABPA), characterized by asthma, peripheral eosinophilia, central bronchiectasis, mucus plugging, and an allergic reaction to *Aspergillus fumigatus*. It is described in detail in Chapter 23. However, other patterns of disease may result from exposure to fungus, including HP, eosinophilic pneumonia, and bronchocentric granulomatosis.

Bronchocentric Granulomatosis

The characteristic histologic abnormality seen in patients with bronchocentric granulomatosis is necrotizing granulomatous inflammation centered around bronchioles and small bronchi (Table 17.10). It may be associated with complete destruction of the airway mucosa and filling of the airway lumen with necrotic material. In asthmatic subjects, bronchocentric granulomatosis is most commonly associated with *Aspergillus*, and fungal hyphae are often present within these lesions. Bronchocentric granulomatosis may also be seen in patients with mycobacterial infection or noninfectious inflammatory diseases such as rheumatoid arthritis and in immunosuppressed patients.

Table 17.10 Bronchocentric Granulomatosis

Necrotizing granulomas centered on bronchioles and bronchi
Hypersensitivity reaction
Peripheral eosinophilia
History of asthma in one-third
Associated with *Aspergillus*, mycobacteria, inflammatory diseases
Nodules, masses, focal consolidation, mucoid impaction
Upper lobe predominance

Bronchocentric granulomatosis is generally considered a hypersensitivity reaction. Patients are usually young; one-third have a history of asthma; and peripheral eosinophilia is seen in half of cases. This process may be associated with ABPA in asthmatic patients, but abnormalities in bronchocentric granulomatosis tend to be more focal than those seen with ABPA. Symptoms are often mild, with fever, cough, chest pain, and hemoptysis.

Chest radiographs may show a nodule or focal area of consolidation. CT findings include mass lesions or lobar consolidation with associated mild volume loss. Mucoid impaction may be present. The abnormalities predominantly involve the upper lobes. Masses and consolidation represent necrotic tissue associated with consolidation or eosinophilic pneumonia.

SUGGESTED READINGS

Adler BD, Padley SP, Müller NL, Remy-Jardin M, Remy J. Chronic hypersensitivity pneumonitis: high-resolution CT and radiographic features in 16 patients. *Radiology*. 1992;185(1):91-95.

Allen JN, Davis WB. Eosinophilic lung diseases. *Am J Respir Crit Care Med*. 1994;150(5 pt 1):1423-1438.

Arakawa H, Webb WR. Air trapping on expiratory high-resolution CT scans in the absence of inspiratory scan abnormalities: correlation with pulmonary function tests and differential diagnosis. *AJR Am J Roentgenol*. 1998;170(5):1349-1353.

Bain GA, Flower CD. Pulmonary eosinophilia. *Eur J Radiol*. 1996;23(1):3-8.

Barnett J, Molyneaux PL, Rawal B, et al. Variable utility of mosaic attenuation to distinguish fibrotic hypersensitivity pneumonitis from idiopathic pulmonary fibrosis. *Eur Respir J*. 2019;54(1):1900531. doi:10.1183/13993003.00531-2019

Buschman DL, Waldron JA Jr, King TE Jr. Churg-Strauss pulmonary vasculitis: high-resolution computed tomography scanning and pathologic findings. *Am Rev Respir Dis*. 1990;142(2):458-461.

Cheon JE, Lee KS, Jung GS, Chung MH, Cho YD. Acute eosinophilic pneumonia: radiographic and CT findings in six patients. *AJR Am J Roentgenol.* 1996;167(5):1195-1199.

Dabiri M, Jehangir M, Khoshpouri P, Chalian H. Hypersensitivity pneumonitis: a pictorial review based on the new ATS/JRS/ALAT clinical practice guideline for radiologists and pulmonologists. *Diagnostics.* 2022;12(11):2874. doi:10.3390/diagnostics12112874

Ebara H, Ikezoe J, Johkoh T, et al. Chronic eosinophilic pneumonia: evolution of chest radiograms and CT features. *J Comput Assist Tomogr.* 1994;18(5):737-744.

Fernández Pérez ER, Travis WD, Lynch DA, et al. Diagnosis and evaluation of hypersensitivity pneumonitis: CHEST guideline and expert panel report. *Chest.* 2021;160(2):e97-e156. doi:10.1016/j.chest.2021.03.066

Gaensler EA, Carrington CB. Peripheral opacities in chronic eosinophilic pneumonia: the photographic negative of pulmonary edema. *AJR Am J Roentgenol.* 1977;128:1-13.

Hansell DM, Moskovic E. High-resolution computed tomography in extrinsic allergic alveolitis. *Clin Radiol.* 1991;43(1):8-12.

Hansell DM, Wells AU, Padley SP, Müller NL. Hypersensitivity pneumonitis: correlation of individual CT patterns with functional abnormalities. *Radiology.* 1996;199(1):123-128.

Hirschmann JV, Pipavath SNJ, Godwin JD. Hypersensitivity pneumonitis: a historical, clinical, and radiologic review. *Radiographics.* 2009;29(7):1921-1938.

Jeong YJ, Kim KI, Seo IJ, et al. Eosinophilic lung diseases: a clinical, radiologic, and pathologic overview. *Radiographics.* 2007;27(3):617-639.

Kang EY, Shim JJ, Kim JS, Kim KI. Pulmonary involvement of idiopathic hypereosinophilic syndrome: CT findings in five patients. *J Comput Assist Tomogr.* 1997;21(4):612-615.

Kim Y, Lee KS, Choi DC, Primack SL, Im JG. The spectrum of eosinophilic lung disease: radiologic findings. *J Comput Assist Tomogr.* 1997;21(6):920-930.

King MA, Pope-Harman AL, Allen JN, Christoforidis GA, Christoforidis AJ. Acute eosinophilic pneumonia: radiologic and clinical features. *Radiology.* 1997;203(3):715-719.

Lynch DA, Newell JD, Logan PM, King TE Jr, Müller NL. Can CT distinguish hypersensitivity pneumonitis from idiopathic pulmonary fibrosis? *AJR Am J Roentgenol.* 1995;165(4):807-811.

Mindell HJ. Roentgen findings in farmer's lung. *Radiology.* 1970;97(2):341-346.

Primack SL, Müller NL. Radiologic manifestations of the systemic autoimmune diseases. *Clin Chest Med.* 1998;19(4):573-586.

Raghu G, Remy-Jardin M, Ryerson CJ, et al. Diagnosis of hypersensitivity pneumonitis in adults: an official ATS/JRS/ALAT clinical practice guideline. *Am J Respir Crit Care Med.* 2020;202(3):e36-e69. doi:10.1164/rccm.202005-2032ST

Remy-Jardin M, Remy J, Wallaert B, Müller NL. Subacute and chronic bird breeder hypersensitivity pneumonitis: sequential evaluation with CT and correlation with lung function tests and bronchoalveolar lavage. *Radiology.* 1993;189(1):111-118.

Silva CI, Müller NL, Lynch DA, et al. Chronic hypersensitivity pneumonitis: differentiation from idiopathic pulmonary fibrosis and nonspecific interstitial pneumonia by using thin-section CT. *Radiology.* 2008;246(1):288-297.

Silver SF, Müller NL, Miller RR, Lefcoe MS. Hypersensitivity pneumonitis: evaluation with CT. *Radiology.* 1989;173(2):441-445.

Uchiyama H, Suda T, Nakamura Y, et al. Alterations in smoking habits are associated with acute eosinophilic pneumonia. *Chest.* 2008;133(5):1174-1180.

Vaglio A, Buzio C, Zwerina J. Eosinophilic granulomatosis with polyangiitis (Churg-Strauss): state of the art. *Allergy.* 2013;68(3):261-273.

Ward S, Heyneman LE, Flint JD, Leung AN, Kazerooni EA, Müller NL. Bronchocentric granulomatosis: computed tomographic findings in five patients. *Clin Radiol.* 2000;55(4):296-300.

Webb WR. Thin-section CT of the secondary pulmonary lobule: anatomy and the image—the 2004 Fleischner lecture. *Radiology.* 2006;239(2):322-338.

Winn RE, Kollef MH, Meyer JI. Pulmonary involvement in the hypereosinophilic syndrome. *Chest.* 1994;105(3):656-660.

Worthy SA, Müller NL, Hansell DM, Flower CD. Churg-Strauss syndrome: the spectrum of pulmonary CT findings in 17 patients. *AJR Am J Roentgenol.* 1998;170(2):297-300.

Chapter 18

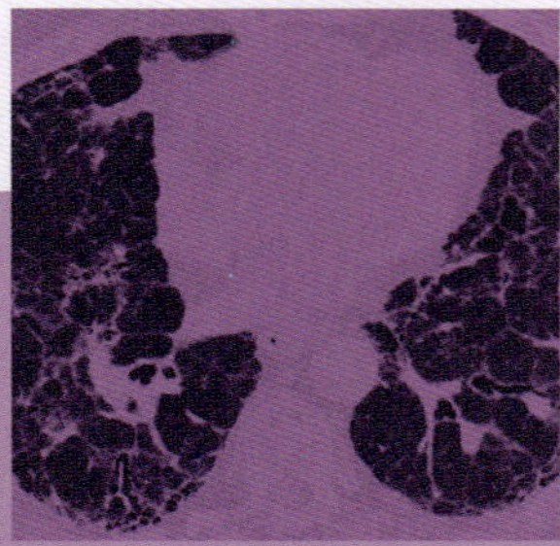

Travis S. Henry

Iatrogenic Lung Diseases: Drug-Induced Lung Disease and Radiation Pneumonitis

DRUG-INDUCED LUNG DISEASE

Many drugs, both therapeutic and illicit, can be associated with lung disease. However, drug-induced lung disease is manifested in a limited number of ways. Specific pathologic reactions occurring with pulmonary drug toxicity include the following:

1. Hydrostatic and increased permeability pulmonary edema
2. Diffuse alveolar damage (DAD) and the acute respiratory distress syndrome (ARDS)
3. Pulmonary hemorrhage
4. Organizing pneumonia (OP)
5. Eosinophilic pneumonia and hypersensitivity reactions
6. Chronic interstitial pneumonitis with fibrosis
7. Systemic lupus erythematosus (SLE)
8. Pulmonary vasculitis and pulmonary hypertension
9. Sarcoid-like reaction
10. Bronchiolitis obliterans

Each of these patterns is characteristically associated with a different group of drugs, although many drugs can result in a number of possible lung reactions, and some overlap between these patterns is common. In most cases, the radiographic appearances of a drug-related lung disease are nonspecific, and the diagnosis must be based on observing a temporal relationship between the administration of a drug and the development of pulmonary abnormalities, and exclusion of other causes for the abnormalities.

Radiographic abnormalities associated with drug-related lung injury vary with the histologic pattern present, and with a few exceptions, the appearance of each pattern appears the same regardless of the drug involved. High-resolution CT (HRCT) is more sensitive than chest radiography in defining the radiographic abnormalities.

Because of the large number of drugs associated with drug reactions, the number of new drugs being introduced in recent years, and the variety of patterns possible, a high degree of suspicion must be maintained when evaluating patients with unexplained lung disease, regardless of what it looks like or what drug treatment is being employed. A recent example underscoring these complexities would be the introduction of targeted molecular therapy and immune checkpoint inhibitors (ICIs). These drugs may cause acute (eg, DAD), subacute (eg, OP, hypersensitivity pneumonitis [HP]), or chronic (eg, nonspecific interstitial pneumonia [NSIP]) type reactions. Prompt recognition of drug-induced lung disease is important because early abnormalities may resolve completely if the drug is discontinued or appropriate therapy is instituted.

The website http://www.pneumotox.com is an excellent source for determining the types of drug reactions associated with a specific drug or the drugs capable of producing a specific toxic reaction. It is highly recommended as a comprehensive database.

Pulmonary Edema

Hydrostatic pulmonary edema may result from drugs affecting the heart or systemic vasculature (Table 18.1). An

Table 18.1 Drugs Associated With Pulmonary Edema

Drugs
Aspirin and salicylates
BCNU
Cocaine
Chlordiazepoxide
Codeine
Cyclophosphamide
Cytosine arabinoside
Heroin
Hydrochlorothiazide
Interleukin-2
Lidocaine
Methadone
Methotrexate
Nitrofurantoin
Nonsteroidal anti-inflammatory drugs
OKT3
Propoxyphene
Tocolytics (ritodrine and terbutaline)
Trimethoprim-sulfamethoxazole
Tricyclic antidepressants

example would be cocaine. Radiographic and HRCT findings are typical of any cause of hydrostatic edema. Pleural effusion may be present.

Increased permeability pulmonary edema also may occur. Onset is usually sudden. Increased permeability pulmonary edema occurring without DAD results in typical findings of pulmonary edema, including interlobular septal thickening (Kerley lines; see Fig. 12.11 in Chapter 12), ground-glass opacity (see Fig. 12.13 in Chapter 12), and to a lesser extent, consolidation. This occurrence is typical of interleukin-2, but many other drugs are capable of causing increased permeability pulmonary edema. These include aspirin, nitrofurantoin, heroin, and cytotoxic agents such as methotrexate, cyclophosphamide, and bis-chloroethylnitrosourea, or carmustine (BCNU). Unlike with hydrostatic edema, pleural effusion is typically absent. Prompt resolution may occur with appropriate treatment.

Diffuse Alveolar Damage

DAD with ARDS can be caused by a variety of drugs, most typically cytotoxic agents (eg, bleomycin, busulfan, and cyclophosphamide), ICIs, nitrofurantoin, and amiodarone (Table 18.2). As with pulmonary edema, onset is usually sudden and occurs within a few days of the onset of chemotherapy.

DAD reflects a more serious lung and capillary endothelial injury than occurs with increased permeability pulmonary edema. The acute or exudative stage of DAD occurs in the first week after injury and is characterized by necrosis of alveolar pneumocytes, edema, hemorrhage, and hyaline membrane formation. Radiographs and CT typically show

Table 18.2 Drugs Associated With Diffuse Alveolar Damage

Drugs
Amiodarone
BCNU
Bleomycin
Busulfan
Chlorambucil
Cyclophosphamide
Cytosine arabinoside
Gold
Immune checkpoint inhibitors
Methotrexate
Mitomycin
Melphalan
Nitrofurantoin
Oxygen
Penicillamine
Tricyclic antidepressants
Vinblastine and vinca alkaloids

extensive bilateral parenchymal consolidation, usually most marked in the dependent lung regions; interlobular septal thickening and Kerley lines are typically absent (Fig. 18.1). Other than a temporal relationship to chemotherapy, there are no clinical or CT findings that allow this appearance to be distinguished from other causes of ARDS. The reparative stage of DAD, characterized by cellular hyperplasia and fibrosis, occurs after 1 to 2 weeks. Depending on the severity of the lung injury, abnormalities may regress, stabilize, or progress to fibrosis and honeycombing.

Pulmonary Hemorrhage

Drug-related diffuse pulmonary hemorrhage is uncommon. Typical causes include anticoagulants, cyclophosphamide, and penicillamine. Hemoptysis may or may not be present (Table 18.3). Radiographic and HRCT findings are typical of pulmonary hemorrhage, with bilateral patchy ground-glass opacity or consolidation (see Chapter 19). Pleural effusion is typically absent.

Organizing Pneumonia

OP has been described with numerous medications, including ICIs, methotrexate, gold, penicillamine, nitrofurantoin, amiodarone, bleomycin, and busulfan (Table 18.4). Symptoms include progressive cough, dyspnea, and fever. Like other causes of OP (see Chapter 14), this pattern is characterized by consolidation or ground-glass opacity that may have a patchy or nodular distribution and may predominate in a peribronchial or subpleural location (Figs. 18.2 and 18.3). Lung nodules with or without the "atoll sign" or "reversed halo sign" may be present (Figs. 18.2A and 18.3). OP tends to predominate in the lower lobes (see Fig. 18.3).

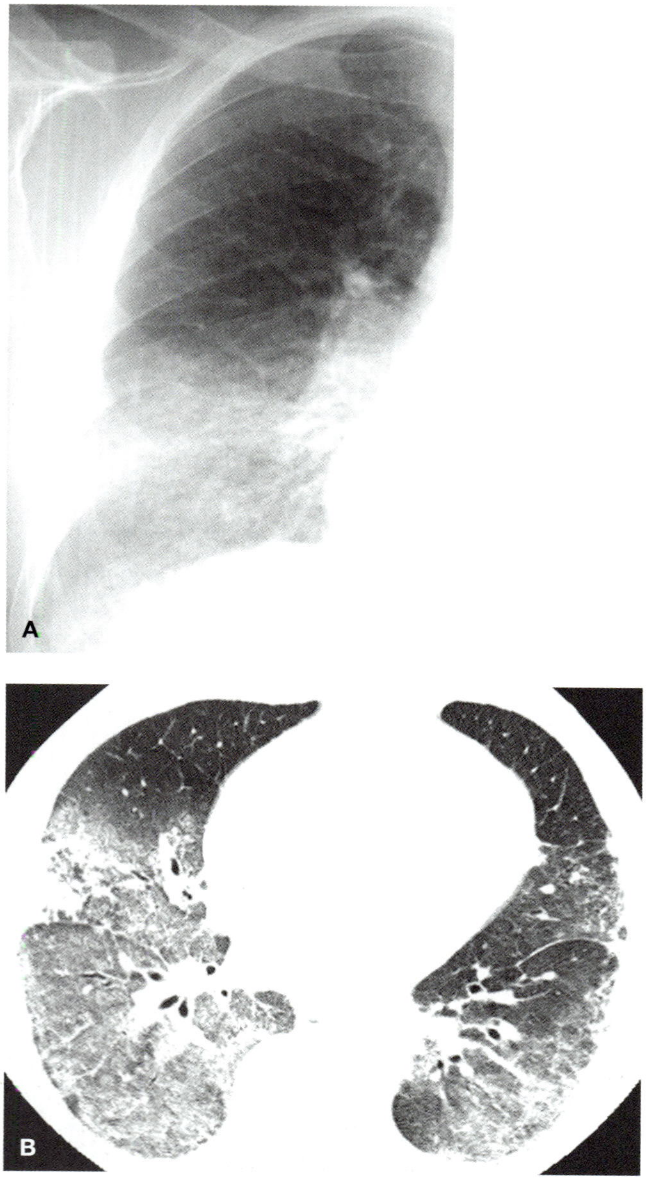

Figure 18.1. Diffuse alveolar damage resulting from treatment with doxorubicin (Adriamycin). **A:** Chest radiograph coned to the right lung shows basilar consolidation. **B:** HRCT shows ground-glass opacity and consolidation with a basal and dependent predominance.

Table 18.3 Drugs Associated With Pulmonary Hemorrhage

Anticoagulants
Amphotericin B
Crack cocaine
Cyclophosphamide
Cytosine arabinoside
Penicillamine
Quinidine

Table 18.4 Drugs Associated With Organizing Pneumonia

Amiodarone
Bleomycin
Busulfan
Cyclophosphamide
Gold
Immune checkpoint inhibitors
Interferon
Methotrexate
Nitrofurantoin
Penicillamine
Sulfasalazine

Hypersensitivity Reactions and Eosinophilic Pneumonia

Hypersensitivity reactions can be attributed to a large number of drugs but are most commonly due to methotrexate, nitrofurantoin, bleomycin, procarbazine, BCNU, cyclophosphamide, nonsteroidal anti-inflammatory drugs, sulfonamides, and ICIs; their presence is unrelated to the cumulative drug dose (Table 18.5).

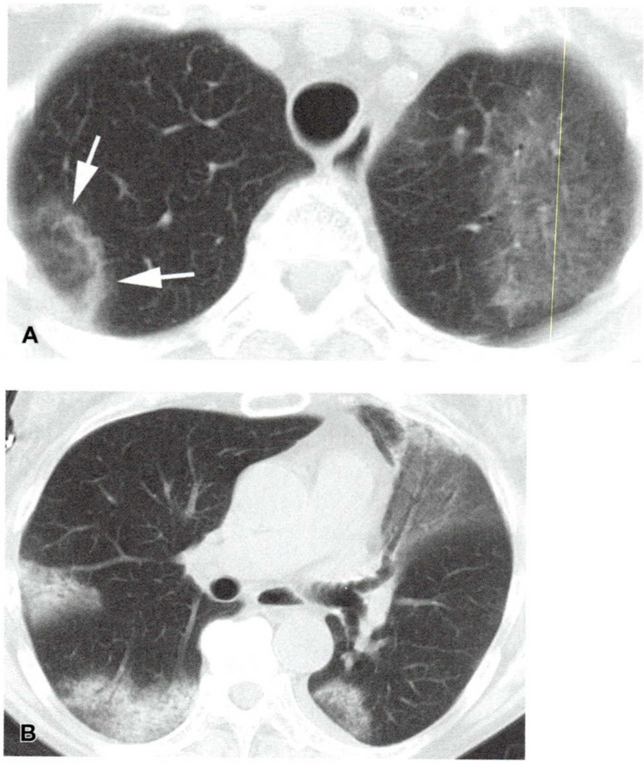

Figure 18.2. Organizing pneumonia (OP) occurring in association with chemotherapy for breast carcinoma. **A:** CT through the lung apex shows ground-glass opacity in the left upper lobe and a ring of ground-glass opacity in the right upper lobe (*arrows*), representing the reversed halo or atoll sign of OP. **B:** CT shows patchy subpleural areas of consolidation and ground-glass opacity typical of OP.

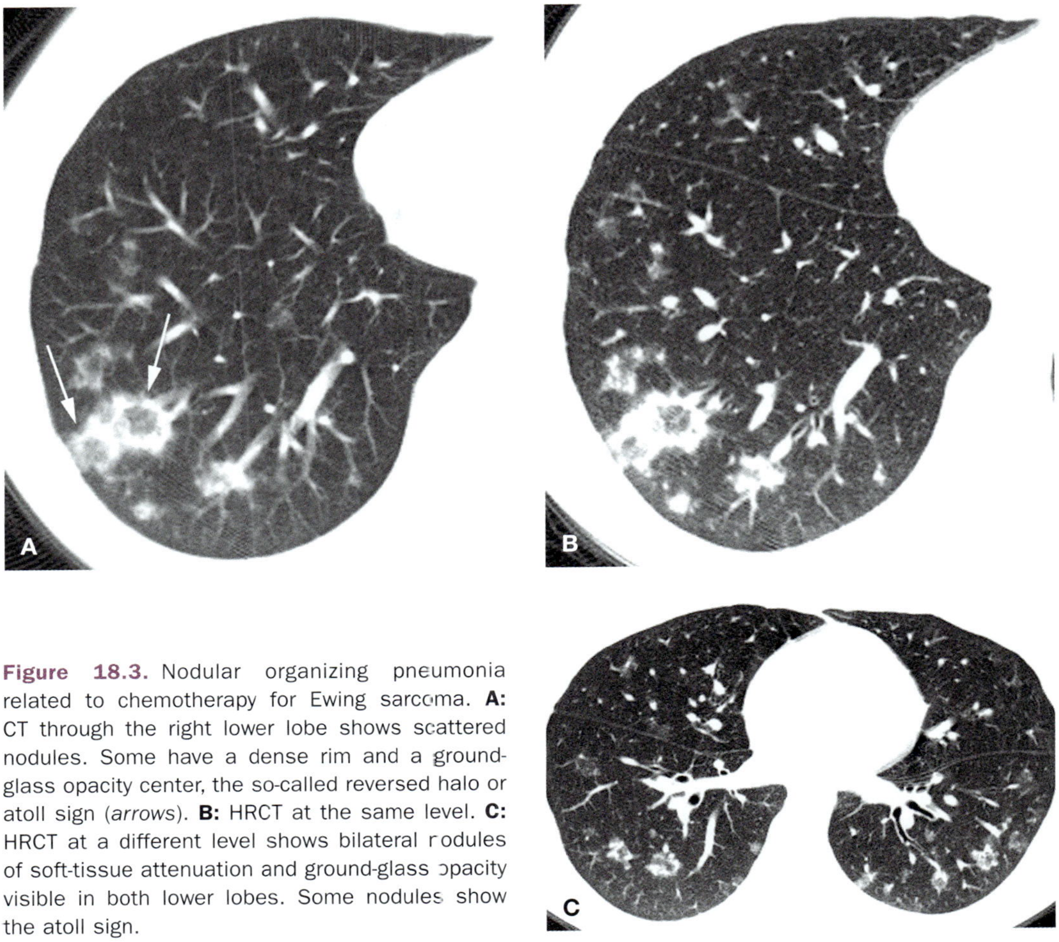

Figure 18.3. Nodular organizing pneumonia related to chemotherapy for Ewing sarcoma. **A:** CT through the right lower lobe shows scattered nodules. Some have a dense rim and a ground-glass opacity center, the so-called reversed halo or atoll sign (*arrows*). **B:** HRCT at the same level. **C:** HRCT at a different level shows bilateral nodules of soft-tissue attenuation and ground-glass opacity visible in both lower lobes. Some nodules show the atoll sign.

Hypersensitivity reactions may have features of simple eosinophilia (Loeffler syndrome), chronic eosinophilic pneumonia, or acute eosinophilic pneumonia. Cough and dyspnea, with or without fever, can be acute in onset or progress over a period of several months following institution of treatment. A peripheral eosinophilia is present in up to 40%. These reactions are characterized on chest radiographs and HRCT by patchy areas of consolidation or ground-glass opacity, which may be chronic or relatively acute, transient, and fleeting. A peripheral and subpleural distribution may be seen.

Chronic Interstitial Pneumonitis and Fibrosis

Both usual interstitial pneumonia and NSIP have been associated with drug injury; in some cases, the pattern may overlap that of OP or DAD. The clinical and radiographic presentations are often identical to those of idiopathic pulmonary fibrosis. A long list of drugs has been implicated in the development of chronic pneumonitis, but this pattern is most commonly the result of cytotoxic chemotherapeutic agents such as bleomycin, busulfan, methotrexate, doxorubicin, and carmustine (BCNU; Table 18.6). Nitrofurantoin, amiodarone, ICIs, gold, and penicillamine are noncytotoxic drugs that can also result in this type of reaction.

Plain radiographs in patients with chronic pneumonitis and fibrosis typically show a mixture of reticulation and consolidation; abnormalities are usually bilateral and symmetric, with a predominant lower lung zone involvement.

The most common pattern seen on HRCT in patients with chronic pneumonitis and fibrosis includes irregular reticular opacities (Fig. 18.4), honeycombing (Fig. 18.5), architectural distortion, and traction bronchiectasis, with or without associated consolidation; ground-glass opacity may be seen in early cases (see Figs. 18.4-18.8). As on chest radiographs, HRCT abnormalities are usually bilateral and symmetric, with a predominant lower lung zone involvement. A peripheral and subpleural distribution of abnormalities is common, particularly in patients with bleomycin toxicity. Patchy fibrosis may be seen in patients receiving nitrofurantoin. The extent of abnormalities depends on the severity of

Table 18.5 Drugs Associated With Eosinophilic Pneumonia and Hypersensitivity Reactions

BCNU
Bleomycin
Cyclophosphamide
Diphenylhydantoin
Erythromycin
Ethambutol
Fluoxetine
Gold
Imipramine
Immune checkpoint inhibitors
Isoniazid
Methotrexate
Nitrofurantoin
Nonsteroidal anti-inflammatory drugs
Para-aminosalicylic acid
Penicillamine
Penicillin
Procarbazine
Sulfasalazine
Tetracycline

lung damage. Mild damage is often limited to the posterior subpleural lung regions of the lower lung zones. In patients with more severe abnormalities, there is greater involvement of the remaining lung parenchyma.

Systemic Lupus Erythematosus

SLE related to drug treatment is indistinguishable clinically and radiographically from idiopathic SLE (Table 18.7). Pleural effusions and pericardial effusions are the most common manifestations.

Table 18.6 Drugs Associated With Chronic Pneumonitis and Fibrosis

Adriamycin
Amiodarone
BCNU
Bleomycin
Busulfan
Chlorambucil
Cyclophosphamide
Gold
Immune checkpoint inhibitors
Methotrexate
Mitomycin
Nitrofurantoin
Penicillamine
Sulfasalazine
Tocainide

Pulmonary Vasculitis and Pulmonary Hypertension

The use of various drugs may result in acute or chronic abnormalities of small vessels within the lung, with histologic abnormalities including pulmonary vasculitis, plexogenic arteriopathy, and pulmonary veno-occlusive disease (Table 18.8).

The radiographic appearances of these vary with the specific abnormalities present. Pulmonary vasculitis may result in an appearance similar to that of pulmonary edema or pulmonary hemorrhage, with patchy or diffuse consolidation or ground-glass opacity. Plexogenic arteriopathy shows findings of pulmonary hypertension, with enlargement of central pulmonary arteries. Pulmonary veno-occlusive disease mimics hydrostatic edema, but with normal heart size. Injection of crushed up tablets (excipient lung disease or IV talcosis) results can cause acute pulmonary hypertension from an angiogranulomatous reaction. On CT, this manifests as diffuse centrilobular nodules and findings of right heart strain (discussed in Chapter 28).

Sarcoid-Like Reaction

Some drugs can produce a systemic granulomatous reaction that is indistinguishable from systemic sarcoidosis both clinically and on imaging (Table 18.9). As with other drug reactions, a temporal relationship between the initiation of treatment and onset of symptoms/imaging findings is the biggest clue. The mechanism for the sarcoid-like reaction is unknown, but patients can present with many manifestations including hilar lymphadenopathy, perilymphatic lung nodules, uveitis, hypercalcemia, or elevated serum angiotensin-converting enzyme levels (see Fig. 18.9). Lesions can show fluorodeoxyglucose uptake on positron emission tomography (PET)-CT. Because many of the drugs that are implicated are used for treatment of cancer, it is important to

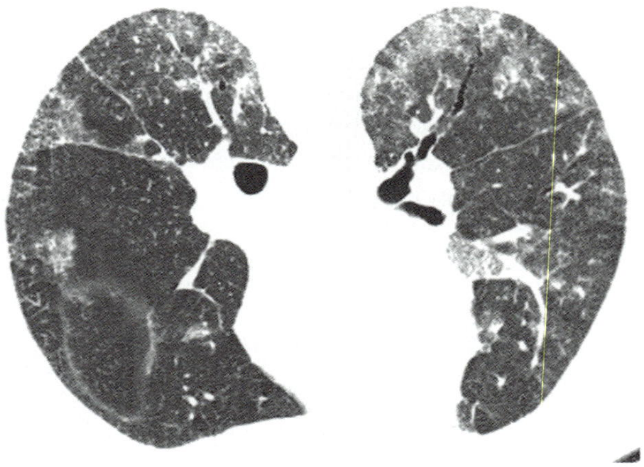

Figure 18.4. Interstitial pneumonia with fibrosis following chemotherapy. Prone HRCT shows subpleural ground-glass opacity and fine reticular opacities. This appearance is consistent with a nonspecific interstitial pneumonia pattern or early usual interstitial pneumonia pattern.

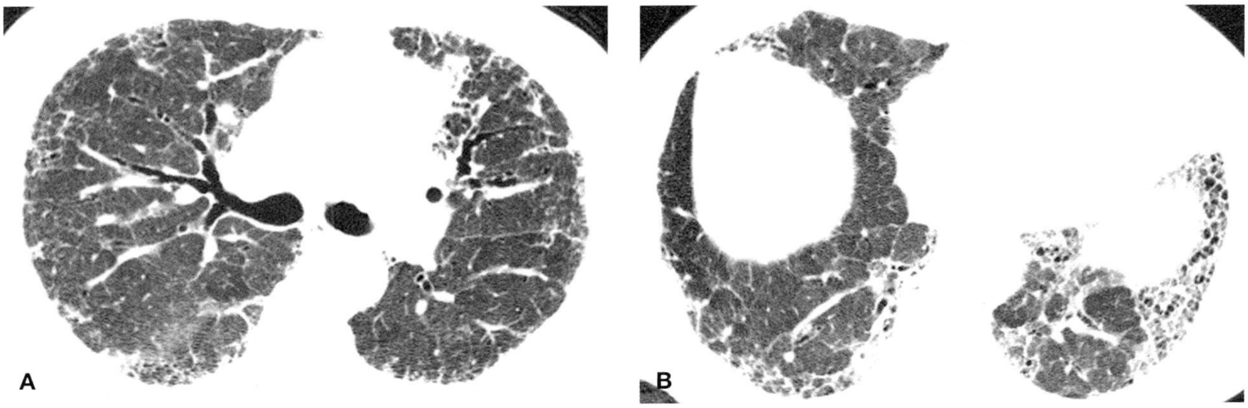

Figure 18.5. Interstitial pneumonia with fibrosis following chemotherapy with methotrexate. **A:** HRCT through the upper lobes shows irregular reticular opacities and traction bronchiectasis. **B:** HRCT through the lung bases shows honeycombing with a subpleural predominance. This appearance is that of usual interstitial pneumonia and is indistinguishable from that of idiopathic pulmonary fibrosis.

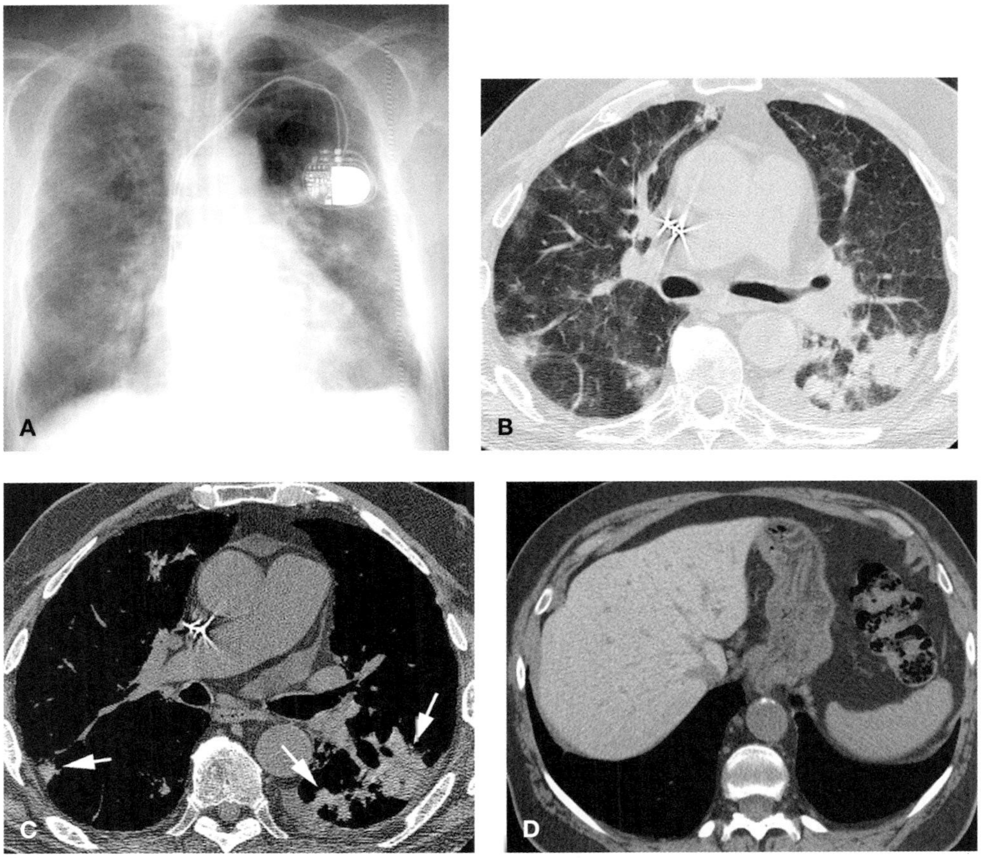

Figure 18.6. Amiodarone treatment with organizing pneumonia (OP). **A:** Chest radiograph shows cardiomegaly, a pacemaker, and patchy lung consolidation. **B:** HRCT shows patchy areas of consolidation and ground-glass opacity in the lung periphery. This appearance is typical of OP. The presence of a small left pleural effusion is not typical of OP but may reflect heart failure. **C:** HRCT with a soft-tissue window shows the areas of lung consolidation to be denser than soft tissue (*arrows*). This is common in patients with amiodarone toxicity. However, dense lung may be seen in any patient on long-term amiodarone treatment who has lung consolidation; dense lung does not imply toxicity. **D:** CT through the upper abdomen shows the liver to be dense.

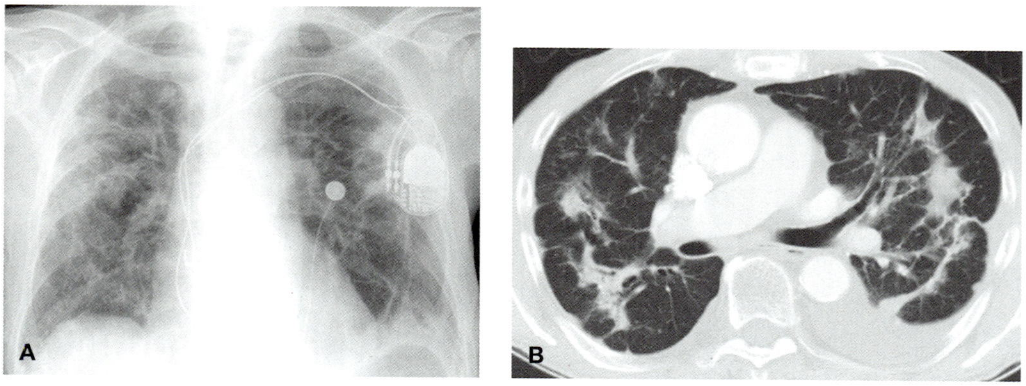

Figure 18.7. Amiodarone treatment with lung fibrosis. **A:** Chest radiograph shows a pacemaker and streaky areas of fibrosis in the peripheral lungs. **B:** HRCT shows irregular reticular opacities, traction bronchiectasis, and nodular areas of consolidation in the lung periphery. This appearance resembles a combination of organizing pneumonia/bronchiolitis obliterans organizing pneumonia and lung fibrosis. The left pleural effusion is likely related to heart failure.

consider sarcoid-like reaction as a possible mimic of metastatic disease in the appropriate clinical context.

Bronchiolitis Obliterans

The least common lung reaction to drugs is bronchiolitis obliterans, a finding described primarily in association with penicillamine therapy for rheumatoid arthritis (Table 18.10). However, the role of penicillamine is controversial, as bronchiolitis obliterans can be seen in patients with rheumatoid arthritis who have not been treated with this drug. Bronchiolitis obliterans has also been seen in patients treated with sulfasalazine. Chest radiographs may show large lung volumes. The abnormalities seen on HRCT consist of bronchial wall thickening and a pattern of mosaic perfusion, similar to that seen with other causes of bronchiolitis obliterans (see Figs. 11.36, 11.38, and 23.25); air trapping on expiratory scans is typically present.

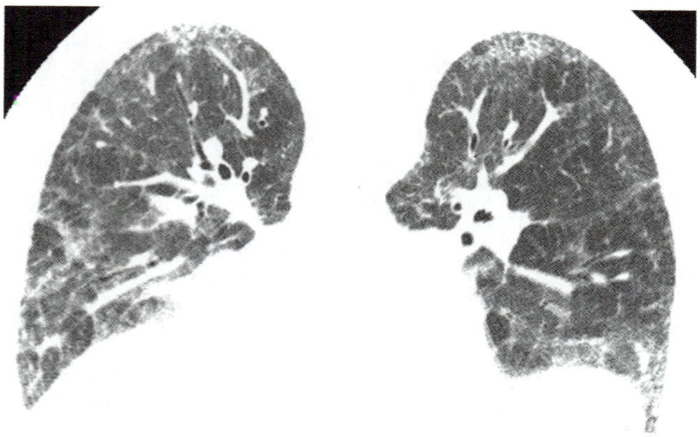

Figure 18.8. Amiodarone treatment with lung fibrosis. Prone HRCT shows peripheral reticular opacities representing nonspecific interstitial pneumonia (NSIP) or usual interstitial pneumonia. The presence of subpleural sparing suggests NSIP.

REACTIONS TO SPECIFIC DRUGS

Drug reactions may occur during treatment with a wide variety of agents. The highest incidence of adverse effects occurs with cytotoxic agents: up to 10% of patients receiving cytotoxic chemotherapeutic agents develop an adverse reaction. Some of the more common drugs to result in significant pulmonary disease are described below, along with drug reactions having a specific appearance, and those that provide examples of a particular pattern.

Commonly used illicit drugs are responsible for similar drug reactions, but lung abnormalities resulting from illicit

Table 18.7 Drugs Associated With Systemic Lupus Erythematosus

Anticonvulsants
Beta blockers
Digitalis
Gold
Hydralazine
Isoniazid
Levodopa
Nitrofurantoin
Nonsteroidal anti-inflammatory drugs
Penicillamine
Penicillin
Phenothiazines
Procainamide
Quinidine
Streptomycin
Sulfonamides
Thiouracil

Table 18.8 Drugs Associated With Pulmonary Vasculitis and Pulmonary Hypertension
Amphetamines (pulmonary hypertension)
Anorectic drugs such as fenfluramine and phenformin (pulmonary hypertension)
Anticonvulsants
Cocaine (pulmonary hypertension)
Hydralazine
Busulfan
Penicillin
Phenothiazines
Quinidine
Sulfonamides
Thiouracil

drug use may also reflect injection of particulate matter (ie, talc) or inhalation of toxic substances.

Amiodarone

Amiodarone is an iodinated drug used in the treatment of refractory cardiac tachyarrhythmias. It accumulates in the liver and lung, where it becomes entrapped in macrophage lysosomes. It results in pulmonary toxicity in 5% of patients.

Pathologic reactions to amiodarone include DAD, OP (see Fig. 18.6), and chronic pneumonitis with fibrosis (see Figs. 18.7 and 18.8). The radiographic patterns of pulmonary reaction to amiodarone vary and include focal or diffuse areas of consolidation, reticular opacities, and less commonly ill-defined nodules or masses (see Fig. 18.6).

Table 18.9 Drugs Associated With Sarcoid-Like Reaction
Immune checkpoint inhibitors
Interferons
Highly active antiretroviral therapy
Pirfenidone
Tumor necrosis factor alpha antagonists

Regions of consolidated lung in patients with amiodarone-related lung toxicity appear denser than soft tissue on unenhanced CT because of their high iodine content (see Fig. 18.6C). However, dense lung may also be seen in any patient on long-term amiodarone treatment who develops lung consolidation or collapse. Patients with amiodarone pulmonary toxicity almost always show increased liver attenuation on CT (see Fig. 18.6D), although this finding is also present in patients treated with amiodarone who do not have drug toxicity.

Aspirin and Salicylates

As many as 5% of asthmatics are sensitive to aspirin; use causes bronchospasm. This may be related to inhibition of prostaglandin synthesis.

Salicylate-induced increased permeability pulmonary edema can occur when the blood salicylate level exceeds 40 mg/dL, particularly in the elderly or in smokers. This may represent a direct toxic effect on capillary permeability. Treatment may require mechanical ventilation; resolution within a week is typical.

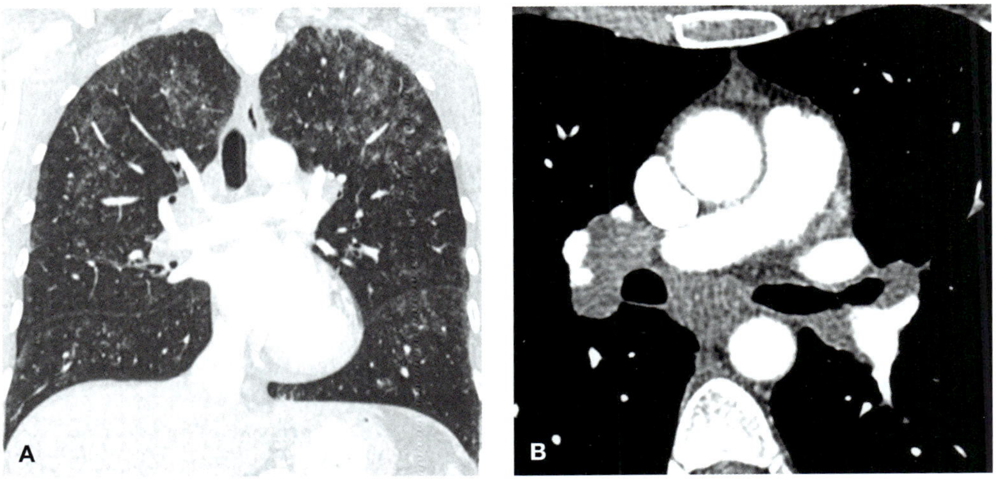

Figure 18.9. Sarcoid-like reaction in a patient undergoing immunotherapy treatment for ovarian cancer. **A:** Coronal CT image shows symmetric bilateral upper lung–predominant nodules in a perilymphatic distribution. **B:** Axial CT image shows symmetric bilateral hilar lymphadenopathy (additional paratracheal and subcarinal lymph nodes not shown). These findings were new from pretreatment scans. Nonnecrotizing granulomas were present on transbronchial biopsy consistent with sarcoid-like reaction and the findings resolved after cessation of therapy.

Table 18.10 Drugs Associated With Bronchiolitis Obliterans
Gold
Penicillamine
Sulfasalazines

Bleomycin

Bleomycin is a cytotoxic drug used in the treatment of lymphomas and some carcinomas. Bleomycin pulmonary toxicity is the most common pulmonary disease related to chemotherapy, with an incidence of about 4%. Toxicity is related to cumulative doses exceeding 400 mg. Associated risk factors for development of lung disease include recent radiation, oxygen therapy, renal disease, and advanced age.

A wide variety of reactions to bleomycin have been reported, including pulmonary edema (see Fig. 12.11 in Chapter 12), DAD with respiratory failure, chronic pneumonitis with fibrosis, OP, and hypersensitivity reactions. Radiographic and CT appearances vary accordingly.

Pneumonitis with pulmonary fibrosis typically presents 1 to 2 months after the onset of treatment with progressive dyspnea and cough. Chest radiographs show reticulation, ground-glass opacity, and sometimes consolidation with a predominant subpleural and lower lobe predominance. With severe or progressive disease, more diffuse involvement of the lower, middle, and upper lungs is typically visible. HRCT is more sensitive than radiographs in detecting early disease. Some abnormalities resolve following cessation of treatment in patients with early disease.

A unique manifestation of bleomycin-related lung toxicity is the presence of multiple pulmonary nodules mimicking the appearance of metastases and having histologic characteristics of OP.

Busulfan

Busulfan is an alkylating agent used in treating chronic myeloproliferative diseases, and clinically recognized lung toxicity occurs in about 5% of cases. It usually results in findings of chronic pneumonitis and fibrosis, OP, or DAD. Radiographic and HRCT findings include patchy or diffuse consolidation or reticulation.

Cocaine and Crack

Use of sympathomimetic agents such as cocaine (or its derivative crack), either by injection or inhalation, may cause hydrostatic pulmonary edema by inducing ischemia-related transient myocardial dysfunction, severe peripheral vasoconstriction with transient left ventricular failure, cardiac arrhythmia, or frank myocardial infarction. Cocaine or crack may also cause acute lung injury with increased permeability pulmonary edema (see Fig. 12.13 in Chapter 12), pulmonary hemorrhage, or pulmonary hypertension. HRCT commonly reveals multifocal ground-glass opacities, occasionally centrilobular in distribution, associated with interlobular septal thickening. Because pulmonary edema, pulmonary hemorrhage, and acute lung injury may be radiographically indistinguishable and may occur in combination, the development of respiratory failure after cocaine or crack use, associated with evidence of bilateral air-space opacities, clearing rapidly following cessation of drug use, has been termed *crack lung*.

Cyclophosphamide (Cytoxan)

Cyclophosphamide is an alkylating agent used in the treatment of a variety of malignancies and autoimmune diseases and is commonly used in combination with other therapeutic agents; pulmonary toxicity occurs in less than 1% of cases. Histologic findings associated with lung injury are similar to those seen in patients with bleomycin toxicity and include chronic pneumonitis and fibrosis, OP, DAD, pulmonary edema, and hypersensitivity reactions. Radiographic appearances vary accordingly.

Heroin and Narcotics

The use of heroin or other narcotics may result in increased permeability pulmonary edema. Possible mechanisms include a toxic effect on the alveolar capillary membrane, effects on the central nervous system with neurogenic edema, hypoxemia, and hypersensitivity. Symptoms of dyspnea typically occur from minutes to a few hours after injection. Radiographs show typical findings of increased permeability edema, with parahilar ground-glass opacity or consolidation, but the appearance may be complicated by associated aspiration. Hemorrhage may also be present. Resolution often occurs within 1 to 2 days.

Immune Checkpoint Inhibitors

ICIs are an ever-expanding list of drugs that recruit the body's immune system to treat some types of cancer. Current targets include inhibitors of PD-1 (eg, pembrolizumab, nivolumab), PD-L1 (eg, atezolizumab, durvalumab), CTLA-4 (eg, ipilimumab), and others. These therapies can cause autoimmune reactions in virtually every organ system in the body; in the chest, they may manifest as myriad forms of lung injury. OP is the most common manifestation of ICI-induced lung injury and is indistinguishable from other causes of OP. DAD, HP, and NSIP are other reported patterns of lung injury.

Interleukin-2

Interleukin-2 is a T-cell growth factor used as an immune system stimulator for treating cancers, particularly melanoma and renal cell carcinoma. It may cause increased permeability pulmonary edema by a direct toxic effect on the capillary endothelium. Symptoms typically begin within 2 to 8 days of the onset of treatment. Radiographs show typical findings of interstitial or air-space edema. Pleural effusion, an unusual finding with increased permeability edema, is common. Clearing occurs within days of drug cessation.

Methotrexate

Methotrexate is a folate antagonist used in the treatment of malignancies and inflammatory diseases. Pulmonary toxicity occurs in 5% to 10% of cases and is unrelated to the duration of treatment or the cumulative dose.

In contrast to many other cytotoxic agents, methotrexate often results in reversible abnormalities. Symptoms usually develop within weeks of the onset of treatment and include fever, cough, and dyspnea. In most cases, the histologic appearance resembles HP or less often OP or DAD; peripheral eosinophilia is present in half of the cases. Chest radiographs show ill-defined reticular opacities, ground-glass opacity, or consolidation. A basal predominance is typical. HRCT usually shows ground-glass opacity as the predominant abnormality. Radiographic abnormalities usually regress following discontinuation of the drug. Some residual fibrosis may be seen. However, fibrosis and honeycombing may result (see Fig. 18.5).

Nitrofurantoin

Nitrofurantoin is an antibiotic used for treatment of urinary tract infections. It may result in either acute or chronic reactions; acute reactions are much more common, accounting for 90% of cases of toxicity. SLE related to nitrofurantoin has also been reported.

Acute nitrofurantoin toxicity is a hypersensitivity reaction and usually begins from 1 day to 2 weeks after initiation of therapy. Symptoms include fever, cough, and dyspnea; peripheral eosinophilia is present in most patients. Chest radiographs show an interstitial abnormality with Kerley lines (ie, pulmonary edema) or consolidation, which may be symmetric or asymmetric. Pleural effusion, usually small and unilateral, is present in one-third of cases. Discontinuation of the drug results in clearing, usually within days.

Chronic nitrofurantoin reaction occurs from 2 months to years after the beginning of continuous treatment. It is unrelated to acute toxicity. Insidious cough and dyspnea are most common; fever is absent, and eosinophilia is uncommon. Radiographs and HRCT show a diffuse reticular abnormality with a basal predominance due to chronic pneumonitis and fibrosis. The appearance closely resembles idiopathic pulmonary fibrosis (Fig. 18.10). Discontinuing the drug should result in some improvement over a period of months. Steroid treatment may also be effective, but mortality is 10%.

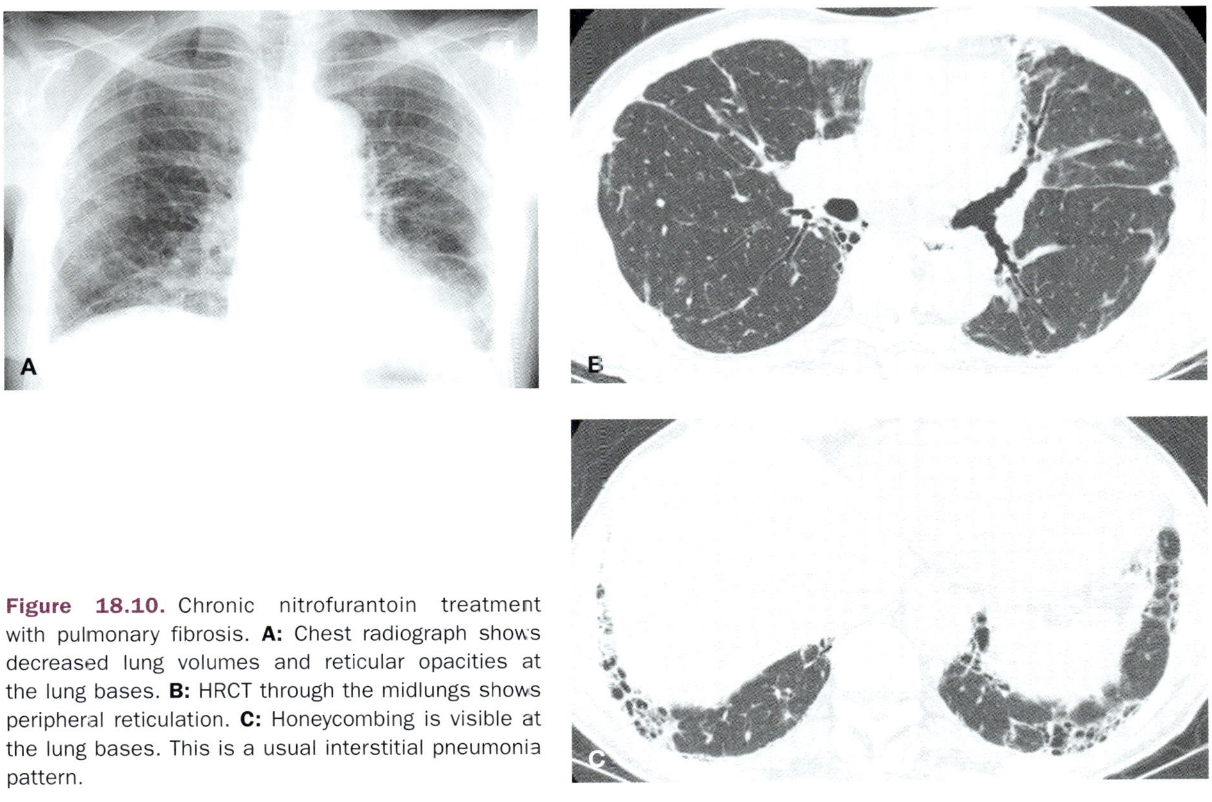

Figure 18.10. Chronic nitrofurantoin treatment with pulmonary fibrosis. **A:** Chest radiograph shows decreased lung volumes and reticular opacities at the lung bases. **B:** HRCT through the midlungs shows peripheral reticulation. **C:** Honeycombing is visible at the lung bases. This is a usual interstitial pneumonia pattern.

Nonsteroidal Anti-inflammatory Drugs

These drugs have been associated with a hypersensitivity reaction with acute onset of dyspnea, cough, low-grade fever, and eosinophilia. They may also be associated with SLE.

OKT3

OKT3 is a monoclonal antibody directed against T cells that is used to treat rejection of solid organ transplants. Pulmonary edema is a common complication in patients who are fluid overloaded prior to the institution of treatment. Consequently, chest radiographs are routinely obtained before treatment begins to exclude preexisting pulmonary edema or heart failure.

Tocolytic Drugs

Tocolytic drugs used to treat premature labor (eg, ritodrine and terbutaline) result in increased permeability pulmonary edema in about 1% of cases. Onset is typically 2 to 3 days after treatment. Increased risk is associated with overhydration, twin gestation, and use of steroids. Rapid recovery is typical.

Tricyclic Antidepressants

Overdose of tricyclic antidepressants may be associated with increased permeability pulmonary edema or DAD with development of ARDS as a direct toxic effect.

RADIATION PNEUMONITIS AND FIBROSIS

Following external beam thoracic radiotherapy, approximately 40% of patients develop radiographic abnormalities, and 7% develop symptomatic radiation pneumonitis.

The development and appearance of radiation lung injury depend on a number of factors, including (1) the volume of lung irradiated, (2) the shape of the radiation fields, (3) the radiation dose, (4) the number of fractions of radiation given, (5) the time period over which the radiation is delivered, (6) prior irradiation, (7) whether chemotherapy is also employed, (8) corticosteroid therapy withdrawal, (9) preexisting lung disease, (10) the type of radiation used, and (11) individual susceptibility.

Generally speaking, radiation is best tolerated by the patient if given in smaller doses, over a long period of time, and to a single lung or a small lung region. For unilateral radiation with fractionated doses, radiographic findings of radiation pneumonitis are seldom detected with doses below 3000 cGy, are variably present with doses between 3000 and 4000 cGy, and are nearly always visible at doses of 4000 cGy. Its likelihood is increased by a second course of radiation, the withdrawal of corticosteroid treatment, and the use of concomitant chemotherapy. Radiographic findings of radiation pneumonitis are usually not associated with symptoms, although low-grade fever, cough, and dyspnea are present in some patients.

Radiation Pneumonitis

Pulmonary abnormalities related to radiation injury have been divided into early and late manifestations. The early stage of radiation lung injury, referred to as radiation pneumonitis, occurs within 1 to 3 months after radiation therapy is completed and is most severe 3 to 4 months following treatment. Radiation pneumonitis is associated with histologic findings of DAD, intra-alveolar proteinaceous exudates, and hyaline membranes. Depending on the severity of lung injury, these abnormalities may resolve completely, but more often they undergo progressive organization, leading eventually to fibrosis.

Radiation Fibrosis

The late stage of radiation-induced lung injury, termed *radiation fibrosis*, develops gradually in patients with radiation pneumonitis when complete resolution does not occur. Radiation fibrosis evolves within the previously irradiated field 6 to 12 months following radiation therapy and usually becomes stable within 2 years of treatment. Histologically, dense fibrosis with obliteration of lung architecture and traction bronchiectasis are present. Patients can present with radiation fibrosis without a previous history of acute pneumonitis.

Radiographic and CT Findings

The hallmark of radiation pneumonitis on radiographs or CT is homogeneous or patchy ground-glass opacity or consolidation corresponding closely to the location of the radiation ports (Fig. 18.11). Abnormalities are typically nonanatomic and do not tend to respect normal lung boundaries such as lobar fissures or lung segments. Volume loss can be seen; this is due to obstruction of bronchioles by inflammatory exudate, loss of surfactant, or both. Large airways are patent, and air bronchograms are commonly visible. Pleural thickening is sometimes seen adjacent to irradiated areas.

Although findings of radiation pneumonitis are characteristically confined to areas of irradiated lung, relatively mild abnormalities (ground-glass opacity or consolidation) are detected outside the radiation portal in as many as 20% of cases, perhaps related to a hypersensitivity reaction or OP (Table 18.11).

Persistence or progression of radiographic or CT abnormalities more than 9 months after treatment likely indicates

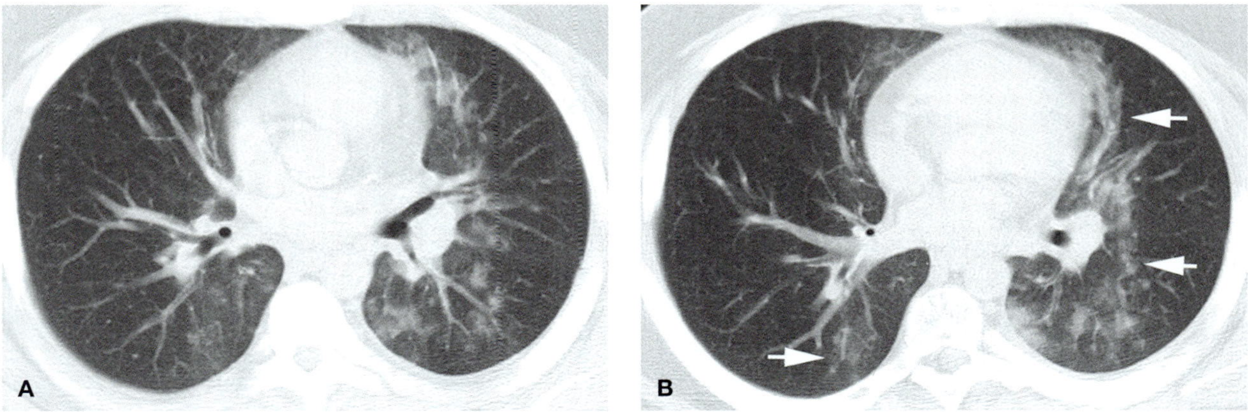

Figure 18.11. Acute radiation pneumonitis. **A:** Patchy areas of ground-glass opacity are visible in a paramediastinal distribution following mediastinal radiation. **B:** The areas of abnormality are nonanatomic but have straight margins corresponding to the radiation ports (*arrows*). Little volume loss is present at this stage.

fibrosis (Fig. 18.12). The development of radiation fibrosis can be recognized by the appearance of streaky opacities, progressive volume loss, progressive dense consolidation (see Figs. 18.12 and 18.13), traction bronchiectasis (see Figs. 18.12B and 18.13), or pleural thickening within the irradiated lung. Fibrosis and volume loss typically result in a sharper demarcation between normal and irradiated lung regions than is seen in patients with radiation pneumonitis (see Figs. 18.12 and 18.13). This gives the abnormal lung regions a characteristically straight and sharply defined edge. Occasionally, the appearance of lung fibrosis mimics honeycombing (Fig. 18.14), although the distribution is related to the radiation ports and is quite different from that of idiopathic pulmonary fibrosis. The adjacent lung may appear hyperinflated and may show bullae. The ipsilateral hemithorax may be reduced in volume (see Fig. 18.13).

Table 18.11 Radiation Pneumonitis and Fibrosis

- Occurrence is multifactorial
- Seldom occurs below 3000 cGy
- Nearly always visible above 4000 cGy
- Radiation pneumonitis
  - 1-3 mo after radiation is completed
  - Most severe 3-4 mo after radiation
  - Diffuse alveolar damage
  - Radiographs and HRCT
    - Homogeneous or patchy ground-glass opacity or consolidation
    - Edges correspond to radiation ports.
    - Abnormalities outside of ports in 20%
- Radiation fibrosis
  - 6-12 mo after radiation is completed
  - Unchanging after 2 y
  - Fibrosis and traction bronchiectasis
  - Radiographs and HRCT
    - Persisting abnormalities after 9 mo
    - Dense consolidation
    - Edges correspond to radiation ports.
    - Traction bronchiectasis typical
    - Honeycombing
    - Ipsilateral volume loss
- Similar by more localized appearances with stereotactic ablative radiotherapy

Although pleural thickening is a common manifestation of radiation, pleural effusions are uncommon. Effusion related to radiation typically develops within 6 months of treatment, in conjunction with radiation pneumonitis, and resolves spontaneously. Rapid accumulation of fluid suggests malignancy.

Mediastinal lymph node calcification, particularly after radiation of lymphomas, the development of thymic cysts, pericarditis, and cardiomyopathy may also be seen.

Stereotactic Ablative Radiotherapy

Stereotactic ablative radiotherapy (SABR), also known as stereotactic body radiotherapy, is a treatment option for patients with stage I non–small cell lung cancer who are unfit for surgery, are medically operable but refuse surgery, or those with adenocarcinomas characterized by lepidic growth. Image-guided SABR is characterized by precise delivery of radiation to a localized region. To date, survival rates are similar to those of surgery, with local control rates of over 90%.

On CT, radiation-induced lung abnormalities after SABR differ from those observed following conventionally radiotherapy. SABR uses complex beam arrangements to conform high-dose regions to the tumor and to create steep

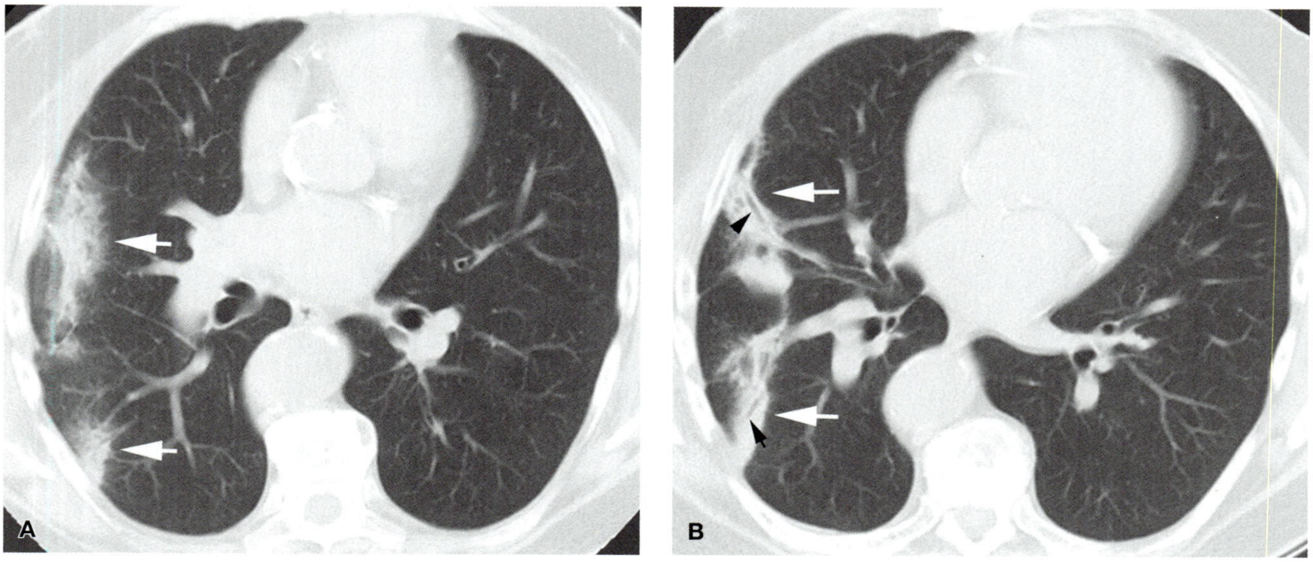

Figure 18.12. Radiation fibrosis 12 months following axillary radiotherapy. **A, B:** CTs at two levels show consolidation in the peripheral lung. The abnormal areas have a straight edge (*white arrows*) due to the port used. Dense consolidation is typical of fibrosis. Traction bronchiectasis (*black arrows*, **B**) indicates that fibrosis is present.

dose gradients around the target volume, with a large volume of lung receiving a low or intermediate dose. Current follow-up relies on CT imaging, with positron emission tomography or biopsy when recurrence is strongly suspected.

Expected CT appearances following SABR include consolidation or ground-glass opacity within the first 6 months after treatment, sometimes associated with an increase in size or density of the lesion, with a pattern of fibrosis emerging 6 months to years after treatment, accompanied by a decrease in lesion size (Fig. 18.15). Increase in size after 1 year suggests recurrence. Although PET standardized uptake value (SUV) may rise immediately post-SABR and may persist for 12 months without recurrence, an SUV greater than 5 is a finding that suggests recurrence.

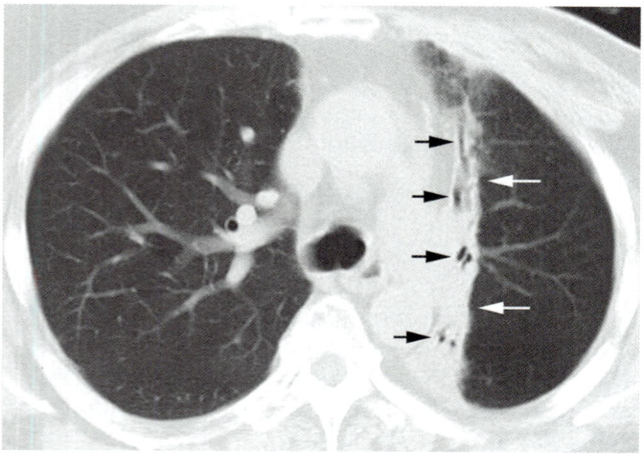

Figure 18.13. End-stage radiation fibrosis. HRCT shows dense paramediastinal fibrosis with a sharp edge (*white arrows*). Traction bronchiectasis (*black arrows*) is extensive. The ipsilateral hemithorax is reduced in volume compared with the opposite side.

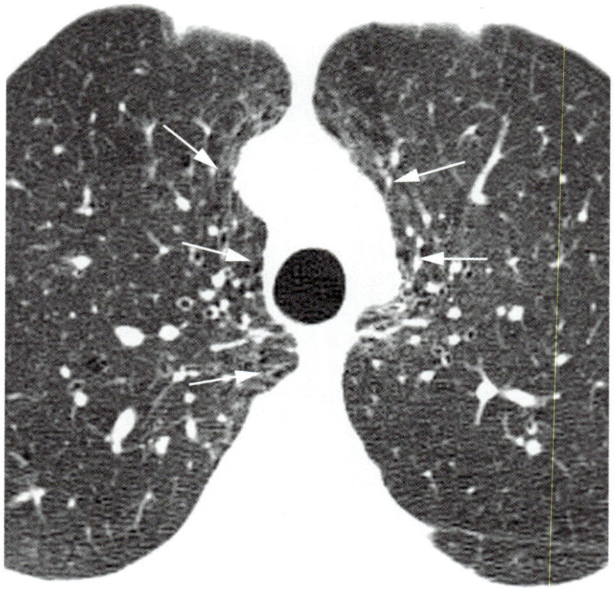

Figure 18.14. Paramediastinal fibrosis following radiation for Hodgkin disease. HRCT shows paramediastinal reticulation, traction bronchiectasis, and honeycombing (*arrows*).

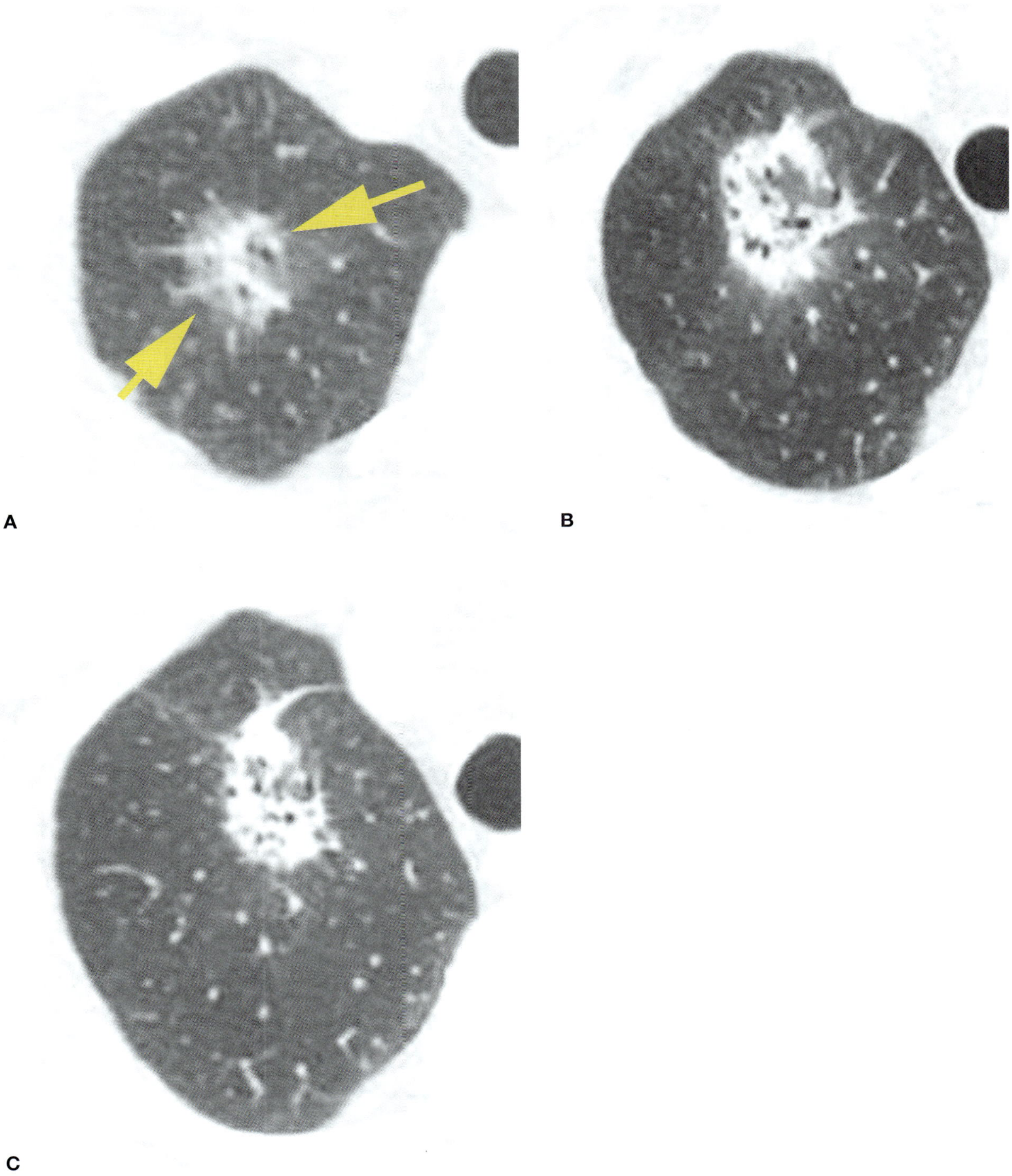

Figure 18.15. Adenocarcinoma treated using stereotactic ablative radiotherapy (SABR). **A:** CT shows a mixed ground-glass and solid nodule in the right apex (*arrows*) consistent with minimally invasive or lepidic predominant adenocarcinoma. **B:** After SABR, the nodule has increased in size and attenuation, associated with radiation pneumonitis. **C:** Subsequently, the nodule is decreased in size because of fibrosis.

SUGGESTED READINGS

Aquino SL, Webb WR, Golden J. Bronchiolitis obliterans associated with rheumatoid arthritis: findings on HRCT and dynamic expiratory CT. *J Comput Assist Tomogr*. 1994;18(4):555-558.

Aronchick JM, Gefter WB. Drug-induced pulmonary disorders. *Semin Roentgenol*. 1995;30(1):18-34.

Bellamy EA, Husband JE, Blaquiere RM, Law MR. Bleomycin-related lung damage: CT evidence. *Radiology*. 1985;156(1):155-158.

Bush DA, Dunbar RD, Bonnet R, Slater JD, Cheek GA, Slater JM. Pulmonary injury from proton and conventional radiotherapy as revealed by CT. *AJR Am J Roentgenol*. 1999;172(3):735-739.

Chopra A, Nautiyal A, Kalkanis A, Judson MA. Drug-induced sarcoidosis-like reactions. *Chest*. 2018;154(3):664-677. doi:10.1016/j.chest.2018.03.056

Cooper JAD, White DA, Matthay RA. Drug-induced pulmonary disease, part 1: cytotoxic drugs. *Am Rev Respir Dis*. 1986;133(2):321-340.

Cooper JAD, White DA, Matthay RA. Drug induced pulmonary disease, part 2: noncytotoxic drugs. *Am Rev Respir Dis*. 1986;133(3):488-505.

Cooper JA Jr. Drug-induced lung disease. *Adv Intern Med*. 1997;42:231-268.

Davis SD, Yankelevitz DF, Henschke CI. Radiation effects on the lung: clinical features, pathology, and imaging findings. *AJR Am J Roentgenol*. 1992;159(6):1157-1164.

Gotway MB, Marder SR, Hanks DK, et al. Thoracic complications of illicit drug use: an organ system approach. *Radiographics*. 2002;22 Spec No:119-135.

Hagan IG, Burney K. Radiology of recreational drug abuse. *Radiographics*. 2007;27(4):919-940.

Huang K, Dahele M, Senan S, et al. Radiographic changes after lung stereotactic ablative radiotherapy (SABR)—can we distinguish recurrence from fibrosis? A systematic review of the literature. *Radiother Oncol*. 2012;102(3):335-342.

Huang K, Senthi S, Palma DA, et al. High-risk CT features for detection of local recurrence after stereotactic ablative radiotherapy for lung cancer. *Radiother Oncol*. 2013;109(1):51-57.

Huang K, Palma DA; IASLC Advanced Radiation Technology Committee. Follow-up of patients after stereotactic radiation for lung cancer: a primer for the nonradiation oncologist. *J Thorac Oncol*. 2015;10(3):412-419.

Johkoh T, Lee KS, Nishino M, et al. Chest CT diagnosis and clinical management of drug-related pneumonitis in patients receiving molecular targeting agents and immune checkpoint inhibitors: a position paper from the Fleischner Society. *Radiology*. 2021;298(3):550-566. doi:10.1148/radiol.2021203427

Kalisz K.R, Ramaiya N.H, Laukamp K.R, Gupta A. Immune checkpoint inhibitor therapy–related pneumonitis: patterns and management. *Radiographics*. 2019;39(7):1923-1937. doi:10.1148/rg.2019190036

Kang KH, Okoye CC, Patel RB, et al. Complications from stereotactic body radiotherapy for lung cancer. *Cancers (Basel)*. 2015;7(2):981-1004.

Kuhlman JE, Teigen C, Ren H, Hruban RH, Hutchins GM, Fishman EK. Amiodarone pulmonary toxicity: CT findings in symptomatic patients. *Radiology*. 1990;177(1):121-125.

Kuhlman JE. The role of chest computed tomography in the diagnosis of drug-related reactions. *J Thorac Imaging*. 1991;6(1):52-61.

Libshitz HI. Radiation changes in the lung. *Semin Roentgenol*. 1993;28(4):303-320.

Logan PM. Thoracic manifestations of external beam radiotherapy. *AJR Am J Roentgenol*. 1998;171(3):569-577.

Movsas B, Raffin TA, Epstein AH, Link CJ Jr. Pulmonary radiation injury. *Chest*. 1997;111(4):1061-1076.

Padley SPG, Adler B, Hansell DM, Müller NL. High-resolution computed tomography of drug-induced lung disease. *Clin Radiol*. 1992;46:232-236.

Pietra GG. Pathologic mechanisms of drug-induced lung disorders. *J Thorac Imaging*. 1991;6:1-7.

Rosenow EC, Myers JL, Swensen SJ, Pisani RJ. Drug-induced pulmonary disease: an update. *Chest*. 1992;102(1):239-250.

Rossi SE, Erasmus JJ, McAdams HP, Sporn TA, Goodman PC. Pulmonary drug toxicity: radiologic and pathologic manifestations. *Radiographics*. 2000;20(5):1245-1259.

Saxon RR, Klein JS, Bar MH, et al. Pathogenesis of pulmonary edema during interleukin-2 therapy: correlation of chest radiographic and clinical findings in 54 patients. *AJR Am J Roentgenol*. 1991;156(2):281-285.

Sridhar S, Kanne JP, Henry TS, Revels JW, Gotway MB, Ketai LH. Medication-induced pulmonary injury: a scenario- and pattern-based approach to a perplexing problem. *Radiographics*. 2022;42(1):38-55. doi:10.1148/rg.210146

Chapter 19

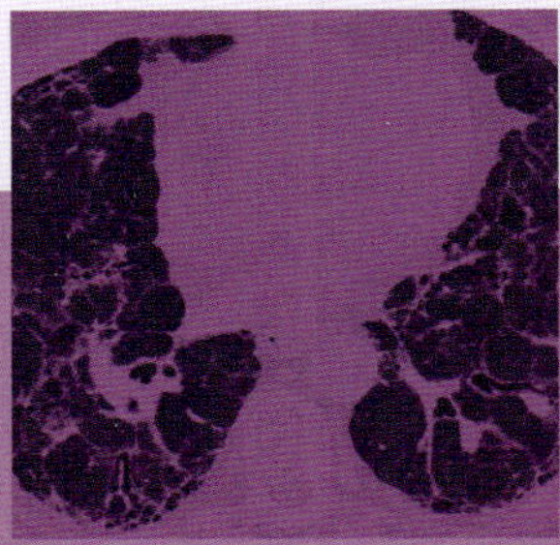

Travis S. Henry

Pulmonary Vasculitis and Diffuse Alveolar Hemorrhage

INTRODUCTION

The term *systemic vasculitis* refers to a variety of clinico-pathological entities, each of which is characterized pathologically by cellular inflammation and destruction of blood vessel walls; the lungs may be involved along with other organs. Pulmonary vasculitis may represent a primary (idiopathic) disorder or may be secondary to other conditions, such as infection, collagen vascular disease, or hypersensitivity disorders. The primary vasculitides are rare.

Systemic vasculitis syndromes have been classified in a number of ways, but none of the proposed systems is ideal or universally accepted. The American College of Rheumatology published the criteria for the classification of vasculitis in 1994, which were reviewed by at an International Consensus Conference in Chapel Hill, North Carolina, and updated it in 2012. The Chapel Hill classification system divides the systemic vasculitis syndromes into three groups based on the size of vessels primarily involved. These are (a) large vessel vasculitis, (b) medium-sized vessel vasculitis, and (c) small vessel vasculitis. Antineutrophilic cytoplasmic antibody (ANCA)-associated small vessel vasculitis, specifically granulomatosis with polyangiitis (GPA), eosinophilic granulomatosis with polyangiitis (EGPA; also Churg-Strauss syndrome), and microscopic polyangiitis (MPA), are the systemic vasculitis syndromes most often associated with pulmonary abnormalities.

Although the Chapel Hill classification has been widely adopted for the description of pulmonary vasculitis, it has been modified by some authors to include Behçet disease (BD) and by others to include primary immune complex–mediated vasculitis and secondary vasculitis resulting in pulmonary capillaritis and diffuse alveolar hemorrhage (DAH).

IgG4-related systemic disease—while not a true vasculitis—can cause numerous manifestations in the thorax and is also reviewed in this chapter. This inclusive classification is reviewed in Table 19.1, listing the most common entities to involve the lung.

Basing the differential diagnosis of pulmonary vasculitis on radiologic findings and patterns has been suggested, at least partially because the clinical presentations of these syndromes overlap. However, the CT features of the vasculitis syndromes also overlap and are of limited utility in diagnosis, without consideration of clinical, laboratory, and pathologic features.

Common manifestations of pulmonary vasculitis include (a) neutrophilic capillaritis with pulmonary hemorrhage, (b) vascular occlusion or thrombosis with lung infarction or ischemia, (c) lung inflammation in association with vascular lesions, and (d) involvement of large arteries with thrombosis, stenosis, or aneurysm formation.

Categories of CT abnormalities used in two diagnostic schemes include (a) localized nodular and patchy opacities, (b) diffuse air-space consolidation or ground-glass opacities due to pulmonary hemorrhage, (c) large pulmonary artery stenosis or aneurysms, and (d) findings of pulmonary hypertension.

LARGE VESSEL VASCULITIS

Large vessel vasculitides predominantly affect the aorta and its largest branches. These vasculitides are suspected when there are signs and symptoms of ischemia.

Giant Cell (Temporal) Vasculitis

Temporal arteritis is relatively common. Affected patients are generally over 50 years of age. Arteries of the head and

Table 19.1 Classification of Pulmonary Vasculitis

Primary Idiopathic Vasculitis
Large Vessel
Giant cell arteritis
Takayasu arteritis
Behçet disease
IgG4
Medium Vessel
Polyarteritis nodosa
Kawasaki disease
Small Vessel (antineutrophilic cytoplasmic antibody)-Associated Vasculitides
Granulomatosis with polyangiitis
Eosinophilic granulomatosis with polyangiitis (Churg-Strauss syndrome)
Microscopic polyangiitis
PULMONARY CAPILLARITIS WITH DIFFUSE ALVEOLAR HEMORRHAGE
Primary Immune Complex–Mediated vasculitis
Goodpasture syndrome
Henoch-Schönlein purpura
Behçet disease
Secondary Vasculitis
Collagen vascular disease
Systemic lupus erythematosus
Rheumatoid arthritis
Mixed connective tissue disease
Polymyositis/dermatomyositis
Scleroderma
Antiphospholipid antibody syndrome
Essential cryoglobulinemia
Inflammatory bowel disease
Lung transplantation
Hypocomplementemic urticarial vasculitis
Drug induced (eg, propylthiouracil, diphenylhydantoin)
Bone marrow transplantation
Paraneoplastic
Infection

neck are typically involved, and the most common symptoms are headache and tenderness in the region of the temporal artery.

Thoracic aortic aneurysm may occur. Large- and medium-sized pulmonary arteries are rarely involved in this disease. CT may show involvement of large pulmonary artery branches, with wall thickening, stenosis, and thrombosis. Generally speaking, giant cell arteritis resembles Takayasu arteritis in its manifestations. Large- and medium-sized pulmonary arteries are rarely involved in this disease. Although upper respiratory symptoms such as cough and hoarseness occur in up to 10% of cases, radiographic correlates are lacking. Some patients show nonspecific radiographic abnormalities such as pleural effusion and diffuse reticular opacities, but what these are due to is unclear.

Table 19.2 IgG4 Related Disease

Vascular Involvement (either arteritis or periarteritis)
Aorta
Pulmonary arteries
Coronary arteries
Carotid arteries and other medium vessels
Nonvascular Involvement
Lung
Mediastinum
Lymph nodes
Orbit
Salivary glands
Pericardium
Pancreas
Bile ducts
Kidney
Retroperitoneum

Takayasu Arteritis

Takayasu arteritis affects large- and medium-sized arteries, most often the aorta and its branches. Females, usually under the age of 40, are affected in 90% of cases. In early disease, pathology shows vessel inflammation and poorly defined necrotizing and nonnecrotizing granulomas; in later lesions, vascular fibrosis and destruction of elastic tissue are present. Pulmonary arteries are involved in 50% of patients. Pulmonary hypertension may occur in late-stage disease, but is seldom severe.

Radiographic abnormalities usually reflect aortic involvement, with aortic contour abnormalities, such as dilatation of the arch, a wavy-appearing descending aorta, and premature aortic calcification. CT and MRI may show concentric aortic wall thickening with aneurysmal dilation and/or narrowing of the aortic lumen or branch vessels.

Central pulmonary artery dilatation may be seen on chest radiographs due to pulmonary hypertension but is relatively uncommon. On CT or MRI, stenosis or obstruction of segmental or smaller pulmonary arteries is often seen in late-stage cases. This may be associated with a patchy decrease in the attenuation of peripheral lung parenchyma (ie, mosaic perfusion), a finding that sometimes is also recognized on chest films. Regional decrease in lung perfusion may be shown using $\dot{V}/\dot{Q}$ scintigraphy.

IgG4-Related Disease

IgG4-related disease (IgG4-RD) is an increasingly recognized immune-mediated systemic disease that is characterized by infiltration of IgG4-positive plasma cells in a variety of organs and vessels in the body (Table 19.2). Large and medium vessel involvement in IgG4-RD is common and can produce either a large vessel vasculitis (eg, aortitis) or a periarteritis (eg, periaortitis). The appearance is similar to Takayasu arteritis on CT and MRI and manifests as wall thickening, inflammation, and aneurysm formation (Fig. 19.1A). The aorta is the most common site of involvement (thoracic and/or abdominal). Pulmonary artery, coronary artery, and arch vessel involvement may also be seen (Fig. 19.1B). Periaortitis has also been described, most commonly in the setting of retroperitoneal fibrosis. Periaortitis is seen as inflammation adjacent to the vessel wall, minimal vascular wall thickening, and minimal luminal narrowing. Both entities can show increased FDG uptake on PET-CT.

Pulmonary and mediastinal manifestations of IgG4-RD are protean. Lung involvement includes nodules or masslike areas of ground-glass opacity and/or consolidation that may mimic malignancy (Fig. 19.1C). Organizing pneumonia, interstitial fibrosis, and airway involvement with bronchovascular thickening have also been described.

The mediastinum is another area of involvement, where IgG4-RD may manifest as lymphadenopathy or rarely fibrosing mediastinitis. Pleural involvement may also be seen in the form of pleural thickening or pleural effusion.

Behçet Disease

BD is a rare systemic large- and small vessel vasculitis likely due to deposition of immune complexes (Table 19.3). It is associated with recurrent oral aphthous ulcers, genital ulcers, uveitis, and skin lesions such as erythema nodosum.

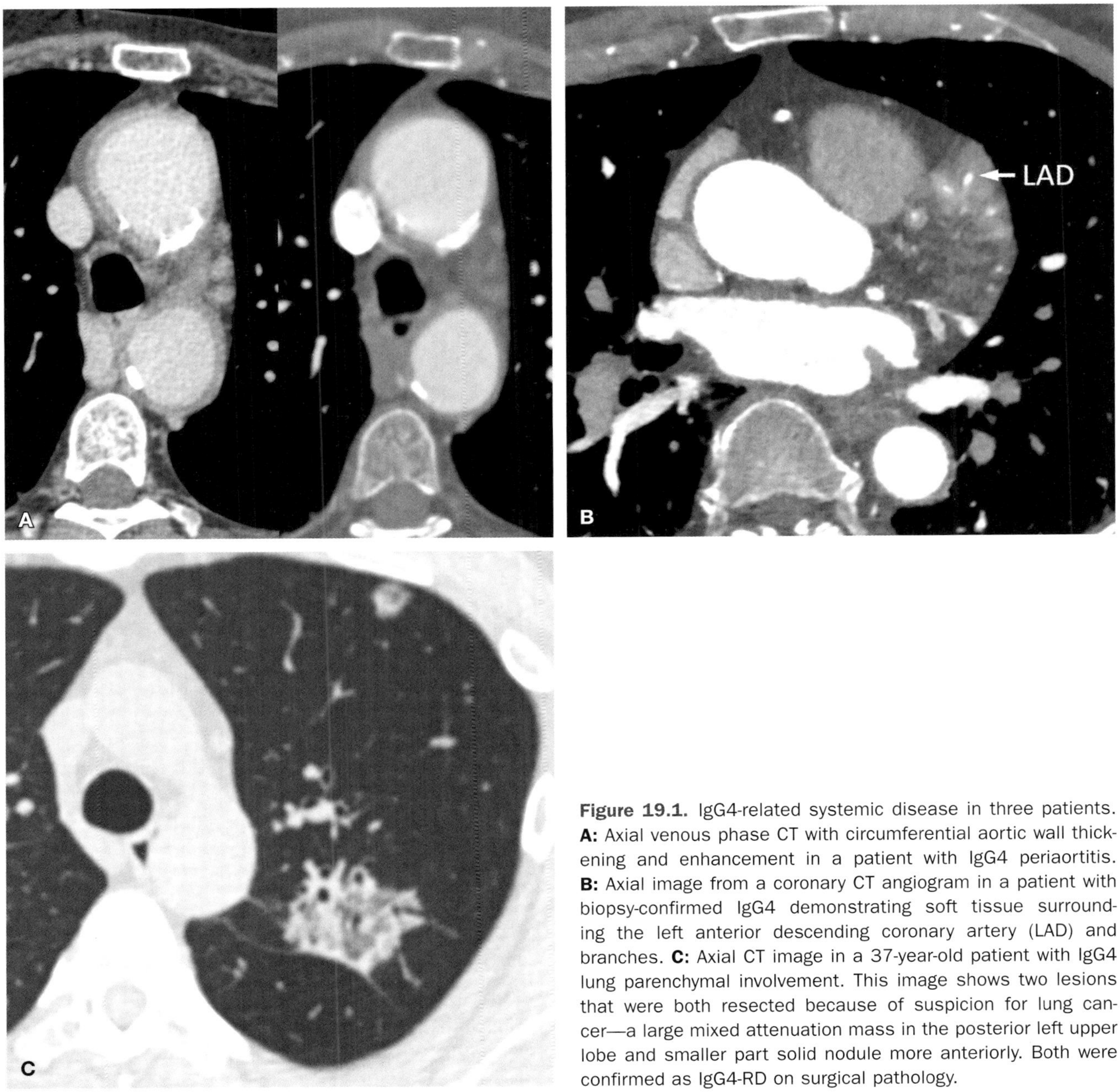

Figure 19.1. IgG4-related systemic disease in three patients. **A:** Axial venous phase CT with circumferential aortic wall thickening and enhancement in a patient with IgG4 periaortitis. **B:** Axial image from a coronary CT angiogram in a patient with biopsy-confirmed IgG4 demonstrating soft tissue surrounding the left anterior descending coronary artery (LAD) and branches. **C:** Axial CT image in a 37-year-old patient with IgG4 lung parenchymal involvement. This image shows two lesions that were both resected because of suspicion for lung cancer—a large mixed attenuation mass in the posterior left upper lobe and smaller part solid nodule more anteriorly. Both were confirmed as IgG4-RD on surgical pathology.

Table 19.3 Behcçet Disease

Young adults
Oral and genital ulcers, uveitis, and skin lesions
Most common in Middle East (Turkey) and Asia (Japan)
Hereditary factors, HLA-5
Vessel thrombosis, vascular obstruction, aneurysms
  Pulmonary artery aneurysm or rupture
  Superior vena cava thrombosis
  Mosaic perfusion
Ground-glass opacities or consolidation due to hemorrhage
Hemoptysis
Variant: Hughes-Stovin syndrome

Other organs and sites are commonly involved, including the joints (arthritis), heart, kidney, gastrointestinal system, and lung.

BD is most common in young adults (20-35 years) and is particularly common in the Middle East and East Asia. A familial incidence suggests hereditary factors, including HLA-5. The vasculitis of BD results in vessel thrombosis, vascular obstruction, aneurysms, and sometimes vessel rupture. Involvement of the lung or intrathoracic vessels occurs in about 5% to 10% of cases.

Pulmonary artery aneurysms, otherwise an uncommon entity, are frequent in BD involving the thorax. These appear as one or more, unilateral or bilateral, rounded hilar or perihilar opacities measuring up to several centimeters in diameter. On CT, these may opacify with contrast, may contain thrombus, or may not opacify because of thrombosis (Fig. 19.2). Poor definition of an aneurysm may be associated with surrounding hemorrhage. Hemoptysis may occur due to leakage or rupture of an aneurysm and may be massive and life threatening. Pulmonary artery aneurysm is thus associated with a poor prognosis.

Pulmonary artery thrombosis and occlusion may be associated with infarctions or focal pulmonary hemorrhage. Diffuse or patchy consolidation may also be seen, likely related to multiple areas of pulmonary hemorrhage.

Thrombosis of the superior vena cava and brachiocephalic veins may occur, resulting in superior vena cava syndrome, mediastinal edema, and widening of the mediastinum, as seen on chest radiographs. Pleural fluid may be seen, representing (1) effusion associated with pulmonary infarction, (2) hemothorax due to rupture of a pulmonary artery aneurysm, or (3) chylothorax due to great vein obstruction.

Hughes-Stovin syndrome, described in the 1950s, is characterized by pulmonary artery aneurysms, superior vena cava thrombosis, and thrombophlebitis. It likely represents BD or a variant of BD.

MEDIUM-SIZED VESSEL VASCULITIS

Polyarteritis Nodosa

Classic polyarteritis nodosa (PAN) typically affects small to medium systemic arteries, resulting in a necrotizing vasculitis. Involvement of arterioles, venules, and capillaries is absent, as is glomerulonephritis. Such abnormalities indicate the presence of MPA, described below, which may otherwise resemble PAN. Pulmonary artery involvement is rare. Pulmonary hemorrhage reported to occur in PAN may represent MPA.

SMALL VESSEL VASCULITIS USUALLY ASSOCIATED WITH ANCA

Small vessel vasculitis primary affects vessels smaller than arteries, such as arterioles, venules, and capillaries.

Granulomatosis With Polyangiitis

GPA, formerly known as Wegener granulomatosis, is a multisystem disease of unknown cause associated with involvement of the upper respiratory tract (nasal, oral, or sinus inflammation), lower respiratory tract (airway or lung), and kidney. Upper respiratory tract involvement occurs in nearly all patients; lung involvement occurs in 90%; glomerulonephritis occurs in 80% (Table 19.4).

Lung disease associated with GPA is characterized by granulomatous inflammation and necrotizing vasculitis. Limited GPA, involving only the lung, may occur.

GPA most commonly affects patients between the ages of 30 and 60 years. Most patients have sinusitis and cough, and hemoptysis is common. Renal disease associated with hematuria, proteinuria, and renal failure is ultimately present in 80% to 90% of patients, but as few as 40% have renal involvement at first presentation (Fig. 19.3). Musculoskeletal symptoms occur in about 30% of patients, usually consisting of arthralgia or arthritis. Neurologic manifestations occur in 20% to 35% of patients. Ocular or skin involvement may also occur.

Lung disease associated with GPA is characterized by a neutrophilic capillaritis, granulomatous inflammation, necrotizing vasculitis affecting small- and medium-sized vessels, and geographic parenchymal necrosis. The presence of serum cytoplasmic antineutrophilic cytoplasmic antibody (C-ANCA) is characteristic and is seen in as many as 90% to 95% of patients with active disease, but a smaller percentage of patients with inactive disease. C-ANCA is primarily associated with antibodies directed against proteinase 3 located in azurophilic granules of neutrophils and monocytes.

Untreated GPA is associated with a poor prognosis, with death usually occurring within 6 months of the onset of renal failure. However, there is a high remission rate following treatment with cyclophosphamide and steroids. Recurrence may be precipitated by infection.

At presentation, chest radiographic abnormalities are visible in 75% of patients with GPA.

Lung Nodules and Consolidation

Multiple lung nodules or masses are most common, being visible in more than half of patients at presentation (see Figs. 19.3 and 19.4). Typically, there are fewer than a dozen nodules visible. In most cases, the nodules are bilateral and widely distributed without predominance in any lung region, but may

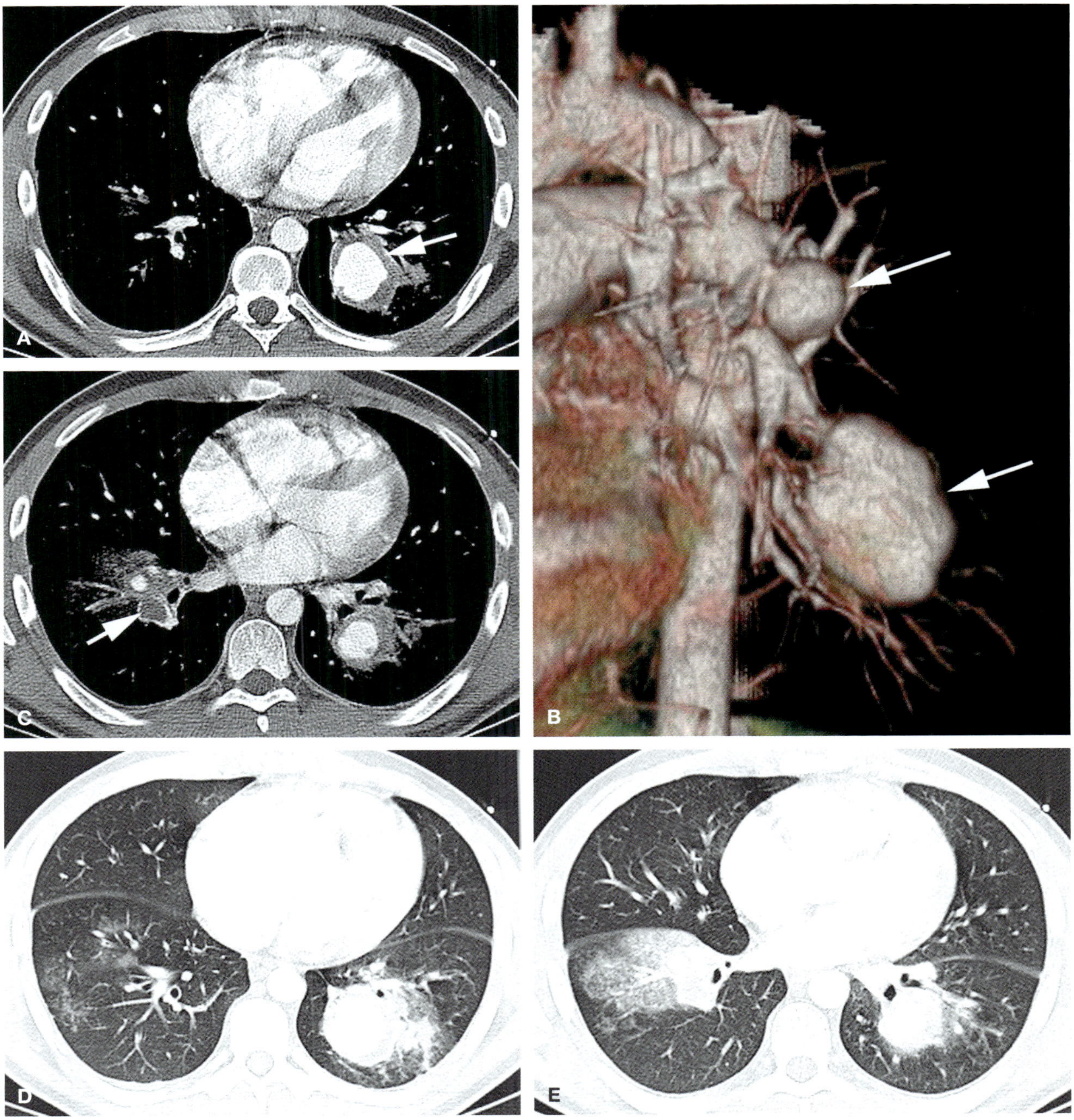

Figure 19.2. Behçet disease in a 25-year-old man with pulmonary artery aneurysms, pulmonary hemorrhage, and frank hemoptysis. **A:** Large left pulmonary artery aneurysm (*arrow*) is partially lined by thrombus and is densely opacified on a volumetric HRCT. **B:** Surface display reconstruction shows two left-sided pulmonary artery aneurysms (*arrows*). **C:** At a different level, an aneurysm is thrombosed (*arrow*). **D:** Lung window scan at the level of (**A**) shows poor definition of the aneurysm because of surrounding hemorrhage. Patchy and centrilobular hemorrhage is also visible in the right lower lobe. **E:** Lung window scan at the level of (**C**) shows right lower lobe hemorrhage. Vessels in the right lower lobe appear smaller than those in the anterior lung. This may be related to thrombosis shown in (**C**). This patient subsequently died as a result of aneurysm rupture.

Table 19.4 Granulomatosis With Polyangiitis

Multisystem disease
- Upper respiratory tract involved in nearly all patients
- Lung involvement occurs in 90%
- Glomerulonephritis occurs in 80%

Ages 30-60 y

Cytoplasmic antineutrophilic cytoplasmic antibody in 90%

Chest radiographs abnormal in 75% at presentation

Multiple nodules and masses
- Usually 2-4 cm
- Cavitation common
- Cavities become thin walled with treatment

Lung consolidation due to hemorrhage

Tracheobronchial involvement
- Tracheal wall thickening
- Subglottic trachea most often involved
- Luminal narrowing

appear peribronchial or peribronchovascular. A solitary nodule or mass may be seen, but this is less common. Masses usually range from 2 to 4 cm in diameter but may be much larger. Masses are round or oval and may be well defined or poorly defined. Calcification of the masses does not occur.

With progression of disease, nodules and masses tend to increase in size and number. With treatment, nodules usually resolve over a period of months. Complete resolution may occur.

Cavitation occurs in approximately 50% of cases (see Figs. 19.3 and 19.4). Cavities are usually thick walled, with an irregular inner margin. Air-fluid levels may be present. Typically, cavitary nodules and masses become thin walled (see Fig. 19.4) and decrease in size with treatment.

Air-space consolidation or ground-glass opacity is the second most common radiographic finding in GPA and may occur with or without associated lung nodules or masses. These areas of consolidation usually represent pulmonary hemorrhage. They may be focal, diffuse, or patchy (Figs. 19.5 and 19.6).

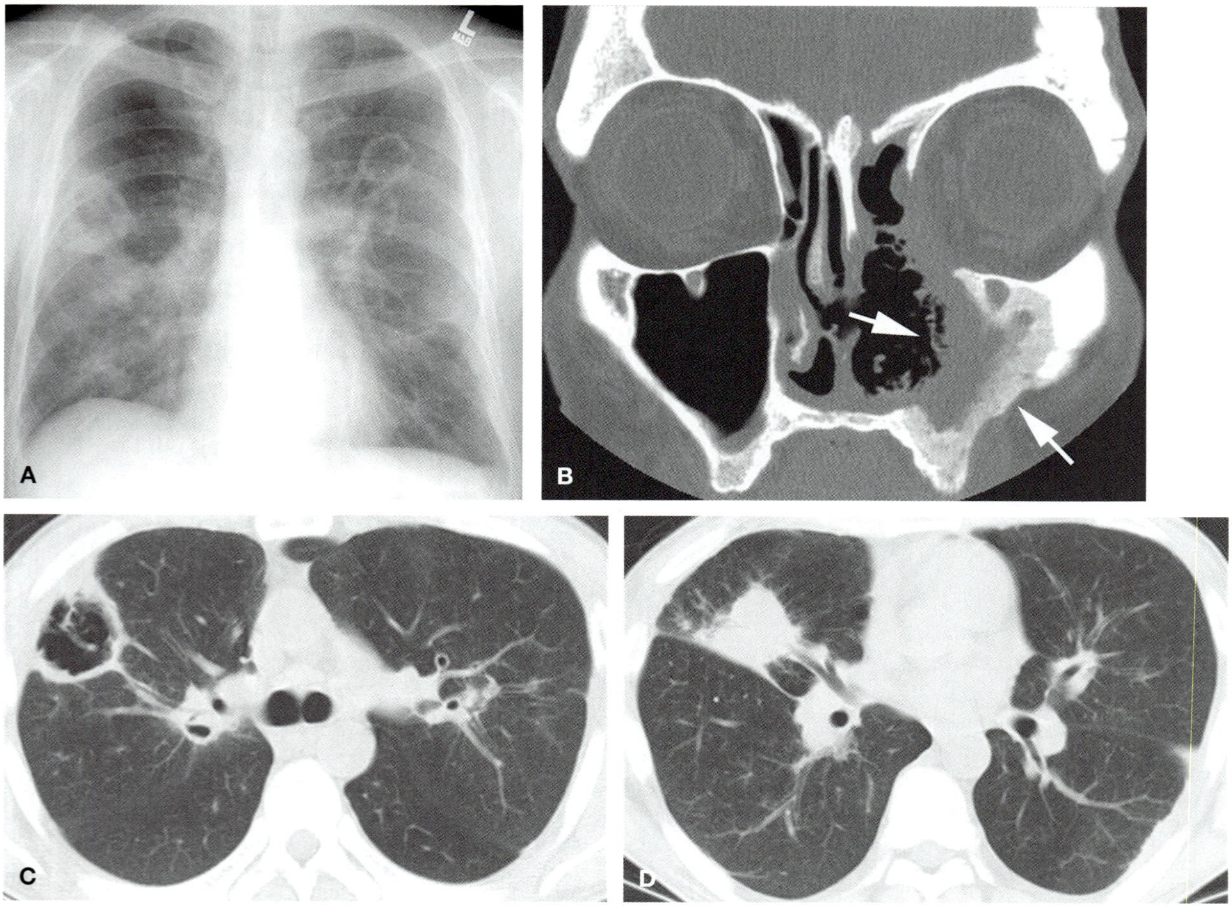

Figure 19.3. Granulomatosis with polyangiitis. **A:** Chest radiograph shows bilateral cavitary lung masses. **B:** Sinus CT shows soft-tissue thickening in the left maxilla with thickening and poor definition of the maxillary wall (*arrows*). **C, D:** Cavitary mass and solid soft-tissue masses are visible on CT.

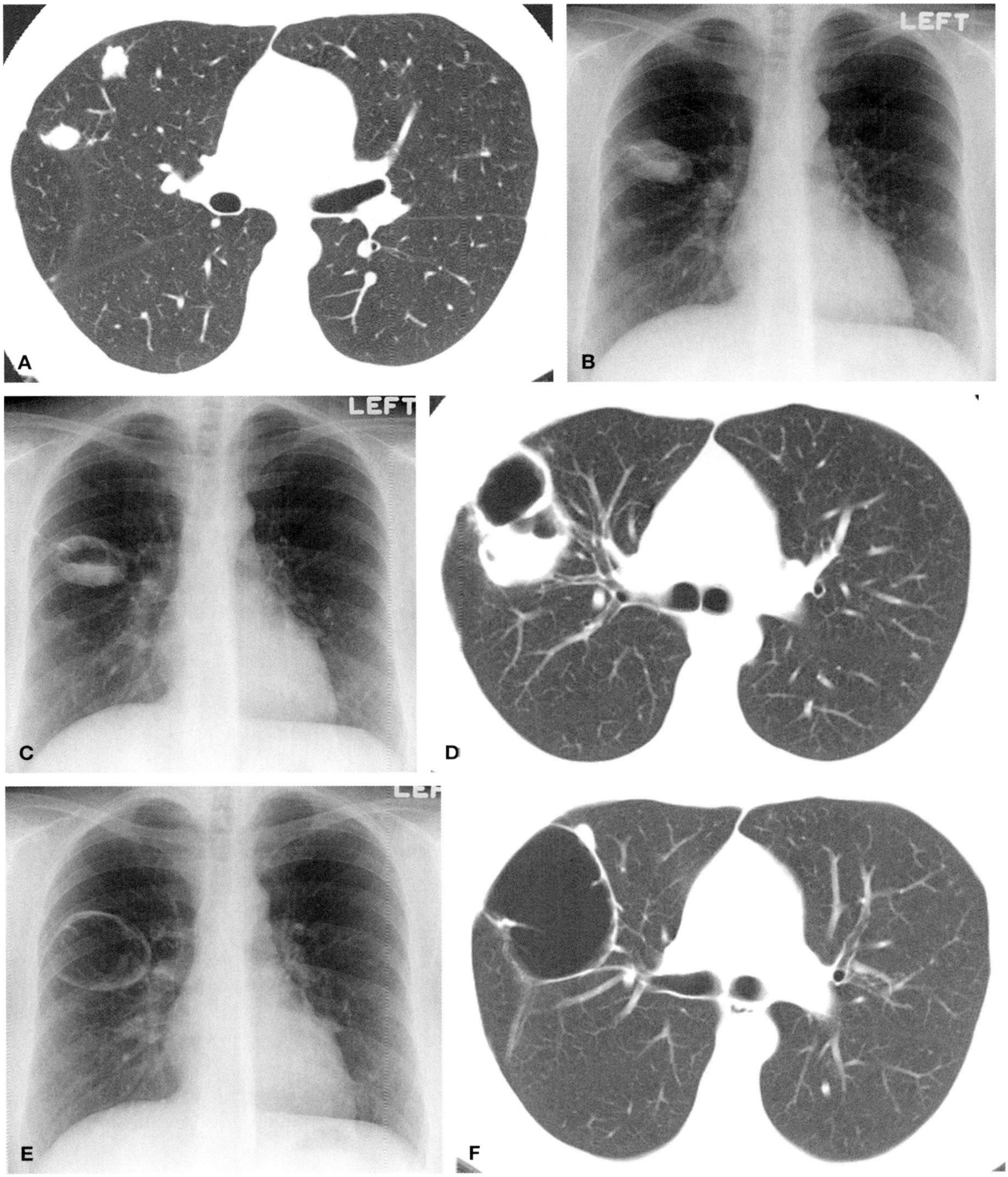

Figure 19.4. Granulomatosis with polyangiitis with progression. **A:** CT shows two small lung nodules. **B:** Chest radiograph 1 year later shows a right upper lobe mass containing an air-fluid level. Other ill-defined nodules are also visible. **C:** Two weeks after (**B**), there was an increase in the size of the right upper lobe mass with progressive cavitation. The cavity is thin walled, and an air-fluid level is again seen. **D:** CT 2 months after (**B**) shows an irregular cavitary mass. **E:** Radiograph 3 months after (**B**) shows a large thin-walled cavity. **F:** CT 5 months after (**B**) shows a persisting thin-walled cavity.

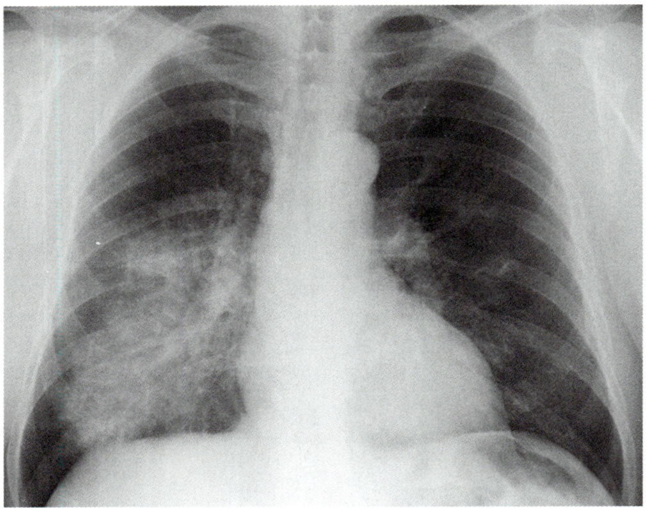

Figure 19.5. Focal pulmonary hemorrhage in granulomatosis with polyangiitis. Focal consolidation is visible in the right lower lobe.

Tracheobronchial Involvement

Tracheobronchial lesions occur in approximately 15% to 25% of patients with GPA. Concentric airway wall thickening due to inflammation, with narrowing of the airway lumen, is present. Involvement of the subglottic trachea is most typical (see Fig. 22.16 in Chapter 22), with variable involvement of the vocal cords, distal trachea, and proximal mainstem bronchi (see Fig. 22.17 in Chapter 22). Lobar or segmental bronchial wall thinking may also be seen. Segmental, lobar, or lung atelectasis may result.

Other Findings

Hilar or mediastinal lymph node enlargement may be seen, but this is uncommon and never an isolated finding. Pleural effusions occur in about 10% of cases. Pleural thickening or effusion may be seen. Centrilobular nodules have been reported, which may reflect vasculitis or hemorrhage. Aortitis has been reported in rare case reports.

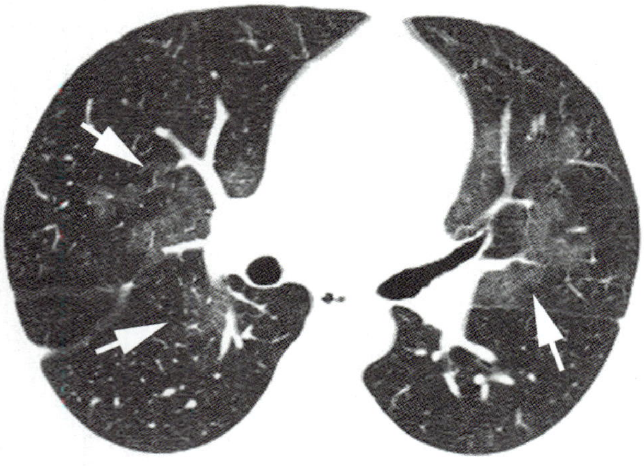

Figure 19.6. Patchy pulmonary hemorrhage in granulomatosis with polyangiitis. Patchy ground-glass opacity is visible on HRCT (*arrows*).

EGPA (Churg-Strauss Syndrome)

EGPA is a necrotizing vasculitis of small- to medium-sized vessels with eosinophilic and granulomatous inflammation. It is also discussed in Chapter 17 (Table 17.9).

In 50% to 75% of patients, EGPA is associated with ANCA, usually P-ANCA (perinuclear pattern), with antibodies directed against a wide variety of intracellular antigens, most frequently myeloperoxidase. EGPA is characterized by a triad of (1) asthma, (2) hypereosinophilia, and (3) necrotizing vasculitis.

EGPA often shows findings of simple pulmonary eosinophilia or chronic eosinophilic pneumonia (ie, peripheral areas of consolidation). CT findings are variable and reflect the different pulmonary manifestations of this disease. Findings include (1) consolidation or ground-glass opacity (60%), which may have a peripheral distribution or be patchy and geographic; (2) pulmonary nodules or masses (20%) ranging from 0.5 to 3.5 cm in diameter, which may contain air bronchograms (Fig. 17.22); (3) bronchial wall thickening or bronchiectasis (35%); and (4) interlobular septal thickening due to pulmonary edema (5%) and associated with cardiac involvement. Although cavitation of nodules or masses may occur, it is much less common than with GPA, which it may resemble clinically and radiographically. EGPA is described in detail in Chapter 17.

Microscopic Polyangiitis

MPA results in systemic necrotizing small vessel vasculitis. Although the histology is similar to classic PAN, involvement of arterioles, venules, and capillaries is not seen in PAN, but occurs in MPA. Also, ANCA (usually P-ANCA) is present in 80%; ANCA is rare in PAN.

MPA typically occurs in middle-aged adults. Glomerulonephritis develops in 90% of patients, and other organs may be involved. Pulmonary hemorrhage related to capillaritis occurs in 25%, associated with dyspnea and hemoptysis. Radiographic findings are typical of pulmonary hemorrhage. Pleural effusion and pulmonary edema are seen in about 10%, likely related to renal disease. Progression to pulmonary fibrosis is rare. Treatment with cyclophosphamide and steroids often results in remission.

DIFFUSE ALVEOLAR HEMORRHAGE

DAH can result from a variety of diseases and insults, and making a specific diagnosis may be difficult. DAH can be associated with the various causes of large, medium, or small pulmonary vessel vasculitis discussed above (GPA, EGPA, MPA, BD) (Figs. 19.5 and 19.6) or the deposition of immune complexes in the walls of small vessels and capillaries. DAH may also be seen in association with pulmonary capillaritis occurring without other manifestations of vasculitis (Table 19.1) and may be seen in patients without capillaritis or other manifestations of vasculitis (Table 19.5).

Table 19.5 Causes of Diffuse Alveolar Hemorrhage Unassociated With Capillaritis

Idiopathic pulmonary hemosiderosis
Systemic lupus erythematosus (some cases)
Goodpasture syndrome (some cases)
Diffuse alveolar damage
Elevated pulmonary venous pressure
Anticoagulation
Coagulation disorders and thrombocytopenia
Inhalation injury, toxic exposures
Barotrauma
Drug-associated disease (eg, chemotherapy)
Illicit drug use (particularly cocaine smoking)
Pulmonary veno-occlusive disease
Pulmonary capillary hemangiomatosis
Lymphangioleiomyomatosis

Radiographic findings in diseases causing DAH are often identical, regardless of its cause. In general, radiographs and high-resolution CT (HRCT) show focal, patchy, or diffuse consolidation or ground-glass opacity in the presence of acute hemorrhage (see Figs. 19.5-19.12). Ill-defined centrilobular nodules may be seen and predominate in some patients (Fig. 19.12); these are sometimes visible on radiographs but are easiest to see on HRCT. Chest radiographs may be normal or show very subtle abnormalities in patients with pulmonary hemorrhage.

Opacities may be diffuse with uniform lung involvement or may show a central and perihilar predominance with relative sparing of the apices, lung periphery, and costophrenic angles. Pleural effusions are not generally associated with pulmonary hemorrhage, although they may be seen in patients with coincident renal failure.

Within a few days of an acute episode of hemorrhage, hemosiderin-laden macrophages begin to accumulate in the interstitium. This occurrence is manifested on chest radiographs by the presence of Kerley lines, which may be seen in isolation or in conjunction with residual consolidation or ground-glass opacity. On HRCT, interlobular septal thickening may replace or be seen in association with ground-glass opacity (Fig. 19.13). Unless further hemorrhage occurs, complete clearing of air-space and interstitial opacities usually occurs within 10 days to 2 weeks of an acute episode of hemorrhage. This is considerably slower than clearing of pulmonary edema, which hemorrhage may closely resemble.

In patients with recurrent episodes of pulmonary hemorrhage, a persistent reticular abnormality may be seen between episodes of bleeding. This reflects interstitial hemosiderin deposition and mild lung fibrosis and has been termed *pulmonary hemosiderosis.*

DAH WITH PULMONARY CAPILLARITIS

Pulmonary capillaritis is characterized by inflammation and neutrophilic infiltration of the alveolar interstitium and pulmonary capillaries, fibrinoid necrosis, disruption of the epithelial-endothelial basement membrane, leakage of red blood cells and neutrophils into the alveolar spaces (ie, DAH), and thrombi within the alveolar capillaries and venules. With time, hemosiderin and hemosiderin-containing macrophages accumulate in the alveoli and interstitium.

Primary Immune Complex–Mediated Vasculitis

Diseases in this category include Goodpasture syndrome, Henoch-Schönlein purpura, and BD (described above).

Goodpasture Syndrome

Antiglomerular basement membrane disease (Goodpasture syndrome) most typically occurs in patients aged 20 to 30; males are affected four times as commonly

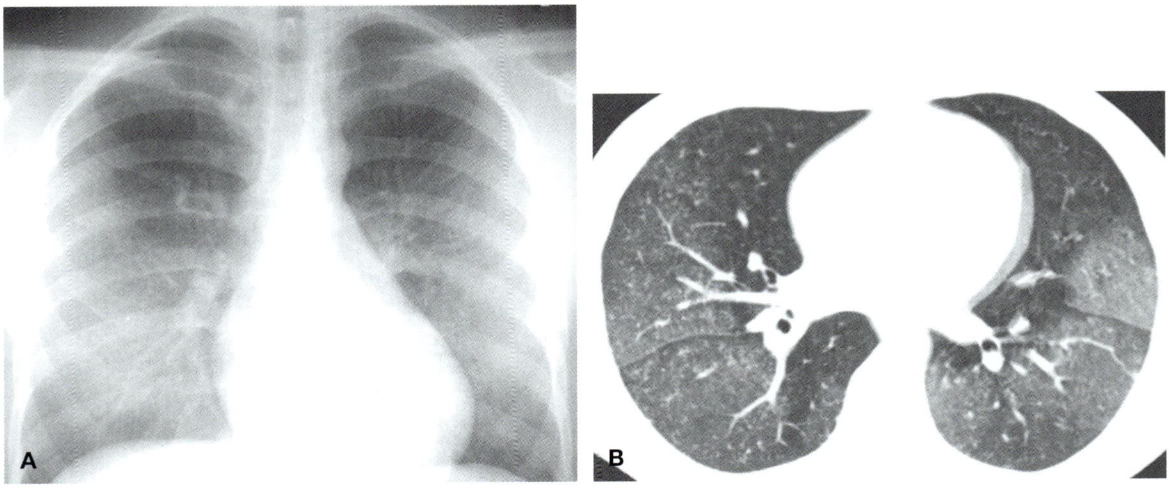

Figure 19.7. Goodpasture syndrome. **A:** Chest radiograph shows a subtle increase in lung opacity. **B:** HRCT shows patchy ground-glass opacity.

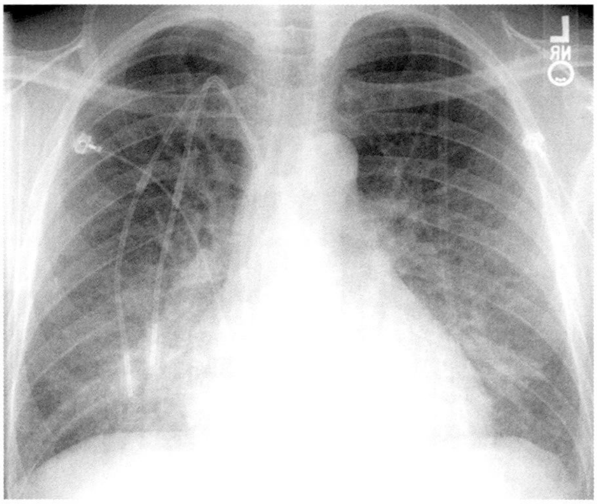

Figure 19.8. Goodpasture syndrome. Chest radiograph shows ill-defined parahilar and lower lobe opacities. The heart appears enlarged because of renal failure and fluid overload, and a dialysis catheter is in place.

as females (Table 19.6). Hemoptysis, usually mild, and anemia are present in 90%. Other symptoms include cough, dyspnea, and weakness. Findings of renal disease are usually but not always present, including hematuria, proteinuria, and renal failure. Antiglomerular basement membrane antibodies are almost always (95%) present in the serum. These antibodies are directed against type IV collagen and cross-react with alveolar basement membrane. Although Goodpasture syndrome does not result in a systemic vasculitis, it may be classified as a small vessel vasculitis because pulmonary capillaritis is present. Renal biopsy shows glomerulonephritis with linear deposition of IgG in the glomeruli.

Although plain radiographs may be normal, they usually show diffuse air-space consolidation or ground-glass opacity, typically bilateral and symmetrical and often with a perihilar predominance (Figs. 19.7A and 19.8). HRCT usually shows consolidation or ground-glass opacity and may be abnormal in the face of subtle plain film findings or normal radiographs (see Fig. 19.7B).

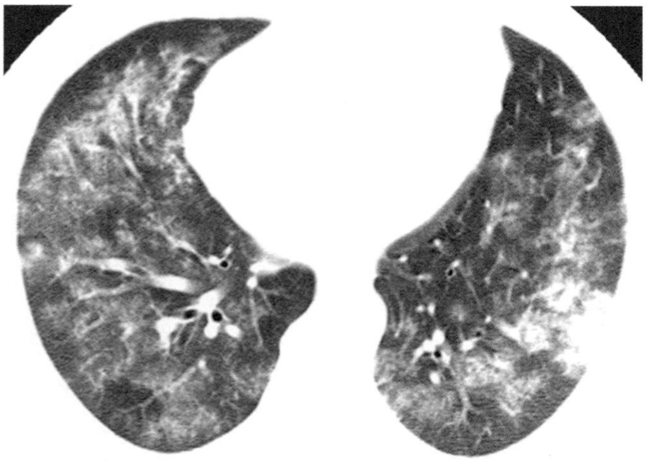

Figure 19.9. Pulmonary hemorrhage in systemic lupus erythematosus with a parahilar predominance. Patchy ground-glass opacities and consolidation are visible.

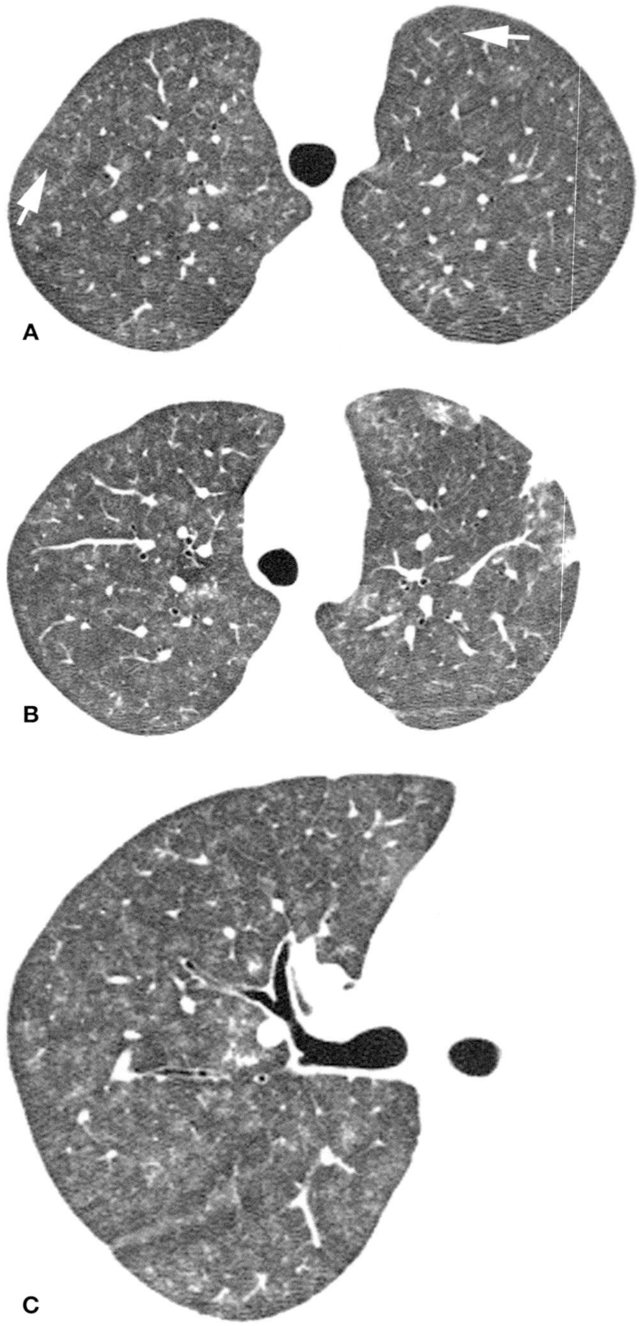

Figure 19.10. Pulmonary hemorrhage associated with systemic lupus erythematosus. **A:** HRCT shows ill-defined centrilobular ground-glass opacities representing hemorrhage. A few thickened interlobular septa are also seen (*arrows*). **B, C:** Centrilobular areas of ground-glass opacity are visible at lower levels. Lobular areas of consolidation (**B**) are also seen.

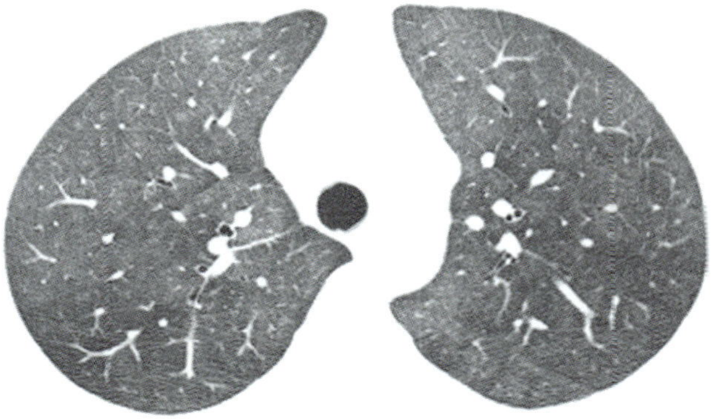

Figure 19.11. Pulmonary hemorrhage in systemic lupus erythematosus. Patchy ground-glass opacity is visible on HRCT.

After an acute episode of hemorrhage, the air-space opacities tend to resolve, being superseded by an interstitial abnormality or septal thickening.

Henoch-Schönlein Purpura

Henoch-Schönlein purpura is characterized by abnormalities of small vessels (capillaries, venules, or arterioles) associated with IgA-predominant deposits. Symptoms include purpura, abdominal pain, gastrointestinal hemorrhage, arthralgia, and glomerulonephritis, although not all are typically present and glomerulonephritis occurs in only 20%. It may occur at any age, but is usually seen in young children and often follows a respiratory tract infection. Relapses are common, but the prognosis is good. Chronic renal failure develops in a small number of cases.

Pulmonary involvement occurs in as many as 5% of patients. Diffuse or patchy consolidation may result from capillaritis and pulmonary hemorrhage. Hemoptysis is often associated. Pleural effusion may be seen.

Secondary Vasculitis

Deposition of immune complexes in the walls of small vessels and capillaries occurs in association with number of diseases or conditions, resulting in capillaritis and pulmonary hemorrhage. Collagen vascular diseases are most common.

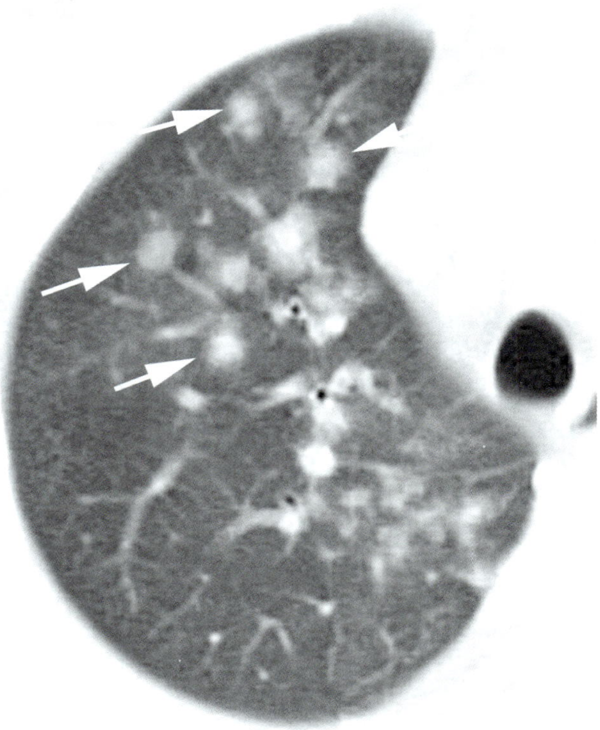

Figure 19.12. Centrilobular nodules in pulmonary hemorrhage. CT scan in a patient with systemic lupus erythematosus and pulmonary hemorrhage shows ill-defined centrilobular nodules (*arrows*).

Collagen Vascular Diseases

Diffuse pulmonary hemorrhage may occur with many collagen diseases, probably associated with circulating immune complexes and small vessel vasculitis. Systemic lupus erythematosus is most common (see Figs. 19.9-19.12).

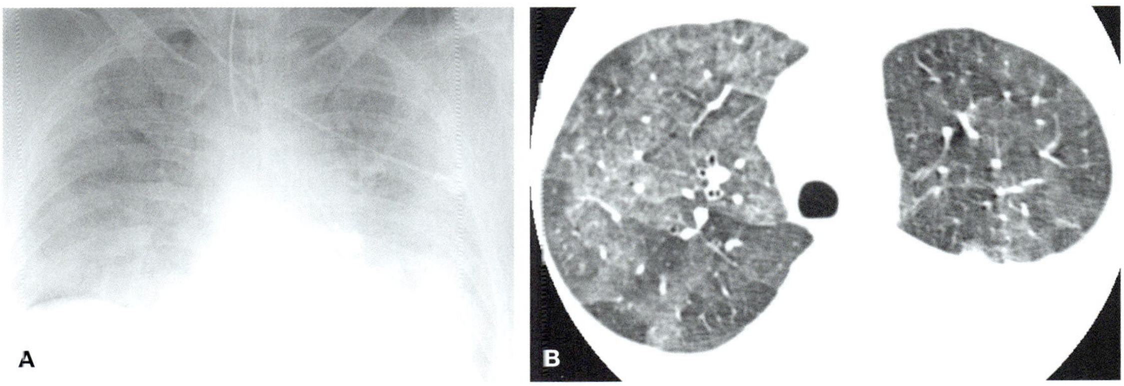

Figure 19.13. Pulmonary hemorrhage associated with leukemia and thrombocytopenia. **A:** Chest radiograph shows ill-defined increased lung opacity. **B:** HRCT shows patchy areas of ground-glass opacity with some thickened interlobular septa. A left pleural effusion is also present.

Table 19.6 Goodpasture Syndrome
Antiglomerular basement membrane antibodies in 95%
Glomerulonephritis
Age 20-30 y
Hemoptysis and anemia in 90%
Consolidation or ground-glass opacity

Hemoptysis often occurs and may be massive. Radiographic and HRCT findings are similar to other causes of diffuse pulmonary hemorrhage. The pulmonary manifestations of the collagen diseases are described in Chapter 15.

Essential Cryoglobulinemia

This disease is characterized by involvement of small vessels with purpura, arthralgia, glomerulonephritis, hepatosplenomegaly, and lymph node enlargement. Serum globulins that precipitate with cold are present. Many cases are related to hepatitis C infection; others are associated with other infections, lymphoma, lymphoproliferative disease, or collagen vascular diseases. Pulmonary disease is uncommon and difficult to characterize. Findings of DAH or a reticular pattern may be seen.

DAH WITHOUT PULMONARY CAPILLARITIS

DAH may be seen in a number of diseases or conditions in which capillaritis is absent (Table 19.5; Fig. 19.13). Histologic findings are largely limited to alveolar hemorrhage and alveolar and interstitial hemosiderin–laden macrophages.

One cause, idiopathic pulmonary hemosiderosis, is included in this chapter because of its resemblance to Goodpasture syndrome.

Idiopathic Pulmonary Hemosiderosis

IPH is a disease of unknown origin characterized by recurrent episodes of diffuse pulmonary hemorrhage without associated glomerulonephritis or a specific serologic abnormality (Table 19.7). Pathologic findings include alveolar hemorrhage, hemosiderin-laden macrophages, and a variable degree of interstitial fibrosis in long-standing cases, but capillaritis is absent. Hemosiderosis and interstitial fibrosis may develop with recurrent episodes of hemorrhage in long-standing cases.

Table 19.7 Idiopathic Pulmonary Hemosiderosis
No serologic abnormalities
No glomerulonephritis
Children or young adults
Associated with exposure to toxic mold, other conditions

IPH most commonly occurs in children under the age of 10 or young adults. In adults, men are affected twice as often as women. IPH is sometimes associated with celiac disease, cow's milk allergy, thyroid disease, or immunoglobulin A gammopathy and has recently been reported in infants with exposure to toxic mold (*Stachybotrys*). Symptoms include cough, hemoptysis, dyspnea, and anemia. The diagnosis is usually made by exclusion. About a quarter of patients die as a result of respiratory insufficiency or cor pulmonale.

Plain radiographic and HRCT findings are similar to those of Goodpasture syndrome. Predominant findings in the acute phase of disease include diffuse ground-glass opacity (Fig. 19.14). On HRCT, ill-defined centrilobular nodular opacities may also be seen. Hemosiderosis and fibrosis may develop with recurrent episodes of hemorrhage.

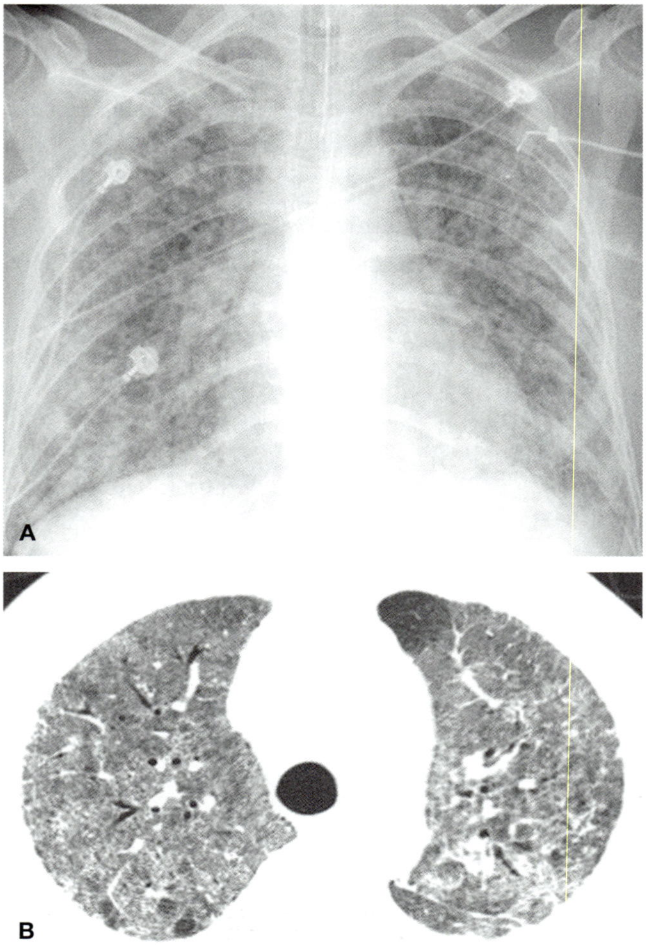

Figure 19.14. Diffuse pulmonary hemorrhage in idiopathic pulmonary hemosiderosis. **A:** Interstitial opacities are visible bilaterally. The appearance is nonspecific. **B:** HRCT in a different patient with pulmonary hemorrhage shows diffuse ground-glass opacity.

SUGGESTED READINGS

Aberle DR, Gamsu G, Lynch D. Thoracic manifestations of Wegener granulomatosis: diagnosis and course. *Radiology*. 1990;174(3 pt 1):703-709.

Brown KK. Pulmonary vasculitis. *Proc Am Thorac Soc*. 2006;3(1):48-57.

Castañer E, Alguersuari A, Gallardo X, et al. When to suspect pulmonary vasculitis: radiologic and clinical clues. *Radiographics*. 2010;30(1):33-53.

Cheah FK, Sheppard MN, Hansell DM. Computed tomography of diffuse pulmonary haemorrhage with pathological correlation. *Clin Radiol*. 1993;48(2):89-93.

Collard HR, Schwarz MI. Diffuse alveolar hemorrhage. *Clin Chest Med*. 2004;25(3):583-592.

Connolly B, Manson D, Eberhard A, Laxer RM, Smith C. CT appearance of pulmonary vasculitis in children. *AJR Am J Roentgenol*. 1996;167(4): 901-904.

Cordier JF, Valeyre D, Guillevin L, Loire R, Brechot JM. Pulmonary Wegener's granulomatosis. A clinical and imaging study of 77 cases. *Chest*. 1990;97(4):906-912.

Feragalli B, Mantini C, Sperandeo M, et al. The lung in systemic vasculitis: radiological patterns and differential diagnosis. *Br J Radiol* 2016;89(1061):20150992. doi:10.1259/bjr.20150992

Hoffman GS, Kerr GS, Leavitt RY, et al. Wegener granulomatosis: an analysis of 158 patients. *Ann Intern Med*. 1992;116(6):488-498.

Ioachimescu OC, Sieber S, Kotch A. Idiopathic pulmonary haemosiderosis revisited. *Eur Respir J*. 2004;24(1):162-170.

Jennette JC, Falk RJ, Andrassy K, et al. Nomenclature of systemic vasculitides. Proposal of an international consensus conference. *Arthritis Rheum*. 1994;37(2):187-192.

Lee KS, Kim TS, Fujimoto K, et al. Thoracic manifestation of Wegener's granulomatosis: CT findings in 30 patients. *Eur Radiol*. 2003;13(1):43-51.

Marten K, Schnyder P, Schirg E, Prokop M, Rummeny EJ, Engelke C. Pattern-based differential diagnosis in pulmonary vasculitis using volumetric CT. *AJR Am J Roentgenol*. 2005;184(3):720-733.

Mayberry JP, Primack SL, Müller NL. Thoracic manifestations of systemic autoimmune diseases: radiographic and high-resolution CT findings. *Radiographics*. 2000;20(6):1623-1635.

Ozer C, Duce MN, Ulubas B, et al. Inspiratory and expiratory HRCT findings in Behcet's disease and correlation with pulmonary function tests. *Eur J Radiol*. 2005;56(1):43-47.

Perugino CA, Wallace ZS, Meyersohn N, Oliveira G, Stone JR, Stone JH. Large vessel involvement by IgG4-related disease. *Medicine*. 2016;95(28):e3344. doi:10.1097/MD.0000000000003344

Primack SL, Müller NL. Radiologic manifestations of the systemic autoimmune diseases. *Clin Chest Med*. 1998;19(4):573-586.

Primack SL, Miller RR, Müller NL. Diffuse pulmonary hemorrhage: clinical, pathologic, and imaging features. *AJR Am J Roentgenol*. 1995;164(2):295-300.

Reuter M, Schnabel A, Wesner F, et al. Pulmonary Wegener's granulomatosis: correlation between high-resolution CT findings and clinical scoring of disease activity. *Chest*. 1998;114(2):500-506.

Seely JM, Effmann EL, Müller NL. High-resolution CT of pediatric lung disease: imaging findings. *AJR Am J Roentgenol*. 1997;168(5): 1269-1275.

Seo JB, Im JG, Chung JW, et al. Pulmonary vasculitis: the spectrum of radiological findings. *Br J Radiol*. 2000;73(875):1224-1231.

Tunaci A, Berkmen YM, Gokmen E. Thoracic involvement in Behcet's disease: pathologic, clinical, and imaging features. *AJR Am J Roentgenol*. 1995;164(1):51-56.

Weir IH, Müller NL, Chiles C, Godwin JD, Lee SH, Kullnig P. Wegener's granulomatosis: findings from computed tomography of the chest in 10 patients. *Can Assoc Radiol J*. 1992;43(1):31-34.

Witte R, Gurney J, Robbins R, et al. Diffuse pulmonary alveolar hemorrhage after bone marrow transplantation: radiographic findings in 39 patients. *AJR Am J Roentgenol*. 1991;157(3):461-464.

Chapter 20

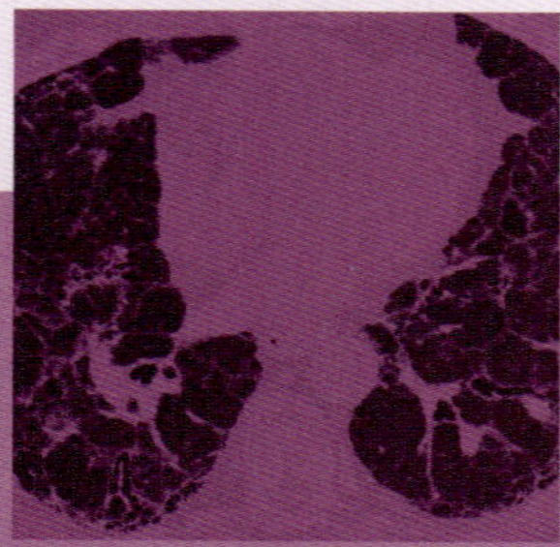

Travis S. Henry

Diffuse Lung Disease Associated With Lipid: Exogenous Lipid Pneumonia and Alveolar Proteinosis

ENDOGENOUS LIPOID PNEUMONIA

Lipoid pneumonia (lung consolidation containing lipids) may be endogenous or exogenous. Endogenous lipoid pneumonia may occur due to bronchial obstruction with accumulation of lipid-rich cellular debris distal to the obstructing lesion; this is sometimes termed "golden pneumonia" because of its yellow color at gross pathology. The term "postobstructive pneumonia" usually suffices for this condition.

EXOGENOUS LIPOID PNEUMONIA

Exogenous lipoid pneumonia results from the chronic aspiration or inhalation of animal-, vegetable-, or petroleum-based oils or fats (Table 20.1). Petroleum-based oil (mineral oil) aspiration is most common, usually associated with its use as a laxative. Responsible animal-based oils (eg, cod liver and shark liver oils, clarified butter) and vegetable-based oils are usually aspirated during ingestion or because of esophageal motility abnormalities with reflux.

Acute aspiration results in an aspiration pneumonia. Chronic aspiration results in lipoid pneumonia associated with variable fibrosis and inflammation. The degree of lung inflammation or fibrosis associated with the aspirated oil is related to the amount of free fatty acid present. Animal fats generally result in more inflammation and fibrosis than vegetable or mineral oils because they are hydrolyzed by lung lipases, releasing fatty acids.

A large quantity of oily material must usually be aspirated over a period of time before symptoms develop. Symptoms include cough, mild fever, and chest discomfort; they are least common with mineral oil aspiration. Fat may be identified in the sputum in some patients.

Radiographic and CT Findings

Consolidation, ill-defined masses, or sometimes findings of fibrosis are seen on chest radiographs (Figs. 20.1A and 20.3A). A lower lobe distribution is typical but not always present. Opacities may be bilateral or unilateral. The radiographic appearance is nonspecific.

CT shows masses that may be well defined or ill defined, or areas of consolidation. As on chest radiographs, these areas tend to have a lower lobe predominance and are often bilateral. A dependent location is also typical. Bronchi may be seen leading to the abnormal areas.

If a large amount of lipid has been aspirated, CT can show areas of low-attenuation consolidation that looks like macroscopic fat (−35 to −75 HU) or low-attenuation regions within larger masses (see Figs. 20.1B-E and 20.2B); this appearance is most common in patients with chronic mineral oil aspiration. Because inflammation or fibrosis accompanies the presence of the lipid material, the CT attenuation of the consolidation or mass need not be low, but often small areas of low-attenuation oil are visible (see Figs. 20.1D and E, and 20.2B). In some patients, necrosis and cavitation are present.

Table 20.1 Exogenous Lipid Pneumonia

Chronic aspiration of animal-, vegetable-, or petroleum-based oils or fats
Esophageal dysmotility or reflux
Variable fibrosis and inflammation
Consolidation or masses
Usually dependent or lower lobe
CT
Well-defined or ill-defined masses
Variable amounts of low-attenuation fat (−35 to −75 HU)
Necrosis or cavitation
Patchy ground-glass opacity or crazy paving

In patients with less severe abnormalities, ground-glass opacity or crazy paving (ground-glass opacity in association with interlobular septal thickening) or centrilobular nodules may also be seen on CT (see Fig. 20.3B). Subpleural pulmonary fibrosis and honeycombing are occasionally encountered. Some resolution of abnormalities is possible with time.

PULMONARY ALVEOLAR PROTEINOSIS

Pulmonary alveolar proteinosis (PAP) is a disease characterized by filling of the alveolar spaces with a PAS-positive proteinaceous, surfactant-like material, rich in lipid. Histologically, this represents the intra-alveolar accumulation of foamy macrophages, along with elevated levels of surfactant proteins and granular debris. The lung interstitium is largely normal, although the lipoprotein may also accumulate within interlobular septa.

Three clinically distinct forms of this disease have been described: (1) *congenital PAP*, accounting for 2% of cases, due to mutations in genes encoding surfactant B or C or the βc chain of the receptor for granulocyte-macrophage colony–stimulating factor (GM-CSF); (2) *secondary PAP*, occurring in association with a wide variety of disorders, including inhalation of silica (acute silicosis or silicoproteinosis) (Fig. 20.6), infection (eg, *Pneumocystis jirovecii*), hematologic and lymphatic malignancies, and immunodeficiency (eg, immunosuppressive treatments, chemotherapy, AIDS); and (3) an acquired form of the disease unassociated with other conditions (*idiopathic/autoimmune PAP*).

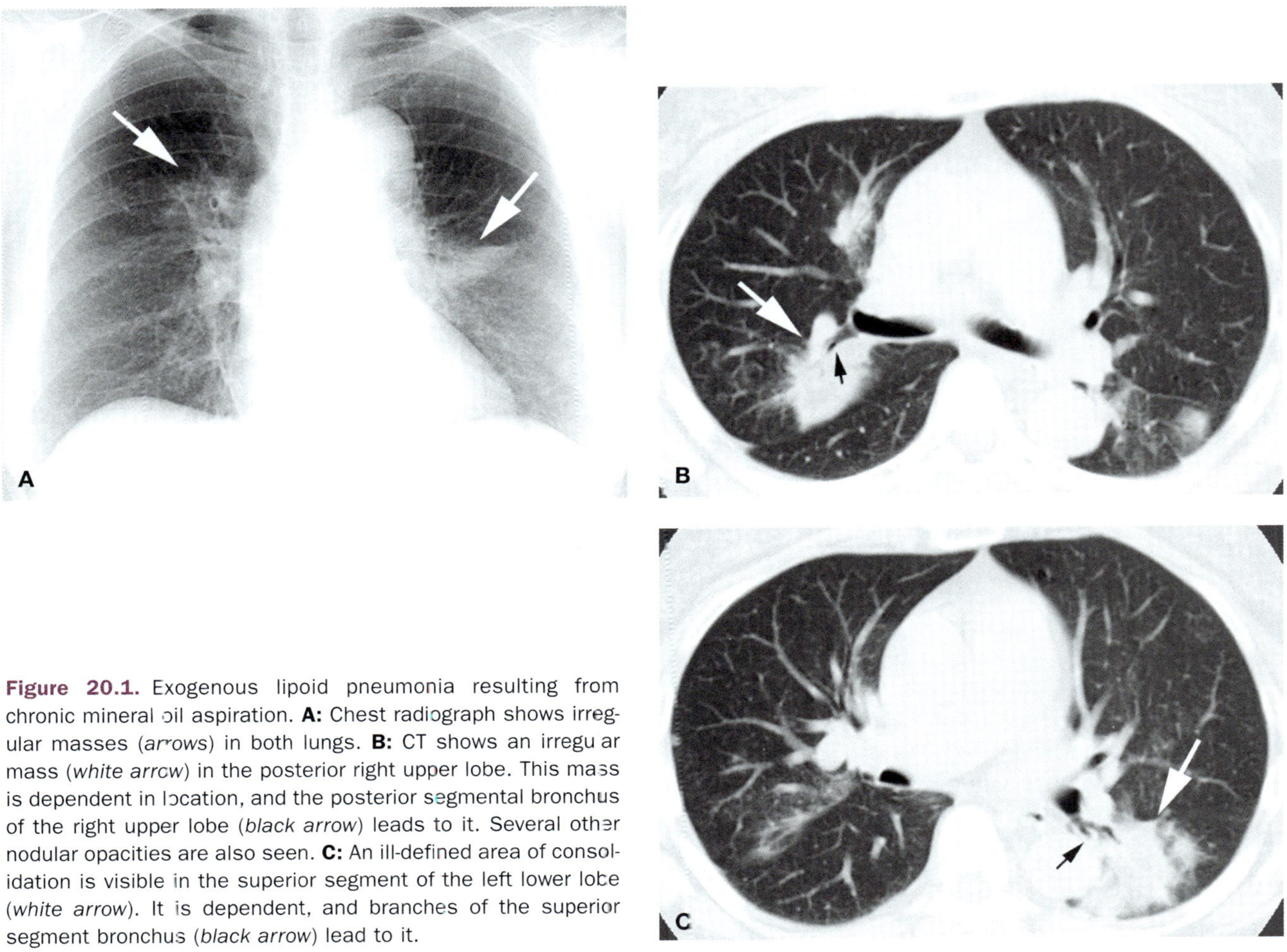

Figure 20.1. Exogenous lipoid pneumonia resulting from chronic mineral oil aspiration. **A:** Chest radiograph shows irregular masses (*arrows*) in both lungs. **B:** CT shows an irregular mass (*white arrow*) in the posterior right upper lobe. This mass is dependent in location, and the posterior segmental bronchus of the right upper lobe (*black arrow*) leads to it. Several other nodular opacities are also seen. **C:** An ill-defined area of consolidation is visible in the superior segment of the left lower lobe (*white arrow*). It is dependent, and branches of the superior segment bronchus (*black arrow*) lead to it.

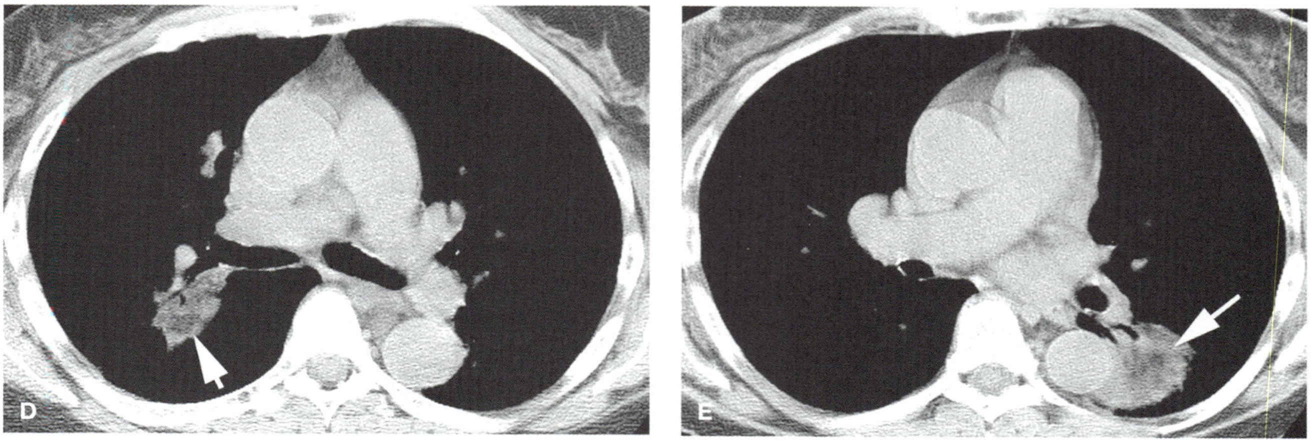

Figure 20.1. (*Continued*) **D, E:** Soft-tissue window scans at the same levels as (**B**) and (**C**) show low attenuation (−75 HU; *arrows*) within these masses.

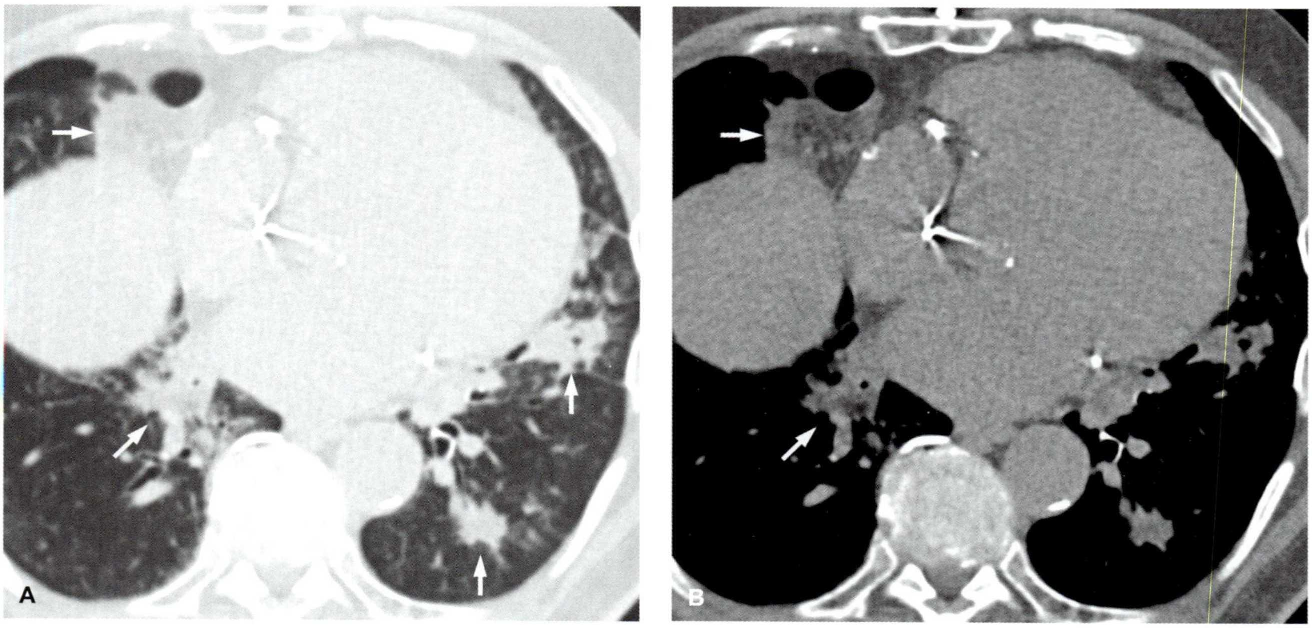

Figure 20.2. Exogenous lipoid pneumonia resulting from chronic mineral oil aspiration. **A:** A: Axial CT at lung windows shows multiple nodular areas of consolidation with irregular margins in the lower lobes (arrows). **B:** Same level of the CT on soft-tissue windows shows that the areas of consolidation contain macroscopic fat, best appreciated in the larger areas within the right lung (arrows).

Idiopathic PAP accounts for nearly 90% of cases. Idiopathic PAP is an autoimmune disease in which autoantibodies block GM-CSF signaling, which prevents macrophages from clearing surfactant from alveoli. The result is a disruption in surfactant homeostasis (Table 20.2).

Patients range in age from a few months to more than 70 years, with two-thirds of patients being between 30 and 50 years old. Symptoms are usually mild and of insidious onset. They include nonproductive cough, fever, and mild dyspnea on exertion. About 30% of patients are asymptomatic.

Radiographic and HRCT Findings

Radiographic manifestations of PAP include bilateral, patchy, diffuse, or parahilar air-space consolidation or hazy ground-glass opacity, which is usually most severe in the lung bases (Figs. 20.4A and 20.5A); dense consolidation and air bronchograms are rare. Although reticular opacities may be seen, they are usually mild. The radiographic appearance often resembles that of pulmonary edema, except for the absence of cardiomegaly and pleural effusion.

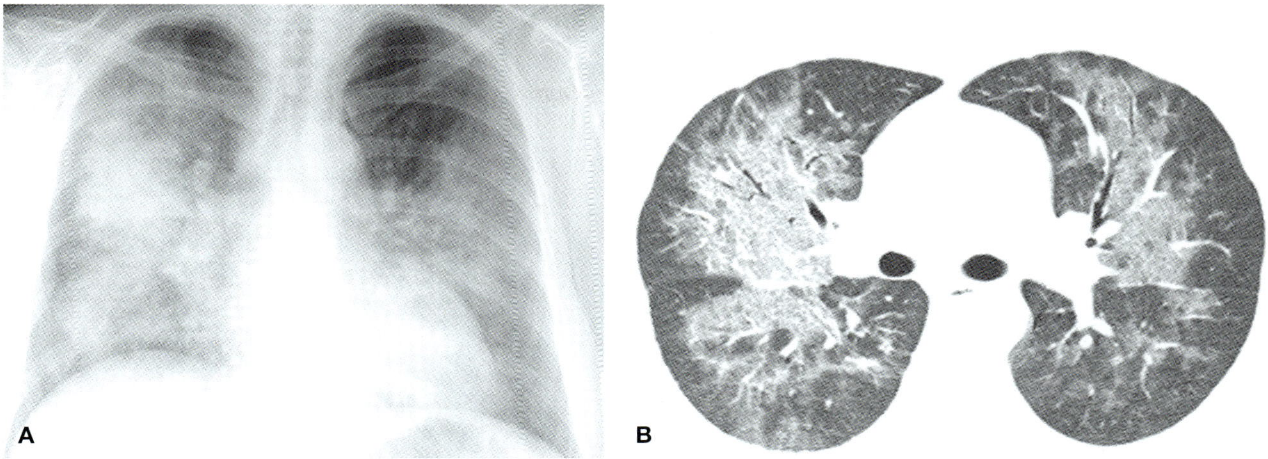

Figure 20.3. Exogenous lipoid pneumonia resulting from mineral oil aspiration. **A:** Chest radiograph shows patchy parahilar consolidation. **B:** HRCT shows ill-defined parahilar consolidation and ground-glass opacity.

High-resolution CT (HRCT) findings (see Figs. 20.4-20.6) in patients with PAP include the following:

1. Bilateral areas of ground-glass opacity
2. Smooth interlobular septal thickening and intralobular lines in lung regions showing ground-glass opacity (ie, crazy paving)
3. Consolidation
4. A patchy or geographic distribution

In many patients, areas of ground-glass opacity or consolidation are sharply demarcated from the surrounding normal parenchyma. In some of these cases, sharply marginated lung opacities appear to represent lobules. The distribution of disease is variable, sometimes being mainly central and sometimes peripheral. It is typically bilateral but may be asymmetrical.

The combination of a geographic distribution of areas of ground-glass opacity and crazy paving is suggestive of alveolar proteinosis in patients with subacute or chronic symptoms (see Figs. 20.4B and D, 20.5, and 20.6). However, this appearance can be seen in other chronic lung diseases, including eosinophilic pneumonia, organizing pneumonia, mucinous adenocarcinoma, and exogenous lipoid pneumonia, and in acute diseases such as pneumonia, pulmonary edema, and pulmonary hemorrhage.

Superimposed infection, often by *Nocardia asteroides*, is a common complication of alveolar proteinosis, resulting in focal areas of dense consolidation or abscess formation (see Fig. 20.6B). *Mycobacterium avium-intracellulare* complex, *Candida*, *Cryptococcus neoformans*, *Aspergillus*, and *P. jirovecii* (*Pneumocystis carinii*) infections have also been reported in patients with PAP.

Autoimmune PAP is primarily treated by whole lung lavage, where the excess intra-alveolar material is washed out. Early clinical trials using inhaled GM-CSF have shown promise as an alternative to lavage in some patients.

Successful treatment is associated with a reduction in the severity of ground-glass opacity, although septal thickening may persist, at least temporarily (see Fig. 20.4E). Prior to the advent of bronchoalveolar lavage, about 30% of patients died of respiratory insufficiency or superimposed infection, but the prognosis has improved considerably. After lavage, many patients remain in remission, but others relapse; patients who relapse require retreatment every 6 to 24 months, and a few become refractory to treatment. In occasional cases where treatment fails, interstitial fibrosis develops.

Table 20.2 Pulmonary Alveolar Proteinosis

Pulmonary Alveolar Proteinosis
PAS-positive lipoproteinaceous material fills alveoli
May be idiopathic, secondary, or congenital
Idiopathic PAP
90% of cases
Autoimmune disease: antibodies to granulocyte-macrophage colony–stimulating factor
Decreased degradation or clearance of surfactant
Secondary PAP
Acute silicosis, immunodeficiency, malignancies, chemotherapy
Symptoms mild and insidious
Superimposed infection with *Nocardia*, *Mycobacterium avium-intracellulare*, and *Pneumocystis jirovecii* (*Pneumocystis carinii*)
Treated with bronchoalveolar lavage
Radiographs show ill-defined opacity, consolidation uncommon
HRCT
Bilateral, patchy, and geographic ground-glass opacity
"Crazy paving" typical
Abnormalities decrease after lavage

PAP, pulmonary alveolar proteinosis.

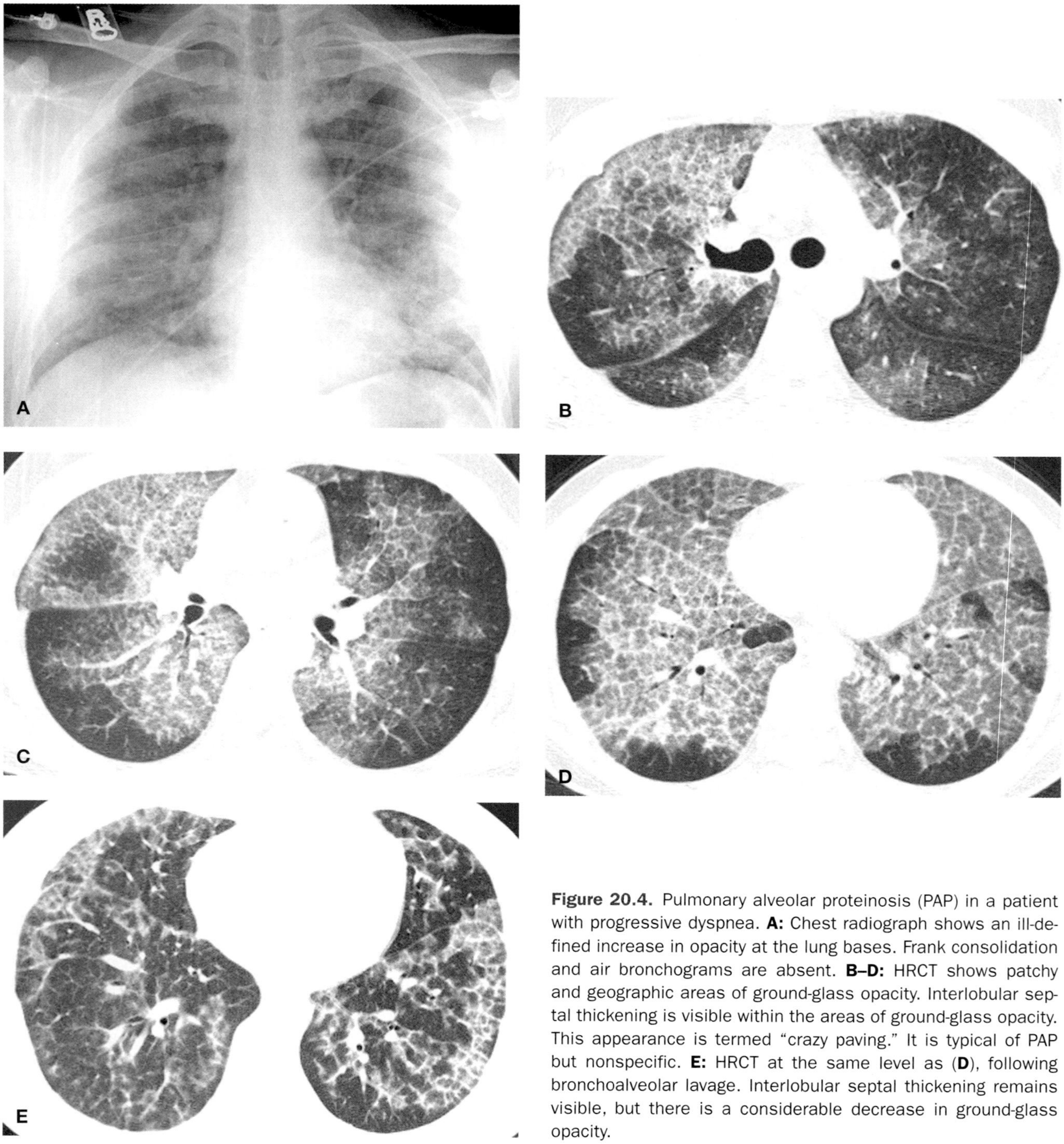

Figure 20.4. Pulmonary alveolar proteinosis (PAP) in a patient with progressive dyspnea. **A:** Chest radiograph shows an ill-defined increase in opacity at the lung bases. Frank consolidation and air bronchograms are absent. **B–D:** HRCT shows patchy and geographic areas of ground-glass opacity. Interlobular septal thickening is visible within the areas of ground-glass opacity. This appearance is termed "crazy paving." It is typical of PAP but nonspecific. **E:** HRCT at the same level as (**D**), following bronchoalveolar lavage. Interlobular septal thickening remains visible, but there is a considerable decrease in ground-glass opacity.

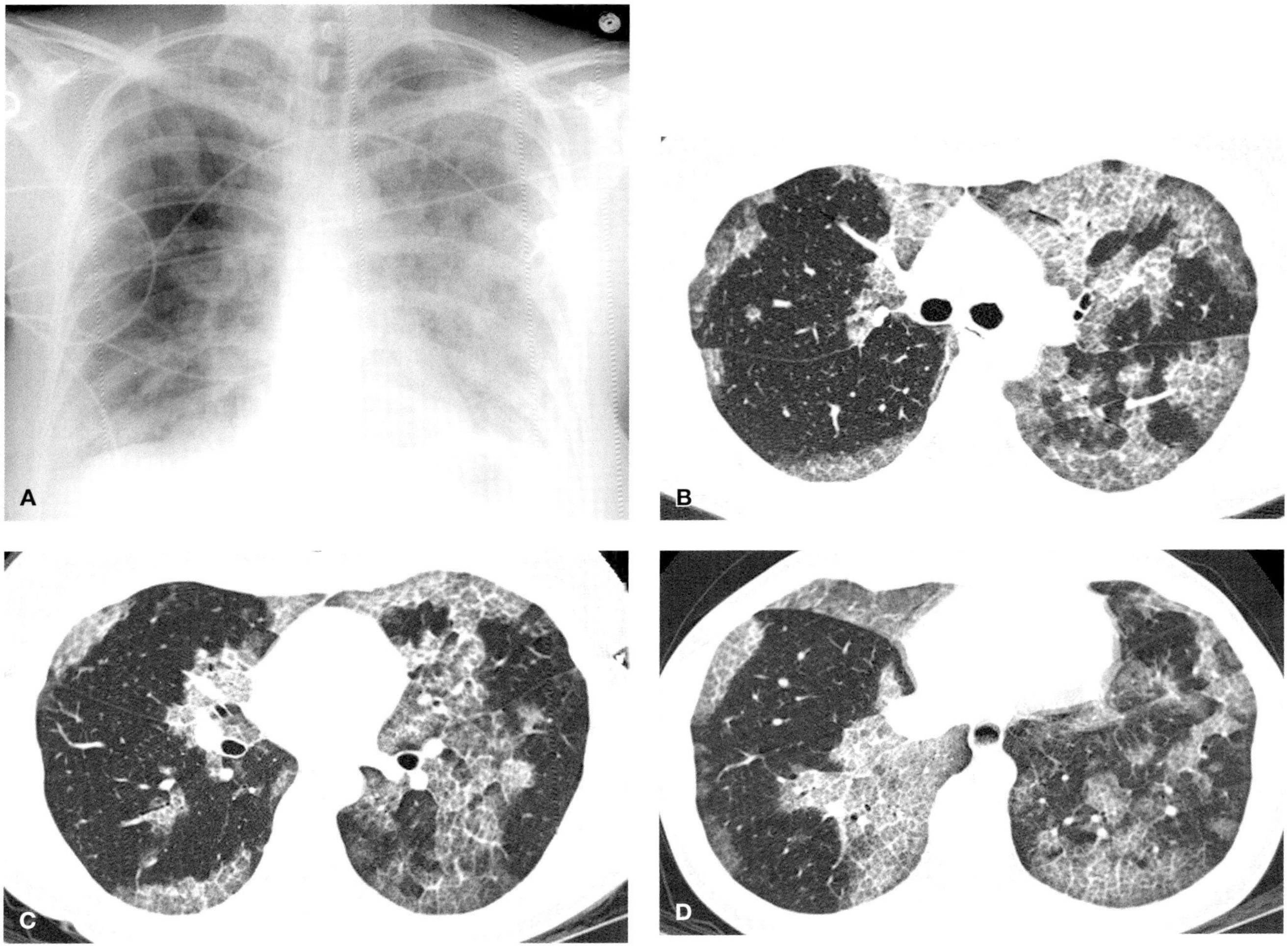

Figure 20.5. Pulmonary alveolar proteinosis in a 40-year-old woman. **A:** Chest radiographs show patchy lung opacity. **B–D:** Patchy areas of ground-glass opacity and associated interlobular septal thickening (ie, crazy paving) are visible. Intervening lung appears normal.

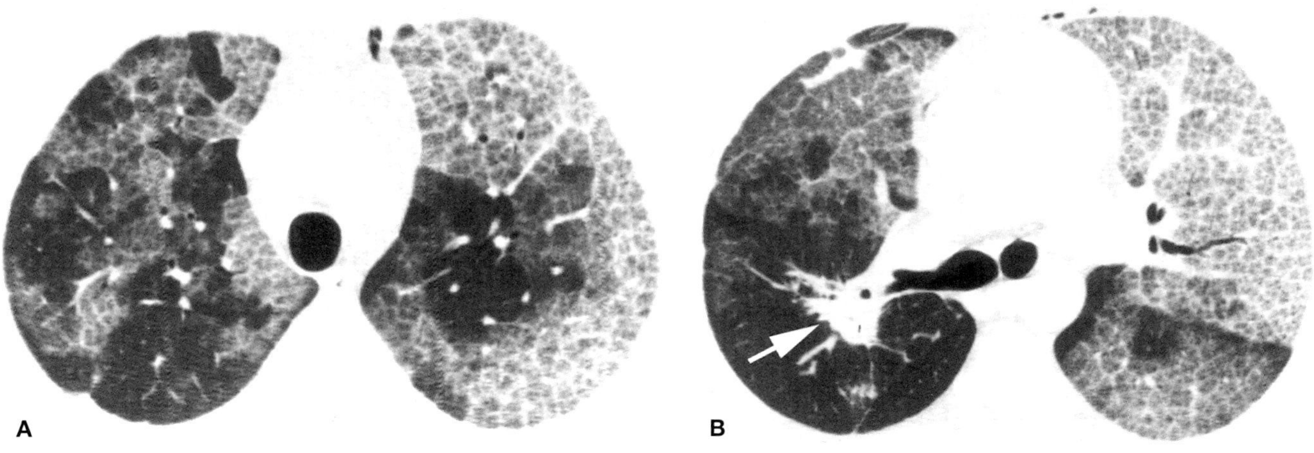

Figure 20.6. Pulmonary alveolar proteinosis in a patient with severe exposure to silica dust (ie, acute silicosis). **A:** HRCT shows patchy and geographic ground-glass opacity with crazy paving. **B:** A focal area of consolidation in the right lung (*arrow*) is due to *Nocardia* infection. Crazy paving is evident.

SUGGESTED READINGS

Franquet T, Giménez A, Bordes R, Rodríguez-Arias JM, Castella J. The crazy-paving pattern in exogenous lipoid pneumonia: CT-pathologic correlation. *AJR Am J Roentgenol.* 1998;170(2):315-317.

Frazier AA, Franks TJ, Cooke EO, Mohammed TLH, Pugatch RD, Galvin JR. From the archives of the AFIP. Pulmonary alveolar proteinosis. *Radiographics.* 2008;28(3):883-915.

Godwin JD, Müller NL, Takasugi JE. Pulmonary alveolar proteinosis: CT findings. *Radiology.* 1988;169(3):609-613.

Guan Y, Zeng Q, Yang H, et al. Pulmonary alveolar proteinosis: quantitative CT and pulmonary functional correlations. *Eur J Radiol.* 2012;81(9):2430-2435.

Hugosson CO, Riff EJ, Moore CC, Akhtar M, Tufenkeji HT. Lipoid pneumonia in infants: a radiological-pathological study. *Pediatr Radiol.* 1991;21(3):193-197.

Johkoh T, Itoh H, Müller NL, et al. Crazy-paving appearance at thin-section CT: spectrum of disease and pathologic findings. *Radiology.* 1999;211(1):155-160.

Lee KS, Müller NL, Hale V, Newell JD Jr, Lynch DA, Im JG. Lipoid pneumonia: CT findings. *J Comput Assist Tomogr.* 1995;19(1):48-51.

Lee KN, Levin DL, Webb WR, Chen D, Storto ML, Golden JA. Pulmonary alveolar proteinosis: high-resolution CT, chest radiographic, and functional correlations. *Chest.* 1997;111(4):989-995.

Prakash UBS, Barham SS, Carpenter HA, Dines DE, Marsh HM. Pulmonary alveolar phospholipoproteinosis: experience with 34 cases and a review. *Mayo Clin Proc.* 1987;62(6):499-518.

Tavare AN, Creer D, Hayward M, Hare SS. Exogenous lipoid pneumonia mimicking multifocal bronchogenic carcinoma. *J Thorac Oncol.* 2015;10(12):1809-1810.

Trapnell BC, Whitsett JA, Nakata K. Pulmonary alveolar proteinosis. *N Engl J Med.* 2003;349(26):2527-2539.

Trapnell BC, Inoue Y, Bonella F, et al, IMPALA Trial Investigators. Inhaled molgramostim therapy in autoimmune pulmonary alveolar proteinosis. *N Engl J Med.* October 22, 2020;383(17):1635-1644. DOI: 10.1056/NEJMoa1913590

Wang BM, Stern EJ, Schmidt RA, Pierson DJ. Diagnosing pulmonary alveolar proteinosis: a review and an update. *Chest.* 1997;111(2):460-466.

Chapter 21

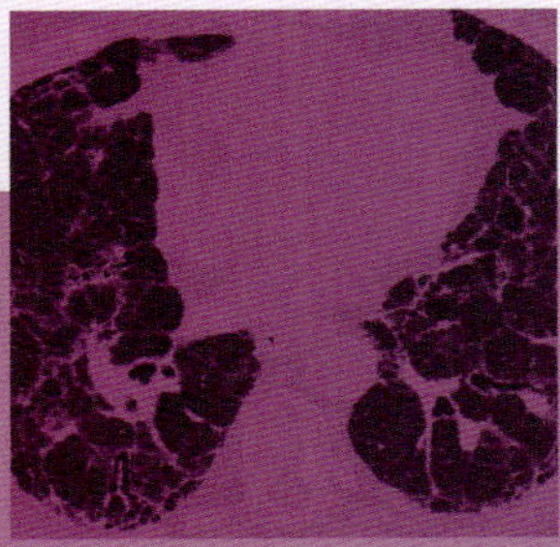

Travis S. Henry

Diffuse Lung Diseases Associated With Calcification

INTRODUCTION

A wide variety of lung diseases may be associated with some degree of lung calcification, most notably granulomatous diseases such as sarcoidosis or prior infection (eg, tuberculosis or histoplasmosis) (Table 21.1).

Several diffuse lung diseases are associated with extensive lung calcification as a common finding or as a primary manifestation of the disease. These are discussed in this chapter.

AMYLOIDOSIS

The term *amyloidosis* refers to a group of conditions characterized by extracellular deposition of abnormal fibrillar protein. Amyloidosis may be classified according to its etiology, the proteins involved, or its primary manifestation (Table 21.2). The first two of these categories overlap, are somewhat confusing, and are reviewed briefly. Classification according to its primary manifestation is most appropriate to the radiologic assessment of amyloidosis and is easiest to remember.

Classification by Etiology

An etiologic classification of amyloidosis includes (1) *primary amyloidosis* (ie, associated with a plasma cell disorder or idiopathic), (2) *secondary amyloidosis* (ie, associated with chronic inflammatory disorders or neoplasms such as Hodgkin disease), (3) *hereditary amyloidosis* (ie, having a genetic basis such as transthyretin amyloidosis), and (4) *senile amyloidosis*, which usually occurs in patients over the age of 70, and commonly involves the heart.

Amyloidosis is also subdivided into systemic forms (ie, diffuse involvement of multiple organs; 80%-90% of cases) or localized forms (ie, focal involvement largely limited to one organ; 10%-20% of cases).

Classification by Specific Proteins

When amyloidosis is classified according to the specific abnormal protein involved, the most important types producing lung disease are amyloid L and amyloid A.

Amyloid L (AL, or light-chain amyloidosis) is the most common form of systemic amyloidosis. It may be either idiopathic or associated with plasma cell disorders (about 90% of cases). The lung is involved in 70% to 90% of patients with AL amyloidosis. Cardiomyopathy almost always is present if the lung is involved. Prognosis generally is poor. AL amyloidosis also may result in localized lung involvement. AL typically occurs in patients in their 50s or 60s.

Amyloid A (AA) occurs as secondary amyloidosis in patients with chronic inflammatory diseases (eg, collagen vascular disease, infections, inflammatory bowel disease, and familial Mediterranean fever) and some neoplasms such as Hodgkin disease. The lung is commonly involved to some degree, but deposits often are small or clinically insignificant. The prognosis is better than that for AL.

Among patients who have pulmonary involvement by amyloid, about 65% have primary systemic amyloidosis (systemic AL), 30% have localized amyloidosis (localized AL), and 5% have secondary amyloidosis (AA).

Classification by Manifestation

From a radiographic standpoint, it is most useful to classify amyloidosis based on the abnormalities it produces. In

Table 21.1 Diffuse or Multifocal Lung Calcification

Infectious diseases
Tuberculosis
Histoplasmosis
Healed varicella pneumonia
Parasitic infections
Sarcoidosis
Silicosis and coal worker's pneumoconiosis
Calcified metastases
Osteogenic and chondrosarcoma
Mucinous adenocarcinoma
Thyroid carcinoma
Amyloidosis
Alveolar microlithiasis
Metastatic calcification
Diffuse pulmonary ossification

Table 21.2 Classification of Amyloidosis

By etiology
Primary amyloidosis—plasma cell disorder or unassociated with underlying disease
Secondary amyloidosis—associated with chronic inflammatory disorders or neoplasm
Heredofamilial amyloidosis
Senile amyloidosis—usually in patients over 70 years
Systemic (diffuse involvement of multiple organs)
Localized (focal involvement largely limited to one organ)
By specific proteins
Amyloid L (AL; light-chain amyloidosis)
Most common
Usually primary amyloidosis
Lung involved in 70%-90%, localized or diffuse
Cardiac involvement
Poor prognosis
Amyloid A
Secondary amyloidosis
Lung involved to a minor degree
Better prognosis
By pulmonary manifestation
Diffuse (alveolar septal) amyloidosis
Usually primary systemic and AL
Dyspnea due to lung or heart disease
Small nodules or reticular opacities
Consolidation
Lymph node enlargement
Calcification common
Localized nodular amyloidosis
Usually primary localized and AL
Usually asymptomatic
Lung nodules, often calcified
Nodules grow slowly
Localized tracheobronchial amyloidosis
Usually primary localized and AL
Tracheal and bronchial narrowing or masses
Calcification common

general, pulmonary amyloidosis is classified into three types: (1) diffuse or alveolar septal amyloidosis, (2) localized nodular amyloidosis, and (3) tracheobronchial amyloidosis.

Diffuse (Alveolar Septal) Amyloidosis

Symptoms of respiratory insufficiency are common with diffuse or alveolar septal amyloidosis and may be related to diffuse lung disease or associated cardiac involvement. This form of amyloidosis is most often related to primary systemic amyloidosis (systemic AL). Diffuse lung involvement is much less common and may be incidental with AA amyloidosis or senile amyloidosis. Occasionally, diffuse alveolar septal amyloidosis reflects localized rather than systemic disease.

The lung may be diffusely involved in the absence of a radiographic abnormality. If radiographs are abnormal, a reticular or reticulonodular pattern typically is seen, usually bilateral and diffuse or with a basal and subpleural predominance (Figs. 21.1 and 21.2A). Focal or patchy areas of consolidation also may be seen. The abnormal areas can calcify or, rarely, show frank ossification. Less often, a small nodular pattern mimicking sarcoidosis or miliary tuberculosis may be seen.

Hilar or mediastinal lymph node enlargement may be seen in patients with AL, either as an isolated finding or in association with interstitial disease; calcification may occur. Cardiac infiltration with heart failure may result in pulmonary edema or pleural effusion.

On high-resolution CT (HRCT), the most common pulmonary manifestations of diffuse parenchymal amyloidosis consist of multiple small nodules, usually ranging from 2 to 4 mm in diameter (see Fig. 21.2B and C), interlobular septal thickening, fine reticular opacities, focal consolidation, foci of calcification within nodules or areas of consolidation (Fig. 21.3), and traction bronchiectasis. A subpleural and basal predominance may be seen.

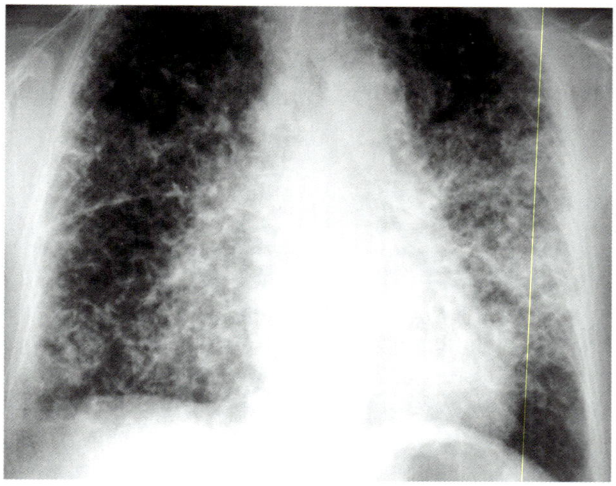

Figure 21.1. Diffuse alveolar septal amyloidosis. A diffuse reticulonodular pattern is visible, with the abnormality predominating at the lung bases. Lung and lymph node calcification is present, and the heart is enlarged.

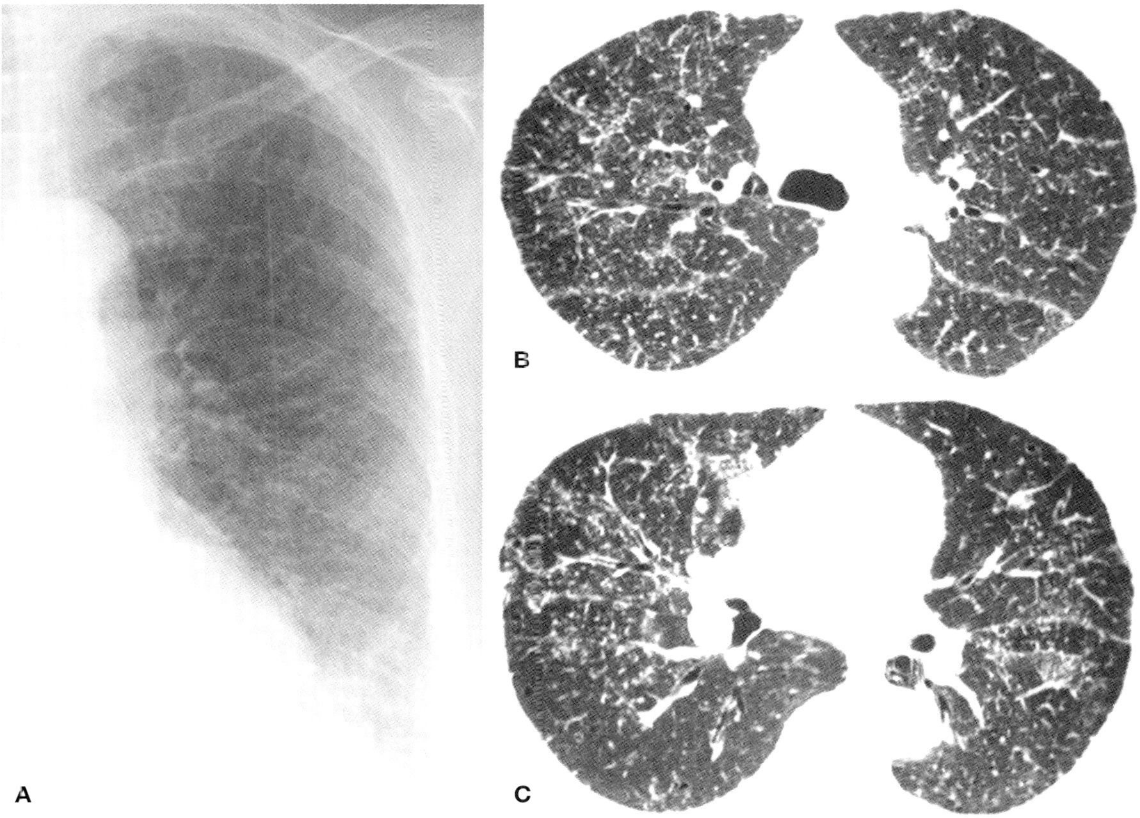

Figure 21.2. Diffuse alveolar septal amyloidosis. **A:** Coned-down view of a PA radiograph shows a reticular pattern within the left lung, with a basal predominance. **B, C:** HRCT shows a diffuse nodular abnormality, with nodules visible in relation to the fissures and interlobular septa.

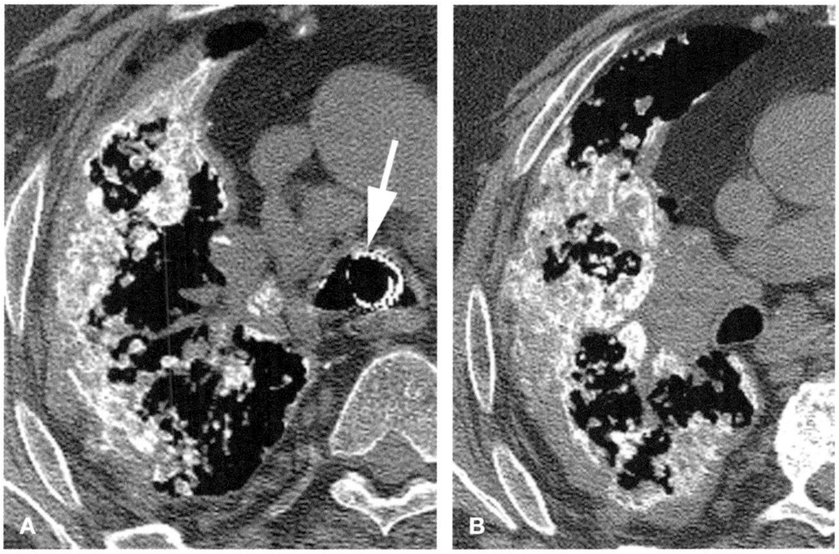

Figure 21.3. Diffuse alveolar septal amyloidosis. **A, B:** HRCTs at two levels show extensive lung consolidation and calcification. A tracheal stent (*arrow* in **A**) is in place because of airway involvement and narrowing.

Progression of the diffuse parenchymal disease typically occurs with time, with an increase in the reticular opacities, septal thickening, the size and number of nodules, the extent of consolidation, and the size and number of calcifications.

As on chest radiographs, other findings seen on CT include lymphadenopathy, lymph node calcification (Fig. 21.4), and pleural effusion. Lymph node enlargement occurs in up to 75% of cases.

The prognosis of patients is usually related to the underlying disease or to involvement of other organs such as the kidney, liver, and heart. In some patients, lung involvement is severe enough to require lung transplantation.

Localized Nodular Amyloidosis

Patients with localized nodular amyloidosis (localized AL) usually are asymptomatic. Localized nodular amyloidosis may manifest as single or multiple lung nodules or masses, usually well-defined and round, elliptical or lobulated, ranging from 0.5 to 5 cm in diameter (Fig. 21.5), with stippled or dense calcification in up to 50% of cases on CT and cavitation in a small percentage. Nodules may grow slowly or remain stable over several years. They are most common in the peripheral lung and in the lower lobes.

Multinodular parenchymal amyloidosis can be seen in patients with Sjögren syndrome and lymphoproliferative diseases, such as mucosa-associated lymphoid tissue lymphoma and lymphoid interstitial pneumonia (LIP). Nodules are sometimes associated thin-walled cystic lesions, which appear to be related to the presence of LIP. A similar appearance is seen in patients with *light-chain deposition disease*. These are discussed in Chapter 25.

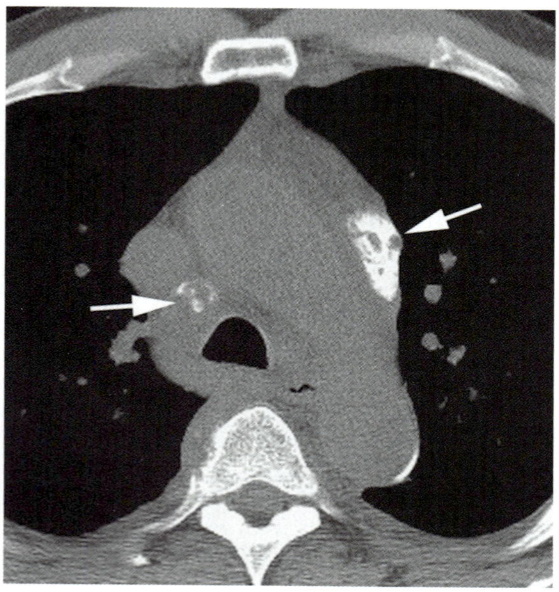

Figure 21.4. Lymph node enlargement and calcification in amyloidosis. Mediastinal lymph nodes (*arrows*) are densely calcified.

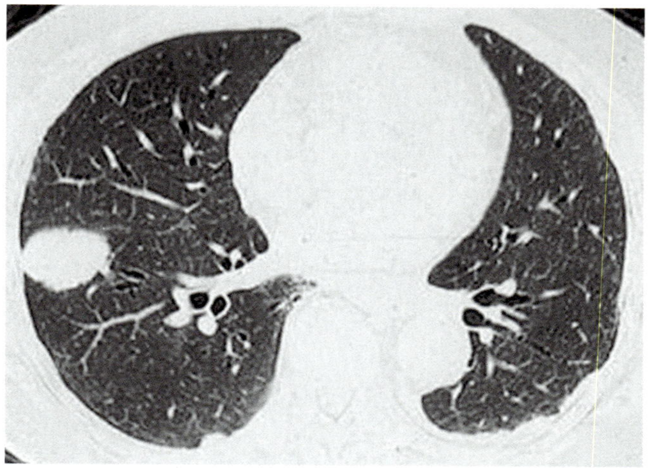

Figure 21.5. Localized nodular amyloidosis. A large right lung nodule is visible. Small subpleural nodules or focal pleural thickening also are seen.

Localized Tracheobronchial Amyloidosis

Localized AL may involve the larynx, trachea, and central bronchi; focal deposits of amyloid within the airway wall or diffuse wall infiltration may be present. Symptoms are common and include hoarseness, stridor, dyspnea, cough, hemoptysis, and recurrent infections. The trachea typically is involved, and concentric or nodular wall infiltration is most common. Calcification is common (Fig. 21.6; also see Fig. 22.20 in Chapter 22).

PULMONARY ALVEOLAR MICROLITHIASIS

Pulmonary alveolar microlithiasis is characterized by the presence of numerous minute calculi (the so-called *microliths* or *calcispheres*) within alveoli (Table 21.3). It is very rare but has a characteristic radiographic appearance.

Histologically, the calcispheres are located largely within the alveolar lumen, although they probably are formed within the alveolar walls. They consist of concentric layers of calcium phosphate. In the early stages of disease, the alveolar walls appear normal, although fibrosis may occur late in the disease process. Emphysema also may be seen, particularly in the apices and subpleural regions.

Microlithiasis may be seen at any age, but most cases occur in patients from 20 to 50 years of age. Two forms have been recognized: *sporadic* and *familial*, predominantly affecting siblings. Microlithiasis occurs because of a gene mutation, resulting in an abnormal protein, which is normally responsible for sodium-dependent phosphate transport in the lungs. The abnormal protein prevents transport of phosphorus ions from the alveolar spaces into type II pneumocytes, which leads in turn to the development of calcospherites within alveoli. Autosomal recessive inheritance of the abnormal gene may occur. Abnormalities of calcium metabolism are absent.

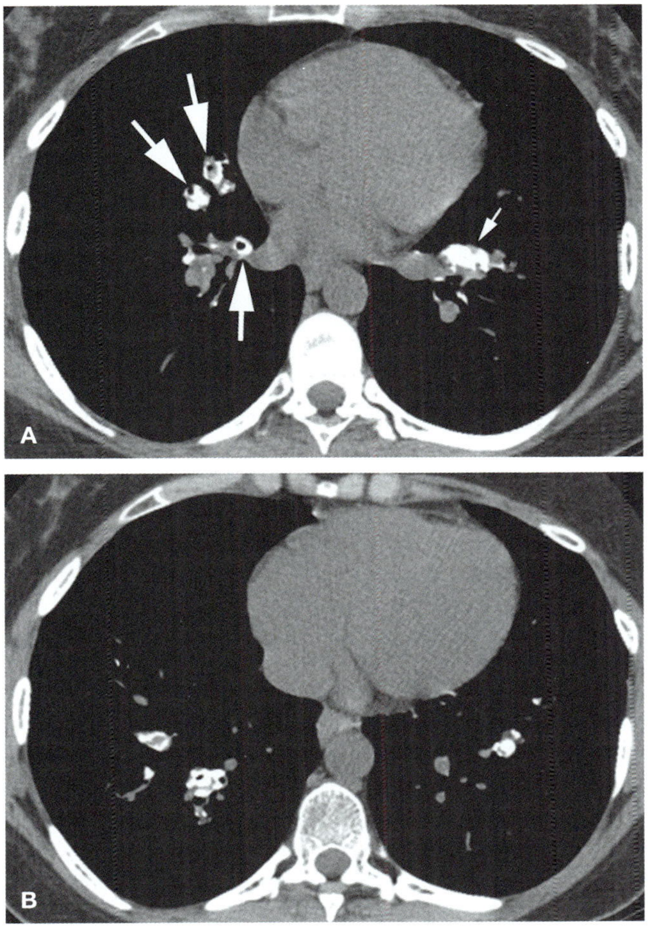

Figure 21.6. Tracheobronchial amyloidosis. **A:** CT shows extensive bronchial calcifications (*large arrows*). Hilar lymph node calcification (*small arrow*) also is present. **B:** Airway calcification due to amyloid deposition also is visible more peripherally.

Table 21.3 Pulmonary Alveolar Microlithiasis

- Calcispheres within alveoli (consist of calcium phosphate)
- Very rare
- 20-50 y of age
- Related to mutation of a gene responsible for phosphate transport in the lung
- Often asymptomatic at diagnosis
- Abnormalities progress slowly
- Radiographs
  - Dense lungs
  - Basal predominance
  - Individual calcified nodules visible
  - Black pleural line
- HRCT
  - Subpleural and perivascular predominance of calcified nodules
  - Black pleural line = emphysema

Patients typically are asymptomatic at diagnosis, despite spectacular radiographic abnormalities. There is a tendency for the abnormalities to progress slowly over a period of several years, although findings may remain stable. Dyspnea may develop with progression of the disease, with other symptoms including hemoptysis and finger clubbing. Although lung fibrosis and cor pulmonale may develop, the prognosis generally is good. There is no treatment.

Radiographs show characteristic findings. Despite their small size, the individual calcispheres may be visible as discrete, dense dots, less than 1 mm in diameter (Fig. 21.7). A basal predominance is typical (see Fig. 21.7). When limited in number, the calcispheres predominate in a subpleural location and in relation to vessels, bronchi, and interlobular septa. When myriad, they become confluent and appear very dense, obscuring the hemidiaphragm, heart, and mediastinal contours. If the lungs are sufficiently dense, the heart may appear relatively lucent, a very unusual finding. Another typical finding on chest radiographs, although it is not always seen, is the so-called *black pleural line*, a stripe of relative lucency at the pleural surface (see Fig. 21.7). Although this feature was thought to be due to sparing of the pleura by the calcispheres, it reflects small subpleural areas of emphysema.

HRCT shows a posterior and lower lobe predominance of the calcifications with a high concentration in the subpleural parenchyma and in association with bronchi and vessels (Figs. 21.8 and 21.9). A perilobular and centrilobular distribution of the calcifications may be seen or calcifications may be associated with interlobular septa. Intraparenchymal emphysema may be seen. Subpleural paraseptal emphysema (ie, the black pleural line) is common (see Fig. 21.9). In children or patients with early disease, ground-glass opacity or reticulation may be the predominant finding; calcifications may be difficult to detect.

Calcification of small interstitial nodules seen on HRCT has a limited differential diagnosis. Multifocal lung calcification, often associated with lung nodules, also has been

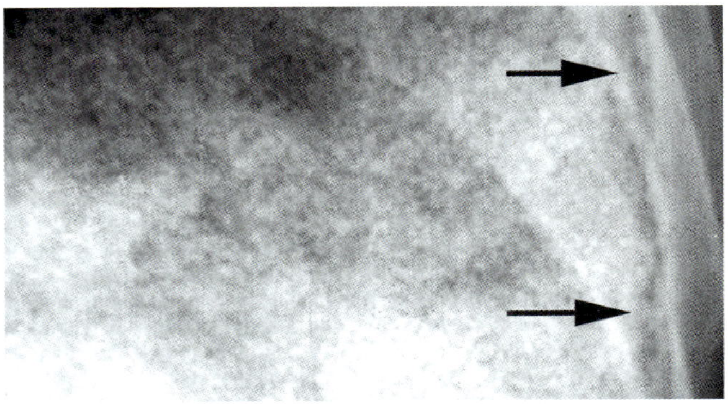

Figure 21.7. Alveolar microlithiasis. Detail view of the left lower lobe in a patient with diffuse lung opacity. Individual dense calcispheres are visible. The subpleural lung appears relatively lucent (*arrows*). This is the so-called black pleural line.

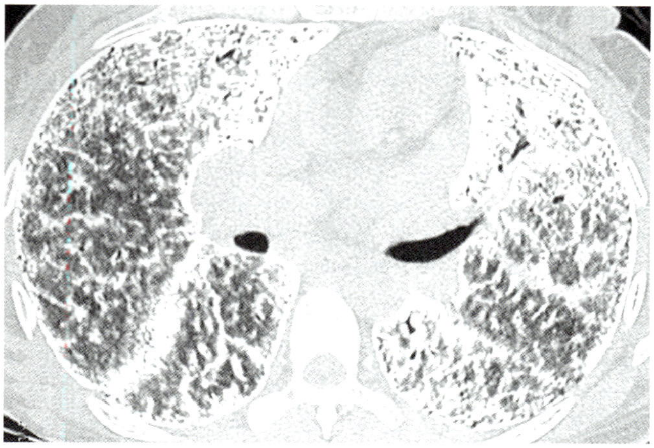

Figure 21.8. HRCT in alveolar microlithiasis. Extensive lung calcification is present with a subpleural and perivascular predominance.

reported in association with amyloidosis, infectious granulomatous diseases such as tuberculosis, sarcoidosis, silicosis, and coal worker's pneumoconiosis, talcosis, and metastatic calcification.

METASTATIC CALCIFICATION

The term *metastatic calcification* refers to the deposition of calcium in soft tissues due to abnormal calcium and phosphate metabolism (Table 21.4). It is associated with hypercalcemia and is most common in patients with chronic renal failure and secondary hyperparathyroidism and in those undergoing chronic hemodialysis.

Metastatic calcification commonly affects the lung; it typically is interstitial, involving the alveolar septa, bronchioles, and pulmonary arteries, and can be associated with secondary lung fibrosis. Patients may be asymptomatic or may have dyspnea. With appropriate treatment of the underlying abnormality, metastatic calcification may resolve.

Abnormalities typically predominate in the lung apices because they are more alkaline than the lung bases, increasing the likelihood of calcium salt precipitation in this region. A higher ratio of ventilation to perfusion in the apices results in a decrease in the partial pressure of CO_2 and a corresponding increase in pH.

Plain radiographs are relatively insensitive in detecting metastatic calcification. In some patients, ill-defined nodules or patchy areas of increased opacity may be seen (Figs. 21.10 and 21.11A). Nodules visible on chest films usually appear to be about 1 to 2 cm in diameter. They may or may not appear to be of calcium density. With progressive disease, these opacities become confluent, mimicking pneumonia. An apical predominance of opacities is typical but not invariable (see Fig. 21.11A).

CT can show areas of ground-glass opacity, consolidation, or calcification in the absence of plain film abnormalities. Numerous fluffy and poorly defined nodules, measuring 3 to 10 mm in diameter, are typical, but opacities can appear focal, centrilobular, lobular, patchy, or diffuse (Figs. 21.11-21.13) and often spare the interlobular septae. Even with HRCT, these opacities may not appear calcified. An apical predominance is common. Calcification of vessels in the chest wall may also be seen.

Radionuclide bone (^{99m}Tc-diphosphonate) scintigraphy (see Fig. 21.12D) is highly sensitive for the detection of metastatic calcification and may show lung uptake when chest films are normal. It may serve to confirm the diagnosis when CT shows typical apical opacities without obvious calcification.

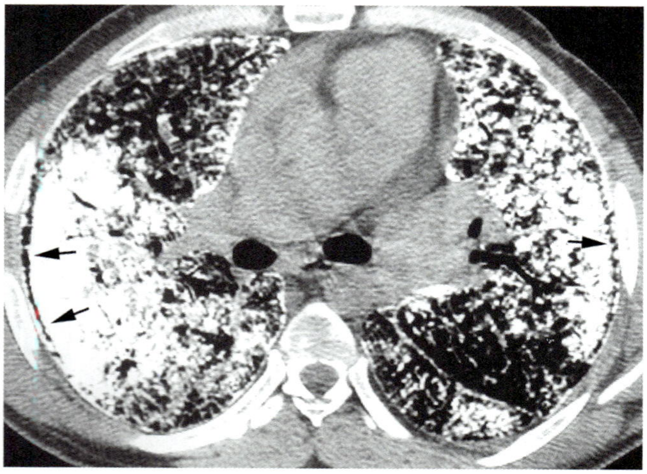

Figure 21.9. HRCT in alveolar microlithiasis. Lung calcification is confluent in some regions and nodular in others. Small areas of emphysema (*arrows*) in the peripheral lung account for the black pleural line.

Table 21.4 Metastatic Calcification

Calcification due to abnormal calcium and phosphate metabolism
Hypercalcemia
- Renal failure
- Secondary hyperparathyroidism
- Chronic hemodialysis

Commonly affects lung
Apices most often involved (more alkaline)
Radiographs
- Nodular opacities or consolidation

HRCT
- Opacities often centrilobular
- May be ground-glass opacity
- May or may not appear calcified

Radionuclide bone (^{99m}Tc-diphosphonate) scintigraphy useful
Opacities may resolve with treatment

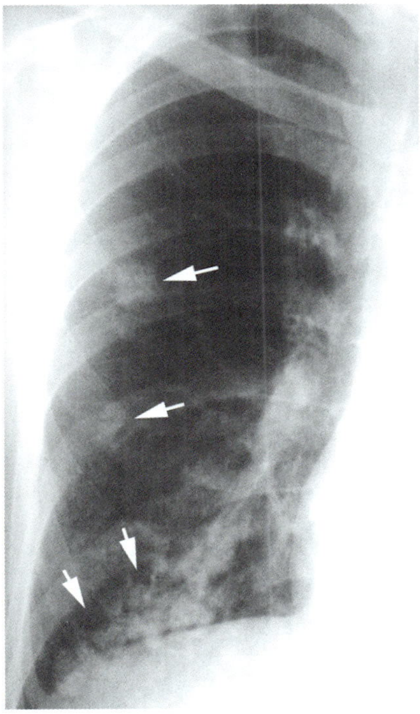

Figure 21.10. Metastatic calcification in a patient with renal disease and secondary hyperparathyroidism. Dense nodular opacities (*arrows*) are visible in the right lung.

DIFFUSE PULMONARY OSSIFICATION

Diffuse pulmonary ossification (DPO) is a rare and intriguing pathological condition wherein bone tissue forms within the lung parenchyma. Notably, there are two distinct subtypes of DPO—nodular and dendriform. It is essential to recognize that these terms, though sometimes used interchangeably in literature, refer to different entities with unique pathologies and imaging characteristics.

Nodular Pulmonary Ossification

Nodular pulmonary ossification (DPO-N) is characterized by the presence of ectopic bone within the alveolar spaces. It is predominantly associated with chronic conditions such as mitral valve disease or chronic left heart failure. The underlying pathogenesis is believed to be related to the development of ossification in areas of hemosiderin deposition and organizing pneumonia, often as a result of chronic pulmonary congestion and edema associated with cardiac conditions.

On computed tomography (CT), DPO-N manifests as calcified micronodules predominantly in the lower lobes, often reflecting the gravity-dependent distribution of edema and hemosiderin in chronic heart failure. These calcified nodules are usually scattered throughout the lung parenchyma. Clinical correlations, particularly the presence of underlying heart conditions, are vital for accurately diagnosing DPO-N.

Dendriform Pulmonary Ossification

Dendriform pulmonary ossification (DPO-D), however, is characterized by the deposition of bone primarily within the interstitial spaces of the lung. The term *dendriform* refers to

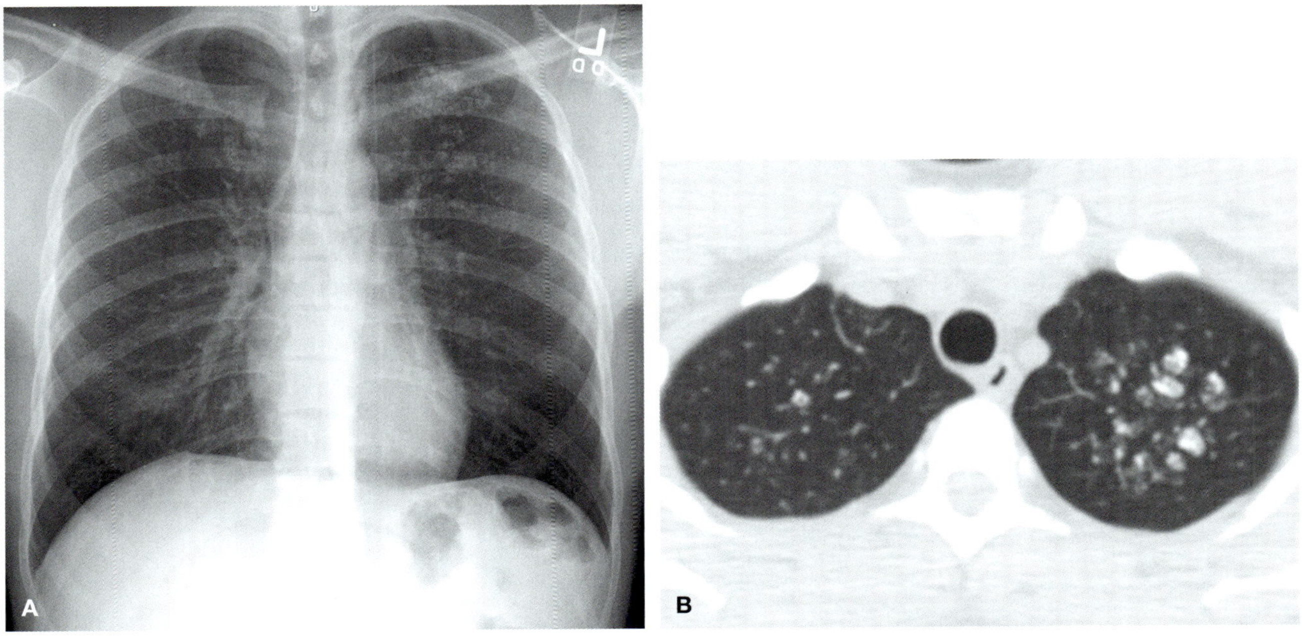

Figure 21.11. Metastatic calcification in renal failure. **A:** Chest radiograph shows ill-defined nodular opacities with an apical predominance with suggestion of calcification at the left lung apex **B:** CT at lung windows shows amorphous nodular opacities in the upper lobes. Calcification is evident even on lung windows.

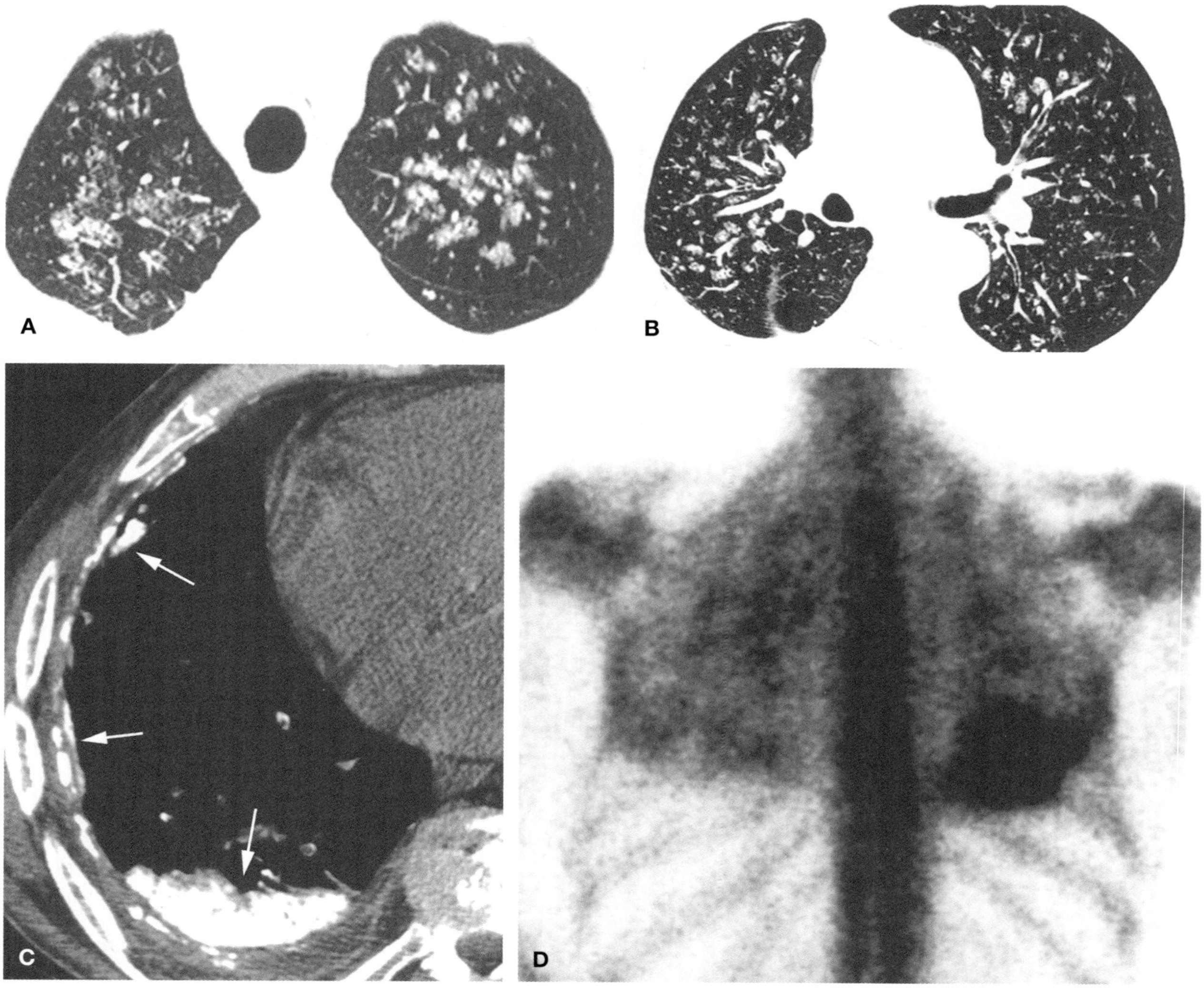

Figure 21.12. Metastatic calcification in renal failure. **A, B:** HRCTs with a lung window setting show nodular opacities in the upper lobes. These opacities appear centrilobular in distribution. They were not obviously calcified on soft-tissue windows. **C:** CT at the lung base shows dense subpleural calcification and calcification of consolidated lung (*arrows*). **D:** Radionuclide bone (^{99m}Tc-diphosphonate) scintigraphy shows extensive isotope uptake within both lungs.

the treelike branching structures that are sometimes seen on imaging. On CT, DPO-D appears as micronodules within the peripheral interstitium that can form branching structures. While ossification is often visible on CT, in some instances, the nodules may be so small that they are below the limits of resolution (Fig. 21.14).

Dendriform ossification is frequently seen in the context of fibrotic lung diseases, especially usual interstitial pneumonia. However, a recent case series described 52 patients who exhibited dendriform ossification in the absence of fibrosis. The patients in this series were predominantly older males, and there seemed to be an association with chronic aspiration. This finding suggests a more diverse etiological basis for DPO-D than previously recognized. DPO-D usually has an indolent course and does not worsen prognosis of underlying fibrosis (when fibrosis is present).

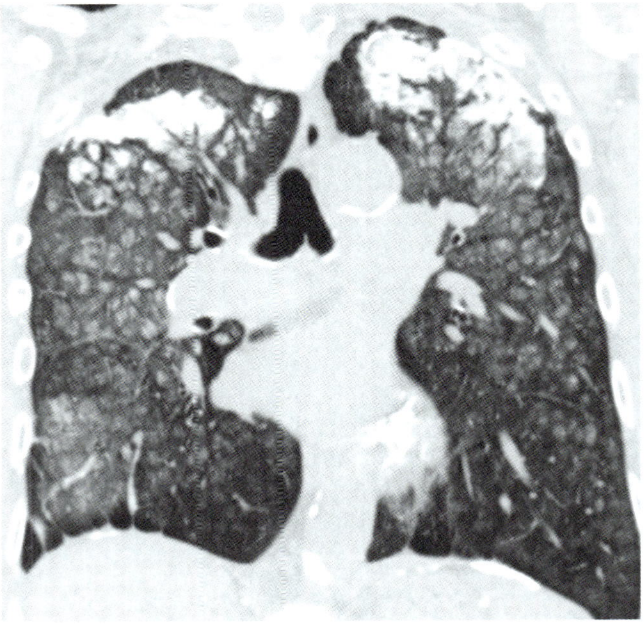

Figure 21.13. Metastatic calcification in renal failure. Coronal HRCT image shows confluent areas of calcification in the upper lobes. The craniocaudal gradient is evident with centrilobular and lobular ground-glass opacities that become less severe more inferiorly. Pleural and vascular calcification is also partially seen.

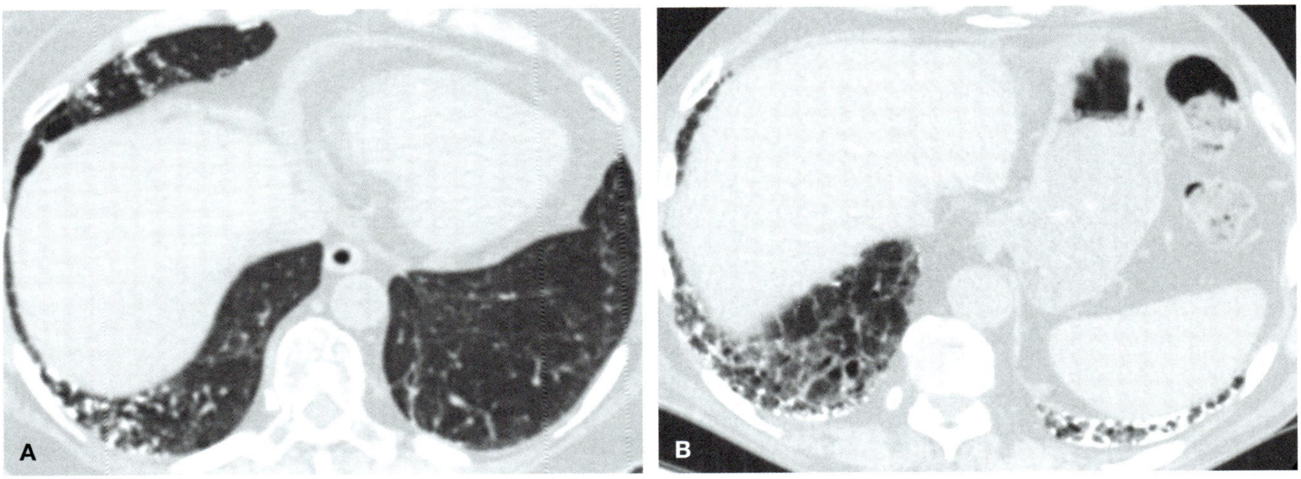

Figure 21.14. Dendriform pulmonary ossification in two patients. **A:** Axial CT from a 72-year-old woman who presented with worsening dyspnea shows asymmetric, clustered, and branching micronodules of calcium attenuation most severe at the right lung base. Note the absence of fibrosis. Surgical lung biopsy confirmed dendriform pulmonary ossification (DPO-D), which was attributed to chronic aspiration. **B:** Axial CT in a patient with DPO-D associated with pulmonary fibrosis. Micronodules of calcium attenuation are similar to those seen in A, but with associated fibrosis in a usual interstitial pneumonia pattern. The patient had a clinical history of idiopathic pulmonary fibrosis.

SUGGESTED READINGS

Aylwin ACB, Gishen P, Copley SJ. Imaging appearance of thoracic amyloidosis. *J Thorac Imaging*. 2005;20(1):41-46.

Ayuso MC, Gilabert R, Bombi JA, Salvador A. CT appearance of localized pulmonary amyloidosis. *J Comput Assist Tomogr*. 1987;11(1):197-199.

Castellana G, Lamorgese V. Pulmonary alveolar microlithiasis. World cases and review of the literature. *Respiration*. 2003;70(5):549-555.

Cluzel P, Grenier P, Bernadac P, Laurent F, Picard JD. Pulmonary alveolar microlithiasis: CT findings. *J Comput Assist Tomogr*. 1991;15(6):938-942.

Colombat M, Stern M, Groussard O, et al. Pulmonary cystic disorder related to light chain deposition disease. *Am J Respir Crit Care Med*. 2006;173(7):777-780.

Colombat M, Mal H, Copie-Bergman C, et al. Primary cystic lung light chain deposition disease: a clinicopathologic entity derived from unmutated B cells with a stereotyped IGHV4-34/IGKV1 receptor. *Blood*. 2008;112(5):2004-2012.

Czeyda-Pommersheim F, Hwang M, Chen SS, Strollo D, Fuhrman C, Bhalla S. Amyloidosis: modern cross-sectional imaging. *Radiographics*. 2015;35(5):1381-1392.

De Almeida RR, Zanetti G, Pereira E Silva JL, et al. Respiratory tract amyloidosis. State-of-the-art review with a focus on pulmonary involvement. *Lung*. 2015;193(6):875-883.

Deniz O, Ors F, Tozkoparan E, et al. High resolution computed tomographic features of pulmonary alveolar microlithiasis. *Eur J Radiol*. 2005;55(3):452-460.

Egashira R, Jacob J, Kokosi MA, et al. Diffuse pulmonary ossification in fibrosing interstitial lung diseases: prevalence and associations. *Radiology*. 2017;284(1):255-263. doi:10.1148/radiol.2017152419

Georgiades CS, Neyman EG, Barish MA, Fishman EK. Amyloidosis: review and CT manifestations. *Radiographics*. 2004;24(2):405-416.

Graham CM, Stern EJ, Finkbeiner WE, Webb WR. High-resolution CT appearance of diffuse alveolar septal amyloidosis. *AJR Am J Roentgenol*. 1992;158(2):265-267.

Gruden JF, Green DB, Legasto AC, Jensen EA, Panse PM. Dendriform pulmonary ossification in the absence of usual interstitial pneumonia: CT features and possible association with recurrent acid aspiration. *Am J Roentgenol*. 2017;209(6):1209-1215. doi:10.2214/AJR.17.18063

Hartman TE, Müller NL, Primack SL, et al. Metastatic pulmonary calcification in patients with hypercalcemia: findings on chest radiographs and CT scans. *AJR Am J Roentgenol*. 1994;162(4):799-802.

Helbich TH, Wojnarovsky C, Wunderbaldinger P, Heinz-Peer G, Eichler I, Herold CJ. Pulmonary alveolar microlithiasis in children: radiographic and high-resolution CT findings. *AJR Am J Roentgenol*. 1997;168(1):63-65.

Jeong YJ, Lee KS, Chung MP, et al. Amyloidosis and lymphoproliferative disease in sjogren syndrome: thin-section computed tomography findings and histopathologic comparisons. *J Comput Assist Tomogr*. 2004;28(6):776-781.

Johkoh T, Ikezoe J, Nagareda T, Kohno N, Takeuchi N, Kozuka T. Metastatic pulmonary calcification: early detection by high-resolution CT. *J Comput Assist Tomogr*. 1993;17(3):471-473.

Korn MA, Schurawitzki H, Klepetko W, Burghuber OC. Pulmonary alveolar microlithiasis: findings on high-resolution CT. *AJR Am J Roentgenol*. 1992;158(5):981-982.

Kuhlman JE, Ren H, Hutchins GM, Fishman EK. Fulminant pulmonary calcification complicating renal transplantation: CT demonstration. *Radiology*. 1989;173(2):459-460.

Lachmann HJ, Goodman HJB, Gilbertson JA, et al. Natural history and outcome in systemic AA amyloidosis. *N Engl J Med*. 2007;356(23):2361-2371.

Lauta VM. Pulmonary alveolar microlithiasis: an overview of clinical and pathological features together with possible therapies. *Respir Med*. 2003;97(10):1081-1085.

Pickford HA, Swensen SJ, Utz JP. Thoracic cross-sectional imaging of amyloidosis. *AJR Am J Roentgenol*. 1997;168(2):351-355.

Seaman DM, Meyer CA, Gilman MD, McCormack FX. Diffuse cystic lung disease at high-resolution CT. *Am J Roentgenol*. 2011;196(6):1305-1311.

Siddiqui NA, Fuhrman CR. Best cases from the AFIP: pulmonary alveolar microlithiasis. *Radiographics*. 2011;31(2):585-590.

Utz JP, Swensen SJ, Gertz MA. Pulmonary amyloidosis. The Mayo Clinic experience from 1980 to 1993. *Ann Intern Med*. 1996;124(4):407-413.

Section Four

Airway Abnormalities

Chapter 22

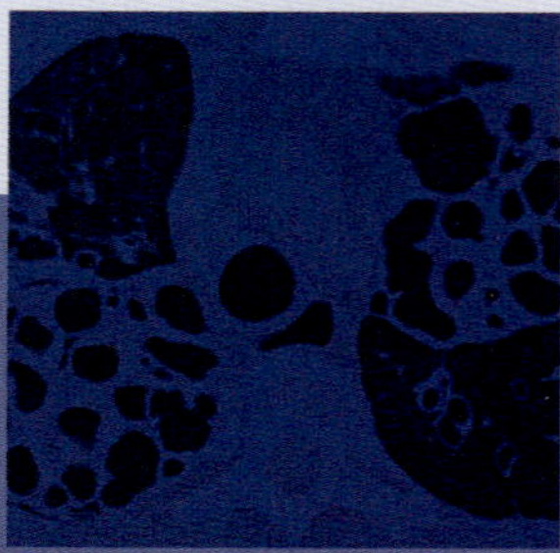

Travis S. Henry

The Trachea

THE NORMAL TRACHEA

The trachea extends from the inferior aspect of the cricoid cartilage (at the level of the sixth cervical vertebra) to the carina (at the level of the fifth thoracic vertebra). It measures from 10 to 12 cm in length. The trachea is divided into extrathoracic and intrathoracic portions at the level it passes posterior to the manubrium; the extrathoracic trachea is 2 to 4 cm in length, while the intrathoracic trachea measures 6 to 9 cm in length. From 16 to 22 horseshoe-shaped bands of hyaline cartilage support the anterior and lateral tracheal walls. The incomplete posterior portion of these rings is bridged by a thin band of smooth muscle and fibrous tissue, the *posterior tracheal membrane* (Fig. 22.1).

The plain film appearance of the trachea is described in Chapter 2. On CT, the trachea usually is round or oval in shape, but it can appear horseshoe shaped, triangular, or like an inverted pear in some normal patients. The tracheal wall is delineated by air in its lumen internally and by mediastinal fat externally and is usually visible as a 1- to 2-mm soft-tissue stripe. The posterior tracheal membrane appears thinner than the anterior and lateral tracheal walls and is variable in shape due to its lack of cartilage; it can appear convex, concave, or flat. The tracheal cartilages may appear calcified or slightly denser than adjacent soft tissue. Calcification of cartilage is most common in older patients and is particularly common in women (Fig. 22.2). In patients with calcified cartilage, little soft tissue is seen in the tracheal wall internal to the cartilage.

Tracheal diameter varies widely in normal subjects. In males, normal tracheal diameter averages 19.5 mm, with a range of 13 to 25 mm (mean $\pm$ 3 SD) in the coronal plane and 13 to 27 mm in the sagittal plane. In females, tracheal diameter is slightly smaller, averaging 17.5 mm and ranging from 10 to 21 mm in the coronal plane and 10 to 23 mm in the sagittal plane. Regardless of diameter, the normal intrathoracic trachea has a relatively circular shape on axial images during a proper inspiratory CT.

On CT performed during or after forced expiration, the posterior tracheal membrane bulges anteriorly, narrowing and, in some cases, nearly obliterating the tracheal lumen (Fig. 22.3). The mean anterior-posterior diameter of the trachea decreases by 30% to 40% during forced expiration due to anterior bulging of the posterior membrane; the transverse diameter decreases by 10% to 20%. The cross-sectional area of the trachea may diminish by more than 50% in normal subjects with forced expiration.

Tracheal Bronchus

A tracheal bronchus represents the origin of all or part (usually the apical segment) of the right upper lobe bronchus from the trachea; its incidence is about 0.1% (see Figs. 9.1 and 9.2 in Chapter 9). Left tracheal bronchus also occurs but is much less common.

ABNORMALITIES ASSOCIATED WITH TRACHEAL NARROWING

Focal tracheal narrowing may be seen with tracheal tumors (Table 22.1), tracheobronchomalacia, tracheal stenosis or stricture, saber-sheath trachea, granulomatosis with polyangiitis (GPA), amyloidosis, sarcoidosis, or tuberculosis (TB) or other infections (Table 22.2).

Diffuse or generalized tracheal narrowing may be seen with TM, saber-sheath trachea, GPA, amyloidosis, tracheobronchopathia osteochondroplastica (TPOP), relapsing polychondritis (RPC), sarcoidosis, and some infections.

Stenting is sometimes used to treat TM, tracheal stenosis, polychondritis, and GPA. Surgery may be employed for localized or focal lesions.

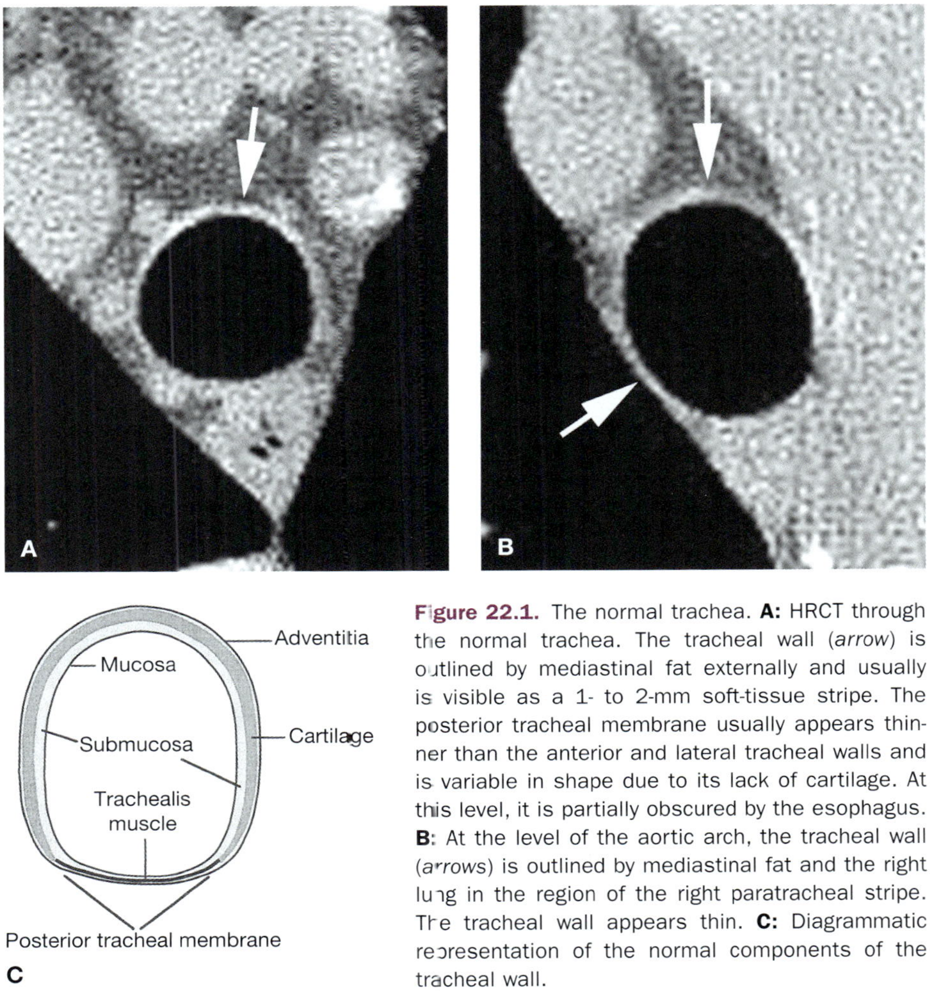

Figure 22.1. The normal trachea. **A:** HRCT through the normal trachea. The tracheal wall (*arrow*) is outlined by mediastinal fat externally and usually is visible as a 1- to 2-mm soft-tissue stripe. The posterior tracheal membrane usually appears thinner than the anterior and lateral tracheal walls and is variable in shape due to its lack of cartilage. At this level, it is partially obscured by the esophagus. **B:** At the level of the aortic arch, the tracheal wall (*arrows*) is outlined by mediastinal fat and the right lung in the region of the right paratracheal stripe. The tracheal wall appears thin. **C:** Diagrammatic representation of the normal components of the tracheal wall.

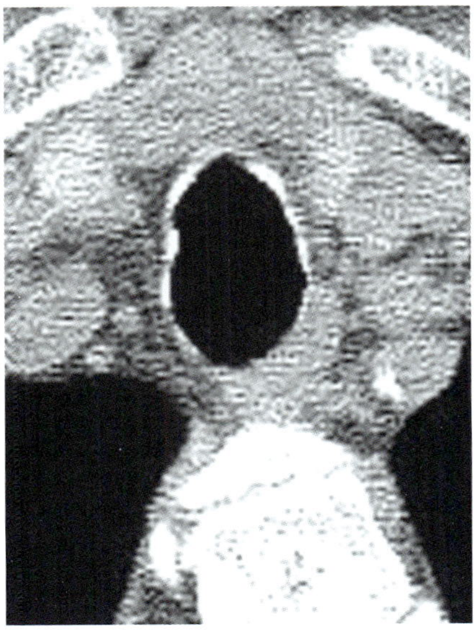

Figure 22.2. Normal calcification of tracheal cartilage in an elderly woman. Discontinuous calcification of the tracheal wall reflects calcification of individual cartilage rings. The tracheal wall appears thin.

Tracheal Tumors

Tumors of the trachea are rare (Table 22.1). Symptoms often are absent or nonspecific (eg, cough, dyspnea), and early diagnosis is difficult. Tracheal tumors tend to be inconspicuous on chest radiographs and may become quite large before they are detected. CT is highly sensitive in detecting tracheal tumors and their extent of spread. Together, squamous cell carcinoma and adenoid cystic carcinoma account for more than 85% of tracheal tumors. Tumors of many other cell types, both epithelial and mesenchymal, may occur in the trachea but are much less common. Ten percent of tracheal tumors are benign.

Squamous cell carcinoma is most common (45%-65% of cases). It is associated with smoking and is multifocal in 10% of cases, often involving the distal trachea; a main bronchus also may be involved (see Figs. 5.37 and 5.38 in Chapter 5). *Adenoid cystic carcinoma* originates from tracheal mucous glands and is most common in the upper trachea (Figs. 22.4 and 22.5). It is less common than squamous cell carcinoma. Adenoid cystic carcinoma often arises from the posterolateral tracheal wall (Figs. 22.5 and 22.6B).

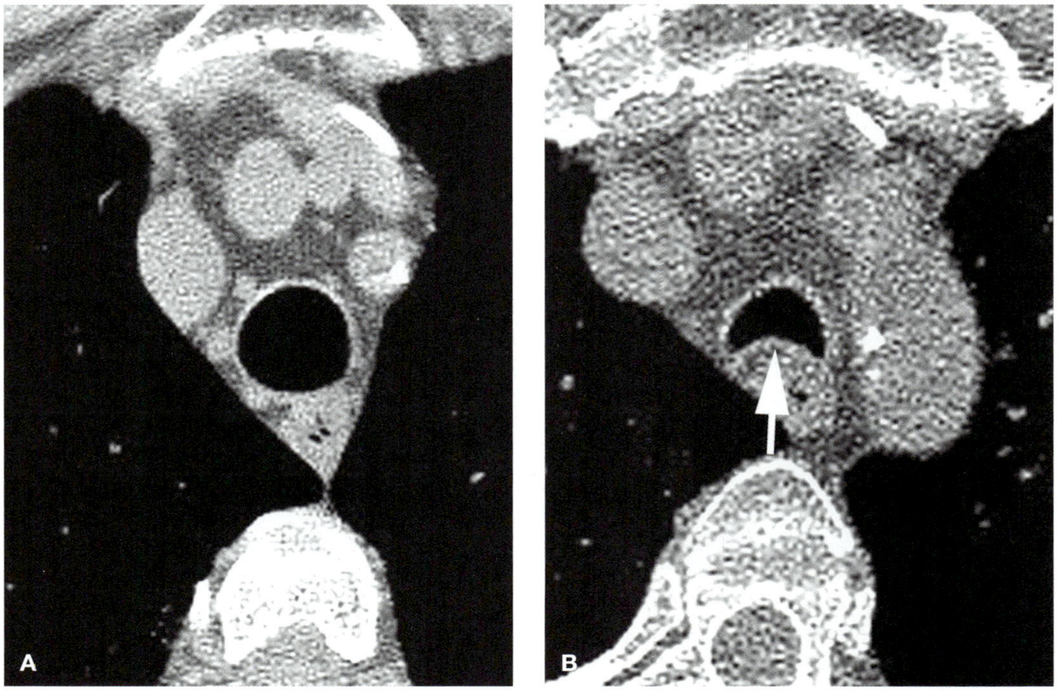

Figure 22.3. Normal expiratory CT. **A:** On inspiration, the trachea has a rounded appearance. **B:** During a dynamic forced expiratory scan, there is anterior bowing of the posterior tracheal membrane (*arrow*). This appearance is normal. Little side-to-side narrowing occurs because of the tracheal cartilage.

Table 22.1 Tracheal Tumors

Primary malignant
Most common (85% of cases)
Squamous cell carcinoma
Adenoid cystic carcinoma
Rare
Other types of bronchogenic carcinoma
Carcinoid tumor
Sarcoma
Lymphoma
Metastatic
Direct invasion most common
Thyroid carcinoma
Laryngeal cancer
Lung cancer
Esophageal cancer
Hematogenous metastases
Melanoma
Breast carcinoma
Colon carcinoma
Kidney carcinoma
Benign
Squamous cell papilloma
Papillomatosis
Hamartoma
Mesenchymal tumors

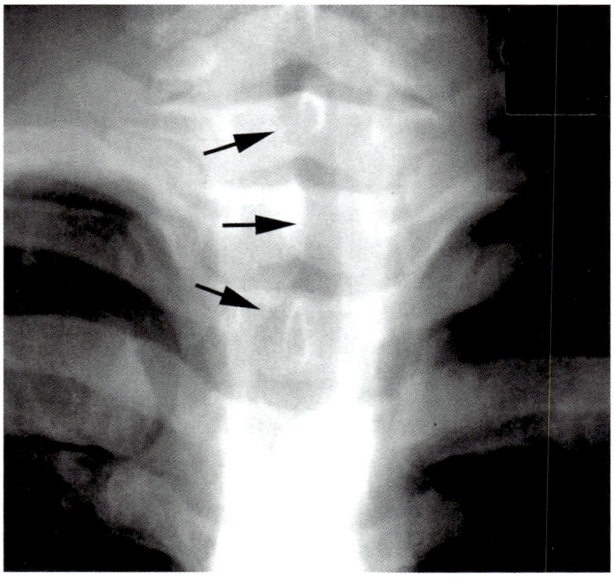

Figure 22.4. Adenoid cystic carcinoma of the proximal trachea. An eccentric narrowing (*arrows*) of the tracheal lumen is caused by a sessile mass arising from the right tracheal wall.

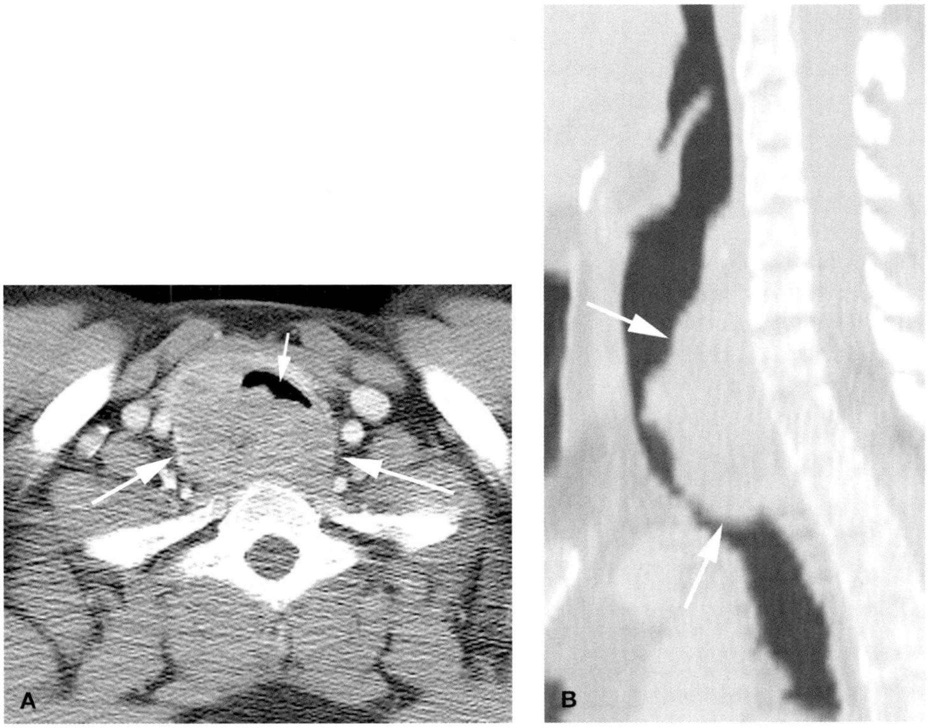

Figure 22.5. Adenoid cystic carcinoma of the trachea. **A:** A large mass (*large arrows*) in the upper trachea markedly narrows the tracheal lumen (*small arrow*) and invades the mediastinum. **B:** On a sagittal reconstruction, the mass (*arrows*) can be seen to arise from the posterior tracheal wall. This location is typical of adenoid cystic carcinoma.

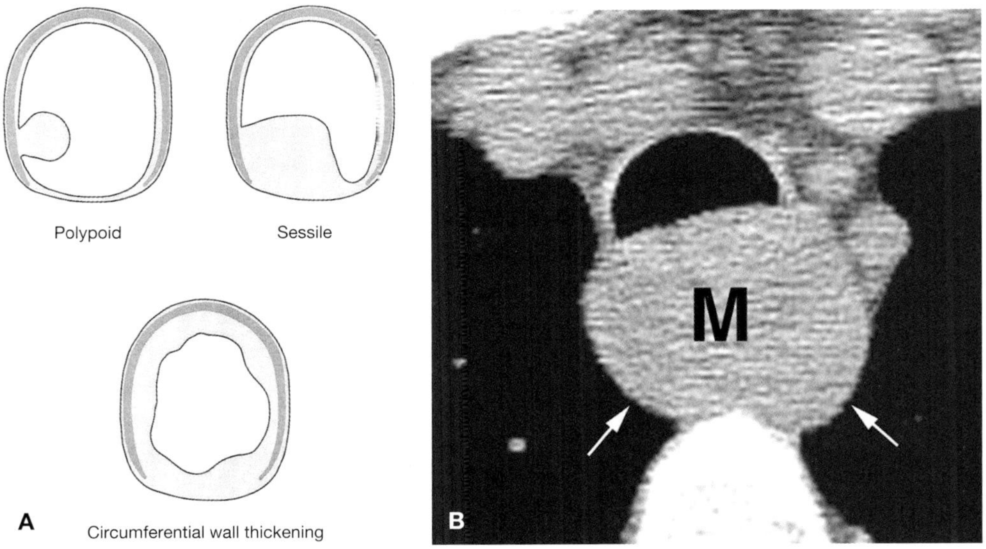

Figure 22.6. CT appearances of primary tracheal tumor. **A:** Tracheal malignancies may appear polypoid, sessile, or circumferential. **B:** Adenoid cystic carcinoma results in a sessile mass (*M*) arising from the posterior tracheal wall and protruding into the tracheal lumen. The mass extends into the adjacent mediastinum (*arrows*).

On CT, a primary malignant tracheal tumor may appear as a polypoid lesion, a focal sessile lesion, eccentric narrowing of the tracheal lumen, or circumferential wall thickening (see Fig. 22.5). Attachment to the tracheal wall may be either broad based (Fig. 22.5) or narrow and pedunculated. CT may underestimate the longitudinal extent of the tumor; submucosal spread may be difficult to see on CT. However, CT is superior to bronchoscopy in evaluating extraluminal spread and the trachea distal to an obstructing lesion that cannot be traversed by a bronchoscope.

Metastases to the trachea may occur via direct extension or by hematogenous spread. Direct extension to involve the trachea most often is secondary to a primary tumor of the lung, larynx, esophagus, or thyroid, or invasion from adjacent lymph nodes. These tumors may compress the trachea, displacing tracheal cartilage inward, or may invade the tracheal lumen, with tumor being seen as abnormal tissue internal to tracheal cartilage (Fig. 22.7; also see Fig. 5.56 in Chapter 5). Hematogenous metastases usually originate from melanoma or from carcinomas of the breast, colon, or kidney. On CT, hematogenous metastases may appear as single or multiple, sessile, or pedunculated endotracheal lesions (Fig. 22.8).

Squamous cell papilloma is the most common benign tracheal tumor. It represents an abnormal proliferation of squamous epithelium and may appear sessile, papillary, lobulated, or polypoid. Solitary papilloma is associated with smoking and is most common in adults. The condition of multiple papillomas (ie, papillomatosis) usually begins in childhood with laryngeal involvement and is associated with human

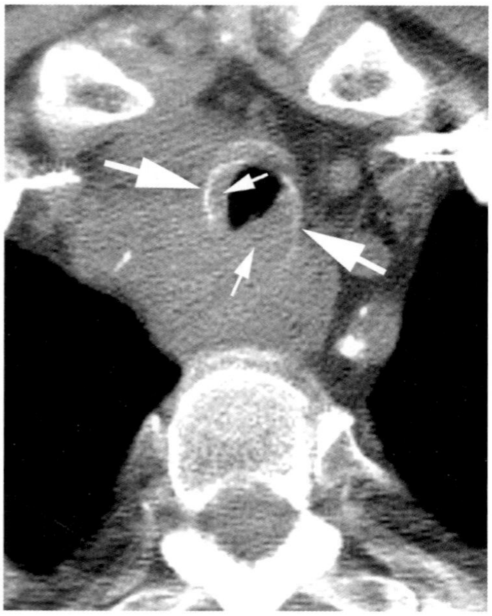

Figure 22.7. Esophageal carcinoma with tracheal invasion. Tumor has invaded the trachea and is seen as soft tissue (*small arrows*) internal to the calcified tracheal cartilage (*large arrows*). The tracheal lumen is narrowed.

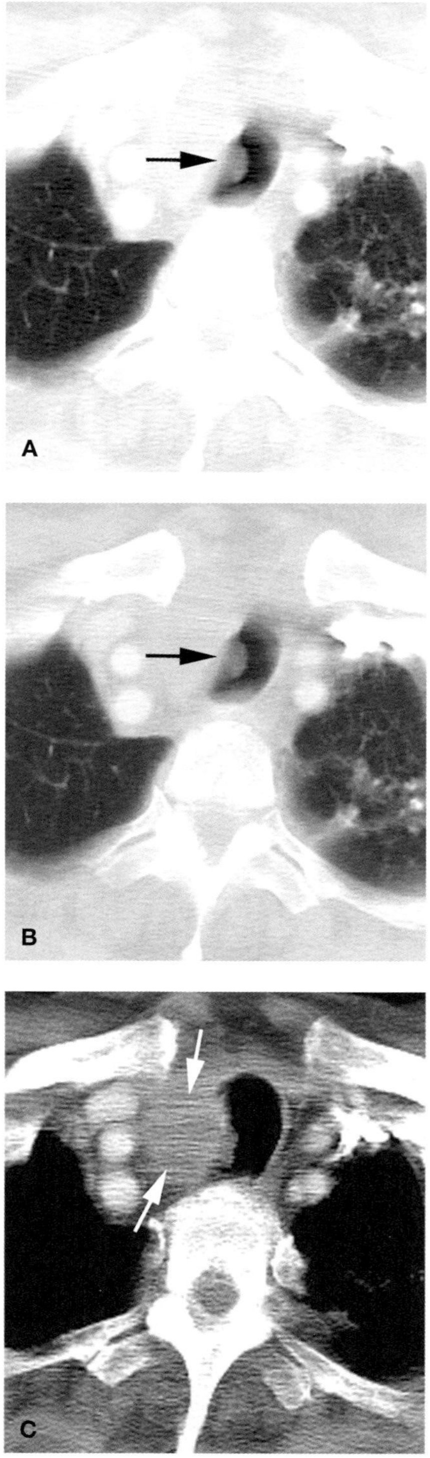

Figure 22.8. Tracheal metastasis. Tracheal metastases may result in tracheal compression with inward displacement of the tracheal wall, an endotracheal mass, or a combination of these findings. **A, B:** There is narrowing of the trachea with an endoluminal mass (*arrow*). **C:** Soft-tissue window at the same level as (**B**) shows a mass involving the right tracheal wall and mediastinal soft tissues (*arrows*).

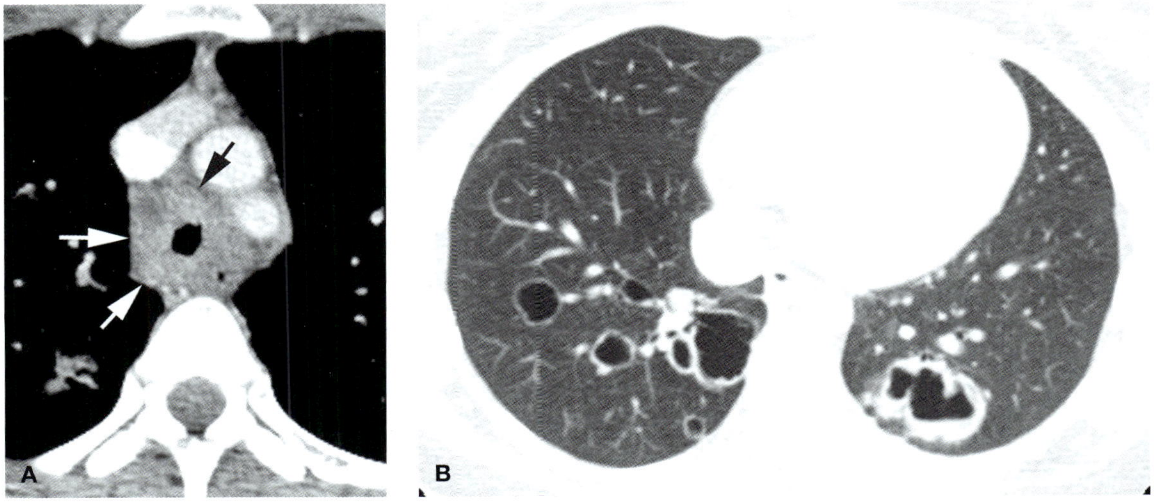

Figure 22.9. Tracheobronchial papillomatosis with tracheal wall thickening. **A:** Concentric thickening of the tracheal wall (*arrows*) is due to diffuse involvement by papillomas. The tracheal lumen is markedly narrowed. **B:** Multiple cystic pulmonary lesions may be seen in some patients with tracheobronchial papillomatosis.

papillomavirus infection. On CT, a solitary papilloma appears as a well-circumscribed nodule that is confined to the tracheal wall and projects into the tracheal lumen; it often shows acute angles where it contacts the tracheal wall. Tracheal cartilage is unaffected. Papillomatosis is characterized by numerous nodules involving the entire length of the trachea (see Fig. 5.25 in Chapter 5) or diffuse thickening of the tracheal wall (Fig. 22.9). Other benign tracheal tumors include hamartoma and tumors of mesenchymal origin such as lipoma or chondroma.

Table 22.2 Nonneoplastic Tracheal Diseases

Disease	Extent	Appearance	Associations
Tracheobronchomalacia	Focal or diffuse	Collapse of tracheal wall (and bronchi) with expiration	Congenital intubation, extrinsic masses, chronic infection, COPD, saber-sheath trachea, polychondritis, tracheobronchomegaly
Tuberculosis	Distal trachea (and main bronchi)	Early: concentric wall thickening Late: stricture or distortion of cartilage	Mediastinal lymph node disease
Post intubation stenosis	Proximal trachea	Early: concentric wall thickening Late: stricture or distortion of cartilage	Malacia may be present
Saber-sheath trachea	Early: thoracic inlet Late: intrathoracic trachea	Side-to-side narrowing, sagittal diameter normal or increased	COPD, chronic cough; malacia may be present
Granulomatosis with Polyangiitis	Focal (subglottic trachea) or diffuse	Concentric wall thickening, cartilage destruction	Occurs in 15%-25% of cases; malacia not often present
Amyloidosis	Focal (nodular) or diffuse	Concentric or nodular wall thickening	Calcification common; malacia is not present
Tracheobronchopathia osteochondroplastica	Diffuse	Calcified submucosal nodules adjacent to tracheal cartilage, nodules spare the posterior membrane	Malacia is not present
Relapsing polychondritis	Diffuse	Thickening of anterior and lateral wall, posterior membrane normal	Arthritis; malacia may be present.
Tracheobronchomegaly (Mounier-Kuhn syndrome)	Diffuse	Increased tracheal diameter (>3 cm), tracheal wall normal or appears scalloped, tracheal diverticula	Cystic bronchiectasis often present; COPD, pulmonary fibrosis, Marfan syndrome, cystic fibrosis, Ehlers-Danlos syndrome, cutis laxa

COPD, chronic obstructive pulmonary disease.

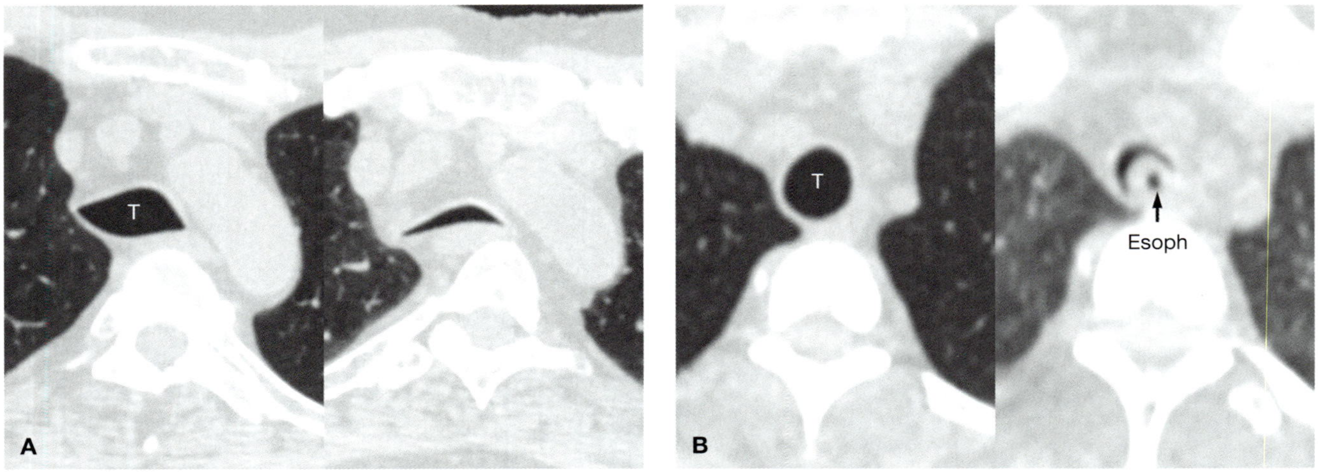

Figure 22.10. Tracheobronchomalacia versus excessive dynamic airway collapse. **A:** Inspiratory and expiratory CT images through the upper thoracic trachea. The trachea (T) has an abnormal configuration during inspiration (left image) due to weakened cartilage. This becomes more pronounced during expiration (right image) with near-complete loss of the lumen. **B:** Inspiratory and expiratory CT images through the upper thoracic trachea. Normal configuration of the trachea (*T*) during inspiration (left image) and near-complete obliteration of the tracheal lumen during exhalation (right image) due to excessive collapse of the posterior membrane of the trachea. The esophagus (*Esoph*) contains air and can create a confusing appearance in this setting.

Tracheomalacia and Excessive Dynamic Airway Collapse

TM and excessive dynamic airway collapse (EDAC) are distinct entities that both result in abnormal expiratory narrowing of the trachea. TM refers to weakness of the tracheal wall, usually due to abnormalities of the tracheal cartilage, associated with excessive collapsibility of the trachea on expiration (Table 22.2). The term *tracheobronchomalacia* is used when bronchi are also abnormally collapsible. TM may be congenital and associated with deficient cartilage, but most often is acquired as a result of intubation injuries, tracheal compression by extrinsic masses or vascular lesions (eg, aortic aneurysm), chronic infection, or chronic obstructive pulmonary disease or in association with saber-sheath trachea, RPC, or tracheobronchomegaly. It may be localized, or it may involve a long tracheal segment.

EDAC is the result of a redundant posterior tracheal membrane that bows forward during exhalation. EDAC is often due to weakening of the smooth muscle fibers. The tracheal cartilage is usually normal except in rare cases where TM and EDAC coexist.

TM and EDAC are reported in at least 5% of patients undergoing bronchoscopy, but these numbers are likely underestimated.

TM and EDAC may result in inefficient cough, retention of secretions, and chronic airway infection and bronchiectasis. Symptoms include recurrent infection, dyspnea, and stridor.

Radiographs or CT on inspiration may show increased or decreased tracheal diameter in patients with TM. The hallmark of TM is a significant decrease in the tracheal diameter or collapse of the tracheal walls with expiration (Fig. 22.10). Tracheal collapse may be diffuse, side to side, or less often anterior to posterior. Historically, a 50% decrease in tracheal diameter or cross-sectional area with expiration was considered indicative of TM, but this degree of tracheal narrowing may be seen in over 70% of normal individuals on dynamic exhalation (see Fig. 22.3). Currently, the degree of stenosis is graded as mild (70%-79%), moderate (80%-89%), and severe (>90%). Treatment is generally reserved for the most severe cases and performed at specialty referral centers.

Tracheal Stenosis

Congenital tracheal stenosis may result from a ring-shaped tracheal cartilage. Acquired tracheal stenosis usually is due to prior intubation or tracheostomy. Progressive dyspnea following extubation typically is present. Inflammation and pressure necrosis of the tracheal mucosa most commonly occur at either the tracheostomy stoma or at the level of the tube balloon, 1 to 1.5 cm proximal to the tube tip; the stenosis usually involves 1.5 to 2.5 cm of the tracheal wall. The extrathoracic trachea most often is involved. Focal narrowing may be seen if the tube tip presses on one part of the tracheal wall, usually the anterior wall.

Acute postintubation stenosis results from edema of the tracheal wall or intraluminal granulation tissue. Plain films may show an eccentric or hourglass-shaped tracheal narrowing. On CT, this may be seen as eccentric or concentric soft tissue internal to normal-appearing tracheal cartilage (Fig. 22.11). The outer tracheal wall has a normal appearance, without evidence of deformity or narrowing. Dynamic expiratory images show little change in tracheal dimensions.

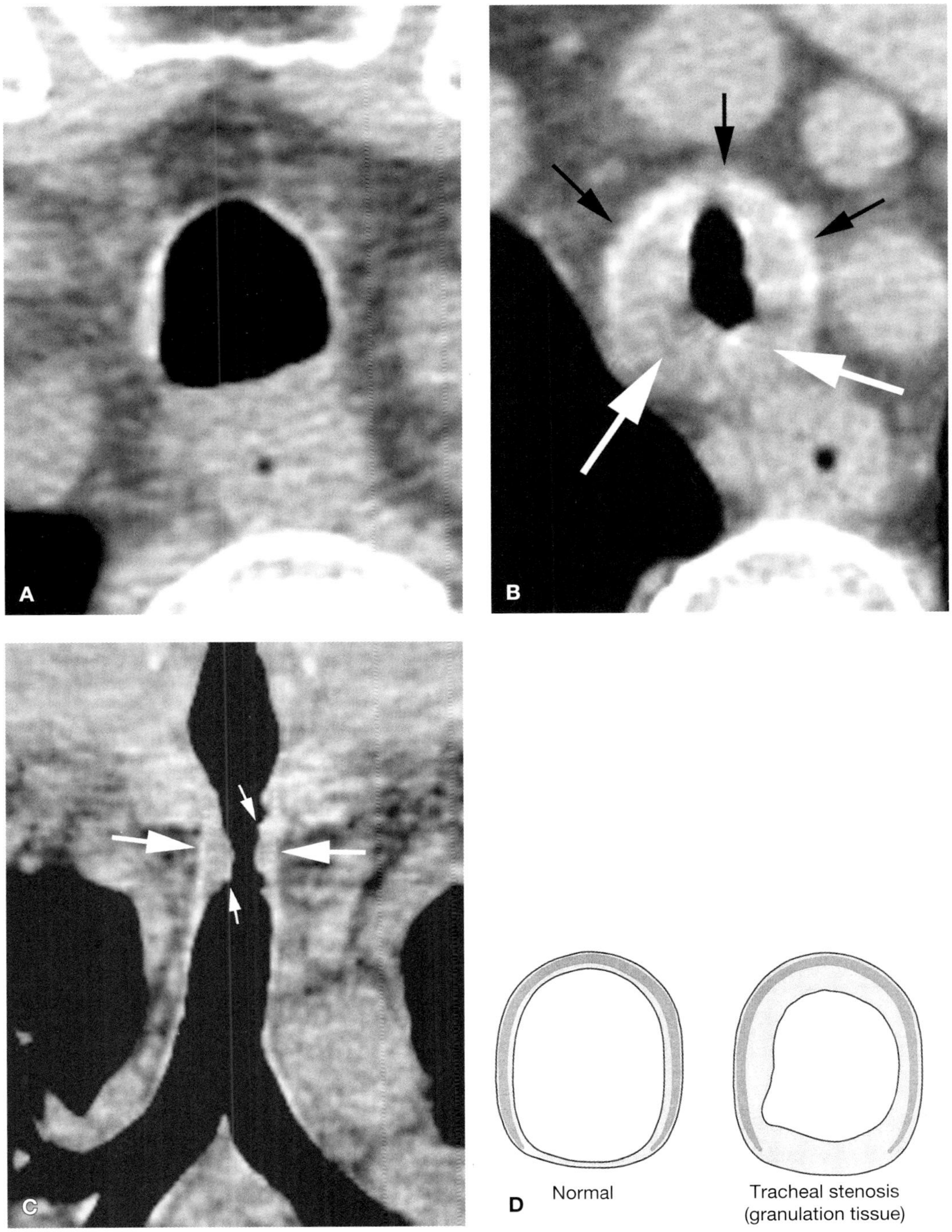

Figure 22.11. Postintubation tracheal stenosis due to granulation tissue. **A:** Near the thoracic inlet, the trachea appears normal. **B:** Below the level shown in (**A**), focal narrowing of the tracheal lumen is associated with increased soft tissue (*white arrows*) within the tracheal lumen. The calcified tracheal cartilage (*black arrows*) appears normal, without evidence of deformity or collapse. **C:** Coronal reconstruction in a patient with an hourglass-shaped tracheal stenosis following intubation. The tracheal wall appears normal (*large arrows*), and granulation tissue is seen narrowing the tracheal lumen (*small arrows*). **D:** Diagrammatic representation of tracheal stenosis due to granulation tissue, compared to the appearance of a normal trachea. (Reproduced with permission of the American Roentgen Ray Society from Webb EM, Elicker BM, Webb WR. Using CT to diagnose nonneoplastic tracheal abnormalities: appearance of the tracheal wall. *AJR Am J Roentgenol*. 2000;174:1315-1321. Copyright© 2000 American Roentgen Ray Society.)

With *chronic postintubation stenosis* or stricture, fibrosis usually is present with deformity of tracheal cartilage and collapse of the tracheal wall. On CT, thickening of the mucosa and submucosa is absent or mild, and deformity of the tracheal cartilage or posterior tracheal membrane accounts for narrowing of the lumen (Figs. 22.12 and 22.13). The area of narrowing may be thin and weblike or long and hourglass shaped. Dynamic expiratory images may or may not show significant malacia. Because of the focal nature of the stenosis, treatment with stenting is useful.

Acute and chronic tracheal or bronchial stenosis may also result from sarcoidosis, histoplasmosis or other fungi, GPA, and inflammatory bowel disease.

Saber-Sheath Trachea

Saber-sheath trachea is common and almost always is associated with chronic obstructive pulmonary disease. It is characterized by a marked decrease in the coronal diameter of the intrathoracic trachea associated with an increase in its sagittal diameter (Fig. 22.14); the extrathoracic trachea is normal. Although it may involve the entire intrathoracic trachea, in its earliest stages, it is visible only at the thoracic inlet. It is thought to be due to chronic injury and malacia of tracheal cartilage due to coughing or increased intrathoracic pressure. The main bronchi are of normal size.

On frontal radiographs, a characteristic side-to-side narrowing of the tracheal lumen is visible beginning at the thoracic inlet (see Fig. 22.14). The right paratracheal stripe, primarily representing tracheal wall, appears normal or slightly increased in thickness. On the lateral radiograph, the tracheal diameter appears normal or slightly increased. If the tracheal diameter on the lateral film measures 1.5 times that seen on the frontal film, saber-sheath trachea is considered to be present.

On CT, there is inward displacement of the lateral portions of the tracheal wall and tracheal cartilage with side-to-side narrowing of the tracheal lumen (Fig. 22.15). The tracheal wall usually is of normal thickness. During forced expiration, CT demonstrates further inward bowing of the tracheal walls in many patients.

Granulomatosis With Polyangiitis

GPA is a systemic vasculitis. In 90% of cases, serum antineutrophil cytoplasmic antibodies characterized by a diffuse granular cytoplasmic immunofluorescent staining pattern (cytoplasmic antineutrophil cytoplasmic antibody) are present.

Tracheobronchial involvement occurs in about 15% to 25% of cases; symptoms are common and include hoarseness, cough, and stridor. Subglottic tracheal involvement is most typical (Fig. 22.16), with variable involvement of the vocal cords, distal trachea, and proximal mainstem bronchi. Abnormalities may be focal or diffuse. Pathologic findings include circumferential airway wall thickening and inflammation and concentric narrowing of the tracheal lumen; mucosal ulceration and destruction of the cricoid or tracheal cartilage are less common. Tracheal involvement may be life threatening, but treatment with stents may be helpful.

Plain radiographs show tracheal narrowing on both the frontal and lateral radiographs; this narrowing may be localized or diffuse. Characteristic CT findings include focal or circumferential thickening of the tracheal wall, an increase in the overall tracheal diameter due to wall thickening, and narrowing of the tracheal lumen (Fig. 22.17). Malacia is not typically seen, but may be present (Fig. 22.18). Proximal bronchi may be involved (Figs. 22.17C and 22.19).

Amyloidosis

Tracheobronchial amyloidosis is rare (see Chapter 21). Symptoms are common and include hoarseness, stridor, dyspnea, cough, hemoptysis, and recurrent infections.

Primary tracheobronchial amyloidosis is usually confined to the airways, with no evidence of concurrent parenchymal disease. Deposits are multifocal or diffuse, being submucosal in location, and involve the length of the trachea; the main bronchi also are commonly affected. On plain radiographs and CT, diffuse tracheobronchial amyloidosis usually leads to concentric or nodular thickening of the tracheal wall (Fig. 22.20). Calcification or ossification is common. Malacia is not present. Rarely, a single localized submucosal nodule is present, resulting in eccentric wall thickening. Multiple isolated lesions also may be seen. Atelectasis may be associated with bronchial involvement. Progression is typical, and bronchoscopic resection of focal lesions or airway stenting may be helpful in some cases.

Tracheobronchopathia Osteochondroplastica

TPOP is a rare, benign disease characterized by the development of cartilaginous and osseous nodules within the submucosa of the tracheal and bronchial walls. It is most typical in men older than 50 and usually is detected incidentally. In some patients, dyspnea, cough, hemoptysis, and wheezing may be present.

Nodules tend to be localized to the submucosa directly associated with the tracheal cartilage, sparing the posterior tracheal membrane (Figs. 22.21 and 22.22). The nodules may consist of cartilage or exostoses occurring in relation to the perichondrium of the tracheal cartilage, or they may be metaplastic, arising in elastic tissue.

Plain radiographs show extensive irregular tracheal and central bronchial calcification. CT findings include thickened cartilage with small irregular nodules along their inner aspect, protruding into the tracheal lumen (Figs. 22.21 and 22.22). The nodules typically measure between 3 and 8 mm in diameter and are usually calcified. The appearance is much more irregular than that seen with normal cartilage calcification. Similar central bronchial calcification also is seen in many patients. No significant decrease in tracheal diameter is seen with forced expiration.

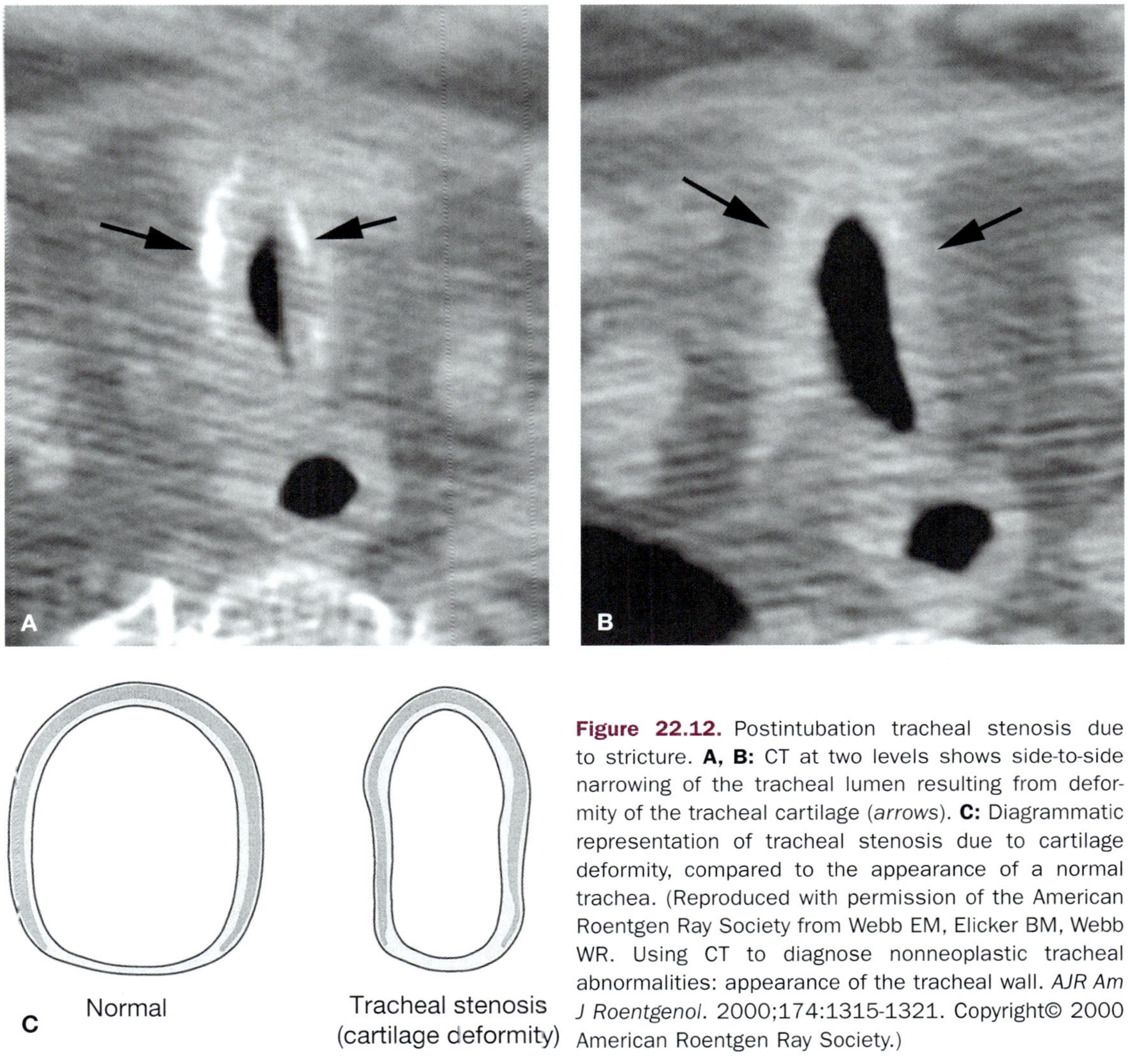

Figure 22.12. Postintubation tracheal stenosis due to stricture. **A, B:** CT at two levels shows side-to-side narrowing of the tracheal lumen resulting from deformity of the tracheal cartilage (*arrows*). **C:** Diagrammatic representation of tracheal stenosis due to cartilage deformity, compared to the appearance of a normal trachea. (Reproduced with permission of the American Roentgen Ray Society from Webb EM, Elicker BM, Webb WR. Using CT to diagnose nonneoplastic tracheal abnormalities: appearance of the tracheal wall. *AJR Am J Roentgenol.* 2000;174:1315-1321. Copyright© 2000 American Roentgen Ray Society.)

Relapsing Polychondritis

RPC is a rare systemic disorder characterized by recurrent episodes of cartilage inflammation most commonly affecting the ear, nose, joints, and the laryngeal and tracheal cartilage. Nonerosive polyarthritis, nasal deformity, and auricular chondritis are characteristic, but need not be present in all cases. The upper airways are affected in more than 50% of cases, and recurrent pneumonia is the most common cause of death. Diffuse tracheal involvement, characterized by a dense inflammatory exudate, is limited to the cartilage and perichondrium and does not affect the mucosa or submucosa. Histologic findings include edema, granulation tissue, cartilage destruction, and, eventually, fibrosis of the tracheal wall. Both the extrathoracic and intrathoracic portions of the trachea are involved. Treatment often requires the use of tracheal and bronchial stents to maintain airway patency.

Plain radiographs usually show cylindrical narrowing of the extrathoracic and intrathoracic trachea and main bronchi (Fig. 22.23). In most cases, CT shows thickening of the anterior and lateral tracheal walls, but the posterior membrane is of normal thickness (Figs. 22.24 and 22.25). Both the inner and outer margins of the thickened tracheal walls are smooth in contour. Collapse of tracheal cartilage may be seen in chronic disease. Narrowing of both the tracheal lumen and the main bronchi is often present. TM is often present (Fig. 22.26).

Infections

A variety of organisms may result in tracheobronchitis, including viruses, bacteria, and fungi (see Chapter 13).

Tuberculosis

TB typically involves both the distal trachea and the proximal main bronchi; isolated tracheal disease is rare. Active inflammation with granulation tissue causes irregular circumferential wall thickening with narrowing of the tracheal lumen. In many cases, tracheal infection results from spread from adjacent lymph nodes, and enlarged mediastinal nodes or

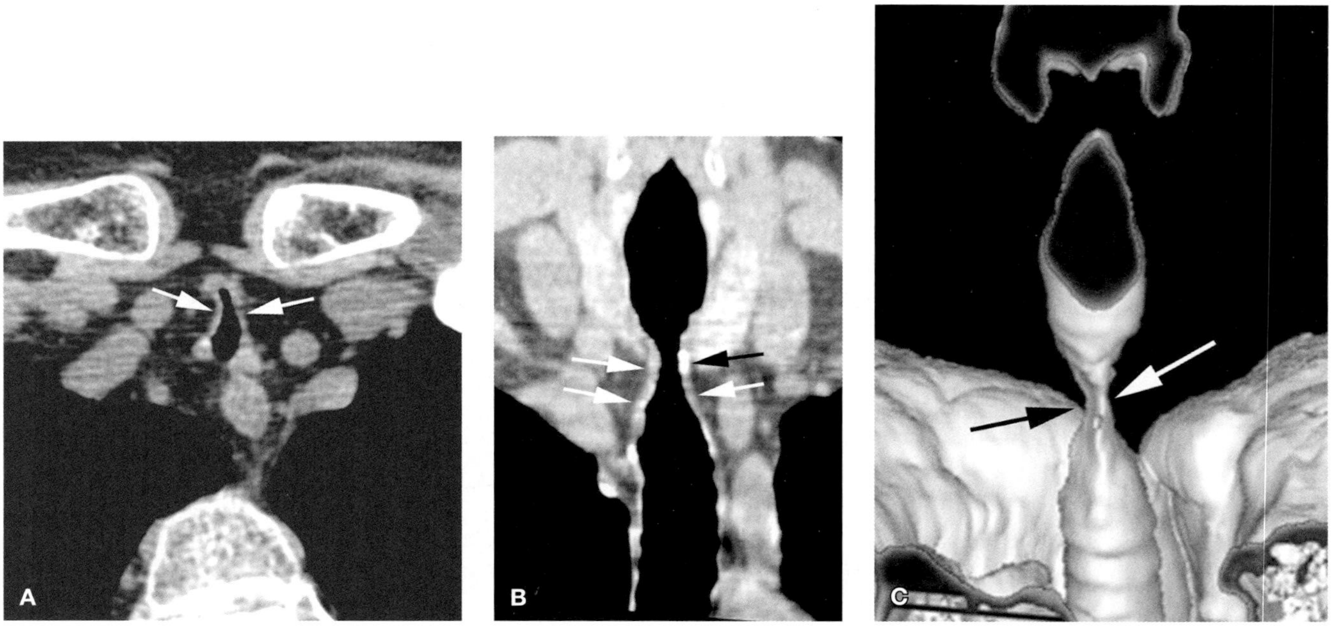

Figure 22.13. Postintubation tracheal stenosis due to deformity of tracheal cartilage. **A:** CT shows side-to-side narrowing of the tracheal lumen resulting from deformity of the tracheal cartilage (*arrows*). The tracheal wall is outlined by mediastinal fat. **B:** Coronal reconstruction shows an hourglass-shaped stenosis, with inward collapse of the tracheal wall (*white arrows*). Calcified tracheal cartilage (*black arrow*) is displaced inward. **C:** Three-dimensional reconstruction shows the hourglass-shaped stenosis (*arrows*).

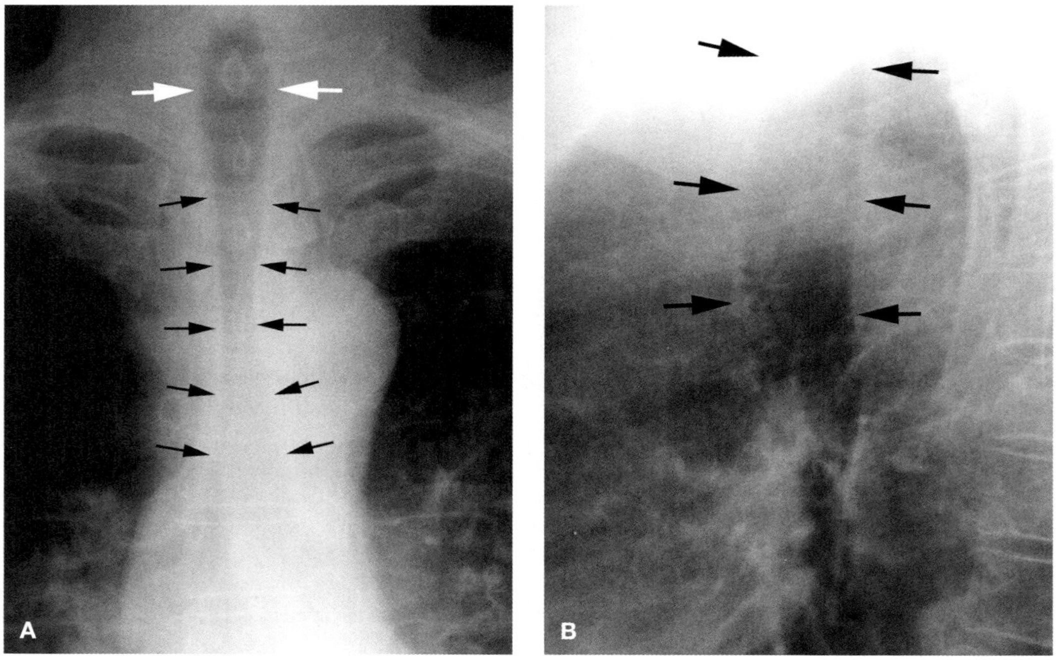

Figure 22.14. Saber-sheath trachea in a patient with chronic obstructive pulmonary disease. **A:** PA chest radiograph shows hourglass-shaped narrowing of the intrathoracic trachea (*black arrows*). The extrathoracic trachea (*white arrows*) appears normal. **B:** In the lateral projection, the tracheal diameter appears normal or increased (*arrows*).

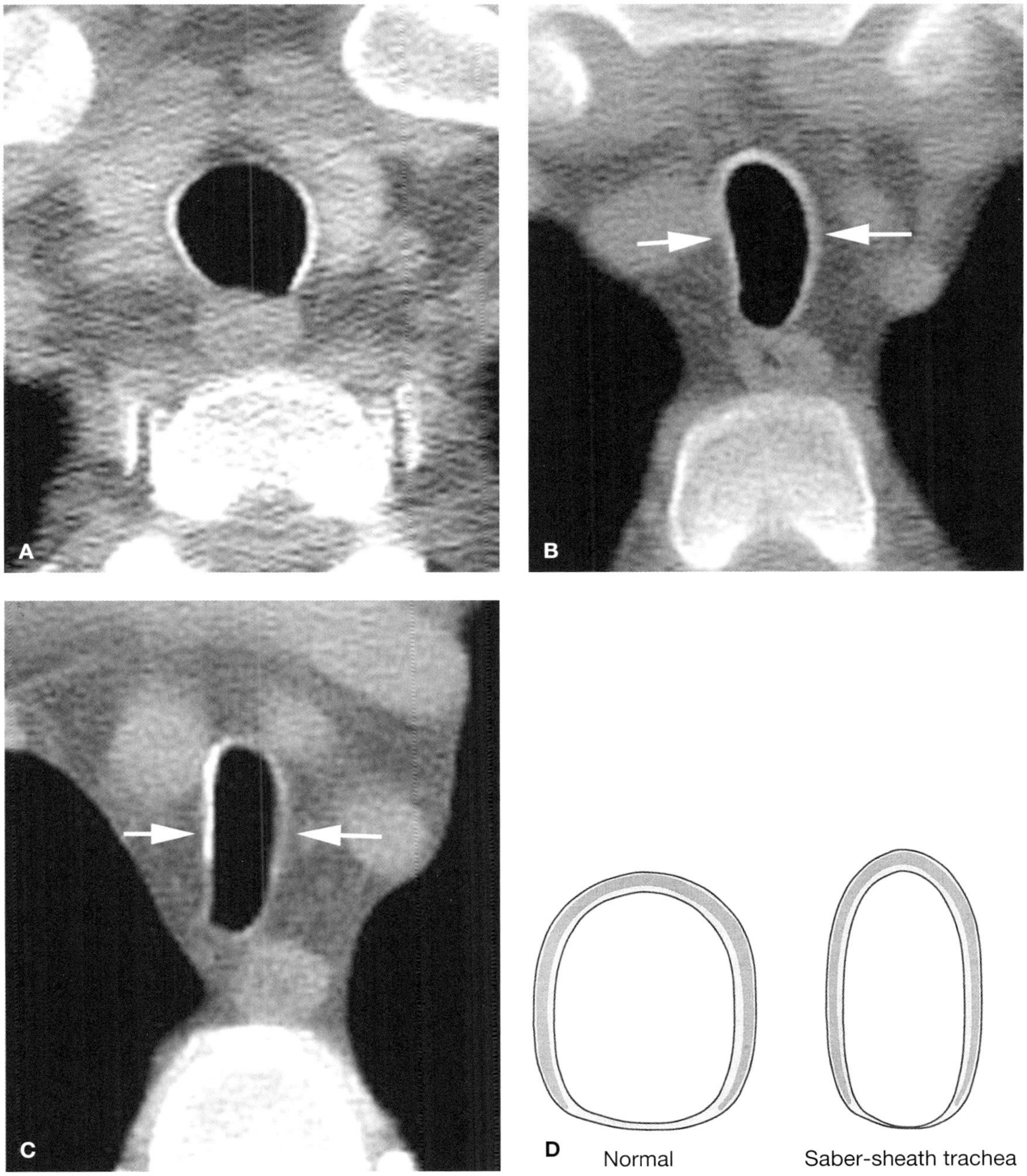

Figure 22.15. Saber-sheath trachea on CT. **A:** The extrathoracic trachea is normal. The tracheal cartilage is calcified and well seen. **B, C:** The intrathoracic trachea at two levels is markedly narrowed from side to side (*arrows*), associated with deformity of the tracheal cartilage. The sagittal tracheal diameter is increased. The tracheal wall is otherwise normal in appearance. **D:** Diagrammatic representation of saber-sheath trachea. (Reproduced with permission of the American Roentgen Ray Society from Webb EM, Elicker BM, Webb WR. Using CT to diagnose nonneoplastic tracheal abnormalities: appearance of the tracheal wall. *AJR Am J Roentgenol*. 2000;174:1315-1321. Copyright© 2000 American Roentgen Ray Society.)

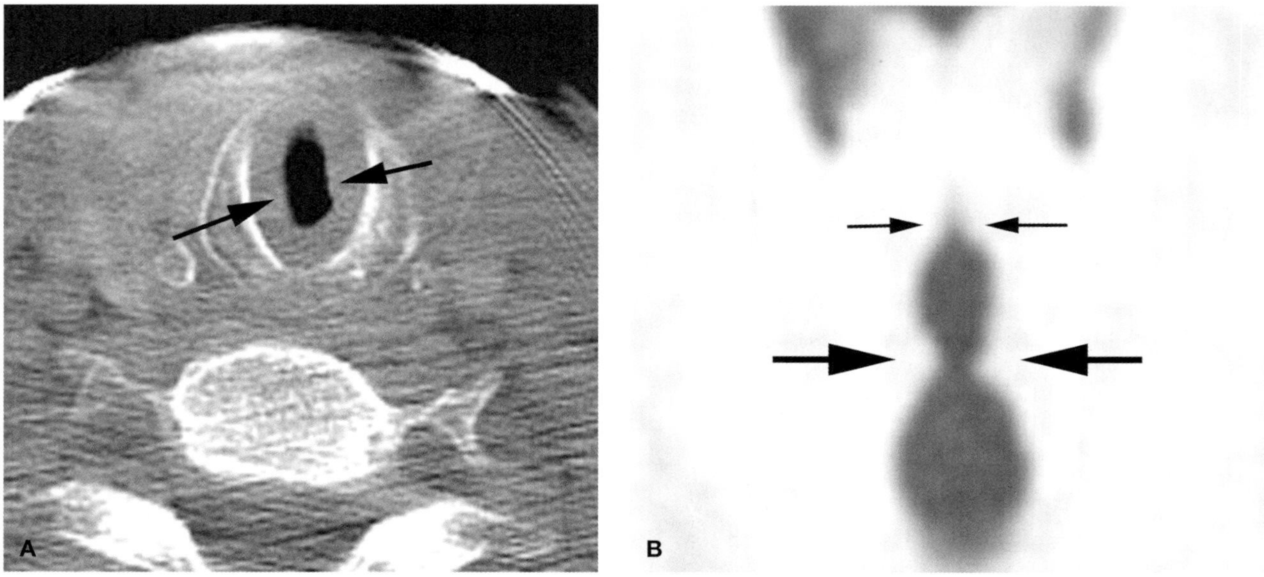

Figure 22.16. Subglottic tracheal stenosis in granulomatosis with polyangiitis (GPA). **A:** Excessive soft tissue (*arrows*) is visible internal to the cricoid cartilage. A tracheostomy is in place below this level. **B:** Coronal reconstruction in subglottic stenosis due to GPA. The focal narrowing (*large arrows*) is just below the level of the vocal cords (*small arrows*).

increased attenuation of mediastinal fat may be seen. Tracheal TB also may occur due to endobronchial spread of infection.

With treatment, wall thickening and tracheal narrowing usually are reversible, although in some patients stricture results, with narrowing of the tracheal lumen in the absence of wall thickening.

Bronchial strictures may be associated with tracheal narrowing. Strictures from TB most often involve the left main bronchus, perhaps because it is longer than the right. CT findings that help to differentiate TB stricture from carcinoma include a long segment of circumferential involvement and the absence of an intraluminal mass.

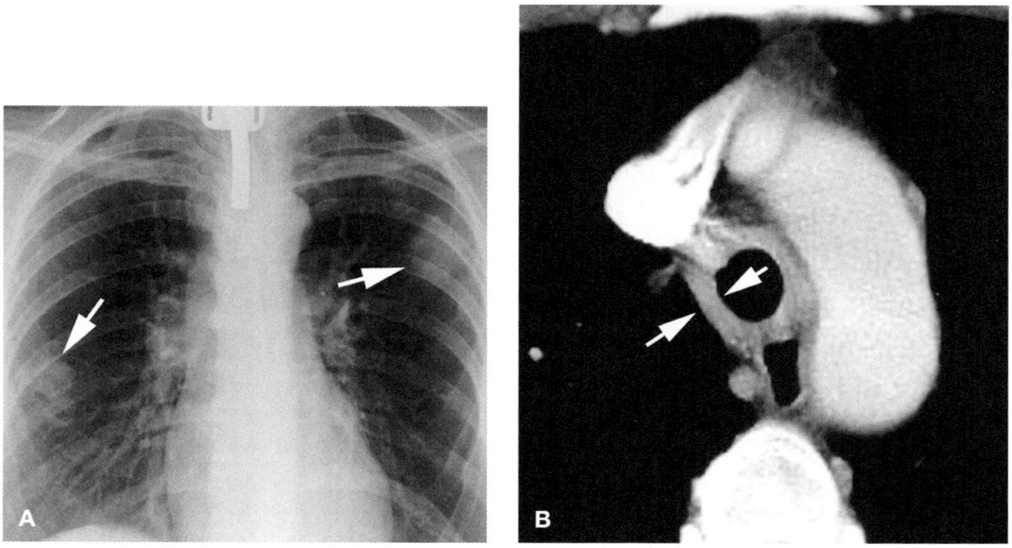

Figure 22.17. Tracheal and bronchial narrowing in granulomatosis with polyangiitis (GPA). **A:** Chest radiograph shows bilateral lung nodules (*arrows*). A tracheostomy is in place. **B:** CT shows tracheal narrowing associated with concentric thickening of the tracheal wall (*arrows*).

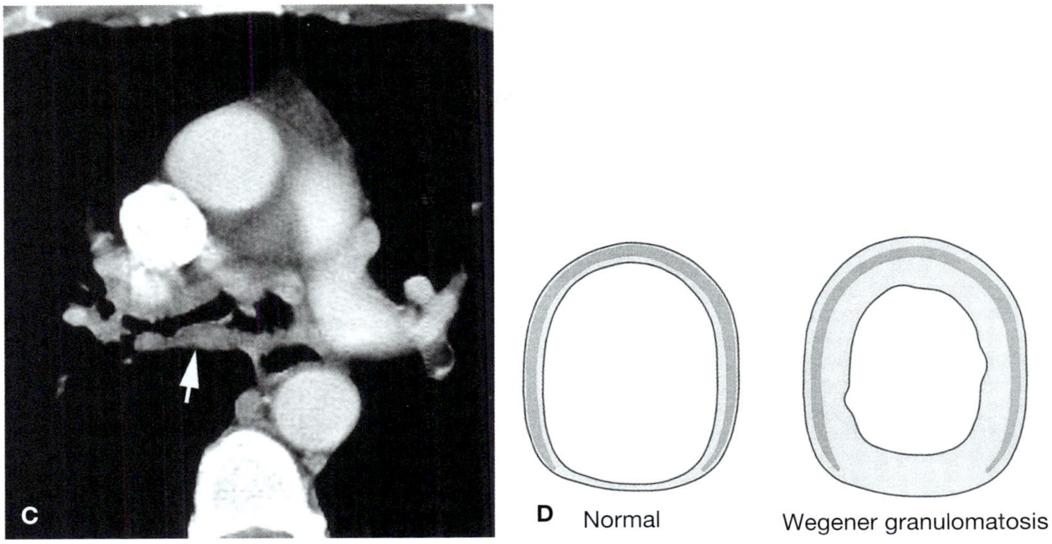

Figure 22.17. *(Continued)* **C:** At the level of the carina, bronchial wall thickening (*arrow*) also is seen. **D:** Diagrammatic representation of abnormalities in GPA. Concentric wall thickening is visible. (Reproduced with permission of the American Roentgen Ray Society from Webb EM, Elicker BM, Webb WR. Using CT to diagnose nonneoplastic tracheal abnormalities: appearance of the tracheal wall. *AJR Am J Roentgenol*. 2000;174:1315-1321. Copyright© 2000 American Roentgen Ray Society.)

Aspergillus *Tracheobronchitis*

About 5% of immunosuppressed patients with invasive aspergillosis develop *Aspergillus* tracheobronchitis. The infection involves the tracheal and/or bronchial walls, resulting in diffuse or focal wall thickening, and narrowing of the tracheal and/or bronchial lumen (Fig. 22.27; Fig. 13.1 in Chapter 13).

Tracheal Scleroma

Scleroma is a granulomatous infection caused by *Klebsiella rhinoscleromatis*, which is localized in the upper airways. It typically involves the nasal and sinus cavities, leading to the term "rhinoscleroma." Laryngeal and trachea involvement may occur in 30%, with granulomatous inflammation and tracheal wall thickening. The disease progresses slowly and

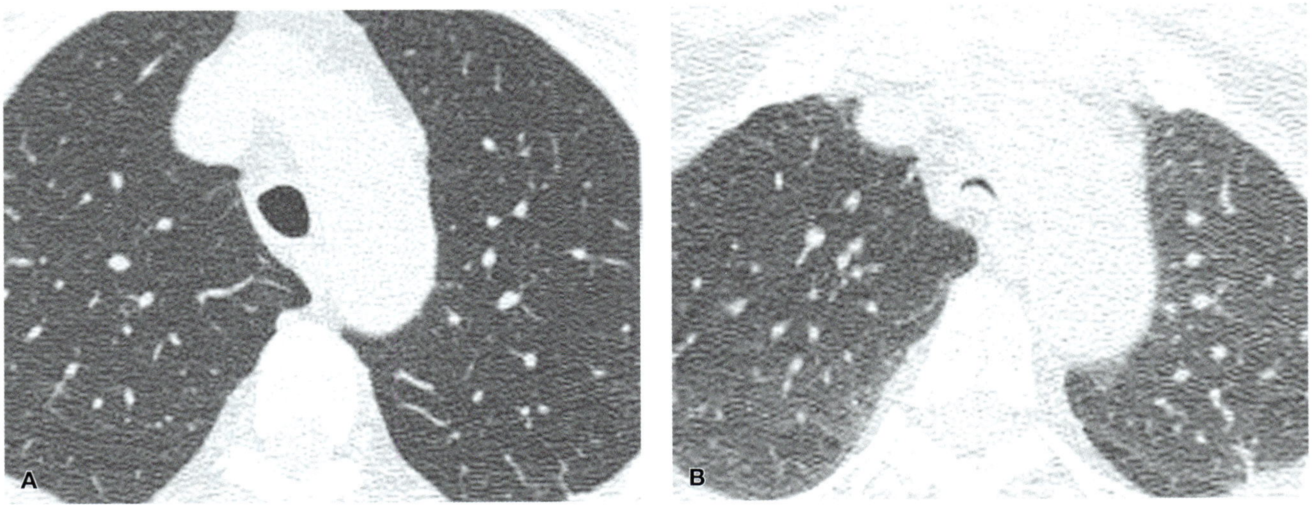

Figure 22.18. Tracheobronchomalacia in granulomatosis with polyangiitis. **A:** CT on inspiration shows the tracheal lumen to be slightly reduced in diameter. **B:** CT during dynamic forced expiration shows flattening of the tracheal cartilage with severe (greater than 90%) reduction in the tracheal cross-sectional area. The patient was symptomatic.

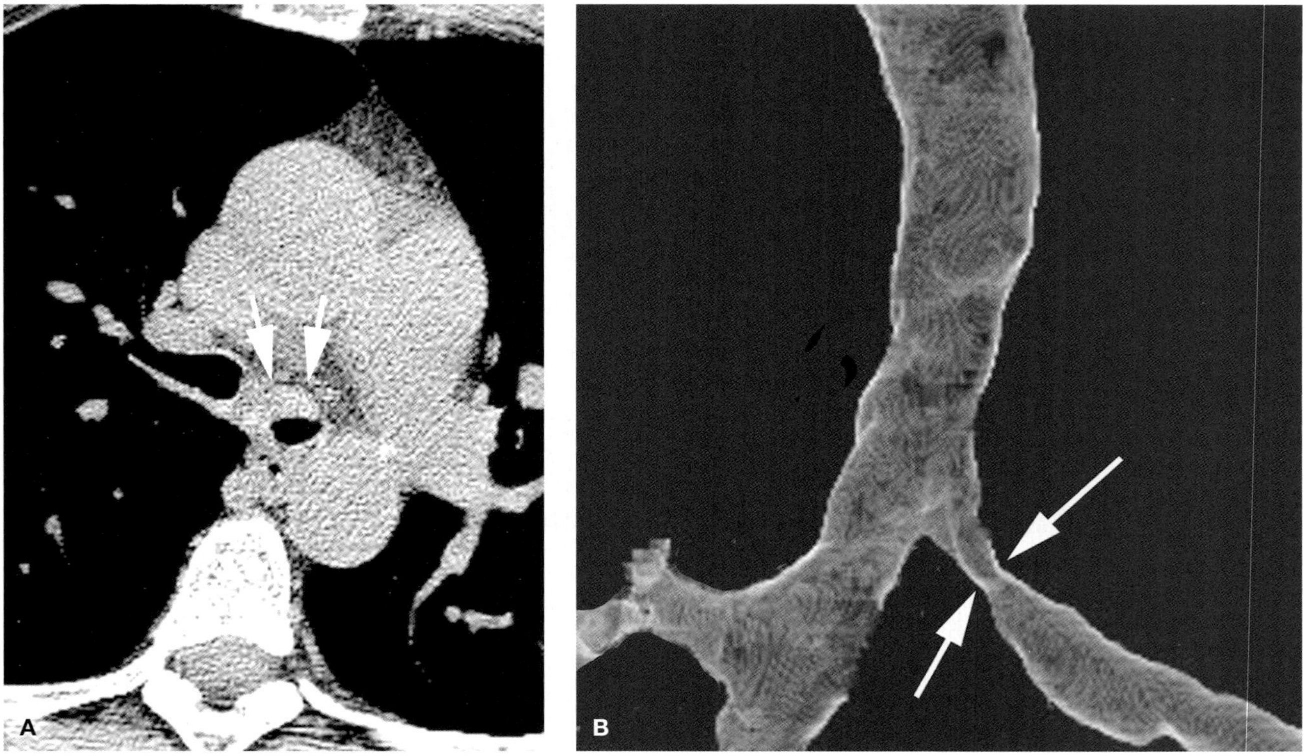

Figure 22.19. Bronchial narrowing in granulomatosis with polyangiitis. **A:** CT shows narrowing of the proximal left main bronchus, associated with thickening of its wall (*arrows*). **B:** Three-dimensional reconstruction shows left main bronchus narrowing (*arrows*). The distal trachea is slightly narrowed.

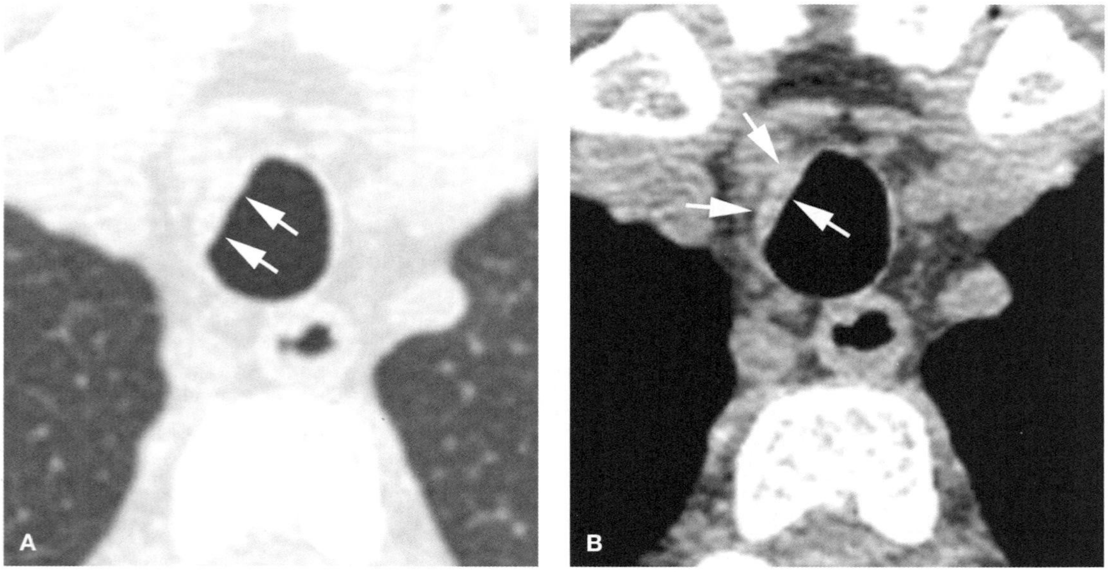

Figure 22.20. Tracheobronchial amyloidosis. CTs through the proximal trachea using lung (**A**) and soft-tissue (**B**) windows show eccentric thickening of the tracheal wall (*arrows*).

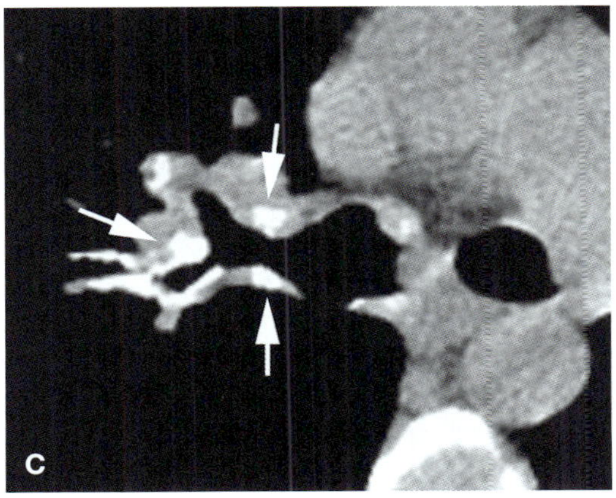

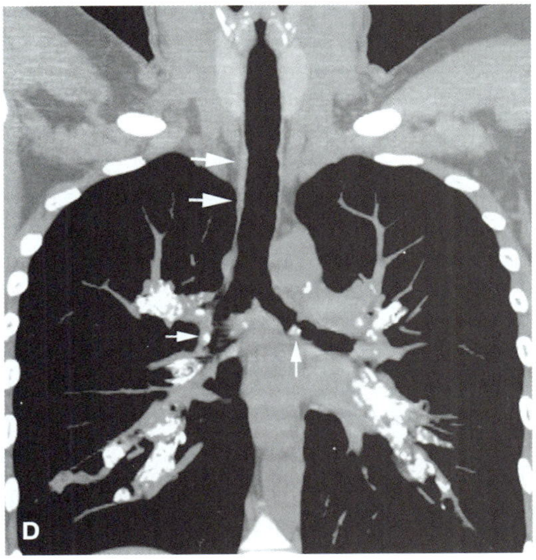

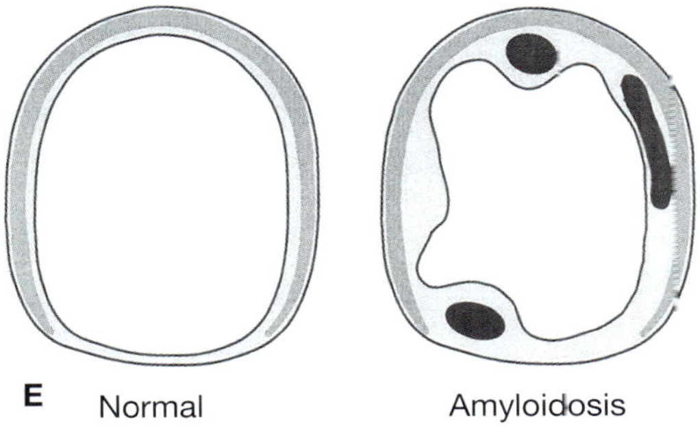

Figure 22.20. *(Continued)* **C:** CT shows nodular thickening and calcification of the walls of the right main and right upper lobe bronchi (*arrows*). **D:** Coronal reformation shows tracheal wall thickening (*large arrows*) and focal thickening and calcification of bronchial walls (*small arrows*). Lymph node calcification also is visible. **E:** Diagrammatic representation of the appearance of the trachea in amyloidosis. Concentric or nodular wall thickening is seen, sometimes with calcification.

is successfully treated using antibiotics. If untreated, it can result in fibrosis and focal or diffuse tracheal narrowing. It is rare in the United States.

ABNORMALITIES ASSOCIATED WITH INCREASED TRACHEAL DIAMETER

Tracheal Diverticulum

Tracheal diverticulum represents a focal herniation of tracheal mucosa through the tracheal wall. Tracheal diverticulum may be seen in normal subjects, although it tends to be associated with chronic obstructive pulmonary disease. It usually is asymptomatic and is detected incidentally.

Tracheal diverticulum most commonly occurs near the thoracic inlet, along the posterolateral right trachea, between the cartilaginous and muscular portions of the tracheal wall (Fig. 22.28). Occasionally, tracheal diverticulum can be seen in other locations and may rarely be multiple. It can appear as an isolated paratracheal air cyst (Fig. 22.28), usually a few millimeters in diameter, or as an air-filled structure communicating with the tracheal lumen (see Fig. 22.28). Tracheal diverticulum is easily seen on CT, but is rarely visible on plain radiographs.

Mounier-Kuhn Syndrome (Tracheobronchomegaly)

Tracheobronchomegaly, also referred to as *Mounier-Kuhn syndrome*, is characterized by marked dilatation of the trachea and mainstem bronchi, often in association with tracheal diverticulosis, recurrent lower respiratory tract infections, and bronchiectasis, which is typically cystic in appearance (see Table 22.2). Tracheobronchomegaly is diagnosed most often in men in their third and fourth decades; it is much less common in women. There may be a history of recurrent respiratory tract infection or chronic cough dating to childhood, but this is not seen in all patients.

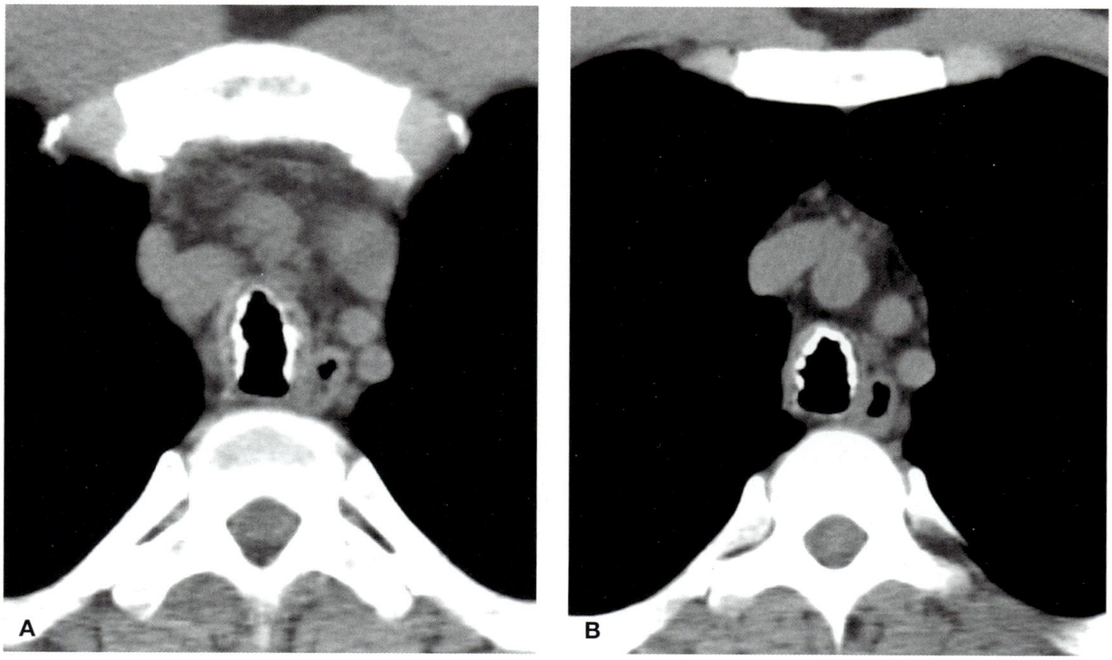

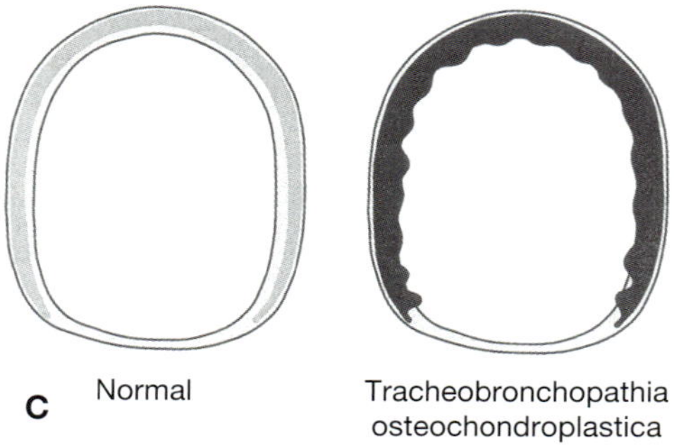

Figure 22.21. Tracheobronchopathia osteochondroplastica. **A, B:** CT at two levels shows nodular thickening and calcification of the anterior and lateral tracheal wall. The posterior tracheal membrane is normal in thickness and devoid of calcifications. **C:** Diagrammatic representation of the appearance of the trachea in tracheobronchopathia osteochondroplastica. Tracheal cartilages are thickened, with small irregular calcific nodules along their inner aspect, protruding into the tracheal lumen. (Reproduced with permission of the American Roentgen Ray Society from Webb EM, Elicker BM, Webb WR. Using CT to diagnose nonneoplastic tracheal abnormalities: appearance of the tracheal wall. AJR Am J Roentgenol. 2000;174:1315-1321. Copyright© 2000 American Roentgen Ray Society.)

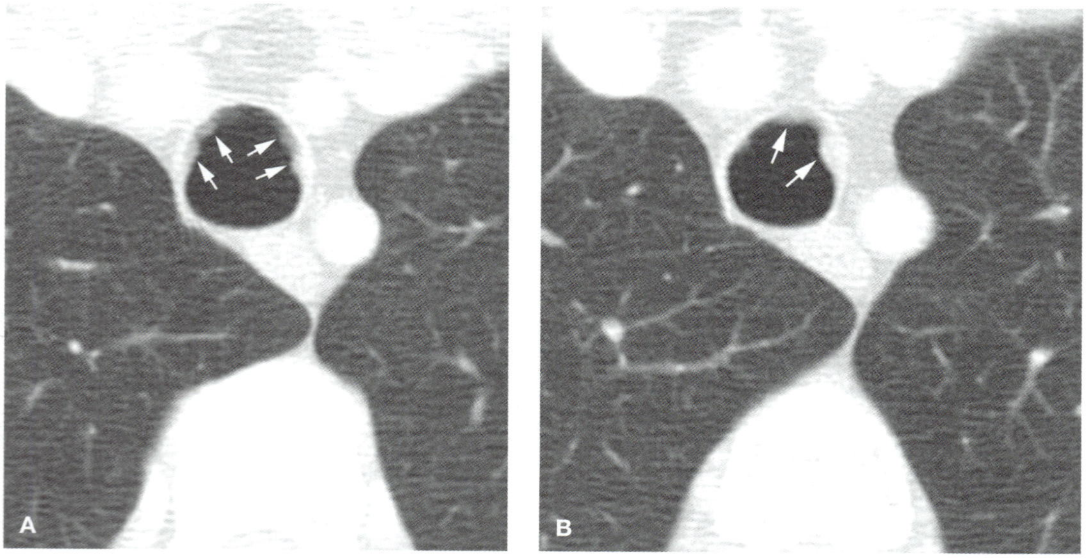

Figure 22.22. Tracheobronchopathia osteochondroplastica. **A, B:** CT at two levels shows nodules (*arrows*) arising from the anterior and lateral tracheal wall, projecting into the lumen. The nodules are uncalcified.

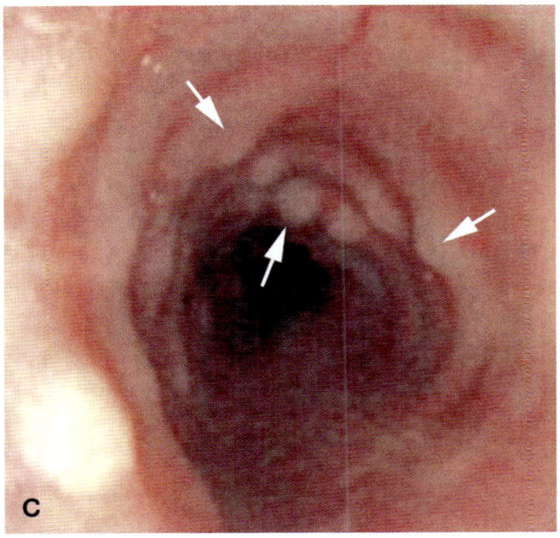

Figure 22.22. *(Continued)* **C:** Photograph at bronchoscopy shows nodules (*arrows*) arising from tracheal cartilage. The posterior trachea is normal.

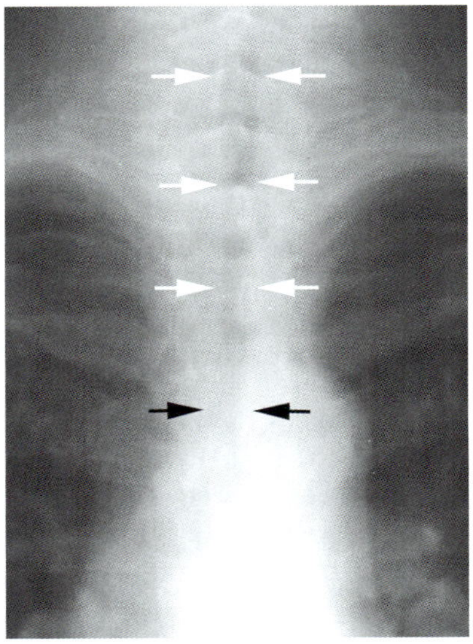

Figure 22.23. Relapsing polychondritis. Chest radiograph shows cylindrical narrowing of the entire trachea (*arrows*).

Although tracheal enlargement is seen in some patients with chronic pulmonary fibrosis or chronic infection, tracheobronchomegaly most likely is congenital in origin Histologic examination of the trachea shows a deficiency of smooth muscle and elastic fibers. A cartilage abnormality undoubtedly is present as well, although this abnormality probably is acquired. Tracheomegaly also may occur in association with other congenital disorders such as Marfan syndrome, cystic fibrosis, Ehlers-Danlos syndrome, and cutis laxa.

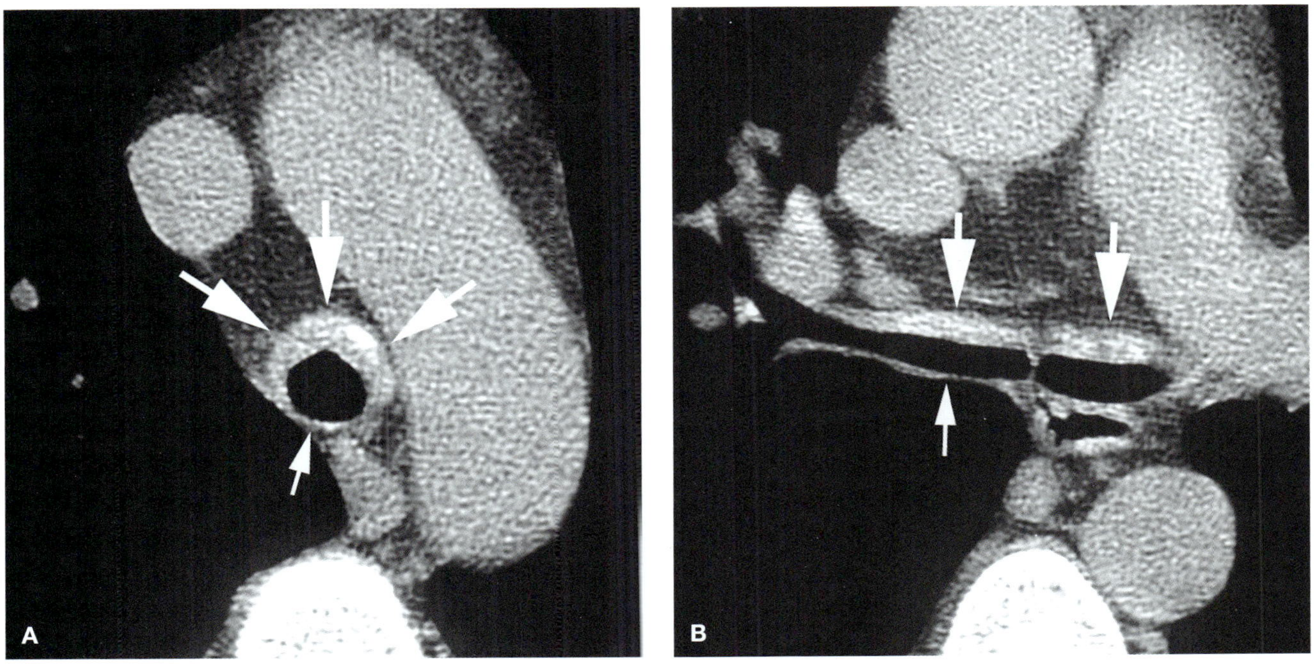

Figure 22.24. Relapsing polychondritis. **A:** CT shows tracheal narrowing. The anterior and lateral tracheal walls (ie, the cartilaginous portions) are thickened (*large arrows*). The posterior tracheal membrane is of normal thickness (*small arrow*). This appearance is characteristic. **B:** Narrowing of the main bronchi also is seen. The anterior bronchial walls are thickened (*large arrows*), while the posterior wall of the bronchus appears normal (*small arrow*).

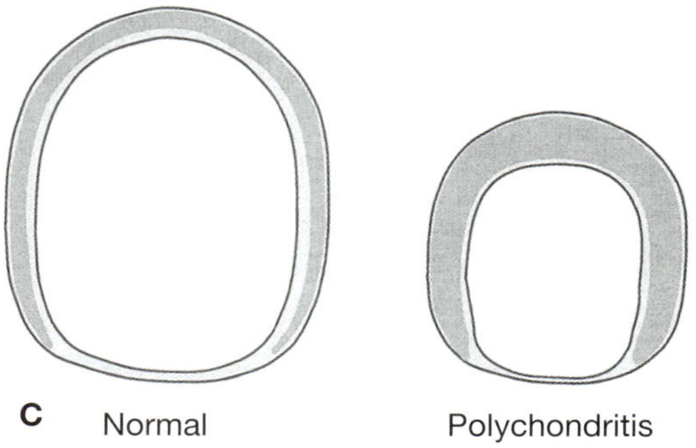

Figure 22.24. *(Continued)* **C:** Diagrammatic representation of relapsing polychondritis. The anterior and lateral tracheal walls are thickened; the posterior tracheal membrane is of normal thickness. (Reproduced with permission of the American Roentgen Ray Society from Webb EM, Elicker BM, Webb WR. Using CT to diagnose nonneoplastic tracheal abnormalities: appearance of the tracheal wall. AJR Am J Roentgenol. 2000;174:1315-1321. Copyright© 2000 American Roentgen Ray Society.)

The diagnosis is based on radiographic findings of increased tracheal and bronchial diameter. Dilatation usually involves the intrathoracic trachea and the first few bronchial divisions (Fig. 22.29). Tracheobronchomegaly may be suggested in a male if the tracheal diameter measured on the frontal and lateral radiographs exceeds 25 and 27 mm, respectively; in a female, it may be suggested if these measurements exceed 21 and 23 mm. The trachea tends to have a corrugated or scalloped contour (see Fig. 22.29) because of mucosa protruding between the tracheal cartilage. On the lateral view, this is visible anteriorly. Frank tracheal diverticula also may be present. Bronchiectasis commonly is present and tends to involve the central bronchi; peripheral airways appear normal.

On CT, a tracheal diameter greater than 3 cm (measured 2 cm above the aortic arch) and diameters of 2.4 and 2.3 cm for the right and left main bronchi have been used to make the diagnosis of tracheobronchomegaly (Figs.

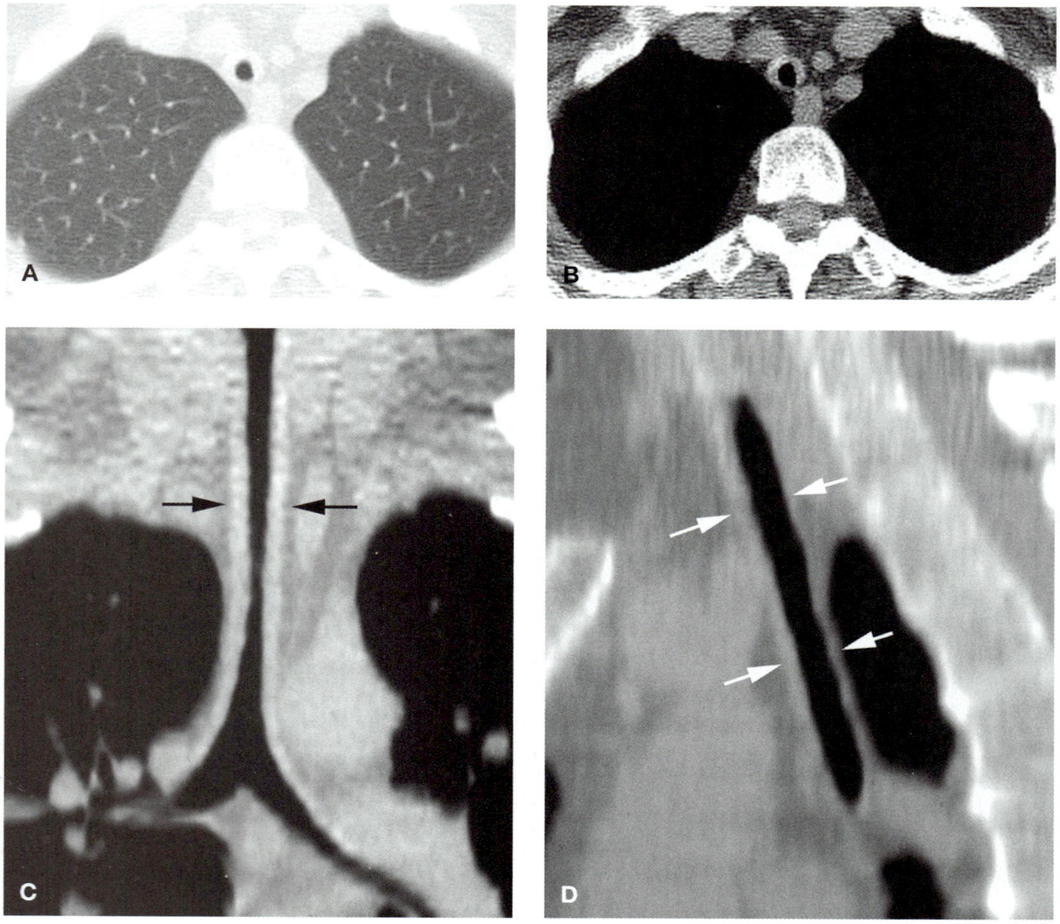

Figure 22.25. Relapsing polychondritis. **A, B:** CT shows marked narrowing of the tracheal lumen, with typical thickening of the anterior and lateral tracheal walls. **C:** Coronal reconstruction shows diffuse narrowing of the trachea with thickening of its lateral walls (*arrows*). **D:** Sagittal reformation shows diffuse narrowing of the trachea (*arrows*).

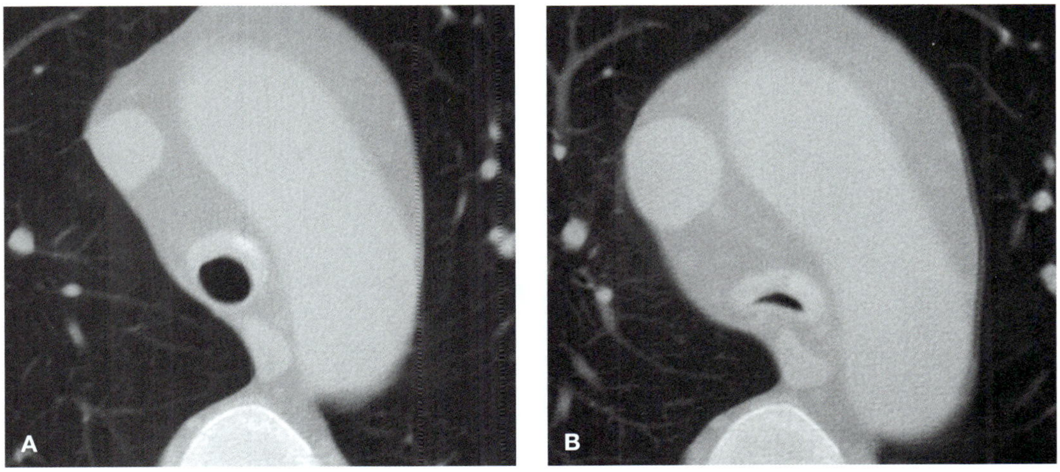

Figure 22.26. Relapsing polychondritis with tracheobronchomalacia. Expiratory CT (**B**) shows significant collapse of the tracheal lumen compared with an inspiratory scan (**A**).

22.30 and 22.31), although these measurements are arbitrary and more conservative than those proposed for use on chest radiographs. Tracheal scalloping is more difficult to see in cross section than on chest films. Diverticula, on the other hand, are more easily seen on CT, typically occurring along the posterolateral tracheal wall. Also common is the finding of a marked tracheal flaccidity or TM on expiratory scans. Cystic bronchiectasis may be seen in the central or parahilar lung regions (Figs. 22.29 and 22.31).

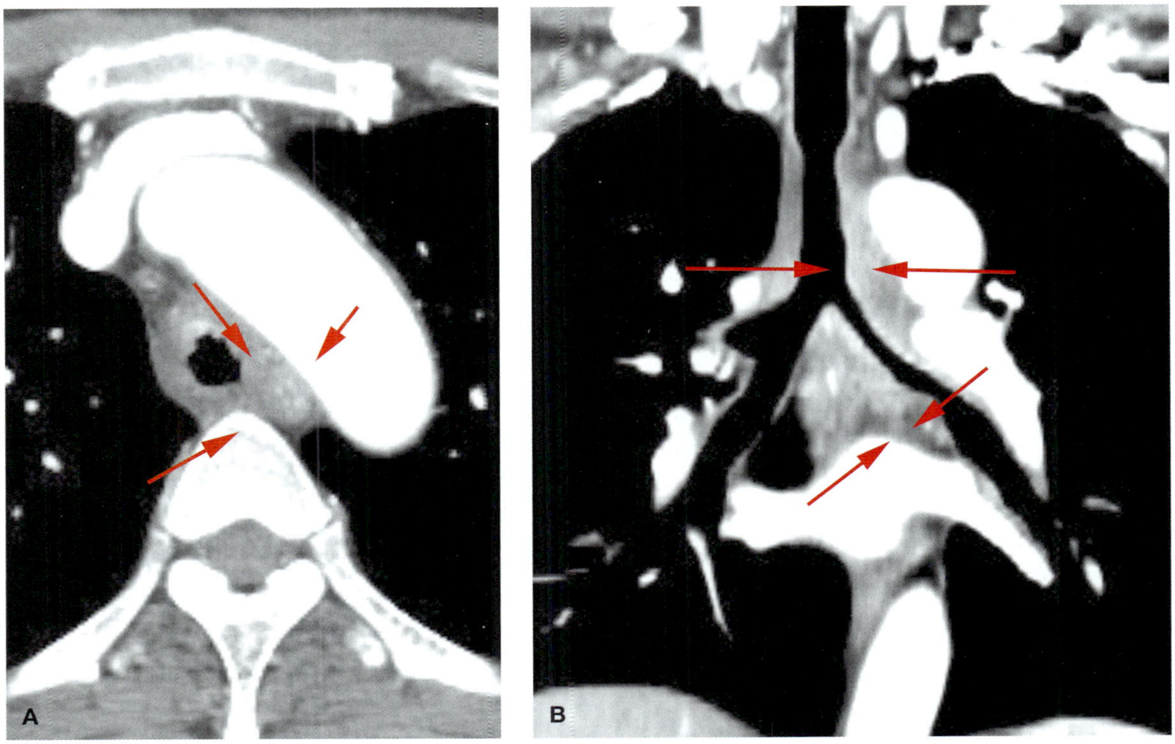

Figure 22.27. *Aspergillus* tracheobronchitis in an immunosuppressed patient with liver transplantation. **A:** Tracheal narrowing is associated with wall thickening (*arrows*). **B:** Coronal CT shows tracheal and left main bronchus wall thickening and narrowing (*arrows*).

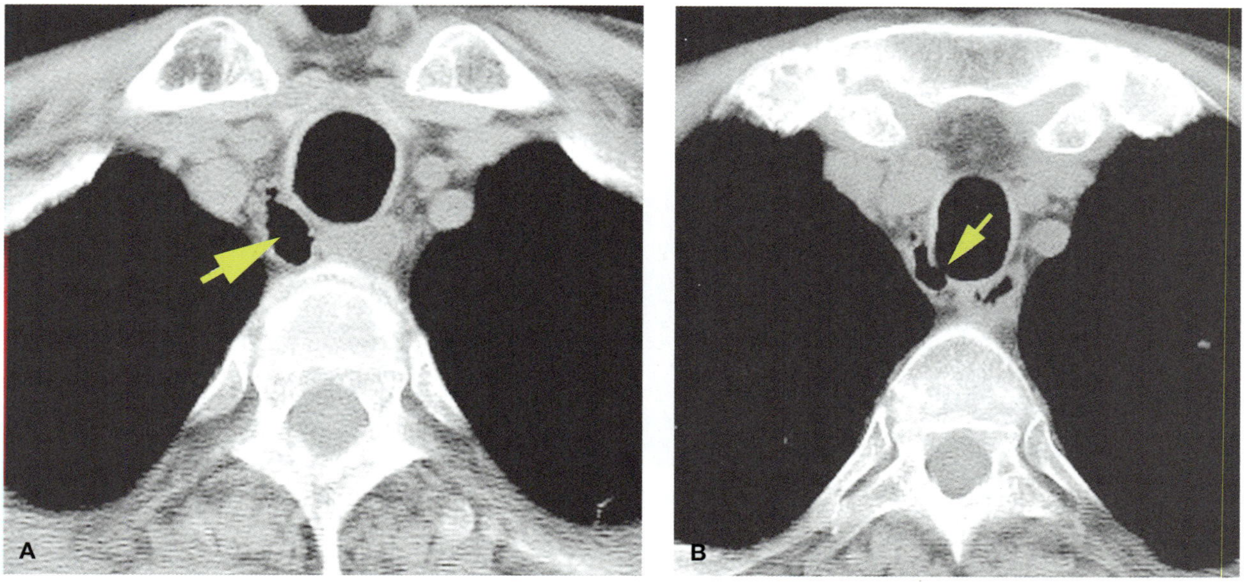

Figure 22.28. Tracheal diverticulum. **A:** A paratracheal air cyst is present in the upper mediastinum, representing a diverticulum (*arrow*). **B:** A defect in the right posterolateral tracheal wall (*arrow*) communicates with the diverticulum.

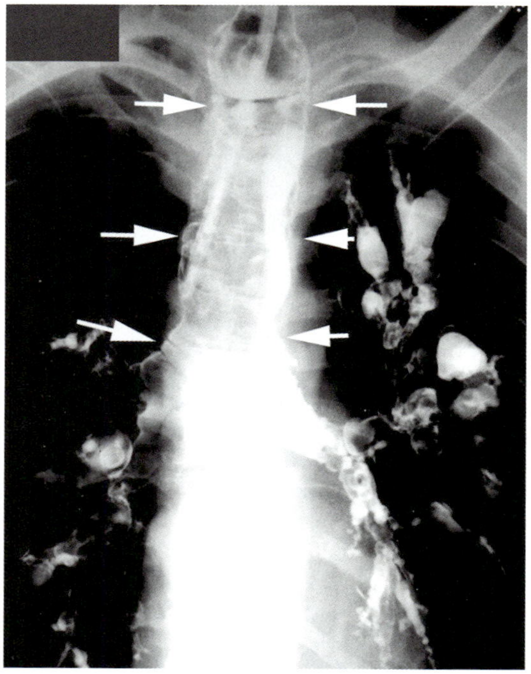

Figure 22.29. Tracheobronchomegaly. A bronchogram shows tracheal dilatation (*arrows*), with the tracheal wall having a corrugated or scalloped contour. Central bronchiectasis also is visible.

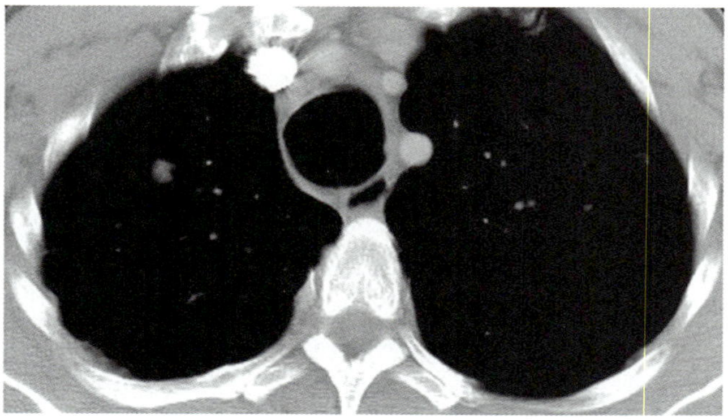

Figure 22.30. Tracheobronchomegaly. CT above the aortic arch shows marked tracheal dilatation. The trachea measures 37 mm in diameter.

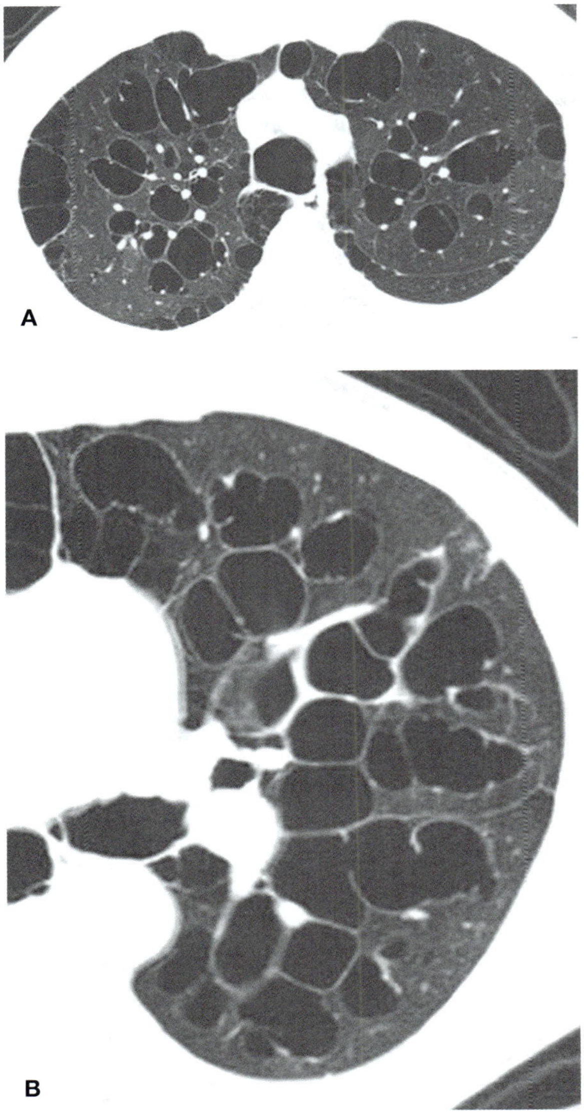

Figure 22.31. Tracheobronchomegaly with bronchiectasis. A: CT above the aortic arch shows tracheal dilatation. The trachea wall has a scalloped appearance. Central bronchiectasis is present, with bullae in the lung periphery. B: The left main bronchus has a scalloped appearance, and cystic bronchiectasis is present.

SUGGESTED READINGS

Aslam A, De Luis Cardenas J, Morrison RJ, et al. Tracheobronchomalacia and excessive dynamic airway collapse: current concepts and future directions. *Radiographics*. 2022;42(4):1012-1027. doi:10.1148/rg.210155

Boiselle PM, O'Donnell CR, Bankier AA, et al. Tracheal collapsibility in healthy volunteers during forced expiration: assessment with multidetector CT. *Radiology*. 2009;252(1):255-262.

Choplin RH, Wehunt WD, Theros EG. Diffuse lesions of the trachea. *Semin Roentgenol*. 1983;18(1):38-50.

Gaafar HA, Gaafar AH, Nour YA. Rhinoscleroma: an updated experience through the last 10 years. *Acta Otolaryngol*. 2011;131(4):440-446.

Gamsu G, Webb WR. Computed tomography of the trachea and mainstem bronchi. *Semin Roentgenol*. 1983;18(1):51-60.

Goo JM, Im JG, Ahn JM, et al. Right paratracheal air cysts in the thoracic inlet: clinical and radiologic significance. *AJR Am J Roentgenol*. 1999;173(1):65-70.

Im JG, Chung JW, Han SK, Han MC, Kim CW. CT manifestations of tracheobronchial involvement in relapsing polychondritis. *J Comput Assist Tomogr*. 1988;12(5):792-793.

Kwong JS, Müller NL, Miller RR. Diseases of the trachea and main-stem bronchi: correlation of CT with pathologic findings. *Radiographics*. 1992;12(4):645-657.

Mariotta S, Pallone G, Pedicelli G, Bisetti A. Spiral CT and endoscopic findings in a case of tracheobronchopathia osteochondroplastica. *J Comput Assist Tomogr*. 1997;21(3):418-420.

Park CM, Goo JM, Lee HJ, Kim MA, Lee CH, Kang MJ. Tumors in the tracheobronchial tree: CT and FDG PET features. *Radiographics*. 2009;29(1):55-71.

Pickford HA, Swensen SJ, Utz JP. Thoracic cross-sectional imaging of amyloidosis. *AJR Am J Roentgenol*. 1997;168(2):351-355.

Prince JS, Duhamel DR, Levin DL, Harrell JH, Friedman PJ. Nonneoplastic lesions of the tracheobronchial wall: radiologic findings with bronchoscopic correlation. *Radiographics*. 2002;22 Spec No:S215-S230.

Roditi GH, Weir J. The association of tracheomegaly and bronchiectasis. *Clin Radiol*. 1994;49(9):608-611.

Screaton NJ, Sivasothy P, Flower CD, Lockwood CM. Tracheal involvement in Wegener's granulomatosis: evaluation using spiral CT. *Clin Radiol*. 1998;53(11):809-815.

Shin MS, Jackson RM, Ho KJ. Tracheobronchomegaly (Mounier-Kuhn syndrome): CT diagnosis. *AJR Am J Roentgenol*. 1988;150(4):777-779.

Stern EJ, Graham CM, Webb WR, Gamsu G. Normal trachea during forced expiration: dynamic CT measurements. *Radiology*. 1993;187(1):27-31.

Webb EM, Elicker BM, Webb WR. Using CT to diagnose nonneoplastic tracheal abnormalities: appearance of the tracheal wall. *AJR Am J Roentgenol*. 2000;174(5):1315-1321.

Chapter 23

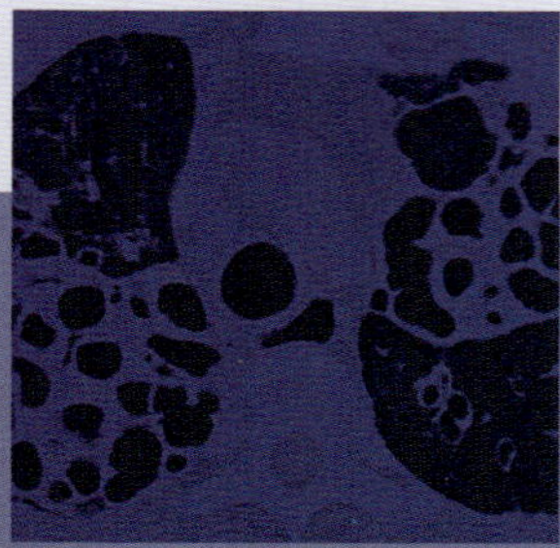

Travis S. Henry

Airway Disease: Bronchiectasis, Chronic Bronchitis, and Bronchiolitis

AIRWAY MORPHOLOGY

Airways divide by dichotomous branching. There are approximately 23 divisions from the trachea to the alveoli.

Bronchi are conducting airways that contain cartilage in their walls. The anatomy of the lobar and segmental bronchi is described in Chapter 3.

Bronchioles are noncartilaginous airways. The largest bronchioles measure about 3 mm in diameter and have walls about 0.3 mm thick. A *terminal bronchiole* is the last purely conducting airway and does not participate in gas exchange. It is approximately 0.7 mm in diameter and gives rise to respiratory bronchioles. A *respiratory bronchiole* is the largest bronchiole with alveoli arising from its walls and, thus, is the largest bronchiole that participates in gas exchange. It gives rise to alveolar ducts and alveoli.

BRONCHIECTASIS

Bronchiectasis is defined as localized, irreversible dilatation of the bronchial tree. Usually, this term is used to refer only to cartilage-containing airways, larger than 2 to 3 mm in diameter.

Etiology

Bronchiectasis has a wide variety of causes (Table 23.1), but in up to 40% of cases, the etiology cannot be determined. Bronchiectasis is commonly associated with acute, chronic, or recurrent infection, particularly infection with bacteria and mycobacteria. Also, bronchiectasis often is present in patients with bronchiolitis obliterans (BO), also known as constrictive bronchiolitis (CB), resulting from viral or mycoplasma infection. Immunodeficiency syndromes including acquired immunodeficiency syndrome (AIDS), abnormalities of mucociliary clearance, structural abnormalities of the bronchial wall, and chronic bronchial obstruction are associated with bronchiectasis, largely because they result in infection.

Noninfectious diseases that result in airway inflammation and mucous plugging, without infection, also can result in bronchiectasis. These include allergic bronchopulmonary aspergillosis (ABPA) and, to a lesser extent, asthma. Bronchiectasis also is seen in patients with BO resulting from chronic rejection following lung transplantation or chronic graft-versus-host disease (GVHD) in patients with bone marrow or solid organ transplantation.

Causes of bronchiectasis having a genetic basis include (1) cystic fibrosis (CF); (2) the dyskinetic cilia (and Kartagener) syndrome (Fig. 23.1); (3) Young syndrome; (4) Williams-Campbell syndrome (congenital deficiency of the bronchial cartilage); (5) Mounier-Kuhn syndrome (congenital tracheobronchomegaly); (6) alpha-1 antitrypsin deficiency; (7) immunodeficiency syndromes, including Bruton hypogammaglobulinemia, IgA, and combined IgA-IgG deficiencies; and (8) the yellow nail lymphedema syndrome (yellow nails, lymphedema, and pleural effusions).

Pathologic Abnormalities

Bronchiectasis usually is associated with bronchial wall thickening, inflammation, destruction of muscular and elastic elements of the bronchial wall, and bronchial and peribronchial fibrosis. Loss of muscular and elastic tissues allows the bronchi to dilate in response to the pull of adjacent tissues (ie, the normal negative interstitial pressure). Ciliated epithelium

Table 23.1 Causes of Bronchiectasis
Infection
Bacteria (*Pseudomonas, Staphylococcus, Bordetella pertussis*)
Mycobacteria (tuberculosis, *Mycobacterium avium-intracellulare* complex)
Virus
Mycoplasma
Immune deficiency states
Congenital (eg, hypogammaglobulinemia)
Acquired (eg, AIDS)
Mucociliary clearance abnormalities
Cystic fibrosis (abnormal mucus)
Dyskinetic cilia syndrome (abnormal cilia)
Young syndrome
Bronchial obstruction
Congenital bronchial atresia
Endobronchial tumor
Bronchial compression by lymph nodes
Bronchial wall abnormalities
Tracheobronchomegaly
Williams-Campbell syndrome
Immune reactions
Allergic bronchopulmonary aspergillosis
Asthma
Lung transplant rejection
Graft-versus-host disease
Proteinase-antiproteinase imbalance
Alpha-1 antitrypsin deficiency
Systemic diseases
Collagen vascular disease
Inflammatory bowel disease

is usually replaced by nonciliated or squamous epithelium. These structural abnormalities of the bronchial wall encourage infection, which, in turn, further damages the bronchi.

Inflammation and fibrosis also are associated with obliteration of small airways and a reduction in the number of bronchial branches, particularly when the disease originates during childhood when the lungs (and airways) are developing.

The affected lung is typically reduced in volume and may be airless. Pulmonary arteries supplying the abnormal lung usually are reduced in number and size, and regional lung perfusion is decreased accordingly.

Clinical Diagnosis

In general, a clinical diagnosis of bronchiectasis is possible only in the most severely affected patients, and differentiation from chronic bronchitis may be difficult. Most patients present with purulent sputum production, recurrent pulmonary infections, fever, weight loss, and sometimes dyspnea. Hemoptysis also is common, occurring in up to 50% of cases, and may be the only clinical finding. Hemoptysis usually is associated with bronchial artery enlargement related to chronic inflammation. Sputum culture often reveals bacterial infection, with common organisms being *Streptococcus pneumoniae*, *Pseudomonas*, *Haemophilus influenzae*, and *Staphylococcus aureus*. *Aspergillus* species and mycobacteria also may be present.

Pulmonary function tests may show airflow obstruction. However, bronchitis, bronchiolitis, or emphysema often accompanies bronchiectasis and may predominate as the cause of obstructive abnormalities.

Classification

Traditionally, bronchiectasis has been classified into three morphologic types: *cylindrical*, *varicose*, and *cystic*. The severity of bronchial dilatation and anatomic abnormalities, and functional abnormalities (to a lesser extent), correlates with these three morphologic classifications. Cylindrical bronchiectasis is associated with the least severe abnormalities, and cystic bronchiectasis is associated with the most severe. However, differentiating between the types of bronchiectasis is less important in clinical practice than is a determination of its extent and distribution of abnormalities. It is important to note that *bronchiectasis* (as described in this chapter) and *traction bronchiectasis* in the setting of pulmonary fibrosis (see Chapter 11) are not interchangeable terms and refer to different mechanisms of airway dilation.

Cylindrical Bronchiectasis

Cylindrical bronchiectasis is characterized by mild bronchial dilatation and lack of bronchial tapering. The dilated bronchi are of relatively uniform caliber and have roughly parallel walls. Often, smaller bronchi are plugged with purulent secretions. The number of bronchial divisions from the carina to the periphery is slightly reduced.

Varicose Bronchiectasis

With increasingly severe abnormalities of the bronchial wall and increasing bronchial dilatation, the bronchi may assume an irregular, beaded or bulbous configuration, referred to as *varicose bronchiectasis*. Usually, peripheral bronchi are obliterated by fibrous tissue. The number of bronchial divisions is reduced significantly.

Cystic Bronchiectasis

With severe bronchiectasis, airways appear ballooned or "cystic" or "saccular," often exceeding 2 cm in diameter. The typical branching appearance of bronchi in areas of bronchiectasis may be difficult to see. The cysts often appear isolated and are not associated with other abnormal airways. Cysts may be

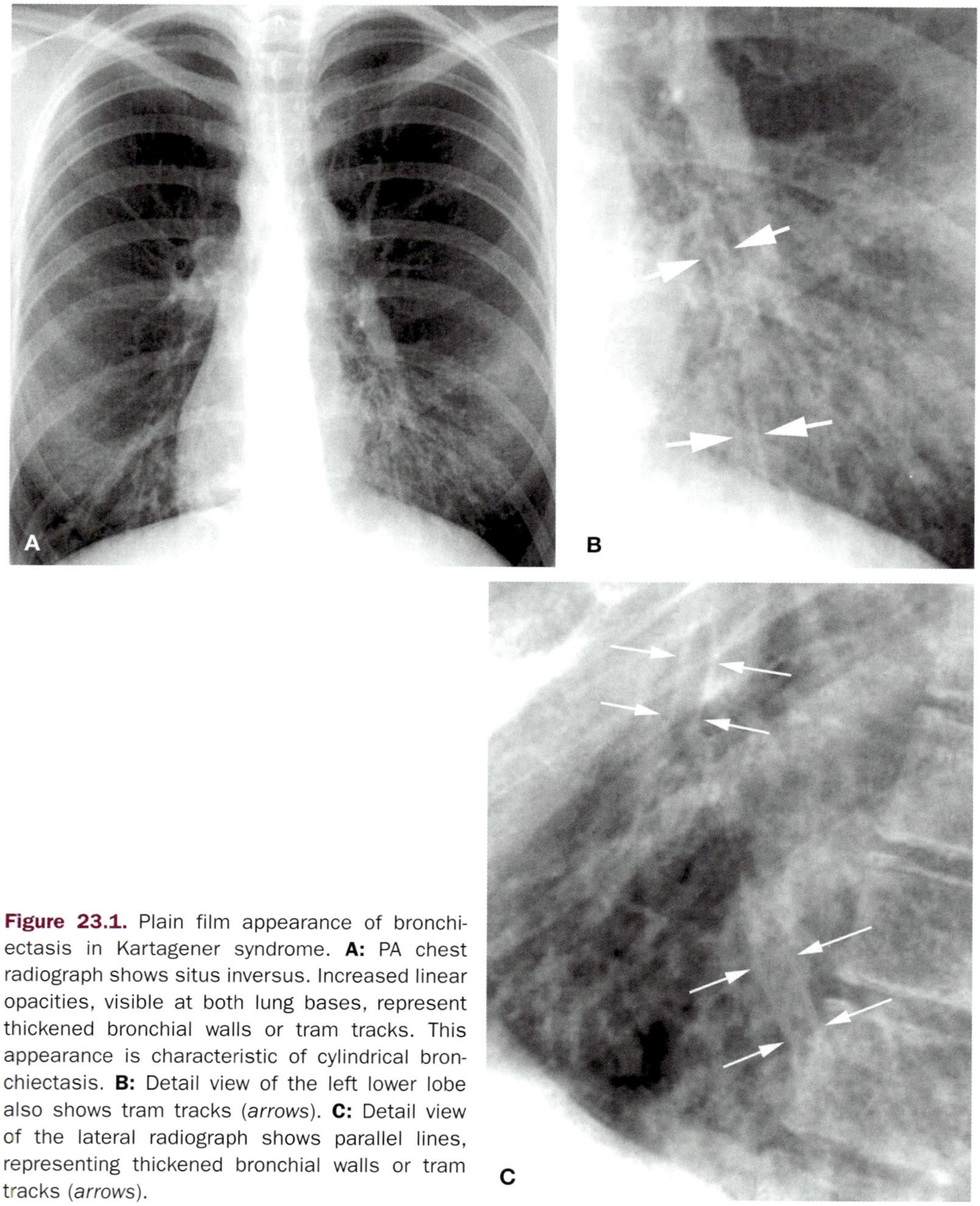

Figure 23.1. Plain film appearance of bronchiectasis in Kartagener syndrome. **A:** PA chest radiograph shows situs inversus. Increased linear opacities, visible at both lung bases, represent thickened bronchial walls or tram tracks. This appearance is characteristic of cylindrical bronchiectasis. **B:** Detail view of the left lower lobe also shows tram tracks (*arrows*). **C:** Detail view of the lateral radiograph shows parallel lines, representing thickened bronchial walls or tram tracks (*arrows*).

seen in a subpleural location. The number of bronchial divisions from the carina to the periphery is markedly reduced.

Bronchography

Although traditionally considered the gold standard for diagnosing bronchiectasis, bronchography is now of historical interest only and has been replaced by CT. However, the same findings that were considered classic indicators of bronchiectasis on bronchography are still used in interpreting CT. These include the following:

1. Proximal or distal bronchial dilatation
2. Abnormal bronchial contours
3. Lack of normal tapering of peripheral airways
4. Reduction in the number of bronchial branches (ie, "pruning")
5. Luminal filling defects due to mucus

Chest Radiograph Diagnosis

Chest radiographs are abnormal in 80% to 90% of patients with bronchiectasis, although findings are often difficult to recognize, and the diagnosis can be suggested in only about 40% of patients. The more severe the abnormality, the easier it is to see and the more likely it is that an accurate diagnosis will be made.

Tram tracks, parallel line shadows representing thickened bronchial walls, are a common finding in bronchiectasis (see Figs. 23.1 and 23.2). They may be the only finding visible

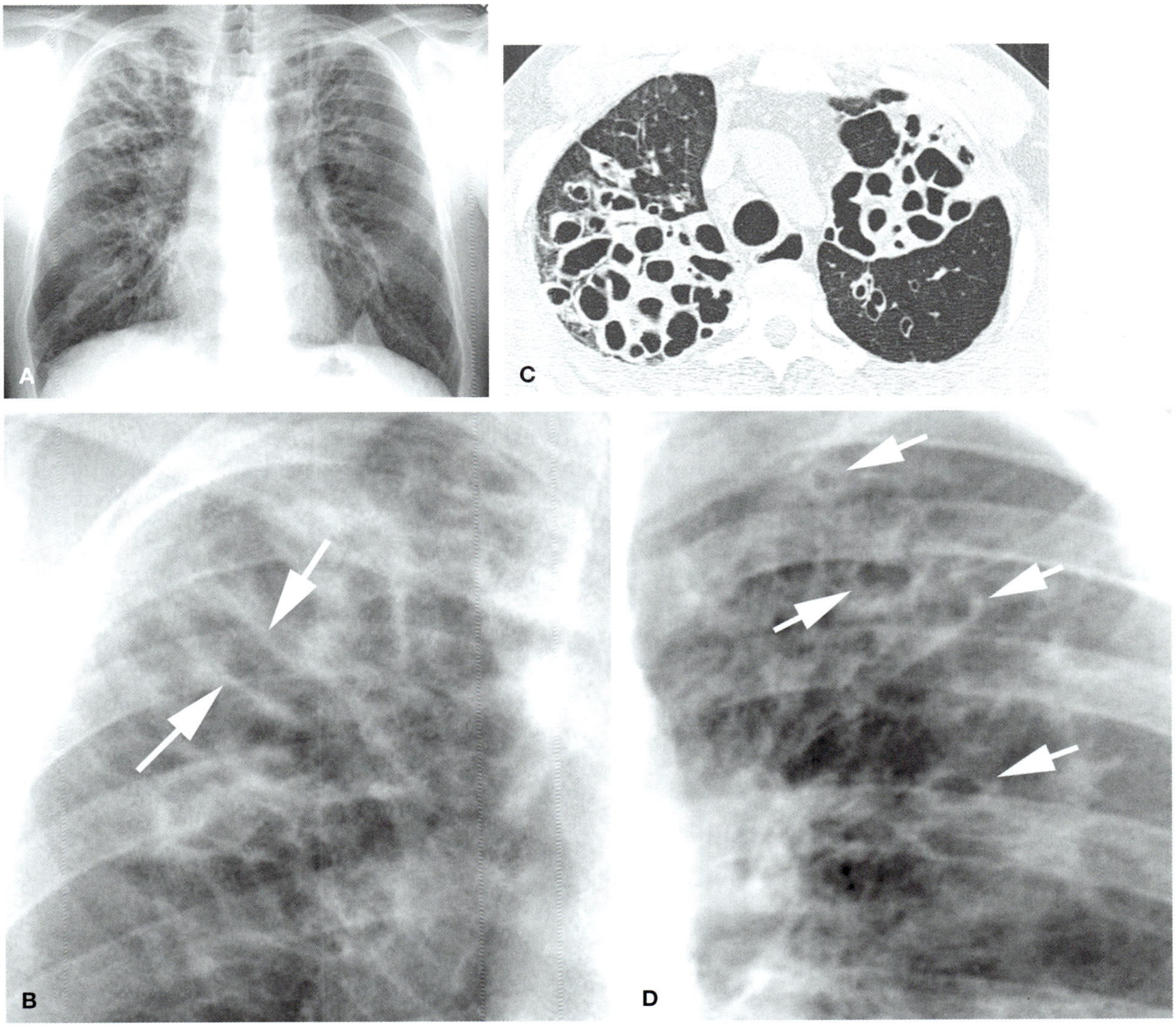

Figure 23.2. Bronchiectasis in cystic fibrosis. **A:** Chest radiograph shows a number of examples of tram tracks and ring shadows in the upper lobes. **B:** Detail view of the right upper lobe shows tram tracks (*arrows*) due to cylindrical bronchiectasis. **C:** HRCT in this patient shows bilateral upper lobe bronchiectasis. **D:** In another patient with cystic fibrosis, ring shadows (*arrows*) indicate bronchiectasis.

in patients with cylindrical bronchiectasis. However, tram tracks also may be seen with bronchial wall thickening in the absence of bronchiectasis and thus are nonspecific. When seen in cross section, thick-walled bronchi appear as ring shadows (Fig. 23.2D).

Recognizing dilatation of bronchi on plain films is more difficult, unless the dilatation is significant or obvious contour abnormalities are present (eg, in varicose bronchiectasis). The dilated bronchi may be visible as irregular, oval, or branching tubular air-filled structures (see Fig. 23.2). When seen in cross section, a dilated bronchus may appear larger than the artery adjacent to it. Mucous plugs or fluid filling the bronchi sometimes is visible and may aid in recognizing them as dilated. Mucous plugs within dilated bronchi may be visible as oval ("finger in glove") or branching ("hand in glove") opacities.

Cystic bronchiectasis results in multiple, air-filled, cystic lesions, which may be thick or thin walled, and clustered, lobar, patchy, or diffuse in distribution. Multiple air-fluid levels often are seen because of infection or retained secretions (see Fig. 10.28 in Chapter 10). Because the cysts communicate with each other through the bronchial tree, air-fluid levels tend to be at about the same height in all the affected cysts but with less fluid present in the upper lobe cysts than in lower lobe cysts (ie, water flows downhill).

Less specific radiographic findings often seen in bronchiectasis include (1) loss of definition of vascular markings in the affected lung, presumably secondary to peribronchial inflammation or fibrosis, (2) increased "lung markings" in the central lung regions, (3) volume loss in the affected lung or lobe, (4) decreased vessel size in the aerated bronchiectatic lung, (5) consolidation of abnormal lung, and (6) compensatory expansion of normal lung.

CT Diagnosis of Bronchiectasis

Thin-slice CT is very accurate in the diagnosis of bronchiectasis with sensitivity and specificity values exceeding 95%. The use of appropriate and consistent window mean and width settings (−600-700/1000-1500 HU) is important. Excessively low or narrow window settings exaggerate bronchial wall thickness.

Specific findings of bronchiectasis indicate that bronchial dilatation is present (Table 23.2). Less specific findings include bronchial wall thickening (diagnosed subjectively or because bronchi are visible in the peripheral lung) and the presence of mucoid impaction or fluid within airways. Ancillary findings, commonly seen in bronchiectasis, include volume loss, mosaic perfusion visible on inspiratory scans, focal air trapping identifiable on expiration scans, "tree-in-bud," and bronchial artery enlargement.

CT Findings of Bronchial Dilatation

Because bronchiectasis is defined by the presence of bronchial dilatation, recognition of increased bronchial diameter is key to the CT diagnosis of this entity. On CT, bronchial dilatation may be diagnosed by an increased bronchoarterial ratio, by detecting a lack of bronchial tapering, and by abnormal bronchial contours.

Table 23.2 HRCT Findings in Bronchiectasis

Specific findings of bronchial dilatation
Increased bronchoarterial ratio
Internal bronchial diameter > adjacent pulmonary artery
"Signet-ring" sign
Lack of bronchial tapering
Contour abnormalities
Cylindrical bronchiectasis—"tram tracks"
Varicose bronchiectasis—"string of pearls"
Cystic bronchiectasis—"cluster of grapes"
Visibility of airways in peripheral 1 cm of the lung
Common nonspecific findings
Bronchial wall thickening
Fluid- or mucus-filled bronchi
Ancillary findings
Volume loss
Mosaic perfusion
Air trapping
Tree-in-bud
Bronchial artery enlargement

Increased Bronchoarterial Ratio

The diameter of a bronchus seen in cross section may be compared to that of the adjacent pulmonary artery by measuring the *bronchoarterial ratio* (the ratio of the internal diameter of a bronchus to that of the adjacent pulmonary artery) (Fig. 23.3A); the bronchoarterial ratio averages about 0.65 to 0.7 in normal subjects.

Bronchiectasis is often considered to be present if the bronchoarterial ratio exceeds 1. However, this may sometimes be seen in the absence of bronchial wall abnormalities in a small percentage of normal subjects, including elderly patients and in patients living at high altitudes (eg, Denver). Usually, true bronchiectasis results in a bronchoarterial ratio greater than 1.5 (Fig. 23.3B). Unless dilatation is obvious, bronchiectasis should not be diagnosed on the basis of an increased bronchoarterial ratio alone. Fortunately, bronchial wall thickening and other abnormalities suggesting disease are typically present in patients with true bronchiectasis.

The association of a dilated bronchus with a smaller adjacent pulmonary artery branch has been termed the *signet ring sign* (Figs. 23.3C and 23.4). This sign is valuable in recognizing bronchiectasis on CT and in distinguishing it from other cystic lung lesions. However, an increased bronchoarterial ratio may reflect the presence of bronchial dilatation (bronchiectasis) or reduction in pulmonary artery size as a consequence of decreased lung perfusion in the affected lung regions. Decreased artery size may accompany bronchiectasis or may be due to other abnormalities.

Lack of Bronchial Tapering

Lack of bronchial tapering may be important in the diagnosis of bronchiectasis, in particular subtle cylindrical bronchiectasis. For this finding to be present, the diameter of the airway should remain unchanged for at least 2 cm distal to a branching point (see Fig. 23.4A, C, and D). Accurate detection of this finding is difficult, however, in the absence of contiguous HRCT sections, especially for vertically or obliquely oriented airways.

Abnormal Bronchial Contours

Bronchiectasis may be classified as cylindrical, varicose, or cystic. Recognition of one of these abnormal contours is diagnostic of bronchial dilatation.

Cylindrical bronchiectasis varies in appearance on CT, depending on whether the abnormal bronchi lie in the scan plane (see Fig. 23.4A, C, and D) or perpendicular to it (Fig. 23.4B). When in the plane of scan, bronchi fail to show normal tapering and are recognizable as "tram tracks."

Varicose bronchiectasis results in more irregular bronchial dilatation with a typical varicose appearance (Fig. 23.5A). The bronchial walls often are irregularly thickened. This diagnosis of varicose bronchiectasis can be made easily only when the involved bronchi course horizontally in the

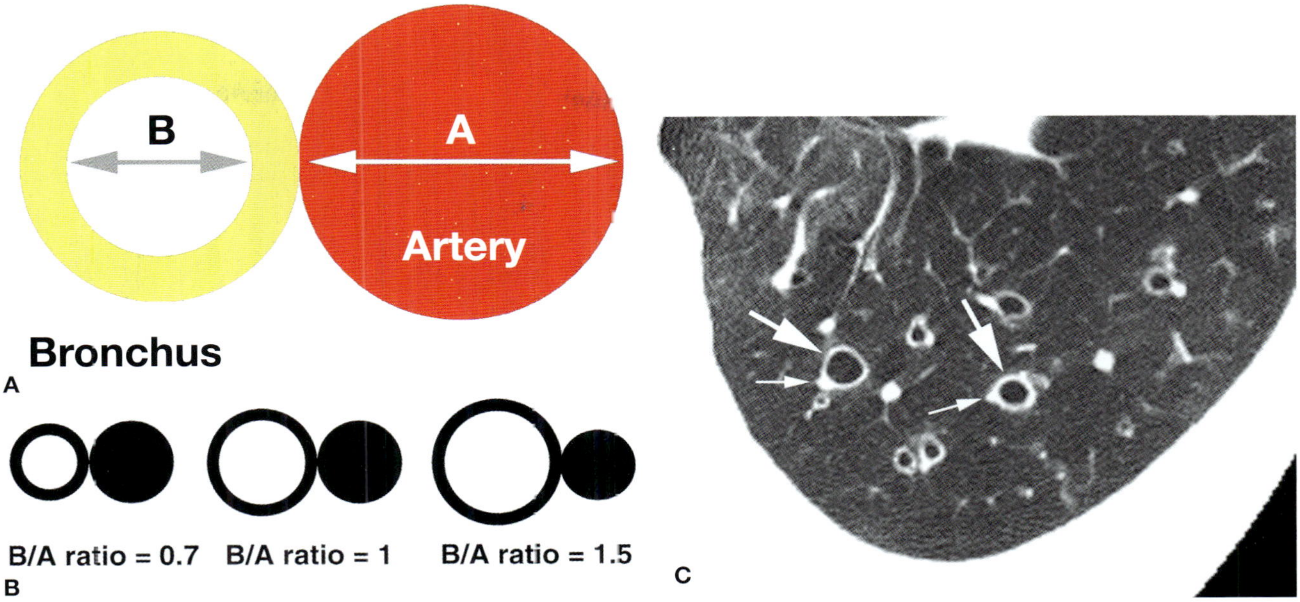

Figure 23.3. Bronchoarterial ratio. **A:** Bronchoarterial (B/A) ratio equals the internal diameter of a bronchus, divided by the diameter of the adjacent pulmonary artery branch. As shown in this diagram, it measures 0.65 to 0.7 in normal patients. **B:** Appearances of a normal B/A ratio (0.70) and B/A ratios of 1.0 and 1.5. A B/A ratio greater than 1 may be seen in some normal patients. A B/A ratio of 1.5 is almost always due to true bronchiectasis. **C:** In a patient with bronchiectasis, HRCT through the left lower lobe shows a number of examples of the signet-ring sign. The signet-ring sign is present when a dilated bronchus (*large arrows*) is associated with a much smaller pulmonary artery (*small arrows*). Bronchial walls are thick.

plane of scan. This appearance has been likened to a "string of pearls." When seen in cross section, the dilated bronchi are visible as thick-walled ring shadows indistinguishable from those of cylindrical bronchiectasis.

Cystic bronchiectasis is characterized by the presence of areas of rounded or cystlike dilation of the airways (see Fig 23.5B). In general, the dilated airways in patients with cystic bronchiectasis are thick walled; however, the cysts may be thin walled. A clear-cut branching appearance of the dilated airways generally may be lacking, and it may be difficult to make the distinction from cystic lung disease in some cases. This appearance has been described as similar to a "cluster of grapes." Air-fluid levels may be seen.

Indirect and Ancillary CT Findings in Bronchiectasis

Bronchial Wall Thickening

Although bronchial wall thickening is a nonspecific finding, it usually is present in patients with bronchiectasis (see Figs. 23.3C and 23.4A and C). Identification of bronchial wall thickening is largely subjective. Because bronchiectasis and bronchial wall thickening often are multifocal rather than diffuse and uniform, a comparison of one lung region to another can be helpful in making this observation (Fig. 23.6). It must be emphasized that using consistent window settings is very important in the diagnosis of bronchial wall thickening; bronchial walls can vary significantly in apparent thickness with different CT window settings.

Visibility of Peripheral Airways

In normal subjects, airways in the peripheral 2 cm of lung are uncommonly seen because their walls are too thin. Peribronchial fibrosis and bronchial wall thickening in patients with bronchiectasis, in combination with dilatation of the bronchial lumen, allow the visualization of small airways in the lung periphery. Bronchi visible within 1 cm of the costal pleural surfaces indicate bronchiectasis (see Figs. 23.4A, 23.5B, and 23.7), but bronchi may be seen within 1 cm of the mediastinal pleural surfaces in normal subjects.

Mucous Impaction and Air-Fluid Levels

The presence of mucus- or fluid-filled bronchi may be helpful in confirming a diagnosis of bronchiectasis (Fig. 23.8). The HRCT appearance of fluid- or mucus-filled airways is dependent on both their size and orientation relative to the scan plane. Larger, mucus-filled airways result in abnormal lobular or branching structures when they lie in the same plane as the CT scan. In cross section, impacted bronchi appear similar to vessels, but on contrast-enhanced scans will be lower attenuation. Since bronchi travel alongside pulmonary arteries, the presence of two side-by-side opacified "tubes" is a clue that one of them is a mucus-filled airway.

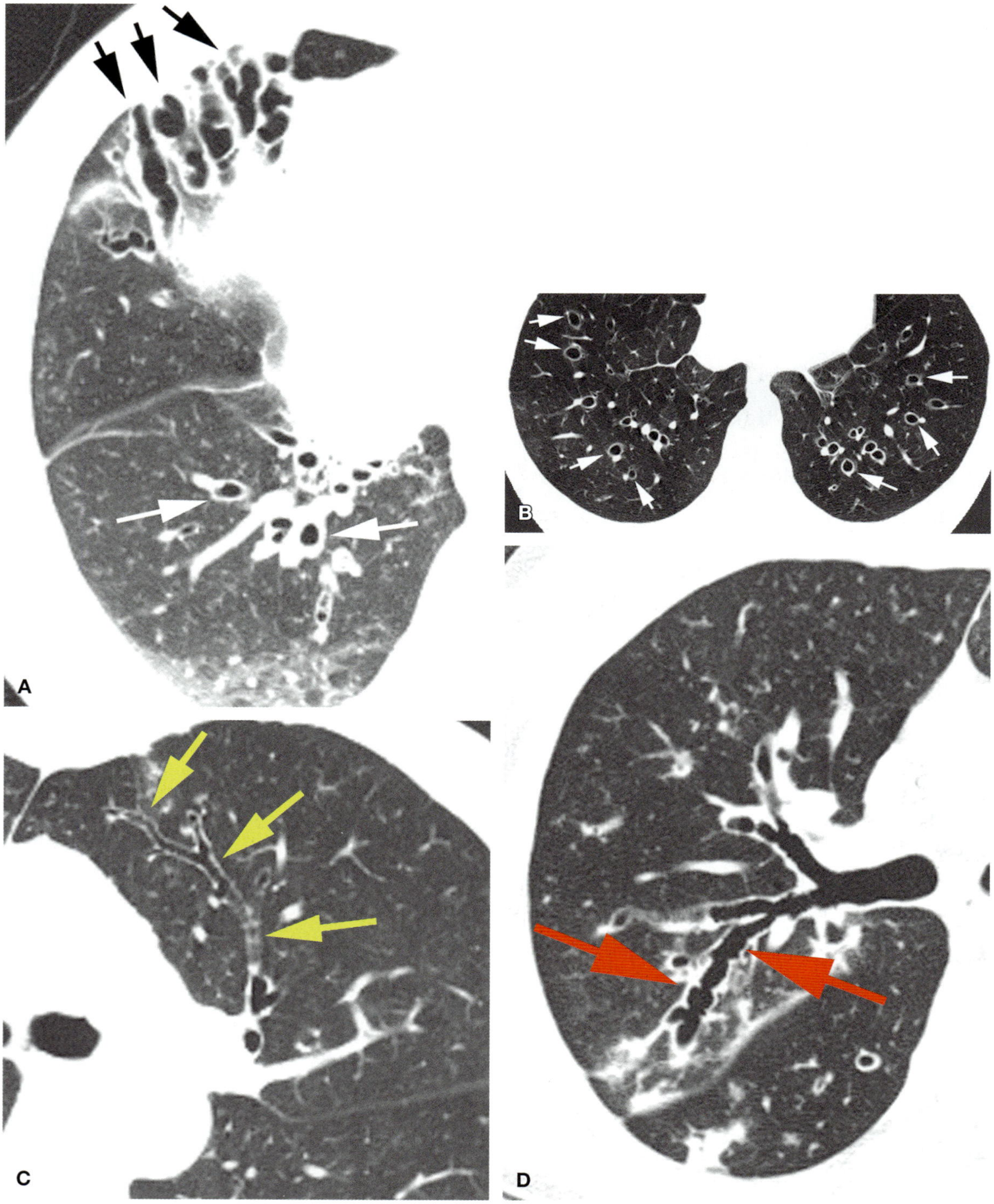

Figure 23.4. CT findings of bronchiectasis in four patients. **A:** CT shows several examples of the signet-ring sign in the lower lobe (*white arrows*). In the right middle lobe, bronchi are seen in the peripheral 1 cm of lung, do not taper, and have a cylindrical appearance (*black arrows*). Bronchial wall thickening is also visible. **B:** Numerous examples of the signet-ring sign (*arrows*) are visible. Note that the bronchus appears much larger than the adjacent artery. **C:** Cylindrical bronchiectasis with lack of bronchial tapering in the lung periphery (*arrows*). **D:** Bronchiectasis in a patient with cystic fibrosis. A dilated bronchus in the right upper lobe (*arrows*) shows a lack of tapering. Examples of the signet-ring sign are also visible.

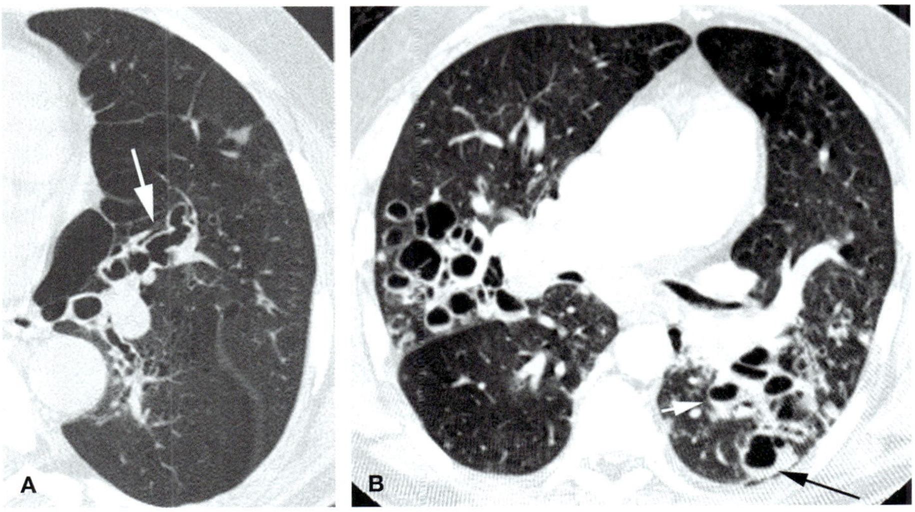

Figure 23.5. Contour abnormalities in bronchiectasis. **A:** Varicose bronchiectasis results in irregular bronchial dilatation (*arrow*). **B:** Cystic bronchiectasis. Air-fluid levels are visible within the abnormal bronchi (*arrows*). The dilated bronchi are visible in the lung periphery.

Patients with cystic bronchiectasis may show fluid levels within the abnormal bronchi (see Fig. 23.5B), due to retained secretions and chronic infection. Air-fluid levels within the multiple cystic spaces are typical, and since they tend to communicate with each other through the bronchi, the air-fluid levels appear similar in height.

Mosaic Perfusion and Air Trapping

Many patients with bronchiectasis also show pathologic findings of small airway disease, either BO or infectious bronchiolitis. Consequently, HRCT findings of small airway disease, such as mosaic perfusion (on inspiratory scans) and focal air trapping (on expiratory scans), are often seen in patients with bronchiectasis.

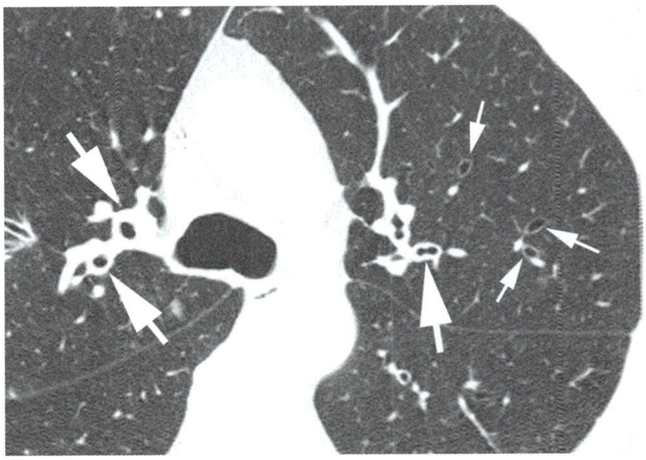

Figure 23.6. Bronchial wall thickening. CT shows several thick-walled bronchi (*large arrows*). Other bronchi show normal bronchial wall thickness (*small arrows*).

Tree-In-Bud

The term *tree-in-bud* refers to the presence of nodular and Y-shaped branching structures, which resemble a budding tree, in the lung periphery (Fig. 23.9; see also Fig. 11.28 in Chapter 11). This appearance generally reflects the presence of dilated, mucus- or pus-filled centrilobular bronchioles (the trunk and branches) associated with small nodular areas of bronchiolar dilatation or peribronchiolar inflammation (the buds at the tips of the branches). This finding is common in patients with airway infection and, therefore, is common in patients with various causes of bronchiectasis. About 90% of patients showing tree-in-bud on CT have an infectious airway disease or aspiration.

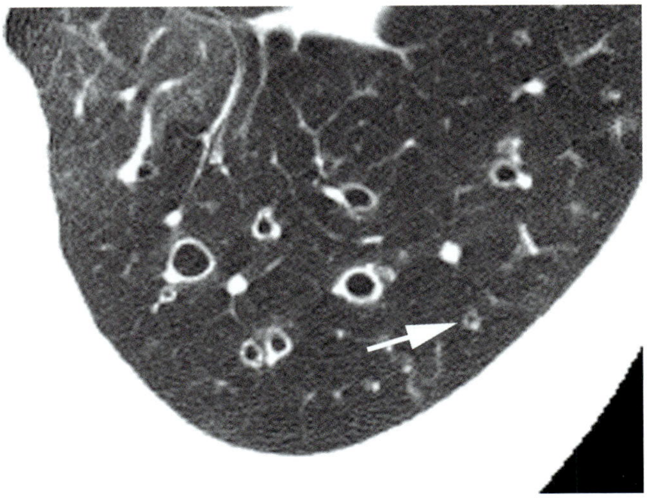

Figure 23.7. Visibility of a peripheral airway as an indication of bronchial wall thickening. In a patient with bronchiectasis, a bronchus (*arrow*) is visible in the peripheral lung. The fact that it is visible indicates that its wall is thickened.

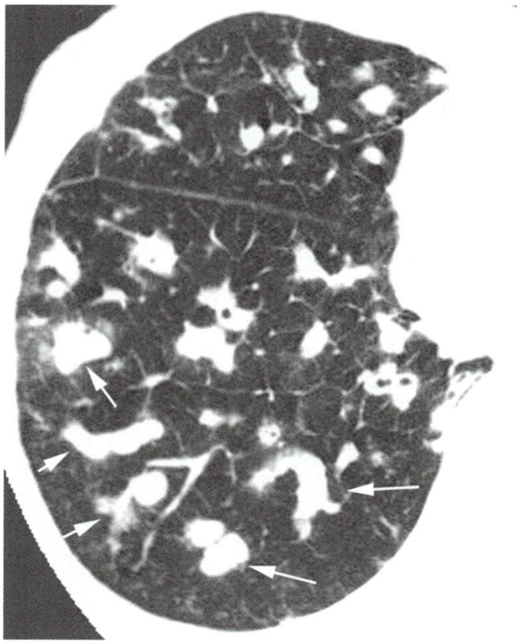

Figure 23.8. Extensive mucous plugging in bronchiectasis. Numerous dilated, opacified bronchi are visible (*arrows*), both along their axis and in cross section.

Systemic Collateral Artery Enlargement

Bronchiectasis and chronic inflammation can recruit enlarged systemic arterial collaterals. Most commonly, these are enlarged bronchial arteries, which can be identified pathologically in most cases of bronchiectasis. Bleeding of these vessels may result in massive and life-threatening hemoptysis. With multidetector CT using thin collimation and contrast infusion, abnormally enlarged bronchial arteries (or other systemic arteries including internal mammary, intercostal, or subclavian artery collaterals) may be identified. If the contrast concentration between the pulmonary arteries and aorta differs, bronchial artery inflow can create flow artifacts that may be mistaken for pulmonary embolism (Fig. 23.10).

Catheter arteriograms also may be used for diagnosis in patients with hemoptysis especially to confirm the source of bleeding, after which systemic artery embolization may be performed as a temporizing or curative treatment in patients with hemoptysis due to bronchiectasis.

Severity of Bronchiectasis

Systems for grading the severity of bronchiectasis using CT have been developed but are not in common clinical use. The severity of bronchiectasis may be related to the diameter of

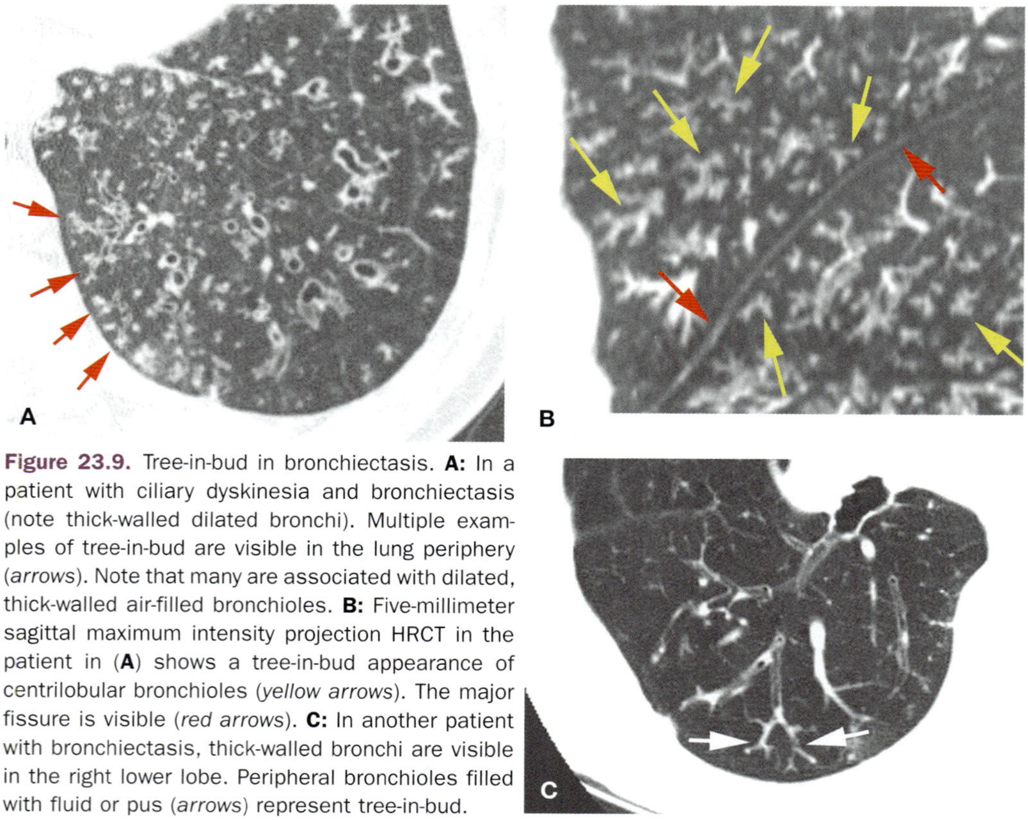

Figure 23.9. Tree-in-bud in bronchiectasis. **A:** In a patient with ciliary dyskinesia and bronchiectasis (note thick-walled dilated bronchi). Multiple examples of tree-in-bud are visible in the lung periphery (*arrows*). Note that many are associated with dilated, thick-walled air-filled bronchioles. **B:** Five-millimeter sagittal maximum intensity projection HRCT in the patient in (**A**) shows a tree-in-bud appearance of centrilobular bronchioles (*yellow arrows*). The major fissure is visible (*red arrows*). **C:** In another patient with bronchiectasis, thick-walled bronchi are visible in the right lower lobe. Peripheral bronchioles filled with fluid or pus (*arrows*) represent tree-in-bud.

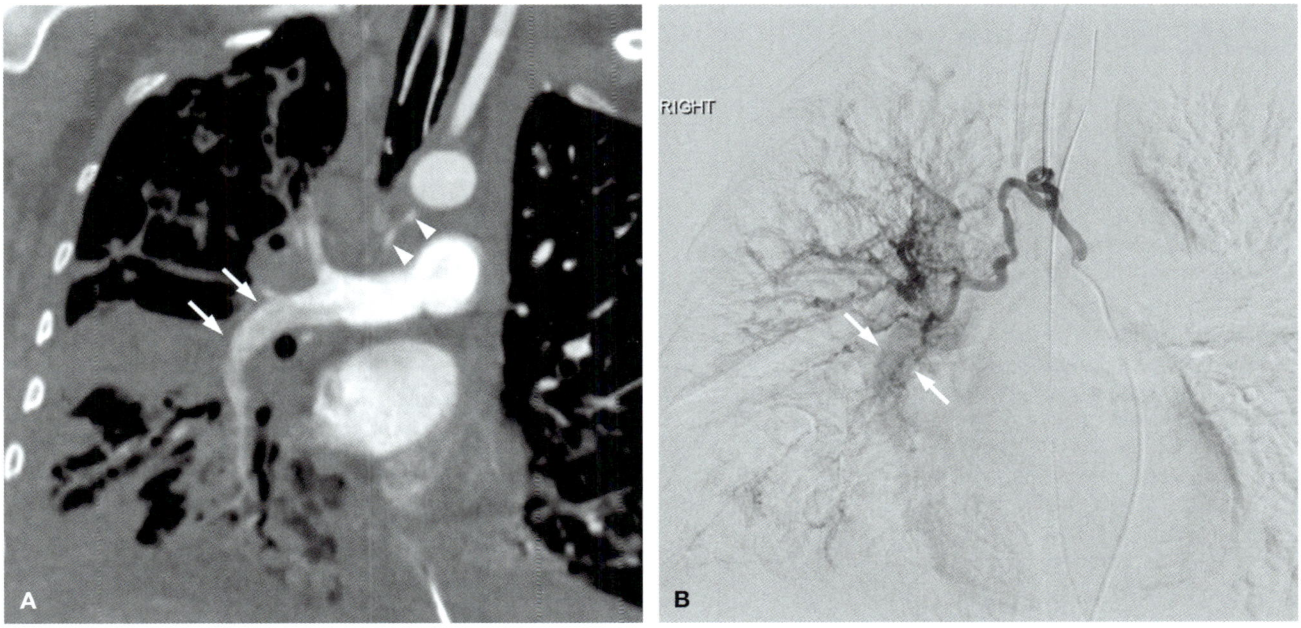

Figure 23.10. Bronchial artery inflow in a 23-year-old patient with bronchiectasis secondary to prior CF. **A:** Oblique coronal image from a CT pulmonary angiogram (CTPA) shows heterogeneous flow in the right pulmonary artery that could be mistaken for pulmonary embolism (*arrows*). Hypertrophied bronchial arteries are also visible (*arrowheads*). **B:** Coronal subtraction image from a catheter angiogram injection of the culprit bronchial artery in the same patient. Note the filling of the pulmonary artery (*arrows*) from the systemic-to-PA fistula responsible for the heterogeneous flow on the CTPA.

the abnormal bronchi. Also, there is a significant correlation between the extent of bronchiectasis and the forced expiratory volume in 1 second and the forced vital capacity (FVC). Furthermore, patients with cystic bronchiectasis are more likely to have infection and purulent sputum than are patients with either cylindrical or varicose bronchiectasis.

Pitfalls in the Diagnosis of Bronchiectasis

Several potential pitfalls in the diagnosis of bronchiectasis should be avoided.

Artifacts due to cardiac or respiratory motion may cause ghosting that can very closely mimic the appearance of tram tracks. Observing other artifacts related to motion helps in identifying them appropriately.

Bronchiectasis is difficult to diagnose with certainty in patients with atelectasis. Normal bronchi dilate in the presence of atelectasis because the collapsed lung results in increased tension on the bronchial wall. Bronchi return to normal size when the collapse resolves. This phenomenon is known as "reversible bronchiectasis" (see Fig. 1.28 in Chapter 1); this term is an oxymoron, since part of the definition of bronchiectasis is that it is irreversible.

Consolidation may obscure vascular anatomy, making assessment of bronchoarterial ratios difficult or impossible.

Bronchiectasis may occur in association with fibrotic lung diseases (ie, "traction" bronchiectasis). Traction bronchiectasis does not represent primary airway disease and is not associated with symptoms of chronic infection. The typical corkscrewed appearance of traction bronchiectasis and its association with obvious fibrosis are diagnostic.

SPECIFIC CAUSES OF BRONCHIECTASIS

In most instances, the radiographic appearance of bronchiectasis is nonspecific and does not allow a determination of its cause. However, a few diseases, discussed in the following sections, require special attention.

Cystic Fibrosis

CF is the most common cause of pulmonary insufficiency in the first 3 decades of life. It results from an autosomal recessive genetic defect in the structure of the CF transmembrane conductance regulator (CFTR), which leads to abnormal chloride transport across epithelial membranes (Table 23.3). The mechanisms by which this leads to lung disease are not entirely understood, but an abnormally low water content of airway mucus is at least partially responsible, resulting in decreased mucus clearance, mucous plugging of airways, and an increased incidence of bacterial airway infection. Bronchial wall inflammation progressing to secondary bronchiectasis is universal in patients with long-standing disease.

Although a single defect in CFTR is responsible for most cases, more than 100 genetic abnormalities may be associated with CF. These CF genotype variants often cause less severe

Table 23.3 Cystic Fibrosis (CF)

Autosomal recessive genetic defect in CF transmembrane conductance regulator
Abnormal chloride transport resulting in abnormal mucus
Bronchiectasis and infection universal
  Pseudomonas (90%)
  Aspergillus (50%)
  Mycobacteria (20%)

Radiographic findings Increased lung volumes Small nodular opacities due to impaction of small airways Bronchial wall thickening or bronchiectasis Mucoid impaction Right upper lobe predominance Atelectasis Cysts (bronchiectasis, abscess cavities, bullae) Pneumomediastinum or pneumothorax Hilar enlargement

HRCT findings
Bronchiectasis
  Central bronchi and upper lobes involved in all cases
  Typically severe (varicose and cystic) and widespread
Bronchial wall thickening
  Central and upper lobe distribution
Mucous plugging
Tree-in-bud
Large lung volumes
Atelectasis
Mosaic perfusion
Air trapping on expiration

disease and thus are more likely to be found in adults who first present with symptoms. Individuals who are carriers of the CF gene may have a selective advantage; they appear to be more resistant to typhoid fever than the general population.

Pulmonary abnormalities may be present within weeks of birth, with the earliest abnormalities being retention of mucus in small peripheral airways, mucous gland hyperplasia, and inflammation. The presence of airway infection is fundamental to the development of CF; the first organisms involved are *S. aureus*, *H. influenzae*, and mucoid *Pseudomonas* species. In adults with CF, *Pseudomonas aeruginosa* predominates (90% of cases), although *Aspergillus* (up to 50% of cases) species and mycobacteria (up to 20% of cases) also may be present. Bronchial wall damage and bronchiectasis occur largely as a result of infection.

In 2019, the introduction of a novel triple combination therapy (elexacaftor/ivacaftor/tezacaftor) targeting certain CFTR gene mutations transformed the treatment of CF patients with eligible mutations. These drugs help to improve the efficiency of the CFTR proteins and have stabilized or reversed symptoms in what was previously a progressive, fatal disease without lung transplant. On imaging, this has resulted in a substantial reduction in the number of infections/acute exacerbations in these patients, with resultant decrease in mucoid impaction and bronchial wall thickening on imaging. Unfortunately, not all CFTR mutations respond to these therapies, and many patients still have progressive disease as described below.

Clinical Presentation

Clinical findings of chronic and recurrent infection in a child, associated with abnormal sweat chlorides, usually are diagnostic. Hemoptysis occurs in more than half of cases because of bronchial artery hypertrophy.

Radiographic Findings

Typical radiographic findings (see Figs. 23.2 and 23.11) can help confirm the diagnosis in patients with symptoms or may be suggestive in patients with an atypical presentation (eg, young adults with CF variants).

Early in the course of disease, plain films are normal. Initial abnormalities include the following:

1. Increased lung volumes due to obstruction of small airways (ie, increased retrosternal space, flattening of the hemidiaphragms)
2. Impaction of small airways, resulting in small nodular or reticular opacities in the lung periphery
3. Accentuated linear opacities in the central or upper lung regions due to bronchial wall thickening or bronchiectasis

The earliest abnormalities in patients with CF are in the right upper lobe. Consequently, early findings may include right upper lobe atelectasis or thickening of the wall of the right upper lobe bronchus, best seen on the lateral radiograph.

In older children and adults, bronchiectasis is typical, often involving bronchi in the central lung regions, that is, *central bronchiectasis*. Dilated bronchi may be cylindrical, varicose, or cystic, depending on the duration and severity of disease. In adult patients and patients with chronic disease, additional abnormalities (see Figs. 23.2 and 23.11) can include the following:

1. Mucoid impaction with oval or branching opacities ("finger in glove" or "hand in glove")
2. Cysts or ring shadows in the upper lobes, representing cystic bronchiectasis, healed abscess cavities, or bullae
3. Atelectasis
4. Pneumothorax (up to 20% of cases)
5. Hilar enlargement due to lymphadenopathy or pulmonary hypertension
6. Pleural thickening (although pleural effusion is uncommon)

In most patients with an established diagnosis of CF, clinical findings and chest radiographs are sufficient for clinical management. A significant exacerbation of symptoms may occur with little visible radiographic change.

CT Findings

CT can demonstrate morphologic abnormalities in patients with early CF who are asymptomatic, have normal pulmonary function, or have normal chest radiographs. In patients with more advanced disease, HRCT also can show abnormalities not visible on chest radiographs, including bronchiectasis and mucous plugging.

On CT and HRCT, bronchiectasis is seen in all patients with advanced CF (Figs. 23.2C and 23.12). Proximal or parahilar bronchi always are involved when bronchiectasis is present, and bronchiectasis is limited to these central bronchi (ie, *central bronchiectasis*) in about one-third of cases. Typically, all lobes are involved, although early in the disease, abnormalities often predominate in the upper lobes; often, abnormalities are most severe in the right upper lobe. The differential diagnosis of central bronchiectasis also includes ABPA, tuberculosis (TB), radiation fibrosis, Mounier-Kuhn syndrome (tracheobronchomegaly), and Williams-Campbell syndrome, although with exception on ABPA, the appearances of these differs significantly from that of CF.

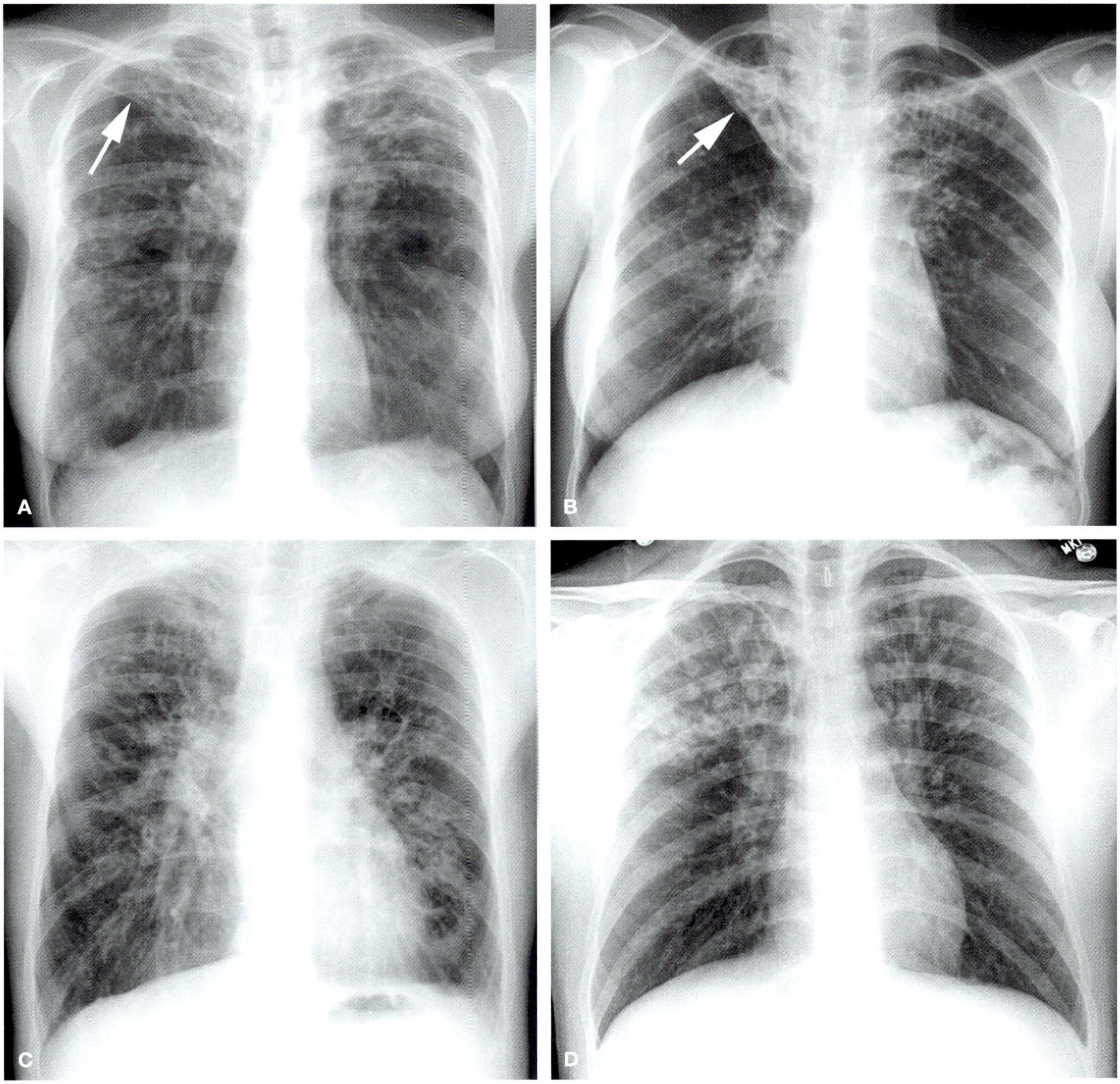

Figure 23.11. Radiographic findings in adults with cystic fibrosis. **A, B:** PA chest radiograph in two different patients shows increased lung volumes. The hila are elevated because of upper lobe volume loss, and the minor fissure (*arrow*) is bowed upward. Increased markings in the upper lobes reflect bronchiectasis. **C:** In this patient, large lung volumes are associated with ring shadows and an increase in markings in the central lung regions, due to bronchiectasis. **D:** Large lung volumes are present. Upper lobe bronchiectasis is present, with ring shadows and branching mucous plugs.

Cylindrical bronchiectasis is most common (95%) on HRCT, but varicose and cystic bronchiectasis are visible in as many as one-third of cases and are more common in advanced cases. Cystic bronchiectasis, abscess cavities, or bullae are visible in half of patients and typically predominate in the subpleural regions of the upper lobes. The name *cystic fibrosis* is sometimes erroneously ascribed to the presence of cystic bronchiectasis; however, the disease derives its name from the characteristic fibrosis and cyst formation within the pancreas on pathologic specimens.

Bronchial wall or peribronchial interstitial thickening also is commonly present in patients with CF. It usually is more evident than bronchial dilatation in patients who have early disease and may be seen independent of bronchiectasis. Thickening of the wall of the proximal right upper lobe bronchi often is the earliest abnormal feature visible on HRCT.

Mucous plugging is visible in one quarter to one half of cases and may be visible in all lobes. Volume loss, collapse, or consolidation can be seen in as many as 80% of patients.

Tree-in-bud (ie, bronchiolar dilatation with associated infection or mucus impaction) often is visible and can be an early sign of disease in children.

Focal areas of decreased lung opacity, representing *mosaic perfusion*, are common (see Fig. 23.12). These may appear to surround dilated, thick-walled, or mucus-plugged bronchi. *Air trapping* often is seen on expiratory scans.

Lung volumes may appear increased on CT, although this diagnosis is rather subjective and may be better assessed on chest radiographs.

Hilar or mediastinal lymph node enlargement and pleural thickening also can be seen, largely due to chronic infection. Pulmonary artery dilatation resulting from pulmonary

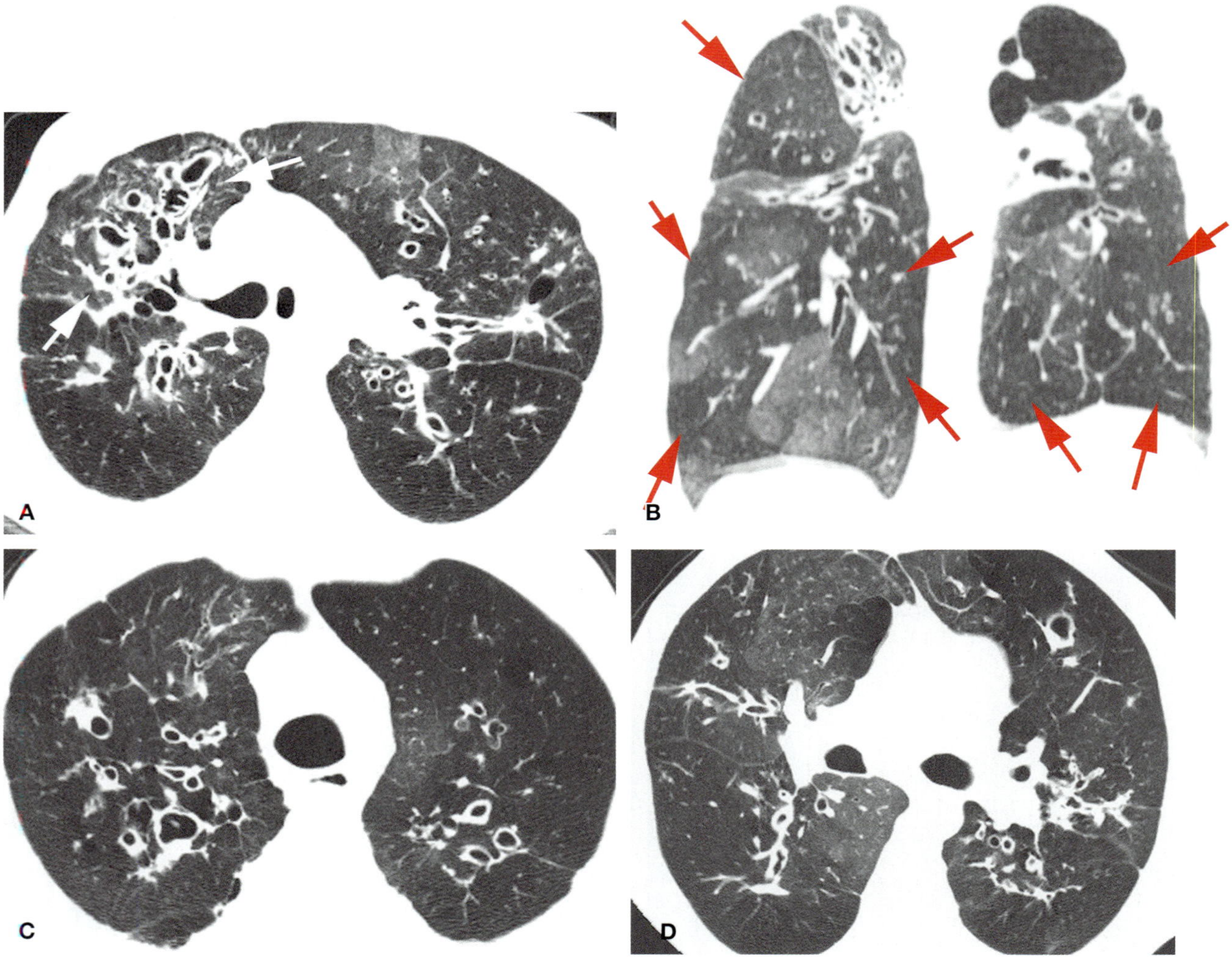

Figure 23.12. HRCT findings in cystic fibrosis (CF). **A:** Parahilar (*central*) bronchiectasis is present (*arrows*), with predominance in the right upper lobe. Patchy areas of lucency reflect mosaic perfusion. Some right upper lobe volume loss is apparent. **B:** In a different patient with CF, coronal CT shows right upper lobe volume loss and bronchiectasis, and left apical lung cysts, associated with multifocal patchy areas of mosaic perfusion (*arrows*) with lung lucency and decreased vessel size. **C, D:** A third patient with CF where central (*parahilar*) bronchiectasis and bronchial wall thickening are present. Mosaic perfusion results in patchy lung opacity with decreased vessel size in the lung periphery.

hypertension also can be seen in patients with long-standing disease.

Allergic Bronchopulmonary Aspergillosis

ABPA reflects a hypersensitivity reaction to *Aspergillus* organisms and characteristically is associated with eosinophilia, symptoms of asthma (eg, wheezing), "central" or "proximal" bronchiectasis, mucoid impaction, atelectasis, and consolidation similar to that seen in patients with eosinophilic pneumonia (Table 23.4). ABPA typically occurs in young adults with a history of asthma or atopy and in 2% to 10% of patients with CF. Asthma may be present for many years before the diagnosis of ABPA.

ABPA results from both type I (IgE-mediated hypersensitivity) and type III (IgG-mediated antigen-antibody complex reaction) immunologic responses to the endobronchial growth of fungal (eg, *Aspergillus*) species.

The type I response results in immediate wheezing when the patient is exposed to *Aspergillus* antigens.

The type III reaction results in bronchial inflammation in response to fungi in the airway, which eventually leads to bronchiectasis. Bronchiectasis usually is varicose or cystic in appearance, central in location (ie, central bronchiectasis), and associated with formation of mucous plugs that contain fungus and inflammatory cells.

Clinical Presentation

Symptoms of ABPA are similar to those of uncomplicated asthma and include wheezing, cough, and dyspnea. Occasionally, fever, hemoptysis, and chest pain may be associated. Expectoration of mucous plugs containing fungus may occur.

Table 23.4 Allergic Bronchopulmonary Aspergillosis

Hypersensitivity reaction to *Aspergillus*
History of asthma or atopy and cystic fibrosis
Type I (IgE-mediated) hypersensitivity results in wheezing
Type III (IgG-mediated antigen-antibody complex) reaction results in bronchiectasis
Radiographic findings
Consolidation (ie, eosinophilic pneumonia)
Central bronchiectasis, upper lobe or widespread
Mucous plugging ("finger in glove")
Increased lung volume
Upper lobe volume loss or scarring
HRCT findings
Central bronchiectasis, widespread
Upper lobe predominance common
Mucous plugging; high-attenuation mucus
Tree-in-bud
Atelectasis
Peripheral consolidation or diffuse ground-glass opacity
Mosaic perfusion
Air trapping on expiration

The diagnosis of ABPA is based on a combination of clinical, laboratory, and radiographic findings. The five essential criteria for diagnosis can be remembered by the acronym *ASPER* and include the following:

1. **A**sthma
2. **S**pecific **S**erum antibodies (IgE and IgG) to *Aspergillus*
3. **P**roximal (central) bronchiectasis
4. **E**levated Ig**E** (greater than 1000 ng/mL)
5. **R**eactive skin test (wheal-and-flare skin reaction to *Aspergillus* antigen)

If proximal (central) bronchiectasis is absent or undetected, a diagnosis of *seropositive ABPA* can be made in the presence of criteria 1, 2, 4, and 5.

Additional criteria, not required for diagnosis, include:

1. Blood eosinophilia
2. Serum precipitins to *Aspergillus* antigen
3. Pulmonary infiltrates on chest radiographs

ABPA typically is characterized by repeated exacerbations. Disease progression may be divided into five phases, although these are not invariable: (1) acute presentation, (2) resolution with clearing of pulmonary abnormalities and decline in serum IgE, (3) recurrence, and (4) development of dependence on corticosteroids, leading in some cases to (5) pulmonary fibrosis.

Radiographic Findings

Patients presenting with an acute exacerbation of ABPA often show consolidation on chest radiographs. Some consolidations are patchy, resembling eosinophilic pneumonia. These may be peripheral or parahilar, surrounding abnormal bronchi. Segmental or lobar consolidation may reflect atelectasis resulting from bronchial obstruction by mucous plugs.

Bronchiectasis is commonly visible with acute or recurrent disease (Figs. 23.13 and 23.14). The abnormal bronchi often are lobar or segmental and, thus, central in location. They may have an oval or branching appearance or may appear round if seen in cross section. Mucous plugs may be seen within the bronchi, outlined by air, or may fill the bronchi, resulting in a "*finger in glove*" or "*hand in glove*" appearance (see Fig. 23.13). The presence of a dilated, thick-walled bronchus sometimes is termed a *bronchocele*, whereas a bronchocele containing a mucous plug may be referred to as a *mucocele*. These tend to have an upper lobe predominance in patients with ABPA.

Lung distal to a mucous plug may be collapsed or may be aerated due to collateral ventilation. Aerated lung may appear hyperlucent and hypovascular due to air trapping. Lung volume may be increased.

The radiographic findings in ABPA (eg, central bronchiectasis with an upper lobe predominance [see Figs. 23.13 and 23.14], mucous plugging, consolidation, large lung volumes) may mimic those of CF. In the later stages of disease, upper lobe scarring and volume loss may mimic prior TB.

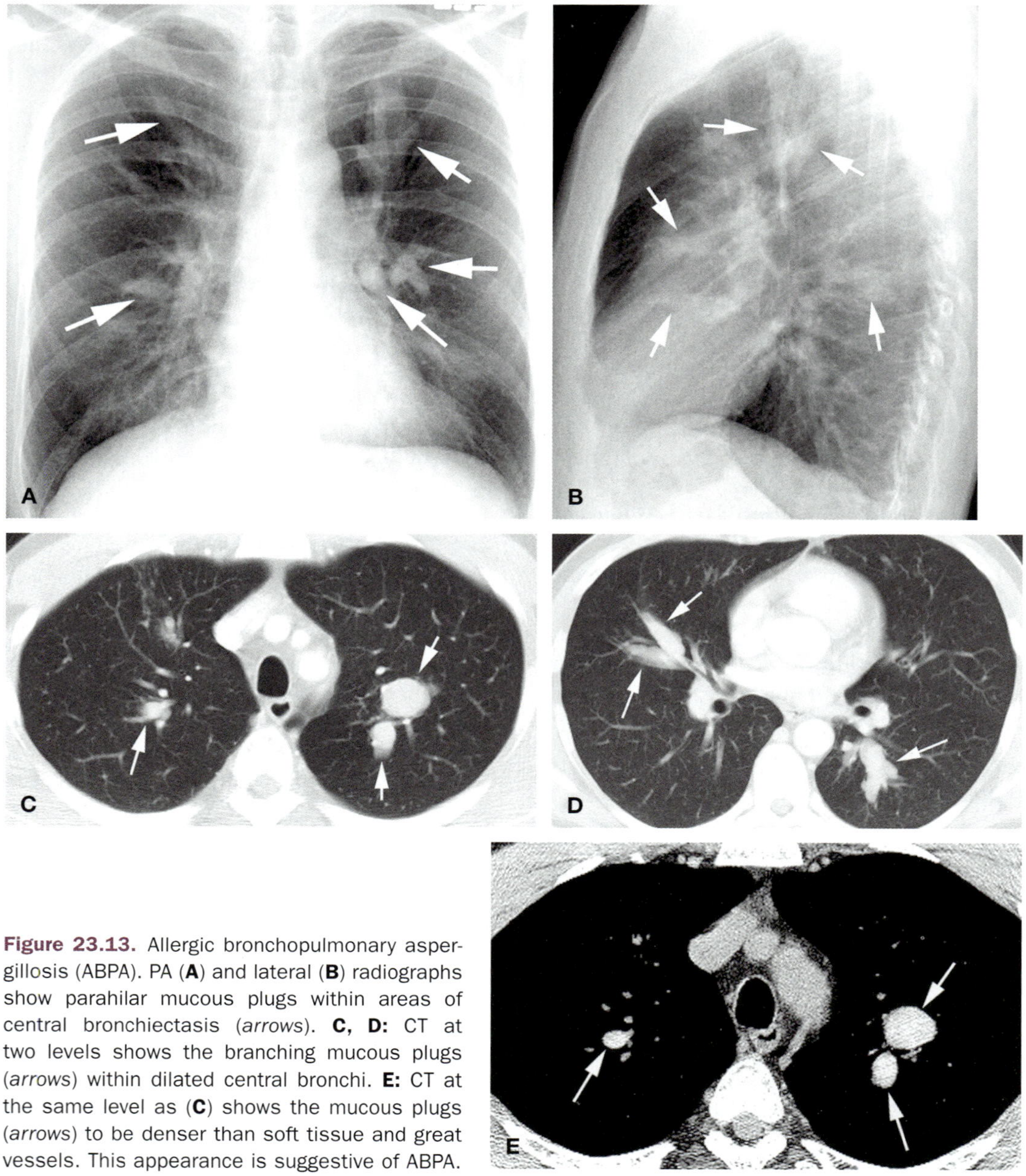

Figure 23.13. Allergic bronchopulmonary aspergillosis (ABPA). PA (**A**) and lateral (**B**) radiographs show parahilar mucous plugs within areas of central bronchiectasis (*arrows*). **C, D:** CT at two levels shows the branching mucous plugs (*arrows*) within dilated central bronchi. **E:** CT at the same level as (**C**) shows the mucous plugs (*arrows*) to be denser than soft tissue and great vessels. This appearance is suggestive of ABPA.

CT Findings

This slice CT is more sensitive than are plain radiographs in detecting airway abnormalities associated with ABPA. HRCT findings include central bronchiectasis (present in 85% of lobes), usually varicose or cylindrical (see Fig. 23.14B), bronchial occlusion due to mucous plugging (see Figs. 23.13C, D and 23.14B-D), and bronchial wall thickening. An upper lobe predominance for these abnormalities is common but not invariable. Ectatic airways sometimes may contain an air-fluid level or an aspergilloma.

In about 25% of cases, mucous plugs in ABPA are greater in attenuation than soft tissue (see Figs. 23.13E and 23.14D); these plugs may be quite dense, measuring more than 100 HU. High-attenuation mucus (HAM) is strongly suggestive of ABPA and is thought to be due to concentration of calcium oxalate or metals by the fungus. HAM plugs also may be seen with bronchial atresia (see Chapter 9).

A tree-in-bud appearance resulting from mucus filling the bronchioles may be seen (Fig. 23.14E), but in most patients with ABPA, the peripheral airways appear normal.

Parenchymal abnormalities including consolidation, collapse, cavitation, and bullae may be identified in as many as 40% of cases, particularly in the upper lobes. Masslike foci of eosinophilic pneumonia may be seen with acute exacerbation. Mosaic perfusion and air trapping may be seen.

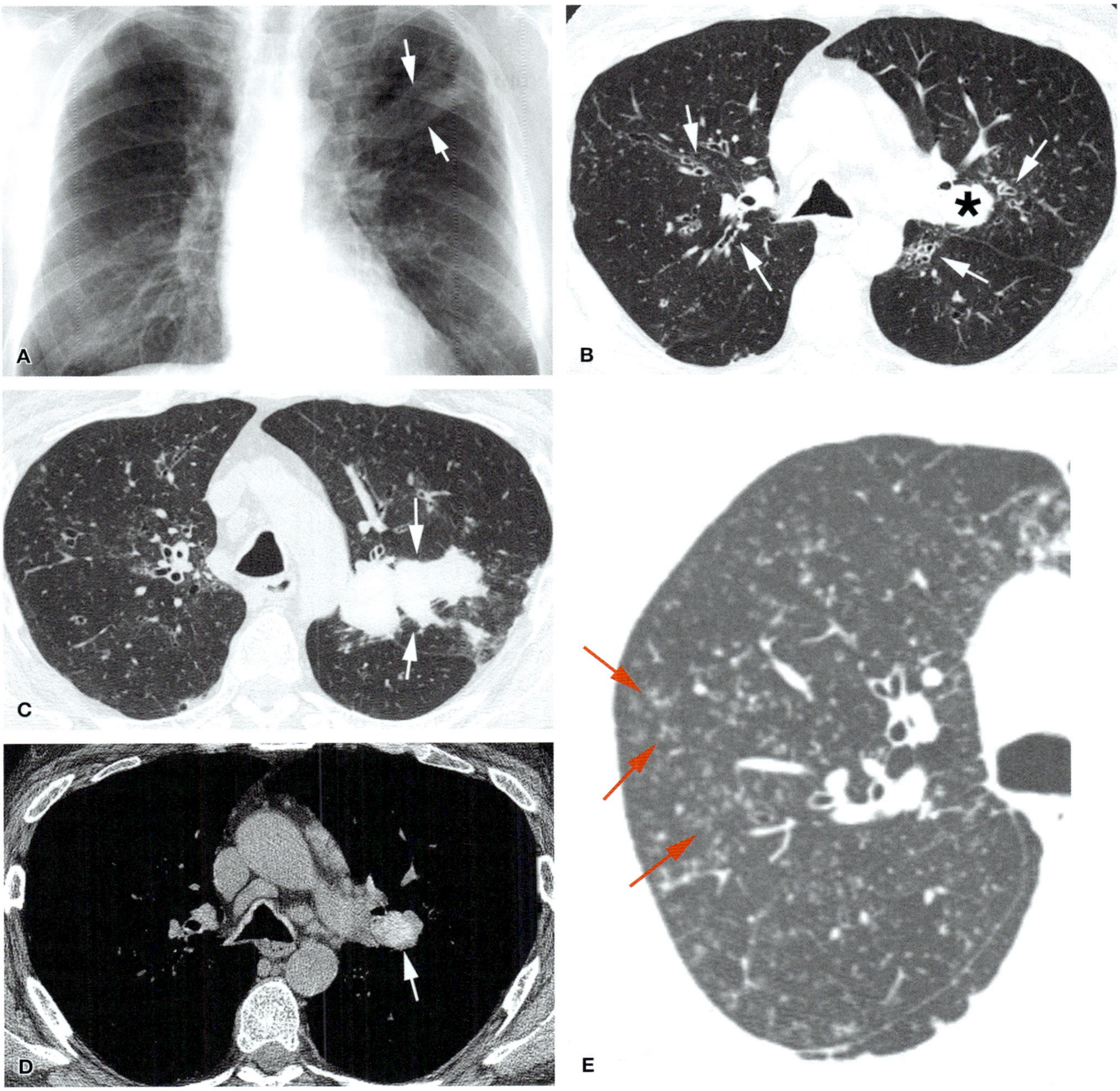

Figure 23.14. Allergic bronchopulmonary aspergillosis (ABPA). **A:** PA radiographs show a mucous plug in the central left upper lobe (*arrows*). **B:** HRCT shows multiple areas of central bronchiectasis and bronchial wall thickening (*arrows*) and a large central mucous plug (*asterisk*). **C:** HRCT slightly above (**B**) shows the branching mucous plug (*arrows*). **D:** CT at the same level as (**B**) shows the mucous plug (*arrow*) to be denser than soft tissue. **E:** HRCT in a different patient with ABPA shows central bronchial wall thickening and mild bronchiectasis, with numerous examples of tree-in-bud in the right lung (*red arrows*).

Asthma

Asthma is characterized by airway inflammation, which is largely reversible (Table 23.5). Pathologically, patients with asthma show bronchial and bronchiolar wall thickening caused by inflammation, infiltration by eosinophils, smooth muscle hyperplasia, edema, and excess mucus production, which can result in mucous plugging. Bronchiectasis may be seen in some patients with long-standing asthma.

Pulmonary function tests show findings of airway obstruction (eg, increased airway resistance, increased total lung volume, increased residual volume, and decreased FVC) during an asthma episode but typically return to normal between attacks.

Table 23.5 Asthma

Reversible airway inflammation and obstruction
Radiographic findings subtle
- Increased lung volume (30%-40%)
- Increased lucency
- Mild bronchial wall thickening (50%)
- Mild hilar prominence

Radiographs most useful in diagnosing complications
- Pneumonia
- Atelectasis
- Pneumomediastinum and pneumothorax

HRCT used to diagnose complications, allergic bronchopulmonary aspergillosis, or emphysema
- Mild bronchial wall thickening or dilatation
- Mucous plugs or tree-in-bud (20%)
- Mosaic perfusion (20%-30%)
- Air trapping on expiration (50%)

Radiographic Findings

Radiographic findings associated with asthma usually are subtle. They include increased lung volume (30%-40%), increased lung lucency, mild bronchial wall thickening (50%), and mild prominence of hilar vasculature due to transient pulmonary hypertension (10%). Bronchiectasis is not usually recognized, but small mucous plugs sometimes can be seen. Associated complications of asthma, although uncommon, include pneumonia, atelectasis, pneumomediastinum, and pneumothorax. Pneumomediastinum is more common than pneumothorax. Radiographic abnormalities generally are more common and more severe in children with asthma.

Plain radiographs are not commonly used to make a diagnosis of asthma; radiographs often are normal, and visible abnormalities in this disease usually are nonspecific. Radiography also has limited usefulness in patients with an established diagnosis of asthma who suffer an acute attack. Correlation between the severity of radiographic findings and the severity and reversibility of an asthma attack usually is poor, and radiographs provide significant information that alters treatment in 5% or less of patients with acute asthma. Although it is difficult to generalize regarding the role of radiographs in adults and children with acute asthma, chest films often are used to exclude the presence of associated pneumonia or other complications when significant symptoms or appropriate clinical or laboratory findings are suggestive.

HRCT Findings

CT is not commonly indicated in the routine assessment of patients with asthma, but it sometimes is used when complications, particularly ABPA, are suspected or in diagnosing emphysema in smokers with asthma.

HRCT shows mild bronchial wall thickening or dilatation of small bronchi (diagnosed by a bronchoarterial ratio slightly greater than 1) in about half of patients with uncomplicated asthma.

Mucoid impaction and tree-in-bud have been reported in as many as 20% of cases and typically clear following treatment.

Mosaic perfusion or diffuse hyperlucency has been observed on inspiratory scans in 20% to 30% of cases. Expiratory CT can show evidence of patchy air trapping in as many as 50% of asthmatic patients.

Although asthma and ABPA can result in similar abnormalities, patients with ABPA have a higher frequency of bronchiectasis (95% vs 30% for asthma), a higher incidence of mucoid impaction, and more severe and extensive abnormalities.

Table 23.6 Dyskinetic Cilia Syndrome and Kartagener Syndrome

Autosomal recessive defect
Abnormal ciliary structure and movement
Abnormal mucociliary clearance
50% have situs inversus: Kartagener syndrome
Sinusitis common
Bilateral bronchiectasis, typically lower or middle lobe

Mycobacterium Avium-Intracellulare Complex Infection

Bronchiectasis predominantly involving the right middle lobe and lingua, in association with lung nodules and tree-in-bud, is characteristic of nontuberculous mycobacterial infection resulting from *Mycobacterium avium-intracellulare* complex (MAC) and is described in detail in Chapter 13. It typically is seen in females older than 60 years.

Dyskinetic Cilia Syndrome and Kartagener Syndrome

Dyskinetic cilia syndrome (DCS) is characterized by abnormal ciliary structure and movement, resulting in abnormal mucociliary clearance and chronic infection (Table 23.6). Bronchiectasis and sinusitis are common manifestations. About half of patients with DCS also have situs inversus. The combination of bronchiectasis, sinusitis, and situs inversus is called *Kartagener syndrome* (see Fig. 23.1).

DCS is an autosomal recessive genetic abnormality with an incidence of about 1 in 20,000 births. Males and females are equally affected. A variety of ultrastructural abnormalities of ciliary microtubules have been reported in association with this syndrome, although in some cases, the cilia appear normal. In men, the syndrome may be associated with immotile spermatozoa and infertility; in females, fertility is not affected. Other congenital abnormalities also may be present. In patients with chronic infections and situs inversus, the diagnosis is not difficult. In the absence of situs inversus, criteria for attributing chronic infection to DCS may include immotile spermatozoa, a family history of DCS, or abnormal cilia on biopsy.

Symptoms of recurrent bronchitis, pneumonia, and sinusitis often date from childhood. Radiographs and CT typically show bilateral bronchiectasis with a basal (lower or middle lobe) predominance. Cylindrical bronchiectasis is most common. Appropriate antibiotic treatment is associated with a normal life expectancy.

Young Syndrome

Young syndrome, also referred to as *obstructive azoospermia*, is characterized by male infertility caused by obstruction of the epididymis, bronchiectasis, and sinusitis. It may resemble DCS clinically, but ciliary abnormalities are absent. The cause is unknown, but it is associated with abnormally viscous mucus. The radiographic appearance of the bronchiectasis is nonspecific.

Syndrome of Yellow Nails and Lymphedema

The syndrome of yellow nails and lymphedema, also known as "yellow nail syndrome," is characterized by (1) slowly growing nails that are thickened, curved, and yellow-green in color; (2) lymphedema, usually of the lower extremities, due to lymphatic hypoplasia; and (3) exudative pleural effusions associated with pleural lymphatic dilatation. It is not necessary for all three manifestations to be present; pleural effusion is least common. Chronic sinusitis, airway infection, and bronchiectasis are present in about half of patients (Fig. 23.15). The syndrome typically presents in adulthood.

Tracheobronchomegaly (Mounier-Kuhn Syndrome)

Tracheobronchomegaly, also referred to as *Mounier-Kuhn syndrome*, is characterized by marked dilatation of the trachea and mainstem bronchi, recurrent lower respiratory tract infections, and bronchiectasis (see Figs. 22.29 and 22.31 in Chapter 22). The finding of central bronchiectasis associated with dilatation of the trachea is diagnostic. It is described in detail in Chapter 22.

Williams-Campbell Syndrome

Williams-Campbell syndrome is a rare type of congenital cystic bronchiectasis due to defective cartilage in the fourth- to sixth-order (central) bronchi. Radiographs and HRCT may show areas of central cystic bronchiectasis with distal regions of abnormal lucency, probably related to air trapping or bronchiolitis (Fig. 23.16). Ballooning of the central bronchi on inspiration and collapse on expiration may occur. These findings are useful in differentiating Williams-Campbell syndrome from other causes of cystic bronchiectasis.

Alpha-1 Antitrypsin Deficiency

In addition to emphysema, bronchiectasis often (40%) is present in patients with alpha-1 antitrypsin deficiency. This correlates well with the fact that approximately 50% of

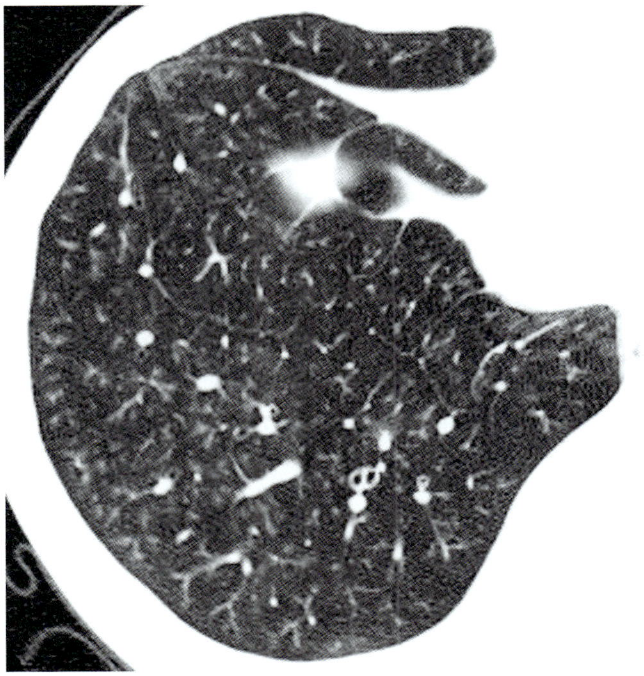

Figure 23.15. Syndrome of yellow nails. HRCT shows tree-in-bud in the right lower lobe, as a manifestation of airway infection.

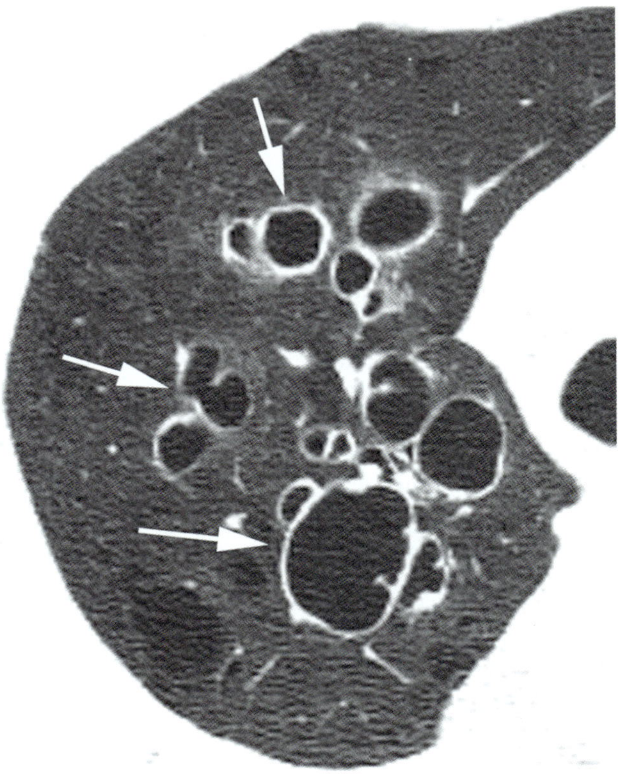

Figure 23.16. Williams-Campbell syndrome with cystic bronchiectasis. Marked cystic bronchiectasis (*arrows*) is visible in the central lung regions.

patients with this deficiency manifest symptoms of airway disease—in particular, chronic sputum production. It is likely that bronchiectasis results from a proteinase-antiproteinase imbalance (also responsible for the emphysema), discussed in Chapter 24.

Bronchiectasis Associated With Systemic Diseases

Bronchiectasis may be an important finding in a number of systemic diseases. Of particular interest are the associations between bronchiectasis and collagen vascular disease and inflammatory bowel disease.

Collagen Vascular Disease

Rheumatoid arthritis (RA) may be associated with a variety of parenchymal abnormalities, including pulmonary fibrosis, organizing pneumonia, respiratory tract infections, BO, and necrobiotic nodules. Airway disease, including both bronchiectasis and bronchiolectasis, may also occur in association with RA (see Fig. 15.7 in Chapter 15). One hypothesis suggests that chronic bacterial infections may trigger an immune reaction in genetically predisposed individuals, leading to RA; bronchiectasis may precede RA by years. It has also been suggested that steroids or immunosuppressive therapy may lead to an increased incidence of respiratory infections.

On HRCT, bronchiectasis is seen in up to 35% of patients with this disease, even when chest radiographs are normal. Other findings include mosaic perfusion on inspiratory scans (20%) and air trapping on expiratory scans (30%). Bronchiectasis may be identified in up to 20% of patients with systemic lupus erythematosus. A similarly high prevalence of airway pathology has also been noted in patients with primary Sjögren syndrome.

Ulcerative Colitis and Inflammatory Bowel Disease

A wide range of airway abnormalities have been identified in patients with ulcerative colitis. In addition to OP and diffuse interstitial lung disease, these include subglottic tracheal stenosis, chronic bronchitis, and chronic suppurative inflammation of both large and small airways (Fig. 23.17). Similar to what is seen in patients with RA, chronic suppurative airway disease may precede, coexist with, or follow the development of inflammatory bowel disease. Unlike other causes of bronchiectasis, chronic suppurative airway disease associated with ulcerative colitis often responds to treatment with inhaled steroids. Bronchiectasis also is associated with Crohn disease.

Airway Disease Related to HIV and AIDS

An accelerated form of bronchiectasis may occur in patients with human immunodeficiency virus (HIV) infection and patients with AIDS. It is likely that bronchiectasis results from recurrent or chronic bacterial airway infection. A wide range of organisms may affect the airways in patients with AIDS, most commonly *H. influenzae*, *P. aeruginosa*,

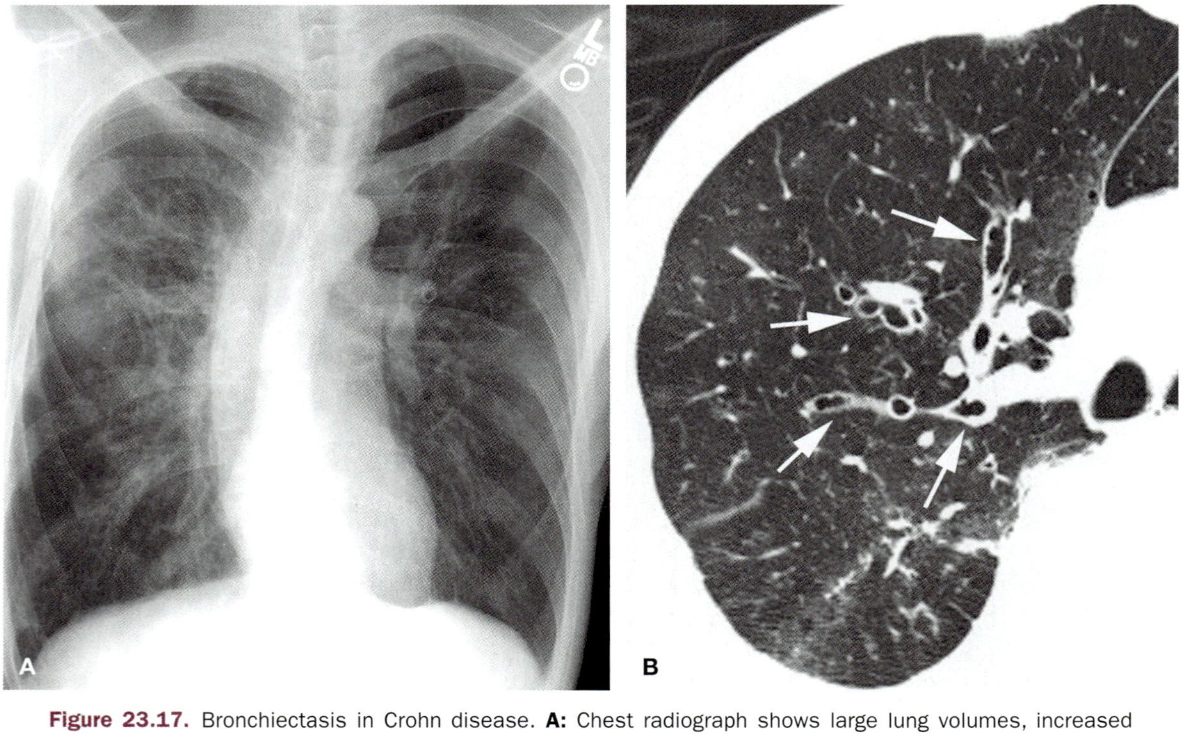

Figure 23.17. Bronchiectasis in Crohn disease. **A:** Chest radiograph shows large lung volumes, increased markings in the central lung, and evidence of bronchial wall thickening, particularly in the upper lobes. **B:** HRCT shows bronchiectasis and bronchial wall thickening (*arrows*).

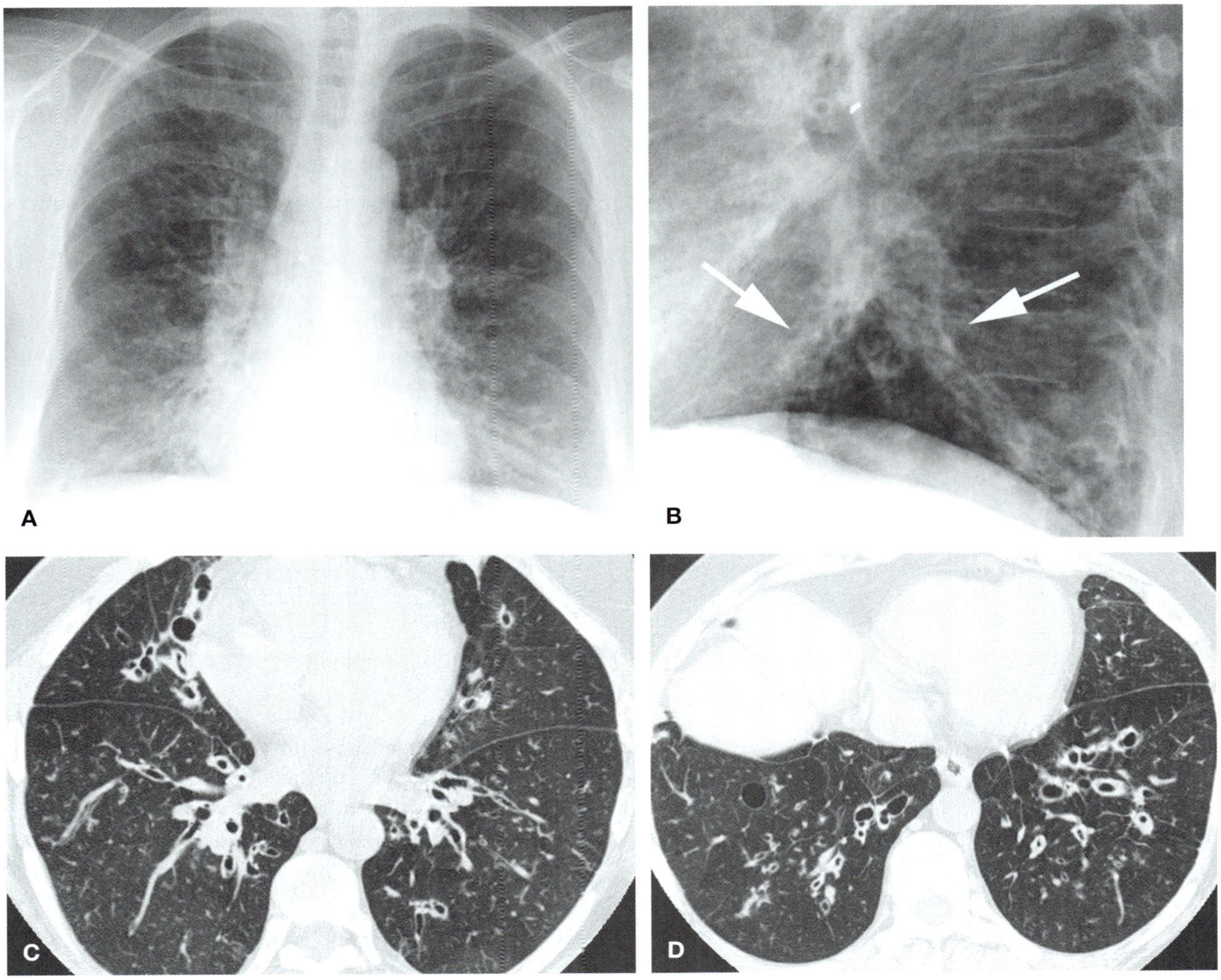

Figure 23.18. AIDS-related airway disease. **A:** PA chest radiograph shows increased opacities at the lung bases. **B:** Detail view of a lateral radiograph shows evidence of bronchial wall thickening in the lower lobes (*arrows*). **C, D:** HRCT through the lung bases shows evidence of bronchiectasis and bronchial wall thickening typical of AIDS-related airway disease.

Streptococcus viridans, *S. pneumoniae*, mycobacteria, and fungi such as *Aspergillus* organisms.

HRCT findings include bronchial wall thickening, bronchiectasis, bronchial or bronchiolar impaction with tree-in-bud, consolidation, and air trapping (Fig. 23.18). A lower lobe predominance is typical, and both lower lobes usually are involved.

About 10% of all reported cases of aspergillosis in AIDS patients will affect the airways. *Aspergillus* infection typically occurs late in the course of HIV infection and usually is associated with corticosteroid use and granulocytopenia. There are several distinct types of airway aspergillosis, including necrotizing tracheobronchitis, airway-invasive aspergillosis, and obstructing bronchopulmonary aspergillosis.

Necrotizing tracheobronchitis and airway-invasive aspergillosis are discussed in Chapters 13 and 22.

Obstructing bronchopulmonary aspergillosis in AIDS patients typically presents with acute fever, dyspnea, and cough associated with the expectoration of fungal casts. It is characterized on CT by the presence of mucoid impaction, typically involving the lower lobe airways. It has been suggested that this form of disease is unique to patients with AIDS.

CT Differentiation of Causes of Bronchiectasis

The reliability of radiographs and CT for distinguishing between different causes of bronchiectasis is limited. However, several general rules apply:

1. Lower lobe bronchiectasis is most typical of childhood infections, chronic infection of any cause, syndromes associated with impaired mucociliary clearance or immunodeficiency (see Figs. 23.18 and 23.19), chronic aspiration, Young syndrome, yellow nails and lymphedema, alpha-1 antitrypsin deficiency, and systemic diseases

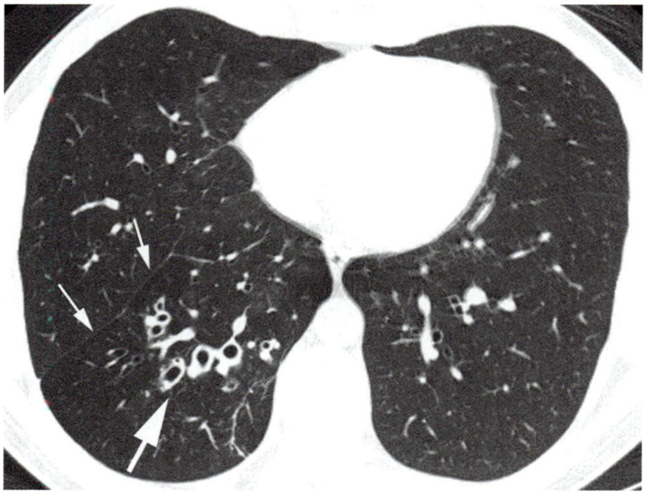

Figure 23.19. Unilateral lower lobe bronchiectasis. Right lower lobe bronchiectasis (*large arrow*) is associated with lower lobe volume loss and posterior displacement of the fissure (*small arrows*). This appearance is most consistent with childhood infection.

(eg, collagen vascular diseases and inflammatory bowel disease). Lower lobe traction bronchiectasis is most common in patients with lung fibrosis, such as usual interstitial pneumonia or nonspecific interstitial pneumonia.

2. Bilateral upper and midlung bronchiectasis is seen most commonly in patients with CF and ABPA (see Figs. 23.2C and Figs. 23.12-23.14). Traction bronchiectasis in the upper lobes may be associated with sarcoidosis, TB, and chronic hypersensitivity pneumonitis.
3. Unilateral upper lobe bronchiectasis is most common in patients with TB (Fig. 23.20).
4. Central bronchiectasis is most common in patients with ABPA and CF (see Figs. 23.12-23.14). Also, it may be seen in tracheobronchomegaly (Mounier-Kuhn syndrome; see Chapter 22) and Williams-Campbell syndrome (Fig. 23.16).
5. Severe and extensive bronchiectasis is most common in patients with ABPA and CF (see Figs. 23.12-23.14).
6. Lobar bronchiectasis suggests infection or bronchial obstruction.
7. Middle lobe and lingular (anterior) bronchiectasis suggests MAC infection. Anterior lung traction bronchiectasis may be seen in patients surviving acute respiratory distress syndrome.

CHRONIC BRONCHITIS

Chronic bronchitis is a poorly characterized condition, which, for lack of a better definition, is considered to be present if the patient has chronic sputum production (productive cough on most days of more than 3 months during 2 successive years) that is not caused by a specific disease such as bronchiectasis or TB.

Morphologic abnormalities in patients with chronic bronchitis include bronchial wall thickening, bronchial smooth muscle hyperplasia, inflammation, mucous gland enlargement, and bronchiolar abnormalities, often referred to as *small airway disease* or *chronic bronchiolitis*. However, specific pathologic criteria for diagnosing chronic bronchitis have proved elusive, and this entity is best thought of as a clinical syndrome without clear-cut anatomic correlates.

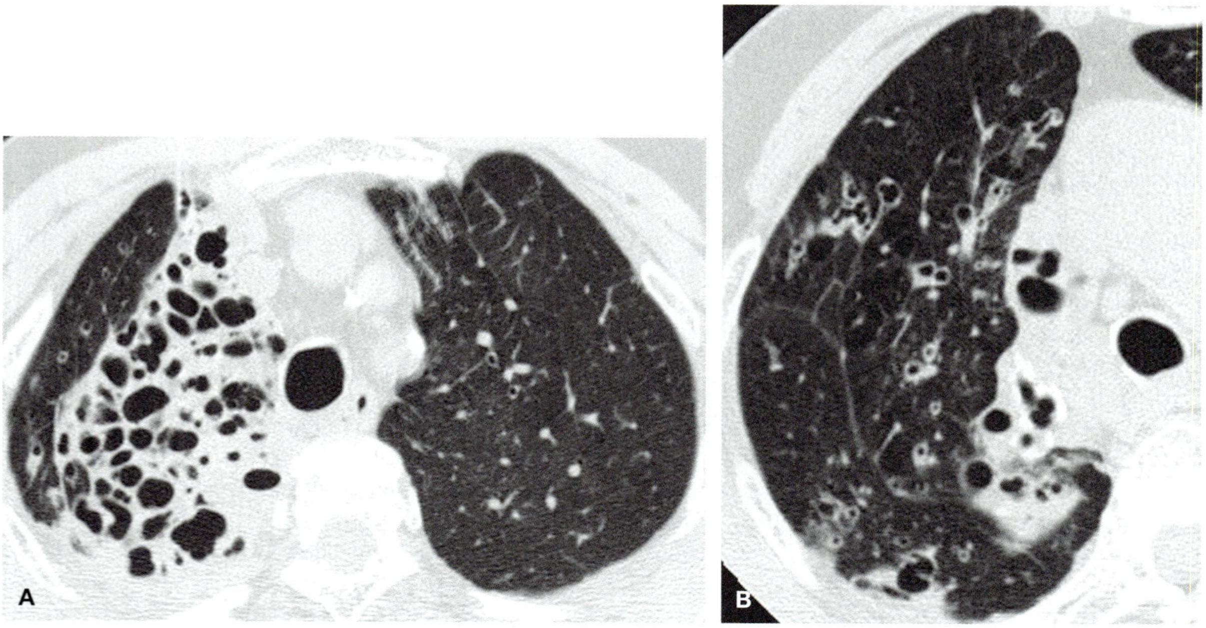

Figure 23.20. Unilateral upper lobe bronchiectasis in tuberculosis. **A:** Right upper lobe bronchiectasis associated with right upper lobe atelectasis is visible on HRCT. The left upper lobe appears normal. **B:** At a lower level, bronchial wall thickening and bronchiectasis are visible.

Chronic bronchitis is largely related to smoking, air pollution, and infection. There is an increased risk in males and in older patients.

Chronic bronchitis does not necessarily result in pulmonary function findings of airflow obstruction, but, because of its common association with chronic bronchiolitis and emphysema, obstructive disease often is present. The occurrence of functional airway obstruction in patients with some combination of chronic bronchitis, chronic bronchiolitis, and emphysema is termed *chronic obstructive pulmonary disease* (COPD). In some patients with chronic bronchitis and COPD, progressive airway obstruction with hypoxemia leads to pulmonary hypertension and cor pulmonale. COPD is discussed in Chapter 24.

Radiographic Findings

Chest radiographs are normal in 40% to 50% of patients considered to have chronic bronchitis. Plain film abnormalities usually are quite subtle and nonspecific, consisting of increased "lung markings," mild bronchial wall thickening, visible as tram tracks or ring shadows, and an overall increase in nonspecific lung markings, sometimes referred to as the "dirty chest." Findings of increased lung volume or hyperlucency usually, but not always, indicate associated emphysema. The presence of "saber-sheath trachea" on a chest radiograph may suggest this diagnosis, although it can be seen with other causes of chronic airway obstruction. Central pulmonary artery enlargement indicative of cor pulmonale may be seen.

CT Findings

On HRCT, findings of emphysema often predominate in patients with symptoms of chronic bronchitis. Some bronchial wall thickening or centrilobular small airway abnormalities, such as tree-in-bud, may be visible on HRCT in patients with clinical findings associated with this entity (Fig. 23.21), but specific HRCT findings usually are lacking. Air trapping may be present on expiratory CT.

CT is generally of more value in excluding causes of chronic sputum production or airflow obstruction, other than chronic bronchitis, such as bronchiectasis or emphysema. The association of emphysema with chronic bronchitis in patients with chronic airflow obstruction (COPD) is discussed in Chapter 24.

BRONCHIOLITIS

Bronchiolitis is a general term used to describe inflammation of the small airways. A number of classifications have been proposed to include the wide spectrum of clinicopathologic conditions associated with bronchiolar inflammation.

Bronchiolitis often is classified by its histologic appearance. However, from a diagnostic standpoint, a radiographic classification is more appropriate and easier to use.

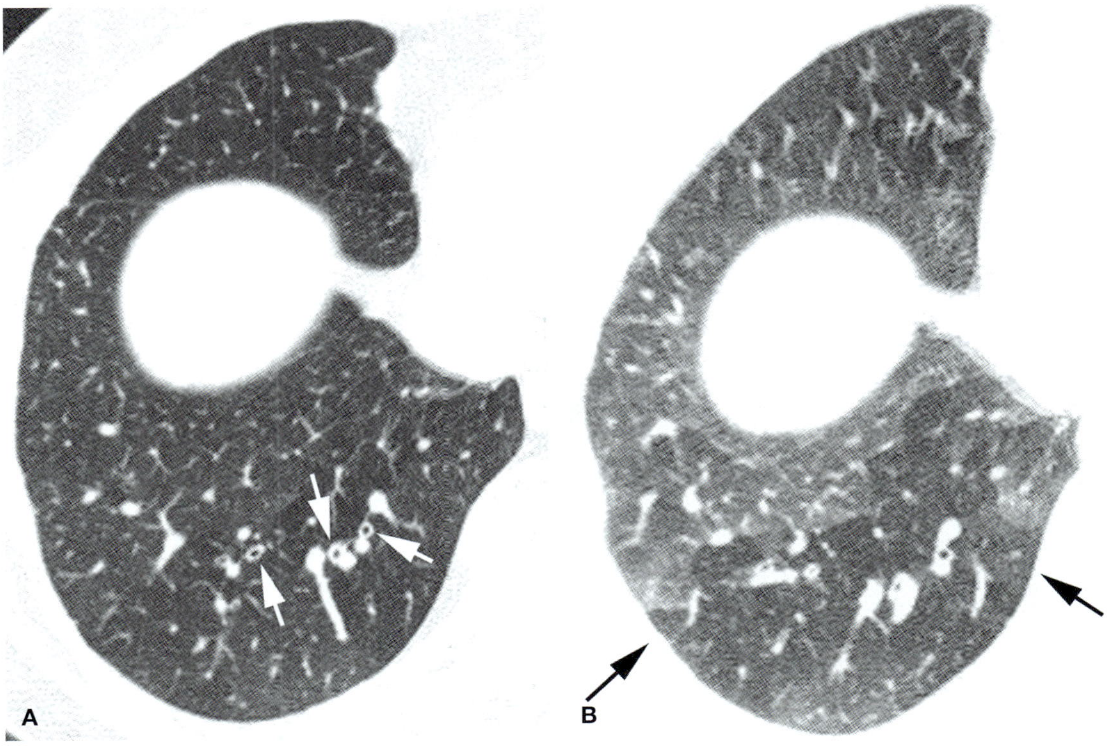

Figure 23.21. HRCT in a patient with symptoms of chronic bronchitis. **A:** Inspiratory scan shows airway wall thickening (*arrows*) in the lower lobe, without evidence of bronchiectasis (ie, bronchial dilatation). **B:** Expiratory scan shows air trapping (*arrows*) in this region.

Histologic Classification of Bronchiolitis

Histologically, bronchiolitis is classified in different ways by different authors, but two entities are recognized consistently (Table 23.7). These include (1) *cellular bronchiolitis* and (2) *CB* or *BO*.

Cellular Bronchiolitis

Cellular bronchiolitis is seen in a diverse group of diseases characterized by inflammation of the bronchiolar wall or bronchiolar lumen, often associated with fibrosis. This classification most commonly includes the following diseases: (1) infectious bronchiolitis (viral, mycoplasma, bacterial, mycobacterial, and fungal), (2) panbronchiolitis, (3) follicular bronchiolitis, (4) bronchiolitis associated with hypersensitivity pneumonitis or other exposures (eg, vaping), (5) bronchiolitis associated with asthma, (6) respiratory bronchiolitis (RB) in smokers, and (7) aspiration.

Constrictive Bronchiolitis (Bronchiolitis Obliterans)

CB (BO) is characterized by the presence of concentric fibrosis involving the submucosal and peribronchial tissues of terminal and respiratory bronchioles, resulting in significant bronchial narrowing or obliteration. It has a variety of causes and is largely irreversible.

Table 23.7 Histologic Classification of Bronchiolar Disease

Cellular bronchiolitis
- Infectious bronchiolitis (viral, mycoplasma, bacteria, mycobacteria, fungus)
- Aspiration bronchiolitis
- Diffuse panbronchiolitis
- Follicular bronchiolitis
  - Primary in lymphoid interstitial pneumonia, collagen disease, immunodeficiency, etc.
  - Secondary in infection
- Hypersensitivity pneumonitis/exposure
- Asthma
- Respiratory bronchiolitis in smokers

Bronchiolitis obliterans (constrictive bronchiolitis)
- Infection (viral, bacterial, mycoplasma)
- Toxic fume inhalation
- Drug treatment
- Collagen vascular disease, particularly rheumatoid arthritis
- Chronic lung transplant rejection
- Bone marrow transplantation with chronic graft-versus-host disease
- Diffuse idiopathic pulmonary neuroendocrine cell hyperplasia
- Idiopathic

Bronchiolitis Syndromes

Infectious Bronchiolitis in Children

Acute bronchiolitis typically is a disease of infants and children less than 3 years of age. It is caused by infection, most often by respiratory syncytial virus or adenovirus, *Mycoplasma pneumoniae*, or *Chlamydia* species. Pathologic examination shows necrosis of the bronchiolar epithelium with a bronchiolar and peribronchiolar inflammatory cell infiltrate and bronchiolar edema. Because of the small size of the bronchioles in young children, significant bronchiolar obstruction often results.

Symptoms include those of upper respiratory tract infection followed by dyspnea, tachypnea, wheezing, and sometimes cyanosis and respiratory failure. Severe symptoms persist for a few days, usually followed by prompt recovery.

Radiographic findings in acute bronchiolitis include hyperinflation, patchy areas of consolidation or atelectasis, streaky perihilar opacities or tram tracks due to bronchial wall or interstitial thickening, and reticular or reticulonodular opacities. HRCT may show mosaic perfusion or air trapping.

Hyperinflation is most specific in making the diagnosis of acute bronchiolitis, but its incidence decreases as the age of the patient increases. Hyperinflation is common in children younger than 2 years and is uncommon in patients older than 5 years. In older patients, findings of patchy consolidation, atelectasis, and reticulonodular opacities predominate.

These abnormalities resolve in nearly all cases, but in a small percentage, bronchiolectasis, BO (CB), and bronchiectasis result. This is most common in patients with adenovirus infection.

Infectious Bronchiolitis in Adults

Infectious bronchiolitis in older children and adults may be associated with a variety of organisms, including those already discussed. Additional organisms that may be responsible include bacteria (eg, *H. influenzae*, *Bordetella pertussis*), atypical mycobacteria such as MAC, TB, and fungi. Infectious bronchiolitis also occurs in association with chronic airway disease such as bronchiectasis, chronic bronchitis and COPD (ie, chronic bronchiolitis), CF, immunodeficiency syndromes including AIDS, or bronchopneumonia.

In adult patients with infectious bronchiolitis, plain radiographs may show evidence of bronchial wall thickening or bronchiectasis, patchy or ill-defined nodular areas of consolidation due to associated bronchopneumonia, and small nodular or reticulonodular opacities. Hyperinflation and air trapping are less common than in young children.

HRCT commonly shows the finding of tree-in-bud (see Figs. 23.9, 23.15, and 23.22; see also Fig. 11.28 in Chapter 11). Tree-in-bud is most typical of bacterial or mycobacterial infections but may sometimes be seen in patients with viral, mycoplasma, or fungal infections. Poorly defined centrilobular nodules or rosettes of nodules are almost always visible in association with tree-in-bud (see Fig. 23.22B); these may represent dilated bronchioles seen in cross-section or nodular areas of peribronchiolar inflammation or pneumonia. Lobular areas of consolidation may accompany the bronchiolar abnormality in patients with "lobular pneumonia" (ie, bronchopneumonia). Bronchial wall thickening or bronchiectasis may be associated.

It is rarely necessary to obtain a biopsy for diagnosis. The presence of tree-in-bud almost always indicates the presence of infection; this finding indicates that "the diagnosis is in the sputum." Viral and mycoplasma infections may result in patchy air trapping in the absence of other findings.

As in children, abnormalities resolve with appropriate treatment in the large majority of patients. As in children, in a small number, bronchiolectasis, BO (CB), and bronchiectasis result.

Aspiration Bronchiolitis

Aspiration bronchiolitis is the consequence of foreign materials in the small airways and may present in acute, chronic, or acute-on-chronic forms. Patients often have risk factors for aspiration (eg, neurologic conditions, oropharyngeal dysphagia, prolonged hospitalization, treated head and neck cancer, prior esophageal or gastric surgery, gastroesophageal reflux disease) and the process may result in a sterile chemical bronchiolitis or infection from aspirated organisms. It is the second most common cause of bronchiolitis behind infection and can be an overlooked clinical diagnosis.

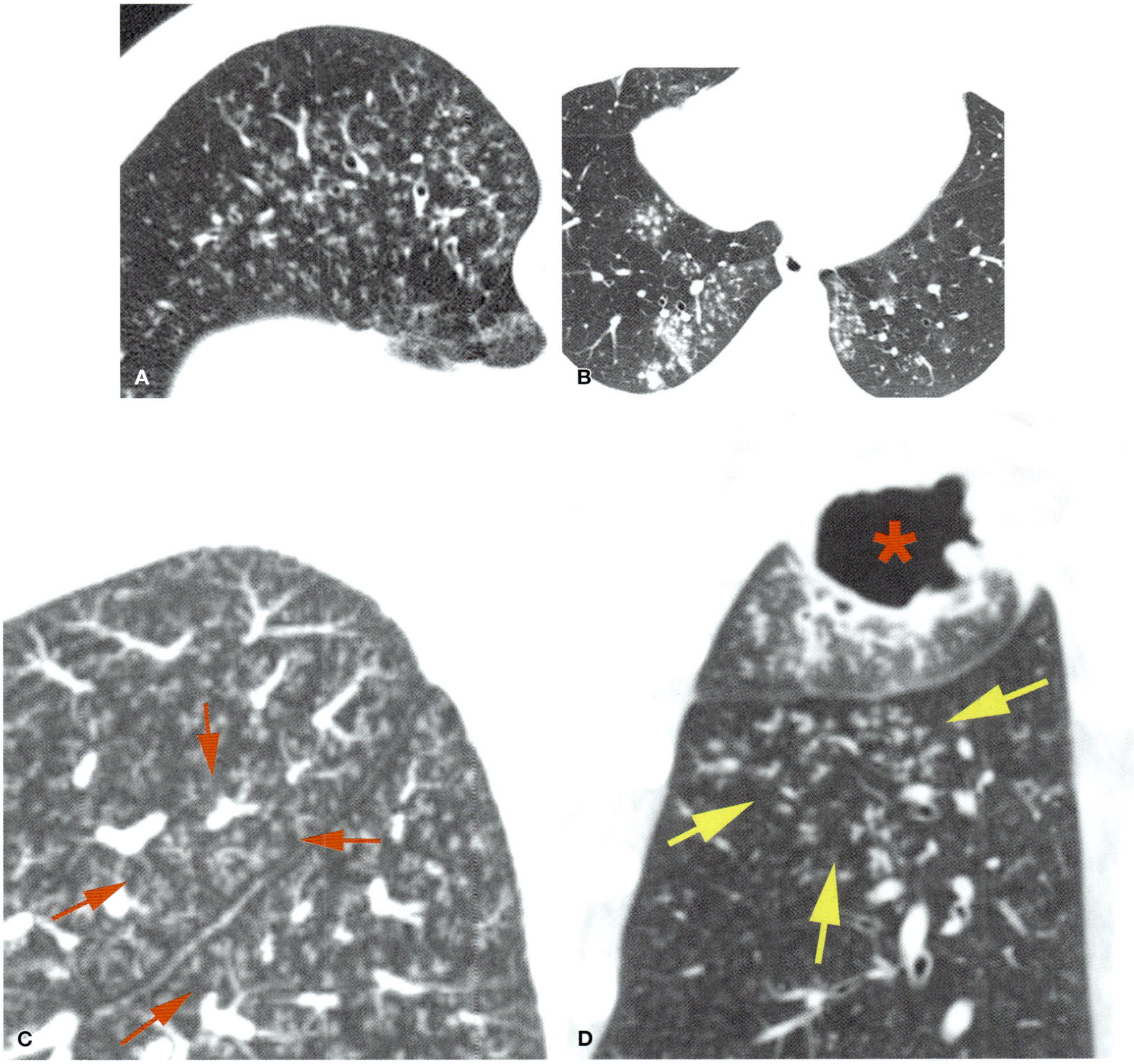

Figure 23.22. Infectious bronchiolitis in four patients. **A:** Detail view of the right left lower lobe from an HRCT in a patient with *Pseudomonas* infection. Many examples of tree-in-bud are visible. **B:** In another patient with bacterial bronchiolitis, ill-defined centrilobular nodules are visible in both lower lobes. **C:** Five-millimeter maximum intensity projection HRCT in an immunosuppressed patient with a viral infection. Extensive tree-in-bud abnormalities are present (*arrows*). **D:** In a patient with cavitary tuberculosis in the right apex (*asterisk*), endobronchial spread of tuberculosis is associated with multiple examples of tree-in-bud (*arrows*).

HRCT findings in the acute setting include tree-in-bud nodules with or without more confluent areas of consolidation that tend to favor the dependent portions of the lungs (Fig. 23.23). Patients may suffer recurrent bouts of aspiration and thus imaging findings may wax and wane. Chronic aspiration may lead to bronchiectasis of the affected lung segments. Ancillary imaging findings such as prior gastric banding, evidence of head and neck cancer treatment, esophageal diverticulum, or hiatal hernia may be clues to the diagnosis of aspiration bronchiolitis.

Diffuse Panbronchiolitis

Diffuse panbronchiolitis (DPB) is a rare disease of unknown etiology that is particularly common in Japan and Eastern Asia but increasingly reported in North America and Europe. It is associated with infection (*H. influenzae*, *P. aeruginosa*, type 1 human T-lymphotropic virus) and genetic susceptibility (including two HLA haplotypes unique to Asians).

DPB typically affects middle-aged patients and is characterized by symptoms of chronic cough, sputum production, and dyspnea. Nearly three quarters of patients have associated sinusitis. The disease is progressive and is marked by frequent episodes of superimposed infection, typically with *P. aeruginosa*. Current therapy requires long-term, low-dose administration of erythromycin. Pulmonary function tests show mild to moderate airflow obstruction. Worsening respiratory failure may occur. In nearly 20% of cases, death occurs within 5 years of the onset of the disease with another 30% of patients dying within 10 years.

Histologically, characteristic findings of DPB include centrilobular, bronchiolar, and peribronchiolar infiltrates of acute and chronic inflammatory cells, associated with bronchiolar dilatation, and intraluminal inflammatory exudates. Lymphoid hyperplasia and accumulations of foamy macrophages are commonly seen. This combination of findings has been referred to as the "unit lesion" of panbronchiolitis and is considered unique to this syndrome. DPB characteristically involves respiratory bronchioles. In a minority of patients, there is also evidence of peripheral bronchiectasis.

Chest radiographs in patients with DPB are nonspecific and usually show small nodular or reticulonodular opacities throughout both lungs and increased lung volumes. Bronchial wall thickening may result in perihilar tram tracks.

HRCT findings in patients with DPB are similar to those of infectious bronchiolitis in adults and include centrilobular tree-in-bud; poorly defined centrilobular nodules; dilated, air-filled, thick-walled centrilobular bronchioles; large lung volumes; and mosaic perfusion or air trapping.

Follicular Bronchiolitis

Follicular bronchiolitis is characterized by a proliferation of lymphoid follicles in the walls of bronchioles and the peribronchiolar interstitium, associated with bronchiolar narrowing. Most commonly, it is an incidental finding in patients with chronic airway disease (eg, bronchiectasis or bronchiolectasis) associated with inflammation or infection. This is termed *secondary follicular bronchiolitis* (Fig. 23.24). In this setting, it often is associated with clinical and radiographic findings of infection (eg, bronchiectasis, tree-in-bud), and its distinction from infectious bronchiolectasis is unnecessary.

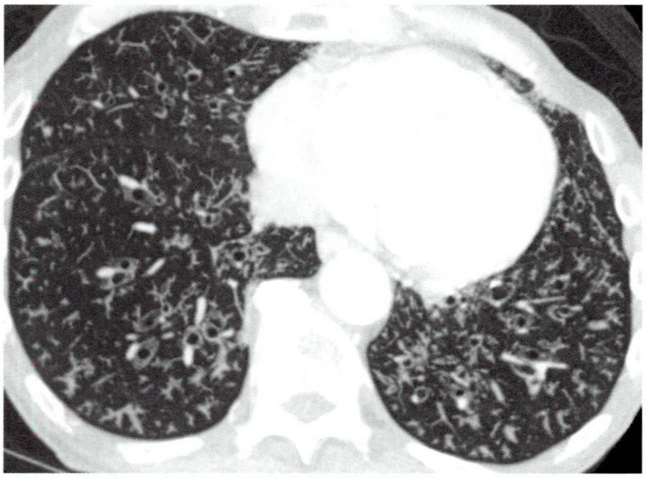

Figure 23.23. Chronic aspiration in a patient with prior head and neck cancer. Axial maximum intensity projection image from a CT shows dependent mucoid impaction, bronchial wall thickening, tree-in-bud nodules, and bronchiectasis from recurrent bouts of acute-on-chronic aspiration. The findings were most severe in the lower lobes and were not present prior to his cancer treatment.

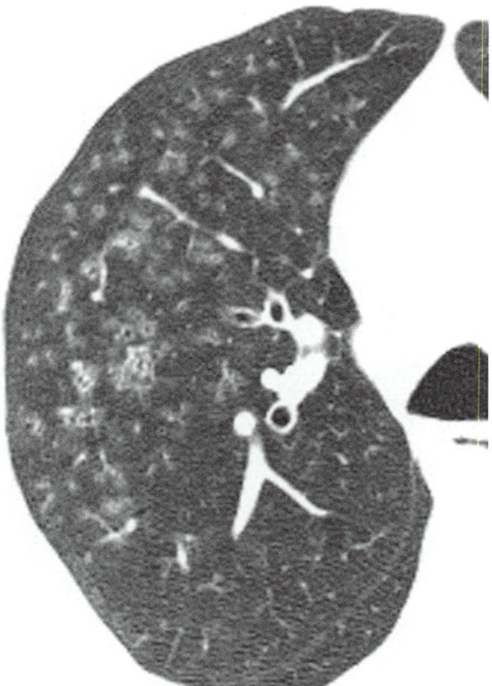

Figure 23.24. Secondary follicular bronchiolitis in a patient with airway infection. HRCT shows ill-defined centrilobular nodules.

Follicular bronchiolitis may also occur in patients with collagen vascular disease such as RA and Sjögren syndrome, immunodeficiency disorders including AIDS, and hypersensitivity reactions. This is termed *primary follicular bronchiolitis*. Primary follicular bronchiolitis is commonly associated with progressive dyspnea, and response to treatment with corticosteroids is variable. In some cases, infection may be associated.

In patients with follicular bronchiolitis, chest radiographs may appear normal or may show a diffuse reticular or reticulonodular pattern. HRCT typically demonstrates tree-in-bud or small nodular opacities in a centrilobular and peribronchovascular distribution. In most cases, these measure 1 to 3 mm in diameter. Larger ill-defined centrilobular or peribronchial nodules of ground-glass opacity may also be seen.

Respiratory Bronchiolitis

RB is part of a spectrum of smoking-related diseases of the airways and lungs, characterized by bronchiolar inflammation, the accumulation of pigmented macrophages within respiratory bronchioles and alveoli, and some degree of fibrosis. This spectrum, in order of increasing severity, includes RB, respiratory bronchiolitis–interstitial lung disease (RB-ILD), and desquamative interstitial pneumonitis (DIP; see Chapter 14).

RB often is an incidental finding on biopsy in asymptomatic smokers. Smokers with RB-ILD have signs and symptoms of diffuse interstitial lung disease and histologically show an exaggerated form of RB, with evidence of more extensive inflammation and fibrosis.

Chest radiographs are normal in most patients with RB or RB-ILD. HRCT may be normal or may show poorly defined centrilobular ground-glass opacities having mid- and upper lung predominance, with or without accompanying larger areas of diffuse ground-glass opacity. Multifocal mosaic perfusion or air trapping may be visible in some patients. Radiographic and HRCT findings in RB, RB-ILD, and DIP are discussed in detail in Chapter 14.

Bronchiolitis Obliterans

BO (CB) is characterized by the presence of concentric fibrosis involving the submucosal and peribronchial tissues of terminal and respiratory bronchioles, resulting in bronchial narrowing or obliteration (Table 23.8). Abnormalities of the large airways such as bronchiectasis may be seen in some cases (see Figs. 11.36 and 11.38 in Chapter 11 and Fig. 15.7 in Chapter 15). Progressive airway obstruction and severe dyspnea, unresponsive to steroid therapy, are typical.

Most commonly, BO results from (1) infection (viral, bacterial, mycoplasma); (2) toxic fume inhalation (eg, nitrogen dioxide or silo-filler's lung, sulfur dioxide, ammonia, chlorine, phosgene, smoke); (3) drug treatment (eg, penicillamine or gold); (4) collagen vascular disease, particularly RA (see Fig. 15.7 in Chapter 15); (5) chronic lung transplant rejection (Fig. 23.25A; see also Fig. 11.38 in Chapter 11); and (6) bone marrow transplantation with chronic GVHD (see Fig. 23.25B). Rarely, it is idiopathic or may be associated with consumption of toxic substances (eg, *Sauropus androgynus*, a plant consumed in Korea) or neuroendocrine hyperplasia. Chest radiographic and CT findings are similar regardless of the cause of BO.

Table 23.8 Bronchiolitis Obliterans (Constrictive Bronchiolitis)

Concentric fibrosis involving terminal and respiratory bronchioles
Bronchiolar obstruction
Variety of causes
Radiographs often nonspecific
Large lung volumes
Increased lucency (60%)
Reduced size of peripheral vessels
Central bronchiectasis (35%)
HRCT findings
Mosaic perfusion, usually patchy in distribution (85%–90%)
Bronchiectasis
Air trapping on expiration, usually patchy in distribution
Air trapping on expiration with normal inspiratory scans
Swyer-James syndrome
Unilateral radiographic abnormalities
Affected lung often reduced in volume

Chest radiographs are normal in one third of cases. Visible abnormalities often are subtle and include hyperinflation, increased lung lucency (60%), peripheral reduction of vascular markings, and findings of central bronchiectasis (35%; see Fig. 11.36 in Chapter 11 and Fig. 15.7 in Chapter 15). Although most patients with BO have bilateral abnormalities, because of the subtle nature of plain film findings in BO, only those with predominantly unilateral disease are easily diagnosed on plain radiographs. This occurrence has been termed the *Swyer-James syndrome* (SJS) (see Fig. 23.26).

HRCT is more sensitive than chest radiographs in detecting abnormalities in patients with BO. In 85% to 90% of cases, HRCT shows focal or multifocal, sharply defined areas of decreased lung attenuation associated with vessels of decreased caliber (ie, *mosaic perfusion*) (see Fig. 23.25; see also Fig. 11.36 in Chapter 11). These areas may be lobar or segmental or may involve individual pulmonary lobules. *Air trapping* is typically visible on expiratory HRCT in areas of lucency (Fig. 23.25; see also Fig. 11.38 in Chapter 11). In some patients with BO, the presence of air trapping on expiratory scans may be the only abnormal HRCT finding. *Bronchiectasis*, both central and peripheral, may be present as well and, when visible, usually occurs in lucent lung regions. Rarely, tree-in-bud or ill-defined centrilobular opacities may be the predominant finding, but recognizable small airway abnormalities usually are inconspicuous in patients with BO.

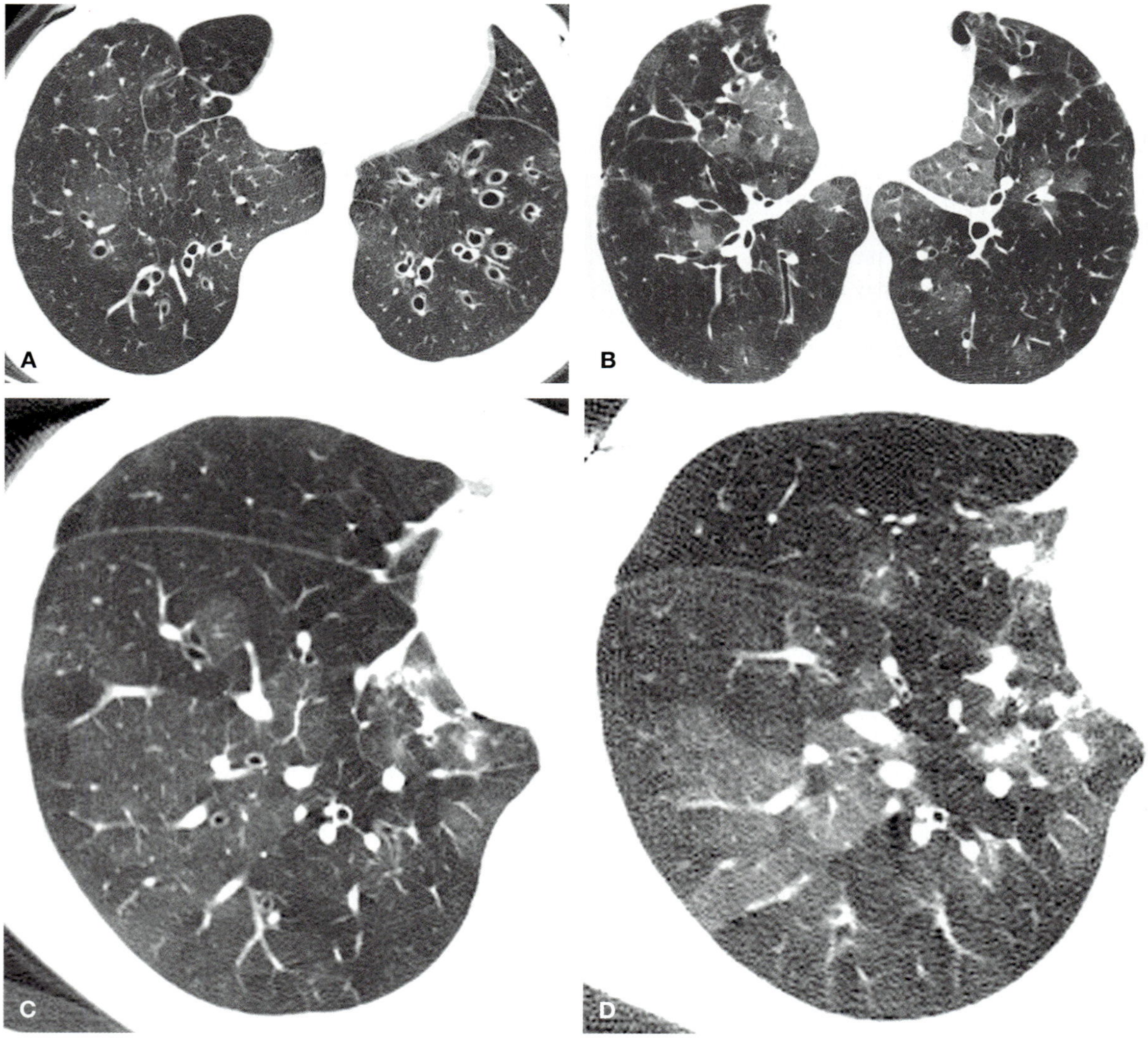

Figure 23.25. Mosaic perfusion and bronchiectasis in two patients with bronchiolitis obliterans. **A:** A patient with chronic lung transplant rejection shows bronchiectasis and mosaic perfusion on HRCT. **B:** In a patient with graft-versus-host disease following bone marrow transplantation, inhomogeneous lung attenuation represents mosaic perfusion. Note the decreased vessel size in lucent lung regions. Mosaic perfusion and air trapping in a patient with bronchiolitis obliterans resulting from smoke inhalation. **C:** Inspiratory HRCT shows subtle mosaic perfusion. There is no evidence of bronchiectasis. **D:** Dynamic expiratory scan shows air trapping indicative of bronchiolitis obliterans.

Swyer-James Syndrome

The SJS (also known as Swyer-James-McLeod syndrome, unilateral emphysema, unilateral lobar emphysema, and unilateral hyperlucent lung) is characterized by predominantly unilateral radiographic findings of BO (Fig. 23.26). It is commonly the result of lower respiratory tract infection, usually in childhood, and due to viral infection, *Mycoplasma* organisms, *B. pertussis*, or TB. Damage to the terminal and respiratory bronchioles leads to incomplete development of alveoli.

SJS was described in the 1950s and has received undeserved attention as a specific entity; its designation reflects the fact that BO was only diagnosable on chest radiographs when it was predominantly unilateral. On CT, BO is usually bilateral; unilateral or predominantly unilateral disease is uncommon. Nonetheless, SJS serves to illustrate the typical plain film features of BO, characterized radiographically by hyperlucency of a lung, lobe, or segment, associated with decreased size of associated pulmonary arteries.

In classic, radiographically diagnosed SJS, (1) the affected lung is decreased in volume because of abnormal development during childhood but may be normal or increased in volume, (2) the ipsilateral pulmonary artery or artery branches are decreased in size, and (3) bronchiectasis may be present. Air trapping is visible on expiratory radiographs. Patients usually are asymptomatic, and the abnormality is detected incidentally. However, dyspnea or recurrent

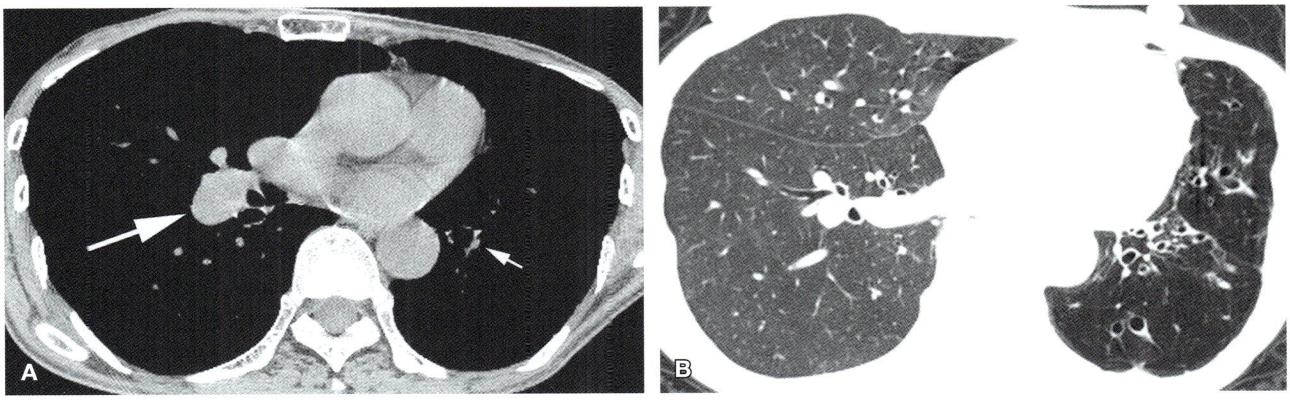

Figure 23.26. HRCT appearance of the Swyer-James syndrome. **A:** CT shows the left pulmonary artery (*small arrow*) to be much smaller than the right (*large arrow*). **B:** The left lung is small and hyperlucent with decreased vessel size. Bronchiectasis also is present, a common finding with bronchiolitis obliterans.

infections may be associated. Ventilation-perfusion scans show matched defects.

CT CLASSIFICATION OF BRONCHIOLITIS

Chest radiographs in patients with bronchiolitis usually appear normal or show nonspecific abnormalities, including ground-glass opacity, poor definition of pulmonary vessels, or ill-defined reticular or nodular opacities. Large lung volumes may be seen, due to air trapping, particularly in patients with BO. Large airway abnormalities such as bronchiectasis may be associated in some cases.

CT and HRCT are of great value in assessing bronchiolar disease (Table 23.9). Direct HRCT signs of bronchiolar disease result from the presence of bronchiolar dilatation, bronchiolar impaction, bronchiolar wall thickening, or peribronchiolar inflammation. The most important indirect signs of bronchiolar disease are mosaic perfusion on inspiratory scans and air trapping on expiratory scans.

Based on the primary HRCT findings present, bronchiolitis may be classified in one of three groups, an approach that is more practical from a diagnostic standpoint than a histologic classification:

1. Bronchiolar disease associated with tree-in-bud
2. Bronchiolar disease associated with centrilobular nodules
3. Bronchiolar disease associated with mosaic perfusion

Bronchiolar Diseases Associated With Tree-In-Bud

The HRCT finding of tree-in-bud is characterized by the presence of centrilobular, branching, or Y-shaped opacities that resemble a budding tree, usually best seen in the lung periphery. A tree-in-bud appearance is most typical of cellular bronchiolitis and in clinical practice almost always (90%) is the result of acute or chronic infection (eg, infectious bronchiolitis, CF, bronchopneumonia, tuberculosis, MAC) or

Table 23.9 Radiographic (HRCT) Classification of Bronchiolar Disease

Bronchiolar diseases with tree-in-bud (TIB)
Typical of cellular bronchiolitis
Usually due to infection
Mycobacterium tuberculosis
Atypical mycobacterial infections (*Mycobacterium avium-intracellulare*)
Bacterial infections (eg, cystic fibrosis; immunosuppressed patients)
Fungal infections (eg, airway-invasive *Aspergillus*)
Viral or mycoplasma infection
Asian panbronchiolitis
Other causes
Aspiration
Follicular bronchiolitis (collagen vascular disease or lymphoid interstitial pneumonitis)
Asthma
Allergic bronchopulmonary aspergillosis
Endobronchial spread of tumor
Bronchiolar diseases with poorly defined centrilobular (CL) nodules
Hypersensitivity pneumonitis
Infectious bronchiolitis (viral, *Pneumocystis carinii* pneumonia)
Respiratory bronchiolitis
Follicular bronchiolitis and lymphoid interstitial pneumonia
Bronchiolar disease associated with decreased lung attenuation
Causes of bronchiolitis with TIB or CL nodules
No associated TIB or CL nodules
Bronchiolitis obliterans (constrictive bronchiolitis)
Hypersensitivity pneumonitis
Respiratory bronchiolitis
Asthma

aspiration. Bacterial and mycobacterial infections are most common in patients with tree-in-bud, but this finding also may be seen with viral, mycoplasma, and fungal infections.

Occasionally, tree-in-bud occurs without infection in patients with asthma, ABPA, BO, follicular bronchiolitis, and endobronchial spread of mucinous adenocarcinoma. Mosaic perfusion on inspiratory scans and air trapping on expiratory scan may be present. Abnormalities of the large airways (eg, bronchiectasis or bronchial wall thickening) also may be seen. Regardless of the associated abnormalities, only a few good examples of tree-in-bud need to be seen in a patient to characterize this pattern.

Mimics of tree-in-bud are uncommon but include intravascular metastasis, vasculitis associated with talcosis in intravenous drug users, and diseases, such as sarcoidosis, which result in centrilobular perilymphatic nodules.

Bronchiolar Diseases Associated With Poorly Defined Centrilobular Nodules

The hallmark of bronchiolar diseases associated with this pattern is the finding of ill-defined centrilobular nodules without associated tree-in-bud. This finding usually results from peribronchiolar inflammation or fibrosis and is associated with a wide range of pathologic entities including cellular bronchiolitis in hypersensitivity pneumonitis, infectious bronchiolitis (particularly in association with viral and *Pneumocystis* pneumonia), RB and RB-ILD, exposures, and lymphoid interstitial pneumonia and follicular bronchiolitis. Despite the large number of diseases included in this category, in most cases, the differential diagnosis is simplified by clinical correlation, including occupational and environmental exposure histories.

Bronchiolar Diseases Associated With Mosaic Perfusion

Bronchiolar diseases associated with mosaic perfusion as a predominant abnormality include BO or cellular bronchiolitis in hypersensitivity pneumonia, RB, and asthma. In patients with cellular bronchiolitis, it may be associated with other findings such as tree-in-bud or centrilobular nodules.

SUGGESTED READING

Agarwal R, Gupta D, Aggarwal AN, Saxena AK, Chakrabarti A, Jindal SK. Clinical significance of hyperattenuating mucoid impaction in allergic bronchopulmonary aspergillosis—an analysis of 155 patients. *Chest.* 2007;132(4):1183-1190.

Akira M, Kitatani F, Lee Y-S, et al. Diffuse panbronchiolitis: evaluation with high-resolution CT. *Radiology.* 1988;168(2):433-438.

Aquino SL, Gamsu G, Webb WR, Kee ST. Tree-in-bud pattern: frequency and significance on thin section CT. *J Comput Assist Tomogr.* 1996;20(4):594-599.

Arakawa H, Webb WR. Air trapping on expiratory high-resolution CT scans in the absence of inspiratory scan abnormalities: correlation with pulmonary function tests and differential diagnosis. *AJR Am J Roentgenol.* 1998;170(5):1349-1353.

Berniker AV, Henry TS. Imaging of small airways diseases. *Radiol Clin North Am.* 2016;54(6):1165-1181. doi:10.1016/j.rcl.2016.05.009

Cartier Y, Kavanagh PV, Johkoh T, Mason AC, Müller NL. Bronchiectasis: accuracy of high-resolution CT in the differentiation of specific diseases. *AJR Am J Roentgenol.* 1999;173(1):47-52.

Chang AB, Masel JP, Masters B. Post-infectious bronchiolitis obliterans: clinical, radiological and pulmonary function sequelae. *Pediatr Radiol.* 1998;28(1):23-29.

Cohen M, Sahn SA. Bronchiectasis in systemic diseases. *Chest.* 1999;116(4):1063-1074.

Dodd JD, Souza CA, Muller NL. Conventional high-resolution CT versus helical high-resolution MDCT in the detection of bronchiectasis. *AJR Am J Roentgenol.* 2006;187(2):414-420.

Friedman PJ. Chest radiographic findings in the adult with cystic fibrosis. *Semin Roentgenol.* 1987;22(2):114-124.

Garg K, Lynch DA, Newell JD, King TE. Proliferative and constrictive bronchiolitis: classification and radiologic features. *AJR Am J Roentgenol.* 1994;162(4):803-808.

Gosink BB, Friedman PJ, Liebow AA. Bronchiolitis obliterans: roentgenographic-pathologic correlation. *AJR Am J Roentgenol.* 1973;117(4):816-832.

Gruden JF, Webb WR, Warnock M. Centrilobular opacities in the lung on high-resolution CT: diagnostic considerations and pathologic correlation. *AJR Am J Roentgenol.* 1994;162(3):569-574.

Helbich TH, Heinz-Peer G, Eichler I, et al. Cystic fibrosis: CT assessment of lung involvement in children and adults. *Radiology.* 1999;213(2):537-544.

Henry TS, Hammer MM, Little BP, et al. Smoke: how to differentiate flow-related artifacts from pathology on thoracic computed tomographic angiography. *J Thorac Imaging.* 2019;34(5):W109-W120. doi:10.1097/RTI.0000000000000429

Howling SJ, Hansell DM, Wells AU, Nicholson AG, Flint JD, Müller NL. Follicular bronchiolitis: thin-section CT and histologic findings. *Radiology.* 1999;212(3):637-642.

Jeong YJ, Lee KS, Koh WJ, Han J, Kim TS, Kwon OJ. Nontuberculous mycobacterial pulmonary infection in immunocompetent patients: comparison of thin-section CT and histopathologic findings. *Radiology.* 2004;231(3):880-886.

Kang EY, Miller RR, Müller NL. Bronchiectasis: comparison of preoperative thin-section CT and pathologic findings in resected specimens. *Radiology.* 1995;195(3):649-654.

King TE. Overview of bronchiolitis. *Clin Chest Med.* 1993;14(4):607-610.

Kligerman SJ, Henry T, Lin CT, Franks TJ, Galvin JR. Mosaic attenuation: etiology, methods of differentiation, and pitfalls. *Radiographics.* 2015;35(5):1360-1380.

Lynch DA, Newell JD, Tschomper BA, Cink TM, Newman LS, Bethel R. Uncomplicated asthma in adults: comparison of CT appearance of the lungs in asthmatic and healthy subjects. *Radiology.* 1993;188(3):829-833.

Lynch DA, Austin JHM, Hogg JC, et al. CT-definable subtypes of chronic obstructive pulmonary disease: a statement of the Fleischner Society. *Radiology.* 2015;277(1):192-205.

Lynch DA. Imaging of small airways diseases. *Clin Chest Med.* 1993;14(4):623-634.

Lynch DA. Imaging of small airways disease and chronic obstructive pulmonary disease. *Clin Chest Med.* 2008;29(1):165-179.

Marquis KM, Raptis CA, Rajput MZ, et al. CT for evaluation of hemoptysis. *Radiographics.* 2021;41(3):742-761. doi:10.1148/rg.2021200150

Martinez S, McAdams HP, Batchu CS. The many faces of pulmonary nontuberculous mycobacterial infection. *AJR Am J Roentgenol.* 2007;189(1):177-186.

McGuinness G, Naidich DP, Leitman BS, McCauley DI. Bronchiectasis: CT evaluation. *AJR Am J Roentgenol.* 1993;160(2):253-259.

Milliron B, Henry TS, Veeraraghavan S, Little BP. Bronchiectasis: mechanisms and imaging clues of associated common and uncommon diseases. *Radiographics.* 2015;35(4):1011-1030.

Müller NL, Miller RR. Diseases of the bronchioles: CT and histopathologic findings. *Radiology.* 1995;196(1):3-12.

Naidich DP, McCauley DI, Khouri NF, Stitik FP, Siegelman SS. Computed tomography of bronchiectasis. *J Comput Assist Tomogr.* 1982;6(3):437-444.

Nishimura K, Kitaichi M, Izumi T, Itoh H. Diffuse panbronchiolitis: correlation of high-resolution CT and pathologic findings. *Radiology.* 1992;184(3):779-785.

Okada F, Ando Y, Yoshitake S, et al. Clinical/pathologic correlations in 553 patients with primary centrilobular findings on high-resolution CT scan of the thorax. *Chest.* 2007;132(6):1939-1948.

Padley SPG, Adler BD, Hansell DM, Müller NL. Bronchiolitis obliterans: high-resolution CT findings and correlation with pulmonary function tests. *Clin Radiol.* 1993;47(4):236-240.

Park CS, Müller NL, Worthy SA, Kim JS, Awadh N, Fitzgerald M. Airway obstruction in asthmatic and healthy individuals: inspiratory and expiratory thin-section CT findings. *Radiology*. 1997;203(2):361-367.

Rossi SE, Franquet T, Volpacchio M, Giménez A, Aguilar G. Tree-in-bud pattern at thin-section CT of the lungs: radiologic-pathologic overview. *Radiographics*. 2005;25(3):789-801.

Shah RM, Sexauer W, Ostrum BJ, Fiel SB, Friedman AC. High-resolution CT in the acute exacerbation of cystic fibrosis: evaluation of acute findings, reversibility of those findings, and clinical correlation. *AJR Am J Roentgenol*. 1997;169(2):375-380.

Shoemark A, Ozerovitch L, Wilson R. Aetiology in adult patients with bronchiectasis. *Respir Med*. 2007;101(6):1163-1170.

Ward S, Heyneman L, Lee MJ, Leung AN, Hansell DM, Müller NL. Accuracy of CT in the diagnosis of allergic bronchopulmonary aspergillosis in asthmatic patients. *AJR Am J Roentgenol*. 1999;173(4):937-942.

Winningham PJ, Martínez-Jiménez S, Rosado-de-Christenson ML, Betancourt SL, Restrepo CS, Eraso A. Bronchiolitis: a practical approach for the general radiologist. *Radiographics*. 2017;37(3):777-794. doi:10.1148/rg.2017160131

Wood BP. Cystic fibrosis: 1997. *Radiology*. 1997;204:1-10.

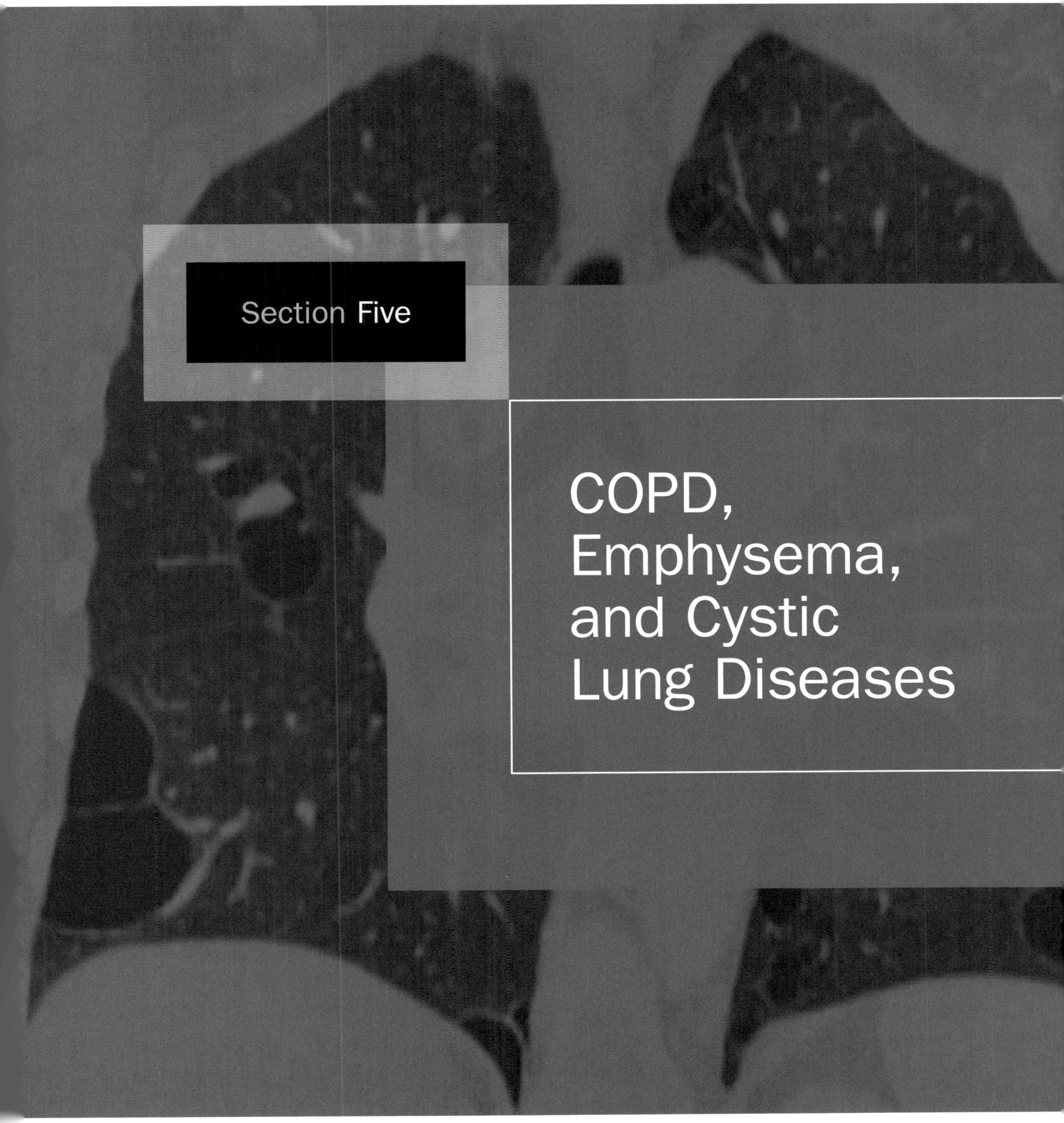

Section Five

COPD, Emphysema, and Cystic Lung Diseases

Chapter 24

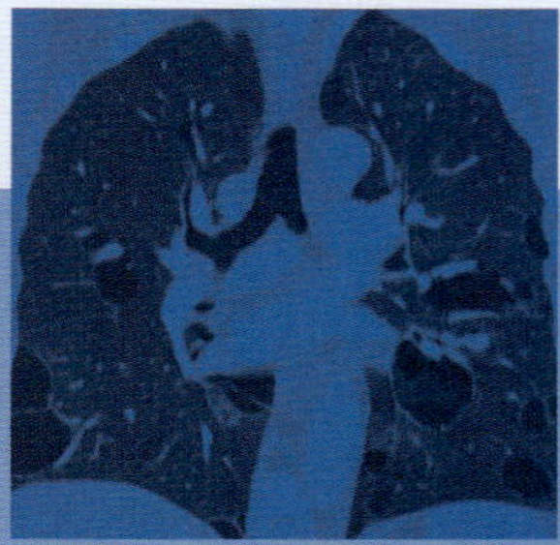

Travis S. Henry

Chronic Obstructive Pulmonary Disease and Emphysema

EMPHYSEMA

As defined by the American Thoracic Society, emphysema is "a condition of the lung characterized by permanent, abnormal enlargement of airspaces distal to the terminal bronchiole, accompanied by the destruction of their walls," but "without obvious fibrosis." Currently, it is estimated that at least 2 million people in the United States suffer from emphysema. It is a significant cause of morbidity and mortality.

PATHOGENESIS OF EMPHYSEMA

It is generally accepted that emphysema results from an imbalance in the dynamic relationship between elastolytic and antielastolytic factors in the lung, usually related to cigarette smoking or enzymatic deficiency. Abnormal or unopposed elastase activity is thought to lead to the tissue destruction that is the primary pathologic abnormality present in patients with this disease.

The proposed mechanisms in the development of emphysema in smokers are as follows:

1. Inhaled tobacco smoke attracts macrophages to distal airways and alveoli (referred to as respiratory bronchiolitis).
2. Macrophages, along with airway epithelial cells, release chemotactic substances that attract neutrophils and induce them to release elastases and other proteolytic enzymes. Macrophages also release proteases in response to tobacco smoke.
3. These elastases have the ability to cleave a variety of proteins, including collagen and elastin. Lung elastin normally is protected from excessive elastase-induced damage by alpha-1-protease inhibitors (alpha-1-antiprotease or alpha-1-antitrypsin) and other circulating antiproteinases.
4. Tobacco smoke tends to interfere with the function of alpha-1-antiprotease.
5. In combination, these interactions result in structural damage in the distal airways and alveoli, leading to emphysema.

Inherited deficiency in alpha-1-antiprotease similarly results in lung destruction and emphysema when neutrophils release elastases and other proteolytic enzymes in response to pulmonary infection.

CLASSIFICATION OF EMPHYSEMA

Emphysema is classified into three types, based on the anatomic distribution of the areas of lung destruction, recently described by the Fleischner Society as (1) *centrilobular emphysema* (*CLE*), also termed proximal acinar or centriacinar emphysema; (2) *panlobular emphysema,* also termed panacinar emphysema; and (3) *paraseptal emphysema,* also termed distal acinar emphysema. The terms *centrilobular, panlobular*, and *paraseptal* are generally accepted and are used to describe these three types of emphysema in the remainder of this chapter. In their early stages, these three forms of emphysema can be easily distinguished morphologically. However, as the emphysema becomes more severe, distinguishing among the types becomes more difficult. *Bullous emphysema* is a nonspecific term used to describe emphysema with a predominant bullous component.

Centrilobular Emphysema

CLE predominantly affects the respiratory bronchioles in the central portions of acini and therefore involves the central portion of secondary lobules. It usually results from cigarette smoking and involves mainly the upper lung zones.

Panlobular Emphysema

Panlobular emphysema involves all the components of the acinus more or less uniformly and therefore involves entire secondary lobules. It is classically associated with alpha-1-protease inhibitor (alpha-1-antitrypsin) deficiency, although it also may be seen without protease deficiency in smokers with confluent CLE, in elderly subjects, distal to bronchial and bronchiolar obliteration, and associated with illicit drug injection (eg, Ritalin lung).

Paraseptal Emphysema

Paraseptal emphysema predominantly involves the alveolar ducts and sacs in the lung periphery, with areas of destruction often marginated by interlobular septa. It can be an isolated phenomenon in young adults, often associated with spontaneous pneumothorax, or can be seen in older patients with CLE. In the recent Fleischner Society description of chronic obstructive pulmonary disease (COPD) subtypes, paraseptal emphysema is classified as mild or substantial, depending on the presence of predominant small (≤1 cm) or large (>1 cm) subpleural lucencies.

Bullae and Bullous Emphysema

Bullae can develop in association with any type of emphysema, but they are most common with paraseptal emphysema or CLE. A *bulla* is a sharply demarcated area of emphysema measuring 1 cm or more in diameter and possessing a wall less than 1 mm in thickness. In some patients with emphysema, bullae can become quite large, resulting in significant compromise of respiratory function; this syndrome is sometimes referred to as *bullous emphysema*. Bullae are most common in a subpleural location, representing foci of paraseptal emphysema associated with air trapping and progressive enlargement.

Irregular Air-Space Enlargement

Irregular air-space enlargement is an additional type of emphysema that occurs in patients with pulmonary fibrosis; this form of emphysema also is referred to as *paracicatricial* or *irregular emphysema*. It commonly is found adjacent to localized parenchymal scars, to diffuse pulmonary fibrosis, and in the pneumoconioses, particularly those pneumoconioses associated with progressive massive fibrosis.

CHRONIC OBSTRUCTIVE PULMONARY DISEASE

The term COPD is currently defined on the basis of pulmonary function test findings of airway obstruction and is characterized by airflow limitation "that is not fully reversible." COPD is a catchall term, which embraces several distinct disease processes, including emphysema, chronic bronchitis, and reversible or (partially) irreversible small airway obstruction. The airflow limitation in COPD, usually associated with cigarette smoking, is typically related to a combination of small airway obstruction and emphysema.

Respiratory symptoms in patients with COPD usually include chronic cough, sputum production, and dyspnea. Although cough and sputum production are largely manifestations of chronic bronchitis in patients with COPD, the relative contributions of airway disease and emphysema to respiratory disability often are difficult to determine. However, therapeutic options for patients with COPD vary considerably depending on whether emphysema or airway abnormalities predominate. The Global Obstructive Lung Disease (GOLD) system has been widely used to identify and classify the severity of airflow limitation in COPD, with GOLD stage I referring to subjects with a ratio of forced expiratory volume in 1 second (FEV_1) to forced vital capacity (FVC) of less than 0.7 but with preserved FEV_1 and GOLD stages II, III, and IV when the FEV_1/FVC ratio is less than 0.7 and FEV_1 is less than 80%, 50%, and 30% of predicted, respectively. Individuals with COPD and identical GOLD stages may have very different pathophysiologic abnormalities, reflected by differing morphologic appearances at computed tomography (CT). Some patients have emphysema, while other patients with similar functional impairment have an airway-dominant abnormality with little or no emphysema being present. These morphologic differences may reflect important differences in the underlying pathophysiology and genomic profile of COPD, although this remains to be determined. Patients with COPD may have markedly varying plain radiographic or CT findings, with emphysema or airway disease being the primary manifestation or with both being present.

Using CT, morphologic abnormalities, such as emphysema, bronchial wall thickening, increased lung volume, and expiratory air trapping, may be assessed and quantitated. Thus, CT has been used to differentiate between airway-predominant and emphysema-predominant COPD in recent research.

The differing appearances of CT abnormalities in patients with COPD have been termed *COPD phenotypes*. These phenotypes are (a) *emphysema-predominant COPD*, (b) *airway-predominant COPD*, and (c) *mixed*.

DIAGNOSIS OF EMPHYSEMA IN COPD

In patients with emphysema, pulmonary function tests usually show findings of chronic airflow obstruction and reduced diffusing capacity. Airflow obstruction in patients with emphysema is due to airway collapse on expiration, resulting largely from destruction of lung parenchyma and loss of airway tethering and support. Abnormal diffusing capacity is due to destruction of the lung parenchyma and the pulmonary capillary bed.

Radiographic Findings

Radiographic abnormalities in patients with COPD are largely the same as those of emphysema. These include (1) increased lung volume and (2) lung destruction (bullae or reduced vascularity). When both findings are used as criteria for diagnosis, a sensitivity as high as 80% has been reported for chest radiographs, although the likelihood of a positive diagnosis depends on the severity of disease. When only findings of lung destruction are used for diagnosis, radiographs are only about 40% sensitive.

Although the accuracy of chest radiographs in diagnosing emphysema is controversial, it can be reasonably concluded from the studies performed that moderate to severe emphysema can be diagnosed radiographically, whereas mild emphysema is difficult to detect.

The presence of increased lung volume, or overinflation, is important in making the diagnosis of emphysema on plain radiographs. However, overinflation is an indirect sign of this disease, and findings of increased lung volume are nonspecific. Such findings can be absent in some patients with emphysema but present in patients who have other forms of obstructive pulmonary disease.

Plain radiographic findings of overinflation (Figs. 24.1 and 24.2; Table 24.1) include the following:

1. Lung height of 29.9 cm or more, measured from the dome of the right diaphragm to the tubercle of the first rib
2. Flattening of the right hemidiaphragm on the lateral projection, with a height of less than 2.7 cm measured perpendicular to a line drawn from the anterior to posterior costophrenic angles
3. Flattening of the right hemidiaphragm on a posteroanterior (PA) radiograph, with the highest level of the dome of the right hemidiaphragm being less than 1.5 cm measured perpendicular to a line drawn between the costophrenic angle laterally and the vertebrophrenic angle medially
4. Increased retrosternal airspace, measuring more than 4.4 cm at a level 3 cm below the manubrial-sternal junction
5. Right hemidiaphragm at or below the level of the anterior end of the seventh rib
6. Sternodiaphragmatic angle measuring 90° or more

Blunting of the costophrenic angles or visible diaphragmatic slips (ie, attachments of the diaphragm to the ribs) on the PA view are common findings in markedly increased lung volume; inversion of the hemidiaphragms may be seen on the lateral view (Fig. 24.2).

The presence of bullae on chest radiographs is the only specific sign of lung destruction caused by emphysema and usually means that paraseptal or severe CLE is present (Fig. 24.3). However, this finding is uncommon and may not reflect the presence of generalized disease. Bullae usually are visible in the lung periphery, have thin walls, and appear

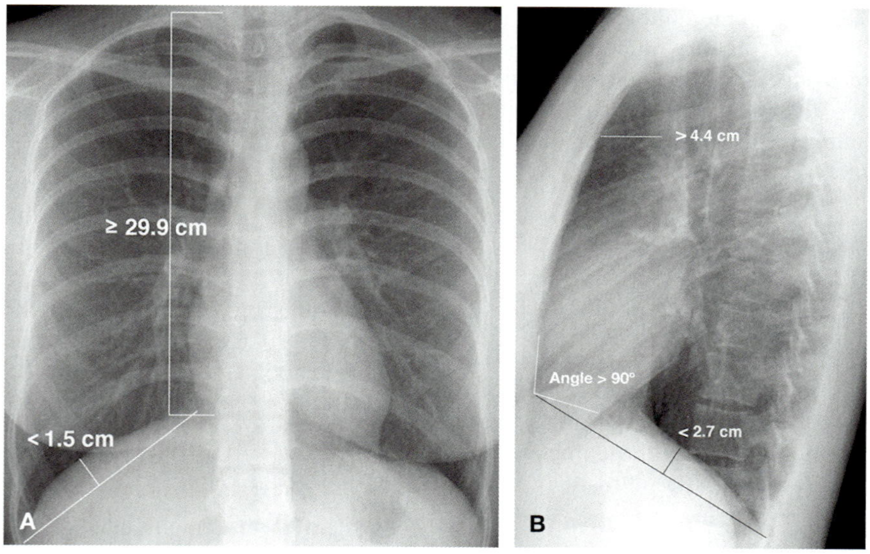

Figure 24.1. Plain film measurements in emphysema. **A:** Plain radiographic findings of emphysema on the PA radiograph include a lung height of 29.9 cm or more, measured from the dome of the right diaphragm to the tubercle of the first rib and flattening of the right hemidiaphragm on a PA radiograph, with the highest level of the dome of the right hemidiaphragm less than 1.5 cm above a perpendicular line drawn between the costophrenic angle laterally and the vertebrophrenic angle medially. **B:** Findings of emphysema on the lateral radiograph include flattening of the right hemidiaphragm, with a height of less than 2.7 cm measured from anterior to posterior costophrenic angles; an increased retrosternal airspace, measuring more than 4.4 cm at a level 3 cm below the manubriosternal junction; and a sternodiaphragmatic angle measuring 90° or more.

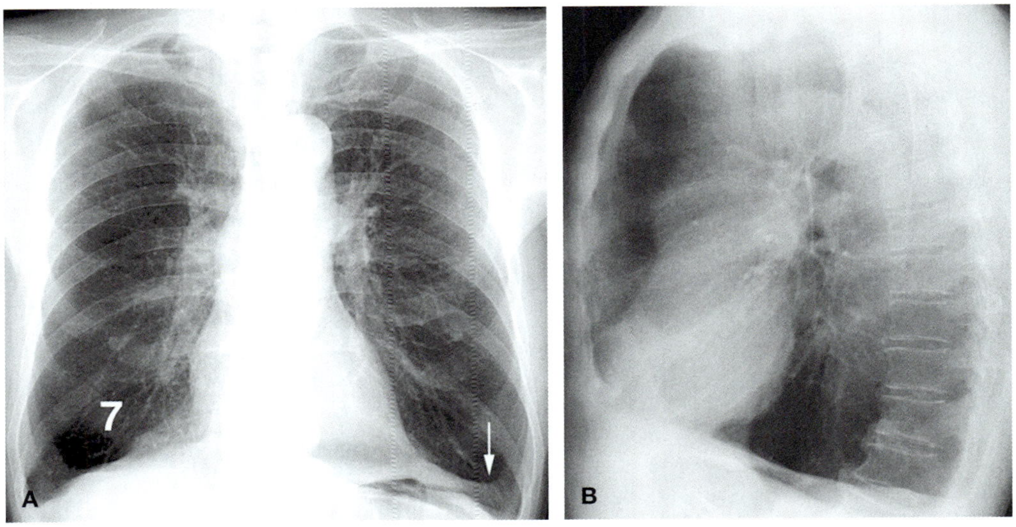

Figure 24.2. Chest radiographs in emphysema. **A:** PA radiograph shows increased lung height with flattening of the diaphragm. The dome of the right hemidiaphragm is below the level of the anterior right seventh rib (7). Blunting of the costophrenic angles is common in increased lung volumes, as are visible diaphragmatic slips (*arrow*) extending to the chest wall. The lungs appear lucent, and vessel size is reduced. Mild prominence of the hila likely reflects pulmonary hypertension. **B:** The lateral view shows increased depth and lucency of the retrosternal space. The diaphragms are flattened and appear inverted (ie, their normal curvature is reversed).

lucent, and lung markings are not seen within them. Lung lucency may reflect the presence of bullae when they are not visible as discrete structures.

A reduction in the size of pulmonary vessels or vessel tapering in the lung periphery also can reflect lung destruction in patients with emphysema (see Fig. 24.2), but this finding lacks sensitivity and can be unreliable. Focal absence or displacement of vessels may reflect the presence of bullae (see Fig. 24.3).

Table 24.1 Radiographic Findings in Emphysema

Increased lung volume
PA view
≥29.9 cm from the dome of the right diaphragm to the first rib
Flattening of the right hemidiaphragm with a height <1.5 cm
Right hemidiaphragm at or below the level of the anterior 7th rib
Blunting of the lateral costophrenic angles
Visible diaphragmatic slips
Lateral view
Flattening of the right hemidiaphragm with a height of <2.7 cm
Increased retrosternal airspace, measuring >4.4 cm
Sternodiaphragmatic angle measuring 90° or more
Blunting of the posterior costophrenic angle
Lung destruction
Bullae
Lung lucency
Decreased vessel size

On chest radiographs, CLE usually shows an upper lobe predominance of increased lucency and decreased vascularity (see Figs. 24.3 and 24.4). In panlobular emphysema, lucency and decreased vascularity usually appear to involve the lung uniformly or have a basal predominance (Fig. 24.5).

Pulmonary hypertension may develop in patients with emphysema and COPD and is associated with shorter survival. The pathogenesis is complex and is the result of many factors including vessel remodeling and hypoxic vasoconstriction. In its early stages, this condition is manifested by dilatation of central pulmonary arteries (see Fig. 24.2). Later, the development of cor pulmonale may result in cardiomegaly and right ventricular enlargement.

HRCT Findings

CT with thick slices is inadequate for the diagnosis of emphysema, but high-resolution CT (HRCT) is highly accurate. On HRCT, emphysema is characterized by the presence of areas of abnormally low attenuation, which can be easily contrasted with surrounding normal lung parenchyma if a sufficiently low window mean (−600 to −700 HU) is used. HRCT is highly accurate in diagnosing emphysema, and findings correlate closely with pathology.

In most instances, focal areas of emphysema can be easily distinguished from lung cysts or honeycombing; with the exception of paraseptal emphysema or bullae, focal areas of emphysema lack distinct walls.

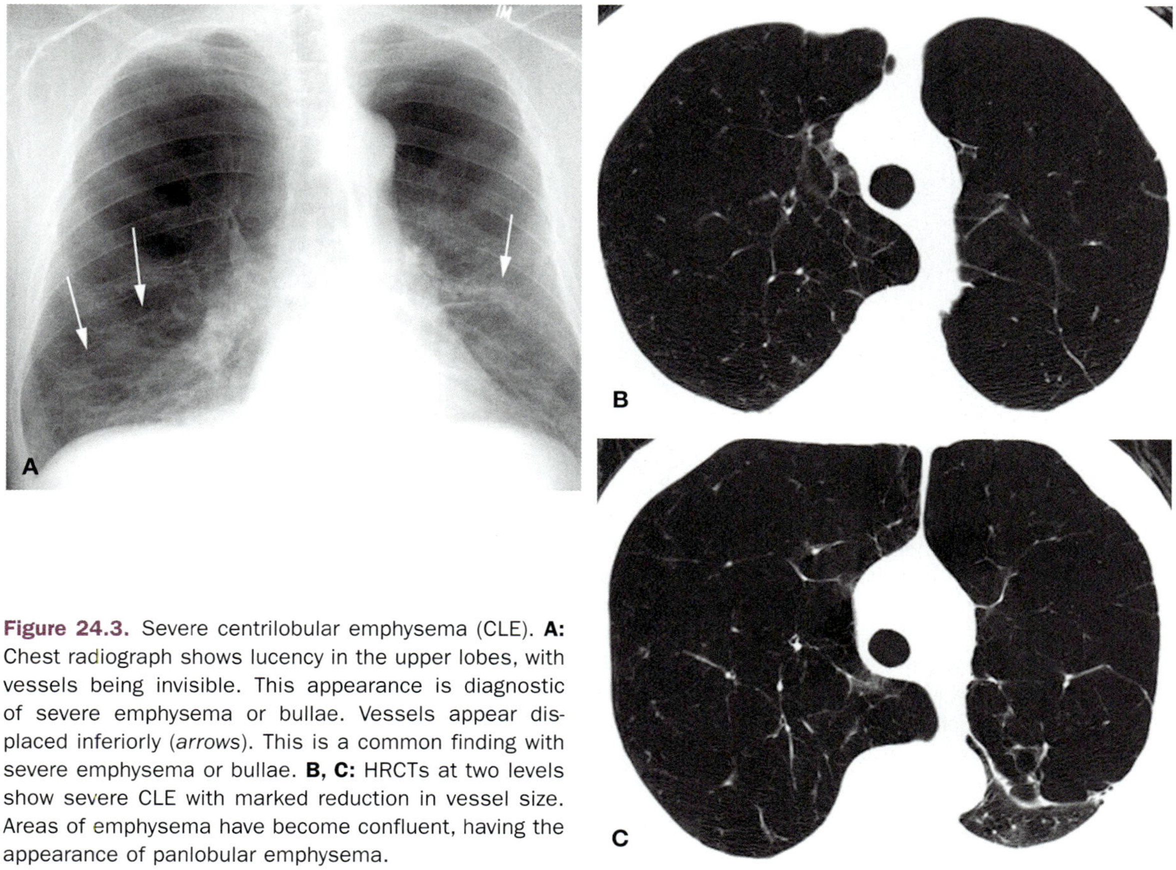

Figure 24.3. Severe centrilobular emphysema (CLE). **A:** Chest radiograph shows lucency in the upper lobes, with vessels being invisible. This appearance is diagnostic of severe emphysema or bullae. Vessels appear displaced inferiorly (*arrows*). This is a common finding with severe emphysema or bullae. **B, C:** HRCTs at two levels show severe CLE with marked reduction in vessel size. Areas of emphysema have become confluent, having the appearance of panlobular emphysema.

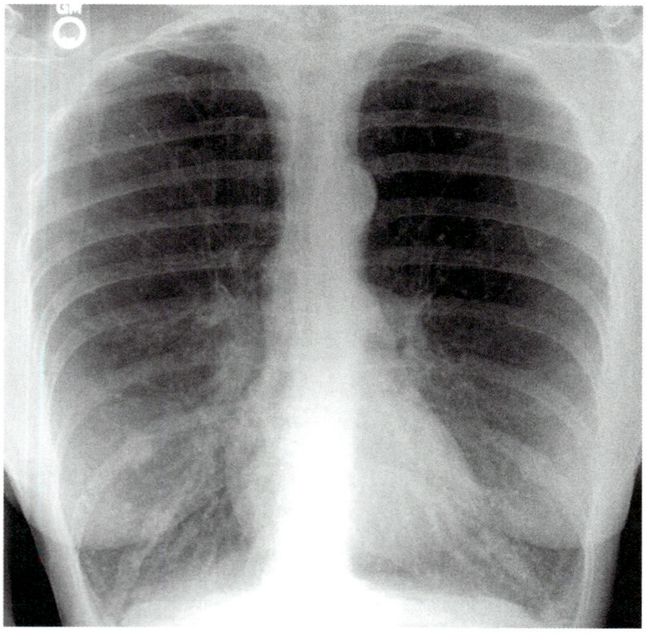

Figure 24.4. Severe centrilobular emphysema. Chest radiograph shows lucency predominating in the upper lobes with reduced vessel size. Vessels are largest at the bases.

Although various CT findings of increased lung volume may also be seen in patients with COPD and emphysema, their identification is usually secondary to the more direct observation of lung destruction characteristic of the various types of emphysema.

Centrilobular Emphysema

CLE of mild to moderate degree is characterized on HRCT by the presence of multiple small, round areas of abnormally low attenuation, several millimeters to 1 cm in diameter, distributed throughout the lung, but usually having an upper lobe predominance (Fig. 24.6; Table 24.2). Areas of lucency often appear to be grouped near the centers of secondary pulmonary lobules, surrounding the centrilobular artery branches. Although the centrilobular location of lucencies cannot always be recognized on CT or HRCT, the presence of multiple, small, areas of emphysema, scattered throughout the lung, is diagnostic of CLE. In most cases, the areas of low attenuation lack visible walls (see Figs. 24.6 and 24.7), although very thin and relatively inconspicuous walls are occasionally seen on HRCT, probably related to surrounding fibrosis. In patients with CLE, bullae may have visible walls (Fig. 24.8), and in association, paraseptal emphysema and subpleural bullae are often seen. With more severe CLE,

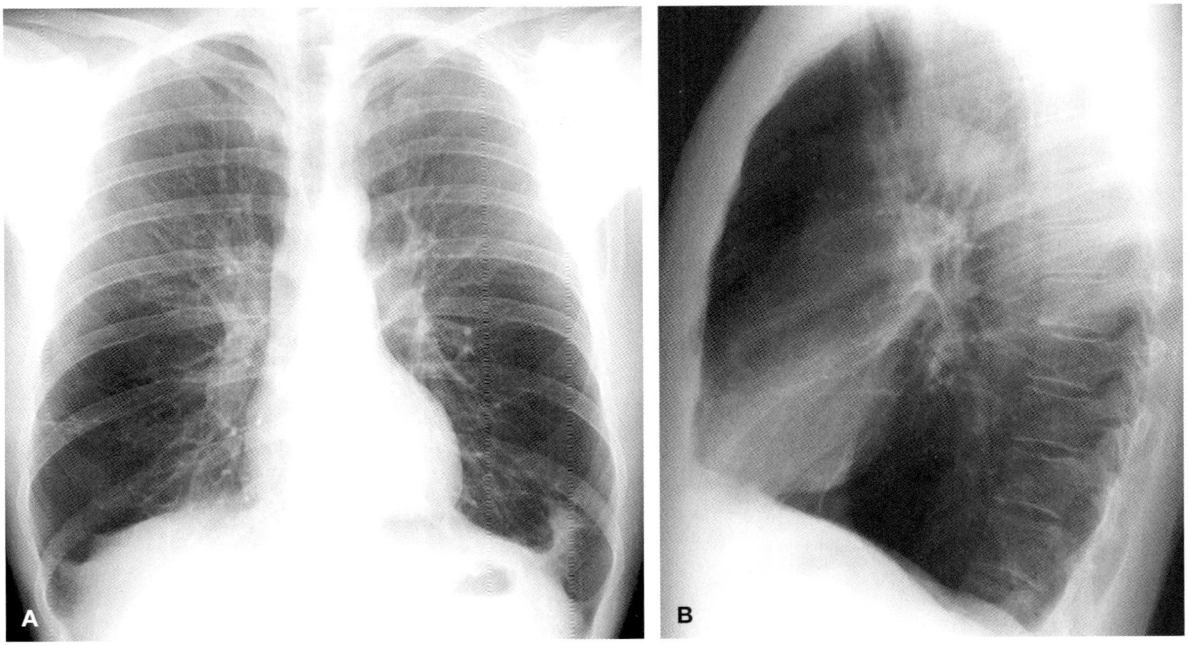

Figure 24.5. Panlobular emphysema in a 34-year-old man secondary to alpha-1-antitrypsin deficiency. **A:** On the PA view, lung volumes are increased. The lungs appear more lucent at the lung bases, and vessel size is greatest in the upper lobes. Diaphragmatic slips are visible. **B:** Findings of emphysema, with increased lung volumes and increased lucency, also are visible on the lateral view. Vessels appear small at the lung bases.

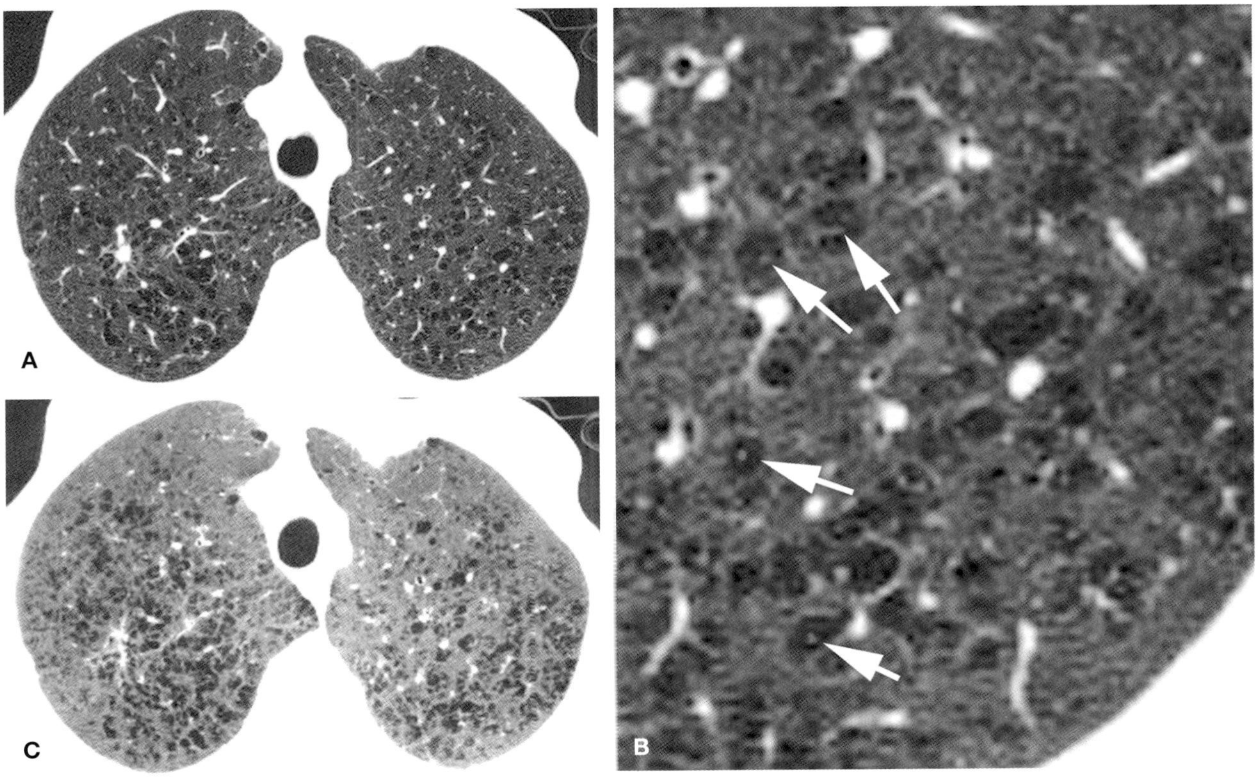

Figure 24.6. HRCT in centrilobular emphysema (CLE). **A:** HRCT through the upper lobes shows multiple small areas of lucency, with a spotty distribution. This is typical of CLE. The individual holes do not have visible walls. A small nodule in the right upper lobe represents a carcinoma. **B:** Coned-down view of the left upper lobe shows the typical appearance of CLE. No walls are visible. Some areas of emphysema are seen to surround small centrilobular arteries (*arrows*). **C:** MinIP image from a stack of five HRCT images shows the typical distribution of CLE.

Table 24.2 Centrilobular Emphysema

Affects the respiratory bronchioles in the central portions of lobules
Cigarette smoking
Upper lobe predominances
Small round areas of low attenuation
Walls usually invisible
Several millimeters to 1 cm in diameter
May be associated with bullae
May become confluent

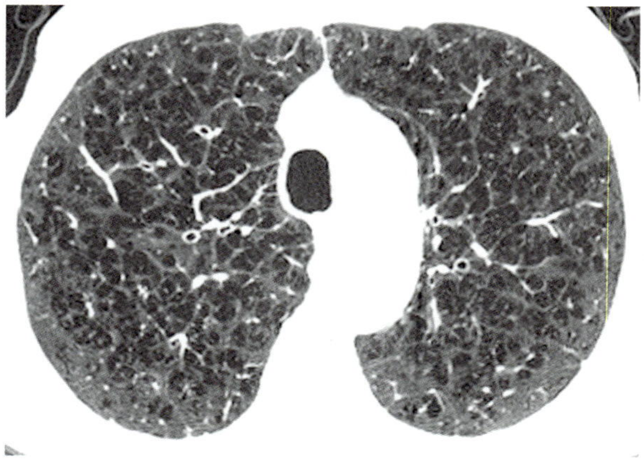

Figure 24.7. Moderate centrilobular emphysema (CLE). Multiple focal lucencies are visible in the upper lobes, without visible walls. This would be classified as moderate CLE using Fleischner criteria.

areas of destruction can become confluent. When this occurs, the centrilobular distribution of abnormalities is no longer recognizable on HRCT (or on pathology). This appearance can closely mimic the appearance of panlobular emphysema, and a distinction between these is of little clinical significance when this occurs (see Fig. 24.3B and C).

A Fleischner Society statement reviewing the CT-definable subtypes of COPD provides the following criteria for reporting the extent of CLE as:

1. *Trace CLE,* minimal centrilobular lucencies occupying less than 0.5% of a lung zone
2. *Mild CLE,* scattered centrilobular lucencies involving 0.5% to 5% of a lung zone
3. *Moderate CLE,* many centrilobular lucencies occupying more than 5% of any lung zone
4. *Confluent CLE,* coalescent centrilobular or lobular lucencies, with lucencies spanning several secondary lobules
5. *Advanced destructive emphysema,* with panlobular lucencies and hyperexpansion of pulmonary lobules

Panlobular Emphysema

Panlobular emphysema is characterized by uniform destruction of the pulmonary lobule, leading to widespread areas of abnormally low lung attenuation (Table 24.3). Involved lung appears abnormally lucent, and pulmonary vessels in the affected lung appear fewer and smaller than normal and may be quite inconspicuous (Figs. 24.9 and 24.10). In contrast to CLE, panlobular emphysema almost always appears generalized or most severe in the lower lobes. Focal lucencies, which are more typical of CLE or paraseptal emphysema, and bullae are relatively uncommon but may be seen in less abnormal lung regions.

In severe panlobular emphysema, the characteristic appearance of extensive lung destruction and the associated paucity of vascular markings are easily distinguished from normal lung parenchyma. However, mild and even moderately severe panlobular emphysema can be very subtle and difficult to detect. Diffuse panlobular emphysema unassociated with focal areas of lung destruction or bullae may be difficult to distinguish from diffuse small airway obstruction and air trapping resulting from bronchiolitis obliterans.

About 40% of patients with alpha-1-antitrypsin deficiency show bronchiectasis or bronchial wall thickening on HRCT. Patients with alpha-1-antitrypsin deficiency are more susceptible to airway damage during episodes of infection than are normal patients because of the same protease-antiprotease imbalance that leads to emphysema.

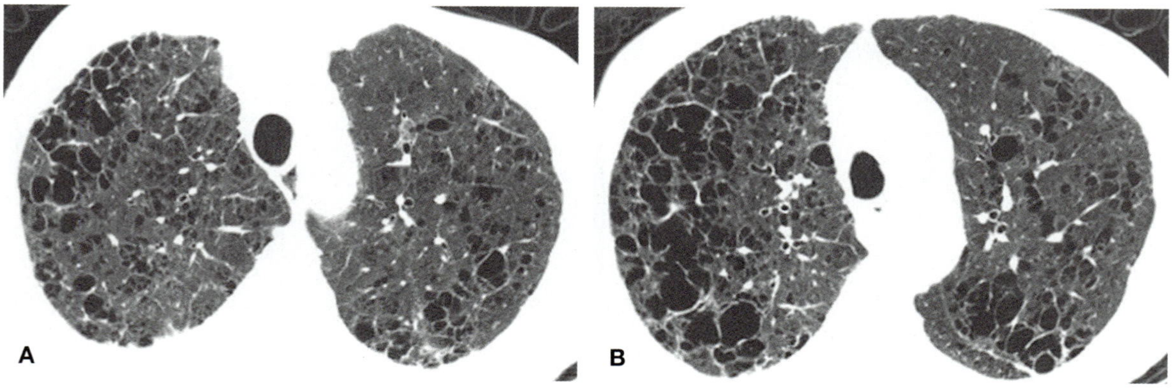

Figure 24.8. Centrilobular emphysema (CLE) with bullae. **A, B:** CLE is visible in the upper lobes. Areas of emphysema larger than 1 cm are bullae. They often have visible walls. Areas of emphysema in an immediate subpleural location represent paraseptal emphysema. Using Fleischner criteria, this would be considered confluent CLE.

Table 24.3 Panlobular Emphysema

Affects the entire lobule
Alpha-1-antitrypsin deficiency or cigarette smoking (rarely IV drug use)
Diffuse or lower lobe predominance
Diffuse decrease in lung attenuation
Focal areas of destruction or bullae usually absent
Reduction in vessel size
May be subtle in its early stages

Paraseptal Emphysema

Paraseptal emphysema is characterized by the involvement of the distal part of the secondary lobule and, therefore, is most striking in a subpleural location (Table 24.4). Areas of subpleural paraseptal emphysema often have visible walls, but these walls are very thin and often correspond to interlobular septa (Fig. 24.11). Even mild paraseptal emphysema is easily detected by HRCT.

Areas of paraseptal emphysema larger than 1 cm in diameter are most appropriately termed *bullae* (see Fig 24.11) Subpleural bullae often are considered to be manifestations of paraseptal emphysema, although they may be seen in all types of emphysema and also as an isolated phenomenon.

HRCT may be useful in the detection of apical subpleural bullae invisible on radiographs in patients with idiopathic spontaneous pneumothorax. This form of pneumothorax occurs most often in tall young adults and is thought to be due to rupture of a subpleural bulla. Apical subpleural emphysema is visible on CT in 80% to 90% of patients with spontaneous pneumothorax.

Although paraseptal emphysema may superficially mimic the appearance of honeycombing, several differences make it possible to distinguish between these entities. Paraseptal emphysema occurs in a single layer at the pleural surface (see Fig. 24.11B and C), whereas honeycombing may occur in multiple layers. Paraseptal emphysema is most severe in the apices (see Fig. 24.11); honeycombing is almost always most severe at the bases. Paraseptal emphysema often is associated

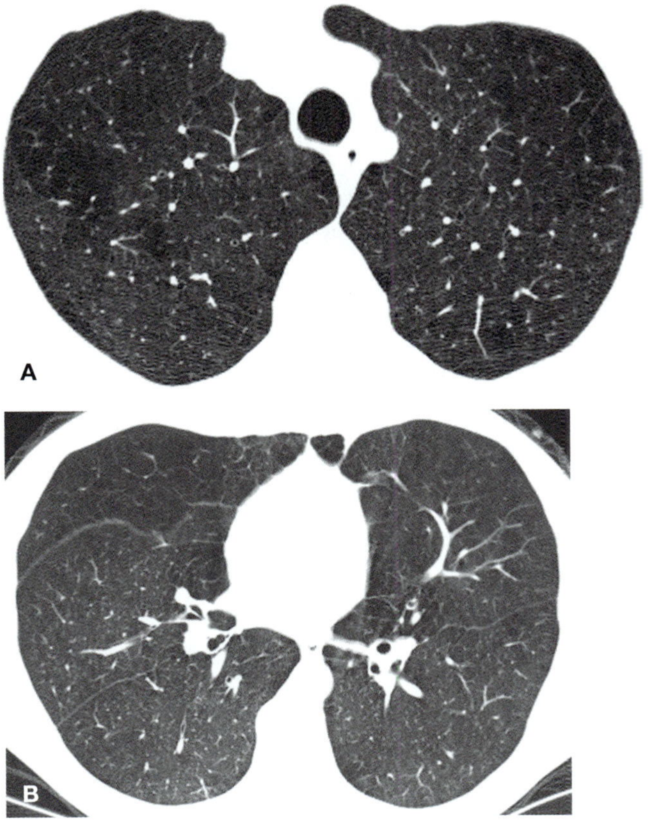

Figure 24.9. Panlobular emphysema in alpha-1-antitrypsin deficiency (same patient shown in Fig. 24.5). HRCT scans through the upper (**A**) and lower (**B**) lobes both show a decrease in lung attenuation and vessel size. Focal lucencies, as seen in centrilobular emphysema, are not present.

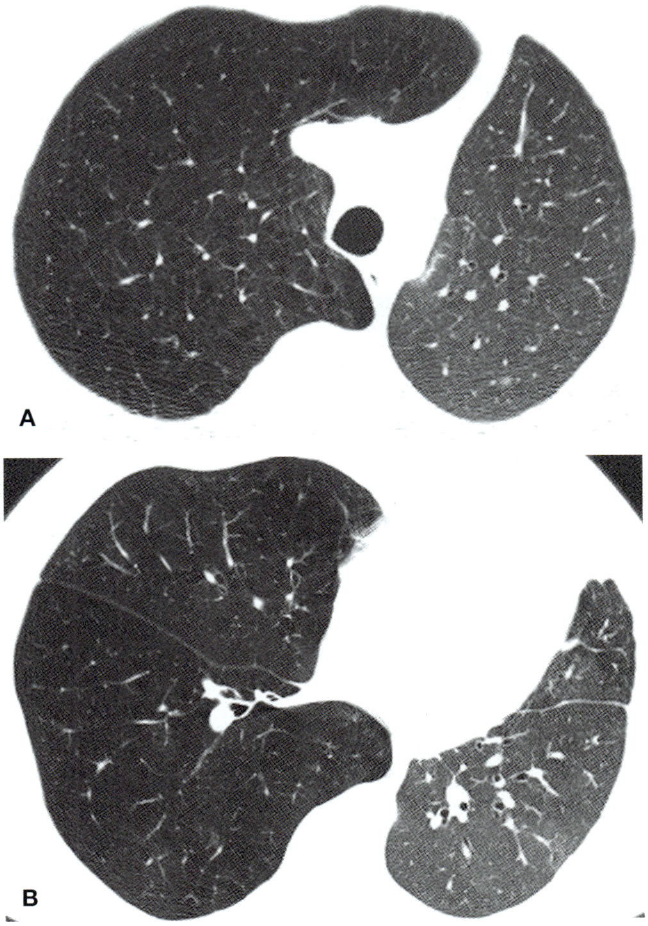

Figure 24.10. Panlobular emphysema in alpha-1-antitrypsin deficiency (right lung) in a patient with a left lung transplant. HRCT scans through the upper (**A**) and lower (**B**) lobes both show decreased lung attenuation and vessel size. The right lung is considerably larger than the (normal) left lung. The normal left lung attenuation, vascular size, and volume may be contrasted with that of the emphysematous lung.

Table 24.4	Paraseptal Emphysema

Affects subpleural lobules
Cigarette smoking or idiopathic
Upper lower predominance
May be associated with centrilobular emphysema
Focal subpleural lucencies marginated by interlobular septae
Bullae common

with cystic spaces larger than 1 cm; such spaces are uncommon with honeycombing.

In the Fleischner Society statement, reviewing CT-definable subtypes of COPD, paraseptal emphysema may be visually quantitated as:

1. *Mild paraseptal emphysema*, with small (≤1 cm) well-demarcated rounded juxtapleural lucencies in a row
2. *Substantial paraseptal emphysema*, with mainly large (>1 cm) juxtapleural cystlike lucencies or bullae involving more than the lung apices

Bullous Emphysema

The term *bullous emphysema* does not represent a specific pathologic entity but refers to the presence of emphysema associated with large bullae (Table 24.5). It usually is seen in patients with centrilobular or paraseptal emphysema (see Figs. 24.8 and 24.11). A syndrome of bullous emphysema, or *giant bullous emphysema*, has been described based on clinical and radiologic features and is also known as "vanishing lung syndrome" or "primary bullous disease of the lung." Giant bullous emphysema often is seen in young males and is characterized by the presence of large, progressive, upper lobe bullae, which occupy a significant volume of a hemithorax and often are asymmetric (Figs. 24.12 and 24.13). Arbitrarily, giant bullous emphysema is said to be present if bullae occupy at least one-third of a hemithorax. Most patients with giant bullous emphysema are cigarette smokers, but this entity may also occur in cannabis smokers or, rarely, nonsmokers.

Typically, bullae increase progressively in size over time. Rarely, bullae may spontaneously decrease in size or disappear, usually as a result of secondary infection or obstruction of the proximal airway. Spontaneous pneumothorax is common.

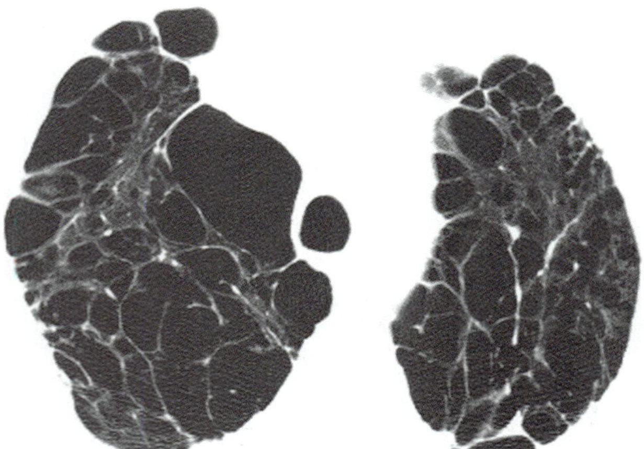
A

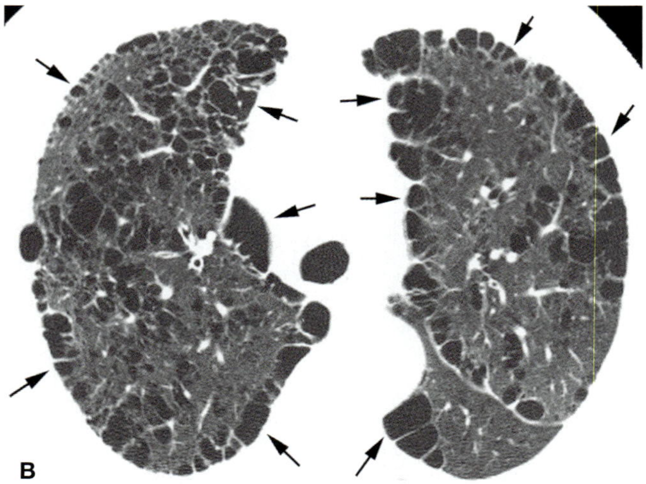
B

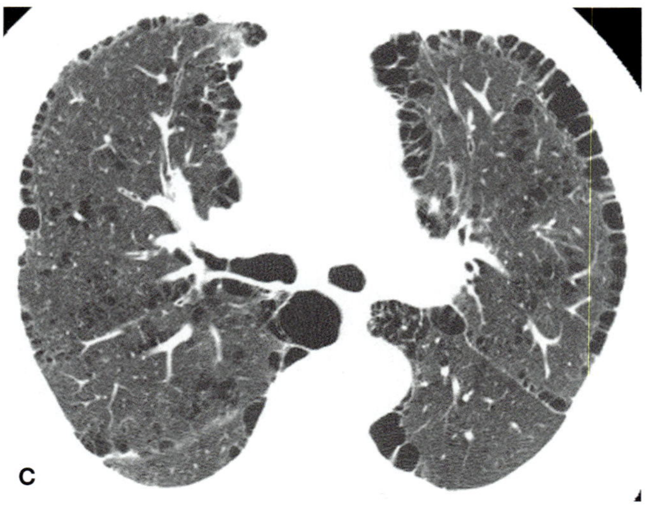
C

Figure 24.11. Paraseptal and centrilobular emphysema in a smoker. **A:** HRCT at the lung apices shows extensive emphysema with bullae. The subpleural bullae represent paraseptal emphysema. **B:** At a lower level, more discrete areas of paraseptal emphysema and subpleural bullae are visible (*arrows*). Emphysema within the central upper lobes is centrilobular. **C:** At a level below that seen in (**B**), the areas of emphysema appear smaller and occur in a single layer.

Table 24.5 Bullous Emphysema
Emphysema associated with bullae
May be seen with paraseptal or centrilobular emphysema
Cigarette and/or cannabis smoking or idiopathic
"Vanishing lung syndrome"
Large bullae
Often upper lobe
Often asymmetric
Compression of normal lung
Bullae increase or sometimes resolve

Quantitative Evaluation of Emphysema

Quantitation of emphysema may be attempted using various measures based on CT lung attenuation, but these are of limited value in clinical practice, and in the absence of dedicated CT attenuation algorithms. As indicated previously, the visual assessment of the type and severity based on an estimation of the extent of lung involvement on CT is also valid, as reviewed in the Fleischner Society statement.

Although routine axial HRCT images usually suffice for evaluating emphysema, minimum intensity projection (MinIP) images may be used, especially in cases with subtle disease. Coronal reconstructions may be useful in showing the distribution of emphysema.

Computer analysis of digital data obtained from CT also has been used to determine the severity of emphysema. The simplest method involves the use of a threshold value below which emphysema is considered to be present and a determination of the percentage of lung below that threshold; this is termed the "density mask" or "pixel index" technique. Normal lung attenuation usually varies from −770 to −875 HU; on HRCT, emphysema is considered to be present if attenuation measures less than −950 HU. Many other measurements have been used in experimental studies.

DIAGNOSIS OF AIRWAY DISEASE IN COPD

Both large and small airway abnormalities may be present in patients with COPD. Although some increase in lung markings may be seen on chest radiographs in patients with COPD, these may be due to mild lung fibrosis, bronchial wall thickening or impaction, or small airway disease. This appearance on chest radiographs has been termed the "dirty chest," because of its nonspecific appearance.

CT Diagnosis of Large Airway Abnormalities in COPD

Bronchial wall thickening is commonly present in heavy cigarette smokers with chronic bronchitis, occurring because of bronchial inflammation and remodeling. It may be recognized on CT as a relative increase in bronchial wall thickness, compared with the diameters of the bronchial lumen or the adjacent pulmonary arteries. However, this diagnosis is largely subjective and associated with substantial interobserver variability. The diagnosis and appearance of chronic bronchitis are reviewed in Chapter 23.

Quantitative CT assessment of airway wall thickness is less subjective but requires more time and effort and appropriate analysis software. Increased thickness of airway walls is associated with COPD, with reversibility of airway obstruction, and with symptoms of chronic bronchitis. In patients with COPD, bronchial wall thickening is an important independent predictor of FEV_1 and the risk of acute exacerbation.

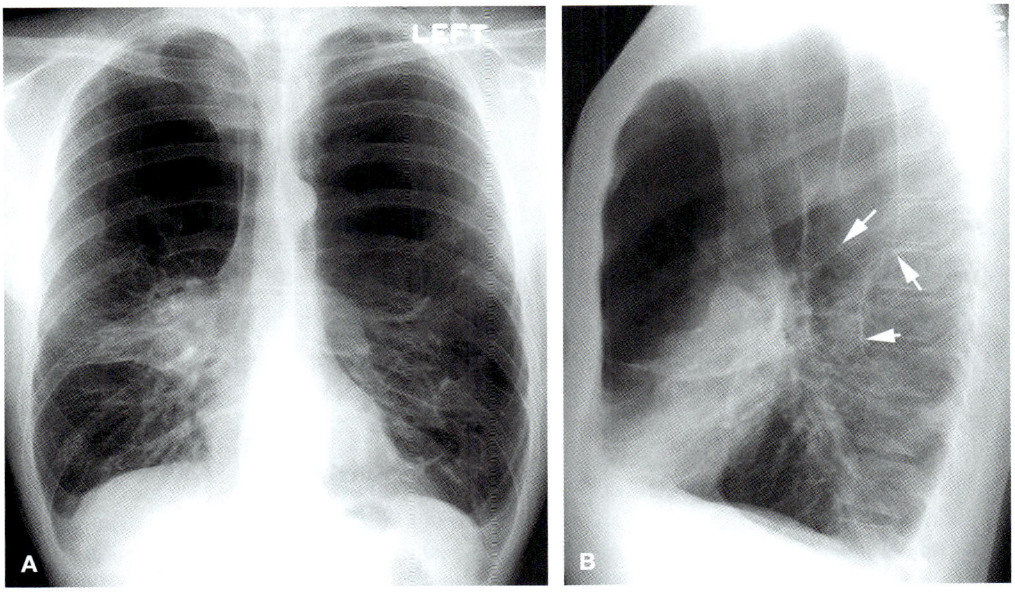

Figure 24.12. Bullous emphysema in a young man. **A, B:** Large bullae are visible in the upper lobes, with displacement of normal lung to the bases. Bulla walls are visible (*arrows* in **B**).

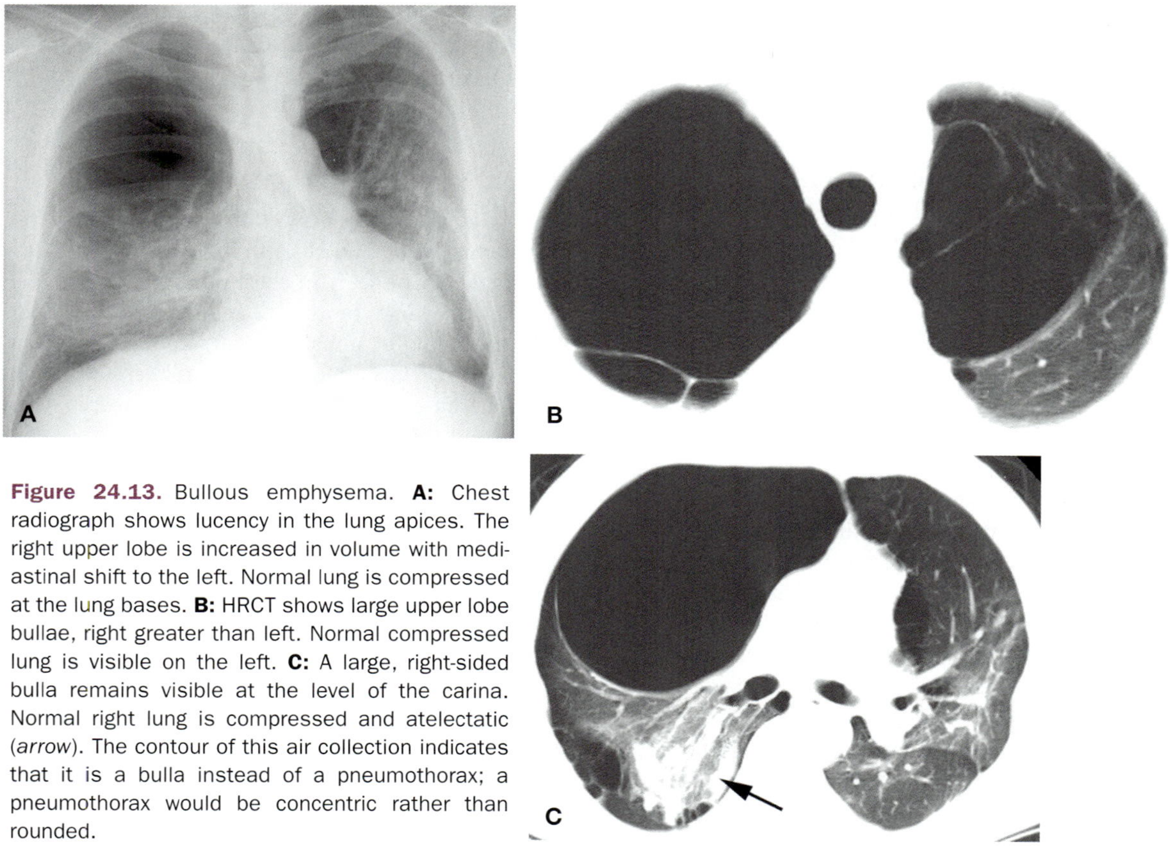

Figure 24.13. Bullous emphysema. **A:** Chest radiograph shows lucency in the lung apices. The right upper lobe is increased in volume with mediastinal shift to the left. Normal lung is compressed at the lung bases. **B:** HRCT shows large upper lobe bullae, right greater than left. Normal compressed lung is visible on the left. **C:** A large, right-sided bulla remains visible at the level of the carina. Normal right lung is compressed and atelectatic (*arrow*). The contour of this air collection indicates that it is a bulla instead of a pneumothorax; a pneumothorax would be concentric rather than rounded.

CT Diagnosis of Small Airway Disease in COPD

Small airway disease is often a major component of both emphysema-predominant and airway-predominant COPD, which also involves larger airways (ie, bronchi). Isolated small airway disease can also occur as a primary abnormality in COPD. Physiologic identification of small airway disease is difficult. CT can be helpful in identifying signs of inflammatory small airway disease and small airway obstruction.

Inflammatory Small Airway Disease

Respiratory bronchiolitis is common in cigarette smokers and in patients with COPD. It results in bronchiolar inflammation with large numbers of bronchiolar and peribronchiolar macrophages containing brown or black "smokers" pigment. Respiratory bronchiolitis in patients with COPD may be visible on CT as poorly defined centrilobular nodules of ground-glass opacity, but abnormalities are often subtle and subject to interpretation.

CLE and bronchial wall thickening are frequent associated findings. The small centrilobular nodules of respiratory bronchiolitis are sometimes associated with patchy areas of ground-glass opacity that reflect respiratory bronchiolitis-interstitial lung disease or desquamative interstitial pneumonia (see Chapters 14 and 23).

Obstructive Small Airway Disease

Obstructive small airway disease is identified by noting the presence of air trapping at expiratory CT and/or by using pulmonary function tests. On expiratory CT in healthy subjects, lung attenuation usually increases in a homogeneous fashion. Air trapping is present if lung attenuation does not increase as expected on expiratory CT. Air trapping may be patchy or diffuse and is common in cigarette smokers. Air trapping and its diagnosis are discussed in Chapters 11 and 23.

Proposed mechanisms of air trapping in COPD include bronchiolar narrowing or obstruction and/or emphysema with loss of the elastic recoil required for normal expiration. In COPD, small airway resistance increases substantially compared to normal subjects, particularly in patients who have minimal emphysematous destruction.

COMPLICATIONS AND EXACERBATION OF EMPHYSEMA AND COPD

Acute complications of COPD include pneumonia, infection of bullae, and pneumothorax. Pneumonia may have a typical appearance, with dense consolidation, but in patients with moderate or severe emphysema, and in patients with bullae, lung consolidation may be heterogeneous with consolidation outlining areas of lung destruction or "holes." In this situation, the lung may have a cystic or "Swiss cheese" appearance; the appearance may mimic cavitation.

The presence of an air-fluid level in a preexisting bulla may indicate infection, hemorrhage, or neoplasm. Thickening of the wall of a bulla may be seen with chronic infection, particularly associated with *Aspergillus*, mycetoma, or neoplasm.

Pneumothorax may occur in patients with emphysema, particularly in the presence of paraseptal emphysema and bullae. COPD is the most common cause of secondary spontaneous pneumothorax (pneumothorax associated with a recognized disease). In some patients with emphysema, it may be difficult to distinguish pneumothorax and bullae on chest radiographs. CT may be valuable in this situation.

Exacerbation of symptoms in patients with COPD may be due to one of these complications. However, exacerbations more often are due to abnormalities not associated with distinct radiographic findings, such as worsening airway infection, increased mucous plugging, and obstruction of small airways. Only about 15% of patients with an exacerbation of COPD show significant abnormal radiographic findings and, based on these abnormalities, treatment is changed in only 5%. It has been recommended that chest radiographs be obtained in patients with an exacerbation of COPD only if there is a history of heart disease or congestive heart failure, intravenous drug abuse, seizures, immunosuppression, other pulmonary disease, or an elevated white blood cell count, fever, chest pain, or edema.

UTILITY OF HRCT IN THE DIAGNOSIS OF EMPHYSEMA AND COPD

HRCT is more sensitive and accurate than plain radiographs in diagnosing the presence, type, and extent of emphysema. Furthermore, HRCT has a high specificity for diagnosing emphysema; emphysema rarely is overdiagnosed in normal individuals or in patients with severe hyperinflation due to other causes.

In clinical practice, however, HRCT rarely is used to diagnose emphysema. Usually, some combination of a smoking history, a low diffusing capacity, airway obstruction on pulmonary function tests, and chest radiographs showing large lung volumes or lung destruction is sufficient to make the diagnosis. However, some patients with early emphysema present with clinical findings more typical of interstitial lung disease or pulmonary vascular disease, namely, shortness of breath and low diffusing capacity, without evidence of airway obstruction on pulmonary function tests or emphysema on chest films. In such patients, HRCT can be valuable in making the diagnosis of emphysema, obviating lung biopsy.

HRCT also can be valuable in the preoperative assessment of patients before surgical treatment of emphysema (eg, bullectomy, lung transplantation, volume reduction surgery, or bronchoscopic lung volume reduction). HRCT has become routine in the evaluation of such patients, both before and after operation, and is used to determine the type, severity, and distribution of emphysema (Fig. 24.14).

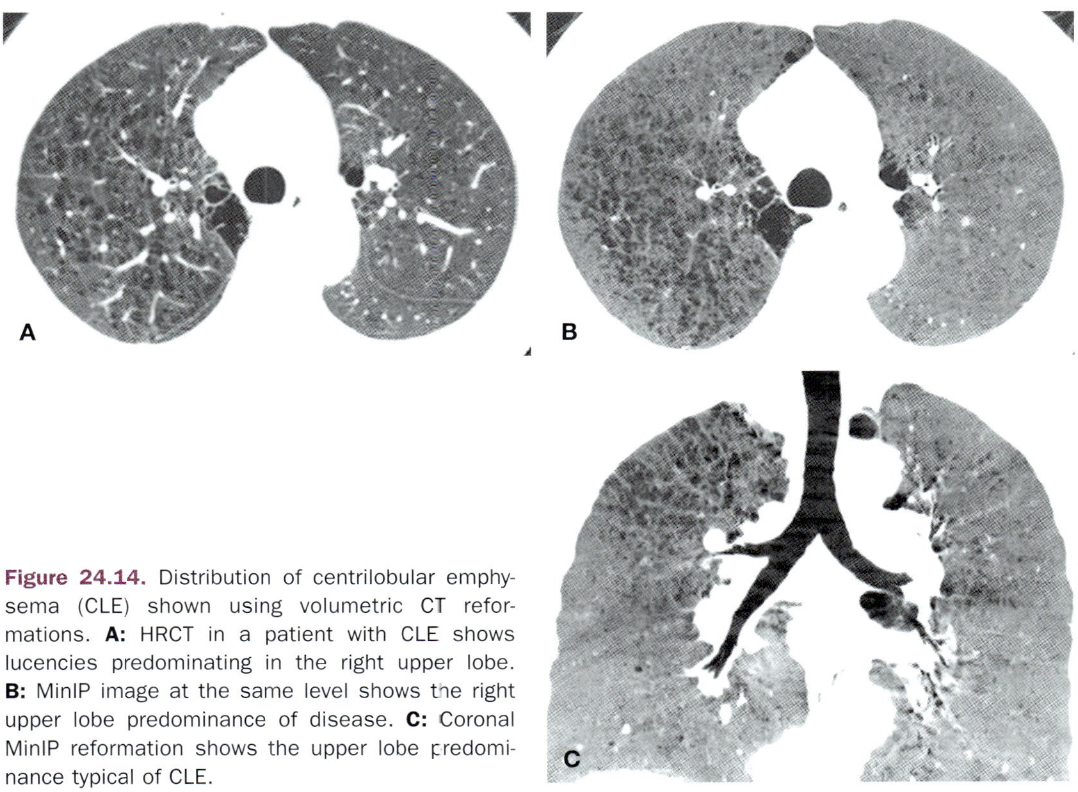

Figure 24.14. Distribution of centrilobular emphysema (CLE) shown using volumetric CT reformations. **A:** HRCT in a patient with CLE shows lucencies predominating in the right upper lobe. **B:** MinIP image at the same level shows the right upper lobe predominance of disease. **C:** Coronal MinIP reformation shows the upper lobe predominance typical of CLE.

SUGGESTED READINGS

American Thoracic Society. Standards for the diagnosis and care of patients with chronic obstructive pulmonary disease (COPD) and asthma. *Am Rev Respir Dis*. 1987;136:225-243.

Arakawa H, Kurihara Y, Nakajima Y, Niimi H, Ishikawa T, Tokuda M. Computed tomography measurements of overinflation in chronic obstructive pulmonary disease: evaluation of various radiographic signs. *J Thorac Imaging*. 1998;13(3):188-192.

Burki NK. Roentgenologic diagnosis of emphysema: accurate or not? *Chest*. 1989;95(6):1178-1179.

Burki NK, Krumpelman JL. Correlation of pulmonary function with the chest roentgenogram in chronic airway obstruction. *Am Rev Respir Dis*. 1980;121(2):217-223.

Fishman A, Martinez F, Naunheim K, et al. A randomized trial comparing lung-volume-reduction surgery with medical therapy for severe emphysema. *N Engl J Med*. 2003;348(21):2059-2073.

Foster WL Jr, Gimenez EI, Roubidoux MA, et al. The emphysemas: radiologic-pathologic correlations. *Radiographics*. 1993;13(2):311-328.

Gevenois PA, de Maertelaer V, De Vuyst P, Zanen J, Yernault JC. Comparison of computed density and macroscopic morphometry in pulmonary emphysema. *Am J Respir Crit Care Med*. 1995;152(2):653-657.

Gevenois PA, De Vuyst P, de Maertelaer V, et al. Comparison of computed density and microscopic morphometry in pulmonary emphysema. *Am J Respir Crit Care Med*. 1996;154(1):187-192.

Global Initiative for Chronic Obstructive Lung Disease. *Global Strategy for the Diagnosis, Management, and Prevention of Chronic Obstructive Pulmonary Disease*. National Heart, Lung, and Blood Institute, World Health Organization; 2008.

Grenier PA, Beigelman-Aubry C, Fetita C, Brillet PY. CT imaging of chronic obstructive pulmonary disease: role in phenotyping and interventions. *Expert Opin Med Diagn*. 2009;3(6):689-703.

Guest PJ, Hansell DM. High resolution computed tomography (HRCT) in emphysema associated with alpha-1-antitrypsin deficiency. *Clin Radiol*. 1992;45(4):260-266.

Han MK, Agusti A, Calverley PM, et al. Chronic obstructive pulmonary disease phenotypes. The future of COPD. *Am J Respir Crit Care Med*. 2010;182(5):598-604.

Han MK, Bartholmai B, Liu LX, et al. Clinical significance of radiologic characterizations in COPD. *COPD*. 2009;6:459-467.

Janoff A. Elastases and emphysema. Current assessment of the protease-antiprotease hypothesis. *Am Rev Respir Dis*. 1985;132(2):417-433.

Klooster K, Slebos DJ. Endobronchial valves for the treatment of advanced emphysema. *Chest*. 2021;159(5):1833-1842. doi:10.1016/j.chest.2020.12.007

Lesur O, Delorme N, Fromaget JM, Bernadac P, Polu JM. Computed tomography in the etiologic assessment of idiopathic spontaneous pneumothorax. *Chest*. 1990;98(2):341-347.

Lynch DA, Austin JHM, Hogg JC, et al. CT-definable subtypes of chronic obstructive pulmonary disease: a statement of the Fleischner Society. *Radiology*. 2015;277(1):192-205.

Matsuoka S, Yamashiro T, Washko GR, Kurihara Y, Nakajima Y, Hatabu H. Quantitative CT assessment of chronic obstructive pulmonary disease. *Radiographics*. 2010;30(1):55-66.

Pratt PC. Role of conventional chest radiography in diagnosis and exclusion of emphysema. *Am J Med*. 1987;82(5):998-1006.

Reich SB, Weinshelbaum A, Yee J. Correlation of radiographic measurements and pulmonary function tests in chronic obstructive pulmonary disease. *AJR Am J Roentgenol*. 1985;144(4):695-699.

Remy-Jardin M, Remy J, Gosselin B, Copin MC, Wurtz A, Duhamel A. Sliding thin slab, minimum intensity projection technique in the diagnosis of emphysema: histopathologic-CT correlation. *Radiology*. 1996;200(3):665-671.

Sherman S, Skoney JA, Ravikrishnan KP. Routine chest radiographs in exacerbations of chronic obstructive pulmonary disease: diagnostic value. *Arch Intern Med*. 1989;149(11):2493-2496.

Slone RM, Gierada DS, Yusen RD. Preoperative and postoperative imaging in the surgical management of pulmonary emphysema. *Radiol Clin North Am*. 1998;36(1):57-89.

Stern EJ, Webb WR, Weinacker A, Müller NL. Idiopathic giant bullous emphysema (vanishing lung syndrome): imaging findings in nine patients. *AJR Am J Roentgenol*. 1994;162(2):279-282.

Sutinen S, Christoforidis AJ, Klugh GA, Pratt PC. Roentgenologic criteria for the recognition of nonsymptomatic pulmonary emphysema: correlation between roentgenologic findings and pulmonary pathology. *Am Rev Respir Dis*. 1965;91:69-76.

The National Emphysema Treatment Trial Research Group. Rationale and design of the National Emphysema Treatment Trial (NETT): a prospective randomized trial of lung volume reduction surgery. *J Thorac Cardiovasc Surg*. 1999;118:518-528.

Thurlbeck WM, Müller NL. Emphysema: definition, imaging, and quantification. *AJR Am J Roentgenol*. 1994;163(5):1017-1025.

Thurlbeck WM, Simon G. Radiographic appearance of the chest in emphysema. *AJR Am J Roentgenol*. 1978;130(3):429-440.

Chapter 25

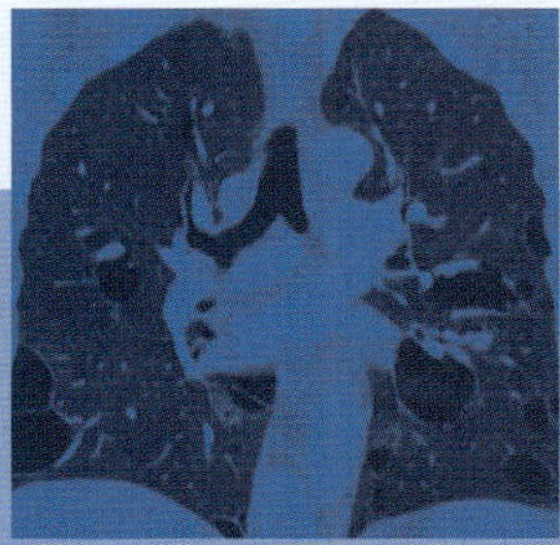

Travis S. Henry

Diffuse Cystic Lung Diseases

INTRODUCTION

A *lung cyst* is a thin-walled, well-defined, air-containing lesion 1 cm or more in diameter, according to Fleischner Society Nomenclature. Cysts may be seen in patients with emphysema (ie, bullae; see Figs. 24.3, 24.8, 24.11, and 24.13 in Chapter 24), honeycombing (ie, large honeycomb cysts; see Fig. 11.17 in Chapter 11), pneumonia (ie, pneumatoceles) (Fig. 25.1), cystic bronchiectasis (ie, dilated bronchi) (Fig. 25.2; see also Figs. 10.28-10.30 in Chapter 10), subacute hypersensitivity pneumonitis, trauma with lung laceration (see Fig. 10.36 in Chapter 10), multiple healing cavities, and some parasitic infections (Table 25.1). The differential diagnosis (see Table 10.6 in Chapter 10) overlaps with that of multiple cavitary masses.

Several lung diseases are characterized by cysts as their primary abnormality. These are rare and include Langerhans cell histiocytosis (LCH), lymphangioleiomyomatosis (LAM), tuberous sclerosis (TS), neurofibromatosis, lymphoid interstitial pneumonia (LIP), protein deposition (eg, amyloid or light-chain deposition disease [LCDD]), Birt-Hogg-Dubé syndrome, and Proteus syndrome. Tracheobronchial papillomatosis, another rare disease, which may be associated with cystic lung lesions, is discussed in Chapter 5.

PULMONARY LCH (PULMONARY HISTIOCYTOSIS X)

The term *LCH* refers to a group of diseases of unknown etiology, most often recognized in childhood, in which Langerhans cells accumulate in one or more organ systems, including bone, lung, pituitary gland, mucous membranes and skin, lymph nodes, and liver. This disease also is known as *histiocytosis X* or *eosinophilic granuloma* (Table 25.2). Lung involvement in LCH is common, seen in 40% of patients, and may be an isolated abnormality. In patients with multisystem disease, other commonly affected sites include bone and the pituitary gland.

In the early stage, pulmonary LCH is characterized by the presence of granulomas containing large numbers of Langerhans cells and eosinophils, resulting in destruction of lung tissue. LCH lesions typically are peribronchiolar in distribution and upper lung predominant. In later stages of the disease, the cellular granulomas are replaced by fibrosis and lung cysts. Although LCH is characterized by a clonal proliferation of cells, it is likely that LCH in adults represents an abnormal immune response to an unidentified antigenic stimulus rather than a neoplasm.

Most patients with pulmonary LCH are young or middle-aged adults (average age, 32 years). Over 90% of adults with LCH are smokers, and this disease is considered to be smoking related in most cases. Common presenting symptoms include cough and dyspnea. Up to 20% of patients present with pneumothorax.

Compared to patients with multisystem disease, the prognosis in patients with isolated pulmonary involvement is good; the disease regresses spontaneously in 25% and stabilizes clinically and radiographically in 50%. In the remaining 25% of cases, the disease follows a progressive downhill course, resulting in diffuse cystic lung destruction. In a small number of cases, death results from either respiratory insufficiency or pulmonary hypertension (PH).

Radiographic Findings

The radiographic findings of LCH include reticular, nodular, and reticulonodular patterns, often in combination (Figs. 25.3 and 25.4A and B); a cystic appearance may mimic honeycombing. Abnormalities usually are bilateral, predominantly involving the middle and upper lung zones, with relative sparing of the costophrenic angles. Lung volumes are

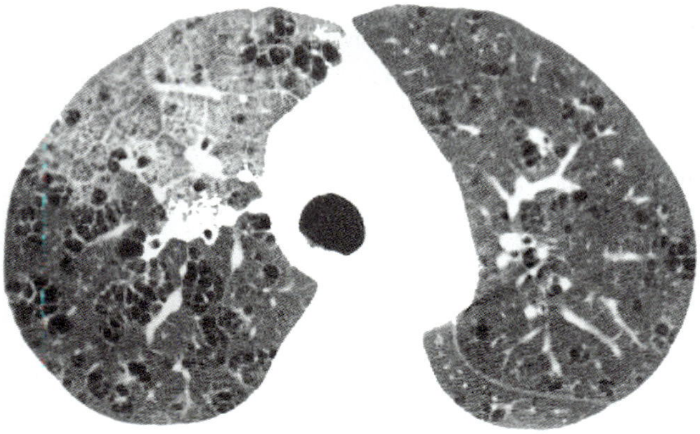

Figure 25.1. Pneumocystis pneumonia with pneumatoceles. Ground-glass opacity representing acute pneumonia is associated with multiple clustered lung cysts. This appearance is common in pneumocystis pneumonia.

characteristically normal or increased (see Fig. 25.4A and B), an unusual appearance in the presence of reticular opacities or honeycombing.

Table 25.1 Multiple Lung Cysts
Bullae
Honeycombing
Pneumonia with pneumatoceles (eg, pneumocystis)
Cystic bronchiectasis
Hypersensitivity pneumonitis (subacute)
Trauma with lung laceration
Healing cavities (eg, abscesses, granulomatosis with polyangiitis [Wegener], cavitary rheumatoid nodules)
Parasitic infections (eg, *Echinococcus*, paragonimiasis)
Langerhans cell histiocytosis
Lymphangioleiomyomatosis
Tuberous sclerosis
Neurofibromatosis
Lymphoid interstitial pneumonia
Sjögren syndrome
Light-chain deposition disease
Birt-Hogg-Dubé syndrome

CT Findings

In almost all patients, HRCT demonstrates cystic airspaces, which are usually less than 10 mm in diameter (see Figs. 25.4-25.6). The lung cysts have walls, which range from being thin and barely perceptible to several millimeters thick. The presence of distinct walls makes it possible to differentiate these cysts from areas of emphysema. Although many cysts appear round, they can also have bizarre shapes, being bilobed or cloverleaf in appearance (see Figs. 25.4-25.6).

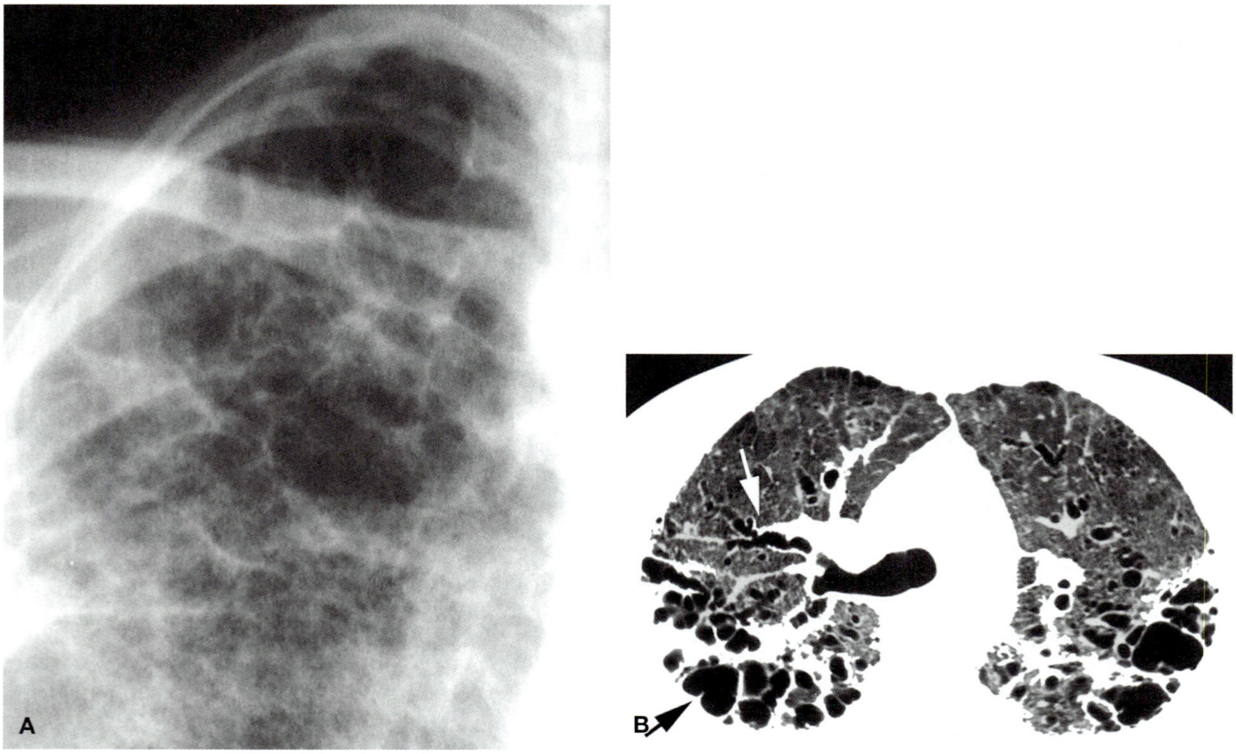

Figure 25.2. Sarcoidosis with extensive upper lobe cystic bronchiectasis. **A:** Detail view of the right upper lobe from a chest radiograph shows a cystic appearance. **B:** HRCT shows cystic bronchiectasis, possibly associated with areas of emphysema. Abnormal bronchi and branching cysts (*arrows*) are a clue to the correct diagnosis.

Table 25.2 Langerhans Cell Histiocytosis
Lung involvement in 40%; may be an isolated abnormality
90% of adult patients are smokers
Granulomas (nodules) in early stages, nodules may cavitate
Lung cysts late in course, irregular in shape
Thick or thin walled
Upper lobe predominance
Spare costophrenic angles
Progression from nodules to cavitary nodules to thick-walled cysts to thin-walled cysts resembling emphysema

Large cysts or bullae (more than 10 mm in diameter) are seen in more than half of the cases; some cysts are larger than 20 mm. True honeycombing, often suggested by the chest radiograph, does not occur.

In some patients, cysts are the only abnormality visible on HRCT, but in many cases, small nodules (usually less than 5 mm in diameter) are also present (see Figs. 25.3 and 25.5). Larger nodules, sometimes exceeding 1 cm, may be seen, but are less common (25%). Nodules can vary considerably in number in individual cases, probably depending on the activity of the disease; nodules can be few in number or myriad. The margins of nodules often are irregular, particularly when there is surrounding cystic or reticular disease. On HRCT, nodules may be centrilobular or random in distribution. Some nodules, particularly those larger than 1 cm in diameter, may show lucent centers, presumably corresponding to small "cavities." These cavities, however, sometimes represent a dilated bronchiolar lumen surrounded by peribronchiolar granulomas and thickened interstitium.

In all but the most severe cases, the lung bases and the costophrenic sulci are relatively spared (see Fig. 25.4). An upper lobe predominance in size and number of cysts is

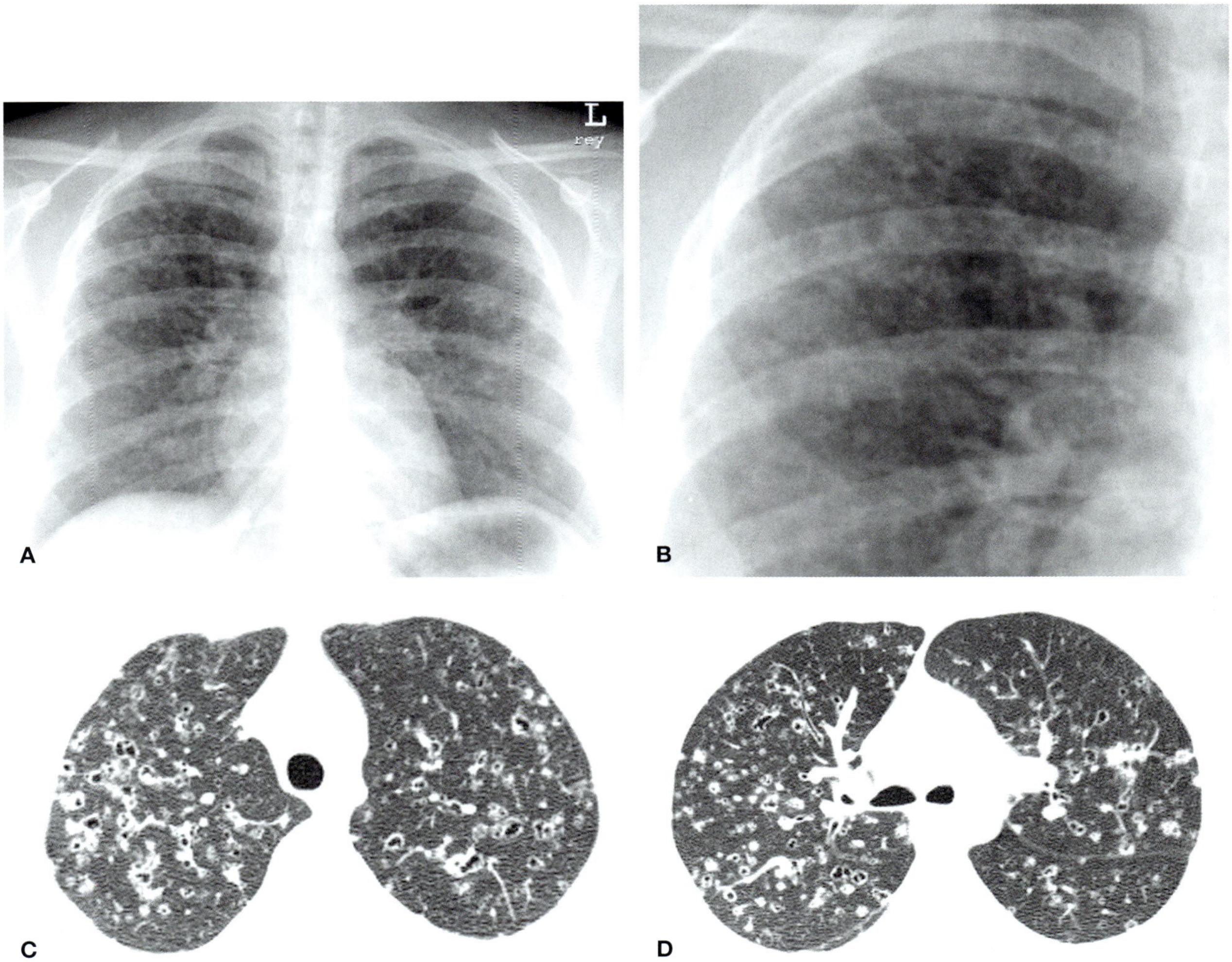

Figure 25.3. Langerhans cell histiocytosis in a 21-year-old smoker. **A:** Chest radiograph shows ill-defined nodules, predominating in the upper lobes. **B:** Detail view of the right upper lobe shows small nodules. **C:** HRCT through the upper lobes shows small nodules, cavitary nodules, and small irregular lung cysts. **D:** HRCT through the mid lungs shows a similar appearance. The lung bases were relatively normal.

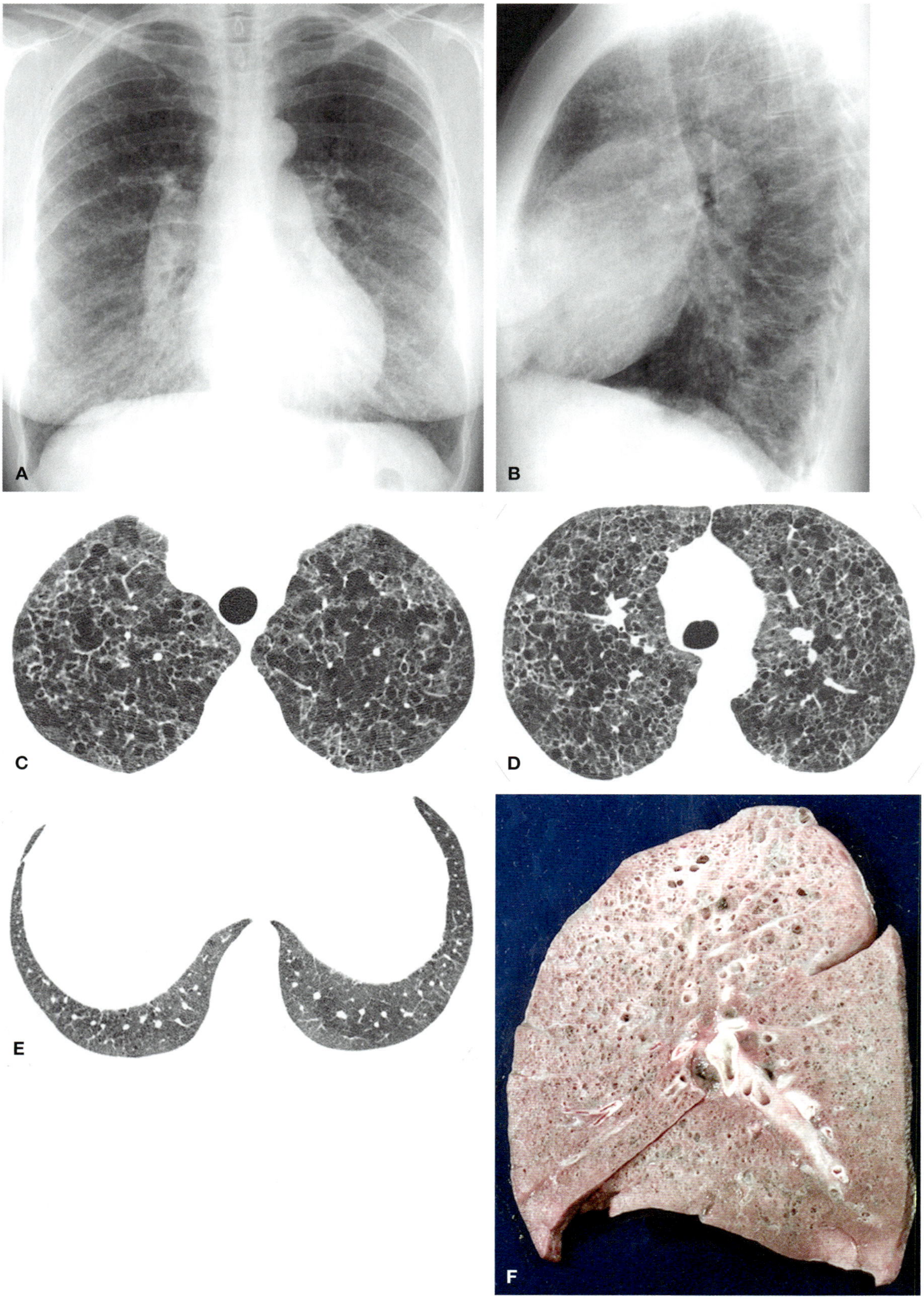

Figure 25.4. Langerhans cell histiocytosis. PA (**A**) and lateral (**B**) chest radiographs show large lung volumes, a fine reticular pattern, and enlarged central pulmonary arteries. **C:** HRCT through the upper lobes shows numerous thin-walled lung cysts, some irregular in shape. **D:** Near the level of the carina, a diffuse cystic abnormality persists. **E:** HRCT shows sparing of the costophrenic angles. **F:** This patient's lung removed at the time of lung transplantation shows cystic lesions with an upper lobe predominance.

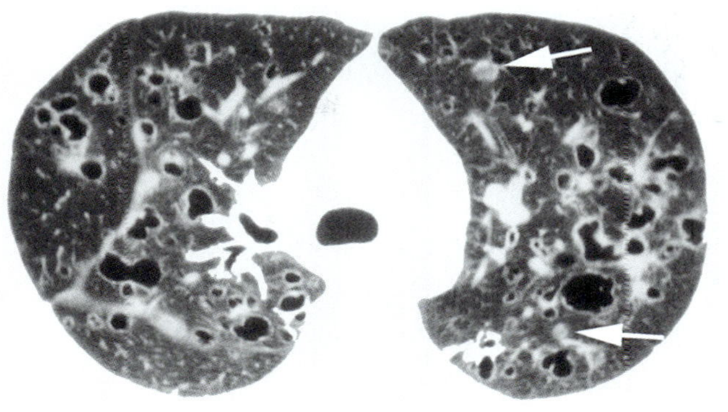

Figure 25.5. Langerhans cell histiocytosis. HRCT shows numerous irregularly shaped cysts in the upper lobes. Nodules (*arrows*) are visible as well.

present in most patients (see Fig. 25.6), and a basal predominance is never observed.

Pulmonary lesions may evolve in a characteristic sequence, beginning with centrilobular nodules, followed by cavitation, the formation of thick-walled cysts, and, finally, thin-walled cysts. Nodular lesions may regress spontaneously or may be replaced by cysts, but cystic lesions, once formed, persist, eventually becoming indistinguishable from diffuse emphysema.

Associated hilar or mediastinal lymph node enlargement or lytic bone lesions also may be present (Fig. 25.7). Severe PH seen in the majority of patients with advanced disease (group 5 PH in the World Health Organization [WHO] classification) may be identified on chest radiograph or CT (Fig. 25.4).

LAM AND TS

LAM is a rare disease characterized by progressive proliferation of perivascular epithelioid cells (PECs) in relation to bronchioles, small pulmonary vessels, and lymphatics in the chest and abdomen (Table 25.3). In the new WHO classification of lung tumors, it is considered to be a low-grade destructive metastasizing malignancy or, in other words, a PEComa. LAM occurs in association with tuberous sclerosis complex (TSC-LAM) or in a sporadic form (sporadic lymphangiomyomatosis [S-LAM]). TSC-LAM is linked to mutations in the tuberous sclerosis genes *TSC1* and *TSC2*, while S-LAM is associated with mutations of *TSC2*. Peribronchiolar PEC infiltration eventually leads to bronchiolar obstruction and destruction of lung parenchyma with formation of isolated lung cysts. Very small nodules (1-3 mm) also may be present, representing focal proliferation of type II pneumocytes. Renal angiomyolipomas are present in 15% of cases.

PEC proliferation also can involve the hilar, mediastinal, and extrathoracic lymph nodes, sometimes resulting in dilatation of intrapulmonary lymphatics and the thoracic duct. Involvement of the lymphatics can lead to chylous pleural effusions or ascites. Proliferation of cells in the walls of pulmonary veins may cause venous obstruction and lead to pulmonary venous hypertension with resultant hemoptysis.

LAM occurs almost exclusively in females of childbearing age. Occasional cases present in postmenopausal women, probably as a result of slow progression.

Most patients present with dyspnea, spontaneous pneumothorax, or cough. The mean time interval from the onset of symptoms to diagnosis is typically 3 to 5 years.

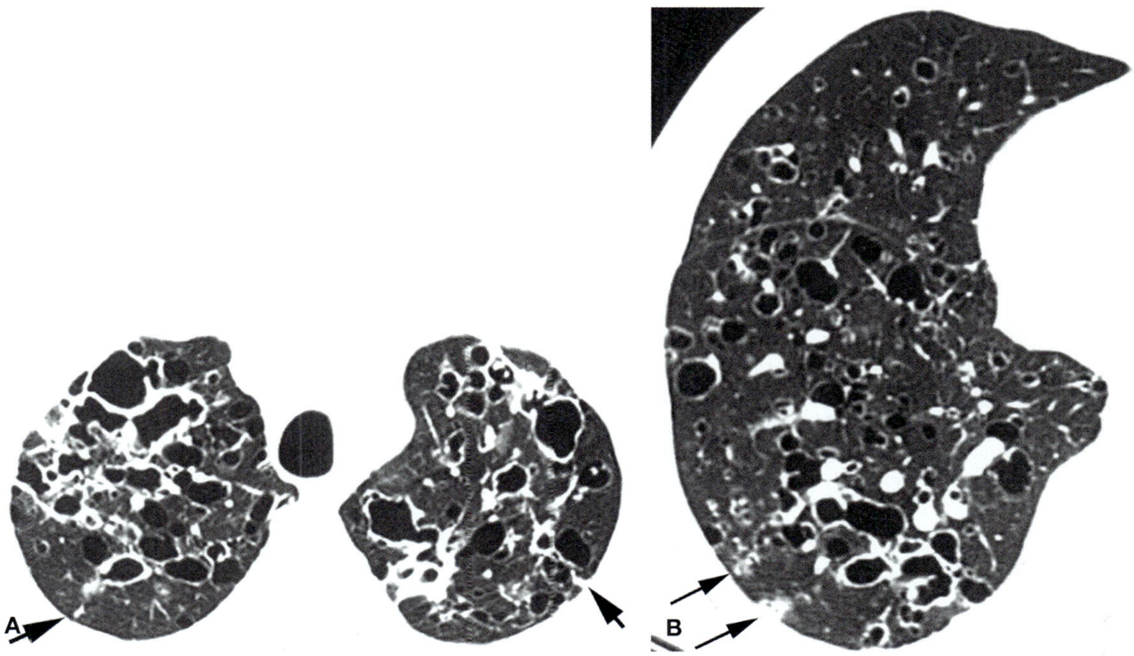

Figure 25.6. Langerhans cell histiocytosis. **A:** HRCT shows numerous irregularly shaped cysts in the upper lobes. The cysts are thick walled. This is characteristic of early disease. Nodules (*arrows*) also are visible. **B:** HRCT at the right lung base shows smaller and less numerous cysts as well as nodules (*arrows*).

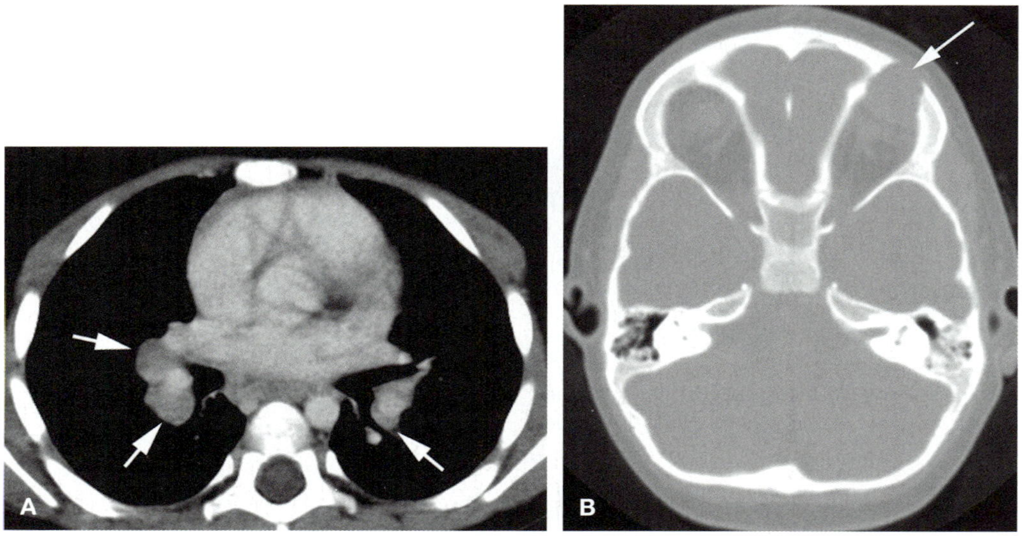

Figure 25.7. Langerhans cell histiocytosis in a 2-year-old child. **A:** Chest CT shows hilar lymph node enlargement (*arrows*). **B:** A lytic lesion (*arrow*) in the skull also is visible.

Sixty percent of patients have chylous pleural effusions; up to 80% have pneumothoraces; and 30% to 40% have blood-streaked sputum or frank hemoptysis. Nearly all patients have abnormal pulmonary function at presentation.

Clinical improvement has been reported following treatment with progesterone, tamoxifen, other antiestrogen agents, radiotherapy, or oophorectomy. Responses to such treatments are variable, however. Progression is typical, and most patients die within 5 to 10 years from the onset of symptoms. As a consequence, LAM is now considered an indication for lung transplantation. The abnormality may recur in the transplanted lung.

Radiographic Findings

On plain radiographs, 80% of patients with LAM show a fine reticular pattern. In patients with advanced disease, a cystic pattern mimicking that of honeycombing may be seen (Figs. 25.8 and 25.9). Lungs usually appear to be diffusely abnormal, with the lung bases involved to the same degree as the apices. As with LCH, lung volumes often appear increased despite the presence of reticulation.

Pleural abnormalities may precede, accompany, or be seen after the recognition of lung disease. About 50% of patients have radiographic evidence of pneumothorax at the time of presentation, and unilateral or bilateral pleural effusion is present in 10% to 20% of cases (see Fig. 25.8). About 10% to 25% of patients have normal-appearing radiographs at presentation despite the presence of lung cysts.

Table 25.3 Lymphangioleiomyomatosis

- Proliferation of immature-appearing smooth muscle cells
- Low-grade destructive metastasizing malignancy (perivascular epithelioid cell tumor)
- Occurs in association with tuberous sclerosis complex (TSC-lymphangioleiomyomatosis), linked to mutations in the tuberous sclerosis genes *TSC1* and *TSC2*
- Women of childbearing age
- Identical to the lung disease seen in tuberous sclerosis
- Cystic lung destruction
- Chylous effusions
- Renal angiomyolipomas are present in 15%
- Lung cysts
  - Round in shape
  - Diffuse distribution
  - Involve the costophrenic angles
- Nodules occasionally seen

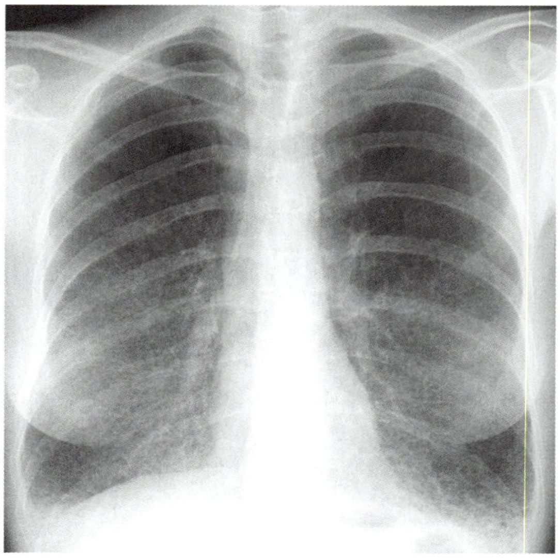

Figure 25.8. Lymphangiomyomatosis. Chest radiograph shows increased lung volume with reticular opacities at the lung bases. Blunting of the costophrenic angles results from chylous effusions.

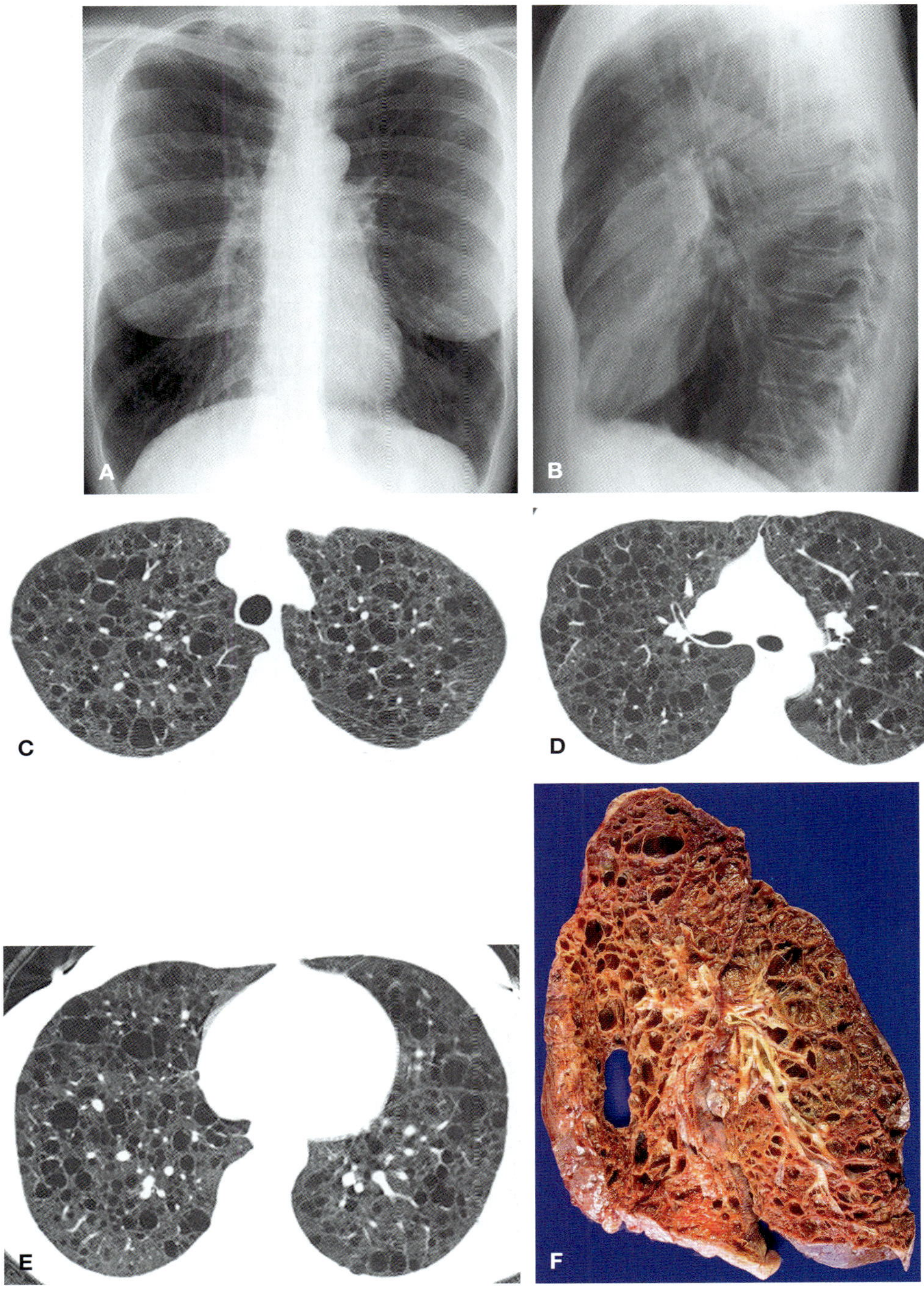

Figure 25.9. Lymphangiomyomatosis. PA (**A**) and lateral (**B**) chest radiographs show large lung volumes and a mild reticular pattern. **C–E:** HRCTs at levels from the apices (**C**) to the lung bases (**E**) show rounded, thin-walled cysts. Distribution is uniform. **F:** This patient's lung, removed at the time of lung transplantation, shows a diffuse cystic abnormality, involving the lung bases to the same extent as the upper lobes.

HRCT Findings

On HRCT, patients with TSC-LAM and S-LAM characteristically show numerous, isolated, thin-walled, rounded lung cysts (see Fig. 25.9). These cysts usually range from 2 to 5 mm in diameter, but may be larger. Their size tends to increase with progression of the disease. In patients with extensive disease in which 80% or more of the lung parenchyma is involved, most cysts are more than 1 cm in diameter. The walls of the lung cysts usually are thin and faintly perceptible. Irregularly shaped lung cysts, as are seen in patients with LCH, are uncommon.

The cysts are most often distributed diffusely throughout the lungs, from apex to base, and no lung zone is spared (see Fig. 25.9); diffuse lung involvement is seen even in patients with mild disease.

In most patients, the lung parenchyma between the cysts appears normal on HRCT. In some cases, however, a slight increase in linear interstitial markings, interlobular septal thickening, or patchy areas of ground-glass opacity also are seen. The latter probably represent areas of pulmonary hemorrhage.

Some patients with TSC-LAM show small lung nodules, ranging from a few mm to 8 mm in diameter, with a random distribution, representing micronodular pneumocyte hyperplasia; this finding is not seen in patients with S-LAM.

In many cases, a specific CT diagnosis may be made when characteristic diffuse, thin-walled, rounded lung cysts are identified in a female of childbearing age.

On HRCT, as with chest radiography, pneumothorax may be associated with cysts in patients with LAM. Other features of LAM include pleural effusion and hilar, mediastinal, and retrocrural adenopathy. Renal angiomyolipomas may be visible on scans through the upper abdomen. These occur in more than 90% of patients with TSC-LAM and in 30% to 50% of patients with S-LAM (Figs. 25.10 and 25.11). Fatty lesions in other organs including the liver and heart may also be seen in some cases (Fig. 25.11). Sclerotic bone lesions (SBLs) can also help differentiate TSC-LAM from S-LAM. These SBLs closely resemble bone islands on CT with dense sclerotic foci within the medullary portion of the bone, and

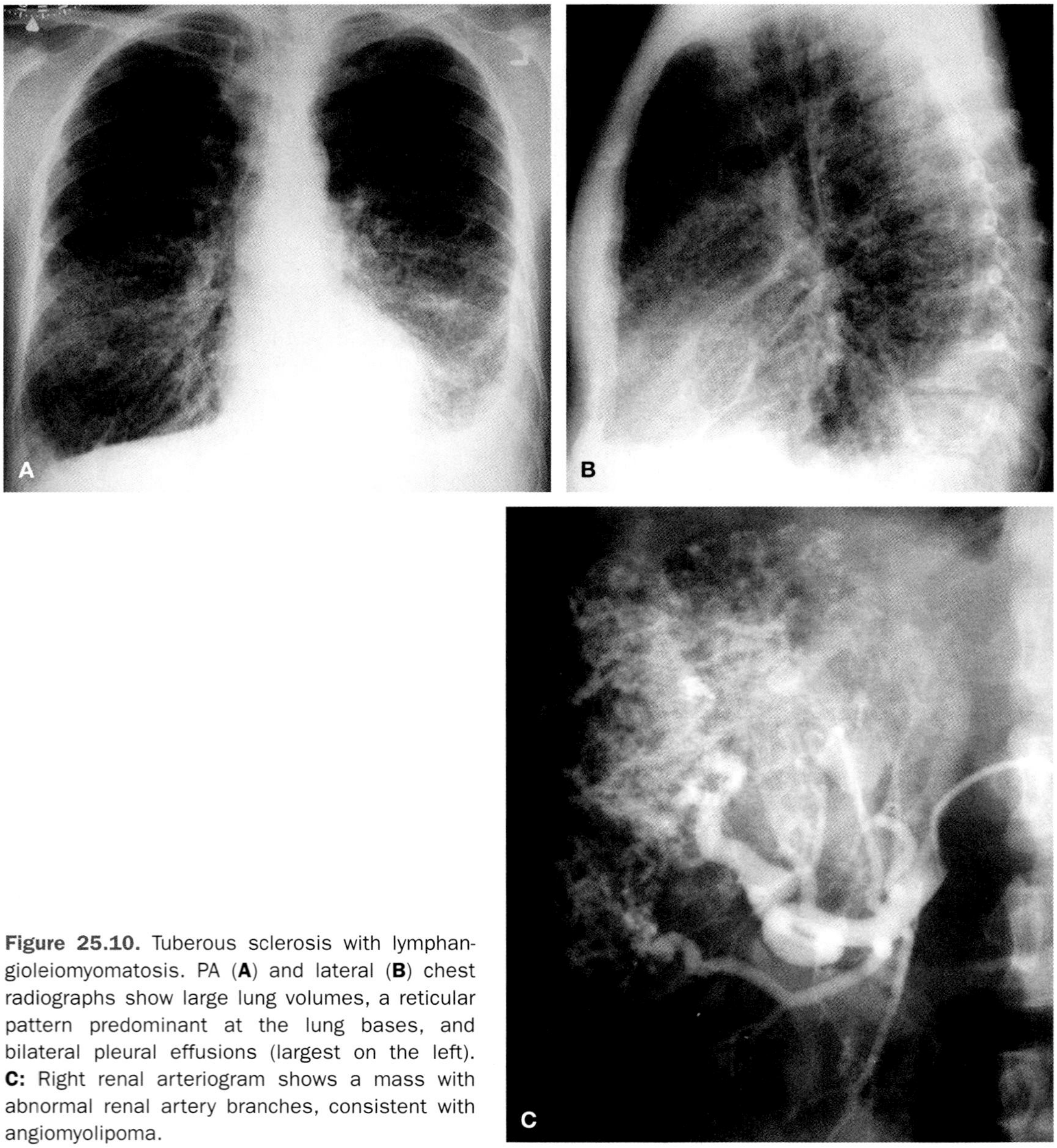

Figure 25.10. Tuberous sclerosis with lymphangioleiomyomatosis. PA (**A**) and lateral (**B**) chest radiographs show large lung volumes, a reticular pattern predominant at the lung bases, and bilateral pleural effusions (largest on the left). **C:** Right renal arteriogram shows a mass with abnormal renal artery branches, consistent with angiomyolipoma.

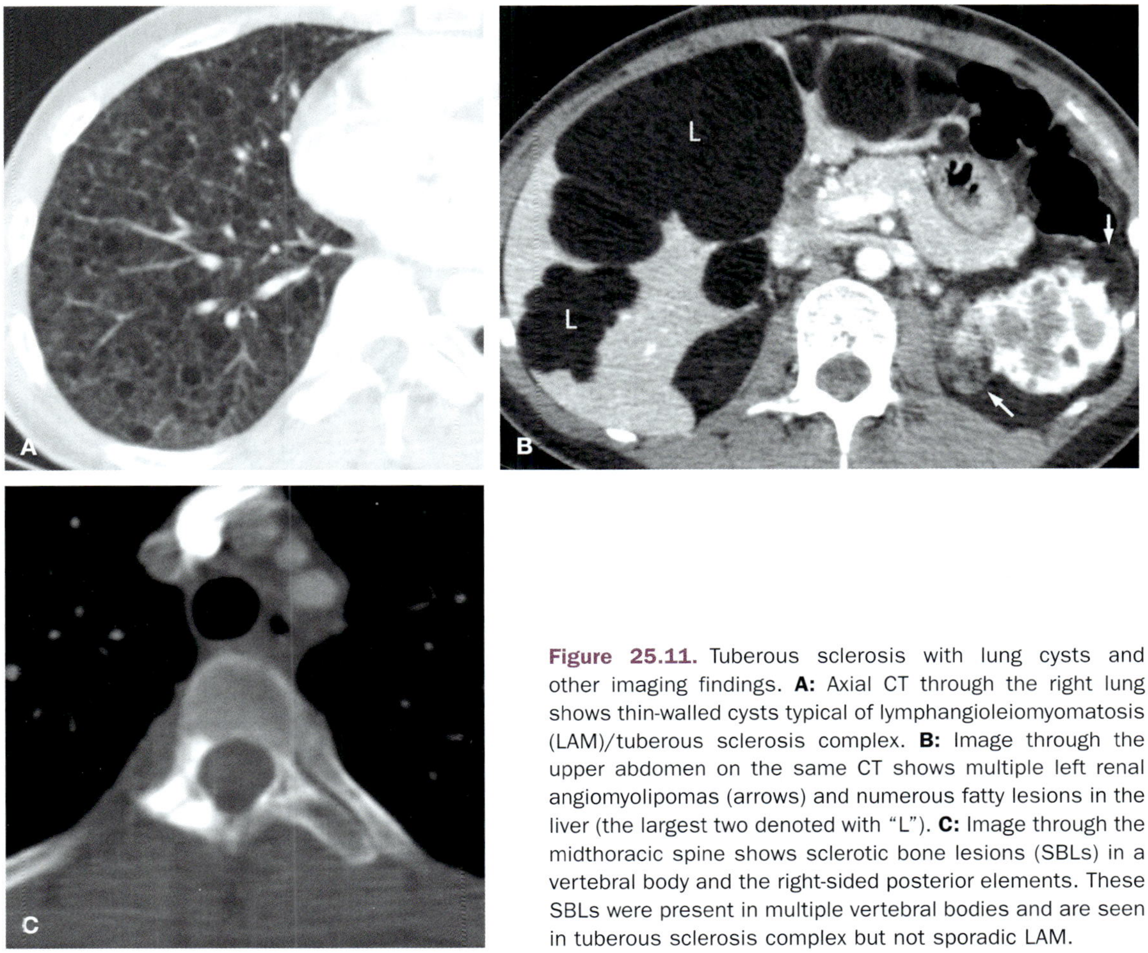

Figure 25.11. Tuberous sclerosis with lung cysts and other imaging findings. **A:** Axial CT through the right lung shows thin-walled cysts typical of lymphangioleiomyomatosis (LAM)/tuberous sclerosis complex. **B:** Image through the upper abdomen on the same CT shows multiple left renal angiomyolipomas (arrows) and numerous fatty lesions in the liver (the largest two denoted with "L"). **C:** Image through the midthoracic spine shows sclerotic bone lesions (SBLs) in a vertebral body and the right-sided posterior elements. These SBLs were present in multiple vertebral bodies and are seen in tuberous sclerosis complex but not sporadic LAM.

the presence of four or more SBLs has a reported specificity of 97% for TSC-LAM (Fig. 25.11).

NEUROFIBROMATOSIS

Neurofibromatosis is a common genetic disorder, affecting about 1 in 3000 individuals. Thoracic manifestations are protean and include the following:

1. Rib abnormalities, including ribbon ribs and rib notching
2. Scoliosis
3. Cutaneous or subcutaneous neurofibromas mimicking the presence of lung nodules on chest radiographs
4. Intercostal or mediastinal neurofibroma or schwannoma (see Figs. 8.64-8.71 in Chapter 8)
5. Paraganglioma
6. Thoracic meningocele (see Fig. 8.74 in Chapter 8)

Lung disease is present in 10% to 20% of adult patients with neurofibromatosis. It is characterized histologically by bullae in the upper lobes and interstitial fibrosis at the lung bases. Patients typically present with dyspnea.

Radiographs usually show upper lobe lucency or bullae, which usually are symmetrical. A reticular pattern, which sometimes is characterized by Kerley B lines, is seen at the lung bases in 50% of cases (Fig. 25.12). Lung volumes typically are increased, with flattening of the diaphragms. HRCT may show isolated cysts or bullae (Fig. 25.13).

LIP, AMYLOID, AND LCDD

LIP is currently included as an idiopathic interstitial pneumonia according to the American Thoracic Society and the European Respiratory Society, but is a broad term that corresponds to a variety of diseases involving lymphoid proliferation, interstitial fibrosis, and cystic lung disease. Moreover, definitions of LIP on histology and radiology vary, leading to further confusion. "Pathologic LIP" has been traditionally defined as a dense interstitial lymphoid infiltrate, including lymphocytes, plasma cells, and histiocytes. These findings correlate with some radiologic features traditionally described in LIP including ground-glass opacity, nodules, consolidation, and interstitial fibrosis. Cystic lung disease, however, usually represents a distinct entity that does not correlate with classic cases of "pathologic LIP" on histologic

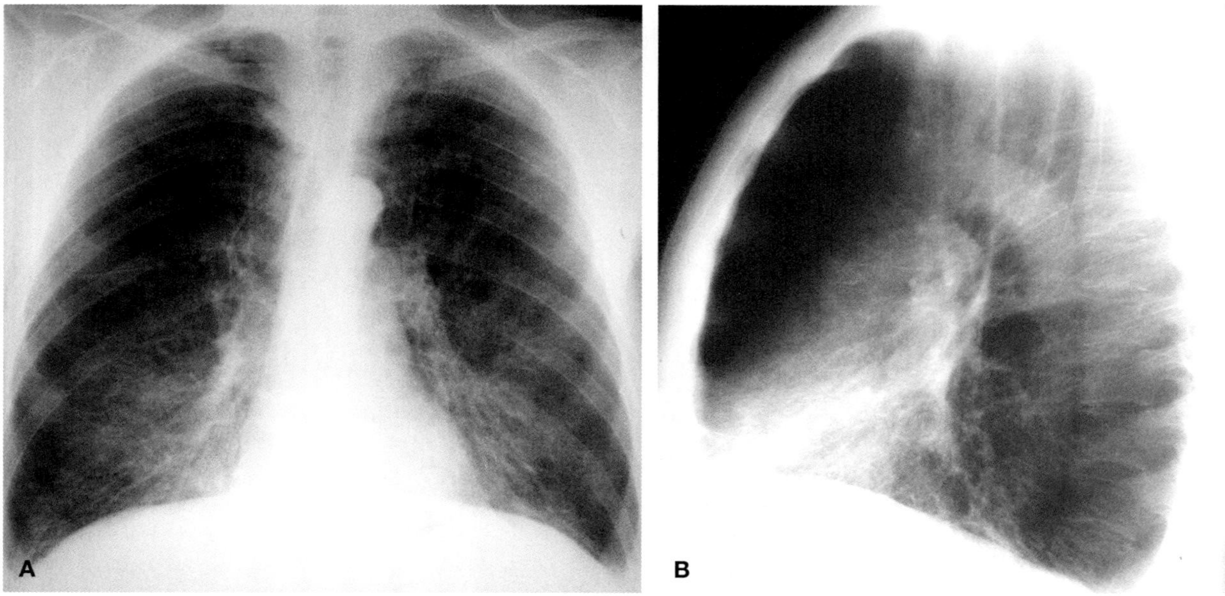

Figure 25.12. Neurofibromatosis. PA (**A**) and lateral (**B**) chest radiographs show large lung volumes with upper lobe lucency and a reticular pattern predominant at the lung bases.

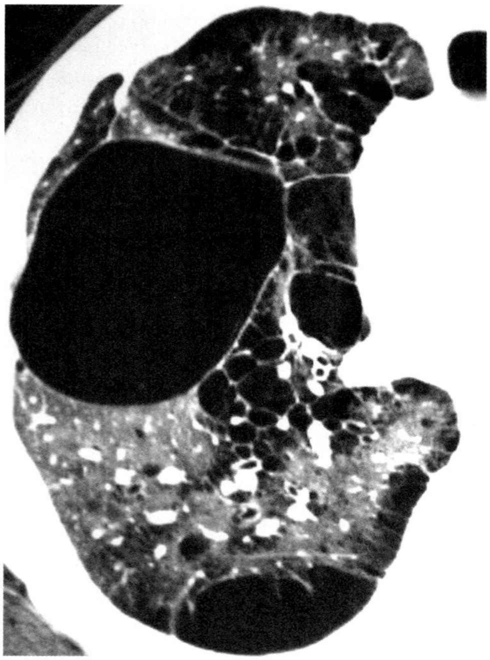

Figure 25.13. Neurofibromatosis. HRCT shows cysts and bullae indistinguishable from emphysema.

analysis. As such, recent groups have proposed a designation of "radiologic LIP" or "autoimmune-related cystic lung disease" to distinguish this unique entity and reduce confusion. This section focuses on the cystic lung disease of "radiologic LIP" (see Chapter 14 for LIP in the context of interstitial pneumonia).

The cysts in "radiologic LIP" are most commonly associated with Sjögren syndrome, but appear similar on imaging to other causes of protein deposition including LCDD and amyloid. While the exact mechanism of cyst formation is unknown, a current theory is that (1) protein deposition recruits macrophages; (2) these macrophages express metalloproteinases; (3) the metalloproteinases cause breakdown of elastin and collagen with subsequent cyst development.

On HRCT, the cysts are typically multiple, thin-walled and seen in relation to pulmonary vessels (see Figs. 14.32, 14.34, and 14.35 in Chapter 14). The cysts may be small or large, round or oval in shape, and tend to be fewer in number than those seen in patients with LCH or LAM. Small areas of calcification/ossification may be seen along cyst walls. Ground-glass opacity nodules that represent areas of lymphoid hyperplasia or MALT lymphoma can also be seen.

Amyloid and LCDD both produce cystic lung disease due to deposition of amyloid protein and non-amyloid light chains in the lungs (see Chapter 21), respectively. LCDD is characterized by the granular deposition of a nonfibrillary amorphous protein along basement membranes and does not bind Congo red as does amyloidosis.

Both entities are associated with protein-producing systemic disorders such as multiple myeloma or a lymphoproliferative disease, especially Waldenström macroglobulinemia. In addition, the kidneys, the liver, and the heart are commonly affected to varying degrees.

Protein deposition almost entirely limited to the lung and not associated with myeloma has also been reported, sometimes in association with Sjögren syndrome (hence the utility of the term "radiologic LIP"). In clinical practice, the CT appearance of cysts in amyloid and LCDD is indistinguishable, and also similar to "radiologic LIP" (Figs. 25.14 and 25.15; Table 25.4).

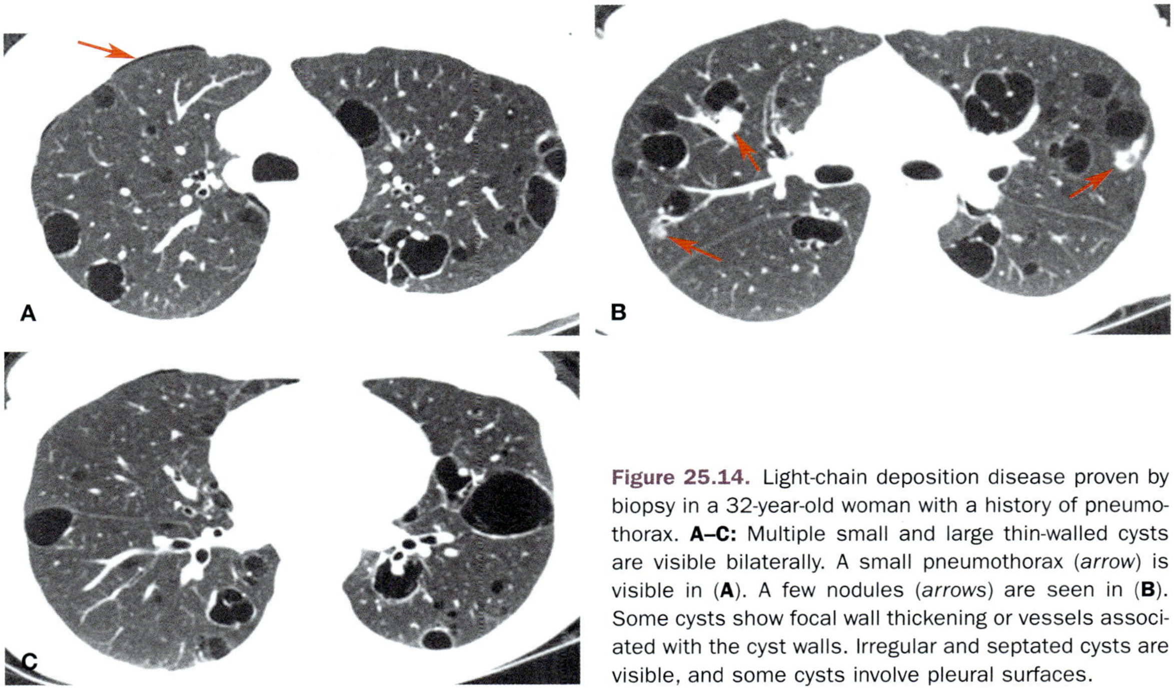

Figure 25.14. Light-chain deposition disease proven by biopsy in a 32-year-old woman with a history of pneumothorax. **A–C:** Multiple small and large thin-walled cysts are visible bilaterally. A small pneumothorax (*arrow*) is visible in (**A**). A few nodules (*arrows*) are seen in (**B**). Some cysts show focal wall thickening or vessels associated with the cyst walls. Irregular and septated cysts are visible, and some cysts involve pleural surfaces.

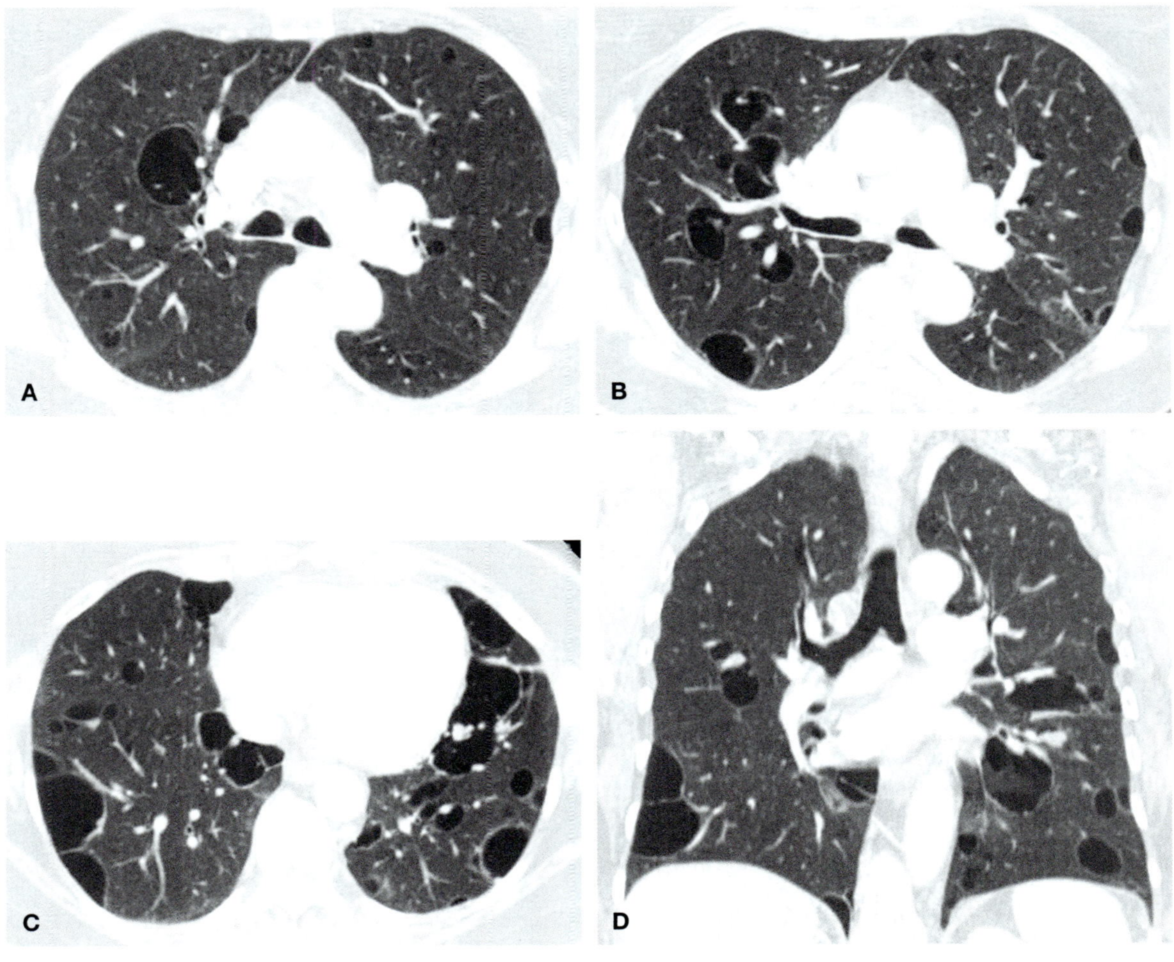

Figure 25.15. Light-chain deposition disease proven by biopsy in a 59-year-old woman. **A–C:** Multiple small and large thin-walled cysts are visible bilaterally. Focal cyst wall thickening or vessels in relation to the cyst walls are visible. Some cysts involve the pleural surfaces, and some appear septated. **D:** A coronal reconstruction shows a basal predominance of the cysts.

Table 25.4 Amyloid and Light-Chain Deposition Disease

Deposition of protein
Often occur in association with multiple myeloma or lymphoproliferative disease
Rarely with lung involvement only
Thin-walled perivascular cysts, usually up to 2 cm or larger
Resemble the appearance of radiologic lymphoid interstitial pneumonia
Cyst walls may have nodular thickening and/or ossification

BIRT-HOGG-DUBÉ SYNDROME

This rare autosomal dominant disorder is characterized by (a) lung cysts; (b) fibrofolliculomas of the skin distributed over the face, neck, and upper trunk; and (c) renal tumors ranging from benign oncocytoma to renal cell carcinoma.

Lung cysts are generally limited in number. Cysts are thin walled, often subpleural in location, and may be rounded or lentiform in shape; they may appear septated (Fig. 25.16).

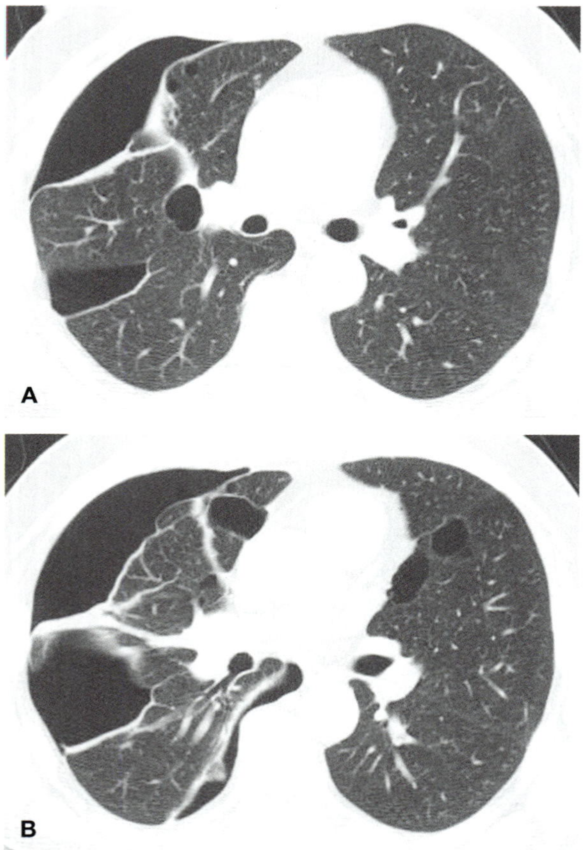

Figure 25.16. Birt-Hogg-Dubé (BHD) syndrome. **A, B:** HRCT images through the mid- and lower thorax, respectively, show several large thin-walled cysts that predominantly involve pleural surfaces and fissures. Histologically, cysts in BHD characteristically extend into both the visceral pleura and interlobular septa. A pneumothorax is also present.

Table 25.5 Birt-Hogg-Dubé Syndrome

Rare autosomal dominant disorder
Lung cysts
Fibrofolliculomas, face, neck, and upper trunk
Renal tumors, benign oncocytoma to renal cell carcinoma
Lung cysts limited in number
Thin walled, often subpleural, may involve fissures
Rounded or lenticular in shape
Cysts are often larger than those in lymphangioleiomyomatosis and Langerhans cell histiocytosis
Predominate and medial lung zones
Pneumothorax

Subpleural cysts, which may involve the fissures, are more frequent than in other cystic diseases (Fig. 25.16). Cysts are often larger than those in LAM and LCH, up to 8 cm in diameter, and predominate in the lower and medial lung zones; bilateral cysts are typical. Pneumothorax may result and can be the initial presentation of the disease. The CT demonstration of lung cysts in a patient with a renal tumor often suggests the diagnosis for the first time (Table 25.5).

SUGGESTED READINGS

Aberle DR, Hansell DM, Brown K, Tashkin DP. Lymphangiomyomatosis: CT, chest radiographic, and functional correlations. *Radiology.* 1990;176(2):381-387.

Adriaensen ME, Schaefer-Prokop CM, Duyndam DA, Zonnenberg BA, Prokop M. Radiological evidence of lymphangioleiomyomatosis in female and male patients with tuberous sclerosis complex. *Clin Radiol.* 2011;66(7):625-628.

Avila NA, Dwyer AJ, Rabel A, Darling T, Hong C-H, Moss J. CT of sclerotic bone lesions: imaging features differentiating tuberous sclerosis complex with lymphangioleiomyomatosis from sporadic lymphangioleiomymatosis. *Radiology.* 2010;254(3):851-857. doi:10.1148/radiol.09090227

Brauner MW, Grenier P, Mouelhi MM, Mompoint D, Lenoir S. Pulmonary histiocytosis X: evaluation with high resolution CT. *Radiology.* 1989;172(1):255-258.

Chu SC, Horiba K, Usuki J, et al. Comprehensive evaluation of 35 patients with lymphangioleiomyomatosis. *Chest.* 1999;115(4):1041-1052.

Colombat M, Stern M, Groussard O, et al. Pulmonary cystic disorder related to light chain deposition disease. *Am J Respir Crit Care Med.* 2006;173(7):777-780.

Egashira R, Kondo T, Hirai T, et al. CT findings of thoracic manifestations of primary Sjögren syndrome: radiologic-pathologic correlation. *Radiographics.* 2013;33(7):1933-1949. doi:10.1148/rg.337125107

Fraune C, Churg A, Yi ES, et al. Lymphoid interstitial pneumonia (LIP) revisited: a critical reappraisal of the histologic spectrum of 'radiologic' and 'Pathologic' LIP in the context of diffuse benign lymphoid proliferations of the lung. *Am J Surg Pathol.* 2023;47(3):281-295. doi:10.1097/PAS.0000000000002014

Furuya M, Nakatani Y. Birt-Hogg-Dube syndrome: clinicopathological features of the lung. *J Clin Pathol.* 2013;66(3):178-186.

Gupta et al., 2015 Gupta N, Vassallo R, Wikenheiser-Brokamp KA, McCormack FX. Diffuse cystic lung disease. Part I. *Am J Respir Crit Care Med.* 2015;191(12):1354-1366.

Gupta N, Vassallo R, Wikenheiser-Brokamp KA, McCormack FX. Diffuse cystic lung disease. Part II. *Am J Respir Crit Care Med.* 2015;192(1):17-29.

Howarth DM, Gilchrist GS, Mullan BP, Wiseman GA, Edmonson JH, Schomberg PJ. Langerhans cell histiocytosis: diagnosis, natural history, management, and outcome. *Cancer.* 1999;85(10):2278-2290.

Jensen L, Howard M. Cystic lung disease from protein deposition: pathogenesis and associated conditions. *Curr Radiol Rep.* 2018;6(3):12. doi:10.1007/s40134-018-0271-y

Johkoh T, Müller NL, Pickford HA, et al. Lymphocytic interstitial pneumonia: thin-section CT findings in 22 patients. *Radiology.* 1999;212(2):567-572.

Johnson SR, Cordier JF, Lazor R, et al.. European respiratory society guidelines for the diagnosis and management of lymphangioleiomyomatosis. *Eur Respir J.* 2010;35(1):14-26.

Kirchner J, Stein A, Viel K, et al. Pulmonary lymphangioleiomyomatosis: high-resolution CT findings. *Eur Radiol.* 1999;9(1):49-54.

Kitaichi M, Nishimura K, Itoh H, Izumi T. Pulmonary lymphangioleiomyomatosis: a report of 46 patients including a clinicopathologic study of prognostic factors. *Am J Respir Crit Care Med.* 1995;151(2 pt 1):527-533.

Lenoir S, Grenier P, Brauner MW, et al. Pulmonary lymphangiomyomatosis and tuberous sclerosis: comparison of radiographic and thin-section CT findings. *Radiology.* 1990;175(2):329-334.

Moore AD, Godwin JD, Müller NL, et al. Pulmonary histiocytosis X: comparison of radiographic and CT findings. *Radiology.* 1989;172(1):249-254.

Müller NL, Chiles C, Kullnig P. Pulmonary lymphangiomyomatosis: correlation of CT with radiographic and functional findings. *Radiology.* 1990;175(2):335-339.

Templeton PA, McLoud TC, Müller NL, Shepard JA, Moore EH. Pulmonary lymphangioleiomyomatosis: CT and pathologic findings. *J Comput Assist Tomogr.* 1989;13(1):54-57.

Tobino K, Hirai T, Johkoh T, et al. Differentiation between Birt Hogg Dube syndrome and lymphangioleiomyomatosis: quantitative analysis of pulmonary cysts on computed tomography of the chest in 66 females. *Eur J Radiol.* 2012;81(6):1340-1346.

Toro JR, Pautler SE, Stewart L, et al. Lung cysts, spontaneous pneumothorax, and genetic associations in 89 families with Birt-Hogg-Dube syndrome. *Am J Respir Crit Care Med.* 2007;175(10):1044-1053.

Section Six

Pleural Abnormalities

Chapter 26

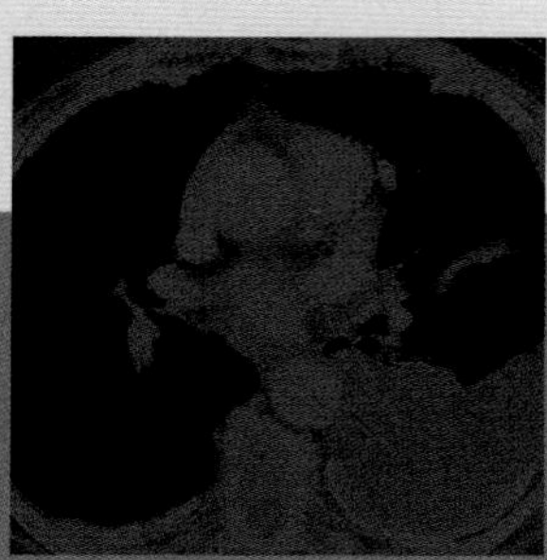

Travis S. Henry

The Pleura and Pleural Disease

INTERLOBAR FISSURES

The interlobar fissures represent invaginations of the visceral pleura that separate or partially separate the lobes of the lung. Recognizing the fissures is essential in the localization and diagnosis of both pleural and parenchymal abnormalities. The fissures are also discussed in Chapter 1.

The Major (Oblique) Fissure

On the left, the major fissure separates the lower lobe from the upper lobe. On the right, it separates the lower lobe from the upper and middle lobes. The major fissures originate posteriorly, above the level of the aortic arch, near the level of the fifth thoracic vertebra, and angle anteriorly and inferiorly, nearly parallel to the sixth rib. They terminate along the anterior diaphragmatic pleural surface of each hemithorax, several centimeters posterior to the anterior chest wall (Fig. 26.1 and Fig. 1.1 in Chapter 1).

Portions of one or both major fissures are almost always visible on the lateral radiograph. A thin triangular opacity representing fat is visible in about 20% of cases, at the point a major fissure contacts the hemidiaphragm. A similar opacity may be seen in the presence of a small amount of pleural fluid. Methods for distinguishing the major fissures on a lateral radiograph are reviewed in Chapter 1.

The major fissures are not clearly seen on frontal radiographs in normal subjects. In 5% to 10% of patients, however, a subtle arcuate opacity (Fig. 26.1) may be seen in the upper thorax, extending superiorly and medially from the lateral chest wall, representing contact of the superior part of the major fissure with the posterolateral thorax; this opacity is likely related to a small amount of fat of fluid entering the fissure. Typically, it is sharply marginated on its undersurface and ill defined superiorly. A similar but more pronounced opacity may be seen with pleural effusion extending into the posterior part of the major fissure.

On computed tomography (CT), the major fissures are oriented obliquely to the scan plane, and because of volume averaging, their appearance is variable and depends on slice thickness.

With thick slices, the fissures themselves are visible in only 40% of cases, although the location of each fissure can usually be inferred because of the presence of an avascular band, several centimeters thick, within the lung parenchyma. These bands appear "avascular" because of the small size of vessels located in the peripheral lung on either side of the fissure.

On CT obtained using thin slices, the major fissures usually appear as thin, well-defined lines surrounded by a plane of relatively avascular lung measuring about 1 cm thick. The orientation of the major fissures varies at different levels (Fig. 1.2 in Chapter 1). In the upper thorax, the major fissures angle posterolaterally from the mediastinum. Within the lower thorax, the major fissures angle anterolaterally from the mediastinum. In nearly 20% of cases, a focal thickening of the fissure is seen on CT just above its point of contact with the diaphragm; this represents fat extending into the fissure.

If a portion of the fissure is invisible on high-resolution CT (HRCT), it likely indicates that the fissure is incomplete with partial fusion of the lobes (Fig. 26.2). Incomplete fissures provide a pathway for collateral ventilation or spread of disease from one lobe to another. The right major fissure is incomplete in 70%, and some degree of fusion is present between the lower lobe and the upper lobe in 70% and between the lower lobe and middle lobe in 50%. On the left, the major fissure has been reported to be incomplete in 40% to 70% of patients.

In some cases, cardiac motion during the scan results in an artifact termed the *double-fissure sign*; when this artifact is present, the fissure is visible in two locations on the same scan separated by a few mm.

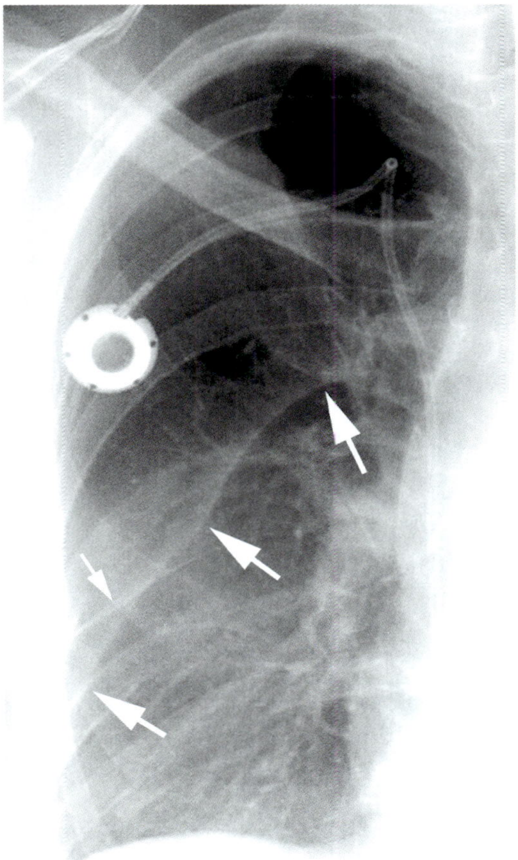

Figure 26.1. Small pleural effusion outlining the posterior right major fissure. The normal location of the major fissure where it contacts the posterolateral chest wall is well shown (*large arrows*). As in this case, it is sharply marginated on its undersurface and ill defined superiorly. The minor fissure is also visible (*small arrow*).

The Minor (Horizontal) Fissure

The minor or horizontal fissure separates the superior aspect of the right middle lobe from the right upper lobe. The minor fissure is incomplete in more than 80% of cases, most often laterally.

On a frontal radiograph, the minor fissure or a portion of the fissure is visible in 50% to 80% of cases, appearing as a roughly horizontal line, generally at or near the level of the anterior fourth rib. Its contour is variable, but its lateral part is often visible inferior to its medial part. Medially, the fissure usually appears to arise at the level of the right hilum and interlobar pulmonary artery.

On the lateral radiograph, the anterior part of the fissure often appears inferior to its posterior part. The posterior part of the fissure may be seen to end at the major fissure or may appear to extend posterior to it.

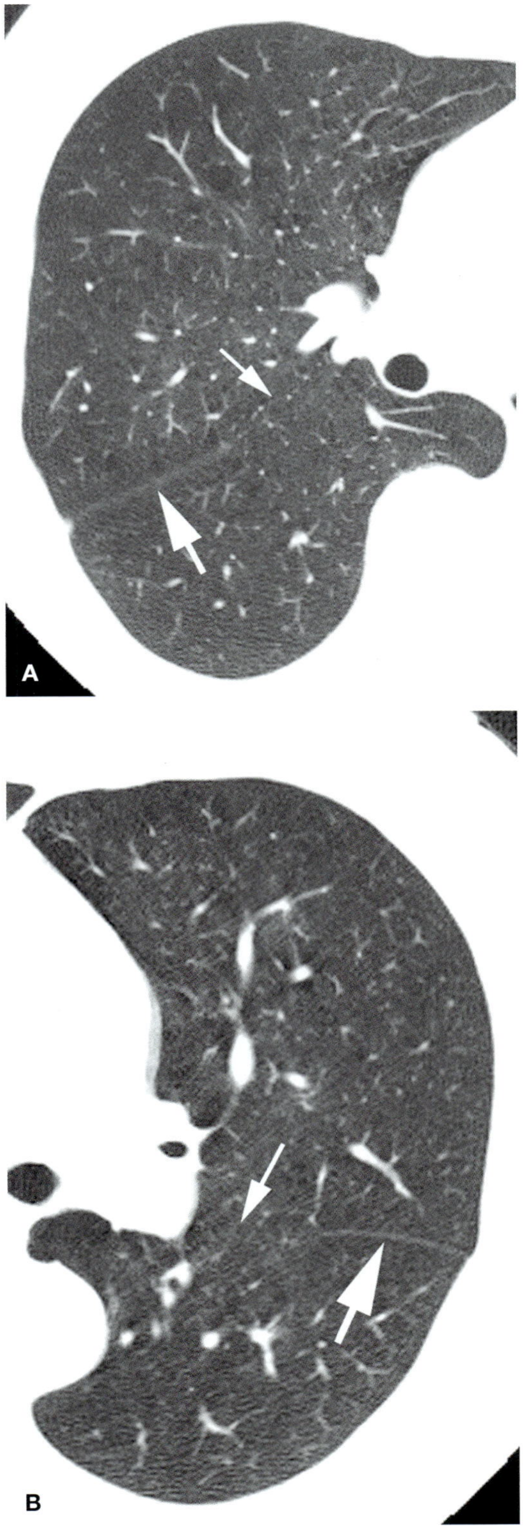

Figure 26.2. Incomplete major fissures. **A and B:** HRCT shows normal-appearing major fissures laterally (*large arrows*). Medially, the fissures are incomplete and invisible on HRCT (*small arrows*).

On CT obtained with thick slices, the minor fissure is rarely visible, as its position generally parallels the scan plane. Characteristically, however, the position of the minor fissure can be inferred because of a broad avascular region in the anterior portion of the right lung, anterior to the major fissure, at the level of the bronchus intermedius. This avascular region represents peripheral lung on each side of the fissure, lying in or near the plane of scan. The avascular region is often triangular, with the one corner of the triangle at the pulmonary hilum and the other two corners laterally. However, there is considerable variation in the appearance of the minor fissure due to variations in its orientation and curvature. In some cases, the avascular plane of the minor fissure appears rectangular, round, or elliptical.

The appearance of the minor fissure on HRCT scans is quite variable (Fig. 26.3 and Fig. 1.2 in Chapter 1). Depending on its orientation and contour, the fissure may appear as (1) a linear opacity, directed from anterior to posterior; (2) a linear opacity extending from medial to lateral, paralleling and anterior to the major fissure (see Fig. 26.3A); (3) a circle or ring (see Fig. 26.3B); or (4) an ill-defined opacity or avascular region resulting from the fissure lying in the plane of scan (see Fig. 26.3C).

Because the minor fissure often angles caudally, from posterior to anterior, the lower lobe, middle lobe, and upper lobe can all be seen on a single HRCT scan (see Fig. 26.3A). If this is the case, the major and minor fissures can have a similar appearance, with the major fissure being posterior and the minor fissure anterior; in this situation, the lower lobe is most posterior, the upper lobe is most anterior, and the middle lobe is in the middle. If the minor fissure is concave caudally, it can appear ring shaped, with the middle lobe in the center of the ring (see Fig. 26.3B).

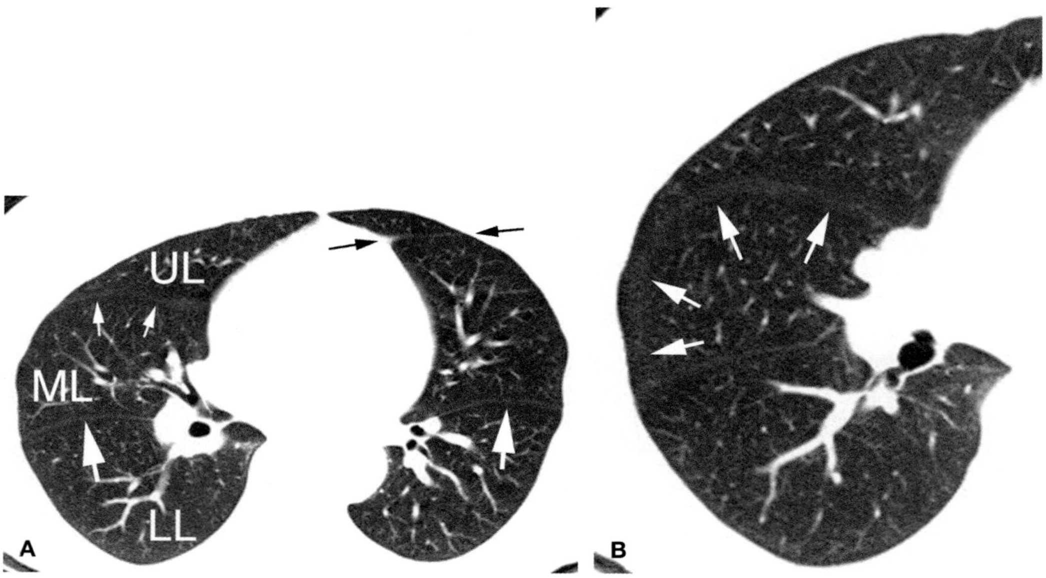

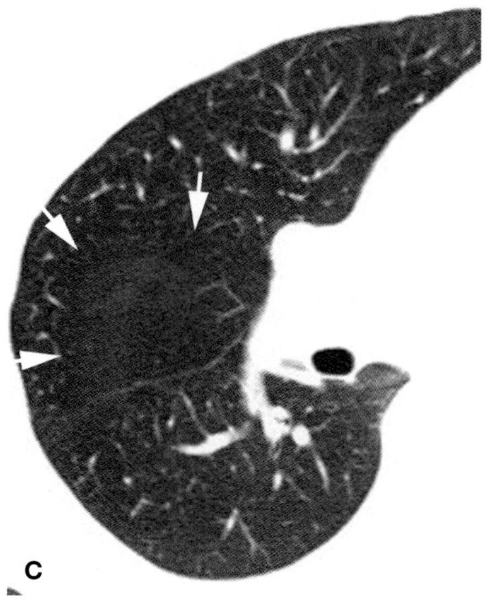

Figure 26.3. CT appearances of the minor fissure. **A:** HRCT through the lung bases shows the major fissures (*large arrows*) and the right minor fissure as a linear opacity extending from medial to lateral (*small white arrows*). The fissures delineate the upper (*UL*), middle (*ML*), and lower lobes (*LL*). A left minor fissure is also visible (*black arrows*), separating the lingula from the remainder of the upper lobe. **B:** At a higher level in the same patient, the minor fissure is visible as an arcuate or ringlike opacity (*arrows*). **C:** Slightly cephalad to **(B)**, the fissure lies in the scan plane. The region of the fissure is visible as an avascular area (*arrows*).

Accessory Fissures

Accessory fissures separate a lung segment or a part of a lobe from the remainder of a lobe; numerous accessory fissures have been identified. As many as 50% of lungs show an accessory fissure, but these are less often visible radiographically.

An *azygos fissure* is present in 1 in 200 subjects, defining the presence of an *azygos lobe* (Fig. 26.4). An azygos lobe represents parts of the apical or posterior segments of the right upper lobe. An azygos fissure and azygos lobe are formed when the azygos vein invaginates the right upper lobe during gestation. The azygos fissure consists of four layers of pleura (two parietal and two visceral) and contains the arch of the azygos vein. On the frontal radiograph, the azygos fissure has a characteristic curvilinear appearance adjacent to the right mediastinum, convex laterally; the azygos vein has a teardrop appearance at the inferior extent of the fissure. The azygos fissure is identifiable on CT as a thin, curved line. It extends from the right brachiocephalic vein, anteriorly, to a position adjacent to the right posterolateral aspect of the T4 or T5 vertebral body (see Fig. 26.4B and C). A left "azygos" fissure, associated with the left superior intercostal vein, is rarely seen.

If the right lung collapses (eg, spontaneous pneumothorax, right lung surgery), the azygos vein can "escape" the azygos fissure and assume its normal position along the mediastinum. This results in an empty azygos fissure on imaging. The empty azygos fissure is a curiosity of little clinical consequence other than indicating prior surgery or pneumothorax (Fig. 26.4D).

The *inferior accessory fissure* separates the medial basal segment of either lower lobe from the remaining basal segments. It is present anatomically in 30% to 45% of lobes. On plain radiographs, this fissure is visible in 10%, extending superiorly and medially from the medial third of the hemidiaphragm. On CT, it is seen in 15% of cases, extending laterally and anteriorly from the region of the inferior pulmonary ligament to join the major fissure (Fig. 26.5).

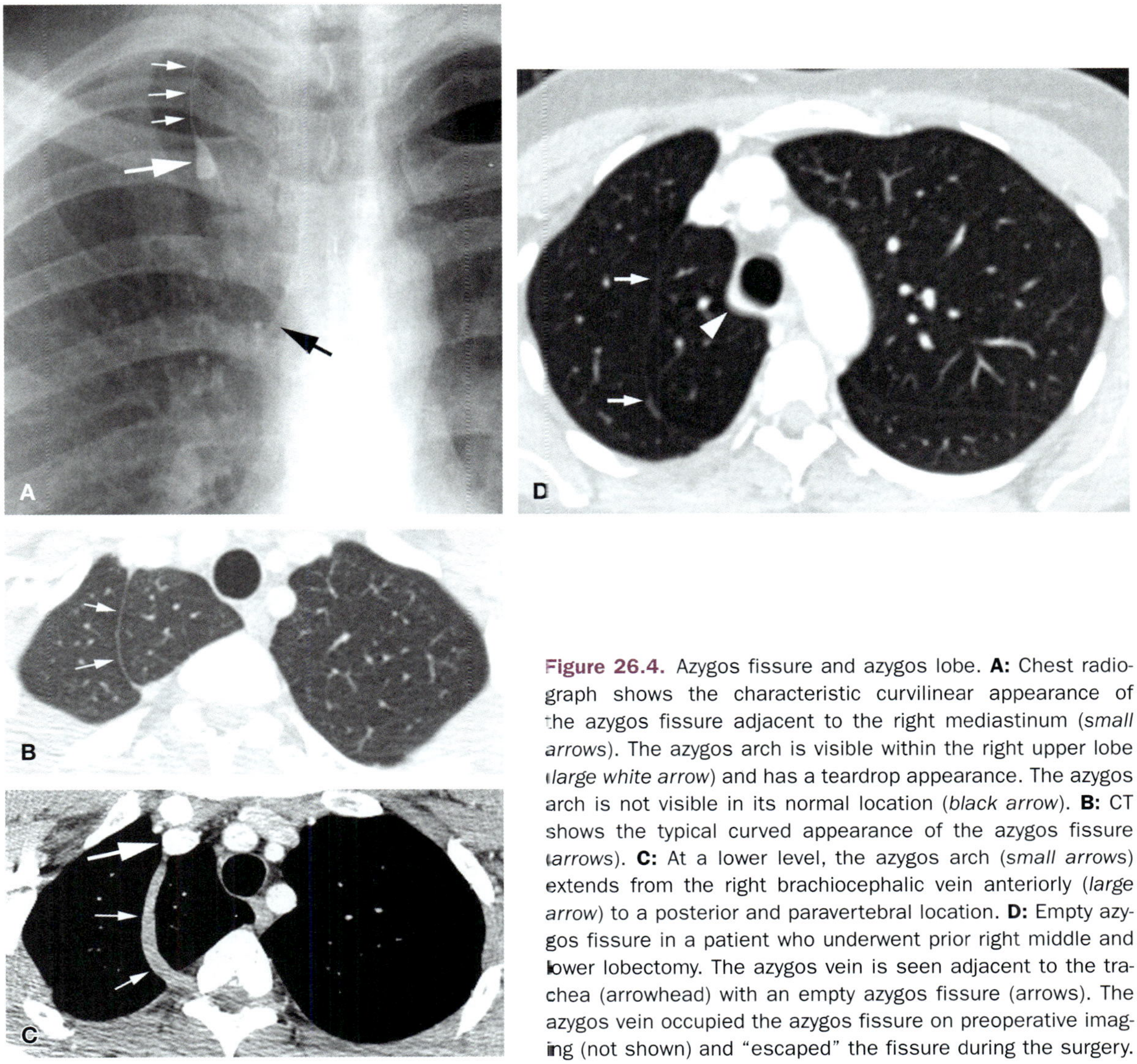

Figure 26.4. Azygos fissure and azygos lobe. **A:** Chest radiograph shows the characteristic curvilinear appearance of the azygos fissure adjacent to the right mediastinum (*small arrows*). The azygos arch is visible within the right upper lobe (*large white arrow*) and has a teardrop appearance. The azygos arch is not visible in its normal location (*black arrow*). **B:** CT shows the typical curved appearance of the azygos fissure (*arrows*). **C:** At a lower level, the azygos arch (*small arrows*) extends from the right brachiocephalic vein anteriorly (*large arrow*) to a posterior and paravertebral location. **D:** Empty azygos fissure in a patient who underwent prior right middle and lower lobectomy. The azygos vein is seen adjacent to the trachea (arrowhead) with an empty azygos fissure (arrows). The azygos vein occupied the azygos fissure on preoperative imaging (not shown) and "escaped" the fissure during the surgery.

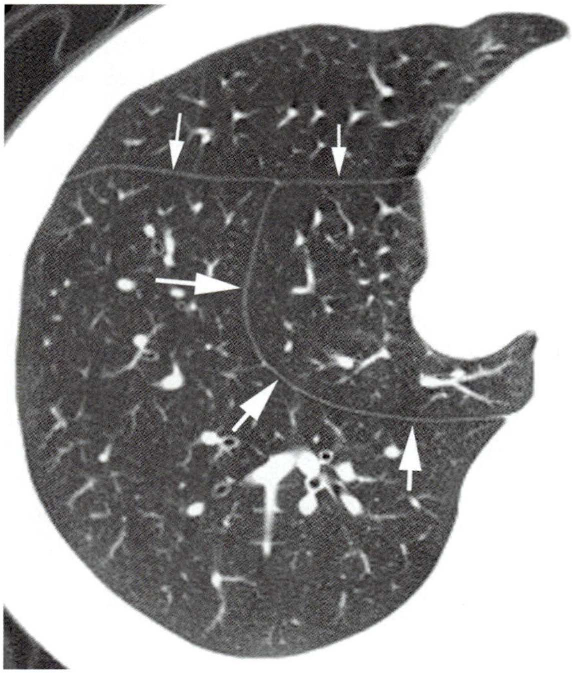

Figure 26.5. Inferior accessory fissure. The fissure (*large arrows*) separates the medial basal segment of the lower lobe from the remainder of the basal segments. The major fissure (*small arrows*) is noted anteriorly.

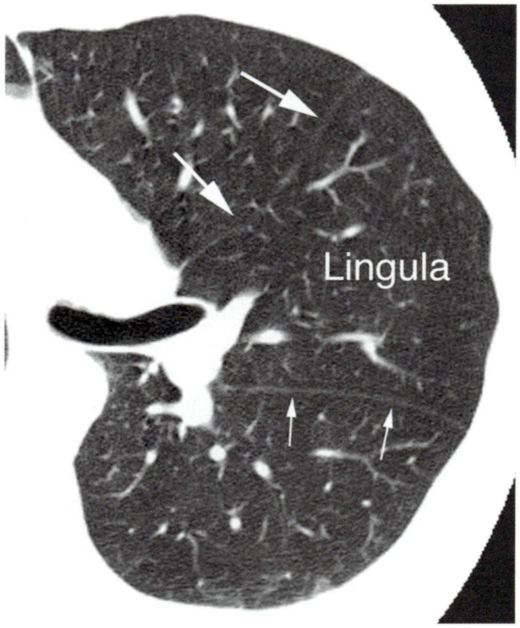

Figure 26.6. Left minor fissure. The minor fissure (*large arrows*) separates the lingular segments from the remainder of the upper lobe. The major fissure (*small arrows*) is also seen.

The *superior accessory fissure* demarcates the superior segment from the remainder of the lower lobe; it is more common on the right. It is seen at about the same level as the minor fissure.

The *left minor fissure* is present anatomically in approximately 10% of normal lungs, separating the lingula from the remainder of the left upper lobe (Figs. 26.3A and 26.6). It is visible on plain radiographs in about 1%, appearing somewhat higher than the right minor fissure.

INFERIOR PULMONARY LIGAMENTS AND PHRENIC NERVES

The right and left inferior pulmonary ligaments each represent a double layer of pleura that serves to anchor the lung to the mediastinum. They are formed as reflections of the visceral pleura lining the medial surfaces of the lower lobes onto the mediastinal pleural surface. They extend inferiorly and posteriorly from just below the pulmonary hila to the diaphragm. The ligaments can terminate before reaching the diaphragm or extend over the medial diaphragmatic surface. They may divide the medial pleural space below the hila into anterior and posterior compartments. The ligaments may also contain systemic vessels supplying the lung.

The inferior pulmonary ligaments are invisible on chest radiographs. On CT, they are visible as very short, thin, linear, or triangular opacities below the level of the right and left inferior pulmonary veins and often adjacent to the esophagus (Fig. 26.7). Although they do not extend into the lung parenchyma, they often appear contiguous with a connective tissue septum in the medial lung, termed the *intersublobar septum* (see Fig. 26.7B). On CT, the inferior pulmonary ligaments are visible in 40% to 70% of cases.

Similar thin lines may be seen on CT, anterior to the inferior pulmonary ligaments, representing pleural reflections over the right and left phrenic nerves (see Fig. 26.7). On the right, this opacity is usually seen lateral to the inferior vena cava (see Fig. 26.7A). The pleural reflections may be seen to extend over the surface of the diaphragm.

THE PLEURAL SURFACES AND ADJACENT CHEST WALL

A number of tissues, arranged in layers, surround the lung and line the inner aspect of the thoracic cavity. Knowledge of their anatomy is helpful in understanding normal radiographic and CT findings and the appearances of pleural diseases (Figs. 26.8 and 26.9).

The combined thickness of the layers of *visceral and parietal pleura* that surround the lung, and the fluid-containing pleural space, is less than 0.5 mm.

External to the parietal pleura is a layer of loose areolar tissue (*extrapleural fat*), which separates the parietal pleura from the endothoracic fascia. This fatty layer is very thin in most locations but can be markedly thickened over the lateral or posterolateral ribs, resulting in extrapleural fat pads several millimeters thick.

The thoracic cavity is lined by the fibroelastic *endothoracic fascia* that covers the surface of the intercostal muscles and

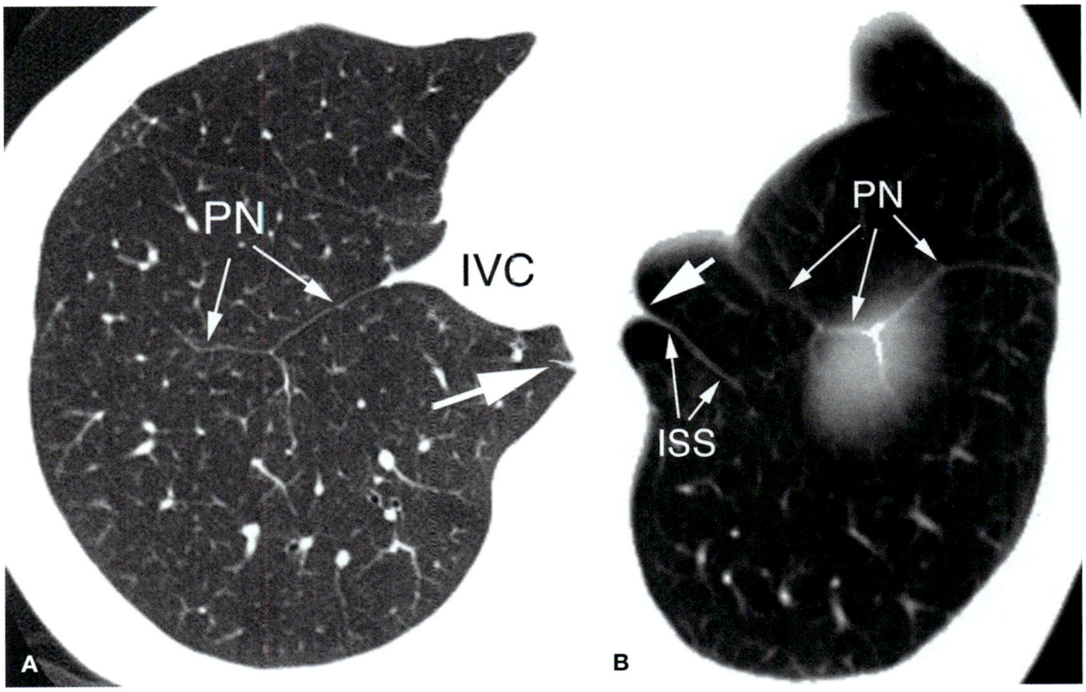

Figure 26.7. The inferior pulmonary ligaments and pleural reflections over the phrenic nerves. **A:** HRCT on the right shows the inferior pulmonary ligament as a thin triangular opacity (*large arrow*) arising in the region of the esophagus. The pleural reflection overlying the right phrenic nerve (*PN*) is seen lateral to the inferior vena cava (*IVC*). **B:** CT on the left shows the inferior pulmonary ligament as a triangular opacity (*large arrow*) lateral to the esophagus. A linear opacity extending from the inferior pulmonary ligament into the lung represents the intersublobar septum (*ISS*). The pleural reflection overlying the left phrenic nerve (*PN*) is seen more anteriorly.

intervening ribs, blends with the perichondrium and periosteum of the costal cartilages and sternum anteriorly, and posteriorly is continuous with the prevertebral fascia that covers the vertebral bodies and intervertebral discs.

External to the endothoracic fascia are the three layers of the *intercostal muscles*. The *innermost intercostal muscle* passes between the internal surfaces of adjacent ribs and is relatively thin; it is separated from the inner and external intercostal muscles by a layer of fat and the intercostal vessels and nerve (Fig. 26.9).

Although the innermost intercostal muscles are incomplete in the anterior and posterior thorax, other muscles (the transversus thoracis and subcostalis) can occupy the same relative plane. Anteriorly, the transversus thoracis muscle consists of

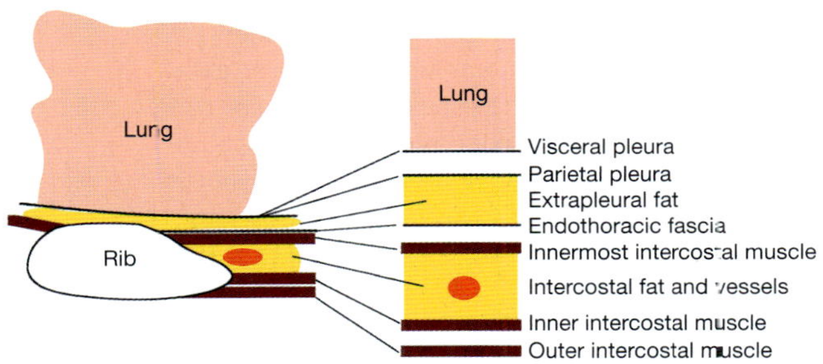

Figure 26.8. Normal structures at the pleural surface.

four or five slips that arise from the xiphoid process or lower sternum and pass superolaterally from the second to sixth costal cartilages. The internal mammary vessels lie external to the transversus thoracis. Posteriorly, the subcostal muscles are thin, variable muscles that extend from the inner aspect of the angle of the lower ribs, crossing one or two ribs and intercostal spaces, to the inner aspect of a rib below.

On CT, in many normal subjects, a 1- to 2-mm-thick soft-tissue stripe is visible in the anterolateral and posterolateral intercostal spaces (the *intercostal stripe*) at the point of contact between the lung and the chest wall (Fig. 26.9). This line primarily represents the innermost intercostal muscle but also reflects the combined thicknesses of visceral and parietal pleura, the fluid-filled pleural space, the endothoracic fascia, and fat layers. Although the pleural layers, fluid-containing pleural space, extrapleural fat, and endothoracic fascia pass internal to the ribs, they are not normally visible in this location. A visible soft-tissue stripe passing internal to the ribs or internal to the intercostal stripe (and separated from it by extrapleural fat) usually represents pleural thickening or pleural effusion.

In the paravertebral regions, the innermost intercostal muscle is anatomically absent. In this location, a very thin line (the *paravertebral line*) is sometimes visible on CT at the lung–chest wall interface; this line represents the combined thicknesses of the visceral and parietal pleura and the endothoracic fascia (Fig. 26.9). A distinct soft-tissue stripe in the

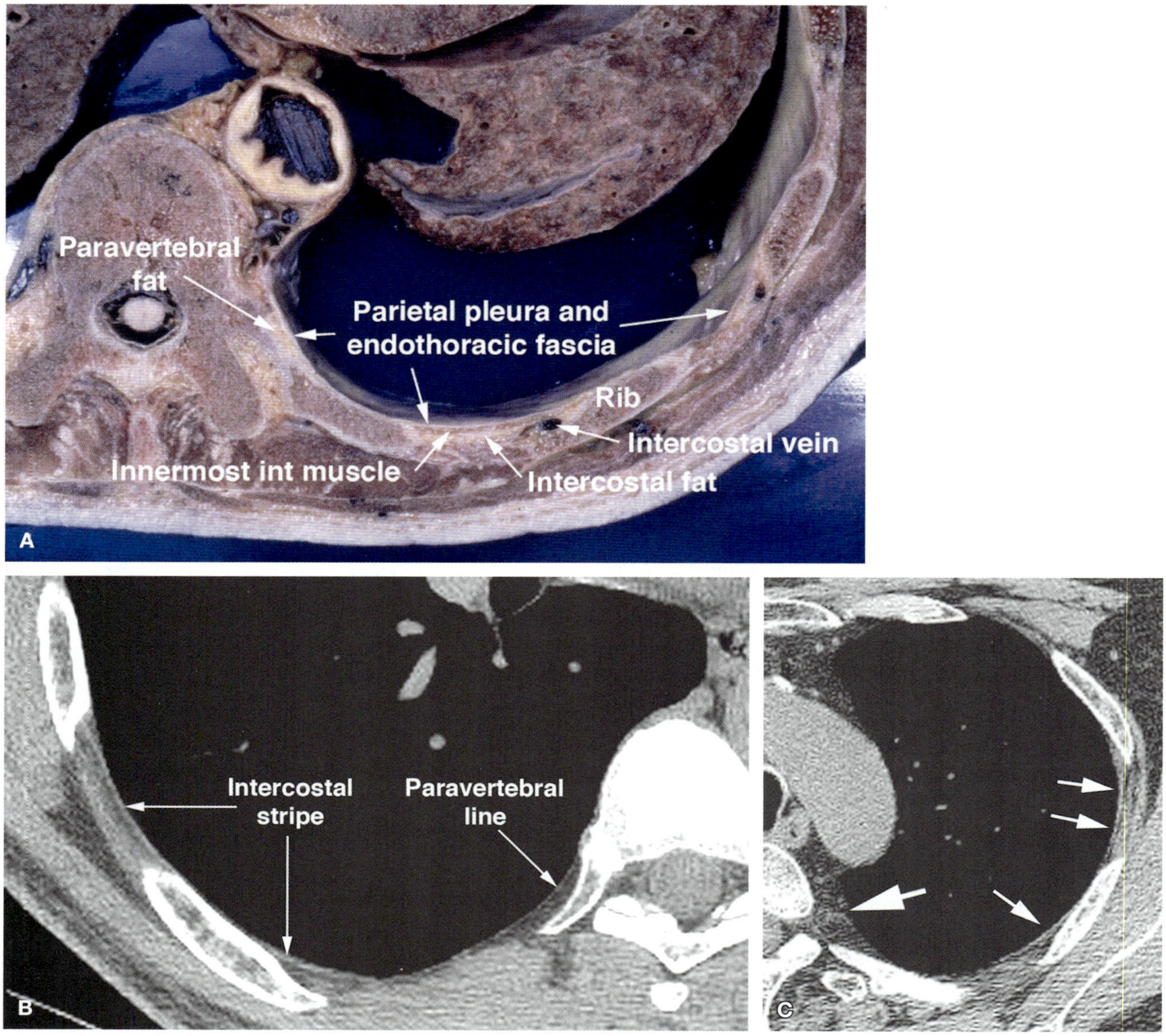

Figure 26.9. Normal anatomy at the pleural surface. **A:** Anatomy of the parietal pleura and chest wall in a section of a cadaver. The parietal pleura and endothoracic fascia are visible as a thin white layer, lining the thoracic cavity. Little extrathoracic fat is present in this example. The innermost intercostal muscle is visible external to the parietal pleura, measuring 1 to 2 mm in thickness. External to this is a layer of fat containing the intercostal vessels and nerve. The intercostal muscles are absent in the paravertebral regions; only parietal pleura, endothoracic fascia, and paravertebral fat are visible. **B:** On HRCT in a normal subject, the intercostal stripe is visible as a thin white line. Although it represents the combined thickness of visceral and parietal pleurae, the fluid-filled pleural space, endothoracic fascia, and innermost intercostal muscle, it primarily represents the innermost intercostal muscle. The intercostal stripe is seen as separate from the more external layers of the intercostal muscles because of a layer of intercostal fat. Posteriorly, the intercostal stripe is visible anterior to the lower edge of a rib. Only a very thin line (ie, the paravertebral line) is visible in the paravertebral region. **C:** In a normal patient, a thin white stripe between adjacent ribs (*small arrows*) represents the intercostal stripe, primarily representing the innermost intercostal muscle. In the paravertebral regions, the innermost intercostal muscle is anatomically absent. In this location (*large arrow*), no definite line is visible.

paravertebral regions usually represents pleural thickening or pleural effusion.

DIAGNOSIS OF PLEURAL THICKENING

Parietal Pleural Thickening

Most causes of "pleural thickening" visible on radiographs or CT primarily affect the parietal pleura. On CT, parietal pleural thickening results in five findings (Fig. 26.10):

1. A stripe of soft-tissue density, 1 mm or more in thickness, internal to the ribs (see Fig. 26.10B and C)
2. A stripe of soft-tissue density, 1 mm or more in thickness, internal to the innermost intercostal muscle and separated from it by a thin layer of extrapleural fat (see Fig. 26.10C)
3. A distinct stripe of soft-tissue density in the paravertebral region, 1 mm or more in thickness (see Fig. 26.10C)
4. Pleural calcification (see Fig. 26.10B-D)
5. Thickening of the normal extrapleural fat layer (see Fig. 26.10B)

Findings of parietal pleural thickening visible on chest radiographs (see Fig. 26.10) include the following:

1. Blunting of the lateral or posterior costophrenic angle (this may also result from pleural effusion)
2. A stripe of soft-tissue density, several millimeters or more in thickness, separating the lung from the adjacent ribs and chest wall, either focal or diffuse (this may also result from pleural effusion)
3. Thickened soft tissue visible internal to the ribs in patients with pneumothorax
4. Pleural calcification
5. An asymmetrical increase in extrapleural fat appearing low in attenuation

Visceral Pleural Thickening

Recognizable visceral pleural thickening almost always occurs in association with parietal pleural thickening and pleural effusion; empyema is the most common cause. Visceral pleural thickening occurring in the absence of parietal pleural thickening is uncommon but may be seen in patients with lung disease, such as lung abscess or diffuse lung fibrosis.

Visceral pleural thickening cannot usually be distinguished from parietal pleural thickening on chest radiographs, although it may appear as any of the following:

1. Thickening of a fissure (this more often reflects pleural effusion)
2. Separation of the lung from the adjacent ribs and chest wall, which may be focal or diffuse, occurring in association with contiguous lung disease (this may also result from parietal pleural thickening or pleural effusion)
3. Thick pleura at the lung surface in patients with pneumothorax

On CT, visceral pleural thickening may appear as either of the following:

1. A distinct stripe of soft tissue at the lung surface in patients with pleural effusion and normal lung parenchyma
2. An enhancing stripe at the lung surface in patients with abnormal lung (thickened visceral pleura often enhances to a greater degree than airless lung)

NORMAL FINDINGS THAT MIMIC PLEURAL THICKENING

Several normal findings can mimic the findings of pleural thickening or effusion.

Normal Fat Pads

Normal extrapleural fat is most abundant over the posterolateral fourth to eighth ribs and can produce fat pads several millimeters thick that extend into the intercostal spaces.

On plain radiographs, the presence of a soft-tissue stripe passing internal to the ribs, thus separating the lung from the chest wall, is generally taken to indicate the presence of pleural thickening or effusion. However, in normal patients with extrapleural fat thickening or fat pads, a similar appearance may be seen.

Pleural disease and fat thickening can usually be distinguished; in contrast to pleural thickening or effusion, normal fat thickening is typically symmetrical and smooth in contour, appears low in attenuation, and is unassociated with costophrenic angle blunting.

Normal extrapleural fat can sometimes be seen on CT internal to the ribs. This appears very low in density and is easy to distinguish from thickened pleura.

The Subcostalis and Transversus Thoracis Muscles

These are invisible on chest radiographs. On CT, a 1- to 2-mm-thick line is sometimes seen internal to one or more ribs, along the posterior chest wall at the level of the heart, representing the subcostalis muscle (Fig. 26.11). This may closely mimic the appearance of focal pleural thickening. The subcostalis muscle is visible in a small percentage of patients.

Anteriorly, at the level of the heart and adjacent to the lower sternum or xiphoid process, the transversus thoracis muscles are nearly always visible on CT internal to the anterior ends of ribs or costal cartilages (see Fig. 26.11).

In contrast to pleural thickening, these muscles are smooth, uniform in thickness, and symmetric bilaterally.

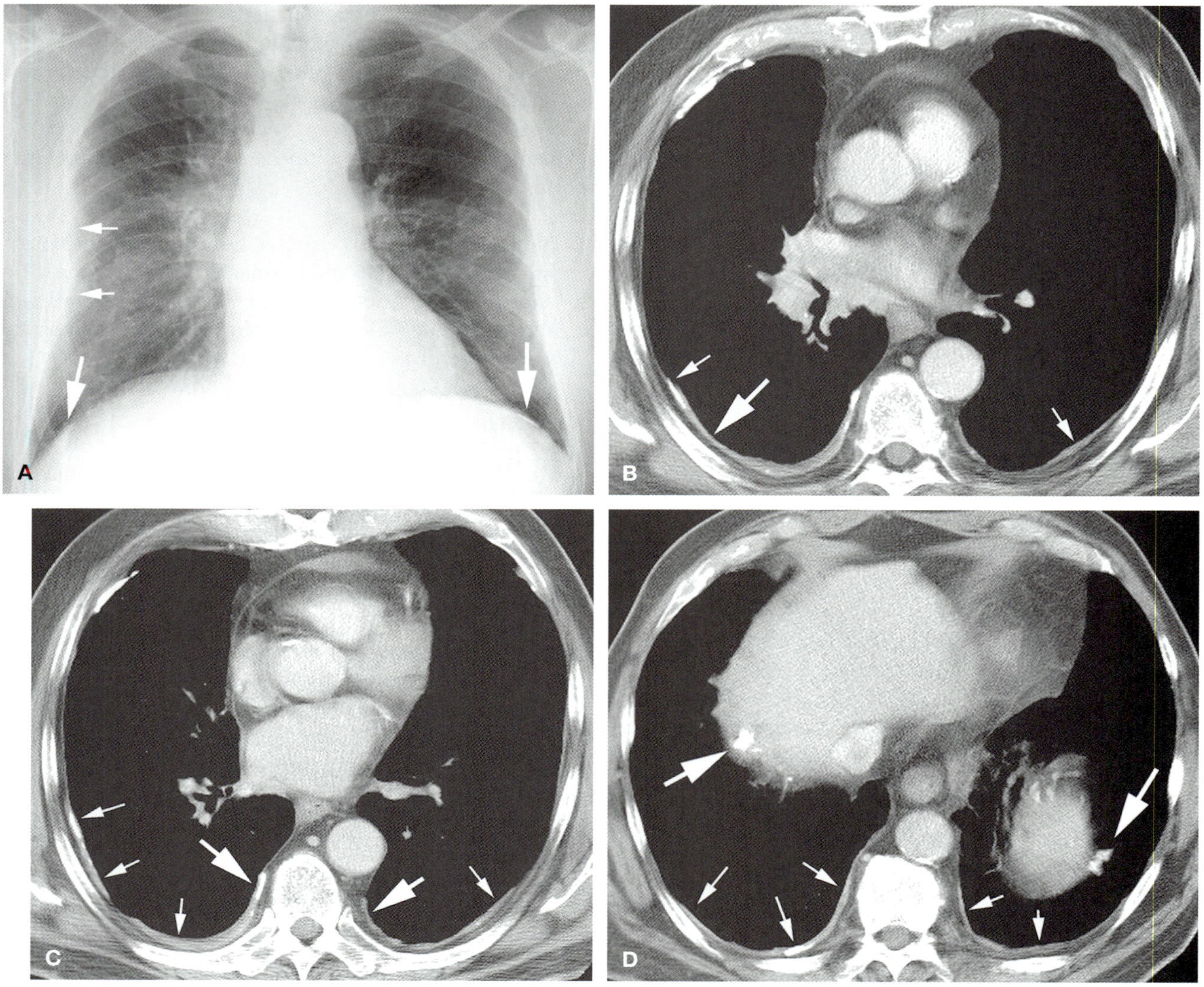

Figure 26.10. Parietal pleural thickening and calcification in asbestos exposure. **A:** Chest radiograph shows thickened pleura separating aerated lung from the adjacent ribs (*small arrows*). Pleural calcification (*large arrows*) is visible on the surface of the hemidiaphragms. **B:** CT shows thickened parietal pleura internal to the ribs (*large arrow*) and internal to the intercostal stripe (ie, innermost intercostal muscle; *small arrows*). In both locations, a layer of thickened extrapleural fat separates the thickened pleura from the chest wall. Pleural calcification is also seen. **C:** Thickened parietal pleura (*small arrows*) is visible internal to the ribs and internal to the intercostal stripe (ie, innermost intercostal muscle). A stripe of density in the paravertebral regions (*large arrows*) indicates pleural thickening. **D:** At the level of the diaphragm, thickened pleura is visible in the paravertebral regions and internal to the ribs (*small arrows*). Calcified pleura on the surface of the hemidiaphragms (*large arrows*) is typical of asbestos exposure.

Paravertebral Intercostal Veins

These are invisible on chest radiographs. On CT, in some normal subjects, segments of intercostal veins seen in the paravertebral regions mimic pleural thickening. Continuity of these opacities with the azygos or hemiazygos veins is sometimes visible, allowing them to be correctly identified (see Fig. 26.11). Also, when viewed using lung window settings, these intercostal vein segments do not indent the lung surface; focal pleural thickening usually does.

DIAGNOSIS OF PLEURAL EFFUSION

Plain Radiographs

Pleural effusion cannot be distinguished from pleural thickening on chest radiographs unless high-density calcification or low-density fat is visible in relation to thick pleura, or air collections are visible within a pleural fluid collection.

The pleural space extends inferiorly, below the visible lung, in relation to the diaphragm and ribs. In upright subjects, pleural

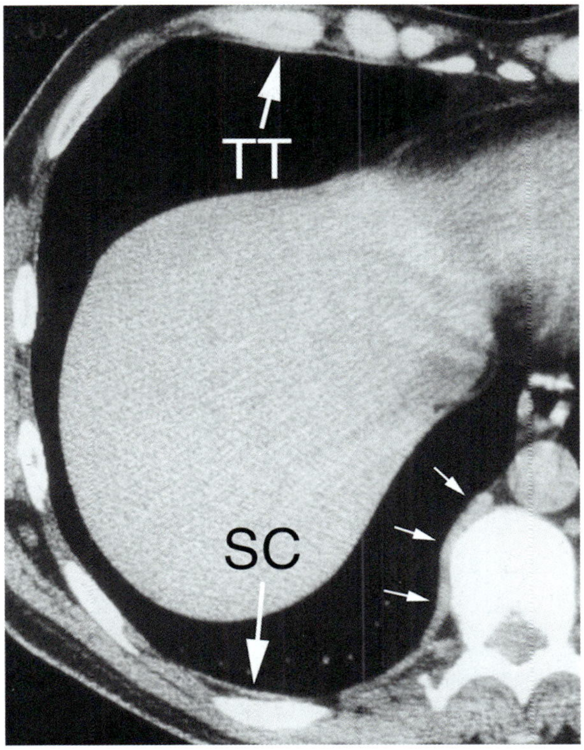

Figure 26.11. Normal findings mimicking pleural thickening. CT shows the subcostalis muscle (*SC*), transversus thoracis muscle (*TT*), and intercostal veins (*small arrows*).

fluid first accumulates in the most inferior portions of the pleural space, including the costophrenic angles and subpulmonic regions. Costophrenic angle blunting is usually the first recognizable plain film finding of pleural fluid (Fig. 26.12A and B).

At least 175 mL of pleural fluid must be present to result in blunting of the lateral costophrenic angle on the frontal radiograph, and as much as 500 mL may be present without recognizable blunting. Blunting of the posterior costophrenic angle on the lateral view requires 75 mL (see Fig. 26.12B). Blunting of the posterior costophrenic angle may sometimes be diagnosed on the frontal view by looking through the shadow of the upper abdominal contents; posterior costophrenic angle blunting results in a sharper lower edge of the lung than normally seen. On a properly performed lateral decubitus film, as little as 10 mL of fluid may be seen. Very small pleural fluid collections, either unilateral or bilateral, are seen in a few normal individuals.

With increasing effusion, fluid may be seen lateral to the lower lobes, separating the lung from adjacent ribs. Because the lung is fixed medially by the hilum and inferior pulmonary ligament, medial pleural fluid collections are usually smaller (Fig. 26.13) and more difficult to recognize. Larger effusions result in a typical meniscus appearance with the level of the fluid and its density appearing greater in the lateral hemithorax. The edge separating the aerated lung from pleural fluid is often sharp and well defined.

Medial fluid collections may be seen when effusions are large. Most often, these accumulate in the posterior gutters, with thickening of the paravertebral stripes. The collections may be triangular, simulating lower lobe collapse.

Pleural fluid often accumulates in the subpulmonic pleural space (*subpulmonic effusion*), allowing the lung base to float superiorly. Subpulmonic fluid collections may be difficult to recognize on frontal radiographs, although some costophrenic angle blunting, a shallow costophrenic angle, or a hazy costophrenic angle is often present. However, greater superior retraction of the lateral lung (likely because the medial lower lobe is fixed by the inferior pulmonary ligament) results in lateral displacement of the diaphragmatic dome or peak, with the lung lateral to the peak angling down sharply (Fig. 26.14). On the left side, 2 cm of separation of the lung base from the top of the stomach bubble is typically taken as evidence of a subpulmonic effusion, but this distance is variable in normal individuals.

On the lateral view (see Fig. 26.14B), a subpulmonic effusion often (1) elevates the posterior lung, flattening its undersurface; (2) insinuates itself into the major fissure, resulting in focal triangular thickening of the fissure; and (3) flattens the inferior contour of the lung anterior to the fissure, which then angles sharply downward.

Fluid may extend into the major or minor fissures. This is usually easy to recognize on the lateral radiographs as fissure thickening. On the frontal radiograph, fluid extending into the posterolateral major fissure typically results in an arcuate opacity, sharply defined medially and inferiorly (see Fig. 26.1). Fluid extending into the lateral aspect of the minor fissure and slightly separating the lobes often results in an opacity resembling a rose thorn (the "thorn sign"; see Figs. 26.12A, 26.13A, and 26.14B).

Large pleural effusions result in significant or complete lung atelectasis (see Fig. 26.13) and result in a mediastinal shift to the opposite side. Downward displacement or inversion of the hemidiaphragm may be recognized on the left because of downward displacement of the stomach bubble.

Supine and semierect radiographs are less sensitive in showing pleural effusion. Signs of effusion on supine radiographs include increased density of a hemithorax due to layering of the effusion posteriorly, blunting of the lateral costophrenic angle, obscuration or poor definition of the hemidiaphragm, and thickening of the paravertebral stripe, usually in the inferior hemithorax, due to accumulation of fluid in the posterior gutters. With large effusions, an apical cap may be seen.

On decubitus radiographs, an increase in separation of the lung from the chest wall indicates the presence of free pleural effusion (see Fig. 26.12C). Lack in change in thickness indicates pleural thickening or loculated pleural effusion.

CT Findings

Pleural effusion usually appears lower in attenuation than does pleural thickening or consolidated or collapsed lung on unenhanced scans and may be distinguished from them. On contrast-enhanced scans, both airless lung and thickened

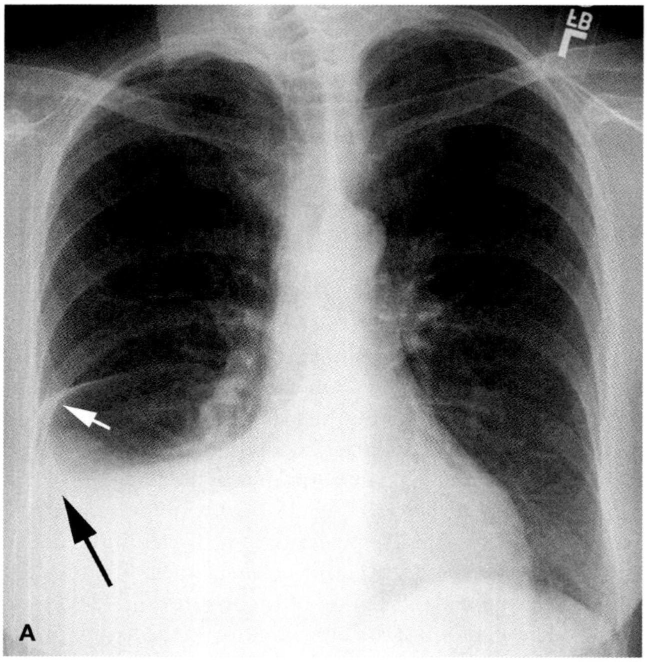

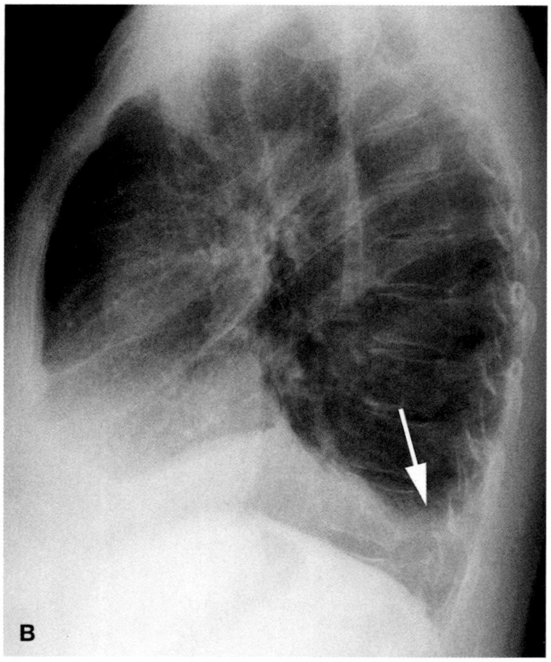

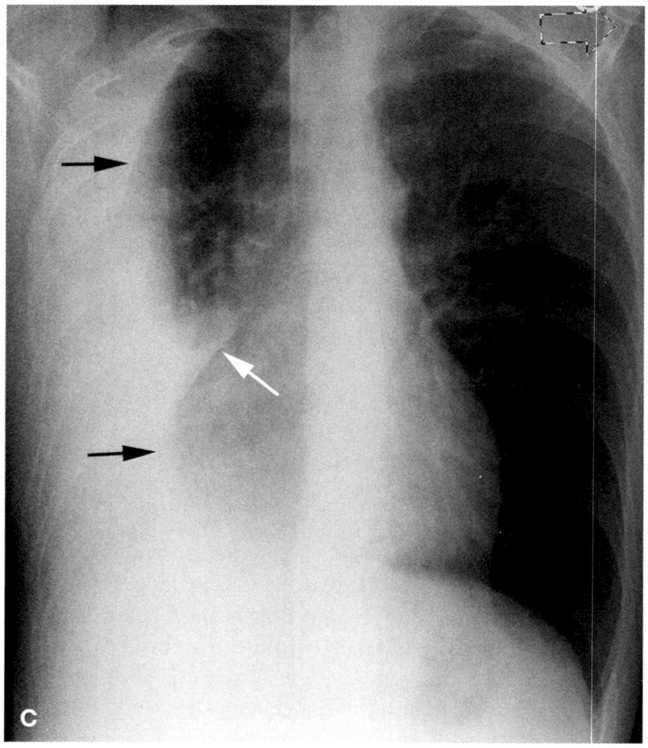

Figure 26.12. Pleural effusion associated with cirrhosis. **A:** Posteroanterior chest radiograph shows blunting of the right costophrenic angle (*black arrow*). This usually indicates that 175 mL of pleural fluid is present. Fluid entering the minor fissure (*white arrow*) resembles a rose thorn. This is termed the "thorn" sign of pleural effusion. **B:** Lateral radiograph shows elevation of the lung base by a subpulmonic fluid collection and blunting of the posterior costophrenic angle (*arrow*). Posterior costophrenic angle blunting occurs with as little as 75 mL of fluid. **C:** Decubitus radiograph shows a large effusion (*black arrows*) separating the aerated lung from the chest wall. Fluid enters the major fissure (*white arrow*).

pleura enhance, and this difference is accentuated (see Fig. 26.13B). Small pleural effusions can be difficult to distinguish from pleural thickening.

In the supine position, free pleural effusion first accumulates in the most dependent part of the pleural space, posterior to the lower lobe. The thickness of a free pleural effusion usually decreases in less dependent parts of the thorax, anteriorly and superiorly. As the effusion increases in size, it becomes thicker and wraps around the lung, extending anteriorly and superiorly and entering the fissures.

When free pleural fluid accumulates, the lung decreases in volume but tends to maintain its normal shape. Thus, a free pleural effusion generally appears crescent shaped on CT. Large effusions often extend into the major fissures, displacing the lower lobes medially and posteriorly. Atelectasis is common in patients with large effusions, and atelectatic lung may be seen floating within the fluid.

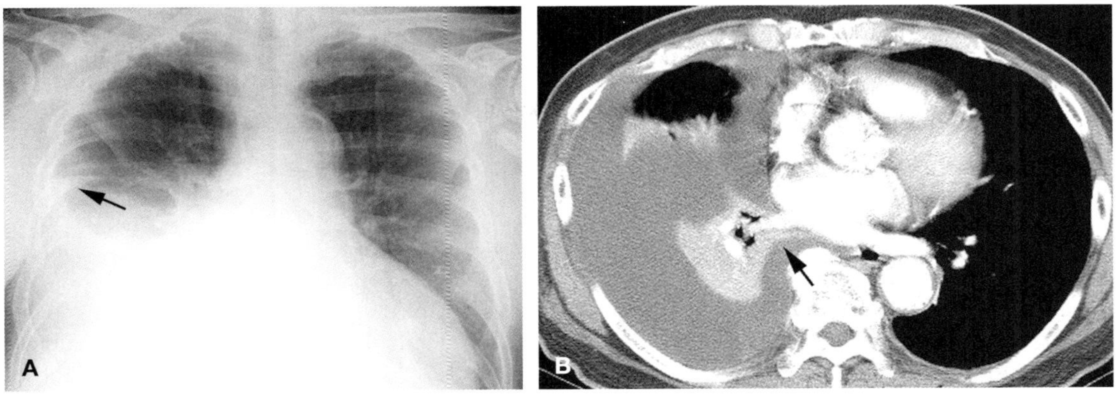

Figure 26.13. Pleural effusion with liver disease. **A:** Chest radiograph shows a large right pleural effusion with costophrenic angle blunting and a thorn sign (*arrow*). **B:** A large effusion is visible on CT. The lower lobe is collapsed. Because the lung is tethered medially by the hilar vasculature and inferior pulmonary ligament (*arrow*), most of the fluid accumulates laterally.

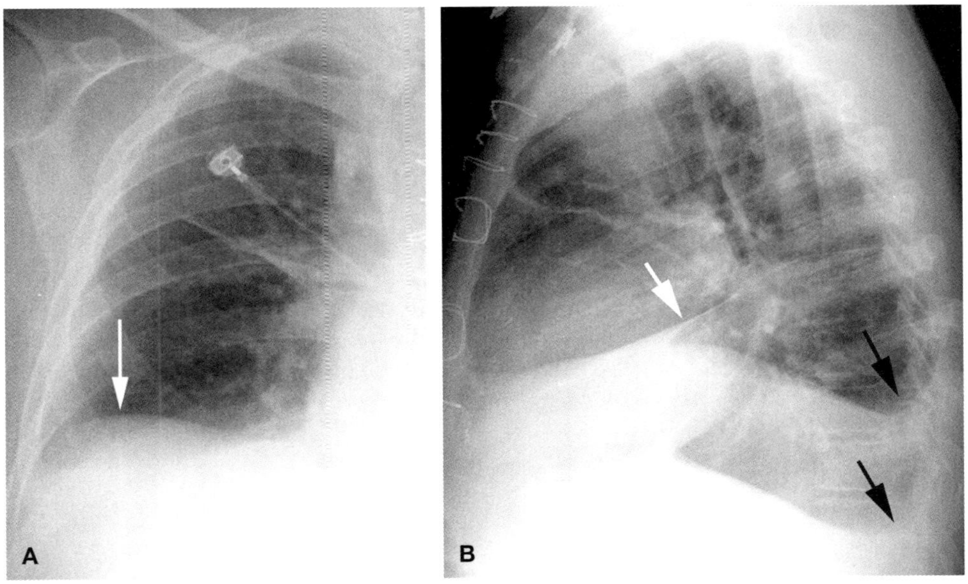

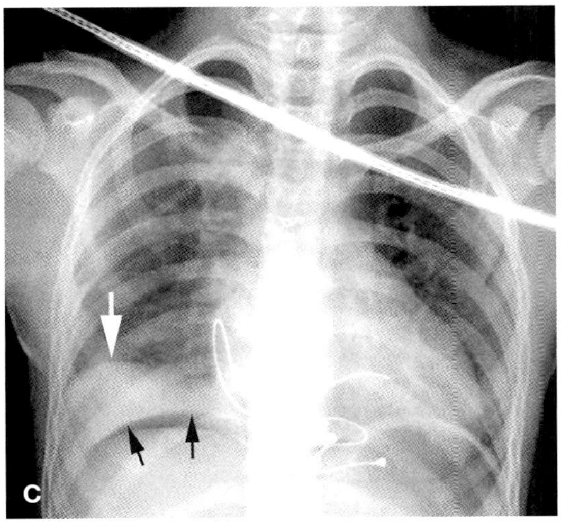

Figure 26.14. Subpulmonic right pleural effusion. **A:** Posteroanterior chest radiograph shows no evidence of costophrenic angle blunting. There appears to be lateral displacement of the diaphragm dome (*arrow*). **B:** Lateral radiograph shows blunting of both costophrenic angles (*black arrows*), and fluid entering the right major fissure, resulting in a thorn sign (*white arrow*). Flattening of the undersurface of the lobes is also typical of subpulmonic effusion. **C:** Subpulmonic effusion in a patient with free abdominal air because of peritoneal dialysis. The free air outlines the undersurface of the right hemidiaphragm (*black arrows*). What appears to represent a laterally displaced dome of the right hemidiaphragm (*white arrow*) represents a subpulmonic effusion.

Pleural Effusion Versus Ascites

Subpulmonic effusion and pleural fluid in the costophrenic angles can be seen below the lung bases on CT and may mimic collections of fluid in the peritoneal cavity. The parallel curvilinear configuration of the pleural and peritoneal cavities at the level of the perihepatic and perisplenic recesses allows fluid in either cavity to appear as a crescentic collection displacing the liver or spleen away from the adjacent chest wall.

However, pleural fluid collections and ascites may be distinguished in several ways.

Pleural fluid collections in the posterior costophrenic angle lie medial and posterior to the diaphragm and cause lateral displacement of the crus (the "displaced crus sign"). Peritoneal fluid collections are anterior and lateral to the diaphragm; lateral displacement of the crus is not visible.

Pleural fluid can also be distinguished from ascites by the clarity of the interface of the fluid with the liver and spleen (the "interface sign"). With pleural fluid, the interface is hazy, whereas with ascites, it is sharp.

Fluid seen posterior to the liver is within the pleural space; the peritoneal space does not extend into this region, the so-called bare area of the liver (the "bare area sign").

The most reliable method for localizing fluid is to identify its relationship to the diaphragm, if it is visible. In patients with both pleural and peritoneal fluid, the diaphragm often can be seen as a uniform, curvilinear structure of muscle density with relatively low-density fluid both anterior and posterior to it. Fluid posterior or lateral to the diaphragm is pleural (the "diaphragm sign").

A large pleural effusion will allow the lower lobe to float anteriorly and lose volume (Fig. 26.15). On CT, the posterior edge of the lower lobe, when surrounded by fluid both anteriorly and posteriorly, can appear to represent the diaphragm (ie, a "pseudodiaphragm"), with pleural fluid posteriorly and ascites anteriorly. Sequential scans at more cephalad levels, however, generally will allow the correct interpretation to be made. Typically, the arcuate density of the atelectatic lower lobe becomes thicker superiorly, is contiguous with the remainder of the lower lobe, and often contains air bronchograms.

LOCULATED FLUID COLLECTIONS

Loculated pleural fluid collections are limited in extent by pleural adhesions. They often occur in association with exudative pleural effusions, high in protein, such as those that occur with empyema. Often they are elliptical or lenticular in shape.

Radiographic Findings

The appearance of loculated pleural fluid on chest radiographs varies with its location and the radiographic projection. Typically, a loculated collection appears sharply marginated when its surface is parallel to the x-ray beam and ill defined when viewed en face (Fig. 26.16A and B). Thus, a collection loculated in the lateral pleural space will appear sharply marginated on the frontal radiograph and ill defined on the lateral film. For a collection loculated anteriorly or posteriorly, the opposite is true.

Localized fluid collections in the fissures may be loculated or may occur in the absence of pleural adhesions. They are most common in patients with congestive heart failure (CHF) and often are transient. Since they mimic the presence of a focal lung lesion, they have been referred to as "phantom tumor" or "pseudotumor." Typically, fluid collections in a fissure are rounded or lenticular and may show a tapering triangular opacity or "beak" at the point at which they merge with the fissure itself (Figs. 26.17 and 26.18).

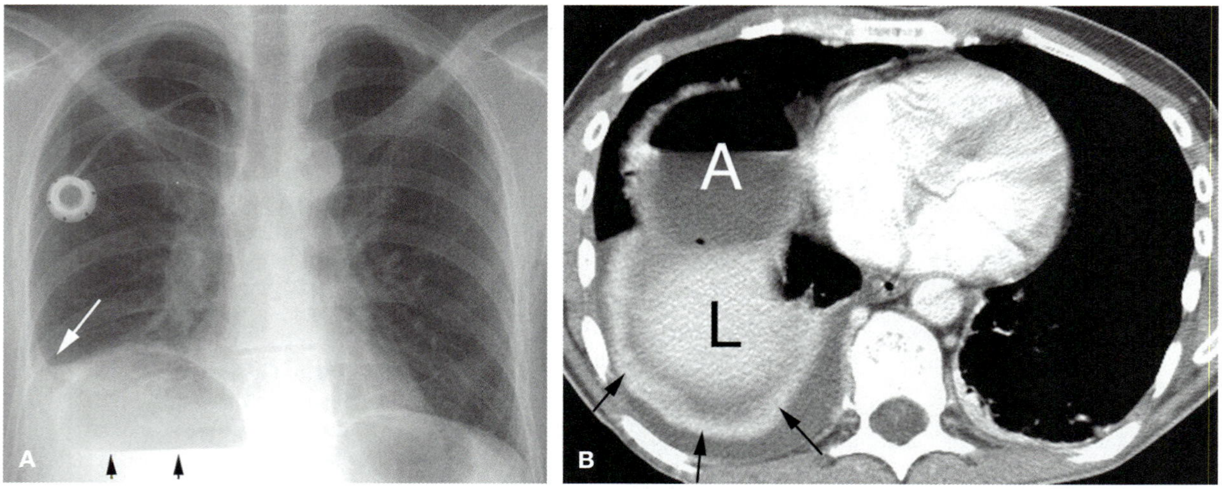

Figure 26.15. "Pseudodiaphragm" with pleural effusion and lower lobe collapse. **A:** Chest radiograph shows costophrenic angle blunting (*white arrow*) due to right pleural effusion. An air-fluid level (*black arrows*) represents a subphrenic abscess. **B:** CT shows the abscess cavity (*A*) in a subphrenic location. The liver (*L*) is also visible at this level. The collapsed lower lobe (*arrows*) surrounded by pleural fluid mimics the hemidiaphragm.

Fluid collections in the minor fissure often appear sharply marginated and lenticular on both posteroanterior and lateral radiographs. Collections in the major fissure may be ill defined on the frontal view.

CT Findings

CT findings of fluid loculation include (1) a localized collection, (2) an elliptical or lenticular shape (rather than crescentic), and (3) a nondependent location (ie, anterior, lateral, or posterolateral; Figs. 26.16C and 26.18-26.20). If air is present within a loculated effusion, multiple septations may be seen, resulting in multiple air bubbles, localized air collections, or air-fluid levels (Fig. 26.21). Loculated effusions are often associated with pleural thickening, best seen with contrast enhancement (see Figs. 26.16C and 26.19). If both the visceral and parietal pleural surfaces are thickened, embracing the fluid collection, the *split pleura sign* is said to be present (see Fig. 26.19).

A focal or loculated collection of pleural fluid in a major or minor fissure can have a confusing appearance on CT images and can be misinterpreted as a parenchymal mass. Careful analysis of sequential images usually will confirm the relationship of the "mass" to the plane of the fissure. If the abnormality is of fluid attenuation, the diagnosis is easier. The edges of the mass may taper to conform to the fissure, forming a "beak," especially if CT with thin collimation is used (see Fig. 26.18). Correlation of CT scans with the plain radiographs can help, particularly for fluid localized in the minor fissure.

CHARACTERIZATION OF EFFUSION: EXUDATES AND TRANSUDATES

Most pleural effusions are classified as exudates or transudates based on their composition. This distinction is usually made at thoracentesis. Other specific causes of pleura effusion are chylothorax and hemothorax.

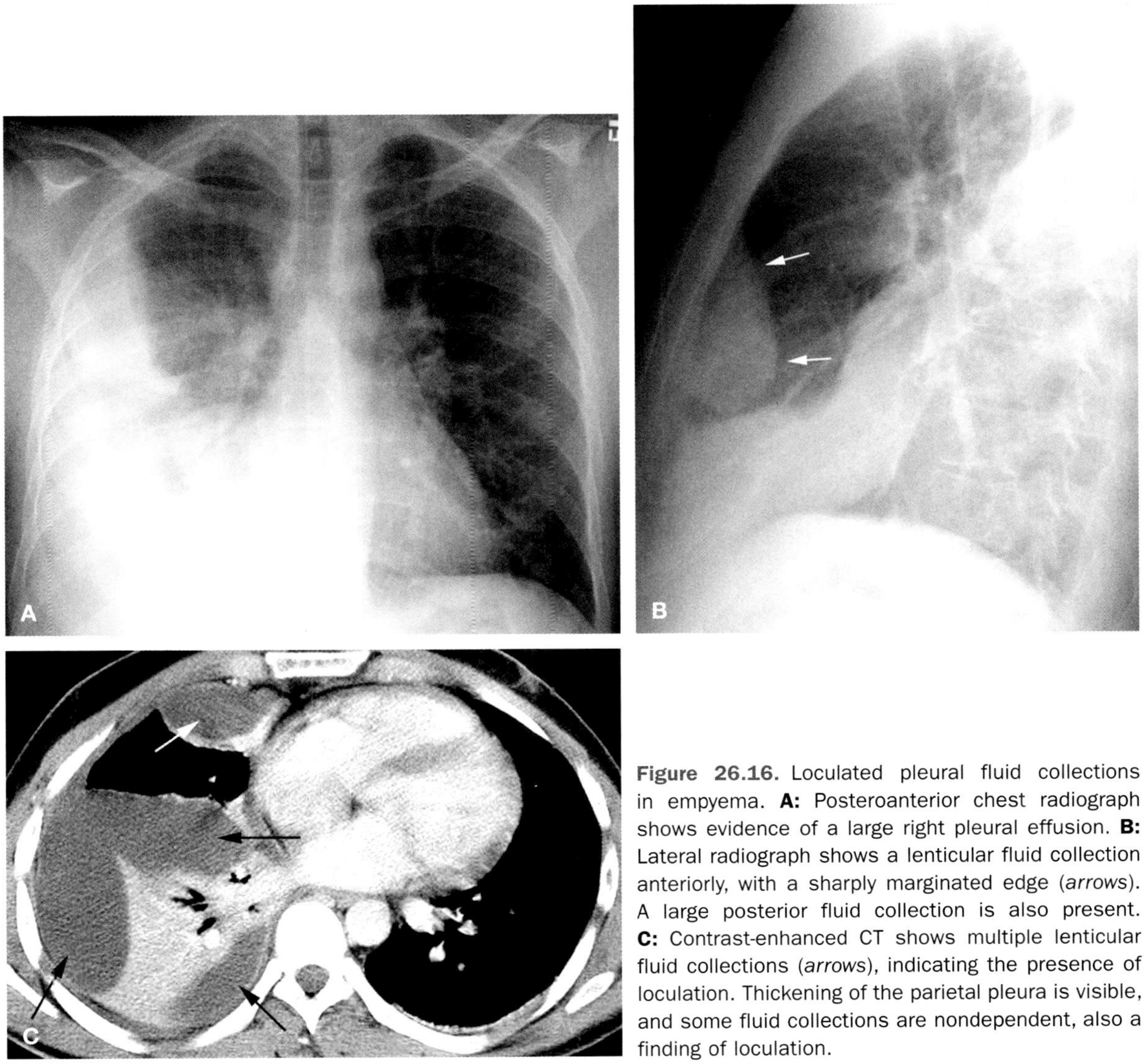

Figure 26.16. Loculated pleural fluid collections in empyema. **A:** Posteroanterior chest radiograph shows evidence of a large right pleural effusion. **B:** Lateral radiograph shows a lenticular fluid collection anteriorly, with a sharply marginated edge (*arrows*). A large posterior fluid collection is also present. **C:** Contrast-enhanced CT shows multiple lenticular fluid collections (*arrows*), indicating the presence of loculation. Thickening of the parietal pleura is visible, and some fluid collections are nondependent, also a finding of loculation.

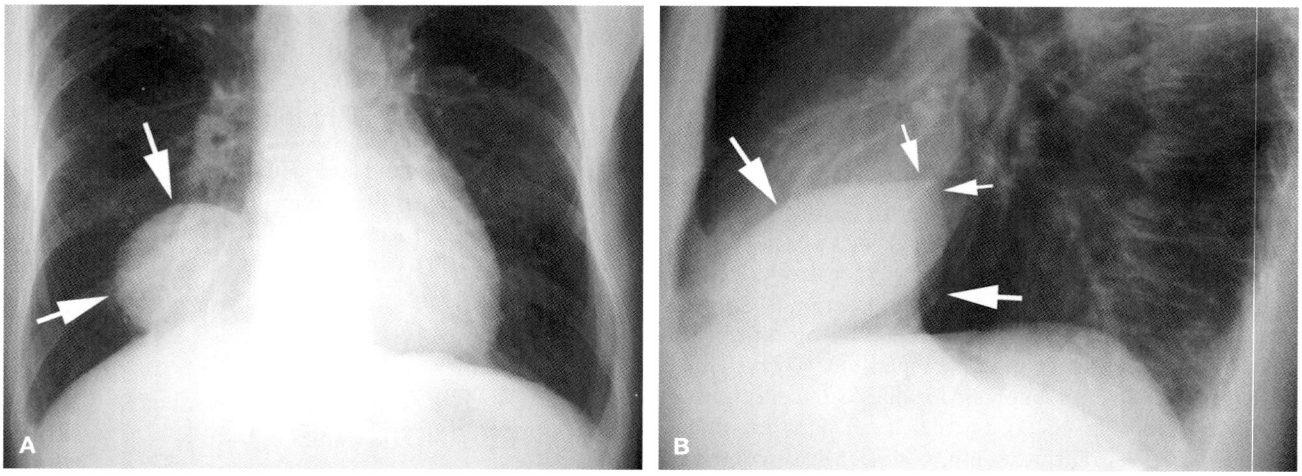

Figure 26.17. Pseudotumor in congestive heart failure. **A:** Chest radiograph shows a rounded opacity (*arrows*) representing fluid localized to the major fissure. **B:** On the lateral view, the collection appears lenticular (*large arrows*). A beak (*small arrows*) is seen at its junction with the major fissure. This collection is resolved later.

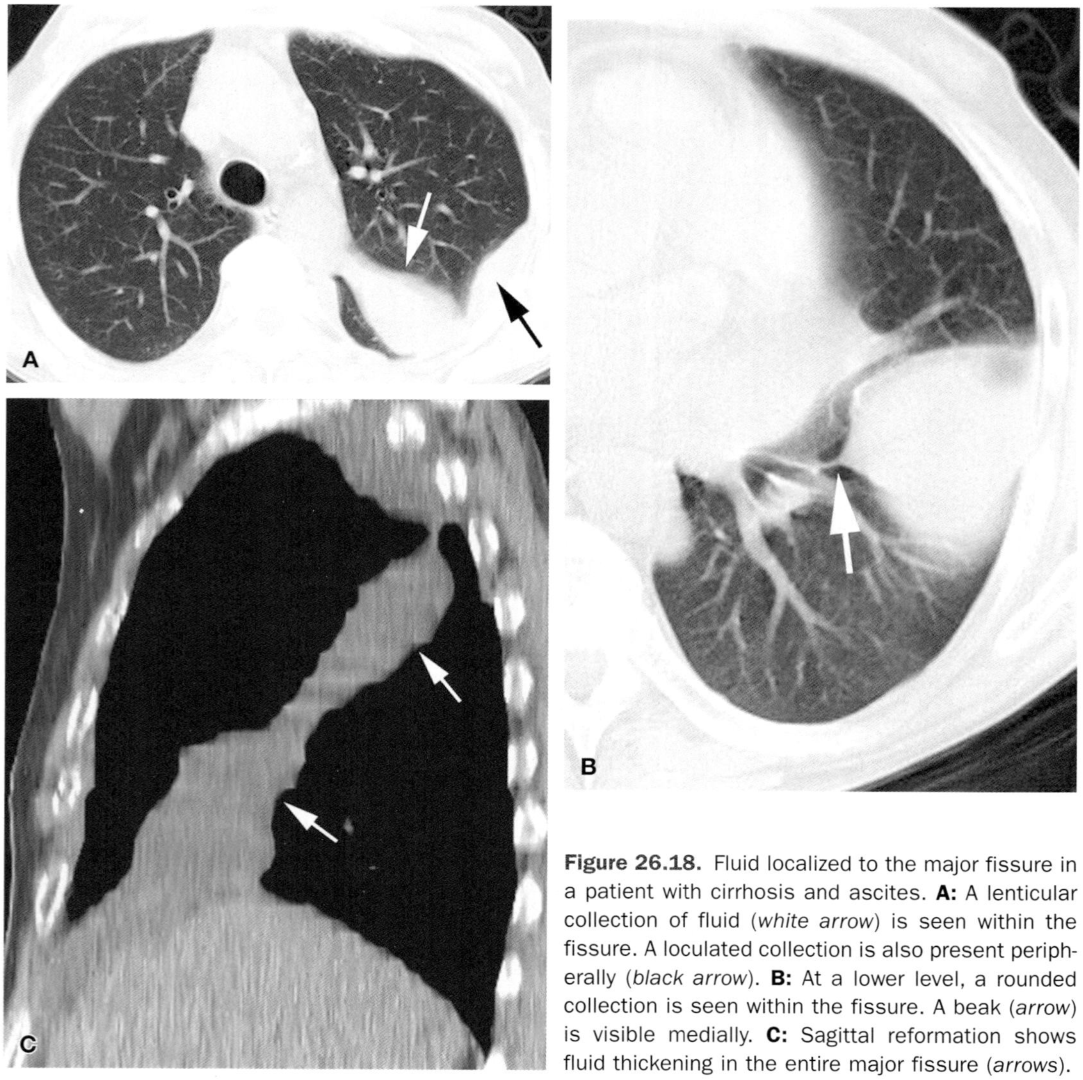

Figure 26.18. Fluid localized to the major fissure in a patient with cirrhosis and ascites. **A:** A lenticular collection of fluid (*white arrow*) is seen within the fissure. A loculated collection is also present peripherally (*black arrow*). **B:** At a lower level, a rounded collection is seen within the fissure. A beak (*arrow*) is visible medially. **C:** Sagittal reformation shows fluid thickening in the entire major fissure (*arrows*).

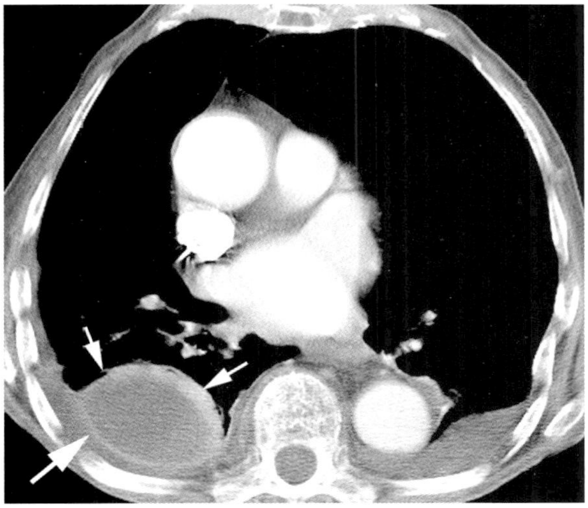

Figure 26.19. Streptococcal empyema. CT shows a loculated, lenticular fluid collection at the right base, associated with thickening of both the parietal (*large arrow*) and visceral (*small arrows*) pleural layers, the so-called split pleura sign. The thickened pleura enhances following contrast infusion. The left pleural effusion is unassociated with pleural thickening and may be an exudate or transudate.

Exudates

Exudative effusion reflects the presence of a pleural abnormality associated with increased permeability of pleural capillaries (Table 26.1). Exudative effusions have a high protein content. According to generally accepted criteria, an exudative effusion meets at least one of the following criteria:

1. A ratio of pleural fluid protein to serum protein higher than 0.5
2. A ratio of pleural fluid lactate dehydrogenase (LDH) to serum LDH that exceeds 0.6
3. A pleural fluid LDH level more than two-thirds the upper limits of normal for serum

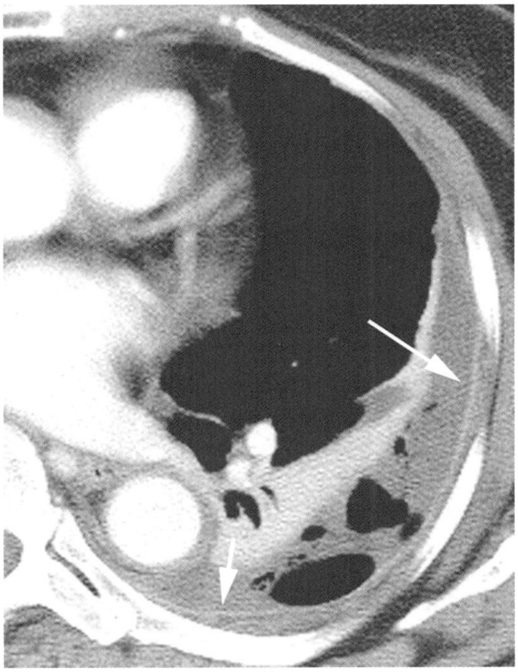

Figure 26.21. Empyema containing air due to thoracentesis. The parietal pleura is thickened (*arrows*). Multiple air bubbles indicate a multiloculated proteinaceous effusion. It may be concluded that this effusion is an exudate. The differential diagnosis of an air-containing fluid collection also included bronchopleural fistula and gas-forming organisms.

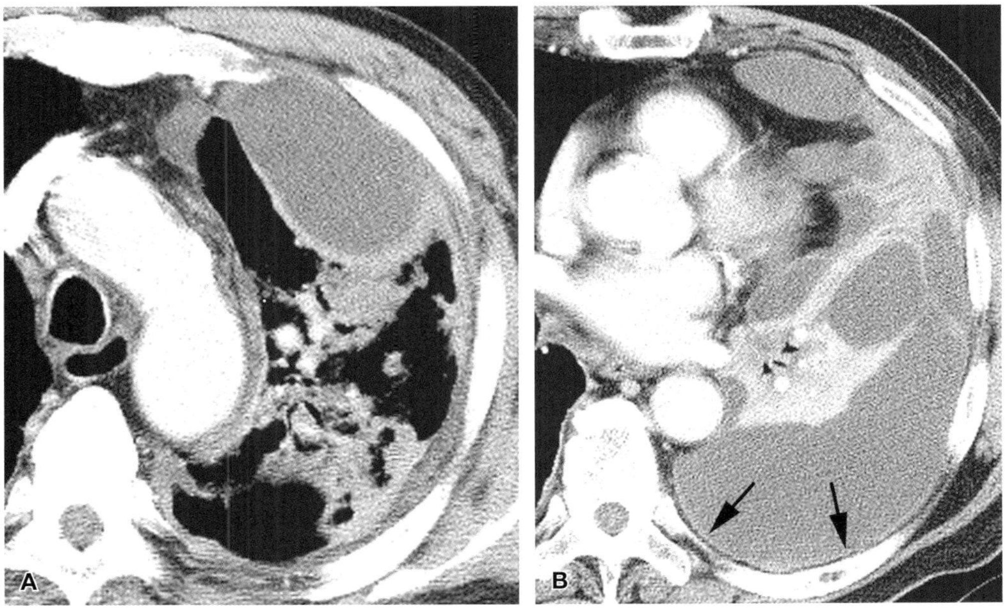

Figure 26.20. Empyema with multiple loculations. **A and B:** CTs at two levels show multiple loculated fluid collections with thickened parietal pleura (*arrows*).

Table 26.1 Causes of Exudative Effusion
Pneumonia (parapneumonic effusion)
Empyema
Tuberculous
Neoplasm
Pulmonary embolism
Collagen vascular diseases
Abdominal diseases (liver, pancreas, surgery, abscess)
Dressler (postpericardiotomy) syndrome
Asbestos exposure
Meigs syndrome
Uremia
Endometriosis
Drug reactions
Radiation

Less specific criteria used to diagnose an exudate include a pleural fluid specific gravity exceeding 1.016 and a pleural fluid protein level exceeding 3 g/dL.

Common causes of exudative effusion include pneumonia with parapneumonic effusion, empyema, tuberculous pleuritis, neoplasm, pulmonary embolism and infarct, collagen diseases such as lupus or rheumatoid arthritis (RA), abdominal diseases (cirrhosis, pancreatitis, abscess, surgery), Dressler (postpericardiotomy) syndrome, asbestos exposure, Meigs syndrome, uremia, endometriosis, drug reactions, and therapeutic radiation.

Transudates

Transudative effusion is unassociated with pleural disease. It usually results from systemic abnormalities causing an imbalance in the hydrostatic and osmotic forces governing pleural fluid formation. A transudative effusion is low in protein and does not meet the criteria for an exudate listed above.

Common causes of a transudative effusion (Table 26.2) include CHF, pericardial disease, cirrhosis, pregnancy and delivery, hypoalbuminemia, overhydration, renal failure, nephrotic syndrome, peritoneal dialysis, and myxedema.

Table 26.2 Causes of Transudative Effusion
Congestive heart failure
Pericardial disease
Cirrhosis
Pregnancy and delivery
Hypoalbuminemia
Overhydration
Renal failure
Nephrotic syndrome
Peritoneal dialysis
Myxedema

Distinguishing Exudate and Transudate

Distinguishing exudate from transudate is important in the differential diagnosis and clinical management of pleural effusion. CT numbers cannot be used to reliably predict the protein content or specific gravity of the fluid and whether it is a transudate or exudate. Most effusions appear to be near water in attenuation on CT, but range up to 20 to 30 HU regardless of their cause. Although the attenuation of exudates may be higher (average 7-17 HU) than transudates (average 10-12.5 HU), there is considerable overlap between the attenuation of exudates and transudates in the 10 to 20 HU range.

However, the appearance of the parietal pleura on contrast-enhanced CT is of value in predicting the nature of a pleural fluid collection. Visibility of the parietal pleura indicates that it is thickened (enhancing pleura is thickened pleura and thickened pleura enhances). The presence of thickened parietal pleura in association with a pleural effusion suggests that the fluid collection is an exudate (see Figs. 26.19-26.21). Parietal pleural thickening is present in about 60% of exudative effusions, and although parietal pleural thickening can be seen in a few patients with transudative effusion, the positive predictive value of this finding in the diagnosis of an exudate is very high (about 95%). Patients with transudative effusions who show pleural thickening on CT often have preexisting pleural disease. If pleural thickening is not visible on CT, an associated effusion may be an exudate or a transudate (see Fig. 26.19).

Note that a venous phase CT is necessary to fully evaluate for pleural thickening. Arterial phase imaging (ie, pulmonary embolism or aortic dissection protocol) may be too early to show pleural enhancement.

Using sonography, the presence of septation, complex nonseptation, or homogeneous echogenicity may be used to predict the presence of an exudate with a sensitivity and positive predictive value of 65% and 100%, respectively. Anechoic effusions may be either transudative or exudative.

If CT shows air within the fluid collection, for whatever reason (usually thoracentesis), and multiple air bubbles or multiple air-fluid levels are visible (rather than a single air-fluid level; see Fig. 26.21), the presence of proteinaceous and multiloculated effusion may be assumed. An exudate may be confidently diagnosed in this setting.

Causes of Pleural Effusion

Abdominal Abscess

Abdominal infections may be associated with ipsilateral pleural effusion. The effusion may be a transudate or exudate. Typical findings include small pleural effusion, elevation of the hemidiaphragm, and lower lobe atelectasis. Subphrenic abscess is associated with pleural effusion in 80% of cases; it may occur on either side. Hepatic abscess is associated with effusion in 20%, typically right sided. Splenic abscess is associated with left-sided effusion in 30%.

Abdominal Surgery

Half of patients who undergo abdominal surgery have a small pleural effusion within the first three postoperative days. Effusions developing after this period likely have another cause. The incidence of pleural effusion is increased in association with upper abdominal surgery, peritoneal fluid, and atelectasis. Orthotopic liver transplantation is almost always associated with right-sided or bilateral effusions.

Asbestos Exposure

Asbestos-related pleural plaques are discussed in Chapter 16. Asbestos exposure can also result in benign exudative pleural effusion in a few percent of exposed individuals. The condition is likely inflammatory in nature and related to the presence of asbestos fibers at the pleural surface. It is dose-related and a relatively early manifestation of disease, usually occurring within 20 years of onset of exposure. Patients are often asymptomatic but may have chest pain. Effusions are usually unilateral and small to moderate in size. They are usually self-limited, lasting a few months, but may be recurrent. Diffuse pleural thickening results in about 20%. Rounded atelectasis may be associated.

Cirrhosis and Ascites

Cirrhosis is associated with pleural effusion (hepatic hydrothorax), but the frequency of effusion is much higher if ascites is present. Effusions are typically right sided or bilateral; isolated left-sided effusions are less common. Most important in the development of effusion is the passage of fluid into the chest through diaphragmatic defects. Reduction in plasma oncotic pressure due to hypoalbuminemia may also contribute to the formation of effusions. The effusions are transudates and may be large.

Collagen Vascular Diseases

Exudative pleural effusion is common in patients with collagen vascular disease, most commonly systemic lupus erythematosus (SLE) and RA.

SLE is associated with pleural effusion in as many as 70% of cases. Arthritis or arthralgia is commonly present. Effusions are usually small and bilateral and are exudates. Pericardial effusion may also be present. Symptoms include pleuritic pain, fever, and dyspnea.

About 5% to 20% of patients with RA have effusion. Effusions are exudates and have a low glucose, a high LDH, and a high rheumatoid factor. Eighty percent of patients with effusion are men, and 80% have subcutaneous nodules. Effusions in RA may be asymptomatic or associated with chest pain. They are usually small, unilateral, and right sided. They may be transient, persistent, or recurrent. Pleural fibrosis may result. Empyema also has an increased incidence in patients with RA.

Congestive Heart Failure

Pleural effusion is present in about half of patients with CHF. CHF is the most common cause of transudative effusion, although exudative effusions may also occur. Pleura fluid accumulates in CHF primarily because pulmonary interstitial (edema) fluid crosses into the pleural space. Bilateral effusions are present in 70% of cases; when unilateral, pleural effusion is more common on the right (20%) than on the left (10%). Although unilateral effusion may be seen, a large unilateral pleural effusion suggests an alternative diagnosis. In a patient with CHF, thoracentesis may be performed for diagnosis if the patient has fever or pleuritic chest pain, if the heart is normal in size, or if the effusion is unilateral or bilateral but asymmetrical.

Dressler Syndrome

Dressler syndrome (also known as postcardiotomy syndrome, postcardiac injury syndrome, and postmyocardial infarction syndrome) occurs in a few patients with myocardial infarction, pericardial or myocardial injury, or cardiac surgery. It typically occurs 2 or 3 weeks following the precipitating episode and is associated with chest pain, fever, dyspnea, and leukocytosis. Radiographs show pleural effusion (85%), lung consolidation (75%), and findings of pericardial effusion (50%). Pleural effusions are exudative and often bloody. They are usually bilateral and small; when unilateral, they are often left sided. Dressler syndrome may be self-limited or recurrent. It is thought to be immunologically mediated. Treatment includes aspirin, nonsteroidal anti-inflammatory drugs, or steroids.

Drug Reactions

A number of drugs may result in pleural effusion, usually exudative. Effusion may be related to the development of drug-related SLE (see Chapter 15), may reflect an allergic reaction, or may be a primary drug effect. Allergic reactions with eosinophilia may be associated with pleural effusion in patients receiving methotrexate or other cytotoxic drugs, nitrofurantoin, propylthiouracil, and muscle relaxants (dantrolene); lung disease is commonly associated. The ergot-based drugs methysergide (migraine treatment) and bromocriptine (Parkinson disease treatment) may cause pleural effusion and fibrosis.

Pleural Endometriosis

Catamenial pleural effusion or hemothorax can be associated with pleural endometrial implants. As with catamenial pneumothorax described below, pleural endometriosis is right sided in 90%, likely related to defects in the right hemidiaphragm that allow passage of endometrium into the thorax. Enhancing pleural nodules and masses, representing the endometrial implants, may be seen in addition to pleural effusion; they may be seen in the abdomen as well. The presence and size of the effusion and the size of masses wax and wane with hormonal changes.

Meigs Syndrome

Meigs syndrome was originally defined as ascites and pleural effusion associated with ovarian fibroma, but the definition has since extended to refer to other ovarian tumors. Pleural effusions are exudative or transudative and occur on the right side (65%), on the left side (10%), or bilaterally (25%); they may be large. Resection of the ovarian tumor results in resolution of the ascites and pleural effusion.

Myxedema

Pleural effusion occurs in as many as half of patients with myxedema, often associated with pericardial effusion. Associated heart failure or renal disease may be contributory. The effusion may be an exudate or transudate.

Neoplasm

Pleural effusion is common in patients with primary or metastatic pleural tumors. Effusions are usually exudative and may be bloody. Malignant effusions are always exudates, but not all exudative effusions in cancer patients are malignant. Exudative effusions in patients with malignancy may reflect pleural involvement by tumor, lymphatic obstruction, or pneumonia. Pleural effusion in patients with malignancy is described in detail below.

Pericardial Disease

Pleural effusion is common in patients with inflammatory pericardial disease. They are left sided in 70%, bilateral in 20%, and right sided in 10%. Left-sided effusion likely predominates because of local inflammation. In patients with constrictive pericarditis, effusions may result from elevated left- or right-sided venous pressures; in this setting, as in patients with CHF, effusions are most often bilateral or right sided.

Pancreatitis

Acute pancreatitis results in effusion in 10% to 20%. Because of the relationship of the pancreatic tail to the left hemidiaphragm, these are usually left sided (70%) or bilateral. They are exudative and often hemorrhagic and often contain high amylase levels.

Chronic pancreatitis may also be associated with a left-sided effusion, which contains high amylase. It is most often left sided (70%) or bilateral. Pseudocyst is commonly present. Associated mediastinal pseudocyst with rupture into the pleural space may result in a pancreaticopleural fistula with a large pleural effusion.

Pancreatic abscess may be associated with pleural effusion containing high amylase levels. It is usually left sided.

Parapneumonic Effusion and Empyema

Pleural effusion is common in patients with pneumonia; this is termed *parapneumonic effusion*. Parapneumonic effusions are typically exudates; they are small and sterile and have normal glucose and pH values. They usually resolve with appropriate antibiotic treatment but may progress to empyema. Empyema is an infected exudative effusion, often requiring tube drainage. These entities are described in detail below.

Pregnancy

Small bilateral transudative pleural effusions are seen in 10% of pregnant women. They are seen for a short time after delivery in up to 25% of women.

Pulmonary Embolism

Pleural effusion occurs in 30% of patients with pulmonary embolism, often associated with infarction. Effusion is more common in patients with the presenting complaint of hemoptysis or pleuritic chest pain (50%) than in those with dyspnea (25%). Exudate is more common (75%) than transudate (25%). They are often unilateral, but this depends on the distribution of emboli. Effusions are usually small and do not increase after 3 days. The majority resolve within a week. Consolidation is associated in half of cases.

Radiation (Therapeutic)

About 5% of patients having chest radiation develop a small exudative pleural effusion in association with radiation pneumonitis. The effusion occurs on the side of radiation and develops within 6 months of radiation. It resolves slowly with time.

Renal Disease

Several manifestations of renal disease may be associated with pleural effusion:

1. Renal failure with overhydration may result in transudative effusion. Acute glomerulonephritis may be responsible for this occurrence. Effusions are usually bilateral.
2. Nephrotic syndrome may result in transudative effusion because of increased hydrostatic pressure and hypoalbuminemia resulting in decreased plasma oncotic pressure. Effusions are often bilateral and subpulmonic in location.
3. Uremia may result in fibrinous pleuritis and a bloody exudative effusion that is often unilateral and large. Fever, chest pain, and dyspnea are often present. Pericardial effusion is often associated. Chronic fibrotic pleural thickening may result.

4. Hydronephrosis may result in retroperitoneal urinoma and ipsilateral pleural effusion. The effusion is a transudate but contains a high creatinine level.
5. Peritoneal dialysis may result in effusion, usually on the right side. Fluid likely enters the pleural space via diaphragmatic defects.
6. Pyelonephritis may rarely cause a unilateral pleura effusion on the side of infection, likely from similar mechanism of spread as described above.

CHYLOTHORAX

Chylous effusion or *chylothorax* contains intestinal lymph (ie, chyle), is high in protein and fatty acid, and is low in cholesterol. It typically appears milky. Chylothorax usually results from disruption of the thoracic duct (25%) or thoracic lymphatic obstruction by tumor (50% of cases). Simple obstruction of the thoracic duct does not result in chylothorax; it may be tied off without the development of chylothorax.

The thoracic duct originates at the cisterna chyli in the upper abdomen and enters the thorax along the right anterior aspect of the spine; it crosses to the left near the level of T6, lying along the left lateral wall of the esophagus, posterior to the descending aorta, and drains into the left brachiocephalic or subclavian vein. Approximately 2 L of chyle passes through the thoracic duct each day, although the volume varies with diet.

Chylous effusion is most common in patients with lymphoma, metastatic neoplasm, or other mediastinal masses (Table 26.3); following thoracic surgery (chylothorax is a complication in about 0.5% of cardiovascular and 4% of esophageal surgeries) or chest trauma (eg, penetrating or nonpenetrating trauma, thoracic vertebral fracture); inflammatory mediastinal lymph node diseases; mediastinal fibrosis; central vein thrombosis/superior vena cava syndrome; lymphangiomyomatosis; chylous ascites; and some congenital abnormalities.

Chylous effusions may be small or massive and unilateral or bilateral. They contain protein in addition to fat and appear to be near water in attenuation on CT (Fig. 26.22). Rarely, chylous effusion measures less than 0 HU in attenuation.

Following chest trauma and duct disruption, chyle typically accumulates in the mediastinum before leading to chylothorax. Mediastinal widening or a localized fluid collection may be seen days before development of the chylothorax. Because the location of the thoracic duct is to the right of midline in the lower thorax and to the left in the upper thorax, injury of the lower duct tends to cause right-sided effusion, while injury to the upper duct causes left-sided effusion. Postsurgical chylothorax is often left sided. Closed trauma usually results in right-sided chylothorax.

Traumatic chylothorax will often resolve over time as the thoracic duct heals. Reduction in lymph flow may be helpful in achieving this result. A pleuroperitoneal shunt may be used. Tube drainage may lead to malnutrition. Ligation of the duct is curative. Chylothorax associated with lymphoma is usually treated with radiation.

Table 26.3 Causes of Chylothorax

Cause	Prevalence (%)
Tumor	50
Lymphoma	35
Other tumor	15
Trauma	25
Surgery	20
Other trauma	5
Miscellaneous	25
Congenital	5
Other	20

Pseudochylous or *chyliform* effusion contains cholesterol but not chyle. It may be seen in patients with chronic inflammatory disease such as tuberculosis or RA or in patients with breakdown of cells presents within a pleural effusion. Pseudochylous effusions are often chronic, being present for years.

HEMOTHORAX

The term "hemothorax" refers to a pleural fluid collection having a hematocrit over 50% of blood hematocrit. On CT, hemothorax results in fluid with high attenuation (usually higher than 50 HU), containing relatively dense clot or a fluid-fluid level, with the densest fluid being in the dependent portion of the pleural space (Fig. 26.23).

Most cases are traumatic, but a select list of entities can result in spontaneous hemothorax. These include rupture

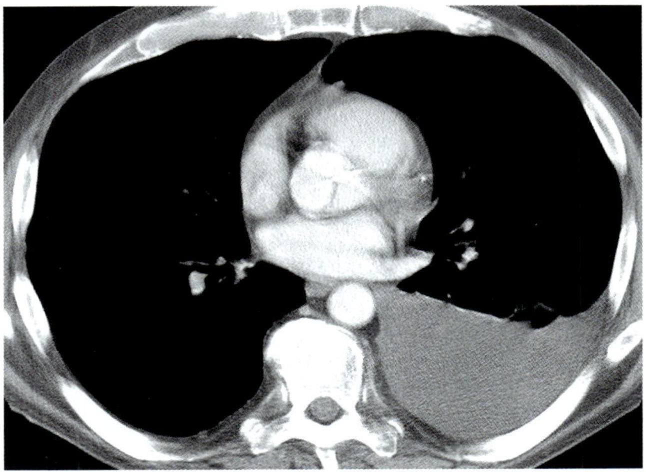

Figure 26.22. Chylous effusion in lymphoma. The effusion is unassociated with pleural thickening and has no distinguishing characteristics.

of an aneurysm or dissection, pulmonary or pleural neoplasm, pneumothorax, coagulopathy, rupture of a pulmonary arteriovenous malformation, and pulmonary or pleural endometriosis.

Treatment includes tube drainage or sometimes thoracotomy for control of bleeding. Empyema may complicate hemothorax. Organization of a hemothorax may result in pleural fibrosis and calcification.

PARAPNEUMONIC EFFUSION AND EMPYEMA

Pleural fluid accumulates in approximately 40% of patients with pneumonia. The term *parapneumonic effusion* is used to describe this occurrence. Parapneumonic effusions are usually classified into three stages. These are (1) the exudative stage (simple parapneumonic effusion), (2) the fibropurulent stage (empyema), and (3) the stage of organization (pleural peel). Progression from one stage to the next does not necessarily occur.

Stage 1 (Exudative Stage): Simple Parapneumonic Effusion

A simple parapneumonic effusion probably results from increased permeability of the visceral pleura occurring in association with pulmonary inflammation in patients with pneumonia (Table 26.4). Effusions in this stage are commonly exudates and are typically small and sterile and have a normal glucose level (more than 40-60 mg/dL) and pH (greater than 7.2).

Parapneumonic effusions usually (1) are small to moderate in size, (2) are dependent in location, (3) do not show evidence of loculation, (4) show a meniscus on plain radiographs, and (5) appear crescent shaped on CT (Fig. 26.24). About 50% of parapneumonic effusions are associated with pleural thickening visible on CT. Visceral pleural thickening and the "split pleura" sign also may be present.

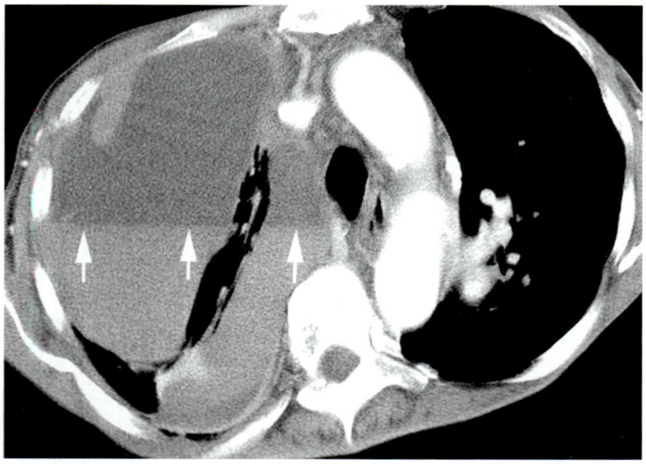

Figure 26.23. Iatrogenic traumatic hemothorax related to thoracentesis. A large right pleural effusion shows a distinct fluid or hematocrit level (*arrows*). The dependent fluid measures in excess of 60 HU.

Simple parapneumonic effusion will usually resolve with appropriate antibiotic treatment of the pneumonia and rarely needs tube drainage. A parapneumonic effusion that requires drainage is termed a *complicated parapneumonic effusion*. A complicated parapneumonic effusion is often an empyema.

Stage 2 (Fibropurulent Stage): Empyema

The term *empyema* is generally used when a pleural effusion is infected, although its true definition necessitates the presence of pus in the pleural space (Table 26.5). Although most empyemas occur in association with pneumonia, approximately 10% are unassociated with obvious lung disease.

Up to 75% of bacterial empyemas result from anaerobic infections or mixed anaerobic and aerobic infections. Common anaerobic organisms include *Bacteroides* species, *Fusobacterium*, anaerobic and microaerophilic cocci, and *Clostridium*. Common aerobic organisms are *Staphylococcus aureus*, *Streptococcus pneumoniae*, *Haemophilus influenzae*, and gram-negative enteric bacilli. Tuberculosis may result in empyema.

Empyema is characterized by the presence of infectious organisms in the pleural fluid, an increase in the size of the effusion, increased white blood cells and polymorphonuclear cells in the fluid, fibrin deposition along the pleural surfaces, a tendency for loculation, decreased glucose levels (less than 40 mg/dL) and pH (below 7.2), and increased LDH (over 1000 IU/L).

In a patient who has pneumonia, the presence of a localized or loculated pleural effusion strongly suggests the presence of an empyema (see Figs. 26.16, 26.19-26.21). On plain radiographs, empyemas often have a lenticular shape and tend to appear larger or better defined in one projection (eg, as seen on the posteroanterior radiograph) than in the other (eg, on the lateral radiograph; see Fig. 26.16). On radiographs, an empyema containing air may be difficult to differentiate from a peripheral lung abscess abutting the chest wall. This distinction can be an important one to make because empyemas are often treated by tube thoracostomy in addition to systemic antibiotics, whereas most lung abscesses require antibiotics only.

Table 26.4 Simple Parapneumonic Effusion

Increased permeability of the visceral pleura
Commonly exudates
Sterile with normal glucose
Small to moderate in size
Dependent in location
No loculation
Meniscus on plain radiographs
Crescentic shape on CT
50% associated with pleural thickening
Resolves with appropriate antibiotic treatment

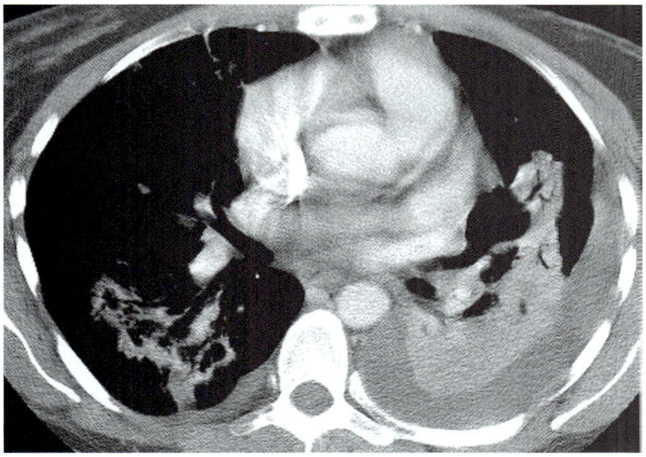

Figure 26.24. Simple parapneumonic effusion. The left pleural effusion is dependent, crescent shaped, small, and unassociated with pleural thickening or findings of location. Bilateral pneumonia and a small right pleural effusion are present.

Classical CT findings of empyema (see Figs. 26.16, 26.19-26.21) include an (1) elliptical or lenticular shape, (2) nondependent location, (3) sharp demarcation from the adjacent lung, (4) the split pleura sign (the enhancing visceral and parietal pleural surfaces are split apart by the fluid collection), (5) smooth pleural thickening of uniform thickness (when enhanced by contrast or outlined by air), and (6) compression of the lung and displacement of adjacent vessels.

In contrast to empyema, lung abscesses (see Figs. 10.10B and 10.40 in Chapter 10) tend to (1) be round, (2) be ill defined, (3) have shaggy walls of irregular thickness, and (4) destroy lung without displacing vessels.

In patients with parapneumonic effusion or empyema, it is common (60% to 80% of cases) to see extrapleural fat thickening on CT when parietal pleural thickening is present. Increased attenuation of the thick extrapleural fat due to edema is less common (30% of cases).

Table 26.5 Empyema

- "Fibropurulent parapneumonic effusion"
- Most empyemas occur with pneumonia
- 10% unassociated with lung disease
- Anaerobic infections or mixed anaerobic and aerobic infections
- Polymorphonuclear neutrophils in the fluid
- Fibrin deposition along the pleural surfaces
- Decreased glucose
- Low pH values (<7.2)
- Increased lactate dehydrogenase (>1000 IU/L)
- Elliptical or lenticular shape on radiographs or CT
- Nondependent location
- Sharp demarcation from the adjacent lung
- "Split pleura" sign
- Air—thoracentesis, bronchopleural fistula, and gas-forming organism
- Empyema necessitates—chest wall involvement, tuberculosis, actinomycosis, etc.

Not all empyemas show classical findings. Many empyemas are crescent shaped and dependent on location, without findings of loculation, and thus are indistinguishable from a simple parapneumonic effusion. Parietal pleural thickening or enhancement is always seen on CT, while visceral pleural thickening or enhancement is seen in half; thus, the split pleura sign is absent in about half of cases.

Bronchopleural Fistula

Bronchopleural fistula (BPF) results from disruption of the visceral pleura, usually in association with lung abscess and empyema. Unless there has been a recent thoracentesis, gas within a pleural fluid collection is presumptive evidence of empyema and a BPF. The presence of a gas-forming organism is less often associated with gas in the pleural space. Rarely, in a patient with lung abscess, the site of BPF (ie, the point of visceral pleural discontinuity) can be demonstrated on CT. BPF is an indication for chest tube drainage.

Empyema Necessitatis

Empyema can involve the chest wall by direct extension; this is termed empyema necessitatis or empyema necessitans. Tuberculosis accounts for about 70% of cases of empyema necessitatis, but other organisms such as *Actinomyces, Nocardia,* and other bacteria or fungi can be responsible. Extensive extrapleural fat thickening, edema or extrapleural fat, and subcutaneous collections of pus can be seen on CT.

Tube Drainage of Empyema

Indications for tube placement in patients with a parapneumonic effusion vary depending on the clinical setting, but one of the following criteria is usually sufficient: (1) thick pus on thoracentesis, (2) positive Gram stain from pleural fluid, (3) positive pleural fluid culture, (4) pleural fluid glucose below 60 mg/dL, (5) pleural fluid pH less than 7.2, (6) LDH greater than 1000 IU/L, or (6) a parapneumonic effusion that does not resolve with antibiotic treatment.

Stage 3 (Organization Stage): Pleural Peel or Fibrothorax

In patients with chronic empyema, ingrowth of fibroblasts and organization can result in extensive pleural fibrosis and the development of an inelastic fibrotic *pleural peel* or *fibrothorax* (Table 26.6). This can cause lung restriction and decreased lung volume ("trapped lung").

Smooth pleural thickening is typically visible on plain radiographs or CT (Fig. 26.25). Extrapleural fat thickening is frequently visible on CT, separating the thickened parietal pleura from the intercostal muscle or rib. Calcification, which usually is focal in its early stages, may become extensive. This is most common with tuberculosis. Chronic pleural effusion may occasionally be high in attenuation because of milk of calcium in the fluid (Fig. 26.26).

A very important finding in diagnosing pleural peel on plain film or CT is reduction in volume of the affected hemithorax (see Fig. 26.25). Loculated fluid collections resulting from active infection may be seen on CT in association with the pleural peel.

In addition to chronic empyema, a pleural peel may result from chronic pleural effusion and inflammation in the absence of infection. This may be seen in patients with collagen vascular diseases, asbestos exposure, uremia, and hemothorax.

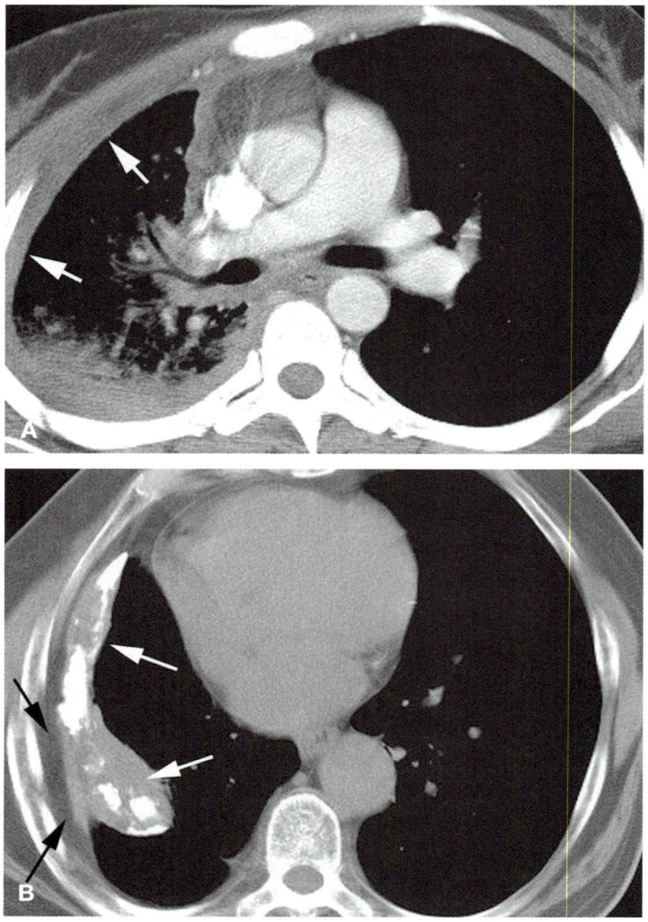

Figure 26.25. Pleural peel in two patients. **A:** In a patient with chronic empyema, smooth pleural thickening is visible (*arrows*) with reduction in volume of the affected hemithorax. **B:** Following tuberculous empyema, there is right pleural thickening and calcification (*white arrows*). Extrapleural fat is thickened (*black arrows*). The volume of the hemithorax is reduced.

Pleural Calcification

Pleural calcification may be associated with pleural fibrosis regardless of its cause. It is seen most commonly with pleural peel in patients with healed tuberculosis or bacterial empyema, hemothorax, or asbestos exposure. Asbestos exposure is bilateral in the majority of cases, whereas the other causes are typically unilateral. When present, it is commonly associated with increased thickness of extrapleural fat.

Talc Pleurodesis

Talc pleurodesis used to treat patients with chronic pleural effusion may mimic the appearance of pleural calcification. Dense accumulations of talc within the pleural space, in association with pleural thickening (Fig. 26.27), are typically seen. Talc is often visible in a clump posteriorly at the lung base.

PLEURAL NEOPLASMS

Neoplasm, either primary or metastatic, is a common cause of pleural mass, pleural effusion, or pleural thickening. Primary pleural tumors have recently been reclassified by the World Health Organization.

Pleural and Extrapleural Masses

Lesions located in the peripheral thorax, in contact with the chest wall, are generally classified as extrapleural, pleural, or parenchymal and are usually characterized radiographically

Table 26.6 Pleural Peel
Chronic empyema
Pleural fibrosis
Restriction of lung function (ie, trapped lung)
Smooth pleural thickening
Reduction in size of hemithorax
Pleural calcification

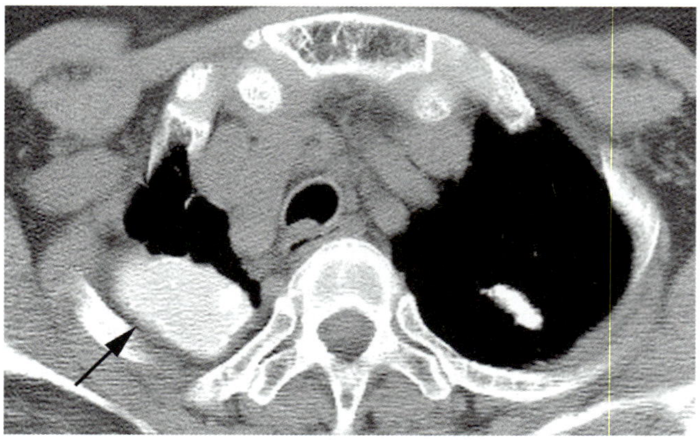

Figure 26.26. Chronic pleural fluid collection in tuberculosis with milk of calcium. CT in a patient with a left upper lobe granuloma shows pleural thickening and high-attenuation pleural fluid (*arrow*) in the right apex.

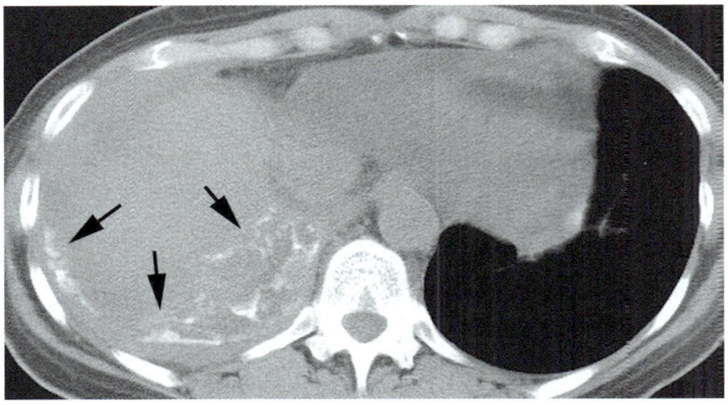

Figure 26.27. Talc pleurodesis. Pleural thickening and dense talc (*arrows*) are visible.

by the angle (either acute or obtuse) formed by the interface between the lesion and the adjacent pleura.

Extrapleural masses usually displace the overlying parietal and visceral pleura, resulting in an obtuse angle between the lesion and the chest wall. Associated abnormalities including chest wall soft-tissue mass or rib destruction may help to confirm the mass as extrapleural. Typically, extrapleural masses are sharply marginated at the point they contact the lung and displace pulmonary vessels away from them. Such masses may be related to rib lesions (tumor or fracture), soft-tissue tumors, infection, or hematoma secondary to trauma.

Pleural masses, arising from the visceral or parietal pleura, usually remain confined to the pleural space and have an appearance similar to that of extrapleural lesions. The presence of an obtuse angle is common unless the lesion is large (Fig. 26.28). Large pleural lesions may have acute angles where they meet the chest wall, although some pleural thickening is often seen adjacent to them. As with extrapleural masses, pleural lesions are sharply marginated and displace pulmonary vessels away from them. Pleural masses or nodular pleural thickening suggests neoplasm, either primary to the pleura (eg, mesothelioma, solitary fibrous tumor [SFT], benign or malignant mesenchymal tumors) or metastatic, although the differential diagnosis includes organized and loculated fluid collections, pleural mesothelial cyst, fibrin ball or thoracolith (see below), splenosis (see below), and asbestos-related pleural plaques (see Chapter 16).

Pulmonary parenchymal masses, when peripheral, may abut the pleura. A peripheral pulmonary lesion typically results in an acute angle with the pleural surface. Lung masses may result in obtuse angles at the chest wall in the presence of pleural invasion. Pulmonary lesions are often ill defined along their inner aspect and may engulf rather than displace vessels. The differential diagnosis of pulmonary masses is long and described elsewhere (see Chapters 5 and 6).

Pleural Effusion With Neoplasm

Pleural effusion is common in patients with pleural malignancy, either primary or metastatic. Such effusions have a variety of causes but are usually exudates.

A *malignant effusion* is one secondary to pleural involvement by tumor and contains malignant cells. The most common causes of malignant effusion are lung cancer and breast cancer. Pleural fluid cytology yield has been reported as positive in 67% to 90% of patients with pleural malignancy, with the highest frequency in patients with adenocarcinoma. Malignant effusions are exudates.

Exudative effusions in patients with malignancy can also reflect the presence of obstructive pneumonia or lymphatic or pulmonary venous obstruction by tumor. This is particularly true of lung cancer; only patients with demonstration of tumor cells in the pleural fluid are considered to have unresectable disease.

Malignant effusions may be small or large and unilateral, bilateral, or asymmetrical. A large unilateral effusion suggests

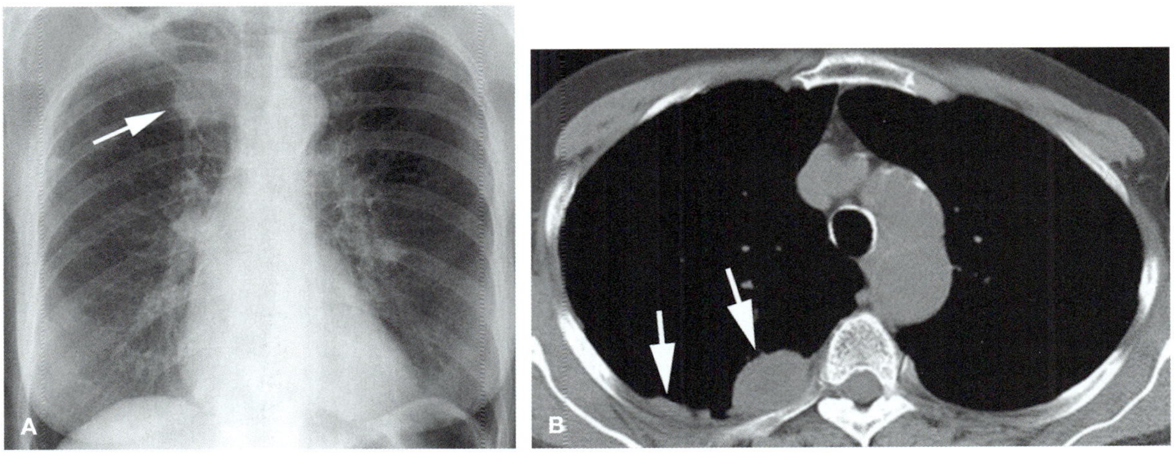

Figure 26.28. Pleural metastases from chondrosarcoma. **A:** Chest radiograph shows a mass at the right apex (*arrow*). **B:** CT shows pleural masses with obtuse angles (*arrows*). No pleural effusion is associated; this is unusual with pleural metastases and implies a slow-growing lesion.

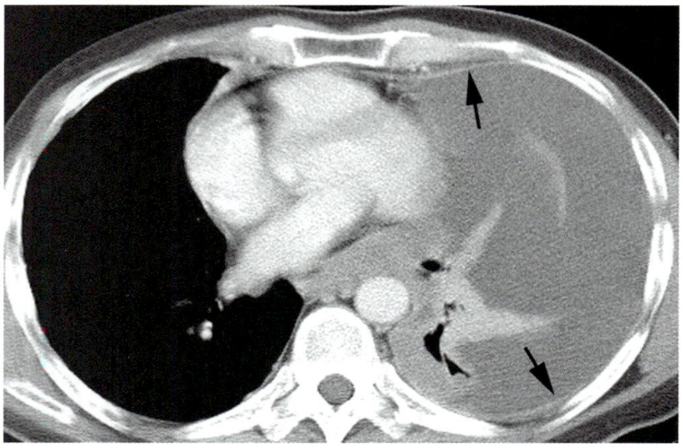

Figure 26.29. Large unilateral malignant effusion. The effusion is large, and the presence of pleural thickening (*arrows*) indicates that it is exudative.

malignancy or infection (Figs. 26.29-26.31). Regardless of their cause, exudative effusions in cancer patients often require treatment by drainage.

Pleural Thickening With Neoplasm

The presence of pleural thickening on CT in a patient with malignancy and pleural effusion indicates the presence of an exudate (see Fig. 26.29), but is of little value in diagnosing malignant effusion. Pleural thickening is seen in 30% of cancer patients with a malignant effusion and 40% of those with a benign effusion. Pleural effusion is usually the only abnormality visible on chest radiographs in patients with malignant effusion. In patients with gross pleural involvement by tumor, nodular pleural thickening may be seen (see Figs. 26.30 and 26.31). Metastatic tumor also may involve the pleural space in a concentric fashion.

The CT findings most specific in diagnosing malignant pleural disease are listed below. If one or more of these findings are considered to indicate malignancy, the overall diagnostic accuracy is about 75%.

1. Nodular pleural thickening (see Figs. 26.30 and 26.31)
2. Circumferential pleural thickening (pleural thickening surrounding the lung; Fig. 26.32)
3. Parietal pleural thickening greater than 1 cm
4. Mediastinal pleural thickening (see Fig. 26.32)

PLEURAL METASTASES

Pleural metastases typically result in pleural effusion. CT may show pleural effusion without pleural thickening, smooth pleural thickening (see Fig. 26.29), localized pleural masses (see Figs. 26.28, 26.30, and 26.31), or gross nodular pleural thickening (see Fig. 26.32). Localized pleural masses strongly suggest metastases. Nodular pleural thickening may be seen with metastatic tumor or mesothelioma. In patients with metastases, gross nodular pleural thickening is most typical of adenocarcinoma, but this is seen in a minority of cases. On chest radiographs, pleural effusion is usually the only visible finding.

In some patients with pleural metastases, particularly from invasive thymoma, pleural metastases may be unassociated with effusion and visible as rounded or lenticular pleural masses. In patients with lung carcinoma abutting the pleural surface, multiple pleural nodules representing direct

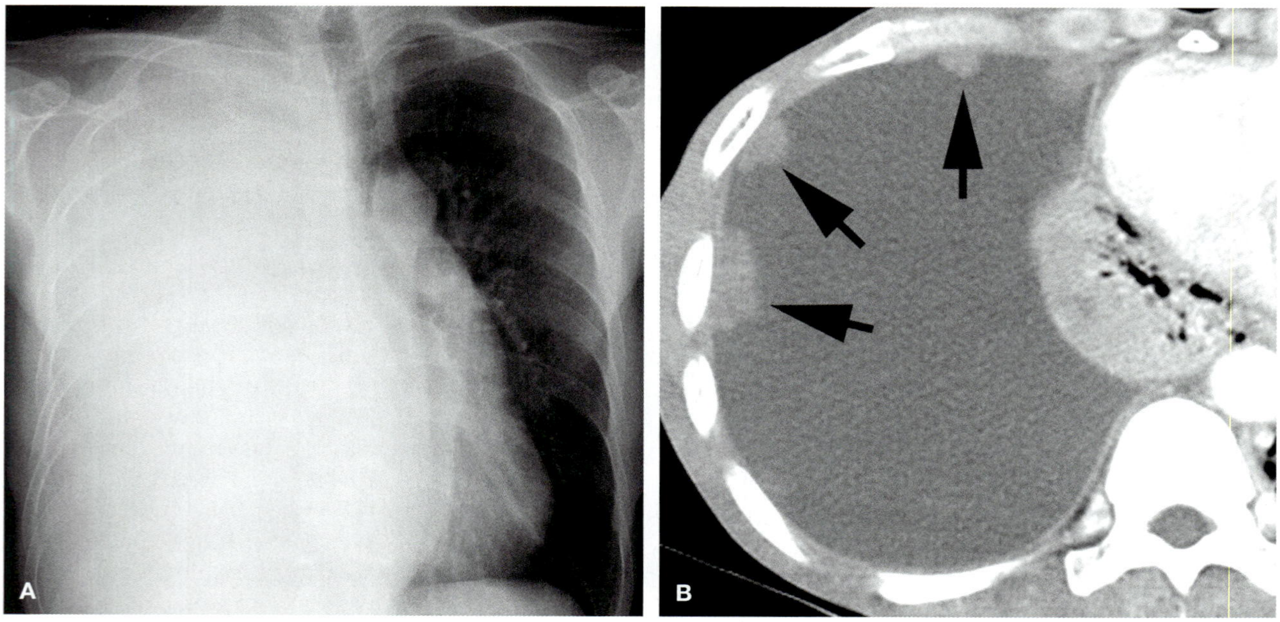

Figure 26.30. Pleural metastases. **A:** Chest radiograph shows a large right pleural effusion with mediastinal displacement to the left. **B:** CT shows nodular pleural thickening (*arrows*) with a large effusion and right lung collapse.

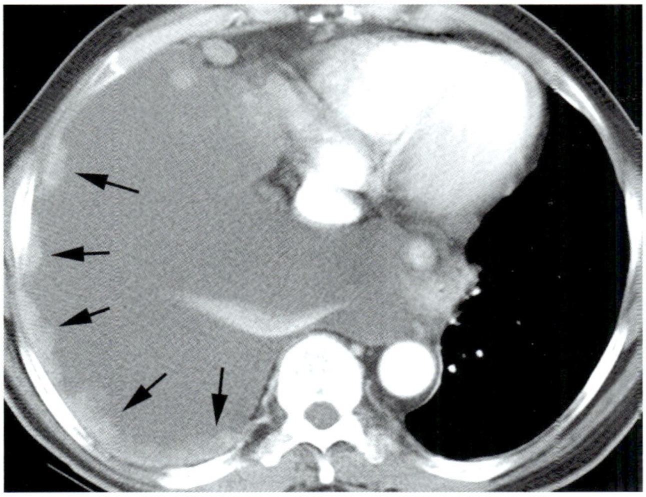

Figure 26.31. Pleural metastasis in colon carcinoma with nodular pleural thickening. Gross nodular thickening of the parietal pleura is present (*arrows*). This appearance strongly suggests malignancy.

pleural invasion can be seen in the absence of pleural effusion, sometimes visible within a fissure (Fig. 26.33).

LYMPHOMA

In patients with lymphoma, particularly those with Hodgkin disease, exudative effusions commonly result from mediastinal lymphatic obstruction and resolve following mediastinal radiation; pleural thickening may or may not be present.

Marked thickening of extrapleural soft tissues may be seen with lymphoma or leukemia, often associated with paravertebral lymph node enlargement. This may result in a rind of soft tissue mimicking the appearance of mesothelioma (see Figs. 7.25 and 7.36 in Chapter 7). This appearance is associated with effusion.

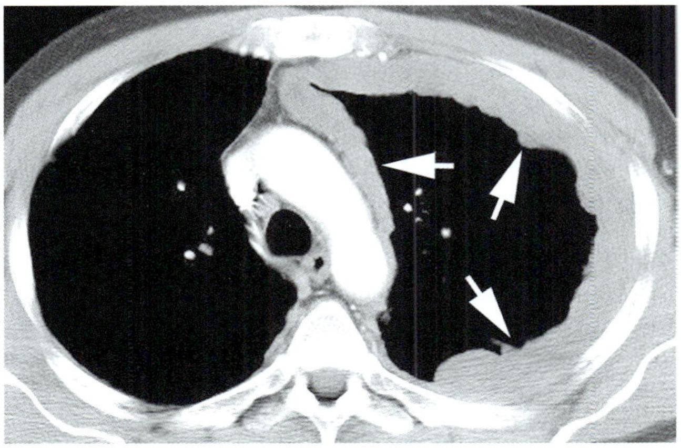

Figure 26.32. Concentric pleural thickening with metastatic adenocarcinoma. Four findings of malignancy are visible: nodular pleural thickening, circumferential pleural thickening (*arrows*), parietal pleural thickening greater than 1 cm, and mediastinal pleural thickening.

MESOTHELIOMA

Mesothelioma (also known as malignant or diffuse mesothelioma) is a highly malignant, progressive neoplasm, arising from mesothelial cells, with an extremely poor prognosis (Table 26.7). In most patients, malignant mesothelioma is related to asbestos exposure. Although mesothelioma is rare in the general population, its incidence in heavily exposed asbestos workers is up to 5% (see Chapter 16 for further discussion of asbestos). A latency period of 20 to 40 years between exposure and development of the tumor is typical. However, with decreasing asbestos exposure over the last 20 years, cases unrelated to asbestos exposure are now common. Mesothelioma is also associated with therapeutic radiation and some specific genetic abnormalities including a familial cancer syndrome associated with a predisposition for mesothelioma, uveal melanoma, renal cell carcinoma, cholangiocarcinoma, and other tumors.

Mean age at diagnosis is 60, but tumors may occur in children. Males are affected 4 times as often as females, but this varies, related to the likelihood of occupational asbestos exposure. Symptoms include chest pain, dyspnea, and weight loss.

Mesothelioma arises in relation to the parietal pleura. It is classified histologically as epithelioid (60% to 80%), sarcomatous (10%), biphasic (mixed epithelioid and sarcomatous; 10% to 15%), or desmoplastic (<2%). The epithelial type has a slightly better prognosis and tends to be associated with pleural effusion. Pleural effusion tends to be small or absent with sarcomatous tumors. Histologic diagnosis of mesothelioma is difficult using pleural fluid cytology, and biopsy is usually required. Special histologic techniques may be needed to distinguish mesothelioma from adenocarcinoma.

Mesothelioma is characterized morphologically by gross and nodular pleural thickening, which can involve the fissures. Hemorrhagic pleural effusion often occurs. Malignant mesothelioma spreads most commonly by local infiltration of the pleura. Hematogenous metastases are present in 50% of patients, although these are usually insignificant clinically.

Radiographic Findings

Plain radiographs may show pleural effusion as the initial abnormality (Fig. 26.34) or concentric and lobulated pleural thickening (Fig. 26.35). This may reflect tumor nodules, multiloculated pleural fluid collections, or both. Thickening of the major fissure is common due to tumor.

Because of pleural thickening and mediastinal infiltration, the involved hemithorax may be normal in volume, without mediastinal shift, despite the presence of a large effusion (the "frozen mediastinum sign"). The hemithorax may also be reduced in volume because of restriction of lung expansion. Asbestos-related pleural thickening or plaques may be seen (see Chapter 16).

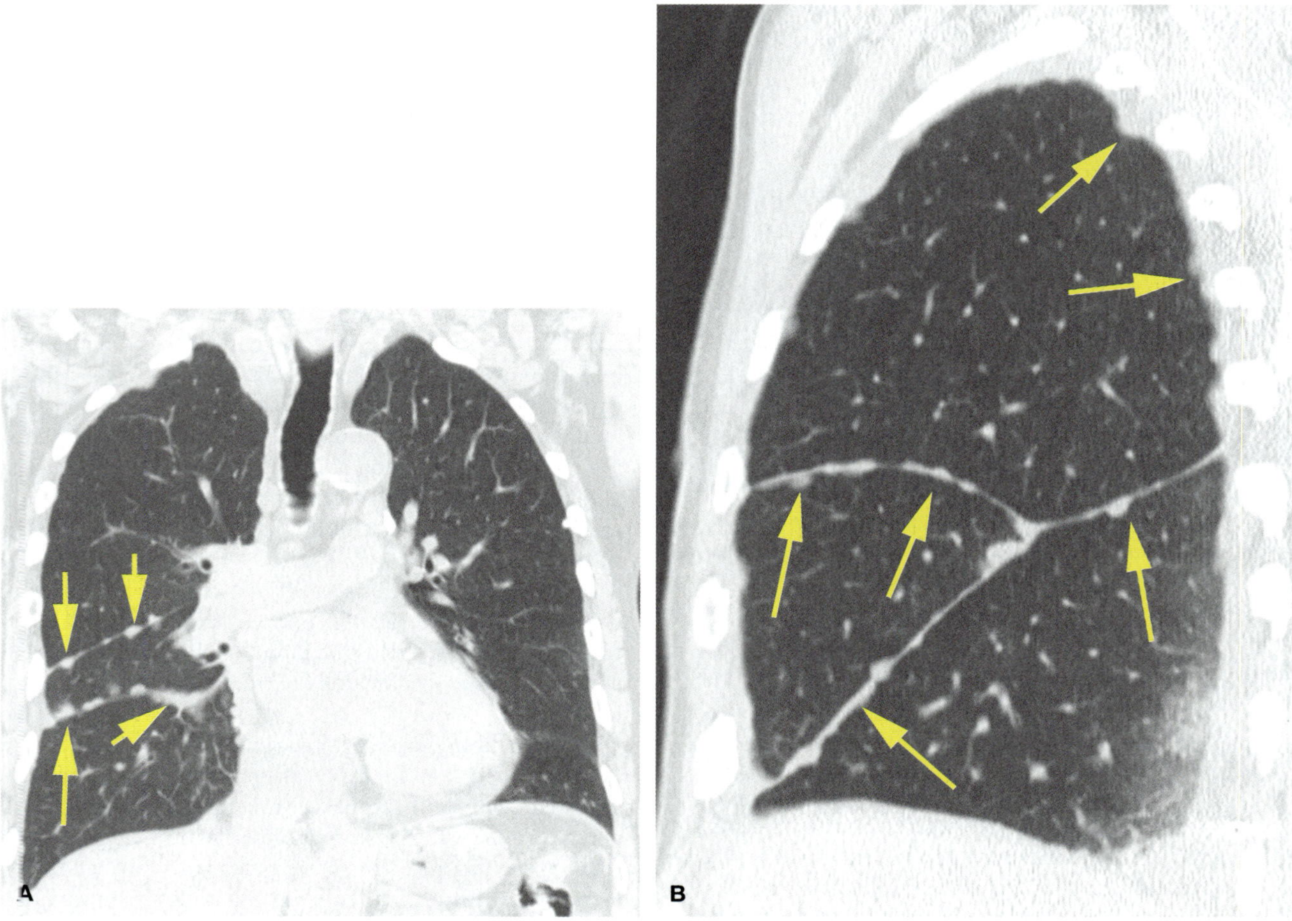

Figure 26.33. Pleural metastases involving fissures. **A.** Coronal CT shows small nodules involving the right major and minor fissures and the peripheral pleural space (*arrows*). **B:** Sagittal CT shows small peripheral pleural and fissural nodules (*arrows*). Only a small associated pleural effusion is visible posteriorly.

CT Findings

Pleural fluid collections are visible on CT in 75% (see Fig. 26.34B). Pleural thickening is seen in 90%. Pleural effusion may be visible in the absence of visible pleural thickening in early disease, but this is uncommon.

Table 26.7 Mesothelioma
Commonly related to asbestos exposure
Other causes: genetic defects, radiation
Incidence up to 5% in heavily exposed subjects
Latency period of 20-40 y
Arises in relation to the parietal pleura
Epithelioid (60%-80%), sarcomatous (10%), or mixed (10%-15%) cell types
Pleural effusion
Concentric and lobulated pleural thickening
Frozen mediastinum sign
Involvement of fissure
Chest wall invasion or distant metastases
Poor prognosis

Nodular concentric pleural thickening is highly suggestive of mesothelioma (Figs. 26.35B and 26.36). However, pleural thickening may also be thin and smooth (Fig. 26.37) or irregular in contour. Localized pleural masses are uncommon. In early disease, pleural thickening may appear discontinuous. As the disease progresses, pleural thickening becomes continuous, it increases in thickness and nodularity, and the amount of fluid may decrease as the pleural layers become fused.

Fluid can be difficult to distinguish from tumor on CT, since tumor nodules can sometimes appear low in attenuation (Fig. 26.38). However, decubitus scans or scans with the patient prone can help to distinguish underlying tumor from free fluid. Enhancement of the pleura after contrast infusion can also help differentiate tumor from adjacent fluid collections. Calcification usually reflects asbestos exposure, but calcification of tumor may be seen.

Although mesothelioma is most frequently visible along the lateral chest wall, mediastinal pleural thickening or concentric pleural thickening is seen with extensive disease. The abnormal hemithorax can appear contracted and fixed (40%), with little change in size during inspiration (see Fig. 26.36). Thickening of the fissures, particularly the lower part

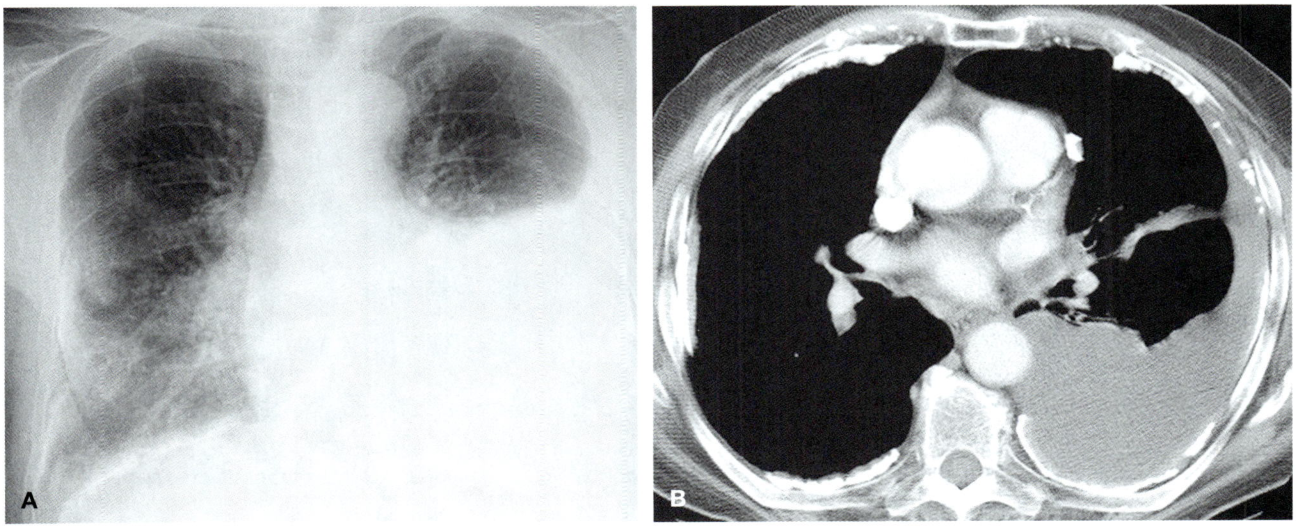

Figure 26.34. Asbestos exposure with mesothelioma. **A:** Chest radiograph shows pleural plaques and a large left pleural effusion. **B:** CT shows extensive pleural plaques and a left pleural effusion without obvious masses. This reflects left-sided mesothelioma.

of the major fissures, can reflect tumor infiltration or associated pleural effusion; involvement of the fissures is seen on CT in 85% (see Fig. 26.36A).

Staging of Mesothelioma

Mesothelioma is staged using a TNM system similar to that used with lung cancer. It is based on a classification adopted by the American Joint Commission on Cancer (AJCC) and the Union for International Cancer Control (UICC) and was most recently updated in 2018 with the 8th edition (Table 26.8). Stage and histologic subtype are the strongest predictors of survival. Patients with stage I, II, III, and IV disease have median survivals of 20, 19, 16, and 11 months, respectively. Stage I-III disease is potentially resectable, while stage IV is generally considered unresectable.

T classification of mesothelioma (T1-T4) is based on the extent of the primary tumor in relation to the ipsilateral pleural surface, without or with invasion of the visceral pleura, mediastinum, chest wall, or diaphragm. N and M criteria are similar to those used for staging of lung cancer.

Extrapleural pneumonectomy may be used for treatment, often in combination with chemotherapy and radiation, and survival may be improved in patients with early disease. PET/CT is of value in determining the respectability of mesothelioma.

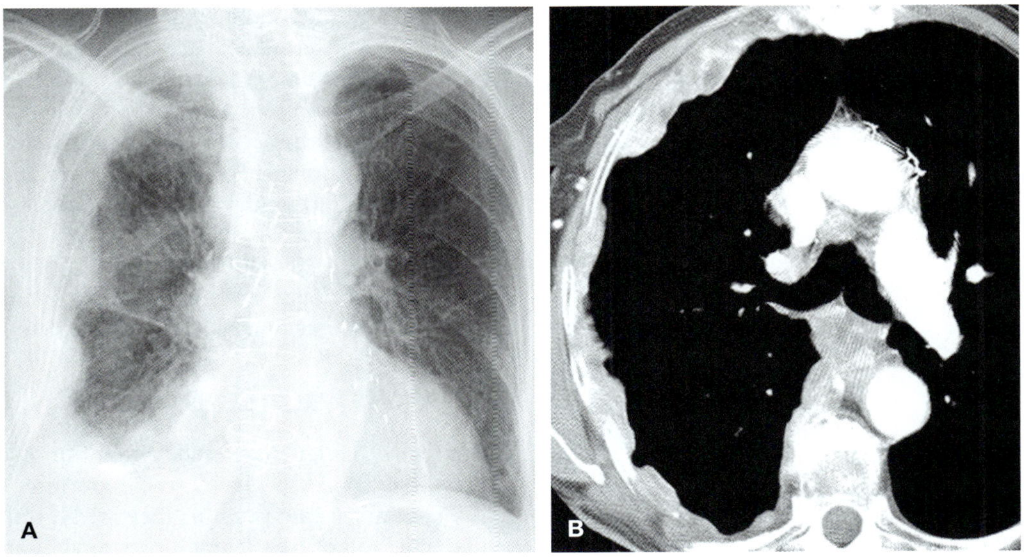

Figure 26.35. Asbestos exposure with mesothelioma. **A:** Chest radiograph shows lobulated right pleural thickening typical of this tumor. **B:** CT shows extensive nodular pleural thickening.

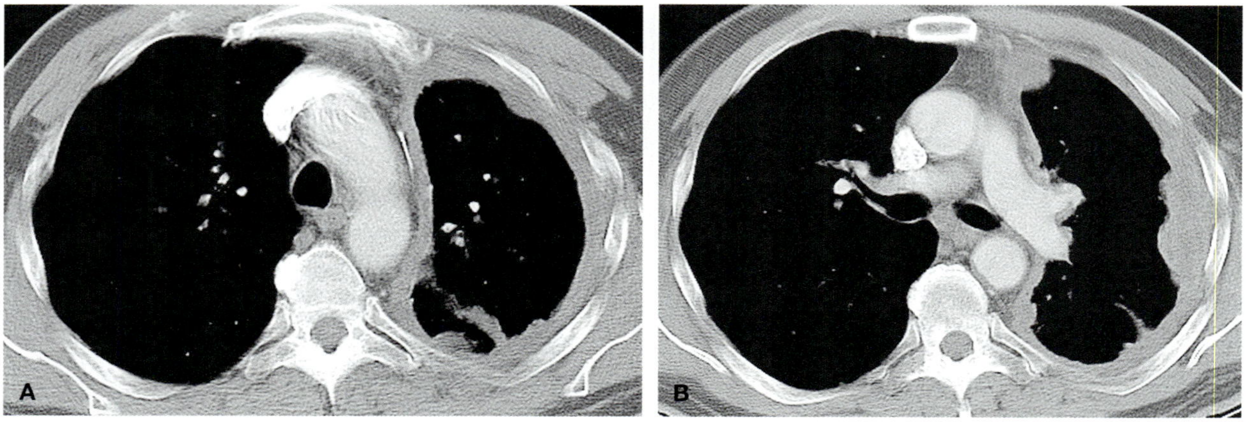

Figure 26.36. Mesothelioma with concentric nodular pleural thickening. **A and B:** CTs at two levels show concentric nodular pleural thickening typical of mesothelioma. Note reduction in volume of the affected hemithorax because of lung restriction.

LOCALIZED MALIGNANT MESOTHELIOMA

Localized malignant mesothelioma is a very rare tumor appearing as a localized pleural lesion, without dissemination, but with microscopic, ultrastructural, and immunohistochemical characteristic, characteristics of malignant mesothelioma. It has a better prognosis than diffuse mesothelioma.

SOLITARY (LOCALIZED) FIBROUS TUMOR OF THE PLEURA

SFT, formerly termed localized fibrous tumor of the pleura, is an uncommon fibroblastic neoplasm, which is most common in the fifth and sixth decades of life. SFT accounts for less than of 5% of primary pleural tumors. Approximately 10% of SFT are malignant, although they have a good prognosis. SFT is unassociated with asbestos exposure (Table 26.9).

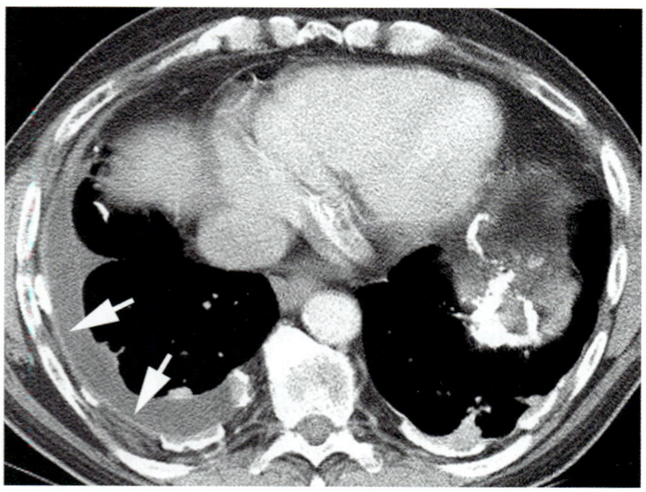

Figure 26.37. Mesothelioma. CT shows mild pleural thickening (*arrows*) and pleural effusion. Extensive pleural plaques from asbestos exposure are also present.

SFT is often detected incidentally on chest radiographs. However, it can be associated with hypoglycemia (5% of cases) due to production of insulin-like growth factor type 2 (IGF-2), hypertrophic pulmonary osteoarthropathy (one-third of cases), or chest pain. These symptoms resolve with resection.

SFT arises from the visceral pleura in 70% and thus can arise within a fissure. It typically appears as a solitary, smooth, sharply defined, often large lesion, contacting a pleural surface (Figs. 26.39 and 26.40). When small, SFT tends to have obtuse angles at the pleural surface; when large, the angles are usually acute. When SFT arises within a fissure, it can mimic the appearance of loculated fluid. A "beak" or "thorn" sign is often visible on plain radiographs in patients with an SFT originating in or projecting into a fissure (see Fig. 26.39). They may also arise on a stalk and move with change in patient position. Pleural effusion is not usually present.

On CT, even if acute angles are visible, some pleural thickening is usually present adjacent to the mass (see Fig. 26.40). This thickening may reflect a small amount of fluid accumulating in the pleural space at the point where the visceral and parietal pleural surfaces are separated by the tumor. Masses may appear homogeneous. Necrosis can result in a multicystic appearance with or without contrast infusion. Large arteries supplying the mass may be seen. Calcification may be present (Fig. 26.41).

Local recurrence after resection occurs in about 10% of cases, and the rate of metastasis is about 5% to 10%.

MESENCHYMAL TUMORS

Benign or malignant mesenchymal tumors (ie, sarcomas) may arise from the pleura. These are rare. Pleural lipoma is a common benign tumor; they are typically 2 to 4 cm in diameter and of fat attenuation. Synovial sarcoma is a relatively common cell type of primary malignancy. Sarcomas tend to appear as large heterogeneous masses with areas of necrosis.

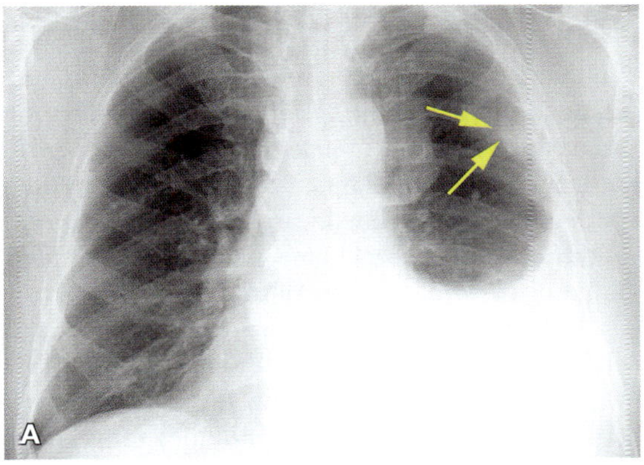

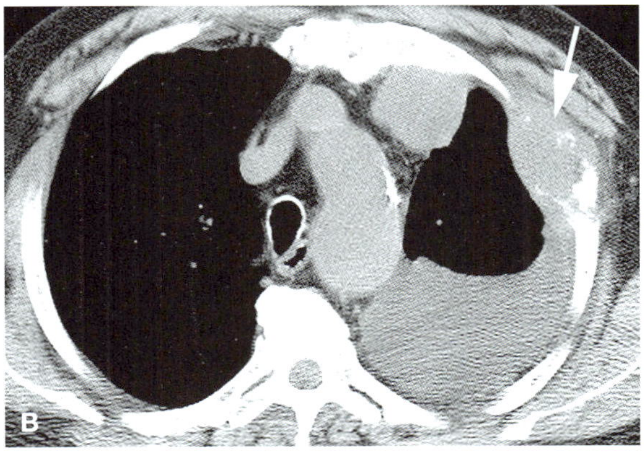

Figure 26.38. Mesothelioma with chest wall invasion. **A:** Chest radiograph shows a large effusion and a peripheral pleural nodule (*arrows*). **B:** The fluid and nodular areas of tumor are difficult to distinguish except for tumor invasion of the chest wall (*arrow*).

Table 26.8 Staging System for Mesothelioma

Primary Tumor	**Description**			
T1	Tumor involves the ipsilateral parietal pleura (including mediastinal and diaphragmatic pleura) with or without involvement of visceral pleura			
T2	Tumor involves any ipsilateral pleural surfaces (parietal, mediastinal, diaphragmatic, and visceral pleura) with at least one of the following features: Confluent visceral pleural tumor (including fissures) Invasion of diaphragmatic muscle Invasion of lung parenchyma			
T3	Tumor involves any ipsilateral pleural surfaces (parietal, mediastinal, diaphragmatic, and visceral pleura) with at least one of the following features: Invasion of endothoracic fascia or mediastinal fat Solitary, resectable focus invading soft tissues of the chest wall Nontransmural pericardial invasion			
T4	Tumor involves any ipsilateral pleural surface with at least one of the following: Diffuse or multifocal chest wall invasion Rib invasion Invasion into peritoneum through diaphragm Invasion of mediastinal organs Direct extension to the contralateral pleura Spine or brachial plexus invasion Transmural invasion of the pericardium (with or without pericardial effusion) or myocardium invasion			
Lymph Nodes				
N0	No regional node metastases			
N1	Metastases in the ipsilateral bronchopulmonary, hilar, or mediastinal lymph nodes (including the internal mammary, peridiaphragmatic, pericardial fat pad, or intercostal lymph nodes)			
N2	Metastases in the contralateral bronchopulmonary, hilar, or mediastinal lymph nodes or ipsilateral or contralateral supraclavicular lymph nodes			
Distant Metastases				
M0	No distant metastases			
M1	Distant metastases			
Stage Grouping	IA	T1	N0	M0
	IB	T2, 3	N0	M0
	II	T1, 2	N1	M0
	IIIA	T3	N1	M0
		T1-3	N2	M0
	IV	T4	Any N	M0
		Any T	Any N	M1

Table 26.9 Solitary Fibrous Tumor
No relation to asbestos exposure
Associated with chest pain, hypoglycemia (5%), and hypertrophic pulmonary osteoarthropathy (35%)
30% malignant; 70% benign
Arises in relation to the visceral pleura
Pleural effusion rare
Focal pleural mass
Good prognosis

FIBRIN BODY AND THORACOLITH

A resolving exudative effusion or hemothorax may deposit a clot of fibrin within the pleural space, termed a *fibrin body, fibrin ball,* or *pleural mouse*. A fibrin body appears as soft-tissue attenuation nodule, usually 1 to 2 cm in diameter. On radiographs or CT, a fibrin body contacts the pleural surface and can move with change in patient position or on follow-up studies (Fig. 26.42). Fibrin bodies typically resolve over time but may remain stable or enlarge.

The presence of a calcified loose body in the pleural space has been termed *thoracolith*. Although various etiologies for thoracolith have been suggested, it most likely represents to fibrin body that has calcified. A thoracolith may range from a few millimeters to a few centimeters in diameter, and as with a fibrin body, it may change in location over time (Fig. 26.43). They are most common on the left side.

THORACIC SPLENOSIS

Thoracic splenosis is a rare condition resulting from simultaneous rupture of the spleen and left hemidiaphragm, with autotransplantation of splenic tissue into the left hemithorax. The splenic implants may be attached to the visceral or parietal pleura, may be located in a fissure, or may be found within the lung parenchyma, likely as a result of lung laceration occurring at the time of trauma.

Thoracic splenosis is usually an incidental finding on chest radiographs or CT, although it is rarely associated with hemoptysis or chest pain. The interval between the initial trauma and detection of nodules ranges from years to decades. Radiographs and CT show sharply marginated, left-sided nodules in contact with the diaphragm or pleural surfaces (Fig. 26.44). Findings of diaphragmatic rupture, splenic rupture, splenectomy, or peritoneal splenosis are usually associated. The radiologic diagnosis can be confirmed by using scintigraphy with ^{99m}Tc sulfur colloid, ^{99m}Tc-labeled heat-damaged erythrocytes, or ^{111}In-labeled platelets.

PNEUMOTHORAX

Pneumothorax is classified as spontaneous or traumatic.

Spontaneous Pneumothorax

A spontaneous pneumothorax is one occurring without associated trauma. These are classified as primary or secondary.

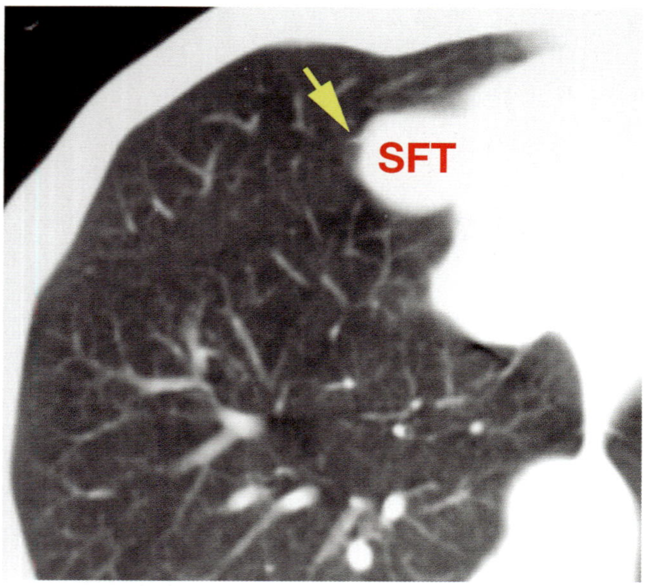

Figure 26.39. Solitary fibrous tumor (SFT) in the right major fissure. The tumor (*SFT*) lies in the plane of the major fissure and shows a small beak (*arrow*) at the point it contacts the fissure. The mass appears smooth and oval.

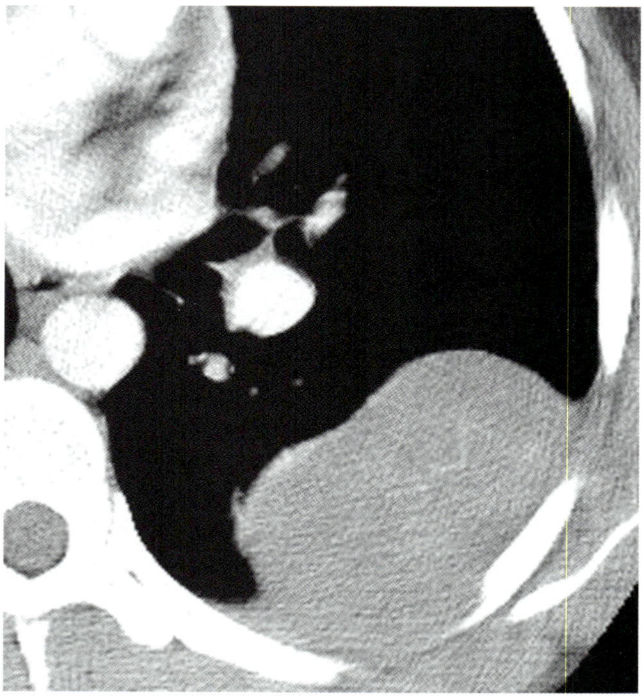

Figure 26.40. Solitary fibrous tumor appearing as a well-defined mass contacting the pleural surface. There is pleural thickening adjacent to the mass.

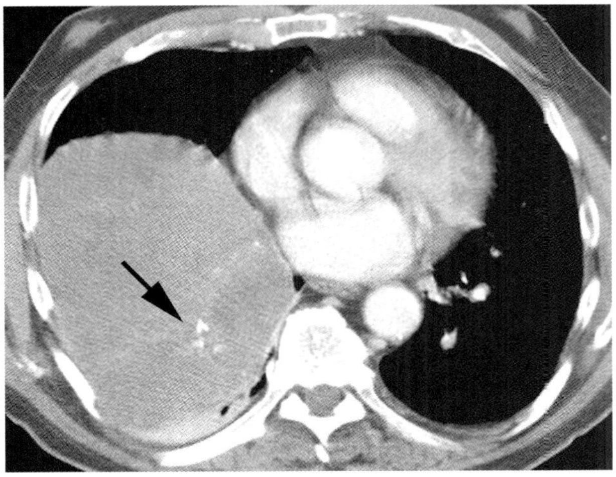

Figure 26.41. Large solitary fibrous tumor in the inferior pleural space. It appears somewhat inhomogeneous in attenuation, and focal calcification is visible (*arrow*).

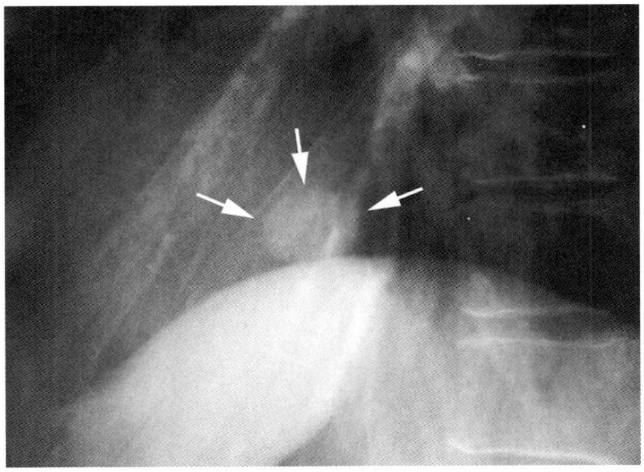

Figure 26.42. Fibrin ball. Coned-down lateral view shows a well-defined small nodular opacity at the pleural surface (*arrows*). This moved within the pleural space.

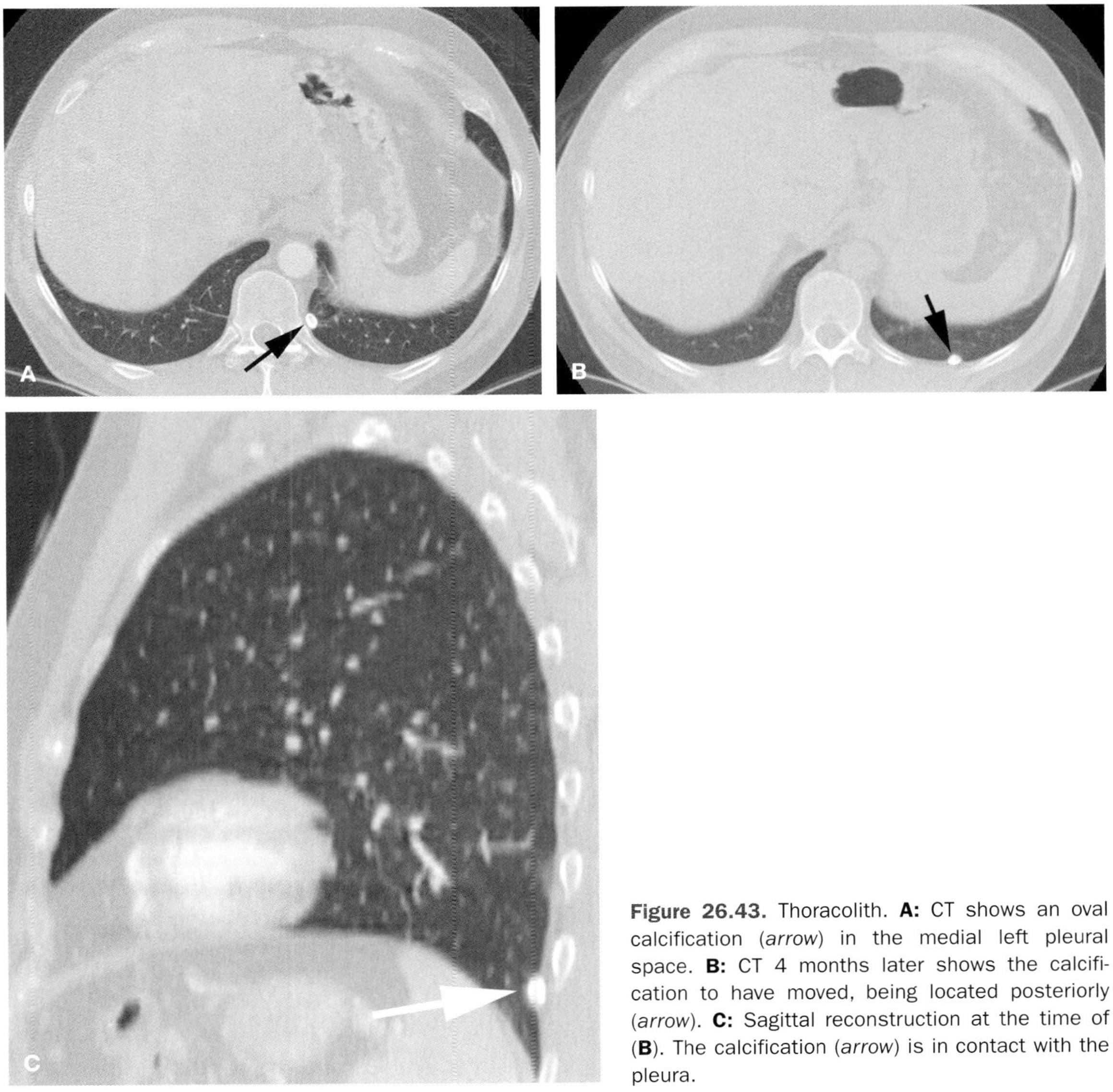

Figure 26.43. Thoracolith. **A:** CT shows an oval calcification (*arrow*) in the medial left pleural space. **B:** CT 4 months later shows the calcification to have moved, being located posteriorly (*arrow*). **C:** Sagittal reconstruction at the time of (**B**). The calcification (*arrow*) is in contact with the pleura.

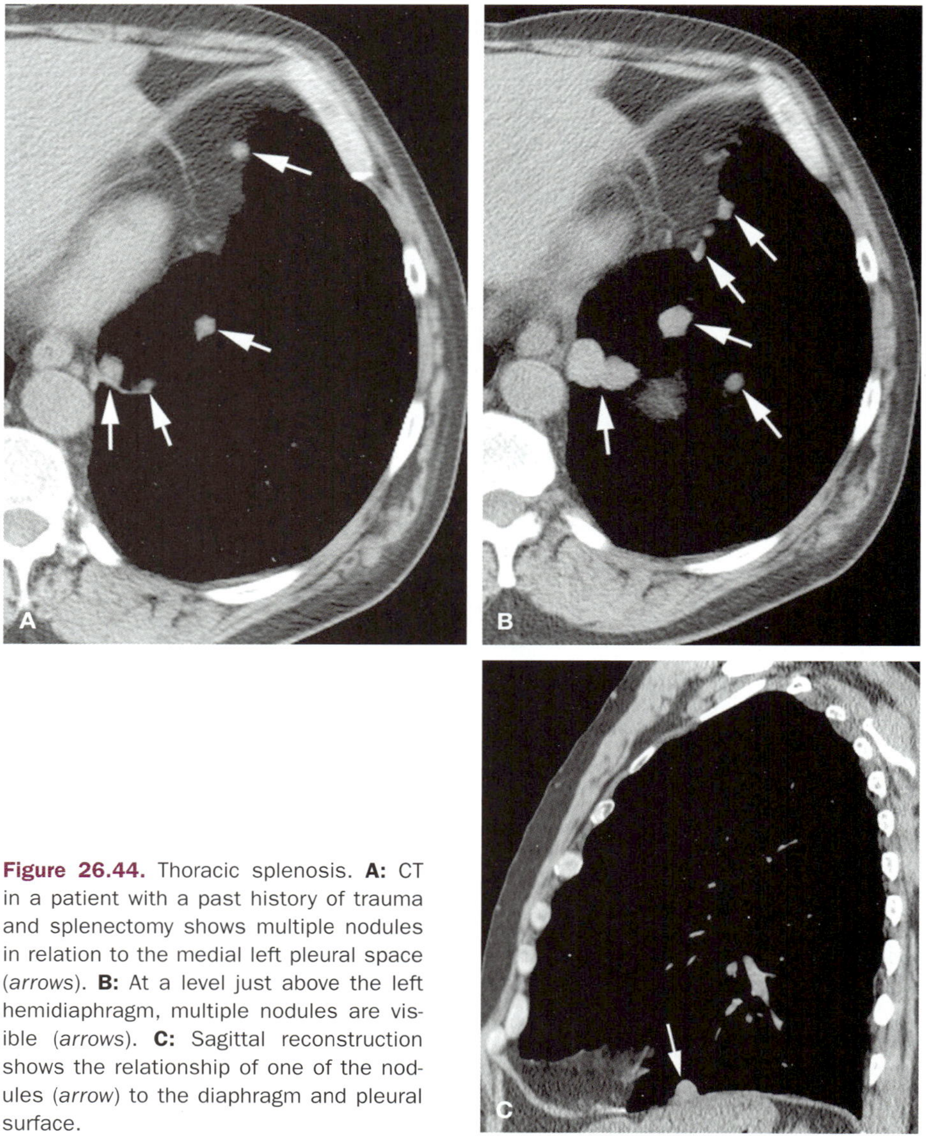

Figure 26.44. Thoracic splenosis. **A:** CT in a patient with a past history of trauma and splenectomy shows multiple nodules in relation to the medial left pleural space (*arrows*). **B:** At a level just above the left hemidiaphragm, multiple nodules are visible (*arrows*). **C:** Sagittal reconstruction shows the relationship of one of the nodules (*arrow*) to the diaphragm and pleural surface.

Primary Spontaneous Pneumothorax

Primary spontaneous pneumothorax occurs without antecedent cause in an otherwise healthy patient. It often occurs at rest and is generally the result of rupture of an apical subpleural bulla or bleb (Fig. 26.45). There is an increased incidence of primary spontaneous pneumothorax in young patients (20-40 years), males (80% of affected patients), tall and thin patients, and smokers (90% are smokers). Pain is common, and a small pleural effusion is present in 10% to 20%, manifested as an air-fluid level. In half of patients, the pneumothorax recurs on the same side; recurrence on the opposite side occurs in 15%.

Secondary Spontaneous Pneumothorax

Secondary spontaneous pneumothorax occurs in patients with underlying lung disease. It is most commonly associated with chronic obstructive pulmonary disease. Other diseases include those associated with lung cysts (eg, histiocytosis, lymphangiomyomatosis, pneumatocele), cavitation (eg, tuberculosis, lung cancer, metastases, lung abscess, septic embolism; Fig. 26.46; see also Fig. 5.44 in Chapter 5), air trapping (eg, asthma, cystic fibrosis), decreased lung compliance (eg, any cause of fibrosis or honeycombing such as usual interstitial pneumonia, radiation, collagen vascular disease, and sarcoidosis), or diseases of connective tissue (eg, Ehlers-Danlos syndrome and Marfan syndrome).

Because of underlying lung disease, patients with secondary spontaneous pneumothorax are often symptomatic. Such pneumothoraces have no specific characteristics, but the underlying lung appears abnormal. Recurrence rates are higher than for primary spontaneous pneumothorax.

Pneumothorax Ex Vacuo

Pneumothorax ex vacuo is a rare cause of secondary spontaneous pneumothorax occurring in patients with acute lobar

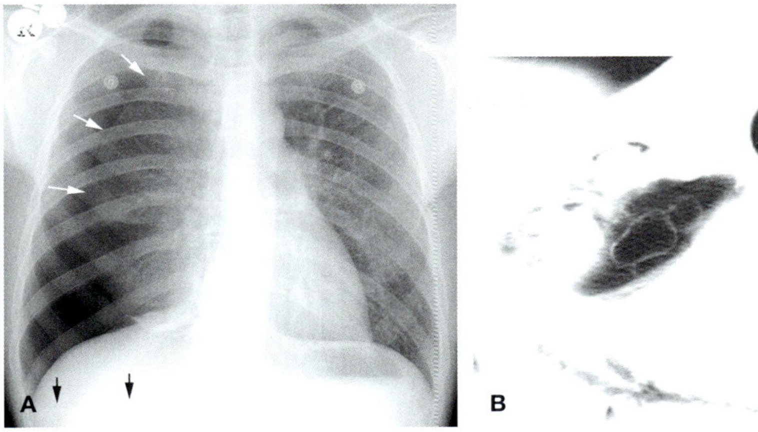

Figure 26.45. Primary spontaneous pneumothorax in a smoker. **A:** Chest radiograph shows a large right pneumothorax (*white arrows*). An air-fluid level (*black arrows*) is visible at the right base. **B:** Follow-up CT shows apical bullae. Subcutaneous emphysema reflects chest tube drainage.

atelectasis, usually due to bronchial obstruction (see Fig. 5.45 in Chapter 5). Sudden collapse results in a rapid decrease in intrapleural pressure adjacent to the collapsed lobe. This in turn results in gas entering into the pleural space from tissue and blood. The resulting pneumothorax is seen adjacent to the collapsed lobe.

Catamenial Pneumothorax and Pleural Endometriosis

The development of pneumothorax coincident with menstruation, the so-called catamenial pneumothorax, is rare. The onset of symptoms is within 48 hours of the onset of menses. It typically occurs in women over 30 years. Most cases (90%) occur on the right side. Recurrence is typical. Two primary mechanisms have been suggested:

1. Air may reach the peritoneum during menses via the vagina, uterus, and fallopian tubes. From there, it may enter the pleural space through defects in the diaphragm, which are most common on the right side, or because of necrotic diaphragmatic implants of endometrium.
2. Endometrial implants may enter the pleural space by the same route, resulting in pleural endometriosis. If endometrial implants involve the visceral pleura and peripheral lung, their breakdown during menstruation may lead to pneumothorax and/or hemoptysis. This mechanism is more likely than the first.

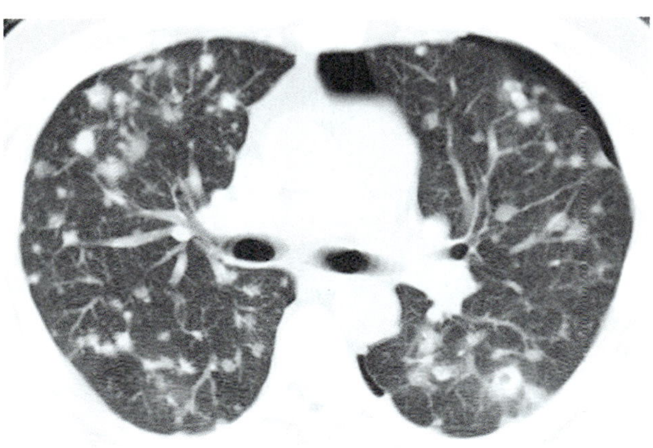

Figure 26.46. Secondary spontaneous pneumothorax in a patient with cavitary metastatic giant cell tumor. Multiple lung nodules and a small left pneumothorax are visible.

Traumatic Pneumothorax

Traumatic pneumothorax refers to pneumothorax caused by chest trauma (penetrating or nonpenetrating, accidental or iatrogenic) or mechanical ventilation. Pneumothorax associated with mechanical ventilation is usually the result of high ventilator pressures; pneumothorax with mechanical ventilation usually occurs because of alveolar rupture, which in turn causes interstitial emphysema, pneumomediastinum, and rupture of the pneumomediastinum into the pleural space. Pneumothorax does not cause pneumomediastinum; it is the other way around. Also, interstitial air may track to a subpleural location, form a subpleural bleb, and rupture directly into the pleural space. Traumatic pneumothorax usually requires chest tube drainage.

Radiographic Findings of Pneumothorax

Upright Patient

In an upright patient, air usually collects first above the lung apex. The visibility of pneumothorax is accentuated on expiration.

The presence of a visible *visceral pleural line* is key in making a definite diagnosis of pneumothorax in an erect patient (Fig. 26.47). In patients with pneumothorax, the visceral pleura is visible as a very thin line at the surface of the lung, with black air in the pleura space above or lateral to it, and air in the lung below or medial to it. Air may enter the fissure, outlining its pleural surfaces.

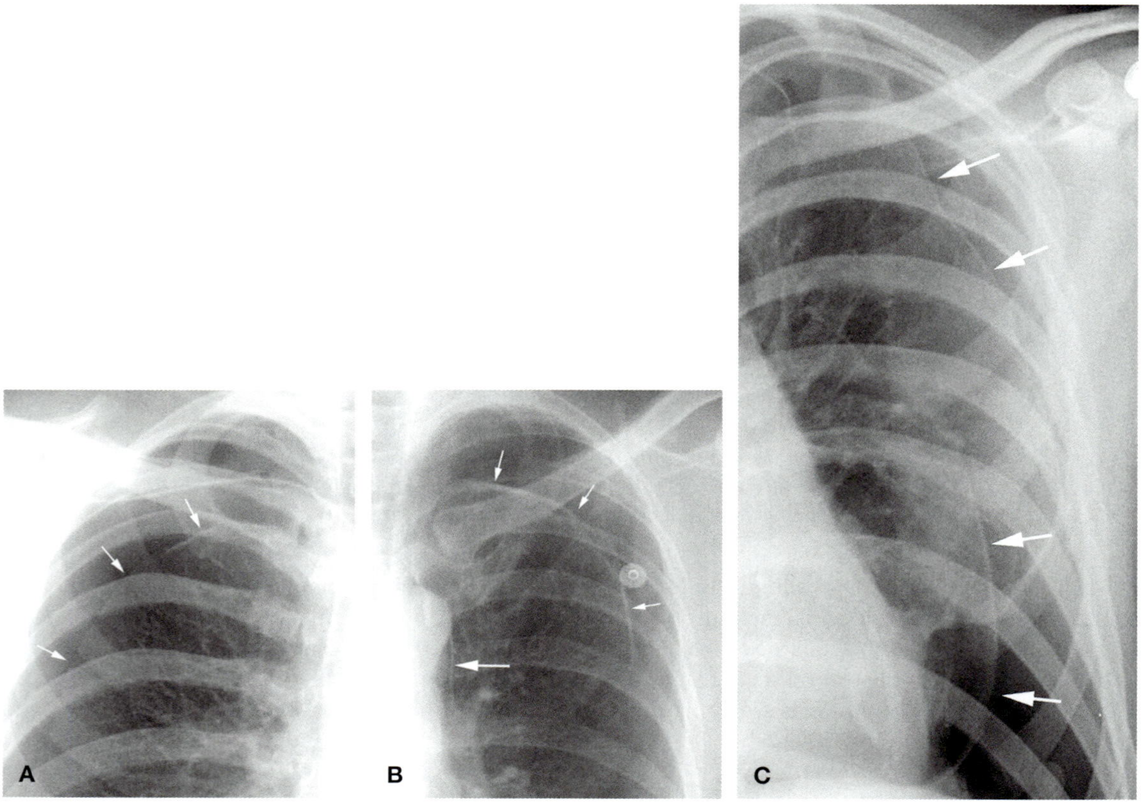

Figure 26.47. Pleural line in pneumothorax in three patients **(A-C)**. **A:** A very thin line (*arrows*; thinnest in the patient in **A**) is visible at the edge of the lung. No lung markings are visible peripheral to it. A pleural line may also be seen medially (*large arrow* in **B**). In **C**, a pleural line (*arrows*) is seen outlining both the upper and lower lobes.

In the absence of underlying lung disease or pleural adhesions, the partially collapsed lung maintains its normal shape. Lung markings are not seen peripheral to the pleural line.

A skin fold may mimic pneumothorax, but a pleural line is not visible, and lung markings may be seen peripheral to it (Fig. 26.48). Pneumothorax increases in relative volume on expiration, although significant pneumothoraces are visible on inspiration (Fig. 26.49).

Distinction of a bulla from a pneumothorax is usually based on shape. Pneumothoraces are typically crescent shaped and taper toward the lung base; bullae are rounded (see Fig. 24.13 in Chapter 24). However, this distinction may be difficult in some cases. Loculated pneumothorax may closely mimic a bulla.

Approximately half of the density of the lung is blood, and when the lung collapses in the presence of pneumothorax, a significant increase in lung density need not be visible. Reduction in lung volume also results in a reduction in lung perfusion. Until the lung becomes very small (Fig. 26.50), its density does not significantly increase.

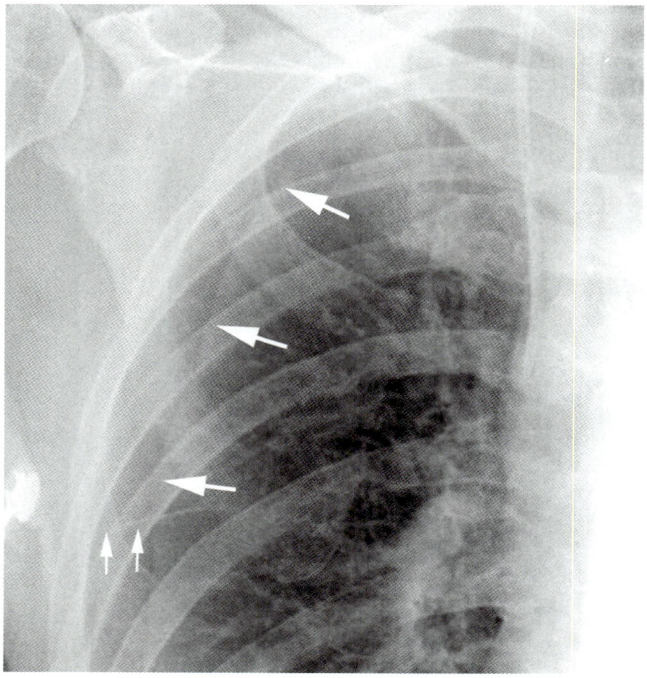

Figure 26.48. Skin fold mimicking pneumothorax. A skin fold (*large arrows*) mimics pneumothorax, but a distinct pleural line is not visible, and lung markings (*small arrows*) may be seen peripheral to it.

Supine Patient

In supine patients, free pneumothorax usually collects within the anterior pleural space. A visceral pleural line may be seen medially in some patients (see Fig. 26.47B), mimicking pneumomediastinum. A subpulmonic pneumothorax with a visible visceral pleural line may be seen at the lung base. Less specific findings of pneumothorax in supine patients include the following:

1. The costophrenic angle may appear abnormally deep and lucent because of air in the anterolateral pleura space, the "deep sulcus sign" (Fig. 26.51).

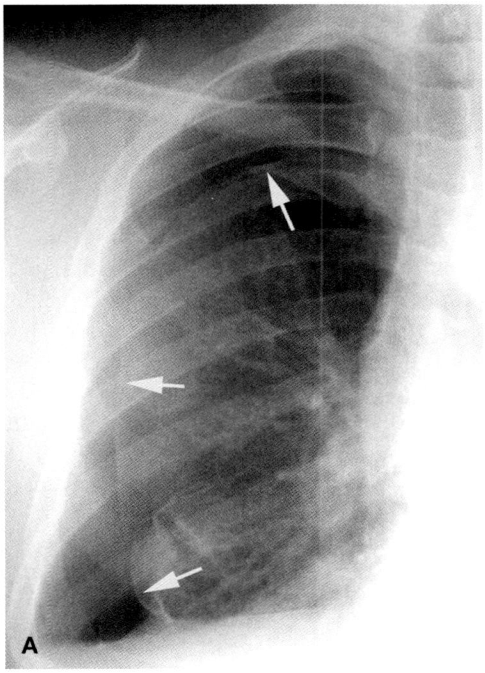

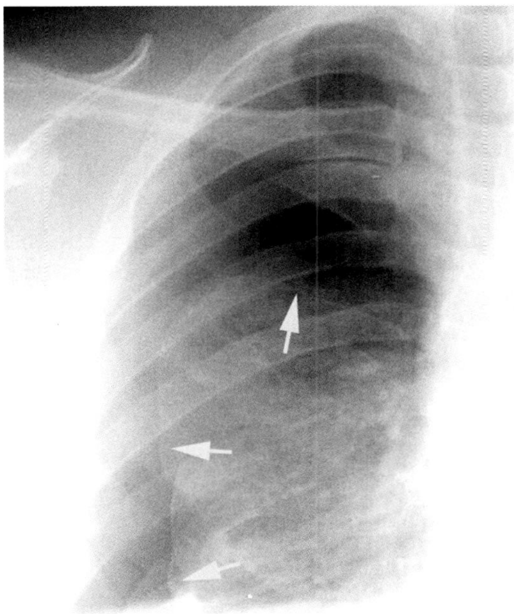

Figure 26.49. Inspiratory and expiratory radiographs in spontaneous pneumothorax. The relative volume of the pneumothorax (*arrows*) is smaller on inspiration **(A)** than on expiration **(B)**.

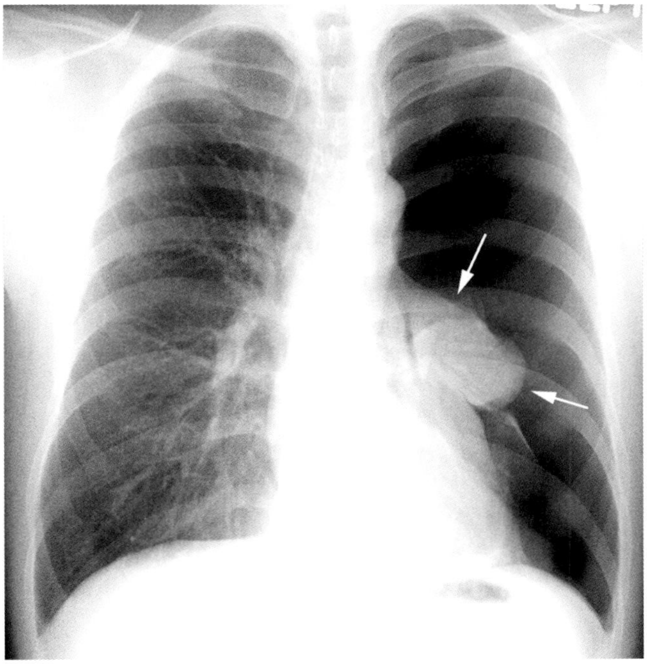

Figure 26.50. Total spontaneous pneumothorax. The left lung is reduced to the size of a fist (*arrows*). At this size, compressed lung tissue causes the lung to be dense. No mediastinal shift is present.

2. Increased lucency over the chest or upper abdomen
3. Visualization of the anterior costophrenic angle as an edge separate from the diaphragm but parallel to it (the "double-diaphragm sign")
4. Increased sharpness of the hemidiaphragm (because it is outlined by air), despite lung disease (see Fig. 26.51)

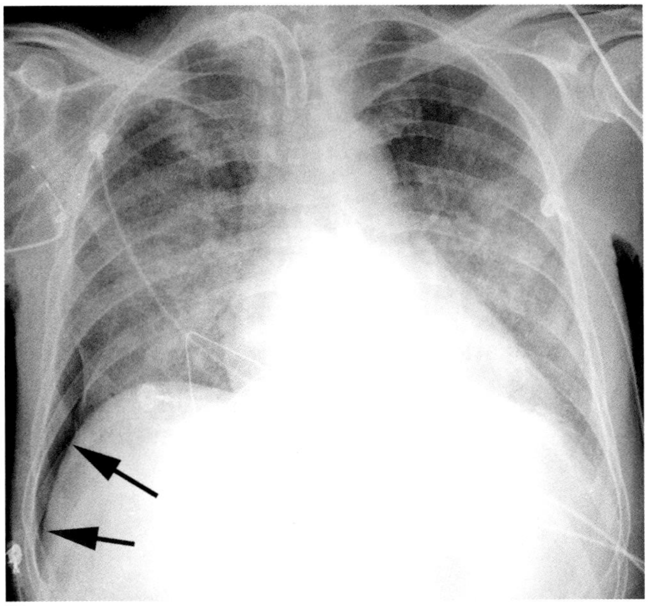

Figure 26.51. The deep sulcus sign in pneumothorax. A supine radiograph in a patient with pulmonary edema shows a right pneumothorax manifested by a deep sulcus (*arrows*) on the right side. The right diaphragm and right heart borders appear sharp despite lung disease at the lung base.

5. Increased sharpness of the cardiac border or mediastinum (because it is outlined by air; see Fig. 26.52)
6. Air in the minor fissure
7. A lumpy appearance at the cardiac apex due to alteration in the shape of the epicardial fat pad in the presence of pneumothorax (Fig. 26.52)

CT Findings of Pneumothorax

Upright expiratory radiographs and CT are similarly sensitive in demonstrating a pneumothorax. CT is considerably more sensitive than supine radiographs in demonstrating pneumothorax.

On CT, a pneumothorax is imaged as air in the pleural space outside the lung and visceral pleura. Even a very small pneumothorax is visible in the anterior pleural space. Its diagnosis is usually straightforward, although differentiating a medial pneumothorax from pneumomediastinum may be difficult in some cases.

Tension Pneumothorax

Tension pneumothorax means that the pressure of intrapleural air exceeds atmospheric pressure, usually throughout the respiratory cycle; it may be life-threatening. True tension pneumothorax is uncommon. It is most often seen in mechanically ventilated patients or patients with chest trauma. Any pneumothorax in a patient on positive pressure ventilation should be considered a tension pneumothorax.

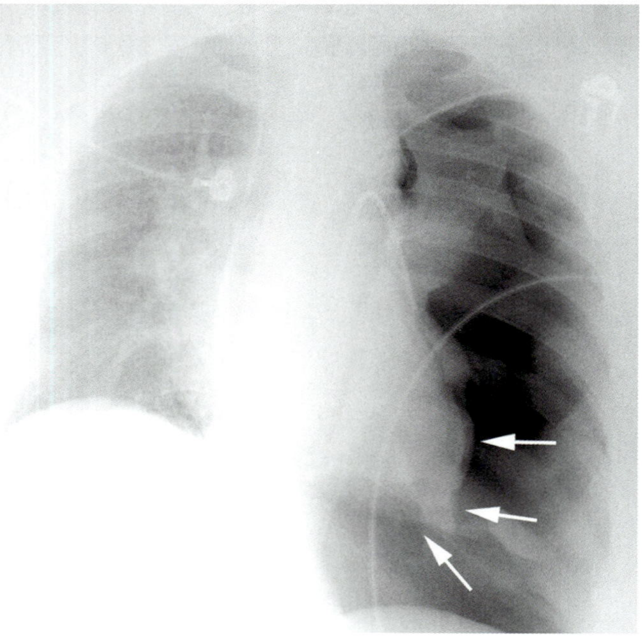

Figure 26.52. Tension pneumothorax with a deep sulcus sign. Left pneumothorax outlines fat at the cardiac apex, giving it a lumpy appearance (*arrows*). The left hemidiaphragm is displaced inferiorly and the mediastinum is shifted to the opposite side.

Tension pneumothorax is difficult to diagnose on chest radiographs. Shift of the mediastinum away from the pneumothorax is not a reliable finding of tension and can be seen with any large pneumothorax. However, this finding in combination with clinical symptoms of circulatory compromise is usually considered diagnostic. Downward displacement or inversion of the hemidiaphragm also suggests tension (see Fig. 26.52).

In a patient with normal lungs, tension pneumothorax usually results in complete lung collapse. However, in the presence of underlying lung disease such as pulmonary edema, pneumonia, or chronic obstructive pulmonary disease, or in patients receiving positive pressure ventilation, complete collapse need not occur. Also, complete lung collapse need not indicate tension (see Fig. 26.50).

Hydropneumothorax

Hydropneumothorax, the combination of fluid and air in the pleural space, is readily diagnosed in the upright position because of the presence of an air-fluid level (see Fig. 26.45). In supine or semierect patients, a visible pleural line or other findings of pneumothorax may be seen in combination with increased pleural density or findings of pleural fluid. A small amount of fluid is seen in 20% to 40% of patients with pneumothorax, regardless of its cause.

Estimating the Size of a Pneumothorax

There is no precise correlation between pneumothorax size and the need for treatment, although a 30% pneumothorax is generally considered to require treatment. Symptoms are more important in determining which patients require treatment, and this depends on both pneumothorax size and underlying lung disease. Nonetheless, an estimate of pneumothorax size is commonly requested.

The size of a pneumothorax may be estimated by using the average interpleural distance (Table 26.10). The distance separating the pleural surface of the lung from the adjacent chest wall (ie, the depth or thickness of the pneumothorax) is measured in three locations (Fig. 26.53). To make these measurements, divide the hemithorax vertically into two halves, from the apex

Table 26.10 Estimating the Size of a Pneumothorax

Average Interpleural Distance (mm)	Percent Pneumothorax	
	Upright Film (%)	Supine Film (%)
10	14	19
20	23	29
30	32	39
40	40	49
50	49	59

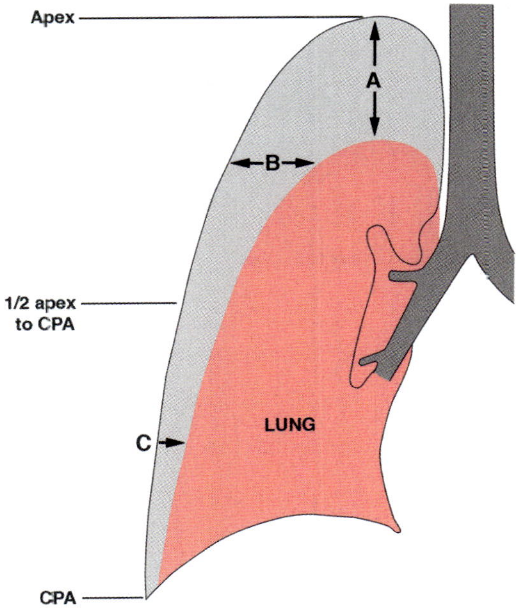

Figure 26.53. Method of calculating average interpleural distance. CPA, costophrenic angle.

of the hemithorax to the costophrenic angle. Then measure the distance between the lung and the lateral chest at the midpoint of both the upper and lower halves; the third measurement is made vertically above the lung apex. The average of these measurements (ie, the average interpleural distance) correlates with pneumothorax size in both upright and supine patients (see Table 26.10). Although the accuracy of this estimate is limited, so is the need to accurately determine the size of a pneumothorax. When reviewing Table 26.10, note that the average interpleural distance in millimeters is approximately equal to the pneumothorax percent in an upright patient; in a supine patient, add 9%.

SUGGESTED READINGS

Abramowitz Y, Simanovsky N, Goldstein MS, Hiller N. Pleural effusion: characterization with CT attenuation values and CT appearance. *AJR Am J Roentgenol.* 2009;192(3):618-623.

Adler BD, Padley SPG, Müller NL. Tuberculosis of the chest wall: CT findings. *J Comput Assist Tomogr.* 1993;17(2):271-273.

Alexander E, Clark RA, Colley DP, Mitchell SE. CT of malignant pleural mesothelioma. *AJR Am J Roentgenol.* 1981;137(2):287-291.

Aquino SL, Chen MY, Kuo WT, Chiles C. The CT appearance of pleural and extrapleural disease in lymphoma. *Clin Radiol.* 1999;54(10):647-650.

Aquino SL, Webb WR, Gushiken BJ. Pleural exudates and transudates: diagnosis with contrast-enhanced CT. *Radiology.* 1994;192(3):803-808.

Berkmen YM, Auh YH, Davis SD, Kazam E. Anatomy of the minor fissure evaluation with thin-section CT. *Radiology.* 1989;170(3 Pt 1):647-651.

Berkmen YM, Davis SD, Kazam E, Auh YH, Yankelevitz D, Girgis FG. Right phrenic nerve: anatomy, CT appearance, and differentiation from the pulmonary ligament. *Radiology.* 1989;173(1):43-46.

Broaddus VC, Light RW. What is the origin of pleural transudates and exudates? [editorial] *Chest* 1992;102(3):658-659.

Choi BG, Park SH, Yun EH, Chae KO, Shinn KS. Pneumothorax size: correlation of supine anteroposterior with erect posteroanterior chest radiographs. *Radiology.* 1998;209(2):567-569.

Choi JA, Hong KT, Oh YW, Chung MH, Seol HY, Kang EY. CT manifestations of late sequelae in patients with tuberculous pleuritis. *AJR Am J Roentgenol.* 2001;176(2):441-445.

Cooper C, Moss AA, Buy JN, Stark DD. CT appearance of the normal inferior pulmonary ligament. *AJR Am J Roentgenol.* 1983;141(2):237-240.

Dynes MC, White EM, Fry WA, Ghahremani GG. Imaging manifestations of pleural tumors. *Radiographics.* 1992;12(6):1191-1201.

Federle MP, Mark AS, Guillaumin ES. CT of subpulmonic pleural effusions and atelectasis: criteria for differentiation from subphrenic fluid. *AJR Am J Roentgenol.* 1986;146(4):685-689.

Godwin JD, Tarver RD. Accessory fissures of the lung. *AJR Am J Roentgenol.* 1985;144(1):39-47.

Godwin JD, Vock P, Osborne DR. CT of the pulmonary ligament. *AJR Am J Roentgenol.* 1983;141(2):231-236.

Halvorsen RA, Fedyshin PJ, Korobkin M, Foster WL Jr, Thompson WM. Ascites or pleural effusion? CT differentiation: four useful criteria. *Radiographics.* 1986;6(1):135-149.

Hulnick DH, Naidich DP, McCauley DI. Pleural tuberculosis evaluated by computed tomography. *Radiology.* 1983;149(3):759-765.

Im JG, Webb WR, Rosen A, Gamsu G. Costal pleura: appearances at high-resolution CT. *Radiology.* 1989;171(1):125-131.

Kawashima A, Libshitz HI. Malignant pleural mesothelioma: CT manifestations in 50 cases. *AJR Am J Roentgenol.* 1990;155(5):965-969.

Lee KS, Im JG, Choe KO, Kim CJ, Lee BH. CT findings in benign fibrous mesothelioma of the pleura: pathologic correlation in nine patients. *AJR Am J Roentgenol.* 1992;158(5):983-986.

Leung AN, Müller NL, Miller RR. CT in differential diagnosis of diffuse pleural disease. *AJR Am J Roentgenol.* 1990;154(3):487-492.

Marks BW, Kuhns LR. Identification of the pleural fissures with computed tomography. *Radiology.* 1982;143(1):139-141.

Mirvis S, Dutcher JP, Haney PJ, Whitley NO, Aisner J. CT of malignant pleural mesothelioma. *AJR Am J Roentgenol.* 1983;140(4):665-670.

Nandalur KR, Hardie AH, Bollampally SR, Parmar JP, Hagspiel KD. Accuracy of computed tomography attenuation values in the characterization of pleural fluid: an ROC study. *Acad Radiol.* 2005;12(8):987-991.

Naylor MF, Karstaedt N, Finck SJ, Burnett OL. Noninvasive methods of diagnosing thoracic splenosis. *Ann Thorac Surg.* 1999;68(1):243-244.

Nickell L, Lichtenberger JP, Khorashadi L, Abbott GF, Carter BW. Multimodality imaging for characterization, classification, and staging of malignant pleural mesothelioma. *Radiographics.* 2014;34(6):1692-1706.

Patz EF, Shaffer K, Piwnica-Worms DR, et al. Malignant pleural mesothelioma: value of CT and MR imaging in predicting resectability. *AJR Am J Roentgenol.* 1992;159(5):961-966.

Proto AV, Ball JB. Computed tomography of the major and minor fissures. *AJR Am J Roentgenol.* 1983;140(3):439-448.

Raasch BN, Carsky EW, Lane EJ, O'Callaghan JP, Heitzman ER. Radiographic anatomy of the interlobar fissures: a study of 100 specimens. *AJR Am J Roentgenol.* 1982;138(6):1043-1049.

Rabinowitz JG, Cohen BA, Mendleson DS. Symposium on nonpulmonary aspects in chest radiology. The pulmonary ligament. *Radiol Clin North Am.* 1984;22(3):659-672.

Rhea JT, DeLuca SA, Greene RE. Determining the size of pneumothorax in the upright patient. *Radiology.* 1982;144(4):733-736.

Rost RC Jr, Proto AV. Inferior pulmonary ligament: computed tomographic appearance. *Radiology.* 1983;148(2):479-483.

Schmitt WGH, Hübener KH, Rücker HC. Pleural calcification with persistent effusion. *Radiology.* 1983;149(3):633-638.

Stark DD, Federle MP, Goodman PC, Podrasky AE, Webb WR. Differentiating lung abscess and empyema: radiography and computed tomography. *AJR Am J Roentgenol.* 1983;141(1):163-167.

Strzelczyka J, Holloway BJ, Pernicanoa PG, Kellya AM. Rolling stones in the pleural space: thoracoliths on CT, and a review of the literature. *Clin Radiol.* 2009;64:100-104.

Travis WD, Brambilla E, Burke AP, et al, eds. *WHO Classification of Tumours of the Lung, Pleura, Thymus and Heart.* 4th ed. International Agency for Research on Cancer (IARC); 2015.

Tyszko SM, Marano GD, Tallaksen RJ, Gyure KA. Best cases from the AFIP: malignant mesothelioma. *Radiographics.* 2007;27(1):259-264.

Villanueva A, Cáceres J, Ferreira M, Broncano J, Pallisa E, Bastarrika G. Migrating azygos vein and vanishing azygos lobe: mdct findings. *AJR Am J Roentgenol.* March 2010;194(3):599-603.

Vix VA. Extrapleural costal fat. *Radiology.* 1974;112(3):563-565.

Waite RJ, Carbonneau RJ, Balikian JP, Umali CB, Pezzella AT, Nash G. Parietal pleural changes in empyema: appearances at CT. *Radiology.* 1990;175(1):145-150.

Wilcox BE, Subramaniam RM, Peller PJ, et al. Utility of integrated computed tomography-positron emission tomography for selection of operable malignant pleural mesothelioma. *Clin Lung Cancer.* 2009;10(4):244-248.

Chapter 27

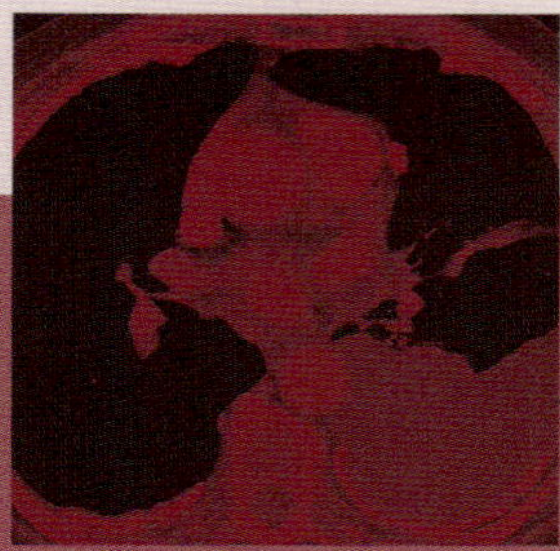

Hamid Chalian • Seyed Ali Nabipoorashrafi • J. David Godwin

The Diaphragm

The diaphragm is the primary muscle of ventilation and the main physical barrier between the thorax and the abdomen. Its dysfunction is an underappreciated cause of dyspnea.

This chapter will start with anatomy, function, and normal imaging findings. Next, it will review the imaging findings in diaphragm dysfunction caused by eventration, paralysis, weakness, and tethering. We will describe how to perform and interpret a meaningful sniff test. Finally, there will be a brief discussion of diaphragmatic hernias and tumors.

ANATOMY

The diaphragm (Fig. 27.1) is musculofibrous, dome-shaped membrane with a peripheral muscular portion and a central fibrous portion, the central tendon. The ratio of central tendon to muscle is typically 10% to 15%. The diaphragm is derived embryologically from the transverse septum anteriorly, the right and left pleuroperitoneal folds posteriorly, the muscular body wall peripherally, and the esophageal mesentery centrally.

The attachments of the diaphragm include the inferior sternum and xiphoid process, the lower six ribs, and their costal cartilages. Posteriorly, medial arcuate ligaments of the diaphragm arch over the anterior psoas muscles and attach to the L1 or L2 vertebral bodies and to the transverse processes of L1. Lateral arcuate ligaments arch over the quadratus lumborum muscles and attach to the transverse processes of L1 and to the midportion of the 12th ribs.

Because the posterior attachments of the diaphragm are lower than the anterior attachments, the posterior muscle fibers are longer and more vertically oriented than the anterior fibers, giving them more power to pull the diaphragm down for inspiration. Another factor that makes the anterior muscle fibers short is that the central tendon is closer to the anterior than to the posterior chest wall.

The central tendon is reinforced by partial fusion with the fibrous pericardium. Under the pericardium, tendinous fiber bands (Fig. 27.1) in the central tendon form an "X" that extends from posterior central tendon to roughly the 10-o'clock and 2-o'clock points on the anterior chest wall. At their ends, the bands fan out and connect with muscle fibers. They form a thick fibrous node at their intersection, which is anterior to the esophagus and to the left of the inferior vena cava (IVC). The bands act to concentrate and focus the forces of contraction of the diaphragm on the node at their intersection, which their arrangement holds in a relatively immovable position. In particular, the bands tie the vigorous downward motion of the posterior diaphragm to the anterior motion of the anterior chest wall. They also resist the stretching of the central tendon that causes eventration, and they create the sharp medial boundary of many eventrations. In an autopsy case, we observed a corresponding band (Fig. 27.2) in the right hemidiaphragm attaching to the anterior chest wall and forming the medial margin of a small eventration.

The crura are downward musculotendinous extensions of diaphragm muscle and tendon that attach to upper lumbar vertebral bodies, disks, and anterior longitudinal ligament. The right crus is broader and longer than the left, attaching to the top three vertebral bodies, whereas the left crus attaches to the top two. Fibers of the right crus loop around the esophageal hiatus, forming a kind of sphincter. The crura are joined in the midline by the fibrous median arcuate ligament.

The hemidiaphragms are innervated by right and left phrenic nerves, which originate from spinal nerves C3-C5.

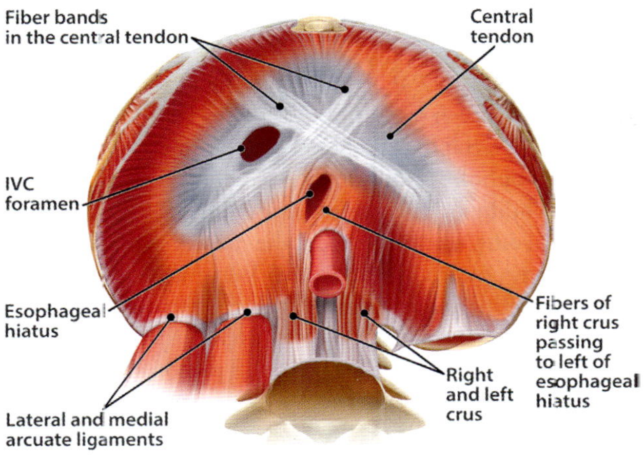

Figure 27.1. Diaphragm anatomy from below. The central tendon is wider on the right than the left. It is reinforced by tendinous fiber bands, which cross near the inferior vena cava (IVC) foramen and the esophageal hiatus. Posterior and lateral muscle fibers are longer and more vertical than anterior fibers, making them more effective at pulling the diaphragm down for inspiration. The crura attach to upper lumbar vertebrae and anterior longitudinal ligament; the right crus is wider and longer than the left; it loops around the esophageal hiatus. The lateral and medial arcuate ligaments cover the anterior quadratus lumborum and psoas muscles, respectively.

The phrenic nerves descend through the lateral compartment of the neck into the thorax along the anterior pericardium, accompanied by pericardiophrenic arteries and veins. The phrenic nerves each divide into three main branches on the superior and inferior aspects of the hemidiaphragms, providing motor and sensory innervation.

Three main hiatuses in the diaphragm allow passage between the thorax and abdomen. The IVC hiatus at the T8 level on the right passes the IVC and branches of the right phrenic nerve. The esophageal hiatus at T10 just to the left of midline passes the esophagus, vagus nerve, and sympathetic nerves. The aortic hiatus at T12 just to the left of midline passes the aorta, thoracic duct, and azygos and hemiazygos veins.

FUNCTION

As the primary muscle of ventilation, the diaphragm contracts and descends during inspiration. In concert with diaphragmatic contraction, the muscles of the abdominal wall relax, and the accessory muscles of respiration (external intercostal, sternocleidomastoid, and scalene muscles) contract, elevating the anterior chest wall and increasing the anteroposterior and lateral diameters of the chest. The expansion of the thoracic cavity draws air into the lungs. When the diaphragm and accessory muscles relax, gravity and the elastic recoil of the lung and chest wall take over; the diaphragm is pulled up and the anterior chest wall is pulled down, shrinking the thoracic cavity and causing exhalation. Contraction of the diaphragm also assists in urination, emesis, and defecation by increasing intra-abdominal pressure. Further, the diaphragm helps prevent gastroesophageal reflux by constricting the esophageal hiatus during inspiration.

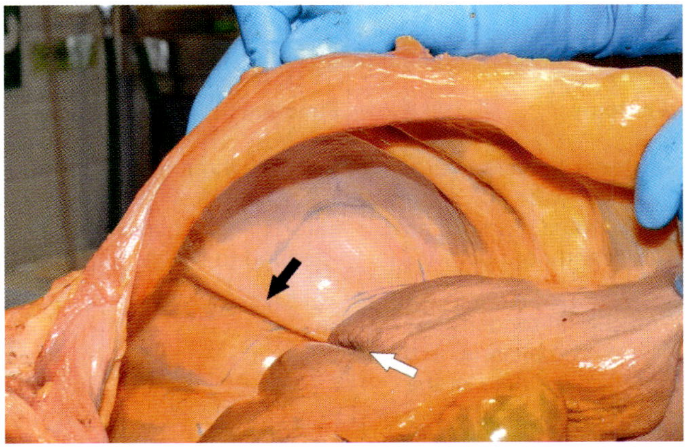

Figure 27.2. Undersurface of diaphragm with diaphragmatic bands and liver grooves. Autopsy photograph of the undersurface of the right hemidiaphragm with prominent band (black arrow) corresponding to the orientation of the anterior fiber band in Figure 27.1. The band has created a deep groove in the liver (white arrow). The band probably consists of muscle fibers near the anterior chest wall and fibrous tissue medially, and it formed the sharp medial margin of a small eventration on CT (not shown). Another muscle band, lateral to the first, has created a second, shallower liver groove. (Used with permission of Radiological Society of North America, from Nason LK, Walker CM, McNeeley MF, et al. Imaging of the diaphragm: anatomy and function. *Radiographics.* 2012;32(2):E51-E70; permission conveyed through Copyright Clearance Center, Inc.)

Again, because posterior muscle fibers are longer and more vertical than anterior fibers, they do most of the work of inspiration. Thus, excursion of the diaphragm is greater posteriorly than anteriorly and over the dome, and lateral fluoroscopy is needed to show it. Table 27.1 summarizes key points of anatomy and function.

NORMAL IMAGING FINDINGS

On radiographs, the right hemidiaphragm is usually higher than the left, particularly anteriorly, and the medial and anterior parts of the diaphragm are normally higher than the lateral and posterior parts (Fig. 27.3). On coronal or sagittal CT images, the dome of the hemidiaphragm is often thin because it consists of central tendon fibers with little muscle (Fig. 27.4), whereas the peripheral diaphragm is thicker because it consists of muscle. The anterior diaphragm is often very thin near its attachments to the sternum (Fig. 27.4). Sometimes muscle fibers of the diaphragm form distinct muscle bundles separated by fibrous tissue (Figs. 27.2 and 27.5). The right crus is usually thicker than the left (Fig. 27.4).

CT assessment of diaphragm muscle thickness is valuable in assessing diaphragm dysfunction. Muscle thickness is assessable anteriorly near the chest wall (Fig. 27.4) and posteromedially along the spine, including the right and left crura. The crus is usually the easiest place to assess muscle

Table 27.1 Anatomic Points and Their Functional Significance

Anatomy	Function
Posterior muscle fibers extend lower and are longer and more vertical than anterior fibers.	Most diaphragmatic motion is posterior. Lateral fluoroscopy is needed to see it.
The central tendon typically makes up 10%-15% of the area of the diaphragm.	
The dome of the hemidiaphragm is often thin, since it consists mostly of central tendon.	Motion of the dome is usually less vigorous than posterior motion.
Tendinous fiber bands in the central tendon form an "X" with intersection under the fibrous pericardium.	They concentrate and coordinate the forces of contraction. They resist the stretching of the central tendon that causes eventration. They form the sharp medial boundary of many eventrations.

thickness. The left crus is almost always thinner than the right and it should be at least 2.5-mm thick at the level of the celiac artery (Fig. 27.4). Thinning of the crus correlates with dysfunction shown by sniff test.

Sometimes the muscle fibers of the diaphragm are separated into bundles, which may be visible as stripes or nodules, depending on their orientation (Fig. 27.5).

As with other skeletal muscle, the muscle of the diaphragm can hypertrophy when made to work against extra resistance. Hypertrophy develops in cases of lung fibrosis, fibrothorax, abdominal distension from obesity, upper airway obstruction, obstructive sleep apnea (Fig. 27.6), stiff person syndrome, and soft-tissue thickening of the chest or abdominal wall in systemic sclerosis or graft-versus-host disease. Hypertrophy can develop from exercise (Fig. 27.7), including weightlifting. One mechanism is tensing the diaphragm against high abdominal pressure caused by wearing a weightlifting belt or by contracting abdominal wall muscles. Other mechanisms are breathing in while in Trendelenburg position or while head standing.

DYSFUNCTION CAUSED BY EVENTRATION, PARALYSIS AND WEAKNESS, AND TETHERING

Abnormal Height

Elevation of one or both hemidiaphragms is usually the first radiographic indication of diaphragm dysfunction caused

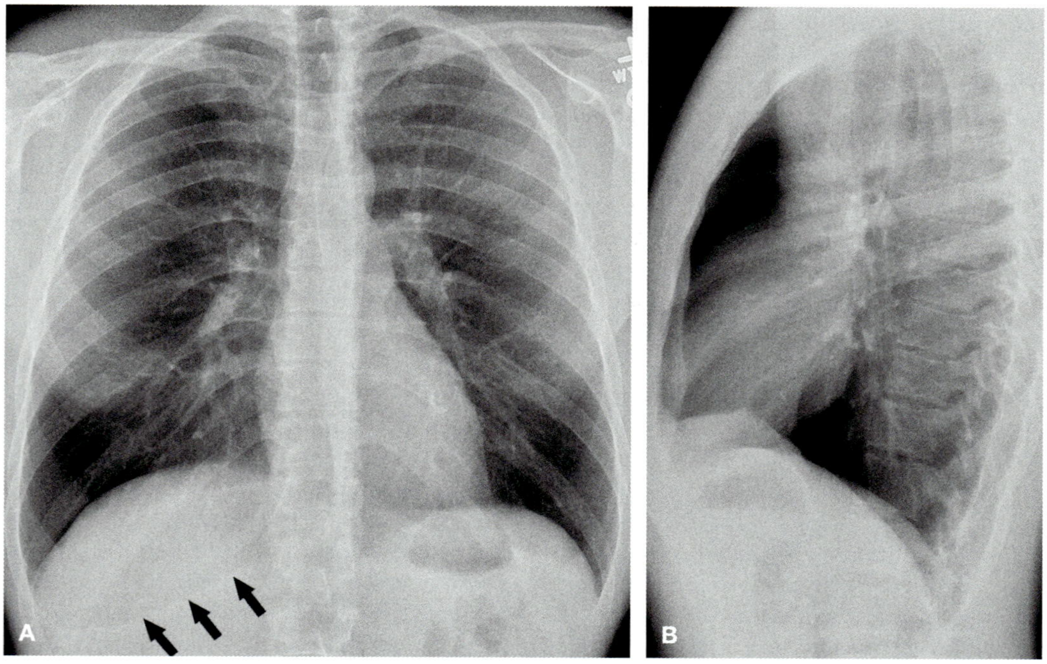

Figure 27.3. Normal diaphragm anatomy on radiographs. **A:** PA and **B:** lateral radiographs. The dome of the right hemidiaphragm is usually higher and more anterior than the left. The diaphragm extends lower posteriorly than anteriorly, and the posterior descent is steeper than the anterior. The posterior sulcus (*arrows*) is sometimes visible on PA view. Medially, it is near the bottom of the T12 vertebral body and slopes down laterally. The anterior aspect of the left hemidiaphragm is obscured on lateral view by the overlying heart.

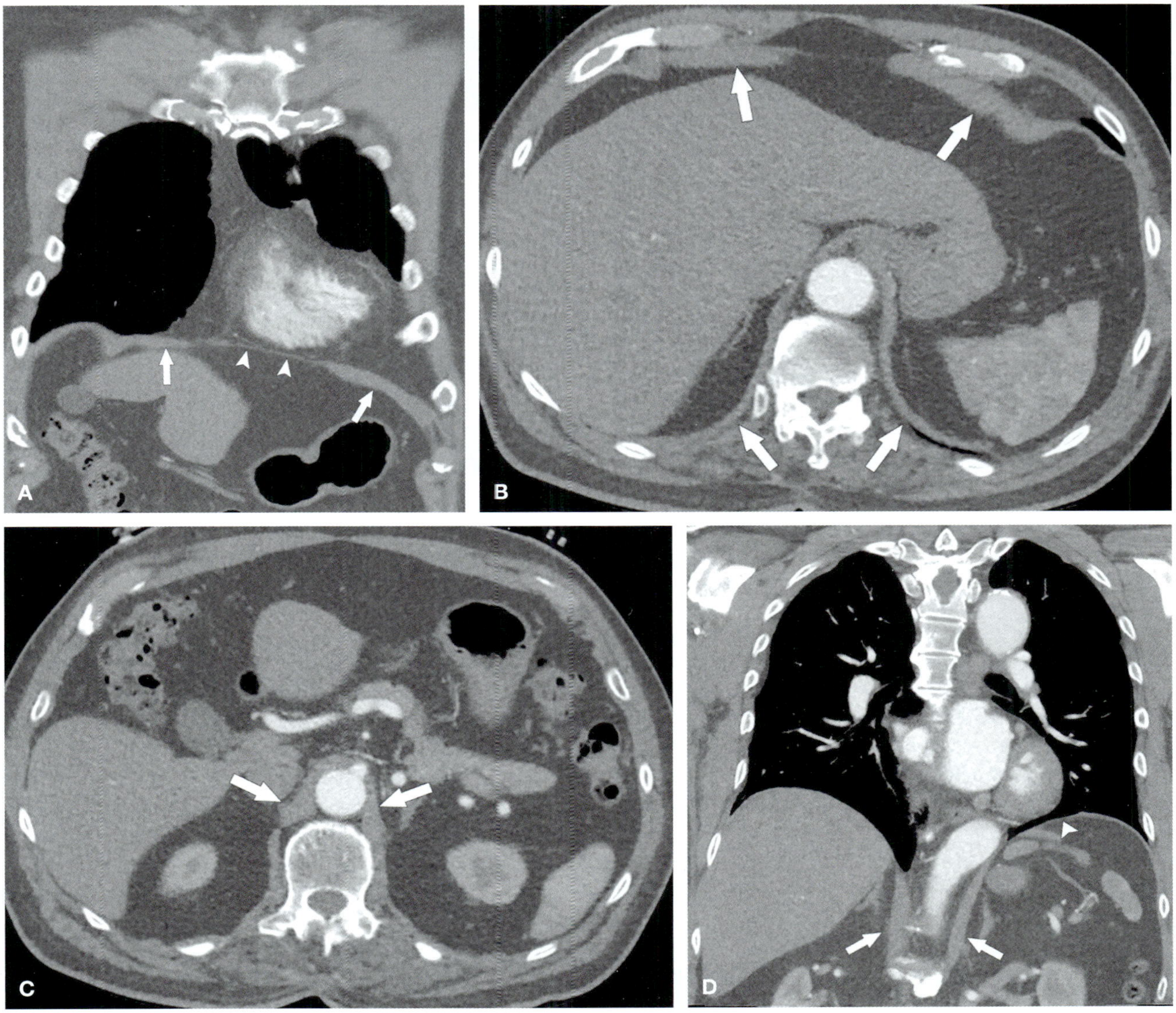

Figure 27.4. Normal anatomy on CT. **A:** Coronal CT near anterior chest wall shows slightly thick anterior diaphragm muscle on both sides (*arrows*). The diaphragm is often very thin medially near the sternum (*arrowheads*). **B:** CT shows the anterior and posterior diaphragm muscle (*arrows*). **C:** CT at the level of the celiac artery shows normal or slightly thickened crura (*arrows*). Crus thickness at this level below 2.5 mm correlates with paralysis as shown by sniff test. **D:** Coronal CT shows the crura (*arrows*) near their attachments to the lumbar spine. The dome of the diaphragm is often thin (*arrowhead*), since it is mostly central tendon with little muscle.

by eventration, weakness, or paralysis, but elevation also has nondiaphragmatic causes. Lung hypoplasia, fibrosis (Fig. 27.8), resection, or atelectasis can elevate the hemidiaphragm by pulling it up. Abdominal distension by obesity (Fig. 27.9), ascites, tumor, hepatosplenomegaly, polycystic disease, or pregnancy can elevate the diaphragm by pushing it up.

Low position of the diaphragm usually has nondiaphragmatic causes, such as pneumothorax, emphysema (Fig. 27.10), bullae, air trapping, or cystic lung disease, such as lymphangioleiomyomatosis. When the diaphragm is low and flat or even concave on its upper surface, its muscle attachments on the anterior ribs can give it a scalloped contour (Fig. 27.10).

Eventration

Etiology and Clinical Presentation

Eventration is a focal elevation of the diaphragm. *Complete* eventration results from embryologic failure of ingrowth of muscle fibers into the developing hemidiaphragm, almost always the left; because of its severity, it is usually diagnosed in early childhood and may be difficult to distinguish from congenital hernia. *Partial* eventration is what is found in adults. It is very common, particularly in older patients, and is usually acquired, through progressive stretching of a weak or unreinforced portion of the

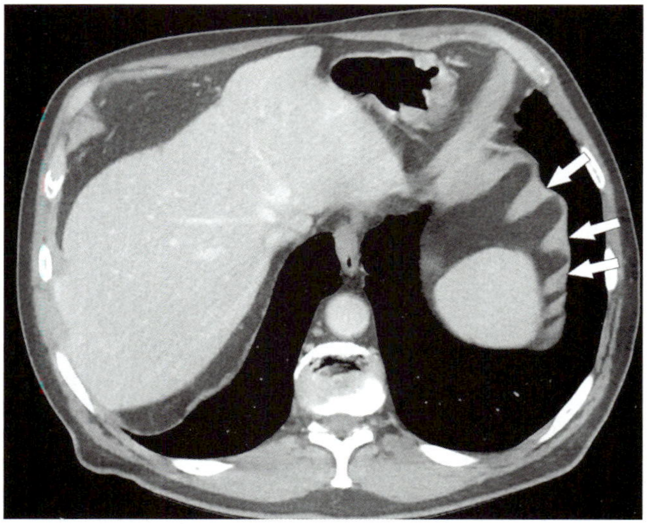

Figure 27.5. **A:** CT shows muscle bundles (*arrows*) near the dome of the left hemidiaphragm, creating a striped or nodular pattern.

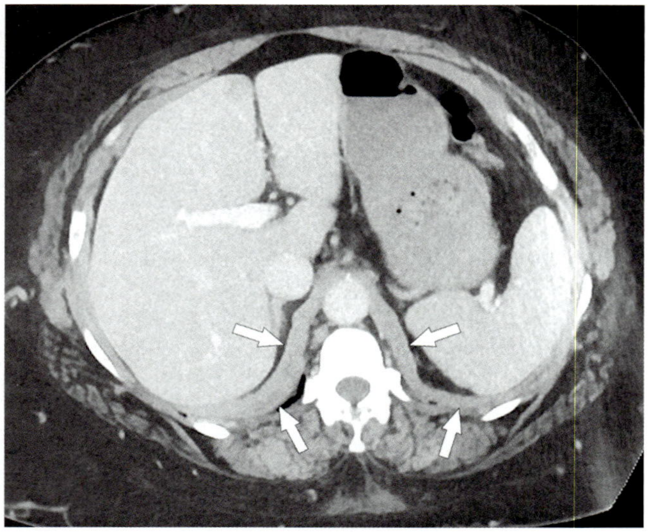

Figure 27.6. Hypertrophy of diaphragm muscle from obesity and obstructive sleep apnea. The crura and posterior diaphragm muscle are hypertrophied (*arrows*) on both sides. Anterior diaphragm hypertrophy was more clearly visible on coronal CT (not shown).

diaphragm, most often the anterior central tendon of the right hemidiaphragm.

One reason that eventration is more common on the right than the left is that the overlying heart and pericardium buttress the anteromedial left hemidiaphragm; when left eventration does occur, its location is usually shifted laterally and posteriorly compared to right eventration. Another reason is that the central tendon, which is more vulnerable to stretching than the muscular portion of the diaphragm, is often wider on the right. The anterior right and left fiber bands in the central tendon resist stretching and create the sharp medial margin shown by many eventrations, particularly on the right.

Abdominal distension by central obesity, ascites, tumor, or polycystic disease promotes eventration, just as it promotes elevation of the diaphragm in general. Once eventration has developed, the thinning of the central tendon is permanent, and the weakened tissue is even more susceptible to further stretching. Thus, eventration may progress, but cannot regress.

In eventration, the stretching of the central tendon shortens the muscle fibers at the periphery, reducing their range of contraction and impairing diaphragm function. This and the loss in lung volume caused by bulging of the hemidiaphragm

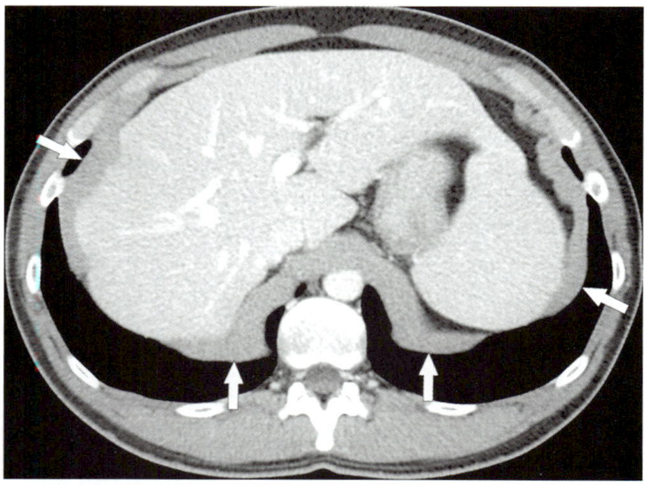

Figure 27.7. Hypertrophy of diaphragm muscle (*arrows*) in a 30-year-old asthmatic man who practiced yoga. It is not known which yoga exercises he performed, but breathing while head standing is one way yoga could lead to hypertrophy. CT shows circumferential hypertrophy of diaphragm muscle. (Courtesy of Blake Niederhauser, MD.)

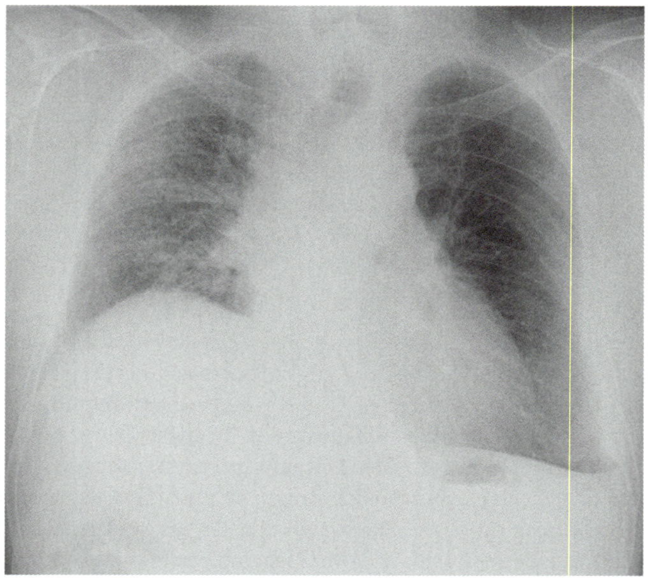

Figure 27.8. Lung fibrosis resulting in an elevated right hemidiaphragm. Chest radiograph shows high right hemidiaphragm due to volume loss from the lung fibrosis. Left hemidiaphragm position has been restored to normal by single left lung transplant.

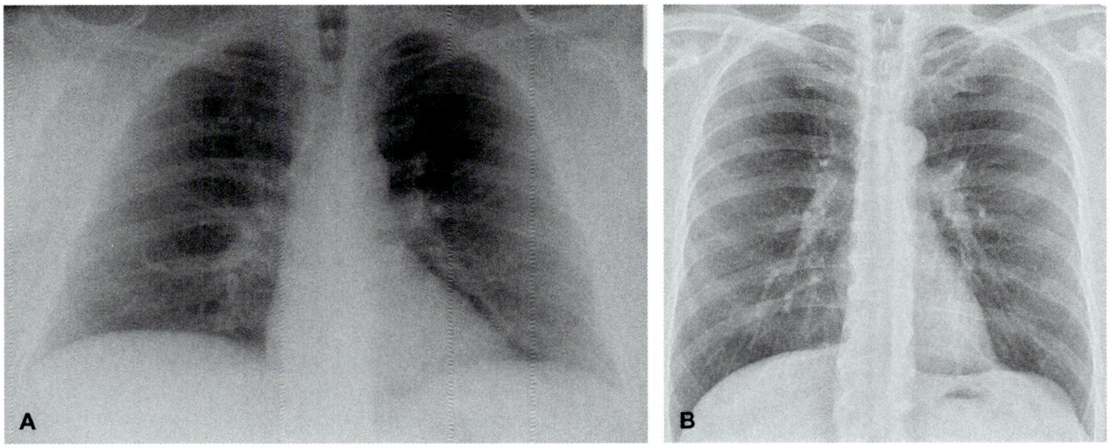

Figure 27.9. Diaphragm elevation caused by abdominal obesity reversed by weight loss. **A:** Radiograph shows high position of the diaphragm caused by intra-abdominal fat. **B:** Radiograph 2 years later after 19 kg weight loss shows gastric band in place and restoration of normal height of diaphragm.

can make larger eventrations symptomatic, with dyspnea and restriction on pulmonary function testing. Table 27.2 summarizes key points about eventration.

Radiographic and CT Findings

On radiographs, eventration can be distinguished in most cases from paralysis of the hemidiaphragm. A small or early eventration may appear as a slightly exaggerated elevation of the dome of the hemidiaphragm (Fig. 27.11). As eventration grows, it usually develops a distinct steeper arc that rejoins the shallower arc of the rest of the hemidiaphragm (Figs. 27.11 and 27.12). On lateral view, the posterior aspect of the hemidiaphragm is usually at normal height, even when the eventration is large (Fig. 27.13); in contrast, a paralyzed hemidiaphragm stays elevated all the way to the posterior chest wall. However, sometimes a large eventration does extend all the way to the posterior chest wall

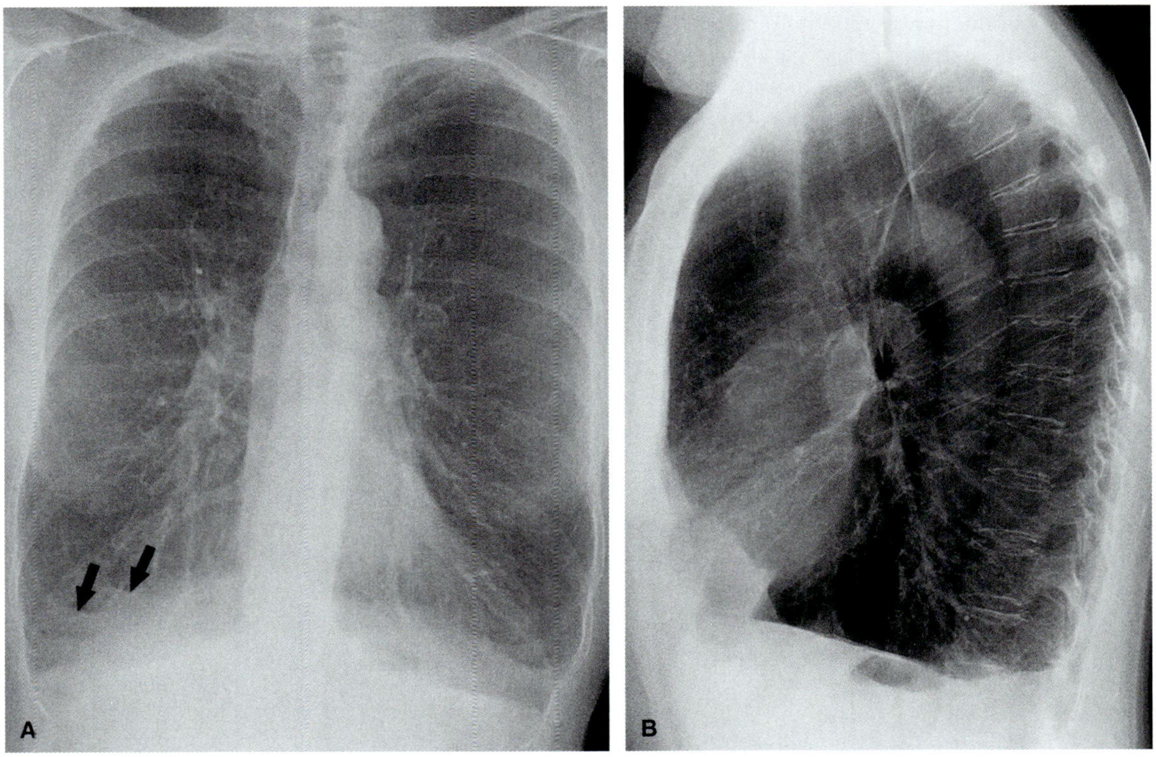

Figure 27.10. Low position of diaphragm caused by chronic obstructive pulmonary disease. **A:** PA radiograph shows low position of the diaphragm, exposing the attachments of muscle slips (*arrows*) to anterior ribs and causing a scalloped contour. **B:** Lateral radiograph shows flattening of both hemidiaphragms.

Table 27.2 Eventration
Caused by stretching and bulging of an unreinforced portion of the central tendon
Usually located anteriorly on the right
Often marginated medially by the anterior fiber band in the central tendon
Promoted by obesity or other cause of increased abdominal pressure
Can grow, but cannot shrink, since stretching of the central tendon is irreversible
Has steeper contour than paralysis or weakness and usually does not extend to posterior chest wall
Eventration can cause dyspnea and restriction because: Bulging of hemidiaphragm reduces lung volume. Stretching of central tendon shortens muscle fibers at the periphery of the hemidiaphragm and reduces their range of contraction.

(Fig. 27.14) and CT evaluation of muscle thickness will be needed to distinguish eventration from paralysis. Another distinguishing feature of eventration is that its arc is often steep, whereas the arc of a paralyzed or weak hemidiaphragm is usually shallow from front to back. Sometimes eventrations are multiple, causing overlapping small bulges between muscle bundles (Fig. 27.15). Often eventration is visible on the posteroanterior or the lateral view, but not both.

On CT, thickness of the crus and anterior muscle of the hemidiaphragm is normal in eventration (unlike in paralysis). However, the dome of the eventration is usually thin because it consists mostly of stretched central tendon with little muscle (Fig. 27.14). Eventration is often marginated medially by the anterior fiber band, as shown in Figure 27.2. If the degree of stretching and redundancy of the central tendon is great enough, the diaphragm may fold back on itself along its medial margin and mushroom above (Figs. 27.16 and 27.17). *This mushrooming should not be mistaken for herniation.* The fiber band can indent the liver, forming a diaphragmatic groove (Figs. 27.2 and 27.17). Adjacent muscle bands may add additional grooves in the liver (Fig. 27.2).

On a sniff test, excursion of the dome of the eventration is reduced on deep inspiration, but excursion of the posterior portion of the hemidiaphragm is usually preserved, as shown by lateral fluoroscopy. On sniffing, the dome may move paradoxically, reflecting its relative weakness.

Paralysis and Weakness

Etiology and Clinical Presentation

Unilateral diaphragmatic paralysis or weakness can result from damage to the phrenic nerve by such causes as tumor, aortic aneurysm, or iatrogenic injury from cardiothoracic surgery, cardioplegia, atrial ablation for atrial fibrillation, or interscalene nerve block. Other causes include trauma, neck surgery, chiropractic manipulation, cervical spondylosis, viral infection (including COVID-19), poliomyelitis, amyotrophic lateral sclerosis (ALS), multiple sclerosis, and inflammatory syndromes, such as Guillain-Barré and Parsonage-Turner (neuralgic amyotrophy). Etiology remains unknown in many cases.

Paralysis or weakness is usually unilateral, but sometimes bilateral. Causes of bilateral hemidiaphragm paralysis include spinal cord injury and neuromuscular disorders, such as ALS and myasthenia gravis. Mediastinal and heart surgery can also cause bilateral hemidiaphragm paralysis.

Symptoms of bilateral dysfunction are always severe, whereas symptoms of unilateral dysfunction may be mild. The patient may experience orthopnea or dyspnea on exertion, on bending forward ("bendopnea"), or when wading in water up to the abdomen or chest ("dyspnea on immersion"). Pulmonary function tests show restriction.

A patient with bilateral hemidiaphragm dysfunction may compensate by using abdominal wall muscles, principally the transverse abdominal muscle, to move the diaphragm passively. Tightening the abdominal wall flattens the abdomen and pushes the diaphragm up, causing expiration; relaxing it allows the diaphragm to fall passively, causing inspiration. We call this *abdominal recruitment.* The patient may not be aware of using it. Recruitment works when the patient is upright, but it is disabled when the patient is supine. On upright fluoroscopy, recruitment can mimic normal diaphragm function, but supine fluoroscopy will reveal the loss of excursion.

Radiographic and CT Findings

On radiographs, the affected hemidiaphragm(s) is usually elevated (Figs. 27.18-27.20) all the way from anterior chest to the posterior chest wall, with a shallower arc than is typical of eventration. There is often atelectasis in the adjacent lung base(s).

CT may show the cause of phrenic nerve dysfunction, such as tumor, lymphadenopathy, aneurysm, or infection. CT may reveal a condition that mimics elevation of the diaphragm such as subpulmonic pleural effusion or tumor.

CT shows thinning of diaphragmatic muscle with weakness or paralysis caused by phrenic neuropathy (Figs. 27.18-27.20), and the degree of thinning is greater with paralysis.

Usually, elevation of a hemidiaphragm without muscle thinning indicates eventration rather than weakness or paralysis. Elevation of both hemidiaphragms without muscle thinning also argues against diaphragm weakness or paralysis and suggests a nondiaphragmatic cause of elevation, such

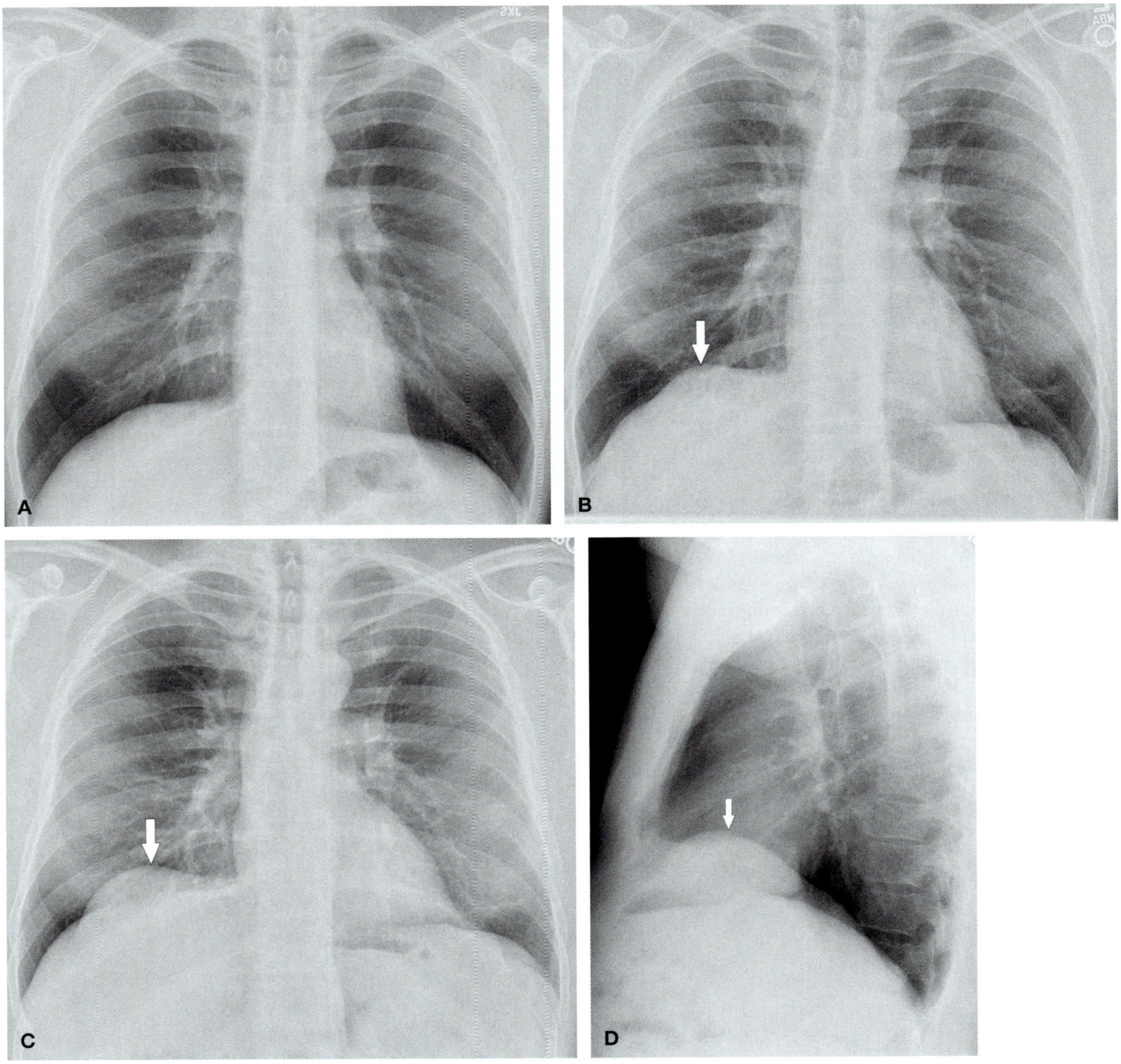

Figure 27.11. Development of small eventration of the right hemidiaphragm. **A:** PA radiograph shows normal contour of right hemidiaphragm. **B:** PA radiograph 6 years later and **C:** PA radiograph 11 years later show growth of right eventration (*arrows*). **D:** Lateral radiograph shows the anterior eventration (*arrow*).

as lung fibrosis or abdominal obesity, as discussed earlier. However, when weakness or paralysis is caused by upper motor neuron disease or myopathy, muscle thickness can be normal despite impaired diaphragm function on the sniff test.

Tethering

Pleural thickening after infection, trauma, or surgery can obliterate the costophrenic angle and fuse the diaphragmatic pleura to the chest wall pleura (Fig. 27.21), restricting the motion of the hemidiaphragm. Fluoroscopy shows focal fixation of the hemidiaphragm to the chest wall, with motion maintained elsewhere. Decortication may be considered to restore mobility.

Functional Imaging—Fluoroscopy of the Diaphragm, the "Sniff Test"

Source: Used with permission of Radiological Society of North America, from Nason LK, Walker CM, McNeeley MF, et al. Imaging of the diaphragm: anatomy and function. *Radiographics*. 2012;32(2):E51-E70; permission conveyed through Copyright Clearance Center, Inc.

Fluoroscopy provides a simple assessment of diaphragm function. Other functional imaging techniques are MRI and

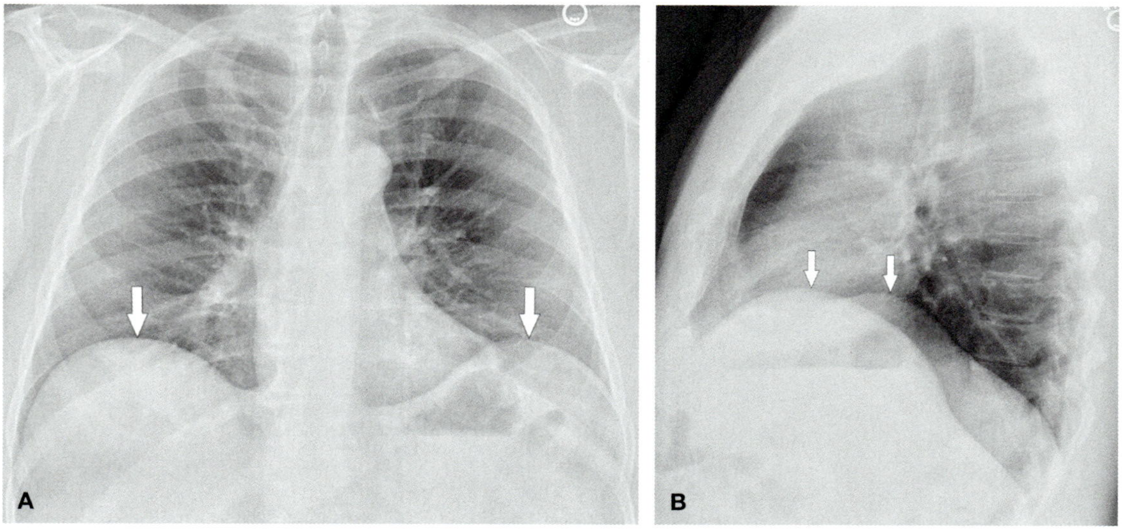

Figure 27.12. Bilateral moderate eventration. **A:** PA and lateral **B:** radiographs show eventrations (*arrows*) of both hemidiaphragms, with the left eventration slightly posterior to the right, as usual.

ultrasonography. MRI can depict anatomy and function without ionizing radiation. Its disadvantages are higher cost and lower availability than CT. Ultrasonography can show not only the motion of the diaphragm but also the thickening of its muscle during inspiration. Lack of radiation and portability make ultrasonography particularly suitable for children and for patients in bed. Its limitations are that some parts of the diaphragm may be blocked from view by intestinal gas and that the whole diaphragm cannot be seen at once.

A meaningful fluoroscopic examination requires more than just sniffing—the most important maneuver is slow deep inspiration. Therefore, our technique incorporates spontaneous quiet breathing, deep inspiration, and sniffing in frontal and lateral views with the patient upright and, when possible, deep inspiration in frontal view with the patient supine. For brevity, we use the term "sniff test" even though we do this comprehensive exam.

By including supine views, our technique can assess bilateral hemidiaphragm paralysis, which sniffing and upright views can miss.

Accuracy of the sniff test (based on sniffing alone) in diagnosing unilateral paralysis is said to be 90%. However,

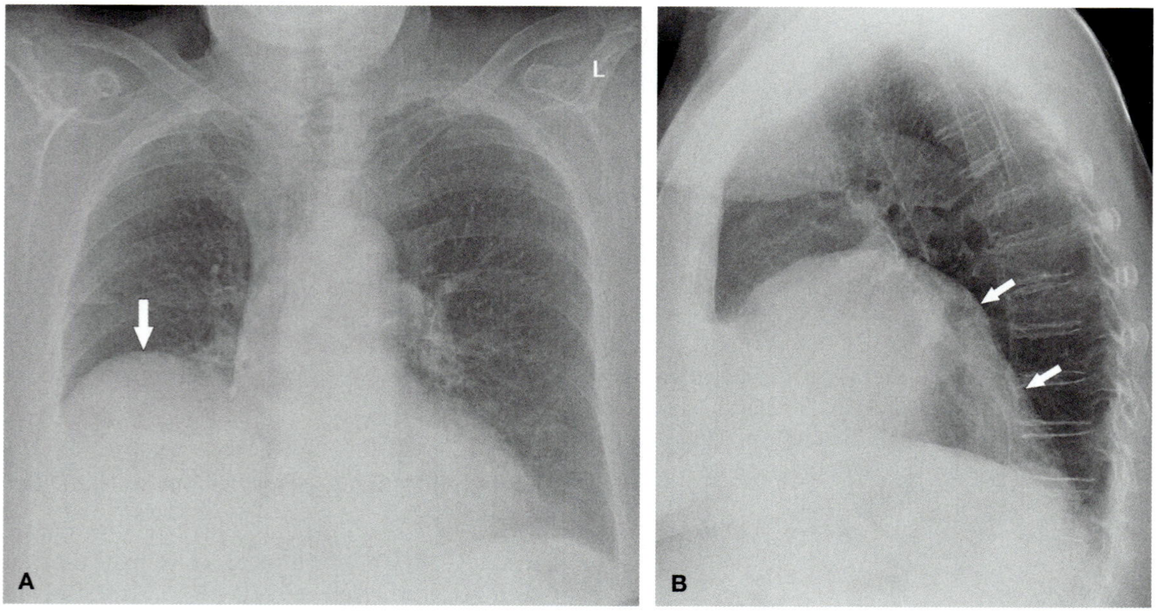

Figure 27.13. Large eventration of the right hemidiaphragm. **A:** and **B:** PA **(A)** and lateral **(B)** radiographs show the large eventration with steep posterior descent (*arrows*) to normal height along the posterior chest wall. With weakness or paralysis, the arc of the elevation is shallower, and elevation extends all the way to the posterior chest wall, as shown in Figure 27.20.

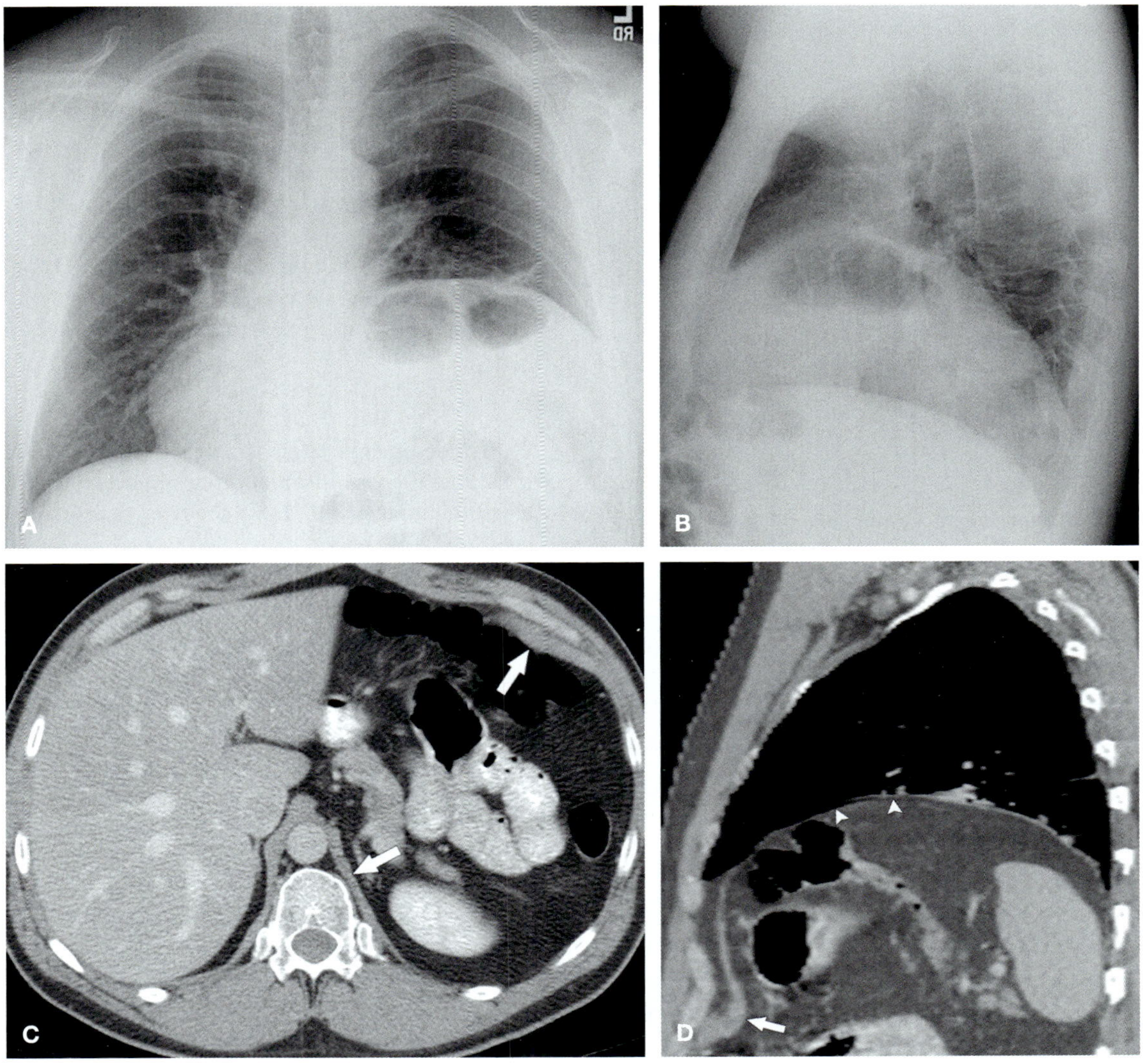

Figure 27.14. Normal muscle thickness on CT helps distinguish large eventration from paralysis. **A:** PA and **B:** lateral radiographs show the large left eventration extending to the posterior chest wall, resembling paralysis. **C:** Transaxial CT and **D:** sagittal CT show normal thicknesses of left crus and of anterior muscle (*arrows*), arguing against paralysis. The dome of the left hemidiaphragm is thin (*arrowheads*), as expected with eventration.

accuracy is difficult to assess, given variation in technique and interpretation and the absence of a gold standard. Our technique for the sniff test gets some validation from its strong correlation with crus thinning in distinguishing paralyzed from nonparalyzed hemidiaphragms.

Principles of the Sniff Test

It is essential for the patient to practice slow, deep breathing and sniffing before fluoroscopy. Detailed instructions are below.

The lateral projection is needed in addition to the frontal projection because the lateral view better shows downward excursion of the posterior diaphragm, which is usually more vigorous than excursion of the dome and anterior diaphragm. In cases of eventration, the lateral projection will show excursion of the posterior diaphragm even if the dome does not move. (In paralysis, this posterior excursion is absent.) Finally, the lateral projection shows the upward motion of the anterior chest wall on inspiration more clearly than the frontal projection does.

Sniffing is not the most important part of the sniff test, and sniffing by itself cannot diagnose paralysis. Instead, paralysis is diagnosed by absence of downward excursion of the hemidiaphragm on slow deep inspiration. Sniffing is a stress test that identifies relative weakness (not just paralysis) of the affected hemidiaphragm. Sniffing pits one hemidiaphragm against the other, akin to arm wrestling. The arm of the stronger opponent moves forward, forcing the arm of the weaker opponent to move backward (ie, paradoxically). The loser's arm is weaker than the winner's, but not paralyzed.

Supine position is essential in evaluating bilateral paralysis and it is another stress test that brings out weakness.

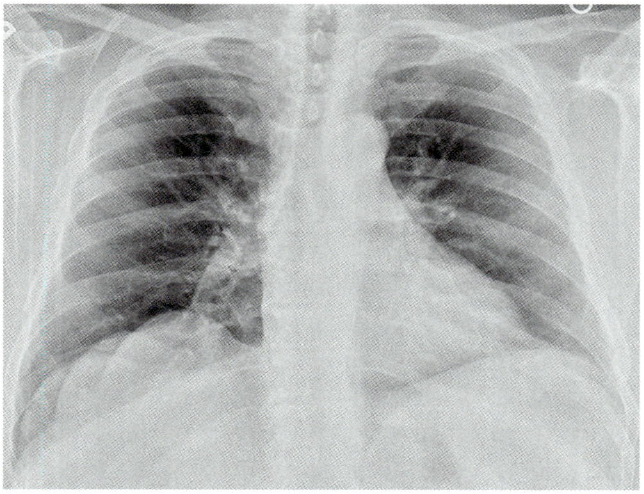

Figure 27.15. Multiple small eventrations of the right hemidiaphragm. PA radiograph shows 3 small eventrations between muscle bundles of the right hemidiaphragm.

Supine position pits the diaphragm against the weight of the abdomen. Supine positioning prevents abdominal recruitment from being mistaken for active diaphragm contraction. Thus, supine positioning is essential if the patient complains of orthopnea (shortness of breath on lying down) or if bilateral hemidiaphragm paralysis or weakness is suspected. We include frontal fluoroscopy with the patient semisupine (45°) on the way to supine position to give the patient a chance to adjust and for us to judge whether the patient will be able to tolerate the fully supine position. If the patient becomes dyspneic, we promptly return the table to upright position.

Technique

We include upright (standing or sitting) frontal and lateral views and then semisupine and supine frontal views. We record the images into PACS for later review and reporting (Fig. 27.21).

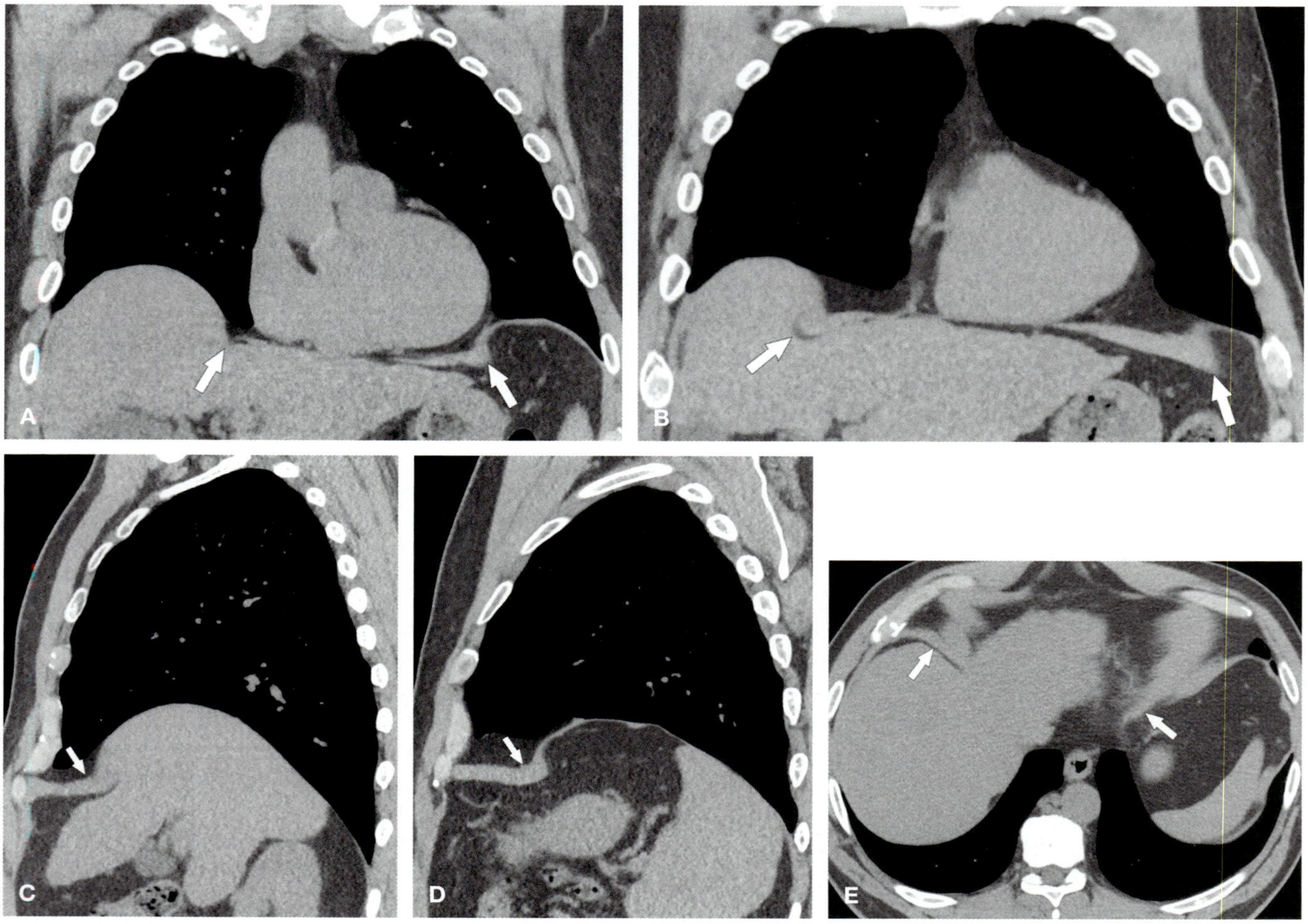

Figure 27.16. Medial margination of right and left eventrations by fiber bands in the central tendon. **A and B:** Coronal CT shows sharp medial margination (*arrows*) of right and left eventrations. In **(B)**, the diaphragm muscle is folded back on itself (*arrows*) at the medial margin of the eventration. **C and D:** Sagittal views also show sharp margins (*arrows*) of the eventrations on the right **(C)** and left **(D)**. **E:** CT shows folding of the diaphragm muscle (*arrows*) at the medial margins of the eventrations. Note that the folds point medially toward the junction of fiber bands, as shown in Figure 27.1.

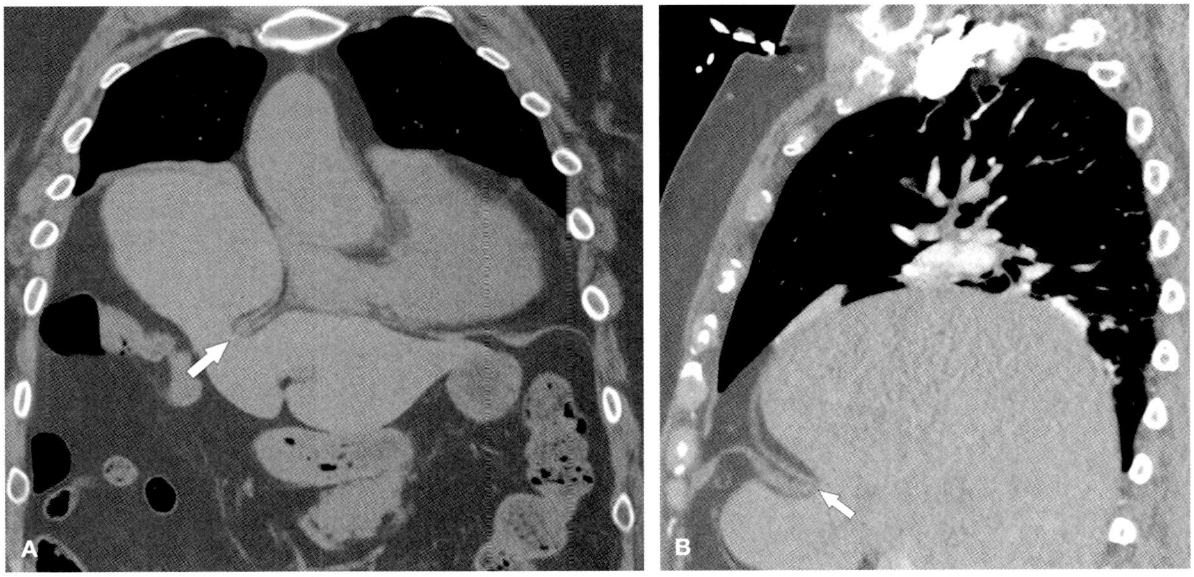

Figure 27.17. Medial margination of right eventration by fiber band in the central tendon with folding of hemidiaphragm and deep groove in liver (*arrow*). **A and B:** Coronal **(A)** and sagittal **(B)** CT shows folded hemidiaphragm at medial **(A)** and anterior **(B)** margin of right eventration, with deep groove in the liver (*arrow*). The large eventration mushrooms above the medial margin (resembling hernia) and contains colon and liver. The liver is displaced and deformed by the eventration.

1. Practice deep slow breathing and sniffing with the patient before performing the sniff test. We do this with the patient sitting or standing before moving to the fluoroscopy table and we do the maneuvers along with the patient. Have the patient take in a slow deep breath with mouth open and then let it out keeping the mouth open and not forcing the breath out or pursing the lips. Practice this slow deep breathing a couple of times. Then practice sniffing. After the patient has exhaled the second slow deep breath, have the patient close their mouth and then suck in through the nose as hard, fast, and long as possible. A long, hard sniff is needed, not a series of short shallow sniffs. Practice the sniff as part of the unit of slow deep inspiration (mouth open), slow expiration (mouth still open), then closing the mouth and sniffing. It often takes several rehearsals of this sequence for the patient to do it smoothly, vigorously, and reproducibly.
2. Move the patient to the upright fluoroscopy table. Collimate to show the entire chest. Observe a couple of quiet spontaneous breaths.
3. Observe a slow, deep breath. Say: "Take in a deep breath… now let it out."
4. Observe a second slow, deep breath and then add the sniff. Say: "Take in a deep breath…now let it out…now close your mouth and sniff!"
5. Repeat steps 3 and 4.
6. Turn the patient for lateral view and raise arms out of the field of view. Repeat steps 3 and 4, ie, observe two quiet

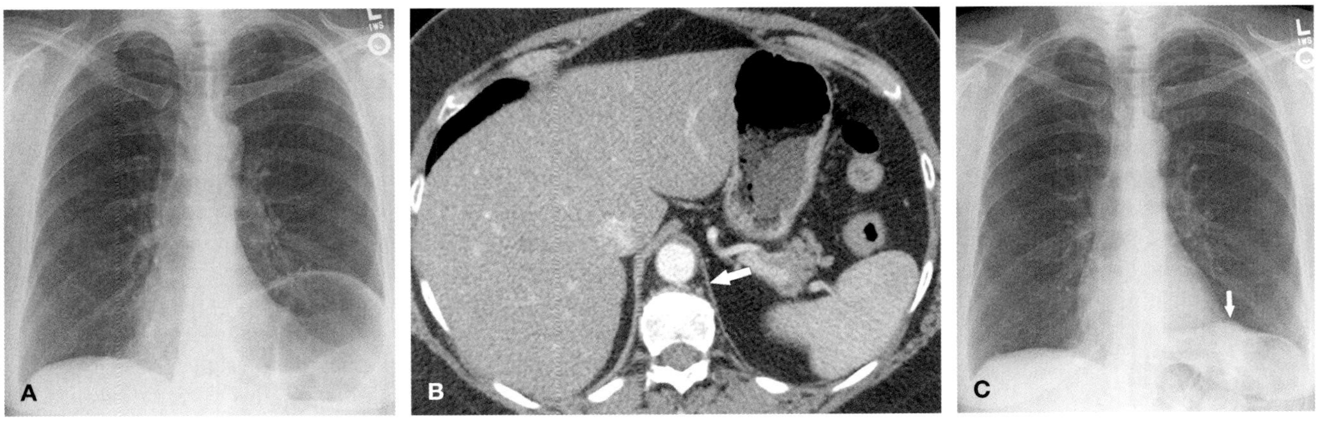

Figure 27.18. Left hemidiaphragm paralysis, probably from neuralgic amyotrophy (Parsonage-Turner syndrome). **A:** Radiograph shows elevation of the left hemidiaphragm, not present on previous radiographs. **B:** CT shows thinning of the left crus (arrow). **C:** Radiograph 1 year after **(A)** shows decreased elevation after plication of the left hemidiaphragm. The plicated tissue forms a ridge (arrow) on the top of the hemidiaphragm.

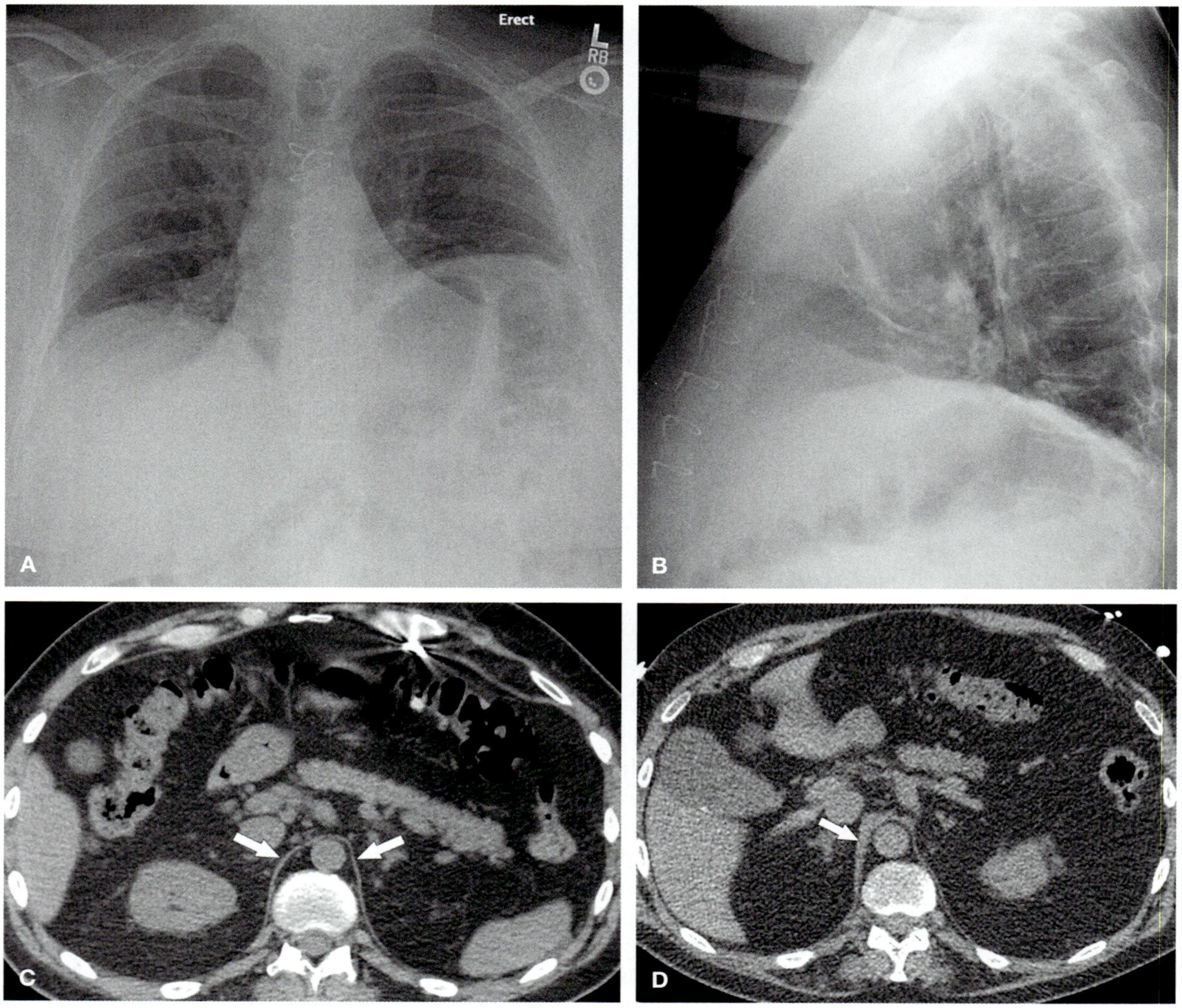

Figure 27.19. Bilateral hemidiaphragm paralysis after heart transplant and pretransplant left ventricular assist device. **A:** PA radiograph shows elevation of both hemidiaphragms and atelectasis in both lung bases. **B:** Lateral radiograph shows shallow arc of both hemidiaphragms and elevation extending to posterior chest wall, as expected with paralysis. **C:** CT shows thinning of both crura (*arrows*). **D:** CT 5 years later shows restoration of right crus thickness (*arrow*), implying recovery of right phrenic nerve.

breaths followed by two deep breaths with sniff after the second exhalation. Repeat.

7. Turn the patient back into frontal position. Observe two quiet breaths followed by two deep breaths and note the resting positions of both hemidiaphragms after quiet exhalation.
8. Tilt the table to the semisupine position (45°). Observe two quiet and two deep breaths and resting positions.
9. Tilt the table to supine position. Observe two quiet and two deep breaths and resting positions.

Interpretation (Table 27.3)

Normal Findings

1. On inspiration, the anterior chest wall moves upward and forward. It is often easier to see chest wall excursion on lateral view. Usually, chest wall excursion is preserved even when diaphragm motion is impaired, as described below.
2. On quiet or deep inspiration, both hemidiaphragms move downward as the anterior chest wall moves upward and anteriorly. Normal excursion on deep inspiration is at least one rib interspace, but motion can be asymmetric and or slightly delayed on one side, typically the right. The excursion of the posterior part of the hemidiaphragm is usually greater than that of the anterior portion of the hemidiaphragm, especially on the right.
3. On sniffing, both hemidiaphragms move downward. The same asymmetry and lag in right hemidiaphragm motion may occur, as in deep inspiration. If sniffing is strong, there may even be transient upward (paradoxical) motion of one hemidiaphragm (usually the right). In supine and

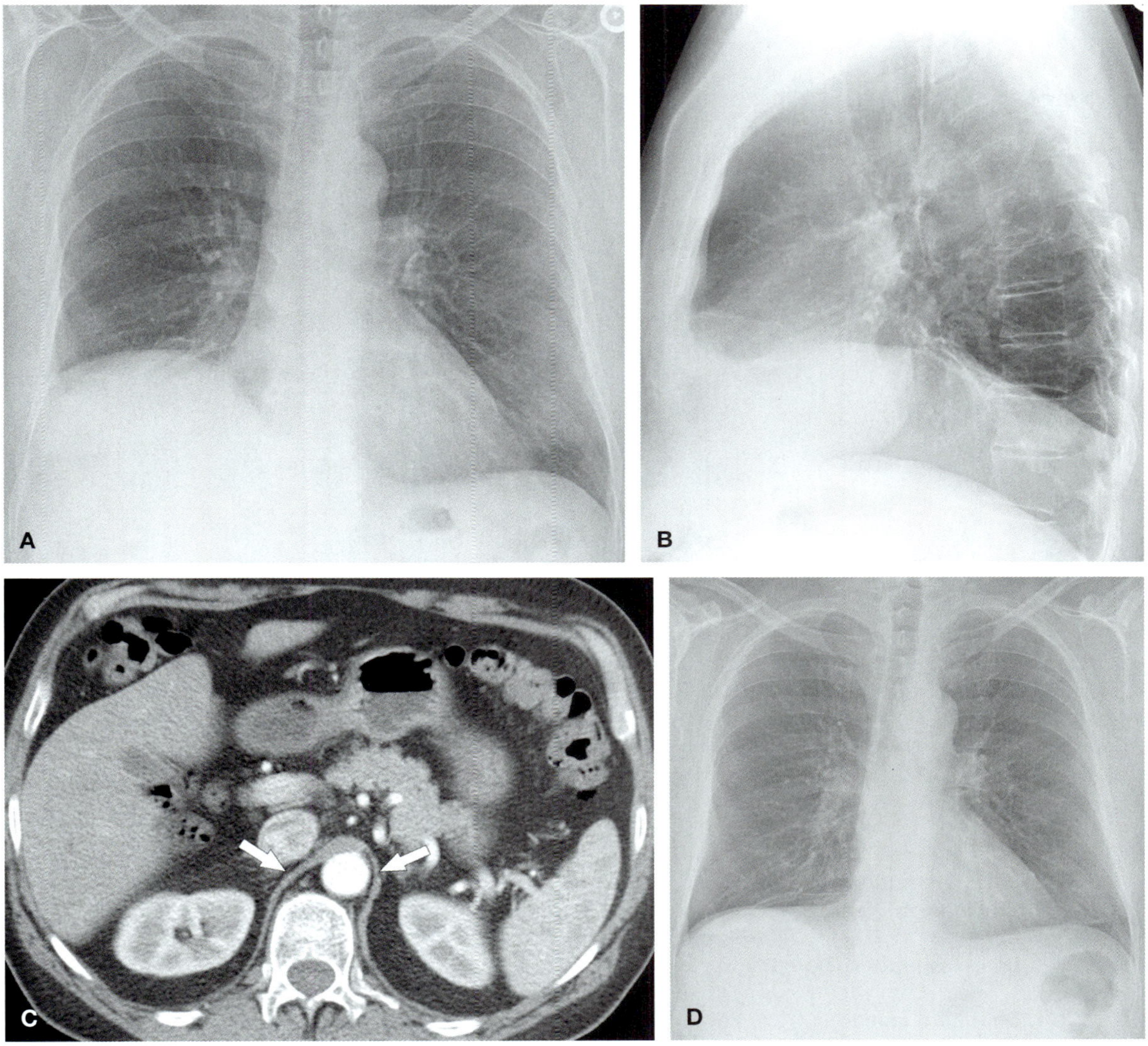

Figure 27.20. Idiopathic weakness, but not complete paralysis, of the right hemidiaphragm. **A:** PA and **B:** lateral radiographs show elevation of the right hemidiaphragm that extends to the posterior chest in a shallow arc, as with paralysis. Sniff test (not shown) showed weakness, but not paralysis of the right hemidiaphragm. **C:** CT shows normal bilateral crus thickness (*arrows*), rather than atrophy, as would occur with paralysis. Preservation of crus thickness suggests potential for recovery. **D:** Radiograph 2 years later shows resolution of elevation of right hemidiaphragm.

semisupine positions, excursion on deep inspiration is usually less than in upright position, but some orthograde excursion is maintained. The resting positions of both hemidiaphragms are usually 1 to 2 cm higher than with the patient upright.

Paralysis of One Hemidiaphragm

1. The paralyzed hemidiaphragm is elevated and there may be atelectasis in the lung base.
2. On deep inspiration, downward excursion is minimal or absent. The paralyzed hemidiaphragm may move upward (paradoxically) on deep or even quiet inspiration. The mediastinum may shift toward the nonparalyzed hemidiaphragm on inspiration.
3. On sniffing, there is usually upward (paradoxical) motion of the paralyzed hemidiaphragm.
4. On inspiration in supine position, any downward excursion on inspiration that might have been present with the patient upright will be further attenuated. The elevation of the resting position of the paralyzed hemidiaphragm may exceed that of the normal hemidiaphragm.

Paralysis of Both Hemidiaphragms

1. Both hemidiaphragms are elevated, and there may be basal atelectasis.
2. On inspiration, both hemidiaphragms may be passively pulled upward (paradoxically) by the normal upward excursion of the anterior chest wall. *It is important to*

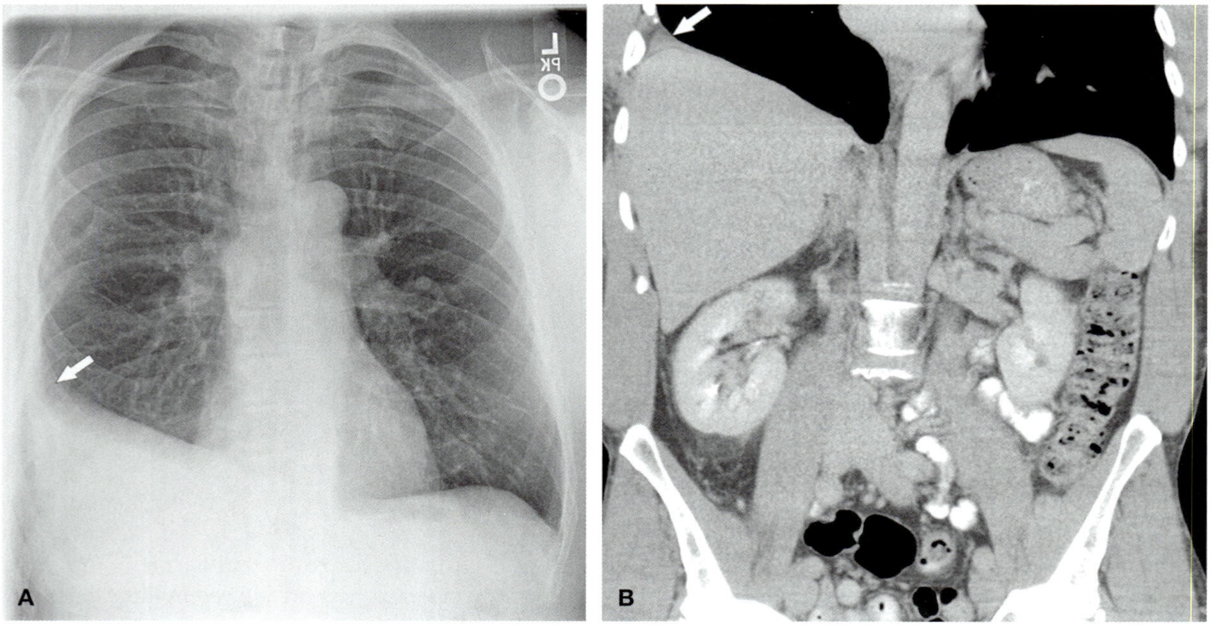

Figure 27.21. Tethering of right hemidiaphragm by pleural adhesion after remote thoracotomy. **A:** The costophrenic angle is elevated and tethered to the right chest wall (*arrow*). The right 7th rib has been resected for thoracotomy. **B:** Coronal CT shows the adhesion (*arrow*) binding the diaphragmatic pleura to the pleura of the lateral chest wall. On fluoroscopy of the diaphragm, the adhesion fixed the right hemidiaphragm to the chest wall, acting like a hinge and restricting diaphragmatic motion.

Table 27.3 Findings on Diaphragmatic Fluoroscopy

Condition	Deep Inspiration (Upright)	Deep Inspiration (Supine)	Sniffing
Normal	Downward motion >1 rib interspace	Downward motion decreased vs upright	Usually downward motion
Unilateral weakness	Downward motion <1 rib interspace	Absent or decreased downward motion vs upright	Either upward or downward motion
Unilateral paralysis	Absent downward motion or upward motion	Absent downward motion	Usually upward motion
Bilateral paralysis	Absent downward motion or bilateral upward motion ****In some cases, abdominal recruitment simulates normal downward motion.***	Absent downward motion ****Supine imaging disables abdominal recruitment that simulates normal downward motion.***	Usually upward motion (from chest wall)
Eventration	Decreased downward motion, sometimes upward movement of eventrated segment	Downward motion decreased vs upright	Downward or upward motion of the affected segment
Tethering by pleural adhesion	Absent downward motion where fixed to the chest wall; normal motion where untethered	Downward motion except where tethered	Downward motion except where tethered

recognize that the diaphragm is paralyzed if it moves in the same direction as the chest wall.

3. On inspiration in upright position, downward excursion of the hemidiaphragms may appear normal if the patient uses abdominal recruitment to passively move the diaphragm. This compensatory mechanism is disabled by supine or even semisupine positioning.
4. On inspiration in supine position, downward excursion of the diaphragm is absent and excursion may be upward (paradoxical), passively following the anterior chest wall. There is excess elevation of the resting position of both hemidiaphragms.

Weakness of One Hemidiaphragm

1. On deep inspiration, downward excursion is less than one rib interspace and excursion may be delayed compared to the normal hemidiaphragm. Paradoxical motion on deep or even quiet inspiration may occur.
2. On sniffing, there may be upward (paradoxical) motion.
3. On inspiration in supine position, excursion may be more attenuated than on the normal side, and there may be excess elevation of the resting position of the hemidiaphragm.

Eventration

1. On deep inspiration, excursion of the eventrated segment is attenuated or even paradoxical. On lateral view, excursion of the dome is abnormal, but excursion of the posterior hemidiaphragm is usually normal, but may be attenuated if the eventration is large.
2. On sniffing, there may be upward (paradoxical) motion of the eventrated segment.
3. On inspiration in supine position, excursion of the dome of the hemidiaphragm may be minimal or absent or even paradoxical. The more normal excursion of the posterior portion of the hemidiaphragm is usually not visible on frontal view. There may be excess elevation of the resting position of the dome.

Tethering

1. On deep inspiration, excursion of the hemidiaphragm is absent at the site of pleural adhesion to the chest wall. Excursion is reduced away from the fixation point.
2. On sniffing, there is no upward motion.

We emphasize that upward (paradoxical) motion of the diaphragm occurs with weakness, paralysis, and eventration, not just with paralysis. Thus, paralysis is not diagnosed by paradoxical motion, but instead on absent downward motion of the diaphragm on slow, deep inspiration.

Table 27.4 summarizes the imaging findings in causes of diaphragm dysfunction.

Treatment

A patient with eventration or a weak or paralyzed hemidiaphragm is usually managed conservatively, at least for a year or year and a half, since some degree of recovery is common (Fig. 27.20). If dysfunction persists, a symptomatic patient with unilateral phrenic nerve dysfunction or large eventration may be treated with plication of the hemidiaphragm, which is often performed thoracoscopically. The thinned tissue of the eventration is gathered into pleats that are sutured together to tighten and lower the hemidiaphragm (Figs. 27.18 and 27.22). Plication is sometimes performed prophylactically when the phrenic nerve is injured during surgery or damaged by tumor in the lung or mediastinum.

Phrenic nerve stimulation may be considered in a case of high cervical spine injury with bilateral hemidiaphragm paralysis, but intact phrenic nerves.

HERNIA OF THE DIAPHRAGM

Herniation of abdominal contents across the diaphragm into the chest has congenital, acquired, traumatic, and iatrogenic causes. Esophageal hiatal hernia is the most common diaphragmatic hernia followed by Bochdalek and then Morgagni hernias.

Hiatal Hernia

The prevalence of hiatal hernia increases with age, from 5% in persons under 40 years, to 30% and 65% in persons from 40 to 59 and 65 to 79 years, respectively. Most hiatal hernias are asymptomatic at the time of diagnosis and are incidental findings on radiographs or CT scans obtained for other reasons. However, hiatal hernia can cause regurgitation, heartburn, or reflux, which can lead to esophageal stricture or even obstruction.

On radiographs, hiatal hernia presents as a retrocardiac mediastinal mass (Fig. 27.23) that obscures the normally well-defined posterior heart border on the lateral radiograph. Hiatal hernia often contains an air bubble and one or more fluid levels. If a large portion of the stomach is herniated, it may undergo volvulus, which manifests as double air bubbles with fluid levels.

CT shows widening of the esophageal hiatus (Fig. 27.23) between the medial right and left crura, which are normally 15 mm or less apart.

Hiatal hernia can be classified into four types based on which structures herniate. The most common (90%-95%) is type I (sliding hernia), in which the gastric body herniates upward into the lower mediastinum along with the gastroesophageal junction, which keeps its position above the stomach. Types II-IV are paraesophageal hernias. In type II (pure paraesophageal hernia), which is uncommon, the gastric fundus herniates into the mediastinum, but the gastroesophageal junction remains below the esophageal hiatus. In type III, the second most common, both the gastroesophageal junction and gastric fundus herniate into the chest. In type IV, an additional viscus, such as the liver, colon (Fig. 27.23), or pancreas, herniates along with the stomach.

Table 27.4 Summary of Diaphragm Dysfunction

Condition	Clinical Condition	Radiologic Findings	Fluoroscopic Findings
Unilateral paralysis	Phrenic nerve dysfunction	• Elevation of paralyzed hemidiaphragm extending to posterior chest wall with shallow arc • Possible basal atelectasis • Crus thinning <2.5 mm	• **Absent or near-absent downward motion on deep inspiration** • Further reduction of downward motion in supine position • Upward (paradoxical) motion on sniffing
Bilateral paralysis	Phrenic nerve dysfunction Spinal cord injury Neuromuscular disorder	• Elevation of both hemidiaphragms extending to posterior chest wall with shallow arc • Possible basal atelectasis • Bilateral crus thinning <2.5 mm	• Absent or near-absent downward motion on deep inspiration in upright position *unless patient uses abdominal muscles* • Possible upward (paradoxical) motion on inspiration from passive following of chest wall • **Absent downward excursion in supine position, which defeats abdominal recruitment** • Possible upward (paradoxical) motion bilaterally on sniffing
Unilateral weakness	Phrenic nerve dysfunction	• Elevation of hemidiaphragm extending to posterior chest wall with shallow arc • Possible basal atelectasis • Mild crus thinning >2.5 mm	• **Reduced (<1 rib interspace), but not absent, downward motion on deep inspiration** • Attenuated excursion on inspiration in supine position • Possible upward (paradoxical) motion during sniffing
Eventration	Usually acquired by stretching of the central tendon by abdominal pressure from obesity, ascites, etc.	• Elevated hemidiaphragm, often with steep contour, not extending to posterior chest wall • No crus thinning	• **Reduced or absent downward motion of eventrated segment of hemidiaphragm on deep inspiration, but preservation of excursion posteriorly** • Possible upward (paradoxical) motion of eventrated segment on sniffing
Tethering	Pleural adhesion binding the diaphragm to chest wall	• Elevation of hemidiaphragm by pleural adhesion to chest wall • Blunting of costophrenic angle • No crus thinning	• **Reduced downward motion at the site of adhesion, often with hingelike motion**

Key diagnostic findings are in bold type. Note that paradoxical motion on sniffing is not diagnostic of paralysis, since it also occurs with weakness and eventration. Note that deep inspiration in supine position is required to diagnose bilateral paralysis.

Bochdalek Hernia

The classic Bochdalek hernia occurs in infants and only rarely in adults. In infants, it is the most common and most serious form of diaphragmatic hernia, with an incidence of about 1 in 2200 live births. Most (75%-90%) are posterolateral on the left, involving the pleuroperitoneal hiatus (foramen of Bochdalek); presumably the liver prevents most right Bochdalek hernias by covering the right pleuroperitoneal canal. When the hernia is large, lung development is impaired and mortality is high, even after surgical treatment.

Because of CT detection of incidental asymptomatic hernias, Bochdalek hernia is now much more commonly found in adults than in infants. The adult version is more likely than the congenital version to be right-sided or bilateral, and it is usually more medial than the location of the pleuroperitoneal hiatus. Adult Bochdalek hernia is probably acquired, given that its prevalence increases with age, from 5% in persons 40 to 49 years old to 15%, and 35% in persons 50 to 69 and over 70 years old, respectively. All these characteristics suggest that the adult version is a different kind of hernia from the neonatal version, involving a different zone of diaphragmatic weakness besides the pleuroperitoneal canal, possibly the medial or lateral arcuate ligament. Despite the differences between the congenital and the adult versions, the term Bochdalek hernia is applied to any posterior hernia in an adult.

On radiographs, adult Bochdalek hernia manifests as a focal bulge or mass along the posterior hemidiaphragm (Figs. 27.24 and 27.25), often posteromedial on either or on both sides. Since it arises from the retroperitoneum, it lacks

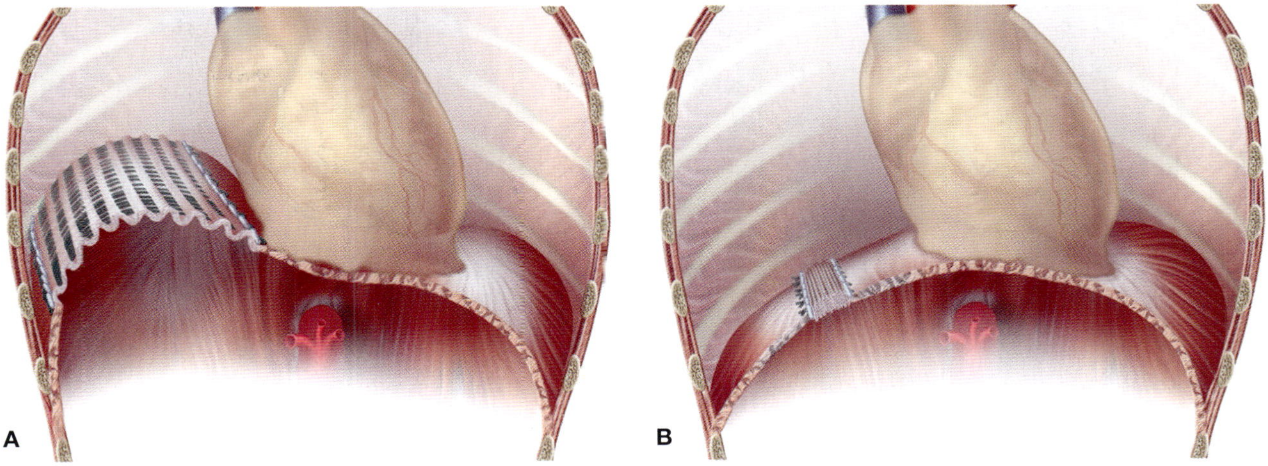

Figure 27.22. Plication of paralyzed right hemidiaphragm. **A:** Sutures buttressed by Teflon pledgets have been placed, forming pleats in the elevated and thinned right hemidiaphragm. **B:** The sutures have been tightened, pulling the pleats together and lowering the right hemidiaphragm. (This is the technique used by Michael S. Mulligan, M.D., who supervised these drawings.) (Reproduced from NASON.)

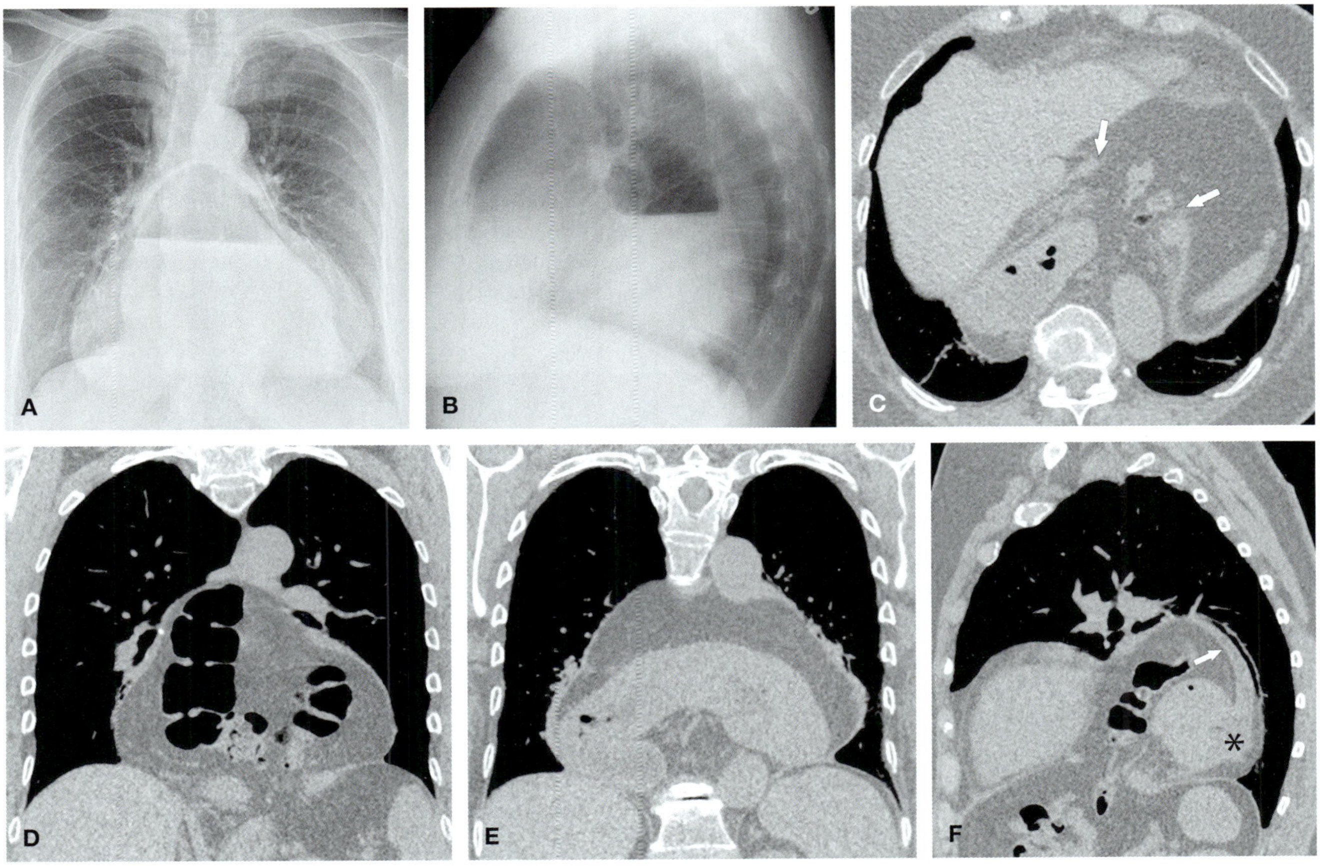

Figure 27.23. Large type IV hiatal hernia containing stomach and colon. **A:** PA and **B:** lateral chest radiographs show large hiatal hernia with fluid level in the stomach, which is inverted by organoaxial volvulus. **C:** CT shows the widened esophageal hiatus (*arrows*). **D:** Coronal CT shows the herniated colon and **(E)** coronal CT posterior to D shows the inverted stomach. **F:** Sagittal CT shows the esophagus (*arrow*) posterior to the hernia with gastroesophageal junction (*) above the diaphragm.

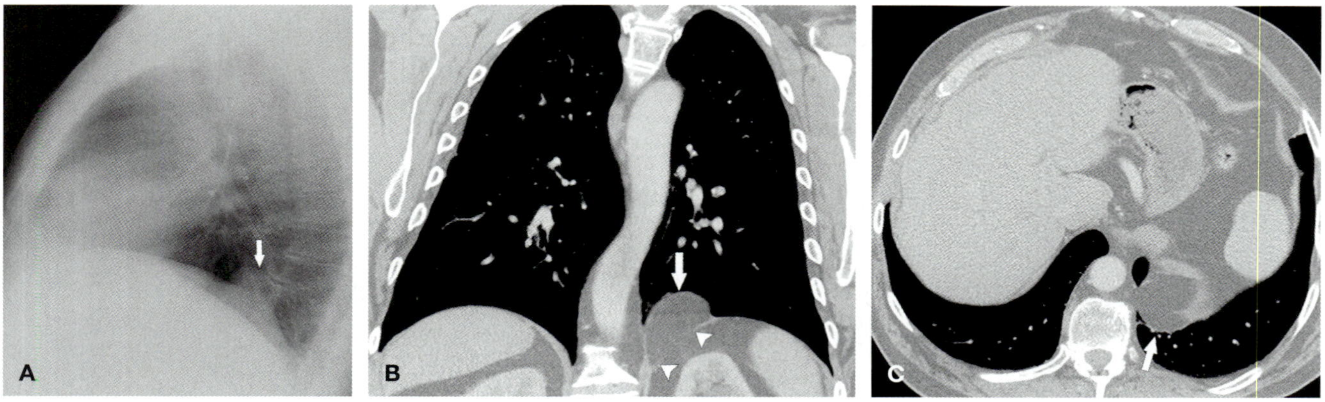

Figure 27.24. **A:** Lateral radiograph shows discrete bulge (*arrow*) along the posterior left hemidiaphragm. **B:** Coronal and **C:** transaxial CT images show the medial bulge (*arrows*) containing perinephric fat. The edges of the defect (*arrowheads*) are visible in **(B)**, along with a small vessel extending into the herniated fat.

a peritoneal sac. It usually contains only perinephric fat, but when large, it can contain kidney, or even stomach or bowel (Fig. 27.25). A small hernia may be contained by the parietal pleura of the diaphragm. However, when a large amount of fat herniates, it is probably free in the pleural space, since it is not contained by a peritoneal sac (Figs. 27.26 and 27.27). Herniated fat in this location can mimic pleural effusion on radiographs (Fig. 27.27).

Morgagni Hernia

Morgagni hernia is less common than hiatal or Bochdalek hernia. It is almost always on the right, probably because the overlying heart prevents herniation through the left parasternal hiatus. Although the diaphragmatic defect is congenital, actual herniation occurs in adult years, promoted by abdominal obesity or other cause of increased intra-abdominal pressure. A peritoneal sac is always present. The abdominal contents that may extend into the hernia are, in descending order, the omentum, colon, stomach, liver, and small intestine. Morgagni hernia is usually asymptomatic, but it can cause epigastric or retrosternal pain, or, if large, shortness of breath.

On radiographs, Morgagni hernia usually manifests as a well-defined smooth convexity in the right anterolateral cardiophrenic angle of the mediastinum (Figs. 27.28 and 27.29). The convexity is centered more medially than the convexity caused by eventration. If the colon enters the hernia, gas and stool may be visible on chest radiographs (Fig. 27.29). CT shows the site of herniation between the costal and sternal attachments of the right hemidiaphragm and shows its contents, usually just omental fat, but sometimes colon, or other abdominal organ (Figs. 27.28 and 27.29).

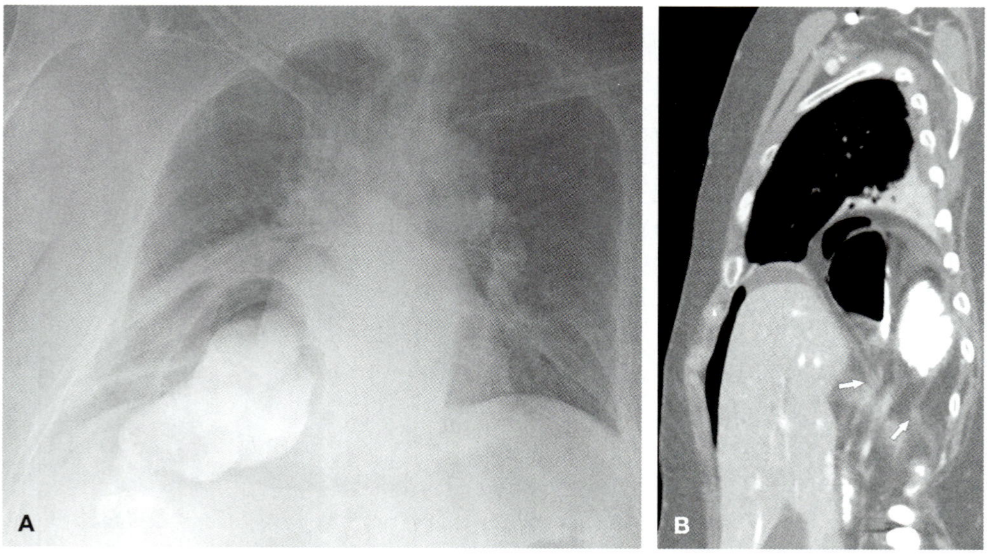

Figure 27.25. Large right Bochdalek hernia containing colon, but not kidney. **A:** AP radiograph shows contrast and gas in large medial right hernia. **B:** Sagittal CT shows edges of defect (*arrows*) in the posterior right hemidiaphragm with herniated colon above.

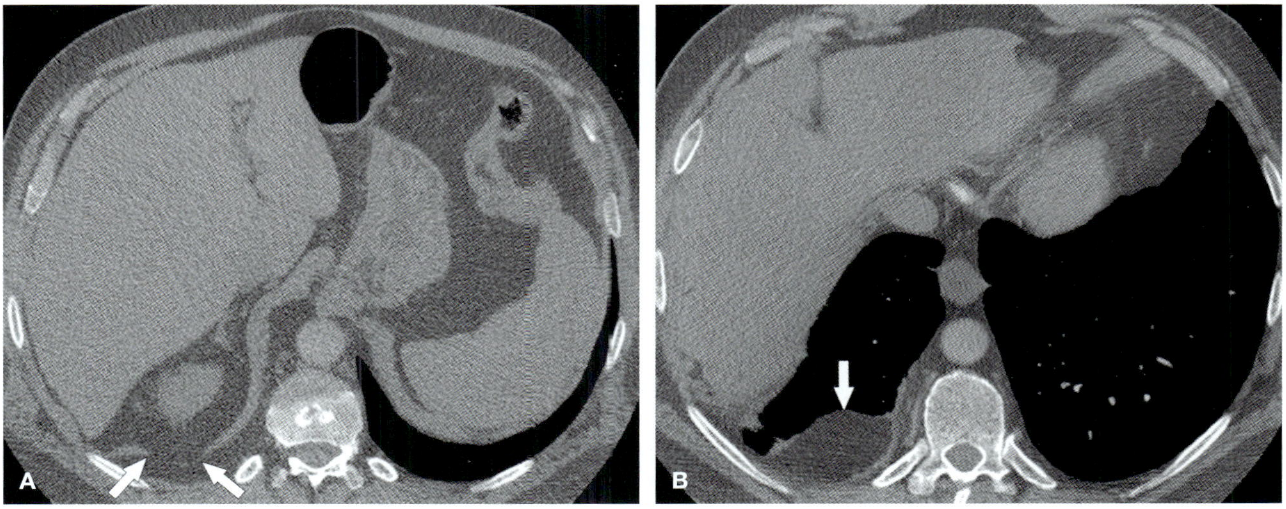

Figure 27.26. Right Bochdalek hernia with fat extruded into pleural space. **A:** CT shows edges of defect (*arrows*) in posterior right hemidiaphragm with fat herniating through. **B:** Herniated fat (*arrow*) in pleural space lies along the posterior chest wall.

Traumatic Hernia

Most traumatic hernias (75%) of the diaphragm are caused by blunt trauma, and hernia (rupture) is found in 1% to 8% of hospital admissions after blunt trauma. The most common site of rupture is the posterolateral left hemidiaphragm, and the mechanism is a sudden increase in intra-abdominal or intrathoracic pressure against a fixed diaphragm. Penetrating trauma causes 25% of traumatic hernias, and the site is variable, depending on the path of the penetrating trauma, which might be from a knife, bullet, or fractured rib.

Traumatic diaphragmatic hernia can have acute or delayed manifestations. Respiratory distress can result from mass effect of the hernia contents entering the thorax, from pneumothorax, or from intrathoracic rupture of a herniated viscus. Strangulation of herniated bowel can cause nausea, vomiting, or obstruction.

On radiographs, traumatic diaphragmatic hernia can be hard to detect (Fig. 27.30). In one study, radiography was diagnostic in 46% (20/44) and suggestive in an additional 18% (8/44) of traumatic left hernias. Chest radiography was strongly suggestive in only 17% (1/6) of right traumatic diaphragmatic hernias. Chest radiography is even less sensitive in penetrating hernia.

Radiographic findings that suggest traumatic hernia include cephalad extension of a nasogastric tube above the expected level of the diaphragm, herniation of the stomach or bowel into the thoracic cavity, obscuration or irregularity of the diaphragmatic contour, greater than 4-cm elevation of the hemidiaphragm compared to the other side, contralateral shift of the mediastinum in the absence of other causes of shift (such as large pleural effusion or pneumothorax), and the collar or hourglass sign, which is focal constriction of the herniated stomach or bowel as it passes through the diaphragmatic defect.

CT is more sensitive than radiography. In one study of 42 confirmed cases of diaphragmatic injury, CT confirmed injury in 57% of the cases with higher accuracy on the left than the right.

Characteristic CT findings are abrupt discontinuity in the hemidiaphragm and herniated abdominal contents in the chest (Figs. 27.30-27.32). Suggestive findings include the *absent diaphragm sign* (obscuration of the diaphragm contour), the *collar or hourglass sign*, and the *dependent viscera sign* (contact between herniated abdominal structures and posterior ribs) (Fig. 27.31).

Focal discontinuity of the diaphragm is found in up to 80% of traumatic hernias. However, its specificity is limited because it can occur in elderly patients without hernias. Herniation of abdominal structures into the chest is more specific and is found in 50% to 60% of hernias. The collar sign is found in 16% to 63% of traumatic hernias. The dependent viscera sign may be the most sensitive CT sign: in a series of blunt trauma cases that underwent emergency laparotomy, it was found in all 4 cases of left and in 5 of 6 cases of right hemidiaphragmatic hernia.

Diagnosis of traumatic hernia may be delayed, even decades after trauma (Fig. 27.32). Symptoms may develop late because the hernia has enlarged or become complicated, as by strangulation.

Iatrogenic Hernia

An iatrogenic hernia is a kind of traumatic hernia. It can arise from laceration during chest or abdominal surgery (Fig. 27.33), from thoracostomy drain placement, from radiofrequency ablation of liver tumors (Fig. 27.34), and from other causes, such as inadequately closing the diaphragmatic defect left after removal of a left ventricular assist device (Fig. 27.35).

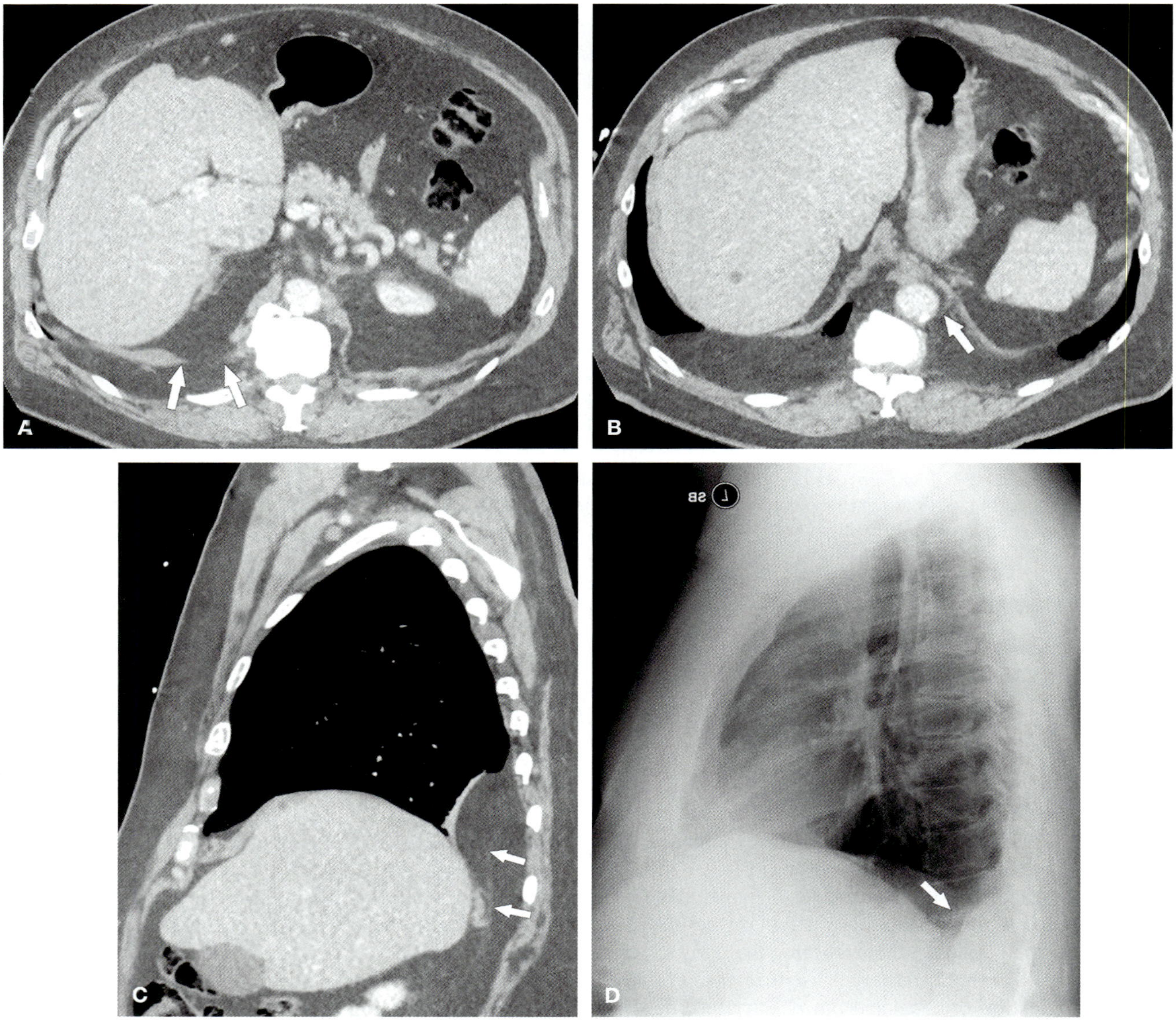

Figure 27.27. Bilateral Bochdalek hernia with herniated fat in pleural space. **A:** CT shows defect (*arrows*) in posteromedial right hemidiaphragm with herniated fat posterior to it. **B:** CT at higher level shows the small medial defect in the posteromedial left hemidiaphragm with small vessel (*arrow*) passing through the defect into the herniated fat. **C:** Sagittal CT shows the herniated fat in the right pleural space with vessel (*arrows*) extending into it from the abdomen. **D:** On lateral radiograph, the extruded fat (*arrow*) mimics bilateral posterior pleural effusion.

One consequence of rupture or hernia of the left hemidiaphragm is splenosis, in which fragments of splenic tissue enter the thorax and grow into one or more splenules along pleural surfaces.

Table 27.5 summarizes the findings in diaphragmatic hernia.

CYSTS AND NEOPLASMS OF THE DIAPHRAGM

Cysts

Both bronchogenic and mesothelial cysts can involve the diaphragm. Mesothelial cysts are easier to explain, given the proximity of the diaphragm to pleural and peritoneal mesothelium. Bronchogenic cysts arise through abnormal budding of the ventral foregut. Most develop in the mediastinum or lung. Ectopic sites such as the diaphragm are rare.

Bronchogenic cyst of the diaphragm (Fig. 27.36) resembles tumor, but may show lower attenuation than soft tissue and it does not enhance with contrast injection; calcifications may be present. More than two-thirds are on the left.

Tumors

Primary tumors of the diaphragm are rare. The most common primary benign tumor is lipoma. The most common primary malignancies are rhabdomyosarcoma and fibrosarcoma.

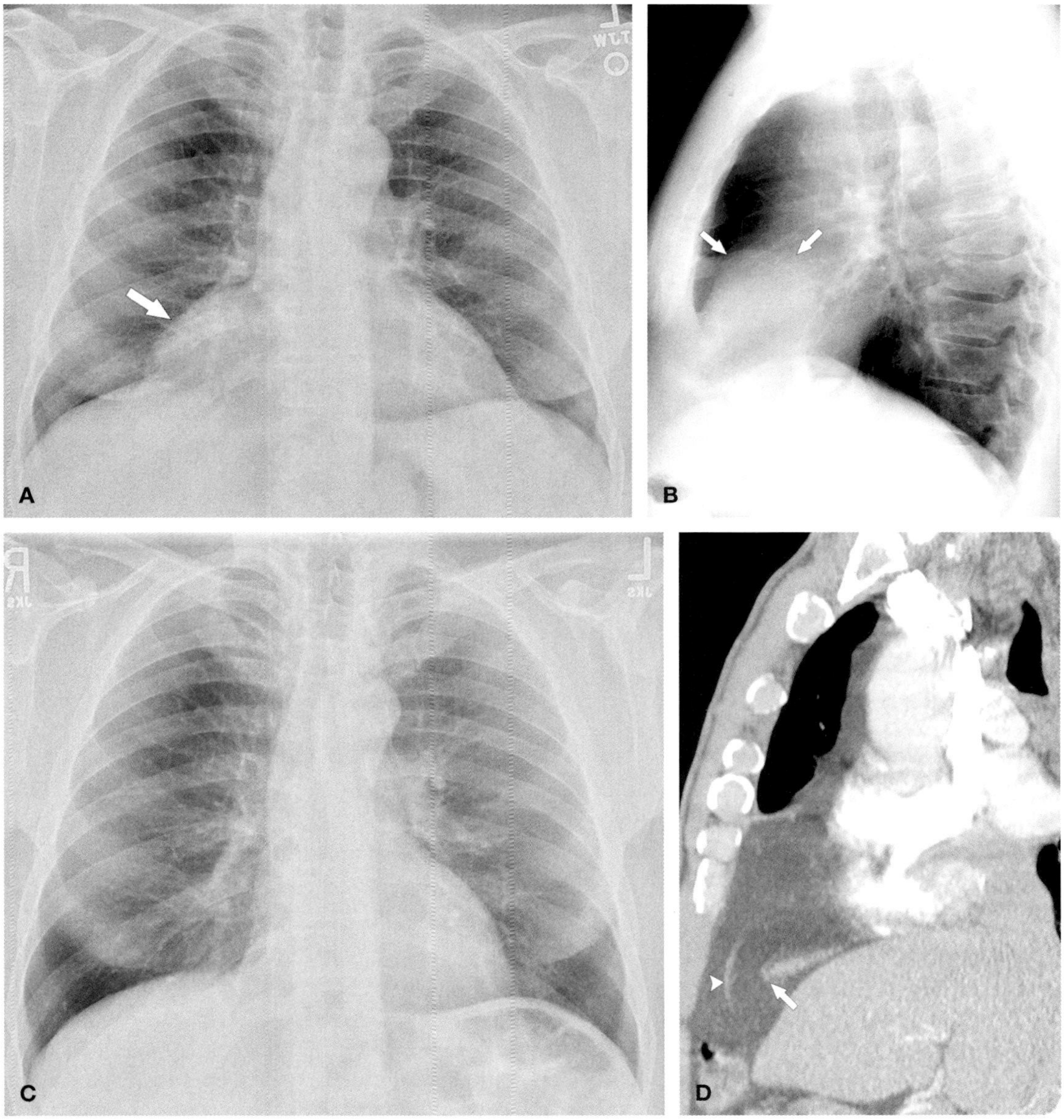

Figure 27.28. Development of small Morgagni hernia. **A:** PA and **B:** lateral radiographs show convexity (*arrows*) in the right anterior cardiophrenic angle that was not present 3 y before **(C)**. **D:** Sagittal CT shows the edge of the defect (*arrow*) with omental fat and blood vessel (*arrowhead*) extending into the anterior mediastinum.

Chest or abdominal pain is the most common clinical manifestation of diaphragmatic tumor. Other possible symptoms are shortness of breath, discomfort, or hiccups.

On CT, lipoma (Fig. 27.37) appears as a well-defined mass with fat attenuation, often in one of the crura. Other diaphragmatic tumors manifest as smooth or lobulated masses with soft-tissue attenuation, sometimes accompanied by pleural effusion.

Secondary tumors are more common than primary tumors. Tumor can involve the diaphragm by hematogenous metastasis or by direct extension from the thorax (eg, mesothelioma) or abdomen (eg, ovarian cancer or hepatocellular carcinoma).

Pleural mesothelioma can infiltrate the hemidiaphragm and extend into the subdiaphragmatic fat and liver (Figs. 27.38 and 27.39). Ovarian cancer can invade the diaphragm from peritoneal implants (Fig. 27.40).

Benign tumors of the diaphragm are usually treated only if symptomatic. Management of malignant tumors depends on the tumor type and treatment options.

Therapy of pleural mesothelioma may involve pleurectomy, or even extrapleural pneumonectomy, in which the lung is removed along with visceral and parietal pleura, hemidiaphragm, and some of the pericardium.

The resected diaphragm is patched with a synthetic membrane, such as polytetrafluorethylene (Gore-Tex, Inc., Flagstaff, AZ). This multilayered membrane traps air and is initially visible as a lucent band on radiographs taken soon after surgery (Fig. 27.41). The lucency fades away in about

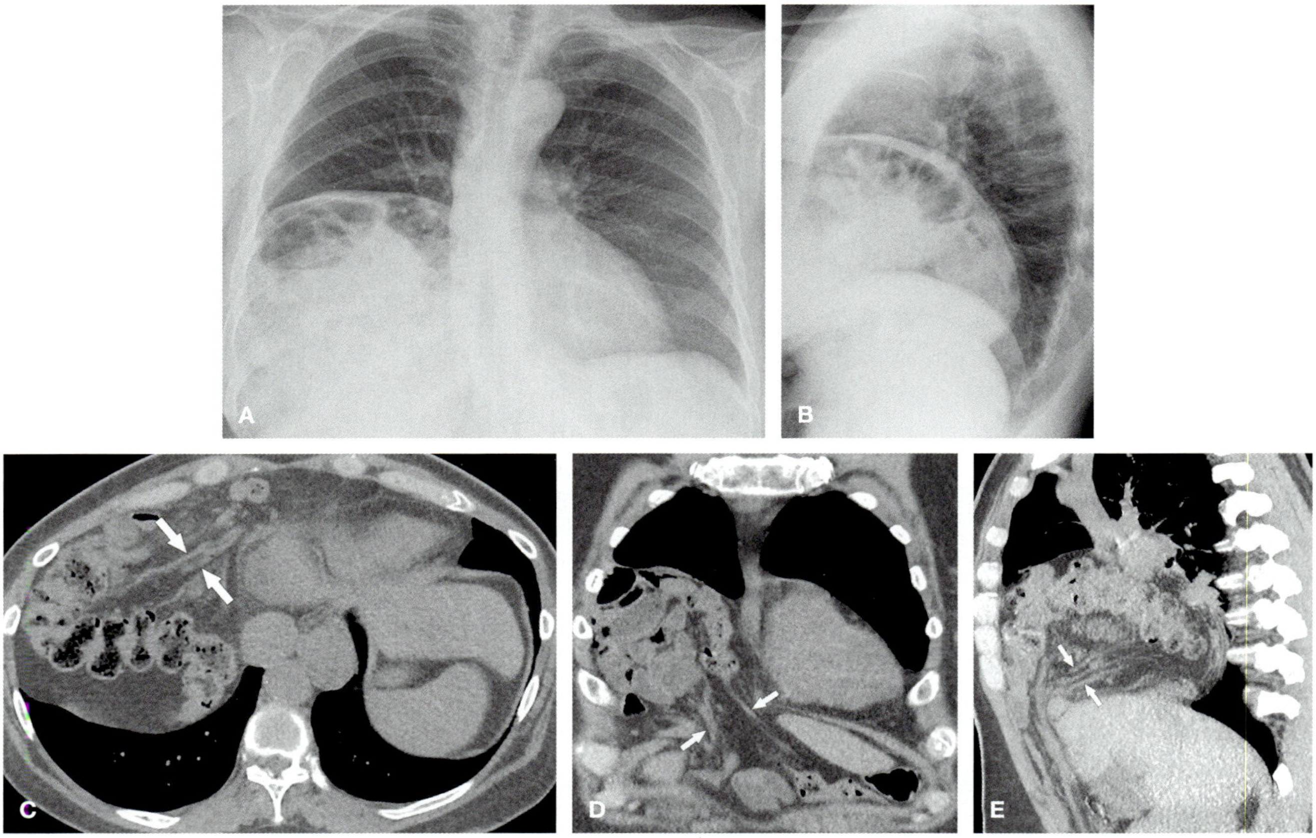

Figure 27.29. Large Morgagni hernia. **A:** PA and **B:** lateral radiographs show colonic gas in large anterior hernia. **C:** Transaxial, **D:** coronal, and **E:** sagittal CT images show vessels (*arrows*) radiating through the anterior diaphragmatic defect, with the colon, small bowel, and omental fat in the hernia.

1 week, after which the prosthesis appears on CT scans as a high-attenuation membrane (Fig. 27.42).

ACKNOWLEDGMENTS

Tess J. Moon, PhD, Professor of Mechanical Engineering (retired), sketched a simple model that clarified the function of the fiber bands in the central tendon of the diaphragm. The University of Washington radiology technologists have brought great skill to performing sniff tests; in particular, Patricia Kieper, RT, has assisted with hundreds of cases, always kept the patient comfortable, solved technical problem on the fly, and trained many coworkers in the art. Medical illustrator Kate Sweeney has again provided illuminating drawings of the diaphragm.

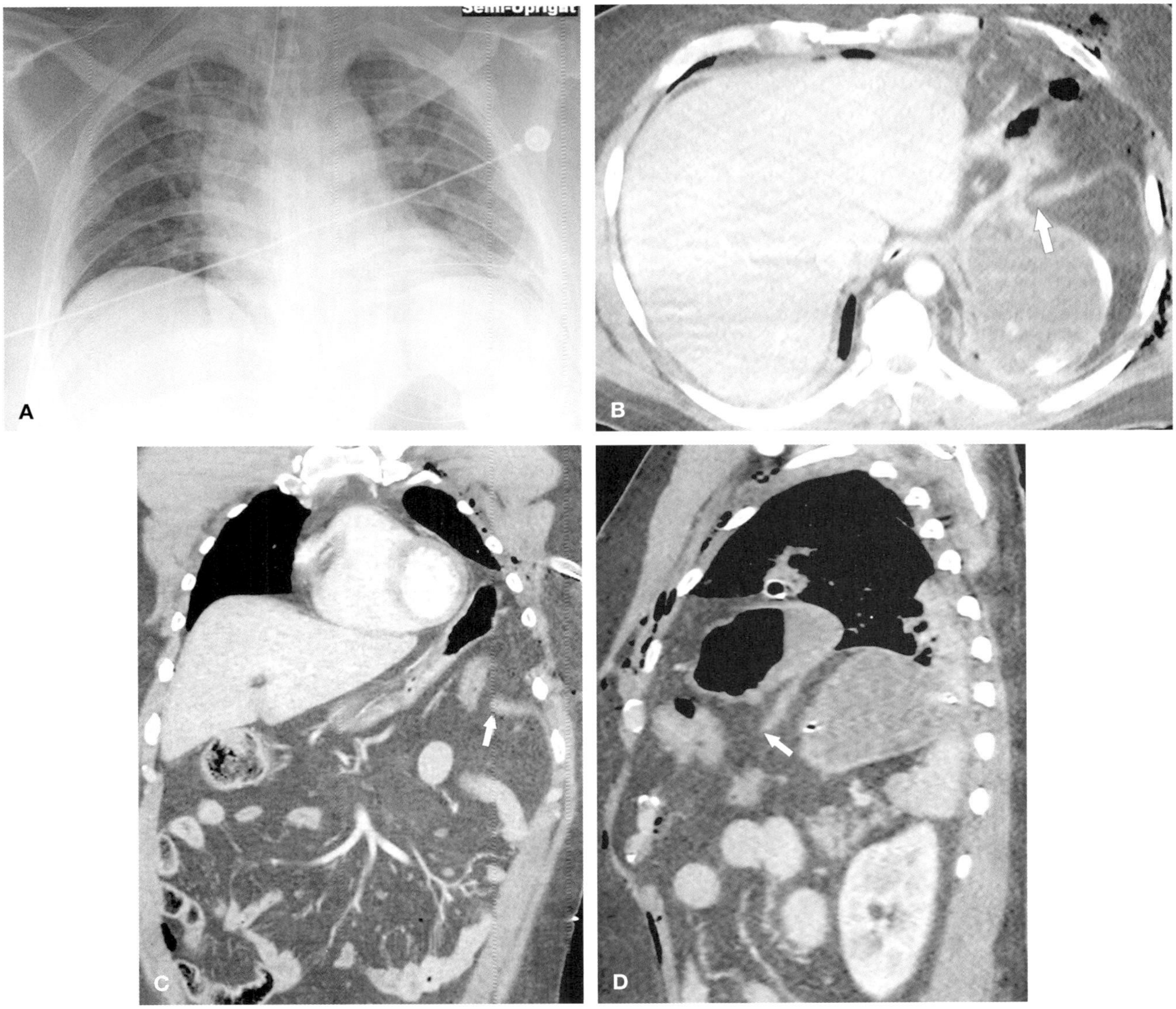

Figure 27.30. Acute rupture (13-cm laceration) of anterior left hemidiaphragm from motor vehicle crash. **A:** Chest radiograph shows apparently normal contour of left hemidiaphragm; the enteric tube in the stomach does not extend above it. **B:** CT shows edge of anterior defect (*arrow*) with narrowing of the segment of stomach extending anteriorly through it, the *collar sign*. **C:** Coronal and **D:** sagittal CT images show the edge of the defect (*arrows*) with the stomach, intestine, and vessels streaming into the anterior chest.

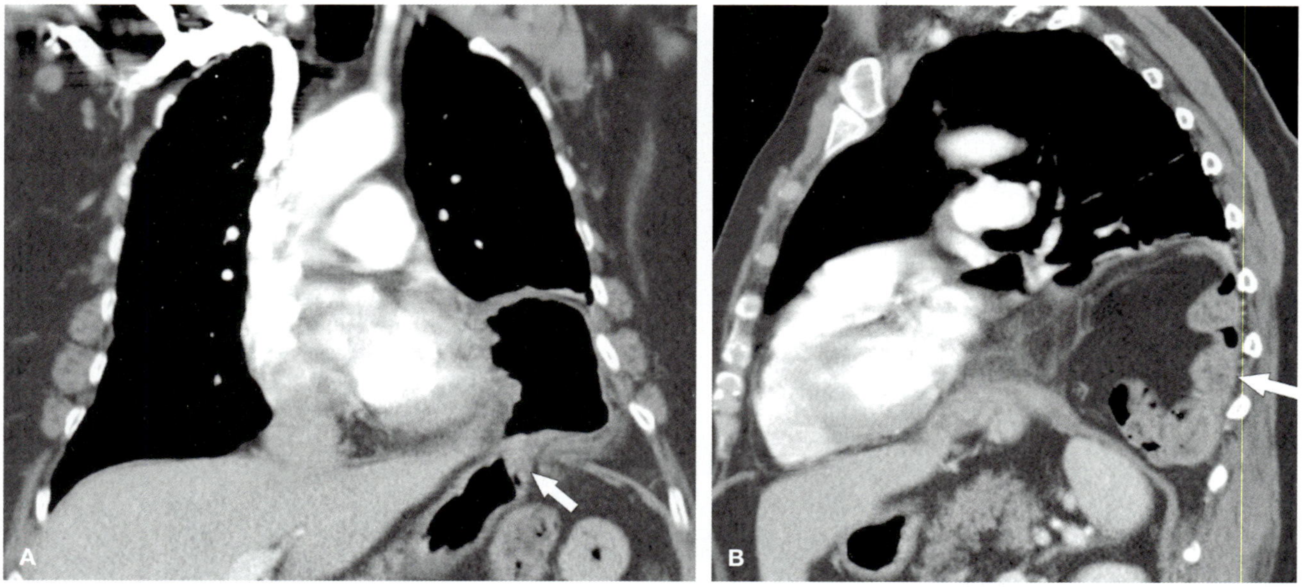

Figure 27.31. Traumatic rupture of left hemidiaphragm. **A:** Coronal CT shows narrowing of the stomach (*arrow*) as it passes through and bulges above the defect in the left hemidiaphragm, the *collar sign*. **B:** Sagittal CT shows herniated colon (*arrow*) lying along the posterior left chest wall, the *dependent viscera sign*.

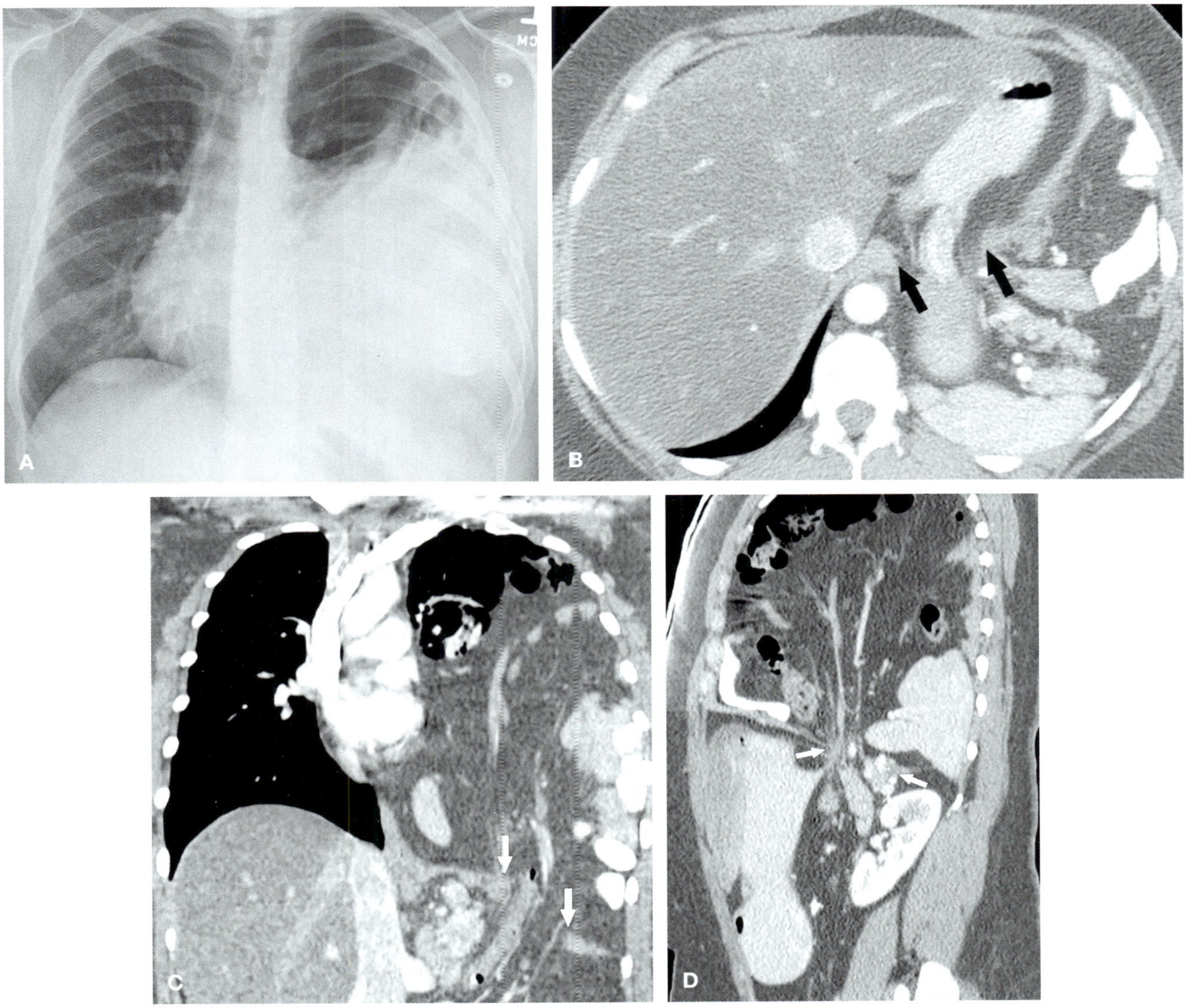

Figure 27.32. Delayed presentation of rupture of left hemidiaphragm from remote childhood trauma in 29-year-old woman. **A:** PA radiograph shows extensive herniation of abdominal contents, including colon, into left hemithorax. **B:** CT shows the edges of the defect (*arrows*) with narrowing of the portion of the stomach passing through (the *collar sign*). **C:** Coronal and **D:** sagittal CT images show the edges of the defect (*arrows*), which is slightly posterior to the midline.

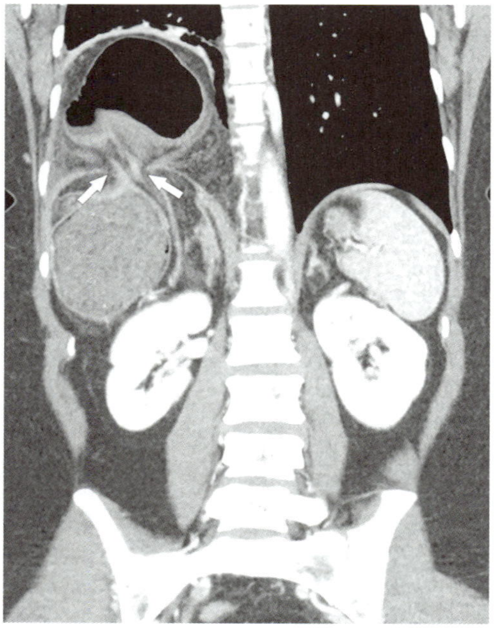

Figure 27.33. Iatrogenic hernia of right hemidiaphragm after partial hepatectomy for liver donation. Coronal CT shows colon and mesenteric fat extending through the defect (*arrows*) with collar sign and distension and fat stranding above. In a second operation, the hernia was reduced and the diaphragmatic defect was repaired.

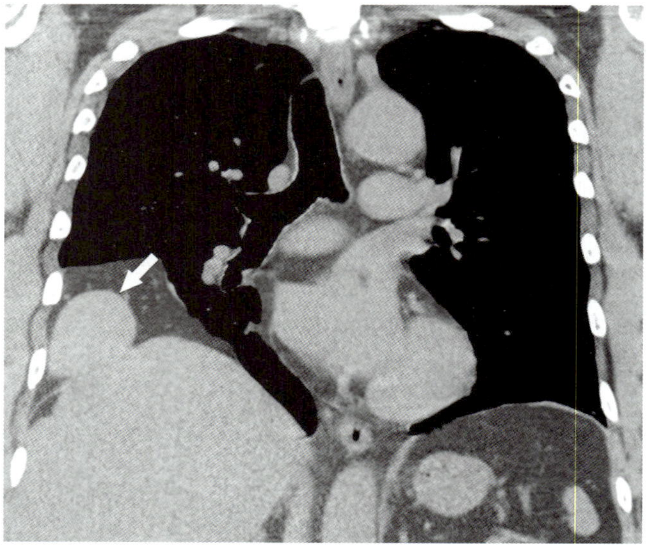

Figure 27.34. Iatrogenic hernia caused by injury to the diaphragm during radiofrequency ablation of hepatocellular carcinoma. Herniated liver (*arrow*) and omental fat bulge through the defect in the right hemidiaphragm.

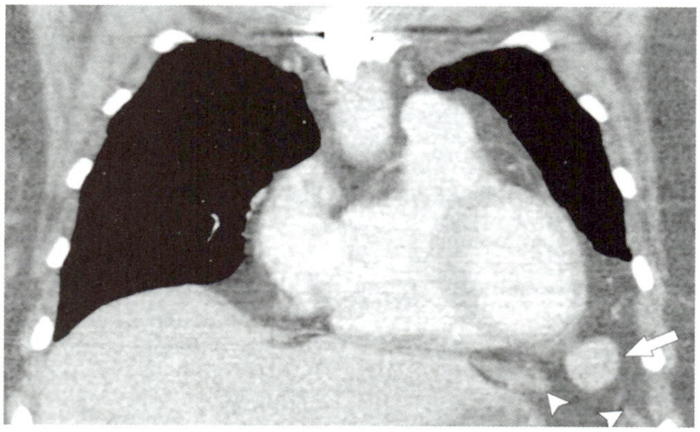

Figure 27.35. Iatrogenic hernia of the left hemidiaphragm from removal of left ventricular assist device from the upper abdomen. A splenule (*arrow*) is surrounded by herniated omental fat just above the defect (*arrowheads*) in the left hemidiaphragm near the cardiac apex.

Table 27.5 Diaphragmatic Hernias

Hernia Type	Clinical	Imaging Findings
Hiatal	Prevalence increases with age Usually asymptomatic Type I: sliding (most common) Type II: pure paraesophageal (rare) Type III: both gastroesophageal junction and gastric fundus herniated (common) Type IV: additional viscus herniated	Retrocardiac mediastinal mass, air bubbles or fluid levels Widened esophageal hiatus on CT Contents of hernia determine type
Bochdalek	**In infants:** Large Posterolateral Almost always on the left Causes respiratory distress and lung hypoplasia **In adults:** Usually small Often posteromedial Mild left predominance Lacks peritoneal sac Frequency increases with age Usually asymptomatic	Focal bulge or mass along the posterior hemidiaphragm Contains perinephric fat, kidney, or even stomach or bowel when large
Morgagni	Less common than hiatal or adult Bochdalek hernia Promoted by increased abdominal pressure from obesity, straining, etc. Herniation is always on the right, between costal and sternal attachments of the hemidiaphragm	Well-defined smooth convexity in the right anterior cardiophrenic angle on radiographs Bulge is more medial than that caused by eventration Usually contains just omental fat, but sometimes with colon or other viscus Colonic gas and stool may be visible on radiographs and CT
Traumatic	Found in 1%-8% of blunt trauma cases Most often posterolateral left hemidiaphragm Can also occur from penetrating trauma	Radiographic findings (insensitive) are: cephalad extension of gastric tube, herniation of stomach/bowel, irregularity or elevation of hemidiaphragm, contralateral shift of mediastinum, collar or hourglass sign of stomach or colon CT findings are: discontinuity of diaphragm, absent diaphragm sign, herniated abdominal contents, collar sign, dependent viscera sign Splenosis may result from left hemidiaphragmatic hernia
Iatrogenic	Can result from surgical or other medical procedure, such as ablation of liver tumor	Radiographs and CT show herniated fat, liver, or other viscus Splenosis may occur

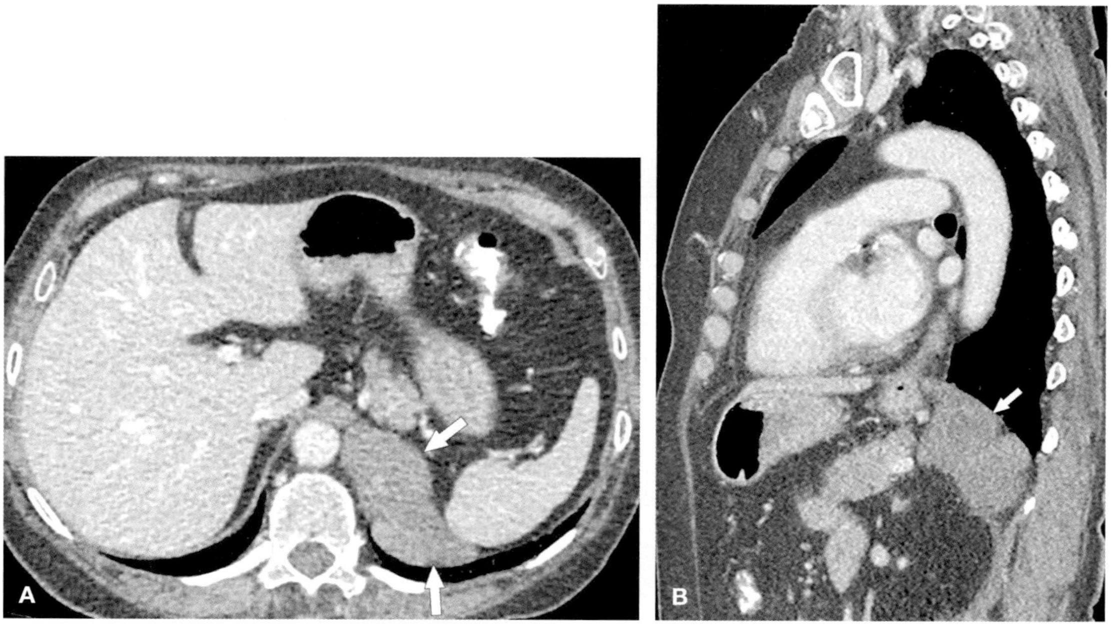

Figure 27.36. Intradiaphragmatic bronchogenic cyst. **A:** Transaxial and **B:** sagittal CT images show a bronchogenic cyst (*arrows*) in the left crus and posteromedial left hemidiaphragm. (Courtesy of Marco Mestas Nuñez, MD.)

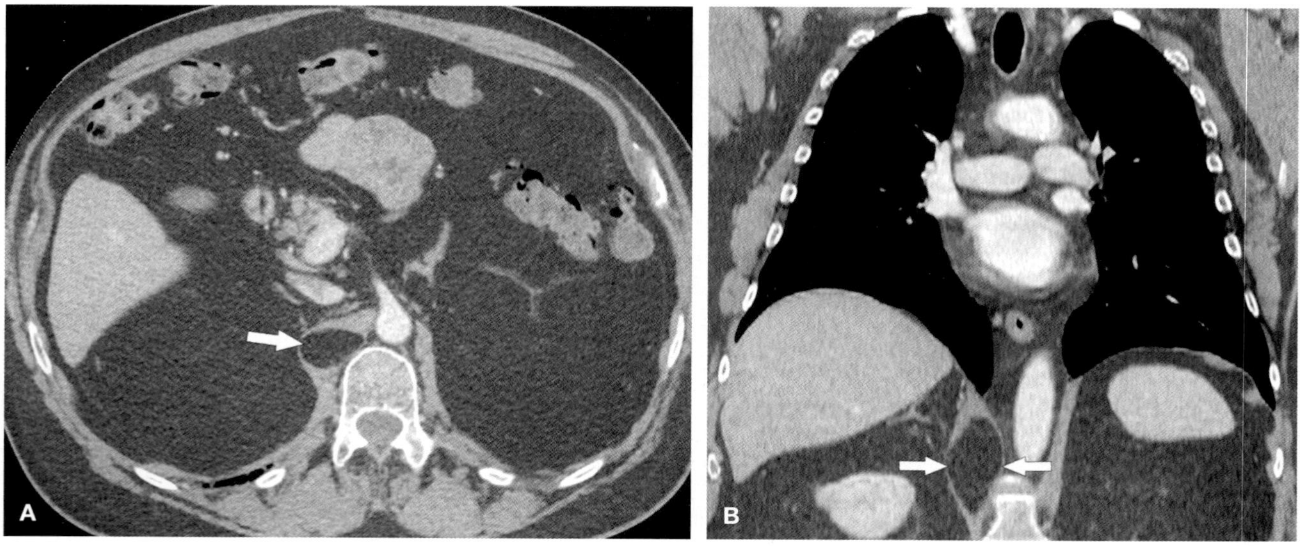

Figure 27.37. Lipoma. **A:** Transaxial and **B:** coronal CT images show a lipoma (*arrows*) in the crus of the right hemidiaphragm with elongation in the vertical axis.

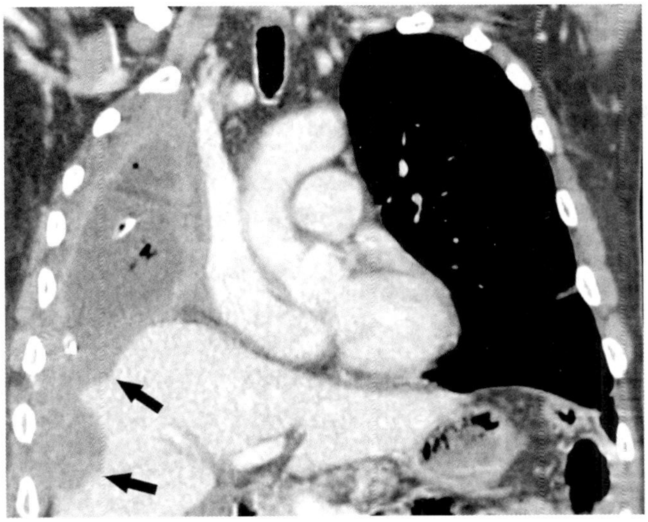

Figure 27.38. Pleural mesothelioma invading the right hemidiaphragm and the liver. Coronal CT shows pleural mesothelioma extending across the hemidiaphragm into the liver (*arrows*).

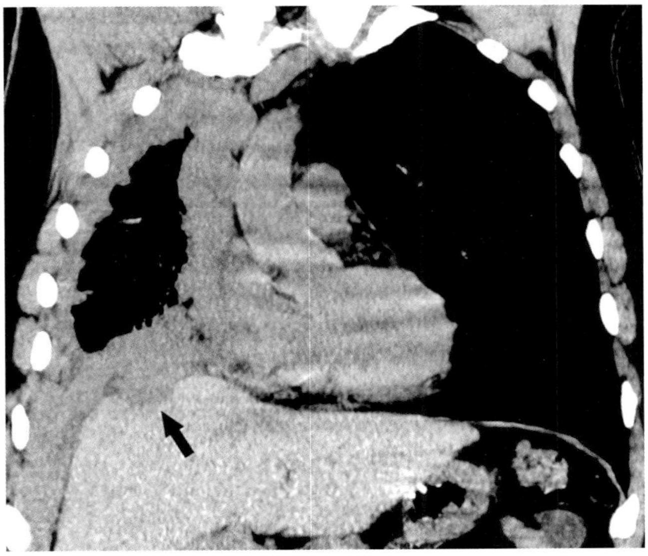

Figure 27.39. Pleural mesothelioma invading right hemidiaphragm and liver. Coronal CT shows thick rind of pleural tumor with infiltration through right hemidiaphragm and subdiaphragmatic fat into liver (*arrow*).

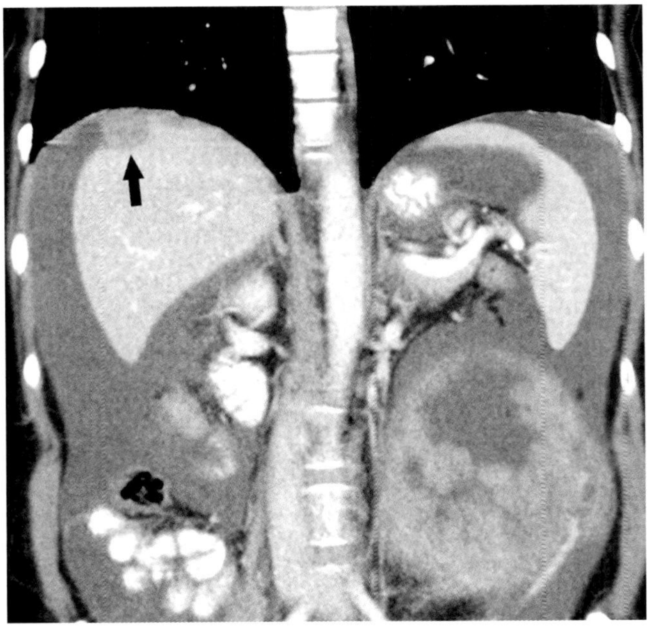

Figure 27.40. Metastatic ovarian cancer adherent to right hemidiaphragm and liver. Coronal CT shows malignant ascites, multiple abdominal masses, and peritoneal metastasis (*arrow*) involving the liver and undersurface of the right hemidiaphragm. A portion of the right hemidiaphragm was resected.

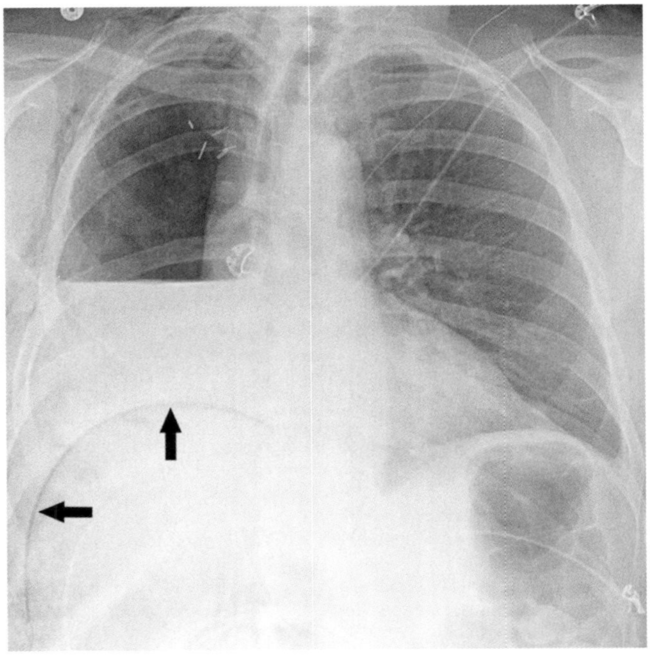

Figure 27.41. Gore-Tex diaphragm prosthesis. The right hemidiaphragm was resected as part of extrapleural pneumonectomy for treatment of mesothelioma. Radiograph a few days after surgery shows curved lucency (*arrows*) caused by air trapped in the Gore-Tex prosthesis. The lucency usually fades within a week of surgery.

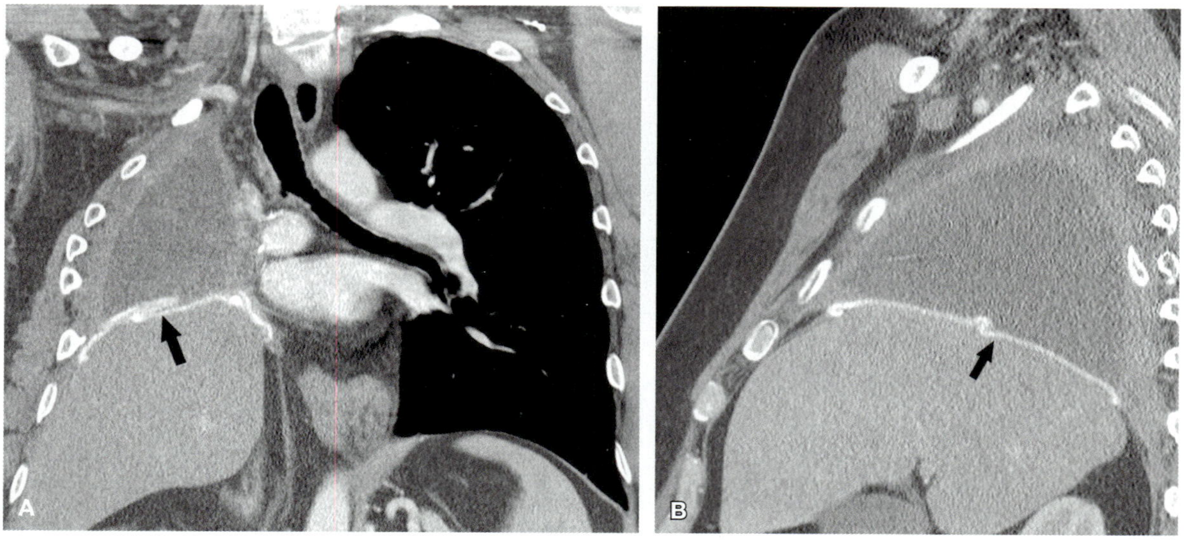

Figure 27.42. Gore-Tex diaphragm prosthesis (different patient from Figure 27.41). **A:** Coronal and **B:** sagittal CT images a few months after extrapleural pneumonectomy for treatment of mesothelioma show the prosthesis (*arrows*) that has replaced the right hemidiaphragm.

SUGGESTED READINGS

Abbara S, Kalan MMH, Lewicki AM. Intrathoracic stomach revisited. *AJR Am J Roentgenol.* 2003;181(2):403-414.

Caskey C, Zerhouni E, Fishman E, Rahmouni A. Aging of the diaphragm: a CT study. *Radiology.* 1989;171(2):385-389.

Celli BR. Respiratory management of diaphragm paralysis. *Semin Respir Crit Care Med.* 2002;23(3):275-281.

Chaturvedi A, Rajiah P, Croake A, Saboo S, Chaturvedi A. Imaging of thoracic hernias: types and complications. *Insights Imaging.* 2018;9(6):989-1005.

Chen IY, Armstrong JD II. Value of fluoroscopy in patients with suspected bilateral hemidiaphragmatic paralysis. *AJR Am J Roentgenol.* 1993;160(1):29-31.

Desir A, Ghaye B. CT of blunt diaphragmatic rupture. *Radiographics.* 2012;32(2):477-498.

Du Plessis M, Ramai D, Shah S, Holland JD, Tubbs RS, Loukas M. The clinical anatomy of the musculotendinous part of the diaphragm. *Surg Radiol Anat.* 2015;37(9):1013-1020.

Gale ME. Bochdalek hernia: prevalence and CT characteristics. *Radiology.* 1985;156(2):449-452.

Gelman R, Mirvis S, Gens D. Diaphragmatic rupture due to blunt trauma: sensitivity of plain chest radiographs. *AJR Am J Roentgenol.* 1991;156(1):51-57.

Groth SS, Rueth NM, Kast T, et al. Laparoscopic diaphragmatic plication for diaphragmatic paralysis and eventration: an objective evaluation of short-term and midterm results. *J Thorac Cardiovasc Surg.* 2010;139(6):1452-1456.

Hoffman RJ, Garner HW, Rojas CA, et al. Atypical causes of dyspnea: a review of neuromuscular and chest wall disorders that compromise ventilation. *J Thorac Imaging.* 2022;37(4):W45-W55.

Kim MP, Hofstetter WL. Tumors of the diaphragm. *Thorac Surg Clin.* 2009;19(4):521-529.

LaRosa DV Jr, Esham RH, Morgan SL, Wing SW. Diaphragmatic hernia of Morgagni. *South Med J.* 1999;92(4):409-411.

McCool FD, Mead J. Dyspnea on immersion: mechanisms in patients with bilateral diaphragm paralysis. *Am Rev Respir Dis.* 1989;139(1):275-276.

McCool FD, Tzelepis GE. Dysfunction of the diaphragm. *N Engl J Med.* 2012;366(10):932-942.

Murray JG, Caoili E, Gruden JF, Evans S, Halvorsen RA Jr, Mackersie RC. Acute rupture of the diaphragm due to blunt trauma: diagnostic sensitivity and specificity of CT. *AJR Am J Roentgenol.* 1996;166(5):1035-1039.

Nason LK, Walker CM, McNeeley MF, Burivong W, Fligner CL, Godwin JD. Imaging of the diaphragm: anatomy and function. *Radiographics.* 2012;32(2):E51-E70.

Nasr A, Fecteau A. Foramen of Morgagni hernia: presentation and treatment. *Thorac Surg Clin.* 2009;19(4):463-468.

Panda A, Kumar A, Gamanagatti S, Patil A, Kumar S, Gupta A. Traumatic diaphragmatic injury: a review of CT signs and the difference between blunt and penetrating injury. *Diagn Interv Radiol.* 2014;20(2):121-128.

Roberts HC. Imaging the diaphragm. *Thorac Surg Clin.* 2009;19(4):431-450.

Shackleton KL, Stewart ET, Taylor AJ. Traumatic diaphragmatic injuries: spectrum of radiographic findings. *Radiographics.* 1998;18(1):49-59.

Shah R, Sabanathan S, Mearns AJ, Choudhury AK. Traumatic rupture of diaphragm. *Ann Thorac Surg.* 1995;60(5):1444-1449.

Sprunt JM, Brown CV, Reifsnyder AC, Shestopalov AV, Ali S, Fielder WD. Computed tomography to diagnose blunt diaphragm injuries: not ready for prime time. *Am Surg.* 2014;80(11):1124-1127.

Standring J. *Respiratory diaphragm and phrenic nerves.* In: *Gray's Anatomy, 42nd Edition. The Anatomical Basis of Clinical Practice.* Elsevier; 2020:1038-1046.e2.

Sukkasem W, Moftah SG, Kicska G, Godwin JD, Pipavath S, Stern E. Crus atrophy: accuracy of computed tomography in diagnosis of diaphragmatic paralysis. *J Thorac Imaging.* 2017;32(6):383-390.

Tarver RD, Conces DJ Jr, Cory DA, Vix VA. Imaging the diaphragm and its disorders. *J Thorac Imag.* 1989;4(1):1-18.

Verhey PT, Gosselin MV, Primack SL, Kraemer AC. Differentiating diaphragmatic paralysis and eventration. *Acad Radiol.* 2007;14(4):420-425.

Section Seven

Great Arteries

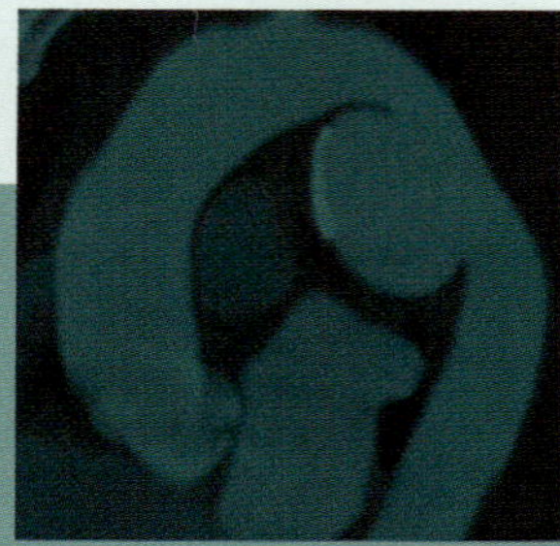

Chapter 28

Clinton E. Jokerst • Michael B. Gotway

Pulmonary Thromboembolic Disease

INTRODUCTION

Deep venous thrombosis (DVT) and pulmonary embolism (PE) represent different ends of the spectrum of a single disease—venous thromboembolism (VTE). VTE is a common problem, affecting between 300,000 and 600,000 people in the United States each year, yet there are many approaches for establishing the diagnosis, and numerous methods for the investigation of VTE may be employed. Familiarity with risk factors for VTE, the clinical presentations of VTE, laboratory evaluation of VTE, and the imaging evaluation of suspected VTE is extremely important for all physicians, particularly radiologists.

CHEST RADIOGRAPHY

Chest radiographic findings of PE have been extensively studied. Although chest radiographs in patients with PE may be completely normal, some abnormality usually is present. Among the patients in the original Prospective Investigation of Pulmonary Embolism Diagnosis I (PIOPED I) study who did not have prior cardiopulmonary disease, chest radiographs were abnormal in 84% of patients with proven PE and 66% of those without PE. However, radiographic abnormalities in the setting of PE generally are nonspecific and transient and do not allow a specific diagnosis of PE. In the proper clinical setting, certain radiographic findings or combinations of findings may suggest the diagnosis of PE and thus serve to direct further imaging to either establish or exclude this diagnosis. However, most commonly, chest radiographs are employed to detect non-VTE causes for clinical situations suggesting PE.

Pulmonary Vascular Abnormalities

Focal peripheral lucency beyond an occluded vessel, often accompanied by mild dilation of the central pulmonary vessels, known as *Westermark sign* (Fig. 28.1), is a very nonspecific finding seen in only 7% to 14% of cases of documented PE in the PIOPED I study. Westermark sign is thought to be caused by embolic obstruction of the pulmonary artery or hypoxic vasoconstriction secondary to ventilation of poorly perfused lung. This sign often is a subtle finding, in many cases not recognized prospectively, and can be mimicked by other common lung diseases, such as emphysema.

Enlargement of the central pulmonary vasculature also may occur with PE and also is frequently subtle and easily overlooked. This finding may be the result of distention of the vessel by thrombus or by acute rise in pulmonary arterial pressure secondary to the presence of distal emboli. Enlargement of the right descending pulmonary artery, occasionally with a "sausage-like" configuration, may be seen in a number of patients with acute PE, and the size and shape of the artery may normalize following resolution of the embolic event. Enlargement of the right descending pulmonary artery is not specific to PE and may result from pulmonary hypertension of any cause.

Pulmonary edema rarely may occur in association with PE. This finding most often is seen in patients with underlying cardiopulmonary disease and may be caused by left ventricular (LV) failure precipitated by PE.

Focal Parenchymal Opacities

Focal parenchymal abnormalities, particularly atelectasis, were the most common chest radiographic abnormalities in patients with PE in the PIOPED I series, occurring in just over two-thirds of the patients. Linear opacities often occur near the lung bases and are thought to represent areas of subsegmental atelectasis related to mucous plugging, to hypoventilation, or, perhaps, to distal airway closure or focal depletion of surfactant. Such opacities commonly are transient; if they persist, they may represent areas of scarring secondary to prior infarction.

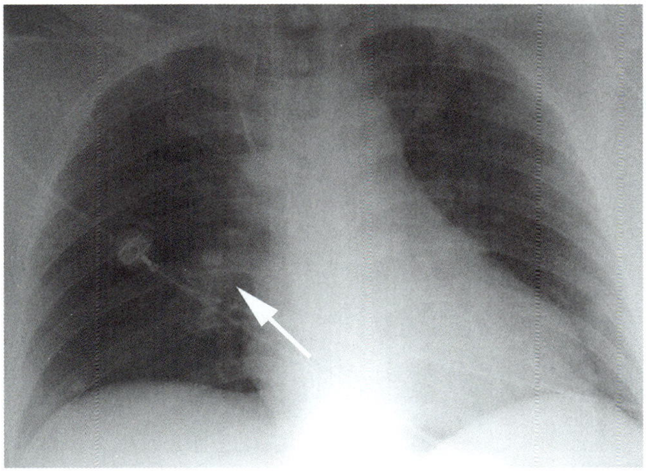

Figure 28.1. Westermark sign. Frontal chest radiograph from a 55-year-old woman with acute onset of shortness of breath following surgery shows increased lucency throughout the right lung with enlargement of the right interlobar pulmonary artery (*arrow*). Acute venous thromboembolism was diagnosed at CT shortly after the chest radiograph was obtained.

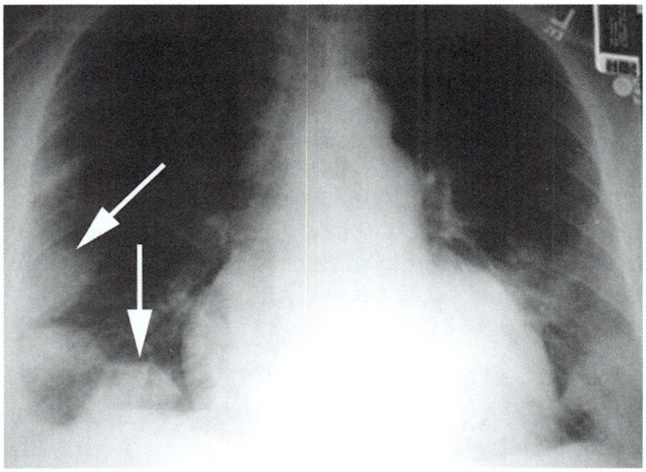

Figure 28.2. Pulmonary infarction. Frontal chest radiograph from a 36-year-old man with abrupt onset of shortness of breath and hemoptysis shows several wedge-shaped, subpleural opacities in the lower lobes bilaterally (*arrows*), representing pulmonary infarction. Note that the rounded and truncated medial borders of the opacities face toward the pulmonary hila. Pulmonary embolism was proven at CT.

Focal air-space consolidation may occur in patients with PE and may represent pulmonary hemorrhage without infarction or true pulmonary infarction with ischemic necrosis of lung tissue. Estimates of the frequency of pulmonary infarction in patients with PE vary from 10% to 60%. Infarction is most likely to occur when diminished cardiopulmonary reserve is present because both the pulmonary and bronchial arterial systems are impaired. Infarcts often are multiple and occur most frequently in the subpleural regions of the lower lobes, usually within 12 to 24 hours of the onset of symptoms. Infarcts are variable in size and often do not show an air bronchogram, a finding that may favor the diagnosis of infarction over pneumonia. Infarcts typically are ill defined but may progress over several days to a discrete focal opacity. The classic description of a pulmonary infarct, the "Hampton hump," is a circumscribed, subpleural opacity with a rounded or truncated convex medial border facing toward the pulmonary hilum (Fig. 28.2). This finding is neither common nor specific, however.

Cavitation within a bland (uninfected) infarct is uncommon. Bland infarct cavitation is more likely when the infarct is larger than 4 cm in diameter. When cavitation occurs, it usually is apparent within 2 weeks of the appearance of the air-space opacity.

When air-space opacities are secondary to pulmonary hemorrhage without infarction, resolution of the abnormality usually is rapid; however, true infarction with ischemic tissue necrosis usually takes weeks or months to resolve, leaving linear scars or occasionally associated with pleural thickening. Resolution of pulmonary infarction has been likened to the "melting of an ice cube," implying that an infarct clears by peripheral dissolution, whereas pneumonia will gradually clear in an irregular, patchy fashion.

Pleural Effusion and Diaphragmatic Abnormalities

Pleural effusion is detected on chest radiography in about half of patients with PE and usually is unilateral and small. When pulmonary infarction occurs, pleural effusions may be larger and hemorrhagic and may take longer to resolve. Diaphragmatic elevation is common in patients with PE, but this finding is nonspecific.

Chest Radiography for the Diagnosis of PE

Chest radiographic abnormalities in patients with PE usually are nonspecific and neither establish nor exclude the diagnosis of PE. The sensitivity and specificity of chest radiography for the diagnosis of PE are only 33% and 59%, respectively. The main value of chest radiographs is for the detection of diagnoses that may clinically simulate PE, such as pneumothorax, pulmonary edema, pneumonia, or rib fractures. In addition, a recent chest radiograph is required for the interpretation of ventilation-perfusion ($\dot{V}/\dot{Q}$) scintigraphy.

LOWER EXTREMITY VENOUS ULTRASOUND

The primary source of PE is thrombosis within the deep venous system of the lower extremities; about 90% of PEs originate from lower extremity DVT. Less common sources of pulmonary emboli include the deep veins of the pelvis, the renal veins, and the veins of the upper extremities. PE arising from DVT in these less common sites often occurs in a suggestive clinical context, whereas up to 50% of lower extremity DVT episodes may be clinically silent. Additionally, DVT often is asymptomatic, even in the presence of clinical evidence of PE. Because the clinical examination is unreliable for the detection of DVT, and the morbidity and mortality related to undiagnosed VTE are significant, much effort has been directed toward the development of accurate methods for DVT detection. DVT detection now largely relies on combinations of D-dimer assays, indirect CT venography (CTV), contrast-enhanced magnetic resonance venography (MRV), and lower extremity ultrasound (US). Owing to its noninvasive nature, availability, ease of performance, and accuracy, lower extremity ultrasonography is in widespread use as the initial diagnostic study in the evaluation of suspected DVT.

Technique

US techniques used in the evaluation of DVT variously include real-time grayscale imaging (with and without compression), continuous-wave and pulsed Doppler, color Doppler imaging, and ancillary techniques, such as the Valsalva maneuver and manual blood flow augmentation. A high-frequency linear array transducer is preferred to provide optimal spatial resolution, but can be supplemented with curved array transducers and harmonic imaging techniques. For larger patients, a lower-frequency transducer may be required to provide adequate tissue penetration to visualize the deep venous system of the lower extremity successfully. The complete lower extremity US examination includes imaging of the lower extremity veins in both longitudinal and transverse planes, utilizing gentle transducer compression at 1 to 2 cm intervals, from the level of the inguinal ligament to the popliteal trifurcation, including the common femoral vein, the superficial femoral vein, the popliteal vein, and the saphenous vein at its junction with the common femoral vein, and extending to the ankle to visualize the posterior tibial and peroneal veins. The complete lower extremity US examination is supplemented with color and spectral Doppler waveform analysis in the common femoral (or iliac) veins bilaterally (to evaluate for symmetry) and popliteal spectral Doppler assessment on the symptomatic side. Additional directed imaging may be employed for symptomatic regions if symptoms cannot be explained by the complete inguinal-to-ankle examination. Abbreviated lower extremity US examinations may be employed in certain circumstances, but are not recommended because limited examinations require a follow-up study in 5 days to safely exclude DVT. Veins appear as tubular, anechoic structures. Although thrombosis occasionally may be seen with grayscale sonography (Fig. 28.3), real-time imaging alone is not sufficient to exclude DVT, because thrombus may have variable echogenicity and often is anechoic, especially when acute; therefore, compression ultrasonography has become the most reliable maneuver to assess for DVT (Fig. 28.4).

The lower extremity venous US examination may be supplemented with a Valsalva maneuver. In response to a Valsalva maneuver, a normal vein dilates to more than 50% of its original diameter as a result of impaired venous drainage upstream from the area sampled, whereas veins with acute thrombus have pathologic changes in their walls that prevent such dilation. Lack of appropriate response to a Valsalva maneuver also may indicate thrombosis or obstruction of more central veins outside the field of view, such as the inferior vena cava (IVC). The Valsalva maneuver requires adequate patient cooperation and generally is limited to assessment of the common femoral vein, which is sufficiently large to demonstrate the caliber changes induced by the altered blood volume caused by the maneuver. Although an abnormal venous response to the Valsalva maneuver supports the diagnosis of DVT when there is a lack of venous compressibility, and a normal response may corroborate the findings of a normal compression US examination, normal or abnormal Valsalva maneuvers alone are not sufficiently sensitive or specific to establish or exclude the diagnosis of DVT.

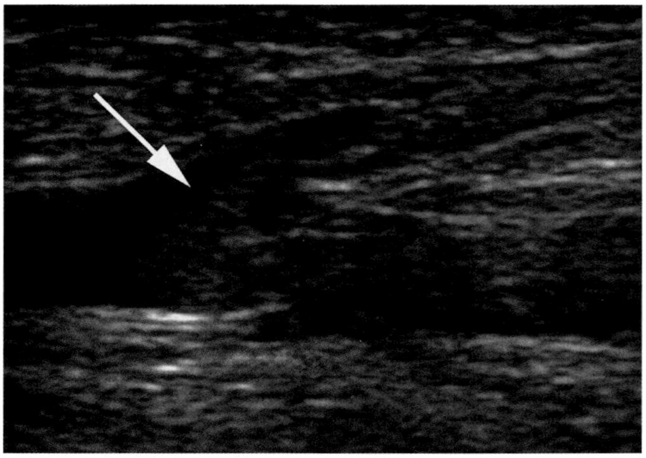

Figure 28.3. Gray-scale ultrasound demonstration of deep venous thrombosis (DVT). Longitudinal image of the common femoral vein at its juncture with the superficial saphenous vein shows echogenic material filling the common femoral vein (*arrow*), consistent with DVT.

Spectral Doppler analysis is particularly useful for vessels that cannot be visualized directly (such as the medial portions of the subclavian veins, the central IVC, the superior vena cava [SVC], and brachiocephalic veins). The spectral Doppler waveform of patent central vessels normally shows respiratory phasicity. A monophasic waveform suggests venous obstruction remote from the point of venous interrogation. This abnormal waveform can indicate central DVT, although stenosis or extrinsic compression of the central veins may result in a similar waveform. The combined use of real-time grayscale and Doppler techniques during venous US analysis is often referred to as venous duplex ultrasound ("duplex US") and is the most commonly employed US exam to assess for extremity venous thrombosis.

For the lower extremity US examination, flow augmentation using spectral Doppler is performed by placing the Doppler gate on the examined vein in the longitudinal plane and manually compressing the calf. A normal response is a rapid rise and fall in blood flow velocity in

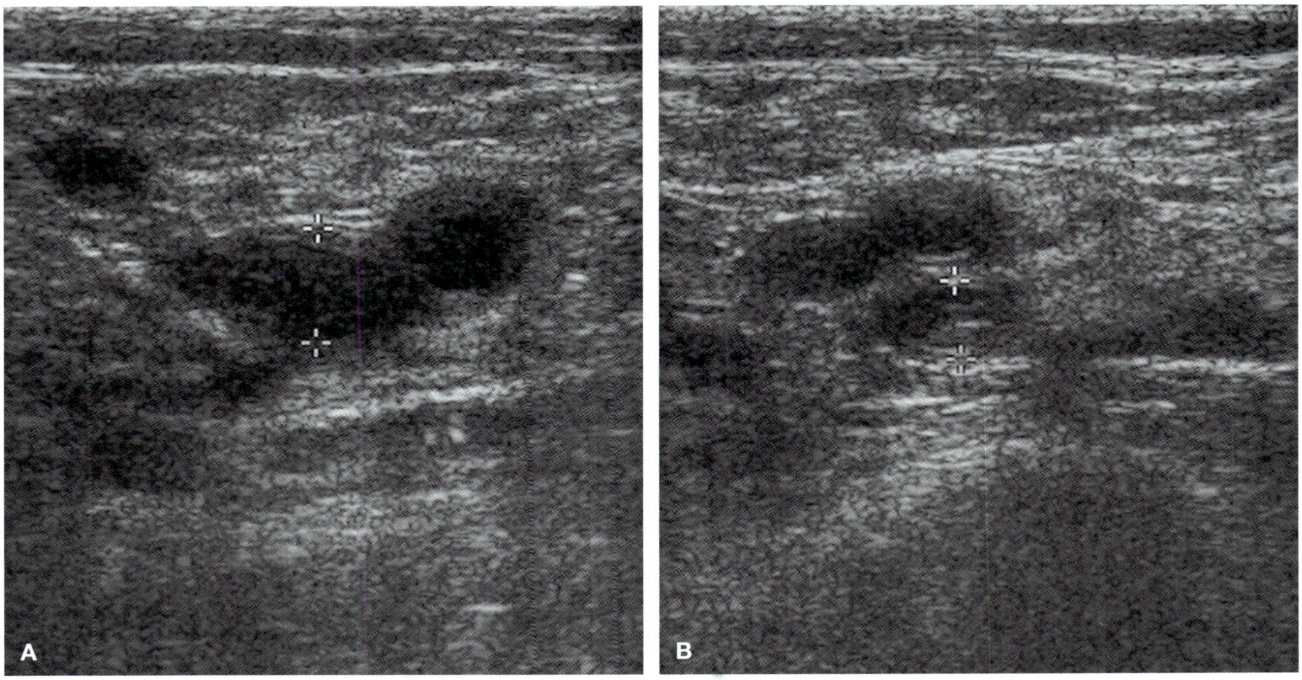

Figure 28.4. Deep venous thrombosis (DVT): compression ultrasonography. **A:** Transverse rest image shows the common femoral vein (indicated by calipers). **B:** Transverse compression image shows that the common femoral vein is not completely compressible (vein marked by calipers), consistent with DVT.

the interrogated vessel. Such a response implies that the venous system is patent between the point of interrogation and the area of manual compression. Lack of a normal response to flow augmentation may indicate nonocclusive thrombus, although this observation is not specific for this diagnosis.

In addition to being an integral part of the complete lower extremity US examination, color Doppler is valuable for identifying deep venous structures and interrogating deep vessels where the application of direct venous compression is difficult, such as the superficial femoral vein in the adductor hiatus and the iliac veins (Fig. 28.5). In patients who may be difficult to image, such as obese or postoperative patients, or those with swollen extremities, color Doppler imaging is a useful tool for identifying and interrogating venous anatomy. Venous thrombosis is shown on color Doppler imaging as absence of color flow within the vessel lumen (Fig. 28.6) at baseline and with augmentation. In patients with clinically suspected DVT and a technically adequate examination, color Doppler imaging demonstrates high sensitivity (95%) and specificity (98%) for the diagnosis of femoropopliteal DVT. However, for asymptomatic, high-risk patients (eg, patients who have recently undergone orthopedic surgery or trauma patients), the sensitivity of color Doppler imaging for the detection of femoropopliteal DVT is lower, perhaps due to the presence of short-segment or nonocclusive thrombus, a relatively high proportion of thrombi limited to the calf veins, or an overall decrease in prevalence of lower extremity DVT in settings where routine DVT prophylaxis is used.

Accuracy of Compression US

The complete lower extremity duplex US examination is a safe strategy for DVT assessment with only a 0.5% 3-month risk for thromboembolic events following a negative examination. Data on the accuracy of duplex US in asymptomatic, high-risk patient populations (eg, following orthopedic surgery) are conflicting, with some older series showing poor sensitivity for lower extremity US (including spectral and color Doppler techniques), but other studies showing better results. Conflicting data may be the result of differences in study design and study populations.

Calf Veins

The importance of diagnosing isolated calf vein thrombosis is controversial. Although many investigators postulate that clinically significant PE does not originate from calf veins, not all sources agree that calf vein thrombosis is self-limited. Older venographic studies have shown that 40% of untreated calf vein thrombi will remain below the knee, 40% will lyse, and 20% may extend into the femoropopliteal system. Once calf vein thrombi extend above the knee, 50% may be associated with abnormal V/Q scintigraphy, indicating possible PE. Many physicians do not treat calf vein thrombosis aggressively, but anticoagulation certainly is warranted for patients with proximal thrombi. Calf vein thrombosis can be demonstrated by detection of proximal DVT extension at serial femoropopliteal imaging with compression US or by direct examination of the calf veins. Outcome studies employing

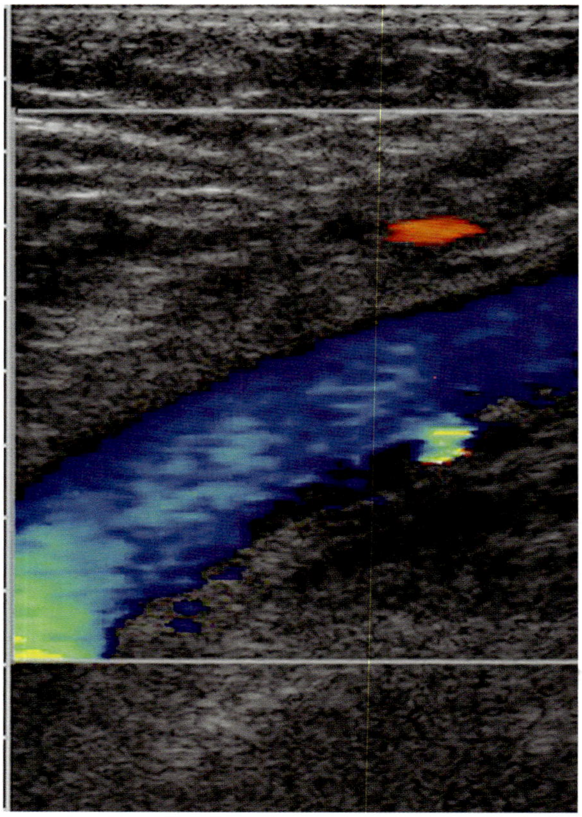

Figure 28.5. Normal venous color Doppler sonography. Longitudinal image of the external iliac vein shows normal color Doppler signal filling the vessel. Color Doppler is useful for the evaluation of venous segments that are not amenable to compression ultrasonography, such as the external iliac vein.

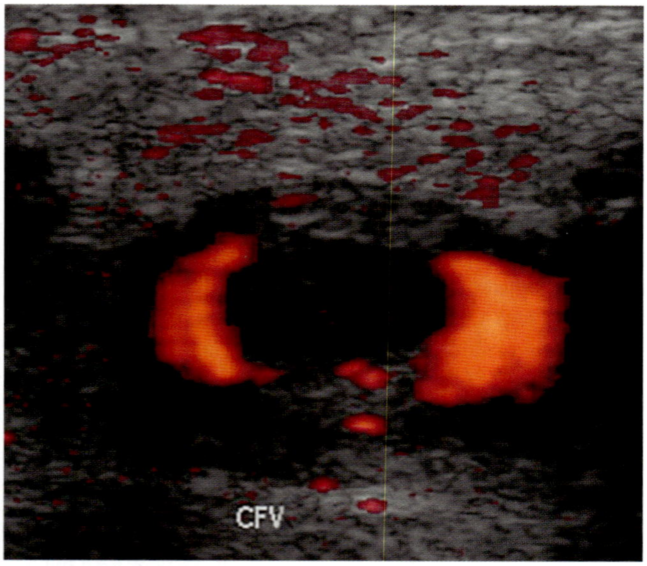

Figure 28.6. Color Doppler ultrasound demonstration of deep venous thrombosis (DVT). Transverse color Doppler image shows exclusion of color Doppler signal from the center of the vein, consistent with DVT.

compression US in symptomatic patients have shown that it is safe to withhold anticoagulation in patients with a negative initial compression US examination, provided that symptoms prompting the initial compression US examination do not persist. If lower extremity symptoms persist following the initial examination, a repeat sonogram should be obtained; a small number of patients with an initially negative examination but persistent symptoms will be found to have femoropopliteal DVT on the subsequent compression US exam, presumably reflecting proximal migration of previously undetected calf vein thrombosis. Patients with isolated calf vein DVT who do not undergo anticoagulation should have a repeat scan in 1 week, and again at 2 weeks if the DVT persists.

The sensitivity of compression US for calf vein DVT is only 56.8% and therefore negative US results do not exclude calf vein thrombosis. Again, color Doppler imaging is a useful adjunct to routine compression US in the evaluation of symptomatic patients with potential calf vein thrombosis. However, the value of duplex US for calf vein thrombosis for asymptomatic high-risk patients remains unestablished.

Upper Extremity Venous Thrombosis

Duplex US is an excellent screening tool for the assessment of potential upper extremity thrombosis. Routine compression US can be utilized in the jugular and brachial venous systems, but the medial aspects of the subclavian veins, the brachiocephalic veins, and the SVC are inaccessible to direct compression. Therefore, interrogation of these vessels requires spectral and color Doppler techniques. Thrombosis may be identified by the absence of color Doppler flow within the vessel lumen, occasionally accompanied by echogenic material completely or partially filling the vessel lumen. Spectral Doppler analysis is particularly valuable in the evaluation of suspected upper extremity thrombosis. The patency of central venous structures that cannot be visualized directly is inferred by the presence of normal respiratory phasicity. Monophasic flow in the jugular or subclavian veins suggests a central venous abnormality such as DVT, stenosis, or extrinsic compression. Familiarity with these methods is important because the incidence of PE in the setting of upper extremity DVT may be as high as 12%. Furthermore, the incidence of upper extremity DVT has risen in recent years, largely due to the increased use of long-term indwelling catheters for total parenteral nutrition, chemotherapy, and other indications.

Compression Ultrasonography in the Evaluation of VTE

Duplex US may be used as an initial study in patients presenting with clinical suspicion of PE with unilateral DVT symptoms. Overall duplex US yields a diagnosis of DVT in 30% to 50% of patients subsequently proven to have PE.

In such instances, anticoagulation may be instituted without further testing. This approach is rapid and inexpensive, avoids the use of ionizing radiation, and is warranted for patients with lower extremity symptoms. However, due to an unacceptably low positive predictive value, duplex US is not recommended by either the American or British Thoracic Societies as a first-line examination for nonpregnant patients suspected of PE, in the absence of lower extremity symptoms. Although 90% of PEs originate in the lower extremity venous system (making it reasonable to begin the evaluation of VTE here), lower extremity venography examinations are negative for DVT for at least one-third or more of patients with proven PE. Nonocclusive thrombus, unrecognized complete embolization of the thrombus without residua in the legs, and thrombus originating in nonimaged venous segments (eg, deep pelvic veins) may account for this apparent discrepancy. So, it is clear that a negative lower extremity duplex US examination is insufficiently sensitive to exclude PE in patients with clinical suspicion of PE.

For patients with nondiagnostic (ie, intermediate- or low-probability) $\dot{V}/\dot{Q}$ scintigraphy results, duplex US may be obtained in an effort to avoid further diagnostic imaging. In this setting, if the duplex US examination is positive, anticoagulation may be instituted without the need for further testing. Duplex US has been shown to be cost-effective when used in this fashion, because only those patients with normal lower extremity duplex US examinations need further evaluation for suspected PE.

$\dot{V}/\dot{Q}$ SCINTIGRAPHY

Scintigraphy has occupied a central role in the evaluation of VTE for more than 3 decades. Although CT scanning has emerged as the initial diagnostic test at many institutions for patients suspected of PE, single photon emission CT (SPECT) $\dot{V}/\dot{Q}$ lung scanning remains in widespread use for the investigation of suspected PE.

Pulmonary Anatomy and Physiology

A basic understanding of normal pulmonary physiology is required to appreciate the alterations in lung function that occur in patients with PE. Reflex pneumoconstriction may occur in alveoli that are ventilated but not perfused (ie, abnormally "high" $\dot{V}/\dot{Q}$); abnormally low carbon dioxide tension elicits this response. However, this reflex is not commonly observed and generally is transient, because patients inhale carbon dioxide from tracheal dead space into the poorly perfused alveoli, and bronchial circulation continues to deliver some carbon dioxide to ischemic alveoli, thus moderating this reflex bronchoconstriction. Abnormalities of ventilation may produce regional alveolar hypoxia, which, in turn, induces reflex pulmonary vasoconstriction. Thus, alveolar hypoxia (ie, areas of abnormally low $\dot{V}/\dot{Q}$) causes redistribution of pulmonary blood flow away from hypoventilated alveoli. These pulmonary responses to alterations in regional ventilation and perfusion provide the basis for $\dot{V}/\dot{Q}$ scintigraphy.

Technique

Ventilation Scintigraphy

The radioactive gas most commonly used for ventilation scintigraphy is xenon-133 (^{133}Xe). ^{133}Xe is an inert gas with a principal photon energy of 81 keV and a physical half-life of 5.2 days. The advantages of ^{133}Xe are that it is relatively inexpensive, is widely available, and allows the acquisition of single-breath, equilibrium, and washout images and provides physiologic evaluation of regional lung volume and ventilation. A disadvantage of ^{133}Xe is its low photon energy (~81 keV), which generally requires that ventilation scans be obtained before perfusion scans. If technetium perfusion images are acquired prior to the ^{133}Xe ventilation study, the downscatter from the technetium-99m (^{99m}Tc) photons (~140 keV principal photon energy) will be detected in the xenon window of the pulse height analyzer and will degrade the ventilation images. If the ventilation study must be performed or repeated after the perfusion study has been completed, ventilation images can be improved if a ^{99m}Tc background image is obtained using the ^{133}Xe window. This background image can then be subtracted from the subsequent ^{133}Xe ventilation images to improve image quality. Performing the perfusion study first can inform the selection of the projection that best shows perfusion defects for the ventilation study, thereby allowing a direct comparison between ventilation and perfusion studies and permitting the omission of the ventilation study if the perfusion scan is normal.

^{133}Xe images are usually obtained in the upright posterior projection to allow evaluation of the largest amount of lung volume. The single-breath image is obtained by having the patient exhale completely and then inhale approximately 5 to 20 mCi (200-750 MBq) ^{133}Xe gas, after which a 15- to 30-second breath-hold is performed to obtain a static image. Then, the patient is instructed to breathe a mixture of the exhaled xenon and oxygen for 3 to 5 minutes, as tolerated, while static equilibrium images are obtained; images thus acquired represent the distribution of aerated lung volume. Finally, washout images are acquired by having the patient breathe fresh air, while serial 15- to 30-second images are obtained for a period of 3 minutes as xenon clears from the lungs. Normal xenon clearance is bilaterally symmetric and usually is complete in 2 to 3 minutes. Areas of delayed clearance may indicate regional air trapping and are commonly seen in patients with obstructive lung disease.

Ventilation imaging can also be performed with aerosols and ^{99m}Tc-labeled ultrafine carbon-labeled nanoparticles, with aerosols now more commonly used for ventilation imaging than radioactive gases. ^{99m}Tc-labeled aerosols have the advantage of the ideal technetium photon energy (~140 keV), widespread availability, ability to image in multiple projections, and optimal half-life, and they do not require the special exhaust systems that must be employed with xenon studies. Disadvantages of aerosols include the inability to obtain single-breath and washout images and, historically, a slightly higher rate of technically inadequate studies compared with xenon imaging. This latter difficulty results from central tracer deposition and inadequate peripheral penetration of the tracer, a problem that is more common in smokers.

The most widely used aerosol is ^{99m}Tc-labeled diethylenetriaminepentaacetic acid (DTPA); ^{99m}Tc sulfur colloid has been used as well. Aerosol imaging is usually performed prior to perfusion imaging because it is more difficult to deliver a larger ^{99m}Tc-labeled aerosol dose than it is to deliver a larger ^{99m}Tc-labeled macroaggregated albumin (MAA) dose, and when the same radiopharmaceutical agent is used for ventilation and perfusion imaging, a three to four times greater count rate is needed for the second study compared with the first study to achieve adequate image quality. A dose of 25 to 35 mCi (900-1300 MBq) of ^{99m}Tc-DTPA is inhaled via nebulizer, and initial images are obtained in the upright position for approximately 300,000 counts/image. Multiple projections may be obtained. The DTPA aerosol is absorbed across the alveolar-capillary membrane with a clearance time of half-life of 45 to 60 minutes, occasionally faster in smokers. When the aerosol study is performed prior to perfusion imaging, only 1 mCi (37 MBq) of activity related to the aerosol is present in the lungs; thus, the aerosol contributes little activity to the perfusion image when 4 to 5 mCi (148-185 MBq) is used for the latter.

Perfusion Scintigraphy

Pulmonary perfusion scintigraphy is performed with ^{99m}Tc-labeled MAA. MAA particles range in size from 10 to 90 μm, allowing them to localize in precapillary arterioles by mechanical blockade. The physiologic effect of pulmonary vascular blockade is usually insignificant, because less than 0.1% of precapillary pulmonary arterioles are occluded. The blockage is temporary because the biologic half-life of ^{99m}Tc-MAA particles in the lungs is only 6 to 8 hours.

About 1 to 5 mCi (37-185 MBq) of ^{99m}Tc-MAA is injected intravenously during quiet respiration, with the patient supine. Supine injections are performed to minimize the normal perfusion gradient between lung apex and base in the upright position and ensure even tracer distribution. Blood withdrawn into the syringe during venipuncture must not be allowed to remain in the syringe, because small blood clots may form. These will be labeled with tracer, and injection of these labeled clots will result in "hot spots" on the perfusion image. The tracer is injected slowly over several respiratory cycles. The number of particles injected ranges from 200,000 to 700,000, with fewer particles employed in children (number of particles injected is a function of age), pregnant women, or patients with right-to-left shunts or pulmonary hypertension. Any further decrease in the number of particles in adults produces tracer inhomogeneity and results in degraded images.

Imaging is performed immediately after tracer injection, preferably with the patient in the upright position to minimize diaphragmatic motion and maximize lung volume. Imaging may be performed in either the supine or decubitus positions, as needed. Imaging is performed with a large field-of-view camera and either a parallel-hole, all-purpose, or diverging collimator. Planar images are obtained in multiple projections (usually anterior, posterior, both posterior oblique, and both lateral projections). Other specialized projections may be obtained as desired. Each projection is acquired for approximately 500,000 to 750,000 counts. The first lateral view is acquired for 500,000 counts, and the opposite lateral view is acquired for the same amount of time needed to obtain the first lateral view.

$\dot{V}/\dot{Q}$ Imaging Using Single-Photon Emission Tomography

Single-photon emission tomography ($\dot{V}/\dot{Q}$/SPECT), without or with CT attenuation correction ($\dot{V}/\dot{Q}$ SPECT/CT), offers improved anatomical information over planar techniques for $\dot{V}/\dot{Q}$ imaging. $\dot{V}/\dot{Q}$ SPECT imaging employs the same agents used for planar $\dot{V}/\dot{Q}$ scintigraphy (using an aerosol for the ventilation portion of the study), with the ventilation study performed before the perfusion portion of the examination. When hybrid imaging is conducted, the low-dose CT scan for attenuation correction is typically performed after the perfusion portion of the study.

Interpretation

A normal ventilation scan shows relatively homogeneous pulmonary tracer activity on the single-breath and equilibrium images. During the washout phase, tracer activity slowly clears, with the bases clearing slightly more slowly than the remainder of the lungs. Clearing usually is complete in 2 or 3 minutes. ^{99m}Tc-DTPA aerosols also demonstrate homogeneous tracer activity from lung apex to base, but unlike xenon scans, the trachea and bronchi normally may be seen. Occasionally, swallowed activity may be detected in the esophagus and stomach.

Normal perfusion scans reveal homogeneous pulmonary tracer activity with predictable defects in the expected locations of the heart, pulmonary hila, and aortic arch, depending on the projection obtained.

Various schemes have been devised to interpret $\dot{V}/\dot{Q}$ scintigraphy. These schemes rely on the principle that PE causes decreased or absent pulmonary blood flow in a portion of lung, producing a perfusion defect. Because the alveoli serving these occluded vessels remain ventilated, a $\dot{V}/\dot{Q}$ "mismatch" is created. Unfortunately, many causes of perfusion defects unrelated to PE exist, and PE itself does not always result in a $\dot{V}/\dot{Q}$ mismatch. Hence, PE is neither diagnosed nor excluded by $\dot{V}/\dot{Q}$ lung scanning; rather, the probability of PE in any given patient is generated by interpretation of the lung scan. These probabilities are based on criteria that evaluate the shape, number, location, and size of perfusion defects on the perfusion scan in combination with the findings on the ventilation lung scan and chest radiograph. Perfusion defects are classified as lobar, segmental, or subsegmental; defects that do not conform to segmental lung anatomy are considered nonsegmental defects. The shape of perfusion defects also is important. Perfusion defects resulting from PE usually are wedge shaped and contact the pleural surface (Fig. 28.7). Defects that do not extend to the pleural surface may show a rim of activity immediately beneath the pleural surface but peripheral to the perfusion defect—a finding known as the "stripe" sign. Such perfusion abnormalities usually are not the result of PE. The number of perfusion defects may also be of some value in determining the likelihood of PE. Solitary perfusion defects usually are not related to PE, whereas multiple subsegmental perfusion defects are associated with PE in up to 50% of cases. The size of a perfusion defect also is significant. Sizes are graded as follows: a small perfusion defect occupies less than 25% of an anatomic lung segment; a moderate perfusion defect represents 25% to 75% of a lung segment; and a large perfusion defect constitutes greater than 75% of an anatomic lung segment. The perfusion scan is interpreted with reference to the chest radiograph, and the size of a perfusion defect is compared to any corresponding chest radiographic abnormality. $\dot{V}/\dot{Q}$ scan patterns can then be classified into one of three patterns: "matched" ventilation and perfusion defects, "mismatched" ventilation and perfusion defects (in which a perfusion defect is present with correspondingly normal ventilation or ventilatory abnormalities less pronounced than the perfusion defect), and a "reverse mismatched" pattern, in which the ventilatory defect is more pronounced than the corresponding perfusion abnormality.

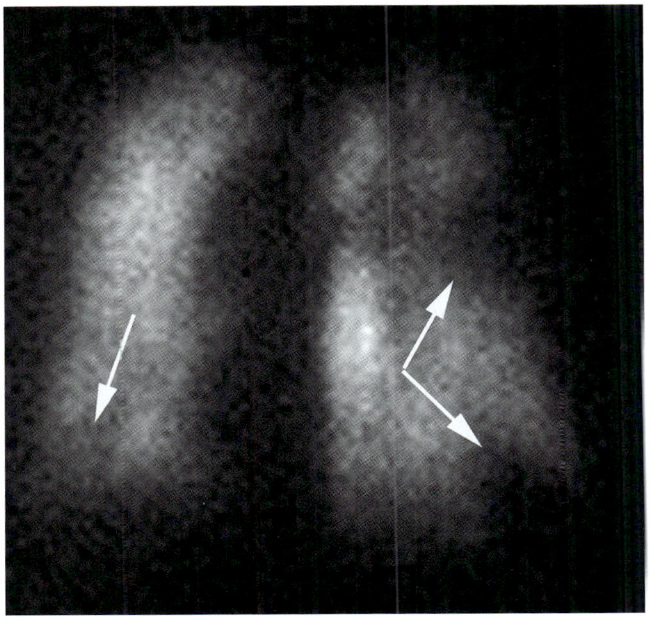

Figure 28.7. High-probability acute pulmonary embolism seen on scintigraphy. Posterior perfusion image shows numerous, segmental, wedge-shaped perfusion defects (*arrows*).

The chief interpretive schemes (McNeil, Biello, PIOPED, revised PIOPED classification schemes) have been divided into four diagnostic categories based on the probability of PE at pulmonary angiography: high-probability, intermediate/indeterminate-probability, low-probability, and normal perfusion scintigraphy. In addition to these categories, the original PIOPED criteria (and subsequently revised PIOPED II criteria) included a very-low-probability group in which the prevalence of angiographically documented PE was 9%. Further attempts to refine these interpretive approaches for $\dot{V}/\dot{Q}$ imaging have resulted in additional classification schemes—the modified PIOPED II and Prospective Investigative Study of Acute Pulmonary Embolism Diagnosis (PISAPED) criteria. In recent years, a trend away from probabilistic reporting schemes toward employing more committed language in a trinary reporting approach as "PE-positive, PE-negative, or indeterminate/nondiagnostic" has gained acceptance. However, to appreciate this more recent trend toward the use of definitive language for $\dot{V}/\dot{Q}$ scintigraphy interpretation, an understanding of the origins of probabilistic reporting schemes developed and refined in the PIOPED series is illustrative.

The Original PIOPED (PIOPED I) Series

The original PIOPED I series represents the largest prospective study examining the role of $\dot{V}/\dot{Q}$ scintigraphy in patients with suspected PE. PIOPED I scan interpretation criteria were designed to provide diagnostic categories that could be applied to all patients studied with $\dot{V}/\dot{Q}$ scintigraphy. The study organization is presented in Figure 28.8. The frequencies of angiographically proven PE for each $\dot{V}/\dot{Q}$ scan category were reported in the PIOPED I series, and familiarity with these data are important for any physician dealing with patients suspected of PE (Fig. 28.8).

The sensitivity for a high-probability scan is only 41% for the detection of PE, but improves to 82% when high- and intermediate-probability scan interpretations are considered together, and further increases to 98% when high-, intermediate-, and low-probability scan results are considered together. However, the specificity of $\dot{V}/\dot{Q}$ lung scans falls from 98% when high-probability scans are considered alone to 52% and 10% when high- and intermediate-probability scan results and high-, intermediate-, and low-probability scan interpretations are considered together, respectively.

The interobserver variability for $\dot{V}/\dot{Q}$ interpretation in the PIOPED I series was 5%, 8%, and 6%, respectively, for high-probability, very-low-probability, and normal $\dot{V}/\dot{Q}$ scan categories. However, the interobserver variability for intermediate- and low-probability scan categories was higher—25% and 20%, respectively.

The positive predictive value of a high-probability scan interpretation in the PIOPED I series in a patient without a prior embolic history was 91%. However, the positive predictive value of a high-probability scan interpretation falls to 74% for patients with prior embolic episodes.

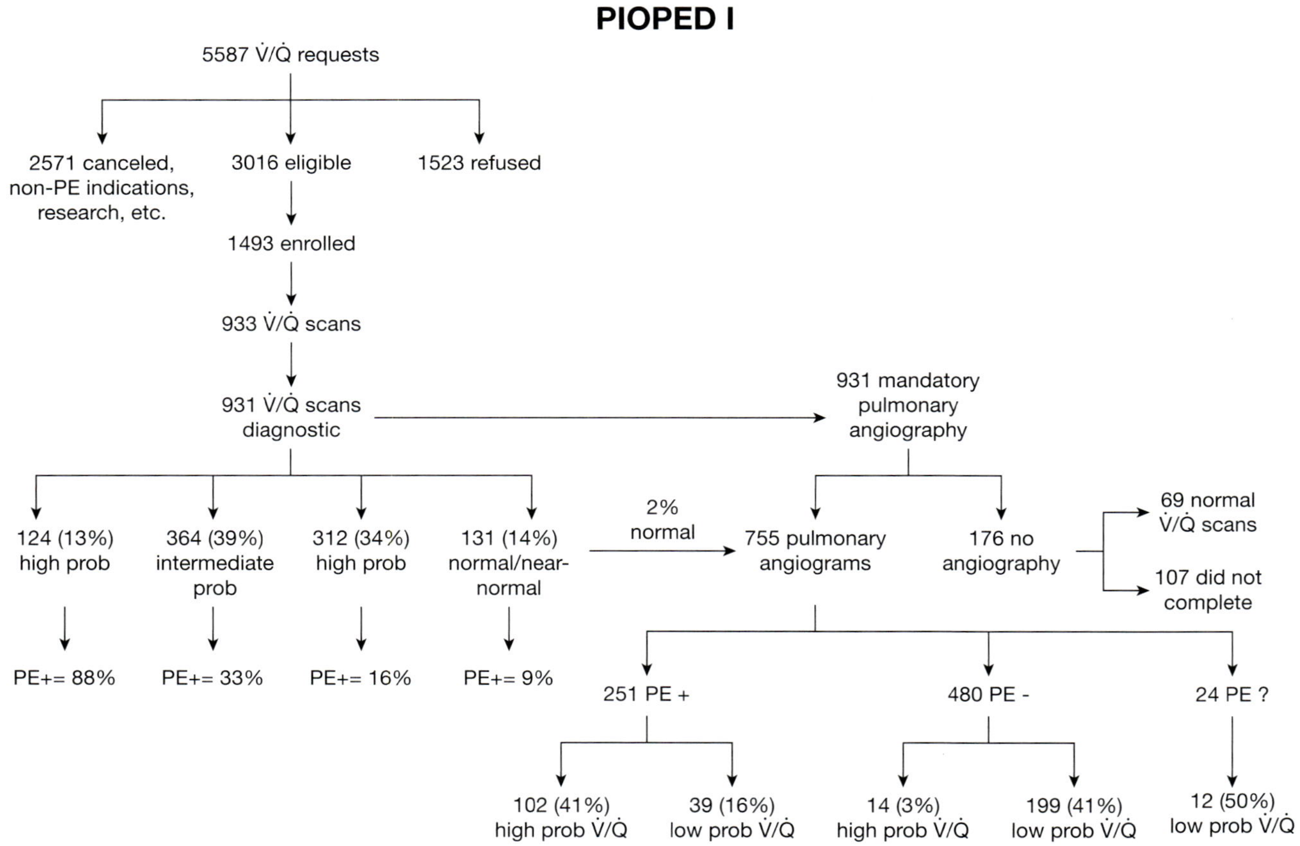

Figure 28.8. Patient recruitment, study workflow, and results in PIOPED I. PE+ = Catheter pulmonary angiograms showing PE for a given V̇/Q̇ scan category. PE, pulmonary embolism; prob, probability.

Integration of Clinical Assessment of PE Probability With Scan Interpretation

The importance of integration of the clinical pretest probability (ie, prior probability) of the likelihood of PE with the V̇/Q̇ scan interpretation was highlighted by PIOPED I (Table 28.1). When a low-probability scan interpretation (angiographically proven PE prevalence of 16%) was combined with a low clinical suspicion for PE (0% to 19% likelihood of PE), the negative predictive value of a low-probability scan increased from 84% to 96% (ie, the prevalence of PE on angiography decreased from 16% to 4%). Similarly, the negative predictive value of a normal/near-normal scan interpretation rose from 91% to 98% when integrated with a low clinical assessment for the likelihood of PE. The positive predictive value of a high-probability scan interpretation increased from 88% to 96% when combined with a high clinical suspicion (80% to 100% likelihood of PE). In contrast, when a high-probability scan interpretation was integrated with a low clinical suspicion for PE, the

Table 28.1 Scan Interpretation and Clinical Assessment of Probability of Pulmonary Embolism

Scan Probability	High (80%-100%)	Intermediate (20%-79%)	Low (0%-19%)
High	96%	88%	56%
Intermediate	66%	28%	16%
Low	40%	16%	4%
Normal/near-normal	0%	6%	2%
Total	68%	30%	9%

positive predictive value of a high-probability scan reading fell from 88% to 56%. Therefore, integration of clinical assessment of the likelihood of PE with scan interpretation results improves the diagnostic accuracy of V̇/Q̇ scintigraphy; this effect of integrated clinical pretest probability with imaging study results has been echoed in subsequent studies, including PIOPED II. Unfortunately, most of the PIOPED I patients had intermediate-probability V̇/Q̇ scan interpretations and intermediate clinical assessments of the likelihood of PE, so most patients did not benefit from this improved diagnostic accuracy and, therefore, required further diagnostic evaluation.

Low-Probability Lung Scans

Outcome studies have shown that most patients with low-probability V̇/Q̇ scan interpretations do well when anticoagulation is withheld, even though the frequency of angiographically proven PE in this setting is known to range from 14% to 30%. This apparent discrepancy may be explained by subclinical, well-tolerated PE. However, patients with poor cardiopulmonary reserve (eg, hypotension, coexistent pulmonary edema, right ventricular [RV] failure, tachydysrhythmias) and low-probability scan interpretations do not necessarily share the same favorable prognosis, and further diagnostic evaluation is required. Furthermore, patients with low-probability scan interpretations and high-probability pretest clinical assessments or significant risk factors for VTE certainly require additional diagnostic evaluation.

V̇/Q̇ Scintigraphy and Obstructive Lung Disease

The clinical diagnosis of PE is even more difficult in patients with obstructive lung disease because the clinical manifestations of PE may easily be misinterpreted as a COPD exacerbation, and laboratory values are not sufficiently sensitive or specific to distinguish acute PE from a COPD exacerbation. Unfortunately, scintigraphy often is abnormal in patients with moderate or severe COPD. Nevertheless, it has been shown that the diagnostic utility of V̇/Q̇ scintigraphy for the evaluation of PE is not diminished in the setting of preexisting cardiopulmonary disease, although intermediate-probability scan interpretations may occur more often in such patients. Furthermore, the diagnostic accuracy of lung scanning in patients with COPD is improved when integrated with the clinical assessment of the likelihood of PE.

Chest Radiography and V̇/Q̇ Scintigraphy

The major role of the chest radiograph in the evaluation of suspected PE is the exclusion of diagnoses that clinically simulate PE, such as pulmonary edema, pneumothorax, pneumonia, and pleural effusion. However, the chest radiograph also is essential for the accurate interpretation of V̇/Q̇ lung scans. An upright posteroanterior and lateral examination, ideally obtained as close as possible to the V̇/Q̇ scan, should be obtained. Perfusion defects substantially larger than corresponding chest radiographic abnormalities are suggestive of PE, whereas perfusion defects substantially smaller than corresponding chest radiographic abnormalities are not commonly associated with PE.

V̇/Q̇ SPECT Imaging

As with other tomographic techniques, V̇/Q̇ SPECT (SPECT-CT when CT is employed for attenuation correction) eliminates the problem of the overlapping anatomy that adversely affects planar scintigraphy, providing better visualization of segmental perfusion defects and improved categorization of perfusion defects as either "vascular" or "nonvascular" categories. Studies have shown both improved sensitivity and specificity for PE diagnosis, as well as reduced "indeterminate" interpretations for V̇/Q̇ SPECT scans compared with V̇/Q̇ scintigraphy. An in-depth review of the technical performance and interpretation of V̇/Q̇-SPECT studies is presented in the Suggested Readings at the end of this chapter.

CATHETER PULMONARY ANGIOGRAPHY IN PATIENTS WITH PE

Catheter pulmonary angiography has served as the gold standard for the diagnosis of PE for decades. Catheter pulmonary angiography traditionally has been indicated whenever a discrepancy between the clinical suspicion for PE and the results of other imaging modalities exists, when V̇/Q̇ scintigraphy is interpreted as high probability but contraindications to anticoagulation are present, or when conditions that may result in false-positive, high-probability V̇/Q̇ lung scans (eg, lung carcinoma, pneumonia) coexist with clinical suspicion for PE. Additionally, pulmonary angiography often is obtained before interventions such as mechanical embolus fragmentation, catheter-directed pulmonary arterial thrombolysis, peripheral venous thrombolytic therapy, or surgical thromboendarterectomy are initiated. Finally, pulmonary angiography has been used to establish the diagnosis of chronic thromboembolic disease in patients with pulmonary hypertension and for the evaluation of hepatopulmonary syndrome. However, the widespread use of CT pulmonary angiography (CTPA) has largely replaced pulmonary angiography for these indications, unless catheter-directed interventions are anticipated.

Relative Contraindications to Catheter Pulmonary Angiography

Iodinated contrast allergy, elevated pulmonary arterial pressure, left bundle branch block, bleeding diatheses, and renal insufficiency are the primary relative contraindications to pulmonary angiography (Table 28.2). Premedication with corticosteroids prior to angiography may be employed for patients who are allergic to iodinated contrast.

Table 28.2 Relative Contraindications to Pulmonary Angiography

Documented contrast material allergies
Elevated right ventricular end-diastolic pressure (>20 mm Hg) and/or elevated pulmonary artery pressure (>70 mm Hg)
Left bundle branch block
Renal insufficiency/failure
Bleeding diatheses

Patients with pulmonary arterial pressures higher than 70 mm Hg and RV end-diastolic pressures (RVEDP) higher than 20 mm Hg have been identified as having a 2% to 3% higher mortality from pulmonary angiography compared to patients with normal or mildly increased pulmonary artery and RVEDP. Despite this, patients with elevated pulmonary arterial pressures often constitute a significant patient population in need of pulmonary angiography. Hence, the presence of increased pressures in the pulmonary circuit is more an indication for selective angiography than an absolute contraindication to the procedure itself.

There is a risk of inducing complete heart block during right heart catheterization in patients with left bundle branch block. Therefore, preprocedural electrocardiographic evaluation should be performed. If left bundle branch block is identified, a temporary pacemaker may be placed before the procedure is performed. Other potential complications, such as hemorrhage at the site of venipuncture, contrast-induced nephropathy, and contrast reactions, can typically be managed with appropriate preprocedural care and, when required, postprocedural supportive measures.

Technique

Standard angiographic preparation and technique are used, including continuous cardiac monitoring. A transfemoral venous approach with standard Seldinger technique is employed when possible, although catheterization may be performed through the internal jugular, subclavian, or brachial veins when required. A vascular sheath may be placed, typically 7 F. A hand injection through the sheath is performed to confirm patency of the IVC. A 6 to 7 F Grollman catheter (Cook, Bloomington, IN), a pigtail catheter with a tip-deflecting wire (or various other specially designed catheters), is used to maneuver across the right heart into the pulmonary arteries. Correlation with prior imaging studies guides which side is the first to be catheterized.

Pulmonary artery pressures should be measured routinely. Right atrial pressure, which approximates RVEDP, also may be measured. For patients with elevated pulmonary arterial pressure or elevated RVEDP, selective catheterization, balloon occlusion, and lower injection rates may be warranted.

Bilateral imaging is obtained in anteroposterior and posterior oblique projections at 3 to 4 images/s for 5 seconds and 1 to 2 images/s thereafter. Subselective catheterization and magnification imaging may supplement the examination. Injection rates of approximately 20 to 25 mL/s for 2 seconds in the main pulmonary artery, 15 to 20 mL/s for 2 seconds in the right and left pulmonary arteries, and 5 to 10 mL/s for 2 seconds in the lobar or segmental pulmonary arteries using digital subtraction angiography typically are employed.

Interpretation

The specificity of catheter pulmonary angiography approaches 100% when a filling defect (Fig. 28.9) or abrupt pulmonary arterial obstruction (Fig. 28.10), with or without outlining of the end of the embolus ("the trailing edge"), is shown in the proper clinical setting. Ancillary criteria that suggest, but are not specific for, the diagnosis of PE include delayed venous return, tortuous vascularity, and decreased pulmonary flow. Angiographic findings in chronic pulmonary thromboembolic disease include pouching, intimal irregularity, tortuosity, webs or bands with poststenotic dilation, abrupt narrowing, and complete vascular obstruction.

Reliability of Catheter Pulmonary Angiography for the Diagnosis of Acute PE

True false-negative catheter pulmonary angiograms are extremely rare. The reported 5% to 10% frequency of false-positive catheter pulmonary angiography reflects a combination of technically limited studies and the influence of the timing of the angiogram relative to the embolic event.

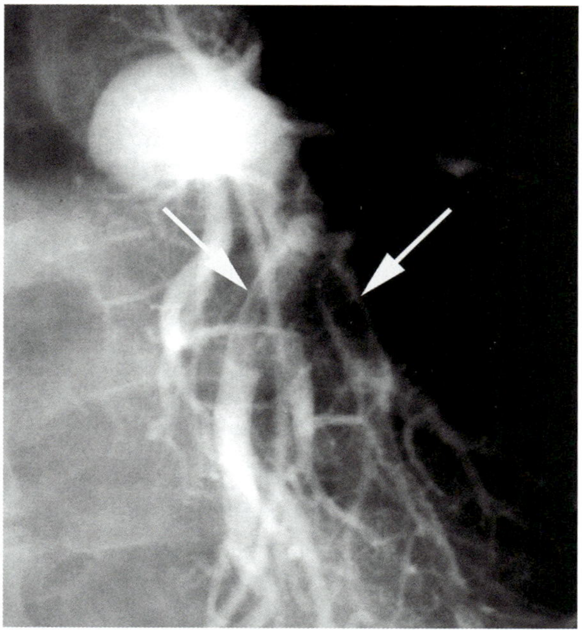

Figure 28.9. Acute pulmonary embolism: filling defects on pulmonary angiography. Left pulmonary angiogram in a 50-year-old man with indeterminate scintigraphy shows intraluminal filling defects (*arrows*) within the segmental vasculature of the left lower lobe.

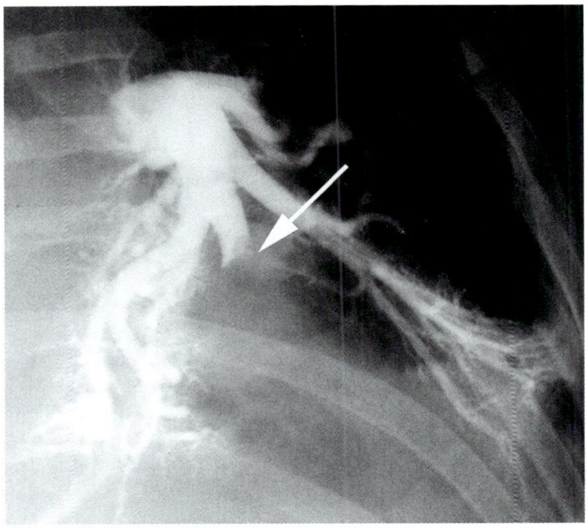

Figure 28.10. Acute pulmonary embolism: abrupt vascular "cut-offs." Left pulmonary angiogram in a 54-year-old man with indeterminate scintigraphy shows abrupt termination of the contrast column (*arrow*) within a segmental left lower lobe artery.

A negative catheter pulmonary angiogram interpretation essentially excludes the diagnosis of clinically significant PE. In the PIOPED I series, only four patients (0.6%) had clinical evidence, including autopsy information, of PE despite negative angiographic results.

Catheter pulmonary angiography, although long considered the reference test for the diagnosis of PE, is an imperfect standard, particularly as regard the detection of small emboli. The interobserver agreement for the detection of pulmonary emboli at catheter pulmonary angiography may approach 10% to 15%, even among experienced angiographers, and is even higher when small (subsegmental) emboli are considered. CTPA has supplanted catheter pulmonary angiography as the reference standard for PE diagnosis.

Complications

Procedure-related fatalities occur in approximately 0.2% to 0.5% of patients undergoing pulmonary angiography. The PIOPED I study showed no statistically significant relation between pulmonary artery pressure and the frequency of complications, although other investigations have shown that patients with elevated pulmonary arterial or RVEDP are at increased risk for complications while undergoing pulmonary angiography. The incidence of fatal and nonfatal complications with catheter pulmonary angiography is quite low due to the use of routine cardiac monitoring; flexible, soft catheters; low-osmolar, nonionic contrast agents; and awareness of the potential hazards of nonselective injections in the presence of elevated pulmonary artery pressures.

Major nonfatal complications occur in about 1% to 3% of examinations, including respiratory distress requiring intubation and resuscitation, cardiac perforation (although this complication was not reported in the PIOPED I series and has nearly been eliminated since the introduction of pigtail catheters), major dysrhythmias, major contrast reactions, renal failure requiring hemodialysis, and hematomas requiring transfusions.

The incidence of minor complications that may occur following pulmonary angiography is about 5%, and complications include contrast-induced renal dysfunction, angina, respiratory distress, contrast reactions that respond promptly to medications and fluids, and transient dysrhythmias.

CT PULMONARY ANGIOGRAPHY

The CT for diagnosis of PE was first described in 1978, but the systematic use of helical single-slice CT (SSCT) for the diagnosis of suspected acute PE was not described until 1992. In a relatively short period of time, iodinated IV contrast-enhanced CTPA (now widely performed as a multislice helical acquisition) has become the study of choice for suspected PE. Further experience has clarified the usefulness of CTPA in the diagnosis of PE and has pointed out its limitations.

Technical Considerations

When scanning a patient suspected of PE, a specific imaging protocol that is designed to optimize diagnostic information is used. Careful attention to numerous scan parameters is essential to ensure high-quality studies and is summarized in Table 28.3; a few considerations will be expanded upon below.

Scanning Range and Direction

Scanning may be performed from the base to apex because respiratory motion, and therefore degradation of scan quality resulting from respiratory motion, is most pronounced in the lung bases. It is, therefore, advantageous to image this area first, should the patient be incapable of suspending respiration. However, given the extreme speed of modern CT scanners (which may image the entire thorax in as little as one second), the impact of the choice of scanning direction is diminished.

Duration of Apnea

Inspiratory apnea is desirable because it results in increased pulmonary vascular resistance and thus promotes pulmonary arterial contrast enhancement. However, patients should avoid performing a Valsalva maneuver as the release of Valsalva can produce dynamics that favor the ingress of unopacified blood from the IVC, resulting in a suboptimal study—the resulting artifact has been referred to as "transient interruption of contrast" and is recognized when appropriate systemic thoracic and pulmonary venous and left-sided cardiac and aortic enhancement is seen in the presence of poor right heart and pulmonary arterial opacification, usually early in the course of the scan, with

Table 28.3 CT Pulmonary Angiography Technical Parameters

Parameter	Technical Performance	Issues
Scanning Direction	Caudal-Cranial Cranial-Caudal	• Caudal-Cranial direction has benefit of suspended respiration in lung region most vulnerable to respiratory motion degradation, also fewer streak artifacts from upper extremity injection • Arms up
Respiration Instruction	"Take a deep breath in and hold it; don't bear down," or "Breathe in, breathe out, stop breathing"	• Avoid Valsalva • Quiet respiration may be employed
Gantry Rotation Time	Minimum	• Exact time depends on CT manufacturer
kVp	Single source ≈ 100-120 kVp Dual Source	• May use automated exposure control if available • Lower kVp produces better vascular contrast; employ
mA		• Use automated exposure control
Contrast Injection Volume	≈60-80 mL	• Volume depends on injection rate, time to peak enhancement, trigger delay, and scan duration • Full concentration (300 mg%) • Quality optimized by patient-specific contrast dosing using weight and/or height
Contrast Injection Rate	≥3 mL/s, up to 5 mL/s	• Followed by saline chaser (3-50 mL) using dual-power injector
Contrast Injection Timing	Manual or automated bolus timing. 20 s fixed delay often suffices if necessary	• Use 120 HU threshold in main pulmonary artery or 150 HU in ascending aorta
Scanning Range	Thoracic inlet through lung bases	• Limit in pregnancy
Detection Collimation	≈1 mm	• Scanner dependent
Reconstruction Increment	≈1 mm	• May overlap
Table Transport Speed	Pitch >1	• "High-pitch" (pitch ≥3) mode may be used on certain DECT systems
Reconstruction	Iterative	• Depends on CT system
Image Reconstruction Kernel	"Sharp" (edge enhancement) for lung window, "soft" for soft-tissue window	• Nomenclature depends on CT manufacturer
Image Postprocessing	Multiplanar reformats	• Maximum intensity projection images for lung nodule detection • Pulmonary blood volume for DECT studies

an upper extremity contrast injection. The patient's ability to maintain apnea may be enhanced by hyperventilation or prebreathing the patient with oxygen prior to scanning. For patients unable to suspend respiration for the entire scan, some investigators have proposed using end-expiratory, as opposed to end-inspiratory, breath-holding, although quiet breathing during the study usually is not problematic. The required apnea duration for modern CTPA acquisitions is very short.

Contrast Concentration and Injection Rates

Intravenous (IV) contrast media with high concentrations of iodine combined with rapid injection rates maximize pulmonary arterial opacification and also allow the use of preloaded syringes and are, therefore, convenient as well as effective.

Saline injections, often referred to as "saline chasers," typically consist of 30 to 50 mL of 0.9% "normal" saline and permit the use of less IV contrast while maintaining excellent image quality. The chaser pushes the end of the contrast bolus, which would normally linger in the upper extremity veins between the IV site and the right heart, into pulmonary circulation. The use of saline chasers requires a dual-syringe power injector, capable of injecting contrast immediately followed by the saline chaser. Given the widespread use of CTPA, even small reductions in the amount of IV contrast required for these studies may produce significant cost savings. The contrast injection must be maintained throughout nearly the entire scan acquisition to avoid contrast washout and consequent flow artifacts in the pulmonary arteries.

Multislice CTPA Findings in PE

Acute PE is diagnosed when an intraluminal filling defect is seen, surrounded to a variable degree by contrast. An acute embolus may appear to be central within a pulmonary artery when seen in cross section (Fig. 28.11A) or may be outlined by contrast when imaged along its axis (Fig. 28.11B); these are the only absolutely reliable signs of acute PE. In some patients with acute emboli, an eccentric thrombus adherent to the vessel wall may be seen, but this finding is more typical in patients with chronic PE. An obstructed artery can be seen as an unopacified vessel, but this finding may also be seen with chronic emboli.

Ancillary Findings in Patients With PE (Fig. 28.12)

Ancillary findings on CTPA that suggest PE include mosaic perfusion, peripheral consolidations, and pleural effusions.

More than 50% of lung parenchymal attenuation on CT is due to pulmonary blood flow. Therefore, any process that alters pulmonary blood flow has the potential to produce visible changes in parenchymal attenuation. Inhomogeneous lung opacity resulting from alterations in pulmonary blood flow has been referred to as *mosaic perfusion*. Although mosaic perfusion is often related to airway-induced alterations in pulmonary blood flow, vascular causes, including emboli, may also produce mosaic perfusion (Fig. 28.12A).

Peripheral consolidations may represent pulmonary hemorrhage with or without pulmonary infarction, particularly when such opacities are wedge shaped and located in the subpleural regions of the lung (Fig. 28.13B and C). Among patients who undergo CTPA, there is a higher incidence of

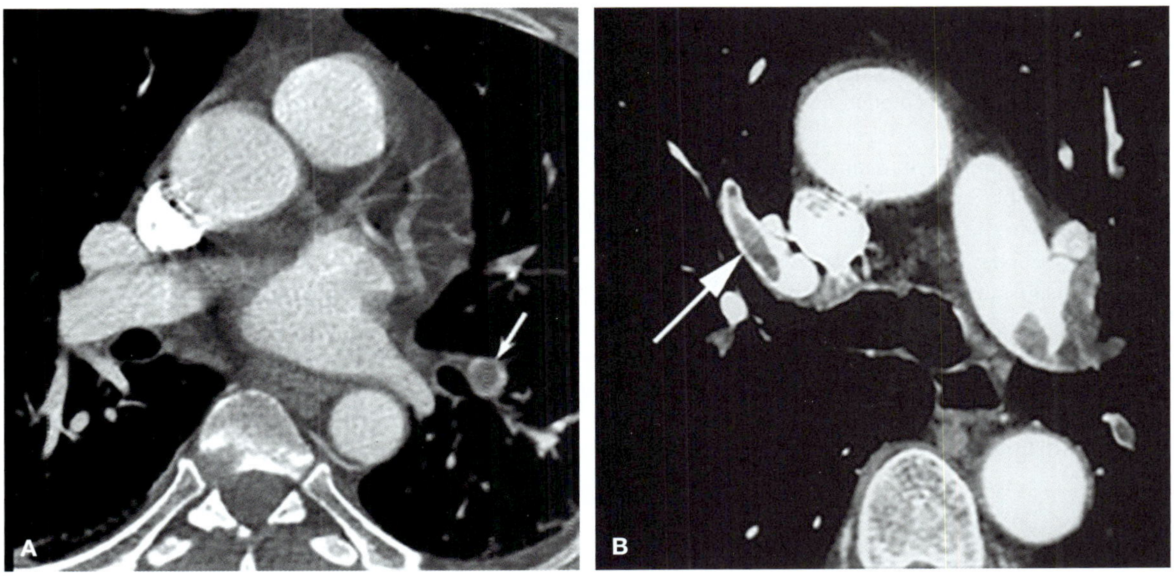

Figure 28.11. Acute pulmonary embolism on CT. **A:** Axial CT pulmonary angiogram in a 60-year-old man with shortness of breath shows a round intraluminal filling defect (*arrow*) within the left lower lobe pulmonary artery. **B:** Axial CT pulmonary angiogram in a 45-year-old man with shortness of breath shows a linear intraluminal filling defect (*arrow*) within the anterior segmental right upper lobe pulmonary artery.

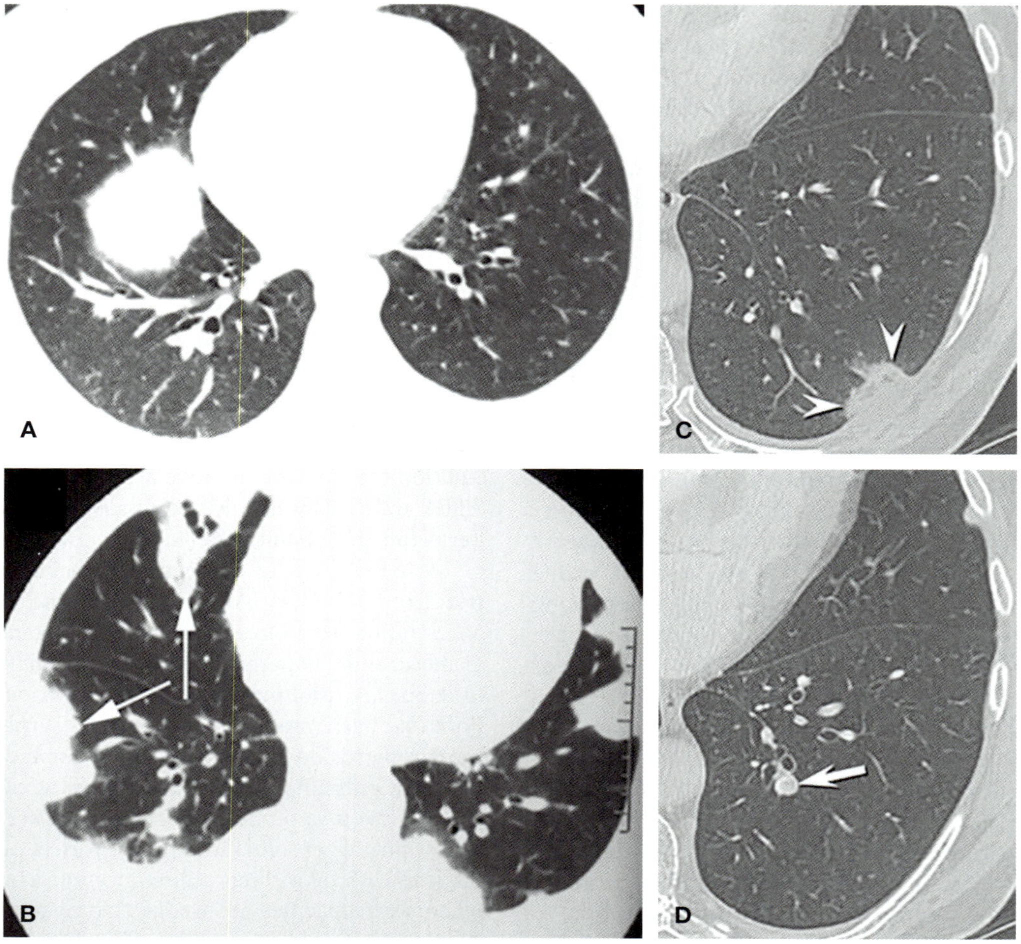

Figure 28.12. Ancillary findings of pulmonary embolism (PE). **A:** Oligemia. Axial CT pulmonary angiogram in a previously healthy 26-year-old man who developed syncope after a neurosurgical procedure shows decreased pulmonary parenchymal attenuation associated with diminished vascular size throughout the left lower lobe. **B:** Pulmonary infarction. Lung windows from a helical CT pulmonary angiogram in a 36-year-old man with proven PE (same patient as Figure 28.2) show bilateral wedge-shaped subpleural opacities (*arrows*) representing pulmonary infarction. **C:** "Reverse ground-glass halo" sign ("atoll" sign). Axial CT shows a subpleural left lower lobe opacity (*arrowheads*) with a truncated apex facing centrally. The opacity consists of ground-glass opacity centrally and consolation peripherally and the opacity is located in a vascular distribution subtended by a vessel with acute PE (*arrow*, **D**).

parenchymal opacities in patients found to have emboli than in those without visible emboli. Unfortunately, peripheral consolidations, even in the setting of suspected PE, rarely are diagnostic by themselves, although a "reverse ground-glass halo" sign ("atoll" sign) may be suggestive in the proper context (Fig. 28.12C).

Pleural effusions often are present in patients with PE, but they also are commonly seen in patients in whom PE is excluded. There are no CT features of pleural effusion that allow the specific diagnosis of PE.

Indirect CTV

Following a CT study for diagnosis of possible PE, indirect CTV of the lower extremities, pelvis, and IVC may be performed without the injection of additional contrast. The entire abdomen, pelvis, and lower extremities, from the symphysis pubis to the tibial plateaus, may be scanned, or the scans may be limited to the pelvic veins and femoropopliteal venous segments. Scans obtained at 3 minutes after the start of contrast injection show opacified veins in the legs and pelvis; thrombi are visible as filling defects within the veins (Fig. 28.14). The addition of CTV to CTPA examinations allows for the assessment of VTE in general in addition to PE. Although several studies have shown that the addition of CTV improves the diagnostic yield for VTE compared to CTPA alone, the technique is not widely practiced and lower extremity imaging in patients suspected of thromboembolic disease is usually performed with US.

Accuracy of CTPA in Diagnosing Acute Embolism

The accuracy of CTPA for diagnosing pulmonary emboli depends on the size of the artery affected and the size of the emboli. Acute emboli in large pulmonary arteries can be diagnosed with an accuracy of 100%. In patients suspected of having massive embolism, CTPA should be diagnostic.

The diagnostic utility of CTPA for the diagnosis of pulmonary emboli is now well established, and CTPA is widely accepted as the first-line technique for the evaluation of suspected thromboembolic disease. Numerous studies have addressed this issue, and most importantly, outcome studies have shown that it is generally safe to withhold anticoagulation for patients with a non-high clinical pretest probability of thromboembolic disease when CTPA results are negative.

One of the largest and best controlled studies of the utility of CT for the diagnosis of PE is the PIOPED II trial. PIOPED II was a prospective, multicenter study designed to determine if CTPA can reliably exclude acute PE and whether the addition of indirect CTV improves the ability to establish or exclude the diagnosis of acute PE. The PIOPED II protocol (Fig. 28.13) used a structured clinical assessment for the pretest likelihood of PE (the Wells score), and patients consented to undergo diagnostic testing, which included CTPA (4, 8, and 16 slice scanners), indirect CTV, V̇/Q̇ scanning, lower extremity US, and, if necessary, catheter pulmonary angiography using digital subtraction technique. A composite reference standard was used to diagnose or exclude PE (Fig. 28.13).

PIOPED II reported a sensitivity and specificity of CTPA of 83% and 96%, respectively, with a negative predictive value of 95%; with the addition of indirect CTV, these values changed to 90%, 95%, and 97%, respectively (Fig. 28.13). As was seen in PIOPED I, the clinical assessment had a strong impact on the predictive value of CTPA. For patients with intermediate or high pretest clinical probability of PE, the positive predictive value of CTPA increased from 86% to 92% and 96%. The negative predictive value of CTPA did not improve much (96%) when combined with a low pretest likelihood because the negative predictive value of CTPA was already high: 95%. However, the negative predictive value of CTPA *fell* from 95% to 60% when combined with a high clinical probability of PE.

The addition of CTV affected the overall reliability for the diagnosis or exclusion of PE. The sensitivity of combined CTPA and CTV increased from 83% to 90% with the addition of CTV. The negative predictive value of combined CTPA and CTV was only marginally improved (97%) from the already high value of 95%.

The PIOPED II trial is important for a number of reasons. First, PIOPED II was a well-controlled study, which addressed numerous assertions published in the clinical literature that studies evaluating the use of CT for PE prior to PIOPED II were plagued with methodological flaws. Second, PIOPED II reinforced the notion that CT imaging for PE—indeed, all PE imaging—is strongly influenced by the pretest probability of disease and, therefore, all PE imaging should be prefaced with the use of structured clinical assessments.

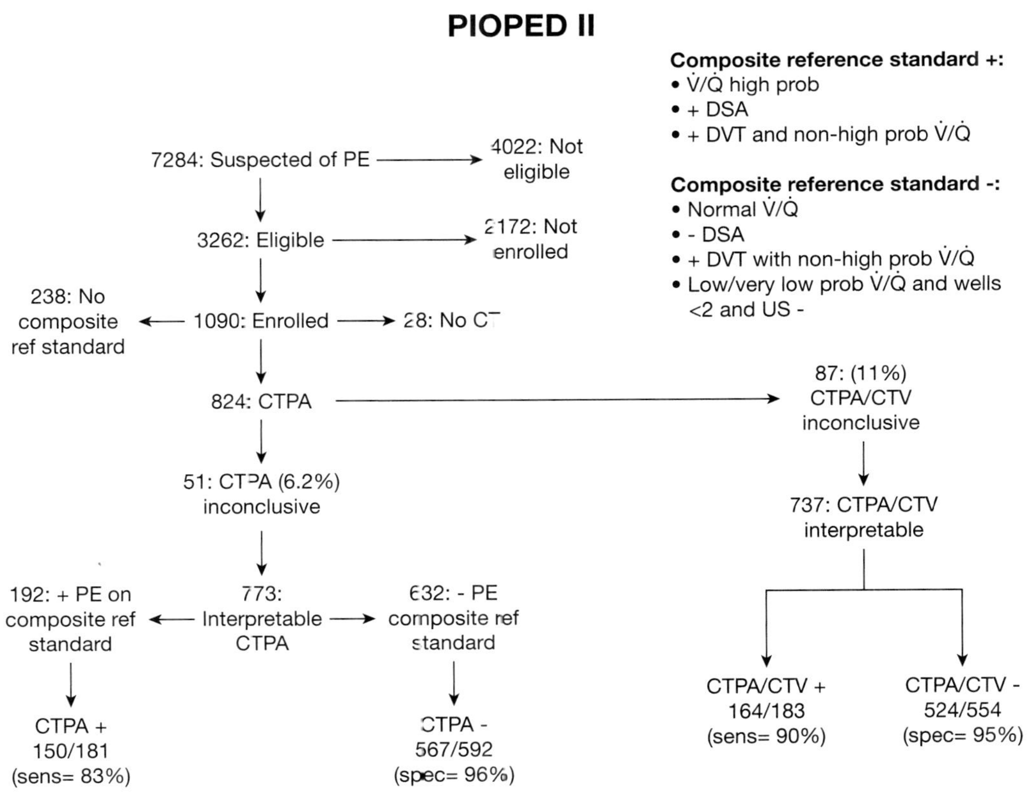

Figure 28.13. PIOPED II. Study workflow and results. PE, pulmonary embolism; prob, probability; ref, reference; sens, sensitivity; spec, specificity.

Unfortunately, despite the evidence that structured clinical assessments (of which there are several, including the Wells score, Geneva score, the revised Geneva score, and others) strongly influence the results of diagnostic imaging in patients with suspected PE, it is still relatively commonplace for CTPA imaging to be ordered without the benefit of formal pretest disease probability assessment. Furthermore, PIOPED II pointed out that when CTPA results and pretest probability are discordant (ie, a negative CT despite high clinical probability for PE and the reverse), CTPA results may be insufficiently reliable and further diagnostic testing may be warranted. Last, PIOPED II reinforced the notion that PE and DVT should be viewed as manifestations of a single disorder—venous thromboembolic disease. As such, the reliability of imaging assessment of suspected PE may be augmented through the use of lower extremity US or indirect CTV to exclude DVT. This approach is of value when CTPA findings and clinical assessment are discordant.

Other fairly large studies, including one large meta-analysis of 3500 patients reported over 15 studies (a mixture of single and multislice CTPA studies), suggest that negative pulmonary CTA results for patients with non–high-probability pretest clinical assessment are sufficient to exclude PE—lower extremity imaging is not required. In other words, the negative predictive value of CTPA for patients with non–high-probability pretest clinical assessment approaches 99%, and anticoagulation may be safely withheld in these patients without the need for lower extremity imaging.

It is interesting to note that some of the initial reluctance to embrace CTPA for the assessment of PE was based on the observation that SSCT's sensitivity may be insufficient to reliably exclude such an important diagnosis. Toward this end, a number of publications in the clinical literature suggested that the SSCT sensitivity for the detection of acute PE is approximately 70%. This number is in part based on comparison of SSCT results to $\dot{V}/\dot{Q}$ scanning or pulmonary angiography, usually in highly selected patient populations. This marginal sensitivity was largely attributed to the presumed inability of SSCT scanning to visualize subsegmental emboli. However, thrombi limited to small vessels are uncommon in patients with PE. Indeed, the highest frequency of isolated subsegmental emboli (30%) and the lowest sensitivity of SSCT (53%) have been reported in patients with nondiagnostic (intermediate- or low-probability) $\dot{V}/\dot{Q}$ scans, whereas the lowest frequency of subsegmental emboli (6%) and the highest accuracy of SSCT are found when unselected patients with suspected PE are studied. Among studies showing the lowest sensitivity rates for SSCT (53% to 63%), a significant number of patients had small thrombi. In such studies, patients had both SSCT and catheter pulmonary angiography, most likely because of nondiagnostic $\dot{V}/\dot{Q}$ radionuclide scans; patients with nondiagnostic scans have a comparatively high prevalence of small emboli.

Recently, it appears that this argument has come full circle. Several publications have expressed concern that CTPA may be *overly* sensitive, detecting small emboli that "do not matter clinically," a situation referred to as "overdiagnosis." This effect offered as an explanation for discordance between CTPA studies and other "gold standards," such as normal or very-low-probability $\dot{V}/\dot{Q}$ scan results or negative catheter pulmonary angiograms. Furthermore, it has also been suggested that the CTPA overdiagnosis of PE accounts for the observation that the number of CTPA examinations, and incidence of PE, has risen dramatically in recent years, but has not been accompanied by a corresponding reduction in PE-related mortality. For those that have intimate familiarity with the diagnosis of PE on CTPA studies, it is well known that very small emboli are readily detectable on high-quality examinations, and when such emboli are confidently seen, negative $\dot{V}/\dot{Q}$ scan or catheter pulmonary angiogram results are of little significance, and it is just as likely that the "gold standard" is in error. Whether or not such emboli should be treated once detected, however, is another matter, and it has been suggested that subsegmental emboli in patients, particularly those with adequate cardiopulmonary reserve, need not be treated in the absence of DVT. Therefore, it is important to recognize that there is a distinction between true "false-positive" CTPA studies (comparatively uncommon) and the detection of small, potentially clinically unimportant, emboli (overdiagnosis) on these examinations. No doubt further research will shed light on which patients with small emboli require anticoagulation and which do not.

The radiologist's job in this effort is to detect the emboli, regardless of size. Since the decision to treat with anticoagulation is not without risk; however, it is important to recognize that CTPA studies should not be "overinterpreted"—this can be a source of false-positive CTPA interpretations. It is often helpful in this effort to provide some estimate of the study quality so that the ordering clinician has some idea of the reliability of the diagnosis. For example, a referring clinician may react to a dictated report stating, "small subsegmental pulmonary embolism identified on a high-quality study," much differently than a report stating, "possible small subsegmental pulmonary embolism identified on a low-quality examination, significantly degraded by respiratory motion." Both reports may be considered "positive" studies, but the latter report conveys the sense to the referring physician that this particular CTPA examination may not be as reliable as the specificity of 95% reported in the literature would suggest. Finally, it must be recognized that the CTPA diagnosis of small emboli can be challenging and one should exercise caution when attempting to diagnose small, isolated, subsegmental pulmonary emboli (sometimes referred to as "solitary" emboli, as some clinical investigators interpret the term "isolated emboli" to refer to the absence of associated DVT, not the number of emboli visualized) because this diagnosis may carry significant implications in the form of potential treatment-related complications. In this circumstance, some investigators have advised obtaining the opinions of additional readers to confirm that the small lesion in question does indeed represent PE.

Comparison of CTPA With Other Modalities

The accuracy of CT for diagnosing PE has been compared to that of planar $\dot{V}/\dot{Q}$ in several studies, and CT has been shown to have a higher sensitivity with similar specificity compared to planar $\dot{V}/\dot{Q}$ scintigraphy. Furthermore, CT provides the additional benefit of suggesting or confirming alternate clinical diagnoses in patients with CT scans interpreted as negative. When together considering positive scans and scans interpreted as negative, but with alternative diagnoses present on scans interpreted as negative, a confident diagnosis may be obtained with CT in 90% or more patients. A recent review of the performance of CTPA, planar $\dot{V}/\dot{Q}$ scintigraphy, and $\dot{V}/\dot{Q}$ SPECT for the diagnosis of acute PE showed that planar $\dot{V}/\dot{Q}$ scanning was inferior to both $\dot{V}/\dot{Q}$ SPECT and CTPA, with little appreciable difference in the diagnostic performance between the latter two, although CTPA was found to be more cost-effective for establishing a final correct diagnosis than either $\dot{V}/\dot{Q}$ approach; note, however, that this analysis was performed in the United Kingdom and therefore may not be readily extrapolated to US practice. $\dot{V}/\dot{Q}$ SPECT was associated with the lowest radiation dose per correct diagnosis, and therefore, this technique could be favored for populations in whom radiosensitivity is of primary concern, such as young and pregnant patients, or for patients in whom CTPA is not feasible.

Several studies have evaluated the accuracy of transthoracic and transesophageal echocardiography with CT for the detection of acute PE. Predictably, transthoracic and transesophageal echocardiograms were found to have a limited accuracy for detecting PE. The major role of echocardiography in the evaluation of patients with PE is not a diagnostic one, but rather is for risk stratification for those patients with proven PE. Several investigators have shown that patients with PE and echocardiographic evidence of RV strain (eg, RV enlargement, RV wall motion abnormalities such as "McConnell sign" (**Video 28.1**), and leftward bowing of the interventricular septum) are at higher risk for death, but whether or not such patients are candidates for more aggressive interventions, such as pharmacologic or mechanical thrombolysis, remains controversial.

Chronic PE

CTPA for chronic pulmonary emboli is reviewed in detail in the context of pulmonary hypertension in Chapter 29 (see Figs. 29.12 and 29.13).

PITFALLS IN CTPA FOR THE DIAGNOSIS OF PE

Awareness of several pitfalls in the diagnosis of acute PE is required for accurate diagnosis. Pitfalls in the CT diagnosis of PE may be divided into anatomic and technical etiologies. Anatomic pitfalls include lymph nodes, pulmonary veins, volume averaging of pulmonary arteries, impacted bronchi, pulmonary arterial catheters (the tip mistaken for a small embolus), cardiac shunts, bronchial artery inflow, and pulmonary arterial sarcoma. Technical causes of pitfalls on CTPA include respiratory and cardiac motion, streak artifacts, improper contrast bolus timing, flow artifacts (including transient contrast interruption), and quantum mottle. A detailed knowledge of normal bronchovascular anatomy is required for accurate interpretation of CTPA studies. Several commonly encountered pitfalls in the CTPA diagnosis of PE are reviewed below and illustrated in Figure 28.14.

Anatomic Pitfalls

Lymph Nodes

Normal peribronchial lymph nodes commonly simulate acute PE on CTPA imaging. Normal nodes appear as soft-tissue structures, which typically are lateral to upper lobe anterior segmental pulmonary arteries but medial in relation to the lower lobe pulmonary arteries. Knowledge of the typical location of lymph nodes makes it possible to discriminate between them and true PE (Fig. 28.14A).

Pulmonary Veins

Pulmonary veins course within connective tissue septa, separate from pulmonary arteries and bronchi, which run together. Knowledge of this anatomic relationship allows one to avoid diagnosing an artifact within a pulmonary vein as acute PE. When a filling defect is encountered, particularly in the peripheral aspects of the lung, if the vessel showing the filling defect is immediately adjacent to a bronchus, the filling defect resides within a pulmonary artery and PE may be diagnosed. If the vessel showing the potential filling defect is not accompanied by a bronchus, it is likely a pulmonary vein, and therefore, PE should not be diagnosed (Fig. 28.14B). Additionally, pulmonary veins may be followed sequentially to their confluence at the left atrium, allowing one to distinguish veins from arteries easily.

Impacted Bronchi

Rarely, a calcified bronchus with mucoid impaction creates the appearance of an intraluminal filling defect surrounded by contrast. Review of lung windows at the appropriate location demonstrates absence of an air-filled bronchus, and review of images with a wider window width may reveal calcification within the bronchial walls, which may superficially simulate IV contrast within a pulmonary artery surrounding an intraluminal filling defect.

Intracardiac and Extracardiac Vascular Shunts

Intracardiac shunts, such as atrial and ventricular septal defects, may result in either left-to-right or, eventually, right-to-left shunting of blood, and asymmetric blood flow following surgical correction for congenital heart conditions may create unusual patterns simulating PE also (Fig. 28.14C). One

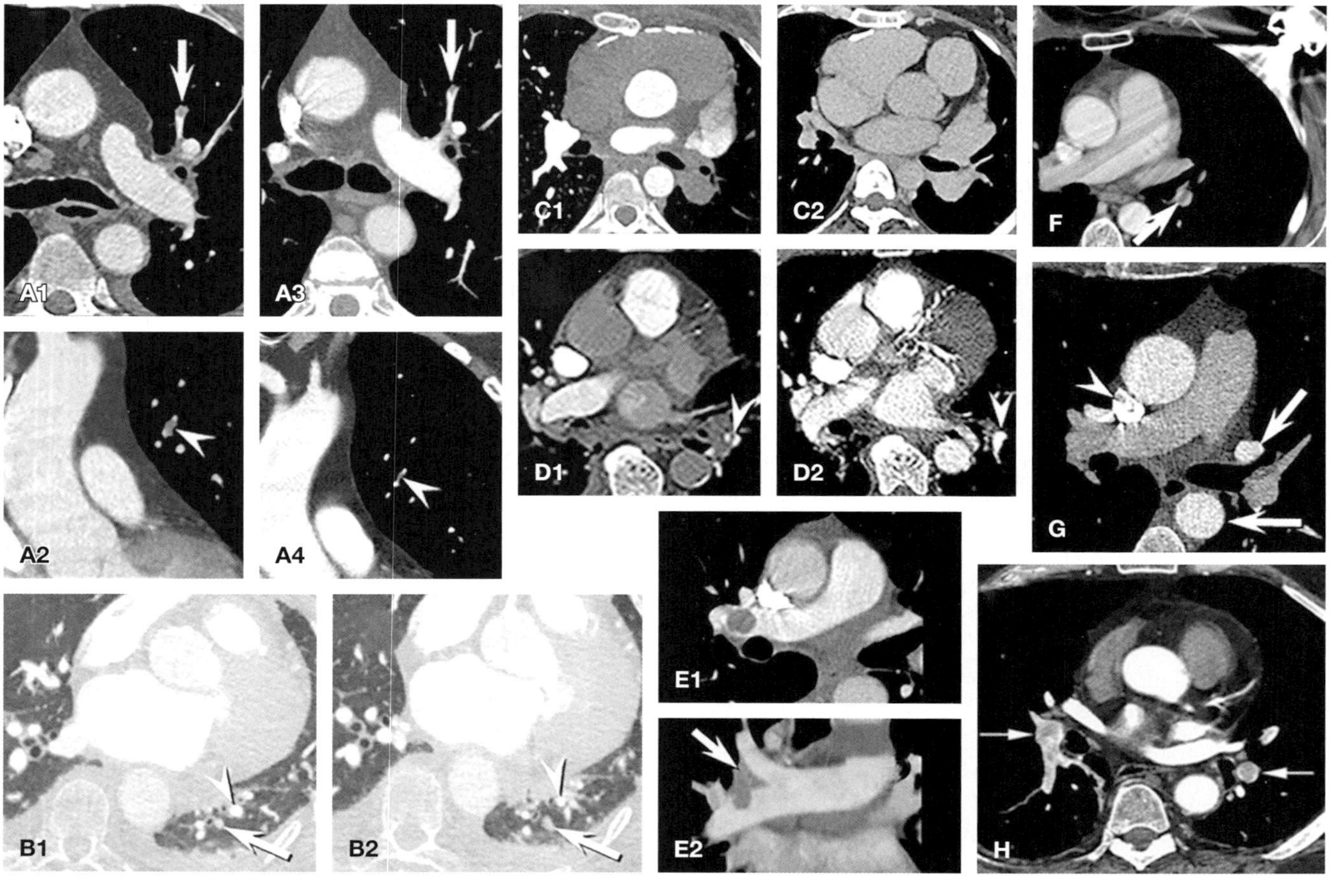

Figure 28.14. Pitfalls in the CTPA diagnosis of pulmonary embolism (PE). **A_1:** Lymph node tissue (*arrow*) misdiagnosed as PE at axial CTPA. The coronal image **(A_2)** shows the lymph node tissue (*arrowhead*) resides between two small pulmonary arteries; lymphoid tissue is commonly found vascular bifurcations. The enhanced pulmonary arteries are visible on either side of the lymph node tissue. Axial and coronal **(A_3 and A_4)** CTPA images 10 ys earlier show lymphoid tissue (*arrow* and *arrowhead*) in the same location. **B:** Diminished enhancement in a pulmonary vein simulating PE. **B_1:** A left lower lobe vessel (*arrow*) shows relatively diminished enhancement compared to adjacent vasculature (*arrowhead*). **B_2:** More caudally, the poorly enhanced vessel (*arrow*) is clearly separate from adjacent bronchi, unlike peripheral pulmonary arteries (*arrowhead*), and can therefore be diagnosed as a pulmonary vein. **C:** Asymmetric pulmonary arterial opacification in a patient with congenital heart disease repair (unilateral Glen procedure connecting the superior vena cava [SVC] to the peripheral right pulmonary artery with Fontan with right atrial appendage anastomosis to the main pulmonary artery supplying the left pulmonary artery). Absent opacification of the left pulmonary artery **(C_1)** could be mistaken for a embolus expanding the vessel. Repeat injection with delay shows the left pulmonary arterial system is patent **(C_2)**. **D:** Bronchial artery inflow. **D_1:** Axial CTPA shows a filling defect within the left lower lobe artery (*arrowhead*); note poor left-sided enhancement. **D_2:** Repeat CTPA with left-sided enhancement shows resolution of the apparent filling defect. E. Pulmonary artery sarcoma. **E_1:** Filling defect resembling PE is present within the right upper lobe artery. **E_2:** Coronal image shows the filling defect (*arrow*) extending through the pulmonary artery into adjacent lymph node tissue as confirmed at resection. F. Streak artifact from a left breast tissue expander creates a filling defect (*arrow*) within the left lower lobe pulmonary artery. **F:** Flow artifact (arrow) in the left pulmonary artery. **G:** Transient contrast interruption. Axial CTPA shows the characteristic features of unopacified blood from the inferior vena cava entering the pulmonary arterial circulation: poor pulmonary arterial opacification in the presence of contrast actively injected (*arrowhead*, SVC) and adequate left-sided enhancement (*arrows*, left superior pulmonary vein and aorta). **H:** Poor bolus timing. Axial CTPA initiated too late following the beginning of the intravenous contrast injection shows apparent filling defects with the right and left lower lobe pulmonary arteries (*arrows*). This artifact is created by laminar flow, which dictates that flow within the center of the vessel is faster than flow at the vessel periphery. In this case, contrast along the periphery of the vessel transited the vessel at a slower pace than blood at the center of the vessel, allowing contrast-enhanced blood at the center of the vessel to wash out before imaging begins. Repeat scanning with the proper contrast injection delay showed no evidence of PE.

of the more common causes of an extracardiac, left-to-right shunting of blood is bronchial arterial hypertrophy induced by chronic pleural and parenchymal pulmonary inflammatory disease. In this circumstance, flow is directed from the bronchial arteries into the pulmonary arteries; such retrograde flow potentially may induce flow artifacts that could create the appearance of low-attenuation defects within the pulmonary arterial system (Fig. 28.14D).

Pulmonary Artery Sarcoma

Pulmonary arterial sarcoma is probably the rarest pitfall in the diagnosis of suspected PE. These tumors are visualized as intraluminal filling defects within the central pulmonary arteries. If recognized preoperatively, the tumor is often mistaken for PE (Fig. 28.14E). The polypoid nature of tumor growth, expansion of the involved pulmonary artery, enhancement of the intravascular tumor itself, and ipsilateral lung nodules may reveal the true nature of the abnormality.

Technical Pitfalls

Respiratory and Cardiac Motion Artifacts

Motion artifacts often result in apparent low-attenuation defects within pulmonary arteries; recognition of the artifact depends on identifying the presence of motion effects on other structures on the same image, often facilitated by review of lung windows. Cardiac motion artifacts usually affect those pulmonary artery branches closest to the LV free wall, medial lingular pulmonary artery branches specifically, and may occur regardless of the patient's ability to suspend respiration. Because motion artifacts can be severe and can render a scan nondiagnostic in quality, every attempt to limit motion degradation should be made. Occasionally, it may be appropriate to repeat a scan after correctable factors have been identified.

Streak Artifact

Streak artifact is encountered when very dense material, such as undiluted injected IV contrast in the SVC or metal, is present within the imaging field of view attenuating photon transmission. Pulmonary artery branches near the SVC, usually anterior and apical branches of the right upper lobe pulmonary artery, are usually involved. Typically, the linear, nonanatomic, radiating configuration of vascular hypodensity is recognizable as artifactual and tracing the artifact to the dense source is confirmatory (Fig. 28.14F).

Mixing and Flow Artifacts

Mixing artifacts result from the entry of unopacified blood into the enhanced imaging volume, as may occur when unopacified IVC blood mixes with opacified blood from the injected upper extremity in the right heart and the heterogeneous contrast opacification then extends into the pulmonary arterial system. Often such artifacts can be recognized by their source just beyond where enhanced and unenhanced vessels meet as well as the poorly marginated nature of the abnormality, in contrast to the circumscribed hypoattenuating margins encountered with PE. One particular flow artifact often encountered at CTPA is transient interruption of contrast; this has been discussed previously (Fig. 28.14G). Regional alterations in blood flow, as may occur when pulmonary resistance is asymmetrically elevated (commonly in the setting of lung disease such as lobar collapse), may also result in heterogeneous contrast opacification that can be mistaken for PE.

Improper Bolus Timing

Accurate evaluation of CTPA requires adequate enhancement of the pulmonary arterial system. Methods for achieving proper bolus timing have been discussed previously. Because laminar flow within vessels dictates that blood flowing within the center of the vessel flows faster than blood at the periphery of the vessel, scanning after the delivery of the contrast bolus may, rarely, create the appearance of a filling defect simulating PE (Fig. 28.14H). If the bolus arrives too late (as may occur in a patient with poor cardiac output or a venous stenosis within the injected extremity), dilute contrast will be present within the pulmonary arterial system once the scan is initiated. Once improper timing is recognized, it usually is corrected easily; the scan may then be performed again with the proper timing.

Quantum Mottle

Quantum mottle, or image noise, may result in unsatisfactory study quality. Mottle is more likely to be encountered if the field of view is small and the collimation is very narrow. To reduce mottle, the field of view should be set properly, and the mA must be increased appropriately. These maneuvers will come at the expense of increased radiation dose.

Incidental Pulmonary Emboli

Incidental pulmonary emboli may be detected in nearly 1.9% to 4.4% of patients undergoing contrast-enhanced thoracic CT for non–embolic-related reasons, often oncologic indications; such patients almost always are at high risk for thromboembolism. This finding may be extremely important and often results in significant changes in patient management.

THE USE OF PULMONARY CTA FOR RISK STRATIFICATION IN PATIENTS WITH ACUTE PE

The "severity" of PE is best approached in terms of PE-related early mortality risk (typically defined as 30-day or in-house mortality) rather than anatomic embolic burden or embolic location. For this reason, some authorities have recommended abandonment of some of the terms that are used below, such as "massive" and "submassive" PE. Rather, the term "hemodynamic instability" is preferred instead of "massive" in the context of PE-related physiologic derangement, and usually indicates PE that is accompanied by cardiac arrest, arterial hypotension, and/or cardiogenic shock. The early mortality related to massive, or high-risk, PE exceeds 15%. Such patients are unstable, and there is general consensus that these patients are appropriately treated aggressively, often with thrombolytic therapy or embolectomy using catheter techniques or surgery. Patients without features of "high-risk" PE (ie, no hemodynamic instability at presentation) are classified as "non–high-risk," including "intermediate-" and "low-risk," patients on the basis of clinical scoring systems that integrate comorbidity and physiologic assessment of PE severity. Patients with intermediate-risk PE (roughly equivalent to submassive PE) are those with an elevated risk severity score and evidence of RV dysfunction at imaging (echocardiography or CTPA) or injury by imaging or biomarkers, such as brain natriuretic peptide and cardiac troponin. Intermediate-risk patients are further classified as "intermediate-high risk"—those with RV dysfunction at imaging *and* elevated biomarkers—versus "intermediate-low risk" patients—those without evidence of RV dysfunction at imaging and normal biomarkers, or one without the other. Patients with low PE severity risk scores are generally regarded as "low-risk."

Generally, normotensive patients with normal RV function are treated only with anticoagulation, typically with excellent results. However, there is controversy regarding the subset of normotensive patients who have evidence of RV dysfunction on imaging studies (typically echocardiography), elevated cardiac biomarkers, and/or electrocardiography (previously referred to as *submassive* PE). The definition of RV dysfunction on echocardiography, often also referred to as *RV strain*, is not standardized and may include RV hypokinesis, dilation of the RV (often defined as an RV/LV cavity ratio of greater than 0.9 or 1 or a RV end-diastolic dimension of greater than 30 mm), straightening or leftward bowing of the interventricular septum, or a number of variables defined by Doppler criteria. Some investigators have shown that normotensive PE patients with one or more of these echocardiographic signs of RV dysfunction have a higher mortality rate when treated with anticoagulation alone compared with hemodynamically stable patients with PE without RV strain. Such patients typically undergo close monitoring to detect early hemodynamic decompensation with the consequent need for rescue reperfusion treatment. Because echocardiography is the primary modality used for the assessment of RV dysfunction, but is insufficiently reliable to diagnose or exclude PE, a number of investigators have explored the possibility that CTPA may be able to simultaneously establish the diagnosis of PE and provide evidence of RV strain in normotensive patients with PE, thereby establishing or excluding the diagnosis of PE and providing management-directing information with a single test.

A number of studies assessing the ability of CTPA to predict PE-related mortality by diagnosing RV strain have been performed and results are conflicting. Some investigators have shown that RV dilation on CTPA (defined as an RV/LV cavity ratio of greater than 0.9 or 1 or straightening or frank leftward bowing of the interventricular septum) predicts PE-related morality at 3 months; other authors have not found such a relationship. Additionally, several investigations have focused on the assessment of a vascular obstruction index (the so-called "clot" scores) as a predictor of PE mortality. Assessment of the degree of vascular obstruction is not possible with echocardiography, and therefore, CTPA may be able to provide incremental prognostic information through embolic load assessment in addition to assessment of RV strain. Results of such investigations, however, are again mixed. Several of the published papers on this topic defined the vascular obstruction index based on scores derived from similar efforts conducted with catheter pulmonary angiography. These assessments provide a numeric score reflecting the number of segmental pulmonary arteries involved with PE, typically with some additional weighting for completely occlusive emboli. Again, some studies have shown that higher vascular obstruction scores are associated with increased mortality in patients with PE, whereas other reports have not found such an association. In the latter studies, elevated vascular obstruction scores may be associated with signs of clinically severe PE, such as admission to the intensive care unit, intubation, or use of vasopressors, but mortality prediction is lacking. Some investigators have attempted to refine the vascular obstruction index by providing a 5-point scale describing the percentage of the cross-sectional vascular area obstructed by emboli. This method of scoring the degree of vascular obstruction has been correlated with echocardiographic signs of severe PE and may have the advantage of a more physiologic description of the hemodynamic effects of PE. One study employing this methodology found that mean pulmonary arterial pressure was significantly elevated in patients with a vascular obstruction score of greater than 50% compared with patients with vascular obstruction scores less than this value.

Most studies assessing the ability of CTPA for risk stratification in patients with PE have not found that main pulmonary artery size is a predictor of adverse outcome.

Ultimately, although some investigations have shown that CT findings of RV strain predict poor outcome related to PE, and other CTPA studies have shown that assessment of the degree of vascular obstruction can also predict PE-related mortality, research in this area has yet to show that findings at CTPA can determine which patients should be treated with anticoagulation alone and which patients should be treated with thrombolytic therapy. As such, it is advisable that radiologists interpreting CTPA examinations be aware of CT findings suggesting RV dysfunction and alert the ordering physician when these features are present, but management of patients with PE cannot be reliably directed on the basis of CTPA findings alone. Toward this end, the RV/LV ratio should be reported on all CTPA studies. Initial evaluation of the use of RV/LV ratios suggested that 4-chamber reconstructions are necessary for accurate assessment, but measurement on axial imaging is probably sufficient. This measurement is performed near the atrioventricular valve planes at the widest transverse diameter of the ventricles, perpendicular to the interventricular septum, which may, or may not, be on the same image (Fig. 28.15). Values ≥ 0.9

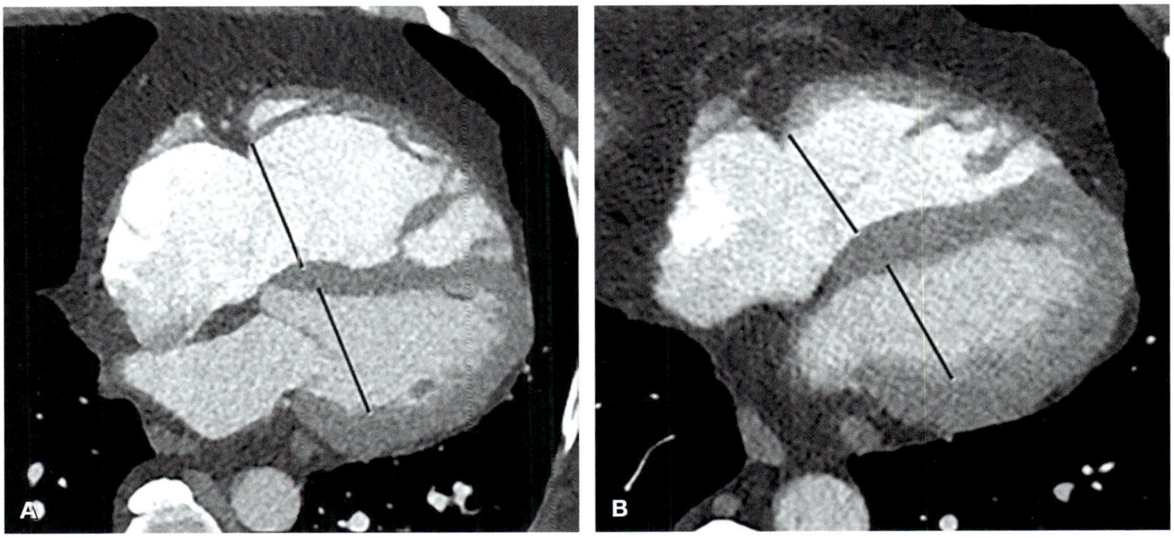

Figure 28.15. Right ventricular dysfunction at CTPA. **A:** Axial CTPA image in a patient with acute PE shows right ventricular enlargement; RV/LV = 1.25. **B:** Axial CTPA 8 months following **(A)** and after catheter-directed thrombolysis shows normalization of the RV/LV ratio (0.89).

initially, and subsequently ≥1, have been considered abnormal and suggestive of right ventricular dysfunction, but use of this threshold results in an unacceptably high number of false positives compared with echocardiography and therefore a threshold of ≥1.1 may strike a better balance between sensitivity and false-positive reduction for diagnosing right ventricular dysfunction at CTPA. In addition to the RV/LV ratio, the shape of the interventricular septum should be noted (**Video 28.2**). While this assessment may be associated with some interobserver variability, straightening or leftward bowing may be another imaging feature of right ventricular dysfunction. Other CTPA features in patients with PE that may be encountered include reflux of contrast into the IVC and hepatic veins, subpleural opacities suggesting hemorrhage or infarction, pleural effusion, and, rarely, oligemia, which have not been shown to reliably contribute to PE outcome prediction.

RADIATION AND PULMONARY CTA: PREGNANT PATIENTS

CTPA is a powerful tool for the investigation of patients suspected of PE and is now recommended as the first-line imaging study for such patients by most authorities on the subject. CTPA does entail use of ionizing radiation, which has been regarded as a limitation of the application of CTPA, particularly in certain patient populations, pregnant patients in particular, but the development of advanced CTPA techniques and application of radiation exposure reduction measures have addressed this concern.

The absorbed radiation dose to the mother during CTPA depends on scanner manufacturer and scan protocol used. The maternal exposure concerns also apply to the fetus, with the additional consideration that the radiation dose to the fetus with CTPA imaging will vary inversely with the gestational age—this is because, as pregnancy progresses, the fetus encroaches upon the maternal upper abdomen and lung bases and is therefore more likely to receive scattered radiation.

As regard the maternal radiation exposure, the risk of the development of radiation-induced breast carcinoma in women is related to the age of exposure and the total radiation dose. It has also been speculated that the female breast could be even more radiation sensitive during and shortly after pregnancy. An increased incidence of breast carcinoma in young women has been suggested in atomic bomb survivors and women who have undergone therapeutic radiation with exposures ≥1 Gy or Sv. In contrast, the effects of low-level radiation (≤100 mSv), the dose range typically associated with medical imaging, are unclear. There is a great deal of controversy regarding the estimation of the incidence of low-level radiation–induced carcinogenesis by extrapolation from patients exposed to higher levels of radiation—the so-called *linear no-threshold* model. Estimates using this model suggest that the lifetime risk of breast carcinoma in a 30-year-old woman exposed to a breast dose of 10 mGy is about 1 in 5000 or a 0.2% increase in relative risk for the development of breast malignancy. With the caveat that the actual radiation dose absorbed by the female breast will vary among different CT scanner manufacturers and CTPA protocols, estimates of the female breast absorbed dose resulting from CTPA range from 10 to 70 mGy (clearly much higher than the average glandular dose of 3 mGy resulting from two-view mammography). In contrast, the dose to the female breast that occurs with planar V/Q scanning is approximately 0.28 to 0.9 mGy.

Regardless of the actual numerical risks for radiation-induced breast carcinogenesis, a number of points are clear:

(1) Radiation has the potential to induce malignancy. (2) The female breast is more susceptible to radiation-induced malignancy when radiation is delivered at a young age. (3) CTPA protocols deliver a substantial amount of radiation to the female breast (the effect being even more pronounced for repeated scans), although recent advancements in CT scanner technology and awareness of radiation exposure reduction methods have significantly mitigated this issue. (4) Physicians, radiologists in particular, must take an active role in reducing the potential for radiation-induced injury.

Estimates of the maternal radiation exposure and fetal absorbed dose from maternal CTPA examinations depend on gestational age and methods for exposure reduction are listed in Table 28.4. And several of these parameters will be expounded upon below.

Decreasing Maternal Radiation Dose

The absorbed radiation dose associated with CTPA can be mitigated, with little to no adverse impact on diagnostic accuracy, by careful manipulation of a number of technical parameters as well as the institution of several dose-reducing and noise-reducing techniques (Table 28.4). These methods will reduce radiation exposure to mother and fetus when pregnant patients undergo CTPA, but these methods can, and should, be applied to essentially any patient undergoing CT imaging. Technical parameters under the radiologists' control that may be modified to reduce the radiation dose associated with CTPA examinations are listed in Table 28.5 and include (1) manual or automated reduction of the product of tube current (mA) and gantry rotation time (seconds),

Table 28.4 Methods for CTPA Dose Reduction

Parameter	Approach	Comment
mA (tube current)	• Manual tube current reduction • Automated exposure control	• Angular (x-axis and y-axis) modulation • Z-axis modulation
kVp (tube potential)	• Reductions have profound effect on exposure and added benefit of increasing vascular attenuation through exploitation of photoelectric effect	• Manual reductions • Automated tube potential
Gantry Rotation Time	• Decreases exposure in a manner roughly equivalent to decreasing tube current	• Maintain minimum for optimal scan acquisition speed and enhanced image quality
Scanning Range	• Limit to aortic arch through lung bases	• Decreases maternal exposure and limiting caudal scan volume decreases fetal exposure
Table Transport Speed	• Pitch typically 1-2 • Some scanner manufacturers offer "high-pitch" mode	• Caution: modern CT scanners often automatically compensate for the dose reduction induced by higher pitch values
Iterative Reconstruction	• Various methods depending on scanner manufacturer	• Replaces filtered back projection • Allows reduction in noise, which allows lower exposure
Filters	• Adaptive filtering: decreases streak artifacts by removing data by high attenuating structures	• Allows reduction in noise, which allows lower exposure
Bismuth Breast Shields	• Reusable radioprotective garments constructed of bismuth • Attenuates low-energy photons within the polychromatic CT x-ray beam that otherwise would contribute to the patient's radiation dose through low-energy photon deposition in the skin and subcutaneous tissues	• Adverse interaction with automated exposure control • Not recommended per the American Association of Physicists in Medicine
Maternal Lead Shielding	• Placed on maternal abdomen caudal to scan range	• Decreases internal scatter to fetus

referred to as *mAs*; (2) manual or automated reduction of the kVp; (3) use of automated tube current modulation; (4) reduction of scan range; (5) increasing the table transport speed/scan pitch; and (6) various dose- and noise-reducing techniques that radiologists may employ to lower the dose associated with CTPA examinations, including use of body shields, the use of noise-reducing filters, and adoption of new scanner technologies, such as noise-reducing image reconstruction software employing iterative and deep learning reconstruction methods as opposed to filtered back projection, which requires higher dose in order to make low-noise, quality images.

Reduction of Tube Current

The amount of radiation applied during a CT scan is usually thought of as the result of the product of the tube current (mA) and the exposure time (the gantry rotation time, or the time the x-ray beam is actually applied to the patient)—this product is often referred to as the tube current-time product or mAs. As a general rule, although the gantry rotation time can be manipulated to adjust radiation dose, it is more rewarding to consistently use a relatively short gantry rotation time to minimize the scan duration and actively manipulate the mA to achieve dose reduction, rather than primarily manipulate the tube rotation time or manipulate both values simultaneously. For CTPA, speed is of the essence, so scanning at a fast pitch, requiring fast rotation time at relatively mA for a given kVp, is preferred.

CTPA examinations typically employ mAs values in the range of 100 to 600 mA, with actual mA values typically ranging from 100 to 400 mA. Tube currents are adjustable over a wide range, typically 20 to 550 mA (some scanners can generate a tube current as high as 1300 mA). Decreasing the mA lowers the radiation dose to the patient in a linear fashion, but simultaneously increases image noise. A number of studies have shown that low-dose thoracic CT protocols can effectively employ very low mA values—as low as 25 mA. However, such studies generally have evaluated scan quality with reference to lung imaging, typically by evaluating the visibility of small nodules or interstitial opacities. Such an approach is successful in the lung due to the high target-to-background ratio intrinsic to the detection of soft-tissue attenuation abnormalities against the low-attenuation background of the lung. Such is not the case for PE imaging, and while reductions in mA are certainly possible, these efforts cannot be as aggressive as with the detection of lung nodules or interstitial lung disease. Studies evaluating the potential for dose reduction through manually reduced mA scanning for CTPA indicate that with all other factors constant, the manual mA value reduction by more than 50% compared with "routine" values may compromise scan quality and could result in an increased rate of nondiagnostic CTPA studies. Newer techniques, particularly adaptive filtering and iterative or deep learning scan reconstruction methods, may allow more aggressive mA reduction through elimination of noise without compromising scan quality. While mA values may be manually manipulated to achieve substantial radiation dose savings, automated reduction in mA values using *automatic exposure controls* (see below) is now routinely available on commercial CT systems and has the benefit of integrating the dose reduction with desired, user-defined image quality, thus maximizing dose savings while ensuring diagnostic quality scans.

Reduction of Tube Kilovoltage

Typical kVp ranges for chest CT examinations are from 90 to 120 kVp depending on scanner manufacturer and patient size. As with mAs, kVp is adjustable, although the allowed adjustments occur in increments and depend on the scanner manufacturer, and the available selections for kVp values are restricted compared with available tube current selections.

The effect of changes in kVp on radiation energy imparted to the patient can be profound as changes in kVp have an exponential effect on radiation exposure, whereas adjustment of other parameters has a linear effect. For example, reducing the kVp from 120 to 80 kVp will decrease the radiation dose by at least 60%, with all other factors held constant. Decreasing the kVp *increases* image contrast but also increases image noise. Overall, the image contrast *decreases* somewhat with reduced kVp scanning because the relative increase in image noise is greater than the relative increase in image contrast. Nevertheless, it has been shown that the "typical" kVp values employed with CTPA can be reduced to 100 kVp and, in some cases, to 70 to 80 kVp while still maintaining diagnostic accuracy. This is because, although the image noise increases with reduced kVp scanning, the reduced kVp value increases the relative contribution by the photoelectric effect to x-ray photon interactions within the patient. This occurs because the reduced kVp lowers the average beam energy to near the k-edge of iodine, favoring the photoelectric effect over Compton scatter. The result is maintenance of, or perhaps slight improvement in, vascular attenuation with contrast-enhanced studies. Experimentally, it has been shown that lowering the kVp from 120 to 140 kVp to 80 kVp increases the attenuation of x-ray photons by a factor of 1.6 and 2, respectively. Therefore, significant dose reductions for CTPA can be realized when reduced kVp protocols are employed. CT manufacturers have introduced *automated tube potential* selection techniques that gather information from the CT topograms and integrate this information with data reflecting user-defined desired image quality to allow the scanner to select the "optimal" tube potential for a patient of a particular size for the CT protocol employed.

Automated Tube Current Modulation

CT scanner technology allows real-time adaptation of the x-ray beam to the shape and thickness of the body part scanned. The cross section of the thorax is roughly elliptical, resulting in less x-ray beam attenuation when the beam traverses the chest in an anteroposterior direction compared with the transverse direction. This difference in shape can be exploited, with reductions in the mA value while the beam is directed in an anteroposterior direction, compared with the mA value employed while the beam is directed in a transverse orientation, resulting in overall dose reduction. This process is referred to as *angular (x-axis and y-axis) modulation*. Angular dose modulation was previously performed based on attenuation of various body parts as estimated by frontal and lateral scout views, but modern CT scanners can now perform this process in real time. Dose savings of 10% to 60% have been reported with this technique. This technology can be further leveraged by decreasing x-ray tube mA while the tube is transiting over certain radiosensitive anatomy, such as the anteriorly over thyroid gland or breast tissue, with a compensatory increase in mA as the tube transits posteriorly, thus decreasing radiation exposure to more radiosensitive tissues. This technique is known as *organ dose management*.

Similar reductions in radiation dose can be achieved in the *z*-axis direction. Modern multislice CT (MSCT) scanners have the ability to modulate the tube current during the scan in the scanning (*z*-axis) direction, allowing images of similar user-selected noise levels independent of patient size and anatomy. This process is known as *z-axis modulation*. *Z*-axis modulation allows for reduced radiation doses when smaller anatomic parts or smaller patients are scanned. Compared with fixed tube current scanning, *z*-axis dose modulation may allow for nearly a one-third reduction in patient dose. Automated exposure control dose reduction methods are commonly combined with iterative or, more recently, deep learning reconstruction techniques (see farther on) to amplify dose savings by reducing image noise and thus maintaining image quality at lower mA, and these two methods can be used in concert with manual or automated kVp reductions for further radiation dose savings.

Dose Reduction for PE Imaging: CTPA Versus Scintigraphy

Any attempts at patient radiation dose reduction should first begin with ensuring that the requested CT is indicated. A number of publications detail the role of noninvasive methods for the evaluation of suspected VTE; such methods include structured clinical assessment for the pretest probability of PE as well as the use of D-dimer measurements. Lower extremity US assessment may be performed for patients suspected of VTE, particularly if lower extremity symptoms are present. Once it is clear that thoracic imaging is required, the choice is usually between CTPA and $\dot{V}/\dot{Q}$ imaging. The average dose for chest CTPA examinations depends on numerous factors as described in Table 28.4, but an "average" absorbed dose for CTPA has traditionally been approximately 5 to 15 mGy. The upper limit of this range reflects dosimetry largely unmodified by active attempts at dose reduction—using a combination of the techniques described in Table 28.4 will result in absorbed doses less than these values and sub-millisievert CTPA exams are now routinely possible with modern CT systems. Planar $\dot{V}/\dot{Q}$ scanning imparts an absorbed dose of approximately 1.4 mSv. Therefore, it is clear that $\dot{V}/\dot{Q}$ scanning imparts a smaller radiation dose to patients than "routine" CTPA studies, but when the latter employs dose reduction strategies, patient radiation doses may be relatively equivalent. However, CTPA enjoys the clear benefit of a "definite" answer in most cases, rather than an assignment of probability of disease, and CTPA offers the potential for identifying nonembolic causes of symptoms prompting PE evaluation. Because of these potentially competing risks and benefits, a number of publications have suggested obtaining $\dot{V}/\dot{Q}$ scans or $\dot{V}/\dot{Q}$ SPECT whenever available in younger patients with relatively few chest radiographic abnormalities—these patients are the most likely group to receive a diagnostic answer from $\dot{V}/\dot{Q}$ scanning. In the PIOPED II series, the planar $\dot{V}/\dot{Q}$ in patients with a normal chest radiograph was diagnostic (high probability or normal/nearly normal) in 52% of patients with suspected PE. However, inpatients, patients with cardiopulmonary disease, and patients with chest radiographic abnormalities stand an increased chance for obtaining nondiagnostic $\dot{V}/\dot{Q}$ scan results, and CTPA is recommended as the initial test for suspected PE in these individuals.

Recommendations for Suspected VTE Evaluation During Pregnancy: Decreasing Fetal Dose

A major consideration when evaluating pregnant patients for suspected PE is the radiation dose imparted to the fetus. Risks to the fetus associated with radiation exposure primarily include neurologic and carcinogenic effects. The risk of neurologic impairment is considered insignificant with fetal exposures less than 100 mGy. However, estimation of the risk of induction of childhood cancer from fetal irradiation is a source of controversy. It has been estimated that the risk of induction of fatal childhood malignancy increases from 1/2000 to 2/2000 for a fetal absorbed dose of 50 mGy. Some data suggest that the risk of carcinogenesis is higher when radiation is delivered during the first trimester compared with the second or third trimesters.

A number of publications have estimated the fetal absorbed dose from CTPA, and it has been recognized that this dose varies depending on the gestational age. Early in gestation (0-3 months), when the embryo or fetus is remotely located from the caudal imaging volume of an CTPA study, the dose to the fetus is minimal—estimates of this dose range from 0.0033 to 0.66 mGy. As gestation progresses, the fetus grows and moves cranially, approaching the caudal aspect of the imaging volume, and therefore is subject to increasing scatter radiation during CTPA or, if the scanning range is carried too caudally, direct irradiation. In the second trimester, fetal doses related to CTPA range from as low 0.0079 mGy to as high as 0.26 mGy. In the third trimester, estimated fetal doses resulting from CTPA range from 0.51 to 0.862 mGy. The first trimester dose ranges represent a combination of SSCT and MSCT studies, with the lower figure reported from SSCT examinations and the higher from MSCT examinations. The wide range in part reflects differences in CT protocols, and, by inference, the profound impact dose-reducing procedures can have. For example, one study combining several dose reduction strategies, including dose modulation, shielding the maternal abdomen with a lead apron, and shortening the caudal imaging volume by 5 cm, allowed a fetal radiation dose savings of more than 50%, with the largest contribution to dose savings provided by trimming the caudal aspect of the imaging volume. The second and third trimester figures quoted above were reported in a SSCT series. One MSCT study estimating fetal doses in the late third trimester indicated a maximal absorbed fetal dose of 0.23 mGy.

The fetal dose attributable to $\dot{V}/\dot{Q}$ scanning (injection of 2 mCi ^{99m}Tc-MAA and inhalation of 10 mCi ^{133}Xe) is approximately 0.32 to 0.36 mGy. $\dot{V}/\dot{Q}$ scanning is often performed using a half dose of ^{99m}Tc-MAA and omission of the ventilation portion of the study for pregnant patients (if the perfusion study is normal) to further reduce maternal and fetal dose, providing a fetal absorbed dose of approximately 0.21 to 0.30 mGy. Therefore, for the most part, CTPA provides a lower fetal radiation dose than $\dot{V}/\dot{Q}$ scanning during the first trimester, a fetal radiation dose nearly equivalent to $\dot{V}/\dot{Q}$ scanning early in the second trimester, and a higher fetal dose than $\dot{V}/\dot{Q}$ scanning later in the second trimester and throughout the third trimester. While the use of fetal radiation dose estimates from SSCT studies cannot be readily applied to multislice CTPA studies, if one applies multiple dose-reducing procedures, it is likely that CTPA fetal doses could approximate, and probably improve upon, SSCT estimates. In particular, reducing the caudal scanning range for pregnant patients has a profound effect on fetal absorbed dose with CTPA imaging because the radiation to the fetus during CTPA is the result of scatter and it decreases according to the square of the distance between the radiation source and the target. Additionally, combining the previously described dose reduction maneuvers should have an additive beneficial effect on fetal dosimetry while still maintaining sufficient scan quality (Fig. 28.16A).

Several other methods of fetal dose reduction are available. The use of lead shielding for the mother results in a lower radiation dose to the fetus and is clearly a simple, readily available maneuver (Fig. 28.16B). The mechanism of fetal dose reduction with the use of a lead apron is due to reduction of external scatter radiation from the CT gantry and collimators. The dose reduction achieved with the use of a lead apron is most pronounced when the patient is circumferentially covered with the apron.

Another innovation capable of reducing fetal dose associated with CTPA is internal barium shielding. Oral administration of a 30% solution of barium sulfate just prior to scanning places an attenuating material—barium—between the caudal imaging volume and the fetus (Fig. 28.16B). In a phantom study, administration of a 30% barium sulfate

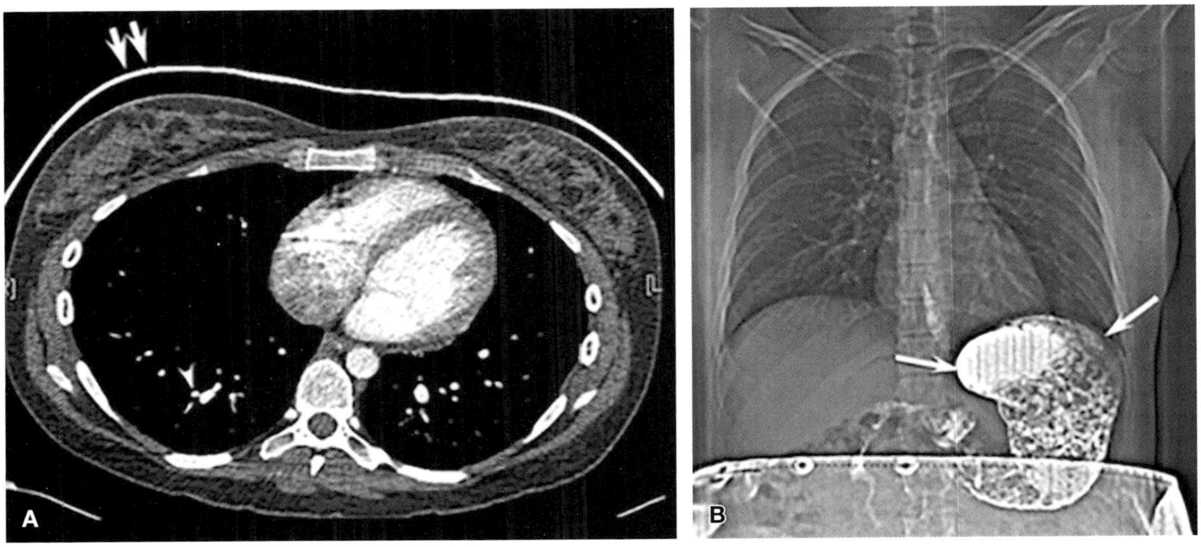

Figure 28.16. Use of multiple dose reduction methods in a pregnant woman undergoing multislice CT pulmonary angiography and combined high-resolution CT (including direct prone inspiratory and supine expiratory imaging) for dyspnea. Without any dose-reducing procedures, and employing "routine" CT parameters, the estimated maternal dose for this scan was 16.28 mGy. After the manual reduction of the mA value by 50% from the original setting, reduction of the kVp from the original value of 120 to 100, and reduction of the scan length, the estimated scan dose was reduced to 6 mGy. **A:** Axial image through the lower lobes shows a good quality examination with clear visualization of subsegmental arteries (*arrowhead*). Bismuth breast shields (*double arrows*) were also applied for this examination—note that these shields do not adversely impact image quality—although recent recommendations do not favor the use of breast shielding for dose reduction optimization. **B:** "Scout view" for the examination shows the use of internal barium shielding (*arrows*) employing a 30% solution of barium sulfate, further reducing scatter radiation to the fetus without compromising scan quality. A lead apron has also been applied.

provided radiation attenuation nearly equal to that of a 1-mm lead sheet.

It should be remembered that the CT scan projection radiograph (topogram, or "scout views") can contribute to fetal dose, particularly if the fetus is directly radiated, and therefore, care should be taken to avoid imaging the fetus directly, and the scout view should be performed only in the posteroanterior projection if possible. Finally, avoiding repeat scanning of the same anatomic region (eg, noncontrast imaging prior to CTPA) should be avoided.

Suspected VTE Evaluation During Pregnancy: Where to Start

Which study should be obtained for suspected PE in pregnant patients? The evaluation should begin with a structured clinical assessment. Lower extremity US may be performed first if lower extremity symptoms are present. If the thorax must be imaged, some investigators favor the initial use of CTPA with dose-reducing procedures, whereas others favor starting with scintigraphy. For example, 69% of the PIOPED II investigators recommend initial investigation with $\dot{V}/\dot{Q}$ scanning, and the American Thoracic Society/Society of Thoracic Radiology recommends that pregnant patients with suspected PE first be imaged with chest radiography to determine which patients should undergo $\dot{V}/\dot{Q}$ scintigraphy and which patients should undergo CTPA, limiting initial CTPA studies to those patients with abnormal chest radiographs or patients with nondiagnostic $\dot{V}/\dot{Q}$ results. With attention to dose reduction, the fetal dose resulting from CTPA will usually be less than that $\dot{V}/\dot{Q}$ scanning. While the maternal dose remains higher with CTPA, even with dose-reducing techniques, the difference should be small when careful attention to technical factors is employed. Further innovations in dose reduction and noise reduction may eventually eliminate dose differences between CTPA and $\dot{V}/\dot{Q}$ scanning all together.

One of the main drivers for the recommendation of CTPA over $\dot{V}/\dot{Q}$> scanning for the evaluation of suspected PE in pregnant patients is the perception that CTPA is more likely to be diagnostic and also provides the ability to identify alternative causes of symptoms that prompted evaluation. The latter is important because the minority of patients who undergo imaging evaluation for suspected PE will actually be diagnosed with PE. Regarding the former, the "nondiagnostic" rate of CTPA is in the range of 5% to 10%, with limited data suggesting that this rate is increased in pregnant patients. The "nondiagnostic" rate of $\dot{V}/\dot{Q}$ scintigraphy in patients with suspected PE has been reported to range from 50% to 70% but has been suggested to be as low as 25% in pregnant patients suspected of PE. Therefore, in pregnant patients suspected of PE, $\dot{V}/\dot{Q}$ scintigraphy remains a useful test and modifications to CTPA protocols to enhance image quality in pregnant patients, including the use of a shallow inspiratory breath-hold (to avoid the transient interruption of contrast artifact) and the injection of high concentration iodinated contrast media at an increased rate and volume, should be employed to overcome the untoward hemodynamic effects pregnancy may exert on CTPA scan quality.

RECENT TECHNOLOGICAL ADVANCES IN CT PE IMAGING: DUAL-ENERGY CT AND ARTIFICIAL INTELLIGENCE

"Dual-energy" CT (DECT) refers to the ability of a CT scanner to create nearly simultaneous images at two x-ray energies. CT manufacturers have approached DECT acquisitions in several different ways, including sequential scanning (initially acquiring a low-energy image followed by a second tube rotation to acquire a higher-energy image), single x-ray tubes capable of rapid kVp switching, dual-source CT simultaneous scanning with two x-ray tubes, one at lower voltage (70-100 kVp) and the other at higher voltage (140-150 kVp), and true "spectral" CT in which a dual layer detector is employed, the superficial layer absorbing lower kVp photons and the deeper layer absorbing higher kVp photons. CT imaging using x-ray beams, each with a distinct energy spectrum, has the ability to favor the photoelectric effect within the material scanned, thus allowing specific characterization and even quantification of the imaged substance. In particular, DECT allows for the "decomposition" of materials, such as water, iodine, silicone, uric acid, and calcium, by characterizing the attenuation changes at different kVps within a given voxel—these substances can thereby be specifically identified and one "subtracted" from the other to create images that highlight features of interest. For example, using DECT for CTPA, the water component of a DECT image can be subtracted from an enhanced acquisition, leaving the iodine component, thus providing a map of the iodine-enhanced blood volume of the lung, which then allows quantification of the distribution and absolute iodine within the pulmonary parenchyma.

DECT technique offers the major advantage of improving suboptimal CTPA acquisitions. Because the low monoenergetic KeV images in a DECT CTPA acquisition approach the K edge of iodine, DECT allows a lower dose of iodinated contrast media to be utilized and reconstruction of the low kVp image set improves pulmonary arterial enhancement, perhaps salvaging an otherwise nondiagnostic study (Fig. 28.17).

DECT CTPA may also provide information somewhat analogous to the perfusion scan of $\dot{V}/\dot{Q}$ scintigraphy because PEs may create "perfusion defects" on DECT images, and it has been suggested that the detection of wedge-shaped perfusion defects may allow improved detection of small emboli by drawing the interpreter's attention to an otherwise overlooked small embolus, improves interobserver agreement, and may even suggest embolic disease not directly visualized at CTPA. Note that the notion of attempting to enhance detection of even smaller emboli conflicts with the concept of the adverse effect of overdiagnosis at CTPA imaging discussed previously. In this vein, it has also been suggested that DECT PE-related perfusion defects could "provide context" to small emboli—conceivably, a small embolus that creates

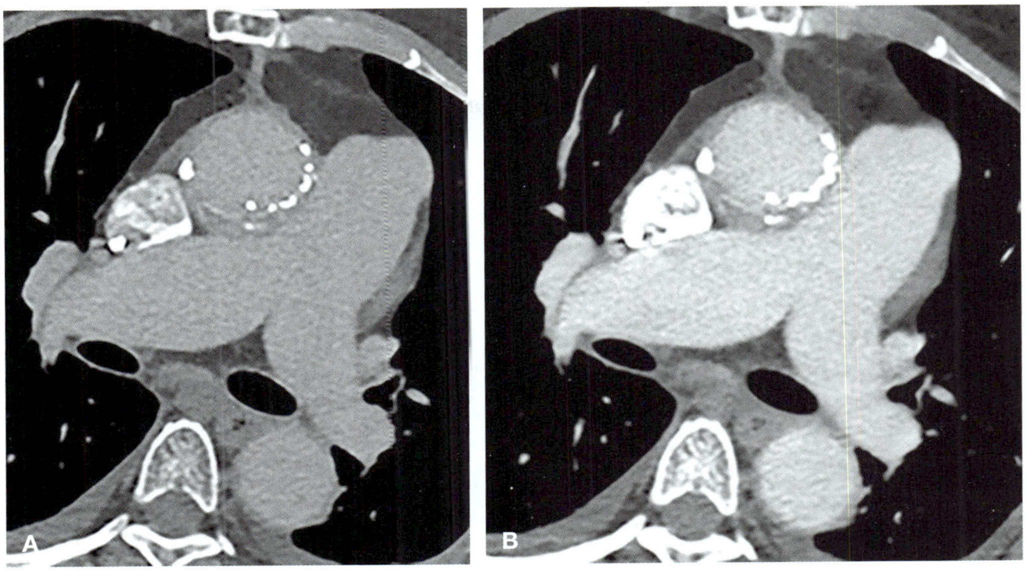

Figure 28.17. Value of dual-energy CTPA technique for salvaging a suboptimal examination. **A:** Axial CTPA image shows poor pulmonary arterial opacification (mean main pulmonary artery [PA] attenuation = 103 HU). **B:** Axial monoenergetic image (70 kVp) reconstructed from the DECT acquisition shows improved pulmonary arterial attenuation (main PA attenuation = 287 HU).

a perfusion defect may be significant enough to warrant therapy, as opposed to a small embolus unassociated with a perfusion abnormality. Note that his concept is unproven, and, furthermore, as with V/Q scintigraphy, some emboli are unassociated with substantial perfusion defects, and not all perfusion defects are the result of embolic disease. Finally, DECT CTPA may play a role in risk stratification and outcome prediction for patients with PE, with some studies indicating that pulmonary blood volume measurements show correlation with arterial obstructive indices and measures of right ventricular dysfunction. Nevertheless, at present, the role of DECT parameters for risk stratification in patients with PE remains speculative.

Artificial intelligence (AI) is a broad term implying efforts in computer programming and development designed to train machines to perform tasks as well or better than humans, particularly tasks that are laborious or repetitive. *Machine learning* can be thought of as a form of AI in which a computer is supplied with programming and large amounts of data to "learn" its own patterns, ultimately extending beyond patterns and limits set by a human programmer, effectively improving from experience. *Deep learning* is a class of machine learning techniques that employs multilayered neural networks. The application of AI to medical tasks is not new, but has exploded in recent years owing to advances in computing power, hardware capabilities, and advances in software sophistication. AI has entered medical imaging at several different levels, ranging from assisting in protocoling examinations, enhancing image acquisition quality (eg, reducing image noise while reducing image reconstruction time), improving the performance of postprocessing software, assisting in decision support analysis, and, perhaps most visibly, providing detection of findings at imaging studies.

For CTPA imaging, several commercially available software programs will, in real time, analyze CTPA datasets for the presence or absence of PE and report results to the interpretation radiologist. Typically, such results are available before the radiologist completes review of the study. The use of AI for PE detection offers the advantage of worklist prioritization (presenting studies with positive detections to the radiologist for more rapid adjudication) as well as a "second reader" function—detecting (Fig. 28.18) and excluding PE. The "second reader" function may prove particularly advantageous given that most CTPA examinations outside academic institutions are interpreted by nonthoracic radiologists. While data regarding the performance of AI for PE detection are limited, the sensitivity for PE detection is greater than 90% and the specific for the AI diagnosis of PE is at least 95%. Nevertheless, both false-positive (Fig. 28.18B also see Figure 28.14A) and false-negative (Fig. 28.18C) detections occur, and AI PE algorithms have not convincingly demonstrated to "outperform" thoracic-trained radiologists. As is the case with human readers, AI algorithms show improved PE detection sensitivity for central compared with peripheral emboli. Future iterations of PE AI detection algorithms may incorporate automated risk stratification for patients with PE by calculating the RV/LV ratio through volumetry and perhaps even "embolic load" scores.

How to Report CTPA Examinations

As with other radiologic examination reports, a structured, or semistructured, reporting scheme for CTPA examinations is advisable. In addition to components common to any chest CT report, essential elements in the CTPA report include a brief description of the technique employed, statement of

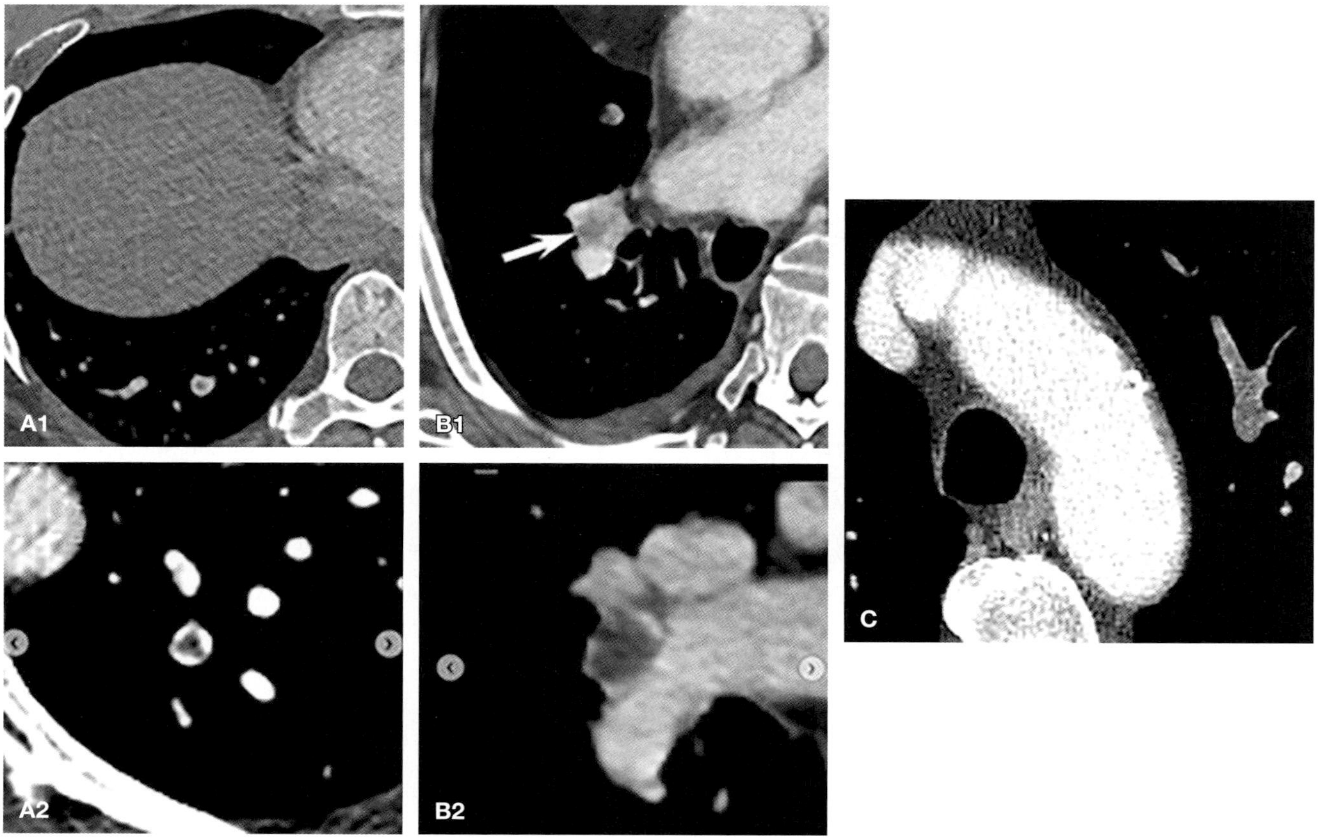

Figure 28.18. Artificial intelligence for pulmonary embolism (PE) diagnosis. **A:** True positive results. **A_1:** Axial CTPA image shows PE within a subsegmental artery, which was also identified by the artificial intelligence (AI) algorithm **(A_2)**. **B:** False-positive results. **B_1:** Axial CTPA image shows a necrotic right peribronchial lymph node *(arrow)*, the patent pulmonary artery is seen posterior to the lymph node. **B_2:** Image from the AI algorithm shows that the necrotic lymph node has been incorrectly identified as PE. Also note the lymph node in Figure 28.14A; this structure was also flagged as PE by the AI algorithm. **C:** Axial CTPA image shows a clear filling defect within an expanded left upper lobe segmental and subsegmental pulmonary artery that was not reported by the AI detection algorithm.

comparison to appropriate previous examinations, and, importantly, a statement of the quality of the examination. The quality statement could be an ordinal scale (eg, excellent, adequate, limited) or could reference the anatomic level to which the pulmonary arteries are adequately opacified (eg, central, lobar, segmental, subsegmental). As the embolic load and PE location have not been conclusively shown to predict patient outcome and management, an exhaustive description of the location and amount of embolic material is not required; it is sufficient to note the most proximal level affected by emboli on each side as well as an estimate of the number of lobes involved by PE. This point is particularly important when CTPA examinations show isolated, or solitary, subsegmental emboli.

The presence or absence of RV dysfunction, as determined by the RV/LV diameter ratio as described previously, or straightening or leftward bowing of the interventricular septum, should be explicitly stated. Ancillary findings suggestive of RV dysfunction, such as enlargement of the main pulmonary artery, great vein dilation, reflux of contrast into the IVC and hepatic veins, and a relatively small left atrium, should be noted as well as their presence may be additive to an impression of RV dysfunction, but when unaccompanied by either an increased RV/LV ratio or abnormal septal curvature, these ancillary findings are less predicative of adverse PE-related outcome and should not engender a firm impression of RV dysfunction. Other findings that may be detected in patients with PE include parenchymal opacities reflecting pulmonary hemorrhage or infarction and pleural effusion should be noted in the report. Images should also make a dedicated attempt to detect embolic material in the right heart chambers (the so-called "embolus in transit," **Video 28.3**) or, exceptionally, PE transit through a patent foramen ovale (Fig. 28.19), as such findings could alter management. The first line of the report impression should be a statement as definitive as possible as regard to the presence or absence of PE with statement of examination quality. If the examination is positive, the second line of the impression should note the presence or absence of RV dysfunction; if negative, the presence of any findings suggesting an alternative explanation for a presentation simulating PE should be offered. When examinations are equivocal for the presence or absence of PE, explicit statements

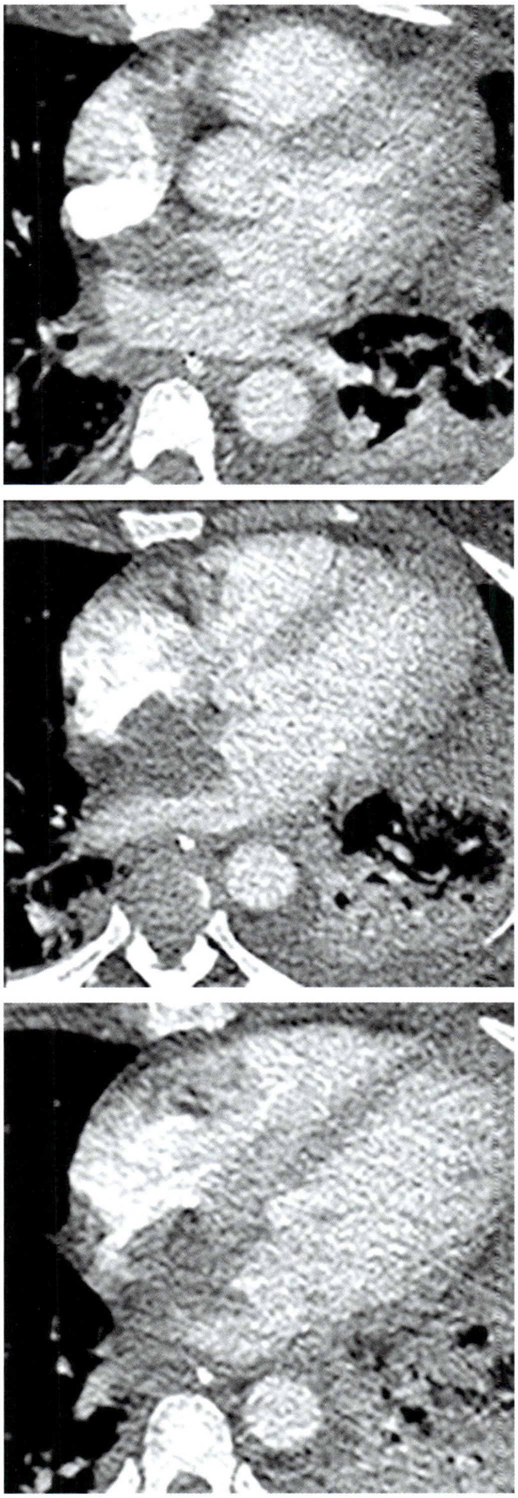

Figure 28.19. Embolus in transit. Axial CTPA images in a patient with acute pulmonary embolism shows an embolus transiting a patent foramen ovale.

regarding recommendations for additional assessment should be provided. The Radiological Society of North America offers a standard CTPA reporting template, and the American Journal of Roentgenology published an expert panel reviewing CTPA reporting; this reference is listed in the Suggested Reading at the end of this chapter.

MAGNETIC RESONANCE IMAGING

MRI of the chest presents significant challenges, including the relative lack of signal due to the paucity of protons within the lungs, susceptibility artifacts resulting from air and soft-tissue interfaces within the thorax, and image degradation from respiratory and cardiac motion. The development of faster and stronger gradients and the evolution of contrast-enhanced magnetic resonance angiography (MRA) have made rapid high-resolution imaging of the thorax and pulmonary vascular system routine, and MRI of the pulmonary vascular system has evolved significantly. Additional techniques for cardiopulmonary imaging—pulmonary perfusion MRI and hyperpolarized 3-helium—also have been investigated and may provide unique diagnostic information. MRV of the pelvis and lower extremities has been shown to be an accurate technique for the diagnosis of DVT and may be combined with the thoracic examination to provide a comprehensive evaluation for patients with suspected VTE.

Techniques

The protocol for 3D MRA varies from institution to institution; the fundamental components integral to an MR PE protocol are presented in Table 28.5. Phased-array coils are used to optimize the signal-to-noise ratio. To aid in breath-holding, the patient can be provided with oxygen by nasal cannula, at a rate of 2 L/min. Gadolinium contrast agent (0.1 mmol/kg), diluted in normal saline for a total injected volume of 30 mL, is administered via an antecubital vein with the use of a power injector (1.5-2 mL/s), or injected at a higher rate (5 mL/s) followed by a 20 mL saline bolus. The scan begins approximately 5 to 10 seconds after the start of the injection of contrast medium when imaging the pulmonary arteries. Timing of the acquisition can be optimized by using bolus triggering when the contrast bolus is seen in the right ventricle or by performing a preliminary acquisition with the use of a test bolus to estimate circulation time. The entire study can be completed in 20 minutes or less. Multiplanar maximum intensity projection reconstructions of the 3D MRA, performed on an offline workstation, often are invaluable for interpretation of the study.

Newer MR techniques that may play a role in PE imaging include MR pulmonary perfusion imaging. MR pulmonary perfusion imaging is a time-resolved technique performed with a fast, 3D low-angle shot (FLASH) gradient-echo sequence with typical sequence parameters including TR = 1.6, TE = 0.6, and a flip angle 25°. Gadolinium contrast (0.5 mmol/mL solution with a dose of 0.125 mmol/kg) is injected at 4 to 5 mL/s followed by a 20 mL saline flush at the same rate. The number of phase-encoding steps depends on the size of the imaging volume, but imaging is very rapid, typically requiring 2 seconds or less. This sequence is repeated a number of times to image the first pass of contrast through the right ventricle and pulmonary arteries, over a period of about 35 to 55 seconds. Patients are asked to suspend respiration as long as possible to minimize diaphragmatic motion.

Both contrast-enhanced MRA and pulmonary perfusion imaging benefit from the introduction of parallel imaging techniques. Parallel imaging allows signal integration from multiple elements within a phased-array receiver coil to accelerate data sampling. This results in improved spatial resolution or volume of coverage, without requiring additional acquisition time. Alternatively, parallel imaging can be used to reduce imaging time (and breath-holding time) by 50% or more. For pulmonary perfusion imaging, parallel imaging may allow for improvements in temporal resolution as well, as improvements in temporal resolution have more relevance for time-resolved imaging than improvements in volume of coverage or spatial resolution. Available parallel imaging techniques include sensitivity encoding (SENSE) and generalized autocalibrating parallel acquisition (GRAPPA). In addition to the basic MR PE protocol components presented in Table 28.5, additional sequences may be prescribed for certain applications. For example, because moving protons create phase shifts proportional to the velocity and the magnetic field gradient strength, phase-contrast imaging can be used to quantify blood flow in the pulmonary arteries, both in and through the acquisition plane. Electrocardiographically gated balanced cine steady-state free precession (SSFP) images create signal within moving blood and therefore provides angiographic images without IV contrast administration, thereby contributing to a multiparametric pulmonary arterial assessment in addition to gradient-echo images and MRA sequences. SSFP sequences can also be employed to assess ventricular function. Additional MR techniques that may prove useful for comprehensive pulmonary vascular evaluation include tissue mapping and late gadolinium enhancement sequences.

Table 28.5 Technique for MRI for Pulmonary Embolism Evaluation

	Basic Parameters	Purpose	Notes
Three-plane single-shot FSE[a] localizers	-	Planning	
Unenhanced T1-weighted 3D SGRE[b]	TR/TE ≈ 2.5-3.2/1-1.5 ms Flip angle = 28°-40°	Determine anatomic coverage	• Coronal plane
Pulmonary arterial phase T1-weighted 3D SGRE	TR/TE ≈ 2.5-3.2/1-1.5 ms Flip angle = 28°-40°	Pulmonary arterial visualization, pulmonary parenchymal perfusion	• Coronal plane • Breath-hold, but can perform free breathing
Immediate enhanced T1-weighted SGRE	TR/TE ˜ 2.5-3.2/1-1.5 ms Flip angle = 28°-40°	Pulmonary arterial visualization	• Coronal plane
Low flip angle–enhanced T1-weighted GRE	TR/TE ≈ 2.5-3.2/1-1.5 ms Flip angle = 15°	Pulmonary arterial visualization, systemic vasculature	• Coronal plane • Allows vessel wall visualization
T1-weighted 2D with fat saturation	TR/TE ≈ 3.8/2.1 ms Flip angle = 28°	Optimal review of non-vascular pathology	• Typically axial plane
Time-resolved MRA	TR/TE ≈ 2.5-3.2/1-1.5 ms Flip angle = 25°	Pulmonary arterial visualization, pulmonary parenchymal perfusion	• Coronal plane
Balanced steady-state free precession	TR/TE ≈ 3/1.5 ms Flip angle = 60°	Excellent vascular depiction, functional imaging if desired	• Free breathing using ECG gating, respiratory triggering, or breath-hold if patient is able • Axial for PE • Cardiac planes for function if desired

[a]*FSE = fast spin echo.*

[b]*SGRE = spoiled gradient-recalled echo.*

Advantages and Disadvantages of MR for Diagnosis of PE

Gadolinium-enhanced 3D MRA has proved its utility for a number of thoracic applications, including diagnosis of PE. Advantages of MRA over CTPA and catheter pulmonary angiography include the use of gadolinium-based contrast agent (rather than iodine) and the lack of ionizing radiation. Unlike iodinated contrast media, gadolinium chelates are not nephrotoxic (at the dose typically used for MRI), and the risk of contrast reaction is very low. Limitations of MRA include a relatively long breath-hold time and the fact that MR is relatively contraindicated in selected patients who may be at risk for PE, including those with pacemakers and certain other devices. Gadolinium chelate contrast agents cross the placenta and are considered class C drugs by the Food and Drug Administration, with reports of rheumatological, inflammatory, and infiltrative skin disorders in exposed neonates. Their use during pregnancy is discouraged, which is unfortunate as MRA would otherwise be an excellent test for pregnant women due to the lack of ionizing radiation. Unenhanced MRA techniques can be employed, but sensitivity suffers. Additionally, while contrast-enhanced MRA was once considered a good option for vascular imaging in patients with renal insufficiency or failure, in whom iodinated contrast-enhanced studies are contraindicated, the association of nephrogenic systemic sclerosis with gadolinium administration in patients with renal insufficiency has tempered the utility of contrast-enhanced MRI techniques in these patients. Furthermore, linear and macrocyclic gadolinium-based chelates have been associated with deposition within the skin, brain, and bones of patients with normal renal function, although the significance of this observation remains undetermined. Finally, pulmonary MR has traditionally been limited by the intrinsic poor signal within lung resulting from low proton density, prominent susceptibility artifact caused by numerous air-tissue interfaces, and cardiac and respiratory motion. Continued advances in scanner hardware (high performance gradients and improved coils), the development of parallel imaging, rapid k-space sampling, view sharing, and ultra-short and zero echo time sequences have mitigated these limitations to a significant extent.

PE Findings on MRI and MRA

MRI and MRA findings of PE depend on the imaging sequence employed. The short T1 signal of methemoglobin in pulmonary emboli produces high signal on T1-weighted imaging. On breath-hold SSFP acquisition sequences, pulmonary emboli usually appear as very-low-signal intensity filling defects within high-signal blood pool, whereas on fast gradient-echo and 3D contrast-enhanced MRA sequences, emboli appear as very-low-signal foci surrounded by high-signal intraluminal contrast (Fig. 28.20).

Much like CTPA, acute PE is diagnosed when an intra-arterial filling defect is identified. Expanded, unenhanced

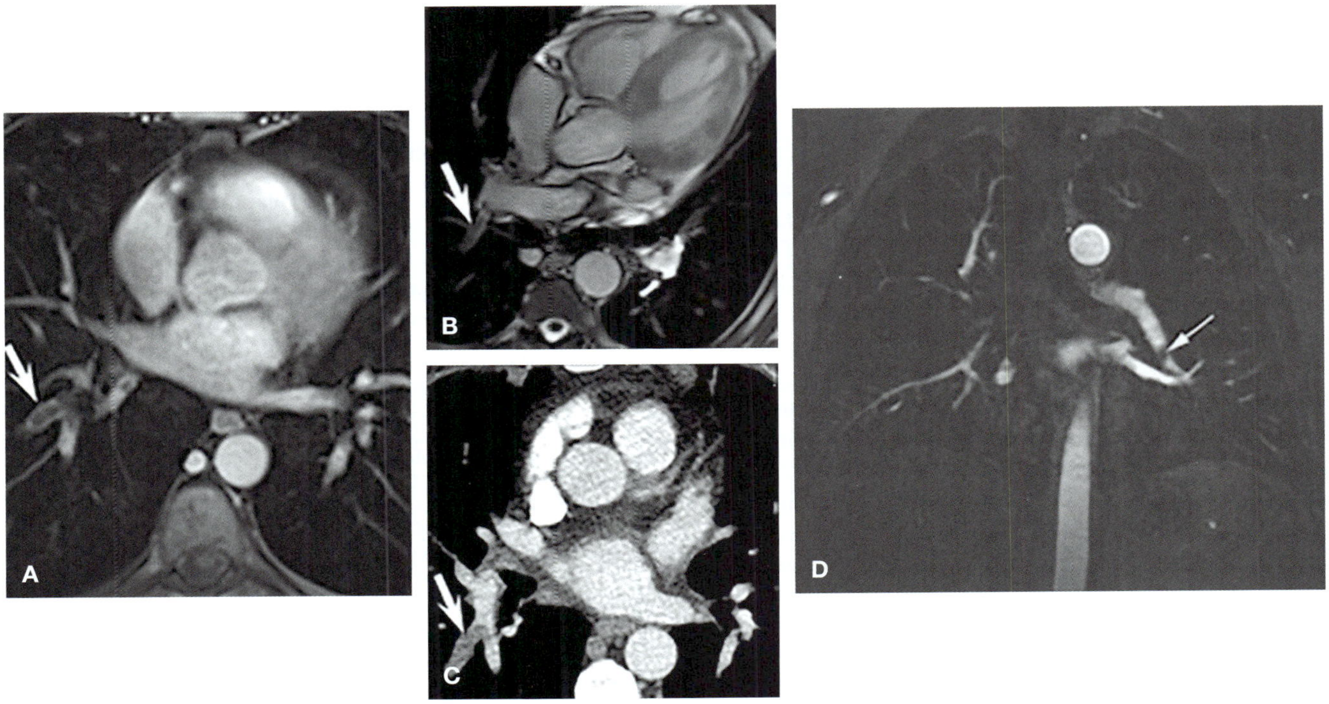

Figure 28.20. Acute pulmonary embolism (PE) on MRI. **A:** Axial fast gradient echo shows an intraluminal filling defect (*arrow*) in the lateral basal segmental right lower lobe pulmonary artery. **B:** Axial steady-state free precession image shows right lower lobe (*arrow*) pulmonary embolism, confirmed at CTPA **(C)**. **D:** Coronal MRA image shows a low-signal filling defect in the left lower lobe pulmonary artery (*arrow*), representing acute PE.

pulmonary arteries also may suggest acute pulmonary embolization. Chronic thromboembolic disease may be suggested when eccentric filling defects (see Figure 29.13) or intravascular webs are identified, often in the presence of an enlarged main pulmonary arterial segment, reflecting pulmonary hypertension.

Accuracy of MRI and MRA for the Diagnosis of PE

Studies examining the utility and accuracy of MR techniques for the diagnosis of PE are smaller and far less numerous than studies detailing other imaging methods used to evaluate patients suspected of PE, particularly CTPA. Nevertheless, data are available from both experimental and clinical studies utilizing MR for the diagnosis of PE. Pooled analysis of the results of several studies shows that the sensitivity for MR techniques for the detection of PE ranges from 75% to 100%, with specificity usually exceeding 90%. Reports of the interobserver agreement of MR examinations for PE have shown good results, although the rate of technically inadequate studies has been slightly higher for MR than for CTPA. In contrast, the PIOPED III trial examined the accuracy of gadolinium-enhanced MRA and MRV for PE diagnosis at seven medical centers and found that 25% of studies were technically inadequate (range among centers, 11% to 52%), primarily related to motion degradation or poor vascular enhancement. The overall sensitivity of MRA for PE diagnosis was 57%, increasing to 78% when focusing only on technically adequate studies; specificity was 99%. Combining technically adequate MRA and MRV increased the sensitivity for PE diagnosis to 92%, but increased the overall technical inadequacy rate. Predictably, MRI/MRA techniques show their highest sensitivity for central emboli, with diminishing sensitivity for smaller emboli, especially for subsegmental PE, a finding echoed in other studies. A limitation of the PIOPED III trial is that this study only examined the accuracy of MRA and MRV for the diagnosis of VTE; other investigations have shown that a multiparametric approach to the MRI diagnosis of PE, with the addition of enhanced 3D gradient-recalled echo, SSFP imaging, and pulmonary perfusion imaging sequences to 3D pulmonary MRA imaging, increases the sensitivity of MRI for PE diagnosis. Furthermore, the MRA techniques employed in PIOPED III utilized older hardware and did not consistently utilize newer features like parallel imaging, so scan times were longer compared to modern approaches, contributing to an increased frequency of motion artifacts and lower spatial resolution in PIOPED III compared with more recent experience. Indeed, data from 675 patients at low to intermediate risk for PE at a single center utilizing modern approaches to PE MRA imaging have shown 6-month outcomes and technical success rate following MR for PE are similar to those following CTPA.

MR Perfusion and Ventilation Imaging of the Lung

Perfusion and ventilation imaging of the lung is now possible. Several methods for pulmonary perfusion imaging exist. Pulmonary perfusion may be performed in combination with 3D MRA, using gadolinium-based contrast agents and a sequence with short TR and TE, in a time-resolved fashion, by employing the first-pass. As contrast enters the imaging volume, regions of diminished perfusion become increasingly apparent as first the vessels and then the pulmonary parenchyma enhance. This technique may allow the demonstration of pulmonary parenchymal perfusion defects as well as the intraluminal emboli producing the perfusion abnormalities in a manner analogous to that described using DECT. MR pulmonary perfusion may also be performed using blood pool agents. Because these agents circulate for a prolonged period of time, perfusion imaging of the lung may be followed by lower extremity and pelvic imaging for potential DVT. Finally, MR pulmonary perfusion may be performed with noncontrast methods, such as Fourier decomposition and arterial spin labeling; the latter technique is capable of distinguishing stationary from moving tissue and thus may provide information on pulmonary blood flow, although both techniques are more prone to artifacts and suffer from inferior signal-to-noise and spatial resolution compared with dynamic contrast-enhanced MRA.

Preliminary techniques for MR ventilation imaging have been studied in recent years. Using hyperpolarized noble gases or molecular oxygen, MR ventilation imaging is now possible. MR ventilation techniques may be combined with MR pulmonary perfusion methods to create a map of pulmonary ventilation and perfusion in a fashion similar to $\dot{V}/\dot{Q}$ scintigraphy. However, experience with these techniques currently is limited, and although they are promising, further technical refinements will be required.

SUGGESTED READINGS

Ahuja J, Palacio D, Jo N, et al. Pitfalls in the imaging of pulmonary embolism. *Semin Ultrasound CT MR*. 2022;43(3):221-229.

Allen BD, Schiebler ML, François CJ. Pulmonary vascular disease evaluation with magnetic resonance angiography. *Radiol Clin North Am*. 2020;58(4):707-719.

Bajc M, Schümichen C, Grüning T, et al. EANM guideline for ventilation/perfusion single-photon emission computed tomography (SPECT) for diagnosis of pulmonary embolism and beyond. *Eur J Nucl Med Mol Imaging*. 2019;46(12):2429-2451.

Farag A, Fielding J, Catanzano T. Role of dual-energy computed tomography in diagnosis of acute pulmonary emboli, a review. *Semin Ultrasound CT MR*. 2022;43(4):333-343.

Le Roux PY, Le Pennec R, Salaun PY, Zuckier LS. Scintigraphic diagnosis of acute pulmonary embolism: from basics to best practices. *Semin Nucl Med*. 2023;53(6):743-751.

Leung AN, Bull TM, Jaeschke R, et al; ATS/STR Committee on Pulmonary Embolism in Pregnancy. American Thoracic Society documents: an official American Thoracic Society/Society of Thoracic Radiology Clinical Practice Guideline—evaluation of suspected pulmonary embolism in pregnancy. *Radiology*. 2012;262(2):635-646.

Metter D, Tulchinsky M, Freeman LM. Current status of ventilation-perfusion scintigraphy for suspected pulmonary embolism. *AJR Am J Roentgenol*. 2017;208(3):489-494.

Miller WT Jr, Marinari LA, Barbosa E Jr, et al. Small pulmonary artery defects are not reliable indicators of pulmonary embolism. *Ann Am Thorac Soc*. 2015;12(7):1022-1029.

Nagle SK, Schiebler ML, Repplinger MD, et al. Contrast enhanced pulmonary magnetic resonance angiography for pulmonary embolism: building a successful program. *Eur J Radiol*. 2016;85(3):553-563.

Needleman L, Cronan JJ, Lilly MP, et al. Ultrasound for lower extremity deep venous thrombosis: multidisciplinary recommendations from the society of radiologists in ultrasound consensus conference. *Circulation.* 2018;137(14):1505-1515.

Pena E, Dennie C. Acute and chronic pulmonary embolism: an in-depth review for radiologists through the use of frequently asked questions. *Semin Ultrasound CT MR.* 2012;33(6):500-521.

Stein PD, Chenevert TL, Fowler SE, et al; PIOPED III Prospective Investigation of Pulmonary Embolism Diagnosis III Investigators. Gadolinium-enhanced magnetic resonance angiography for pulmonary embolism: a multicenter prospective study (PIOPED III). *Ann Intern Med.* 2010;152(7):434-W143.

Stein PD, Woodard PK, Weg JG, et al. Diagnostic pathways in acute pulmonary embolism: recommendations of the PIOPED II investigators. *Radiology.* 2007;242(1):15-21.

Tan S, Nance JW, Haramati LB, et al. Pulmonary CTA reporting: AJR expert panel narrative review. *AJR Am J Roentgenol.* 2022;218(3):396-404.

Chapter 29

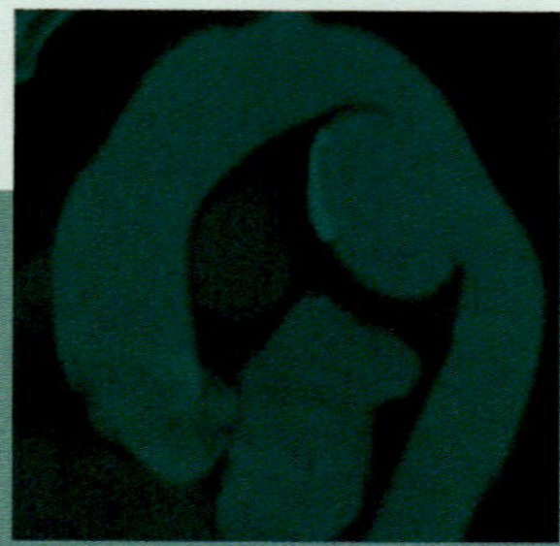

Clinton E. Jokerst • Michael B. Gotway

Pulmonary Hypertension

ANATOMY AND PHYSIOLOGY OF THE PULMONARY CIRCULATION

The pulmonary circulation consists of two parallel networks: the pulmonary arterial circulation and the bronchial arterial circulation. Pulmonary arteries carry deoxygenated blood to the alveoli for gas exchange. On the way, they course along the lobar, segmental, and subsegmental airways to the level of the respiratory bronchioles. Small pulmonary arteries from the subsegmental level to the terminal bronchioles possess a thick muscular media and range from 50 to 1000 μm in size, progressively losing much of their arteriolar media muscle as well as their external elastic membrane. By the level of the respiratory bronchioles and alveolar ducts, they are termed *pulmonary arterioles*, and range in size from 10 to 150 μm. These vessels ramify further within the alveolar walls to form a rich capillary network. Capillary blood collects in venules, which coalesce progressively to form veins, which course within the interlobular septa, eventually to empty into the left atrium.

The bronchial circulation, accounting for about 1% of the systemic cardiac output, originates from the thoracic aorta or intercostal arteries. Bronchial arteries, averaging two per lung, course within the pulmonary hila along the mainstem bronchi to the level of the terminal bronchiole and form a plexus extending from the adventitia through to the submucosa of the associated airway and adjacent pulmonary artery (PA). Bronchial arteries freely anastomose with pulmonary arteries, primarily at the capillary and postcapillary levels.

Unlike the tracheobronchial system, in which the major component to airflow resistance is located within the large airways, the major site of resistance to pulmonary arterial blood flow is located at the small muscular pulmonary arterial and arteriolar level. Caliber changes in the vessels at this level regulate pulmonary arterial pressure and are critical for optimizing ventilation and perfusion matching.

The pulmonary circulation is a low-pressure system—the mean arterial pressure is approximately one sixth that of the systemic circulation. This low pressure is maintained at a relatively consistent level even with large increases in pulmonary blood flow such as may occur with exercise. This is possible because when the body is at rest, numerous pulmonary capillaries normally are not perfused; these capillaries are "recruited" when increased pulmonary blood flow must be accommodated.

PATHOGENESIS OF PULMONARY HYPERTENSION

Definitions

Pulmonary hypertension (PH) has been recently redefined at the 6th World Symposium on PH in Nice in 2018 as a resting mean pulmonary arterial pressure (mPAP) > 20 mm Hg at rest as measured by right heart catheterization. The revised definition also stipulates that pulmonary vascular resistance (PVR) be ≥3 Wood Units (WU) for all forms of PH not due to postcapillary PH. Note that the most recent revision of the European Society of Cardiology and European Respiratory Society define the pulmonary vascular resistant upper normal limit at ~2 WU; the recommendations from this body have not yet been harmonized with the forthcoming World Symposium on PH (scheduled in 2024). Pulmonary venous hypertension, or postcapillary PH, is present when pulmonary venous pressure, usually approximated by measurement of the pulmonary (capillary) arterial wedge pressure (PAWP), exceeds 15 mm Hg. In contrast, precapillary PH is present when mPAP is >20 mm Hg at rest with PAWP ≤ 15 mm Hg and PVR ≥ 3 WU.

Pathogenesis of PH

Several mechanisms may produce a decrease in the total number of small pulmonary arteries, thereby increasing PVR and producing elevated pulmonary arterial pressure. These mechanisms include intraluminal arterial occlusion, muscular contraction of small pulmonary arteries (70-500 μm) and arterioles (20-70 μm), vascular remodeling with wall thickening, or conditions that produce pulmonary venous hypertension. Several of these mechanisms may be operative simultaneously in a patient with PH.

The pulmonary vascular endothelium responds to changes in oxygen tension, transmural pressure, and pulmonary blood flow and participates actively in the regulation of pulmonary arterial pressure through the elaboration of various vasoactive substances, such as prostacyclin, nitrous oxide, and endothelin. These agents have a direct effect on pulmonary vascular smooth muscle tone (promoting relaxation and vasodilation) and may directly affect platelet function. Abnormalities in endothelial cell function or injuries to these cells may be the fundamental derangement that ultimately produces the structural vascular changes observed in patients with PH.

Various histopathological abnormalities may be observed in patients with PH varying somewhat depending on the cause of hypertension. In general, regardless of the specific cause of the PH, the pulmonary arteries become dilated, occasionally to the point of being considered aneurysmal. Pulmonary arterial atherosclerosis, although occasionally present to a mild degree in the larger pulmonary arteries of normal adults, may be extensive in patients with PH and commonly involves small arteries. PH-related pulmonary arterial atherosclerosis pathologically appears similar to atherosclerosis in systemic arteries, although complicating features, such as necrosis, ulceration, and calcification, are relatively uncommon. Thickening of the muscular media of small pulmonary arteries is a common feature in many causes of PH and usually results from a combination of muscular hyperplasia and hypertrophy. Often, extension of muscular tissue into arterioles that normally contain no muscle, or "arterialization," may be observed in patients with PH.

The term *pulmonary plexogenic arteriopathy* refers to a constellation of histopathological vascular changes that is often encountered in patients with pulmonary arterial hypertension (PAH), including patients with hepatic disease, connective tissue disorders, congenital cardiovascular disease, and some medications previously prescribed for weight loss. Less commonly, plexogenic arteriopathy may be encountered in patients with other causes of PH. Histopathological features present in pulmonary plexogenic arteriopathy include a combination of fibrinoid necrosis, dilation lesions, plexiform lesions, intimal fibrosis, and vasculitis. Plexiform lesions affect small muscular arteries ranging in size from 100 to 200 mm, usually near vascular branch points, and consist of a focally dilated muscular vessel with a disrupted internal elastic membrane that contains very narrow vascular channels interspersed with fibroblasts and connective tissue. Plexiform lesions are characteristic of prolonged severe PH.

CLASSIFICATION OF PH

Numerous classification schemes have been developed to categorize the causes of and associations with PH. One common method classifies PH into precapillary and postcapillary etiologies (Table 29.1). In 1998, during the Second World Symposium on PH held in Evian, France, a new clinical classification system for PH emerged. The impetus for the new classification system for PH was to provide a scheme that groups diseases and conditions associated with PH according to similarities in the pathophysiologic mechanisms, clinical presentation, and treatment options. Such a classification system has obvious advantages for standardizing diagnostic approaches, conducting clinical trials, determining the effectiveness of therapy, and assessing prognosis in patients with PH. Revisions to this classification system have been undertaken approximately every 5 years since. The latest, from Nice in 2018, is presented in Table 29.2. This 6th World Symposium on PH recognizes five major categories of PH.

The 2018 Nice PH classification system is used in this chapter since it reflects the most comprehensive and advanced approach to the diagnosis, assessment, and treatment of PH.

Table 29.1 Precapillary and Postcapillary Classification of Pulmonary Hypertension

Precapillary Etiologies	Postcapillary Etiologies
1 Primary pulmonary hypertension 2 Pulmonary hypertension associated with: 2.1 Hepatic disease 2.2 HIV infection 2.3 Drugs and toxins 3 Congenital cardiovascular disease 4 Chronic thromboembolic disease 5 Nonthrombotic embolization 5.1 Neoplastic emboli 5.2 Particulates and foreign material 5.3 Parasites 6 Chronic alveolar hypoxia 6.1 Chronic obstructive pulmonary disease 6.2 Interstitial lung disease 6.3 Hypoventilation syndromes 7 Pulmonary capillary hemangiomatosis	1 Left-sided cardiovascular disease: 1.1 Mitral stenosis 1.2 Cor triatriatum 1.3 Aortic valvular disease 1.4 Cardiac tumors 2 Extrinsic pulmonary venous compression 3 Fibrosing mediastinitis 4 Pulmonary veno-occlusive disease

This system is in common use by the experts and physicians referring patients to radiologists for imaging assessment of PH. Although seemingly complex compared to PH classification systems previously used in the radiology literature, the five major disease classifications in the 2018 Nice classification broadly group the causes of PH in a fashion that is relevant to imaging and has the added benefit of providing subclassifications that serve as a reminder that PH can be associated with a number of conditions affecting various organ systems. Compared with the previous 2013 Nice classification, the major change in the 2018 Nice PH classification is the change of the definition of PH as resting mPAP from ≥25 mm Hg to >20 mm Hg at rest as measured by right heart catheterization, with the additional requirement of an increase in the PAWP and/or PVR to exclude patients with high cardiac output as a cause for elevated mPAP. The classification of PH is otherwise like the 2013 Nice approach, with some minor revisions. The 2018 Nice 6th World PH Symposium recognized the prognostic importance of elevated mPAP as a biomarker for worse outcomes in various settings and had advanced a new treatment algorithm for PAH.

GENERAL IMAGING MANIFESTATIONS

The characteristic finding of PH on chest radiography, CT, or MRI is dilation of the central pulmonary arteries with rapid tapering of the pulmonary vessels as they course peripherally, known as pulmonary arterial "pruning." This pattern is present in PH regardless of etiology.

Chest radiography may reveal enlargement of the main PA segment and dilation of the right and left main and interlobar pulmonary arteries in patients with PH of any etiology (Fig. 29.1A-D). It has been suggested that PH may be diagnosed on chest radiography if the transverse diameter of the right interlobar PA, measured from the lateral aspect of the vessel to its medial portion adjacent to the bronchus intermedius, exceeds 15 mm in women and 16 mm in men (Fig. 29.1A). Similarly, an enlarged left PA may also indicate the presence of PH. The left PA is best measured on the lateral radiograph from the orifice of the left upper lobe bronchus to the posterior aspect of the vessel; when this measurement exceeds 18 mm (Fig. 29.1B), PH probably is present. Chest radiographs may show the enlarged central pulmonary arteries rapidly tapering peripherally, referred to as pruning (Fig. 29.1E). Chest radiography may also show right-sided cardiac enlargement, manifesting as increased density occupying the retrosternal space on the lateral radiograph (Fig. 29.1F). Pulmonary parenchymal abnormalities associated with PH may be evident at chest radiography, particularly group II (left-sided heart disease), group III (obstructive or fibrotic lung disease), and some group V diseases (such as sarcoidosis).

The main PA cannot be measured on chest radiography, but it is measured easily on CT or MRI. A body of literature has addressed to ability of main PA measurement to predict

Table 29.2 Updated Clinical Classification of Pulmonary Hypertension

1. Pulmonary arterial hypertension (PAH)
- 1.1 Idiopathic PAH
- 1.2 Heritable PAH
  - 1.2.1 Bone morphogenetic protein receptor type 2 germline mutations
  - 1.2.2 Activin receptor–like kinase type 1 (endoglin) mutations, with or without hereditary hemorrhagic telangiectasia, endoglin, caveolin-1, others
  - 1.2.3 Unknown
- 1.3 Drug and toxin induced
- 1.4 Associated with:
  - 1.4.1 Connective tissue disease
  - 1.4.2 HIV infection
  - 1.4.3 Portal hypertension
  - 1.4.4 Congenital heart disease
  - 1.4.5 Schistosomiasis
- 1.5 PAH long-term responders to calcium channel blockers
- 1.6 1′ Pulmonary veno-occlusive disease and/or pulmonary capillary hemangiomatosis
- 1.7 1″ Persistent pulmonary hypertension of the newborn

2. Pulmonary hypertension secondary to left heart disease
- 2.1 PH due to left heart failure with preserved LVEF
- 2.2 PH due to left heart failure with reduced LVEF
- 2.3 Valvular disease
- 2.4 Congenital/acquired cardiovascular conditions leading to postcapillary PH

3. Pulmonary hypertension secondary to hypoxia and/or lung disease
- 3.1 Obstructive pulmonary disorders
- 3.2 Restrictive lung disease
- 3.3 Other pulmonary diseases with a mixed restrictive and obstructive pattern
- 3.4 Hypoxia without lung disease
- 3.5 Developmental disorders

4. PH due to pulmonary arterial obstruction
- 4.1 Chronic thromboembolic PH
- 4.2 Other pulmonary artery obstructions

5. Pulmonary hypertension with unclear multifactorial mechanisms
- 5.1 Hematologic disorders: chronic hemolytic anemia, myeloproliferative disorders
- 5.2 Systemic and metabolic disorders: sarcoidosis, Langerhans cell histiocytosis, glycogen storage disease, Gaucher disease, neurofibromatosis
- 5.3 Others: chronic renal failure with or without hemodialysis, fibrosing mediastinitis
- 5.4 Complex congenital heart disease

HIV, human immunodeficiency virus; LVEF, left ventricular ejection fraction; PH, pulmonary hypertension.

Reproduced with permission of the © ERS 2024: Simonneau G, Montani D, Celermajer DS, et al. Haemodynamic definitions and updated clinical classification of pulmonary hypertension. Eur Respir J. *201924;53(1):1801913. doi: 10.1183/13993003.01913-2018*

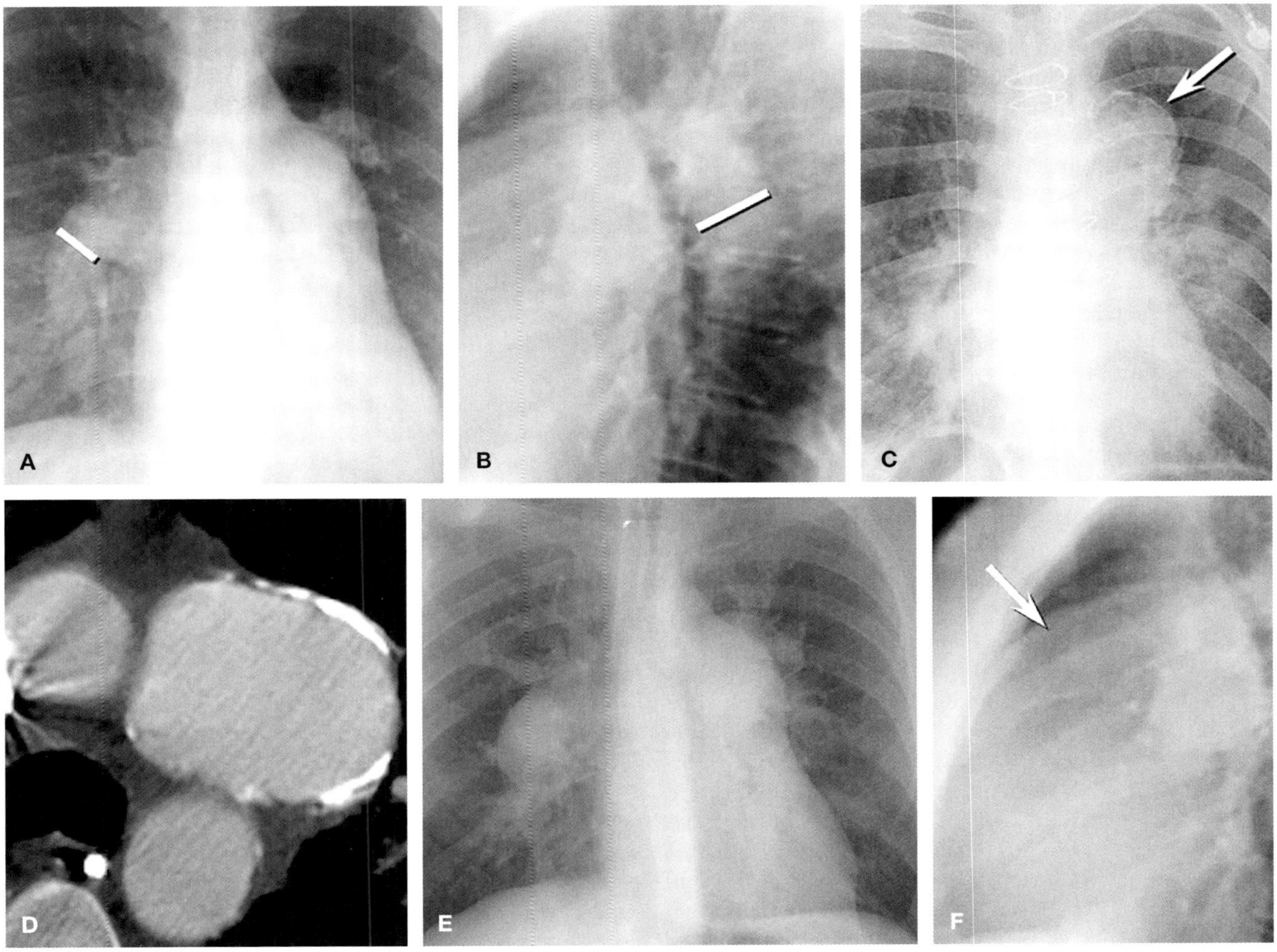

Figure 29.1. Chest radiographic findings of pulmonary hypertension (PH). Pulmonary arterial enlargement measurement. **A:** Using the frontal chest radiograph, PH is suggested if the transverse diameter of the right interlobar pulmonary artery, measured from the lateral aspect of the vessel to its medial portion adjacent to the bronchus intermedius (*line*), exceeds 15 mm in women and 16 mm in men (patient with idiopathic pulmonary arterial hypertension [PAH]). **B:** The left pulmonary artery is measured on the lateral radiograph from the orifice of the left upper lobe bronchus to the posterior aspect of the vessel (*line*). **C:** Curvilinear calcification of a dilated main pulmonary artery (*arrow*), confirmed at CT, which also shows pulmonary arterial wall calcification **(D)**, in a patient with Down syndrome and congenital heart disease. **E:** Vascular pruning. Frontal chest radiograph in a patient with portopulmonary PH shows enlarged central pulmonary arteries rapidly tapering peripherally. **F:** Enlargement of the right ventricle manifesting as increased retrosternal space opacity (*arrow*) in a patient with idiopathic PAH.

PH, with conflicting results. In general, main PA diameter correlates with mPAP, but absolute measurement cutoff values for diagnosing PH show variable accuracy, owing to differences in diagnostic criteria and reference standards for establishing PH, variable patient populations studied (eg, age, sex, body surface area, presence of lung disease, etc.), the chronicity and severity of PH, as well as how the main PA measurement is performed. Traditionally 29 mm has been regarded as the upper size limit for a normal main PA segment on axial CT or MR images. When the main PA segment exceeds this size (Fig. 29.1A), PH is usually, but not invariably, present. However, PH may be present in patients with a main PA segment that is normal in size, particularly when the mPAP duration elevation is short, as in patients with acute respiratory distress syndrome, or in patients with mild PH, as often occurs in interstitial lung or obstructive pulmonary disease. Furthermore, the accuracy of this main PA measurement cutoff value has not been adequately validated following the change in the 2018 World Symposium on PH threshold from mPAP ≥25 mm to ≥20 mm Hg. It must also be noted that an enlarged main PA can be set in patients *without* PH, particularly patients with fibrotic lung disease. Recognizing the variable performance of main PA measurement accuracy for PH diagnosis, the Fleischner Society has advocated scaling the main PA measurement threshold according to the risk (low, intermediate, high) of PH. For patients at low risk for PH, a main PA diameter threshold measurement of >34 mm is suggested for diagnosing PH, whereas thresholds of 32 and 30 mm are suggested for diagnosing PH in patients at intermediate (connective tissue disease, portal hypertension, HIV, previous pulmonary embolism, etc.) and high (eg, left heart disease, obstructive pulmonary disease, interstitial lung disease, etc.) risk, respectively, for PH.

Rather than measuring the main PA, one may compare the size of the main PA with the ascending aorta near the base of the heart. If the main PA is visibly larger than the aorta, elevated pulmonary pressure is usually present (Fig. 29.2A and B) although this approach is not applicable in the presence of ascending aortic dilation.

When PH is prolonged and severe, calcification of the pulmonary arteries (Figs. 29.1D and 29.2B) may occur. This usually affects the main, right, or left pulmonary arteries and, less commonly, the lobar pulmonary arteries. This finding usually, but not invariably, is associated with irreversible vascular disease. Eccentric filling defects, reflecting mural thrombus or eccentric emboli, may be encountered at CT in patients with PH. Other CT features suggestive of PH include right heart enlargement (Fig. 29.2C), right ventricular (RV) hypertrophy (Fig. 29.2D), and distension of the inferior vena cava (IVC) with reflux of injected contrast into the IVC and hepatic veins (Fig. 29.2E). Recently, attention has been directed toward atrial and ventricular measurements to determine the presence of elevated mPAP. Chamber volumetry, even using ungated CT scans, has been shown to be of value for predicting elevated right heart pressure, particularly when such measurements are expressed as ratios such as RV/left ventricular (LV) diameter or volume. Additionally, when the main pulmonary is enlarged and the segmental PA-to-bronchus ratio exceeds 1:1 in ≥3 pulmonary lobes (Fig. 29.2F), PH is likely present. Pulmonary parenchymal findings that may be encountered in patients with PH include foci of centrilobular ground-glass opacity (Fig. 29.2G), and often nodular and angiocentric—the latter may reflect plexogenic lesions, cholesterol granulomas, or hemorrhage; "corkscrew" peripheral pulmonary arteries (Fig. 29.2H); and mosaic perfusion (Fig. 29.2I and J). Certain lung parenchymal findings that may be seen in PH, such as interlobular septal thickening, subpleural opacities reflecting previous infarction (Fig. 29.2J), airway disease, and features of alveolitis or fibrosis, may suggest a particular PH etiology and will be discussed in the context of such lesions. Rarely, PA dissection may occur in patients with PH (Fig. 29.2K).

Although chest radiography and CT scanning often suggest the presence of PH, echocardiography is the most used examination for noninvasive assessment of possible PH. Echocardiography provides noninvasive estimation of pulmonary arterial pressures and allows detailed morphologic evaluation of the right ventricle. Echocardiography is also very useful for the assessment of LV morphology and function as well as valvular function. Echocardiography also is used for the assessment of the hemodynamic changes in the pulmonary arterial circulation in response to a variety of challenges, such as exercise or pharmacologic agents; this technique is termed *stress echocardiography*. Echocardiography does have some limitations, particularly difficulty obtaining appropriate acoustic windows in patients with emphysema or obesity, as well as operator dependence. Also, the complex anatomical shape of the right ventricle can make the echocardiographic assessment of RV dimensions challenging. It is worth noting that echocardiography is often used to estimate PA systolic pressure, but this estimate requires the presence of a tricuspid regurgitant jet, which may be absent in a significant fraction of PH patients. The echocardiographic estimate of PA systolic pressure ultimately carries only a moderate correlation with right heart catheterization measurement of pulmonary arterial pressure. Therefore, echocardiography is used to screen for PH, but is not a reliable method for diagnosing PH nor for categorizing PH phenotypes.

MRI can provide functional information equivalent to that available from echocardiography (including stress echocardiography), such as direction and velocity of blood flow and detection and quantification of shunt. MRI provides this information while also providing the specific anatomic information that is attainable from CT, such as main PA and RV size (Fig. 29.3A and B). Cardiac MR also shows features suggesting elevated PA pressure, such as straightening and leftward bowing of the interventricular septum (Fig. 29.3C). Nonischemic foci of delayed enhancement, particularly at the RV insertion points (Fig. 29.3D), may be encountered. MR also allows assessment of RV wall thickness and function. The RV ejection fraction is an important prognostic indictor for PH patients (Fig. 29.3F and G). More recent studies using MR for the diagnosis of PH have noted that features such as the interventricular septal angle, PA pulsatility, ventricular mass index, pulmonary contrast transit times, and a visual scoring system of artifacts due to slow pulmonary blood flow (average pulmonary blood flow velocity is inversely correlated with PA pressure) using ECG-gated spin-echo double inversion recovery sequence are capable of distinguishing PH and non-PH patients. The technical aspects of the MR examination for patients with suspected PH are beyond the scope of this review but are reviewed in detail in several excellent sources in the Suggested Reading at the end of this chapter. MRI provides excellent depiction of characteristics suggesting PH, and some MRI features have shown prognostic significance for patients with PH, including RV volumes (particularly RV end-systolic volume index), RV ejection fraction, and RV stroke volume index. Despite this, noninvasive imaging findings have not replaced the need for right heart catheterization to establish the diagnosis and severity of PH; in particular, right heart catheterization is required to identify patients with idiopathic PAH (IPAH) that are likely to benefit from calcium antagonist therapy.

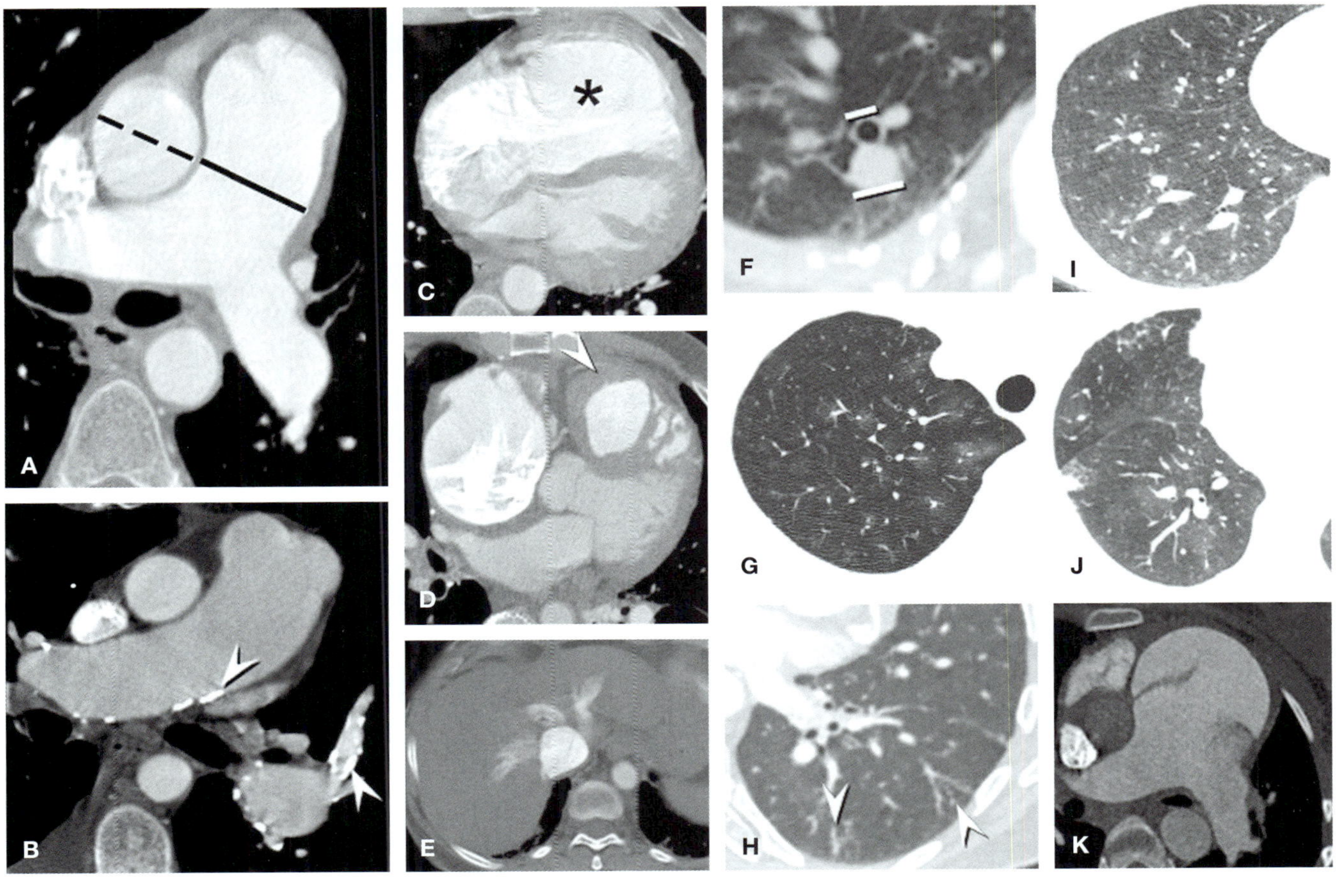

Figure 29.2. A-K: CT findings of pulmonary hypertension (PH). **A:** Pulmonary arterial enlargement measurement (*solid line*; transverse dimension 36 mm, larger than aorta at same level, *dashed line*). **B:** Enlarged pulmonary artery with wall calcification (*arrowhead*) representing atherosclerosis in a patient with idiopathic pulmonary arterial hypertension (PAH). **C:** Enlarged right ventricle (*) in a patient with HIV-related PAH. **D:** Right ventricular hypertrophy (*arrowhead*) in a patient with PAH related to congenital heart disease. Right atrial dilation is also evident. **E:** Reflux of injected intravenous contrast into a dilated inferior vena cava and hepatic veins. **F:** Enlarged peripheral pulmonary arteries manifesting as a decreased broncho-arterial ratio. **G:** Poorly defined ground-glass opacity nodules with a perivascular distribution in a patient with idiopathic PAH. **H:** "Corkscrew" vessels (*arrowheads*) in a patient with congenital heart disease. **I:** Inhomogeneous lung attenuation representing mosaic perfusion in a patient with acute cor pulmonale due to neoplastic thrombotic microangiopathy resulting from breast cancer. **J:** Peripheral nodular opacity reflecting previous infarction in a patient with chronic thromboembolic PH. **K:** Severely enlarged main pulmonary artery with dissection.

Imager's Approach to PH

The radiologist typically encounters PH in one of three ways:

1. One or more of the aforementioned imaging features suggestive of PH is detected and the diagnosis of PH must be confirmed or refuted;
2. Clinical features known to represent risk factors for PH are detected at imaging and the presence of PH must be sought; or
3. The clinical indication for the study has established the presence of PH and imaging features suggesting that the potential etiology for the PH should be sought, or at least certain PH phenotypes excluded.

Regarding 1 and 2, the imaging findings of PH have been reviewed above, and we will now turn to the individual disorders associated with PH using the classification approach advocated by the 6th World Symposium on PH in Nice in 2018 with special attention to imaging findings that may suggest a particular etiology for PH.

PAH (WHO GROUP 1)

PAH is a syndrome that results from restriction of blood flow through the pulmonary arteries, leading to increased PVR and eventually to right heart failure. PAH can usually be attributed to an imbalance between vasodilating agents and vasoconstricting agents, with a relative paucity

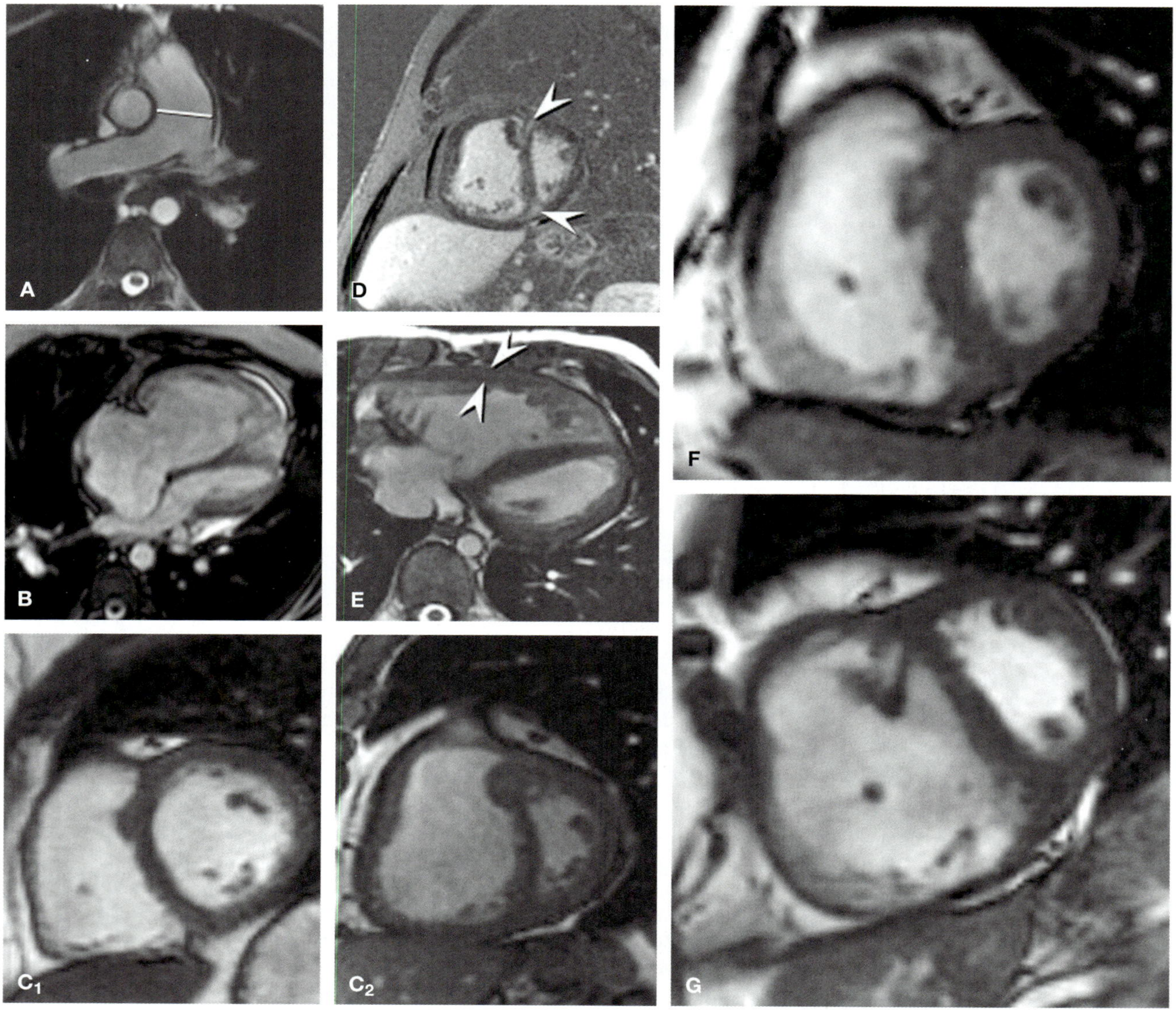

Figure 29.3. MR findings of pulmonary hypertension (PH) in pulmonary arterial hypertension (Group 1). **A:** Axial steady-state free precession image shows main pulmonary arterial enlargement (*line*; transverse dimension 37 mm also larger than aorta at same level). **B:** 4-chamber steady state free precession image shows right ventricular enlargement with interventricular septal flattening. **C_1 and C_2:** Short-axis steady-state free precession image in a patient with mild PH (**C_1**, mean pulmonary arterial pressure [mPAP] = 24 mm Hg) shows normal interventricular septal curvature, whereas leftward bowing of the interventricular septum is present in a patient with severe group 1 PH (**C_2**, mPAP = 58 mm Hg). **D:** Late gadolinium enhancement short-axis image shows ventricular insertion point delayed enhancement (arrowheads). **E:** 4-chamber steady-state free precession image shows right ventricular free wall hypertrophy (6 mm; between *arrowheads*. Normal is <4 mm). Patient with Eisenmenger syndrome (note that right ventricle is only moderately enlarged). **F:** Short-axis steady-state free precession image shows right ventricular enlargement with mild interventricular septal flattening (right ventricular ejection fraction = 49%). **G:** Short-axis steady-state free precession image 9 y after (F) shows marked right ventricular enlargement with leftward displacement of the interventricular septum with a "D"-shaped left ventricle (right ventricular ejection fraction = 16%).

of prostacyclin and nitric oxide synthase expression and an increase in expression of vasoconstrictive compounds, such as endothelin-1 and thromboxane A_2. A relative procoagulant state is present. Also, inflammatory mediators, such as certain proinflammatory cytokines and autoantibodies, may also abound, suggesting that inflammation may play a role in the development of PAH in some patients.

The inciting factors are not always clearly known, but the pathological progression of PAH has been well characterized. Arterial medial hypertrophy, intimal proliferation and fibrosis, necrotizing arteritis, and plexiform lesions are manifestations of the progressive obliterative pulmonary vasculopathy. Superimposed organized thrombi may be present. As outlined in Table 29.2, PAH consists of several subcategories, including IPAH, heritable (familial) PAH, and PAH associated with a number of conditions, including drugs and toxins and several systemic conditions.

Etiology and Pathogenesis of PAH

The prevalence of PAH is ~15 per million, perhaps greater by some estimates. IPAH is the most common form of PAH and affects women more commonly than men. IPAH represents patients with sporadic disease (no family history of PH) and no identifiable risk factors. The term *primary PAH*, formerly in wide use, encompasses what is now considered IPAH, heritable PAH, and anorexigen-induced PAH. Heritable PAH (formerly referred to as familial PAH in the Evian-Venice/World Health Organization classifications of PH) may be associated with several genetic derangements, including mutations in bone morphogenetic protein receptor 2 and activin receptor–like kinase type 1, the latter most commonly coexisting with hereditary hemorrhagic telangiectasia. In recent years, a number of new genetic mutations that are associated with PAH, including mutations in the transforming growth factor (TGF)-β super family, such as activin-like receptor kinase 1, endoglin, and mothers against decapentaplegic 9, have been identified, as have other mutations affecting non–TGF-β genes, such as the gene coding for caveolin-1 and the gene encoding the potassium channel KCNK3. Heritable PAH accounts for less than 10% of cases of PAH. PAH is also associated with several other conditions, including exposures to certain drugs or toxins, connective tissue diseases, human immunodeficiency virus (HIV) infection, congenital heart diseases associated with systemic-to-pulmonary shunts, portal hypertension, and schistosomiasis. Among the drug or toxic causes of PAH, potential etiologic agents are classified according to the strength of the evidence supporting their causal role in the development of PAH as "definite" such as appetite suppressants, benfluorex (used to treat diabetes and metabolic syndrome), and dasatinib or "possible" such as cocaine, phentermine, and interferons, among others.

PAH is associated with connective tissue diseases but is best established in the setting of systemic sclerosis. Progressive systemic sclerosis produces changes in the vasculature more commonly than rheumatoid arthritis or systemic lupus erythematosus and, therefore, has a higher association with PH. The incidence of PH in patients with systemic sclerosis ranges from 5% to 19%. PH in patients with systemic sclerosis is a marker for poor prognosis. PAH is not the only cause of elevated pulmonary arterial pressure in patients with systemic sclerosis—obviously, myocardial dysfunction (group 2 PH) and fibrotic lung disease (group 3 PH) may contribute to PH. It is important to note that PAH in patients with systemic sclerosis, and possibly other connective tissue diseases (particularly systemic lupus erythematosus, Sjögren syndrome, mixed connective disease, polymyositis, and rheumatoid arthritis), may occur independently of coexistent pulmonary and cardiac disease.

PAH is a rare complication of HIV infection and shares close similarities with IPAH in clinical, histopathological, and hemodynamic findings. The cause of PAH in patients with HIV infection is unknown, but humoral or indirect viral effects are suspected because the presence of viral DNA or the HIV virus itself has not been isolated from the pulmonary vascular endothelium.

Untreated congenital heart defects, particularly those with left-to-right shunting, may develop PAH. Prolonged exposure of the pulmonary vasculature to increased blood flow and pressure results in arteriopathy, which eventually leads to persistently elevated PVR. The histopathological changes in PAH associated with congenital heart disease are similar to IPAH. Ultimately, pulmonary arterial pressure may rise sufficiently to produce shunt reversal and cyanosis—this situation is referred to as Eisenmenger syndrome.

PAH may be associated with portal hypertension—the so-called portopulmonary hypertension. The prevalence of PH in the setting of portal hypertension based on hemodynamic studies has been estimated at 2% to 6%. While liver disease is the primary condition associated with portal hypertension, the defining risk factor for portopulmonary hypertension is the presence of portal hypertension itself, not hepatic disease. The proposed mechanism for the development of PH in patients with portal hypertension is thought to be the incomplete hepatic degradation of humoral factors that exert vasoconstricting and inflammatory effects on the pulmonary circulation. While portopulmonary hypertension may be associated with autoimmune hepatitis and female sex, some studies have not found a sex predilection and not infrequently the diagnosis of portopulmonary hypertension is established in patients without a known cause for hepatic disease. Other causes of elevated pulmonary arterial pressures are often present in patients with liver disease and portal hypertension, such as increased circulating fluid volume, a hyperdynamic circulatory state, and diastolic dysfunction, but, unlike portopulmonary hypertension, these conditions are uncommonly associated with elevated PVR. Because the causes of PH in patients with portal hypertension may be multifactorial, right heart catheterization is required to establish the diagnosis of portopulmonary hypertension.

PAH may occur in patients with schistosomiasis, particularly those with hepatosplenic involvement. Schistosomiasis may be the most common cause of PAH worldwide and is discussed farther on.

Clinical Presentation

Patients with PAH usually present with dyspnea on exertion. Other presenting symptoms include fatigue, syncope, chest pain, and, occasionally, cough. Raynaud phenomenon may be present in certain patients, particularly those with PH associated with connective tissue diseases such as systemic lupus erythematosus and progressive systemic sclerosis.

PAH is about 2 to 5 times more common in women than men, with this ratio influenced by age, etiology of PAH, and geography. A mean age of diagnosis of 37 years has been noted previously, but recent data suggest that the age range of PAH may be evolving, and the disease is increasingly reported in older patients—a more recent PH registry study noted a mean age of PAH diagnosis of 56 years.

Portopulmonary hypertension usually occurs in the setting of cirrhosis and very rarely in patients with noncirrhotic portal hypertension due to portal fibrosis or multifocal nodular hyperplasia, although most patients with cirrhosis do not develop PAH. However, the rate may be higher when considering patients with severe cirrhosis, such as those awaiting liver transplantation. PAH associated with cirrhosis improves slowly following liver transplantation.

Patients with HIV-associated PH have a presentation similar to that of patients with PAH. Patients are often still relatively immunocompetent—in most, the CD4 count is above 200 cells/mL at presentation. Prior to the era of highly active antiretroviral therapy (HAART), PAH associated with HIV survival was poor, but with the advent PAH-specific treatment, survival has improved considerably. It is unclear if HAART positively impacts PAH-related mortality in HIV, but HAART has clearly improved overall survival in these patients, allowing other causes of PH, such as cardiac (group 2) and pulmonary disease (group 3), to supplant PAH as the leading cause of PH in these patients.

The prognosis of untreated PAH is generally poor with a mean survival of 2.8 years, but has improved over the last several decades with treated PAH patients now surviving for 10 years, or more, following initial diagnosis. Survival rates vary among the conditions associated with PAH, being comparatively worse in patients with systemic sclerosis and relatively better in patients with congenital heart disease. Factors that predict poor survival in patients with PAH include poor exercise capacity, advanced World Health Organization functional class, RV dysfunction, elevated right atrial pressure, presence of systemic sclerosis, elevated brain natriuretic peptide, and low cardiac output.

Imaging Manifestations

Chest imaging in patients with PAH shows enlargement of the main, right, and left pulmonary arteries (Figs. 29.1 and 29.4), often with enlargement of the right ventricle and right atrium.

High-resolution CT (HRCT) may show that the peripheral pulmonary arteries are substantially larger than usual (Fig. 29.5). CT (Fig. 29.2), MR, MR perfusion, and functional MR techniques (Fig. 29.3) will show pulmonary arterial enlargement and other features of PH as well.

HRCT may demonstrate inhomogeneous lung opacity, representing the presence of differential pulmonary parenchymal perfusion. The regions of decreased pulmonary parenchymal attenuation represent areas of mosaic perfusion, and the vessels in these regions of lung are often visibly smaller than their counterparts in regions of increased lung attenuation. Although airway diseases may result in a similar pattern of mosaic perfusion, vascular and airway causes of mosaic perfusion may be distinguished using postexpiratory imaging. When due to airway diseases, differences in lung attenuation become accentuated with postexpiratory imaging, whereas a proportional increase in attenuation in areas of both increased and decreased attenuation is expected for patients with pulmonary vascular disease.

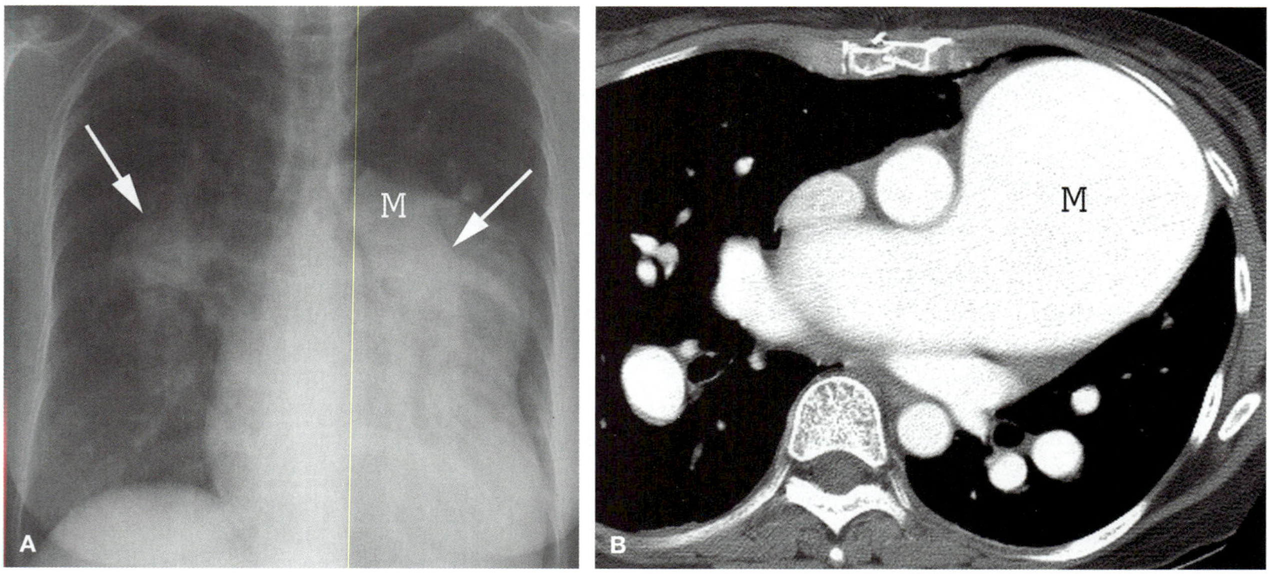

Figure 29.4. Pulmonary hypertension: pulmonary arterial enlargement. **A:** Frontal chest radiograph shows massive enlargement of the main pulmonary artery (*M*) and bilateral interlobar pulmonary arteries (*arrows*) in a patient with Eisenmenger syndrome. **B:** CT shows massive enlargement of the main pulmonary artery (*M*).

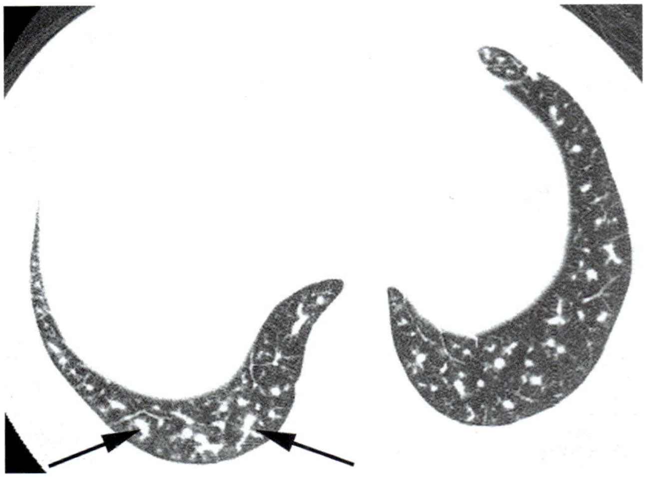

Figure 29.5. Pulmonary arterial hypertension: enlargement of peripheral pulmonary arteries. Axial CT through the lung bases in a patient with fenfluramine-induced pulmonary hypertension shows that the peripheral pulmonary arteries are abnormally large (*arrows*).

Occasionally, HRCT shows centrilobular ground-glass opacities in patients with PH (Fig. 29.2G), representing foci of hemorrhage or cholesterol granulomas.

Ventilation/perfusion (V-Q) scintigraphy commonly is abnormal in patients with PAH and often is interpreted as having low probability for pulmonary thromboembolism.

Catheter pulmonary angiography in patients with PAH shows tapering peripheral vessels with a "corkscrew" appearance, occasionally with visualization of subpleural collateral vessels.

In general, many of the conditions associated with PAH are indistinguishable radiographically from one another. In patients with connective tissue disease, associated PAH may show evidence of fibrotic lung disease, although the presence of relatively mild fibrotic lung disease does not predict that PH will be mild. Occasionally, other thoracic findings associated with connective tissue diseases, such as a dilated esophagus in systemic sclerosis or connective tissue–associated pulmonary findings, may be seen. However, patients with congenital cardiovascular disease associated with PAH may have very specific imaging findings that allow an accurate diagnosis. Also, imaging is often used for serial evaluation and assessment of therapy in these patients. Therefore, PAH associated with congenital cardiovascular disease merits further discussion.

Congenital Cardiovascular Diseases: Systemic-to-Pulmonary Shunts

Etiology and Pathogenesis

Intracardiac and extracardiac systemic-to-pulmonary shunts (left-to-right shunts), such as ventricular septal defects, atrial septal defects, partial anomalous pulmonary venous return, and patent ductus arteriosus, produce increased blood flow through the pulmonary arterial bed. This increased pulmonary arterial flow produces persistently increased vasomotor tone within the pulmonary arteries and eventually may lead to the development of pulmonary plexogenic arteriopathy and irreversible vasculopathy. Eventually, the systemic-to-pulmonary shunting may reverse, producing a pulmonary-to-systemic shunt (Eisenmenger syndrome).

Clinical Presentation

Many patients with congenital cardiovascular disease and systemic-to-pulmonary shunts are asymptomatic. Among patients who do experience symptoms, palpitations, fatigue, shortness of breath, and dyspnea on exertion commonly are reported. Cardiac failure may ensue in some patients. Physical examination may reveal suggestive cardiac murmurs.

Imaging Manifestations

Chronic increase in pulmonary flow causes the stereotypical imaging changes associated with PH—increased size of the pulmonary trunk and central pulmonary arteries (Fig. 29.1D), diminished peripheral vessel caliber (pruning), and RV chamber dilatation and possibly hypertrophy (Fig. 29.2D). Other associations include pulmonic and tricuspid regurgitation, right atrial dilatation, and fibrosis at the RV insertion points on delayed enhanced imaging from cardiac MRI. It is important to note, however, that decreasing, or relatively normal, chamber size can represent increasing pulmonary pressures with progression toward Eisenmenger physiology as pulmonary pressures overcome systemic pressures and there is reversal of intracardiac shunting (right-to-left) (Fig. 29.3E).

CT may display calcification (Figs. 29.1D and 29.2B) and thrombus within the main pulmonary arteries secondary to high pressure and turbulent flow within the affected vessels, and also provides a direct view of abnormal vascular connections such as atrial septal defects, partial anomalous pulmonary venous return (Fig. 29.6), and patent ductus arteriosus.

MRI, in addition to revealing dilated pulmonary arteries and enlargement of the right ventricle, quantifying shunt, and providing assessment of ventricular function also may directly show abnormal atrial or ventricular connections (Fig. 29.7A) as well as abnormal intravascular signal, such as flow jets between vascular chambers of different pressure (see Fig. 29.7B).

Pulmonary Veno-occlusive Disease and/or Pulmonary Capillary Hemangiomatosis (WHO Group 1′)

Pulmonary veno-occlusive disease (PVOD) and pulmonary capillary hemangiomatosis (PCH) have repeatedly undergone reclassification in prior systems, but are now grouped together because both conditions share similar histopathological features, clinical presentations, and risk factors for disease development, and are regarded as different manifestations of the same process. These risk factors include mutations in the bone morphogenetic protein receptor 2

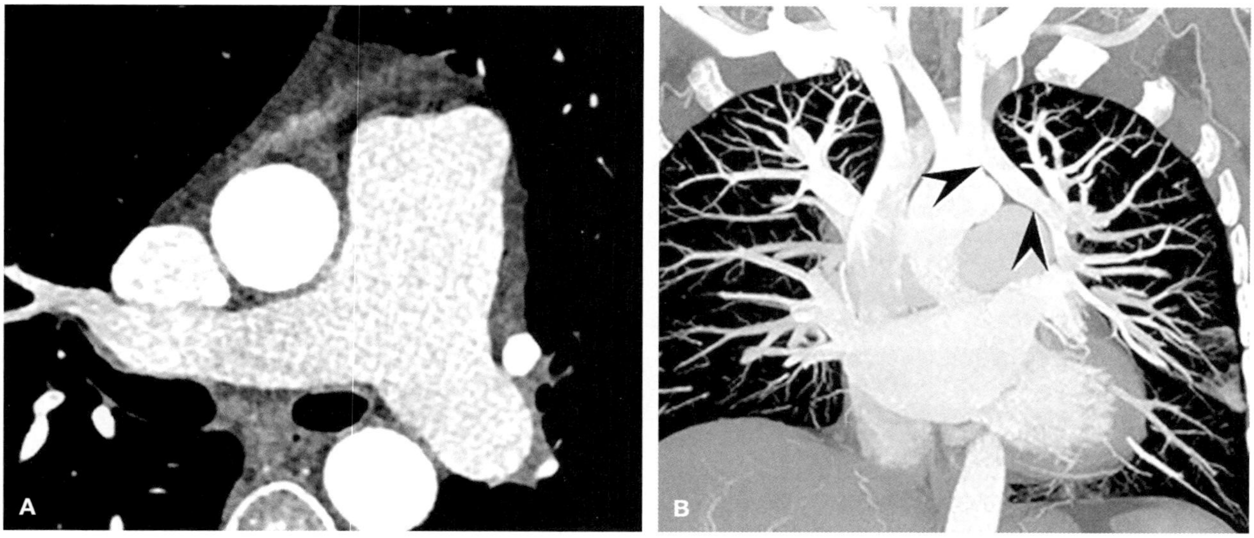

Figure 29.6. Pulmonary hypertension due to congenital cardiovascular disease. **A:** Axial image from a CTA examination shows enlargement of the main pulmonary artery (35 mm); ascending aorta measures 28 mm. **B:** Coronal maximum intensity projection image shows left upper lobe partial anomalous pulmonary venous return (*arrowheads*) emptying into the left brachiocephalic vein.

and eukaryotic translation initiation factor 2 alpha kinase 4 (EIF2AK4) gene, drugs (bleomycin, carmustine, and cisplatin, among others), toxic exposures, and stem cell marrow transplantation. Both immunologic mechanisms and viral infections have been implicated as potential etiologies in this disorder as well, although most cases are idiopathic.

A characteristic hemodynamic feature of PVOD/PCH is normal PAWP (normal ≤12 mm Hg) with normal left atrial and LV function and pressures. Pathology along the PVOD spectrum affects the venous bed in a patchy distribution, which may produce some variability in wedge pressure measurements. Occasionally, elevations in PAWP are reported, but as a general rule, PAWP measurements are normal in patients with PVOD/PCH and do not differ from patients with other forms of PAH. Histopathologically, hemosiderosis with fibrous intimal obliteration of pulmonary venules with acute or recanalized thrombi is present in patients with PVOD. Plexiform lesions are typically absent.

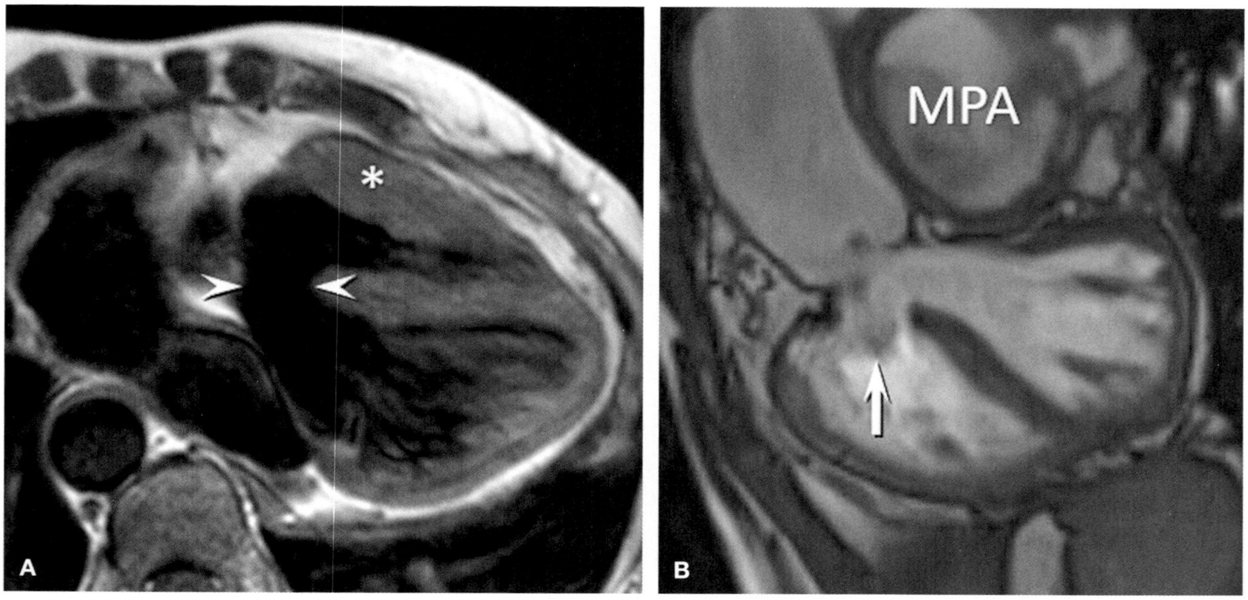

Figure 29.7. Pulmonary hypertension due to congenital cardiovascular disease. **A:** Axial T1-weighted spin-echo image shows a supracristal ventricular septal defect (*arrowheads*). Note significant right ventricular hypertrophy (*). **B:** Coronal cine image shows a low-signal flow jet within the right ventricle (*arrow*), confirming left-to-right shunting through the ventricular septal defect. Note massively dilated main pulmonary artery (MPA).

Histopathologically, abnormalities in patients along the PCH spectrum involve the small pulmonary arteries, pulmonary venules, and pulmonary capillaries. Proliferating capillaries are present and may invade small pulmonary arteries, veins, and alveolar septa, but this process occurs in a patchy fashion, resulting in normal PAWP measurements. Progressive scarring with in situ thrombosis develops, with pulmonary infarcts occurring as a result of vascular obliteration.

PVOD/PCH histopathologically shows evidence of pulmonary hemosiderosis, interstitial edema, and dilation of the lymphatic systems, as well as pulmonary vascular intimal fibrosis and medial hypertrophy. The common presence of the latter two features contributed to the classification of PVOD and PCH together as a condition associated with PAH (group 1). PVOD/PCH share similarities with PAH, such as reports of a familial association. However, there are important differences between PAH and PVOD/PCH, particularly as regards imaging features and treatment. For this reason, PVOD/PCH continues to be included under group 1 (PAH) in the 2018 6th World Symposium on PH classification scheme, but as a separate subcategory, group 1' (one prime) (Table 29.2).

Clinical Presentation

The PVOD spectrum of PVOD/PCH is a rare disorder occurring in approximately 0.1 to 0.2 per million individuals. Patients with PVOD present with chronic, progressive dyspnea, and malaise, usually during childhood and adolescence, but a second age peak between 60 and 80 years is recognized. It is important to distinguish between patients presenting with PVOD/PCH and those with interstitial lung disease because therapy for interstitial lung disease–induced PH is vasodilation, which could precipitate pulmonary edema, sometimes fatal, in patients with PVOD/PCH. The prognosis for PVOD is poor, with most patients dying within 3 years of diagnosis.

The PCH spectrum of PVOD/PCH is also a rare disorder, said to present at a mean age of 29 years, usually affecting patients between 20 and 40 years of age, although the disorder has been reported in the pediatric population as well. Disease onset is often insidious, with affected patients usually complaining of cough, dyspnea, and weight loss. Less commonly, patients may present with fever, upper respiratory tract infection, or even hemothorax. In pediatric patients, thrombocytopenia may occur. Mean survival in patients with PCH is approximately 3 years, with patients often dying of cor pulmonale. Lung transplantation is the definitive therapy for both PVOD and PCH.

Imaging Manifestations

Chest radiography in patients with the PVOD spectrum of PVOD/PCH shows features typical of PH but evidence of increased pressure pulmonary edema often is present as well (Fig. 29.8A and B). Left atrial enlargement and redistribution of blood flow into the upper lobes are absent, making it possible to distinguish PVOD/PCH from mitral stenosis. HRCT shows normal or small central pulmonary veins, patchy, dependent ground-glass opacity, smoothly thickened interlobular septa, lymphadenopathy, and pleural effusions. Ground-glass opacity centrilobular nodules and, more rarely, panlobular ground-glass opacity are common.

V-Q scintigraphy in patients with PVOD/PCH shows patchy perfusion, most likely secondary to superimposed PAH, but the pattern can occasionally simulate thromboembolic disease. Pulmonary angiography shows stigmata of PH, including enlarged pulmonary arteries with peripheral pruning, but with delayed filling of the central pulmonary veins and a prolonged parenchymal enhancement phase. These latter findings are secondary to the obstruction present in the venous system.

Chest radiography in patients with the PCH spectrum of PVOD/PCH may show diffuse reticular or nodular opacities; interlobular septal thickening is seen less commonly and favors the presence of the PVOD spectrum of PVOD/PCH. When interlobular septal thickening is present in patients with PCH, it is usually less pronounced than that seen in patients along the PVOD spectrum. The typical findings of PH are also present. Pleural effusions are also reportedly less common with the PCH spectrum of PVOD/PCH compared with PVOD. HRCT may show diffuse, poorly defined, centrilobular ground-glass opacities (Fig. 29.8C and D) with some areas of hypoattenuation, reflecting oligemia. Smooth or nodular interlobular septal thickening may be present. Areas of ground-glass opacity may reflect foci of alveolar hemorrhage.

PH SECONDARY TO LEFT HEART DISEASE (WHO GROUP 2)

PH due to left heart disease is defined as rest mPAP >20 mm Hg with PAWP >15 mm with normal or reduced cardiac output. The most commonly encountered left-sided cardiovascular causes of pulmonary venous hypertension are LV systolic or diastolic dysfunction, aortic stenosis, aortic regurgitation, mitral stenosis, or an obstructing intra-atrial tumor or thrombus. In patients with left-sided tumor or thrombus, the size of the obstructing lesion correlates with the degree of PH. Overall, left-sided cardiac disease is probably the most common cause of PH.

Secondary PH arises when increased pulmonary venous pressure requires elevated arterial pressure to promote forward flow. The pathophysiologic mechanism of PH in patients with left heart disease includes an increase in LV filling pressure transmitted to the pulmonary circulation, pulmonary arterial endothelial dysfunction (resulting in vasoconstriction), arterial and/or venous remodeling, RV dilation and dysfunction with tricuspid regurgitation, and altered RV-PA coupling. The histopathological changes in the arterial system, therefore, are caused secondarily by the increased venous pressure and include medial hypertrophy, intimal

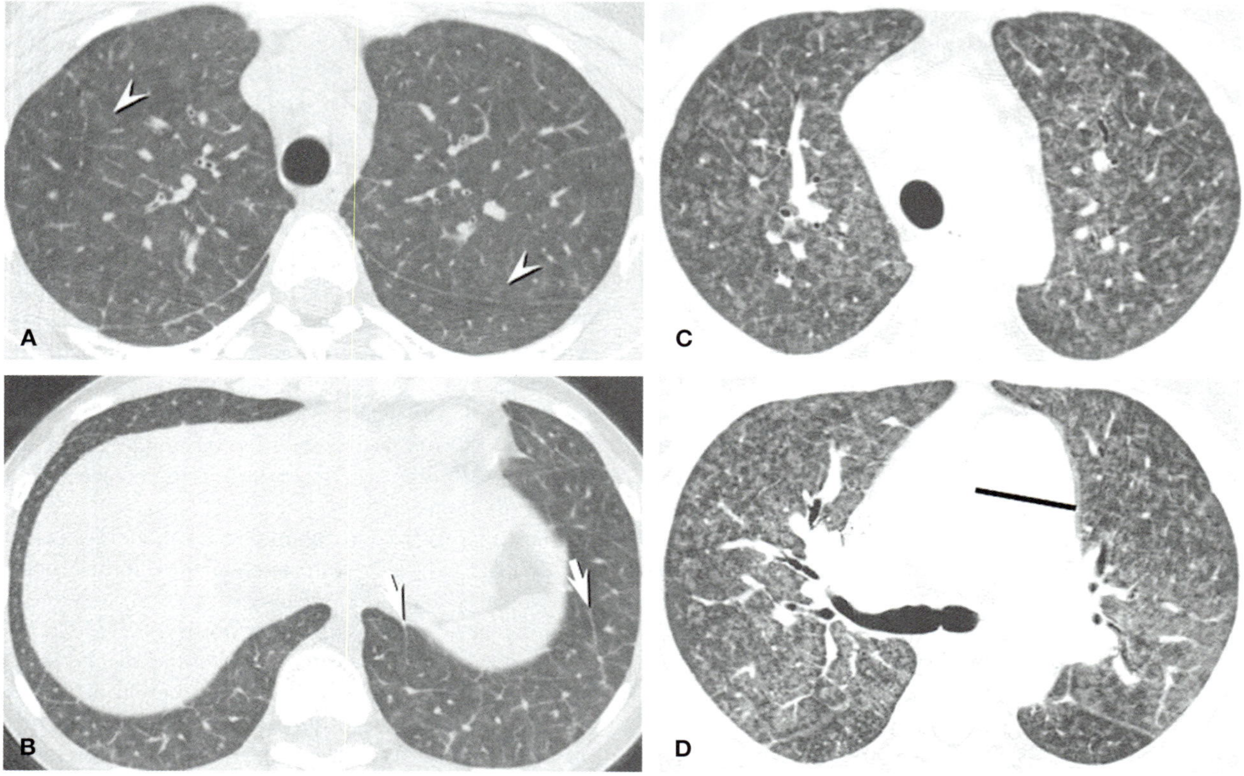

Figure 29.8. Pulmonary veno-occlusive disease and pulmonary capillary hemangiomatosis. **A and B:** Pulmonary veno-occlusive disease with pulmonary hypertension in a 22-year-old man shows patchy, poorly defined areas of faintly nodular ground-glass opacity (*arrowheads*) with basilar smooth interlobular septal thickening (*arrows*). **C and D:** Pulmonary capillary hemangiomatosis and PH shows multifocal bilateral poorly defined centrilobular ground-glass opacity nodules. The main pulmonary artery (*line*) is enlarged.

fibrosis, and in situ thrombosis, with plexiform lesions typically lacking. Histopathological specimens from the venous system show medial hypertrophy, interstitial thickening and edema, hemosiderosis, and, occasionally, venous infarction. Usually, there is no significant gradient between the elevated pulmonary arterial pressure and the PAWP, and PVR is normal or near normal; this situation reflects postcapillary PH (Table 29.1). In some patients, pulmonary arterial pressure rises disproportionately to left atrial pressure in patients with PH due to left heart disease, probably as a result of increased pulmonary vasomotor tone and/or vascular remodeling (PVR >3 WU; note that the most recent European Society of Cardiology and European Respiratory Society PH guideline statement uses a PVR threshold of ≥2 WU), resulting in a situation in which the diastolic PA pressure is elevated "out of proportion" to the PAWP. This phenomenon occurs in 25%, or perhaps more, of patients with group 2 PH and is also referred to as "combined precapillary and postcapillary PH."

Clinical Presentation

PH due to left heart disease is the most common form of PH. The clinical presentation of PH due to left heart disease is variable and depends on the specific disorder under consideration. Chronic left-sided cardiac diseases often present with progressive shortness of breath and exercise intolerance; chest pain, syncope, cough, and lower extremity edema may also be present.

Imaging Manifestations

Chest radiographs and thoracic CT (Fig. 29.9) show the characteristic findings of pulmonary venous hypertension manifesting as pulmonary vascular "cephalization," and possibly findings of interstitial edema, interlobular septal thickening (Kerley A and B lines), thickening of the fissures, peribronchial cuffing, and pleural effusion, with or without air-space opacity representing alveolar edema. Depending on the cardiac disorder present and the severity of disease, cardiomegaly with specific chamber enlargement may be present.

Some left-sided cardiovascular diseases have radiographic features that may allow a specific diagnosis with chest radiography or CT. Mitral stenosis may result in ossific micronodules within the pulmonary parenchyma, often with visible left atrial and especially atrial appendage enlargement.

Echocardiography is the imaging method most commonly used for the evaluation of left-sided cardiac disease. Echocardiography provides useful functional cardiac

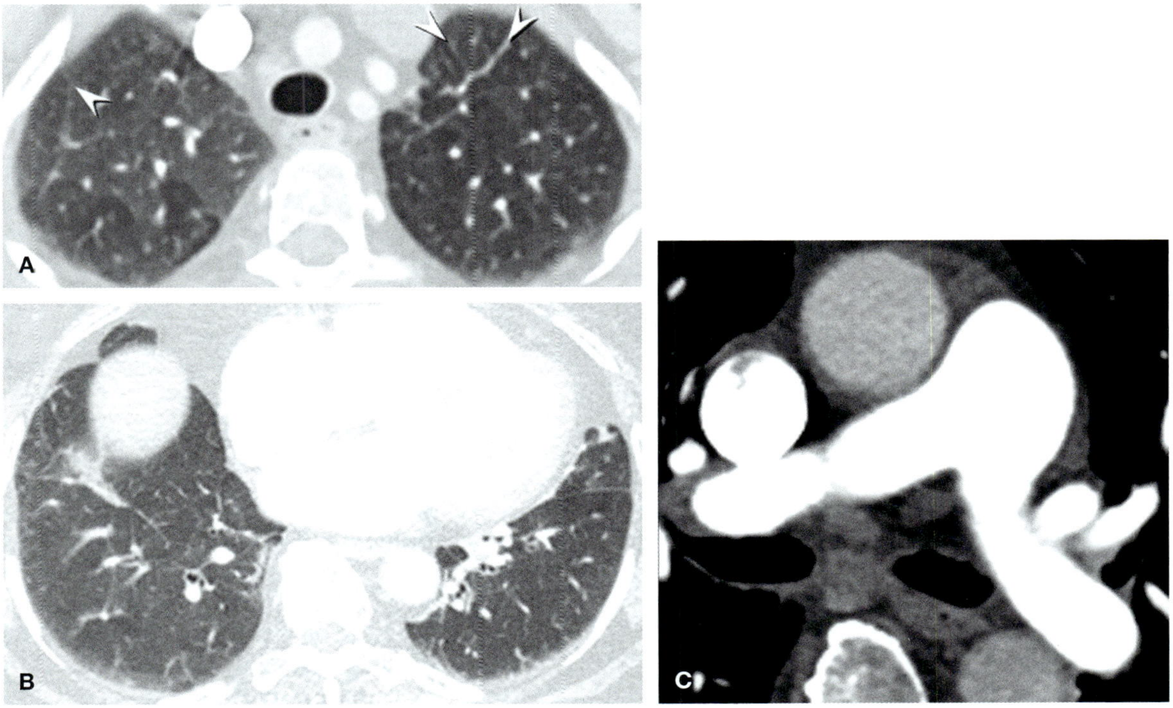

Figure 29.9. Pulmonary hypertension due to left heart disease. **A-C:** Axial CT images show mild upper lobe venous distension and interlobular septal thickening (*arrowheads*). Biatrial enlargement is present and the main pulmonary artery is mildly enlarged (34 mm; ascending aorta 32 mm). Cardiac MRI showed normal biventricular function and size. Echocardiography showed elevated right ventricular systolic pressure of 73 mm Hg as well as moderately elevated left ventricular filling pressures, and right heart catheterization showed mean pulmonary arterial pressure = 38 mm Hg, pulmonary capillary wedge pressure = 22 mm Hg, and pulmonary vascular resistance = 3.3 WU. The findings are consistent with heart failure with persevered ejection fraction.

information, such as estimates of chamber volume and pressure, stroke volume, and ejection fraction, as well as features of PH, such as elevated RV/LV ratio, LV eccentricity index, right atrial area, and the RV forming the cardiac apex.

MRI is also useful for the assessment of left heart disease and may provide data similar to echocardiography as regards cardiac function, chamber volumes, and severity of valvular disease.

PH SECONDARY TO HYPOXIA AND/OR LUNG DISEASE (WHO GROUP 3)

Etiology and Pathogenesis

PH may result from several mechanisms that eventually lead to alveolar hypoxia. Etiologies of chronic alveolar hypoxia that may produce PH include chronic obstructive pulmonary disease (COPD, including emphysema and bronchiectasis), interstitial lung diseases, sleep-disordered breathing, alveolar hypoventilation disorders, chronic high-altitude exposure, and some developmental disorders. All these disorders produce hypoxia, with or without associated acidosis, through V-Q mismatching, shunt, or alveolar hypoventilation. Other associated conditions, such as polycythemia, destruction of the alveolar-capillary membrane, systemic arterial flow through bronchial artery–PA anastomoses, and pulmonary thromboemboli, also may play a role in chronic alveolar hypoxia-induced PH.

Chronic Obstructive Pulmonary Disease

COPD refers to a heterogeneous, variably progressive, range of pulmonary disorders resulting from a cycle of injury and repair after prolonged oxidative inhalational exposure. The term COPD typically includes emphysema and chronic bronchitis, which share the characteristic of airflow obstruction on forced expiration. The histopathological changes associated with PH associated with COPD include pulmonary vascular remodeling, including intimal thickening with a reduction in pulmonary vascular cross-sectional area. V-Q mismatching is the primary mechanism of hypoxemia in COPD, and regional alveolar hypoxia physiologically results in hypoxic vasoconstriction and increased resistance in the pulmonary arterial vasculature. The PH that results from this sequence of events is exacerbated by the alveolar-capillary destruction present in patients with COPD. Various biological mechanisms may play a role in the development of PH in patients with COPD, and some investigators feel that severe PH may be a disorder that occasionally presents in patients with COPD as much as it is a condition resulting from COPD. Regardless, the presence of PH in patients with COPD is associated with impaired exercise tolerance and decreased survival compared to patients without COPD, and the presence of PH, even if mild, may be a more adverse prognostic finding than the severity of lung disease.

The prevalence of PH in patients with COPD is uncertain but is related to disease severity. In most patients with COPD, PH is mild (mPAP <35 mm Hg) and treatment is directed at COPD itself rather than PH. PH is more likely to occur, and be clinically significant, in COPD patients when airflow limitation is severe. The onset of severe PH (>35 mm Hg or, as some investigators believe, PVR >5 WU; this same definition is used for PH with interstitial lung disease), in the patient with COPD is associated with a poor prognosis, with a 5-year survival of 10% in patients with mean PA pressures greater than 45 mm Hg. The PAWP pressure has been found to be elevated in a number of PH patients with COPD, suggesting that left heart disease significantly contributes to PH in COPD patients.

Interstitial Lung Disease

The interstitial lung diseases are a heterogeneous group of pulmonary disorders characterized by inflammatory and fibrotic destruction of the pulmonary parenchyma. PH is common among patients with interstitial lung diseases, and its prevalence has been estimated between 8% and 15% at initial diagnosis, to 30% in advanced, and up to 60% of end-stage patients with idiopathic pulmonary fibrosis (IPF). PH associated with interstitial lung diseases is produced in part by chronic hypoxemia. Fibrotic restriction of pulmonary vessels, limiting their distensibility, and reduction of the vascular surface area also may play a role, resulting in increased PVR. As mentioned earlier, in the case of connective tissue diseases, the development of PH may be related to immunologic mechanisms. Pulmonary arteriolar vasoconstriction is present, mediated by hypoxia, and is associated with vascular inflammation, eventually producing pulmonary vascular remodeling; plexiform lesions are typically absent. Thrombotic angiopathy and perivascular fibrosis may present. Examination of explanted lungs in patients with IPF shows thickening of the walls of pulmonary arteries and veins associated with luminal narrowing in areas of dense fibrosis but narrowing and obliteration of venules and small veins may also be found in areas without dense fibrosis. Much like COPD, the presence of PH in patients with interstitial lung disease, even if mild, may be a more adverse prognostic finding than the severity of lung disease.

The correlation between measurements of lung function and HRCT fibrosis scores and severity of PH is poor in patients with IPF, implying that there is more to the development of PH that the mere degree of pulmonary fibrotic disease would predict. The ability of thoracic CT to predict PH (mPAP > 25 mm Hg in studies conducted prior to the revised definition of PH from 2018 6th World Symposium on PH in Nice) in patients with IPF has been questioned by some investigators, whereas others have found that main PA size and the ratio of the size of the main PA to the ascending aorta are predictive of PH regardless of PH etiology. Using an abnormal threshold measurement of the main PA of ≥29 mm, the sensitivity of this measurement for the detection of elevated pulmonary arterial pressure on right heart catheterization may approach or even exceed 90%, but at the expense of insufficient specificity and negative predictive value. Increasing the abnormal threshold improves specificity but inevitably compromises sensitivity.

Sleep-Disordered Breathing (Hypoventilation Syndromes)

Sleep-disordered breathing (some investigators prefer the term "hypoventilation syndromes") includes several sleep-related breathing disorders, such as central sleep apnea, obstructive sleep apnea, and nocturnal hypoxemia. The prevalence of sleep-disordered breathing may be as high as 4% among middle-aged men. Obstructive sleep apnea is an increasingly common cause of PH, present in 20% to 40% with obstructive sleep apnea, typically resulting in mild PH.

Sleep-disordered breathing results in chronically depressed PO_2 and elevated PCO_2. The chronic hypoxemia produces pulmonary arterial vasoconstriction and increased pulmonary arterial resistance, and subsequent vascular remodeling, resulting in PH. Sleep-disordered breathing is also associated with other cardiovascular diseases, and left atrial hypertension often contributes to PH in these patients.

Clinical Presentation

The clinical presentation of both COPD and interstitial lung diseases is dominated by the presence of the lung disease, and PH may not be recognized until cor pulmonale develops. Sleep-disordered breathing is often suggested by the presence of load snoring, daytime sleepiness, and poor-quality or restless sleep.

Imaging Manifestations

The appearance of PH associated with COPD on chest radiography is like that of PH from any other cause. The presence of abnormally large lung volumes and other stigmata of COPD are key to diagnosing obstructive lung disease as the cause of PH (Fig. 29.10). Basilar reticulation and diminished lung volumes suggest interstitial lung disease in patients with PH (Fig. 29.11). HRCT is more sensitive and specific than chest radiography for the diagnosis of PH associated with either COPD or interstitial lung disease. No specific imaging features allow the diagnosis of sleep-disordered breathing—the diagnosis is usually established based on clinical and laboratory assessment. Often such patients are obese, but little else on imaging allows the diagnosis of sleep-disordered breathing to be suggested. PH in this setting has the same imaging features on chest radiography and thoracic CT as other causes of PH.

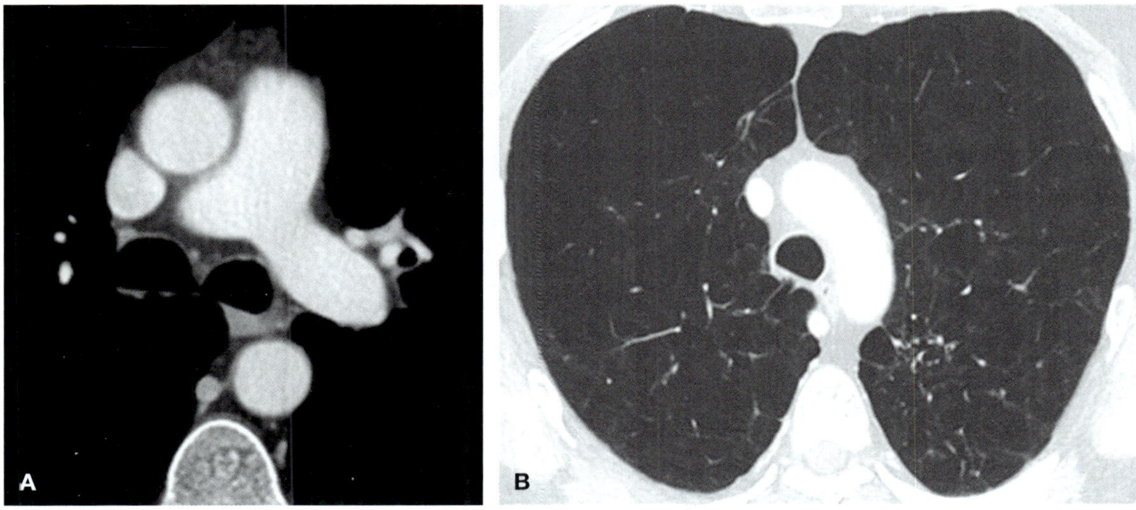

Figure 29.10. Pulmonary hypertension due to hypoxia and/or lung disease: chronic obstructive pulmonary disease in a 48-year-old man awaiting transplant. **A:** Axial enhanced CT shows a normal caliber main pulmonary artery and **(B)** severe advanced destructive emphysema. Right heart catheterization showed mean pulmonary arterial pressure = 25 mm Hg, pulmonary capillary wedge pressure = 16 mm Hg, and pulmonary vascular resistance = 5.2 WU.

CHRONIC THROMBOEMBOLIC PH (WHO GROUP 4)

Etiology and Pathogenesis

Chronic thromboembolic PH (CTEPH) represents a group 4 lesion in the 6th World PH Symposium classification system and is defined as precapillary PH (mPAP >20 mm Hg with PAWP ≤15 mm Hg at right heart catheterization) in the presence of organized or flow-limiting thrombi/emboli in the elastic pulmonary arteries for ≥3 months of effective anticoagulation.

Thromboemboli have numerous sources, including the deep veins of the pelvis and thigh, the right atrium, indwelling catheters, or septic thromboemboli in patients with endocarditis involving the tricuspid or pulmonic valves. Emboli commonly are multiple and bilateral, with a predilection for the right pulmonary circulation. Acute thromboembolic disease can produce transient pulmonary arterial pressure elevations, but sustained elevations are more likely to be a consequence of chronic thromboembolic disease. The incidence of CTEPH has previously been estimated at 1% to 5% of patients following acute pulmonary embolization, usually within 2 years of the initial embolic episode.

Thromboemboli induce PH by occluding the pulmonary vascular bed. This occlusion may result from numerous repeated small thromboembolic episodes, a few large embolic episodes that fail to completely resolve, or the development of in situ thrombosis within small vessels and proximal migration of thrombosis without actual embolization from deep venous sources. There are data to suggest that the latter mechanism plays a role in the development of CTEPH in some patients. Ultimately, an imbalanced or ineffective fibrinolytic system leads to the development of PH via cytokine-mediated pulmonary arterial scarring resulting from lysis of pulmonary thromboemboli. This scarring may occur after only one thromboembolic episode. Frequent abnormalities of the coagulation or fibrinolytic systems that may be found in patients with CTEPH include the presence of anticardiolipin antibody and elevated levels of factor VIII. In general, prothrombotic states are not consistently observed in patients with CTEPH. This suggests that the problem in patients with CTEPH is not recurrent embolic episodes, but the inability to resolve an embolic episode once it has occurred.

Pathologically, chronic emboli may organize, forming vascular channels interspersed with connective tissue. Fibrous bands and webs, representing organizing thrombi, are seen, often in association with fresh thrombi. The elevated pulmonary pressures also produce the characteristic histopathological changes of medial hypertrophy, intimal proliferation, and luminal obliteration, often in association with atherosclerosis. Plexogenic lesions are occasionally present.

Clinical Presentation

Patients at high risk for the development of chronic thromboembolic disease (note: the *chronic thromboembolic disease* refers to patients with postembolic exercise intolerance attributable to postthromboembolic pulmonary arterial obstruction, after at least 3 months of therapeutic anticoagulation, but without PH, and should be distinguished from CTEPH) include patients with cancer, chronic cardiac or pulmonary disease, and some clotting disorders, among a number of other conditions, none considered predictive

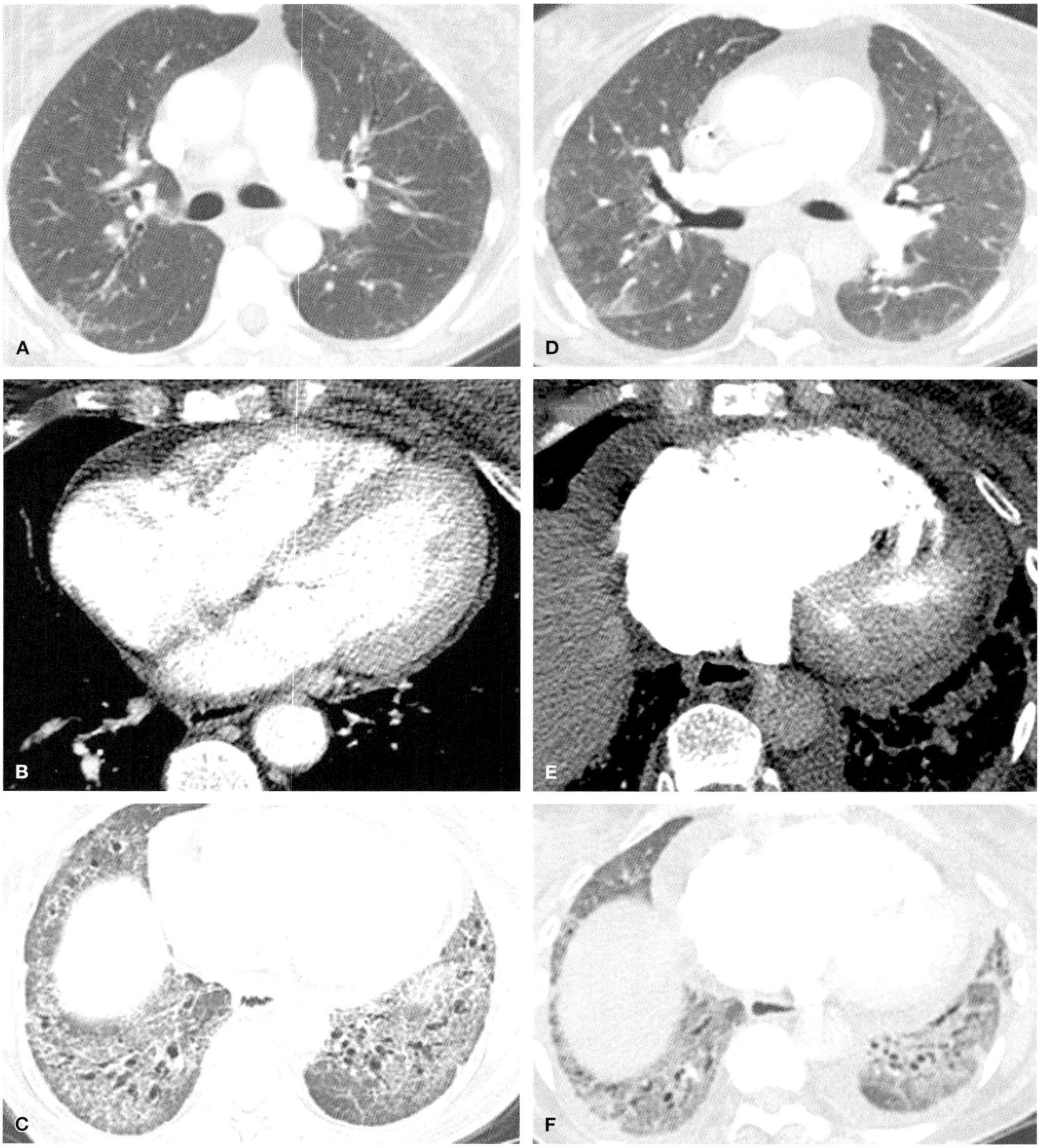

Figure 29.11. Pulmonary hypertension (PH) due to hypoxia and/or lung disease: exacerbation of PH in a patient with scleroderma. **A-C:** Axial CT shows the characteristic appearance of nonspecific interstitial pneumonia. The main pulmonary artery is borderline enlarged (31 mm, equal to ascending aorta) and the right atrium is enlarged, whereas the right ventricle is not clearly enlarged and septal curvature appears normal. Right heart catheterization showed mean pulmonary arterial pressure (mPAP) = 34 mm Hg, pulmonary capillary wedge pressure (PAWP) = 8 mm Hg, and pulmonary vascular resistance (PVR) = 4.8 WU. **D-F:** Axial CT 3 mo later when the patient developed worsening dyspnea, lower extremity edema, and hypoxemia shows the main pulmonary artery has not measurably changed in size (31 mm) although there is now clear enlargement of the right atrium and right ventricle, with leftward bowing of the interventricular septum and new pericardial fluid. Repeat right heart catheterization showed mPAP = 62 mm Hg, PAWP = 32 mm Hg, and PVR = 12 WU.

enough to advocate routine surveillance for the development of chronic thromboembolic disease. Patients with CTEPH often complain of progressive dyspnea and exercise intolerance and occasionally chest pain, cough, and syncope. Patients with chronic thromboembolic disease have a poor prognosis. Without proper treatment, the 5-year survival rate is only 30% when mPAP exceeds 40 mm Hg in patients with CTEPH.

The treatment of CTEPH depends on the location and extent of embolic burden within the pulmonary circulation. If thromboemboli are shown within the lobar arteries or more proximally, the patient may be a candidate for surgical pulmonary thromboendarterectomy. Thromboemboli distal to the proximal segmental vessels usually are not amenable to surgical resection, and oral anticoagulation is the preferred treatment.

Surgical pulmonary thromboendarterectomy is an effective treatment for patients with CTEPH providing significant improvement in symptoms and pulmonary hemodynamics. However, surgical pulmonary thromboendarterectomy can be associated with a mortality approaching 10%, and another 10% to 15% of patients who undergo the procedure may fail to have substantial reductions in PVR. It has been suggested that a postoperative residual PVR of greater than 500 dyn s cm^{-5} is associated with a mortality of just over 30% in patients undergoing surgical pulmonary thromboendarterectomy, whereas the mortality for these patients is less than 1% when the postoperative PVR falls below 500 dyn s cm^{-5} following surgery. Preoperative imaging assessment may be important for segregating those patients who stand a chance of deriving a benefit from surgical pulmonary thromboendarterectomy from those who will not. When visible central thromboemboli are present on CTPA, it is more likely that patients will have improvements in PVR following pulmonary thromboendarterectomy. However, the amount of central thromboembolic material does not necessarily correlate with mPAP, and some patients with central disease will not respond well to surgical pulmonary thromboendarterectomy, whereas others without central disease may have favorable results with surgery. The cause of this discrepancy is uncertain but suggests that factors other than mere vascular obstruction are at play in the development of CTEPH.

Balloon pulmonary angioplasty (BPA) is an emerging interventional technique that may be employed for the treatment of inoperable CTEPH patients or patients in whom PH persists or recurs following endarterectomy. BPA has been shown to improve right heart function and exercise capacity and decrease PVR, although serious complications, including fatalities, have been reported.

Imaging Manifestations

Chest radiography may be normal early in the course of the development of CTEPH. Later, the characteristic findings of PH, including enlargement of the main, right, and left pulmonary arteries, are seen. Subpleural opacities representing recent or remote pulmonary infarction may be encountered.

V-Q scintigraphy often is interpreted as high probability in patients with CTEPH, although scintigraphy may underestimate the degree of hemodynamic derangement associated with CTEPH. Furthermore, in the original Prospective Investigation of Pulmonary Embolism Diagnosis (PIOPED I) series, the positive predictive value of a high-probability V-Q scan interpretation fell from 91% to 74% for patients with a prior history of thromboembolic disease, representing a loss of specificity in the high-probability scan interpretation. Other studies have shown that normal V-Q scintigraphy results exclude CTEPH with a high degree of certainty, whereas, as discussed below, negative results on CTPA do not exclude this diagnosis, nor do they always establish or exclude the possibility of a favorable response to surgical intervention in patients with CTEPH. For this reason, some investigators have recommended that V-Q scintigraphy should remain the primary noninvasive imaging method for the investigation of suspected CTEPH, with positive results typically followed by CTPA. It is likely, however, that a multiparametric approach, combining V-Q scintigraphy and CTPA examinations, may provide the optimal ability to detect CTEPH and guide management for these patients.

CTPA is an important study for the evaluation of suspected CTEPH (Fig. 29.12) not only for the assessment of the location of embolic material but for the exclusion of competing diagnosis for abnormal V-Q scintigraphy results. Eccentric filling defects adjacent to the vessel wall, representing organizing thrombi, are characteristic of chronic thromboembolic disease. These thrombi may calcify. The eccentric nature of organizing thrombi may be shown to advantage with multiplanar reformatted imaging. Organizing thrombi may undergo recanalization, in which case CTPA will show small foci of contrast within an occluded vessel. Linear intraluminal filling defects representing intravascular webs also may be seen. Abrupt narrowing of pulmonary arteries with reduction in arterial diameter is common in patients with CTEPH, and CTPA also may show markedly hypertrophied bronchial arteries in these patients.

Dual-energy CT (DECT) generates maps of regional iodine density in the pulmonary parenchyma surrogate for pulmonary parenchymal perfusion, offering the opportunity to simultaneously asses for the presence and level of thromboembolic disease as well as directly image pulmonary blood flow derangements in CTEPH patients (Fig. 29.12I). DECT assessment of altered pulmonary blood volume correlates fairly well with perfusion deficits at V-Q scintigraphy, and it has been suggested that DECT is capable of differentiating PAH from peripherally distributed thromboembolic disease in PH, although the assessment of suspected CTEPH still typically begins with scintigraphy. DECT iodine map agreement with scintigraphy.

HRCT may show bilateral, geographically distributed inhomogeneous lung density in patients with CTEPH

(Fig. 29.12G), representing mosaic perfusion. The vessels within the regions of decreased pulmonary parenchymal attenuation often are visibly smaller than their counterparts in the areas of normal or increased parenchymal attenuation. Such perfusion abnormalities may be demonstrated with DECT (Fig. 29.12I). Small foci of subpleural consolidation (Fig. 29.2J), representing areas of prior pulmonary infarction, also may be evident.

Enlarged bronchial arteries may occur in response to chronic RV outflow tract or pulmonary arterial obstruction. Occasionally, transpleural collateral vessels, derived from the intercostal arteries, may also develop in this situation. Under normal conditions, bronchial arterial flow compromises about 1% of the cardiac output and does not contribute to gas exchange. However, with pulmonary arterial obstruction, significant enlargement of bronchial vessels may occur, and

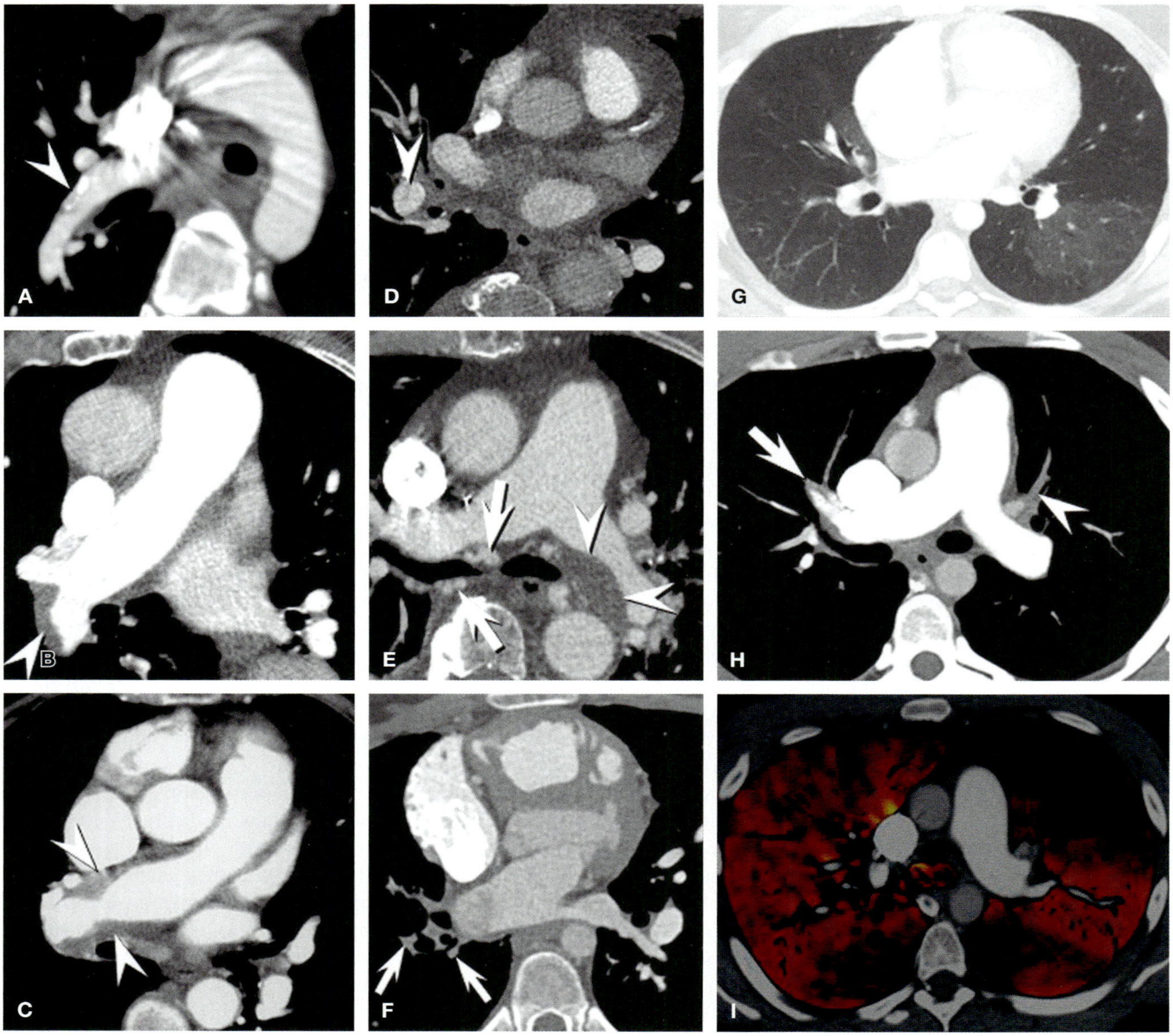

Figure 29.12. Pulmonary hypertension due to chronic thromboembolic pulmonary hypertension: CT imaging spectrum. **A:** Eccentric calcified filling defect in the right upper lobe pulmonary artery (*arrowhead*). **B:** Eccentric thromboembolism (*arrowhead*) right interlobar pulmonary artery. **C:** Eccentric partial filling defects (*arrowheads*) reflecting recanalized right interlobar pulmonary artery. **D:** Intravascular web (*arrowhead*). **E:** Hypertrophied bronchial arteries (*arrows*) and left pulmonary artery eccentric filling defect (*arrowheads*). **F:** Severely stenosed left lower lobe segmental arteries (*arrows*). **G:** Geographic inhomogeneous lung attenuation reflecting mosaic perfusion. **H:** Occluded left upper lobe (*arrowhead*) and right upper lobe (*arrow*) arteries. **I:** Multifocal decreased perfusion, particularly in the left upper lobe corresponding to the obstructed left upper lobe artery seen in (**H**), on dual-energy pulmonary blood volume image.

flow through the bronchial arterial circulation can account for as much as 30% of the cardiac output. In this situation, enlarged bronchial arteries develop anastomoses with small pulmonary arteries distal to sites of pulmonary arterial obstruction. The CTPA findings of abnormal bronchial arterial enlargement include extensive arterial tortuosity and proximal bronchial arterial diameters greater than 2 mm (Fig. 29.12E). Bronchial artery enlargement in patients with CTEPH has been associated with a good response to surgical pulmonary thromboendarterectomy. Enlarged bronchial arteries are more commonly seen in patients with CTEPH than patients with nonembolic causes of PH, and the presence of these vessels tends to favor chronic PE over acute PE.

RV enlargement and hypertrophy are readily visible on CTPA studies in patients with CTEPH. Leftward bowing of the interventricular septum may also be present. When the tricuspid annulus dilates, tricuspid regurgitation may develop and is associated with reflux of injected intravenous contrast into the IVC and hepatic veins; however, these findings can be seen as a result of increased right heart pressures in the absence of significant tricuspid valvular dysfunction also. Nonspecific CTPA findings in patients with CTEPH include mild lymphadenopathy, pericardial effusion, and mild pericardial thickening.

The anatomic findings of CTEPH on MRI and magnetic resonance angiography (MRA) (Fig. 29.13) are similar to those on CT. Chronic, organized thrombi appear as very low-signal foci adjacent to the vascular wall on T1-weighted double inversion recovery "black blood", gadolinium-enhanced MRA, and steady-state free precession images. Vascular webs and stenoses and hypertrophied bronchial arteries may be visible. MRI has the added utility of accurate assessment of RV performance, and improvements in RV ejection fraction and peak systolic pulmonary arterial flow velocity may be seen in patients with CTEPH treated with thromboendarterectomy. Additionally, velocity-encoded cine phase-contrast MRI has been used to assess the degree of bronchopulmonary shunt volume through hypertrophied bronchial arteries before and after surgical pulmonary endarterectomy—reduction of bronchopulmonary shunt volume represents a favorable response to surgical therapy in patients with CTEPH.

Catheter pulmonary angiography (typically using digital subtraction technique) typically shows vascular tortuosity, webs, bands, stenoses, "pouching defects," and abrupt vascular cutoffs or occlusions in patients with CTEPH. Catheter pulmonary angiography is rarely employed for diagnostic purposes in CTEPH, but rather as part of hemodynamic and surgical eligibility assessment and is still regarded as the gold standard for determining if thromboemboli are surgically accessible. Although some centers with expertise for CTEPH treatment may offer thromboendarterectomy for patients with distal segmental or subsegmental disease, in general, pulmonary thromboendarterectomy is reserved for patients with thromboemboli in the main, right or left, interlobar, lobar, and/or segmental pulmonary arteries.

NONTHROMBOTIC PULMONARY ARTERIAL EMBOLIZATION

Nonthrombotic emboli to the pulmonary arterial circulation may produce PH. Potential etiologies include tumor emboli, particulates such as mercury and talc, and parasites.

Tumor Embolization

Etiology and Pathogenesis

PH resulting from microvascular obstruction caused by tumor emboli is considered here because tumor embolization shares a common theme with particulate and parasitic embolization: nonthrombotic pulmonary embolization. Note that pulmonary tumor thrombotic microangiopathy is classified as a group 5 lesion (Pulmonary Hypertension with Unclear or Multifactorial Mechanisms) in classification system advanced by the 6th World Symposium on PH in Nice in 2018 (see Table 29.2).

As many as 25% of patients with a solid malignancy may have microemboli that lodge in the pulmonary circulation. The most common etiology of tumor microembolization is gastric cancer, but breast (Fig. 29.14), lung, ovarian, renal, hepatocellular, and prostate cancers also may produce tumor emboli. Most emboli preferentially occlude small arteries and arterioles with the exception of atrial myxomas and renal carcinomas, which may form larger, more centrally located, thromboemboli.

Histopathological specimens in patients with pulmonary tumor embolization show visible tumor within pulmonary arteries (Fig. 29.14E), often accompanied by lymphangitic tumor, organizing thrombi, pulmonary infarction, and intimal fibrosis. Larger vessels may be affected, although small, peripherally located pulmonary arteries (at the centrilobular artery level) may be affected as well. Occasionally, myxoid intimal hyperplasia may be present and may induce arteriolar obliteration. This situation has been referred to as *thrombotic tumor microangiopathy*.

Clinical Presentation

Because tumor emboli are quite small, symptoms related to tumor embolization are uncommon. If the embolic load is great enough, patients may present with dyspnea on exertion, hypoxemia, chest pain, cough, syncope, and even right-sided heart failure.

Imaging Manifestations

Chest radiographs in patients with intravascular tumor embolization often are normal, but sometimes they may resemble pulmonary lymphangitic carcinomatosis.

In addition to the characteristic findings of PH (Fig. 29.14A-C) and thromboembolism described previously, thoracic CT of patients with tumor emboli may reveal lymphadenopathy, lymphangitic carcinomatosis, and peripheral, wedge-shaped opacities representing infarction. When emboli affect larger vessels, such as subsegmental arteries,

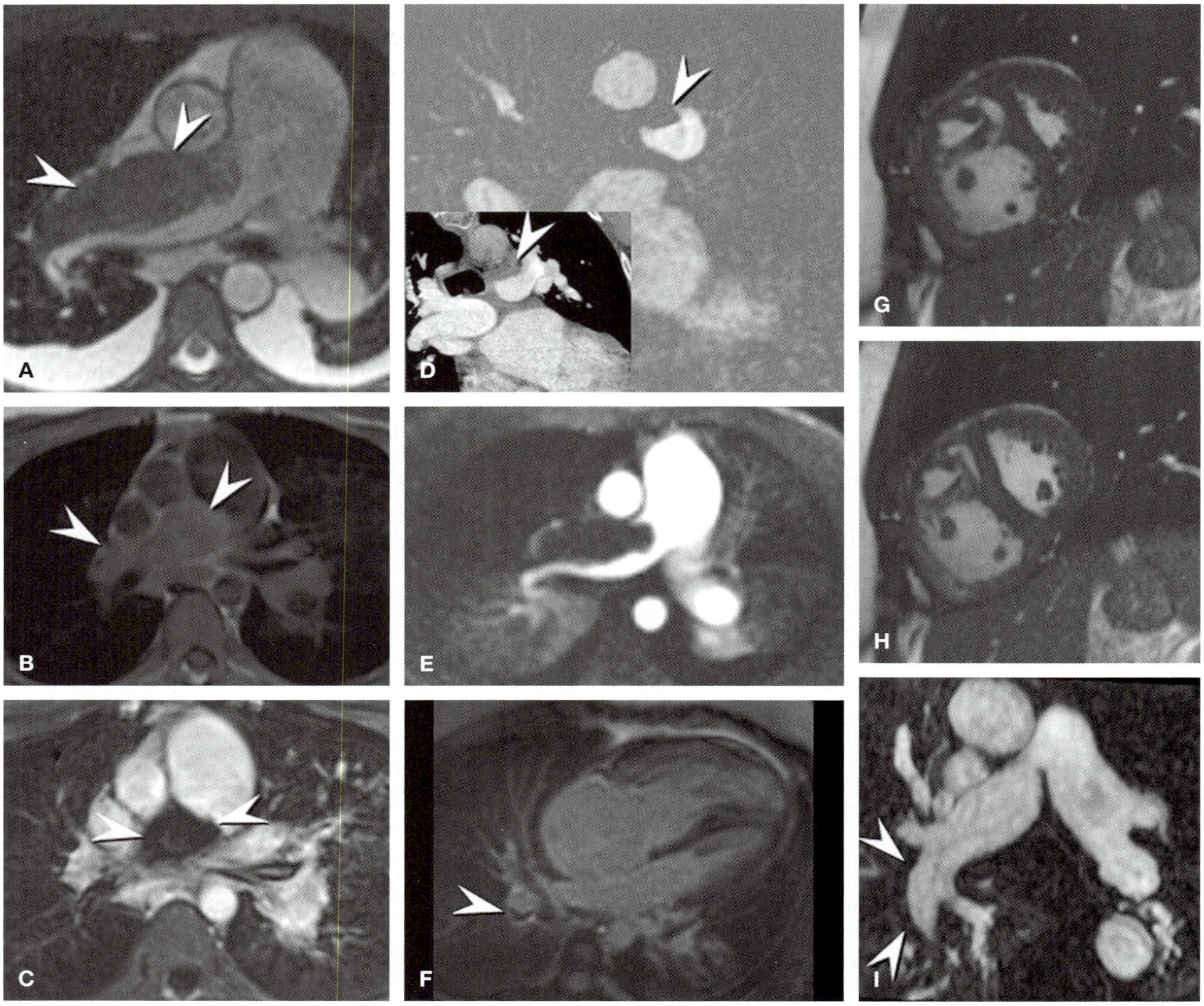

Figure 29.13. Pulmonary hypertension due to chronic thromboembolic pulmonary hypertension: MRI findings. **A:** Eccentric right pulmonary artery thromboembolism (*arrowheads*) on axial steady-state free precession image (mean pulmonary arterial pressure [mPAP] = 42 mm Hg, pulmonary capillary wedge pressure = 10 mm Hg, and pulmonary vascular resistance = 10.8 WU). **B:** Axial T1-weighted double inversion recovery "black blood" image shows intermediate signal in the right pulmonary artery (*arrowheads*) at the site of thromboembolism. **C:** (Same patient as **B**) Axial enhanced fast gradient-echo image shows a hypointense filling defect in the proximal right pulmonary artery (*arrowheads*). **D:** Eccentric partial filling defect (*arrowhead*) in the left pulmonary artery on coronal MRA, correlated with CT (inset). **E:** Multifocal pulmonary hypoperfusion on enhanced first-pass imaging (the MR equivalent of oligemia at CT). Note enlarged main pulmonary artery and right pulmonary artery partial filling defect. Same patient as **A**. Patient underwent endarterectomy. **F:** Eccentric filling defect in the right lower lobe artery (*arrowhead*) on 4-chamber delayed enhancement imaging. **G:** Leftward systolic interventricular septal motion reflecting elevated pulmonary artery pressure (mPAP = 55 mm Hg); relatively normal septal curvature in diastole **(H)**. **I:** Eccentric filling defect in the right lower lobe pulmonary artery (arrowheads) on axial MRA.

CT may reveal a "beaded" appearance of these vessels. When smaller vessels are affected (at the centrilobular level), beading and nodularity may be observed, and the affected vessels may assume a branching configuration, resembling "tree-in-bud," or, more rarely, oligemia (Fig. 29.14C).

Lung scintigraphy may reveal subsegmental unmatched perfusion defects (Fig. 29.14D), indistinguishable from thromboembolic disease. Pulmonary angiography may show a delayed arterial phase, intravascular filling defects with a beaded appearance, and peripheral pruning.

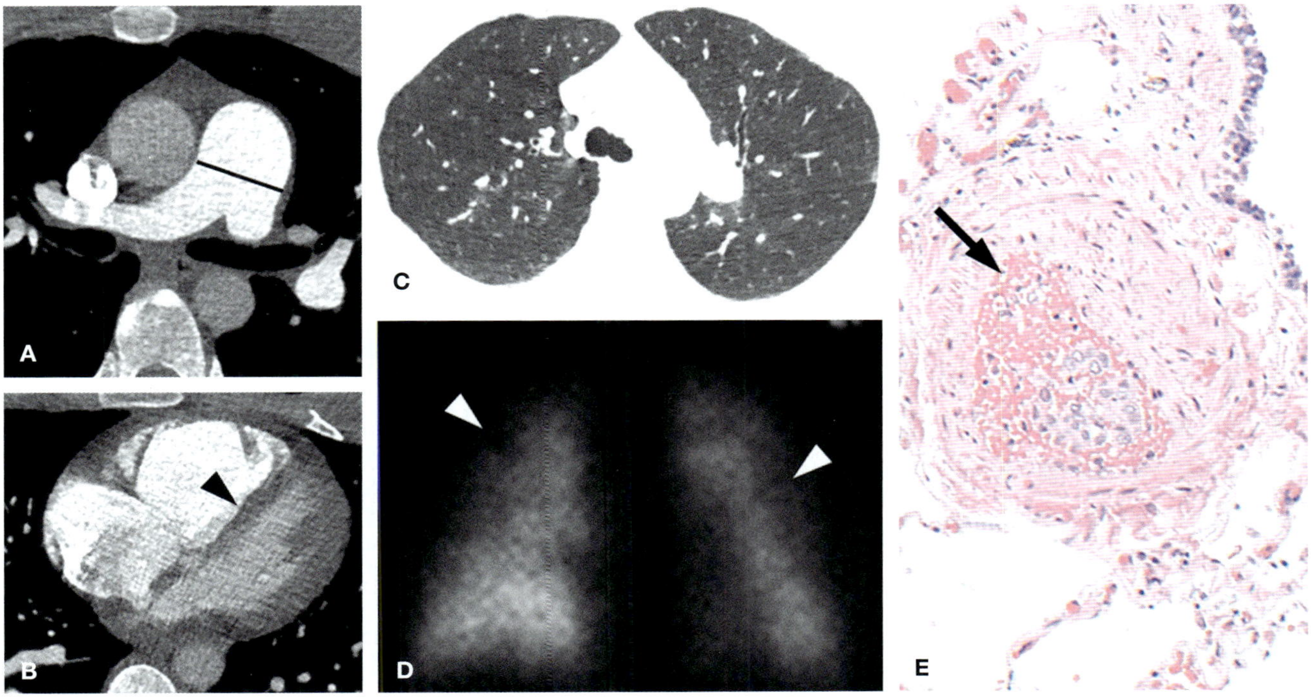

Figure 29.14. **A-E:** Pulmonary hypertension with right ventricular failure resulting from pulmonary arterial embolization from breast malignancy. **A and B:** Axial soft-tissue windows from a CTPA study shows enlargement of the main pulmonary artery (*line*) and leftward bowing of the interventricular septum (*black arrowhead*). **C:** Lung window image from the CTPA examination shows subtle, bilateral inhomogeneous lung opacity representing oligemia caused by small pulmonary arteriolar tumor emboli. **D:** Frontal planar ^{99m}Tc-labeled macroaggregated albumin perfusion study shows small, subpleural, bilateral perfusion defects (*white arrowheads*). **E:** Histopathologic specimen obtained at autopsy shows tumor emboli from breast malignancy within a small pulmonary arteriole (*arrow*).

Particulate Embolization

Etiology and Pathogenesis

Intravascular mercury embolization may produce PH. After injection, mercury embolizes small vessels and eventually migrates from the vessel into the surrounding pulmonary interstitium, where the metal elicits an inflammatory, granulomatous response that produces vascular obstruction and, eventually, PH.

Excipient lung disease (also known by numerous other names; the term "excipient" denotes an inactive additive substance used as a vehicle for medication delivery, and hence is the favored term) results from the intravascular injection of substances such as talc, microcrystalline cellulose, and cornstarch, which are insoluble fillers used as binding agents in several oral medications. When intravenous drug users abuse medications containing these substances, they intravenously inject a suspension containing crushed tablets intended for oral use, thereby embolizing small pulmonary arterioles with the insoluble material. This material may migrate from the vessels into the surrounding pulmonary interstitium, where its presence elicits a foreign body granulomatous response. Vascular thrombosis with recanalization, medial arterial hypertrophy, fibrosis, and refractile talc particles are present in histopathological specimens.

Clinical Presentation

Mercury may be injected into the vascular system accidentally or intentionally. Intentional mercury injection most often represents a suicide attempt.

Excipient lung disease may produce few symptoms, but patients may present with chronic, progressive shortness of breath, dyspnea on exertion, and cough. Symptoms may progress even after cessation of drug abuse.

Imaging Manifestations

On chest radiography, mercury embolization appears as fine, branching, symmetric, very dense nodules representing intra-arterial mercury deposits. Metal deposits also may collect within the heart, particularly at the apex of the right ventricle.

Chest radiographs in patients with excipient lung disease show diffuse, bilateral, small nodular opacities about 1 to 2 mm in diameter throughout the lung parenchyma. Perihilar conglomerate masses associated with fibrosis, producing retraction of lung parenchyma and relative hyperlucency in the lower lung, may be seen in some patients.

CT may demonstrate numerous, small centrilobular micronodules (which may show a branching configuration) with or without patchy ground-glass opacity. Upper lobe fibrotic opacities, resembling progressive massive fibrosis, may be present. These fibrotic opacities may show high attenuation due to the presence of talc.

Parasitic Embolization

Etiology and Pathogenesis

PH resulting from schistosomiasis is considered a group 1 lesion (PAH) in the 2018 World Symposium on PH classification (see Table 29.2), but is discussed here since parasitic embolization shares similar pathophysiological mechanisms to other nonthrombotic pulmonary emboli. Cardiopulmonary schistosomiasis most often is the result of infection with *Schistosoma mansoni* (see Chapter 12, pages 452-453), which is endemic in the Middle East, Africa, and South America. There usually is a latency period of 5 years or more after the onset of infection before cardiopulmonary disease develops. Secreted ova migrate to the lungs via portal-systemic collaterals and lodge within medium-sized muscular arteries and arterioles. Within the pulmonary circulation, the eggs elicit an inflammatory reaction that results in medial hypertrophy, granuloma formation, intimal hyperplasia, collagen deposition and fibrosis, and obliterative arteritis. An associated eosinophilic alveolitis may be present.

Clinical Presentation

Presenting symptoms of parasitic embolization include hepatosplenomegaly, symptoms of right heart failure, dyspnea, and cough. Patients with cardiopulmonary schistosomiasis always have cirrhosis and portal hypertension.

Imaging Manifestations

Chest radiography in patients with parasitic embolization shows findings consistent with PH. Small nodules, representing parasitic granulomas, may be evident. Pulmonary infarction rarely is seen with parasitic embolization.

HRCT may demonstrate nodules, interstitial prominence and thickening, and ground-glass opacity associated with the classic findings of PH.

PH WITH UNCLEAR OR MULTIFACTORIAL MECHANISMS (WHO GROUP 5)

Various, seemingly disparate, conditions may produce PH and are classified under group 5 in the 6th World Symposium on PH in Nice in 2018 as "pulmonary hypertension with unclear and/or multifactorial mechanisms." PH in these conditions shares the same imaging characteristics as other causes of PH, although some of the diseases in this category may show thoracic imaging findings suggestive of a particular disorder. The specific imaging features of such disorders have been reviewed elsewhere.

The first subcategory of group 5 in the 2018 6th World Symposium on PH classification of disorders producing PH (Table 29.2) includes hematological disorders, such as myeloproliferative diseases and chronic hemolytic anemias, including sickle cell disease and β-thalassemia. polycythemia vera, essential thrombocytosis, chronic myeloid leukemia, and splenectomy. A number of mechanisms may result in PH in patients with these conditions, including high cardiac output, congestive heart failure, asplenia, or mechanical pulmonary arterial obstruction due to circulating megakaryocytes. Other systemic conditions included in group 5 include sarcoidosis, Langerhans cell histiocytosis, and rare disorders, such as glycogen storage diseases, Gaucher disease, and neurofibromatosis. In patients with sarcoidosis, postulated mechanisms producing PH include capillary bed destruction due to fibrosis, PA and venous compression by lymphadenopathy, and granulomatous inflammation directly involving the pulmonary vessels, particularly the veins. Elevated pulmonary arterial pressure in patients with end-stage Langerhans cell histiocytosis is not uncommon and may be related to a combination of pulmonary parenchymal destruction with associated hypoxemia and vasculopathy (Fig. 29.15).

Various mechanisms for the development of PH in rare group 5 lesions include hypoxemia, pulmonary parenchymal disease, portocaval shunts (in the case of type Ia glycogen storage disease), and capillary blockade by Gaucher cells. The mechanisms by which thyroid disorders may produce PH are unclear, but an association between autoimmune thyroid disease and PAH raises the possibility of a linked genetic pathogenesis.

Additional group 5 subcategories in the 2018 Nice classification includes patients with PH and chronic renal failure with hemodialysis, fibrosing mediastinitis, and complex congenital heart disease. Among these disorders, fibrosing mediastinitis may present with suggestive thoracic imaging findings and is discussed in detail.

Fibrosing Mediastinitis

Fibrosing mediastinitis represents a progressive proliferation of collagenous and fibrous tissue throughout the mediastinum, producing encasement and compression of mediastinal structures. Granulomatous infections, particularly *Histoplasma capsulatum* and *Mycobacterium tuberculosis*, are among the most common causes of fibrosing mediastinitis.

The deposition of fibrous tissue in fibrosing mediastinitis commonly affects relatively deformable structures, such as the superior vena cava, the trachea and central airways, the pulmonary arteries, the pulmonary veins, and the esophagus. PH may be produced by fibrous encasement of either the pulmonary arteries or draining pulmonary veins. The

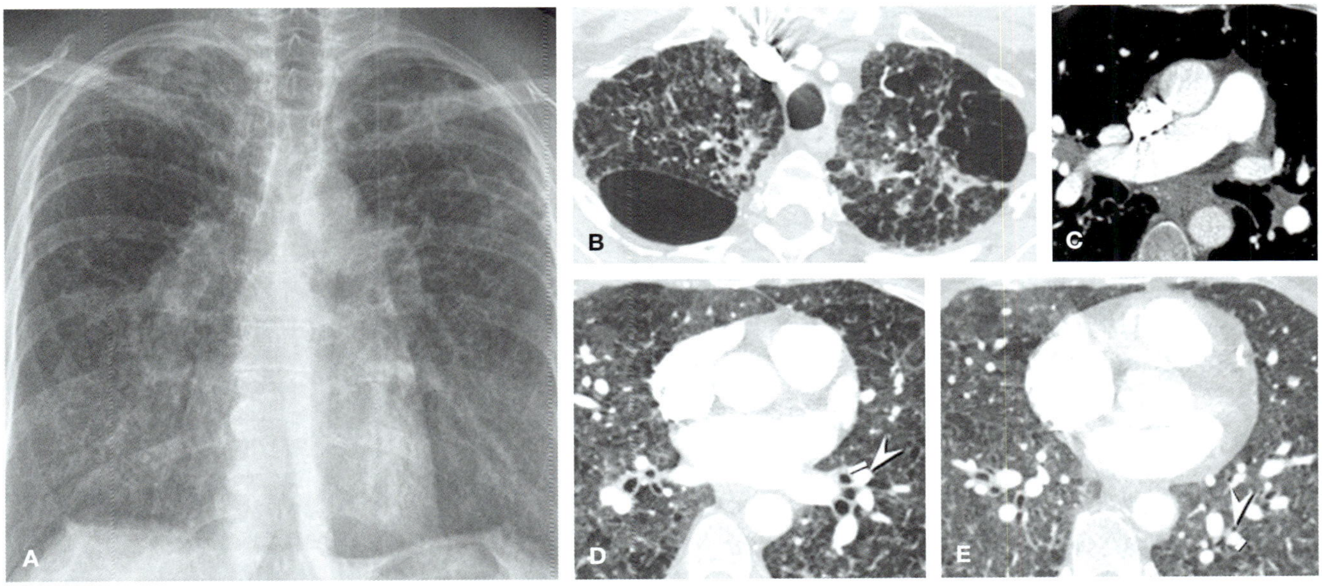

Figure 29.15. **A-E:** Pulmonary hypertension (PH) in pulmonary Langerhans cell histiocytosis. **A:** Frontal chest radiography shows large lung volumes and bilateral central pulmonary arterial enlargement with a background of reticular and cystic change. **B:** Axial chest CT shows severe confluent hypoattenuation consistent with advanced smoking-related changes, although patient was a lifelong nonsmoker. Tissue sampling showed pulmonary Langerhans cell histiocytosis. **C:** Main pulmonary artery is normal in size (24 mm Hg) and smaller than ascending aorta. However, segmental pulmonary arteries (lines, **D** and **E**) are larger than their accompanying airways (*arrowheads*), suggesting PH. Right heart catheterization showed mean pulmonary arterial pressure = 40 mm Hg, pulmonary capillary wedge pressure = 9 mm Hg, and pulmonary vascular resistance = 6.54 WU.

former produces precapillary PH, which often is mistaken for chronic thromboembolic disease, and the latter produces postcapillary PH. Pulmonary venous obstruction is patchy in distribution, producing wide variations in PAWP measurements, although the wedge pressure usually is elevated. Cardiac catheterization reveals normal left heart size and pressures.

Fibrosing mediastinitis produces histopathological changes characteristic of venous hypertension, including medial hypertrophy, septal thickening secondary to edema, hemosiderin-laden macrophages, venous infarction, and the typical vascular changes of PH. Thrombi may be found within affected veins.

The predominant symptoms of fibrosing mediastinitis depend on the structures most severely involved. Patients often present with nonspecific symptoms of pulmonary venous hypertension such as dyspnea and hemoptysis. The treatment for the disorder is limited; if focal fibrosis of a pulmonary vein is diagnosed, surgical treatment or stenting may be effective. Corticosteroids have shown limited efficacy in reversing the disease.

Chest radiographs often show a widened mediastinum with hilar prominence and calcified lymph nodes. Findings of pulmonary venous hypertension, including interlobular septal thickening and alveolar edema, may be present. Fibrosing mediastinitis may result in airway stenoses, which may cause lobar volume loss.

CT reveals extensive infiltration of the mediastinum with abnormal soft tissue. Fibrosing mediastinitis due to *H. capsulatum* usually produces extensive lymph node calcification, which is readily identified with CT. Contrast-enhanced CT may show extensive collateral vein formation due to fibrotic involvement of systemic thoracic veins such as the superior vena cava or azygos vein. PA compression may be visualized directly. Pulmonary venous infarcts, appearing as subpleural, wedge-shaped consolidations, may be seen in patients with pulmonary venous involvement. V-Q scintigraphy may show focal unmatched perfusion defects. Unilateral lack of perfusion of one lung has been reported in patients with fibrosing mediastinitis.

Pulmonary angiography findings vary depending on the location of obstruction. If the arterial circulation is affected primarily, asymmetric narrowing of the pulmonary arteries will be present. When pulmonary veins are affected primarily, venous phase angiography will show stenoses, dilation, or obstruction, often near the junction of the affected vein and the left atrium.

SUGGESTED READINGS

Alabed S, Garg P, Johns CS, et al. Cardiac magnetic resonance in pulmonary hypertension-an update. *Curr Cardiovasc Imaging Rep*. 2020;13(12):30.

Altschul E, Remy-Jardin M, Machnicki S, et al. Imaging of pulmonary hypertension: pictorial essay. *Chest*. 2019;156(2):211-227.

Aluja Jaramillo F, Gutierrez FR, Díaz Telli FG, et al. Approach to pulmonary hypertension: from CT to clinical diagnosis. *Radiographics*. 2018;38(2):357-373.

Frazier AA, Galvin JR, Franks TJ, Rosado-DeChristenson ML. From the archives of the AFIP: pulmonary vasculature—hypertension and infarction. *Radiographics*. 2000;20(2):491-532.

Galiè N, McLaughlin VV, Rubin LJ, Simonneau G. An overview of the 6th world symposium on pulmonary hypertension. *Eur Respir J*. 2019;53(1):1802148.

Humbert M, Kovacs G, Hoeper MM, et al; ESC/ERS Scientific Document Group. 2022 ESC/ERS Guidelines for the diagnosis and treatment of pulmonary hypertension. *Eur Heart J*. 2022;43(38):3618-3731.

Peña E, Dennie C, Veinot J, Muñiz SH. Pulmonary hypertension: how the radiologist can help. *Radiographics*. 2012;32(1):9-32.

Rajaram S, Swift AJ, Condliffe R, et al. CT features of pulmonary arterial hypertension and its major subtypes: a systematic CT evaluation of 292 patients from the ASPIRE Registry. *Thorax*. 2015;70(4):382-387.

Chapter 30

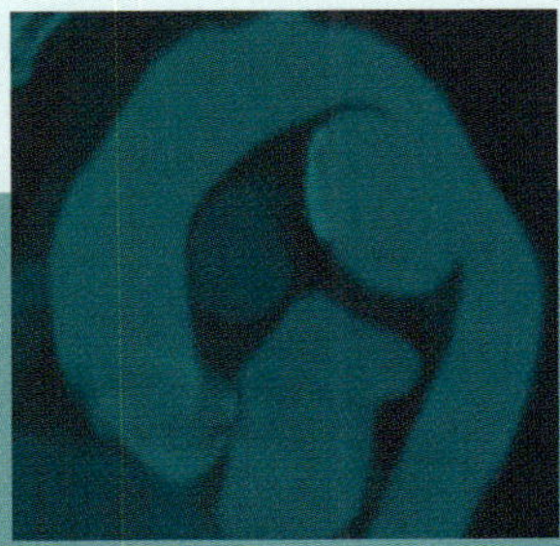

Bradley D. Allen • Karen G. Ordovas

CT and MRI of the Thoracic Aorta

INTRODUCTION

The thoracic aorta is best evaluated with cross-sectional imaging. Computed tomography angiography (CTA) is commonly used in the acute setting because of its availability and speed, along with its unique ability to diagnose nonaortic disease, whereas surveillance imaging of known aortic pathology can be performed with either CTA or magnetic resonance angiography (MRA). Other imaging modalities that may identify aortic disease are the chest X-ray and transesophageal echocardiography (TEE), but neither one offers a complete assessment of the thoracic aorta. If aortic dilation is suspected or partially imaged with X-ray or TEE, further evaluation with cross-sectional imaging should be performed for a more comprehensive assessment.

Aortic dissection and rupture are high-mortality events and are the central focus of CTA evaluation of the thoracic aorta for acute chest pain. Along with the related pathologies of intramural hematoma and penetrating aortic ulcer (PAU), these life-threatening diseases are termed the *acute aortic syndromes*. We will discuss the clinical context in which these disorders often present, their key imaging findings and significance, as well as management options.

Surveillance imaging can be appropriate in some instances of acute aortic syndromes and is the mainstay of clinical management of aortic dilation and smaller aortic aneurysms. The common theme of surveillance imaging is that elective aortic repair is performed at a threshold aortic diameter or interval growth rate. We will review strategies for making accurate and reproducible aortic diameter measurements and consider some of the new functional imaging techniques that can reveal more of the complexity of aortic disease than conventional anatomic analysis alone.

Endovascular management of aortic disease has advanced considerably in the last decade. Aortic stent grafting has been increasingly used with promising long-term results, and transcatheter aortic valve repair (TAVR) is now commonly used in many patients with severe and symptomatic aortic stenosis who are not optimal surgical candidates. New CTA protocols and more involved aortic measurements are needed for preprocedural planning, particularly for TAVR evaluation. We will highlight these techniques and address some of the challenging issues that frequently arise with aortic imaging, including the need for cardiac-gated studies, imaging with renal failure, and the value of noncontrast evaluation.

IMAGING TECHNIQUES

CTA and MRA are the principal modalities for aortic imaging. The advantages of CT are its speed, ease of use, and lack of operator dependence. At many institutions, CT is the examination of choice for the evaluation of acute aortic pathology. However, for serial evaluation, MR has several advantages: absence of ionizing radiation, avoidance of iodinated contrast agent, dynamic imaging, and a wider range of soft tissue contrast that allows the delineation of vascular and perivascular structures. In this section, we will discuss the utilization trends of CT and magnetic resonance imaging (MRI) in the evaluation of aortic pathology and introduce general imaging protocols.

Computed Tomography Angiography

A typical aortic protocol in the setting of acute chest pain or the postoperative aorta includes a noncontrast series in addition to the CTA. Thick slices (5 mm) are sufficient for the noncontrast scan, the purpose of which is to evaluate for intramural hematoma and/or to identify dense surgical material that could be misconstrued as contrast on the CTA. Delayed postcontrast imaging may be added for the evaluation of aortic rupture or endoleaks if thoracic endovascular aortic repair (TEVAR) was performed.

Modern 64-slice or better scanners generate slice thicknesses of less than 1 mm, which provide excellent spatial resolution and allow for high-quality reconstructed images. While a pitch of 1.375 to 2 allows a large volume of coverage to be obtained rapidly, recent studies have demonstrated that adequate image quality can be obtained with significant reduction of radiation dose with high-pitch CTA of the aorta using dual-source CT (pitch values up to 3.4). Iodinated contrast volumes of approximately 80 to 140 mL are injected at a rate of 3 to 5 mL/s for optimal arterial enhancement. A standard scan delay of 25 seconds after the start of injection will usually suffice for CTA. However, patients with diminished cardiac function or an unsuspected stenosis of the injected vein may require longer delays to achieve optimal opacification. Automatic bolus detection and triggering software is now commonly used to optimize contrast opacification.

Motion is one of the main challenges of aortic imaging. Respiratory and other patient motion are minimized with the rapid imaging acquisition of modern CT scanners. Electrocardiographic (ECG) gating can reduce motion at the aortic root and is central to TAVR evaluation. Prospective ECG gating is preferable to retrospective gating because it reduces radiation exposure, but with cardiac arrhythmias and patient motion, stair-step artifacts may be seen (Fig. 30.1). High-pitch helical scanning with prospective ECG triggering can often provide adequate cardiac motion control with shorter breath-holds and lower radiation dose. This option should be considered when available, especially in young patients and in patients who may have difficulty with breath holding for longer ECG-gated acquisitions (Fig. 30.2).

Increased awareness of the risks of ionizing radiation in medical imaging in recent years has influenced CT protocols. Best practices for the reduction of radiation exposure in aortic imaging include the use of automatic tube current modulation, optimization of field of view, high-pitch helical scanning, and avoidance of unnecessary imaging. Iterative data reconstruction techniques permit the acquisition of diagnostic-quality images at lower radiation dose. Alternatives to ionizing radiation such as MRI may also be appropriate, particularly in young patients or those who will undergo serial aortic imaging.

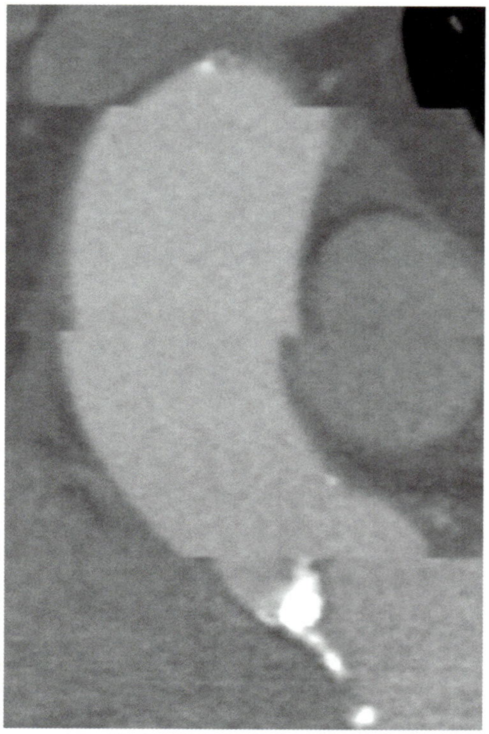

Figure 30.1. Stair-step artifact on cardiac-gated computed tomography angiography for transcatheter aortic valve planning.

Magnetic Resonance Imaging

The three most useful MRI sequences for evaluation of the thoracic aorta are: (1) bright blood steady-state free precession (SSFP) cine; (2) contrast-enhanced three-dimensional MR angiography (CEMRA), and (3) black-blood double inversion fast spin echo (Fig. 30.3). With respect to the long axis of the aorta, images can be acquired parallel (sagittal oblique) or perpendicular (transverse). ECG gating must be used for black blood and SSFP cine acquisitions, and should also be utilized in most CEMRA to provide cardiac motion control adequate for aortic root evaluation.

SSFP sequences render the blood pool homogeneously bright without the need for gadolinium-based contrast agent (GBCA). SSFP can also be used to provide dynamic cine images for valve or cardiac assessment. SSFP sequences are especially useful for aortic evaluation because they demonstrate intraluminal pathology as a “filling defect” in the bright blood pool. Slow flow and turbulent flow can result in signal perturbation and are potential sources of artifact. SSFP is a type of gradient echo (GRE) acquisition and is especially sensitive to magnetic field inhomogeneities and associated susceptibility artifact. When susceptibility artifacts are anticipated, such as in patients with cardiac implantable electronic device (CIED) or after aortic repair with metallic components SSFP images are likely to be low quality and alternative imaging with CE MRA or black-blood sequences may provide a better depiction of anatomy (Fig. 30.4).

Noncontrast MRA sequences using SSFP-based bright blood imaging are another potential solution in patients with contraindications to CT and MR contrast agents. These techniques are generally longer, “free-breathing” acquisitions that utilize both respiratory compensation and ECG-gating to achieve adequate motion control. In addition to being noncontrast, the fact that these techniques do not require breath-holding can be advantageous in many patients with cardiopulmonary diseases.

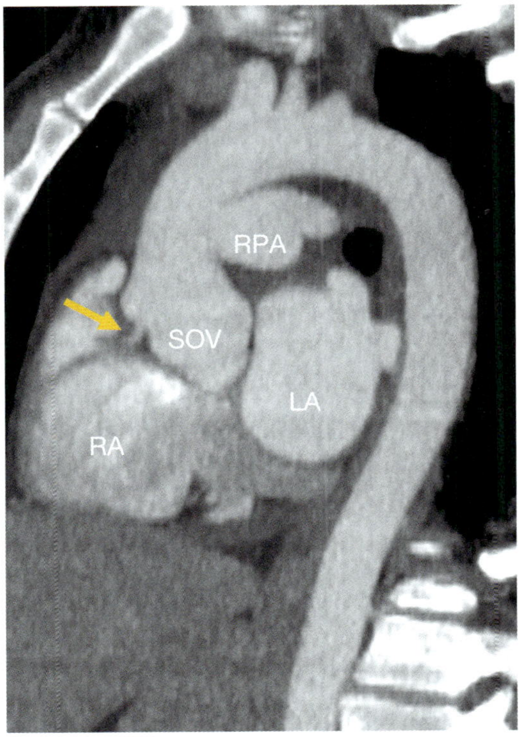

Figure 30.2. High-pitch helical prospective ECG triggered computed tomography angiography maximal intensity projection demonstrating a high origin of the right coronary artery (yellow arrow). ECG, electrocardiographic; LA, left atrium; RA, right atrium; RPA, right pulmonary artery; SOV, sinuses of Valsalva.

MRA with intravenous gadolinium chelate contrast agent relies on the T1-shortening effect of gadolinium to produce high-signal intensity in blood vessels, thereby avoiding flow-related artifacts. Timing of the acquisition can be optimized by using real-time imaging for bolus detection or by performing a preliminary acquisition employing a test bolus. Cardiac gating is generally recommended to provide adequate cardiac motion control (Fig. 30.5), especially for evaluation of the ascending aorta in acute aortic syndrome or the aortic root in patients with hereditary thoracic aortic disease.

For black-blood imaging, a double inversion recovery pulse sequence is used to suppress the signal of flowing blood, making the aortic lumen black. This technique can be especially useful in patients with aortitis with edematous and thickened aortic wall. Luminal signal is not completely suppressed, however, when there is slow flow, leading to artifacts. Other limitations of black-blood imaging are the need for multiple breath holds and static imaging, limiting aortic evaluation to a single time point. The black-blood pulse sequence utilizes a spin echo approach for spin refocusing and this technique is less prone to susceptibility artifact relative to SSFP or GRE pulse sequences.

There is an increasing need to image patients with MR conditional pacemakers/defibrillators, aortic valve prosthesis, and other implantable prostheses. As discussed above, SSFP sequences are more artifact-prone in these circumstances. Especially in patients with CIED, dedicated low specific absorption rate protocols that account for institutional

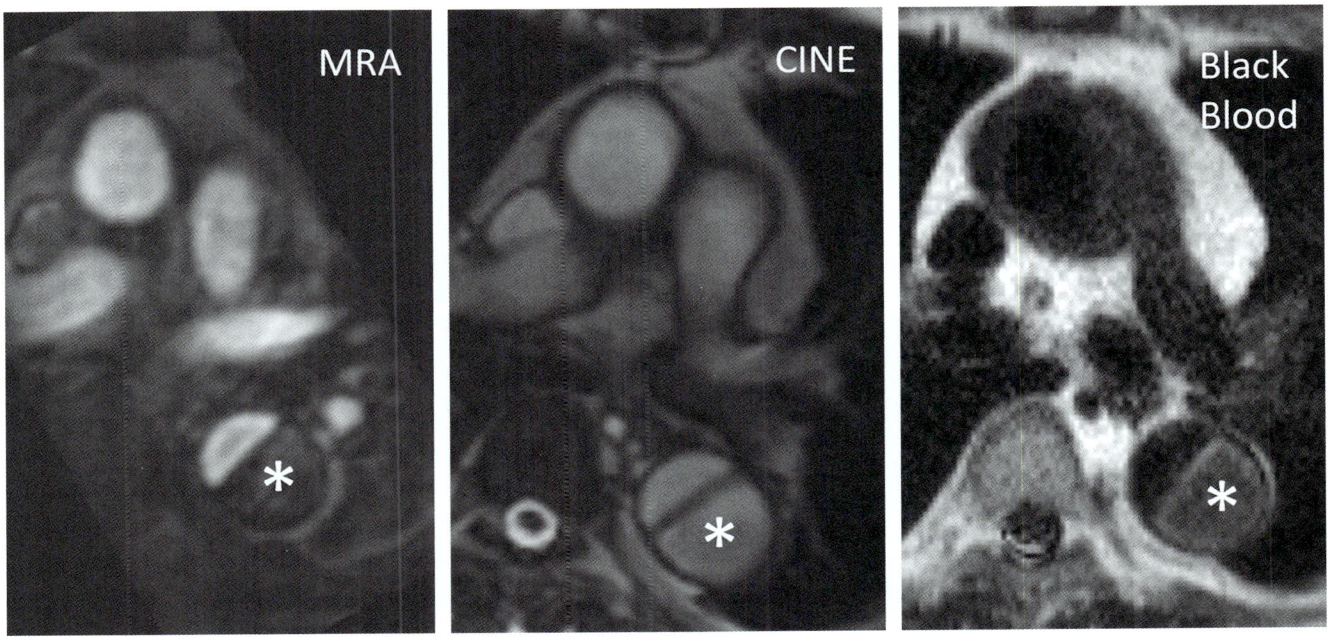

Figure 30.3. First-pass contrast-enhanced magnetic resonance angiography is analogous to computed tomography angiography where the smaller true lumen in this type B dissection is enhanced relative to the false lumen (*asterisk*). Bright blood steady-state free precession cine (CINE) relies on intrinsic signal within the blood pool, and thus both true and false lumen are equally bright. Black-blood double inversion fast spin echo (Black Blood) is designed to nullify signal in fast-flowing blood but demonstrates signal in slow or stagnant blood flow, explaining why there is an increased signal in the false lumen here.

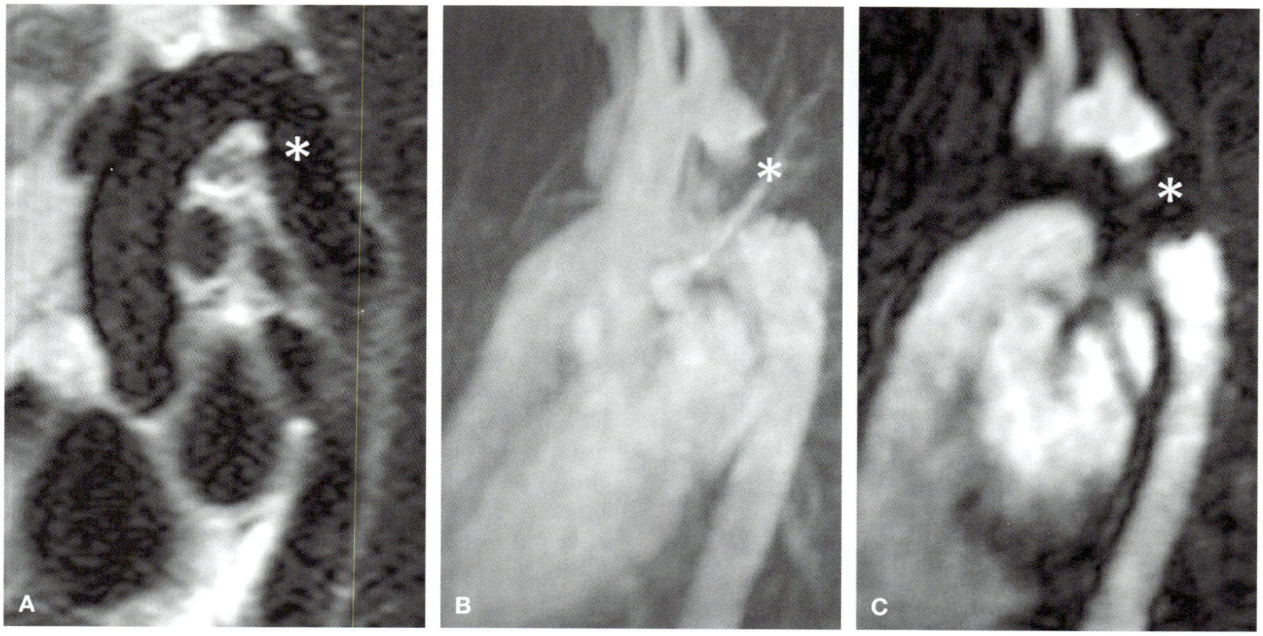

Figure 30.4. Because black-blood imaging **(A)** employs a spin echo sequence, which can provide a better depiction of anatomy when susceptibility artifacts are anticipated, such as in this patient after stent repair of aortic coarctation (*asterisk*). Gradient echo sequences like magnetic resonance angiography [maximum intensity projection in **(B)** and sagittal slice in **(C)**] are severely limited by the susceptibility artifact caused by the aortic stent.

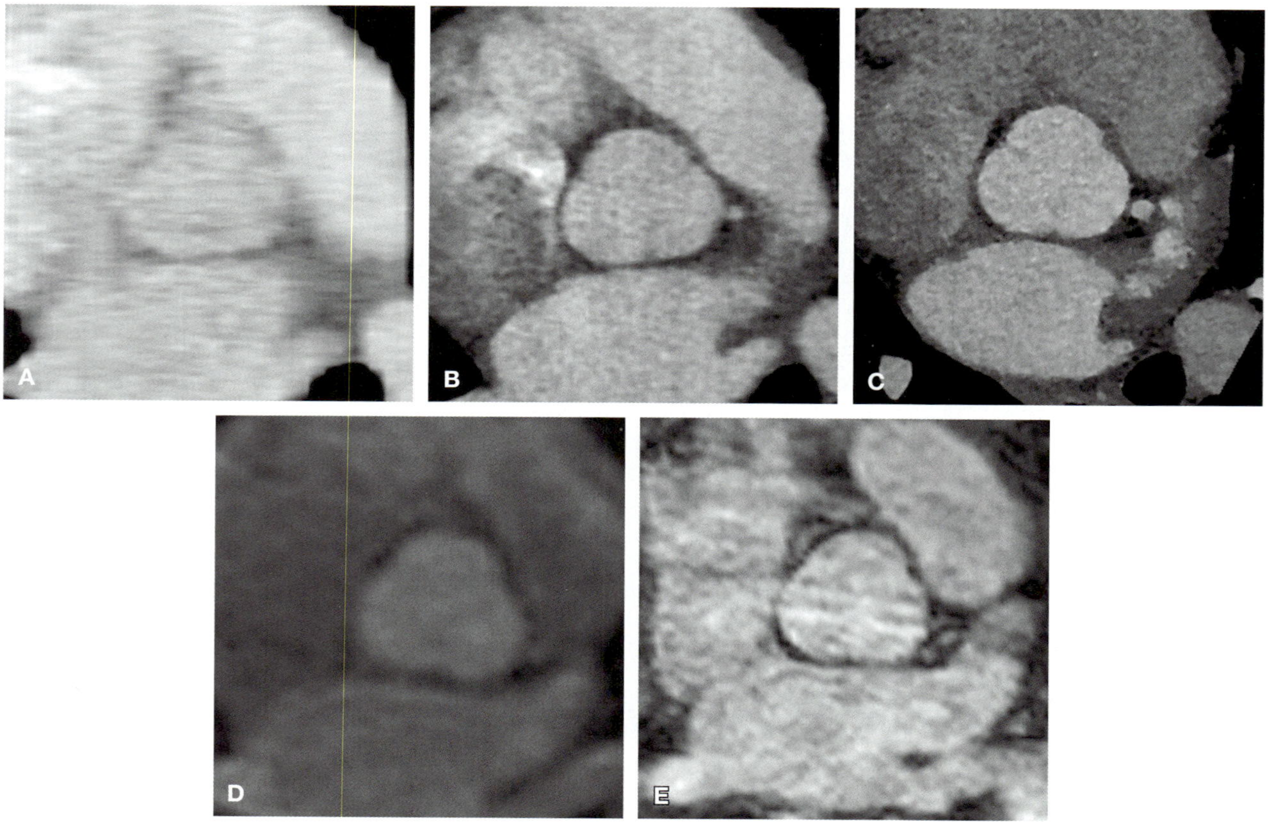

Figure 30.5. Aortic root evaluation in a 38-year-old man with ascending aortic aneurysm using **(A)** nongated CT Chest, **(B)** high-pitch helical prospectively ECG triggered CTA, **(C)** ECG-Gated CTA, **(D)** ECG gated contrast-enhanced MRA, **(E)** respiratory and ECG gated steady-state free precession MRA. CTA, computed tomography angiography; ECG, electrocardiographic; MRA, magnetic resonance angiography.

policy and expert guidance are necessary to ensure safe and effective imaging of these patients.

Renal failure makes aortic imaging challenging with both CT and MRI. Concerns regarding nephrogenic systemic fibrosis (NSF) have limited the utilization of certain GBCA for MRA. The American College of Radiology recognizes several GBCAs as Group II agents which are associated with a low risk of NSF and can generally be safely used in most patients with reduced renal function. Alternative MRI contrast agents that do not carry a risk of NSF have been explored such as the ultrasmall superparamagnetic iron oxide (USPIO) particle ferumoxytol (see "Emerging Trends" section).

ACUTE AORTA

In this section, we will discuss the imaging of acutely symptomatic aortic pathology including trauma/aortic rupture and the *acute aortic syndromes*, which encompass intramural hematoma, PAU, and aortic dissection. CT is the primary imaging modality used to evaluate acute aortic syndromes. Surveillance imaging of chronic aortic pathologies, where MR is more frequently employed, will be discussed in the following section.

Traumatic Aortic Injury

Traumatic aortic injury (TAI) is usually the result of severe deceleration, such as a high-speed motor vehicle collision or a fall from height. TAI may result in aortic rupture leading to exsanguination and immediate death in 80% to 90% of patients (Figs. 30.6 and 30.7). Among patients with TAI who survive the initial trauma, the mortality of untreated TAI may be as high as 1% per hour for the first 48 hours. The most common site of TAI is the aortic isthmus (90%). The reason for this preponderance of injury at the isthmus is that the aorta is tethered here by the ligamentum arteriosum, focusing on the shearing forces experienced during a rapid deceleration injury at this location. Other sites to consider are the great vessel origins (5% to 10%), the aortocardiac junction (1%), and the descending aorta at the diaphragmatic hiatus (1% to 3%).

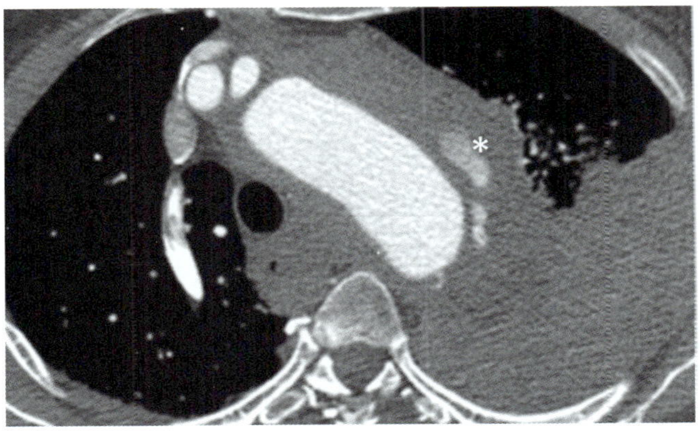

Figure 30.6. Aortic rupture with traumatic aortic injury as evidenced by active extravasation of contrast into the mediastinum (*asterisk*) with hemorrhage throughout the mediastinum and left pleural space.

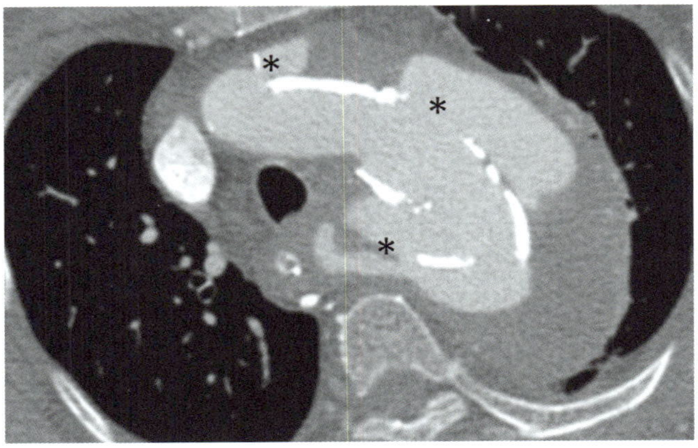

Figure 30.7. Aortic rupture with traumatic aortic injury as evidenced by clear disruption of the calcified aortic wall (*asterisk*) and both contrast and blood throughout the mediastinum.

Imaging of Traumatic Aortic Injury

CTA has replaced catheter angiography in the assessment of TAI. CTA findings of TAI can be classified as direct or indirect. A common direct finding of TAI is a pseudoaneurysm at the aortic isthmus (Fig. 30.8). A congenital ductus diverticulum may be a mimicker of aortic pseudoaneurysm;

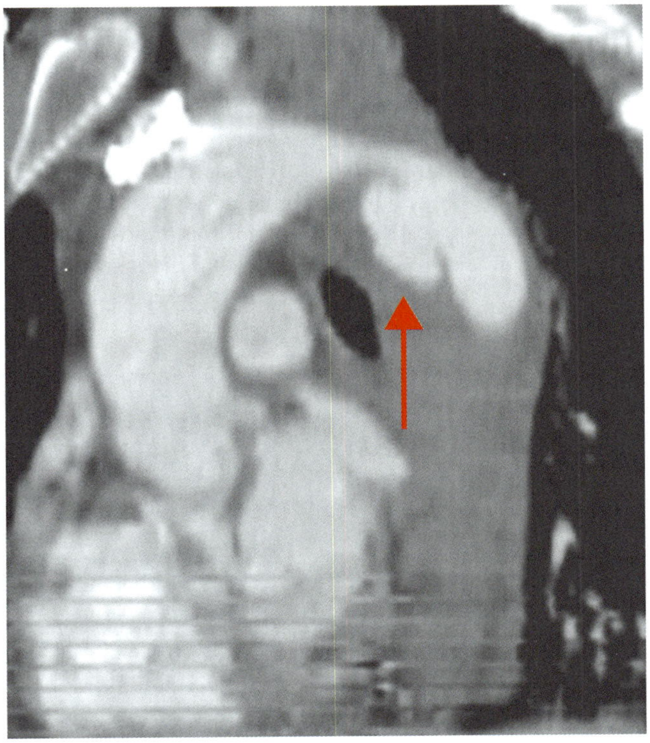

Figure 30.8. The most common site of traumatic aortic injury is the aortic isthmus where the aorta is tethered by the ligamentum arteriosum. In this case of traumatic aortic injury, a pseudoaneurysm (*red arrow*) is seen at this location.

however, this benign finding can usually be distinguished by its smooth border and obtuse angles with the wall of the aorta (Fig. 30.9). Extravasation of contrast is a rarely seen direct sign of TAI. Other direct signs are an intimal flap or irregularity. Subtle aortic injuries or isolated intimal injuries are now more commonly seen with high spatial resolution CTA. Patients with direct findings of TAI are usually treated by urgent endovascular repair or surgery.

The indirect sign of TAI is mediastinal hematoma, but this is a problematic finding because it more commonly results from benign injury of small mediastinal vessels or adjacent fractures than from TAI. When a mediastinal hematoma is noted, its relationship to the aorta should be determined. Hematoma that is in direct contact with the aorta (ie, not separated by a fat plane) is more likely the result of aortic injury. In contrast, mediastinal hematoma that is separated from the aorta by an intact fat plane is often due to venous bleeding (Fig. 30.10).

Acute Aortic Syndromes

Acute aortic syndrome is a term for the overlapping clinical presentations of aortic dissection and the related pathologies of intramural hematoma and PAU/pseudoaneurysm. In this section, we will introduce each of these pathologies, discuss the typical imaging appearance, and briefly address treatment strategies. Follow-up of previously diagnosed or repaired acute aortic syndromes will be discussed in the following section.

Aortic Dissection

Aortic dissection is a separation of the aortic wall that results from a tear in the intima. Blood extends through the intimal disruption into the media, displacing the intima inward. The dissection may reenter the lumen at one or more sites of fenestration. Typically blood flows through both the true and false channels, although the false channel is sometimes thrombosed. The most common entry points for aortic dissection are just distal to the sinuses of Valsalva and just beyond the origin of the left subclavian artery. In older patients (>40 years old), the single most common predisposing factor for aortic dissection is hypertension. Younger patients (<40 years old), in contrast, are likely to have genetic aortopathy, frequently associated with connective tissue disorder such as Marfan syndrome or bicuspid aortic valve.

Aortic dissection can be classified by the Stanford or DeBakey systems, both of which are based on the location of the dissection and the presence or absence of ascending aortic involvement. Stanford type A dissections involve the ascending aorta, whereas type B dissections involve the descending aorta only, originating beyond the left subclavian artery origin. The DeBakey system divides dissections into three types: type I involves the ascending aorta and extends into the descending aorta; type II involves the ascending aorta only; and type III involves the descending aorta only, beyond the origin of the left subclavian artery (Fig. 30.11).

Aortic dissection involving the aortic arch has been a source of controversy. A unified classification system was recently proposed in order to align radiology terminology with the surgical literature and suggests the classification of aortic arch lesions without the involvement of the ascending aorta as Stanford type B dissections with aortic arch involvement.

There are four life-threatening complications of type A (I and II) dissection: pericardial hemorrhage and tamponade; aortic valve rupture and acute aortic insufficiency; coronary artery dissection and myocardial infarction; and carotid artery dissection and stroke. Patients with type A dissection usually undergo immediate surgery. Type B dissections, on the other hand, have been traditionally managed with medical therapy alone, although stent grafting is now increasingly used with good results. Recent studies have demonstrated decreased 5-year mortality in patients with type B dissection treated with TEVAR compared to medical management.

Thrombosis of the false channel and remodeling of the thoracic aorta can occur in some patients. Persistent false

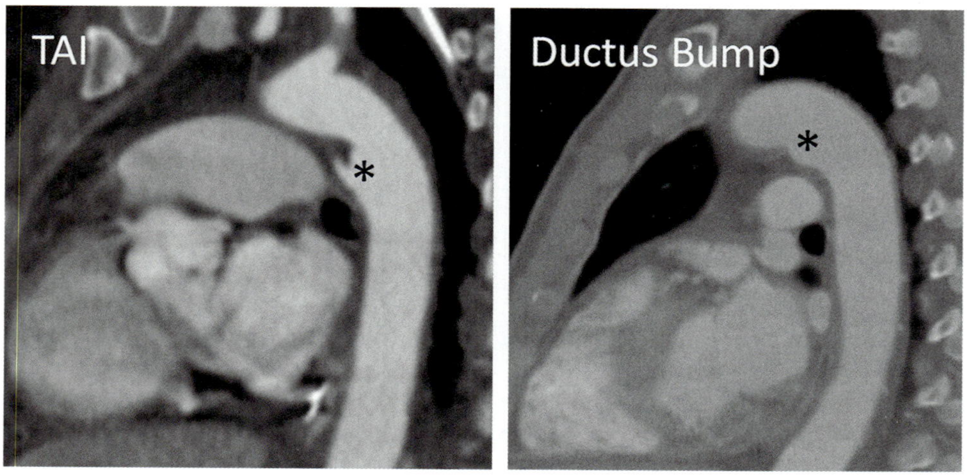

Figure 30.9. Traumatic aortic injury results in sharp and acute angles at the aortic isthmus (*asterisk*), whereas a congenital ductus diverticulum (ductus bump) can usually be distinguished by its smooth border and obtuse angles with the wall of the aorta (*asterisk*).

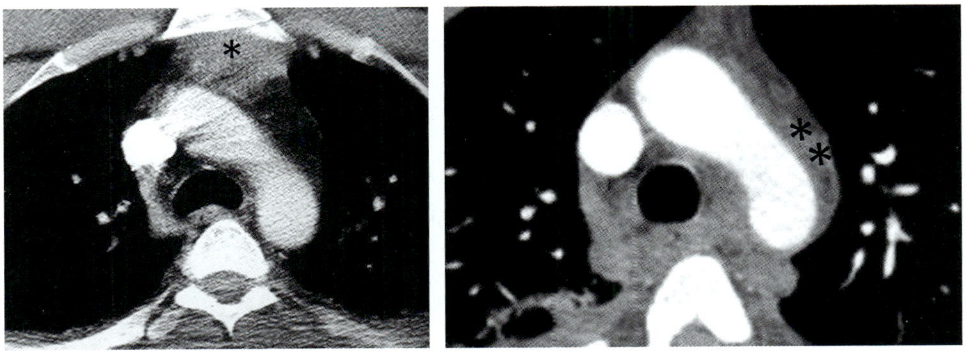

Figure 30.10. Mediastinal hematoma that is separated from the aorta by an intact fat plane (**left**, *single asterisk*) is likely benign, and often due to venous bleeding, whereas hematoma in direct contact with the aorta (**right**, *two asterisk*) is more likely the result of traumatic aortic injury.

lumen patency years following aortic dissection have been shown to be associated with a poor prognosis, including increased mortality and requirement for surgical repair. The presence of multiple false lumens, also known as the "multibarreled" aorta, has been shown to be a very poor prognostic sign. Patients with multibarreled aorta demonstrate a significantly lower survival rate compared to patients with only one false lumen, also called the "double-barreled" aorta (Fig. 30.12).

Limited intimal tear (LIT) is an increasingly recognized subtype of acute aortic syndrome. Similar to aortic dissection, LIT is characterized by a tear in the intimal layer of the aorta. However, in the case of LIT, the tear does not result in significant dissection of blood into the media, but often has a small focal bulge or contour irregularity (Fig. 30.13). Recognizing this entity as a cause of acute chest pain is important as studies suggest similar 30-day and 5-year outcomes as other causes of acute aortic syndrome.

Imaging of Aortic Dissection

Beyond establishing the diagnosis, the goals of imaging are to identify the extent of involvement and provide accurate classification; identify the entry tear location; determine if arch vessels or coronary arteries are involved and if they arise from true or false lumen; assess the patency of the false lumen; and assess for complications including pericardial hematoma, which can result in tamponade and is an indication for immediate surgery. Noncontrast images are useful for demonstrating high attenuation intramural hematoma (discussed in the next section) or thrombosis of the false lumen. Noncontrast images may also show inward displacement of

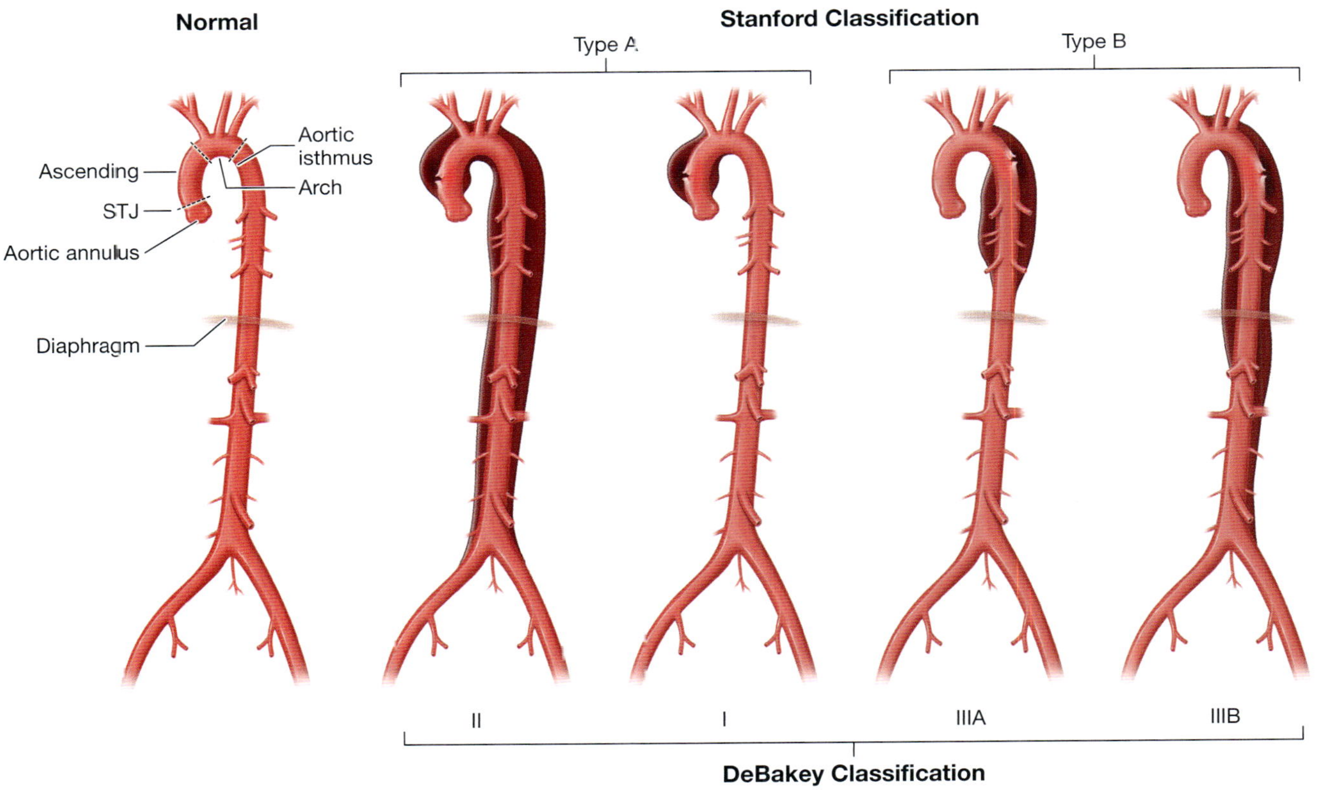

Figure 30.11. Two commonly used classification systems for aortic dissection. STJ, sinotubular junction.

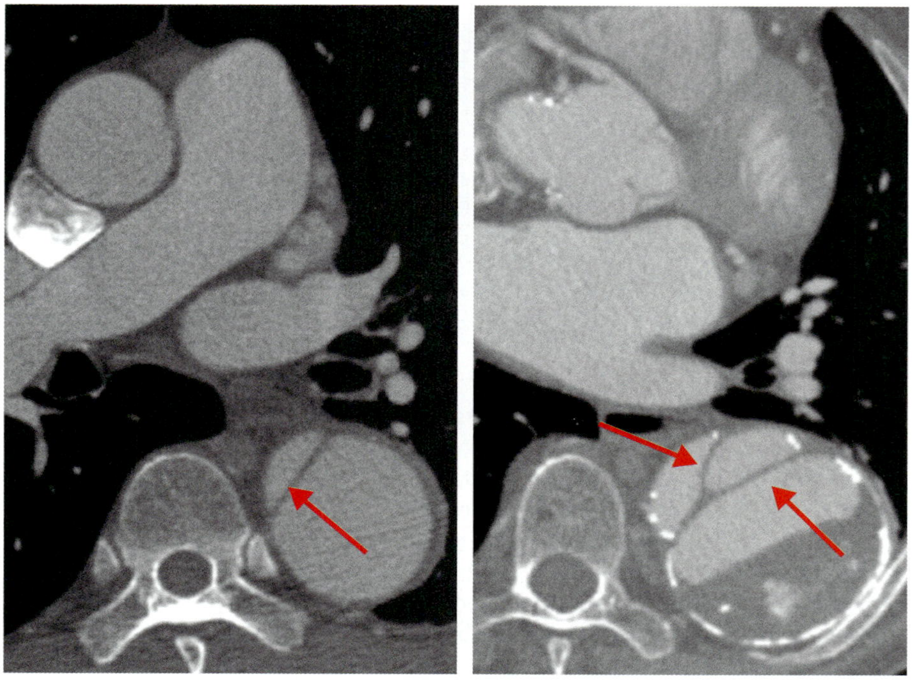

Figure 30.12. Double-barreled (**left**, *red arrow*) versus multibarreled (**right**, *red arrows*) aortic dissection.

intimal calcification. The most reliable finding for the diagnosis of dissection on CTA is the presence of an intimal flap separating the true and false channels (Fig. 30.14).

By MRI, the definitive diagnosis of dissection also requires the identification of the intimal flap. MRA is similar to CTA with early arterial enhancement in the true lumen relative to the false lumen. SSFP cine images rely on intrinsic signal, rather than IV contrast, and will have bright signal in both the true and false lumens if they are patent. Absence of signal can be seen with slow flow or thrombus. Black-blood imaging may reveal an intimal flap between the flow void in the true and false channels if there is rapid flow in the false channel, or elevated signal in the false channel if there is slow flow (Fig. 30.3).

Differentiating between the true and false channels can sometimes be challenging. Relative size may be useful, as the true lumen is typically smaller compared to the false lumen. The dynamic change of the lumens, if evident, is very useful for identifying the true lumen: It will increase in size with systole and flatten with diastole. A pathognomonic sign of the false lumen that is occasionally seen is the "cobweb sign," or remnants of the torn-up aortic media through the false lumen. When the dissection flap appears as a circular or oval

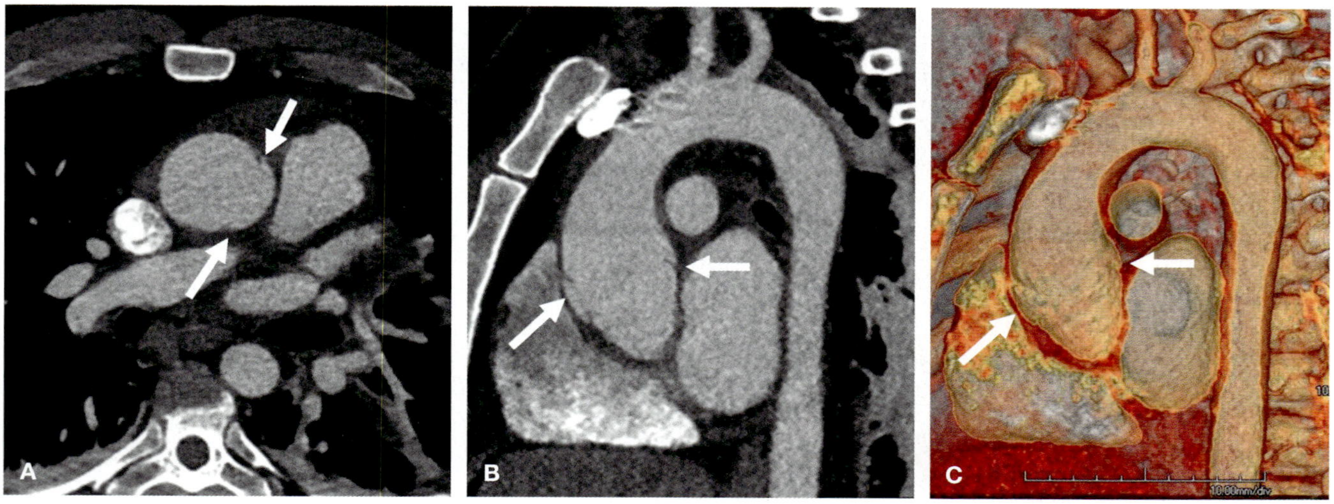

Figure 30.13. A 37-year-old man with a history of hypertension presenting with substernal chest pain radiating to the back. On imaging, a limited intimal tear (*white arrows*) with associated focal bulge of the ascending aorta. A and B show this region on axial **(A)** and sagittal oblique **(B)** CT angiography. Panel C uses cinematic rendering to better visualize the contour abnormality. (Images provided by Dr. Jody Shen, Stanford University.)

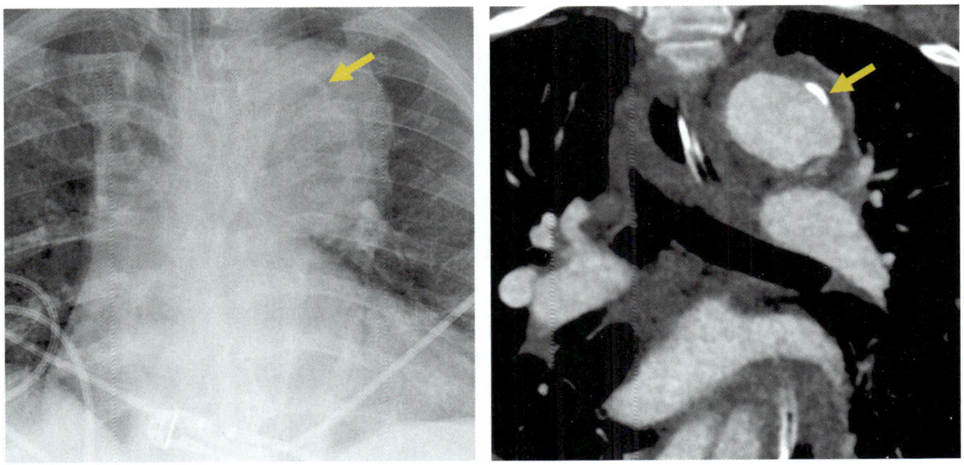

Figure 30.14. Displaced intimal calcifications (*yellow arrow*) in type B aortic dissection on chest radiograph (left) and computed tomography angiography (right).

structure within the center of the aorta, the center of the circular/oval structure represents the true lumen (Fig. 30.15).

Surveillance imaging is used to monitor the progression of disease either postrepair or in patients for whom the intervention is deferred. For chronic type B dissection, delayed aortic repair is indicated when the overall aortic size surpasses 5.5 cm.

Intramural Hematoma

Intramural hematoma (IMH) is bleeding within the media of the aortic wall. It has been suggested that IMH may be caused by rupture of the vasa vasorum, the arteries that supply the aortic wall. However, increasingly, data suggests that IMH is caused primarily by small intimal tears that are not resolved by imaging. If the intima does not rupture, causing a frank dissection, an intramural hematoma is generated (Fig. 30.16). Management of intramural hematoma is similar to that of aortic dissection and depends upon the location (Table 30.1). While intramural hematoma can progress to dissection or spontaneously resolve, the most common long-term sequela of intramural hematoma is aortic aneurysm or pseudoaneurysm.

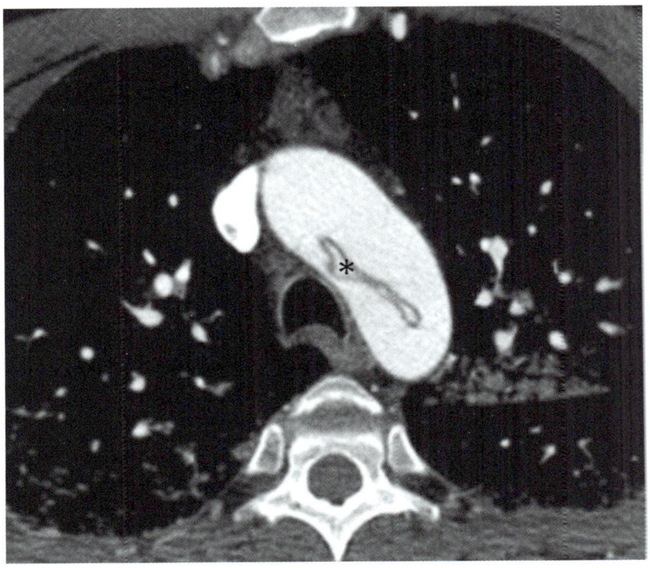

Figure 30.15. Extreme case of aortic dissection with circumferential detachment of the intima with a small and distorted true lumen centrally (*asterisk*).

Imaging of Intramural Hematoma

Noncontrast CT is particularly useful in the diagnosis of IMH. Although the crescent-shaped high-density thickening of the aortic wall may be appreciated on contrast-enhanced images, the finding is often more conspicuous on noncontrast images (Fig. 30.17). Noncontrast images can also be useful for distinguishing atherosclerotic plaque from IMH (Fig. 30.18). IMH is diagnosed on MR T1-weighted black-blood images by the presence of intermediate- or high-signal-intensity material within the wall of the aorta. MRI may be used in the follow-up of IMH in those cases where surveillance is elected rather than intervention (Fig. 30.19).

Penetrating Aortic Ulcer/Pseudoaneurysm

Development of a PAU occurs when atherosclerotic plaque burrows into the vessel wall, disrupting the internal elastic lamina and extending into the media. PAU most commonly occurs in the mid–descending thoracic aorta. This is in contrast to the more common *ulcerated plaque*, which is an asymptomatic ulceration of atherosclerotic plaque without penetration of the internal elastic lamina (Fig. 30.20). The saccular progression of contrast beyond the media contained only by adventitia and surrounding fibrous tissue is defined as a pseudoaneurysm (Fig. 30.21). Aortic pseudoaneurysms (aka false aneurysms) are saccular in configuration and extend well beyond the vessel wall. The three major causes of aortic pseudoaneurysms are PAU, trauma (as previously discussed), and infection (called mycotic pseudoaneurysms) (Fig. 30.22).

Mycotic pseudoaneurysms result from an infection of the aortic wall following the involvement of the vasa vasorum

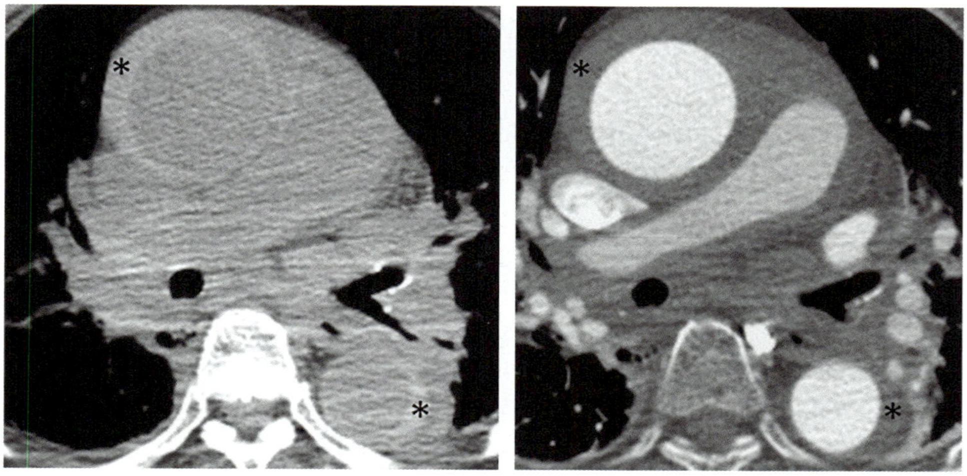

Figure 30.16. Intramural hematoma imaged with noncontrast CT (**left**, *asterisk*) and computed tomography angiography (**right**, *asterisk*). Note how the crescentic high density in the aortic wall at the convexity is more conspicuous on the noncontrast evaluation.

by septic emboli. Etiologies of mycotic pseudoaneurysm include septic emboli from intravenous drug use and indwelling catheters, infection of prosthetic valves, or infection of atherosclerotic plaque. Common infectious agents include *Salmonella*, *Staphylococcus aureus*, streptococci, tuberculosis, and fungi, such as Candida and *Aspergillus*. As they are at high risk for rupture, mycotic pseudoaneurysms are often repaired.

Imaging of PAU/Pseudoaneurysm

Unlike the more common ulcerated plaque, a PAU usually causes a contour abnormality of the aorta because it penetrates into the vessel wall. The aorta will no longer have a circular margin but instead bulge in the direction of involvement (Fig. 30.20). A pseudoaneurysm will also have an asymmetric bulging of the aortic contour, but the characteristic finding of this pathology is a saccular outpouching beyond the outer vessel wall with a narrow neck. Sometimes it is difficult to determine if a lesion extends into the vessel wall (PAU) or beyond the wall (pseudoaneurysm) with imaging alone. As there is a continuum between a PAU and pseudoaneurysm, this type of intermediate lesion should, at minimum, be followed at a close interval, with intervention recommended should a frank pseudoaneurysm develop (Fig. 30.21).

SURVEILLANCE IMAGING

Surveillance imaging is most commonly used to follow aortic dimensions. When threshold diameters are met, elective intervention should be considered, as the risk of disease progression is greater than the risk of surgical repair or other intervention. Follow-up aortic imaging may also be used for the acute aortic syndromes, as discussed in the previous section. In this section, we will review surveillance imaging goals and guidelines for dilated aortas, as well as the role of imaging in the diagnosis and management of aortic vasculitis and neoplasms.

Thoracic Aortic Aneurysm

Surprisingly, an accurate definition of normal aorta size and aorta aneurysm is not straightforward. The traditional definition of aneurysm is a vessel with a diameter that is 1.5 times larger than normal. This definition of aneurysm does not hold for the aortic root or ascending aorta. Importantly, normal dimensions vary by biological sex and body size, and indexed aortic measurements or aorta volumes may be better suited to capture this variability. True aneurysms are fusiform in shape and most frequently occur secondary to atherosclerosis. Other etiologies of true aneurysms include hypertension, connective tissue disorders such as Marfan

Table 30.1 High-Risk Features of Intramural Hematoma According to the 2022 AHA/ACC Guidelines for the Diagnosis and Management of Aortic Disease

Type A IMH	Type B IMH	Both Type A and Type B IMH
• Max aortic diameter >45-50 mm • IMH thickness ≥10 mm • Intimal disruption with ulcer-like projection of ascending aorta or arch • Pericardial effusion	• Max aortic diameter >47-50 mm • IMH thickness ≥13 mm • Intimal disruption with ulcer-like projection of descending aorta in acute phase • Increasing or recurrent pleural effusion	• Progression to dissection • Increasing aortic diameter • Increasing hematoma thickness

IMH, intramural hematoma.

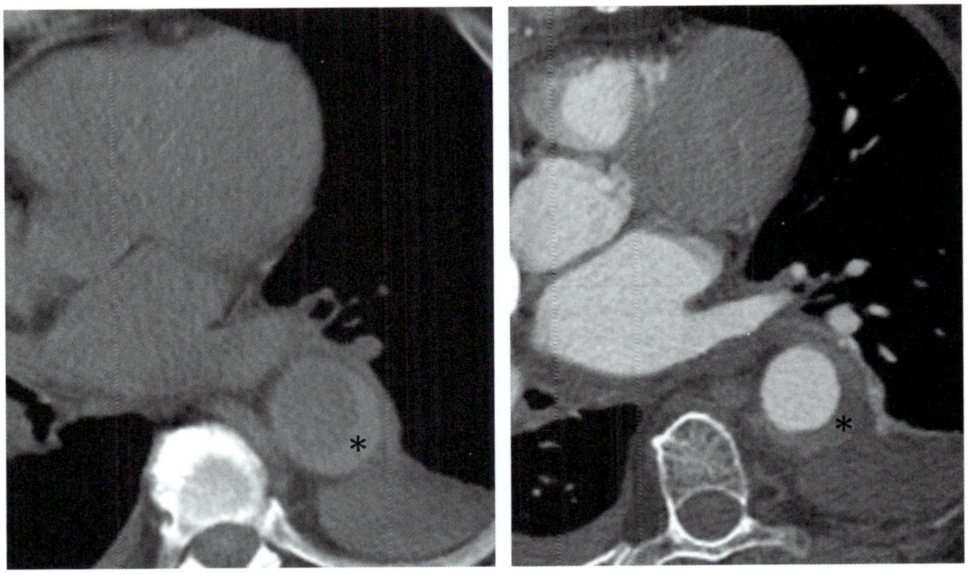

Figure 30.17. Noncontrast CT (**left**) versus computed tomography angiography (**right**) for evaluation of an intramural hematoma (*asterisk*) in the mid–descending thoracic aorta.

syndrome, nonsyndromic aortopathies such as bicuspid aortic valve, vasculitis, and valve-related aortic disease.

In general, aortic diameter greater than 4 cm is termed *dilation*, and this definition is useful for screening ascending aorta size on axial images at the level of the main pulmonary artery. Some authors suggest that *aneurysm* can be used for an aortic diameter greater than 5 cm. However, because normal and high-risk aorta dimensions are not consistent across patients' subgroups, it is more important and clinically relevant to provide accurate aortic dimensions and their change over time rather than summary terminology. In most instances, using the terms *dilated* or *non-dilated* along with reference measures allows for simplification and consistency of reporting across most patient cohorts. In general, the term ectasia should be avoided.

Elective repair of aortic aneurysms has a lower mortality rate than emergent repair, making regular surveillance and planned repair the preferred approach to management. Guidelines for the management and repair of fusiform aortic aneurysms are based on symptoms, aortic size, and rate of growth. Aortic diameters are the key determinant of risk (Table 30.2). For example, when the aortic diameter exceeds 6 cm, the risk of rupture in the next 5 years is greater than 30%. In the most recent guidelines, in patients with sporadic aorta aneurysms, elective repair is recommended at diameters of 5.5 cm or greater in the ascending aorta. For both the aortic arch and descending thoracic aorta, diameter equal to or greater than 5.5 cm is the size threshold for surgical intervention.

Size thresholds for elective repair differ in patients with heritable thoracic aortic disease and in patients who are already undergoing aortic valve interventions. For example, in Marfan syndrome, repair may be performed at aortic diameters of 4.5 to 5 cm. Patients with bicuspid aortic valve may undergo aortic valve replacement and ascending aortic repair at a diameter of 4.5 cm. Turner syndrome is another example of a patient subgroup at increased risk for aortic complications. Because they are typically small,

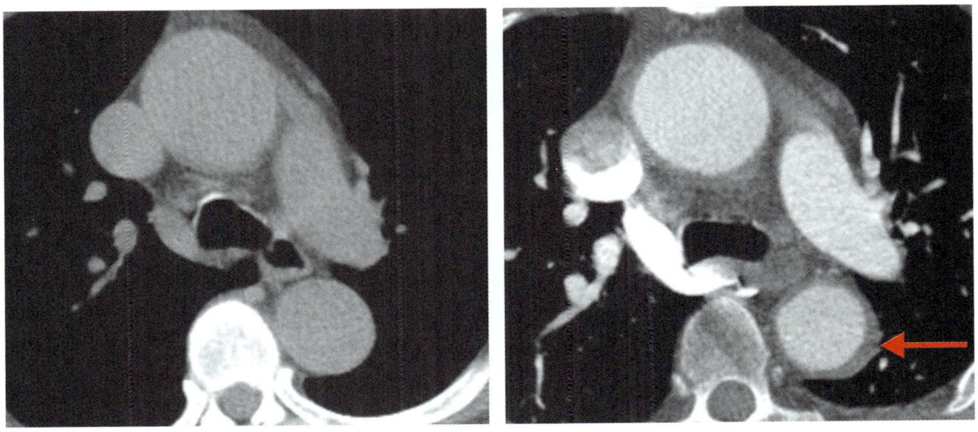

Figure 30.18. A possible small intramural hematoma seen on the computed tomography angiography (**right**, *red arrow*) does not demonstrate high density on the noncontrast CT (**left**) and is thus consistent with atherosclerotic plaque.

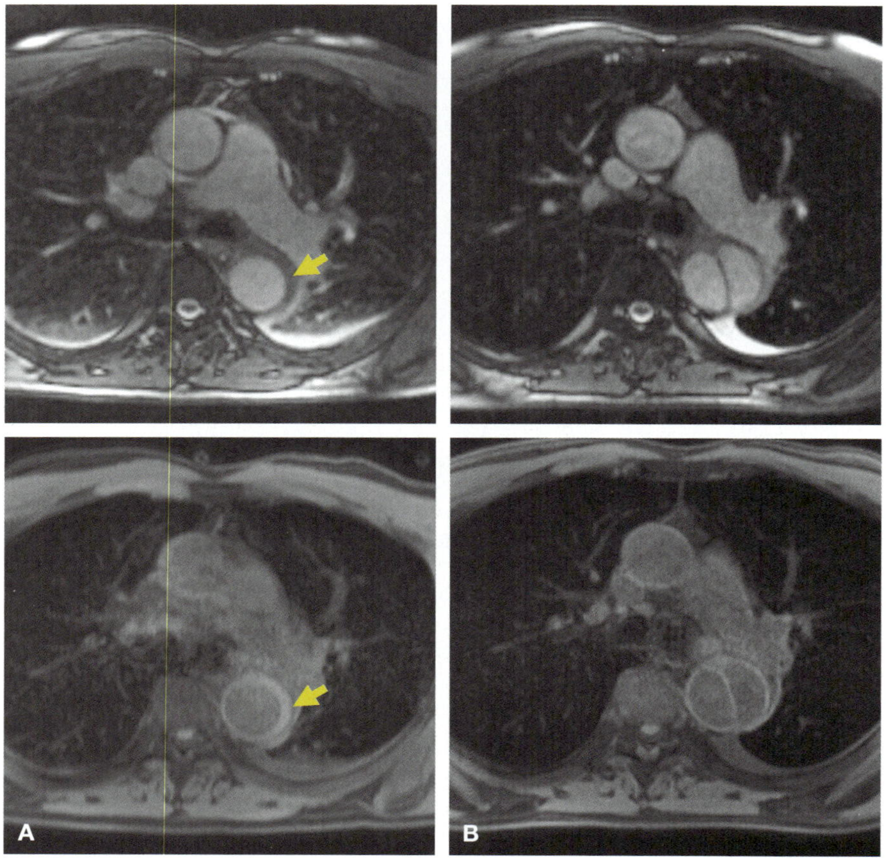

Figure 30.19. Magnetic resonance angiography of the thoracic aorta in a 64-year-old man with type B intramural hematoma at baseline (**panel A**, *arrows*) which progressed to type B aortic dissection 1 month later (**panel B**). Top images: balanced steady-state free precession. Bottom images: T1 weighted fat suppressed.

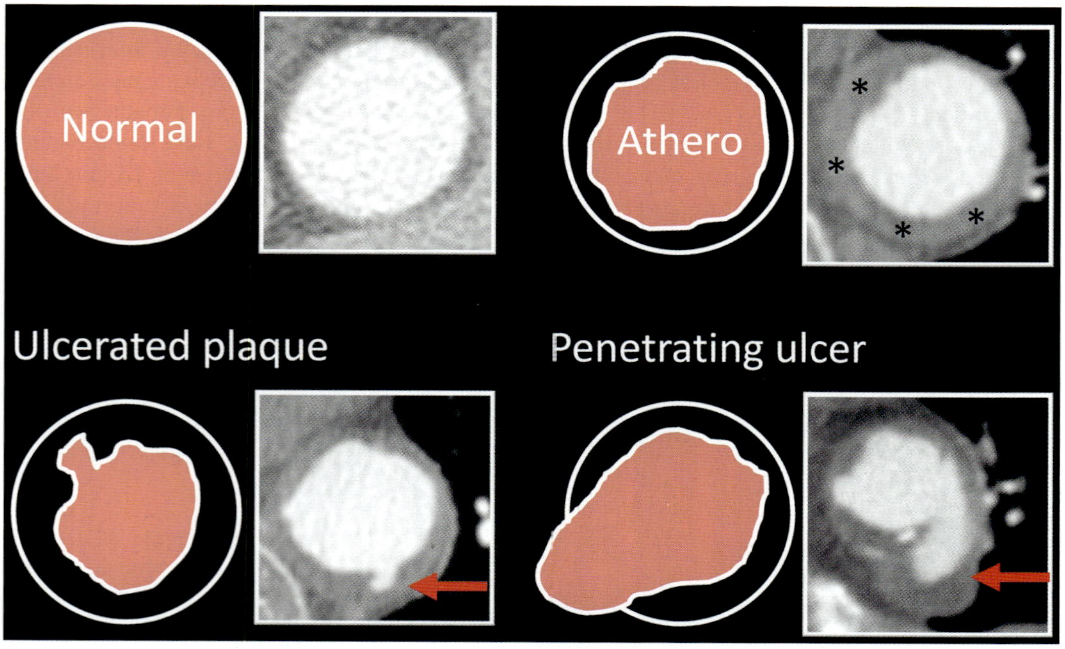

Figure 30.20. Ulcerated plaque versus penetrating aortic ulcer. The *white circle* in the diagram represents the internal elastic lamina of the aortic wall. Atherosclerosis with or without ulcerated plaque does not violate this *circle*, and the outer contour of the corresponding CTA images is not disrupted. A penetrating ulcer, however, violates the *circle* and borrows into the media of the aortic wall. Asymmetric bulging of the outer contour on the CTA is evident. CTA, computed tomography angiography.

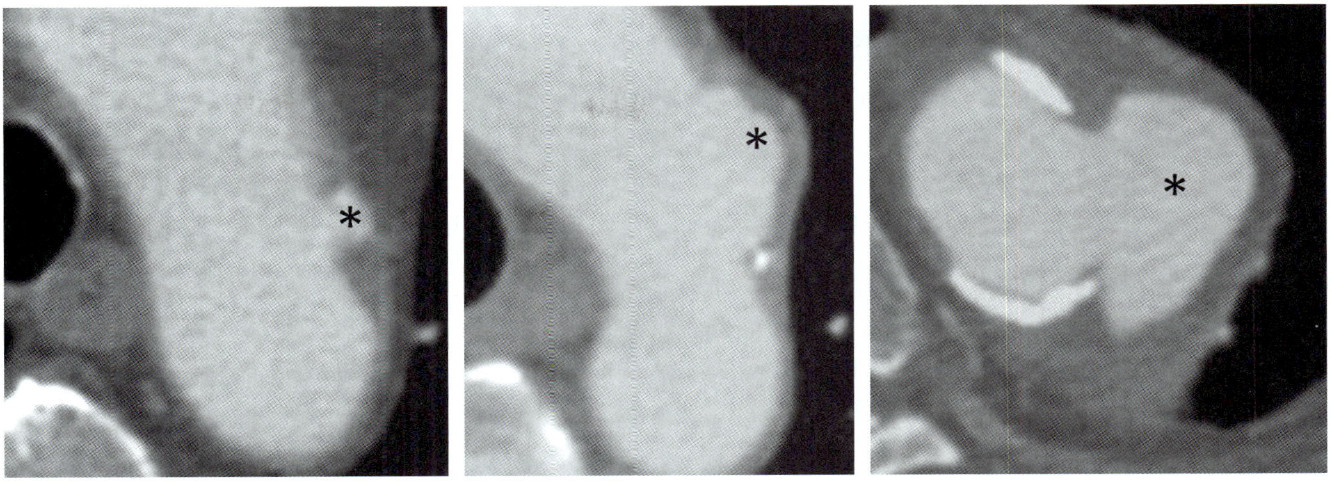

Figure 30.21. Penetrating aortic ulcer versus pseudoaneurysm. At the ends of the spectrum, a distinction between a process that extends into the vessel wall (penetrating aortic ulcer, **left**) versus a saccular outpouching beyond the vessel wall (pseudoaneurysm, **right**) can be made. For intermediate lesions (**center**), defining the extent of disease is challenging. They should, at minimum, be followed closely because they are at higher risk for progressing to frank pseudoaneurysms.

absolute aortic diameters are problematic in Turner syndrome patients, and diameters normalized by body surface area (BSA) better represent patient-specific risk.

Rapid aortic growth rate is another factor in the decision to perform elective repair. The mean growth rate for thoracic aortic aneurysms is low (1 mm per year or less). With fast growth rates of 3 mm per year for two consecutive years or 5 mm or more in 1 year, repair is generally recommended.

Imaging of Thoracic Aortic Aneurysm

The goals of imaging are to determine the maximum diameter, extent of involvement, and any findings that may suggest rapid progression or impending rupture. The concept of measuring aortic diameter is straightforward but can be challenging in practice. Measurements perpendicular to the aorta centerline are needed for reliable and reproducible

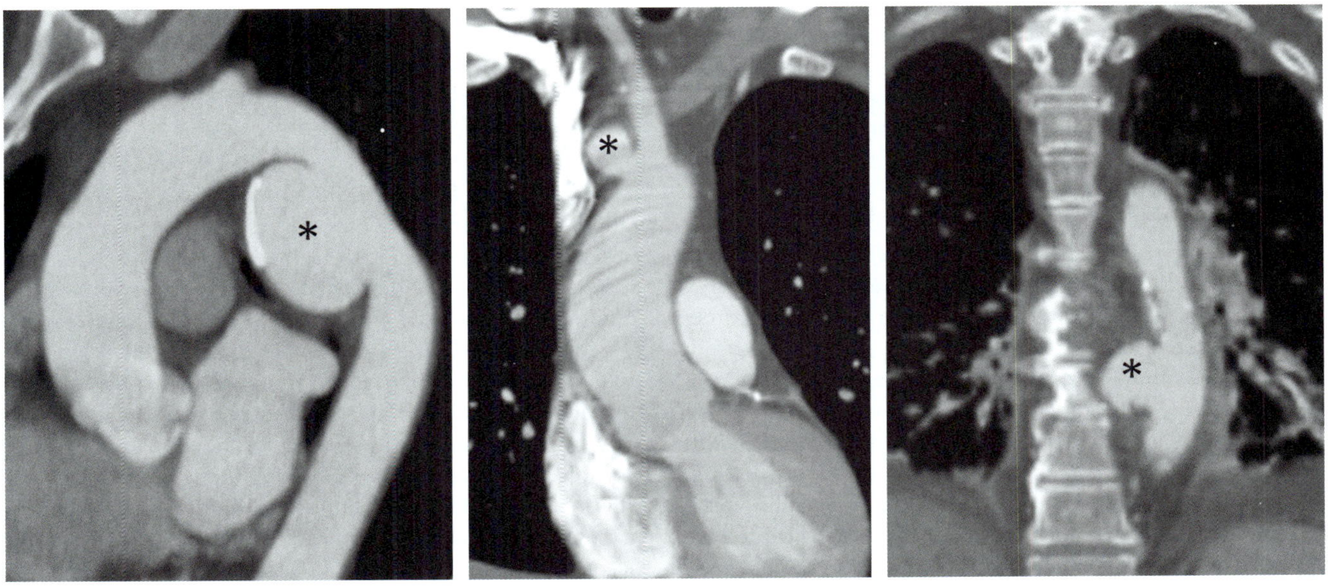

Figure 30.22. Characteristic computed tomography angiography images for the three etiologies of pseudoaneurysms (*asterisk*): trauma at the aortic isthmus (**left**); infection in a young intravenous drug user at an atypical location for both trauma and atherosclerosis (**center**); and atherosclerosis with a penetrating ulcer progressing to a pseudoaneurysm in the descending thoracic aorta (**right**).

Table 30.2 Aorta Size and Growth Rates Thresholds for Considering Surgical Intervention

Etiology of Aortic Aneurysm	Recommendation for Surgical Intervention	Growth Rate
Sporadic aortic aneurysm	≥5.5 cm	Rapid if >0.5 cm growth in 1 year Or >0.3 cm per year in 2 consecutive years
Non-syndromic heritable aortic aneurysm	≥5.0 cm Or ≥4.5 cm[a]	Rapid if >0.3 cm growth per year
Marfan syndrome	≥5.0 cm Or ≥4.5 cm[a]	
Loeys-Dietz syndrome	≥4.5 cm Or ≥4.0 cm[a]	
Ehlers-danlos syndrome	No data available. Increased risk of bleeding due to vascular fragility. Multidisciplinary Aortic- Team and shared-decision-making	
Turner syndrome	ASI [aortic diameter (cm^2)/BSA (m^2)] is recommended. ASI ≥2.5 cm/m^2 plus risk factors +	

The table shows the growth rate among heritable and non-heritable aortic diseases. ASI, aortic size index; BSA, body surface area.

[a]For heritable aortic diseases, specific clinical and historical risk factors may change risk assessments.

Used with permission from Hamid A, Gupta M, Rajiah PS, Abbara S, Hanneman K, Allen BD. The current and future role of imaging of thoracic aortic disease: a North American Society for cardiovascular imaging commentary on the 2022 AHA/ACC guidelines for the diagnosis and management of aortic disease. Int J Cardiovasc Imaging. *2024;40(1):5-14.*

assessment. Multiplanar reformatted images are required to accurately define the perpendicular plane and should always be used for aorta surveillance imaging. These measurements should be made at standard anatomic landmarks (Fig. 30.23) in all patients undergoing surveillance imaging as well as at the site of maximal aorta diameter (if the maximum diameter is not at a standard location). Measurements should be reported as "maximal diameter" x "diameter perpendicular to maximal diameter" and measured from the inner wall to the inner (I-I) wall of the aorta (Fig. 30.23). When aortic wall abnormalities are present, outer wall-to-outer (O-O) wall contours can be used. Several different techniques may be used to measure the diameter at the sinuses of Valsalva and there is currently no absolute consensus. In general, the same approach should be used for all patients and all follow-up imaging, and reports should include current and prior aortic diameters as well as measurement techniques such as I-I versus O-O measurements (particularly if not standard). For screening purposes, axial measurements of the ascending aorta can be performed at the level of the right pulmonary artery, where an axial plane is perpendicular to the trajectory of the ascending aorta. However, axial diameter is not a precise assessment of aorta size and should not be considered to document vessel growth on follow-up studies.

Both CTA and MRA may be used for surveillance of dilated aortas. Due to the absence of ionizing radiation, MRA is preferred in some settings, particularly for serial follow-up in high-risk young patients, such as those with Marfan's or Turner syndromes. The shape of an aortic aneurysm can suggest the underlying etiology. For example, pronounced involvement of the aortic root (annuloaortic ectasia) is characteristic of Marfan syndrome. Patients with bicuspid aortic valve typically have asymmetric dilation of the convexity of the ascending aorta.

Aortic mural thrombus is another important finding, especially in patients who present with peripheral embolization. Mural thrombus may be seen in larger aneurysms and sometimes in regions of atherosclerosis. CTA readily depicts the location and morphology of aortic thrombus and atherosclerotic plaque, which typically appears as low-density material adjacent to the aortic wall. TEE is frequently used for the specific investigation of aortic thrombus but is limited by acoustic windows. Involvement of the ascending aorta and arch may be more effectively identified with CTA. MRI black-blood sequences may also be useful, but slow flow can produce artifactual intraluminal signal. Steady-state free precession cine and/or contrast-enhanced MRA may be needed to differentiate slow flow from thrombus. In cases of mural thrombus, the aorta should be measured from the outer aspect of the aorta (O-O) as opposed to just the opacified portion of the lumen. In the setting of aneurysm rupture, CT and MR may demonstrate periaortic or mediastinal

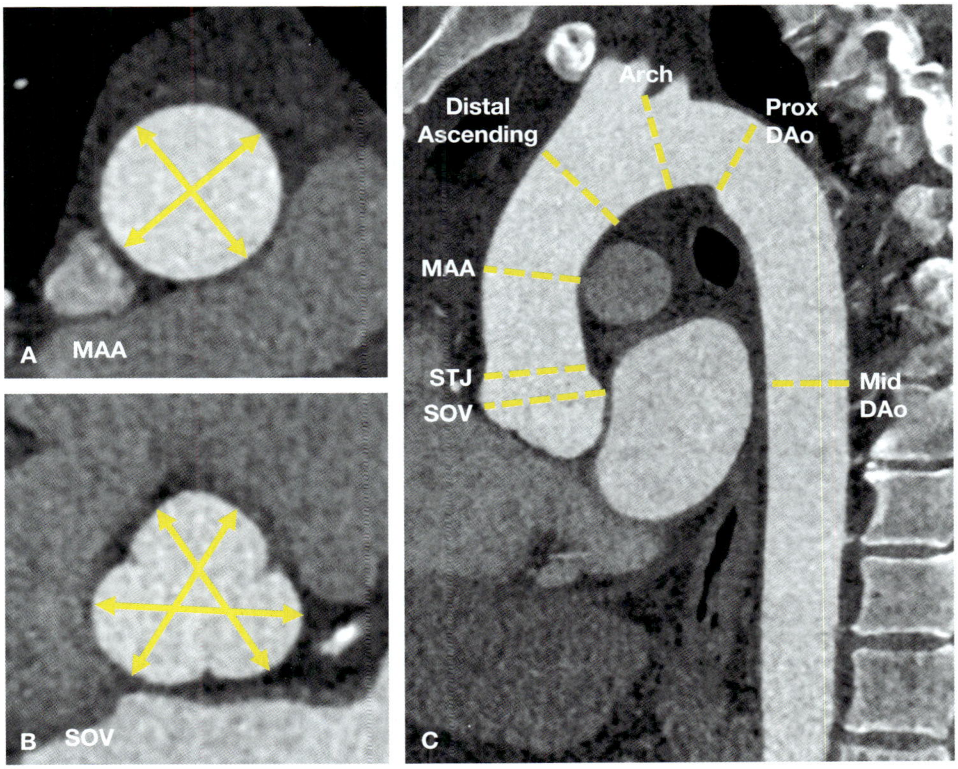

Figure 30.23. Suggested measurement approach **(A and B)** and standardized anatomic locations **(C)** for comprehensive aorta evaluation. For the mid-ascending aorta **(A)** and all tubular portions of the aorta, measurement should be performed in a double oblique fashion, inner-to-inner diameter, and reported as "maximum diameter" x "diameter perpendicular to maximum." For the sinuses of Valsalva **(B)**, the measurement in this example is performed using a sinus-to-sinus approach but other techniques including sinus-to-commissure measurement can be utilized. Dao, descending aorta; MAA, mid ascending aorta; SOV, sinuses of Valsalva, STJ, sinotubular junction.

hematoma. Although rarely seen, early-contained rupture may be evidenced by the "draped aorta" sign: indistinctness of the posterior aortic wall or close alignment of the posterior wall with the adjacent vertebral bodies.

Aortitis

Aortitis is defined as inflammation of the aortic wall. Imaging findings consist of arterial narrowing and luminal irregularity, wall thickening, and dilation or aneurysm formation. Complications include progressive luminal stenosis and structural weakening of the aortic wall that can lead to dissection or rupture. MRI may afford clearer depiction of the aortic wall thickening and enhancement than CTA (Fig. 30.24). Fluorodeoxyglucose positron emission tomography (FDG-PET) may also be used to identify active inflammation.

Common causes of noninfectious aortitis are giant cell arteritis, Takayasu's arteritis, and aortic inflammation associated with other systemic diseases. Symptoms of acute aortitis include malaise, low-grade fevers, arthralgias, and myalgias. Typical laboratory abnormalities are elevated erythrocyte sedimentation rate and elevated C-reactive protein. Medical treatment is primarily corticosteroids, which are administered to suppress inflammation. Symptomatic vascular lesions and critical stenoses are treated with angioplasty/stenting or surgery during periods of disease remission to reduce the incidence of complications.

Giant Cell Aortitis

Giant cell arteritis is the most common autoimmune condition associated with aortitis. The disease mainly involves the thoracic aorta and is emerging as an important cause of ascending thoracic aortic aneurysm in the elderly. Patients with giant cell arteritis are 17 times more likely to develop a thoracic aortic aneurysm than the general population. Noninvasive imaging is used to identify and characterize the severity of large vessel involvement, monitor the course of disease, and disclose the presence of subclinical active inflammation.

Takayasu's Arteritis

Takayasu arteritis is a large vessel vasculitis that affects the aorta, its main arterial branches, and the coronary and pulmonary circulation. There can be diffuse involvement of the

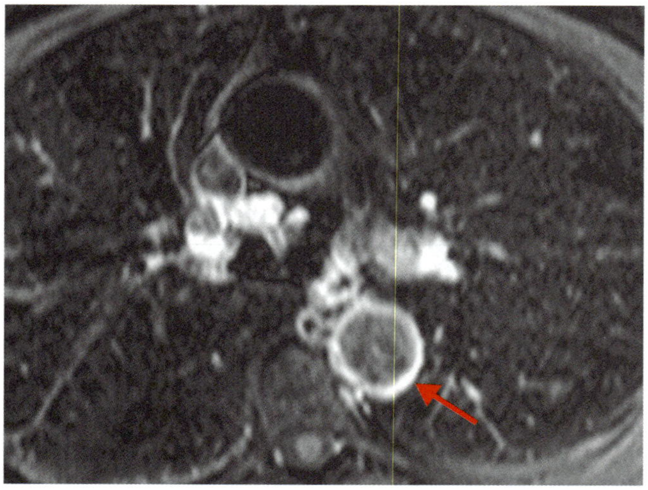

Figure 30.24. Postcontrast, fat-saturated black-blood images demonstrate avid enhancement of a thickened descending thoracic aortic wall (*red arrow*) in this patient with giant cell arteritis.

aorta with or without isolated disease of individual branch arteries. The branch vessels most frequently affected are the subclavian (90%), carotid (45%), and vertebral (25%) arteries.

Aortic Neoplasms

Primary vascular neoplasms of the aorta are very rare and include angiosarcoma and spindle cell sarcoma. These tumors may manifest as an irregular mass projecting into the vessel lumen. CTA and MRI can define the intraluminal and perivascular extent of the neoplasm.

Staging CT and MRI can show involvement of the aorta by mediastinal tumor or bronchogenic carcinoma, which renders the tumor inoperable. Findings that suggest aortic involvement by tumor are irregular thickening of the aortic wall, intraluminal mass, and tumor extending around more than 180° of the aortic circumference.

PERIPROCEDURAL IMAGING

In this section, we will discuss open and endovascular repair techniques for the thoracic aorta, including the role of preoperative imaging, the expected postoperative appearance of the aorta, and the imaging appearance of common postoperative complications.

Open Surgical Repair

Selection of the appropriate surgical technique for repair of the thoracic aorta is primarily affected by anatomic considerations: the status of the aortic valve, portions of the aorta that are involved, and the extent of repair that is required. Patients' functional status and medical comorbidities are also major considerations in the decision to proceed with open versus endovascular repair.

Periprocedural Imaging

The graft material used for open aortic repair is slightly denser than the native aorta on CT, but it is the hyperdense felt rings that are used to reinforce the proximal and distal anastomoses that are most conspicuous on CT. Felt pledgets are also used to reinforce aortic cannulation sites and can be misconstrued as a pseudoaneurysm or PAU on contrast-enhanced images (Fig. 30.25). CT imaging protocols of postoperative patients should include noncontrast as well as postcontrast sequences to properly identify the prosthetic material and avoid inadvertently mistaking these normal structures with postprocedural complications such as intramural hematoma or aortic leak. MR protocols of postoperative patients should take into account the potential for susceptibility artifact from surgical material. Black-blood imaging may be useful in this regard as described in the "Imaging Techniques" section.

Open surgical repair involving the aortic root may require reimplantation of the coronary arteries. To reduce

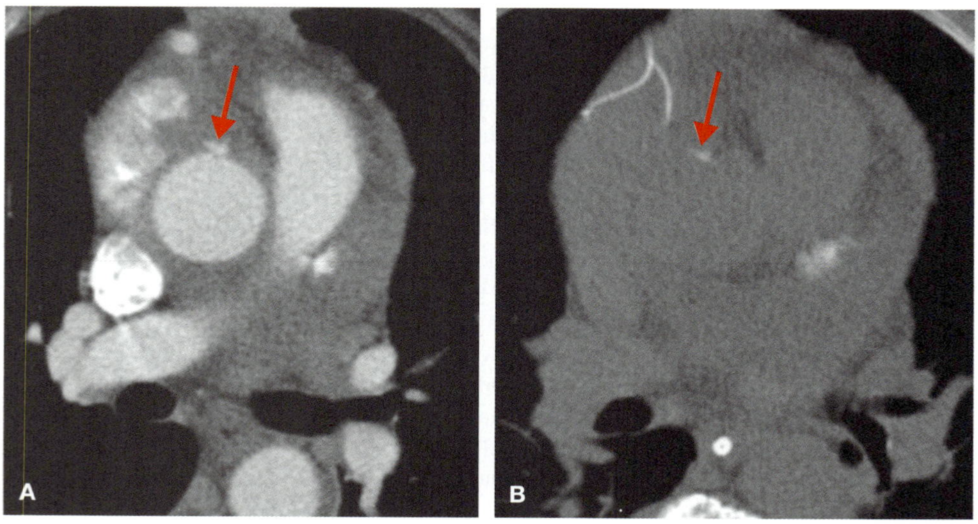

Figure 30.25. On the computed tomography angiography, an apparent penetrating aortic ulcer is noted (**A**, *red arrow*). When the noncontrast CT is reviewed (**B**, *red arrow*), this region is intrinsically dense and represents a felt pledget at the site of an arterial cannula used for cardiopulmonary bypass.

complications arising from coronary artery reimplantation, buttons of tissue surrounding and including the native coronary artery ostia are removed and reanastomosed to the graft material. On postprocedural imaging, the normal coronary buttons may demonstrate focal, triangular outpouching at the coronary artery ostia, which should not be mistaken for an aneurysm.

The presence of small amounts of air in the mediastinum is normal for days following open repair (Fig. 30.26). Increase in the amount of gas over time and persistence of gas for more than 10 to 14 days following repair, however, is suspicious for perigraft infection and/or fistulas. Fluid may surround the aorta and graft material in the immediate postoperative period but should progressively decrease over time. Large volumes of periaortic fluid, growth of the fluid collection, and/or persistence following repair are also concerning for infection.

Acute Complications

Immediate perioperative mortality and embolic events following open thoracic aortic repair occur in 5% to 15% of cases in the literature. Other serious complications following aortic repair occur including postoperative infection (as discussed above), failure of the graft anastomosis/anastomotic dehiscence (Fig. 30.27) or a growing pseudoaneurysm followed by rupture (Fig. 30.28) occurs rarely, in approximately 2% of cases.

Thoracic Endovascular Aortic Repair

TEVAR has been increasingly used in the last decade. Thoracic stent grafts have a stainless steel or nitinol skeleton with a polyester fabric covering. The proximal or distal ends of most stents have an uncovered skeletal section, for better fixation without occlusion of aortic side branches. Ideally, a landing zone of normal aorta about 15 mm above and below the diseased aorta is desired for optimal stent graft fixation and seal. However, the left subclavian artery origin can be covered if there is a short proximal landing zone. This may be accompanied with a subclavian artery bypass procedure if compromise to the vertebrobasilar system, left internal mammary (LIMA) coronary artery bypass grafts, or left upper extremity arterial supply is anticipated.

Periprocedural Imaging

Preprocedural imaging delineates the location and configuration of the aortic pathology, determines whether a patient is a stent graft candidate, and aids in the selection of the appropriate type and size of the stent. CTA may also be useful in identifying the location of the artery of Adamkiewicz and the contour of the proximal and distal landing zones. Usually, a stent device is selected with a diameter 10% to 15% greater than at the proximal and distal landing zones. Imaging of the abdominal aorta, iliac arteries, and proximal femoral arteries is also necessary to detect significant kinking or stenosis that could limit endovascular access.

Lifelong surveillance following TEVAR is recommended, with CTA as the preferred modality, although MRA may be performed if nitinol stents were used. Follow-up imaging protocols vary, with surveillance typically performed at 1, 6, and 12 months and then annually.

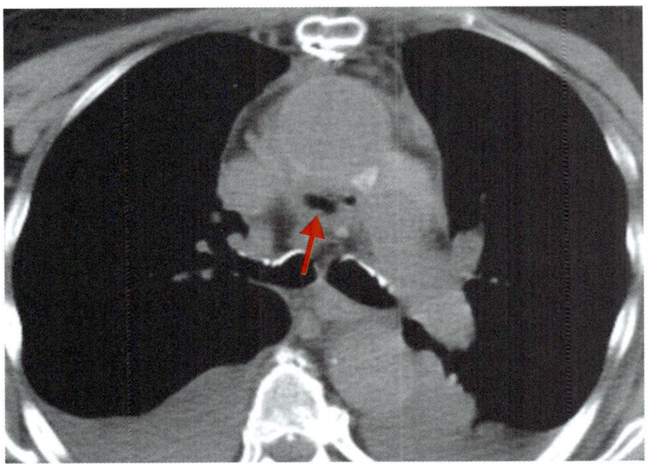

Figure 30.26. Small pockets of air (*red arrow*) can be seen adjacent to surgical aortic repair for up to days after the procedure.

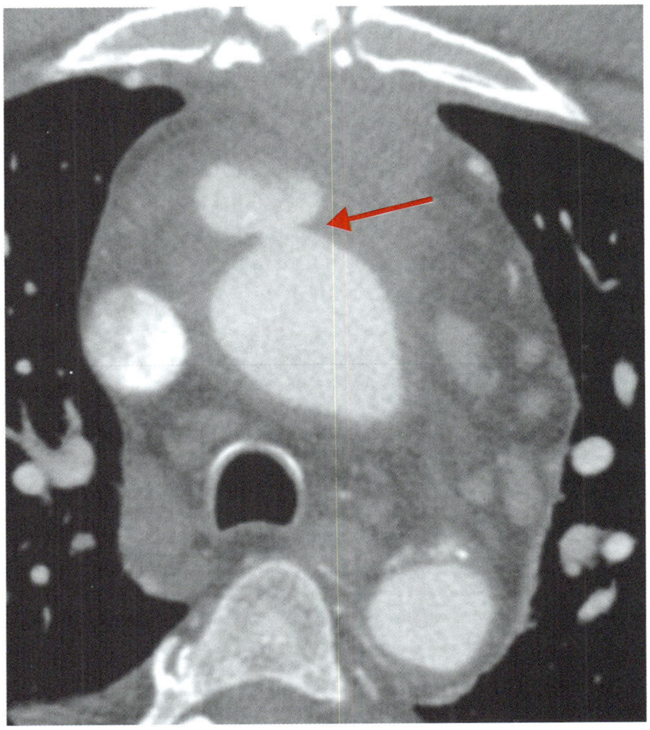

Figure 30.27. Postoperative complication. Aortic dehiscence is seen at an arterial cannulation site in the ascending aorta (*red arrow*).

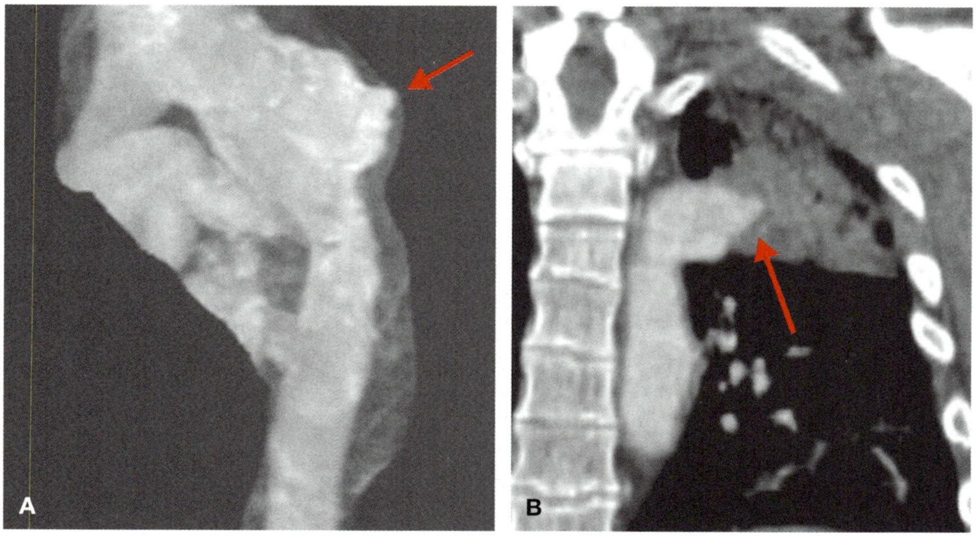

Figure 30.28. After surgical repair of the distal aortic arch for traumatic aortic injury, a beak-like progression is noted on a magnetic resonance angiography (**A**, *red arrow*). On follow-up computed tomography angiography (**B**, *red arrow*), rupture has occurred at this site with hemorrhage seen through the adjacent left upper lobe.

Acute TEVAR Complications

Complications of TEVAR include endoleaks, stent migration/collapse, and aortoenteric fistula. Endoleaks refer to blood flow within the excluded aortic sac, outside the stent graft lumen (Table 30.3; Fig. 30.29). Type I endoleaks usually do not resolve spontaneously and should be repaired. Type II endoleaks occur uncommonly in the chest and are usually caused by retrograde flow through bronchial, intercostal, or left subclavian arteries. Incomplete coverage of the left subclavian artery is associated with a high risk of endoleak. Note that persistent retrograde false lumen flow from the abdominal aorta should not be considered as an endoleak but should be specifically described in imaging reports.

Stent graft fixation depends on outward radial force on the aortic wall, supplemented by barbs in some devices. Inadequate early fixation or subsequent aortic remodeling may lead to loss of this fixation and migration and/or collapse of the stent. Aortoenteric fistula is a communication between the aorta and adjacent bowel that may develop as a postoperative complication following aortic stent graft repair or due to aortic inflammation (Fig. 30.30). Treatment characteristically involves the exclusion of the infected graft/segment and bypass grafting.

Table 30.3 Classification of Endoleaks

I	Attachment site leak
	A. Proximal
	B. Distal
II	Collateral vessel leak(s)
	A. Single vessel
	B. Two or more vessels
III	Graft failure, junctional leak, or disconnection fabric disruption
	A. Junctional separation (modular devices)
	B. Endograft defect
IV	Graft-wall porosity (rare)
V	Endotension

Transcatheter Aortic Valve Replacement

Patients with severe and symptomatic aortic stenosis who are not surgical candidates because of medical comorbidities now can undergo endovascular repair, termed TAVR, with much-improved survival compared to the alternative of medical therapy. Imaging with CTA is crucial for the success of this procedure.

Periprocedural Imaging

Appropriate sizing of stented aortic prostheses is best achieved with cardiac-gated CTA of the aortic root during systole. Accurate valve measurements are needed as undersizing may lead to paravalvular regurgitation or device embolization, while oversizing can cause rupture. The diameter, circumference, and area measurements of the aortic valve annulus should be made at the hinge points at the base of the aortic leaflets, with a typical annulus having an oval shape (Fig. 30.31). The distance from the coronary artery ostia to the valve leaflets is also important to evaluate in order to avoid coronary occlusion.

Diameters perpendicular to the centerline of the of common femoral and iliac arteries is performed to ensure adequate minimal luminal diameter and vessel course to allow sheath access. In cases where these diameters are below the minimal threshold of 5 mm, measurements of upper extremity or carotid access sites are often required. Vascular complications including dissection, vessel perforation, or occlusion following insertion of vascular access sheaths are an important source of postoperative morbidity, occurring in 6% to

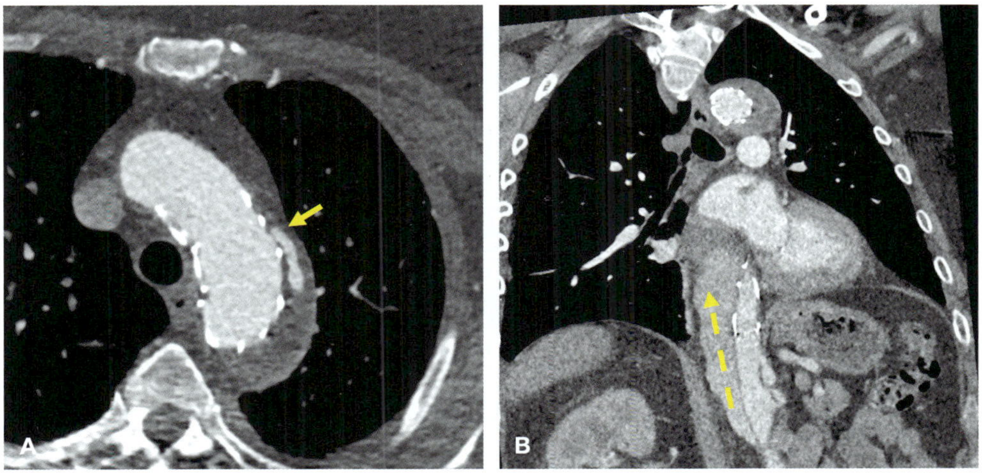

Figure 30.29. Examples of residual false lumen filling after thoracic endovascular aortic repair. Panel A demonstrate a Type III endoleak. Panel B demonstrates retrograde filling of the false lumen the abdominal aorta dissected segment. This finding would not be classified as an endoleak.

17% of TAVR procedures. Up to 35% of potential TAVR candidates have unfavorable peripheral access, the majority of which is due to insufficient vessel size. Identification of small peripheral access diameter, significant peripheral atherosclerosis, vessel tortuosity, and kinking of the peripheral arteries with CTA is key to minimize complications.

EMERGING TRENDS

Aortic diameters are a simple but powerful means of risk stratifying patients and determining when elective aortic intervention is most likely to be of benefit. Yet aortic dilation is a manifestation of disease, not the driver of disease. Advanced aortic imaging techniques now offer a glimpse into potential drivers of aortic disease, including inflammation and adverse hemodynamics. In this section, we will briefly touch on some of the emerging trends in advanced aortic imaging.

New MRI Contrast Agents

Conventional gadolinium-based MRI contrast agents are extracellular and thus require careful bolus timing for optimal vascular imaging. Blood pool agents, however, provide a plateau of vascular signal that allows imaging without the limitations of bolus timing.

In patients with renal failure who cannot undergo gadolinium-enhanced MRI imaging due to the risk of NSF, USPIO contrast agents such as ferumoxytol are an appealing option. As ferumoxytol is an intravenous treatment for

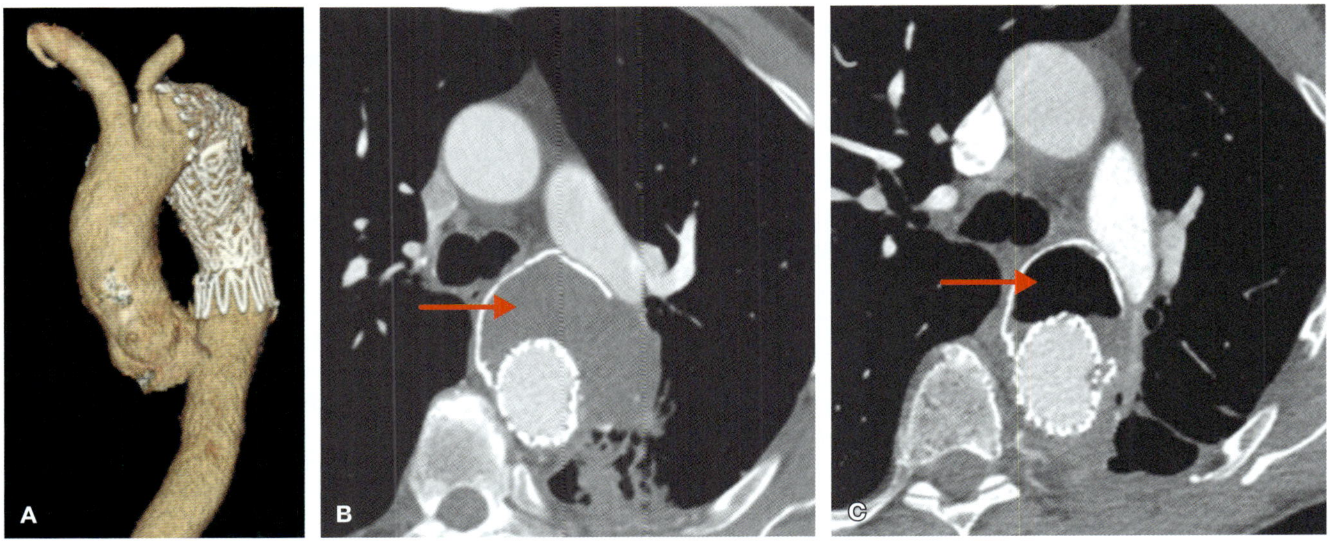

Figure 30.30. A stent graft has been placed in the proximal descending aorta for exclusion of a focal aneurysm **(A)**. The excluded aneurysm appears thrombosed on immediate follow-up imaging (**B**, *red arrow*). Months later, air is seen through the excluded aneurysm (**C**, *red arrow*), an ominous finding. An infected aorta-esophageal fistula was found soon thereafter.

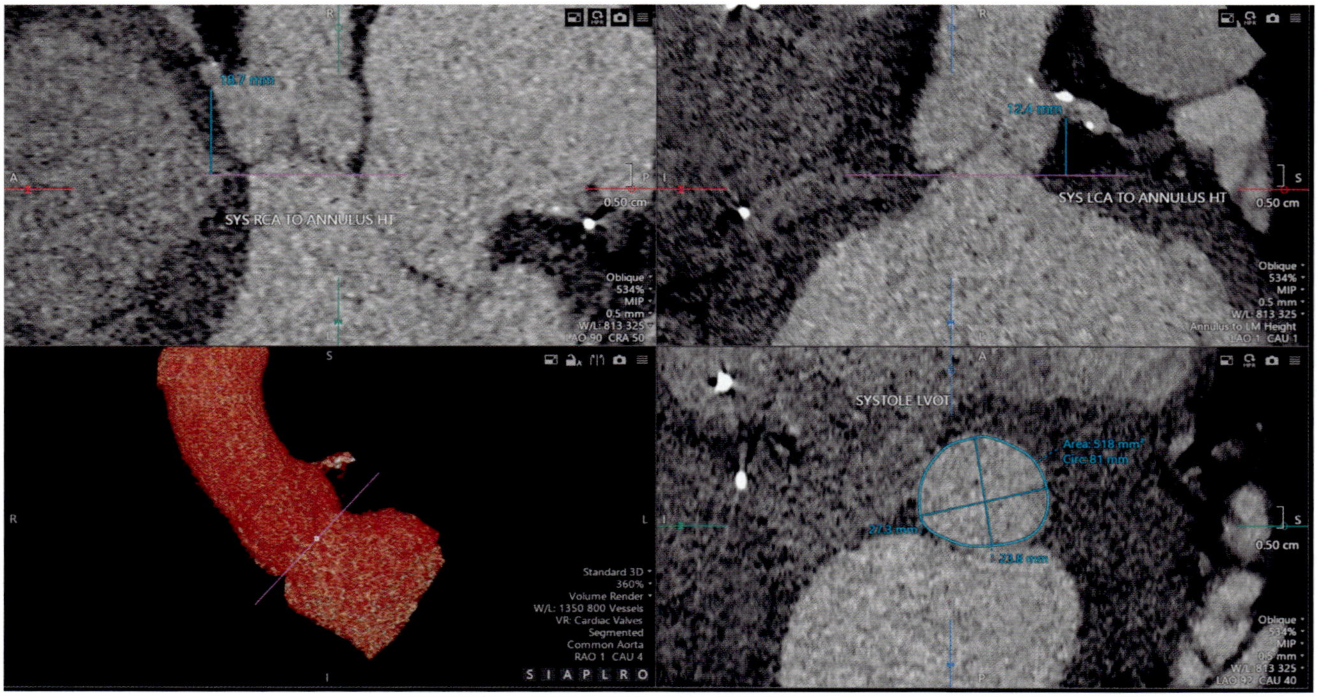

Figure 30.31. CT transcatheter aortic valve repair measurements derived using dedicated software. The bottom right frame shows aortic annular circumference, area, and diameter measurements and the level of the annular plane while the top left and top right images show the coronary heights from the annular plane. The bottom left images show the three-dimension orientation of the annular plane. LCA, left coronary artery; LVOT, left ventricular outflow tract; Purple line: annular plane; RCA, right coronary artery; SYS, systolic phase.

iron deficiency anemia in the context of chronic kidney disease, it is safe for patients with renal failure. It also exhibits a long blood pool phase and considerable T1 shortening, making it an attractive positive contrast vascular imaging agent. Because of the long half-life, imaging can be performed many hours after injection with persistent arterial and venous signal. This property makes ferumoxytol a reasonable contrast choice in patients who may be challenging for accurate contrast bolus timing and breath-holding such as children. It also allows imaging to be repeated if image quality is poor. The main downside of ferumoxytol contrast agent is the risk of anaphylaxis during rapid injection. As a result, ferumoxytol injection should always be a slow infusion, and dynamic or time-resolved MRA is generally not possible.

PET Imaging

Metabolic imaging with FDG-PET, in combination with anatomic assessment (CT or MRI), has been used for the evaluation of inflammatory diseases of the aorta. The ability of FDG-PET to determine which patients with aortitis have active inflammation can inform medication regimens, as well as the timing of surgical interventions. Occasionally, FDG-PET can identify active aortic inflammation or infection not obvious on anatomic imaging (Fig. 30.32). Other PET agents are being explored for vascular imaging. Sodium fluoride (NaF) PET affords the ability to detect microcalcifications in unstable atherosclerosis. Agents that target integrins such as arginine-glycine-aspartic acid (RGD) peptide RGD-PET have shown promise in revealing vascular inflammation and neoangiogenesis.

Flow Imaging

Pathologic blood flow contributes to the progression of vascular disease but is challenging to characterize with noninvasive imaging. Advances in phase-contrast MRI in the last decade have made imaging of 3D dynamic blood flow feasible in about 10 minutes. The technique has been termed 4D Flow MRI and allows both qualitative and quantitative assessment of blood flow and related parameters including wall shear stress, turbulence, and relative pressure. Potential clinical applications include streamlining conventional 2D phase-contrast analysis with a single MRI sequence and new approaches for risk-stratifying patients for progressive aortic disease. One promising new application is the use of 4D Flow for assessing the flow velocity and wall shear stress in the ascending aorta to identify patients at increased risk for valve-related aortic disease (Fig. 30.33). In type B aortic dissection, there is increasing interest in 4D flow MRI-derived quantification of entry tear, true lumen, and false lumen hemodynamics can help identify patients at high risk of aorta growth and need for intervention (Fig. 30.34).

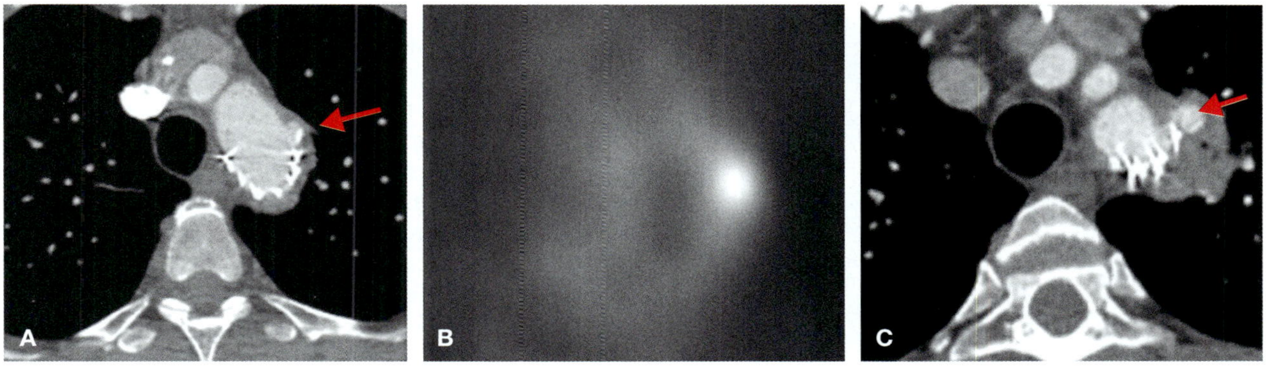

Figure 30.32. FDG-PET reveals active disease that is difficult to identify by CTA. A small wall irregularity is noted on CTA at the proximal margin of a stent graft (**A**, *red arrow*). FDG-PET demonstrates focal avidity at this location **(B)**. Follow-up imaging 5 days later reveals rapid progression of disease at this location with a clear pseudoaneurysm on CTA (**C**, *red arrow*), which was determined to be mycotic. CTA, computed tomography angiography. FDG-PET, Fluorodeoxyglucose positron emission tomography.

ARTIFICIAL INTELLIGENCE IN THORACIC AORTA ASSESSMENT

As in all radiology, artificial intelligence (AI) tools and techniques are increasingly being explored and applied in patients with thoracic aorta disease. Because of the important role of aortic dimensions in diagnosis and risk stratification, most aorta AI applications have focused on accurate aorta segmentation and diameter measurement. Numerous AI-based tools have been developed, predominantly for CTA, that can provide automated measurements at standard anatomic locations and some of these tools are now commercially available. Fewer tools exist for MRA at this time but will likely be developed over the next several years. AI-driven automated aorta measurement can be very impactful in several aspects of clinical care. At the most basic level, automated measurements can save time for physicians or technologists who need to perform these measurements on many patients per day. These tools also make it easier to perform more advanced assessments such as aortic volumes or indexed dimensions that may better assess aortic risk relative to simple diameter measurements. Perhaps most importantly, use of these tools should lead to more consistent and reproducible aorta measurements that allow for more accurate size and growth assessment without potential biases introduced by human-performed measurements. As researchers and vendors develop and commercialize these

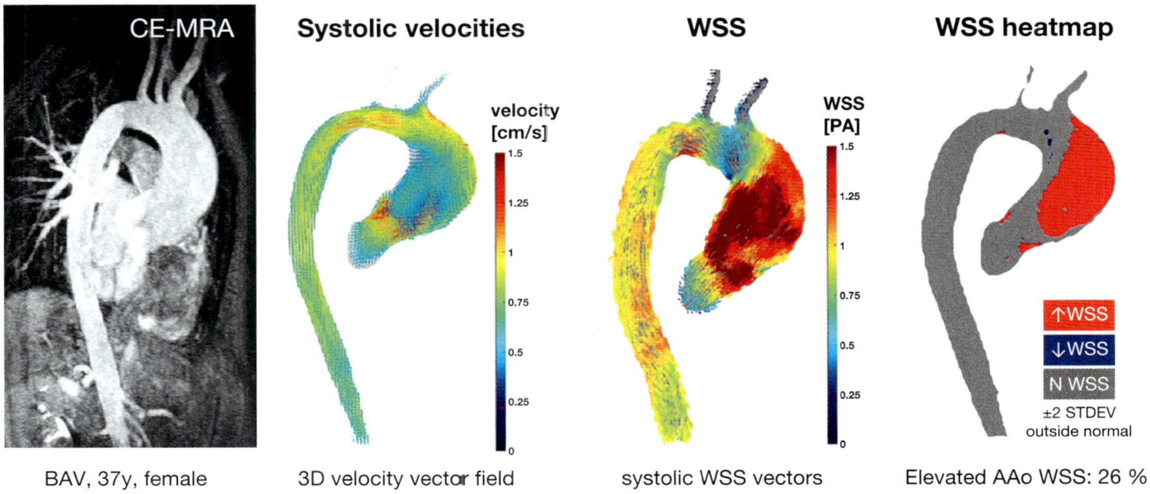

Figure 30.33. Anatomic and hemodynamic assessment in a 37-year-old woman with bicuspid aortic valve. The contrast-enhanced MRA maximal intensity projection shows a dilated ascending aorta. Advanced hemodynamic analysis from 4D flow MRI quantifies systolic velocity and wall shear stress (WSS) throughout the aorta. The WSS heatmap demonstrates % of the aortic area with abnormal WSS compared to age and gender matched group of healthy control patients. Elevated WSS has been shown to correlate with higher aortic growth rates in BAV patients. Image courtesy of Dr. Michael Markl, Northwestern University. MRA, magnetic resonance angiography.

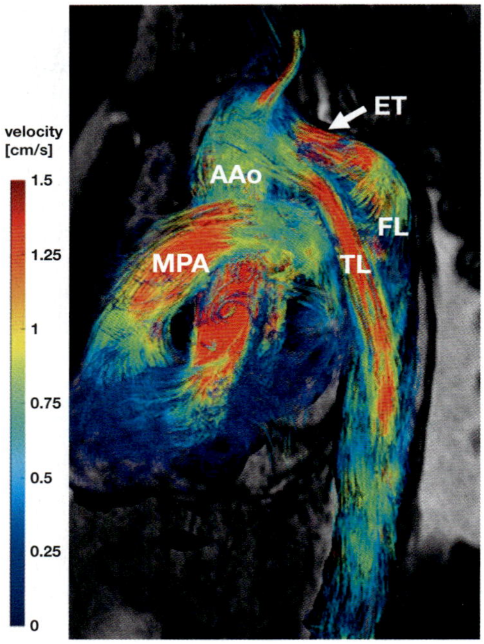

Figure 30.34. 4D flow magnetic resonance imaging in a patient with type B aortic dissection demonstrating large volume of high-velocity flow through the entry tear into the false lumen. Aao, ascending aorta; MPA, main pulmonary artery; TL, true lumen.

products, end-users must insist that guideline-driven standards are followed, for example, accuracy of standard anatomic location detection and use of I-I or O-O techniques as appropriate.

Similarly for aortic dissection, accurate assessment of aortic size still tends to drive decisions. AI tools that can detect, segment, and measure the overall aorta size as well as the true and false lumens are actively being developed. This problem is more complex than standard aorta measurements because of the large degree of variability of aortic dissection anatomy, particularly related to the false lumen location and degree of thrombus. Therefore, in general, significantly larger amounts of training data are needed for models attempting to address this issue. However, there are commercial products currently available that can accurately detect and classify aortic dissection, including some that can function "in line" on the scanner. The ability of these tools to detect dissection before a human review the images allow for more rapid triage by radiologists or other members of aorta treatment teams which can be crucial for expedited treatment, especially in centers that may not have surgeons readily available for aortic interventions.

Aorta hemodynamic assessment is also an important target for AI-driven applications. As in standard anatomic aorta assessment, hemodynamic assessment with 2D or 4D phase contrast imaging generally requires accurate aorta segmentation. An important difference in hemodynamic assessment is that the segmentation is ideally time-resolved meaning multiple phases must be segmented, and additional data processing steps are often needed to account for background offsets for example. When performed manually, these tasks are very time-consuming and have limited their use in clinical practice. AI tools are being developed that accurately and efficiently perform these tasks, and some of these tools have already been incorporated into commercial products. It is likely that future iterations will provide hemodynamic assessments such as peak velocity and flow "in line" from the scanner. Automated tools that allow for advanced hemodynamic assessment such as wall shear stress in more patients will more efficiently provide data that can determine how these measurements and analysis tools will fit into the clinical evaluation of patients with aorta disease.

SUGGESTED READINGS

Bhave NM, Nienaber CA, Clough RE, Eagle KA. Multimodality imaging of thoracic aortic diseases in adults. *JACC Cardiovasc Imaging.* 2018;11(6):902-919.

Bossone E, Eagle KA. Epidemiology and management of aortic disease: aortic aneurysms and acute aortic syndromes. *Nat Rev Cardiol.* 2021 May;18(5):331-348.

Elefteriades JA, Mukherjee SK, Mojibian H. Discrepancies in measurement of the thoracic aorta: JACC review topic of the week. *J Am Coll Cardiol.* 2020;76(2):201-217. doi:10.1016/j.jacc.2020.03.084

Evangelista A, Mukherjee D, Mehta RH, et al, International Registry of Aortic Dissection IRAD Investigators. Acute intramural hematoma of the aorta: a mystery in evolution. *Circulation.* 2005;111(8):1063-1070.

Fleischmann D, Afifi RO, Casanegra AI, et al, American Heart Association Council on Cardiovascular Radiology and Intervention; Council on Arteriosclerosis, Thrombosis and Vascular Biology; Council on Clinical Cardiology; and Council on Cardiovascular Surgery and Anesthesia. Imaging and surveillance of chronic aortic dissection: a scientific statement from the American Heart Association. *Circ Cardiovasc Imaging.* 2022;15(3):e000075.

Hope MD, Hope TA, Zhu C, et al. Vascular imaging with ferumoxytol as a contrast agent. *AJR Am J Roentgenol.* 2015;205(3):W366-W373.

Isselbacher EM, Preventza O, Hamilton Black J III, et al, Peer Review Committee Members. 2022 ACC/AHA guideline for the diagnosis and management of aortic disease: a report of the American Heart Association/American College of Cardiology Joint Committee on clinical practice guidelines. *Circulation.* 2022;146(24):e334-e482.

Mussa FF, Horton JD, Moridzadeh R, Nicholson J, Trimarchi S, Eagle KA. Acute aortic dissection and intramural hematoma: a systematic review. *JAMA.* 2016;316(7):754-763.

Steenburg SD, Ravenel JG, Ikonomidis JS, Schönholz C, Reeves S. Acute traumatic aortic injury: imaging evaluation and management. *Radiology.* 2008;248(3):748-762.

Wolak A, Gransar H, Thomson LE, et al. Aortic size assessment by noncontrast cardiac computed tomography: normal limits by age, gender, and body surface area. *JACC Cardiovasc Imaging.* 2008;1(2):200-209.

Zilber ZA, Boddu A, Malaisrie SC, et al. Noninvasive morphologic and hemodynamic evaluation of type B aortic dissection: state of the art and future perspectives. *Radiol Cardiothorac Imaging.* 2021;3(3):e200456.

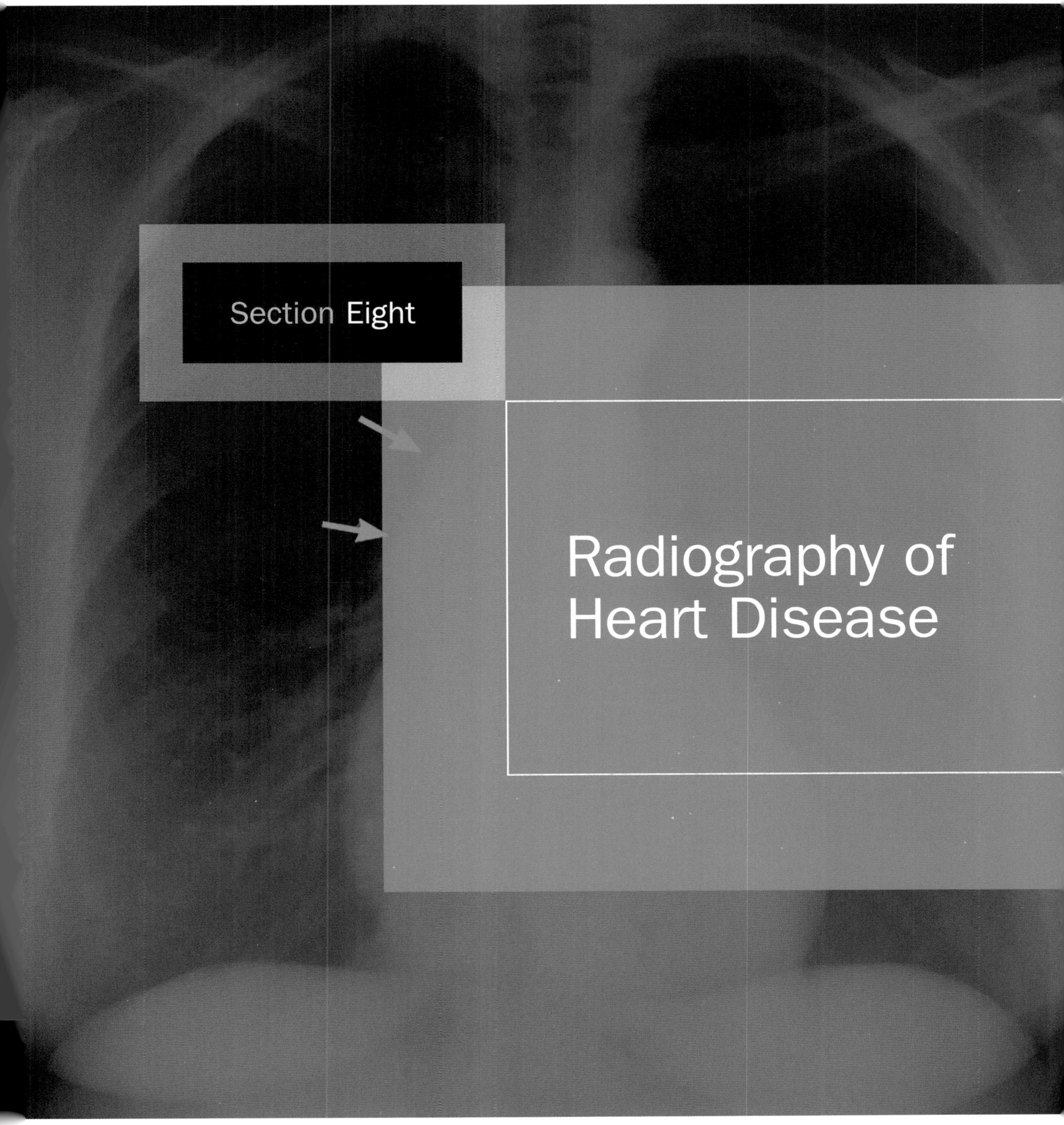

Section Eight

Radiography of Heart Disease

Chapter 31

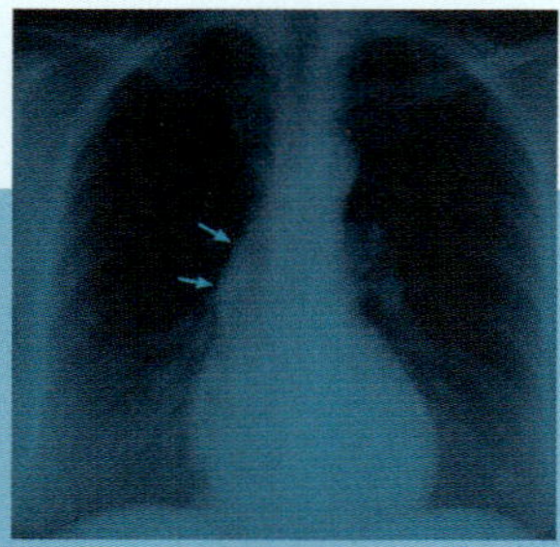

Karen G. Ordovas • Charles B. Higgins

Radiography of Acquired Heart Disease

INTRODUCTION

The thoracic radiograph is one of the earliest points of departure in the evaluation of heart disease. It may provide the first indication that cardiac disease is present, but more frequently, it is used to determine the severity of known or suspected disease. The severity of some cardiac diseases is readily reflected on the thoracic radiograph, while other significant diseases cause little or no alterations in the pulmonary vessels or cardiac silhouette. Consequently, the thoracic radiograph may have only limited value in the assessment of some diseases, while in others, it may serve as one of the most sensitive and reliable gauges of the course of the disease. The propensity of various cardiac diseases to cause substantial cardiomegaly serves as the major dividing line in our system for cataloging acquired heart disease.

APPROACH TO THE CHEST X-RAY IN ACQUIRED HEART DISEASE

A systematic approach is directed toward discerning the pertinent findings from the radiograph and, for each finding, narrowing the array of diagnostic considerations. A free-floating approach places one into the unnecessary jeopardy of failing to examine salient features of the cardiovascular anatomy.

A five-step systematic approach permits the orderly examination of the thoracic radiograph, and at each step, it is possible to narrow the diagnostic possibilities (Figs. 31.1 and 31.2). A radiographic classification of acquired heart disease is used in association with this five-step examination (see Fig. 31.2; Table 31.1).

The five steps in the examination of the thoracic radiograph in patients with suspected cardiac disease are (1) thoracic musculoskeletal structures, (2) pulmonary vascularity, (3) overall heart size, (4) specific chamber enlargement, and (5) great arteries (ascending aorta, aortic knob, main pulmonary arterial segment).

Thoracic Musculoskeletal Structures

Examination of the thoracic wall discloses evidence of prior operations, such as rib or sternal deformities or sternal wire sutures. Sternal deformities such as pectus may serve as a clue to cardiac lesions associated with it, such as Marfan's syndrome and mitral valve prolapse, or perhaps, the deformity is responsible for a cardiac murmur or even symptoms caused by cardiac compression. Narrow anteroposterior diameter of the thorax can be caused by a straight thoracic spine (straight-back syndrome) or pectus excavatum. A narrow anteroposterior diameter is defined as a distance between the sternum and the anterior border of the vertebral body that measures less than 8 cm and a ratio of the transverse diameter (determined by frontal view) to the anteroposterior diameter (determined by lateral view) exceeding 2.75. The anteroposterior diameter is the maximum diameter from the undersurface of the sternum to the anterior border of the vertebral body.

Pulmonary Vascularity (Pulmonary Edema)

There are three steps in assessing pulmonary vascularity: the type of abnormality (pulmonary arterial overcirculation versus pulmonary venous hypertension [PVH]), the severity of the pulmonary vascular abnormality, and determination of the symmetry, asymmetry, or even focal nature of the abnormality. In patients with acquired heart disease, the type of abnormality is usually PVH. The major signs of

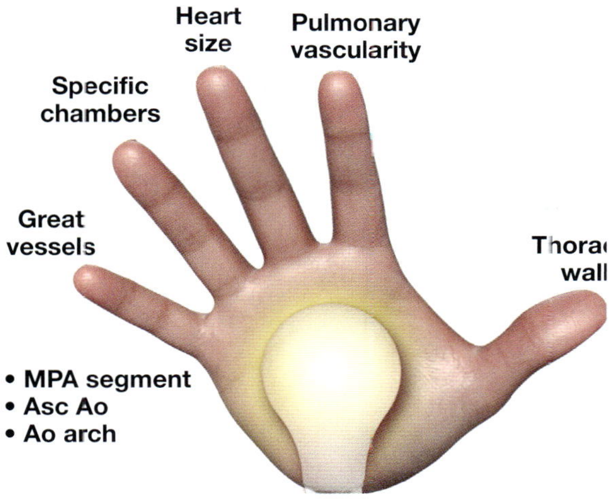

Figure 31.1. Five-step approach to analysis of the thoracic radiograph in cardiac disease.

PVH are equalization or larger diameter of the upper compared to the lower lobe vessels; loss of prominence or clear visualization of the right lower lobe pulmonary artery; prominence of the interstitial markings, especially the appearance of Kerley's A and B lines; indistinctness of the pulmonary vascular margins and/or hilar vessels; loss of the right hilar angle; and alveolar filling (Figs. 31.3-31.6). After repeated episodes of pulmonary edema in long-standing cases of mitral valve disease, permanent interstitial lines or ossific nodules may appear. Ossific nodules are small foci of bony metaplasia that appear in the lungs only after multiple episodes of edema and chronic PVH. Foci of hemosiderin may form fibrotic nodules in patients with multiple episodes of edema as well as after multiple episodes of pulmonary hemorrhage.

Table 31.1 Radiographic Classification of Acquired Heart Disease

Small Heart (C/T < 0.55)	Large Heart (C/T > 0.55)
Aortic stenosis	Aortic regurgitation
Arterial hypertension	Mitral regurgitation
Mitral stenosis	Tricuspid regurgitation
Acute myocardial infarction	High output states
Hypertrophic cardiomyopathy	Congestive cardiomyopathy
Restrictive cardiomyopathy	Ischemic cardiomyopathy
Constrictive pericarditis	Pericardial effusion
	Paracardiac mass

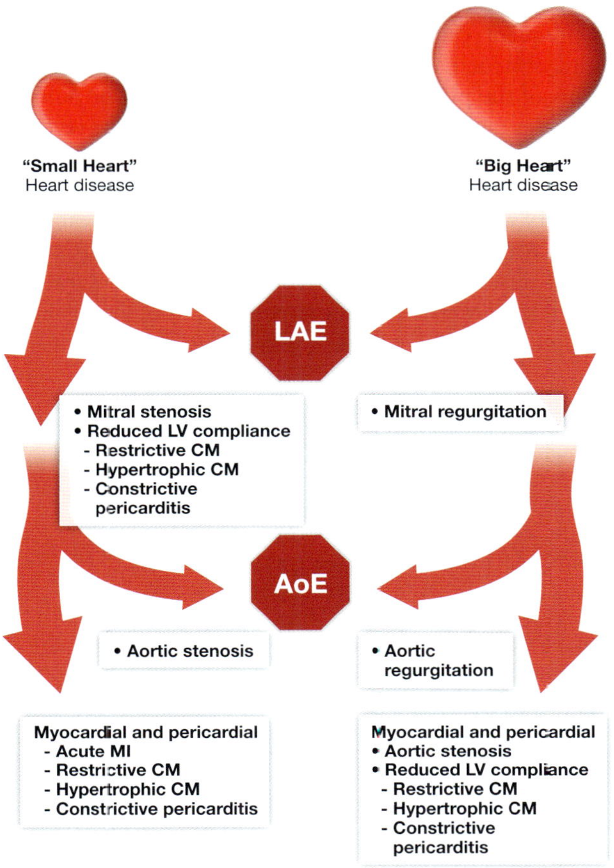

Figure 31.2. Diagnostic pathway for the identification of the hemodynamically predominant cardiac lesion. Signposts gleaned from the thoracic radiograph guide the analysis.

The severity of PVH can be gauged by the signs observed. The radiographic severity of PVH can be divided into three grades: grade I (redistribution of pulmonary blood volume), grade II (interstitial pulmonary edema), and grade

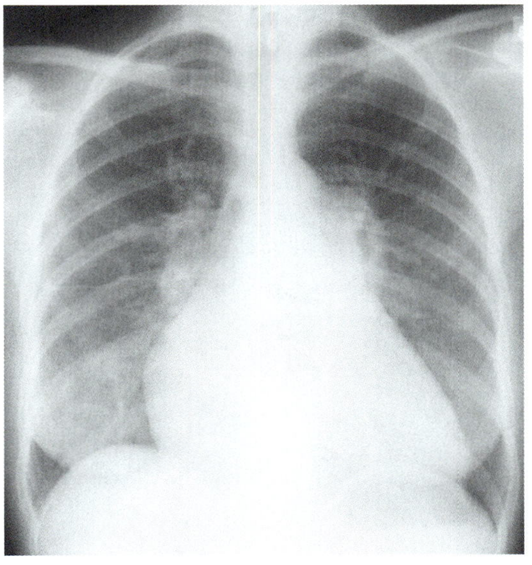

Figure 31.3. Pulmonary venous hypertension in mitral valve disease. Radiograph demonstrates redistribution of pulmonary blood flow (upper lobe vessels larger than lower lobe vessels) indicating grade I pulmonary venous hypertension. There is cardiomegaly and straightening of the upper left cardiac border indicative of left atrial enlargement.

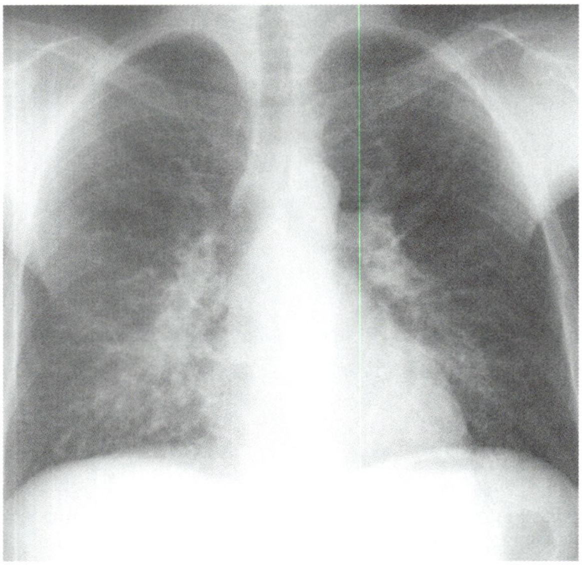

Figure 31.4. Interstitial pulmonary edema after acute myocardial infarction. Radiograph demonstrates interstitial pulmonary edema with Kerley's B lines, indistinct vascular margins, and peribronchial cuffing.

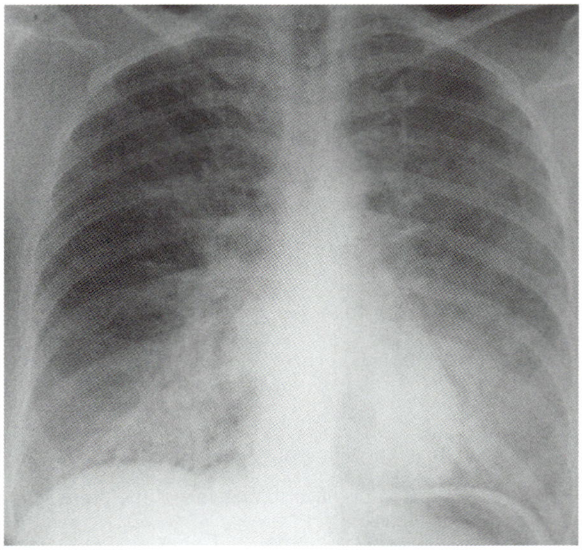

Figure 31.6. Alveolar pulmonary edema with normal heart size in a patient with left atrial myxoma obstructing the mitral valve.

III (alveolar pulmonary edema; Table 31.2). The pulmonary venous pressure (or mean left atrial wedge pressure) associated with edema varies depending on whether the cardiac dysfunction is acute or chronic (Table 31.3). The venous pressure in chronic disease is approximately 5 mm Hg greater for each grade of PVH compared to that in acute disease.

Asymmetric PVH

Asymmetric distribution of PVH or pulmonary edema raises a number of diagnostic possibilities (Table 31.4; Fig. 31.7). The most frequent cause of such asymmetry is probably gravitational; patients with heart disease frequently sleep lying on their right side because of consciousness of the prominent left-sided pulsation (prominent point of maximum impulse in the presence of cardiomegaly). The next most frequent cause is underlying lung disease such as chronic obstructive pulmonary disease, which obliterates portions of the pulmonary vascular bed. Edema or pulmonary venous distention appears in the normal or less severely abnormal portions of the lungs. Unilateral pulmonary edema may occur contralateral to an occluded or severely stenotic pulmonary artery. Such unilateral edema might appear contralateral to a pulmonary embolism, or a pulmonary artery stenosis caused by congenital anomalies (branch pulmonary arterial stenosis, proximal interruption, or agenesis of a pulmonary artery) or acquired diseases (bronchogenic

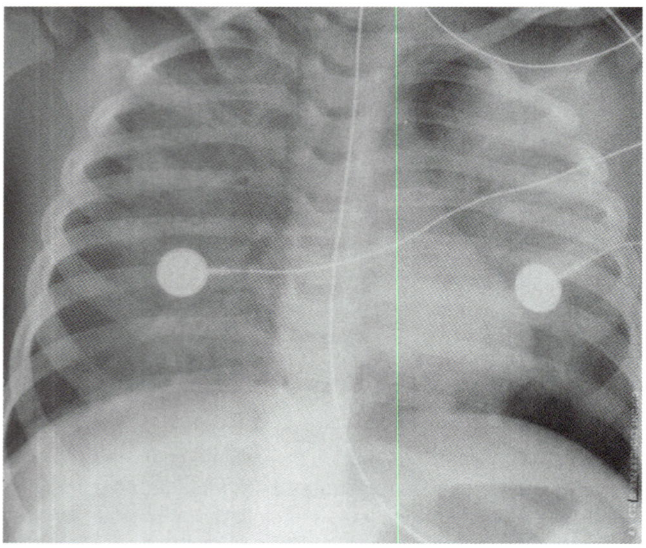

Figure 31.5. Noncardiac pulmonary edema. Alveolar pulmonary edema with normal heart size in a child after drowning.

Table 31.2 Signs of Pulmonary Ventricular Hypertension by Grade of Severity

Grade I: vascular redistribution
- Equal upper and lower lobe vessels
- Larger upper lobe vessels

Grade II: interstitial edema
- Kerley's A or B lines
- Increased prominence of "interstitial markings"
- Peribronchial cuffing
- Loss of the hilar angle
- Enlargement and indistinctness of hila
- Subpleural edema (increased thickness of pleura)
- Loss of visibility of much of the descending branch of the right pulmonary artery

Grade III
- Confluent acinar shadows (pulmonary alveolar edema)
- Perihilar alveolar filling
- Lower lobe or more generalized alveolar filling

Table 31.3 Correlates of Left Atrial Pressure (Mean)[a] and Pulmonary Vascular Hypertension Grade

	Left Atrial Pressure	
	Acute Disease (Myocardial Infarction)	**Chronic Disease (Mitral Stenosis)**
Grade I	12-19 mm Hg	15-25 mm Hg
Grade II	20-25 mm Hg	25-30 mm Hg
Grade III	25 mm Hg	30 mm Hg

[a]Left atrial mean pressure is usually inferred from the mean pulmonary wedge pressure. Correlation between left atrial pressure and radiographic signs of pulmonary edema is only fair because of phase lag between rapid pressure changes and slower changes in radiographic alterations.

carcinoma, Takayasu's arteritis, fibrosing mediastinitis, mediastinal tumors). Unilateral edema is infrequently used by unilateral obstruction of pulmonary veins caused by mediastinal or lung tumors, primary and secondary tumors of the heart and pericardium, mediastinal fibrosis, and complications of the Mustard procedure and other procedures used in congenital heart disease. Finally, pulmonary edema induced by reinflation of a collapsed lung or after thoracentesis must be considered.

Pulmonary edema may occur in the absence of underlying cardiac disease. Such noncardiogenic edema is usually due to damage to the alveolar-capillary membrane, causing a leak of fluid into the lung at normal or near-normal pulmonary venous pressure and capillary oncotic pressure. A partial list of the many settings in which this occurs is shown in Table 31.5.

Overall Heart Size

Acquired heart disease can be divided into two groups, depending on the presence or absence of substantial cardiomegaly. "Small heart" heart disease is associated with a normal heart size or only mild cardiomegaly. For the sake of our discussion, we set a cardiothoracic (CT) ratio of less than 0.55 as consistent with this group of lesions. The choice of 0.55 is obviously somewhat arbitrary. The CT ratio is calculated using the convention of measuring the thoracic diameter as the distance from the inner margin of the ribs at the level of the dome of the right hemidiaphragm and the cardiac diameter as the

Table 31.4 Unilateral Pulmonary Edema

- Gravitational
- Chronic lung disease (emphysema)
- Unilateral pulmonary arterial obstruction
  - Thromboembolic disease
  - Extrinsic obstruction of pulmonary artery
  - Lung cancer, thoracic aortic aneurysm, mediastinal fibrosis
- Unilateral pulmonary venous obstruction
  - Left atrial tumor
  - Mediastinal tumor encasing pulmonary veins
  - Mediastinal fibrosis
- Reexpansion pulmonary edema
  - Postpneumothorax, postthoracentesis

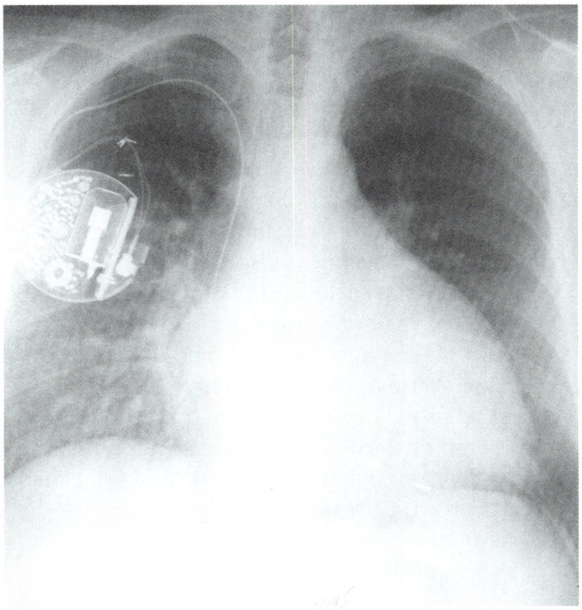

Figure 31.7. Asymmetric pulmonary edema. Unilateral pulmonary edema in a patient with a metastatic tumor selectively obstructing the right pulmonary veins. Note the increased density of the right lower lung field.

Table 31.5 Noncardiogenic Pulmonary Edema

- Drowning
- Asphyxia
- Upper airway obstruction
- High altitude
- Increased intracranial pressure
- Reexpansion pulmonary edema
- Noxious gases
  - Smoke inhalation
  - Nitrous dioxide (silo filler's disease)
  - Sulfur dioxide
  - Others
- Drugs
  - Aspirin
  - Valium, librium, barbiturates, heroin, cocaine, methadone
- Poisons—parathion
- Blood transfusion reaction
- Contrast media reaction
- Adult respiratory distress syndrome

horizontal distance between the most rightward and most leftward margins of the cardiac shadow. The second group, called "big heart" heart disease, is characterized by substantial cardiomegaly (CT ratio greater than 0.55).

The pathophysiologic factors associated with "small heart" heart disease are pressure overload and reduced ventricular compliance. The pathophysiologic factors associated with "big heart" heart disease are volume overload and myocardial failure. Pericardial effusion also is included in this group.

The cardiac lesions included in the two groups are listed in Table 31.1. The major pressure overload types of acquired lesions are aortic and mitral stenosis and hypertension. The major volume overload types of acquired lesions are aortic, mitral, and tricuspid regurgitation and high output states. The most common cardiac diseases that cause reduced left ventricular (LV) compliance or resistance to full expansion of the ventricles are acute myocardial infarction (MI), hypertrophic cardiomyopathy, restrictive cardiomyopathy, and constrictive pericardial disease.

Specific Chamber Enlargement

It is not until the fourth step in the examination of the chest x-ray that attention should be directed to determine specific chamber enlargement. A critical observation is the identification of left atrial enlargement. It is also useful to determine which ventricle is enlarged or if both ventricles are enlarged. It is sometimes not possible to clearly determine the type of ventricular enlargement on the thoracic radiograph. The radiographic signs observed with enlargement of each of the cardiac chambers are given below.

Left Atrial Enlargement

1. Right retrocardiac double density. Distance from the middle of the double density (lateral border of the left atrium) to the middle of the left bronchus is less than 7 cm in greater than 90% of normal subjects and greater than 7 cm in 90% of patients with left atrial enlargement, proven by echocardiography (Fig. 31.8). In cases of severe left atrial enlargement, the left atrial border may extend further to the right than the right atrial border (Fig. 31.9).
2. Enlargement of the left atrial appendage. This is seen as a bulge along the left cardiac border just beneath the main pulmonary artery segment (see Figs. 31.8 and 31.9). Using the left bronchus as an orientation point, the bulge above it is the main pulmonary artery segment, while the bulge at the level of and/or just below the left bronchus is the left atrial appendage.
3. Splaying of the carina and/or elevation of the left bronchus (Fig. 31.10).
4. Horizontal orientation of the distal portion of the left bronchus.
5. Posterior displacement of the left upper bronchus (see Fig. 31.10). On the lateral radiograph, the circular shadow of the right upper lobe and left bronchi is located within the tracheal air column. Left atrial enlargement causes displacement of the left bronchus posterior to this level and beyond the plane of the trachea ("walking man sign").

Right Atrial Enlargement

1. Lateral bulging of the right heart border on the posteroanterior radiograph (see Fig. 31.10).
2. Elongation of the right heart border on the posteroanterior view. A rough rule is that a right atrial border exceeding 60% in length of the mediastinal cardiovascular shadow is a sign of substantial right atrial enlargement (Fig. 31.11).

Left Ventricular Enlargement

1. On the posteroanterior view, leftward and downward displacement of the cardiac apex. The vector of enlargement of the LV is leftward and downward compared with the vector of right ventricular enlargement, which is leftward only or perhaps leftward plus upward (Figs. 31.12 and 31.13).
2. On the lateral view, the posterior border of the heart is displaced posteriorly. The Hoffman-Rigler sign is measured 2.0 cm above the intersection of the diaphragm and the

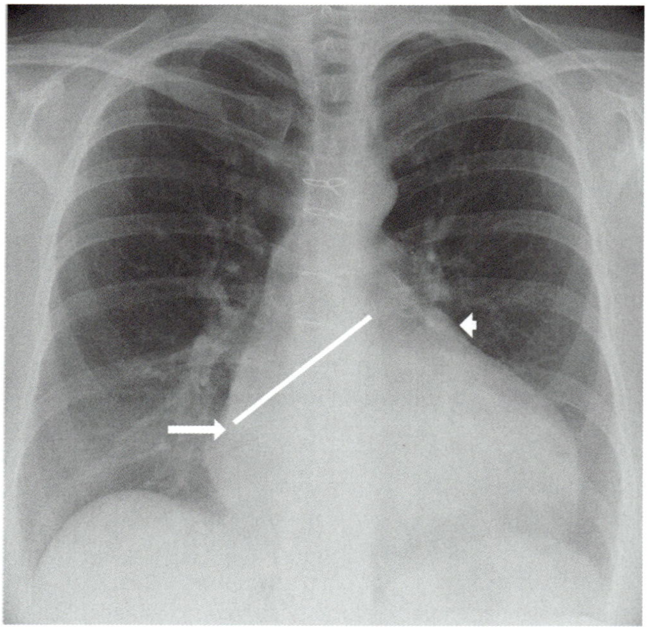

Figure 31.8. Mitral stenosis causing left atrial enlargement. Subtle convexity along the upper left cardiac border is caused by enlargement of the left atrial appendage (*arrowhead*). Note right retrocardiac double density (*arrow*) caused by enlargement of the left atrial chamber. The left atrial dimension is the length of a line (*white line*) from the middle of the double density to the medial border of the left bronchus. A value greater than 7 cm indicates left atrial enlargement.

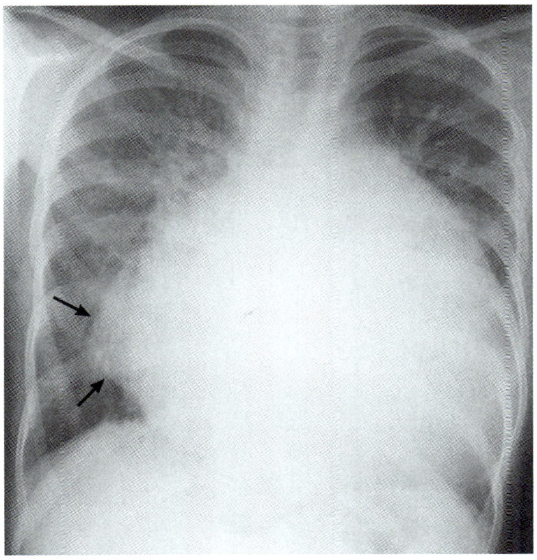

Figure 31.9. Mitral regurgitation. There is cardiomegaly and marked left atrial enlargement with pulmonary ventricular hypertension. The left atrium is enlarged to the extent that it forms the right heart border on the frontal view (*arrow*).

inferior vena cava. A positive measurement for LV enlargement is a posterior border of the heart extending more than 1.8 cm behind the inferior vena caval shadow at this level.

Right Ventricular Enlargement

1. On the posteroanterior view, the left border of the heart is enlarged directly laterally or laterally and slightly superiorly (see Fig. 31.12). In some instances, this causes the apex to be displaced superiorly ("upward tipped apex"; Fig. 31.14); in the extreme form, this causes a "boot shape" (see Fig. 32.28).
2. On the lateral view, the retrosternal space is encroached upon by the enlarged right ventricle. Right ventricular enlargement is inferred by contact of the right heart border over greater than one-third of the sternal length. A prominent convexity to the anterior border rather than the usual straight surface is an early sign of right ventricular enlargement.

Signposts for Cardiac Valvular Lesions

There are three signposts on the thoracic radiograph that direct attention to a certain cardiac valve:

1. Left atrial enlargement
2. Ascending aortic enlargement
3. Right atrial enlargement

These signs point specifically to the following:

1. Mitral valve (left atrium)
2. Aortic valve (ascending aorta)
3. Tricuspid valve (right atrium)

Using our classification system ("big heart" vs "small heart" heart disease) and applying the signpost, we can analyze the thoracic radiograph in accordance with the flow diagram shown in Figure 31.2. This schema obviously works well for diseases causing typical alterations in the chest x-ray. Of course, a specific cardiac lesion does not always cause typical features because of other associated abnormalities or because the lesion is very mild or has been present for insufficient time to alter the cardiac morphology to a degree discernible on the thoracic radiograph.

The schema can be briefly described by considering the chest x-ray that shows a normal heart size or mild cardiomegaly in a patient with significant heart disease. This means that the lesion likely causes pressure overload (hypertension, aortic stenosis, or mitral stenosis) or reduced LV compliance. If the left atrial signpost is present, then attention is directed

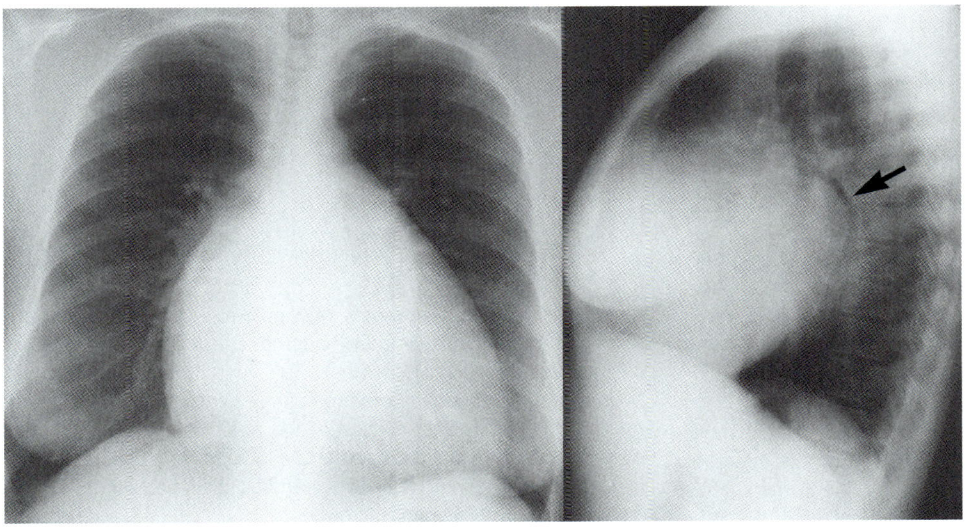

Figure 31.10. Mitral and tricuspid regurgitation. Frontal (left) and lateral (right) radiographs show prominent double densities on both sides of the spine due to marked left atrial enlargement. Right atrial enlargement is shown by the elongation of the right-sided convexity on the front view. Prominent upper left cardiac border on frontal view is caused by dilatation of the right ventricular outflow region. Lateral view shows posterior displacement of the left bronchus (*arrow*) by the enlarged left atrium and obliteration of the retrocardiac space by right ventricular enlargement.

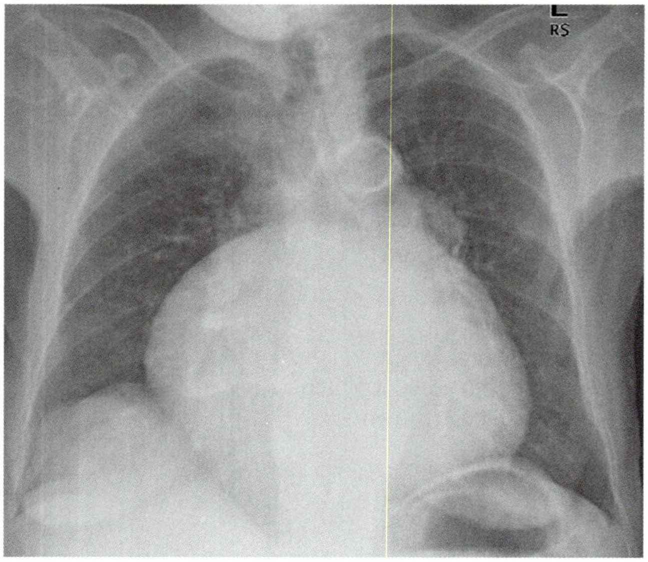

Figure 31.11. Tricuspid regurgitation. Severe right atrial enlargement is evident by the elongation of the right atrial shadow. The length of the right atrial border exceeds 60% of the height of the mediastinal cardiovascular structures.

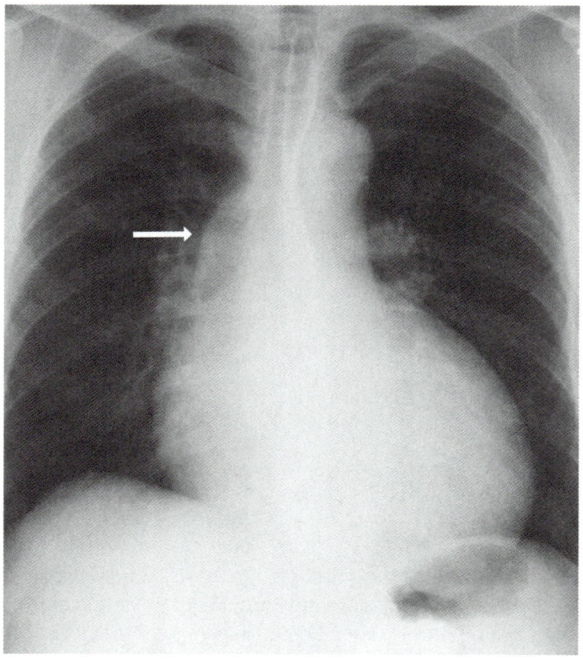

Figure 31.13. Aortic regurgitation. The ventricular contour is enlarged along a left inferolateral vector, causing the apex to droop over the left hemidiaphragm. Concavity along the upper left cardiac border indicates that the right ventricle is not enlarged. There is enlargement of the ascending aorta (*arrow*).

to the mitral valve (see Fig. 31.8). The diagnosis should be either mitral valvular stenosis or resistance to left atrial emptying. Diseases that significantly reduce LV compliance (and increase LV diastolic pressure) cause resistance to left atrial emptying and thereby induce left atrial enlargement. Diseases that may reduce LV compliance are hypertrophic cardiomyopathy, restrictive cardiomyopathy, and constrictive pericardial disease. Acute MI may also reduce LV compliance, but usually, this has not been present for a sufficient time to cause left atrial enlargement. LV hypertrophy from any cause can reduce LV compliance if it is sufficiently severe.

If the ascending aorta is enlarged, then this signpost points to the aortic valve, indicating aortic stenosis (Fig. 31.15). Systemic hypertension can produce a similar appearance, although it usually causes enlargement of the entire thoracic aorta rather than the ascending aorta alone. If no signposts are present, then the diagnosis is unlikely to be a

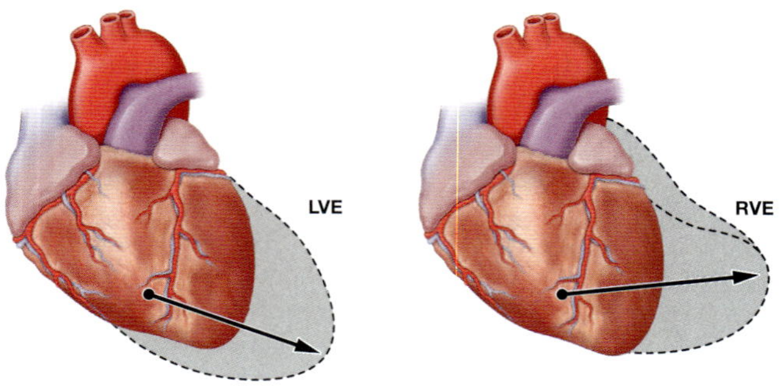

Figure 31.12. "Vectors of enlargement" for the left and right ventricles. For left ventricular enlargement, the vector is directed leftward and caudal. For right ventricular enlargement, the vector is directed leftward or leftward and slightly cranial.

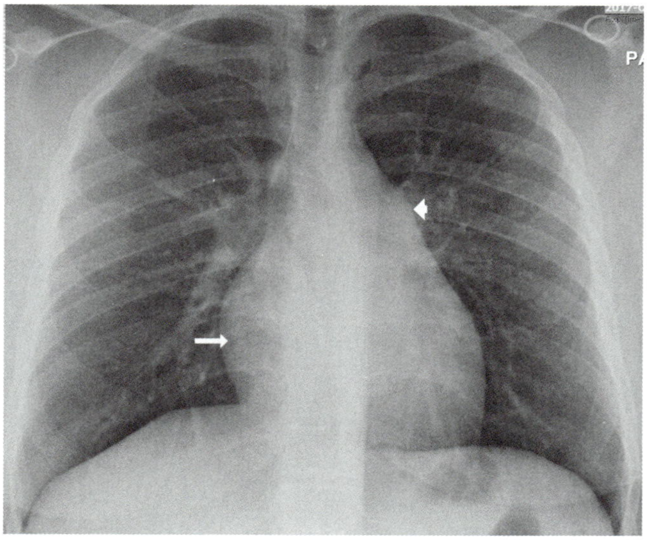

Figure 31.14. Mitral stenosis with pulmonary arterial hypertension and interstitial pulmonary edema. Cardiomegaly is caused by right ventricular enlargement. The vector of enlargement of the ventricle is directly lateral, indicating right ventricular enlargement. The most lateral portion of the apex is located above the diaphragm. Left atrial enlargement is indicated by double density (*arrow*). Pulmonary arterial hypertension is indicated by pulmonary arterial enlargement (*arrowhead*).

valvular lesion. The absence of signposts should direct attention to a disease directly afflicting the myocardium or pericardium, such as acute MI, hypertrophic cardiomyopathy, restrictive cardiomyopathy, and constrictive pericardial disease. However, even these latter diseases sometimes induce left atrial enlargement, as stated above.

The schema for a patient with substantial cardiomegaly proceeds along the following path. The big heart suggests that there is either a volume overload lesion (valvular regurgitation) or myocardial failure or pericardial effusion. High output states are certainly a volume overload and can cause substantial cardiomegaly, but sometimes they cause only mild cardiomegaly. If left atrial enlargement is noted, then the signpost points to mitral regurgitation (Fig. 31.16). If the ascending aorta is enlarged in "big heart" heart disease, then this signpost points to aortic regurgitation (see Fig. 31.13). If the right atrium is enlarged, then this signpost points to tricuspid regurgitation (see Fig. 31.11). Acquired pulmonic regurgitation is rare, except as a consequence of operation for right ventricular outflow obstruction, and is not considered in this schema. If no signposts are present, then the favored diagnostic considerations are congestive (dilated) cardiomyopathy or pericardial effusion.

RADIOGRAPHIC FEATURES OF SPECIFIC CARDIAC LESIONS

Aortic Stenosis

Aortic stenosis is a pressure overload lesion for which the compensatory mechanism is concentric LV hypertrophy (Table 31.6). Concentric LV hypertrophy causes a slight reduction in the volume of the LV but little increase in the overall cardiac size. Consequently, aortic stenosis, for much of its natural history, is a disease that is clearly "small heart" heart disease. There is little or no cardiac enlargement. The characteristic radiographic feature is enlargement of the ascending aorta (see Figs. 31.15, 31.17, 31.18). The pulmonary vascularity is also generally normal for much of the course of aortic stenosis. However, in the decompensated phase of aortic stenosis, there may be evidence of PVH due to LV failure. Occasionally, when LV hypertrophy has reduced LV compliance considerably, there may also be signs of PVH even in the absence of LV enlargement.

Hypertension

Hypertensive heart disease is a pressure overload lesion and consequently is associated with a normal heart size for much of the compensated phase of this disease (Table 31.7; Fig. 31.19). The severity or even the presence of LV hypertrophy cannot be reliably determined from the thoracic radiograph.

Mitral Stenosis

The features of a thoracic radiograph are frequently diagnostic for mitral stenosis (see Figs. 31.8 and 31.14). Likewise, the radiograph provides considerable insight into the severity of mitral stenosis. While mitral stenosis is a pressure overload lesion that causes little increase in overall heart size during the early phase of the disease, it does produce characteristic enlargement of the left atrium and the left atrial appendage and produces signs of PVH (Table 31.8).

Hypertrophic Cardiomyopathy

The chest radiograph is neither specific nor sensitive for the diagnosis of hypertrophic cardiomyopathy. More than 50% of patients with hypertrophic cardiomyopathy

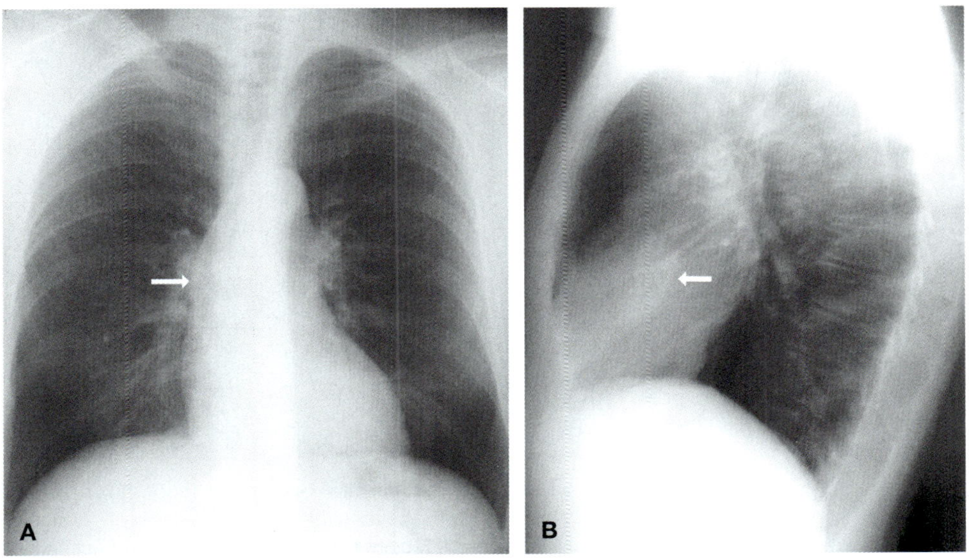

Figure 31.15. Aortic stenosis with calcification in 43-year-old man. Frontal radiograph **(A)** shows a nearly normal appearance except for the enlargement of the ascending aorta (*arrow*). Lateral view **(B)** demonstrates heavy calcification (*arrow*) of the aortic valve (*arrow*).

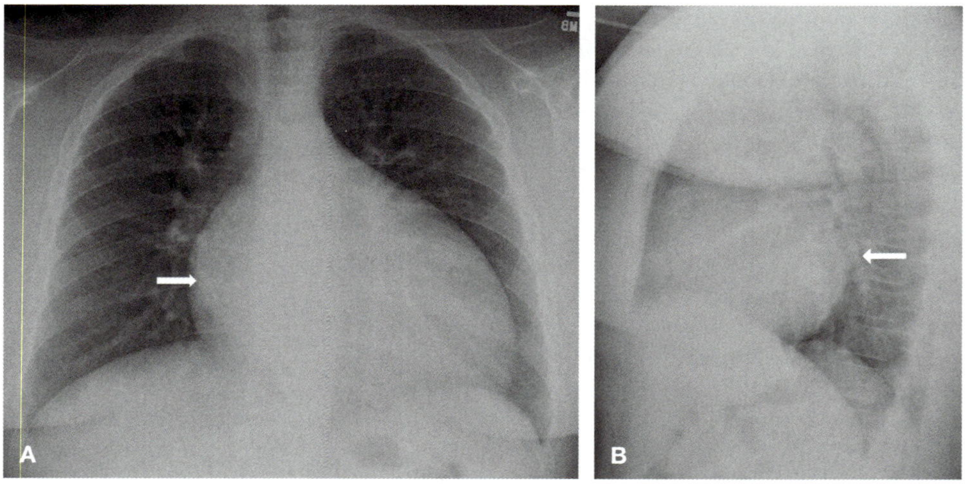

Figure 31.16. Mitral regurgitation. Frontal radiograph **(A)** shows an enlarged cardiac size with left atrial enlargement as evidenced by a right double density (*arrow*). Lateral radiograph **(B)** confirms the left atrial enlargement by displaying posterior bulging of the cardiac contour with displacement of the left lower bronchus (*arrow*).

have a normal chest x-ray. In a few patients, there is some abnormality of the chest x-ray, which is usually relatively vague and not particularly indicative of this disease. Since some patients with hypertrophic cardiomyopathy have a reduction in LV compliance, the radiograph sometimes demonstrates PVH. The PVH is usually relatively mild. The overall heart size is generally normal. In patients with reduced LV compliance, left atrial size may be increased. Approximately 30% of patients with symptomatic hypertrophic cardiomyopathy have associated mitral regurgitation. Because of the mitral regurgitation, there again is a proclivity to left atrial enlargement. A few patients have a squared appearance of the left cardiac border. This is caused by a prominent evagination on the upper left cardiac border. This focal enlargement is a consequence of extreme enlargement of the upper or outflow portion of the ventricular septum (Table 31.9).

Restrictive Cardiomyopathy

Restrictive cardiomyopathy is a relatively rare disease that may occur in an idiopathic form or maybe the form of cardiomyopathy that is a consequence of various infiltrative diseases of the LV. Types of infiltrative processes of the LV that may produce restrictive cardiomyopathy include sarcoidosis, hemochromatosis, and amyloidosis.

During the early stage of restrictive cardiomyopathy, the cardiac size is within normal limits. Restrictive cardiomyopathy has as its main physiologic deficit a reduction of LV compliance. Because of the reduced compliance, there is frequently an elevation in pulmonary venous pressure, which of course is reflected on the chest radiograph as various degrees of PVH (Figs. 31.20 and 31.21). Likewise, because of the reduced LV compliance, there is a rise in left atrial pressure, which may cause a left atrial enlargement to be visible on the radiograph. Because the major radiographic features of this disease are PVH and left atrial enlargement, the plain radiograph may mimic the appearance of mitral stenosis.

Table 31.6 Salient Radiographic Features of Aortic Stenosis
Enlargement of the ascending aorta due to poststenotic dilatation
Mild or no cardiomegaly in compensated stage
Substantial cardiomegaly occurs only after myocardial failure has ensued
No pulmonary venous hypertension or pulmonary edema is seen during most of the course of this disease
Calcification of aortic valve may be discernible on radiograph but is more readily shown on cardiothoracic

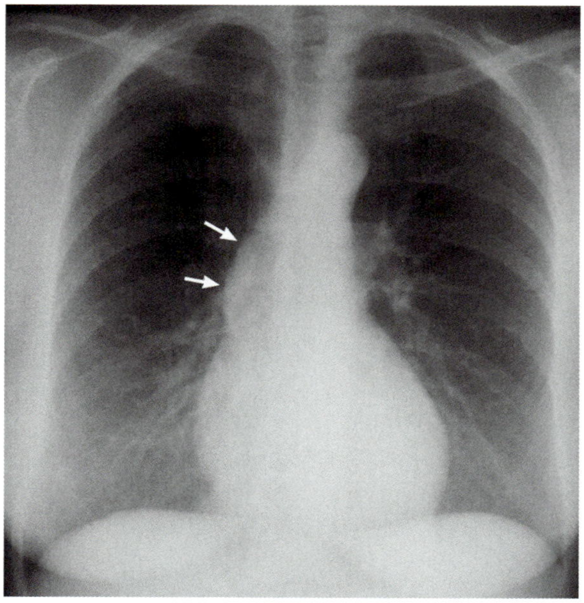

Figure 31.17. Aortic stenosis. Frontal radiograph shows normal cardiac size and normal pulmonary vascularity. The sole abnormality in this 40-year-old subject is the enlargement of the ascending aorta (*arrows*). The posterior aortic arch is normal in size.

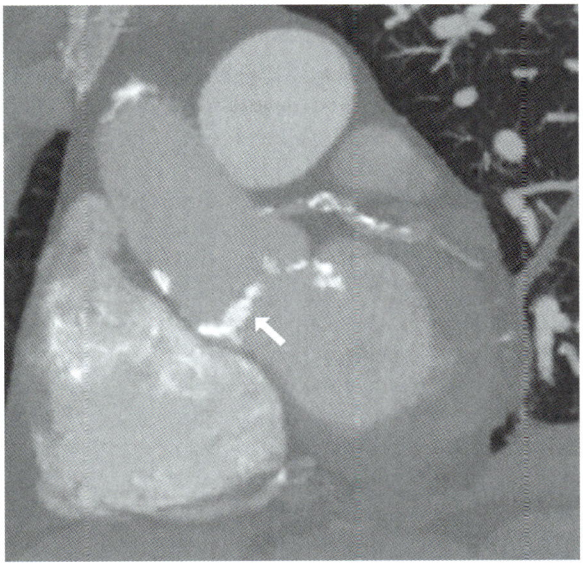

Figure 31.18. Aortic calcifications on CT. Oblique coronal maximum intensity projection of a CT angiogram shows severe aortic valve leaflet calcifications (arrow), consistent with aortic valve stenosis. CT, cardiothoracic.

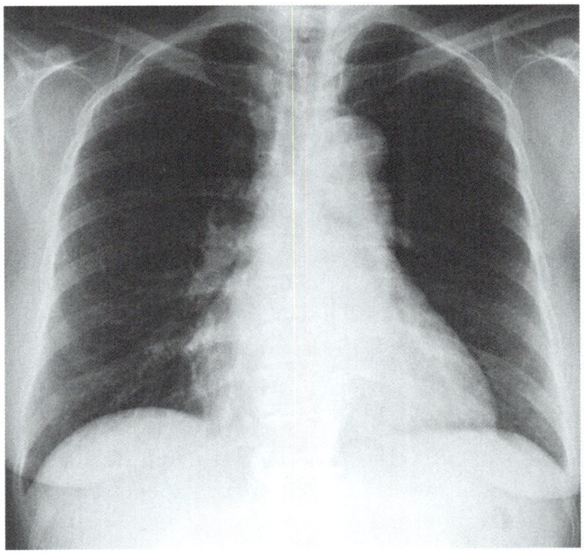

Figure 31.19. Systemic hypertension. Frontal view shows borderline cardiomegaly and prominence of the entire thoracic aorta.

In advanced disease, there is frequently some degree of LV enlargement, which along with the left atrial enlargement usually results in a mild to moderate cardiomegaly (see Fig 31.21). However, in some patients, the restrictive cardiomyopathy may progress to congestive cardiomyopathy, which is associated with considerable cardiomegaly and LV enlargement (Table 31.10).

Acute Myocardial Infarction

The plain radiograph is obtained in the emergency room for most patients with an acute MI. The initial chest x-ray or a chest x-ray within the first 24 hours after the onset of acute MI is normal in approximately 50% of patients with initial acute MI. In the other 50% of patients, the most frequent finding is some degree of PVH or pulmonary edema, along with a normal heart size (Fig. 31.22). The major physiologic deficit in the early phase of acute MI is an abrupt decrease in LV compliance, which results in an increase in pulmonary venous pressure. The increase in pulmonary venous pressure is reflected on the chest x-ray by varying degrees of PVH or pulmonary edema. It is unusual for the patient with a first acute MI, even when the infarction is severe and eventually lethal, to have cardiomegaly or perceptible LV enlargement.

The plain chest x-ray does provide some insight into the severity of the acute MI. The degree of PVH on the plain radiograph within the first 24 hours and the early and late survival rates after the initial MI. The plain radiograph may also be useful in demonstrating complications of acute MI, such as cardiac rupture; pericardial effusion; LV aneurysm, both true and false; papillary muscle rupture; and intractable congestive heart failure.

Table 31.7 Salient Radiographic Features of Arterial Hypertension

- Enlargement of the thoracic aorta—ascending, arch and descending aorta
- Mild or no cardiomegaly until the onset of myocardial failure
- No pulmonary edema or pulmonary venous hypertension until the occurrence of diastolic dysfunction due to severe left ventricular hypertrophy or myocardial failure

Table 31.8 Salient Radiographic Features of Mitral Stenoses

- Pulmonary venous hypertension or edema is present
- Pulmonary edema may be observed intermittently
- Mild cardiomegaly is seen in isolated mitral stenosis
- Enlargement of the left atrium is characteristic
- Enlargement of the left atrial appendage is frequent and suggests a rheumatic etiology
- Right ventricular enlargement indicates some degree of pulmonary arterial hypertension or associated tricuspid regurgitation
- Enlargement of the pulmonary arterial segment is indicative of associated pulmonary arterial hypertension
- Right ventricular enlargement in the absence of prominence of the main pulmonary artery suggests associated tricuspid regurgitation. The right atrium is also enlarged with tricuspid regurgitation
- The ascending aorta and aortic arch are usually inconspicuous in isolated mitral stenosis. Even slight enlargement of the thoracic aorta raises the question of associated aortic valve disease

Table 31.9 Salient Radiographic Features of Hypertrophic Cardiomyopathy

Normal in most patients
Mild cardiomegaly and pulmonary venous hypertension in a minority of patients
Left atrial enlargement can be caused by associated mitral insufficiency or reduced left ventricular compliance
In the obstructive form (subaortic stenosis), ascending aortic enlargement is infrequent.
Left ventricular enlargement may occur in end-stage disease

Some patients with a true LV aneurysm demonstrate a normal chest x-ray. However, in many patients, there is evidence of an abnormal cardiac configuration, especially an abnormal evagination along the midportion of the left cardiac border or in the region of the cardiac apex (Fig. 31.23). The abnormal contour generally occurs in these sites because the most frequent location of a true LV aneurysm is the anterolateral wall or the apical wall of the LV. Calcification of the anterolateral region of the LV is suggestive of LV aneurysm (Fig. 31.24). Calcification of an infarct is more readily displayed on CT (Fig. 31.25).

An abnormal evagination that is localized to the posterior wall or the diaphragmatic wall of the LV should raise the possibility of a false LV aneurysm (Fig. 31.26). While only approximately 5% of true LV aneurysms involve the upper diaphragmatic and posterior wall, these sites are the most frequent ones for false LV aneurysm. Consequently, an abnormal contour or a double density localized to these sites should raise the consideration of this diagnosis. The differentiation of a false aneurysm from a true aneurysm becomes important because of the known propensity of false aneurysms to be complicated by late rupture. Other plain radiographic signs of a false aneurysm are an aneurysm that is extremely large with a prominent projection of the posterior or diaphragmatic surface of the heart (see Fig. 31.26) and an increase in the size of the aneurysm in sequential studies. A false aneurysm is more frequently associated with occlusion of either the circumflex or right coronary artery, while a true aneurysm is most frequently associated with occlusion of the left anterior descending coronary artery.

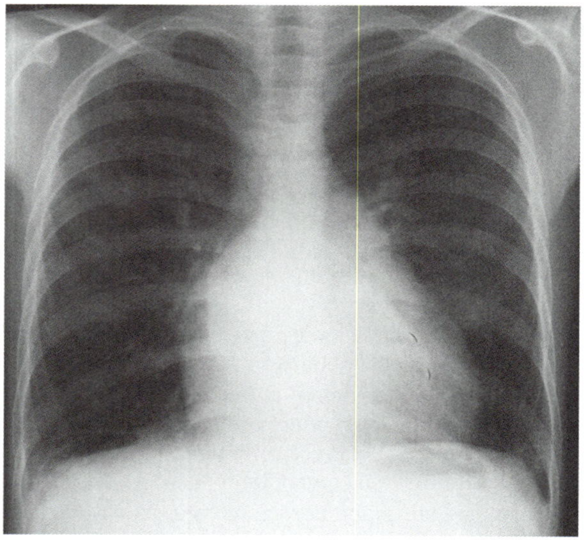

Figure 31.20. Restrictive cardiomyopathy. Normal cardiac size with left atrial enlargement.

Papillary muscle rupture is a dramatic event that usually induces severe and many times intractable pulmonary edema. Partial rupture of the papillary muscle, resulting in less severe mitral regurgitation, may produce a moderate degree of mitral regurgitation and less severe or even no evidence of pulmonary edema. The dramatic radiographic findings in acute papillary muscle rupture are pulmonary edema with little increase in left atrial size or cardiomegaly. If the patient survives beyond several weeks or months, then varying degrees of left atrial enlargement and cardiomegaly may be present.

Postinfarction rupture of the ventricular septum may produce a radiographic appearance very similar to that of acute mitral regurgitation. The radiographic signs of acute ventricular septal defect include an increase in the prominence of the pulmonary arteries (ie, pulmonary arterial overcirculation), usually pulmonary edema, and mild degrees of cardiomegaly. Again, if the patient tolerates the episode and survives for several weeks to months, then the degree of cardiomegaly may be more considerable, and there may even be signs of left atrial enlargement.

Dressler's syndrome, another complication of acute MI, occurs within the first weeks to months after an acute MI. This is an autoimmune response to various antigens that are released during acute MI. This autoimmune response involves the pericardial and pleural surfaces, eventuating in pericardial and pleural effusions. Chest radiographs in this syndrome demonstrate an increase in cardiac size as a consequence of the pericardial effusion, along with evidence of unilateral or bilateral pleural effusions (Table 31.11).

Constrictive Pericarditis

Constrictive pericarditis is a disease that is being encountered with increasing frequency. Currently, the major causes are iatrogenic. The most frequent inciting factor is postoperative bleeding associated with cardiac surgery, especially coronary revascularization procedures. The second most frequent inciting factor is mediastinal irradiation; the third most common cause is repeated episodes of viral pericarditis. Uremic pericardial disease may also eventuate in constrictive pericarditis, but usually, this disease produces an effusive/constrictive type of pericardial disease. In Third World countries, tuberculosis continues to be a major cause of constrictive pericarditis.

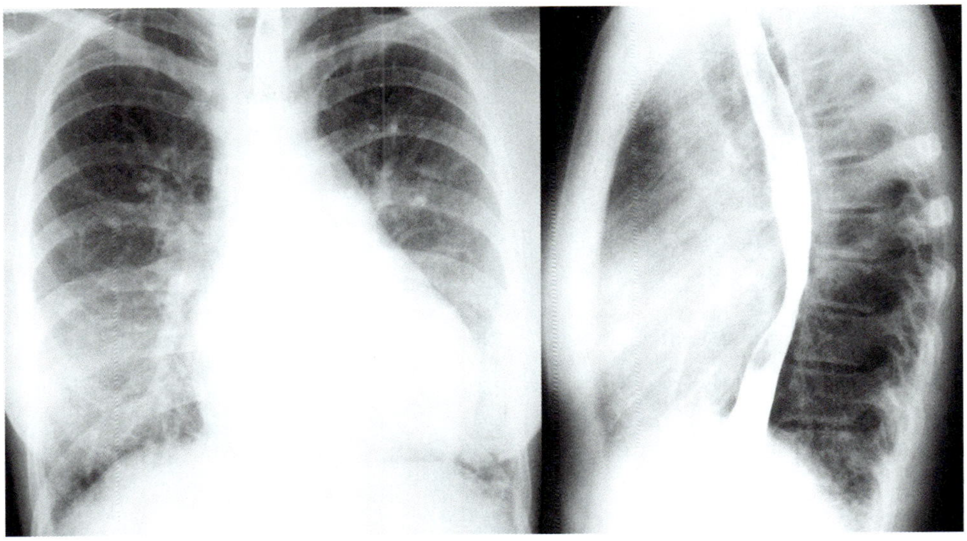

Figure 31.21. Restrictive cardiomyopathy. Frontal (left) and lateral (right) radiographs show interstitial pulmonary edema and left atrial and right ventricular enlargement.

The plain radiograph is frequently but not always abnormal in patients with hemodynamically significant constrictive pericarditis. Because of pericardial constriction, there is a restriction to left atrial emptying during diastole, with a subsequent rise in left atrial and pulmonary venous pressures. The rise in pulmonary venous pressure is reflected on the chest radiograph by signs of PVH, such as redistribution and interstitial or alveolar pulmonary edema. The overall cardiac size is usually normal, or there is only mild cardiomegaly. Frequently, there is left atrial enlargement but normal ventricular size. Recognition of pericardial calcification supports or may initially suggest the diagnosis of constrictive pericarditis (Fig. 31.27; Table 31.12).

"BIG HEART" HEART DISEASE

Aortic Regurgitation

Aortic regurgitation is characterized on the plain radiograph by a substantial degree of cardiomegaly, which is due predominantly to LV enlargement (see Figs. 31.12 and 31.28). A signpost pointing to the aortic valve is present in this disease, consisting of enlargement of the ascending aorta, aortic knob, and usually the descending thoracic aorta. As opposed to aortic stenosis, the enlargement of the thoracic aorta involves the aortic knob as well as the ascending aorta. Consequently, "big heart" heart disease with the aortic signpost is indicative of aortic regurgitation.

The severity of aortic regurgitation is reflected on the plain radiograph. Since this is a volume overload lesion, the extent of the increase in the volume of the heart is related to the severity and the duration of aortic regurgitation. For most of the course of aortic regurgitation, the pulmonary vascularity is normal. Consequently, the presence of PVH in a patient with aortic regurgitation is indicative of LV failure and is frequently associated with end-stage aortic valve disease (Table 31.13).

Table 31.10 Salient Radiographic Features of Restrictive Cardiomyopathy

Pulmonary venous hypertension is typical
Pulmonary edema may occur intermittently
Normal heart size or mild cardiomegaly in most patients
Left atrial enlargement
Left atrial appendage is typically not enlarged
Moderate to severe cardiomegaly can ensue in end-stage disease

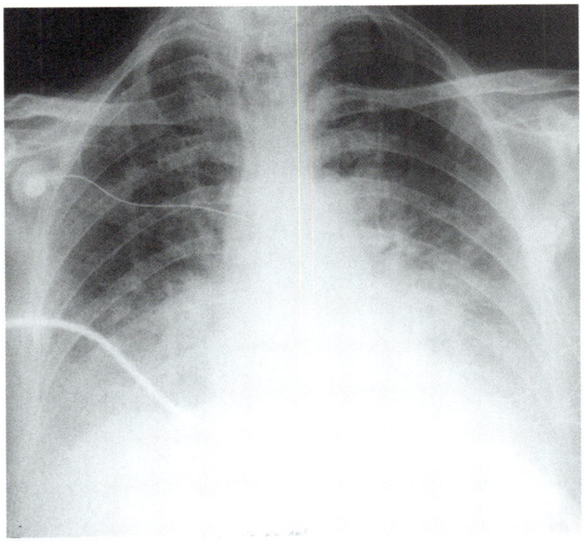

Figure 31.22. Acute myocardial infarction with alveolar pulmonary edema. Note alveolar filling in perihilar regions and lower lobes with normal heart size.

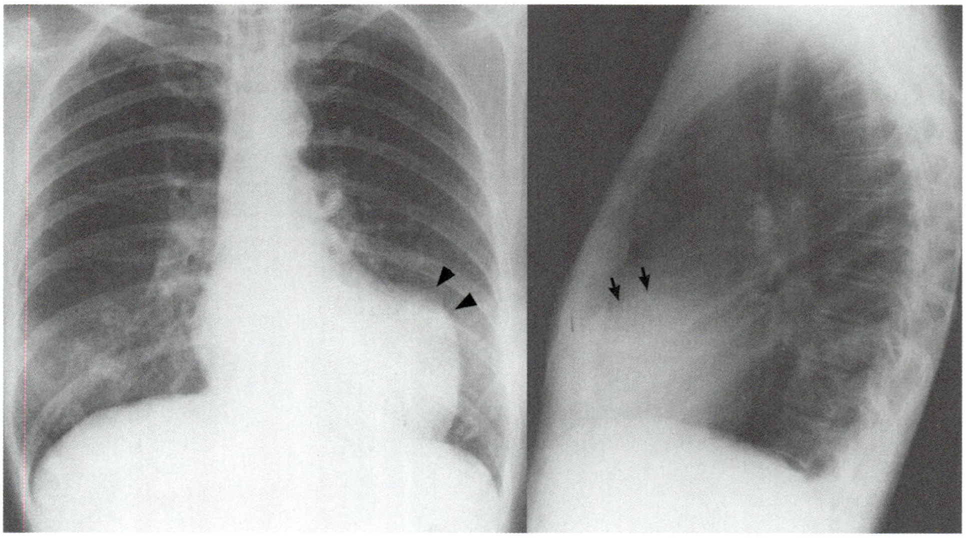

Figure 31.23. True left ventricular aneurysm complicating myocardial infarction. Frontal (left) and lateral (right) views. Abnormal evagination of left cardiac border (*arrowheads*) is typical for an aneurysm involving the anterolateral and/or apical segment of the left ventricle. Lateral view demonstrates an anterior double density (*arrows*), characteristic of an anterolateral aneurysm.

Mitral Regurgitation

The plain radiograph in mitral regurgitation shows variable degrees of PVH, cardiomegaly, left atrial enlargement, and LV enlargement (see Figs. 31.9, 31.10, 31.16) and sometimes signs of right-sided chamber enlargement (see Fig. 30.10). In the presence of isolated mitral regurgitation, the ascending aorta is relatively small. Consequently, recognition of prominence of the ascending aorta in a patient with isolated mitral valve disease raises the prospect of associated aortic valve disease.

The left atrial appendage is generally enlarged in patients who have a rheumatic etiology of the mitral regurgitation (see Fig. 31.8). On the other hand, the left atrial appendage is frequently not enlarged in patients who otherwise have left atrial enlargement of nonrheumatic etiology.

The severity of PVH in mitral regurgitation is generally less than in isolated mitral stenosis. Most patients with compensated mitral regurgitation have minimal or no signs of PVH. A practical axiom is that mitral stenosis causes PVH that is prominent in relation to the degree of left atrial enlargement, whereas mitral regurgitation is associated with left atrial enlargement that is out of proportion to the expected severity of PVH. Patients with mixed mitral stenosis and mitral regurgitation may have both very substantial left atrial enlargement as well as prominent signs of PVH. The giant left atrium can be associated with either mitral stenosis or regurgitation but is more frequently caused by the latter. The right border of the left atrium may even extend beyond the border of the right atrium rather than causing a right retrocardiac double density (see Fig. 31.9).

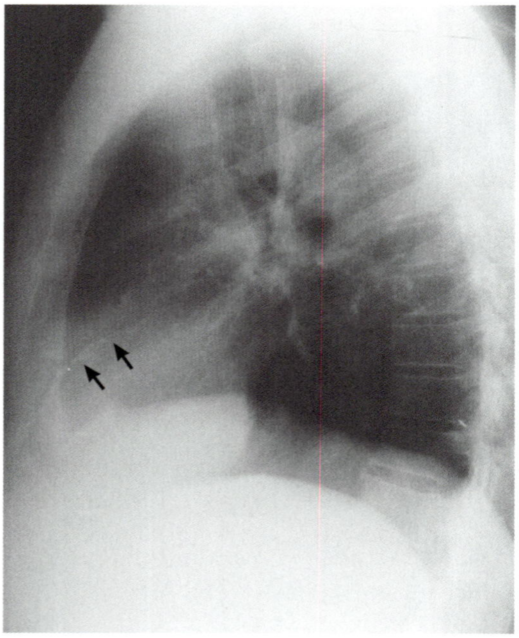

Figure 31.24. Calcified apical left ventricular aneurysm. Lateral thoracic radiograph shows calcification (*arrows*) on the anteroapical region of the left ventricle.

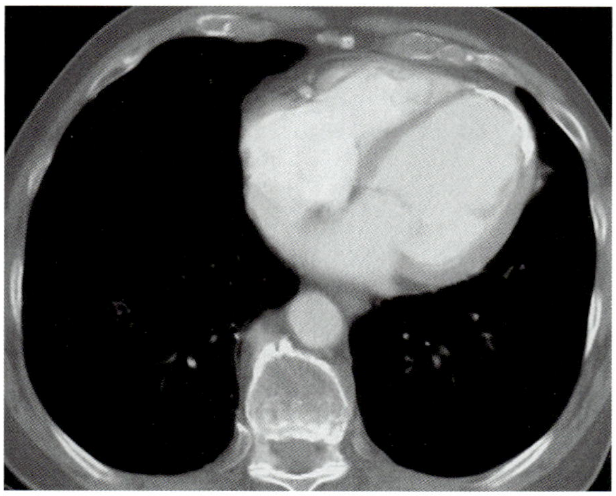

Figure 31.25. Cardiothoracic scan shows mural calcification at the site of an old apical myocardial infarction.

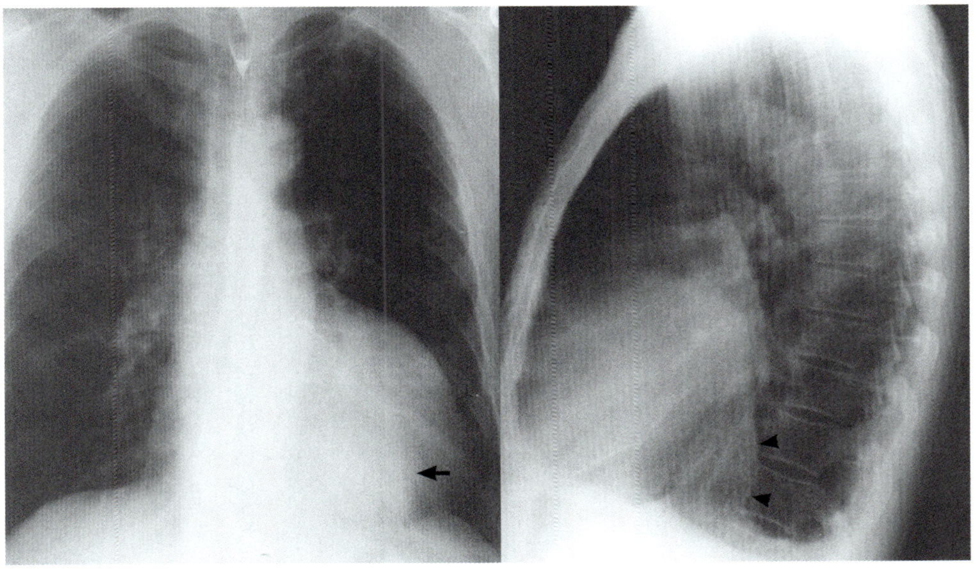

Figure 31.26. False left ventricular aneurysm complicating myocardial infarction. Frontal (left) and lateral (right) radiographs show left retrocardiac density (*arrow*) on the frontal view and large posterior evagination (*arrowheads*) of left ventricular contour on the lateral view. Large size and posterior location are characteristics of false aneurysm.

The plain radiograph may be useful in assessing the severity of mitral regurgitation. Because this is a volume overload lesion, the overall heart size may be a reasonable indicator of the severity of regurgitation. Likewise, the overall heart size may be of some prognostic use in patients undergoing mitral valve replacement. In general, patients with lesser degrees of cardiomegaly demonstrate a greater 5-year survival rate after replacement of the mitral valve (Table 31.14).

Tricuspid Regurgitation

The signs of tricuspid regurgitation may be difficult to discern on the plain radiograph. Signs of right atrial enlargement are frequently dubious and not sharply discriminated from normal. Indeed, there must be substantial right atrial enlargement before it is possible to recognize its occurrence. In general, the best sign of right atrial enlargement is the elongation of the right atrial border (see Fig. 31.11). The radiographic signs of tricuspid regurgitation are normal or perhaps reduced prominence of the pulmonary vascularity, cardiomegaly, right atrial enlargement, and occasionally signs of superior vena caval and especially inferior vena caval enlargement (see Figs. 31.10 and 31.11).

Cardiomegaly, with the signpost of right atrial enlargement, would indicate the likely diagnosis of tricuspid regurgitation. The cardiac contour in patients with tricuspid regurgitation may be similar to that of congestive cardiomyopathy and pericardial effusion. The most extreme cardiomegaly is seen with severe tricuspid regurgitation of long duration; it can cause the "wall-to-wall" heart (Fig. 31.29; Table 31.15).

Table 31.11 Salient Radiographic Features of Acute Myocardial Infarction

Normal chest x-ray in about 50% of first acute infarctions

Normal heart size with pulmonary venous hypertension or pulmonary edema in about 50% of first acute infarctions

Cardiomegaly is usually indicative of acute infarction in a patient with history of previous infarctions

Cardiomegaly maybe indicative of ischemic cardiomyopathy

Signs of complication of acute myocardial infarction

- Intractable pulmonary edema may occur with papillary muscle rupture (mitral regurgitation) or ventricular septal rupture (left to right shunt)
- Enlarged cardiac silhouette may be caused by pericardial effusion
- Abnormal cardiac contour may be a sign of true (bulge of the anterolateral or apical regions); or false (bulge of the posterior or diaphragmatic regions) aneurysms

Dilated Cardiomyopathy

The radiographic appearance in dilated cardiomyopathy is relatively nonspecific. There is usually some degree of PVH and substantial cardiomegaly (Figs. 30.37 and 30.38). Characteristically, the cardiomegaly exists without the presence of signposts to the aortic, mitral, or tricuspid valve. Consequently, substantial cardiomegaly ("big heart" heart disease), without radiographic signposts, should raise the diagnostic consideration of dilated cardiomyopathy. Of course, a similar appearance can exist with pericardial effusion. The most frequent cause of dilated cardiomyopathy is ischemic heart disease. Dilated cardiomyopathy can also be genetic in etiology, related to cardiotoxicity, or idiopathic, among other causes (Table 31.16).

Pericardial Effusion

The cardiac configuration in pericardial effusion is relatively nonspecific. It has been assumed that the presence

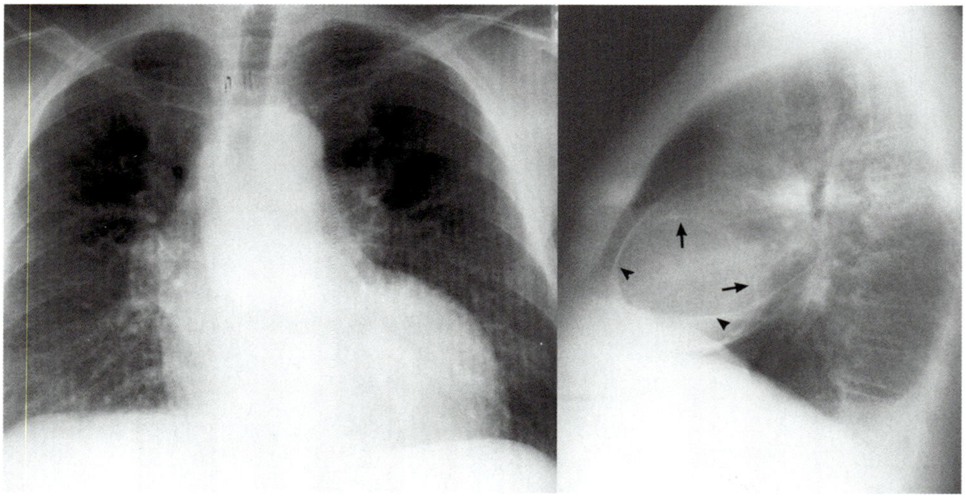

Figure 31.27. Constrictive pericarditis. Frontal (left) and lateral (right) radiographs demonstrate pericardial calcification. The calcification involves the atrioventricular (*arrows*) and the interventricular (*arrowheads*) grooves.

of substantial cardiomegaly in the absence of signs of PVH should be a clue to the presence of pericardial effusion (Figs. 31.30 and 31.31). This radiographic appearance is actually quite nonspecific. Similar to the appearance of dilated cardiomyopathy, the cardiac configuration is that of cardiomegaly without a radiographic signpost. A specific appearance providing a diagnosis of pericardial effusion is relatively infrequent in this entity. The so-called water-bottle appearance of the heart is nonspecific and difficult to recognize. The "fat pad" sign seen on the lateral radiograph does permit identification but occurs in only a few patients (see Fig. 31.30). The varying density sign is also sometimes present on the frontal radiograph (see Fig. 31.31). This consists of a lesser density at the periphery of the cardiac contour compared to the central portion of the cardiac contour. The cause of this varying density is that the x-ray beam encounters only fluid toward the periphery of the pericardial effusion, while in the center of the pericardial effusion, the radiographic beam must pass through both waters anteriorly and the cardiac substance more centrally.

With the frequent use of echocardiography, large pericardial effusions are being encountered less frequently. The

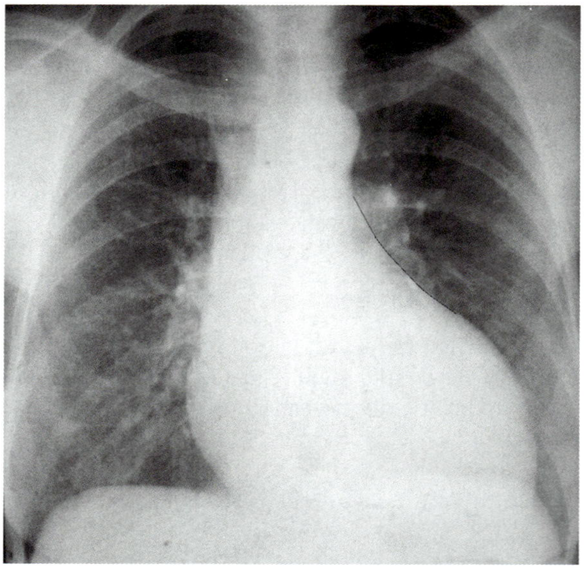

Figure 31.28. Aortic regurgitation. Frontal radiograph shows marked cardiomegaly with the displacement of the ventricular contour laterally and caudally, indicating left ventricular enlargement. The ascending aorta and the contour of the posterior aortic arch are enlarged. Concavity (broken line) along the upper left cardiac border indicates no right ventricular enlargement.

Table 31.12 Salient Radiographic Features of Constrictive Pericarditis
Pulmonary venous hypertension
Normal heart size or mild cardiomegaly
Left atrial enlargement may be discernible
Flattened cardiac contours are pathognomonic but infrequently observed
Calcification of the cardiac margin, especially the atrioventricular and interventricular grooves

Table 31.13 Salient Radiographic Features of Aortic Regurgitation
Absence of pulmonary venous hypertension or pulmonary edema until late in the course of this lesion
Moderate to severe cardiomegaly
Left ventricular enlargement
Enlargement of the ascending aorta and aortic arch

Table 31.14 Salient Radiographic Features of Mitral Regurgitation
Variable degree of pulmonary venous hypertensive or pulmonary edema (less severe than with mitral stenosis)
Moderate to severe cardiomegaly
Left ventricular enlargement
Left atrial enlargement
Enlargement of left atrial appendage

presence of any degree of pericardial effusion can be easily recognized by echocardiography (Table 31.17).

Paracardiac Masses

Enlargement of the cardiac contour may not always be indicative of cardiac enlargement itself or pericardial effusion. One must also consider the infrequent possibility that the enlargement represents a cardiac or paracardiac mass (Fig. 31.32). Such consideration should be prompted by the recognition of an unusual cardiac contour. The various causes of paracardiac masses are legion, but considerations are pericardial cysts, paracardiac tumors such as lymphoma and germinal cell tumor, cardiac tumors such as rhabdomyoma or various sarcomas, metastasis to lymph nodes within the pericardiophrenic angle, eventration or hernia of the diaphragm, neural tumors of the phrenic nerve, and various types of skeletal muscle tumors arising from the diaphragm. The diagnosis of the paracardiac mass can be readily made by CT and even more precisely with gated MRI.

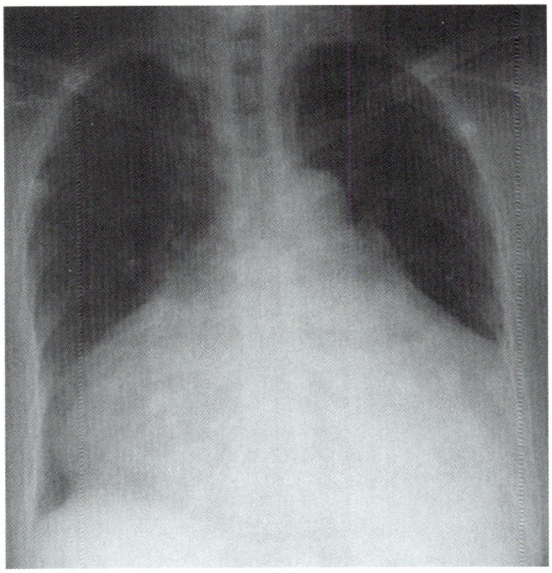

Figure 31.29. Tricuspid regurgitation. The features of this lesion are diminished pulmonary vascularity, marked cardiomegaly, and right atrial and right ventricular enlargement. The severe enlargement of the right-sided chamber produced the 'wall-to-wall heart."

Table 31.15 Salient Radiographic Features of Aortic Regurgitation
No pulmonary venous hypertension or pulmonary edema (isolated tricuspid regurgitation)
Pulmonary venous hypertension or edema indicates associated mitral valve disease
Moderate to severe cardiomegaly
Right ventricular enlargement
Right atrial enlargement

ABNORMAL CARDIAC CONTOURS

Enlargement of the Main Pulmonary Arterial Segment

Enlargement of the main pulmonary arterial segment is usually due to enlargement of the main pulmonary artery itself (Fig. 31.33). There are a number of causes of enlargement of the main pulmonary artery (Table 31.18).

Enlargement of the main pulmonary artery segment is the main indicator of pulmonary arterial hypertension (see Fig. 31.33). Severe pulmonary hypertension may cause calcification of the central pulmonary arteries (Fig. 31.34). Whenever one recognizes enlargement of the main pulmonary artery segment in a patient with no known pulmonary valvular disease, the differential diagnosis of pulmonary hypertension must be considered. The differential diagnosis of pulmonary hypertension should lead to a systematic organization of the diagnostic possibilities. There are six diagnostic categories for pulmonary hypertension: (1) pulmonary hypertension resulting from PVH, (2) pulmonary hypertension resulting from left-to-right shunts resulting in pulmonary arteriolar disease (arteriolopathy), (3) pulmonary hypertension resulting from obliteration of the pulmonary vascular bed from chronic lung disease, (4) pulmonary hypertension resulting from obliteration of the pulmonary vascular bed as a consequence of pulmonary embolic disease or schistosomiasis, (5) pulmonary hypertension due to obliteration of pulmonary venous drainage in chronic veno-occlusive disease, and (6) primary pulmonary hypertension. Radiographic signs that permit the differential diagnosis of the various causes include recognition of the following:

1. Signs of PVH would indicate the likelihood that the pulmonary hypertension is secondary to PVH.

Table 31.16 Salient Radiographic Features of Dilated Cardiomyopathy
Pulmonary venous hypertension or pulmonary edema may be but is not invariably present
Moderate to severe cardiomegaly
Left ventricular enlargement
Left atrial enlargement is infrequently evident but can be caused by mitral regurgitation caused by left ventricular enlargement

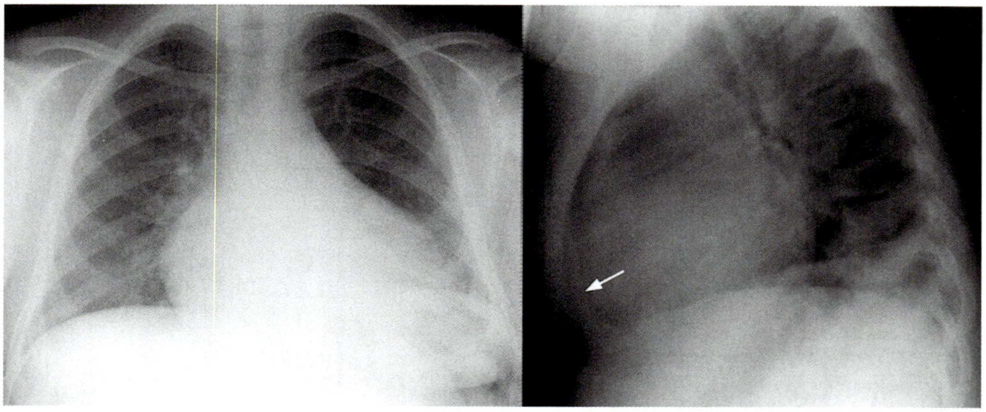

Figure 31.30. Pericardial perfusion. "Fat pad" sign is shown on lateral view (right). A stripe of water density (*arrow*) separates two fat layers on the outer surface of the parietal pericardium and beneath the visceral pericardium.

2. Signs of chronic lung disease such as chronic obstructive pulmonary disease or interstitial lung disease would indicate this as the etiology.
3. Asymmetric pulmonary vascularity or signs of pulmonary scarring might indicate the presence of chronic thromboembolic disease.
4. Marked enlargement of the central pulmonary arteries or signs of enlargement of the specific cardiac chambers may indicate the presence of a previous left-to-right shunt that has resulted in Eisenmenger's syndrome.

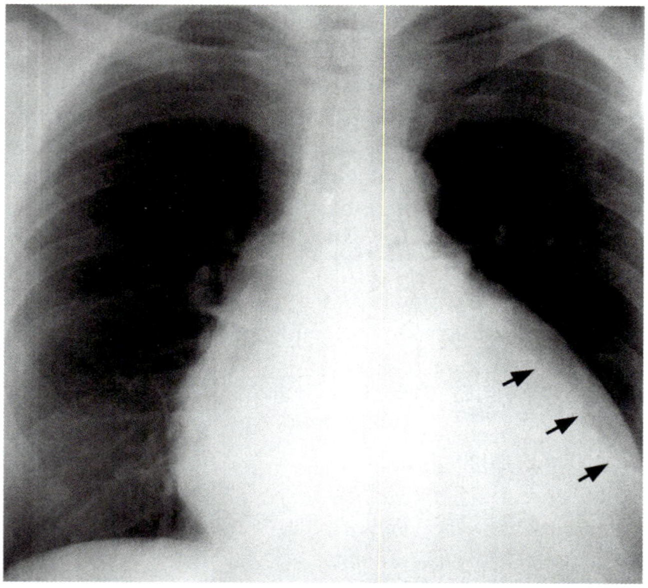

Figure 31.31. Pericardial perfusion. Varying cardiac density sign caused by transition of density near the margin of the cardiac silhouette (*arrows*).

Cardiac Calcification

Calcification in the central cardiovascular structures is frequent and is an important diagnostic sign. In a few instances, calcification of a specific shape and location is pathognomonic for a disease. The various cardiovascular calcifications include the following:

1. Ascending aortic calcification. This is most frequently observed on the right anterolateral margin of the ascending aorta in elderly individuals, especially in the presence of aortic valve disease.
2. Mitral annular calcification (Fig. 31.35). This is a dense C-shaped calcification in the region of the mitral valve. It may be a causative factor of mitral regurgitation. It is frequently observed in apparently normal elderly patients.
3. Aortic annular calcification, a circular calcification in the region of the aortic valve. Extension of this calcification into the region of the conducting system can produce complete heart failure.
4. Valvular calcification (aortic and mitral). Calcification of the aortic valve of sufficient density and extent to be visualized on the radiograph (see Fig. 31.15) is nearly always

Table 31.17 Salient Radiographic Features of Pericardial Effusion

No pulmonary venous hypertension or pulmonary edema
Moderate to severe enlargement of cardiac silhouette
Associated pleural effusion is not uncommon
Specific features, such as "fat pad" and/or "variable density" signs, are infrequently evident (see Figs. 30.39 and 30.40)

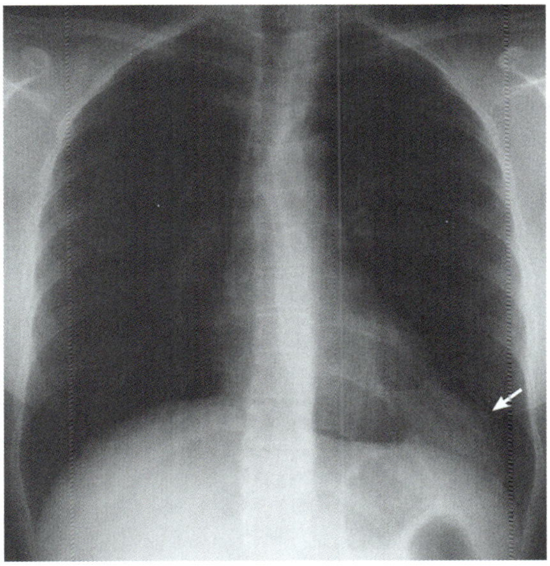

Figure 31.32. Pericardial cyst. Frontal radiograph shows a mass (*arrow*) adjacent to the cardiac apex.

associated with hemodynamically important aortic stenosis (gradient more than 50 mm Hg).

5. Coronary arterial calcification. Coronary arterial calcification is frequently observed by fluoroscopy or CT. It must be both dense and extensive to be recognized on the thoracic radiograph.
6. LV mural calcification. This is most frequently located in the anterolateral or apical regions of the LV and marks the site of a transmural MI or aneurysm (see Figs. 31.24 and 31.25).

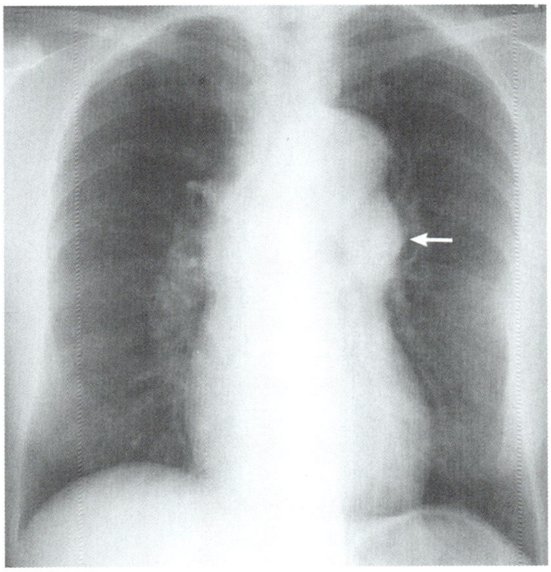

Figure 31.33. Marked dilatation of the pulmonary artery (*arrow*) due to Eisenmenger syndrome caused by patent ductus arteriosus. The main pulmonary artery and aortic arch are moderately enlarged.

Table 31.18 Enlargement of Main Pulmonary Artery: Etiology

Pulmonary arterial hypertension
Excess pulmonary blood flow (left to right shunts, chronic high output states)
Valvular pulmonic stenosis
Pulmonary regurgitation
Congenital absent pulmonary valve (aneurysmal pulmonary artery)
Absence of left pericardium
Aneurysm of pulmonary artery
Idiopathic dilatation of pulmonary artery

7. Pericardial calcification is indicative of constrictive pericarditis. It is located usually in the interventricular or atrioventricular grooves of the heart (see Fig. 31.27).
8. Unusual sites of calcification may represent intracardiac tumor (left atrial myxoma), pericardial tumor (dermoid), or healed granulomas (myocardial tuberculoma).

APPLICATIONS OF ARTIFICIAL INTELLIGENCE

Artificial intelligence tools for the detection of cardiac abnormalities in chest radiograph are currently available, mostly focused on the detection of cardiomegaly. The main

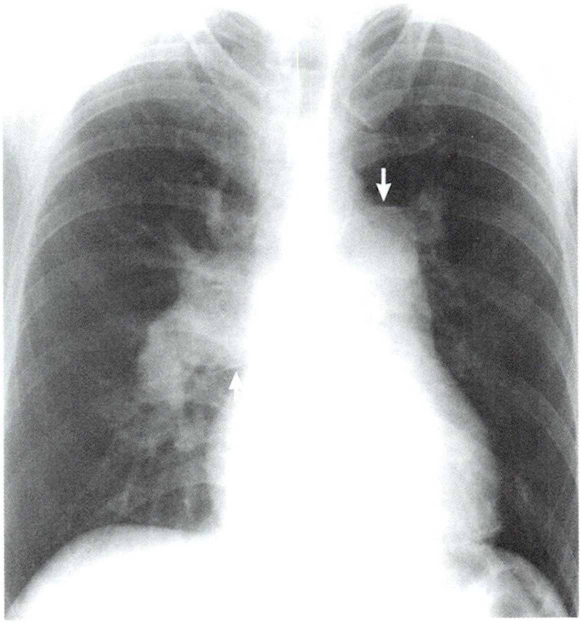

Figure 31.34. Pulmonary arterial hypertension due to Eisenmenger's complex; the underlying lesion was an atrial septal defect. Frontal view shows the markedly enlarged main (*arrow*) and right pulmonary arterial segments. There is calcification (*arrow*) in the pulmonary arteries consistent with a systemic arterial pressure level in the pulmonary circulation.

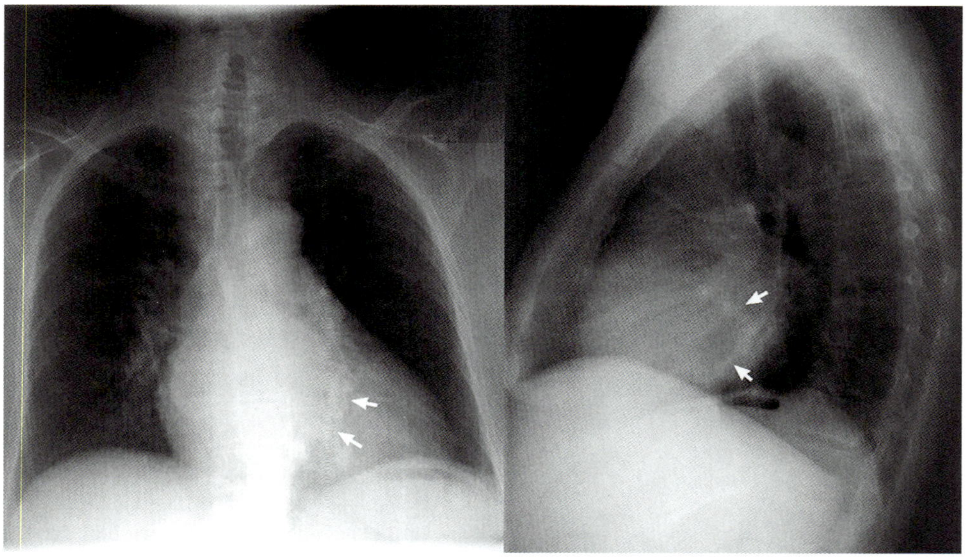

Figure 31.35. Mitral annular calcification. Frontal (left) and lateral (right) views show a C-shaped calcification (*arrows*) in the mitral annulus.

clinical applications pertain to the detection of potential cardiac disease in large databases of chest radiographs obtained for other purposes in patients without suspected heart disease. There are also algorithms design for the detection of coronary calcifications on chest radiograph, which could inform the need for further cardiovascular assessment.

SUGGESTED READINGS

Higgins CB. *Essentials of Cardiac Radiology and Imaging*. JB Lippincott; 1992.

Miller SW. *Cardiac Radiology: The Requisites*. Mosby-Year Book; 1996.

Skorton DJ, Shelbert HR, Wolf GL, et al. *Cardiac Imaging*. WB Saunders; 1996.

Steiner RM. Radiology of the heart and great vessels. In: Braunwald E, Zipes DP, Libby P, eds. *Heart Disease*. 16th ed. WB Saunders; 2001.

Chapter 32

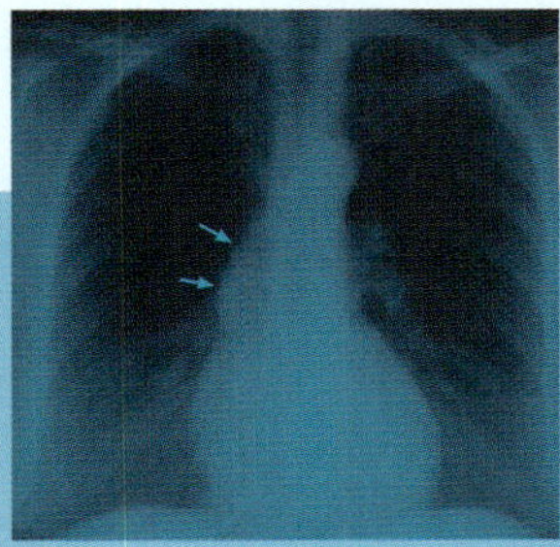

Karen G. Ordovas • Charles B. Higgins

Radiography of Congenital Heart Disease

INTRODUCTION

The radiographic diagnosis of congenital heart disease (CHD) can be seen as a confusing and difficult topic because of the myriad of congenital heart lesions that exist. Assessment of the plain radiograph can usually provide only a notion of the generic type of congenital heart lesion rather than a clear indication of specific lesions. An approach that is cognizant of the realistic insights possible from the plain radiograph must be pursued. Such an approach should be based on the observations on the radiograph that can be made with some degree of certitude and in which there is minimal ambiguity. Such an approach should also take advantage of the clinical information upon which one can rely. The presented classification system for radiographic diagnosis of CHD depends on a few clinical observations and a few findings on the radiograph that can be made with reasonable reliability.

CLINICAL-RADIOGRAPHIC CLASSIFICATION OF CONGENITAL HEART DISEASE

This classification depends on two pieces of clinical data: (1) whether patient is cyanotic or noncyanotic and (2) presents symptoms of congestive heart failure, such as dyspnea, tachypnea, tachycardia, and frequent respiratory infections. The salient radiographic findings are (1) increased or normal/decreased pulmonary arterial vascularity and (2) cardiomegaly or normal/nearly normal heart size.

This classification system permits most major lesions involving right-to-left or left-to-right shunts to be classified into four categories (Table 32.1). A fifth group consists of patients with primarily pulmonary venous congestion (Table 32.2). Therefore, when interpreting the chest x-ray, the physician should attempt to decide which class or category of congenital heart lesions exists. The decision on the specific lesion is usually based on the statistical frequency of a particular cardiac lesion within one or more groups. Based on the clinical and radiographic findings, there are five groups of congenital heart lesions. The groups and criteria used in this classification system are as follows:

Group I: left-to-right shunts

Noncyanotic: Sometimes symptoms of pulmonary congestion or congestive heart failure.

Radiographic signs of pulmonary arterial overcirculation (Fig. 32.1)

Group II: right-to-left shunts with little or no cardiomegaly

Cyanosis.

Decreased or normal pulmonary arterial vascularity and little or no cardiomegaly (Fig. 32.2)

Group III: right-to-left shunts with cardiomegaly

Cyanosis.

Radiographic evidence of normal or decreased pulmonary blood flow and cardiomegaly (Fig. 32.3)

Group IV: admixture lesions (ie, both right-to-left and left-to-right shunts)

Cyanosis.

Radiographic evidence of increased pulmonary arterial vascularity and usually cardiomegaly (Fig. 32.4)

Table 32.1 Classification of Shunt Lesions

Group I lesions: acyanotic; pulmonary arterial overcirculation
Atrial septal defect
Partial anomalous pulmonary venous connection
Atrioventricular septal defect (endocardial cushion defect)
Ventricular septal defect
Patent ductus arteriosus
Other aortic level shunts (eg, ruptured sinus of Valsalva aneurysm, aorticopulmonary window)
Group II lesions: cyanotic; decreased pulmonary vascularity, no cardiomegaly
Tetralogy of Fallot
Transposition with pulmonic stenosis and VSD
Double-outlet right ventricle with pulmonic stenosis and VSD
Double-outlet left ventricle with pulmonic stenosis and VSD
Single ventricle (univentricular atrioventricular connection) with pulmonic stenosis
Corrected transposition with pulmonic stenosis and VSD
Pulmonic atresia with intact ventricular septum, type I
Pulmonic stenosis with atrioventricular septal defect
Hypoplastic right ventricle syndrome
Some types of tricuspid atresia (large atrial septal defect and pulmonary stenosis or atresia)
Group III lesions: cyanotic; decreased pulmonary vascularity; cardiomegaly
Ebstein's anomaly
Pulmonary stenosis (critical) with atrial septal defect or patent foramen ovale
Some types of tricuspid atresia (restrictiveatrial septal defect)
Pulmonary atresia with intact ventricular septum, type II
Transient tricuspid regurgitation of the newborn
Group IV lesions: cyanotic; pulmonary arterial overcirculation
Transposition of great arteries
Truncus arteriosus
Total anomalous pulmonary venous connection
Tricuspid atresia
Single ventricle (univentricular atrioventricular connection)
Double-outlet right ventricle
Double-outlet left ventricle
Atrioventricular septal defect (complete form)
Hypoplastic left heart syndrome
Pulmonary arteriovenous fistulae

ASD, atrial septal defect; VSD, ventricular septal defect.

Table 32.2 Group V Lesions

Pulmonary venous hypertension (congestion)
Cardiomegaly disproportionate to pulmonary vascularity
Nonstructural heart disease in newborns
Asphyxia
Hypervolemia, hyperviscosity
Overhydration
Twin-twin transfusion
Maternal-fetal transfusion
Excess stripping of the cord
Paroxysmal atrial tachycardia
Heart block
Hypoglycemia
Hypocalcemia
Hydrops fetalis
Systemic hypertension
Structural heart disease in newborns
Hypoplastic left heart syndrome
Total anomalous pulmonary venous connection, type III
Coarctation of the aorta
Critical aortic stenosis
Endocardial fibroelastosis
Anomalous origin of the coronary artery from the pulmonary artery
Intrauterine myocarditis

It is frequently difficult to distinguish between normal and diminished pulmonary vascularity. This observation can be greatly simplified, however, when one remembers that normal pulmonary vascularity, as gleaned from the radiograph in a patient with cyanosis, can be equated with decreased pulmonary vascularity in the presented classification. Consequently, the major observation on the radiograph in terms of pulmonary vascularity in the cyanotic patient is to determine whether the pulmonary vascularity is increased. Normal or diminished pulmonary vascularity in a patient with cyanosis indicates that the lesion produces a right-to-left

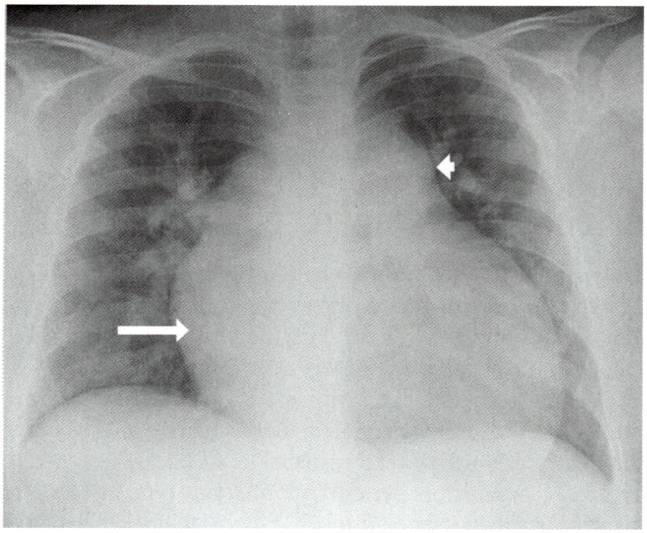

Figure 32.1. Patent ductus arteriosus. Note pulmonary arterial overcirculation and cardiomegaly. Pulmonary arterial overcirculation is indicated by prominent hilar vessels. There is a left atrial double density (*arrow*) and enlarged aortic arch (*arrowhead*).

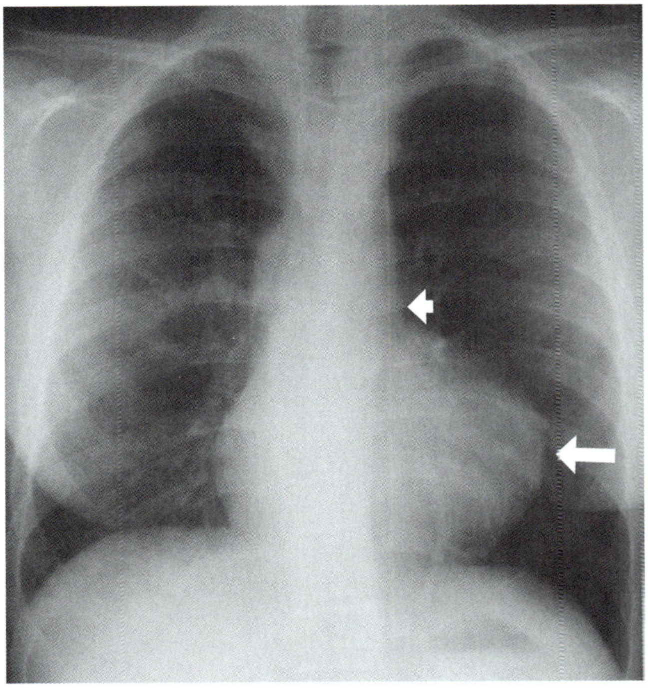

Figure 32.2. Tetralogy of Fallot. Note decreased pulmonary vascularity without cardiomegaly. The main pulmonary arterial segment is concave (*arrowhead*), and the hilar vessels are small. The apex is situated high above the diaphragm (*arrow*).

shunt. Increased pulmonary vascularity in a cyanotic patient indicates that there is an admixture lesion; the cyanosis is indicative of right-to-left shunting, whereas the increased pulmonary vascularity is a sign of left-to-right shunting.

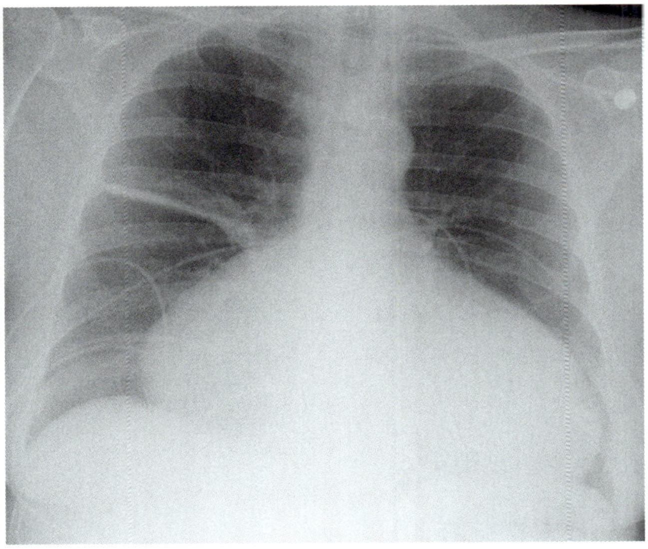

Figure 32.3. Ebstein's anomaly. Note decreased pulmonary vascularity with cardiomegaly. Hilar vessels are small, and segmental pulmonary arteries are hardly visible, especially in the upper lobes. Vector of enlargement of the apex of the heart is directly lateral, indicating right ventricular enlargement.

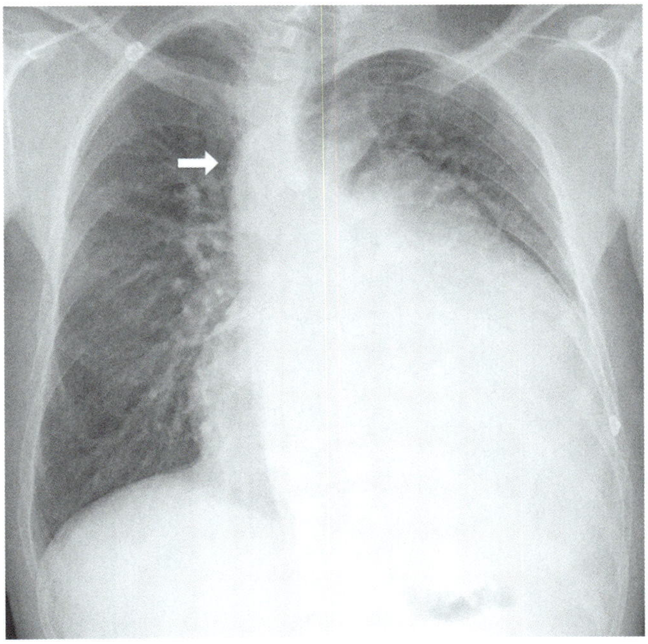

Figure 32.4. Truncus arteriosus, type I. Note pulmonary arterial overcirculation in the presence of cyanosis and cardiomegaly. There is an enlarged aorta with right arch (*arrow*).

GROUPS OF CONGENITAL HEART LESIONS

Group I – Left-to-Right Shunt

Group I contains all of the left-to-right shunts; consequently, this is the group into which most patients with congenital heart disease are classified. The criteria that place a patient within this category are for the most part dependent on the clinical recognition of the absence of cyanosis with the subsequent demonstration on the chest radiograph of increased pulmonary arterial vascularity (see Figs. 32.1 and 32.5-32.8). The degree of cardiomegaly is usually in proportion to the increase in pulmonary vascularity. The left-to-right shunts are volume overload lesions. Consequently, there is frequent cardiomegaly, and this cardiomegaly should in general be in proportion to the prominence of the pulmonary vascularity.

Two imaging signposts can be used when navigating the diagnostic pathway to help distinguish among the various types of left-to-right shunts (see Fig. 32.7). The first of these is the left atrium. Left atrial enlargement indicates that the predominant lesion is not an atrial-level shunt but rather a VSD or a patent ductus arteriosus (PDA). The atrial septal defect and partial anomalous pulmonary venous connection lack both of these signposts (see Fig. 32.5). The next signpost is the aortic arch. A prominent aortic arch distinguishes between the PDA and the VSD. The aortic arch usually has a normal dimension or is small in VSD (see Fig. 32.6), whereas PDA is associated with a prominent aortic arch (see Fig. 32.1). In infants, prominence of the aortic arch may be difficult to recognize, so this signpost may not always be useful. Consequently, since a VSD is a more frequent lesion, this should be the diagnosis

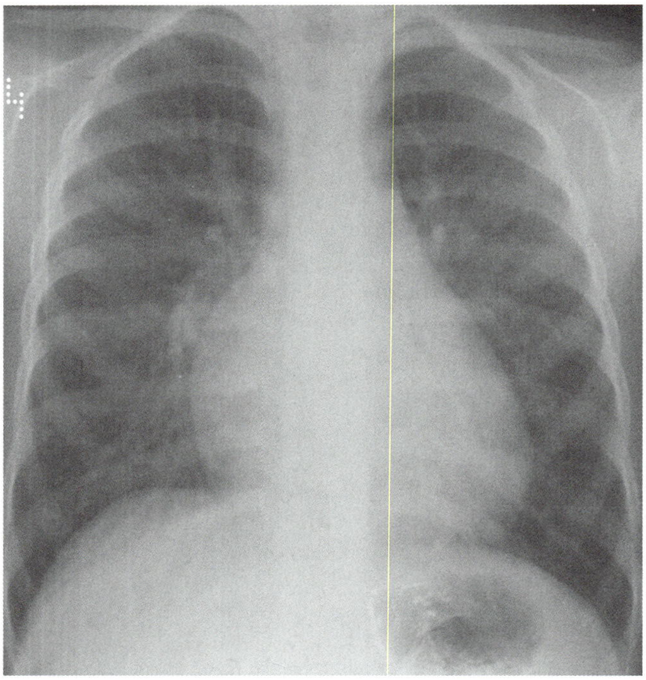

Figure 32.5. Atrial septal defect. Pulmonary arterial overcirculation is shown by large hilar and segmental pulmonary arteries. The absence of left atrial enlargement, indicated by no double density in the heart-heart border, is characteristic for an atrial-level shunt.

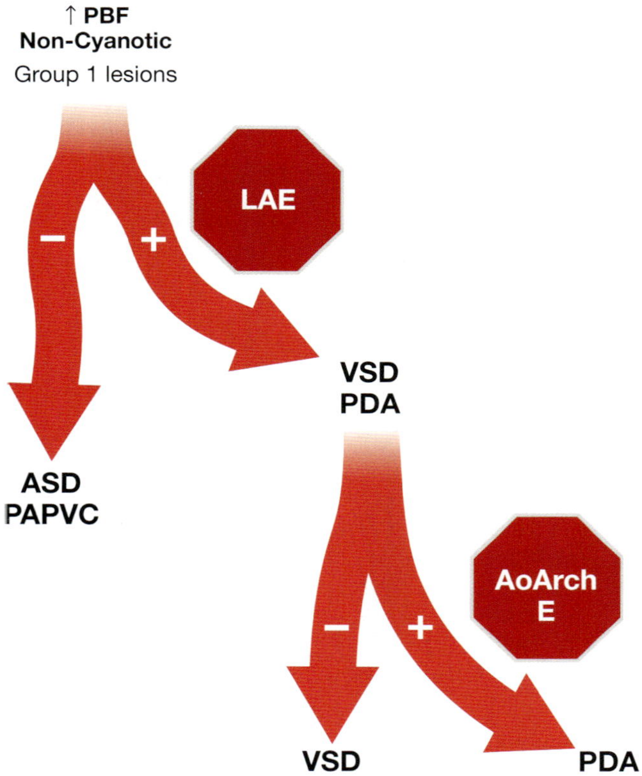

Figure 32.7. Signposts on the diagnostic pathway of left-to-right shunts.

when there is left atrial enlargement and no clearly discernible enlargement of the aortic arch. An exception to this rule is in the premature infant, where a PDA is statistically by far the most frequent congenital heart lesion. The radiograph of the premature infant with PDA usually does not disclose signs of left atrial and aortic arch enlargement.

The plain radiograph may be useful in determining the severity and progression of left-to-right shunts. The severe volume overload with large left-to-right shunts causes pulmonary venous congestion or pulmonary edema in addition to pulmonary arterial overcirculation (see Fig. 32.8). In individuals with large left-to-right shunts, there should also be substantial cardiomegaly.

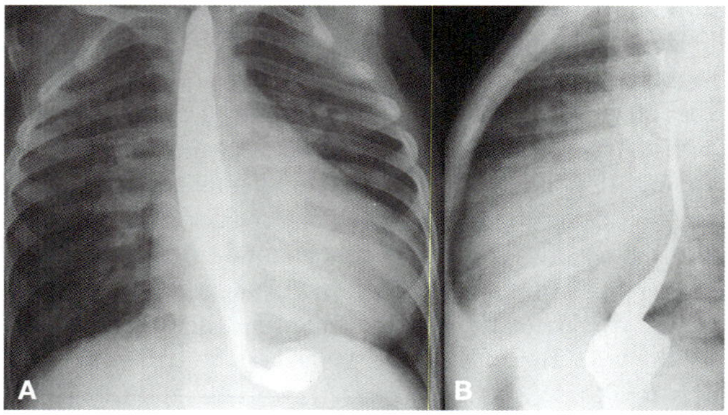

Figure 32.6. Ventricular septal defect. Frontal **(A)** and lateral **(B)** views. Pulmonary arterial overcirculation is evidenced by shunt vessels and prominent hilar vessels. Heart size is increased in proportion to overcirculation. Left atrial enlargement is evidenced by double density (*arrow*) in the frontal view and posterior displacement of the left bronchi (*arrowhead*) in the lateral view.

Group II – Pulmonary Blood Flow Obstruction

A lesion is included in group II when there is cyanosis and the plain radiograph demonstrates diminished or normal

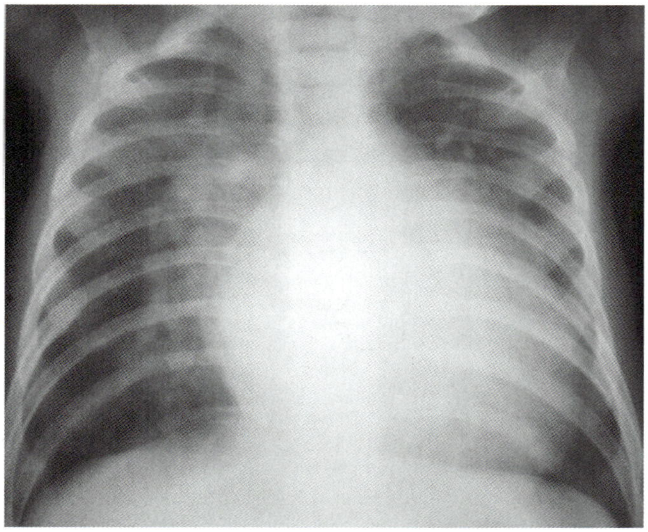

Figure 32.8. Ventricular septal defects. Large-volume left-to-right shunt causing pulmonary edema, severe pulmonary arterial overcirculation, and cardiomegaly. Indistinct hilar and segmental arteries on the right side are caused by interstitial edema.

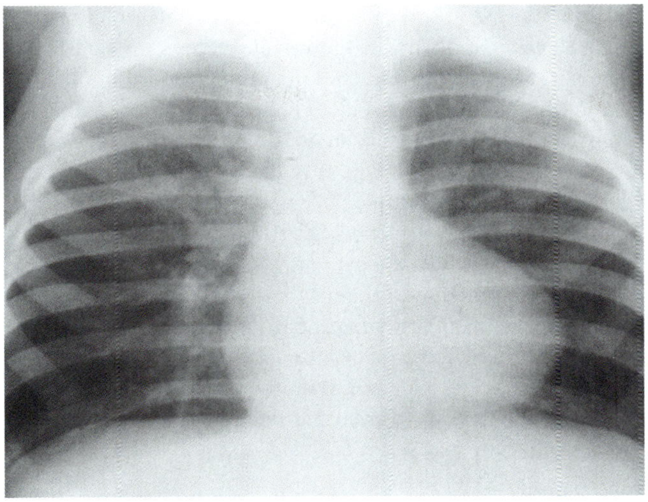

Figure 32.9. Tetralogy of Fallot. Note pulmonary oligemia with more diminished vascularity on the left, especially the left upper lobe. Normal heart size and concave pulmonary artery segment are characteristic features in the infant.

pulmonary vascularity and the absence of substantial cardiomegaly (see Figs. 32.2, 32.9, 32.10). The pathophysiology that produces this constellation of findings involves a nonrestrictive intracardiac shunt and a severe obstruction to pulmonary blood flow. The nonrestrictive intracardiac shunt permits equalization of the pressures between two chambers, and this prevents substantial enlargement of the right ventricle. Consequently, there is usually little or no cardiomegaly.

Statistically, the most frequent lesion in group II is tetralogy of Fallot. The remaining diagnostic considerations are, for the most part, variants of tetralogy of Fallot. Some examples of these lesions are transposition of great arteries (TGA) with severe pulmonary stenosis and unrestrictive VSD and double-outlet right ventricle with severe pulmonic stenosis and an unrestrictive VSD. Table 32.1 provides a reasonably complete list of the differential diagnostic considerations in group II. However, the plain radiograph infrequently permits a specific diagnosis to be chosen from among this myriad of lesions.

An example of the importance of the size of the intracardiac defect is in patients with tricuspid atresia. The patient with tricuspid atresia with a large atrial septal defect demonstrates little or no cardiomegaly (Fig. 32.11). On the other hand, the patient with tricuspid atresia with a restrictive atrial septal defect experiences substantial right atrial enlargement, which results in cardiomegaly. Consequently, the former patient would be classified in group II, and the latter patient in group III. Please note that tricuspid atresia can be classified in group IV when there is an associated increase in pulmonary blood flow, which is caused by either a large left-to-right shunt at the ventricular septal level or the concurrence of transposition of the great vessels, which occurs in approximately 30% of these patients.

Group III – Tricuspid Lesions

Group III lesions differ from group II lesions by the radiographic observation of cardiomegaly (see Figs. 32.3 and 32.12-32.14). These patients have cyanosis, normal or decreased pulmonary vascularity and a substantial degree of cardiomegaly. The cardiac chamber that is frequently

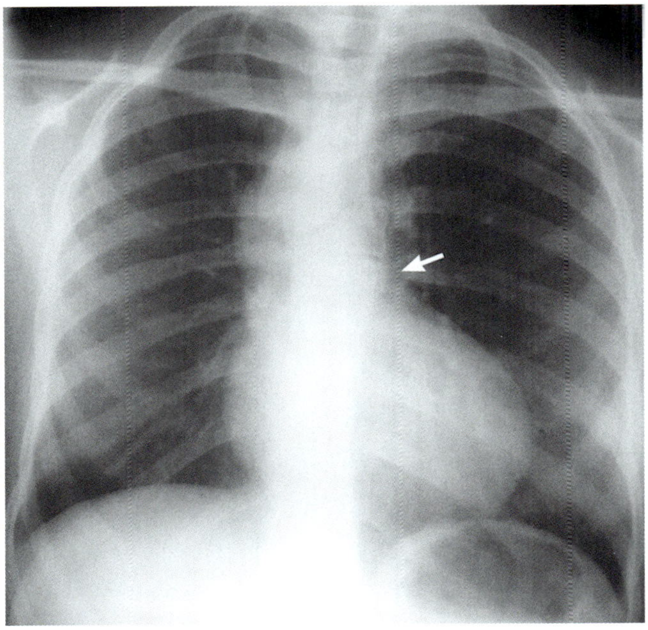

Figure 32.10. Pulmonary atresia with ventricular septal defect (severe tetralogy of Fallot). Pulmonary oligemia, absent main pulmonary artery segment (*arrow*), and normal heart size are characteristic features. There is a right aortic arch.

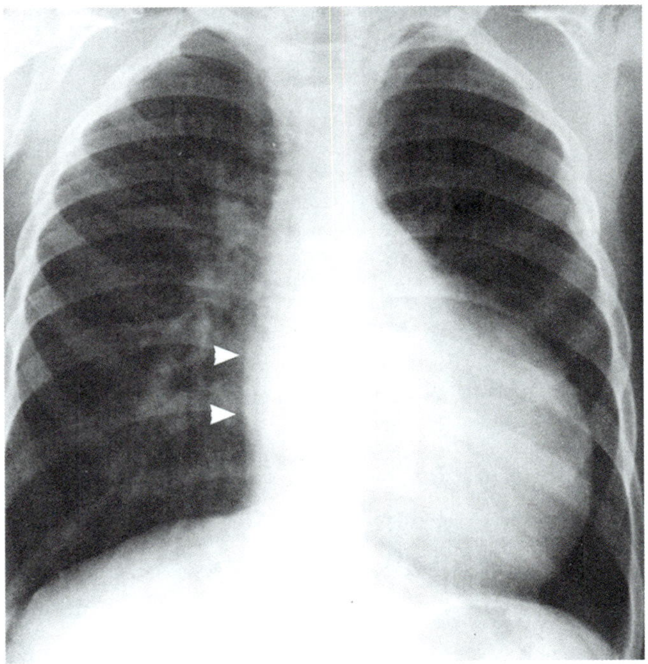

Figure 32.11. Tricuspid atresia with large (nonrestrictive) atrial septal defect. There is decreased pulmonary vascularity and only mild cardiomegaly. Note the flattened right atrial border (*arrowheads*), which is characteristic for this lesion when there is a large nonrestrictive atrial septal defect.

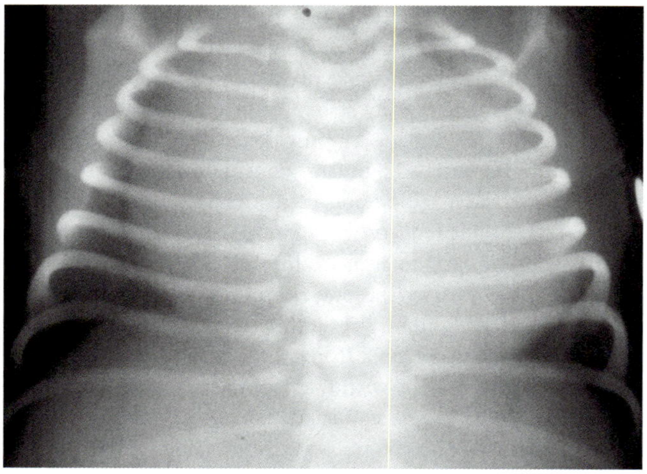

Figure 32.12. Pulmonary atresia with intact ventricular septum, type II. Substantial tricuspid regurgitation in association with this anomaly (type II) causes right-sided chamber enlargement, especially right atrial enlargement.

enlarged in this lesion is the right atrium. Many of the patients in this category have substantial tricuspid regurgitation, which is a major pathogenetic mechanism of the right atrial enlargement and cardiomegaly. The "wall-to-wall" heart (extension from the right to the left chest wall) should prompt the diagnostic consideration of a lesion causing tricuspid regurgitation.

In the older child and adult with this constellation of findings, the most likely diagnosis is Ebstein's anomaly (see Fig. 32.13).

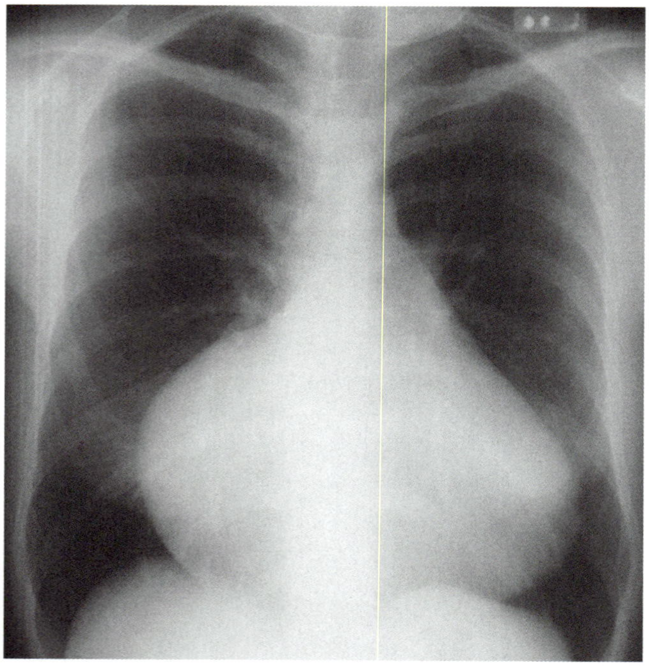

Figure 32.13. Ebstein's anomaly in an adult. Note decreased pulmonary vascularity and marked cardiomegaly. The prominent bulging and elongation of the right heart border are indicative of severe right atrial enlargement.

Uhl's anomaly is a rare cause of a cardiac configuration similar to Ebstein's anomaly. In the infant, there is no statistically dominant diagnostic consideration in this category, but the following lesions must be considered in the differential diagnosis: severe ("critical") pulmonary stenosis with an atrial septal defect or patent foramen ovale, type II pulmonary atresia with intact ventricular septum, tricuspid atresia with a restrictive atrial septal defect, and Ebstein's anomaly. Another unusual diagnosis in this category, which appears only in the neonatal period, is tricuspid regurgitation of the newborn (see Fig. 32.14). In this entity, there is frequently substantial cardiomegaly, diminished pulmonary blood flow, and cyanosis within the first few days of life. However, with reduction in pulmonary vascular resistance over time, the amount of tricuspid regurgitation decreases and the cardiomegaly may resolve.

Group IV – Admixture Lesion

A lesion is included in this group when the radiograph displays pulmonary arterial overcirculation in the presence of cyanosis. The heart size is usually increased, but cardiomegaly is not a necessary feature for patients to be included in group IV. The observation of increased pulmonary vascularity in a patient with cyanosis is an incongruous finding and should alert the observer to the presence of an admixture lesion rather than a strictly left-to-right shunt. An aid to remembering the major diagnoses in this category is the letter T. The most common diagnosis in this category is TGA, which is the most frequent cyanotic congenital heart lesion at birth (Fig. 32.15). The other diagnostic considerations are truncus arteriosus (Fig. 32.4), total anomalous pulmonary venous connection (Fig. 32.16), tricuspid atresia, and single ("tingle") ventricle. Double-outlet right

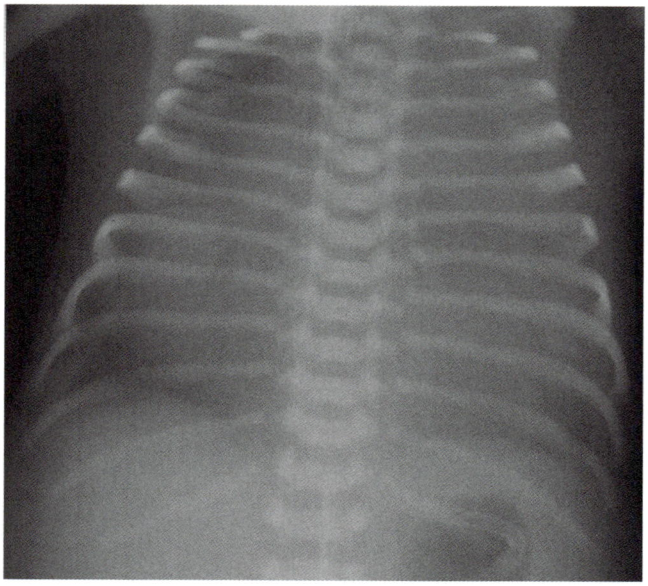

Figure 32.14. Tricuspid regurgitation of the newborn. Pulmonary vascularity is decreased, and marked cardiomegaly is present due to right-sided chamber enlargement. Extreme cardiomegaly producing the "wall-to-wall" heart is usually due to severe tricuspid regurgitation.

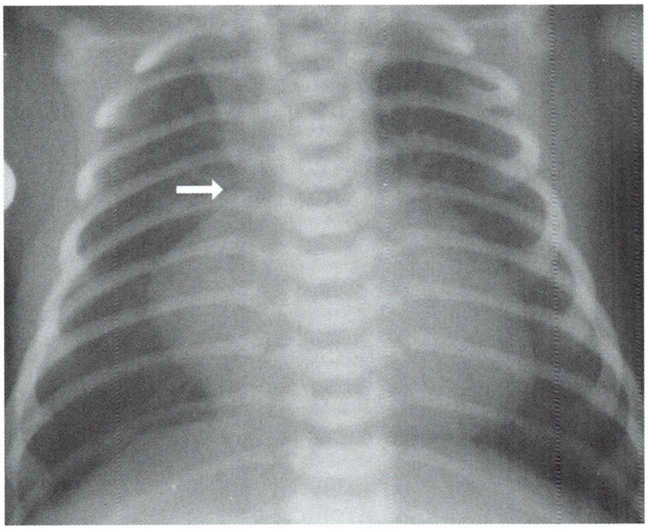

Figure 32.15. Transposition of the great arteries. Pulmonary arterial overcirculation and an ovoid heart with a narrow base (vascular pedicle) of the heart (*arrow*) are characteristic features

ventricle and double-outlet left ventricle are also considered in this category, but these can be brought to mind when one thinks of TGA since these lesions are essentially hybrids of TGA.

GROUP V - PULMONARY VENOUS CONGESTION

A fifth group of congenital lesions are those that produce predominantly pulmonary venous congestion and alter the pulmonary venous vascularity rather than the pulmonary arterial vascularity. Patients with these lesions may have shunts, but inclusion in group V requires that the predominant pathophysiologic event is pulmonary venous congestion (Figs. 32.17-32.19; see Table 32.2).

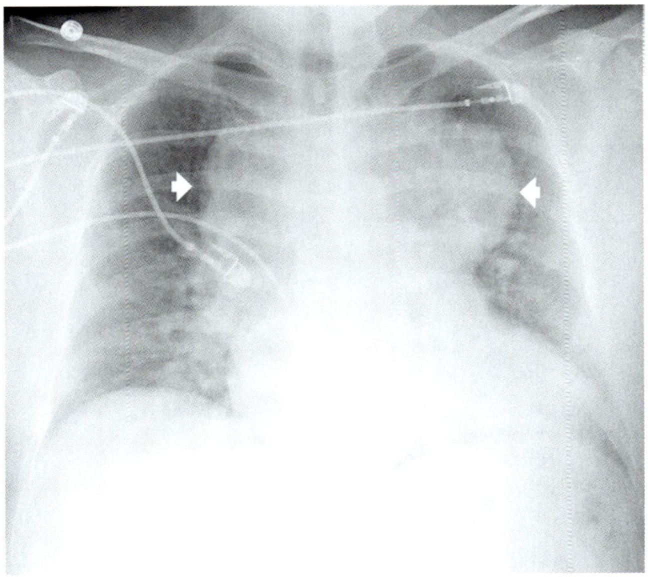

Figure 32.16. Total anomalous pulmonary venous connection, supracardiac type (type I). Note pulmonary arterial overcirculation and cardiomegaly. Enlargement of supracardiac region (*arrowheads*) is caused by an enlarged left-sided vertical vein and a dilated right superior vena cava; it is characteristic of this anomaly.

The clinical features of the group V lesions are a lack of cyanosis and frequently severe symptoms of heart failure. These usually consist of dyspnea, tachypnea, and tachycardia. The salient radiographic findings are indistinctness of the pulmonary vascularity, especially in the perihilar area, or interstitial pulmonary edema (see Figs. 32.17 and 32.19). Another observation that places a lesion into this group is disproportionately prominent cardiomegaly in comparison to the prominence of pulmonary vascularity (see Figs. 32.17 and 32.18).

The lesions included in this category are listed in Table 32.2. The statistical frequencies of the lesions in this category are also important in deciding on the diagnosis. Diagnosis in this category includes conditions that produce reversible stresses upon the heart of the newborn as well as structural cardiac lesions. Lesions in this category tend to present at certain times after birth; for instance, the nonstructural causes of pulmonary venous congestion or edema usually present within the first day or two of life. Abnormalities that may be encountered within the first day of life include severe anemia (hydrops fetalis), asphyxia, hypocalcemia, hypoglycemia, abnormalities of heart rate and rhythm, hypervolemia, and intrauterine myocarditis. Pulmonary venous congestion with substantial cardiomegaly presenting in the first day or so of life is a feature of hypoplastic left heart (Fig. 32.22). Pulmonary venous congestion with an essentially normal heart size presenting within the first day or so of life is the feature of total anomalous pulmonary venous connection, infradiaphragmatic type, with obstruction (see Fig. 32.20). In the infant presenting with these features between 1 and 3 weeks of age, statistically, the most frequent diagnosis is

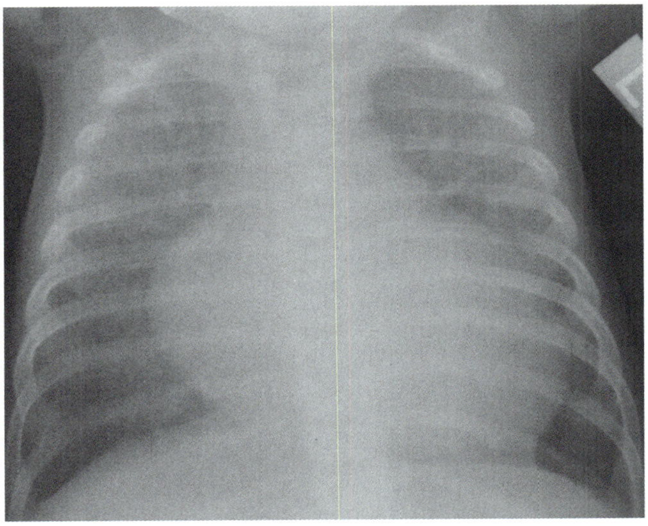

Figure 32.17. Endocardial fibroelastosis. Pulmonary edema and cardiomegaly are characteristic features of group V lesions.

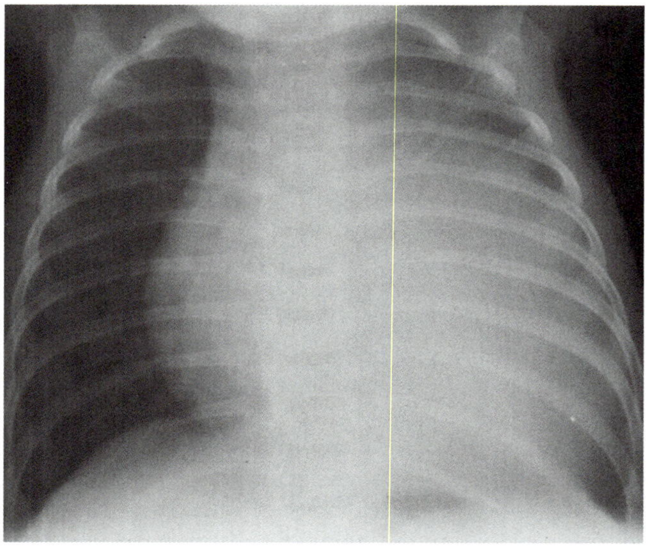

Figure 32.18. (previous Figure 31.20) Anomalous origin of the left coronary artery from the pulmonary artery. Cardiomegaly is disproportionate to pulmonary vascularity in a noncyanotic infant. Left atrial enlargement (right retrocardiac double density) is caused by mitral regurgitation from papillary muscle infarction.

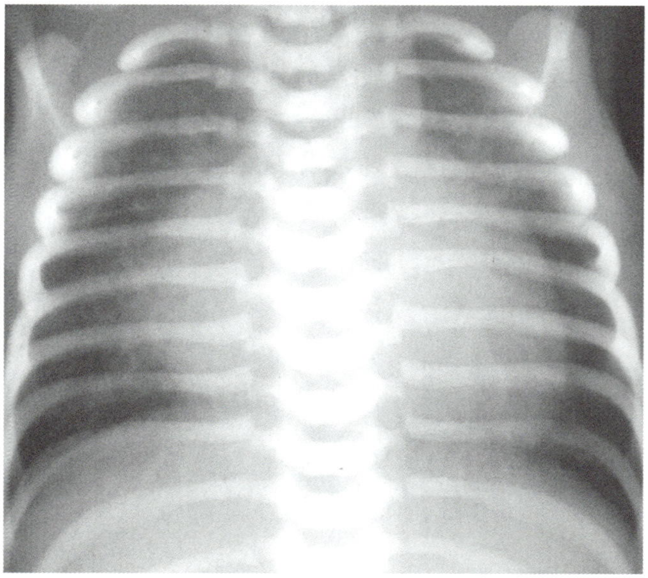

Figure 32.20. Hypoplastic left heart. Note pulmonary venous congestion and edema and cardiomegaly. Prominent right atrium and ventricle and posterior aortic arch are characteristic features of this lesion.

coarctation of the aorta (Fig. 32.21). Rib notching is not evident in infants with coarctation.

SPECIFIC LESIONS: SALIENT RADIOGRAPHIC FEATURES

Acyanotic

Atrial Septal Defect and Partial Anomalous Pulmonary Venous Connection

There are four types of atrial septal defects: secundum (most frequent), primum, sinus venosus (superior and inferior vena caval locations), and coronary sinus (least frequent). The primum type is usually part of an atrioventricular septal defect (AVSD), which was formerly called endocardial cushion defect. In addition, a patent foramen ovale exists in many children with congenital heart disease, and the foramen may be stretched in the setting of elevated right-sided pressures. The defects are named according to their position in the atrial septum: ostium secundum in the region of the fossa ovalis, which is approximately the middle of the septum; primum in the lower part of the septum and bordering on the atrioventricular valves; and sinus venosus in either the upper part of the septum and bordering on the ostium of the superior vena cava or the lower septum and bordering on the ostium of the inferior vena cava (see Fig. 38.3). A rare type of defect occurs

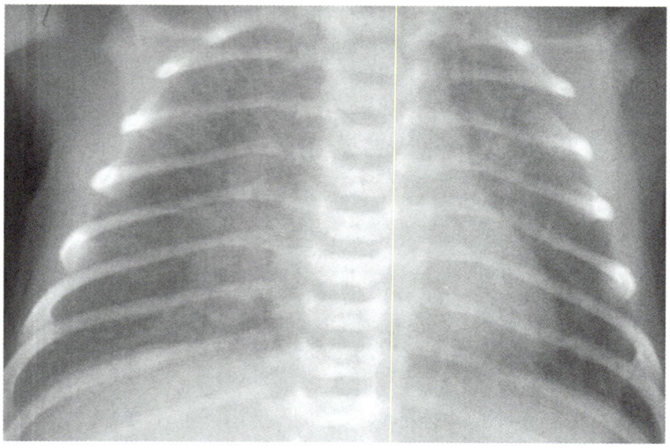

Figure 32.19. Total anomalous pulmonary venous connection, type III. Radiograph shows pulmonary edema and normal heart size.

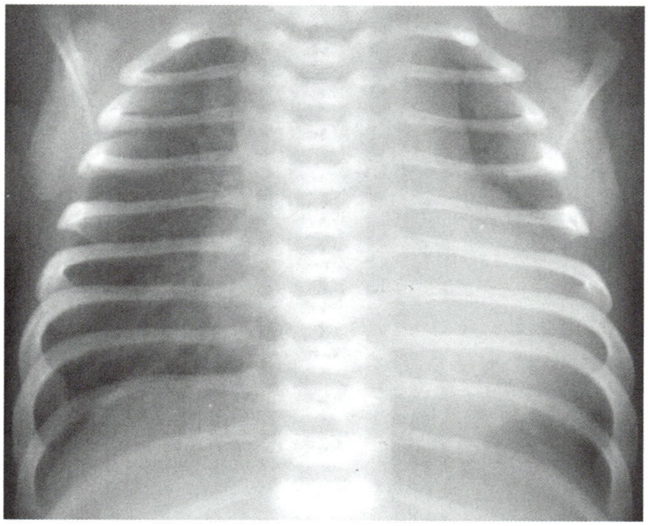

Figure 32.21. Severe coarctation of the aorta in a newborn. There is marked cardiomegaly with pulmonary edema.

with absence of the wall separating the coronary sinus from the left atrium, so that the associated left superior vena cava enters into the left atrium. The coexistence of large primum and secundum defects constitutes a common atrium.

The isolated atrial septal defect and partial anomalous pulmonary venous connection are left-to-right shunts. A stretched foramen ovale or atrial septal defect may permit predominant right-to-left shunting in complex lesions with severe right-sided obstruction (ie, tricuspid atresia). The volume of shunting across an interatrial communication usually depends on the size of the defect and the relative distensibility of the two ventricles. The wall of the right ventricle is more distensible than the left ventricle during diastole, so blood preferentially flows toward the right ventricle at this time. However, obstruction of flow into or out of the right ventricle can reverse this pattern. A large atrial septal defect is defined as one that results in equalization of pressure between the atria (Tables 32.3-32.6; Figs. 32.5 and 32.22).

Atrioventricular Septal Defect (Endocardial Cushion Defect)

The embryonic endocardial cushions contribute to the development of the medial portions of the mitral and tricuspid valves, the primum atrial septum, and the inlet portion of the ventricular septum. Defects in this region have been called endocardial cushion defects but more recently have received the name **atrioventricular septal defects** (AVSDs). The fundamental lesion is a common atrioventricular valve and variable deficiency of the primum atrial septum and the inlet ventricular septum. The atrioventricular valve in this anomaly has five leaflets, with two of the leaflets spanning the ventricular septum and the opening to both ventricles. The spanning leaflets are the anterior and posterior bridging leaflets. If there is a tongue of tissue connecting the anterior and posterior bridging leaflets and this tongue is attached to the crest of the inlet ventricular septum, then incomplete forms of the defect result. The anomaly exists in a complete form with a single atrioventricular valve, primum atrial septal defect, and inlet VSD with no connecting tissue exists between the bridging leaflets.

The most common incomplete lesion is a primum atrial septal defect and a "cleft" in the mitral valve, causing varying degrees of mitral regurgitation. Because the primum atrial septal defect is situated immediately above the cleft, mitral regurgitation may traverse the defect and enter the right atrium. Consequently, the left atrium may not be enlarged even in patients with substantial mitral regurgitation (Table 32.7; Figs. 32.23 and 32.24).

Ventricular Septal Defect

VSDs have been characterized by their location in the septum: perimembranous, outlet, inlet, and trabecular (see Fig. 38.12). Defects in the perimembranous and outlet regions have also been described in relation to the crista supraventricularis of the right ventricle as infracristal (more frequent) and supracristal (doubly committed) types. While any perimembranous or outlet VSD can cause aortic regurgitation, the supracristal type frequently causes prolapse of the right sinus of Valsalva and aortic regurgitation. Prolapsed sinus

Table 32.3 Salient Radiographic Features of Atrial Septal Defect

Pulmonary arterial overcirculation: Generally a 2:1 shunt must exist before pulmonary plethora is universally present. About 50%-60% of patients with less than 2:1 shunt have only mild or no evident pulmonary plethora. Pulmonary edema rarely occurs in the simple atrial septal defect
Enlargement of the right atrium
Enlargement of the right ventricle
Enlargement of the main and hilar pulmonary arterial segments: In older subjects, the right pulmonary artery is sometimes especially prominent
Small ascending aorta and aortic arch
Small superior vena caval shadow

Table 32.4 Salient Radiographic Features of Atrial Septal Defect With Pulmonary Arterial Hypertension

Enlarged main and central pulmonary arteries
Disparity in enlargement of the central and lobar arteries to peripheral arteries
Calcification of main or central pulmonary arteries
Onset of severe pulmonary arterial hypertension may be associated with reduction in degree of cardiomegaly or normal heart size.
Cardiomegaly may be persistent because of tricuspid insufficiency caused by severe pulmonary hypertension.

Table 32.5 Salient Radiographic Features of Partial Anomalous Pulmonary Venous Coarctation

Pulmonary arterial overcirculation: This may be apparent or more severe only in the lung with anomalous drainage
Enlargement of the right atrium
Enlargement of the right ventricle
Enlargement of the main and hilar pulmonary arterial segments
Small ascending aorta and aortic arch
Enlargement of the superior vena cava, azygos vein, coronary sinus, or other systemic veins, depending on the site of connection
Prominent left superior vena cava
Abnormal course of pulmonary veins through the lung or in relation to mediastinal margins

Table 32.6 Salient Radiographic Features of Scimitar Syndrome

Enlarged curved vascular structure coursing medially toward the right diaphragm: This structure enlarges in diameter as it approaches the diaphragm
Dextroposition of the heart
Hypoplasia of the right lung

tissue may reduce the size or obliterate the septal defect. The outlet defect may be caused by malposition of the outlet septum, resulting in a small right ventricular outflow region and an aorta overriding the septal defect (tetralogy of Fallot). VSDs are not uncommonly multiple. Multiple defects in the trabecular septum may produce a "Swiss cheese septum."

A small VSD is one in which the diameter or cross-sectional area is less than that of the aortic annulus. A large or nonrestrictive defect has a diameter or cross-sectional area exceeding the aortic annulus. A nonrestrictive defect permits the equalization of pressures in the two ventricles. Isolated VSD causes a left-to-right shunt in which the volume is determined by the cross-sectional area of the defect and pulmonary vascular resistance. With large defects, shunting is not restricted by the defect but is controlled only by pulmonary vascular resistance. With low pulmonary vascular resistance, the volume of the shunt is large, causing severe pulmonary overcirculation and eventually pulmonary edema and elevated left ventricular end-diastole pressure. With higher resistance, the flow is less severe and there is pulmonary arterial hypertension. Increased pulmonary vascular resistance and pulmonary arterial hypertension may be due to pulmonary arteriolar constriction (reversible) or arteriolopathy (irreversible).

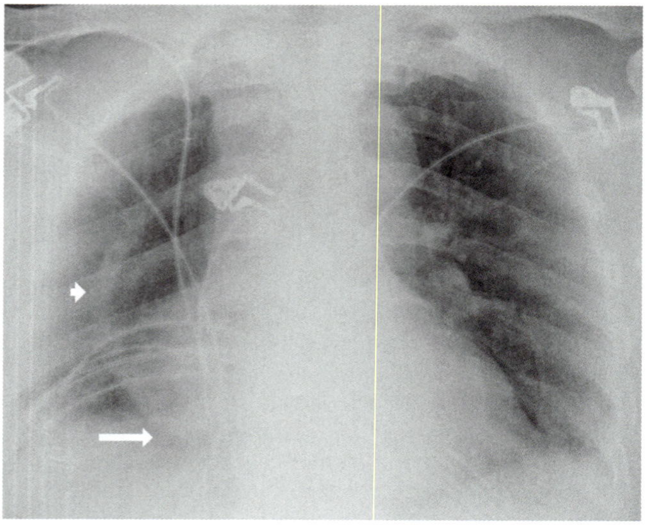

Figure 32.22. Scimitar syndrome. Radiograph showing a scimitar vein (*arrowhead*) connecting to the IVC near the right diaphragm (*arrow*), and a small right lung.

Table 32.7 Salient Radiographic Features of Atrioventricular Septal Defect

Skeletal features of trisomy 21, such as 11 ribs, double manubrial ossification center, and tall vertebral bodies
Pulmonary arterial overcirculation: This is severe in the complete forms and may be associated with pulmonary edema. Concurrent pneumonia is frequent in the complete form, especially in the child with mongolism
Enlargement of the right atrium: The superior margin of the right atrium is frequently prominent
Enlargement of the right ventricle
Enlargement of the main and central pulmonary arterial segments
Left atrial enlargement may be present but is generally not severe and may be absent despite mitral regurgitation
Small thoracic aorta
A cleft mitral valve without a primum defect (rare) produces the radiographic configuration of mitral regurgitation

Most isolated VSDs close spontaneously. The process of closure is frequently marked by a ventricular septal aneurysm. The aneurysm usually consists of portions of the septal leaflet of the tricuspid valve adherent to the rim of the defect; a hole may develop in the adhesed leaflet. Although the supracristal defect may be obstructed by the prolapsed sinus of Valsalva, it does not actually close. The inlet VSD (part of the AVSD) rarely closes spontaneously.

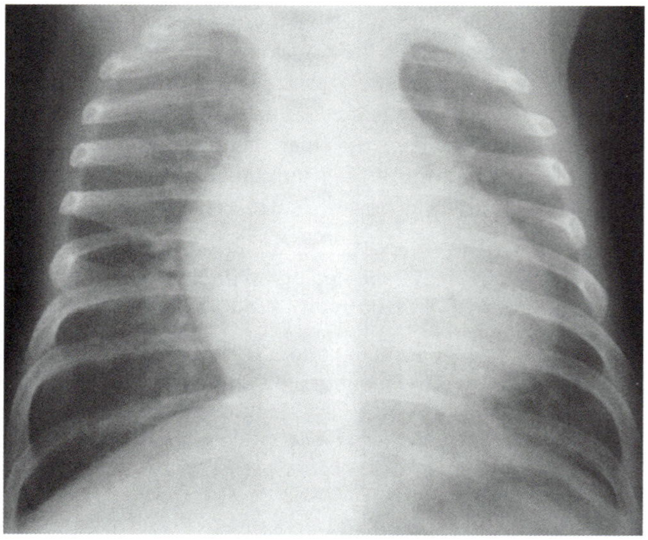

Figure 32.23. Atrioventricular septal defect/primum atrial septal defect. Radiography shows pulmonary arterial overcirculation and cardiomegaly due to right atrial and ventricular enlargement. The vector of ventricular enlargement is laterally and superiorly, causing the apex to be located high above the diaphragm. Prominent bulging of the upper right atrial border is a feature of primum atrial septal defects.

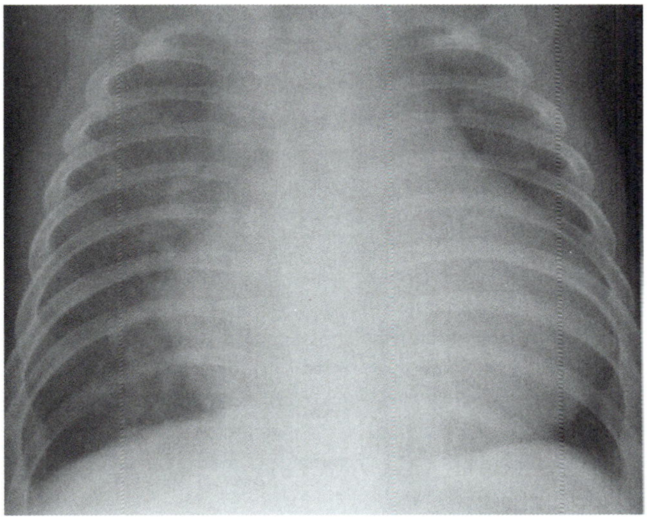

Figure 32.24. Atrioventricular septal defect (atrioventricular canal). Pulmonary arterial overcirculation and cardiomegaly due to right atrial and ventricular enlargement are present. There is elongation of the right atrial border, indicating substantial right atrial enlargement.

In the early postpartum period, pulmonary vascular resistance has not declined completely to adult levels, and the elevated resistance limits the left-to-right shunting through large defects. Pulmonary arteriolar resistance tends to reach a nadir 4 to 6 weeks postnatally and pulmonary overcirculation peaks. Because of the process of gradual closure and a relative decrease in the defect due to cardiac growth, the defect is physiologically maximal during the first year of life. Since VSD is a volume overload lesion and the volume overload is directly related to the excess pulmonary blood flow, cardiac enlargement is proportional to the degree of overcirculation (Table 32.8; see Figs. 32.6 and 32.9).

Table 32.8 Salient Radiographic Features of Hemodynamically Significant Ventricular Septal Defect

Pulmonary arterial overcirculation: With large shunts, pulmonary edema is frequent during infancy
Enlargement of the left atrium: This may not be easy to identify during infancy
Enlargement of either or both ventricles
Enlargement of the main and central pulmonary arterial segments
Disproportionate enlargement of central pulmonary arteries compared with peripheral vasculature suggests the Eisenmenger's complex but can also be observed with very large shunts. Pulmonary arterial calcification can occur in Eisenmenger's complex
Small thoracic aorta: Right aortic arch is alleged to occur in about 2% of ventricular septal defects

Patent Ductus Arteriosus

The ductus arteriosus connects the proximal descending aorta to the proximal left pulmonary artery just beyond the pulmonary arterial bifurcation. With mirror-image right aortic arch, the ductus usually connects the distal left innominate artery to the left pulmonary artery. With non–mirror-image right arch (retroesophageal left subclavian artery), the ductus connects the proximal right descending aorta to the proximal left pulmonary artery and causes a vascular ring.

PDA closes within the first day of life in full-term neonates, but persistent PDA is frequent in the premature infant. Significant left-to-right shunting in a premature infant during the early neonatal period is nearly always due to PDA. The shunt is predominantly left to right and causes pulmonary overcirculation and, if severe, pulmonary edema. However, right-to-left shunting across a PDA may be encountered in neonates if the pulmonary vascular resistance fails to decline from fetal levels (persistent fetal circulation).

PDA occurs as an isolated anomaly but also frequently in association with other simple and complex anomalies. There is a propensity for the triplex of PDA, coarctation of the aorta, and VSD to occur. PDA is also frequently present in cyanotic lesions with severe obstruction to pulmonary blood flow, such as pulmonary atresia. The PDA is life-sustaining in these instances but cannot be relied upon to maintain pulmonary blood flow because it may severely constrict or obliterate over time.

Table 32.9 Salient Radiographic Features of Hemodynamically Significant PDA

Pulmonary arterial overcirculation
Enlargement of the left atrium
Enlargement of the left ventricle
Enlargement of the aortic arch: While this may not be evident with infants, it is an invariable feature in the older child and adult. It may also be possible to identify prominence of the ascending aorta and lateral displacement of the descending aorta
Enlargement of the main and central pulmonary arterial segments: This tends to be less prominent than in atrial septal defect
Abnormal contour of the posterior aortic arch and proximal descending aorta: In many normal subjects, there is a localized dilatation of the aorta at the site of attachment of the ligamentum arteriosus, the aortic spindle (also called infundibulum). This aortic spindle is enlarged in patients with patent ductus arteriosus. The combined shadows of the posterior arch and aortic spindle cause apparent elongation, prominence, or atypical contour of the aortic knob. The aorticopulmonary window may be obliterated or convex due to the PDA
Calcification in the aorticopulmonary window due to calcification of the walls of the ductus in older individuals

The large-caliber PDA may conduct a large left-to-right shunt because a gradient exists between the aorta and pulmonary artery throughout the cardiac cycle. Flow through the PDA is controlled by the caliber of the ductus and pulmonary vascular resistance. The volume overload (excess pulmonary blood flow) causes enlargement of the left atrium and left ventricle. The left-to-right shunt continually recirculates to the lungs, left atrium, left ventricle, ascending aorta, and aortic arch (Fig. 31.1). The volume experienced by the left-sided chamber causes an elevated left ventricular diastolic pressure. With large shunts, the excess blood flow and elevated left ventricular diastolic pressure eventuate in pulmonary edema. The excess flow and elevated pulmonary venous pressure may cause considerable pulmonary arterial hypertension, which induces right ventricular hypertrophy. The eventual outcome of the process is pulmonary arteriolopathy and Eisenmenger's syndrome (Tables 32.9 and 32.10; Fig. 32.25).

Aorticopulmonary Window

This rare anomaly is a large connection between the ascending aorta and the main pulmonary artery. Both semilunar valves are present, and this feature distinguishes the lesion from truncus arteriosus. This lesion usually causes a large left-to-right shunt and pulmonary edema in early infancy.

The physiology of this lesion is similar to PDA but is invariably severe, so nearly all cases present during early infancy. This lesion is almost never encountered in childhood or adult life. If an untreated patient is rarely encountered beyond infancy, irreversible pulmonary arterial hypertension is present.

The radiographic features should resemble PDA if the patient survives beyond infancy. The usual radiographic appearance is severe pulmonary overcirculation and pulmonary edema. The ascending aorta and main pulmonary arterial segment are more prominent than for PDA in the infant.

Table 32.10 Salient Radiographic Features of Patent Ductus Arteriosus With Pulmonary Arterial Hypertension

- Enlarged main and central pulmonary arteries
- Disparity in enlargement of the central and lobar arteries compared with peripheral arteries
- Calcification of main or central pulmonary arteries
- Calcification of the ductus (tracklike calcification in the aorticopulmonary window)
- Onset of pulmonary arterial hypertension is usually accompanied by a decrease in cardiomegaly or normal heart size
- Enlargement of the aortic arch and proximal descending aorta

Congenital Sinus of Valsalva Aneurysm and Fistula

The aneurysm begins as a funnel-shaped outpocketing at a congenital weakness at the junction of the aortic media and annulus fibrosis of the aortic valve. Congenital aneurysm arises from the right coronary sinus and noncoronary sinus. Aneurysms of the right coronary sinus rupture into the right ventricle or right atrium, while those of the noncoronary sinus rupture into the right atrium. This entity should be distinguished from diffuse aneurysmal dilatation of the sinuses, which occurs in Marfan's syndrome. A large acute rupture may cause intractable pulmonary edema. All fistulas to the right heart cause volume overload of the left heart since there is volume overload of the downstream chambers. Depending on the site of rupture, volume overload of the right ventricle, right atrium, or both also occurs. These lesions may also be associated with aortic regurgitation and perimembranous or supracristal VSD.

Coronary Arteriovenous Fistula

This is a fistula or angiodysplasia from a coronary artery to a coronary vein, coronary sinus, right atrium, right ventricle, or pulmonary artery. There may be multiple sites of communication. The involved coronary artery is usually dilated and tortuous. The right coronary artery is involved more frequently and most frequently enters the right atrium or ventricle. The shunt is usually small and does not produce recognizable pulmonary overcirculation or volume overload enlargement of the heart.

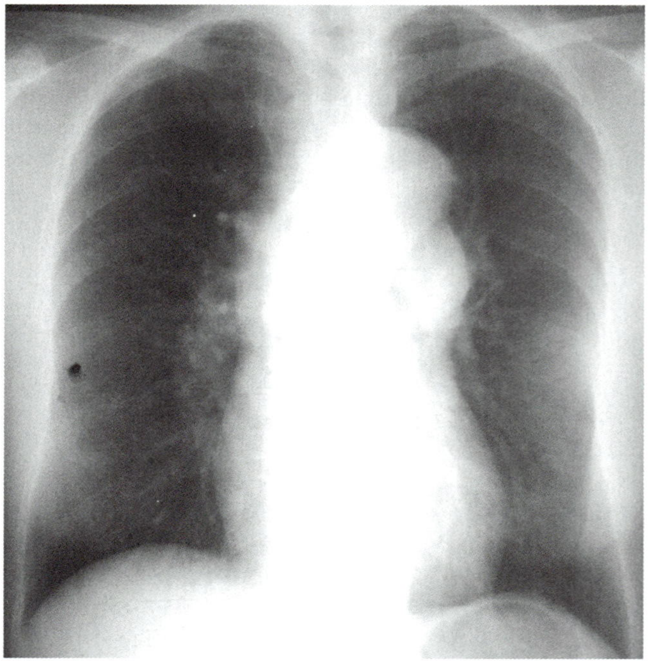

Figure 32.25. Patent ductus arteriosus. Thoracic radiograph shows no pulmonary arterial overcirculation but instead reveals attenuated peripheral vessels, normal heart size, and markedly enlarged main pulmonary.

Pulmonary arterial overcirculation and cardiomegaly are usually not evident. The ectatic coronary artery is infrequently discernible on the thoracic radiograph. Ectasia of the circumflex coronary artery may cause a localized bulge in the upper left cardiac margin in the region near the site of the left atrium on the frontal radiograph. Calcification rarely occurs in the ectatic coronary artery.

Cyanotic

Tetralogy of Fallot

The major components of this anomaly are caused by a displacement of the outlet septum (conal septation) toward the right ventricle, resulting in a diminutive right ventricular outflow region and failure of alignment of the outlet portion with the remainder of the ventricular septum. The latter abnormality causes a large VSD (infracristal), and the aorta is located immediately over the defect. Consequently, right ventricular blood is ejected directly into the aorta. There is a reciprocal relationship between the aortic and pulmonary arterial diameters; the ascending aorta is substantially enlarged in the presence of severe pulmonic stenosis and pulmonic atresia. The VSD is nonrestrictive, so pressures are equal in the ventricles. Multiple VSDs may occur in this anomaly.

The obstruction to pulmonary blood flow is frequently diffuse and exists at multiple levels, causing subvalvular, valvular, and supravalvular stenoses. There is invariably infundibular stenosis. The annulus and proximal pulmonary artery are usually hypoplastic. The stenosis may involve the entire outflow region and may include severe hypoplasia of the segmental and intraparenchymal pulmonary arteries. The extreme form of tetralogy is pulmonary atresia with a nonrestrictive VSD. Branch pulmonary arterial stenosis, especially at the origin of the left pulmonary artery, may cause asymmetric pulmonary blood flow. However, even in the absence of branch stenosis, preferential flow occurs to the right lung due to the orientation of the right ventricular outflow tract. A right aortic arch is present in about 20% of patients with tetralogy; the incidence is about 25% with pulmonary atresia and VSD (extreme form of tetralogy).

The physiology of the anomaly consists of reduced pulmonary blood flow and arterial desaturation. Because of the reduced blood flow through the lungs, the left-sided cardiac chambers are small. Radiographic features are shown in Tables 32.11 and 32.12 and Figs. 32.2, 32.9, 32.10, 32.26, 32.27.

Early in life, the thoracic radiograph may not be typical, but it becomes characteristic later. Regression of the thymus reveals the concave main pulmonary artery segment, which is characteristic for tetralogy of Fallot.

After surgical repair of tetralogy, a number of radiographic findings may be identified, such as aneurysm of a right ventricular outflow patch; asymmetry of pulmonary

Table 32.11 Salient Radiographic Features of Tetralogy of Fallot

Decreased pulmonary vascularity: Normal vascularity in a cyanotic individual is equated with decreased vascularity since the distinction between normal and mildly decreased vascularity is frequently difficult
Normal or nearly normal cardiac size
Right ventricular enlargement or prominence: This may cause an uplifted cardiac apex
Concave or absent main pulmonary arterial segment
Small hilar pulmonary arteries: This may be most evident on the lateral view
Asymmetric pulmonary vascularity is frequent, especially because of associated branch pulmonary artery stenosis
Prominent ascending aorta and aortic arch
Right aortic arch (20%-25% of cases)

Table 32.12 Salient Radiographic Features of Tetralogy of Fallot With absent Pulmonary Valve

Decreased distal pulmonary vascularity
Aneurysmal enlargement of the main and central pulmonary arteries
Cardiac size variable, depending on the severity of pulmonary regurgitation

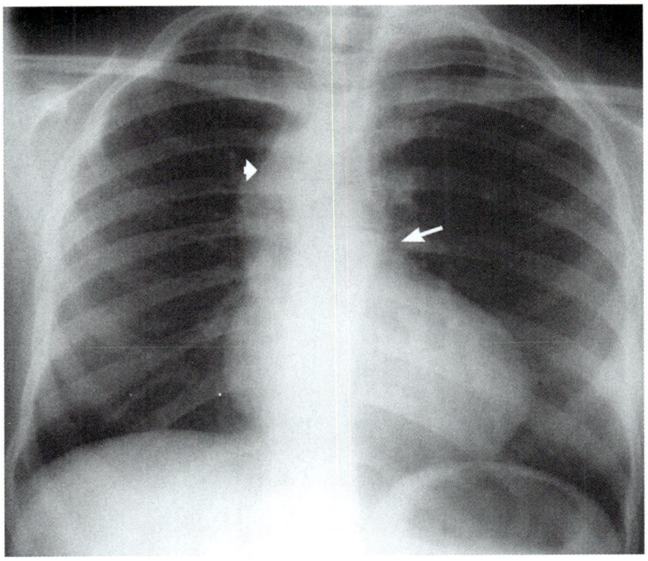

Figure 32.26. Tetralogy of Fallot. Radiograph shows reduced pulmonary vascularity, normal heart size, right ventricular prominence, concave main pulmonary arterial segment (*arrow*), and right aortic arch (*arrowhead*).

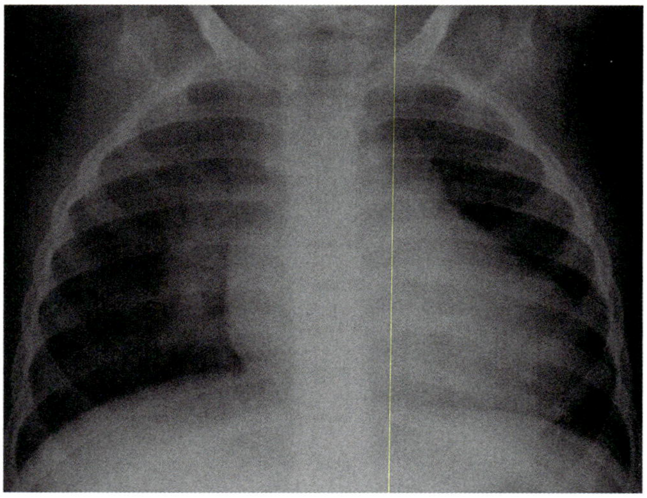

Figure 32.27. Tetralogy of Fallot with absent pulmonary valve in infant. Aneurysmal dilatation of main and right pulmonary arterial segments is diagnostic of this anomaly. Note the disparity in size of the right hilar arterial region and the peripheral segments of the pulmonary arteries.

vascularity due to persistent branch pulmonary arterial stenosis; and progressive right ventricular enlargement due to pulmonary regurgitation complicating a transannular patch (Fig. 32.28). Pulmonary arterial overcirculation can develop when a hemodynamically significant residual VSD exists after successful repair of outflow stenosis.

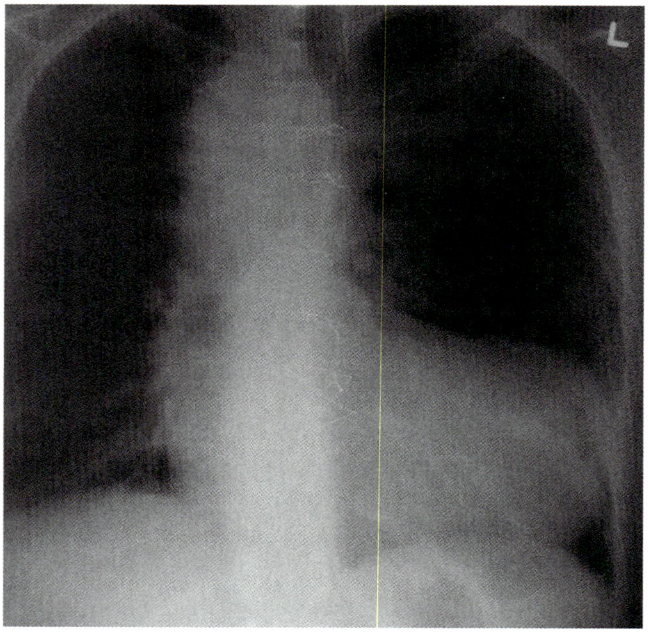

Figure 32.28. Tetralogy of Fallot with severe pulmonary regurgitation several years after repair. The cardiomegaly is caused by marked right ventricular enlargement, as indicated by the uplifted apex (*arrow*). Note the right aortic arch (*arrowhead*) creating the appearance of a the "boot-shaped" heart.

Transposition of Great Arteries

TGA is one of several abnormalities of arterioventricular connection. The others are double-outlet right ventricle, double-outlet left ventricle, and truncus arteriosus. All of these anomalies are admixture lesions, all produce cyanosis, and in the absence of obstruction to blood flow, all are associated with pulmonary arterial overcirculation.

In TGA, the aorta arises from the right ventricle and the pulmonary artery arises from the left ventricle. The base of the aorta is positioned anterior to pulmonary artery. If the aorta lies to the right of the pulmonary artery, the name d-TGA (dextro-TGA) applies, while if the aorta lies to the left of the pulmonary artery, the name l-TGA (levo-TGA) applies. If the aorta is directly anterior to the pulmonary artery, the term a-TGA (antero-TGA) is sometimes used.

The physiologic consequence of TGA is pulmonary arterial overcirculation and cyanosis due to the combination of left-to-right and right-to-left shunts (admixture lesion). Because the pulmonary and systemic circulations are parallel, most of the blood ejected by the left ventricle into the pulmonary artery is recirculated. The severity of overcirculation is usually greater in the presence of VSD and reduced in the presence of pulmonic stenosis. Cardiac size increases in relation to the pulmonary overcirculation. Pulmonary arterial hypertension and arteriolopathy tend to ensue early in life in children with TGA. Pulmonary arteriolopathy and fixed hypertension do not uncommonly develop at 6 to 12 months of age in children with TGA with VSD.

TGA is the most frequent cyanotic heart lesion. Without surgical intervention, most of the infants would die in the first year of life.

The radiographic appearance is influenced a great deal by the associated lesions. TGA is the most frequent anomaly causing pulmonary overcirculation in a cyanotic infant (see Fig. 32.15). The presence of significant pulmonic stenosis produces a radiographic appearance similar to tetralogy of Fallot (ie, decreased pulmonary vascularity and normal heart size in a cyanotic infant). The radiographic appearance during the first day or first few days of life may not be characteristic, since a prominent thymus conceals the narrow great vessel region and pulmonary blood flow is still limited by high pulmonary vascular resistance persisting from intrauterine life. After thymic involution in the stressed newborn, the narrow base of the heart becomes evident (Table 32.13; see Fig. 32.15).

Corrected Transposition (l-TGA)

Corrected transposition consists of arterioventricular transposition and atrioventricular discordance. The aorta originates from the right ventricle, and the right ventricle is inverted with connection to the left atrium. There is an l-ventricular loop with the morphologic right ventricle to the left of the morphologic left ventricle. Thus, blood flow in the central circulation is corrected; pulmonary venous

Table 32.13 Salient Radiographic Features of Transposition

Pulmonary arterial overcirculation: Asymmetry of pulmonary flow, greater on the right side, is sometimes apparent.
Pulmonary edema is frequent, especially in the presence of a VSD or PDA.
Cardiomegaly: A cardiothoracic ratio exceeding 0.58 constitutes cardiomegaly in the neonatal period.
In newborns, specific chamber enlargement is difficult to identify. In older children, there is left atrial and right ventricular enlargement.
Narrow vascular pedicle: The great vessels are usually but not invariably inconspicuous. The ascending aorta occupies a more medial position than normal and is hidden in the mediastinum. Likewise, the pulmonary artery lies medially within the mediastinum, so a typical main pulmonary arterial segment is not present. Thus, there is the incongruity of pulmonary arterial overcirculation with a small or absent main pulmonary arterial segment. Infrequently, even in complete TGA, the aorta lies to the right or left of the pulmonary artery, causing a normal or even increased width of the pedicle.
Right aortic arch occurs in about 5% of patients with TGA, usually in association with pulmonic stenosis and VSD.
In the presence of pulmonic stenosis and VSD, there is decreased pulmonary vascular size and normal heart size, producing an appearance similar to tetralogy of Fallot.

ASD, atrial septal defect; TGA, transposition of the great arteries; VSD, ventricular septal defect.

blood flows to the left atrium, to the right ventricle, and into the aorta. Most patients with corrected transposition have significant additional cardiac anomalies. The most frequent ones are pulmonic stenosis, VSD, Ebstein's anomaly (tricuspid regurgitation into the left atrium), and complete heart block (Table 32.14; Fig. 32.29).

Table 32.14 Salient Radiographic Features of Corrected Transposition

Prominent convexity of upper left cardiac border: The convexity may extend nearly to the arch or merely involve the base of the heart.
Ascending aortic shadow on the right is not visible
Crossing of the edge of the ascending aorta and the lateral edge of the proximal descending aorta.
Conspicuous absence of a convex main pulmonary arterial segment even in the presence of pulmonary arterial overcirculation: Sometimes there is upward tilt of the right and downward tilt of the left pulmonary artery
Left atrial enlargement can be caused by pulmonary overcirculation caused by the ventricular septal defect or by tricuspid regurgitation caused by Ebstein's anomaly.

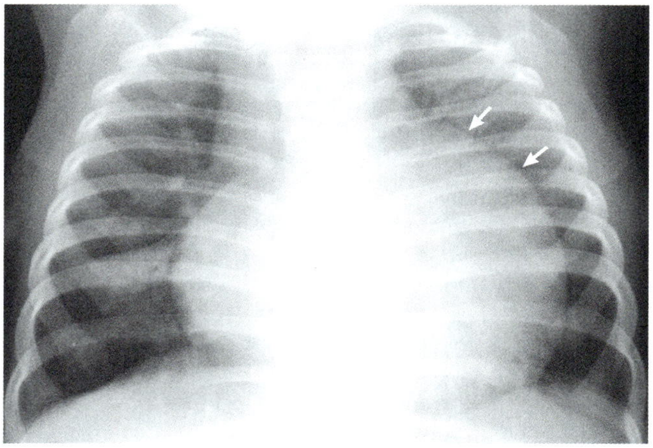

Figure 32.29. Corrected transposition of great arteries (l-ventricular loop with l-TGA). There is a prominent elongated convexity (*arrows*) of the upper left cardiac border.

Double-Outlet Right Ventricle

Double-outlet right ventricle is an anomaly in which more than 50% of both great vessels originate from the right ventricle. The aorta is positioned further to the right of the pulmonary artery and originates completely from the right ventricle, while the pulmonary artery may originate entirely from the right ventricle or have a biventricular origin (Taussig-Bing malformation). A VSD is always present, and other associated anomalies are frequent. The physiology of double-outlet right ventricle is determined to a great degree by the position of the VSD. A VSD oriented to the aortic valve (subaortic VSD) causes preferential flow from the left ventricle into the aorta and is frequently associated with significant pulmonic stenosis, resulting in physiology and radiographic appearance similar to tetralogy of Fallot. In the absence of pulmonic stenosis, preferential left ventricular to aortic flow may make cyanosis minimal. A VSD located beneath the pulmonic valve (Taussig-Bing malformation) causes preferential flow from the left ventricle into the pulmonary artery and consequently severe pulmonary arterial overcirculation. The right ventricular outflow is preferentially into the aorta; consequently, there is also cyanosis. Coarctation or interruption of the aortic arch is sometimes associated with the subpulmonic VSD. A large VSD may be situated beneath the origin of both great vessels (doubly committed VSD) or may be displaced away from both origins (noncommitted VSD). The great arteries tend to be side by side at the base of the heart, but either vessel can be located more anteriorly.

This is an admixture lesion that causes the combination of cyanosis (right-to-left shunt) and pulmonary arterial overcirculation (left-to-right shunt). The severity of pulmonic stenosis and the position of the VSD initially determine the relative severity of the two shunts.

Double-outlet left ventricle is an exceedingly rare anomaly in which both arteries originate from a morphologic left ventricle. The presentation and radiologic appearance are similar to double-outlet right ventricle (Tables 32.15 and 32.16; Fig. 32.30).

Table 32.15 Salient Features of DORV Without Significant Pulmonic Stenosis

Pulmonary arterial overcirculation: it is one of the causes of cyanosis and pulmonary arterial overcirculation
Cardiomegaly.
Enlargement of the left atrium, left ventricle, and right ventricle: distinction between left and right ventricle enlargement during infancy is usually inconclusive.
Widened great artery pedicle due to side-by-side position of the aorta and pulmonary artery: This is not always evident. It can be a distinguishing feature when compared to the appearance of d-TGA.
Prominent main pulmonary arterial segment: this can also be a distinguishing feature for DORV in comparison with d-TGA.
Signs of coarctation or interruption of the aortic arch.

DORV, double-outlet right ventricle; TGA, transposition of the great arteries.

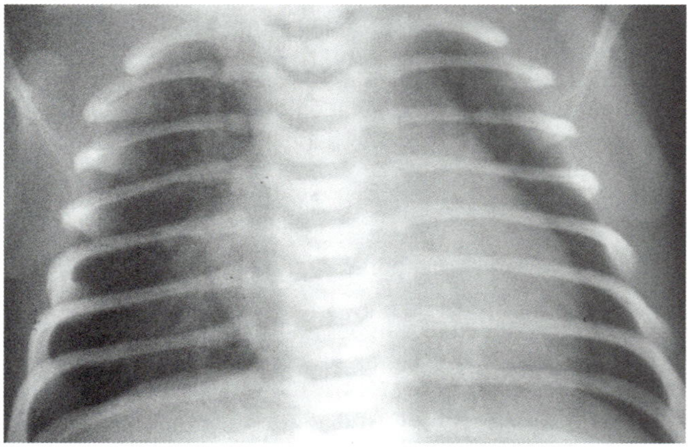

Figure 32.30. Double-outlet right ventricle. Note pulmonary arterial overcirculation and cardiomegaly. Prominent great vessel region is shown in contradistinction to narrow great vessel region as seen in dextro-transposition of great arteries.

Tricuspid Atresia

Tricuspid atresia is the absence of a direct connection of the right atrium to the right ventricle. The atresia can be due to a membrane or a ridge of muscle between the chambers. An atrial septal defect or patent foramen ovale is always present. Other associated lesions are frequent and are usually important in determining the physiology and clinical presentation. The most frequently associated lesions are TGA, VSD, and pulmonic stenosis. A classification of tricuspid atresia is based on the presence or absence of these associated lesions. Tricuspid atresia without TGA can be (1) with pulmonary atresia and no VSD, (2) with pulmonary stenosis and a small restrictive VSD, or (3) with no pulmonary stenosis and a large nonrestrictive VSD. Tricuspid atresia with TGA can be (1) with pulmonary atresia and a large VSD, (2) with pulmonary stenosis and a large VSD, or (3) with no pulmonary stenosis and a large VSD.

The most common form is tricuspid atresia with pulmonic stenosis and normally related great arteries and restrictive VSD. TGA is present in about 30% of patients with tricuspid atresia. It is usually associated with VSD and no pulmonic stenosis.

When the VSD is large and the pulmonary stenosis mild or nonexistent, there is pulmonary overcirculation. This is the situation both for normally related arteries and TGA. Restriction of pulmonary blood flow usually exists at pulmonic valvular and subvalvular levels or at a restrictive VSD. A small atrial septal communication also limits pulmonary flow and additionally causes the right atrium to enlarge. Despite obstruction to the right atrial outlet, the right atrium usually does not dilate since a large interatrial communication causes the right atrium to function as a venous conduit similar to the vena cava (Table 32.17; Figs. 32.11 and 32.31).

Table 32.16 Salient Radiographic Features of double-outlet right ventricle With Pulmonic Stenosis

Decreased pulmonary vascularity
Normal or nearly normal cardiac size
Right ventricular prominence
Inconspicuous main pulmonary arterial segment
Right aortic arch in about 10%-15% of patients

Table 32.17 Salient Radiographic Features of Tricuspid Atresia

With normally related great vessels, VSD, and pulmonic stenosis, the appearance is similar to tetralogy of Fallot. There is decreased pulmonary vascularity, small central pulmonary arteries, and normal or nearly normal heart size. A distinguishing feature from tetralogy, if discernible, is prominence of the left atrium and left ventricle and flat right atrial border.
With TGA, VSD without pulmonic stenosis, the typical feature of d-TGA, is present. There is pulmonary overcirculation, cardiomegaly, and a narrow vascular pedicle. A distinguishing feature may be the right atrial border. The right atrial border (right atrial enlargement) is frequently prominent in d-TGA, but it is not prominent or even flat in tricuspid atresia when the interatrial communication is large.
With a small (restrictive) interatrial communication, the right atrium may enlarge considerably. The right atrium enlarges to the extent of causing considerable cardiomegaly as depicted on the frontal radiograph.
Tricuspid atresia with TGA is sometimes associated with left juxtaposition of the atrial appendages: the right atrial appendage extends posteriorly behind the great arteries and lies above the left atrial appendage. This causes a prominent upper left cardiac border and flattening of the right cardiac border.

VSD, ventricular septal defect; TGA, transposition of the great arteries.

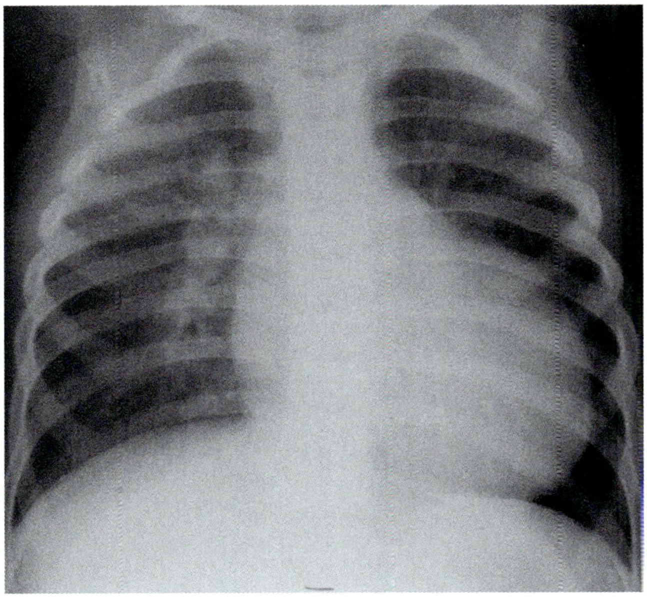

Figure 32.31. Tricuspid atresia with transposition of great arteries. Radiograph shows the narrow base of the heart that is characteristic for transposition. Flat right atrial border is a feature of tricuspid atresia with nonrestrictive atrial septal defect.

Single Ventricle

Single ventricle consists of a predominant ventricle that receives both atrioventricular valves (double-inlet ventricle) and a tiny remnant portion of the other ventricle. A more specific term for most of the anomalies grouped under this title is *univentricular atrioventricular connections.* The great arteries can both originate from the dominant ventricle, or one may originate from the small ventricle. The dominant ventricle can be either the left or right.

Single ventricle is frequently associated with an abnormality of arterioventricular connection, such as TGA or double-outlet right ventricle. Normally, related great vessels are uncommon with single ventricle. The left ventricular type of single ventricle is frequently associated with an inverted right ventricular outlet chamber and l-TGA. The dominant ventricle communicates with the outlet chamber through a "bulboventricular foramen."

The physiology is determined to a substantial degree by associated obstruction of the outflow to the pulmonary artery or aorta. There is an admixture of systemic and pulmonary venous blood in the dominant ventricle, so both cyanosis and pulmonary overcirculation occur. The presence and severity of the pulmonary overcirculation are regulated by pulmonary stenosis. If pulmonary stenosis is severe, the physiology and clinical presentation are similar to tetralogy of Fallot. If obstruction to pulmonary blood flow is not present, then the physiology and clinical presentation are similar to transposition. The physiology of the common ventricle is identical to a large VSD, which is really the proper designation for this lesion (Table 32.18; Fig. 32.32).

Table 32.18 Salient Radiographic Appearance of Single Ventricle

With normally related arteries and no pulmonic stenosis, the appearance is like a VSD or d-TGA, depending on the preferential streaming in the ventricle. There is pulmonary overcirculation and cardiomegaly.
With significant pulmonic stenosis and normally related great arteries, the appearance is reduced pulmonary vascularity and normal or nearly normal heart size. The appearance is similar to tetralogy of Fallot.
With d-TGA, the appearance can be typical of d-TGA. Pulmonary blood flow may be increased or decreased.
With l-TGA, the appearance can be typical of l-TGA. Pulmonary blood flow may be increased or decreased. A notch along the upper left cardiac border may be due to the intersection of the contour of an inverted right ventricular outlet chamber with the dominant ventricle.

VSD, ventricular septal defect; TGA, transposition of the great arteries.

Truncus Arteriosus

Truncus arteriosus is a single trunk originating from the heart and supplying the pulmonary, systemic, and coronary arteries. The truncus straddles a large VSD. It is an admixture lesion, with both left-to-right and right-to-left shunts. Two classification systems for truncus arteriosus are extant currently. The older and more familiar one was proposed by Collett and Edward in 1949. The types are grouped according to the site of origin of the pulmonary arteries from the truncus (Table 32.19; Fig. 32.33).

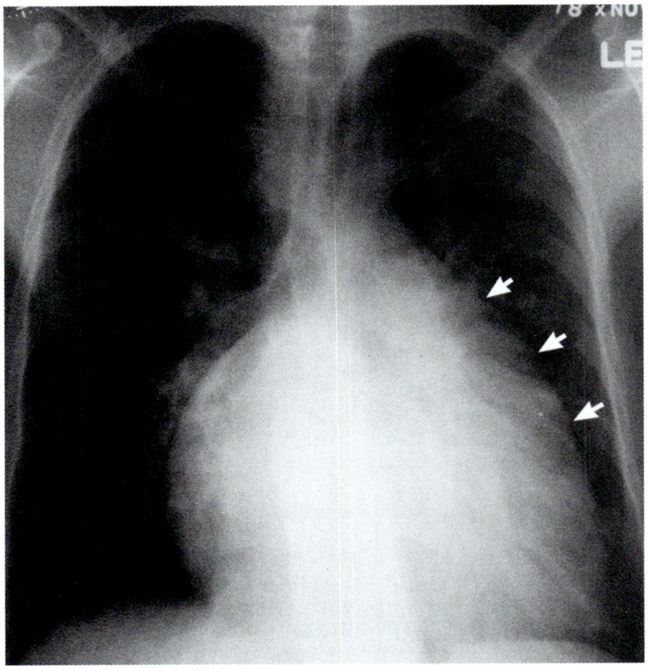

Figure 32.32. Single ventricle with inverted outlet chamber (l-loop) and levo-transposition of great arteries. Prominent convexity of upper left cardiac border represents the inverted right ventricle outlet chamber (*arrows*) and the l-transposed ascending aorta.

Table 32.19 Two Classification Systems for Truncus Arteriosus

Type	Description
Grouped according to the site of origin of the pulmonary arteries from the truncus	
I	A main pulmonary artery originates from the proximal portion of the truncus, usually from the left posterolateral aspect.
II	Right and left pulmonary arteries have individual origins from the posterior aspect of the truncus.
III	One of both pulmonary arteries arises from the lateral aspect of the truncus.
IV	No pulmonary arteries arise from the ascending truncus (aorta) but rather from the descending aorta. This type is not really a truncus arteriosus but rather pulmonary atresia with VSD and major pulmonary blood flow from bronchial and other systemic arteries originating from the descending aorta.
Classification of Van Praagh and Van Praagh	
I	Common pulmonary artery arises from the truncus.
II	Right and left pulmonary arteries arise separately from the truncus.
III	Absence of one pulmonary artery, other pulmonary artery arises from the ductus.
IV	Common pulmonary artery arises from the truncus with arch interruption.

The truncal valve can have two to five cusps. The valves with numbers of cusps more or less than three are frequently incompetent, and truncal insufficiency can be severe. Hemitruncus is not infrequent; one pulmonary artery originates from the ascending aorta, and the other arises directly from the right ventricle. Stenosis at the origin of the right and/or left pulmonary arteries is common, especially in types II and III of Collett and Edwards. Consequently, asymmetry of blood flow occurs with this anomaly. A right aortic arch is common (Tables 32.20 and 32.21).

The physiology is characterized by excess pulmonary blood flow and frequent volume overload of especially left-sided chambers. This is one of the lesions causing pulmonary arterial overcirculation in a cyanotic patient. Congestive heart failure and pulmonary edema are common.

Total Anomalous Pulmonary Venous Connection

All pulmonary veins connect to a systemic venous structure or the right atrium directly in this anomaly. This is another

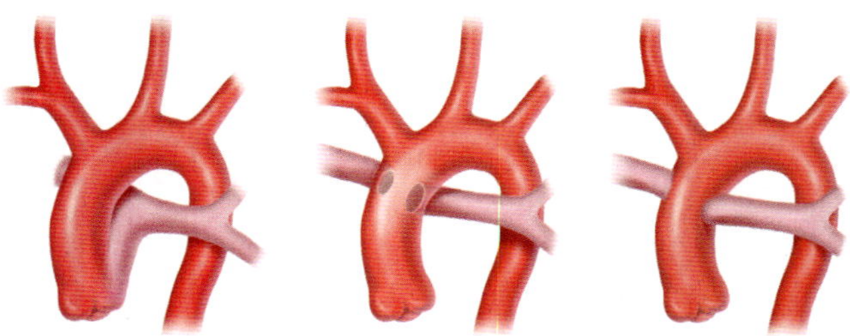

Figure 32.33. The types of truncus arteriosus: type I, single origin of main pulmonary artery; type II, separate origins of left and right pulmonary arteries from dorsal aspect of the truncus; type III, separate origins of left and right pulmonary arteries from the left and right side of the truncus. (Reprinted with permission from Lee EY. Pediatric Thoracic Imaging. Wolters Kluwer, 2018. Figure 4-30.)

admixture lesion. Generally, the pulmonary veins form a central confluence before entering the systemic venous site. Infrequently, they do not all join together and may drain to different sites. This anomaly is divided into three types based on the site of pulmonary venous drainage.

In the supracardiac type, connections are to the left innominate vein, right superior vena cava, or azygos vein. A left-sided vertical vein connects the pulmonary venous confluence to the left innominate vein. The cardiac type has

Table 32.20 Salient Radiographic Features of Truncus Arteriosus

- Pulmonary arterial overcirculation: asymmetry of flow is not uncommon, even to the extent of plethora on one side and oligemia on the other.
- Pulmonary venous hypertension or edema is frequent, especially in type I.
- Cardiomegaly: the heart size is frequently, but not always, proportionate to the pulmonary overcirculation. Cardiomegaly may also be related to truncal insufficiency.
- Four-chamber enlargement may be present.
- Enlargement of the left atrium and left ventricle is generally identified.
- Prominent main pulmonary arterial segment (type I) or reduced main pulmonary arterial segment (type II or III): in type I, the left pulmonary artery has a higher position than usual and a comma-shaped configuration ("hilar comma") as it curves upward and leftward.
- Right aortic arch in about 35% of patients
- Dilated ascending aorta: there are two cyanotic lesions that are frequently associated with a large ascending aortic shadow: one causes decreased pulmonary vascularity (tetralogy of Fallot) and the other causes increased pulmonary vascularity (truncus arteriosus).

Table 32.21 Frequency of Right Aortic Arch in Congenital Heart Disease

Abnormality	Frequency (%)
Tetralogy of Fallot	20
Pulmonary atresia with ventricular septal cefect	25
Truncus arteriosus	35
Double-outlet right ventricle	12
Tricuspid atresia	10-15
Transpos tion of great arteries	5-8
Ventricular septal defect	2

connections to the right atrium or coronary sinus. In the infracardiac type, the connection is below the diaphragm to the portal vein or one of its branches, ductus venosus, or hepatic vein. In this type, a long vein courses from the pulmonary venous confluence and through the esophageal hiatus to its site of infradiaphragmatic connection. Pulmonary venous drainage is always obstructed with this type because of a variety of mechanisms, including narrowing or stenosis of the connecting vein at its site of connection with the systemic vein or the systemic vein itself. The need for pulmonary venous blood to pass through the hepatic sinusoids has also been held to be an additional site of obstruction. However, portal venous pressure is not higher than pulmonary venous pressure in normal individuals. Infrequently, total anomalous pulmonary venous connection above the diaphragm is associated with pulmonary venous obstruction.

The physiology of total anomalous pulmonary venous connection depends on whether pulmonary venous obstruction exists. Mixing systemic and pulmonary venous blood occurs in the right atrium, and there is an obligatory right-to-left shunt of mixed venous blood through an interatrial connection. The size of the communication determines the volume of the flow to the left heart. Preferential flow from the right atrium is usually to the right ventricle and pulmonary artery, causing a large volume of recirculated blood. In total anomalous pulmonary venous connection above the diaphragm, the volume of pulmonary blood flow is very high and is the major feature, while cyanosis may be mild. The volume overload of the lungs may be so great that pulmonary edema occurs.

In total anomalous pulmonary venous connection with obstruction, the major feature is pulmonary venous hypertension and edema. The flow to the lungs is not very great. Because there is less pulmonary venous blood to mix with the desaturated systemic venous blood, cyanosis is conspicuous. Total anomalous pulmonary venous connection can occur in association with a number of other cardiac anomalies. It is a frequent lesion in patients with the asplenia syndrome (Tables 32.22 and 32.23; Fig. 32.34).

Table 32.22 Salient Radiographic Features of TAPVC Without Venous Obstruction

- Pulmonary arterial overcirculation. Pulmonary venous hypertension and edema may be present with extreme volume overload.
- Cardiomegaly. This is usually proportionate to the pulmonary arterial overcirculation.
- Enlargement of the right atrium and right ventricle
- The enlarged systemic vein into which drainage occurs or the anomalous connecting vein may be visible as the "snowman appearance," dilated right superior vena cava, or dilated azygos vein or coronary sinus.

TAPVC, total anomalous pulmonary venous connections.

Table 32.23 Salient Radiographic Features of TAPVC With Venous Obstruction

- Pulmonary edema
- Normal heart size
- Prominence of the right atrium and, less frequently, right ventricle
- Infrequently, the connecting vein can be identified on the lateral view in a position behind the heart. A barium swallow may show an anterior impression on the esophagus.

TAPVC, total anomalous pulmonary venous connections.

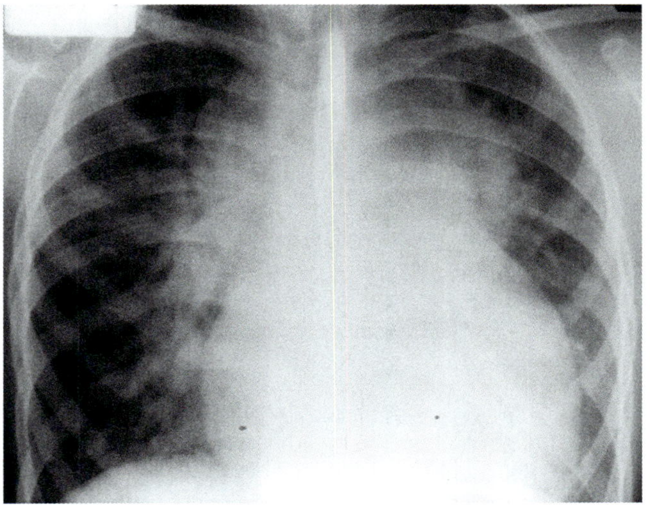

Figure 32.34. Total anomalous pulmonary venous connection, supracardiac type (type I). Note pulmonary arterial overcirculation, cardiomegaly, and enlargement of the superior mediastinum ("snowman" appearance). The snowman is caused by the dilated vertical vein connecting to the left innominate vein (left-sided enlargement) and the dilated superior vena cava (right-sided enlargement).

Ebstein's Anomaly

Ebstein's anomaly is a deformity of the tricuspid valve in which one or more leaflets are displaced into the inflow portion of the right ventricle. The leaflets have lines of attachment to the right ventricle of varying length. The displacement into the right ventricle and the deformity of the valve cause tricuspid regurgitation, and the mural attachments in the right ventricle may cause obstruction to pulmonary blood flow. The septal and posterior leaflets are involved, while the anterior leaflet usually has a normal attachment to the atrioventricular ring. A small to substantial portion of the inflow region of the right ventricle has a thin wall and lacks ventricular myocardium (atrialization of the right ventricle). A patent foramen ovale or secundum atrial septal defect is present in about 80% of cases.

The physiologic consequence of the lesion is nearly always tricuspid regurgitation and usually a small-volume right-to-left shunt. Cyanosis may be absent or very mild. Occasionally, the major effect is tricuspid obstruction, due to limitation of the atrioventricular inlet to only narrow slits in the displaced leaflets of the valve. In this circumstance, the right-to-left shunt is more severe. In the 20% or so of patients without an interatrial communication, cyanosis is not present (Table 32.24; Fig. 32.3).

Pulmonary Atresia With Intact Ventricular Septum

Pulmonary atresia with intact ventricular septum exists in two forms: hypoplasia of the right ventricle and tricuspid valve with little or no tricuspid regurgitation (type I) or a normal or enlarged right ventricle with significant tricuspid regurgitation (type II). This entity is distinct from pulmonary atresia with VSD (extreme form of tetralogy of Fallot).

The physiology of this lesion is reduced pulmonary blood flow so that the volume of fully oxygenated blood entering the left atrium is small. The shunting of nearly all systemic venous blood occurs through the interatrial communication. There is admixture of desaturated and oxygenated blood in the left atrium. Because the volume of pulmonary venous blood is reduced, cyanosis is severe. Blood reaches the lung by a PDA and/or bronchial arteries (Tables 32.25 and 32.26).

Table 32.24 Salient Radiographic Features of Ebstein's Anomaly

Decreased pulmonary vascularity

Cardiomegaly

Enlarged right atrium: The right heart border is elongated, with a prominent convexity.

Enlargement of the right ventricle. The right ventricle is less conspicuous than the atrium.

Main pulmonary arterial segment and hilar segments are small. However, the right ventricular outflow tract may produce a prominent bulge just caudal to the pulmonary arterial segment on the frontal view.

Small thoracic aorta

Table 32.25 Salient Radiographic Features of Type I Pulmonary Atresia

Decreased pulmonary vascularity.

Normal cardiac size or only slight cardiomegaly.

Concave main pulmonary arterial segment and small hilar pulmonary arteries.

Uplifted apex: This appearance may be due to left ventricular enlargement in the presence of a diminutive right ventricle.

Thoracic aorta can be enlarged.

Pulmonic Stenosis

Pulmonary valvular stenosis exists in two distinct syndromes. The most frequent type presents in an innocuous manner with mild symptoms, a systolic murmur, and a slightly abnormal thoracic radiograph. Infrequently, infants present with severe symptoms and marked cardiomegaly. The severity of the valvular stenosis is so great that the right ventricle dilates markedly and right ventricular failure ensues. Because of the elevated right-sided diastolic pressure, there is considerable right-to-left shunting across a secundum atrial septal defect or stretched foramen ovale. When the stenosis is so severe that right ventricular failure occurs, the entity is called critical pulmonary stenosis (Tables 32.27 and 32.28; Fig. 32.35).

Hypoplastic Left Heart

This lesion consists of several or all of the following features: hypoplastic ascending aorta, severe aortic stenosis or atresia, hypoplastic left ventricle (thick wall and diminutive cavity), and mitral atresia. The coronary arteries are perfused by right-to-left flow across a PDA and retrograde into the ascending aorta. An atrial septal communication is present so that admixture of pulmonary and systemic venous blood occurs in the right atrium. Consequently, there is volume overload of the right-sided chambers and excess pulmonary blood flow. The usual clinical presentation is severe congestive heart failure in the first few days of life (Table 32.29; see Fig. 32.20).

Coarctation of the Aorta

Coarctation of the aorta is a narrowing of the distal aortic arch and/or proximal descending aorta due to a discrete fibromuscular ring or a long- or short-segment tunnel narrowing

Table 32.26 Salient Radiographic Features of Type II Pulmonary Atresia

Decreased pulmonary vascularity

Cardiomegaly

Right atrial and right ventricular enlargement

Small pulmonary arterial segment

Thoracic aorta may be enlarged

Table 32.27 Salient Features of Compensated Valvular Pulmonic Stenosis

Normal pulmonary vascularity
Normal cardiac size
Right ventricular enlargement or prominence: This is usually detected initially on the lateral view as a prominent convexity of the anterior cardiac border or filling of the retrosternal space
Poststenotic dilatation of main pulmonary arterial segment
Dilated and usually laterally displaced left pulmonary artery

of the aortic isthmus. There may also be hypoplasia of the posterior portion of the aortic arch. The coarctation usually occurs adjacent to the site of attachment of the ligamentum arteriosus and distal to the left subclavian artery. The coarctation is infrequently proximal to the origin of the left subclavian artery. The coarctation can extend into the origin of the left subclavian artery, causing stenosis of this artery. Both of these situations cause lower arterial pressure in the left compared to the right pulmonary artery. Anomalous origin of the right subclavian artery (retroesophageal right subclavian artery) from a site distal to the coarctation causes lower arterial pressure in the right arm.

Coarctation may be associated with a wide variety of congenital lesions, but two occur with noticeable frequency: PDA and VSD. The triad of coarctation, VSD, and PDA has been called the coarctation syndrome and is especially frequent when the lesion presents in early infancy. A bicuspid aortic valve occurs in a high percentage of patients.

The physiology is hypertension in arteries originating proximal to the site of coarctation and reduced blood flow to arteries arising below the coarctation. If the coarctation occurs proximal to the site of origin of one of the subclavian arteries, then there is hypertension in only one arm and rib notching on only the side with hypertension. The numerous causes of rib notching are listed in Table 32.30. The 4th to 8th ribs are the ones usually notched; the 3rd and 9th ribs are less frequently notched. The notching consists of scalloped regions on the undersurface of the posterior portion of the ribs. The posterior upper surface is infrequently involved. Sclerosis may outline the scalloped sites. Rib notching is unusual in patients younger than 5 years of age. Rib notching depends on the origin of the ipsilateral subclavian artery proximal to the site of the coarctation. Coarctation proximal to the left subclavian arterial origin causes right-sided rib notching only, while an anomalous origin of the right subclavian artery from a site below the coarctation produces unilateral left-sided notching.

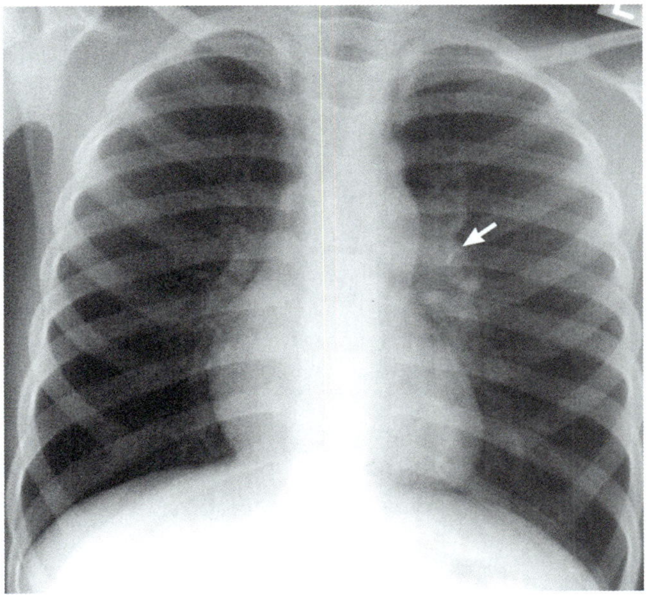

Figure 32.35. Valvular pulmonic stenosis. Radiograph shows enlargement of the main and left pulmonary arterial (*arrow*) segments. The descending branch of the left pulmonary artery is frequently very prominent.

Hypertension usually causes left ventricular hypertrophy but may induce left ventricular dilatation and failure if extremely severe. Left ventricular dilatation, myocardial failure, and pulmonary edema are most likely to occur in early infancy (Tables 32.31 and 32.32; Fig. 32.36).

Interruption of Aortic Arch

The arch can be interrupted at any of three sites: beyond the left subclavian artery (type A), between the left subclavian and left common carotid arteries (type B), and between the innominate artery and left carotid artery (type C). Types A and B occur with approximately equal frequency; type C is rare. The right subclavian artery sometimes originates

Table 32.28 Salient Radiographic Features of Critical Pulmonic Stenosis

Decreased pulmonary vascularity
Cardiomegaly
Enlargement of the right atrium and ventricle
Enlarged main pulmonary arterial segment

Table 32.29 Salient Radiographic Features of Hypoplastic Left Heart

Pulmonary arterial overcirculation and/or pulmonary edema
Cardiomegaly
Prominent right-sided chambers, especially the right atrium
Because of the patent ductus, the aortic arch may be prominent

Table 32.30 Cause of Rib Notching

Aortic obstruction
- Coarctation of the aorta
- Interruption of the aorta
- Acquired obstruction of the aorta: Takayasu's aortitis, atherosclerotic obstruction, etc.
- Unusual causes of coarctation: neurofibromatosis, Williams syndrome, rubella syndrome

Subclavian arterial obstruction
- Blalock-Taussig shunt (upper two ribs)
- Takayasu's arteritis (usually unilateral)
- Atherosclerosis

Severely reduced pulmonary blood flow
- Tetralogy of Fallot
- Pulmonary atresia
- Tricuspid atresia
- Unilateral absence or atresia of a pulmonary artery
- Pulmonary emphysema
- Chronic pulmonary thromboembolic disease
- Superior vena canal obstruction

Vascular shunts
- Pulmonary arteriovenous shunt
- Intercostal arteriovenous shunt
- Intercostal to pulmonary arterial shunt
- Intercostal neuroma
- Poliomyelitis (upper margin)
- Hyperparathyroidism

Modified from Felson B. Chest Roentgenology. *Philadelphia: WB Saunders; 1973.*

ectopically as a fourth aortic branch in this anomaly, which is called a type B2 interruption. In this circumstance, hypertension is confined to the carotid arteries.

This lesion can exist in an isolated form but usually is associated with VSD and PDA. There is an association with double-outlet right ventricle with subpulmonic VSD (Taussig-Bing malformation (Table 32.33; Fig. 32.37).

Table 32.31 Salient Radiographic Features in Compensated Coarctation

- Rib notching
- Retrosternal undulating soft tissue due to dilated tortuous internal mammary arteries (site of collateral flow)
- Abnormal appearance of the aortic arch
- A notch on the proximal descending aorta followed by poststenotic dilatation causes a figure-3 sign on the aorta and a reverse figure-3 sign on the barium-filled esophagus
- Left ventricular prominence
- Prominent ascending aorta
- A duplicated aortic "knob" may be caused by tortuosity of the posterior arch and proximal descending aorta causing kinking of the aorta: This is called pseudocoarctation of the aorta when no pressure gradient exists

Table 32.32 Salient Radiographic Features in Decompensated Coarctation

- Pulmonary venous hypertension or edema.
- Cardiomegaly
- Left ventricular enlargement.
- Pulmonary arterial overcirculation is present, with associated ventricular septal defect and patent ductus arteriosus.
- Rib notching is not present during infancy.
- The aortic knob is usually not characteristic during infancy. The only sign may be lateral displacement of the descending aortic stripe.

Aortic Stenosis

Congenital aortic stenosis is caused by a bicuspid aortic valve, unicuspid and unicommissural, or dysplastic valves. It may be so severe as to induce intractable left ventricular failure in the neonate (critical aortic stenosis). Stenosis also occurs at the subvalvular (discrete membranous or tunnel forms) and supravalvular sites (Tables 32.34 and 32.35; Fig. 32.38).

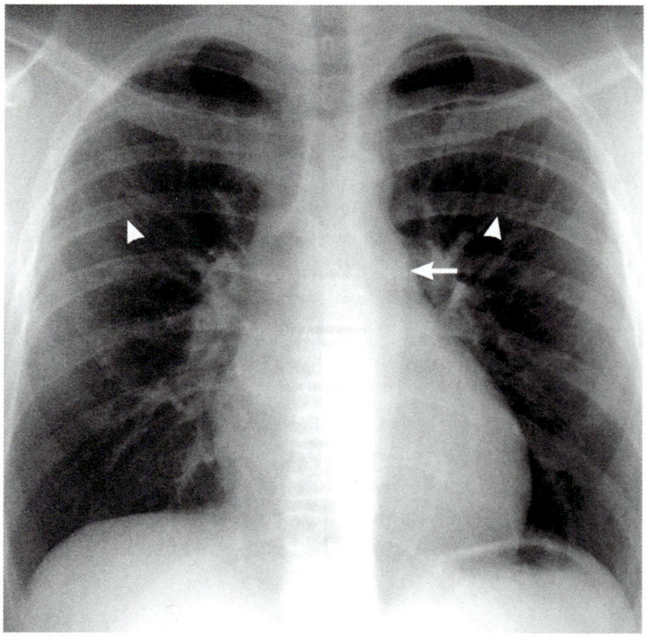

Figure 32.36. Coarctation of the aorta. Abnormal contour of arch and proximal descending aorta. The duplicated aortic knob is due to poststenotic dilatation (*arrow*) in the proximal descending aorta. There is outward displacement of the lateral margin of the descending aorta. A figure-3 configuration is caused by the notch at the site of the coarctation with poststenotic dilatation. Rib notching is present (*arrowheads*).

Table 32.33 Salient Radiographic Features of Interruption of Aortic Arch

Isolated variety has the appearance as described for coarctation.

Interruption with ventricular septal defect and patent ductus arteriosus causes pulmonary arterial overcirculation and usually severe pulmonary edema with cardiomegaly.

The trachea is sometimes identified to lie exactly in the midline, and there is no indentation on the trachea.

If a patent ductus arteriosus is present, the posterior arch may be prominent yet the trachea, not indented, lies exactly in the midline.

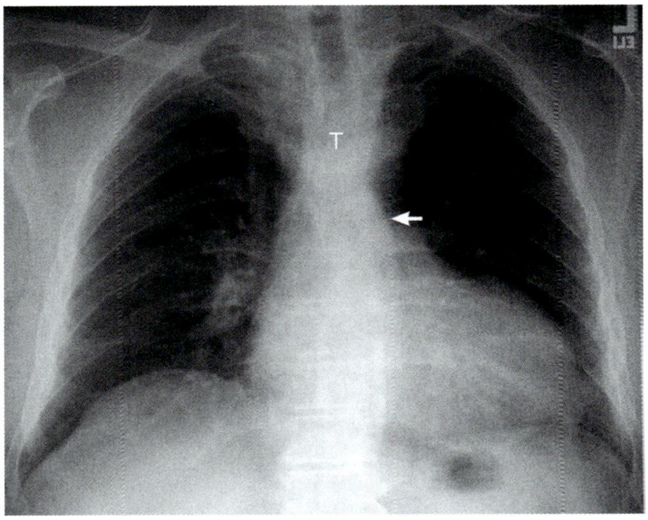

Figure 32.37. Interruption of the aortic arch as an isolated anomaly. Radiographs show midline trachea and dilated proximal descending aorta (*arrow*) below the narrow site of interruption.

Table 32.34 Salient Radiographic Features in Uncomplicated Aortic Stenosis

Normal heart size.

Enlargement of the ascending aorta: This occurs in valvular stenosis and about half of patients with discrete membranous subvalvular stenosis.

Ascending aorta is small in supravalvular form.

Table 32.35 Salient Radiographic Features of Critical Aortic Stenosis

Pulmonary venous hypertension or edema

Cardiomegaly

Left ventricular enlargement

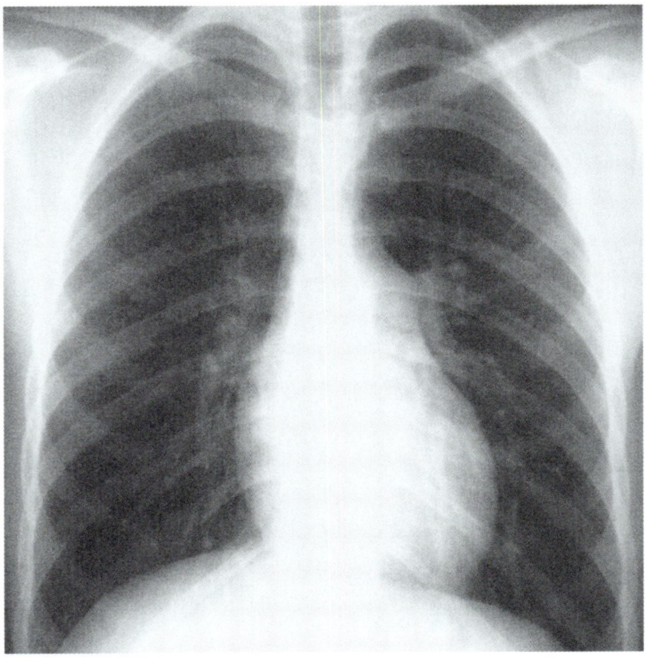

Figure 32.38. Supravalvular aortic stenosis. Concavity is seen in the region occupied by the ascending aorta.

SUGGESTED READINGS

Elliott LB. *Cardiac Imaging in Infants, Children, and Adults.* JB Lippincott; 1991.

Higgins CB. Radiography of congenital heart disease. In: Higgins CB, ed. *Essentials of Cardiac Radiology and Imaging.* JB Lippincott; 1992:49.

The Brant and Helms Solution: Fundamentals of Diagnostic Radiology. 3rd ed. Lippincott Williams & Wilkins; 2003.

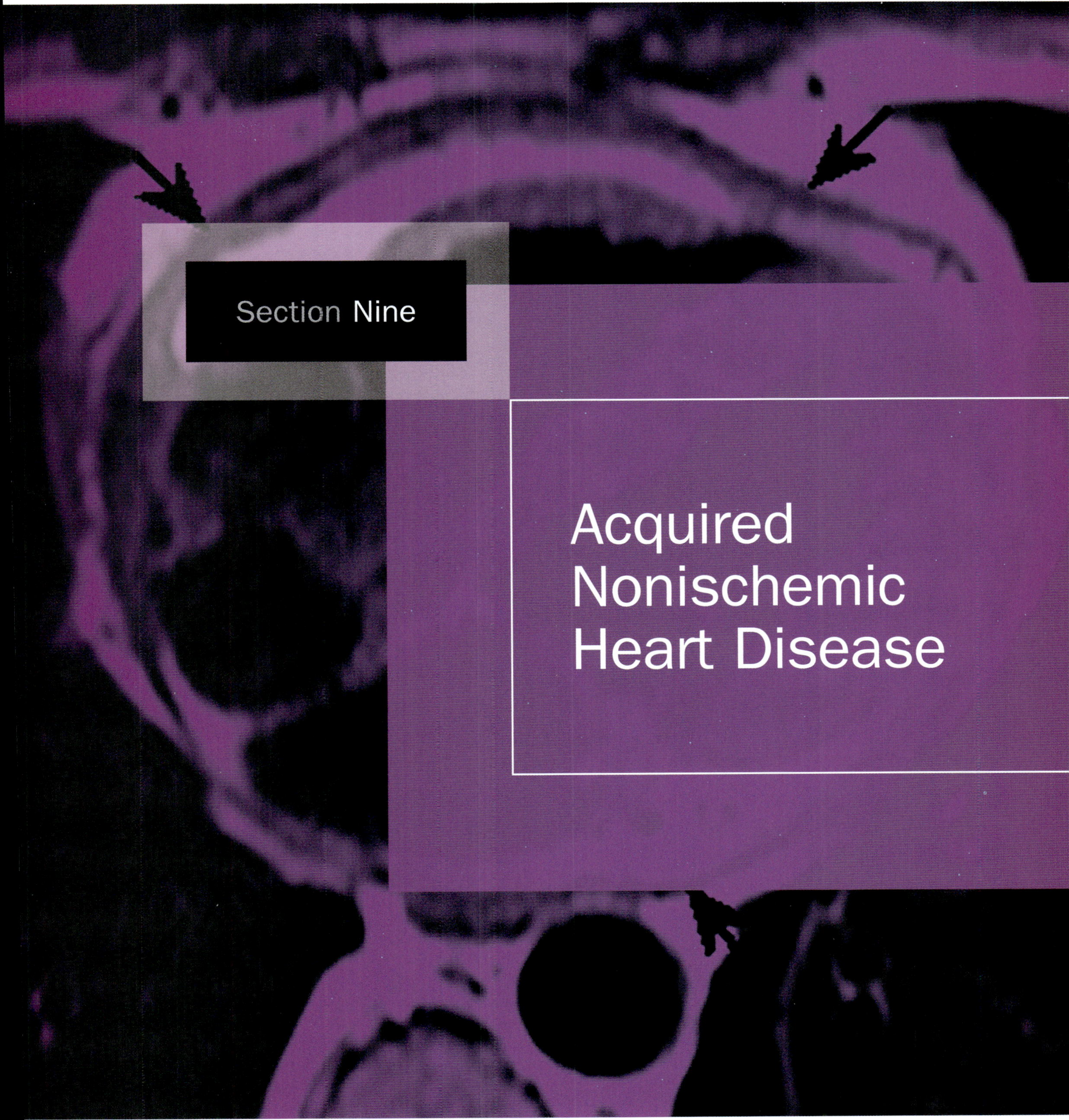

Section Nine

Acquired Nonischemic Heart Disease

Chapter 33

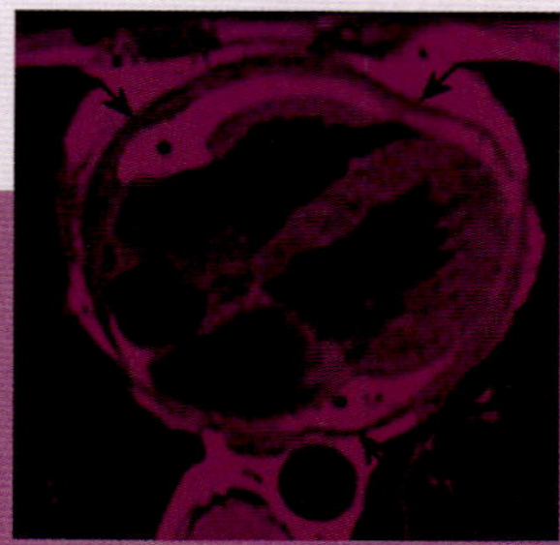

Daniel Ocazionez • Karen G. Ordovas

Valvular Heart Disease

INTRODUCTION OF IMAGING MODALITIES

The goals of imaging in valvular heart disease are as follows:

1. Identification of stenosis or insufficiency of one or more valves.
2. Estimation of the pressure gradient (or valve orifice area) and severity of regurgitation (regurgitant fraction).
3. Quantification and sequential monitoring of chamber volumes, mass, and function.
4. Determination of response to therapy.

Echocardiography is the first-line imaging modality for the evaluation of valvular heart disease. For the most part, it provides definitive diagnoses and assessment of severity of valvular dysfunction. The echocardiographic aspects of valvular heart disease are the topic of a number of chapters in other textbooks. The current role of angiography in valvular heart disease is the exclusion of significant coronary artery disease before surgery or as a contributing factor for heart failure in these patients. Currently, noninvasive imaging of coronary arteries by multidetector cardiac computed tomography angiography (CCTA) has almost replaced coronary angiography for these purposes.

All valvular lesions exert a stress on the supporting ventricle or atrium. Valvular stenosis exerts a pressure overload in the chamber, which involves the compensatory mechanism of myocardial hypertrophy. Regurgitation exerts a volume overload in the chamber, which may lead to chamber dilatation. Eventually, these compensatory mechanisms are dissipated, and in the advanced stage of valvular heart disease, myocardial failure and low cardiac output state ensue.

Chest radiograph is usually the first imaging modality used to evaluate patients with suspected valvular heart disease. Although there is significant overlap in the radiographic appearance of different valvular heart diseases, some imaging findings are quite suggestive of a specific diagnosis. The most common example is the presence of left atrial enlargement in patients with mitral regurgitation, and the presence of ascending aorta dilatation in patients with aortic stenosis. A detailed approach to x-ray interpretation in acquire heart disease can be found in Chapter 31.

Cardiac magnetic resonance (CMR) can be used to identify valvular dysfunction and to assess the effect of the lesion on ventricular volumes, mass, and function. In addition to identifying stenosis and regurgitation, the gradient across stenotic valves and volume of valvular regurgitation can be quantified. Sequential CMR studies can be used for monitoring the severity of the valvular lesion and ventricular function over time and in response to therapy.

Cine MR imaging is the preferred sequence to identify abnormal flow jets across a dysfunctional valve. It consists of multiple gradient echo or balanced steady-state free precession (SSFP) images in which the blood under normal flow conditions has bright (white) signal intensity. SSFP is the preferred sequence nowadays given the high speed of acquisition. High-velocity flow jet, such as occurs with the flow across a valvular stenosis or the retrograde flow across a regurgitant orifice, produces a signal void (low-signal region within the bright signal of the blood pool). The currently employed SSFP cine sequence mitigates the signal void of high-velocity flow. Therefore, the size of the flow jet in SSFP images should not be used to determine severity of the valvular lesion.

Quantification of ventricular mass and function can be done precisely from a three-dimensional set of cine MR images that can be acquired in any plane. In contrast to echocardiography, CMR does not rely on geometric assumptions or calculations based on partial sampling of the cardiac volume. Typically, a set of contiguous tomograms encompassing the entire heart from the apex to the bifurcation of the pulmonary artery is acquired. Cine MR images typically are acquired at 16 or more phases of the cardiac cycle. These images can be laced together and displayed in a cinematic format. When viewed in the cinematic format, it is possible to assess global right ventricular (RV) and LV function and to assess wall thickening and motion to define regional myocardial function. The optimal technique for maximizing contrast between blood and myocardium is the use of b-SSFP sequences—true fast imaging with steady precession, balanced fast-field echo.

Cine MR imaging can also be used for calculation of right and left atrial (LA) size. These are usually performed on both vertical long-axis and horizontal long-axis planes during peak ventricular systole, using either biplanar or monoplanar methodology similar to that performed with echocardiography.

Ventricular cavity volumes are simply calculated as the sum of the cavity area times the slice thickness (Fig. 33.1). Interobserver variabilities for left ventricular (LV) end-diastolic volume and LV end-systolic volume have been shown to be very small. Mass measurements are highly accurate, with excellent interstudy and interobserver variabilities for LV mass of less than 5%. Because interstudy variabilities of ventricular volumetric and mass measurements by cine MR imaging are small, this technique is ideal for serial imaging while monitoring the effectiveness of therapy in patients with aortic stenosis.

<u>Velocity encoded cine (VEC) MRI</u> is the most useful sequence for quantification of valvular regurgitation or stenosis. It measures the phase shifts that accumulate as hydrogen nuclei move through a magnetic field gradient relative to stationary tissues. The net phase shifts of protons within various voxels are displayed in gray levels, in proportion to the degree of phase shift. Because the magnitude of phase shift is basically proportional to motion over time, VEC MRI can be used to measure flow velocity along the plane of encoded velocity. The velocity-encoding direction can be selected in any orientation or in all three dimensions. Reconstruction of VEC data provides a magnitude image (anatomic information) and a phase image (velocity information in selected encoded direction; Fig. 33.2A). The cross-sectional area of the vessel can be measured by drawing a region of interest on the magnitude image. The same region of interest is then applied on the corresponding phase image, where spatial mean velocity is measured. The product of area and spatial mean velocity provides the instantaneous flow volume for a specific time frame of the cardiac cycle. Integration of all instantaneous flow volumes throughout the cardiac cycle (usually 16 or more phases) gives volume flow per heartbeat (see Fig. 33.2B). This technique has been validated in vitro with flow phantoms and in vivo by comparing flow measurements in the pulmonary artery and the aorta with left and right stroke volumes measured by cine MRI in healthy volunteers.

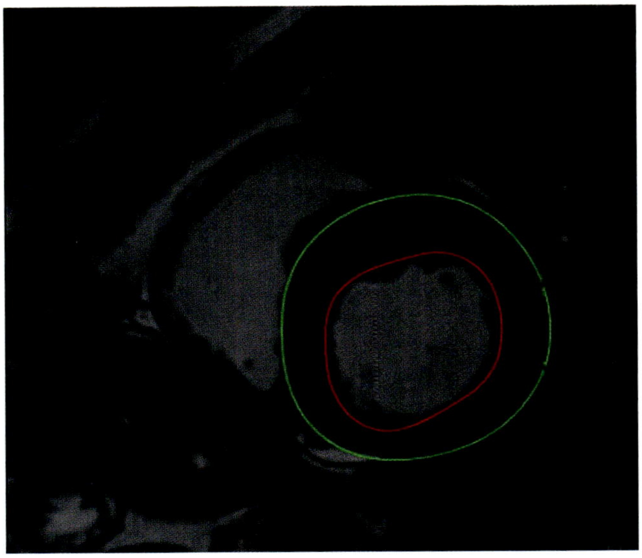

Figure 33.1. Short axis steady state free-precession image shows method for volumetric quantification with cardiac magnetic resonance. Stack images are obtained encompassing the entire heart. The red line delineates the endocardial contour outlining the chamber area for one slice. Quantification software calculates the volume of the chamber by multiplying area by slice thickness and adding the volumes from all slices that contain the chamber in question. Green light delineates the epicardial contour which outlines the myocardial and chamber volumes. Subtracting the red area from the green area provides the myocardial volume, which is multiplied by a constant to yield myocardial mass.

CCT has emerged as a critical tool for anatomic assessment of cardiac valves mostly for planning and postprocedure assessment of surgical or transcatheter valvular interventions such as transcatheter aortic valve replacement and mitral valve replacement. The high spatial resolution and ability for cardiac gating allows for precise measurement of the valvular annulus and structures around it to guide selection of appropriate devices. Depiction of amount of calcification in valvular stenotic leaflets and annuli are great applications of CCT in valvular heart disease. CCT can also be used for quantification of chamber size and function, but echocardiography and CMR are best for this application.

AORTIC STENOSIS

Aortic stenosis usually is described at three anatomic levels: supravalvular, valvular, and subvalvular. The classification of the types of aortic stenoses is presented in Table 33.1.

<u>*Supravalvular aortic stenosis*</u> is nearly always a congenital anomaly, either as an isolated lesion or as part of Williams' syndrome. The supravalvular narrowing has roughly three configurations: focal constriction at the sinotubular junction (hourglass configuration) with poststenotic dilation of the mid and distal ascending aorta, focal membrane at the sinotubular junction, and tubular narrowing from the sinotubular junction to just below the origin of the innominate artery. Williams' syndrome is characterized by hypercalcemia, elfin facies, variable mental retardation and characteristic personality ("cocktail party personality"), hypertension, and additional peripheral arterial stenoses. Concomitant cardiovascular lesions variably associated with supravalvular aortic stenosis include (1) aortic and pulmonary valvular stenoses,

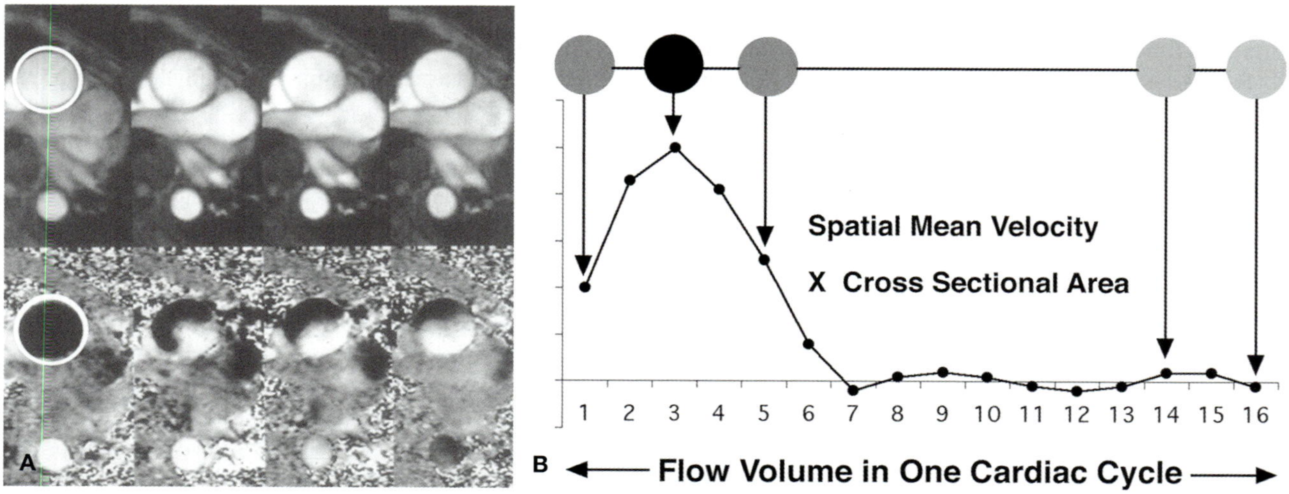

Figure 33.2. A: Four magnitude **(top)** and phase **(bottom)** images acquired during the cardiac cycle to measure blood flow in the aorta. Regions of interest are drawn around the aorta on magnitude images to measure cross-sectional area and around phase images to measure spatial average velocity. Volumetric flow is the product of cross-sectional area and spatial average velocity. **B:** Schematic diagram of aortic blood flow versus time curve during an average cardiac cycle. Each point on the curve is derived from a pair of images acquired at 16 time points during a cardiac cycle.

(2) peripheral pulmonary arterial stenoses, (3) diffuse hypoplasia of the aorta, (4) discrete stenoses of branches of the aortic arch and abdominal aorta, and (5) stenoses at the origin of the coronary arteries. However, the coronary arteries usually are ectatic because they originate below the obstruction at the sinotubular junction and are thereby subjected to elevated pressure. Rarely, supravalvular stenosis is acquired.

Table 33.1 Classification of Aortic Stenosis

Supravalvular
Congenital
Hourglass shape
Membranes or fibrous diaphragm
Diffuse
Acquired (aortitis; operative scarring)
Valvular
Congenital
Bicuspid
Unicuspid
Primitive (dysplastic)
Annular hypoplasia
Acquired
Rheumatic
Degenerative
Subvalvular
Congenital
Membranous
Fibromuscular tunnel
Extra mitral valve tissue
Idiopathic hypertrophic subaortic stenosis (hypertrophic cardiomyopathy—asymmetric type)

This can be a sequela of aortitis. Another possible cause is exaggerated scarring at the site of aortotomy performed for aortic valve replacement.

Valvular aortic stenosis may have either a congenital or an acquired etiology. The most common congenital cause is a bicuspid aortic valve. A less common cause is a unicuspid valve; this type of valve causes more severe stenosis, usually presenting in the first year of life. A rarer pathology is the primitive valve, usually consisting of a hypoplastic annulus containing a ring of gelatinous tissue. This lesion also presents most often during infancy. Rheumatic valvular aortic stenosis commonly occurs in association with mitral stenosis or regurgitation. Degenerative aortic stenosis is now the most frequent cause of calcific aortic stenosis in the adult. Although degenerative aortic stenosis once was considered to be a result of premature fibrosis and calcification of a bicuspid aortic valve, it is now also recognized as degeneration of tricuspid aortic valves in elderly patients. The bicuspid aortic valve degenerates into hemodynamically significant aortic stenosis in the fourth and fifth decade; the tricuspid aortic valve degenerates into hemodynamically significant stenosis usually after the sixth decade. With the aging of the population, this type of aortic stenosis is becoming the most commonly encountered type. All types of acquired aortic stenosis are characterized by heavy calcification (calcific aortic stenosis).

Subvalvular Aortic Stenosis

Congenital subvalvular aortic stenosis is most commonly caused by a thin membrane situated within 1 cm beneath the aortic cusps. Other types consist of a discrete fibromuscular ring or tunnel-like narrowing of the left ventricular outflow tract (LVOT). Redundant gelatinous tissue attached to the anterior mitral valve leaflet also may rarely cause subvalvular stenosis, either alone or as part of an endocardial cushion anomaly. Muscular subaortic stenosis is caused by the asymmetric basal form of hypertrophic cardiomyopathy. It is usually due to the combination of asymmetric hypertrophy of the basal septum and systolic anterior motion of the anterior leaflet of the mitral valve.

Chest Radiograph

The findings on chest x-ray in **valvular aortic stenosis** depend on the severity and level of the obstruction and the age at presentation (Chapter 31). The x-ray image in infants presenting with symptoms of heart failure is characterized by pulmonary edema and cardiomegaly. Cardiomegaly without pulmonary edema may also occur. On the other hand, x-rays in older children and adults may display only enlargement of the ascending aorta. In the presence of severe LV hypertrophy (reduced ventricular compliance) or with the onset of myocardial failure, pulmonary venous hypertension or edema may become evident. This usually occurs late in the natural history of uncomplicated valvular aortic stenosis. The extent and density of aortic valvular leaflet calcification roughly parallel the severity of the stenosis in adults before the seventh decade. On the other hand, ascending aortic dilation does not correlate with severity of stenosis and may be substantial with a nonobstructive bicuspid valve.

Supravalvular aortic stenosis may cause a narrow base of the heart with inconspicuous ascending aortic region (right superior mediastinum; see Chapter 31). With **subvalvular aortic stenosis**, enlargement of the ascending aorta often is not evident on the chest x-ray. Ascending aortic enlargement is discernible in about 50% of patients with the membranous type of subvalvular stenosis.

Cardiac Magnetic Resonance

CMR can be used to identify the presence and quantify the severity of aortic valve stenosis. It can also demonstrate associated abnormalities such as ascending aorta dilatation and left ventricular hypertrophy. A summary of MRI abnormalities in aortic stenosis can be seen on Table 33.2.

Identification of Aortic Stenosis - Aortic stenosis is identified using cine MR images, usually in the left ventricular outflow tract or coronal plane. Cine images show an area of signal loss distal to the valve during systole (Fig. 33.3). At moderately increased velocities, the flow jet has decreased signal, but at very high velocities, the center of the jet shows high signal while the periphery may show a signal void (Fig. 33.4). The central hyperintensity corresponds to the vena contracta.

Estimation of the Valve Gradient—The valve gradient is estimated using velocity-encoded cine, usually with an acquisition plane aligned to the direction of blood flow (in plane). The peak velocity can be identified within the voxels of the phase image by placing a region of interest around the jet (Fig. 33.6). Peak systolic jet velocities over 5.0 m/s have been measured with this technique in patients with aortic stenosis. Using the measurement of peak velocity by VEC MR imaging, the pressure gradient can be estimated by the modified Bernoulli equation as $\Delta P = 4V^2$, where ΔP = pressure drop across the stenosis (mm Hg) and V = peak velocity (m/s). An example of the use of VEC to estimate the gradient across valvular aortic stenosis as derived from VEC measurement of a peak velocity of 4 m/s looks like this:

$$\Delta P = 4V^2$$
$$\Delta P = 4(4)^2$$
$$\Delta P = 64 \text{ mm Hg}$$

Table 33.2 CMR Features of Valvular Aortic Stenosis

1. Thickening and limitation of systolic excursion of cusps
2. ± Bicuspid aortic valve
3. High-velocity jet (central increased signal and peripheral signal void) on cine—SSFP
4. Dilatation of proximal ascending aorta
5. Symmetric increase in LV wall thickness (≥12 mm)
6. Increase in LV mass—measured at end diastole on cine—SSFP in short-axis plane
7. Hyperdynamic LV contraction in compensated state

LV, left ventricular; SSFP, steady-state free precession.

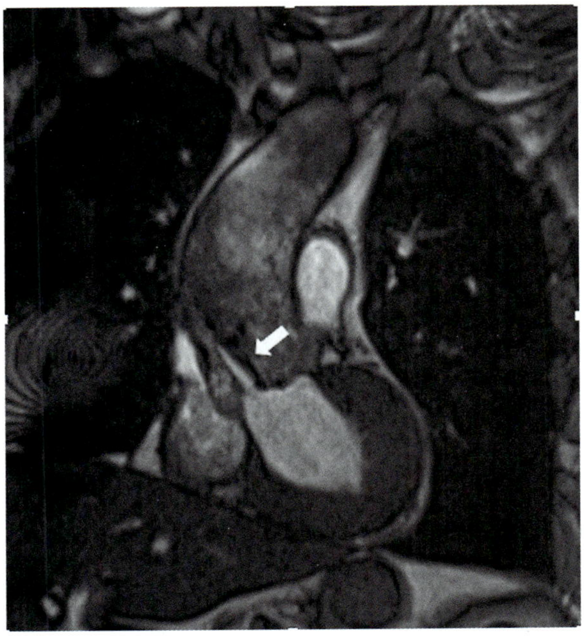

Figure 33.3. Cine steady-state free precession magnetic resonance image and supplemental video in the coronal plane during systole demonstrates a signal void emanating from the aortic valve in a patient with valvular aortic stenosis (arrow). Note the post-stenotic dilatation of the ascending aorta.

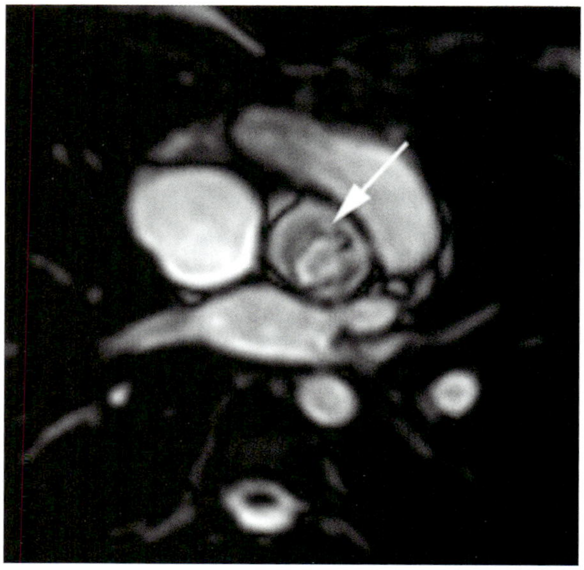

Figure 33.4. Cine magnetic resonance image and supplemental video parallel to the aortic valve orifice shows a high-intensity flow jet (*arrow*) and thickened aortic valve leaflets in a patient with aortic stenosis.

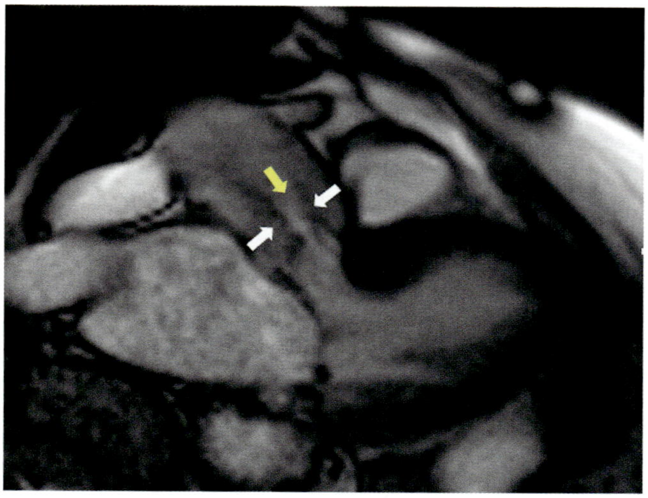

Figure 33.5. Cine steady-state free precession magnetic resonance image and supplemental video in the left ventricular outflow tract plane in systole shows a flow jet starting at the level of the aortic valve and extending to the ascending aorta. Periphery of the flow jet shows low signal intensity (white *arrows*), and center of the flow jet (yellow arrow) shows increased signal intensity (vena contracta).

However, it should be noted that this measurement by VEC has limitations. The number of images reconstructed for a cardiac cycle may lack temporal resolution for capturing the exact instant when peak velocity occurs. The direction of flow encoding may differ from the flow direction of the jet. These limitations can be minimized by using three-dimensional flow encoding, but this further reduces temporal resolution. Therefore, echocardiography is considered a superior method for calculation of pressure gradient across a stenotic valve.

Calculation of the Aortic Valve Orifice Area - The estimated gradient is dependent on the stroke volume, ejection time, and aortic pressure. It provides an incomplete assessment of severity of aortic stenosis. Indeed, depression of LV myocardial contractile state may cause the gradient to decline when heart failure ensues in end-stage decompensated aortic stenosis. Consequently, it is important to determine the aortic valve area which can be performed with CMR (Figs. 33.7 and 33.8). Severe AS is defined as an

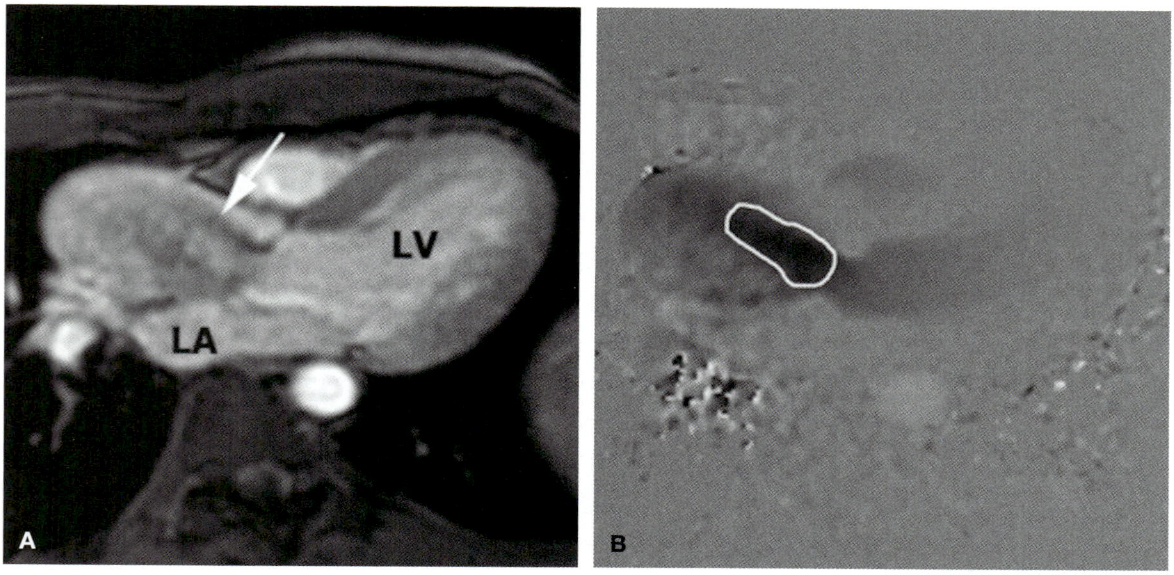

Figure 33.6. Magnitude **(A)** and phase **(B)** images from velocity-encoded cine magnetic resonance sequence on the left ventricular outflow tract plane in systole show a flow jet (*arrow*) in the ascending aorta starting at the level of the aortic valve, consistent with aortic stenosis. A manual region of interest outlines the area containing the peak velocity in the phase image. LA, left atrium; LV, left ventricle.

aortic valve area less than 1.0 cm^2 (less than 0.60 cm^2/m^2). Cine views parallel to the aortic valve annulus can show the number of valve leaflets, excursion of leaflets, and the aortic valve orifice (Fig. 33.8). These images can be used to measure the maximum aortic valve area. The orifice area can also be measured with VEC MRI by acquiring a through plane image at the level of the origin of the flow jet (Fig. 33.7). As an alternative, application of the continuity equation on VEC MRI profiles in the LVOT (velocity measured below the valve) and aorta (Ao) (just above the valve in the aorta) can also be used. The velocity time integral (VTI) is measured for systolic forward flow in both planes (planes perpendicular to LVOT and Ao. The aortic valve area A (centimeters squared) is given by:

$$A_{Ao} = A_{LVOT}\left(\frac{VTI_{LVOT}}{VTI_{Ao}}\right)$$

where A_{LVOT} = LVOT area in cm^2, VTI_{LVOT} is LVOT VTI, and VTI_{Ao} is A_O VTI.

Quantification of Chamber Volumes, Mass, and Function - Patients with moderate to severe aortic stenosis may develop global hypertrophy of the LV, which can be quantified with cine MR images by calculation of left ventricular wall mass. Advanced aortic stenosis may progress to systolic dysfunction and enlargement of the LV, which can also be quantified with cine MR.

Evaluation of Ascending Aorta - In patients with aortic stenosis, there is usually poststenotic enlargement of the proximal ascending aorta (greater than 4.0 cm or 2.2 cm/m^2) (Fig. 33.3). This is especially so for some types of bicuspid aortic valves as these patients have abnormal aortic wall composition (aortopathy). The dimensions of the ascending aorta can be initially made and monitored with cine MR imaging in the axial plane or a plane perpendicular to the long axis of the ascending aorta. However, magnetic resonance angiography with or without contrast is the prefer method for quantification of aortic size.

Cardiac Computed Tomography

The most common finding of aortic stenosis on CCT is extensive calcifications of the aortic valve leaflets. The degree of aortic calcification is associated with the degree of stenosis, particularly in women. CT planimetry can also be performed for measurement of the maximum aortic valve orifice area by displaying peak systolic images in a plane aligned to the tip of the leaflets following the same principles described for CMR imaging. CCT is particularly useful to interrogate complications after aortic valve interventions. Perivalvular lesions such as abscess in endocarditis can be clearly delineated (Fig. 33.9). The use of 4DCT is also an excellent adjuvant in cases of prosthetic valvular dysfunction and can show abnormalities such as in hypoattenuated leaflet thickening (Fig. 33.10), Detailed review of CCT for planning and following up aortic valve interventions is shown in Chapter 42.

AORTIC REGURGITATION

Aortic regurgitation imposes a volume overload on the left ventricle as a consequence of retrograde flow across the aortic valve during diastole. Because of the excessive diastolic volume, the left ventricle becomes dilated. Regurgitation may be caused by lack of coaptation of the valvular cusps, annular dilatation, or ascending aortic dilatation. Aortic

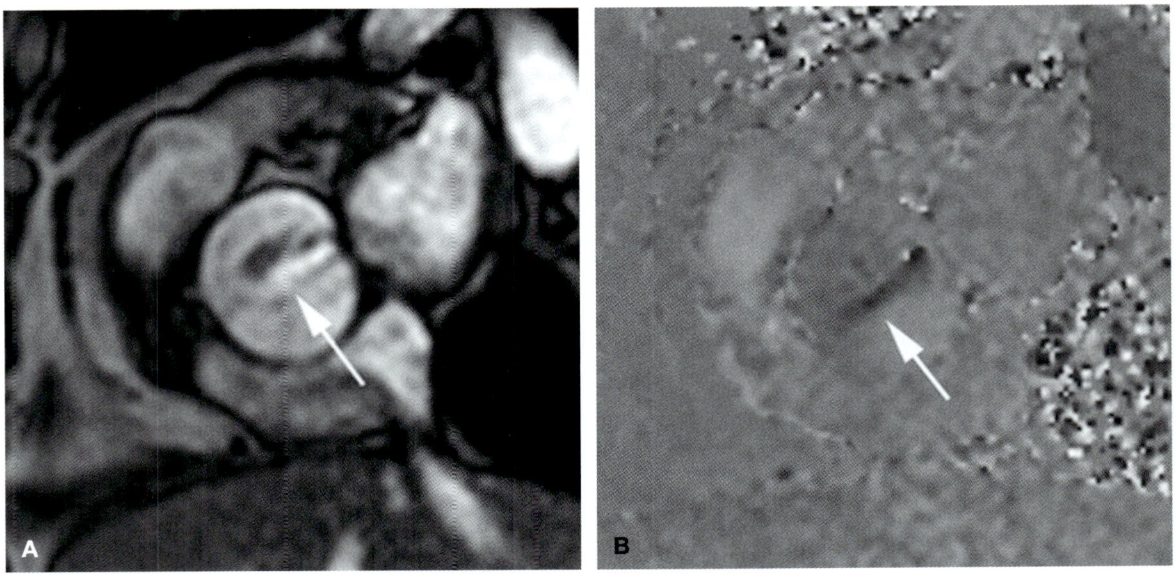

Figure 33.7. Magnitude **(A)** and phase **(B)** images from velocity-encoded magnetic resonance sequence parallel to the aortic valve orifice show the blood flow (*arrows*) across the maximum opening of the valve at peak systole. The valve area was measured as 0.9 cm^2 (0.45 cm^2/m^2).

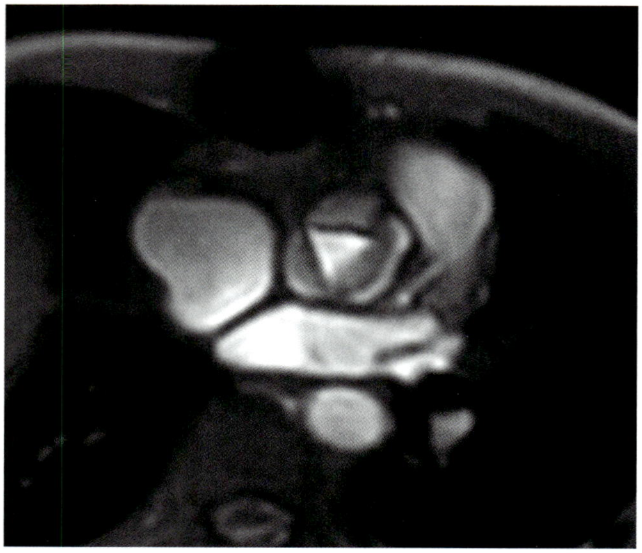

Figure 33.8. Aortic stenosis of tricuspid aortic valve. Cine MR image and supplemental video in aortic valve orifice plane show mild limitation of execution of cusps at peak systole.

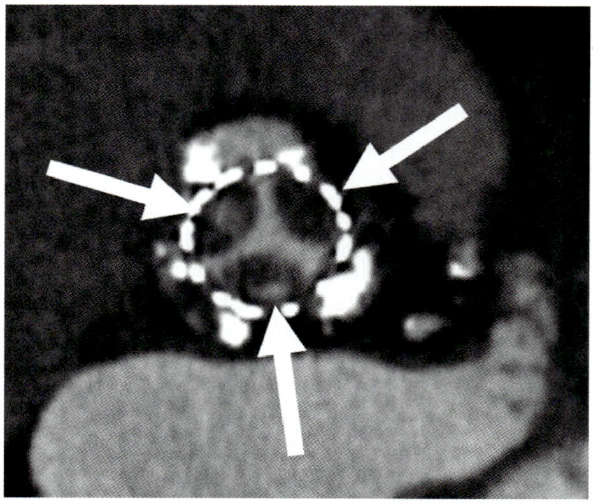

Figure 33.10. Hypoattenuated leaflet thickening. Axial contrast enhanced CT image at the level of the aortic root in this patient status post transcatheter aortic valve replacement demonstrating diffuse hypo-attenuated thickening of the aortic valve leaflets (white arrows) consistent with thrombosis.

regurgitation has a number of possible etiologies (Table 33.3); moreover, it may be a component of several systemic diseases and inherited syndromes (Table 33.4). With some causes, there may be abnormalities at more than one site (eg, Marfan syndrome, annuloaortic ectasia, and relapsing polychondritis).

Chest Radiograph

Findings on chest x-ray are governed by the severity and chronicity of aortic regurgitation and whether there is associated pathology of the ascending aorta (see Chapter 31).

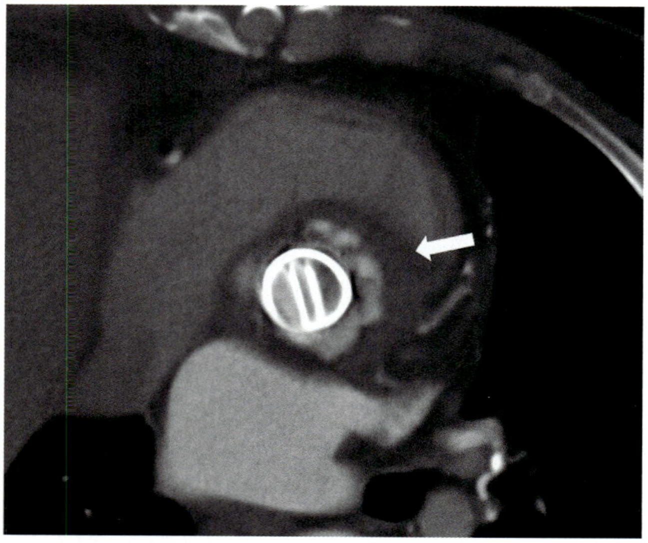

Figure 33.9. Prosthetic aortic valve abscess. Axial CT contrast enhanced image showing prosthetic aortic valve with diffuse periprosthetic thickening and phlegmonous changes (arrow).

The typical features of chronic regurgitation are (1) absence of pulmonary venous hypertension or edema, (2) cardiomegaly due to LV enlargement, and (3) ascending aorta and arch enlargement. Pulmonary venous hypertension and edema usually occur late in the natural history of chronic aortic regurgitation and signify the onset of myocardial failure. On the other hand, acute regurgitation such as occurs with infective endocarditis may produce severe pulmonary edema even with normal cardiac size.

Table 33.3 Etiology of Aortic Regurgitation

Aortic cusps abnormality
Bicuspid aortic valve
Rheumatic disease
Infective endocarditis
Supracristal ventricular septal defect
Syphilis
Aortic annulus abnormality
Aortoannular ectasia
Systemic hypertension
Marfan syndrome
Aortic dissection (type A)
Ankylosing spondylitis
Relapsing polychondritis
Ascending aorta abnormality
Aortoannular ectasia
Marfan syndrome
Ehlers-Danlos syndrome
Loeys-Dietz syndrome
Aortic dissection (type A)
Relapsing polychondritis
Ascending aortic aneurysm

Table 33.4 Systematic Diseases or Inherited Syndromes Associated With Aortic Regurgitation

Inherited syndromes
Marfan syndrome
Ehlers-Danlos syndrome
Loeys-Dietz syndrome
Osteogenesis imperfecta
Pseudoxanthoma elasticum
Systemic diseases
Rheumatoid arthritis
Rheumatoid variants
Ankylosing spondylitis
Psoriatic arthritis
Reiter's syndrome
Relapsing polychondritis
Giant cell aortitis
Syphilis (luetic aortitis)

Cardiac Magnetic Resonance

CMR is used to identify the presence and quantify the volume of aortic regurgitation. It also is used to monitor the effect of regurgitation on LV volumes, mass, and function (Table 33.5).

Identification of Aortic Regurgitation—Cine MR imaging demonstrates the regurgitant jet as a signal void. This signal void emanates from the closed aortic valve and projects into the left ventricle during most or all of the diastolic period (Fig. 33.11).

Quantification of Regurgitant Volume - Cine MR imaging can be used for assessment of regurgitant volume by determining RV and LV stroke volumes. In the normal subject, RV stroke volume is nearly equivalent to LV stroke volume. Stroke volumes are calculated from a stack of MR images as the difference between end-diastolic and end-systolic volumes of each ventricle. The regurgitant volume can be calculated by the difference between RV and LV stroke volumes. These calculations are valid only for patients with a single regurgitant valve. In patients with combined aortic and mitral regurgitation, this method assesses the total regurgitant volume of the left side of the heart. Aortic regurgitant fraction is calculated as the regurgitant volume divided by the LV stroke volume.

Table 33.5 CMR Features of Aortic Regurgitation

1. Diastolic signal void starting at closed aortic valve on cine MRI
2. Increased LV stroke volume (effective stroke volume + regurgitant volume)
3. Increased LV end-diastolic and end-systolic volumes
4. Forward (stroke volume) and retrograde flow (regurgitant volume) on VEC (phase contrast) MRI

CMR, cardiac magnetic resonance; LV, left ventricular; VEC, velocity encoded cine.

VEC MRI can also be used to calculate the regurgitant volume and regurgitant fraction of the aortic valve. This assessment can be done in two different ways. First, the regurgitant volume can be assessed by the difference between the systolic flow in the ascending aorta (LV stroke volume) and the systolic flow in the main pulmonary artery (RV stroke volume). The two-stroke volumes are calculated from time-integrated measurements of flow volumes during systole on imaging perpendicular to the proximal ascending and another perpendicular to the main pulmonary. Aortic regurgitant volume is the value of: LV stroke volume – RV stroke volume.

VEC MRI can discriminate between antegrade and retrograde flow during the cardiac cycle, enabling retrograde flow to be measured directly to quantify regurgitation. For example, bright voxels in the ascending aorta during systole indicate antegrade flow, whereas dark voxels in diastole represent retrograde flow caused by aortic regurgitation (Fig. 33.11). High accuracy and interstudy reproducibility ($r = 0.97$) of VEC MRI measurement of retrograde diastolic flow in the ascending aorta have been found in patients with chronic aortic regurgitation. Diastolic retrograde aortic flow equals aortic regurgitant volume (Fig. 33.12). The measurements of regurgitant volume and fraction by this method correlate closely with volumetric cine MRI measurements. Measurement of regurgitant volume by this has a high interstudy reproducibility, which allows for follow-up and monitoring response to therapy in patients with aortic regurgitation. The severity of regurgitation of the aortic valve is based on the regurgitant fraction: less than 15% (mild); 15% to 30% (moderate); >30% (severe).

Quantification of Chamber Volumes, Mass, and Function—Cine MRI can disclose the typical effect of aortic

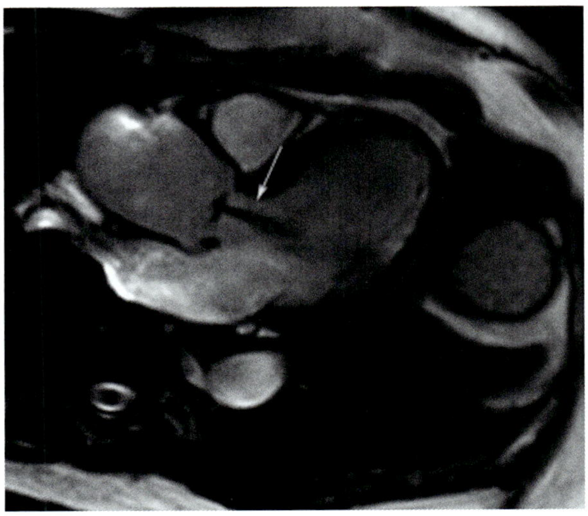

Figure 33.11. Aortic regurgitation Cine magnetic resonance image and supplemental video in left ventricular outflow tract plane in diastole. Balanced fast-field echo image in mid diastole shows signal void (*arrow*) emanating from aortic valve.

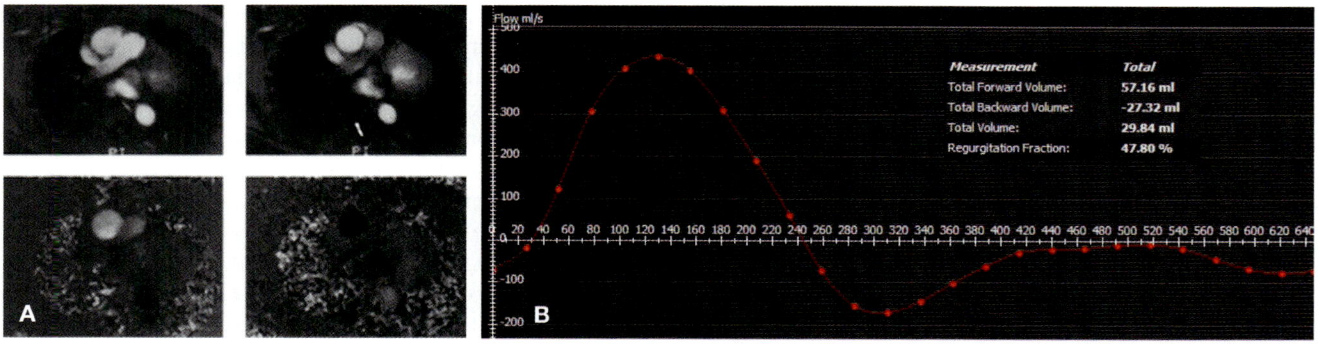

Figure 33.12. A: Velocity-encoded cine magnetic resonance images in the axial plane in aortic regurgitation. Magnitude **(top)** and phase **(bottom)** images in systole **(left)** and diastole **(right)**. Note that on the phase images antegrade flow in systole is represented by bright voxels, whereas retrograde flow (aortic regurgitation) in diastole is represented by dark voxels in the ascending aorta. **B:** A flow versus time curve derived from image pairs at 16 phases of the cardiac cycle shows negative values (retrograde flow) in diastole. The area under the curve with negative values is the volume of aortic regurgitation which was calculated at 48%.

regurgitation on the left ventricle. According to the severity of regurgitation, there is an increase in LV end-diastolic and end-systolic volumes. Although LV wall thickness may be within the normal range (less than 12 mm at end-diastole), the total LV mass may be increased substantially because of the increase in end-diastolic volume (mass = mean wall thickness × end-diastolic volume). Cine MRI demonstrates elevated LV stroke volume. The total stroke volume consists of the effective stroke volume and regurgitant volume. During the compensated phase of aortic regurgitation, the effective stroke volume remains in the normal range.

The following formulas are relevant for aortic regurgitation assessment:

$$\text{Total LV stroke volume} = \text{effective stroke volume} + \text{regurgitant volume}$$

$$\text{Regurgitant volume} = \text{LV stroke volume} - \text{RV stroke volume}$$

$$\text{Regurgitant fraction} = \frac{\text{regurgitant volume}}{\text{total LV stroke volume}}$$

Cardiac Computed Tomography

The main application of CCT for the assessment of aortic regurgitation is to provide accurate measurement of the aortic valve annulus for surgical or transcatheter intervention planning. Although volumetric and functional assessment can be done with CCT, CMR and echocardiography are preferred given lack of radiation and need for contrast media.

MITRAL STENOSIS

Mitral stenosis usually is acquired and nearly always caused by rheumatic fever. It is the salient lesion of rheumatic heart disease. Other etiologies are rare; these include congenital valvular, subvalvular (parachute mitral valve), or supravalvular stenoses; left atrial myxoma; and exuberant mitral annular calcification. Mitral stenosis often is accompanied by a variable degree of mitral regurgitation.

Mitral stenosis causes elevated left atrial pressure throughout diastole. Elevation of pulmonary venous pressures may follow, which leads to pulmonary arterial hypertension if severe and sustained. In long-standing mitral stenosis, pulmonary arterial hypertension may be severe, and pulmonary regurgitation eventually ensues across a dilated pulmonary annulus. The right ventricle eventually dilates, causing tricuspid regurgitation from a dilated annulus.

Chest Radiograph

The chest x-ray provides good insight into the severity of mitral stenosis by showing the relative severity of pulmonary venous hypertension (see Chapter 31). In mild disease, there may be only equalization or reversal of the diameter of upper and lower lobe pulmonary vessels (cephalization). In more severe disease or with an imposed hypervolemic state, interstitial pulmonary edema or alveolar pulmonary edema becomes evident. Interlobular septal thickening (Kerley B lines) usually is a sign of interstitial edema but may become permanent as a consequence of fibrosis or deposition of hemosiderin after multiple episodes of pulmonary edema. Rarely, high-density nodules (ossific nodules) in the lower lobes may be a consequence of multiple episodes of alveolar pulmonary edema and hemorrhage.

In compensated mitral stenosis, only mild cardiomegaly or normal heart size is seen. The left atrium invariably is enlarged, causing a right retrocardiac double density. A convexity on the upper left cardiac border in the frontal view indicates enlargement of the left atrial appendage. This finding nearly always is evident in rheumatic mitral stenosis. Enlargement of the pulmonary arterial segment and right heart indicates pulmonary arterial hypertension.

Enlargement of the right heart in the absence of pulmonary arterial enlargement usually indicates concomitant rheumatic tricuspid regurgitation. The ascending aorta and aortic arch are characteristically small in isolated mitral valve disease. Even slight prominence of the thoracic aorta should raise suspicion of associated rheumatic aortic valve disease.

Cardiac Magnetic Resonance

CMR can be used to identify mitral valvular stenosis and any associated mitral regurgitation; estimate the gradient across the valve; and quantify chamber volumes, mass, and function (Table 33.6).

Identification of Mitral Stenosis—Cine MR images demonstrate a signal void emanating from the opened mitral valve in ventricular diastole and projecting into the left ventricle (Fig. 33.13). This signal void is depicted well on images acquired in the vertical or horizontal long-axis planes. Associated mitral regurgitation appears as a signal void projected into the left atrium during systole. Likewise, signal voids may be recognized in right-sided cardiac chambers if there is any associated pulmonary or tricuspid regurgitation.

Estimation of the Valve Gradient—VEC MRI is rarely used for this purpose. It can be acquired in a plane perpendicular or parallel to the stenotic jet to sample the peak velocity of the jet of mitral stenosis. The diastolic phase image containing the highest velocities can be selected. Then, the voxels with peak velocity on that phase image can be sought for calculation of pressure gradient using the modified Bernoulli equation as previously described. In general, the MR method is expected to underestimate the pressure gradient compared with Doppler echocardiography because it has a lesser sampling rate. Comparative studies have shown a good correlation between the two techniques, but the CMR method has tended to underestimate the gradient.

Quantification of Chamber Volumes, Mass, and Function—Cine MR images are performed for quantification of LV volumes, mass, and function. As discussed earlier, cine MR imaging is a highly accurate and reproducible method of monitoring LV function. Isolated mitral stenosis usually is associated with smaller-than-average LV volumes and normal ejection fraction.

Quantification of left atrial size with CMR is usually performed for a comprehensive hemodynamic assessment of mitral stenosis severity. In severely dilated left atria, the presence of intracavitary thrombus can also be depicted as an intracavitary low signal lesion in cine MR.

Table 33.6 CMR Features of Mitral Stenosis

1. Diastolic signal void (or hyperintensity) emanating from mitral valve in diastole on cine MRI
2. Thickened and limited excursion of leaflet on cine MRI
3. Left atrial enlargement
4. Normal LV end-diastolic and end-systolic volumes
5. High-velocity flow on VEC (phase contrast) cine MRI

CMR, cardiac magnetic resonance; LV, left ventricular; VEC, velocity encoded cine.

Cardiac Computed Tomography

The most important application of CCT for mitral stenosis is the depiction of thickness and extent of mitral leaflet calcifications and precise dimensions of the mitral valve annulus. This information is important for the selection and guidance of interventional approaches. CCT can also provide accurate left atrial volume for severity assessment of mitral regurgitation. Intracavitary thrombi can also be identified when left atrium enlargement is present, depicted as a filling defect usually in the area of the appendage. Delayed CCT images can be helpful to differentiate a real LA thrombus from slow flow artifact.

MITRAL REGURGITATION

Mitral regurgitation may be caused by an abnormality of any portion of the mitral apparatus or by LV dilatation. The dysfunction may involve one or more of several components: leaflets, chordae, anterior and posterior papillary muscles, or annulus. The etiologies of mitral regurgitation are presented in Table 33.7.

Chronic mitral regurgitation produces LA and LV enlargement. Pulmonary venous hypertension or edema usually is less severe than mitral stenosis. Pulmonary arterial hypertension is less common and less severe than stenosis.

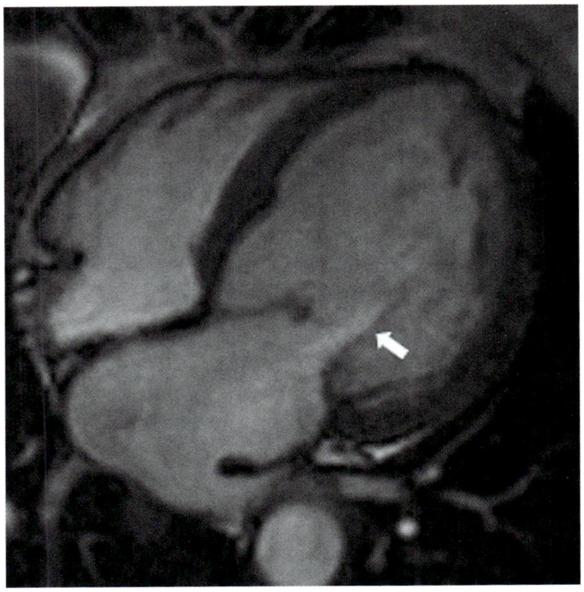

Figure 33.13. Mitral stenosis. Cine b-steady-state free precession magnetic resonance image and supplemental video in the horizonal long axis (4-chamber) plane during diastole demonstrates thickened leaflets and signal void (white arrow) emanating from the mitral valve.

Acute onset of mitral regurgitation such as with chordal or papillary muscle rupture in the setting of myocardial infarction imposes sudden onset of pulmonary venous hypertension with no time for compensating mechanisms to become operative. Severe pulmonary edema may ensue as a result. In this event, the left atrium and ventricle are normal in size.

Mitral annular calcification occasionally is the sole cause of regurgitation. The cause of the calcification usually is unknown, but such calcification occurs more often in hypertension, aortic stenosis, hypertrophic cardiomyopathy, hyperlipidemia, and hypercalcemia.

Chest Radiograph

The radiographic features of mitral regurgitation are regulated by the duration and severity of the lesion and associated lesions of the mitral and other valves (see Chapter 31). Isolated chronic mitral regurgitation is a volume overload lesion that causes LA and LV enlargement. In the absence of myocardial failure, the degree of cardiomegaly bears a rough relation to the severity of regurgitation. Signs of pulmonary venous and arterial hypertension are less prominent than with mitral stenosis. Nonrheumatic causes of mitral regurgitation usually do not cause radiographically discernible enlargement of the left atrial appendage. Acute onset of mitral regurgitation is characterized by pulmonary edema with a normal heart size. Rupture of the posterior papillary muscle or associated chordae may cause focal or more severe pulmonary edema of the right upper lobe.

Mitral valve prolapse is observed in about 5% of the population. Pathologically, it is caused by myxomatous degeneration of the mitral valve leaflets and chordae tendineae. Some patients with prolapse have mitral regurgitation, which often is mild. However, one complication that may occur—rupture of a chordae tendineae—can induce severe regurgitation. Other complications include supraventricular and ventricular arrhythmias, bacterial endocarditis, and cerebral emboli.

Table 33.7 Etiology of Mitral Regurgitation

Leaflet distortion or perforation
Rheumatic carditis
Myxomatous degeneration (mitral valve prolapse)
Bacterial endocarditis
Asymmetric form of hypertrophic cardiomyopathy
Left atrial tumor (myxoma)
Congenital (parachute mitral valve; cleft mitral valve)
Systemic lupus erythematosus
Chordae
Myxomatous degeneration (spontaneous chordal rupture)
Traumatic (weight lifting, etc.)
Bacterial endocarditis
Papillary muscle
Rupture from acute infarction
Dysfunction during myocardial ischemia
Congenital (parachute mitral valve)
Annulus
Annular dilation with left ventricular enlargement
Annular (periannular) calcification
Myxomatous degeneration

Cardiac Magnetic Resonance

CMR can be used to identify mitral regurgitation, quantify the regurgitant volume, and measure LV volumes, mass, and function (Table 33.8).

Identification of Mitral Regurgitation - Cine MR images in the axial, horizontal long axis, or vertical long axis can be employed to demonstrate the signal void caused by the flow jet of mitral regurgitation. The signal void originates at the closed valve in systole and is directed into the left atrium (Fig. 33.14).

Identification of Mitral Valve Prolapse - It is easy to distinguish mitral valve prolapse from flail. **Prolapse** is ballooning of the middle of the valve 2 mm beyond the annulus during systole; the tips of the leaflets to which the chordae attach do not pass beyond the annulus (Fig. 33.15). **Flail** is indicated by passage of the tips of the mitral leaflets beyond the annulus and into the left atrium during systole.

Quantification of Mitral Regurgitation - Mitral regurgitation is quantified using VEC MRI acquired in a plane parallel to and near the mitral annulus, usually in the ventricular size. Calculating mitral regurgitation directly from this method is complicated by through plane motion of the mitral annulus during the cardiac cycle. Another more robust approach involves measuring LV diastolic inflow across the mitral annulus and systolic outflow in the proximal ascending aorta (Fig. 33.16). In normal subjects, these values are equivalent, and each represents a measurement of stroke volume (Fig. 33.17). In mitral regurgitation, the diastolic mitral inflow exceeds the systolic aortic outflow; the difference represents the regurgitant volume (Fig. 33.16). Any concomitant aortic regurgitation invalidates this approach unless an additional VEC MR measurement is used for quantification of aortic regurgitation.

Using cine MR images, mitral regurgitation can be quantified by comparison of ventricular stroke volumes. The stroke volume of the left ventricle exceeds the stroke volume of the

Table 33.8 CMR Features of Mitral Regurgitation

1. Systolic signal void (or hyperintensity) into the left atrium during systole
2. Left atrial enlargement
3. Increased LV end-diastolic and end-systolic volumes
4. Mitral inflow greater than aortic outflow on VEC (phase contrast) MRI

CMR, cardiac magnetic resonance; LV, left ventricular; VEC, velocity encoded cine.

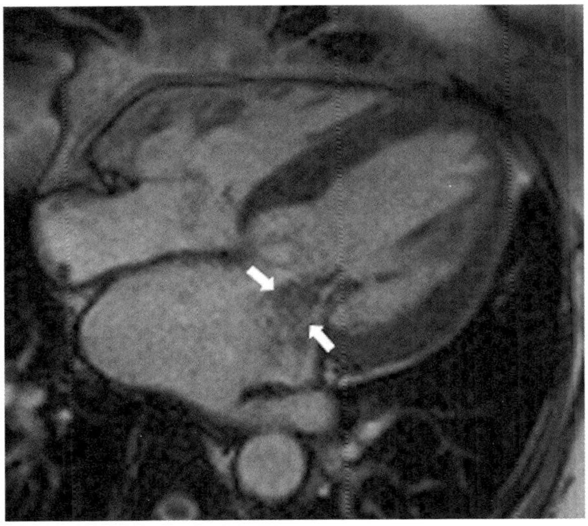

Figure 33.14. Mitral regurgitation. Cine b-steady-state free precession magnetic resonance image and supplemental video in the horizonal long axis (4-chamber) plane during systole demonstrates a signal void (white arrow) emanating from the mitral valve.

right ventricle by a volume equal to the mitral regurgitant volume. This method is valid only for isolated mitral regurgitation; it does not apply in the presence of a regurgitant lesion of the right ventricle or aortic regurgitation, unless additional VEC MR sequences are performed to interrogate those valves.

The following formulas are relevant to calculations in mitral regurgitation:

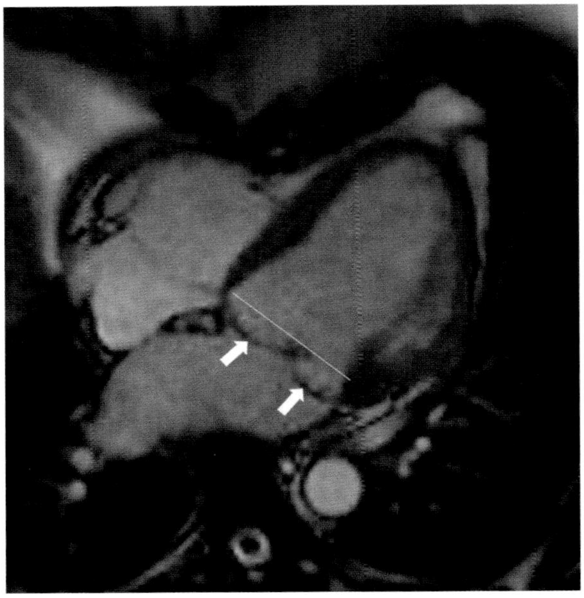

Figure 33.15. Mitral valve prolapse. Cine b-steady-state free precession magnetic resonance image and supplemental video in the horizonal long axis plane during systole demonstrates bi-leaflet mitral valve prolapse (white arrows) below the annular plane (yellow line).

$$\text{Stroke volume} = \text{end-diastolic volume} - \text{end-systolic volume}(\text{volumetric method})$$

$$\text{Mitral regurgitant volume} = \text{LV stroke volume} - \text{RV stroke volume}(\text{volumetric method})$$

$$\text{Mitral regurgitant fraction} = \frac{\text{regurgitant volume}}{\text{LV stroke volume}(\text{volumetric method})}$$

$$\text{Mitral regurgitant volume} = \text{mitral inflow} - \text{aortic outflow}(\text{VEC method})$$

$$\text{Mitral regurgitant fraction} = \frac{\text{regurgitant volume}}{\text{mitral inflow}(\text{VEC method})}$$

Quantification of Chamber Volumes, Mass, and Function—Similar to aortic regurgitation, the hemodynamic severity of mitral regurgitation can be assessed by calculation of left ventricular size and function. Chronic severe lesions lead to significant LV enlargement and decreased systolic function. Because of the precision and reproducibility of LV volumetry using cine MR images, this technique is optimal for monitoring LV volumes and function to assess therapy or to define criteria for surgical intervention. Left atrial enlargement can also be quantified with CMR and adds to the severity assessment of mitral regurgitation.

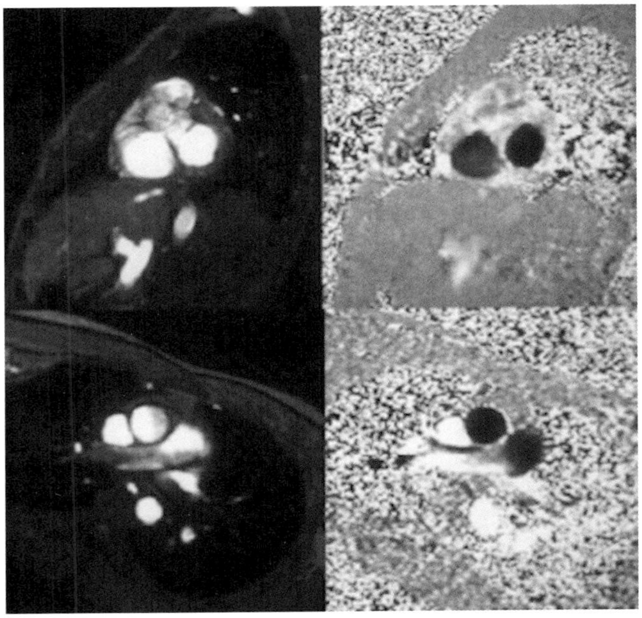

Figure 33.16. Magnitude **(left)** and phase **(right)** images at the mitral annulus **(top)** and at the proximal ascending aorta (**bottom**). These are used to measure inflow and outflow of the left ventricle. Inflow exceeds outflow volume by the mitral regurgitant volumes.

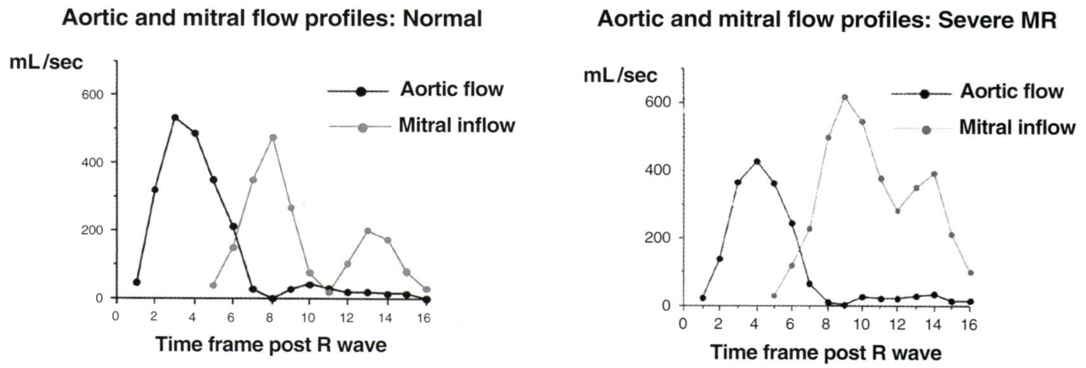

Figure 33.17. Flow versus time curve for proximal aorta (left ventricular outflow) and mitral valve (left ventricular inflow) in a normal subject and a patient with mitral regurgitation. The area under the inflow curve is considerably greater than the area under the outflow curve in the patient with mitral regurgitation.

Cardiac Computed Tomography

In patients with mitral regurgitation, the main role of CCT is to delineate the presence and extent of mitral annular calcifications (MAC). Patients with severe mitral annular calcification may pose challenges for surgical mitral valve replacement. The assessment of MAC including quantification using the new grading classification is of utmost importance and has been associated with mitral valve dysfunction, arrythmias, and endocarditis (Fig. 33.18). The presence of associated caseous degeneration of the mitral valve can be easily assessed (Fig. 33.19).

Pulmonary Stenosis

Pulmonary stenosis results when egress of blood from the right ventricle is obstructed. It can be divided into four types, depending on the level of obstruction: valvular, supravalvular, subvalvular, and midventricular. Pulmonary stenosis usually is a congenital anomaly.

Pulmonary stenosis is rarely caused by rheumatic disease. The etiology of pulmonary stenosis is given in Table 33.9. A more detailed review of pulmonary stenosis is seen in Chapters 37 and 38

Chest Radiograph

The typical feature of valvular pulmonic stenosis is enlargement of the main and left pulmonary arterial segments. In the absence of an associated intracardiac defect, there is no oligemia. Obstruction at any level may cause RV enlargement. The radiographic features of congenital pulmonic stenosis are discussed in Chapter 32.

Cardiac Magnetic Resonance

Cine MRI demonstrates the signal void caused by the flow jet of pulmonic stenosis. The site of origin of the signal void indicates the level of obstruction. A signal void originating at the valve and projecting into the pulmonary artery indicates valvular pulmonic stenosis. CMR can be used to exclude other causes of stenosis such as tumors or hypertrophic cardiomyopathy.

VEC MRI can be used to estimate the gradient across the stenotic valve, although it usually underestimates the severity of stenosis as discussed above. Cine MR imaging is the most accurate technique for assessment of right ventricular volumes, function, and mass. Right ventricular mass is typically elevated in patients with pulmonary valve stenosis, usually

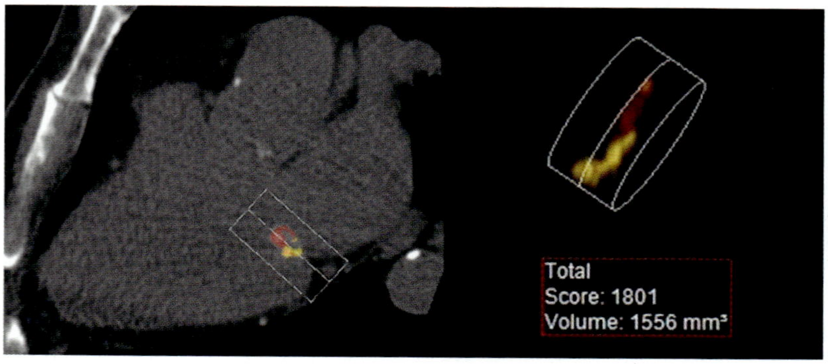

Figure 33.18. Mitral annular calcification. Noncontrast CT image in the left ventricular outflow tract plane demonstrating mitral annular calcification with calcium score measurements.

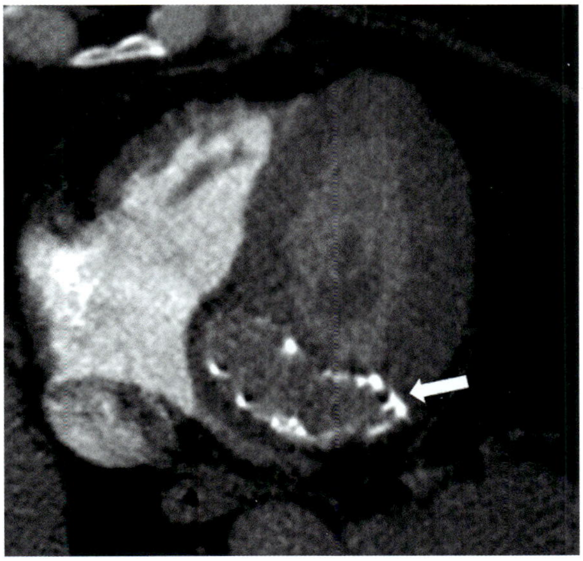

Figure 33.19. Caseous calcification of the mitra annulus. Axial CT contrast enhanced image showing diffuse peripheral calcification of the mitral annulus with expansion and internal hypodensity (*arrow*).

with a combination of increased ventricular wall thickness and hyper-trabeculation. RV mass is usually calculated as the mass of the RV free wall (the septum is assigned to the left ventricle by convention).

Cardiac Computed Tomography

CCT is an excellent technique for depiction of pulmonary artery enlargement in the setting of pulmonary stenosis. Assessment of pulmonary valve leaflets is rarely done with CCT, but calcifications could be obviated with this technique and may be missed on echocardiography or CMR. Pre-procedure assessment for pulmonary valve transcatheter or surgical intervention can be done with CCT and are discussed thoroughly on another chapter.

PULMONARY REGURGITATION

Pulmonary regurgitation most often is caused by pulmonary arterial hypertension. It can occur as a congenital anomaly in which the pulmonary valve is absent. It nearly always occurs after pulmonary valvuloplasty and surgical correction of tetralogy of Fallot. Pulmonary regurgitation can be severe after repair of tetralogy and over many years can cause severe RV dilatation and failure. Many patients with pulmonary regurgitation also have tricuspid regurgitation as a result of RV dilatation.

Chest Radiograph

The major feature of pulmonary regurgitation is enlargement of the main pulmonary arterial segment, central pulmonary arteries, and right ventricle.

Table 33.9 Etiology of Pulmonary Stenosis

Valvular Stenosis
Congenital
- Central perforated diaphragm
- Bicuspid valve
- Dysplastic valve
- Hypoplastic annulus
- Tetralogy of Fallot

Acquired
- Rheumatic carditis
- Carcinoid syndrome

Supravalvular
Congenital
- William's syndrome
- Tetralogy of Fallot

Acquired
- Surgical (banding, etc.)
- Carcinoid syndrome
- Rubella syndrome
- Behçet's disease
- Takayasu's arteritis

Subvalvular
- Congenital
- Isolated infundibular narrowing
- Tetralogy of Fallot

Acquired
- Infundibular hypertrophy (hypertrophic cardiomyopathy)
- Tumor

Midventricular
Anomalous muscle bundles (double-chamber right ventricle)

Cardiac Magnetic Resonance

Cine MRI demonstrates a diastolic signal void emanating from the pulmonary valve and projecting into the right ventricle (see Chapter 38). VEC MRI is frequently used to quantify the volume of pulmonary regurgitation. Currently, it is used to monitor the regurgitant volume of patients after the repair of tetralogy of Fallot. The total regurgitant volume of valvular regurgitation on the right side of the heart (pulmonary and tricuspid regurgitation) can be measured as the difference between RV and LV stroke volumes employing volumetric measurements of cine MR images. However, pulmonary regurgitation is usually assessed using VEC MRI (see Chapter 38). If the volume of pulmonary regurgitation is measured directly by VEC MRI in a plane perpendicular to the main pulmonary artery, tricuspid regurgitant volume can be assigned as the difference between the regurgitant volume measured by the volumetric and flow techniques. The volumetric technique gives the total right-sided regurgitant volume; VEC MRI measurement in the pulmonary artery gives pulmonary regurgitant volume only.

Cine MRI is the most precise noninvasive method that can quantify RV volumes, mass, and function. The accuracy and reproducibility of CMR for RV volumetric analysis is superior to that of echocardiography, particularly when the RV is severely enlarged.

Cardiac Computed Tomography

CCT has little applications for the assessment of pulmonary regurgitation. Although not usually the preferred imaging method for this purpose, it can provide precise RV volumes and function, with good agreement with echocardiography. Depiction of severely dilated pulmonary arteries when present, and potential mass effect in adjacent coronary arteries or airways, is the main advantage of CCT in this clinical scenario.

TRICUSPID STENOSIS

Acquired tricuspid stenosis is uncommon in comparison with stenosis of left-sided valves. Congenital tricuspid stenosis is rare in comparison with congenital pulmonary stenosis. Other causes of tricuspid stenosis are rare (Table 33.10).

Chest Radiograph

The major feature of chest radiograph in tricuspid stenosis is isolated right atrial (RA) enlargement. Enlargement of the right atrium may be difficult to discern on the chest x-ray. The superior vena cava and azygos vein may also be dilated.

Cardiac Magnetic Resonance

Cine MRI demonstrates the flow jet across the stenotic tricuspid valve in diastole, coursing from the tricuspid leaflets into the RV. The severity of right atrial enlargement can be assessed by cine MR in the horizontal long-axis plane. VEC MRI may be used to measure the peak velocity and thereby estimate the peak pressure gradient, although it is rarely used given superiority of echocardiography for this application.

Cardiac Computed Tomography

CCT has limited applications in patients with tricuspid stenosis. It is a useful method when delineation of valve annulus and leaflet calcifications is desired, particularly for surgical planning. Precise measurement of right atrial size can also be obtained with CCT.

Table 33.10 Etiology of Tricuspid Stenosis
Congenital
Rheumatic carditis
Carcinoid syndrome
Right ventricular or atrial tumors
Pericardial and paracardiac tumors (compression of tricuspid annulus)
Focal constrictive pericarditis (constriction of the tricuspic annulus)
Tricuspid annular (periannular) calcification

TRICUSPID REGURGITATION

Chest Radiograph

Tricuspid regurgitation produces cardiomegaly with RA and RV enlargement, which may be difficult to distinguish from other chamber enlargement on radiographs. The most remarkable degree of cardiomegaly may occur with chronic severe tricuspid regurgitation. A cardiac silhouette extending from one lateral chest wall to the other ("wall to wall") usually is due to severe tricuspid regurgitation. This lesion does not produce pulmonary venous hypertension or edema. In severe cases, the pulmonary vascularity may appear attenuated.

Cardiac Magnetic Resonance

Cine MRI demonstrates a systolic signal void into the right atrium emanating from the tricuspid valve in systole (Fig. 33.20). Cine MRI also is used to quantify RV volumes, mass, and function. RA size can also be determined. With isolated tricuspid regurgitation, the stroke volume of the right ventricle exceeds that of the left ventricle by a volume equal to that of the tricuspid regurgitant volume. VEC MR is rarely used for measurement of tricuspid regurgitation due to reasons similar to those related to mitral regurgitation quantification as described above. Utilizing a combination of volumetric cine MR analysis and VEC MR is the most reliable method for quantification of tricuspid regurgitation on CMR.

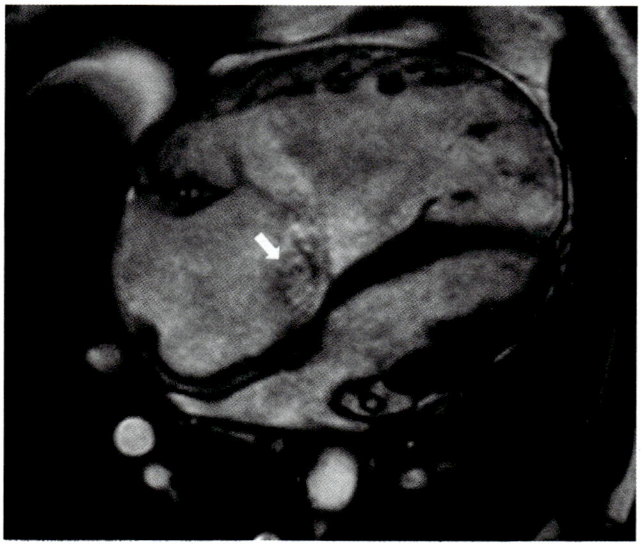

Figure 33.20. Tricuspid regurgitation. Cine b-steady-state free precession magnetic resonance image and supplemental video in the horizonal long axis (4-chamber) plane during systole demonstrates a signal void (white arrow) emanating from the tricuspid valve.

Cardiac Computed Tomography

CCT can be used for precise measurement of the tricuspid valve annulus, which can be used for planning surgical or transcatheter interventions.

Artificial Intelligence in Valvular Heart Disease

Clinical applications of artificial intelligence (AI) including machine learning (ML) are promising not only in the early diagnosis of valvular heart disease but also in the treatment decision, procedure planning, and postprocedure monitoring. The use of AI in cardiovascular imaging (echocardiography, CT and MRI) in the setting of valvular heart disease includes the use of automated measurements and volumes using deep learning segmentation and modeling to increase reproducibility and speed therefore improving efficiency. The accurate serial assessment of velocities and dimensions is crucial in the management of valvular heart disease as there are major determinants for intervention which can affect prognosis. Also, deep learning algorithms can help in the improvement of image quality depending on different patient conditions.

SUGGESTED READINGS

Boegaert J, Taylor AM. Valvular heart disease. In: Higgins CB, de Roos A, eds. *MRI and CT of Cardiovascular System*. 3rd ed. Lippincott Williams & Wilkins; 2013:196.

Caruthers SD, Lin SJ, Brown P, et al. Practical value of cardiac magnetic resonance imaging for clinical quantification of aortic valve stenosis: comparison with echocardiography. *Circulation*. 2003;108(18):2236-2243.

Didier D, Ratib O, Lerch R, Friedli B. Detection and quantification of valvular heart disease with dynamic cardiac MR imaging. *Radiographics*. 2000;20(5):1279-1301.

Dulce MC, Mostbeck GH, O'Sullivan M, Cheitlin M, Caputo GR, Higgins CB. Severity of aortic regurgitation: interstudy reproducibility of measurements with velocity-encoded cine MR imaging. *Radiology*. 1992;185(1):235-240.

Friedrich M, Schulz-Menger J, Dietz R. Magnetic resonance to assess the aortic valve area in aortic stenosis. *J Am Coll Cardiol*. 2004;43(11):2148-2149.

Koo HJ, Yang DH, Oh SY, et al. Demonstration of mitral valve prolapse with CT for planning of mitral valve repair. *Radiographics*. 2014;34(6):1537-1552. doi:10.1148/rg.346130146

Morris MF, Maleszewski JJ, Suri RM, et al. CT and MR imaging of the mitral valve: radiologic-pathologic correlation. *Radiographics*. 2010;30(6):1603-1620. doi:10.1148/rg.306105518 –.

Thoenes M, Agarwal A, Grundmann D, et al. Narrative review of the role of artificial intelligence to improve aortic valve disease management. *J Thorac Dis*. 2021;13(1):396-404. doi:10.21037/jtd-20-1837

Xu B, Kocyigit D, Wang TKM, et al. Mitral annular calcification and valvular dysfunction: multimodality imaging evaluation, grading, and management. *Eur Heart J Cardiovasc Imaging*. 2022;23(3):e111-e122. doi:10.1093/ehjci/jeab185

Chapter 34

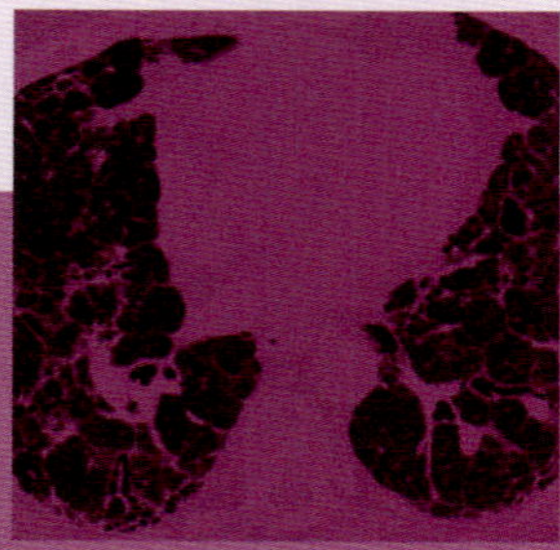

Kate Hanneman • Karen G. Ordovas

Myocardial Diseases

INTRODUCTION

Cardiac magnetic resonance imaging (MRI) is considered the reference standard for quantification of ventricular size and function. Although echocardiography is often the first-line imaging test for assessment of suspected myocardial disease, cardiac MRI provides incremental information on myocardial tissue characterization. In comparison with echocardiography, the three-dimensional data sets available with MRI also provide a more precise and reproducible method for qualifying ventricular volumes, mass, and function. Cardiac CT can also be used for assessment of ventricular size and function and tissue characterization with techniques such as late iodine enhancement, but is performed for evaluation of suspected myocardial disease less frequently unless there is a contraindication to MRI. MRI tissue characterization techniques including late gadolinium enhancement (LGE) and newer parametric mapping techniques can help diagnose specific myocardial diseases and may also be useful for prognostication and monitoring longitudinal changes over time.

TECHNIQUES

The ECG-gated spin-echo (SE) or black blood acquisitions were initially used to demonstrate the morphology of the ventricles and pericardium. Sharp demarcation of the endocardium is achieved on turbo SE images with preparatory double-inversion recovery pulses applied to vitiate the signal of the blood pool (Fig. 34.1). However, SE or black blood images are now infrequently used. Contrast-enhanced T1-weighted inversion recovery–prepared fast gradient sequences are used to demonstrate focal differential (hyperenhancement) enhancement of sites of inflammation, ischemic injury, or fibrosis associated with some myocardial diseases (Fig. 34.2). T2-weighted images are applied to demonstrate myocardial edema. Parametric mapping images can be constructed based on signal decay curves for T1, T2, and T2* times (Fig. 34.3).

Cine MR images are acquired for the purpose of quantifying ventricular volumes, mass, function, and strain. Cine MR images are now usually acquired using balanced steady-state free precession sequences. A set of these images at multiple levels encompassing the heart provides a volumetric data set for the direct measurement of the end-diastolic, end-systolic, and stroke volumes, mass, and ejection fraction of both the left ventricle and right ventricles. The balanced steady-state free precession techniques represented by true fast imaging with steady precession, fast imaging employing steady-state acquisition, and balanced fast field-echo sequences provide a homogeneous bright signal of the blood pool throughout the cardiac cycle and relatively high temporal resolution in a short acquisition period (Fig. 34.4). Cine MRI sequences are usually acquired in the cardiac short-axis plane covering both ventricles from base to apex and in multiple long-axis planes for the assessment of ventricular volumes and function. On cine MR images, valvular regurgitation associated with cardiomyopathies or subvalvular stenosis accompanying some forms of hypertrophy cardiomyopathy may be recognized by a signal void (high-velocity jet flow; Fig. 34.5). High-velocity flow can also cause a circumscribed jet of high signal when the velocity is below a certain threshold.

Velocity-encoded cine (VEC; phase-contrast) MRI can be used to measure blood flow into the aorta or pulmonary artery to quantify the left ventricular (LV) or right ventricular (RV) stroke volume, respectively. It has also been used for direct measurement of the volume of valvular regurgitation, which may accompany some cardiomyopathies.

Late gadolinium-enhanced (LGE)-MRI involves the application of an inversion recovery or phase-sensitive inversion sequence at a delay time after administration of a gadolinium

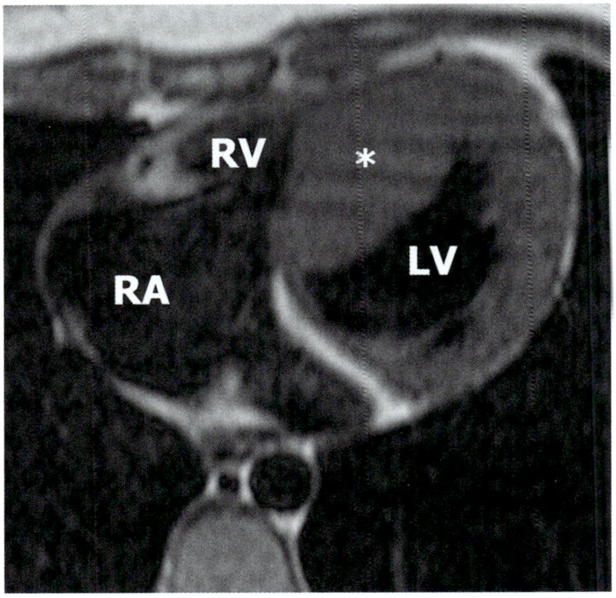

Figure 34.1. Asymmetric hypertrophic cardiomyopathy. T1-weighted spin-echo image in the axial plane shows asymmetric thickening of the ventricular septum (*asterisk*) with a more normal thickness of the left ventricular (*LV*) lateral wall. *RV*, right ventricle; *RA*, right atrium.

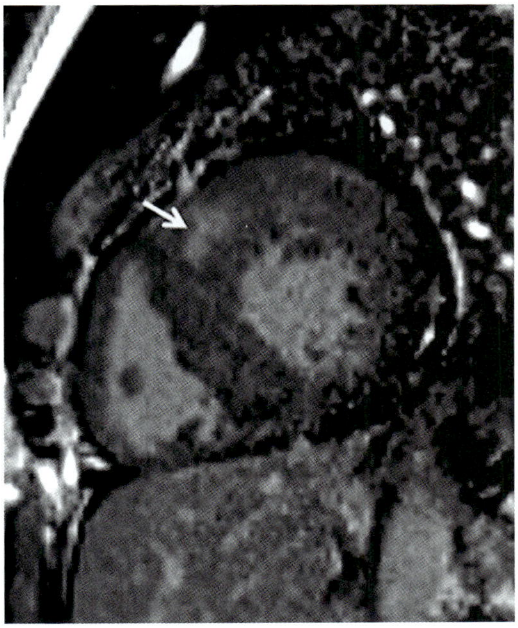

Figure 34.2. Late gadolinium-enhanced (LGE) image in the short-axis plane in a patient with hypertrophic cardiomyopathy demonstrates patchy areas of LGE within the hypertrophied ventricular septum (arrow).

chelate (0.1-0.2 mmol/kg). The delay time is typically 10 to 15 minutes after injection and the inversion time is set to null the signal of normal myocardium. Abnormal myocardium appears bright in contrast to normal myocardium (Fig. 34.2). The abnormal bright region can be due to edema, necrosis, fibrosis, or various infiltrates, which expand the extracellular space of the myocardium.

T1 mapping is a newer technique that can be useful for visualization and quantification of diffuse myocardial tissue changes including interstitial fibrosis (Fig. 34.3). Native T1 mapping refers to acquisition of T1 maps without contrast or precontrast. Postcontrast T1 maps can also be acquired but should not be interpreted in insolation as they are highly dependent on contrast kinetics. However, they are needed

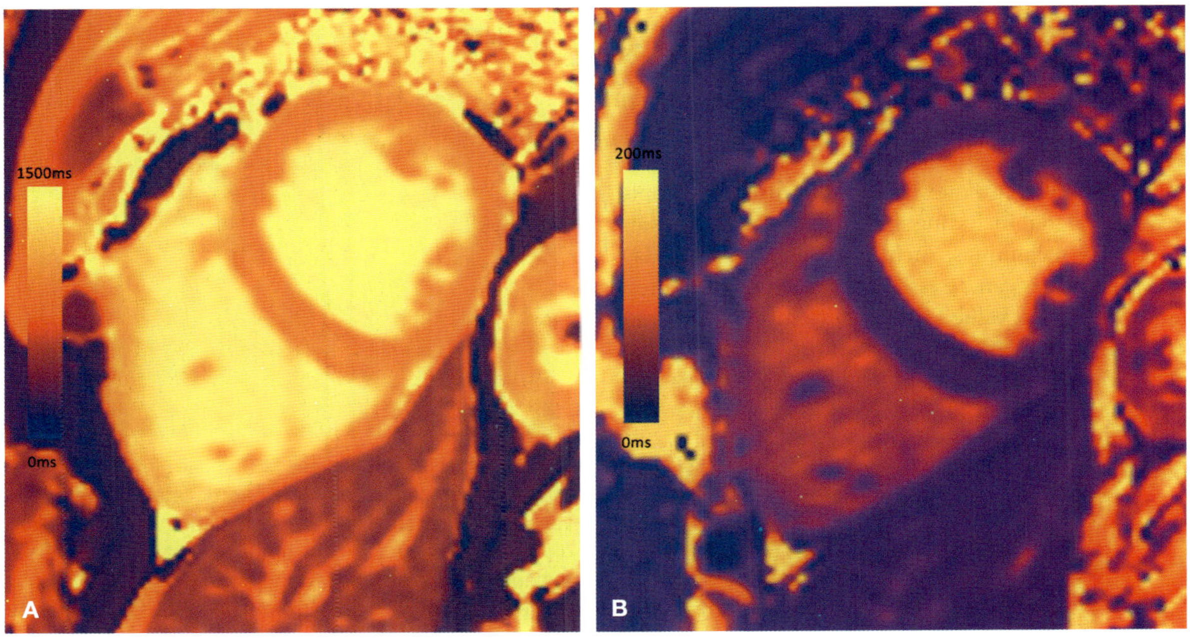

Figure 34.3. Parametric native T1 (**A**) and T2 (**B**) maps in a healthy control with color scales.

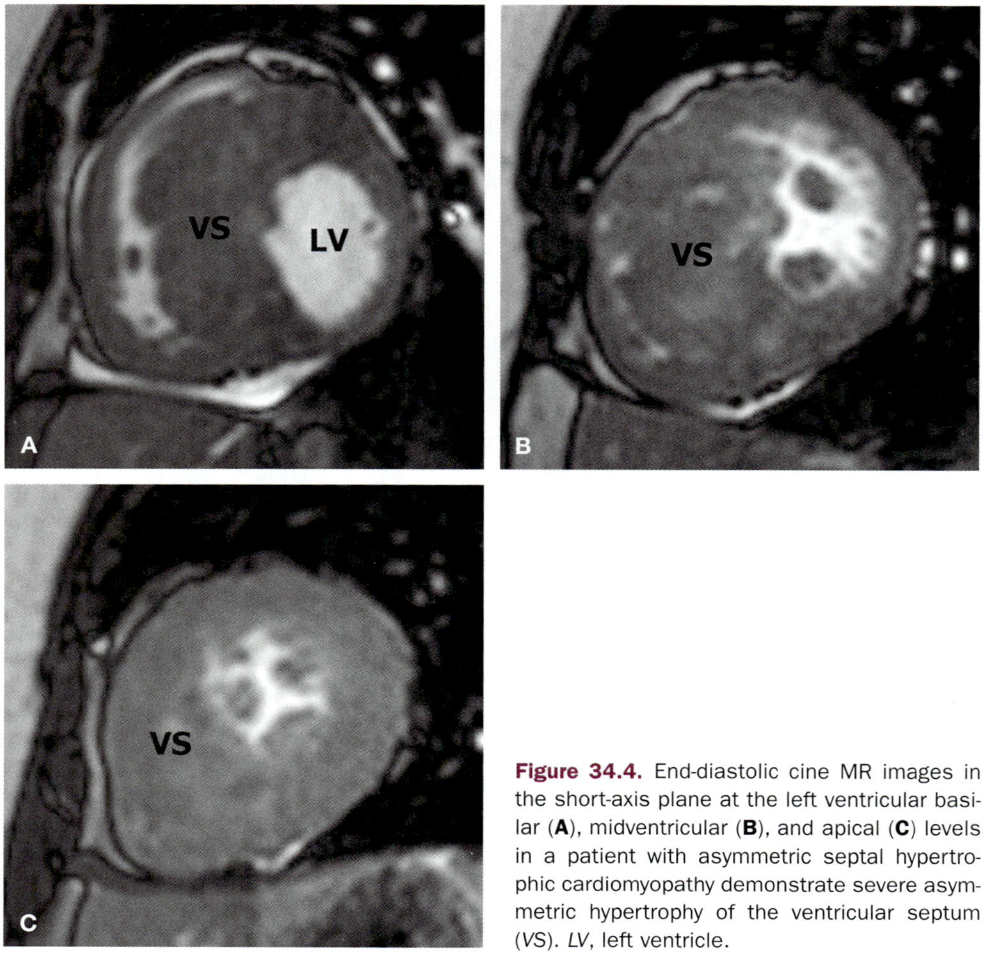

Figure 34.4. End-diastolic cine MR images in the short-axis plane at the left ventricular basilar (**A**), midventricular (**B**), and apical (**C**) levels in a patient with asymmetric septal hypertrophic cardiomyopathy demonstrate severe asymmetric hypertrophy of the ventricular septum (*VS*). *LV*, left ventricle.

and useful for calculation of myocardial extracellular volume (ECV) according to the formula:

$$\lambda = c \cdot T = \frac{c}{f} = \frac{1600 \text{ m/s}}{1.6 \text{ MHz}} = \frac{1.6 \cdot 10^3 \text{ m/s}}{1.6 \cdot 10^6 /\text{s}} = 10^{-3} = 1 \text{ mm}$$

There are several techniques that can be used to sample the T1 recovery signal including inversion recovery and saturation recovery techniques, such as MOLLI and SASHA, respectively. T1 values can be assessed as a region of interest or as an average global value for the entire myocardium. T1 values are high in the setting of edema, fibrosis, and infiltration and are low in the setting of fat and iron. T1 values are much higher at 3T compared to 1.5T and also vary depending on the sequence used.

T2 and T2* mapping can be acquired using a similar principle. High T2 values are specific for edema. T2 and T2* values are low in the setting of iron. T2* values are typically measured at the interventricular septum for the assessment of myocardial iron. T2 and T2* values are much higher at 1.5T compared to 3T and also vary depending on the sequence used.

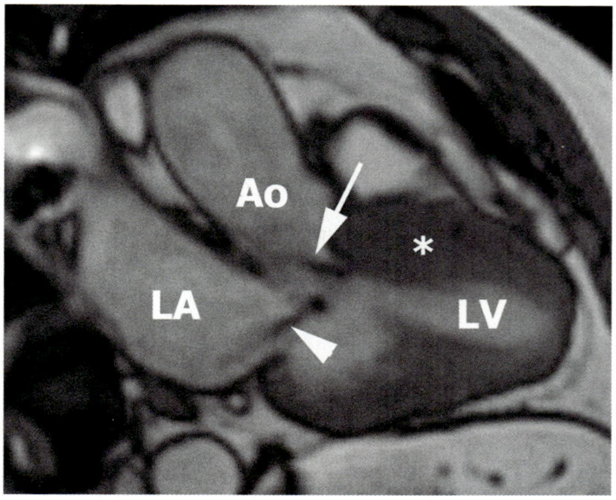

Figure 34.5. Systolic cine MR image in the left ventricular outflow tract plane shows subaortic stenosis due to a thick ventricular septum (*asterisk*) in a patient with hypertrophic cardiomyopathy. Note the flow jet (*arrow*) starting at the level of the subaortic stenosis and extending to the ascending aorta (*Ao*). There is also a flow jet (*arrowhead*) consistent with associated mitral regurgitation. *LV*, left ventricle; *LA*, left atrium.

CLASSIFICATION OF CARDIOMYOPATHIES

According to the consensus of the World Health Organization and the International Society and Federation for Cardiology, cardiomyopathies are defined as diseases of the myocardium associated with cardiac dysfunction. Based on pathophysiologic features, they are often divided into four main categories: dilated, hypertrophic, restrictive, and arrhythmogenic cardiomyopathy (ACM) (Table 34.1). Cardiomyopathies caused by pathologic substances or cells infiltrating the myocardium are called infiltrative cardiomyopathies such as amyloid.

Dilated Cardiomyopathy

This entity is characterized by dilation and impaired contraction of the left or both ventricles. End-systolic and end-diastolic volumes are increased, whereas stroke volume and ejection fraction are decreased. Mild to moderate mitral regurgitation and tricuspid regurgitation are frequently associated with the ventricular enlargement. The wall thickness of the left ventricle is usually within the normal range but mass is frequently elevated. There are many causes of dilated cardiomyopathy (DCM) (Table 34.2). However, many cases have no identifiable cause (idiopathic). The most common cause of DCM is myocardial ischemia secondary to coronary artery disease in which the degree of myocardial dysfunction is frequently not explained by the obvious extent of myocardial infraction. Hypertension, viral diseases, alcoholism, diabetes, obesity, and several toxins can also lead to DCM. There is increasing recognition of inherited causes of DCM including variants in the gene encoding titin (TTN).

Hypertrophic Cardiomyopathy

A variety of distribution patterns of inappropriate myocardial hypertrophy develop in the absence of an obvious hemodynamic stress (increased afterload), such as aortic stenosis or systemic hypertension (Fig. 34.5; Table 34.3). Hypertrophic cardiomyopathy (HCM) is genetically transmitted in about half of the cases and follows an autosomal dominant inheritance pattern with variable penetrance. Possible manifestations are symmetric or concentric involvement of the entire left ventricle or both ventricles or asymmetric hypertrophy of the upper septum, midportion of the ventricular septum, midcavity, or apex. A large registry of cardiac MRI in patients with HCM has characterized phenotypic presentations of the disease that includes the following subtypes: localized basal septal hypertrophy, reverse curvature septal hypertrophy, apical HCM, concentric (symmetric) HCM, and mid-cavitary obstruction with apical aneurysm.

Some subtypes of HCM, usually asymmetric septal hypertrophy, are associated with left ventricular outflow tract (LVOT) obstruction. The hallmark of obstructive HCM is dynamic subvalvular aortic stenosis (Fig. 34.6). During diastole, the LVOT appears normal or slightly narrowed because of the presence of basal septal hypertrophy. Increasing stenosis develops during systole as the anterior leaflet of the mitral valve moves in an anterior direction toward the septum, thereby narrowing the outflow tract. Apical hypertrophy is less prevalent but has a distinct phenotype. This type of HCM is characterized by lack of normal apical tapering with frequent apical cavity obliteration and development of apical fibrosis and aneurysms in some patients. Midventricular type involves hypertrophy of the middle of the LV with mid-cavitary obliteration in systole causing high wall tension in the isolated LV apex, which also may lead to aneurysmal formation. Concentric (symmetric) HCM is also recognized and may be a particularly severe form. Involvement of the right ventricle may be a feature of the disease in infants and children.

Restrictive Cardiomyopathy

This entity is characterized by impaired ventricular filling secondary to myocardial diastolic stiffness. Flow into the

Table 34.1 Classification of Cardiomyopathies

Dilated cardiomyopathy
Hypertrophic cardiomyopathy
Restrictive cardiomyopathy
Arrhythmogenic cardiomyopathy

Table 34.2 Some Etiologies of Dilated Cardiomyopathy

Ischemic
Familial and inherited
Alcohol
Cocaine
Postmyocarditis
Drug toxicity (doxorubicin)
Cobalt (beer drinkers' cardiomyopathy)
Metabolic (eg, carnitine deficiency, thiamine deficiency, scurvy)
Endocrine (eg, acromegaly, myxedema, thyrotoxicosis, etc.)
Postpartum (peripartum)
Tachyarrhythmia
Idiopathic

Table 34.3 Phenotypes of Hypertrophic Cardiomyopathy

1. Asymmetric septal
   - Obstructive
   - Nonobstructive
2. Concentric
3. Apical
4. Midventricular

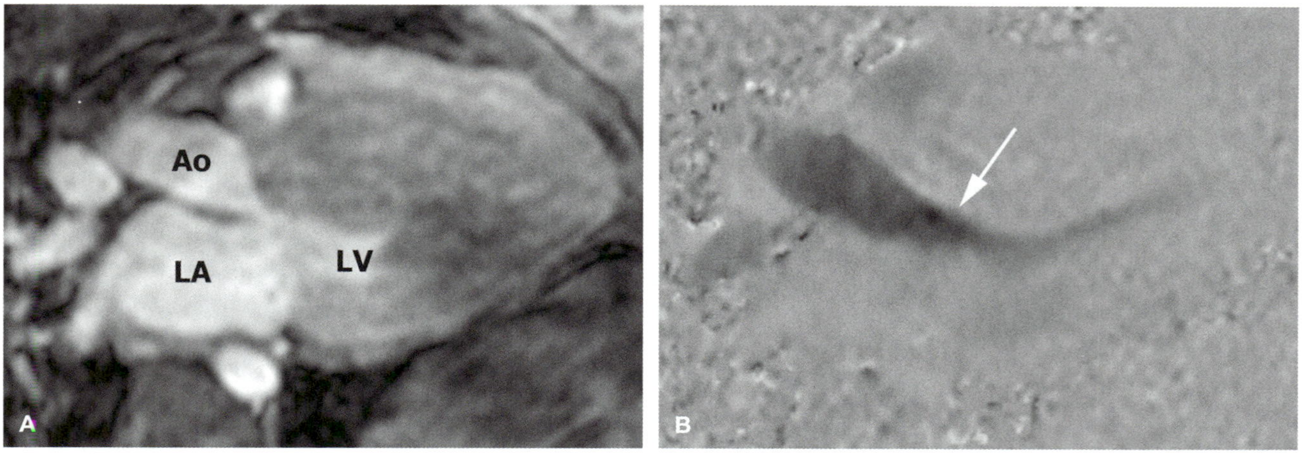

Figure 34.6. Magnitude (**A**) and phase (**B**) images of velocity-encoded cine sequence in the left ventricular outflow tract. Note the flow jet (*arrow*) starting at the subaortic region, consistent with flow acceleration. *LV*, left ventricle; *LA*, left atrium; *Ao*, aorta.

ventricles is rapid during early diastole; it then plateaus, and little filling takes place in late diastole. End-diastolic pressure is elevated in both ventricles, whereas systolic function is normal or only slightly reduced. Tropical endomyocardial fibrosis and Loeffler eosinophilic endomyocardial fibrosis are classified as types of restrictive cardiomyopathy. Loeffler endocarditis is associated with hypereosinophilia. Degranulation of endomyocardial eosinophils is suspected to be responsible for focal necrosis and subsequent fibrosis and for the formation of mural thrombus. Increased stiffness of the ventricular walls and reduction of the cavity by organized thrombus contribute to the restrictive filling pattern. Tropical endomyocardial fibrosis, a different entity with a peak geographic distribution in equatorial Africa, is not associated with hypereosinophilia. In this disease, fibrosis of the apex and subvalvular regions leads to restrictive cardiomyopathy. Glycogen storage diseases, radiation fibrosis, and certain infiltrative diseases, such as amyloidosis, can also cause restrictive cardiomyopathy. Many cases of restrictive cardiomyopathy are idiopathic.

Specific cardiomyopathies are myocardial diseases that are associated with a specific cardiac or systemic disease. Hemochromatosis, sarcoidosis, amyloidosis, and hypertensive or metabolic cardiomyopathy are examples of specific cardiomyopathies. DCM can also result in inflammation, for example, after myocarditis or sarcoidosis, or end-stage infiltrative cardiomyopathy, for example, in severe iron overload (Fig. 34.7).

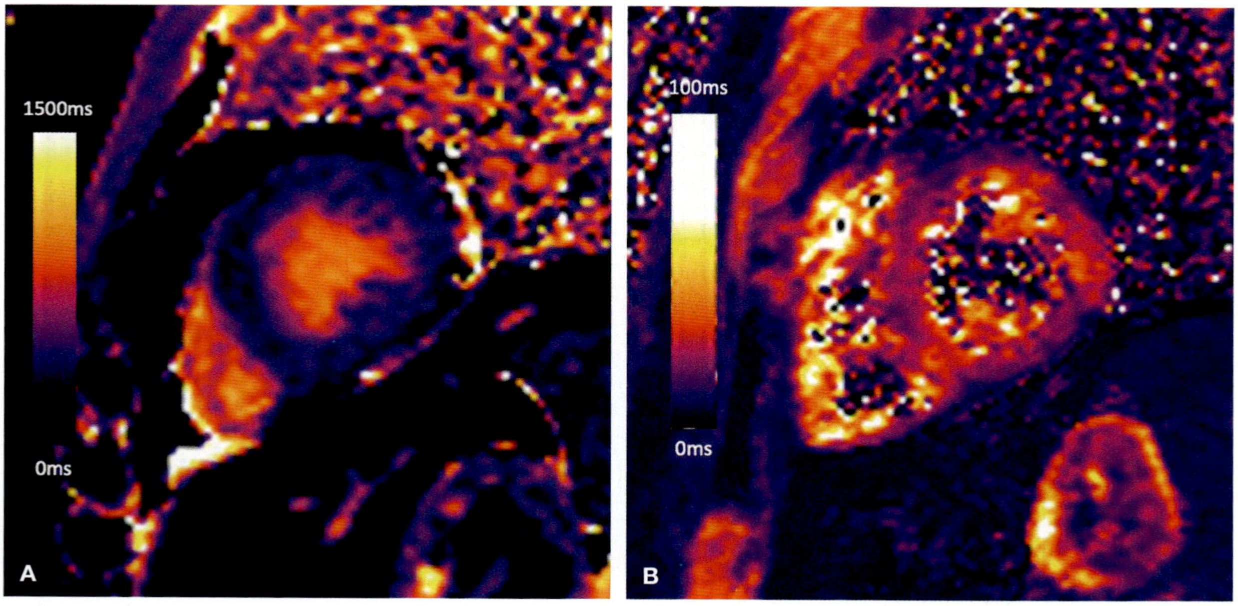

Figure 34.7. Native T1 (**A**) and T2* (**B**) maps in a patient with thalassemia major and iron overload. Native T1 and T2* maps in a mid-ventricular short-axis plane demonstrates low T1 and T2* values in keeping with iron deposition.

Table 34.4 Types of Restrictive and Infiltrative Diseases of the Myocardium and Endocardium

1. Amyloidosis
2. Loeffler eosinophilic endocarditis
3. Endomyocardial fibrosis
4. Hemochromatosis
5. Glycogen storage diseases
6. Mucopolysaccharidoses
7. Anderson-Fabry disease
8. Gaucher disease

Infiltrative cardiomyopathy refers solely to the histopathologic mechanism of infiltration of myocardial tissue (Table 34.4).

IMAGING FEATURES

Dilated Cardiomyopathy

The morphologic characteristics of DCM are clearly depicted on cine MRI (Figs. 34.8 and 34.9; Table 34.5). Morphologic changes include enlargement of the left ventricle and sometimes the right ventricle and atria. The thickness of the LV wall usually remains normal. The MRI features in DCM are often nonspecific, so that the various underlying causes cannot be distinguished. However, it is usually possible to distinguish between ischemic and nonischemic forms of DCM. In most cases of nonischemic DCM, the wall thickness of the left ventricle is uniform; no regional wall thinning is recognized. If the cardiac dilation is caused by prior myocardial infarction and ischemia, usually one or more regional areas of severe wall thinning with or without ventricular aneurysm are seen. MRI may demonstrate localized ventricular dilation after occlusion of a major coronary artery rather than global dilation; the latter is characteristic of DCM. LGE-MRI may be used to demonstrate regional hyperenhancement in a subendocardial or transmural distribution at the site of prior myocardial infarction to distinguish patients with ischemic cardiomyopathy (Fig. 34.10). Patients with idiopathic DCM can have LGE, which is often linear, in a mid-wall pattern especially in the septum (Fig. 34.11). The presence of mid-wall LGE indicates a poorer long-term prognosis and increased risk for ventricular arrhythmias (see section on LGE for Risk Assessment in Nonischemic Myocardial Diseases). Mural LV thrombus can be readily identified on cine MR images and on LGE images (Fig. 34.12).

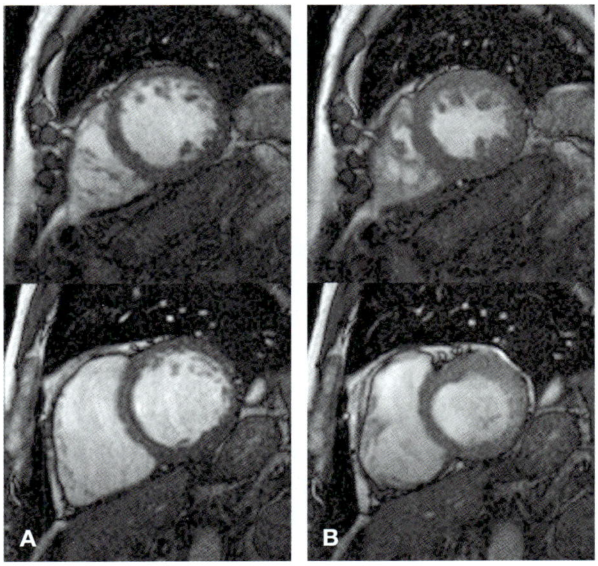

Figure 34.8. Cine MR images at two levels at end diastole (**A**) and end systole (**B**) in a patient with dilated cardiomyopathy.

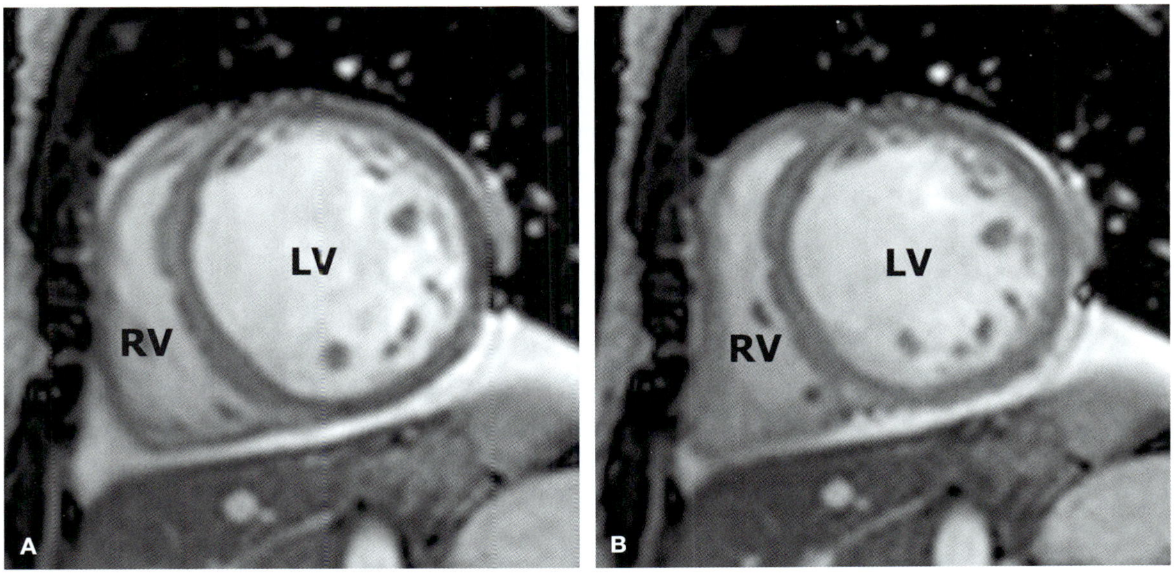

Figure 34.9. Short-axis cine MR images in the end diastole (**A**) and end systole (**B**) demonstrate a severely enlarged left ventricle (*LV*) with poor systolic function. *RV*, right ventricle.

Table 34.5 Imaging Features of Dilated Cardiomyopathy

1. Increased LV end-diastolic volume
2. Increase LV end-systolic volume
3. Decreased LV stroke volume
4. Decreased LVEF
5. Normal LV wall thickness
6. Ischemic or nonischemic patterns of LGE
7. High T1 mapping values

LGE, late gadolinium enhancement; LV, left ventricular; LVEF, left ventricular ejection fraction.

Ventricular mass, ventricular wall thickness, and ventricular volumes can be quantified with cine MRI to determine the severity of DCM. Cine MRI measurements of LV volumes, mass, and ejection fraction in DCM are highly reproducible and particularly useful for monitoring LV dimensions and function over time. Because of its high degree of accuracy and reproducibility, MRI can be used to monitor the effect of treatment in individual patients and in clinical studies to assess the efficacy of new therapeutic interventions. For example, significant decreases in LV systolic volume, wall stress, and mass and increase in ejection fraction have been shown in DCM after angiotensin-converting enzyme inhibitor treatment and other therapies.

Although the right ventricle is usually less dilated and its systolic function is less severely impaired, RV diastolic abnormalities, such as an increased time to peak filling rate, have been detected using cine MRI and VEC (phase-contrast) cine MRI. The profile of diastolic inflow velocity measured in the region of the tricuspid valve is flattened in comparison with that in healthy volunteers. It is suspected that the altered morphology and function of the left ventricle causes functional changes in RV filling.

Hypertrophic Cardiomyopathy

The initial diagnosis of HCM is often established by echocardiography (Table 34.6). The typical diagnostic feature is maximum end-diastolic LV wall thickness of 15 mm or greater. However, in patients with a family history, a maximum wall thickness of 12 mm is sufficient for diagnosis in the absence of a cause for hypertrophy, such as hypertension, aortic stenosis, or extreme isometric exercise. Of note, in apical forms of HCM, maximum end-diastolic wall thickness might not exceed 12 to 15 mm and therefore assessment of morphology and associated imaging features is important.

MRI enables a precise delineation of the pattern and extent of hypertrophic myocardium in HCM (see Figs. 34.1-34.5, and 34.13-34.17). The major clinical roles of MRI are to evaluate unusual forms of hypertrophy and assess for the presence and extent of myocardial fibrosis using LGE and T1 mapping (Figs. 34.17 and 34.18). Another indication for MRI is sequential monitoring of LV mass and LGE extent, which are adverse prognostic indicators. See section (below) on LGE for Risk Assessment in Nonischemic Myocardial Diseases.

A comprehensive examination, which also addresses the functional impact of the hypertrophy, includes measurement of the LV mass, volume, and ejection fraction by cine MRI. In HCM, the end-systolic and end-diastolic wall thicknesses

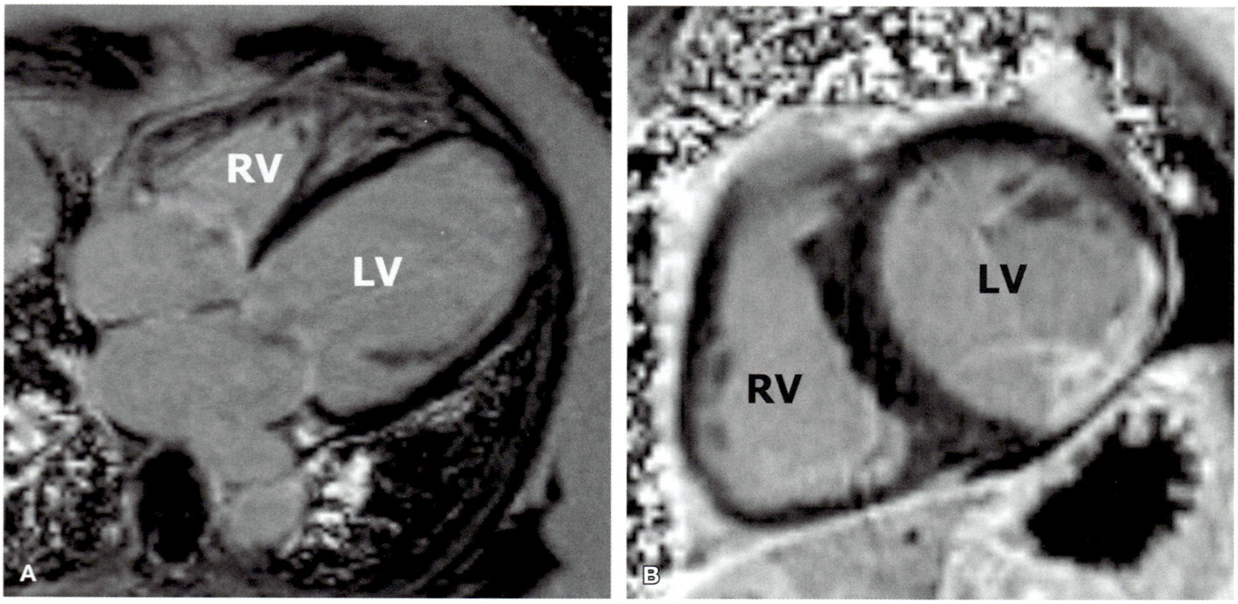

Figure 34.10. Late gadolinium-enhanced image in two different patients. **A:** No delayed enhancement in a 4-chamber plane image of a patient with idiopathic dilated cardiomyopathy (same patients as in Fig. 34.8). **B:** Short-axis image with transmural delayed enhancement in the inferolateral wall, consistent with prior myocardial infarction in a patient with ischemic dilated cardiomyopathy. *LV*, left ventricle; *RV*, right ventricle.

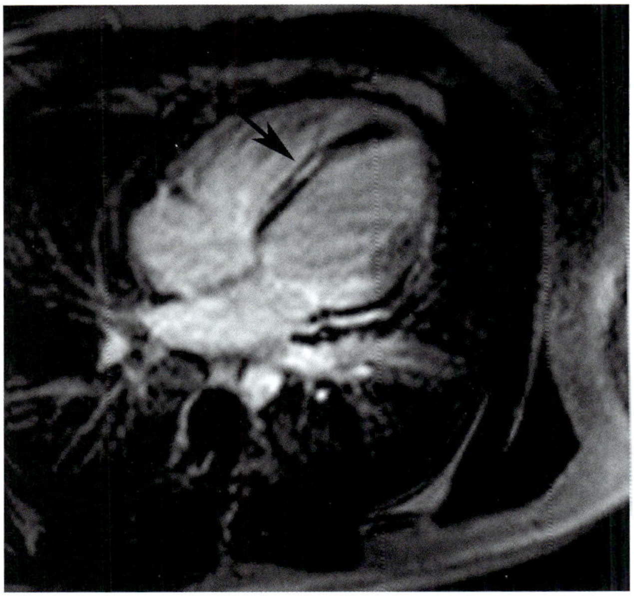

Figure 34.11. Idiopathic dilated cardiomyopathy with linear mid-wall ventricular late gadolinium enhancement (LGE). LGE image in 4-chamber plane shows linear mid-wall enhancement (*arrow*).

are increased (see Figs. 34.1 and 34.15). The total LV mass is variably increased in HCM.

In addition to defining the location and severity of hypertrophy, MRI can differentiate between obstructive and non-obstructive HCM. In the obstructive form, a jet flow in the narrowed outflow tract causes a signal void on GRE and balanced steady-state free precession images (Figs. 34.5 and 34.6). A possible outflow tract gradient can be quantified by velocity mapping at sites proximal and distal to the stenosis.

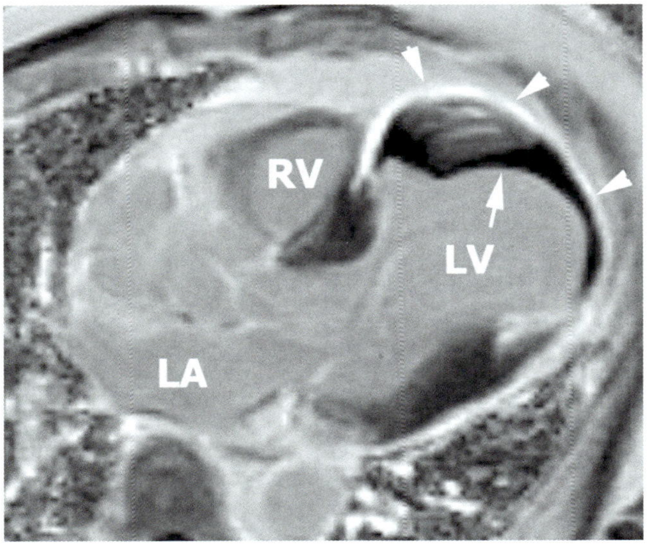

Figure 34.12. Late gadolinium-enhanced (LGE) image in a 3-chamber long-axis plane shows transmural apical LGE (*arrowheads*) and left ventricular thrombus (*arrow*) in a patient with ischemic cardiomyopathy consistent with prior myocardial infarction. *LA*, left atrium; *LV*, left ventricle; *RV*, right ventricle.

Table 34.6 Imaging Features of Hypertrophic Cardiomyopathy

1. Normal LV end-diastolic volume
2. Normal or reduced LV end-systolic volume
3. Normal or increased LVEF
4. Increased LV wall thickness (>15 mm)
5. Asymmetric or symmetric increased LV wall thickness
6. LGE involving hypertrophied myocardium and ventricular hinge points
7. Myocardial crypts
8. Left ventricular outflow tract obstruction

LGE, late gadolinium enhancement; LV, left ventricular; LVEF, left ventricular ejection fraction.

VEC (phase-contrast) cine MR images in the LVOT plane can be employed to interrogate the ensemble of flow velocities at the site of the subvalvular flow jet (Fig. 34.6). The peak velocity can be used to estimate the subaortic gradient in obstructive HCM using the modified Bernoulli equation (peak pressure gradient = 4 × [peak velocity]^2). Additionally, mitral regurgitation, which is frequent in HCM, can be detected by cine MRI. It causes a signal void that projects into the left atrium during systole on cine MR images and is often posteriorly directed. The volume of mitral regurgitation can be quantified either by calculating the difference in stroke volumes of the two ventricles (in the absence of a shunt or other valvular regurgitation) or by measuring the difference in the inflow and outflow volumes of the left ventricle by means of VEC (phase-contrast) cine MRI (see Chapter 33).

Myocardial-tagged cine MRI has shown a disordered pattern of the regional myocardial contraction and twisting of the left ventricle in HCM. Wall motion in the hypertrophic septum and cardiac rotation in the posterior region of the left ventricle are often reduced. Longitudinal and circumferential shortening of the ventricles is also reduced. At the same time, ventricular torsion is increased and thickening of the myocardium is more heterogeneous than in healthy volunteers.

Because of its high accuracy and reproducibility in quantifying LV mass, MRI has the potential to monitor the response to therapy in HCM. Septal ablation has been used in patients with obstructive HCM to cause scarring of the hypertrophic tissue and thereby reduce the gradient in the LVOT (see Fig. 34.16). MRI has defined the size of scarring and demonstrated a continuous improvement in the size of the outflow tract area during follow-up. Myocardial LGE is frequent and usually progresses over time. LGE is usually present in hypertrophic areas of myocardium and has been shown to reflect replacement fibrosis. A characteristic site of hyperenhancement is the ventricular septum near its junction with the anterior ventricular wall, and anterior and/or inferior ventricular hinge points (Fig. 34.19). Elevated native T1 and ECV have also been demonstrated even in areas of myocardium remote from LGE, likely reflecting interstitial fibrosis.

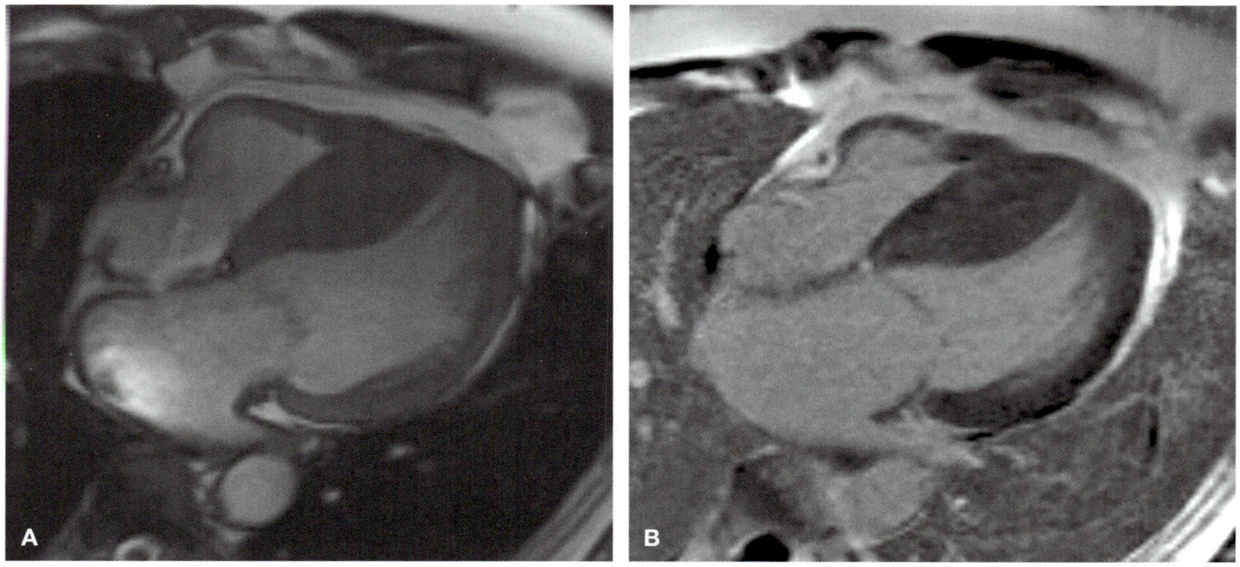

Figure 34.13. End-diastolic cine (**A**) and late gadolinium-enhanced (LGE) (**B**) cardiac MR images in 4-chamber plane in a genotype-positive patient with asymmetric septal hypertrophic cardiomyopathy demonstrating a reverse septal curvature morphology of wall thickening and patchy nonischemic pattern LGE.

Cine MRI may show abnormalities in regional LV morphology in patients with a certain genotype for HCM but without phenotypic expression of hypertrophy. Typical features include myocardial crypts extending from the endocardium into the myocardium usually in the posterobasal region and posteroseptal region of the LV.

An unusual variant of HCM can present clinically with restrictive physiology and symptomatology. The ventricles are small in volume, while the atria are markedly dilated; these are morphologic features more characteristic of restrictive cardiomyopathy. Sites of LGE of regional myocardium may be present.

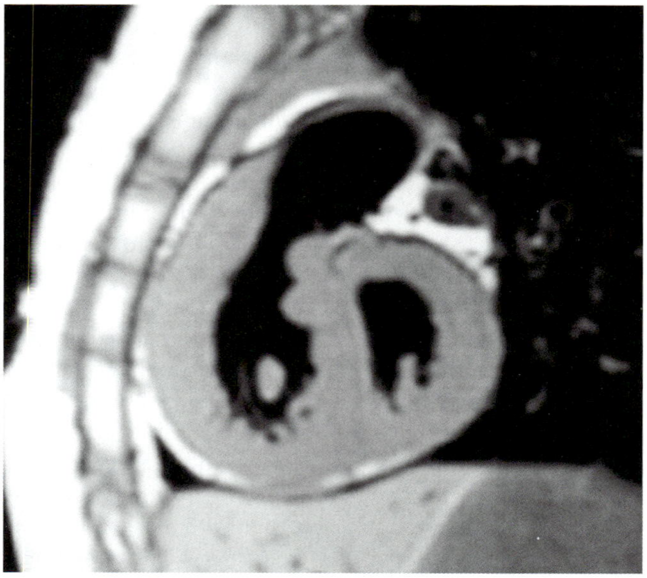

Figure 34.14. ECG-gated spin-echo sagittal image of a young child with the concentric form of hypertrophic cardiomyopathy that more severely affects the right ventricle.

MRI can provide prognostic information in HCM. The major prognostic features are the severity of regional wall thickening, overall LV mass, and presence and overall extent of LGE.

Restrictive Cardiomyopathy

The etiologies of restrictive cardiomyopathy are multiple including amyloidosis and endomyocardial fibrosis. The main purpose of MRI and CT in patients with restrictive cardiomyopathy is to differentiate this entity from constrictive pericarditis, which presents with a similar clinical picture. The differential diagnosis is essential because constrictive pericarditis can be treated effectively with surgical resection of the pericardium, whereas treatment of restrictive cardiomyopathy is guided by the underlying etiology. In constrictive pericarditis, the pericardium is nearly always thickened, whereas restrictive cardiomyopathy does not have this feature.

MRI and CT can demonstrate pericardial thickening reliably. CT can also disclose calcification of the pericardium, a feature that is highly suggestive of constrictive pericarditis. The diagnostic accuracy of MRI for differentiating between these two diseases was greater than 90% in a series of symptomatic patients.

The MRI features of restrictive cardiomyopathy, which are characteristic but nonspecific, are caused by impaired diastolic filling of the ventricles (Table 34.7). Impaired diastolic expansion of the ventricles causes dilation of the atria, inferior and superior vena cavae, and hepatic veins. Furthermore, stasis of blood in the atria leads to a high

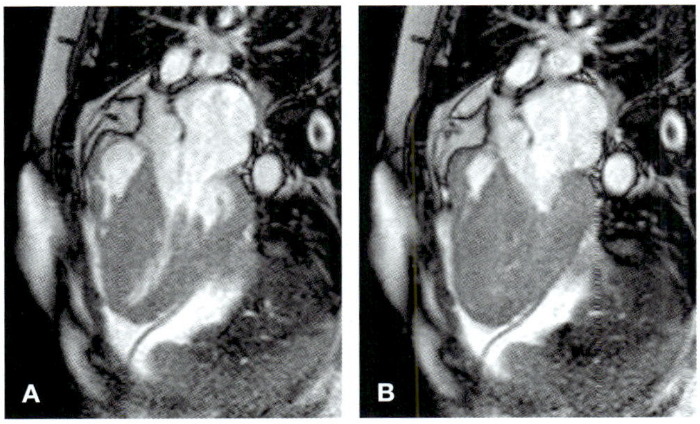

Figure 34.15. Three-chamber long-axis cine MR images in diastole (**A**) and systole (**B**) in obstructive hypertrophic cardiomyopathy. Note severe septal hypertrophy in diastole and cavity obliteration in systole. (Courtesy of Scott Flamm.)

signal intensity in the atrial cavities on SE images. A very characteristic morphologic pattern of restrictive cardiomyopathy revealed on MRI and CT is markedly enlarged right and left atria in the presence of normal-sized or small ventricles.

Cine MRI demonstrates low normal or reduced LV ejection fraction (LVEF). The restrictive filling pattern of the ventricles can be quantified and monitored during therapy by measuring the diastolic flow across the mitral and tricuspid valves with VEC (phase-contrast) cine MRI. Evaluation of possible atrioventricular valve regurgitation in patients with restrictive cardiomyopathy can be performed with cine MRI or VEC cine MRI. LGE imaging shows myocardial enhancement in a characteristic distribution in some myocardial diseases associated with restrictive physiology such as amyloidosis (Fig. 34.20) and endomyocardial fibrosis, but is nonspecific in others such as sarcoidosis (Fig. 34.21).

Endomyocardial Fibrosis

Endomyocardial fibrosis, of which Loeffler eosinophilic endomyocardial form is most frequent in temperate climates, is a rare disorder. It usually causes restrictive physiology but, in the tropics, it can exist as a form which nearly obliterates the ventricular chamber(s) (obliterative cardiomyopathy).

In endomyocardial fibrosis, areas of circumscribed myocardial fibrosis have been detected as areas of low signal intensity on T1- and T2-weighted images. The ventricular walls may be severely thickened by the deposition of subendocardial fibrotic tissue, which causes a narrowing of the cavities and contributes further to the decreased diastolic ventricular filling. Mural thrombus adjacent to the subendocardial fibrous is a characteristic feature; both may be displayed on SE or cine MR images.

Cine MRI may show reduced ventricular volumes and ejection fraction(s). Apical wall thickness is characteristically increased; the apex of one or both ventricles is attenuated or obliterated. Atrioventricular regurgitation is present in cine MRI and may be severe.

LGE-MRI shows characteristic subendocardial enhancement of either ventricle or both. However, the wall is thickened rather than thinned as would be expected with subendocardial enhancement associated with old (chronic) myocardial infarction. Moreover, the distribution of LGE may not correspond to the distribution territory of a specific coronary artery.

SPECIFIC INFILTRATIVE CARDIOMYOPATHIES

Amyloidosis

The most common types of amyloidosis to involve the heart are immunoglobulin light chain and transthyretin amyloidosis. Interstitial deposition of amyloid fibrils causes thickening of the atrial and ventricular walls and the atrioventricular valve leaflets (Fig. 34.22). Very few diseases cause thickening of the right atrial wall so this is a relatively specific feature of cardiac amyloidosis. Severe amyloid deposition in the ventricular myocardium often results in wall thickening of the LV and thereby produce morphologic features simulating those of HCM. However, these two entities can be differentiated by divergent ventricular contraction. In contrast to the hyperdynamic ventricular contraction characteristic for HCM, the systolic contraction is impaired in amyloidosis.

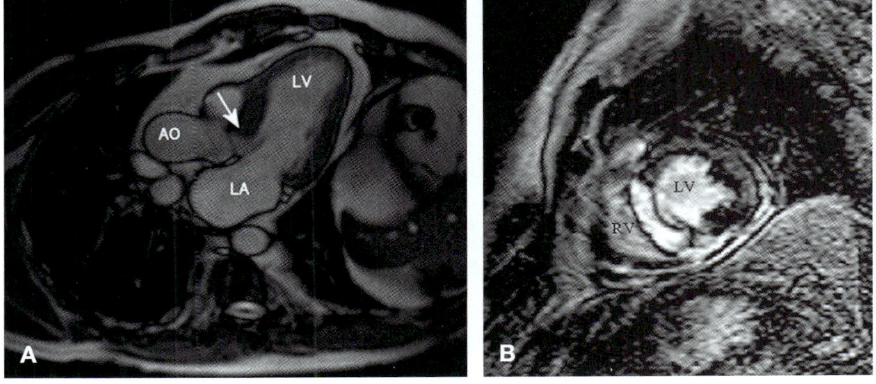

Figure 34.16. Asymmetric hypertrophic cardiomyopathy. **A:** The left ventricular outflow plane shows septal hypertrophy (*arrow*). **B:** After septal ablation (alcoholic injection into septal artery), an inversion recovery gradient-echo short-axis image taken 10 minutes after administration of gadolinium chelate shows delayed enhancement of the induced septal infarction. *Ao*, aorta; *LA*, left atrium; *LV*, left ventricle; *RV*, right ventricle.

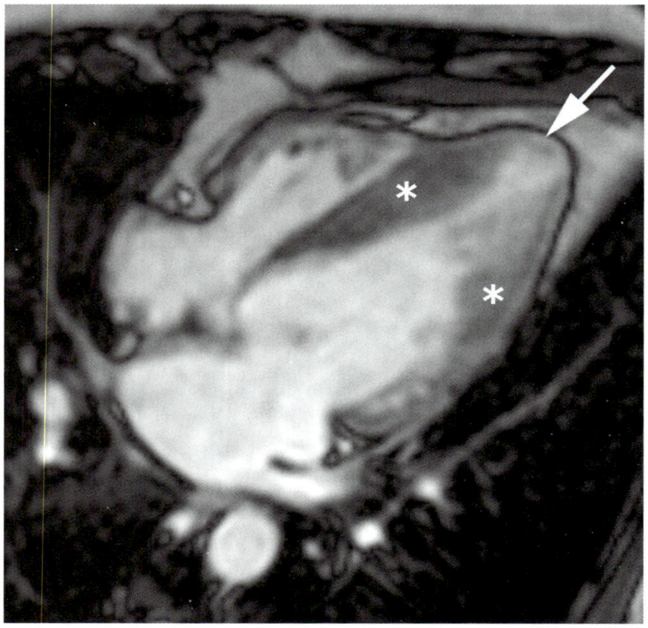

Figure 34.17. Cine MR image in the 4-chamber long-axis plane in a patient with mid-ventricular and apical type of hypertrophic cardiomyopathy shows myocardial hypertrophy (*asterisks*) at the midventricular level involving both septal and lateral walls and a focal aneurysm at the left ventricular apex (*arrow*).

The ejection fraction and systolic wall thickening are depressed. Amyloidosis most commonly leads to restrictive cardiomyopathy with dilated atria (Table 34.8).

A characteristic pattern of delayed gadolinium enhancement of the myocardium is observed on LGE-MRI in most patients with cardiac amyloidosis. This most characteristic (diagnostic) pattern is subendocardial hyperenhancement around the entire circumference of the LV (Fig. 34.22). Other patterns include diffuse LGE and difficulty nulling the myocardium. Hyperenhancement may also be recognized in the right atrial and RV walls and in the atrioventricular valves and tips of papillary muscles (Figs. 34.22 and 34.23). Other typical features on LGE-MRI include very dark blood pool and RV enhancement (Fig. 34.23).

An ensemble of multiple inversion times may be employed to determine the nulling point of the amyloid infiltrated myocardium compared to cavitary blood. Normally with increasing inversion time, the blood pool nulls before the myocardium. In amyloidosis, the myocardium nulls before or coincident with the blood pool (Fig. 34.20). Delayed enhancement in amyloidosis is mostly due to expansion of the extracellular space due to amyloid fibrils. Native T1 and ECV are typically dramatically elevated in cardiac amyloidosis (Fig. 34.24). Native T1 mapping is particularly useful if amyloidosis is suspected, but there is a contraindication to administration of gadolinium-based contrast.

Sarcoidosis

Sarcoidosis is an inflammatory multisystem granulomatous disease that can involve the heart. Patients often present with arrhythmias or heart block.

Sarcoidosis can be manifested in the myocardium with typical granulomas and can cause restrictive cardiomyopathy. Only 5% of patients with systemic sarcoidosis have clinical evidence of cardiac involvement, but it is found at

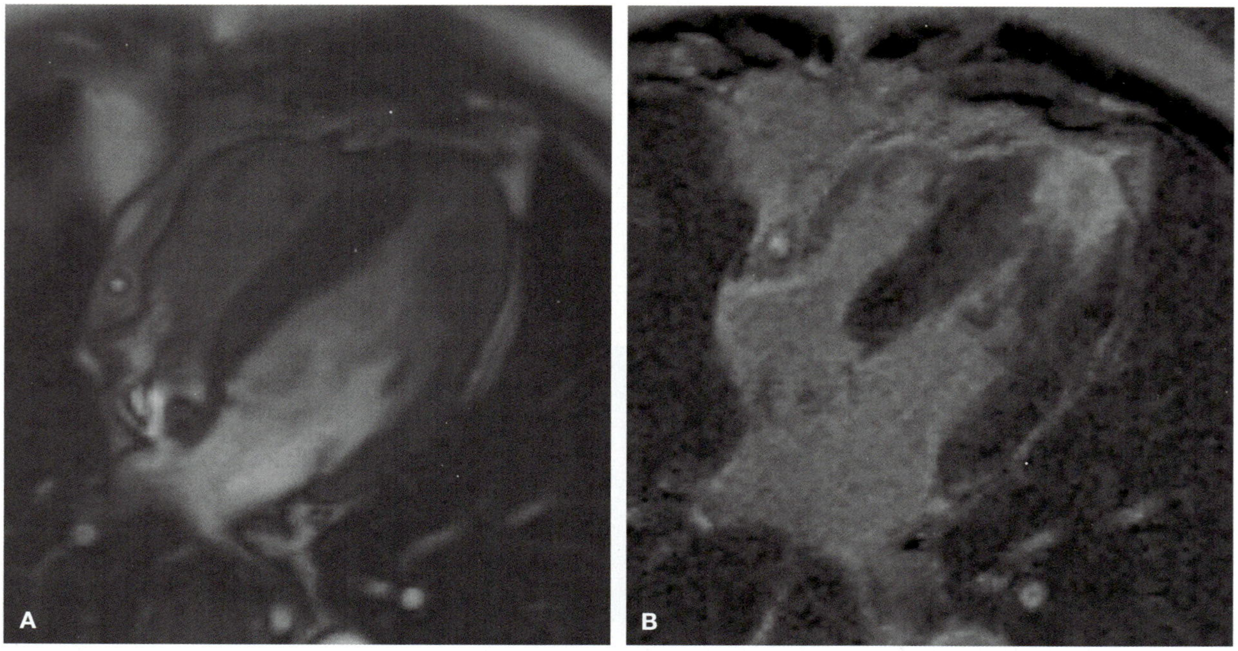

Figure 34.18. End-diastolic cine (**A**) and late gadolinium-enhanced (LGE) (**B**) cardiac MR images in 4-chamber plane in a patient with apical hypertrophic cardiomyopathy demonstrating marked wall thickening at the left ventricular apex (spade-shaped configuration) and moderate intensity transmural LGE at the hypertrophied apical myocardium.

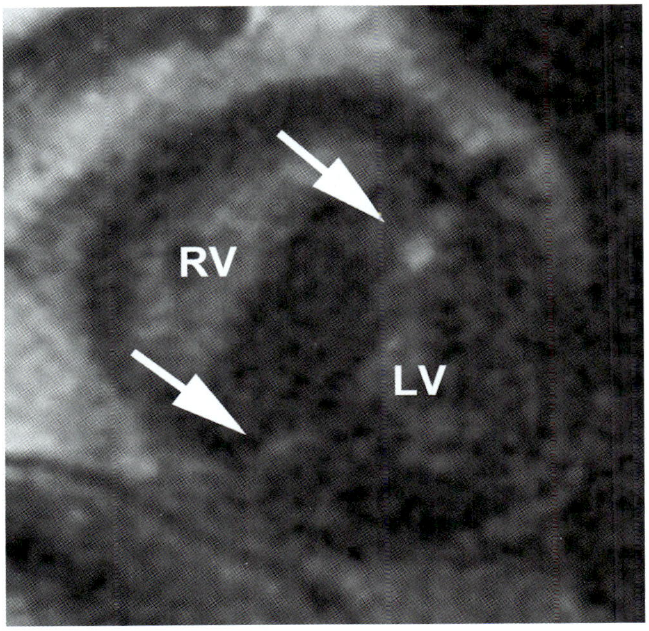

Figure 34.19. Hypertrophic cardiomyopathy. Late gadolinium-enhanced image in the short-axis plane shows hyperenhancement at the ventricular hinge points, at the sites of connections (*arrows*) of ventricular septum to anterior and posterior walls of the LV and RV. *LV*, left ventricle; *RV*, right ventricle.

Table 34.7 Imaging Features of Restrictive Cardiomyopathies

1. Normal or mild increase in LV volumes
2. Decrease in LVEF
3. Markedly enlarged right and left atria
4. Normal pericardial thickness
5. Normal or increased LV wall thickness
6. Nonischemic LGE of myocardium in some
7. Pleural and pericardial effusions

LGE, late gadolinium enhancement; LV, left ventricular; LVEF, left ventricular ejection fraction.

autopsy in 20% to 30% of such patients. Cardiac symptoms are highly suggestive of myocardial involvement in patients with systemic sarcoidosis. In patients with clinical manifestations of myocardial sarcoidosis who do not have systemic disease, however, the diagnosis is challenging, and myocardial biopsy is usually required for confirmation. Because distribution of the infiltration is patchy, nondirected biopsy is associated with false-negative results. Fluorodeoxyglucose–positron emission tomography demonstrates focal uptake in the myocardium at sites of active disease.

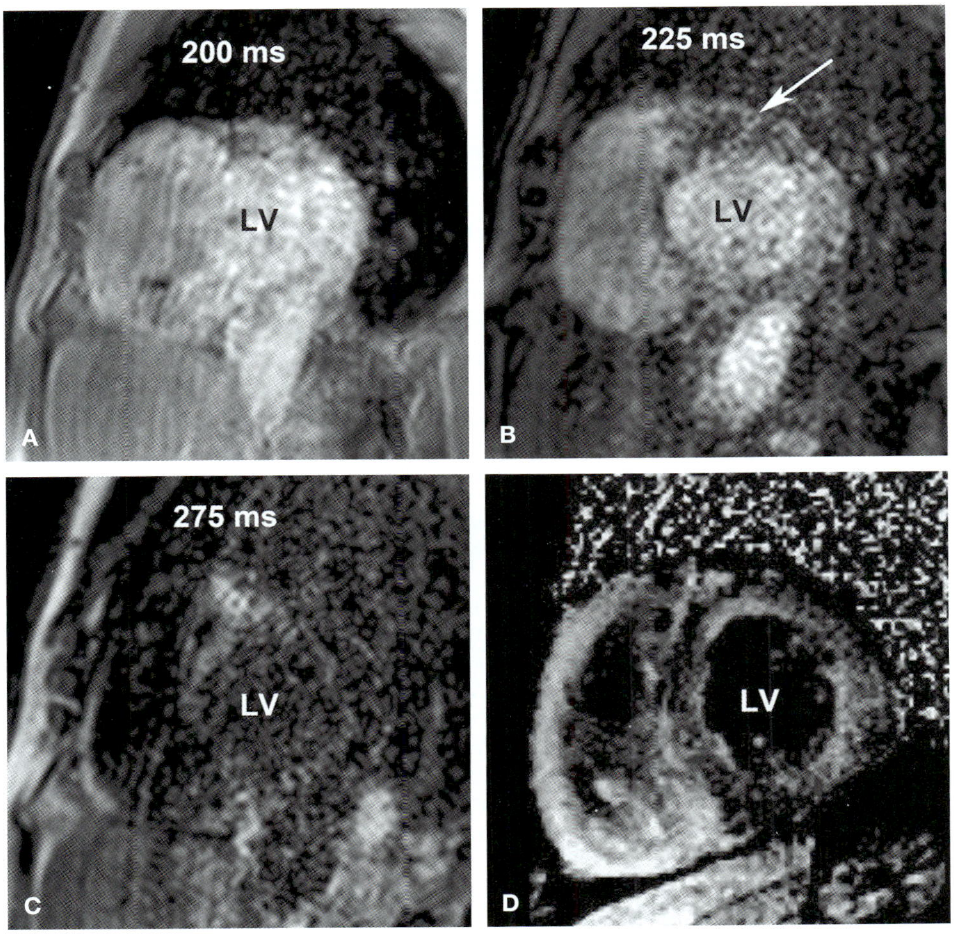

Figure 34.20. Series of increasing inversion times for short-axis IRGRE images (**A, B**) shows the myocardial signal starting to null (*arrow*) before cavitary blood. (**C**) Higher-resolution late gadolinium enhancement at optimal inversion time for nulling normal myocardial signal (**D**) demonstrates circumferential subendocardial hyperenhancement. Note signal of cavitary blood is nulled with normal myocardium. The near simultaneous nulling of blood pool and normal myocardium is characteristic for cardiac amyloidosis. *IRGRE*, inversion recovery gradient echo; *LV*, left ventricle.

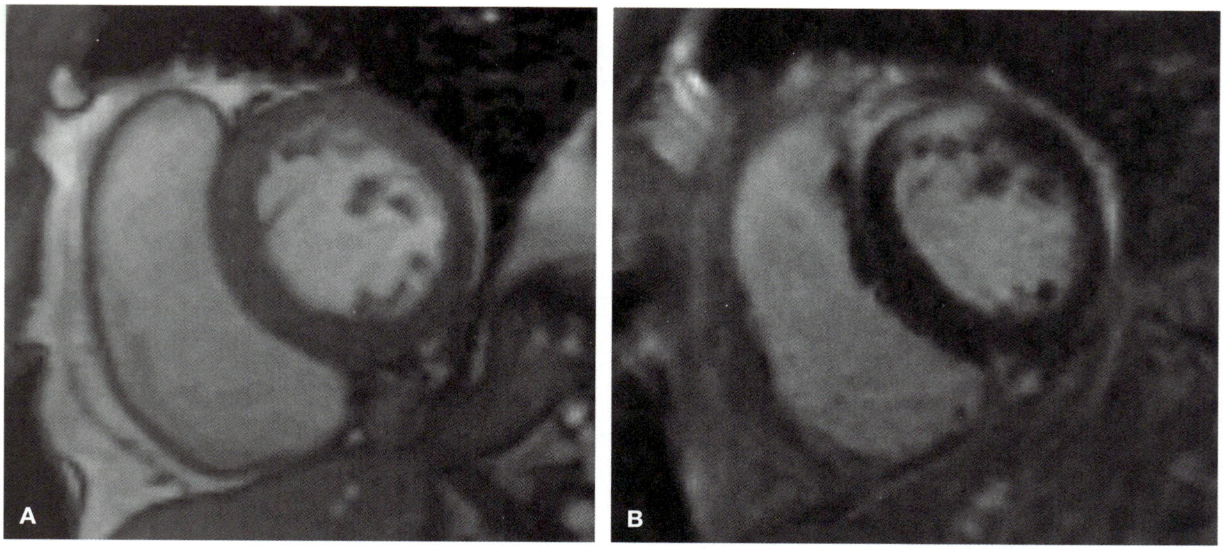

Figure 34.21. Cine MR image (**A**) in the short-axis plane in a patient with cardiac sarcoidosis show mild left ventricular (LV) wall thickening and dilation. Late gadolinium-enhanced (LGE) image in the short-axis plane (**B**) shows mid-wall nodular LGE at the LV anterior wall.

Cine MRI usually demonstrates reduced LV and/or RV ejection fraction (Table 34.9). There may be global or regional LV hypokinesis (Fig. 34.21). Less commonly, the cine MRI features mimic a restrictive cardiomyopathy as described above.

LGE-MRI shows sites of postinflammatory fibrosis or sarcoid activity as hyperenhancement, which are often nodular or patchy with a predilection for the basal anterior septum, often extending into the RV and LV anterior wall (Fig. 34.21).

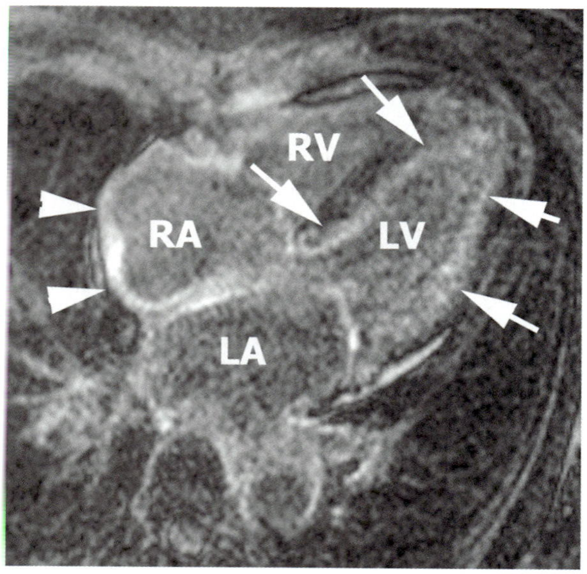

Figure 34.22. Late gadolinium-enhanced (LGE) image in the 4-chamber long-axis plane shows global subendocardial hyperenhancement (*arrows*) on the left ventricle (*LV*) of a patient with cardiac amyloidosis. Note the right atrial wall thickening and delayed enhancement (*arrowheads*) characteristic of cardiac amyloidosis. *RA*, right atrium; *LA*, left atrium; *RV*, right ventricle.

After the granulomas have regressed, postinflammatory scars may persist. These can be delineated as regions of diminished or absent wall thickening or as regions of diastolic wall thinning and regions of delayed enhancement on LGE-MRI (Table 34.10).

The presence and extent of LGE has prognostic significance in cardiac sarcoidosis. The presence of LGE is associated with ventricular arrhythmias and cardiac death.

Fabry Disease

Fabry disease is an X-linked inherited lysosomal storage disease resulting in accumulation of glycosphingolipids in multiple organs including the heart. Men typically have more severe involvement but women are also affected due to X-inactivation. Cardiac involvement can mimic morphologic and clinical features of HCM although the typical pattern of wall thickening is concentric. LGE characteristically occurs in a mid-wall pattern at the basal to

Table 34.8 Imaging Features of Cardiac Amyloidosis

1. Normal or mild increase in LV volumes
2. Mild to severe decrease in LVEF
3. Increased LV wall thickness (usually concentric)
4. Increase in atrial wall thickness
5. Normal pericardial thickness
6. LGE—usually LV circumferential subendocardial
7. Delayed hyperenhancement of RV and atria
8. Elevated native T1 and ECV

ECV, extracellular volume; LGE, late gadolinium enhancement; LV, left ventricular; LVEF, left ventricular ejection fraction.

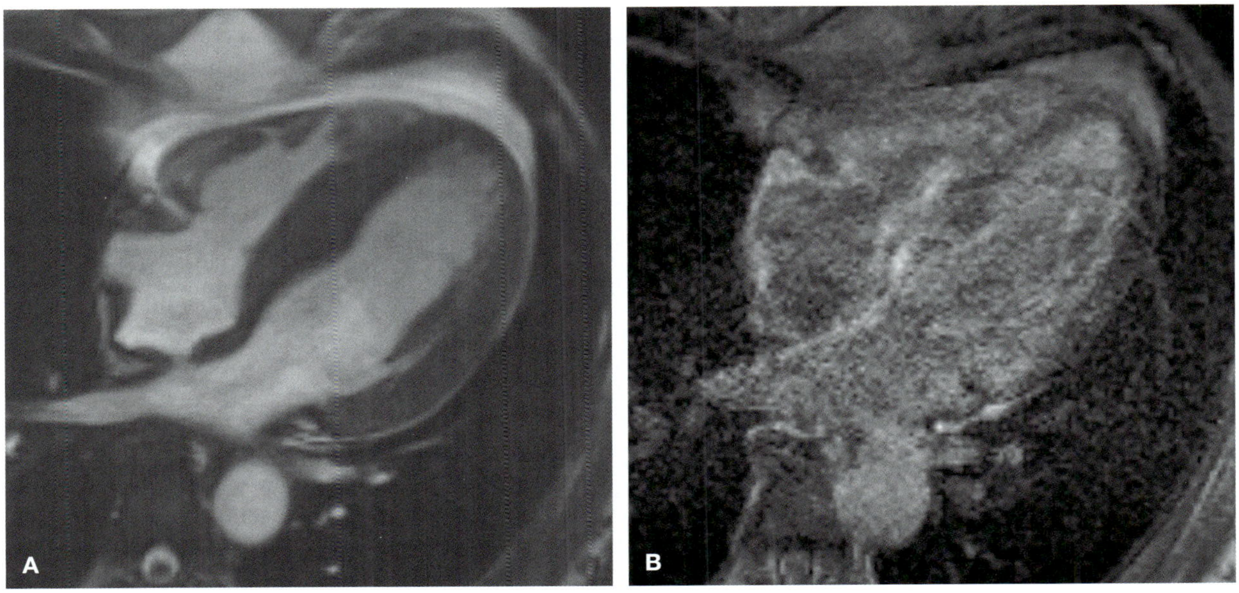

Figure 34.23. End-diastolic cine (**A**) and late gadolinium-enhanced (LGE) (**B**) cardiac MR images in 4-chamber plane in a patient with cardiac amyloidosis demonstrating marked left ventricular wall thickening and extensive subendocardial enhancement to diffuse LGE involving both ventricles and both atrial walls with dark blood pool.

mid-inferolateral wall (Fig. 34.24). Native T1 values are reduced at the septum reflecting glycosphingolipid accumulation. However, areas with LGE typically reflect fibrosis and therefore regional elevation of native T1 is often seen at the inferolateral wall corresponding to the area with LGE (Fig. 34.25).

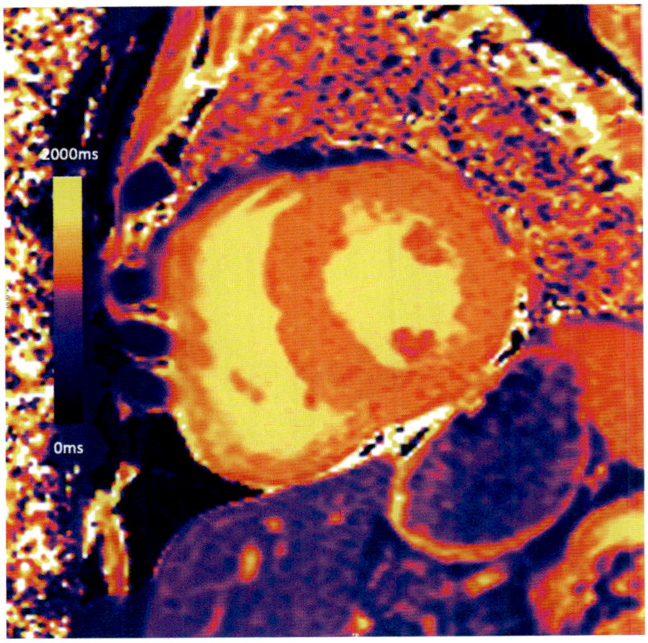

Figure 34.24. Native T1 map in a patient with cardiac amyloidosis (same patient as Fig. 34.23). Native T1 map in a mid-ventricular short-axis plane demonstrates diffusely elevated T1 values.

Danon Disease

This is a rare inherited lysosomal storage disorder. It usually affects men early in life causing heart failure, skeletal myopathy, and neurocognitive impairment. In the heart, there is often severe concentric wall thickening with reduced LV function. LGE is often extensive but typically spares the septum, which is distinct from the pattern typical in HCM.

Hemochromatosis

Hemochromatosis may be primary or secondary. Primary hemochromatosis is an inherited autosomal recessive disease. Secondary hemochromatosis develops mainly secondary to repeated blood transfusions required to treat thalassemia major. In primary hemochromatosis, iron is deposited in the liver and pancreas, but the spleen remains normal. This characteristic distinguishes primary from secondary hemochromatosis, in which iron is also deposited in the spleen. Increased iron deposition in the cardiac myocytes

Table 34.9 Imaging Features of Cardiac Sarcoidosis

1. Nodular foci of high signal on T2-weighted images or focal high T2 mapping values
2. Nodular or linear foci of myocardial LGE
3. LGE on RV side of ventricular septum
4. May have increased wall thickness and decreased LV function

LGE, late gadolinium enhancement; LV, left ventricular; RV, right ventricular.

Table 34.10 Myocardial Abnormalities Associated With Late Gadolinium Enhancement

1. Acute and chronic myocardial infarction
2. Acute myocarditis
3. Hypertrophic cardiomyopathy
4. Dilated cardiomyopathy
5. Restrictive cardiomyopathy (some cases—usually infiltrative type)
6. Amyloidosis
7. Sarcoidosis
8. Fabry disease
9. Endomyocardial fibrosis
10. Postoperative and adult congenital heart disease

in hemochromatosis causes diastolic and systolic cardiac dysfunction and ventricular dysrhythmias. After an initial asymptomatic period, cardiopathy caused by iron overload initially presents as diastolic dysfunction with a restrictive filling pattern. When the iron overload reaches a critical level, systolic functional abnormalities occur, and the disease can take the form of a DCM.

Iron reduces T1 and T2 relaxation times due to local magnetic field inhomogeneities, causing myocardial signal intensity to be reduced (see Fig. 34.11). The amount of signal decrease on T2-weighted images correlates with the iron level in tissue but not with serum iron levels. MRI is a valuable tool for noninvasively estimating the iron concentration in the heart and for monitoring therapy.

Table 34.11 Imaging Features of ACM

1. Myocardial fibrofatty changes
2. Focal wall thinning
3. Regional akinesis or dyskinesis
4. Global hypokinesis and reduced ejection fraction of RV and/or LV
5. RV and/or LV dilation
6. Myocardial LGE

ACM, arrhythmogenic cardiomyopathy; LGE, late gadolinium enhancement; LV, left ventricle; RV, right ventricle.

Assessment for myocardial dysfunction caused by myocardial iron deposition is most effectively done using a cine MRI acquisition in the short-axis plane in order to calculate the LVEF. A specialized T2* (star) sequence is done, which produces an array of images at varying T2 delays. From this acquisition, a T2* value can be calculated. A value below 20 milliseconds at 1.5T is considered indicative of iron deposition in the myocardium. Native T1 mapping is also useful for assessment of myocardial iron although less commonly integrated in clinical practice.

Arrhythmogenic Cardiomyopathy

ACM was initially described as an RV disease, hence the term arrhythmogenic RV cardiomyopathy. However, ACM is now recognized to have right-dominant, left-dominant, and biventricular phenotypes. ACM has characteristic features on SE and cine MRI (Table 34.11). Typical findings are fatty

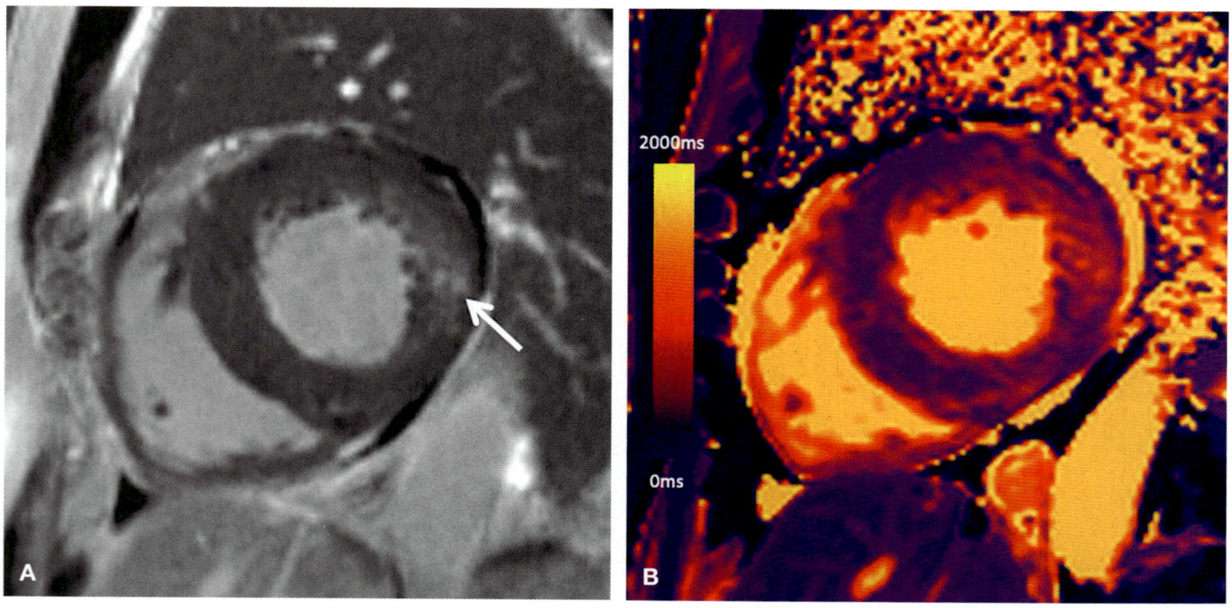

Figure 34.25. Late gadolinium-enhanced (LGE, **A**) and native T1 map (**B**) cardiac MR images in short-axis plane in a patient with Fabry disease demonstrating marked concentric left ventricular wall thickening with patchy mid-wall LGE at the basal inferolateral wall (*arrow*) and low native T1 values at the interventricular septum but mildly elevated T1 values at the basal inferolateral wall corresponding to the area of LGE.

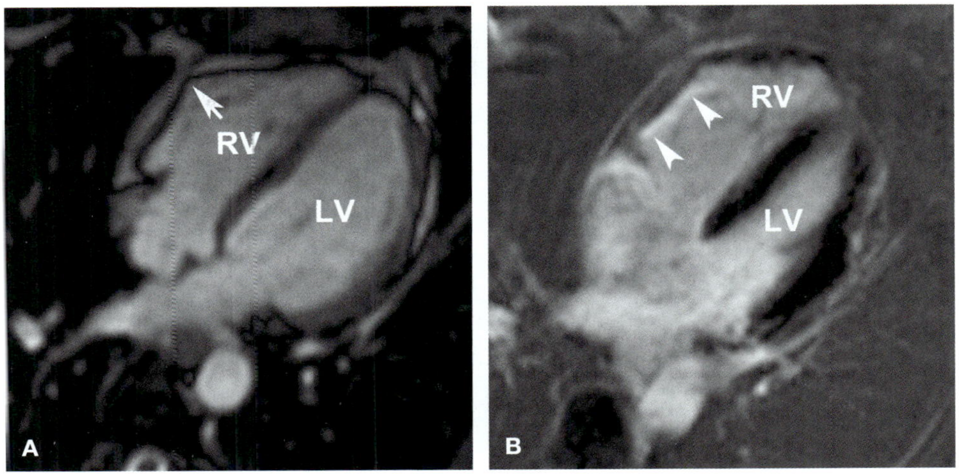

Figure 34.26. Arrhythmogenic cardiomyopathy with RV involvement, right dominant type. Cine (**A**) and late gadolinium-enhanced (**B**) images show wall thinning and dyskinesis (*arrow*) of RV free wall and hyperenhancement (*arrowheads*). *LV*, left ventricle; *RV*, right ventricle.

deposition in the RV free wall and subepicardial LV reflected by chemical shift artifact on cine imaging or on T1-weighted imaging. However, fat in the RV wall can be a normal finding so that this observation is unreliable for the diagnosis of ACM. Another feature is regional bulging or thinning of the RV free wall (Figs. 34.26 and 34.27). Additional morphologic features include focal sacculations, aneurysms, ventricular dilation, and systolic dysfunction. LGE-MRI can demonstrate RV free wall and subepicardial LV LGE (Figs. 34.26 and 34.28). In left-dominant ACM associated with desmosomal mutations, a characteristic ringlike pattern of nearly circumferential subepicardial LGE has been described.

Findings on MRI can be highly suggestive of the diagnosis of ACM. However, the diagnosis is not definitely established by MRI findings alone; the MRI features are used in association with clinical and electrophysiologic findings to establish the diagnosis. Moreover, MRI studies may be equivocal for the diagnosis, and MRI cannot be relied upon to exclude early stages of this disease.

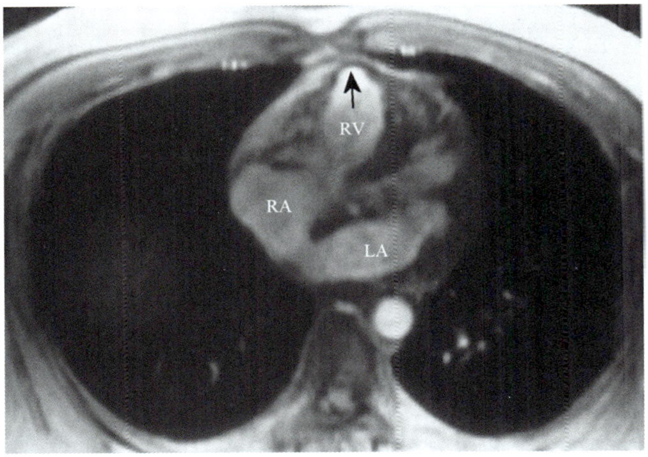

Figure 34.27. Cine MR image shows regional dyskinesis (*arrow*) of the right ventricle in a patient with arrhythmogenic cardiomyopathy with RV involvement, right dominant type. *LA*, left atrium; *RA*, right atrium; *RV*, right ventricle.

Myocarditis

Typical presenting symptoms include chest pain, shortness of breath, and palpitations. Profound dysfunction of the ventricles may occur. Most cases of myocarditis are triggered by viral infections. Other causes include autoimmune disease and vaccination (including mRNA-based COVID-19 vaccinations in a minority of individuals). Endomyocardial biopsy is rarely performed for diagnosis due to the patchy nature of the disease and invasiveness of the procedure.

MRI is a useful noninvasive test for diagnosing myocarditis and monitoring longitudinal changes over time (Table 34.12). Because of the interstitial edema, the T2 relaxation time is increased, so that the signal may be increased on T2-weighted images or T2 maps. LGE is frequent, most often in a subepicardial pattern (Fig. 34.29). A linear mid-wall septal pattern is less frequent but is associated with worse prognosis. When a patient with a presumptive diagnosis of myocarditis is assessed, the imaging findings must be interpreted in relation to the clinical symptoms and signs.

Cine MRI typically shows global LV hypokinesis and sometimes also RV hypokinesis (Fig. 34.30). Some LV segments may show more severe dysfunction than others. The LV and sometimes RV volumes are increased and ejection fractions are usually severely reduced in the acute phase. LVEF and function may show recovery in days to weeks. In a minority of patients, the LV function may remain depressed. LGE typically decreases in extent, but can also resolve or persist at follow-up (Fig. 34.30).

Chagas disease is caused by the protozoan *Trypanosoma cruzi*. Cardiac involvement is frequent. This infection is characterized by acute, intermediate, and chronic phases. In chronic Chagas disease, the heart is the most frequently affected organ, and lymphocytic infiltration can be observed. Regions of focal inflammation are reflected as focal myocardial LGE. The regional distribution of LGE is typically inferolateral basal and apical. Apical aneurysm of the left ventricle is a characteristic finding of chronic Chagas disease. LGE is seen more frequently in more advanced diseases and worse clinical statuses.

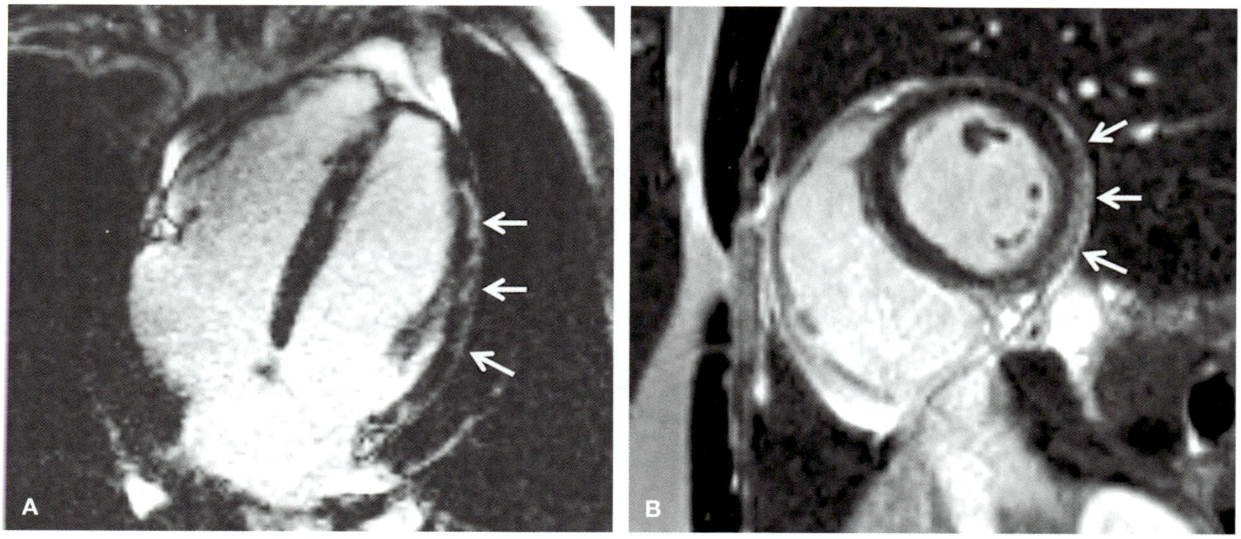

Figure 34.28. Late gadolinium-enhanced (LGE) cardiac MR image in 4-chamber plane (**A**) and mid-ventricular short-axis plane (**B**) in a patient with left dominant arrhythmogenic cardiomyopathy demonstrating extensive subepicardial left ventricular LGE predominantly involving the lateral wall (arrows).

LGE for Risk Assessment in Nonischemic Myocardial Diseases

LGE-MRI provides risk assessment in several nonischemic myocardial diseases. These include HCM, DCM, and sarcoidosis.

LGE-MRI is important in risk assessment in patients with HCM. Patients with HCM and any degree of myocardial LGE have much higher risk of nonsustained ventricular tachycardia. In addition to an increased incidence of arrhythmias, LGE is also associated with decreased LV function and sudden cardiac death.

The extent of LGE in patients with HCM increases over time. LGE extent >15% of LV myocardium may be useful in supporting an indication for ICD placement.

LGE-MRI is also associated with worse prognosis in patients with DCM. The extent of fibrosis depicted on LGE images has been associated with increased interventricular dyssynchrony in DCM. Patients with LGE have more future adverse cardiac events including cardiac death.

The presence and extend of LGE has prognostic significance in cardiac sarcoidosis. The presence of LGE has been related to deleterious alteration in ventricular volumes and function, ventricular arrhythmias, and severity of mitral regurgitation.

Table 34.12 Imaging Features of Myocarditis

1. Regional wall motion abnormalities
2. Decreased LV ± RV ejection fraction.
3. Focal LGE—most often subepicardial
4. Mid-wall septal LGE associated with worse prognosis
5. Corresponding high T2 in area of LGE in acute myocarditis
6. ± Pericardial effusion and enhancement (if associated pericarditis)

LGE, late gadolinium enhancement; LV, left ventricular; RV, right ventricular.

Cardiac Noncompaction

Noncompaction refers to increased noncompacted or hypertrabeculated myocardium relative to the normal compacted myocardium (Fig. 34.31). Excessive trabeculation has been proposed more recently as an alternative term. It can be

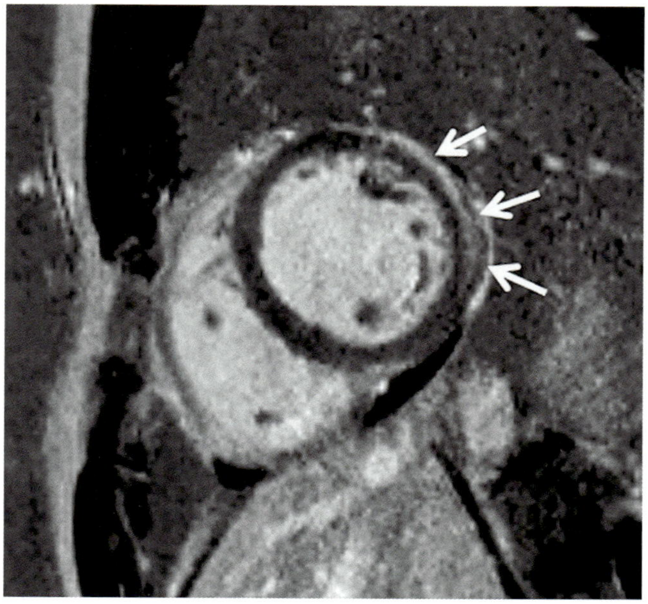

Figure 34.29. Late gadolinium-enhanced (LGE) cardiac MR image in short-axis plane in a patient with myocarditis demonstrates subepicardial left ventricular LGE at the mid-ventricular anterior and inferior lateral wall (arrows).

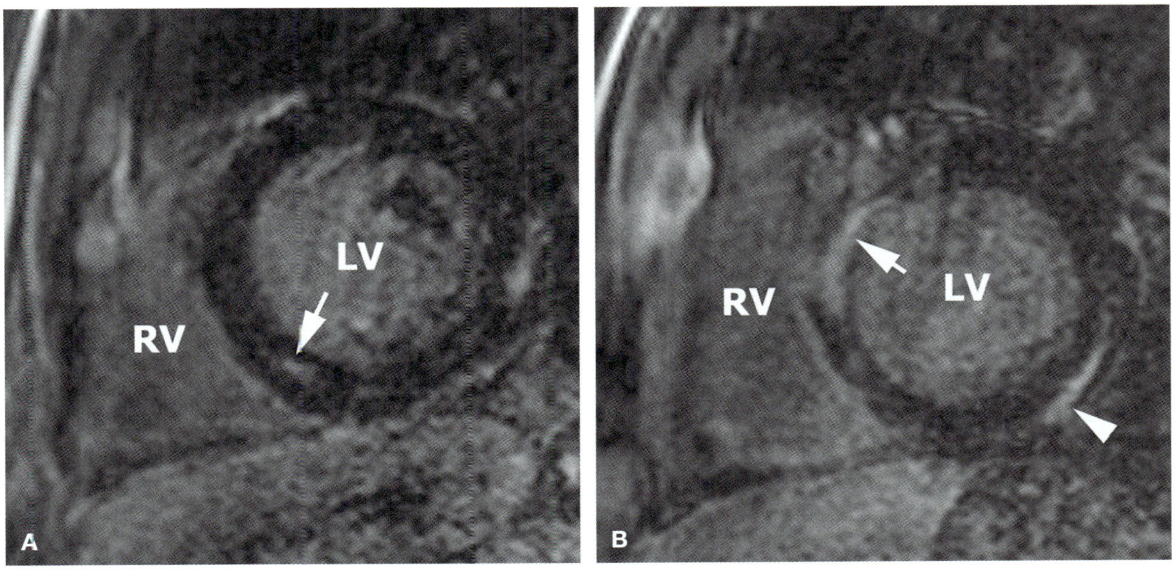

Figure 34.30. **A, B:** Late gadolinium-enhanced images at two short-axis planes show mid-wall (*arrow*) and subepicardial (*arrowhead*) hyperenhancement in a patient with myocarditis. *RV*, right ventricle; *LV*, left ventricle.

associated with heart failure and cardiac death. However, the presence of excessive trabeculation by itself does not define the presence of cardiomyopathy. Management should be guided by symptoms.

Heart Transplantation and Transplant Rejection

Measuring the ventricular volume, myocardial mass, and ejection fraction with cine MRI can be used to monitor the morphology and function of a transplanted heart.

Acute rejection is one of the main causes of death during the first year after transplantation. Historically, repeat biopsy was used to evaluate for transplant rejection although more recently noninvasive testing has been introduced, including molecular techniques and imaging. Cardiac MRI parameters that have been proposed for transplant monitoring include T2 mapping, T1 mapping, LGE, wall thickness, and perfusion.

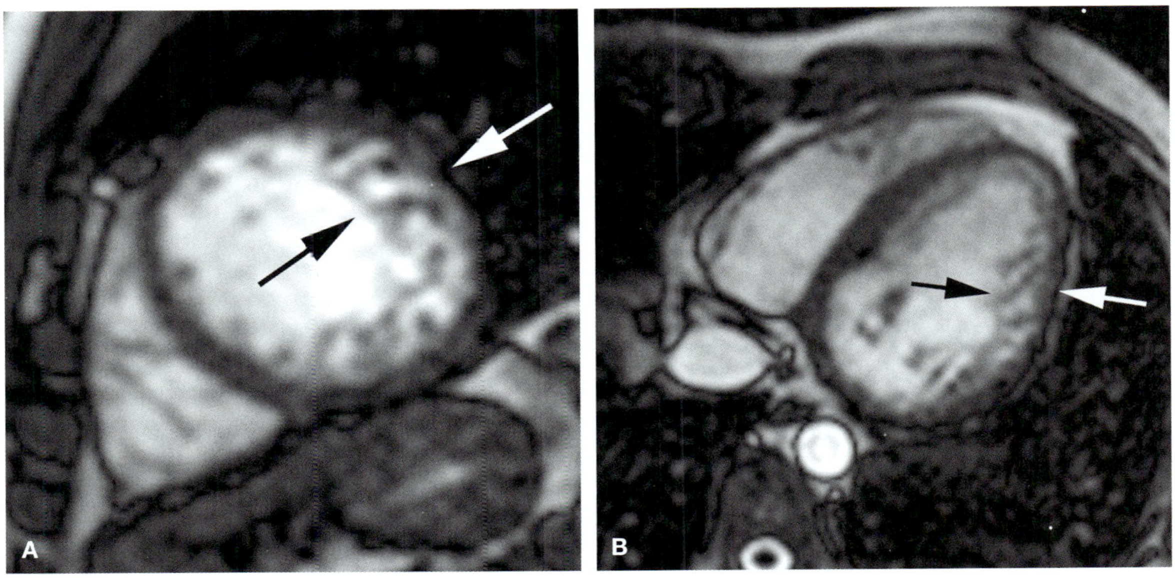

Figure 34.31. Short-axis (**A**) and axial (**B**) cine MR images at end diastole in a patient with myocardial partial noncompaction. Note the prominent myocardial trabeculation in the lateral wall (*black arrow*) with adjacent thinning of the compacted myocardium (*white arrow*).

MYOCARDIAL INVOLVEMENT IN SYSTEMIC DISEASE

There is increasing recognition that many systemic diseases can involve the heart including autoimmune diseases such as systemic lupus erythematosus. Other rheumatologic diseases that can result in cardiac changes include rheumatoid arthritis and psoriatic arthritis. In general, cardiac involvement leads to worse prognosis in patients with systemic diseases. Importantly, the treatment from these diseases can also negatively impact the heart such as in the setting of long-term Plaquenil therapy for lupus, which can lead to anti-malarial induced cardiomyopathy in a minority of patients.

SUGGESTED READINGS

Aitken M, Chan MV, Urzua Fresno C, et al. Diagnostic accuracy of cardiac MRI versus FDG PET for cardiac sarcoidosis: a systematic review and meta-analysis. *Radiology*. 2022;304(3):566-579. doi:10.1148/radiol.213170

Corrado D, Perazzolo Marra M, Zorzi A, et al. Diagnosis of arrhythmogenic cardiomyopathy: The Padua criteria. *Int J Cardiol.* 2020;319:106-114. doi:10.1016/j.ijcard.2020.06.005

Ferreira VM, Schulz-Menger J, Holmvang G, et al. Cardiovascular magnetic resonance in nonischemic myocardial inflammation: expert recommendations. *J Am Coll Cardiol.* 2018;72(24):3158-3176. doi:10.1016/j.jacc.2018.09.072

Neubauer S, Kolm P, Ho CY, et al; HCMR Investigators. Distinct subgroups in hypertrophic cardiomyopathy in the NHLBI HCM registry. *J Am Coll Cardiol.* 2019;74(19):2333-2345. doi:10.1016/j.jacc.2019.08.1057

Warnica W, Al-Arnawoot A, Stanimirovic A, et al. Clinical impact of cardiac MRI T1 and T2 parametric mapping in patients with suspected cardiomyopathy. *Radiology*. 2022;305(2):319-326. doi:10.1148/radiol.220067.

Weng Z, Yao J, Chan RH, et al. Prognostic value of LGE-CMR in HCM: a meta-analysis. *JACC Cardiovasc Imaging.* 2016;9(12):1392-1402. doi:10.1016/j.jcmg.2016.02.031

Chapter 35

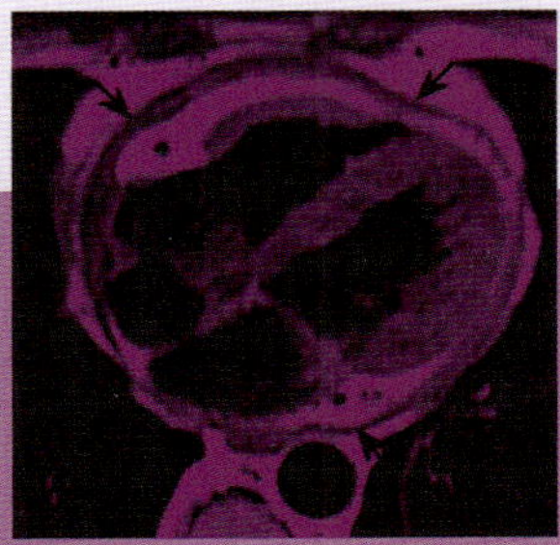

Tushar Kumar • Gautham Reddy • Karen G. Ordovas

Pericardial Diseases

INTRODUCTION

Pericardial disease may be primary and involve the pericardium alone. It is also frequently a manifestation of a wide variety of systemic diseases or secondary to other cardiovascular diseases. There are several imaging techniques that are effective for the diagnosis of pericardial diseases. Asymptomatic abnormalities of the pericardium are occasionally identified on computed tomography (CT) of the thorax. However, the imaging modality of choice for initial evaluation of patients with suspected pericardial effusion is transthoracic echocardiography. This widely available and relatively low-cost method has a high accuracy for detection of pericardial effusion and signs of tamponade. It is also a good method for guiding diagnostic or therapeutic pericardiocentesis. The main limitation of echocardiography in pericardial diseases is its inability to assess the entire pericardial extension. It is also not very accurate for depiction of pericardial thickening, because echogenicity of the pericardium is similar to adjacent tissues.

Major indications for further investigation of pericardial effusion with CT or magnetic resonance imaging (MRI) are identification of loculated effusion, evaluation of complicated pericardial effusion (hemorrhagic vs nonhemorrhagic), measurement of pericardial thickness, assessment of enhancement of the pericardium, and characterization of pericardial masses.

CT and MRI provide excellent delineation of the mediastinal anatomy, with high soft-tissue contrast and spatial resolution. The visualization of the entire chest can also give important information for differential diagnosis and extent of pericardial diseases. Both methods provide some information on tissue characterization, which is useful for the diagnosis of pericardial masses and pericardial inflammation.

CT is the best method for depiction of pericardial calcification, a finding suggestive of constrictive pericarditis in the appropriate clinical setting. CT-guided pericardiocentesis can be used for the management of loculated pericardial effusions. Electrocardiogram-gated cardiac CT can eliminate the artifacts related to cardiac motion but is usually not necessary for the evaluation of pericardial abnormalities.

MRI has the advantage of avoiding iodinated contrast media and ionizing radiation as well as providing clear distinction between pericardial fluid and layers. Cine MRI can usually differentiate a small pericardial effusion from pericardial thickening, which can be misinterpreted by CT. The major indication for MRI in pericardial disease is the measurement of pericardial thickness, which is useful for diagnosis of constrictive pericarditis in patients with constrictive/restrictive physiology.

TECHNIQUES

Multidetector cardiac CT imaging with cardiac gating is ideally used to assess pericardial anatomy and cardiac function with adequate temporal and high spatial resolution. However, nongated multidetector CT is usually adequate for diagnosis of pericardial disease.

MRI studies with morphologic and functional sequences allow a complete evaluation of the pericardium with high soft-tissue contrast and spatial resolution. It is particularly useful for evaluation of pericardial effusion, constriction, inflammation, masses, and congenital anomalies. Images of the entire pericardium can be acquired with a few breath holds or during free breathing.

Turbo T1-weighted spin-echo (SE) images are usually acquired at least in the axial and coronal planes for morphologic assessment of the pericardium. SE images and inversion

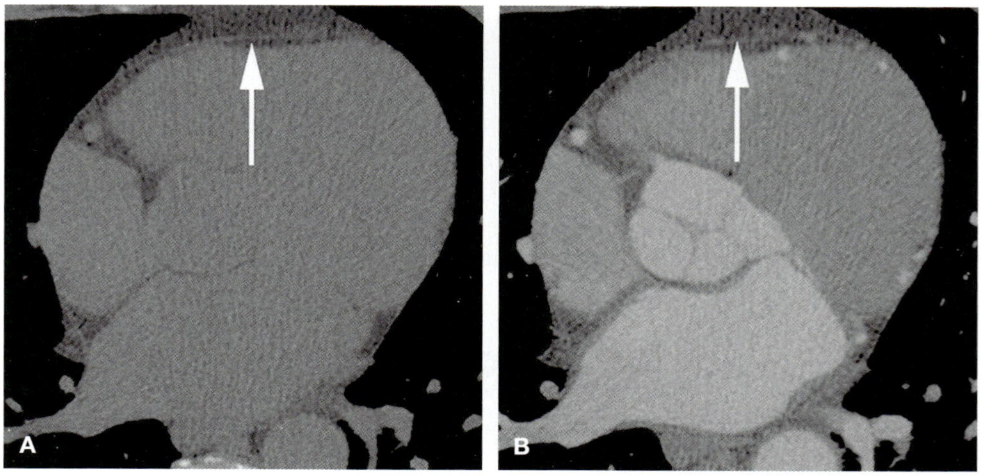

Figure 35.1. Normal pericardium on CT. Cardiac-gated axial images before (**A**) and after (**B**) iodinated contrast media show normal appearance of a thin pericardium, best seen adjacent to the right ventricular free wall (arrows).

recovery images can be obtained early and late after the administration of gadolinium chelates to detect enhancement caused by inflammatory processes of the pericardium. Cine MR images using gradient echo sequences (GRE) or steady-state free precession sequences are acquired to evaluate ventricular function, ventricular sliding motion over the pericardium, and diastolic ventricular septal motion.

NORMAL PERICARDIUM AND PERICARDIAL RECESSES

The pericardium is a compliant sac that envelops the heart and the origin of the great vessels. It is attached to the sternum anteriorly and to the diaphragm inferiorly. The left atrium is only partially covered by the pericardium. Parietal pericardium consists of fibrous tissue with an inner layer of mesothelial cells that reflect in the regions of pericardial attachment and cover the surface of the heart, forming the visceral pericardium. On MRI and CT studies, the normal pericardium is usually less than 2 mm thick (Figs. 35.1 and 35.2). A thickness greater than 4 mm is considered abnormal. CT can overestimate pericardial thickness in the presence of isodense effusion. Visualization of the pericardium on both CT and MRI is possible because of its position between two fat planes (epicardial and pericardial). Although the pericardium is visible over the right cardiac chambers in most studies, it may not be visible over the lateral and inferior walls of the left ventricle.

The pericardial cavity normally contains up to 50 mL of serous fluid that distributes diffusely around the heart surface and inside the pericardial recesses. The complex configuration of the pericardial cavity can be understood as two connected complex spaces surrounding the heart and great vessels. The first region surrounds the proximal two-thirds of the ascending aorta and pulmonary artery out to its bifurcation and is known as the transverse sinus (Fig. 35.3). The second region surrounds the attachment of the inferior vena cava (IVC), superior vena cava (SVC), and pulmonary veins, delineating a cul-de-sac behind the left atrium called oblique sinus (Fig. 35.4A). The pericardial cavity has several

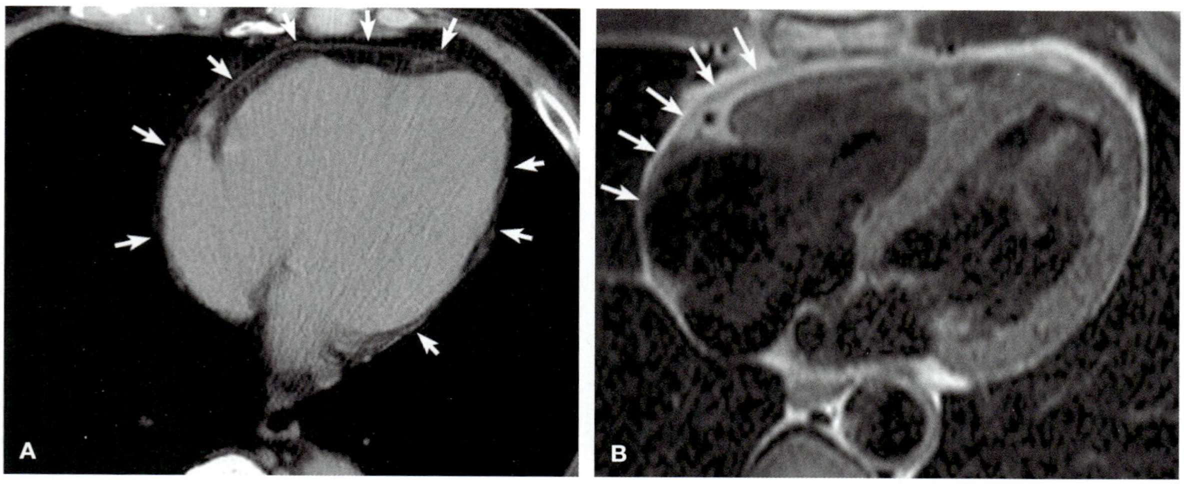

Figure 35.2. Normal pericardium. CT (**A**) and axial T1-weighted spin-echo images (**B**) show the normal appearance of the pericardium (arrows).

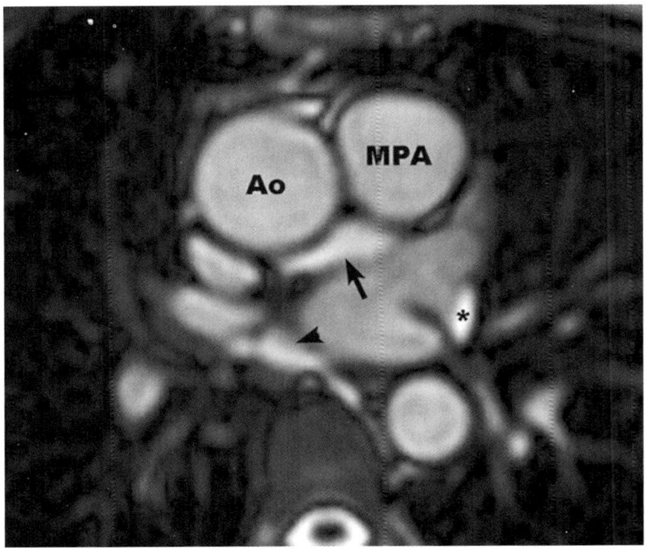

Figure 35.3. Transverse sinus of the pericardium. Axial cine MR image at the level of the main pulmonary artery (MPA) and ascending aorta (Ao) shows the transverse sinus of the pericardium (arrow). Note that the pericardial fluid inside the sinus has the same signal intensity of the flowing blood. Also shown are the oblique sinus (arrowhead) and left pulmonic vein recess (asterisk).

recesses that can be recognized on CT and MR images: these are the superior and inferior aortic recesses, left and right pulmonic recesses, posterior pericardial recess, left and right pulmonary vein recesses, and postcaval recess (Figs. 35.4B and 35.5).

Knowledge of the cross-sectional anatomy of the pericardial recesses is essential for its differentiation from lymph nodes or abnormalities of adjacent mediastinal structures. In the setting of malignancy, a misinterpretation of a normal recess as lymphadenopathy could lead to inappropriate staging of tumors. Normal pericardial fluid resides in the recesses of normal individuals. Fluid is invariably observed in one or more recesses on CT and MRI in the absence of a pericardial effusion. Occasionally, one of the recesses can be much more prominent than the others, increasing the chances of misinterpretation (Fig. 35.6).

One or more recesses may be particularly prominent in some normal subjects.

The pericardium is composed of fibrous tissue and appears dark on T1- and T2-weighted SE images (Fig. 35.2B). In the area of the right ventricle (RV), it is located between the bright mediastinal and subepicardial fat, which provides a natural high level of contrast, so that the sensitivity for the visualization of the pericardium in this region is 100%. In regions adjacent to the lung, the natural contrast is lower, so that the sensitivity for visualization in the area of the lateral wall of the left ventricle is lower. The thickness of the pericardium on MR images ranges from 1 to 3 mm. Anatomic studies have shown the thickness of the pericardium to be in the range of 0.4 to 1 mm. The relative overestimation on MRI has been presumed to result from motion-induced signal loss of the normal pericardial fluid, which cannot be readily distinguished from the pericardium itself. Pericardial thickness depends also on the anatomic level and increases toward the diaphragm. This

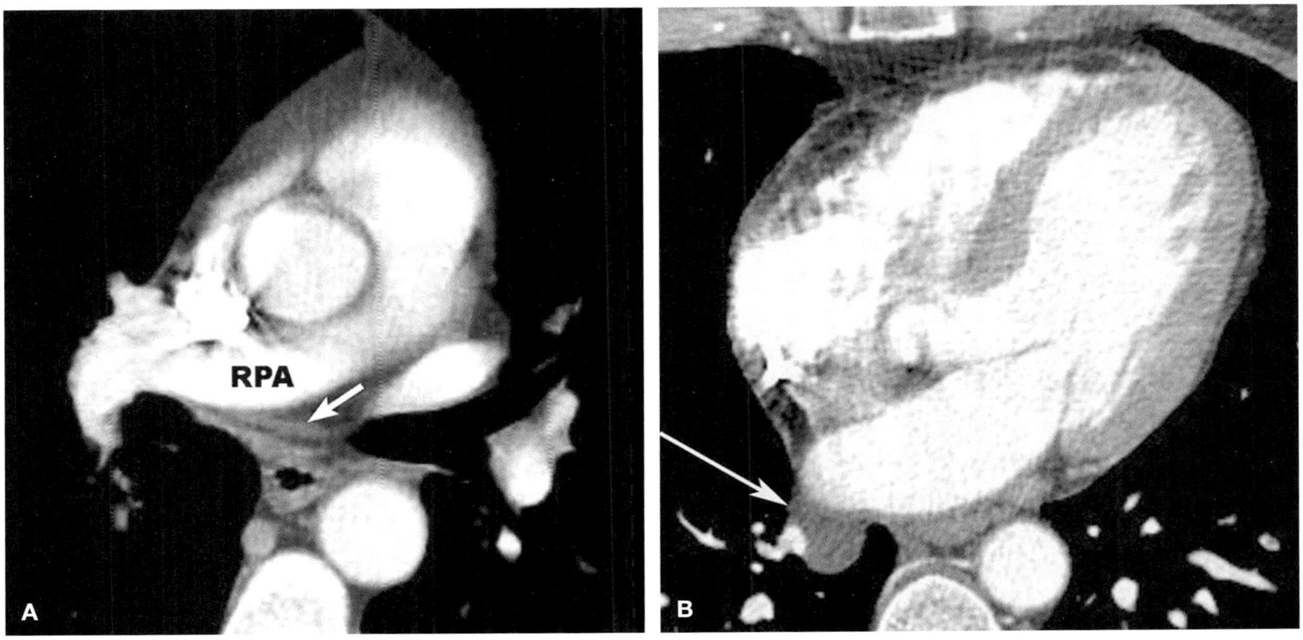

Figure 35.4. A: Oblique sinus of the pericardium. Contrast-enhanced CT image at the level of the right pulmonary artery (RPA) shows fluid inside the oblique sinus of the pericardium (arrow). Note that a fat plane separates this pericardial sinus from the anterior esophageal wall. **B:** Contrast-enhanced CT scan shows small pericardial recess around right inferior pulmonary vein (arrow).

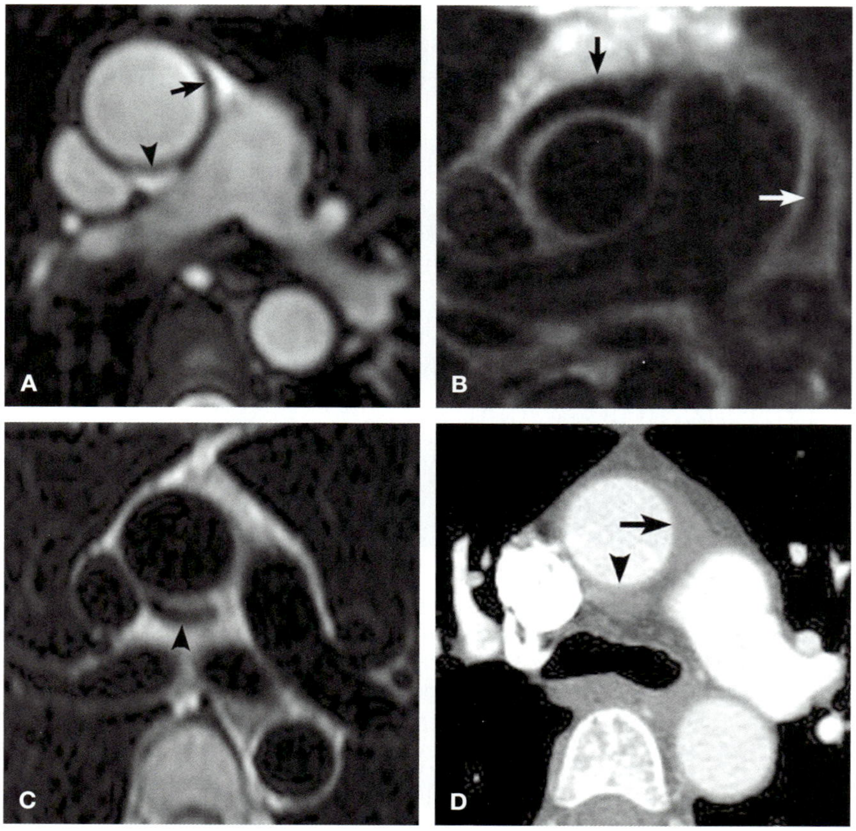

Figure 35.5. Pericardial recesses. Axial cine MR (A) and axial SE (B) images at the level of the pulmonary artery bifurcation show the anterior (black arrow) and posterior (arrowhead) portions of the superior aortic recess and the left pulmonic recess (white arrow). Axial SE image (C) and contrast-enhanced CT (D) at the level of the left pulmonary artery also show the anterior (arrow) and posterior (arrowhead) portions of the superior aortic recess.

effect results from the ligamentous insertion of the pericardium into the diaphragm and from its tangential direction to the imaging plane. Consequently, the measurement of pericardial thickness is most reliable at the midventricular level.

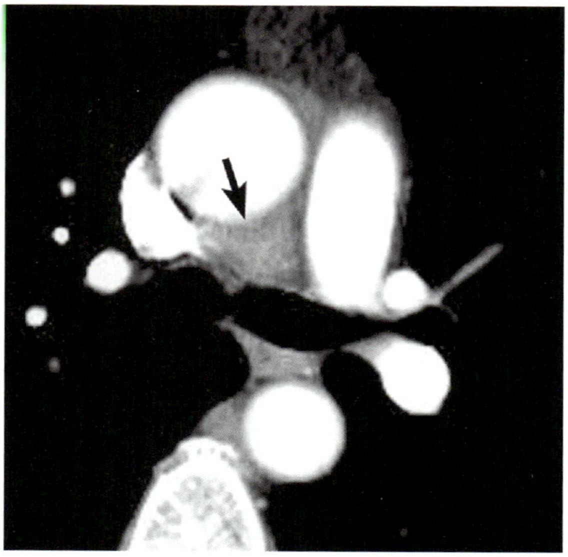

Figure 35.6. Prominent superior aortic recess. Contrast-enhanced CT at the level of the carina shows more than usual volume of pericardial fluid inside the posterior portion of the superior aortic recess (arrow).

PERICARDIAL EFFUSION

The pericardial space normally contains 10 to 50 mL of fluid. In most normal subjects, pericardial fluid can be identified in the pericardial recesses on CT and MRI. The numerous etiologies of pericardial effusion are listed in Table 35.1. In many cases, the etiology is never established. The effusion is recognized as an incidental finding on echocardiography, CT, or MRI. Imaging is essential to verify the presence, extent,

Table 35.1 Etiologies of Pericardial Effusions

1. Acute pericarditis (including myopericarditis)
2. Effusive-constrictive pericarditis
3. Congestive heart failure
4. Collagen vascular diseases (especially systemic lupus erythematosus)
5. Uremia
6. Postmyocardial infarction (Dressler syndrome)
7. Postpericardiotomy syndrome
8. Trauma
9. Aortic dissection—type A
10. Drug reaction
11. Myxedema
12. Chylopericardium
13. Neoplastic (pericardial metastases, frequently hemorrhagic)
14. Idiopathic

and severity of the fluid; for differentiating transudative versus exudative effusion; to exclude underlying inflammation; to evaluate effects on functioning of heart; and to guide pericardiocentesis.

The procedure of choice for evaluation of the presence and size of pericardial effusion is transthoracic echocardiography. Collections of fluid within the pericardial cavity can represent transudate or exudates. The latter include serous, fibrinous, purulent, and hemorrhagic or (rarely) chylous pericardial effusion.

Simple pericardial effusion (transudate) has a density close to water on CT (Fig. 35.7). The typical appearance on MRI is low signal on T1-weighted SE and high-signal intensity on T2-weighted SE, cine GRE, and steady-state free precession sequences (Fig. 35.8).

Differentiation of transudate from exudates is usually not possible based on imaging appearance alone. However, increased fluid density and heterogeneity on CT suggest exudates; on MRI, intermediate signal on T1-weighted SE images suggests exudates (Fig. 35.9).

Causes of increased CT attenuation of pericardial effusion include hemopericardium, malignancy, purulent exudates, or less likely hypothyroid-related effusion.

The appearance of pericardial hematoma depends on the age of the pericardial blood. Acute hemopericardium has a high density on CT, whereas subacute hematomas present with a heterogeneous density (Fig. 35.10). MRI of acute pericardial hematoma shows a high-signal intensity on SE T1-weighted sequences (Fig. 35.11A) and a low-signal intensity on cine GRE images. Subacute and chronic hematomas are usually heterogeneous with both high- and low-signal intensity regions on T1-weighted images, but odd hematomas may be homogenously low intensity (Fig. 35.11). Distinguishing features of pericardial hematoma compared to nonhemorrhagic effusion are summarized in Table 35.2.

Chylous effusion is extremely rare. It has been described as a low-density pericardial collection on CT.

Small amounts of pericardial fluid can be misinterpreted on CT imaging because of similar appearance to pericardial thickening. MRI can distinguish between the high T2 signal intensity of a small simple effusion and the adjacent low signal of normal parietal pericardium. However, small volume of fluid and pericardium may be indistinguishable on SE MRI and thereby simulate pericardial thickening. Pericardial effusion shows no increase in signal on T1-weighted images after administration of gadolinium chelate. This feature aids in distinguishing between pericardial fluid and pericardial or myocardial tumor on T1-weighted SE images. CT and MRI are very sensitive for the detection of generalized or loculated pericardial effusions. CT and MRI can detect pericardial effusion as small as 30 mL. Both provide information on the location of pericardial effusion and are especially effective for demonstrating loculated effusions (Fig. 35.11A). Because of uneven distribution, the total fluid volume cannot be calculated from the width of the pericardial space by applying a simple formula. However, a semiquantitative estimation can be obtained by measuring the width of the pericardial space in front of the RV. A moderate effusion of 100 to 500 mL fluid is associated with a width of more than 5 mm. Loculated effusion occurs when fluid is trapped by adhesions between the parietal and visceral pericardium. MRI is more sensitive than echocardiography in detecting loculated effusion because of its wide field of view.

ACUTE PERICARDITIS

Acute pericarditis is an inflammation of the pericardium due to a multiple etiologies (Table 35.3), of which the most frequent is viral. Pericarditis can manifest early after infarction, affecting about 10% of patients, particularly those with

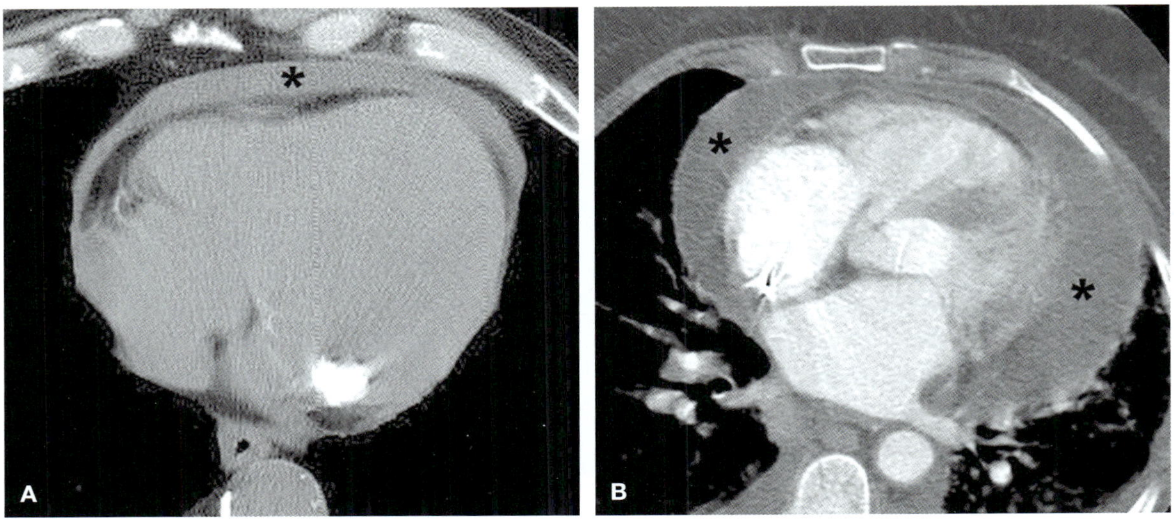

Figure 35.7. Pericardial effusion on CT. CT image (**A**) demonstrates homogeneous small pericardial effusion with water density (asterisk). Contrast-enhanced CT (**B**) shows a large pericardial effusion (asterisks).

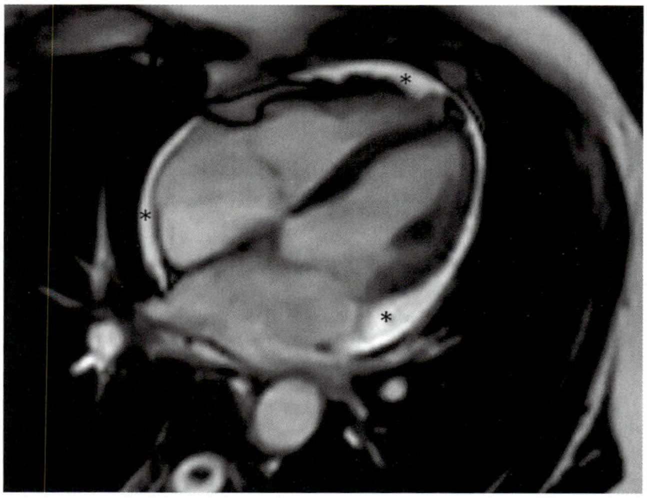

Figure 35.8. Pericardial effusion on MRI. High-signal intensity of the effusion (asterisks) is observed on axial cine MR image.

transmural infarction (referred to as "epistenocardiac pericarditis"). It is important to distinguish this condition from late postinfarction pericarditis, known as Dressler syndrome. Acute postinfarction pericarditis is closely tied temporally to the acute event, resulting from the spread of inflammation related to the infarct. In contrast, Dressler syndrome has an autoimmune origin and lacks a close temporal connection with the initial myocardial infarction.

The diagnostic features of pericarditis in cross-sectional imaging are effusion and thickened pericardium. The thickening of the pericardium is due to fibrinous exudates and edema. Although a variable amount of pericardial fluid is usually present, "dry pericarditis" (also known as pericarditis sicca) may be seen as well. Acute pericarditis is often accompanied by some degree of myocarditis.

The thickened pericardium and effusion can be identified on CT and MRI (Fig. 35.12). After contrast media administration, the pericardium shows various levels of enhancement (Fig. 35.12). Enhancement of the pericardium is best demonstrated on SE MRI using fat saturation technique (Fig. 35.13). The diagnostic features of acute pericarditis are summarized in Table 35.4.

Pericarditis has the potential to advance into chronic sclerosing pericarditis, marked by the deposition of fibroblasts and collagen. This progression may culminate in end-stage chronic pericarditis leading to hemodynamic effects on myocardial relaxation, where the pericardium becomes stiff and constricts the heart, resulting in a condition known as constrictive pericarditis.

CARDIAC TAMPONADE

Cardiac tamponade is a potentially life-threatening condition necessitating immediate intervention. It arises from accumulation of fluid, blood, pus, or gas in the pericardial space, elevating pericardial pressure. This elevation can result in compression of cardiac chambers, impeding diastolic filling, and leading to diminished cardiac output, which may manifest as hypotension, tachycardia, and in severe cases, progress to cardiogenic shock.

Due to limited stretching capacity of pericardial layers, the rapid buildup of a relatively small volume of fluid can lead to a significant increase in pericardial pressures, potentially resulting in a life-threatening situation within minutes of onset. However, a gradual accumulation of a substantial volume of fluid (up to 2 L of more) may not markedly affect ventricular filling. The diagnosis of pericardial tamponade is a clinical one that is usually confirmed with echocardiography. Nevertheless, radiologists should be acquainted with the appearance on CT and MR images, even though their diagnostic role in acute cardiac tamponade is typically restricted.

Typical imaging features of cardiac tamponade are (1) diastolic RV collapse with flattening of the free wall; (2) inversion of the interventricular septum; (3) compression of the

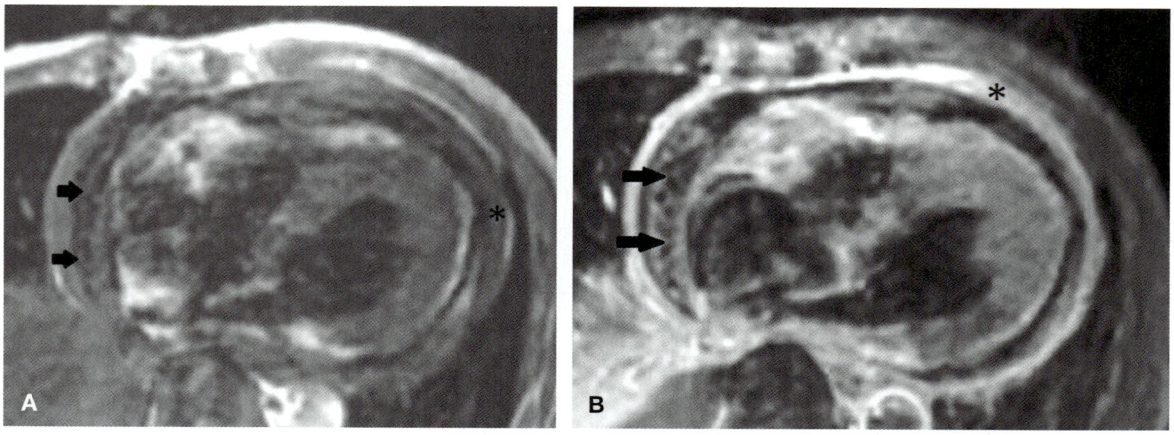

Figure 35.9. Pericardial exudate. SE MR images in the axial noncontrast (**A**) and postcontrast (**B**) images show a heterogeneous pericardial effusion with areas of intermediate signal in the fluid (arrows). A thickened pericardium is also visible (asterisk), consistent with an inflammatory process.

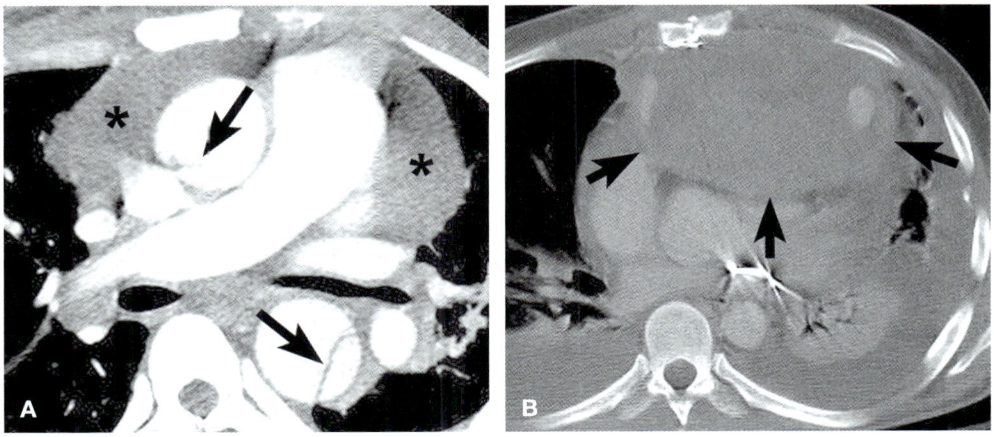

Figure 35.10. Pericardial hematoma on CT. Contrast-enhanced CT at the level of the right pulmonary artery (**A**) shows a type A aortic dissection (arrows) associated with a high-density pericardial effusion (asterisks) consistent with acute hemopericardium. CT image at the level of the base of the heart (**B**) in another patient after cardiac surgery shows a large heterogeneous collection on the anterior aspect of the pericardium (arrows). Note the compression of the right ventricle by the hematoma.

right atrium; (4) exaggerated respiratory variation in mitral and tricuspid inflow as a consequence of increased ventricular coupling; and (5) distention of SVC, IVC, and hepatic veins with associated diastolic flow reversal and reflux of contrast into azygos vein and IVC on contrast-enhanced CT images.

CONSTRICTIVE PERICARDITIS

Constrictive pericarditis is due to progressive pericardial fibrosis, which impedes diastolic ventricular expansion and is a nonspecific reaction to various conditions (Table 35.5). Currently, constrictive pericarditis is most often a sequela

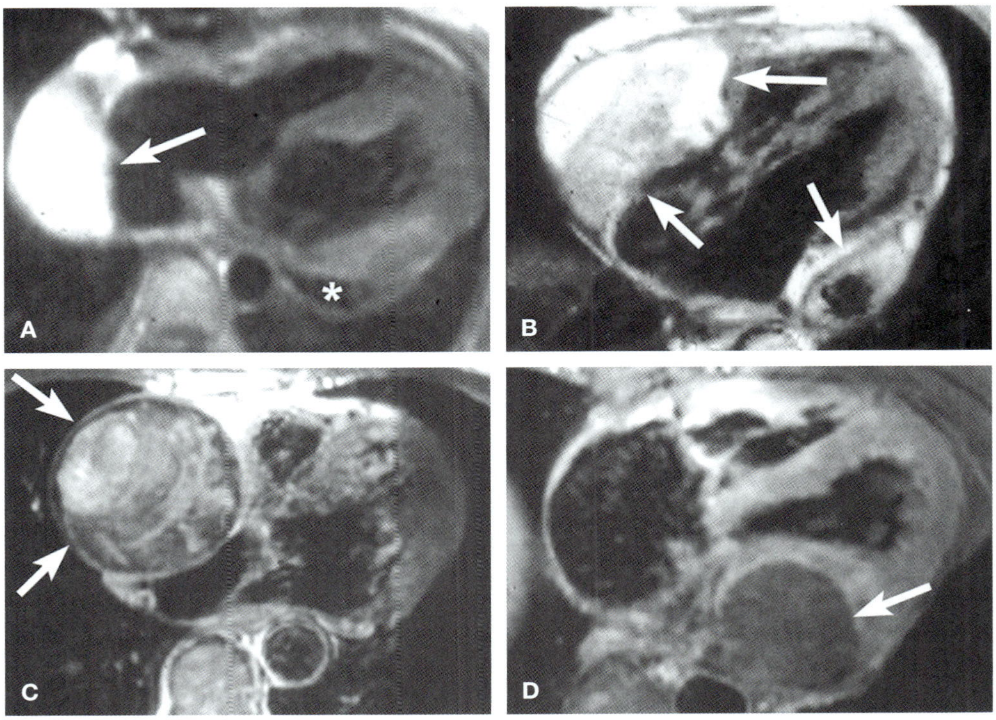

Figure 35.11. MRI appearance of pericardial hematoma. Axial SE MR images at the midventricular level show different ages of pericardial blood. The homogeneous high-intensity collection adjacent to the right atrium (arrow) is an acute hematoma (**A**). Note the low intensity of simple pericardial effusion at the left side of the cavity (asterisk). Subacute pericardial hemorrhage with areas of low- and high-signal intensity is shown in loculated (**B, C**) pericardial hematomas (arrows). The homogeneous low-intensity collection compressing the left ventricle (**D**) is a typical presentation of an old chronic hematoma (arrow).

Table 35.2 Hemorrhagic Versus Nonhemorrhagic Pericardial Effusion

Hemorrhagic effusion

1. High density on CT (higher than 40-45 density units)
2. High intensity on T1-weighted spin-echo MRI
3. Heterogeneous (high, medium, low) on T1-weighted spin-echo MRI
4. Heterogeneous or low signal on gradient-echo (cine MR) and balanced steady-state free precession (cine MR) images
5. Low signal on all types of MRI sequences (old loculated pericardial hematoma)

Nonhemorrhagic effusions

1. Low (water density) on CT (usually <20 density units)
2. Low signal (less than myocardium) on T1-weighted spin-echo images
3. Homogeneous high signal on T2-weighted spin-echo images
4. Homogeneous high signal on gradient-echo (cine MR) and balanced steady-state free precession (cine MR) images

Table 35.3 Etiologies of Acute Pericarditis

1. Infection
   a. Viral (coxsackie A, coxsackie B, echovirus, adenovirus, hepatitis B, herpes virus, parvovirus, AIDs, etc.)
   b. Bacterial (staphylococcal, streptococcal, pneumococcal, etc.)
   c. Fungal (histoplasmosis, coccidioidomycosis, candidiasis, aspergillosis, cryptococcosis, etc.)
   d. Tuberculosis
2. Acute myocardial infarction
3. Acute myocarditis (myopericarditis)
4. Neoplastic (especially lymphoma, melanoma, lung cancer, breast cancer, leukemia)
5. Radiation
6. Collagen vascular diseases (especially systemic lupus erythematosus, rheumatoid arthritis, scleroderma, mixed connective tissue disease)
7. Sarcoidosis
8. Systemic diseases (amyloidosis, Behçet disease, inflammatory bowel disease)
9. Drug reaction (Adriamycin, hydralazine, procainamide, diphenylhydantoin, methysergide)
10. Postmyocardial infarction (Dressler syndrome)
11. Postpericardiotomy syndrome
12. Thoracic trauma
13. Idiopathic

of cardiac surgery in Europe and North America. However, tuberculous pericarditis remains a leading cause of constrictive pericarditis in developing countries.

The risk of constrictive pericarditis after acute pericarditis is relatively low in viral or idiopathic acute pericarditis (0.5%) but is relatively frequent in purulent and tuberculous pericarditis, particularly in patients with an incessant course and large pericardial effusions.

As a result of inflammatory processes, fibrosis of the pericardium and/or pericardial adhesions may occur, sometimes with concomitant calcifications. The less compliant pericardium impedes ventricular and/or atrial filling, depending on the extent of the disease. Another consequence of the rigid pericardium is ventricular interdependence. Because the free walls of ventricular chambers have restricted expansion during diastole, the volumetric capacity of one ventricle is strictly related to the filling of the opposite-sided ventricle. Therefore, minimal and instantaneous differences in ventricular filling result in diastolic ventricular septal motion toward the left ventricle.

There are four different presentations of constrictive pericarditis: acute inflammatory, effusive-constrictive, adhesive-constrictive, and chronic fibrous. The CT and MRI morphologic features are summarized in Table 35.6. The classic picture is classified as chronic fibrous constrictive pericarditis and consists of fibrotic changes with or without associated calcifications consequent to a previous chronic inflammatory process (Fig. 35.14). Adhesive constrictive pericarditis is characterized by the presence of fibrous bridges between the parietal and visceral pericardium and is usually related to previous suppurative or caseous pericarditis (Fig. 35.15). Acute inflammatory constrictive pericarditis presents as an acute pericarditis with marked thickening of the pericardium associated with constrictive physiology (Fig. 35.16). The inflammatory process can resolve completely or become a chronic constriction. Effusive-constrictive pericarditis is subacute constrictive pericarditis mainly involving the visceral pericardium and associated with a chronic pericardial effusion (Fig. 35.17). It is usually recognized when constrictive physiology remains after drainage of the pericardial effusion.

Various patterns of distribution have been described including global, right-sided, left-sided, and focal (Fig. 35.18). The focal type usually involves the atrioventricular groove and thereby may impede right atrial and, less frequently, left atrial emptying (Fig. 35.18). Note enlargement of the IVC.

The distinction between constrictive pericarditis and restrictive cardiomyopathy is difficult clinically because both diseases present with symptoms of diastolic heart failure and frequently have similar findings of increased and equalized atrial and ventricular diastolic pressures on both sides of the heart on cardiac catheterization. This differentiation is crucial for the patient's management because constrictive pericarditis is treated surgically and has a good prognosis, whereas restrictive cardiomyopathy is treated medically and has a poor outcome.

CT and MRI are the methods of choice for measuring pericardial thickness. MRI has a reported accuracy of 93%

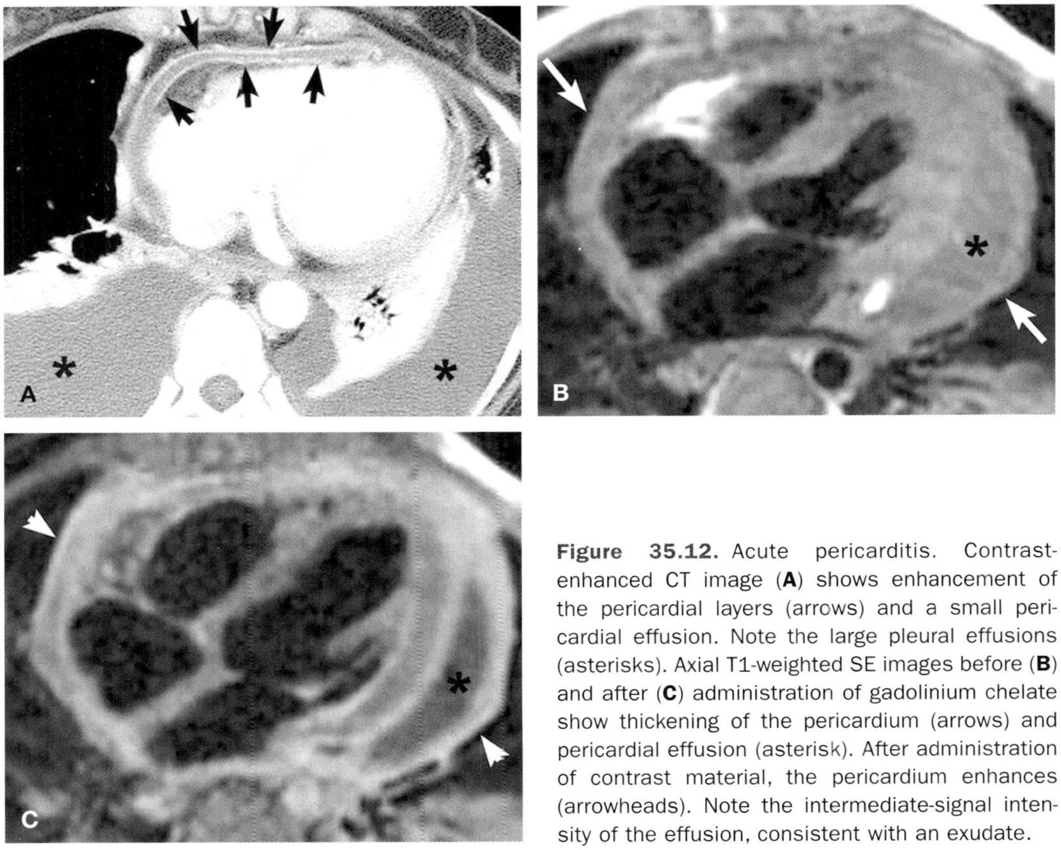

Figure 35.12. Acute pericarditis. Contrast-enhanced CT image (**A**) shows enhancement of the pericardial layers (arrows) and a small pericardial effusion. Note the large pleural effusions (asterisks). Axial T1-weighted SE images before (**B**) and after (**C**) administration of gadolinium chelate show thickening of the pericardium (arrows) and pericardial effusion (asterisk). After administration of contrast material, the pericardium enhances (arrowheads). Note the intermediate-signal intensity of the effusion, consistent with an exudate.

for the diagnosis of constrictive pericarditis based on the presence of pericardial thickness (≥4 mm) in the appropriate clinical setting. It is important to emphasize that rarely constrictive pericarditis can occur with normal pericardial thickness. An advantage of CT is its high sensitivity for detection of pericardial calcification, a finding highly suggestive of constrictive pericarditis (Fig. 35.14).

Other morphologic characteristics that can be visualized in constrictive pericarditis are the presence of adhesions between visceral and parietal pericardium, tubelike configuration of one or both ventricles, enlargement of one or both atrium, and enlargement of SVC and IVC.

Cine MRI with high temporal resolution can depict ventricular septal motion toward the left ventricle in early diastole (Fig. 35.19). Previously described on echocardiography, this finding is related to the characteristic increased ventricular interdependence present in constrictive pericarditis (**Video 35.1**). This finding also has high sensitivity and specificity for the diagnosis of constrictive pericarditis.

Cine MRI usually shows normal right and left ventricular ejection fractions and normal wall motion in constrictive pericarditis. It may also demonstrate the loss of normal sliding motion of the ventricle over the pericardium. The functional features of constrictive pericarditis on cine MRI are summarized in Table 35.7.

Late gadolinium-enhanced MRI shows enhancement of the pericardium in constrictive pericarditis due to fibrosis

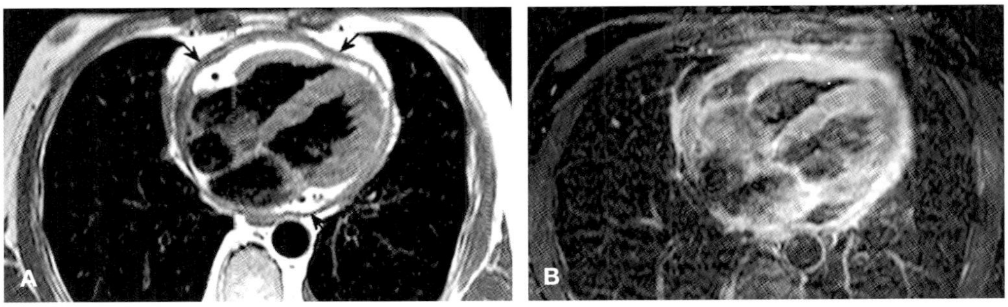

Figure 35.13. Acute pericarditis; T1-weighted spin-echo images before (**A**) and after (**B**) gadolinium chelate administration. Thickened pericardium (arrows) is markedly enhanced by the contrast.

Table 35.4 CT and MRI Features of Acute Pericarditis

1. Pericardial effusion
   a. Water density on CT
   b. Low intensity on T1-weighted spin-echo MRI
   c. High intensity on cine MRI
2. Thickened pericardium on CT and MRI (>4 mm thickness)
3. Early contrast enhancement of pericardium on CT and MRI
4. Delayed gadolinium enhancement of pericardium ± epicardial myocardium on delayed inversion recovery gradient-echo MRI sequence (10-15 min after gadolinium administration)
5. Possible early enhancement of pericardial inflammatory deposits and adhesions on gadolinium-enhanced T1-weighted spin-echo MRI (usually with fat saturation)

particularly if there is persistent inflammation (Fig. 35.20). This imaging technique is an inversion recovery GRE sequence acquired at 10 to 15 minutes after administration of gadolinium chelate (0.1-0.2 mmol/kg) with inversion time optimized to null signal of normal myocardium (typically 225-275 ms). Hyperenhancement on late gadolinium-enhanced images has been seen with both fibrosis alone and fibrosis with residual inflammation. A different contrast-enhanced method is used to show pericardial inflammation alone (edema); this consists of fat-saturated T1-weighted SE imaging within the first minute after injection of gadolinium chelate (Fig. 35.16).

More recently, myocardial tagging has been proposed as a mean of identifying constrictive pericarditis. Cardiovascular magnetic resonance (CMR) myocardial tagging uses certain image slice to create a grid-like pattern of saturated areas, which helps in evaluation of deformation of the grid over the cardiac cycle. It can hence be used to evaluate immobility and adherence of the pericardial-myocardial interface. Finally, phase contrast (PC) images has been utilized to measure abnormalities in blood flow related to constriction. CMR phase contrast assesses the forward flow and rate of flow from vena cava to right heart during ventricular systole and can demonstrate abnormal phase-velocity map that suggests constrictive pericarditis.

Table 35.5 Etiologies of Chronic Constrictive Pericarditis

1. Postcardiac surgery (most frequent cause in advanced industrialized nations)
2. Idiopathic (nearly as frequently as 1—probably due to previous episode(s) of viral pericarditis)
3. Postradiation
4. Tuberculosis (still most frequent cause in Third World nations)
5. Fungal and parasitic infections
6. Chronic renal failure (complication of uremic pericarditis)
7. Collagen vascular diseases (especially systemic lupus erythematosus and rheumatoid arthritis)
8. Neoplastic infiltration (encasement) of pericardium
9. Asbestosis (very rare)

Table 35.6 CT and MRI Features of Constrictive Pericarditis Morphologic

1. Acute inflammatory constrictive
   a. Pericardial thickness ≥4 mm
   b. ±Effusion
   c. Early contrast enhancement of pericardium
2. Effusive-constrictive
   a. Pericardial thickness ≥4 mm
   b. Effusion
   c. ±Adhesions between parietal and visceral pericardium
   d. Early contrast enhancement of parietal and visceral pericardial
3. Chronic fibrous constrictive
   a. Pericardial thickness ≥4 mm
   b. No effusion
   c. No early contrast enhancement
   d. Enhancement of thickened pericardium on delayed (10-15 mm after gadolinium) inversion recovery gradient-echo MR images
4. Adhesive constrictive (very rare)
   a. Pericardial thickness >4 mm
   b. Adhesions between visceral and parietal pericardium
   c. Adhesions between pericardium and other surrounding mediastinal tissues
5. Cardiac chamber configuration (types 1-3)
   a. Dilated right atrium and inferior vena cava
   b. Normal size or small right ventricle
   c. Tunnel-shaped right ventricle
   d. Sigmoid-shaped ventricular septum

ABSENCE OF PERICARDIUM

Pericardial defects are rare and usually asymptomatic congenital abnormalities. The defect can be partial or complete and usually on the left side. CT and MRI can depict herniation of cardiac structure through the defect. Discontinuation of the pericardial line can occasionally be detected in the partial form. The most reliable signs of complete absence of the left pericardium are interposition of lung between the aorta and main pulmonary artery, in the aortopulmonary window, and a rotation of the cardiac axis to the left side (Fig. 35.21).

The usual presentation is in an asymptomatic person with an abnormal chest radiograph with a configuration of the chest suggestive of complete or partial absence of pericardium. A possible complication is bulging of the left atrial appendage and base of the heart through the defect. The edges of the defect can compress the left coronary artery when the base of the left ventricle herniates through the partial defect

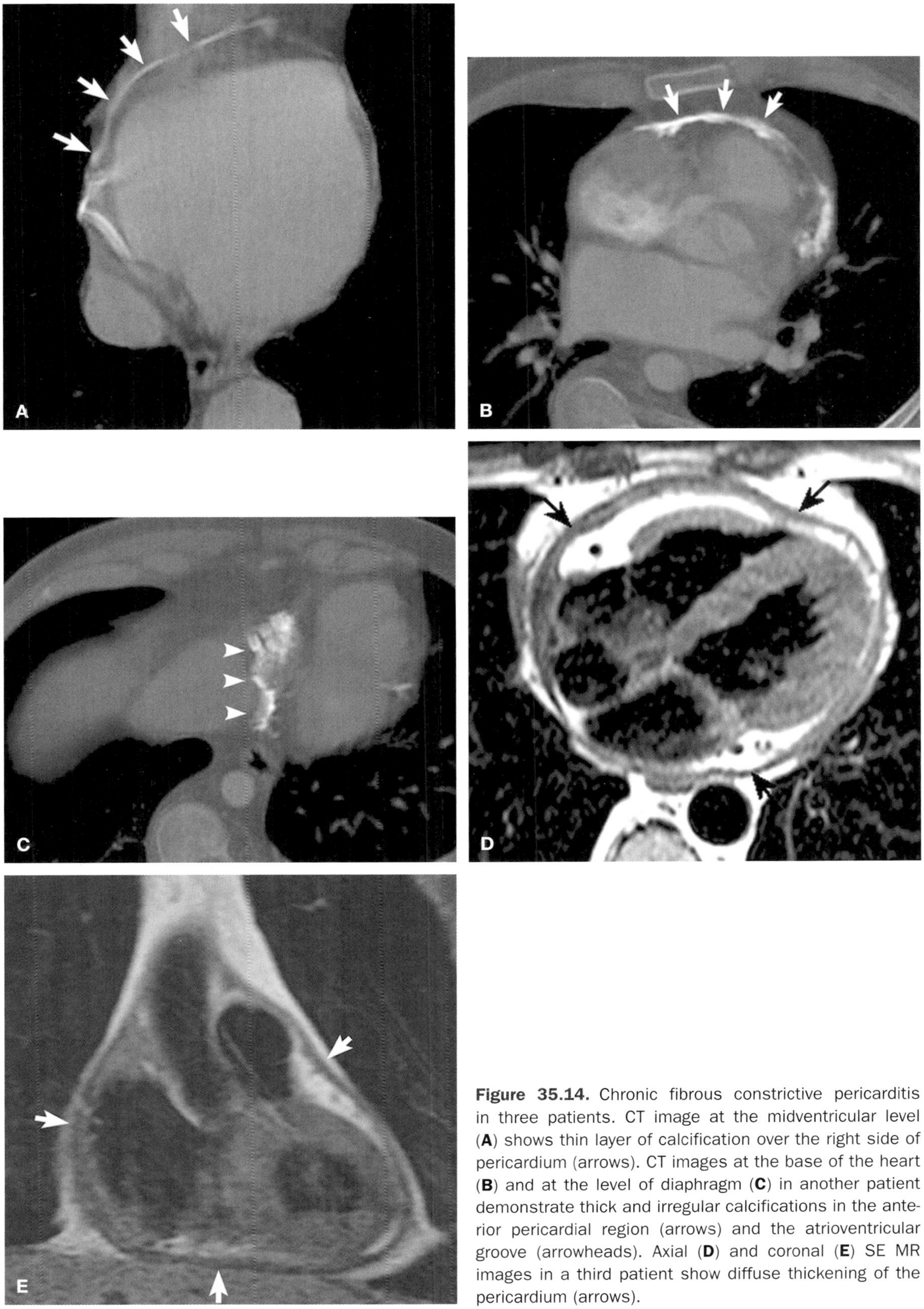

Figure 35.14. Chronic fibrous constrictive pericarditis in three patients. CT image at the midventricular level (**A**) shows thin layer of calcification over the right side of pericardium (arrows). CT images at the base of the heart (**B**) and at the level of diaphragm (**C**) in another patient demonstrate thick and irregular calcifications in the anterior pericardial region (arrows) and the atrioventricular groove (arrowheads). Axial (**D**) and coronal (**E**) SE MR images in a third patient show diffuse thickening of the pericardium (arrows).

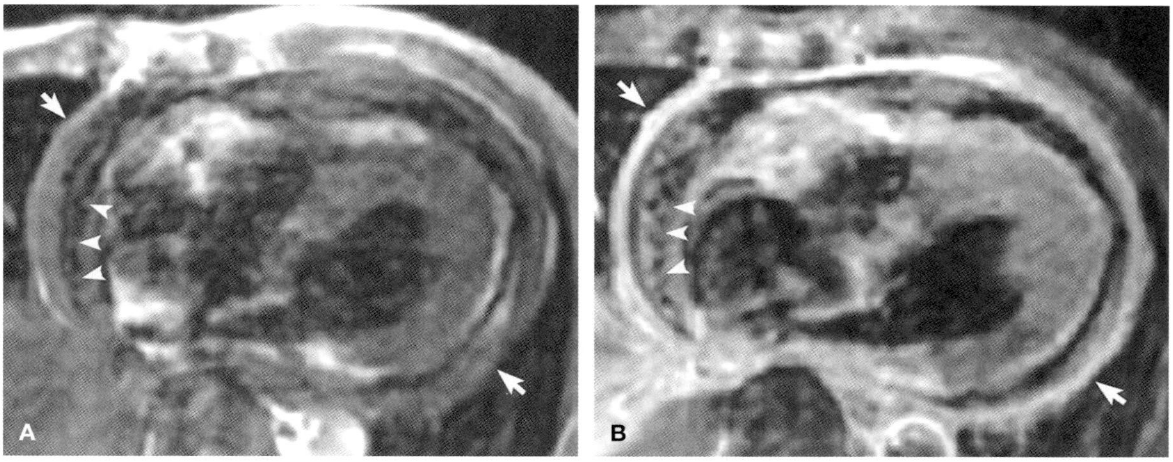

Figure 35.15. Adhesive constrictive pericarditis. Axial SE images at the midventricular level before (**A**) and after (**B**) administration of contrast media show a diffusely thick and irregular pericardium (arrows) and pericardial effusion with heterogeneous signal intensity. Note the presence of adhesions between the pericardial layers (arrowheads). After the administration of gadolinium chelate, there is enhancement of the pericardium and adhesions in this patient with chronic pericardial tuberculosis.

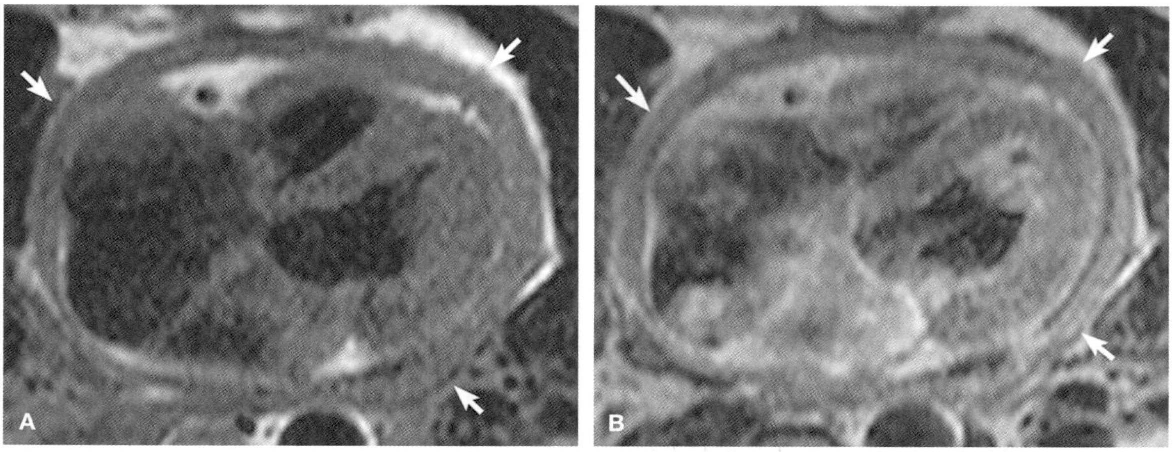

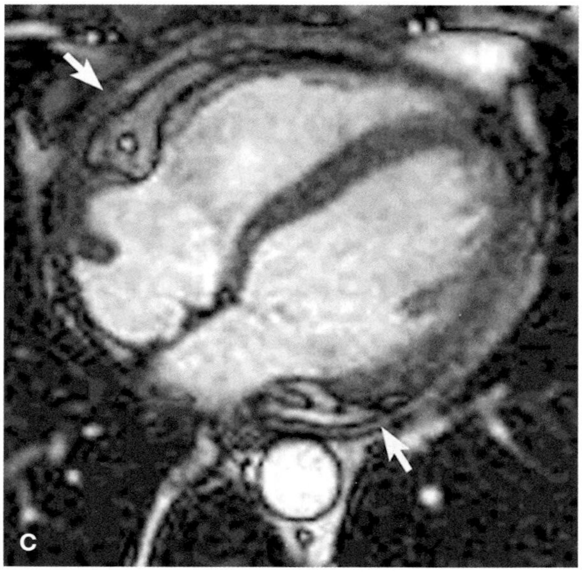

Figure 35.16. Acute inflammatory constrictive pericarditis. Axial SE images before (**A**) and after (**B**) administration of gadolinium chelate show thickening of the pericardium, with diffuse pericardial enhancement after the administration of contrast media (arrows). Cine MR image (**C**) at the same level shows a thick pericardium with intermediate-signal intensity (arrows).

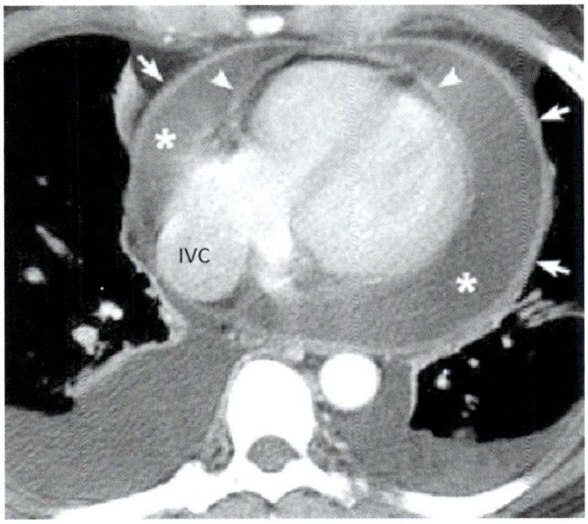

Figure 35.17. Effusive-constrictive pericarditis. Contrast-enhanced CT at the midventricular level shows thickening and enhancement of both the visceral (arrowheads) and parietal (arrows) pericardium associated with a large pericardial effusion (asterisks). IVC, inferior vena cava.

causing myocardial ischemia, ventricular arrhythmias, or sudden death. Because of the herniation, one or more of the major coronary arteries are compressed against the edge of the defect.

PERICARDIAL CYSTS AND DIVERTICULA

Pericardial cysts are caused by developmental abnormalities and are alleged to occur when a small portion of the pericardium is pinched off during embryonic development. Pseudocyst of the pericardium may develop after surgical pericardiotomy. Ninety percent of pericardial cysts are located in the cardiophrenic angles (70% on the right and 20% on the left side). However, they can occur anywhere in the pericardium, and a pericardial cyst at an unusual location sometimes cannot be distinguished from a thymic or bronchogenic cyst. Pericardial cysts usually do not communicate with the pericardial cavity. In contrast, diverticula have a narrow communication with the pericardial cavity. With increase or decrease in pericardial fluid, diverticula can change in size.

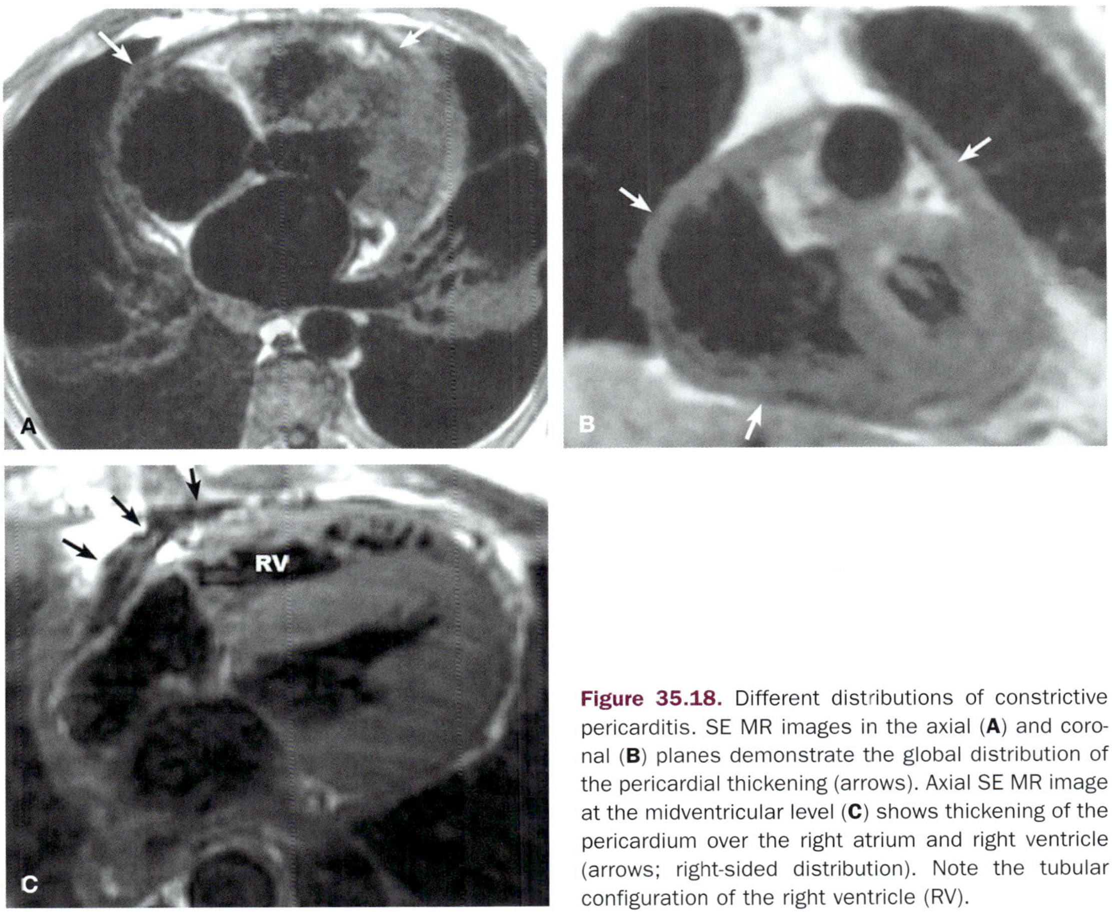

Figure 35.18. Different distributions of constrictive pericarditis. SE MR images in the axial (**A**) and coronal (**B**) planes demonstrate the global distribution of the pericardial thickening (arrows). Axial SE MR image at the midventricular level (**C**) shows thickening of the pericardium over the right atrium and right ventricle (arrows; right-sided distribution). Note the tubular configuration of the right ventricle (RV).

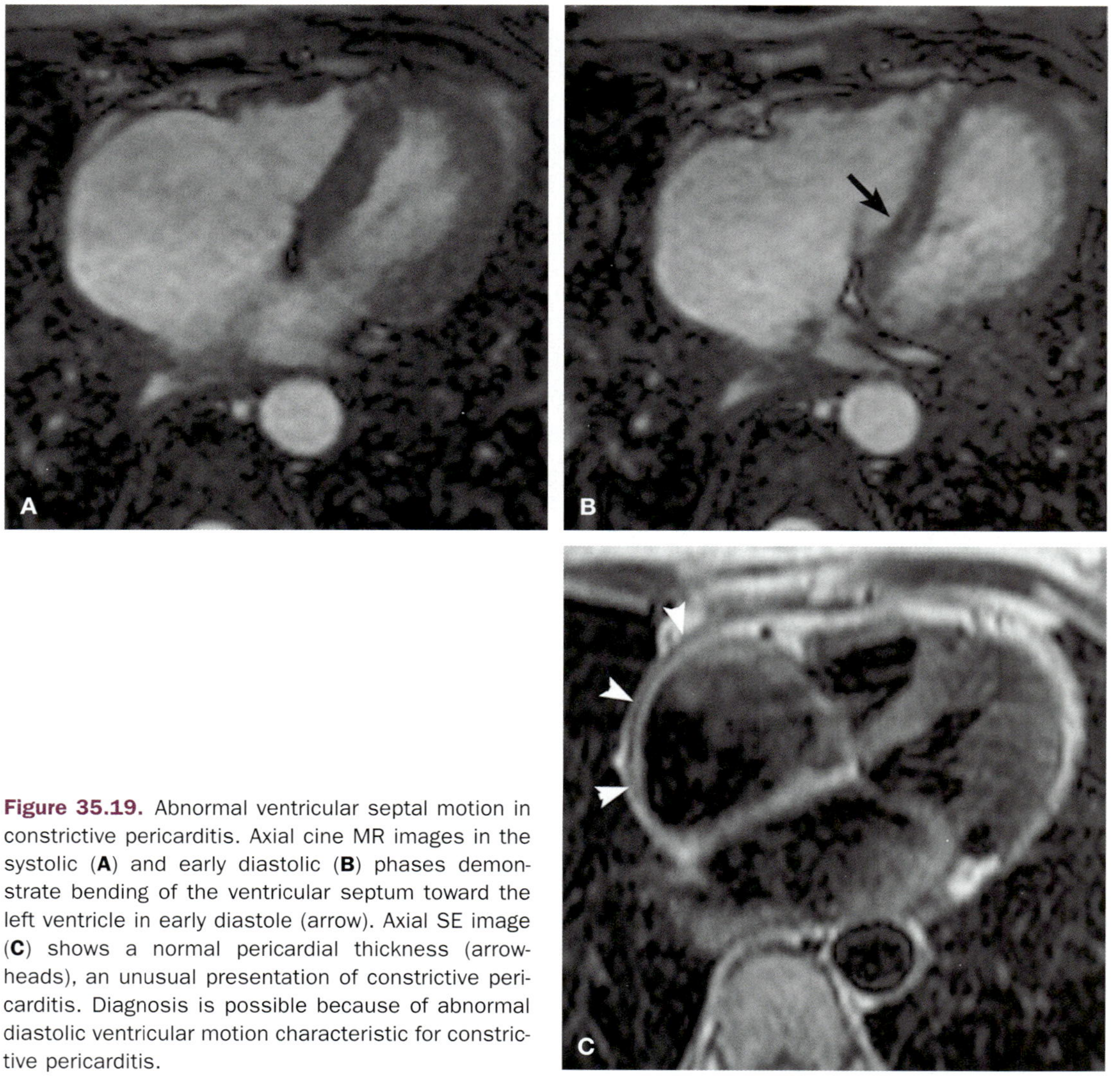

Figure 35.19. Abnormal ventricular septal motion in constrictive pericarditis. Axial cine MR images in the systolic (**A**) and early diastolic (**B**) phases demonstrate bending of the ventricular septum toward the left ventricle in early diastole (arrow). Axial SE image (**C**) shows a normal pericardial thickness (arrowheads), an unusual presentation of constrictive pericarditis. Diagnosis is possible because of abnormal diastolic ventricular motion characteristic for constrictive pericarditis.

A cyst filled with simple fluid (low protein content) appears dark on T1-weighted images and homogeneously bright on T2-weighted images (Fig. 35.22). The cyst does not enhance after the administration of gadolinium chelate. If the cyst is filled with blood or highly proteinaceous fluid (almost 40% of cysts), it is bright on T1-weighted images. The pericardial rim is visible with the characteristic low signal intensity of the pericardium. On CT, cysts have water density typically (Fig. 35.23). However, the density may approach solid tissue if the cyst contains highly proteinaceous fluid (40%).

Table 35.7 Functional Features of Constrictive Pericarditis on Cine MRI

1. Early diastolic leftward bowing of inlet ventricular septum (cine MRI in axial or horizontal long-axis planes)
2. Ventricular septal bounce in diastole
3. Sigmoid shape of ventricular septum in diastole
4. Normal right and left ventricular ejection fractions

PERICARDIAL HEMATOMAS

Pericardial hematomas occur most frequently as a sequela of cardiac or coronary surgery. Rarely, they are caused by transcatheter interventional procedures or blunt or penetrating thoracic trauma. Loculated subacute or chronic hematomas can mimic pericardial tumors on thoracic radiography or echocardiography. On T1-weighted SE images, the signal intensity is characteristic (Fig. 35.11). There is mixed high to low intensity for subacute hematomas due to various components of the clot. With old hematomas, the signal is very low on T1 and T2 SE images. Hematomas have low signal on cine MR images and do not enhance on SE images after gadolinium.

PERICARDIAL TUMORS

Although pericardial cysts and diverticulae are common, other primary pericardial lesions are rare, with mesothelioma being the most common malignant tumor. Sarcoma, lipoma, hemangioma, dermoid, and teratoma can also occur

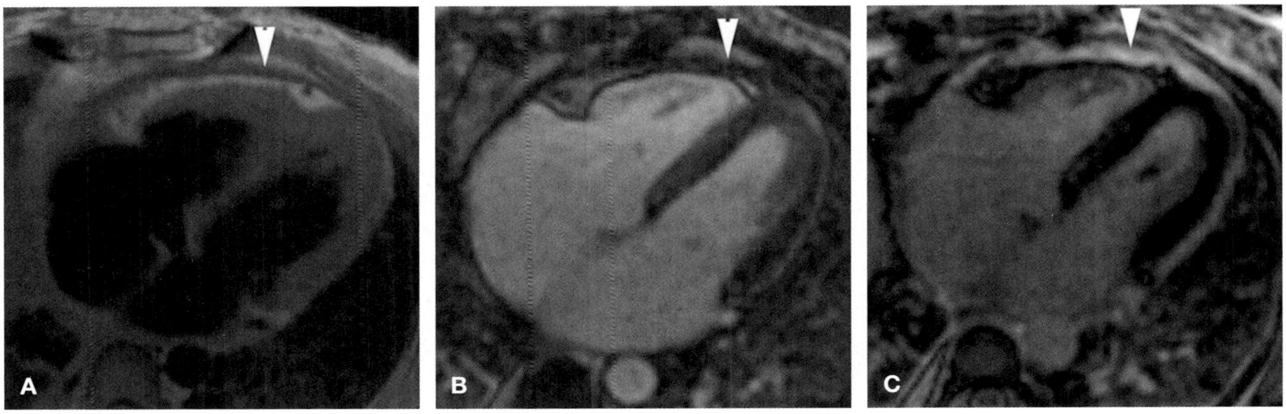

Figure 35.20. Delayed enhancement in constrictive pericarditis. Axial black-blood image (**A**), inversion recovery turbo field echo immediately after gadolinium (**B**) and 15 minutes after the contrast (**C**). Note the thick pericardium without early contrast enhancement but intense hyperenhancement on the delayed images (arrowheads) consistent with chronic fibrotic form or fibrosis with residual inflammation of constrictive pericarditis. Greater intensity of this enhancement may indicate cases that will respond to anti-inflammatory therapy.

in the pericardium (see Chapter 36). Pericardial mesothelioma most commonly occurs in men during the 5th to 7th decades and can be either benign or malignant. Imaging features of malignant pericardial mesotheliomas may include pericardial thickening, effusion, and masses with possible invasion of adjacent structures.

Secondary tumors of the pericardium are far more common. These occur from local invasion of lung and mediastinal malignancies and from distant metastases. Lymphomas, melanomas, lung, and breast carcinomas are the most common primary tumors that involve the pericardium (Fig. 35 24).

Chest radiograph can demonstrate irregular cardiac contour with cardiac/mediastinal enlargement. CT adds value in defining the location of the tumor, differentiating cystic and solid lesions, and overall staging. ^{18}F-FDG–PET/CT can help with differentiation of a tumor from mimics such as complex collections and is useful for staging and to assess for potential recurrence of disease. MRI further helps in characterizing the type of tumor and the relationship with adjacent structures. Assessment of cardiac function and features of pericardial constriction can be done with MRI by using real-time cine steady-state free precession.

Most neoplasms have medium-signal intensity on T1-weighted SE images and high-signal intensity on T2-weighted SE images. Melanoma is an exception with characteristic high intensity on T1-weighted images.

Pericardial hemorrhagic effusion caused by a malignant primary or secondary tumor of the heart or pericardium can be recognized by MRI and CT, and confirmed by ultrasound-guided pericardiocentesis. An incidental hemorrhagic effusion should raise suspicion for pericardial malignancy. Pericardial metastases can also be recognized as enhancing nodules or masses on the visceral or parietal pericardium after administration of contrast media (Fig. 35.25).

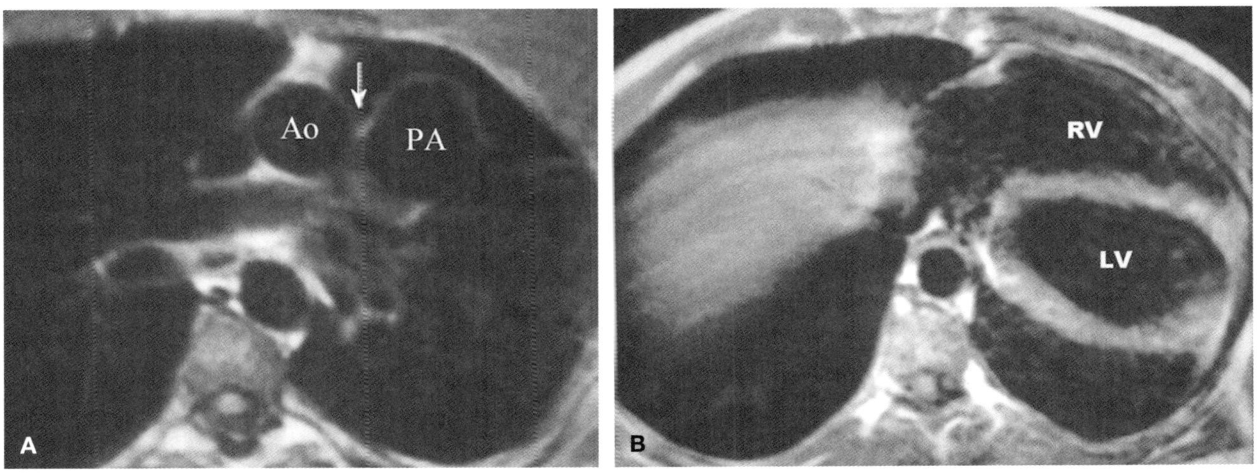

Figure 35.21. Absence of pericardium. Axial SE images at the level of the great vessels (**A**) and ventricles (**B**). There is interposition of the lung between the aortic knob and the main pulmonary artery (arrow) associated with a leftward shift of the heart. Ao, aorta; FA, pulmonary artery; RV, right ventricle; LV, left ventricle.

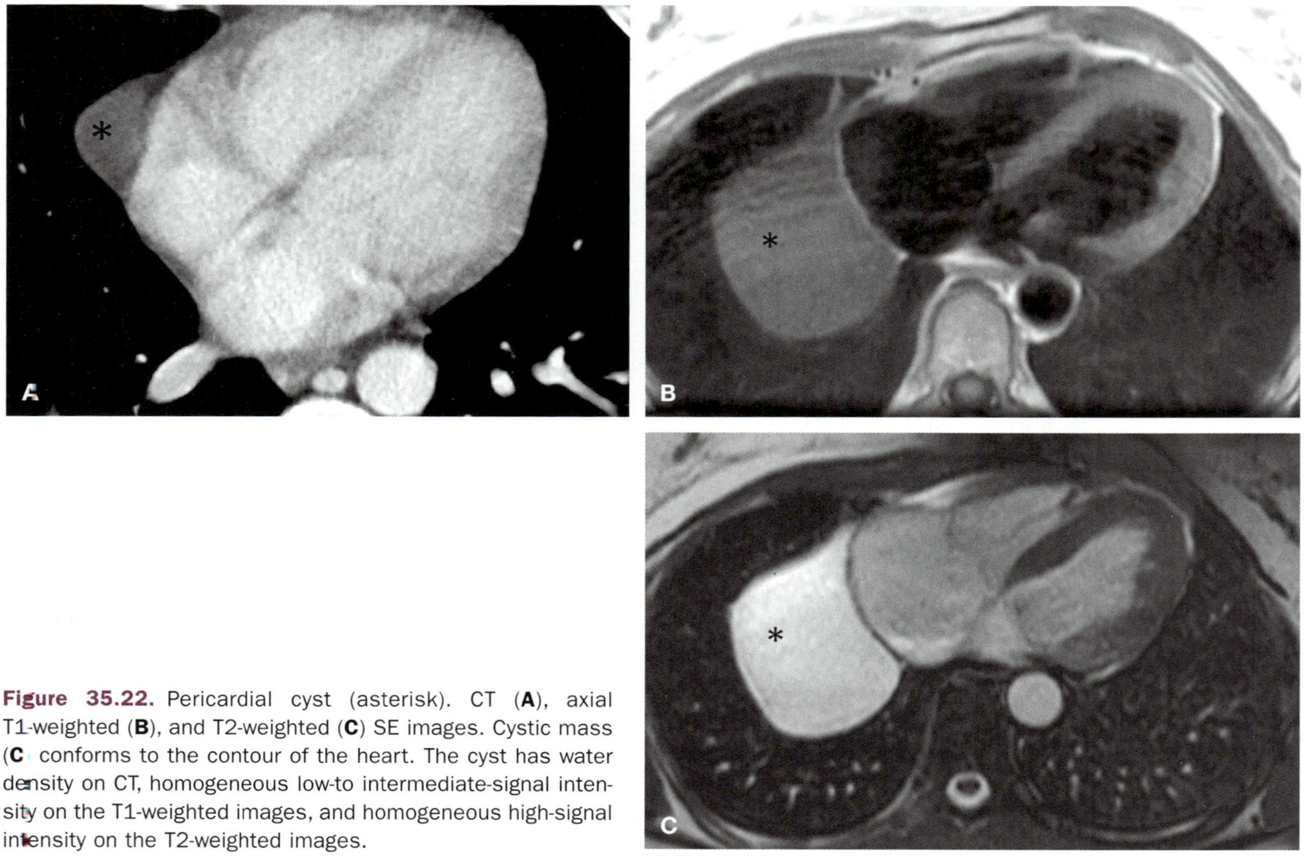

Figure 35.22. Pericardial cyst (asterisk). CT (**A**), axial T1-weighted (**B**), and T2-weighted (**C**) SE images. Cystic mass (**C**) conforms to the contour of the heart. The cyst has water density on CT, homogeneous low-to intermediate-signal intensity on the T1-weighted images, and homogeneous high-signal intensity on the T2-weighted images.

The signal intensity of masses such as cyst, lipoma, hemangioma, and melanoma metastases is very characteristic and therefore allows for a high probability of a histologic diagnosis based on MRI (see Chapter 36). However, definitive differentiation between benign and malignant tumors is frequently not possible based on imaging alone. Detection, evaluation of the tumor extension, and differentiation between benign and malignant appearance are the most important roles of cross-sectional imaging in this setting.

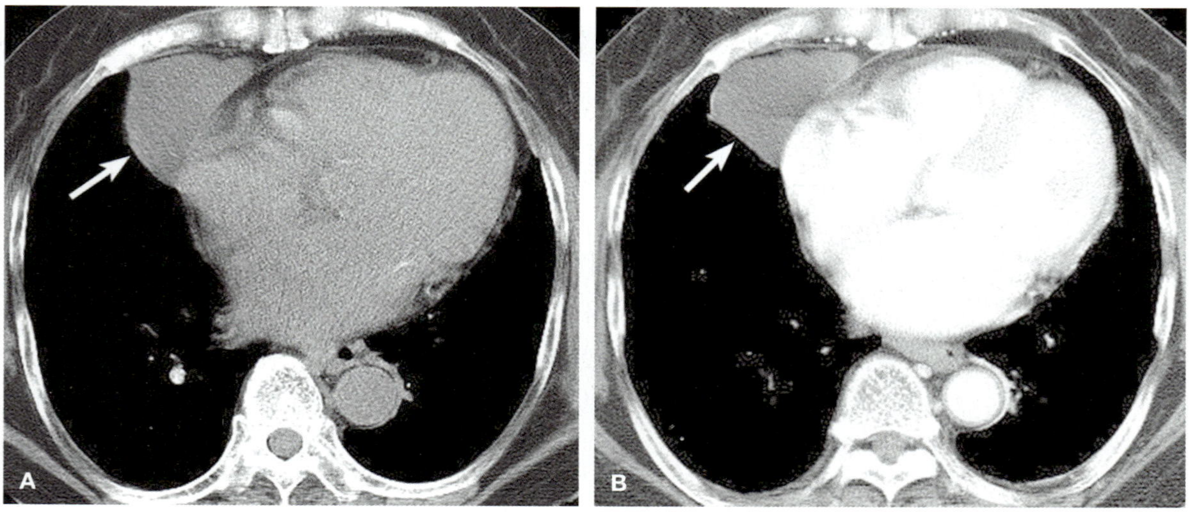

Figure 35.23. Pericardial cyst. CT images before (**A**) and after (**B**) the administration of contrast media show a homogeneous mass at the right cardiophrenic angle with water attenuation (arrow). No enhancement is observed in the postcontrast image.

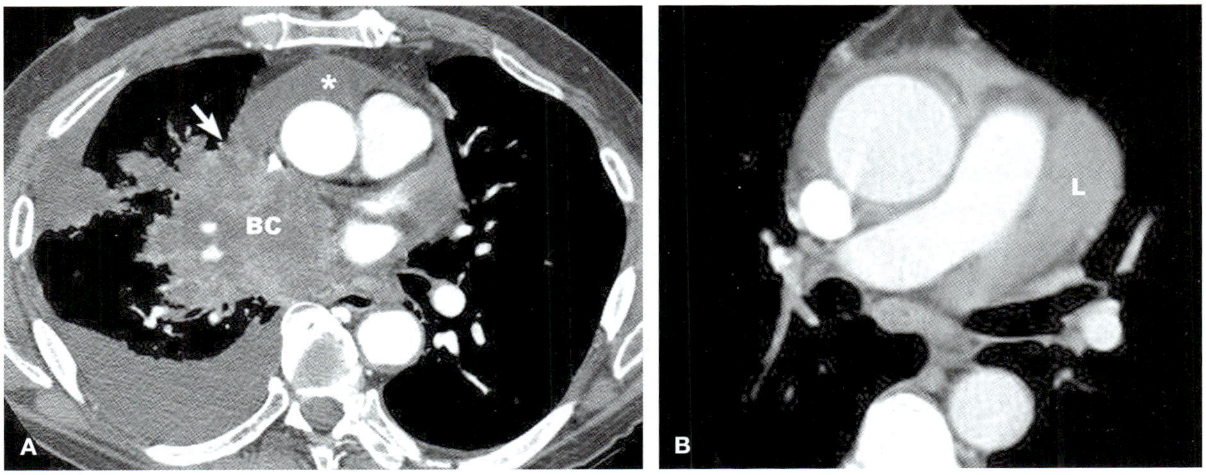

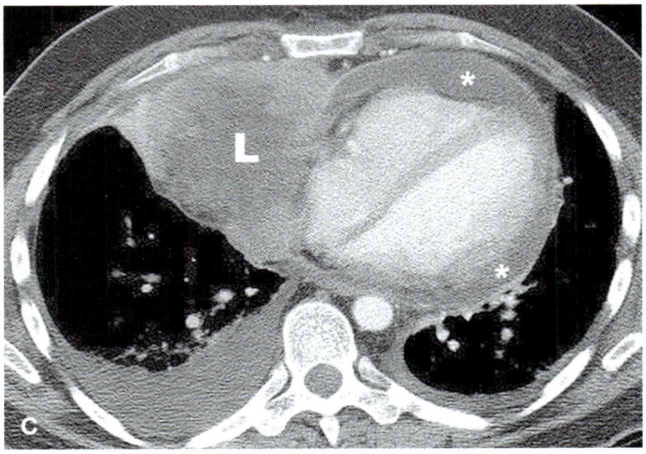

Figure 35.24. Pericardial neoplastic invasion in three patients. Contrast-enhanced CT at the level of the great vessels (**A**) shows invasion of the pericardium by a bronchogenic carcinoma (BC). Note obliteration of the pericardial line (arrow) and pericardial effusion (asterisk). Contrast-enhanced CT at the level of the right pulmonary artery (**B**) in another patient shows a mediastinal lymphoma (L) involving the pericardial cavity. Contrast-enhanced CT at the midventricular level (**C**) in a third patient demonstrates another invasive lymphoma (L) obliterating the adjacent pericardial line, with an associated pericardial effusion (asterisks).

THE ROLE OF ARTIFICIAL INTELLIGENCE IN PERICARDIAL IMAGING

The main developments in the field of artificial intelligence for pericardial disease relate to the creation of algorithms that can automatically detect large pericardial collections. The goal of such functionality is to detect potential life-threatening pericardial disease and help imagers prioritize timely interpretation of such studies.

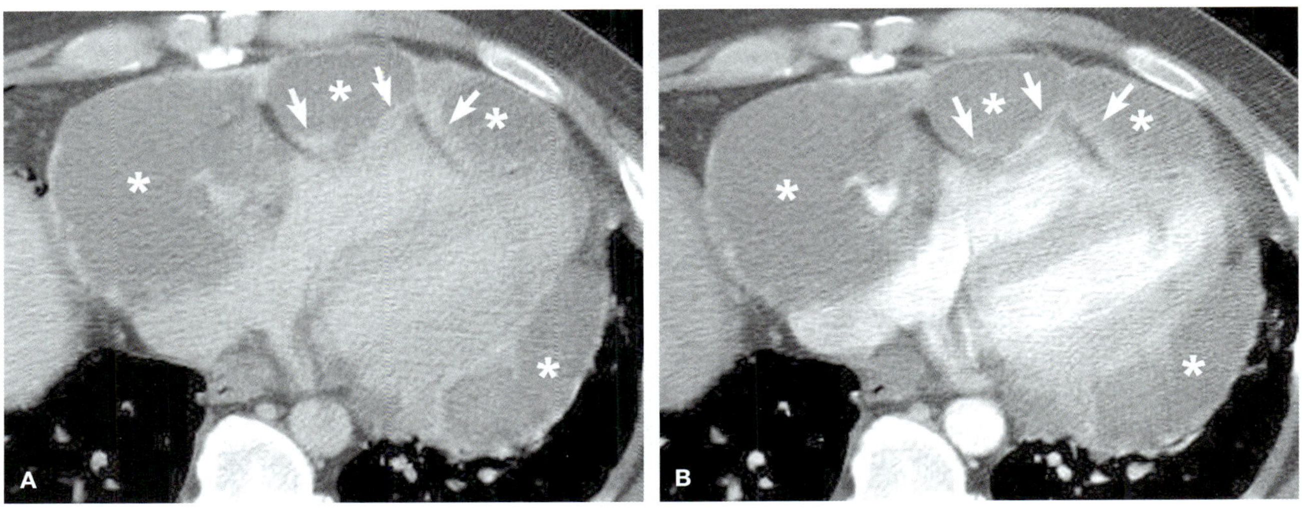

Figure 35.25. Pericardial metastases. CT images before (**A**) and after (**B**) administration of contrast media show a loculated pericardial effusion (asterisks). There are enhancing pericardial nodules on the visceral pericardium (arrows).

SUGGESTED READINGS

Feng D, Glockner J, Kim K, et al. Cardiac magnetic resonance imaging pericardial late gadolinium enhancement and elevated inflammatory markers can predict the reversibility of constrictive pericarditis after antiinflammatory medical therapy: a pilot study. *Circulation*. 2011;124(17):1830-1837.

Giorgi B, Mollet NR, Dymarkowski S, Rademakers FE, Bogaert J. Clinically suspected constrictive pericarditis: MR imaging assessment of ventricular septal motion and configuration in patients and healthy subjects. *Radiology*. 2003;228(2):417-424.

Maui T, Frick S, Higgins CB. Constrictive pericarditis and restrictive cardiomyopathy: evaluation with MRI. *Radiology*. 1992;182:369-373.

Reinmüller R, Gröll R, Lipton MJ. CT and MRI of pericardial disease. *Radiol Clin N Am*. 2004;42:587-601.

Spodick DH. Pericardial diseases. In: Braunwald E, Zipes D, Libby P, eds. *Heart Disease*. 6th ed. WB Saunders; 2001:1823-1876.

Chapter 36

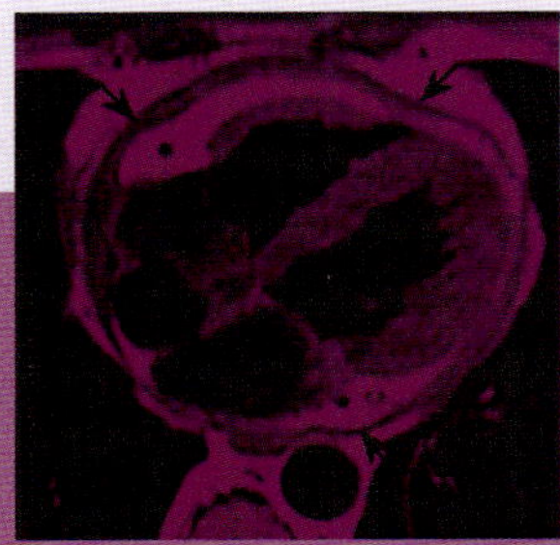

Carole Dennie • Karen G. Ordovas

Cardiac and Paracardiac Masses

INTRODUCTION

The goals of cross-sectional imaging in the evaluation of cardiac masses are the following:

1. Identify an intracardiac or paracardiac mass.
2. Recognize the precise location, extent, and relationship to adjacent structures.
3. Distinguish between tumor and thrombus.
4. Distinguish between primary and secondary tumor if possible.
5. Identify features that suggest a malignant tumor.

The term *mass* is used rather than *tumor* in this chapter because the most frequent mass within a cardiac chamber is a thrombus rather than a tumor. Primary cardiac tumors are rare. Secondary cardiac tumors, either metastatic or representing direct extension of primary tumors of another organ, are about 40 times more frequent than primary cardiac tumors.

Cardiac computed tomography (CCT) and cardiac magnetic resonance (CMR) can help determine the presence and extent of cardiac and paracardiac tumors. These modalities, especially CMR, can also sometimes characterize the tissue of the mass. CMR is most frequently used for assessment of cardiac masses given its superior ability for tissue characterization, whereas CCT adds value in delineating involvement of adjacent small vascular structures and delineating calcific components.

Because of a wide field of view that encompasses the cardiovascular structures, mediastinum, and adjacent lung simultaneously, CCT and CMR can display the intracardiac and extracardiac extent of tumors. In addition, the ability to image in multiple planes makes CMR especially suited for the demarcation of the spatial relationship of a mass to the various cardiac and mediastinal structures. Multiplanar CMR images and multiplanar reconstructions using CCT and newer CMR imaging techniques overcome the volume-averaging problem at the diaphragmatic interface encountered with a solely transaxial imaging plane. These features permit a clear delineation of the possible infiltration of a mass lesion into cardiac and adjacent mediastinal structures. CMR also allows for the assessment of functional parameters such as ventricular wall thickening, ejection fraction, or flow velocity, which aid in characterizing the impact of a tumor on cardiac function.

In clinical practice, CMR and CCT are most often used to verify or exclude a possible mass initially detected by echocardiography. Echocardiography clearly depicts cardiac morphology and provides an assessment of functional parameters. However, the effectiveness of transthoracic echocardiography is limited by the acoustic window, which varies considerably with patient body habitus. Echocardiographic image quality may be severely decreased by the presence of obesity or chronic obstructive pulmonary disease. Transesophageal echocardiography overcomes this problem but adds invasiveness. The soft-tissue contrast achieved with echocardiography also remains limited in comparison to CMR and CCT. In general, pericardial involvement and infiltration of the myocardium can be better visualized with CMR and CCT.

Tissue characterization of cardiac masses with CMR based on specific T1 and T2 relaxation times is possible to a limited degree. Nevertheless, definitive differentiation between benign and malignant tumors is frequently not possible. Most cardiac tumors have low to intermediate signal intensity on T1-weighted images and high signal intensity on T2-weighted images. However, the combination of imaging characteristics of a cardiac mass, such as location, signal intensity on T1- and T2-weighted images, possible early and late hyperenhancement after the administration of paramagnetic contrast agents, and possible suppression of signal with the application of a fat saturation technique, may render a specific tissue diagnosis highly probable in some cases.

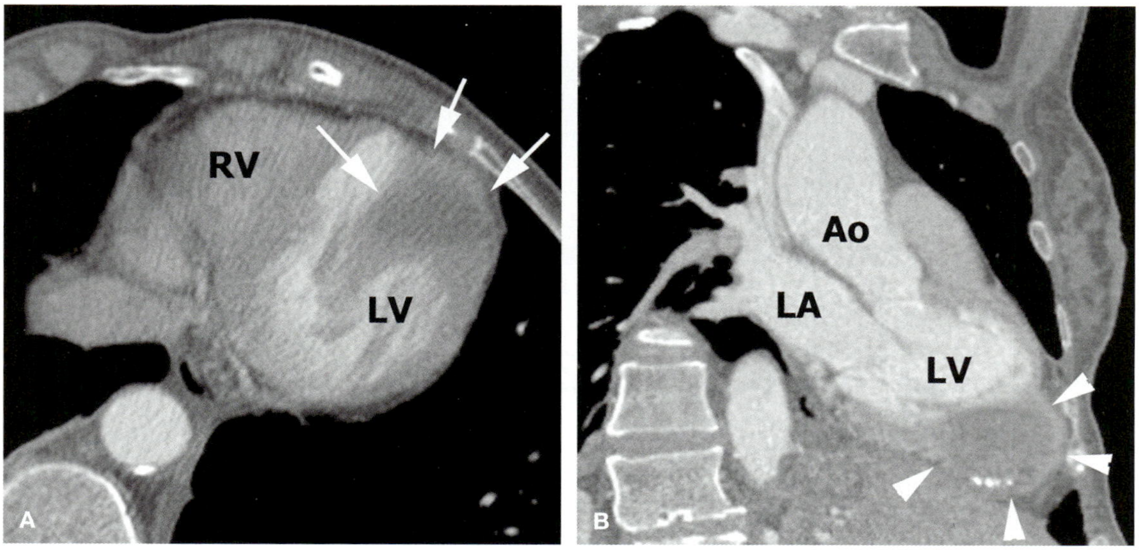

Figure 36.1. Contrast-enhanced CT in the axial plane (**A**) shows a low-density left ventricular mass involving the apex (*arrows*). Coronal reconstruction from the CT (**B**) better demonstrates the relationship of the mass (*arrowheads*) with the left ventricular apex. Note the peripheral rim of high density with some calcifications surrounding the lower density central mass (fibroma). *Ao*, aorta; *LA*, left atrium; *LV*, left ventricle; *RV*, right ventricle; .

TECHNIQUES

Cardiac Computed Tomography

Multidetector CCT scans in the axial plane after contrast enhancement are used to identify and determine the extent of masses (Fig. 36.1). For this evaluation, ECG-gated CT acquisitions are used and are particularly helpful for evaluation of an intracardiac mass. Collimation is usually 0.5 to 0.625 mm. Reconstruction of volumetric data in the sagittal, coronal, or oblique plane may be useful. Additionally, image reconstructions in standard cardiac planes such as short axis, vertical long axis, and horizontal long axis may add value when multimodality assessment with echocardiography and CMR is performed. Positron emission tomography (PET)/CT can also be used to indicate metabolic activity, which helps determine the likelihood of a malignant nature of intracardiac and paracardiac tumors (Fig. 36.2).

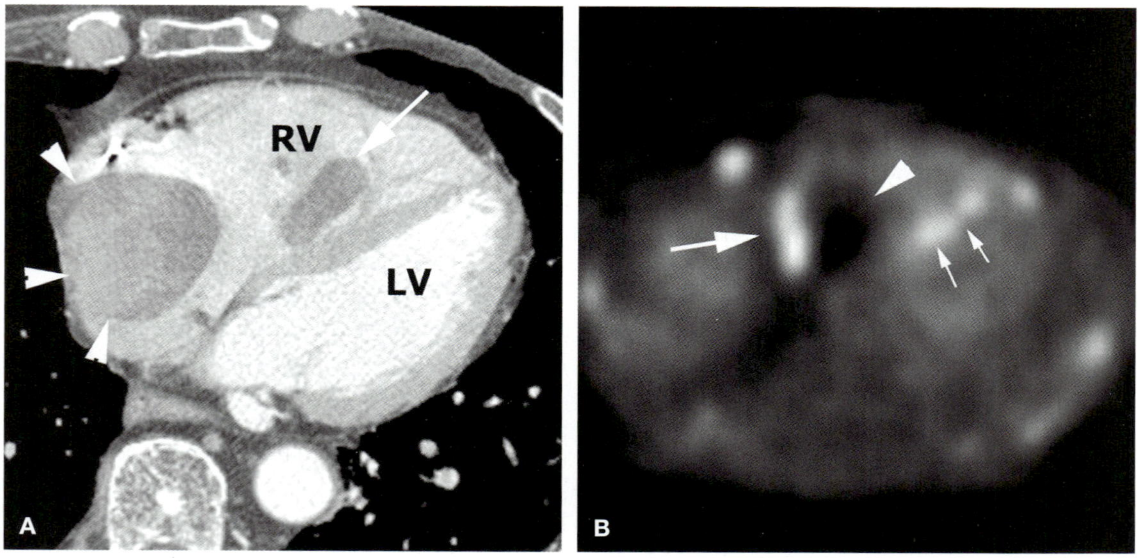

Figure 36.2. A: Axial contrast-enhanced CT image shows a right atrial mass (*arrowheads*) with a wide point of attachment to the wall. Note a second mass (*arrow*) within the right ventricle (*RV*). **B:** PET scan in the axial plane shows avid uptake of FDG in part of the atrial mass (*large arrow*) and in the ventricular mass (*small arrows*) in this patient with metastatic thyroid cancer. Note that part of the atrial mass (*arrowhead*) has no uptake due to tumor necrosis. *LV*, left ventricle.

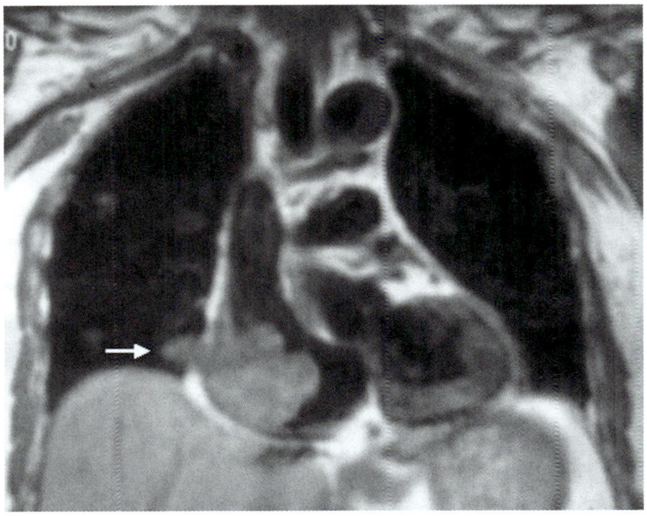

Figure 36.3. Angiosarcoma. ECG-gated spin-echo image in the coronal plane shows a large tumor in the right atrium extending through the atrial wall (*arrow*). The wide field of view of the coronal plane demonstrates the extent of this angiosarcoma.

Cardiac Magnetic Resonance

Steady-state free precession (SSFP) cine images of the entire chest are usually the first sequence obtained to identify a suspected cardiac mass and define the best imaging plane for additional acquisitions aimed at tissue characterization. With the SSFP sequence, the blood pool appears bright (white blood) and most cardiac tumors appear of the same signal intensity to or brighter than normal myocardium, although thrombus shows a characteristic low signal intensity. In addition to offering important information on cardiac mass signal characteristics, SSFP cine images provide valuable information regarding the movement of the cardiac mass relative to cardiovascular structures. A targeted CMR examination is usually recommended including acquisitions of the area of interest in axial, sagittal, and/or coronal planes and standard cardiac planes to delineate the regions that are displayed suboptimally in the axial plane, such as the diaphragmatic surface of the heart. Coronal images facilitate the evaluation of masses involving the aortopulmonary window and pulmonary hila and mediastinal masses that extend through the cervicothoracic junction. The wide field of view afforded by sagittal and coronal images can readily display the extent of tumors (Fig. 36.3). Images can also be obtained in standard cardiac planes.

ECG-gated T1-weighted spin-echo (SE) images with a double inversion pulse to null the signal of the blood pool (black blood images) are usually obtained, with and without fat saturation. Contrast between intramural tumor and normal myocardium may be low on nonenhanced T1-weighted images. Therefore, T1-weighted images immediately after intravenous contrast media may help differentiate and delineate normal myocardial tissue from an enhancing intramural tumor. T2-weighted black blood images can also delimit the contrast between myocardium and tumor tissue, which usually has a longer T2 relaxation time, and delineate possible cystic or necrotic components of a mass. The comparison of signal intensities of a mass lesion on T1-weighted and T2-weighted images may to a certain degree allow for tissue characterization. For example, lipomas have relatively high signal intensity on T1-weighted images and moderate signal intensity on T2-weighted images and show signal drop if a fat saturation pulse is applied (Fig. 36.4). Cystic lesions (filled with simple fluid) have low signal intensity on T1-weighted images and high signal intensity on T2-weighted images (Fig. 36.5). The administration of gadolinium-based intravenous contrast media may also facilitate tissue characterization. Early hyperenhancement of tumor tissue with CMR contrast agents indicates a high degree of vascularization of the mass. Late gadolinium enhancement (LGE, 10-15 min after injection) on inversion recovery turbo field-echo sequence (late gadolinium enhancement sequence) indicates enlarged extracellular space of tumor tissue in comparison with normal myocardium (Fig. 36.6).

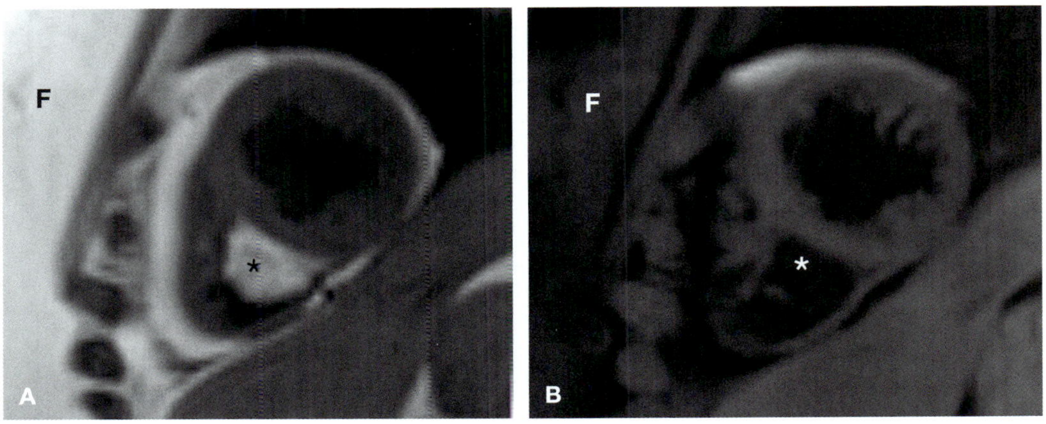

Figure 36.4. Cardiac lipoma (*). **A:** T1-weighted spin-echo (SE) short-axis image shows a high intensity mass in the right ventricle abutting the interventricular septum. It has the same signal intensity as subcutaneous fat (F). **B:** T1-weighted fat-saturated SE short-axis image shows loss of signal intensity within the mass similar to subcutaneous fat (F).

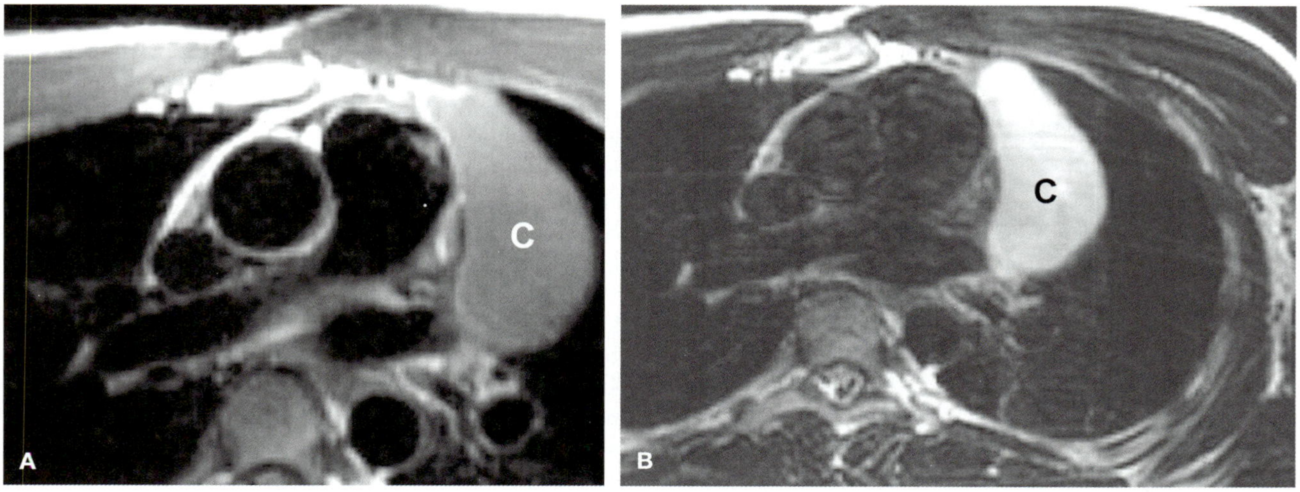

Figure 36.5. Pericardial cyst. ECG-gated spin-echo T1-weighted (**A**) and T2-weighted (**B**) images of a pericardial cyst (*C*). The simple fluid in the cyst has typical low signal on T1-weighted and homogeneous high signal on T2-weighted images.

LOCATION OF CARDIAC AND PARACARDIAC MASSES

1. Intracavitary
2. Intramural
3. Intrapericardial—outer contour of pericardium with compression of adjacent cardiac chamber
4. Paracardiac or mediastinal (Fig. 36.7)

BENIGN PRIMARY CARDIAC TUMORS

About 80% of primary cardiac tumors are benign (Table 36.1). Although these tumors do not metastasize or invade locally, they may lead to significant morbidity and mortality by causing arrhythmias, valvular obstruction, or embolism. An intramyocardial location can interfere with normal conduction pathways and produce arrhythmias, obstruct coronary blood flow, or diminish compliance or contractility through replacement of myocardium. Both benign and malignant tumors have characteristic sites of origin (Table 36.2).

Myxoma

Myxoma is the most common benign cardiac tumor. It is located in the left atrium in 75% of cases and in the right atrium in 20% of cases. Multiple atrial myxomas may occur rarely, especially in Carney syndrome. This tumor is usually spherical, but the shape may vary during the cardiac cycle

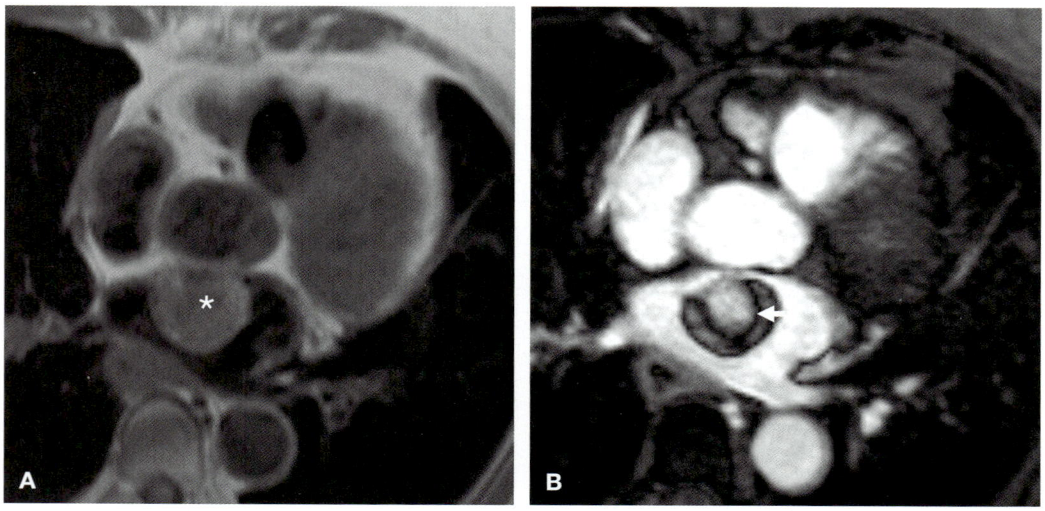

Figure 36.6. Left atrial myxoma (*). **A:** ECG-gated spin-echo T1-weighted axial image depicts a round mass in the left atrium attached to the atrial septum. **B:** A late gadolinium-enhanced image show hyperenhancement of the center of the tumor (arrow). The postcontrast image uses fat saturation.

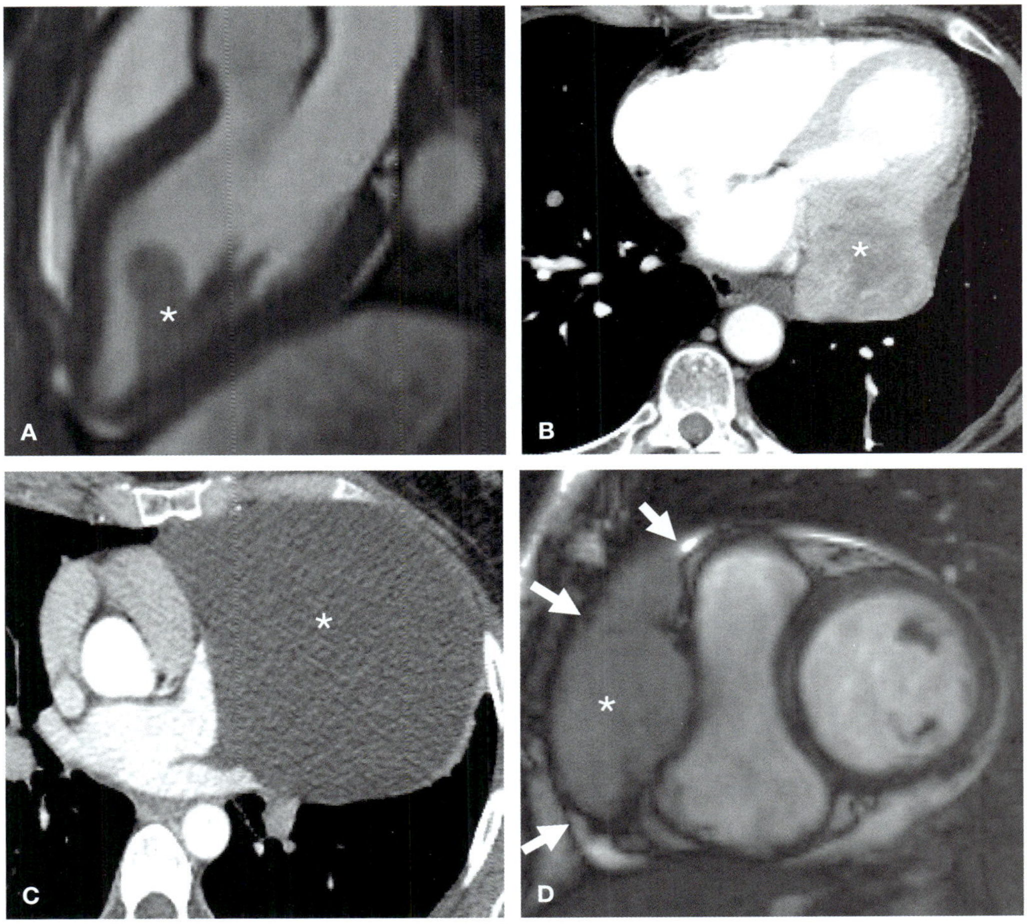

Figure 36.7. Location of masses on CT and MR—(**A**) intracavitary, (**B**) intramural, (**C**) paracardiac, and (**D**) pericardial. The masses are depicted by an asterisk The arrows highlight the the contiguity of the mass with the pericardial surface.

because of its gelatinous consistency. Left atrial myxomas are typically attached by a narrow pedicle to the area of the fossa ovalis (Fig. 36.8A). Infrequently, myxomas have a wide base of attachment to the atrial septum (Fig. 36.8B). However, a wide mural attachment is more frequently encountered with malignant tumors. The extent of attachment may be difficult to assess for large tumors, which fill nearly the entire cavity so that they are compressed against the septum (Fig. 36.8C). As a result, the tumor appears to have broad contact with the atrial septum on static magnetic resonance (MR) and CT images. Myxomas can grow through a patent foramen ovale and extend into both atria, a condition that has been described as a "dumbbell" appearance. CMR cine images permit the evaluation of tumor motion and may help to identify the site and length of attachment of the tumor to the wall or walls of the cardiac chambers. With this technique, myxomas have been shown to prolapse through the funnel of the atrioventricular valve (Fig. 36.9) or into the corresponding ventricle during diastole. Rarely, myxoma can be seen in unusual locations (Figs. 36.10 and 36.11).

Table 36.1 Primary Benign Cardiac Tumors

Myxoma
Usually attached to atrial septum
Most frequently in left atrium
Lipoma or lipomatous hypertrophy of atrial septum
Papillary fibroelastoma
Usually attach to valve (aortic valve most frequent)
Rhabdomyoma
Most common tumor in children
Fibroma
Pheochromocytoma
Hemangioma

Usually, myxomas display intermediate signal intensity (isointense to the myocardium) on T1-weighted SE images. On T2-weighted SE images, myxomas usually have higher signal intensity than myocardium. However, myxomas with very low signal intensity have also been observed. Fibrous stroma, calcification, and the deposition of paramagnetic

Table 36.2 Typical Sites of Origin of Cardiac Tumors

Tumor	Site(s)
Myxoma	Left atrium 75%; right atrium 20%
Lipoma	Right atrium; atrial septum
Papillary fibroelastoma	Fibroelastoma aortic valve 30%; mitral valve 2%; pulmonary valve 13%; tricuspid valve 17%
Rhabdomyoma	Left and right ventricular myocardium
Fibroma	Right ventricular wall and ventricular septum
Paraganglioma	Peri-left atrium; retroaortic; aorticopulmonary window
Hemangioma	Any cardiac chamber
Angiosarcoma	Right atrium, right atrioventricular groove, pericardial cavity
Rhabdomyosarcoma	Ventricular myocardium
Lymphoma	Right atrium

iron following interstitial hemorrhage can reduce the signal intensity of the tumor on both T1- and T2-weighted SE images. Most myxomas show increased signal intensity after the administration of gadolinium-based contrast media on T1-weighted images and on late gadolinium enhancement images (Fig. 36.6 and 36.11), which is probably secondary to an increased interstitial space and, therefore, a larger distribution volume of the contrast agent within the tumor than in normal tissue.

Lipoma and Lipomatous Hypertrophy of the Atrial Septum

Lipomas are reported to be the second most common benign cardiac tumor in adults but may actually be the most common. They may occur at any age but are encountered most frequently in middle-aged and elderly adults. Lipomas consist of encapsulated mature adipose cells. The tumor consistency is soft and may grow to a large size without causing symptoms. Lipomas tend to be epicardial in location but can arise from any layer of the heart (Fig. 36.4). They typically have a broad base of attachment. Lipomas have the same signal intensity as subcutaneous and epicardial fat on all CMR sequences. Because fat has a short T1 relaxation time, lipomas have high signal intensity on T1-weighted images, which can be suppressed with fat-saturating pulse sequences (Fig. 36.4). Usually, they appear with homogeneous signal intensity but may have a few thin septations. They do not enhance after the administration of contrast. On T2-weighted images, lipomas have intermediate signal intensity. CT reveals their homogeneous fat attenuation (Fig. 36.12).

Lipomatous hypertrophy of the atrial septum is common and is alleged to be a cause of supraventricular arrhythmias. It is defined as a deposition of fat in the atrial septum around the fossa ovalis that exceeds 2 cm in transverse diameter. It spares the fossa ovalis, a characteristic feature that is clearly delineated on CMR and CT (Fig. 36.13), which helps differentiate this entity from a lipoma. Lipomatous hypertrophy has the same cellular composition as lipoma but may contain brown fat. Unlike lipomas, lipomatous hypertrophy is not encapsulated and infiltrates through the tissue of the atrial septum. Fatty tissue may extend from the septum into both atria and even along the superior vena cava to a considerable degree. Signal intensity on CMR and density on CT are similar to that of lipomas.

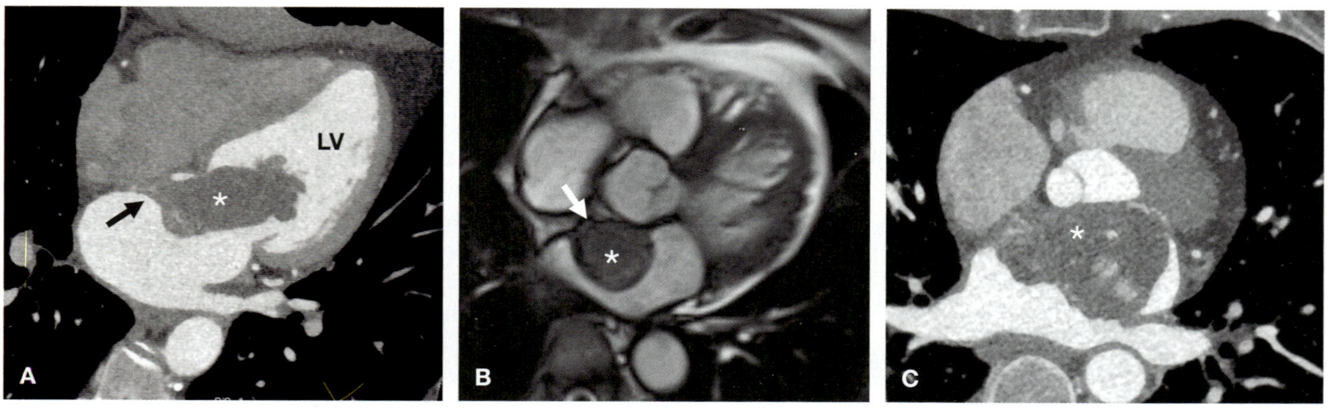

Figure 36.8. Left atrial myxoma (*). **A:** 4-chamber cardiac CT angiography image shows a lobulated mass in the left atrium attached to the fossa ovalis by a stalk (arrow) protruding through the mitral valve into the left ventricle (LV). **B:** Axial steady-state free precession cine MR image in a different patient depicts a spherical mass in the left atrium attached with a broad base of attachment to the atrial septum (white arrow). **C:** Axial prospective ECG-triggered cardiac CT angiogram illustrates a large tumor almost completely filling the left atrium.

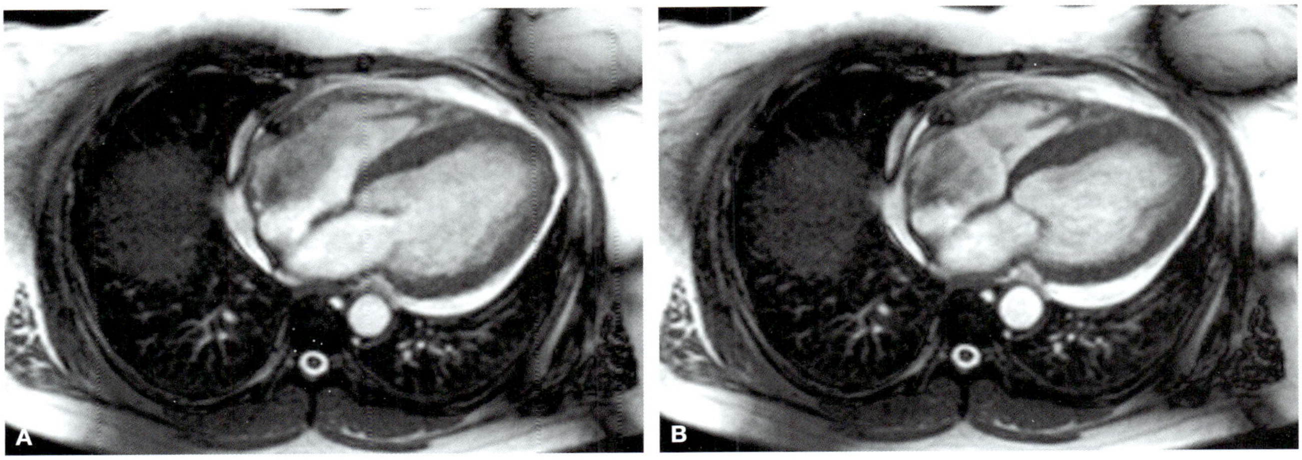

Figure 36.9. Myxoma. Cine MR images (balanced steady-state free precession) in the axial plane display a right atrial myxoma in diastole (**A**) and systole (**B**). The motion of the tumor is evident with movement into the tricuspid valve during diastole.

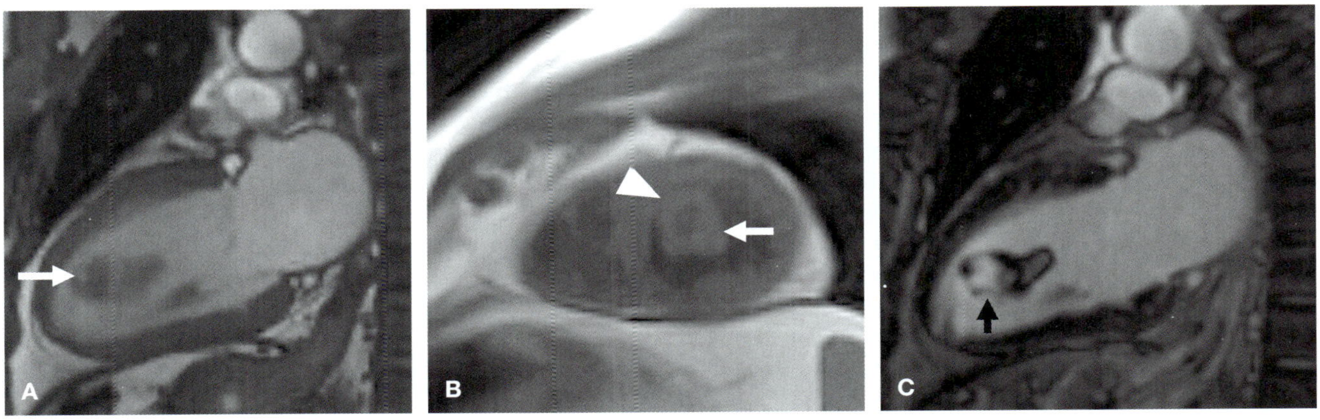

Figure 36.10. Left ventricular myxoma. 2-chamber cine (**A**), short-axis T1-weighted spin-echo (**B**), and late gadolinium-enhanced (**C**) images show a mass (white arrows) with a wide base attachment to the interventricular septum (arrowhead) that demonstrates central enhancement on the late gadolinium image (black arrow).

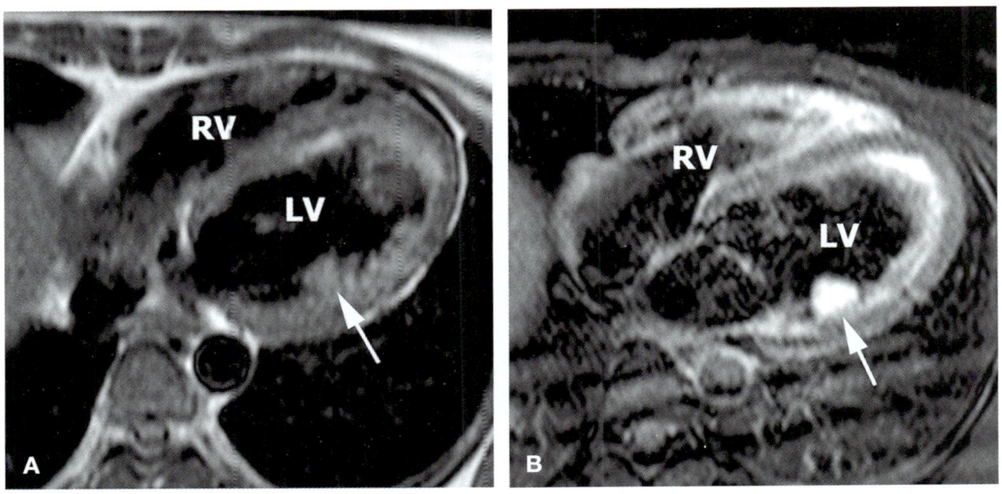

Figure 36.11. Left ventricular myxoma. T1-weighted axial spin-echo images before (**A**) and after (**B**) the administration of gadolinium chelate show a tumor (arrow) with a wide point of attachment to the left ventricular (LV) endocardium. Tumor markedly enhances after contrast media. Fat saturation was used after gadolinium. RV, right ventricle.

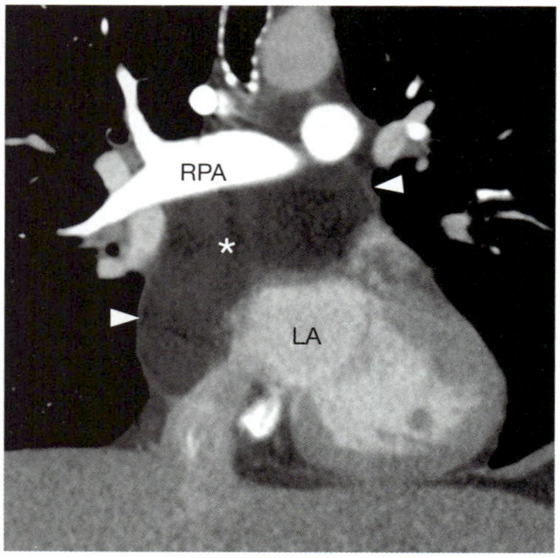

Figure 36.12. Lipoma (*). Coronal reformat from a CT angiogram depicts a thinly encapsulated (arrowheads) fat density mass above the left atrium (LA) and below the right pulmonary artery (RPA).

Papillary Fibroelastoma

Papillary fibroelastomas constitute about 10% of benign primary cardiac tumors. These tumors consist of avascular fronds of connective tissue lined by endothelium. Papillary fibroelastomas are attached to the valves by a short pedicle in approximately 90% of cases. They usually do not exceed 1 cm in diameter. Papillary fibroelastomas have been found on the aortic (29%), mitral (2%), pulmonary (13%), and tricuspid (17%) valves. Right-sided tumors usually remain asymptomatic. Symptoms associated with fibroelastomas are related to embolization of thrombi, which may accumulate on the tumor. Because of their high content of fibrous tissue, they have low signal intensity on T2-weighted images. The diagnosis of these valvular tumors is challenging because of their small size, low contrast relative to the blood pool on SE images, and location on the rapidly moving valves. CT may be helpful to localize these lesions due to its higher spatial resolution, but tissue characterization of the lesion is limited (Fig. 36.14A). On cine SSFP sequences with improved homogeneity of the bright blood pool, signal visualization of valve motion during the cardiac cycle can be excellent, so visualization of small masses attached to valves can be depicted. Cine SSFP MRI can be used to assess the effect of valvular tumors on valve function; a flow jet may be identified caused by either obstruction or regurgitation.

In most cases, signal intensity characteristics after the administration of gadolinium contrast media are difficult to evaluate, so the differential diagnosis between thrombus and tumor may not be feasible. However, these lesions are frequently bright on late gadolinium enhancement sequence due to high fibrotic content (Fig. 36.14B).

Rhabdomyoma

Rhabdomyomas are the most common cardiac tumors in children, representing 40% of all cardiac tumors in this age group. Thirty to fifty percent of rhabdomyomas occur in patients with tuberous sclerosis. Rhabdomyomas may vary in size and are frequently multiple. They are characterized by an intramural location and involve the left and right ventricles (RV) equally. Small, entirely intramural tumors may be difficult to identify. Larger tumors distort the shape of the myocardial wall or may bulge into the cavity. Larger tumors can also distort the epicardial contour of the heart. Rhabdomyomas may have a signal intensity that is similar to normal myocardium on SE images and may display hyperenhancement after the administration of gadolinium contrast.

Fibroma

Fibroma is the second most common benign cardiac tumor in children. It is a connective tissue tumor that is composed of fibroblasts interspersed among collagen fibers. It

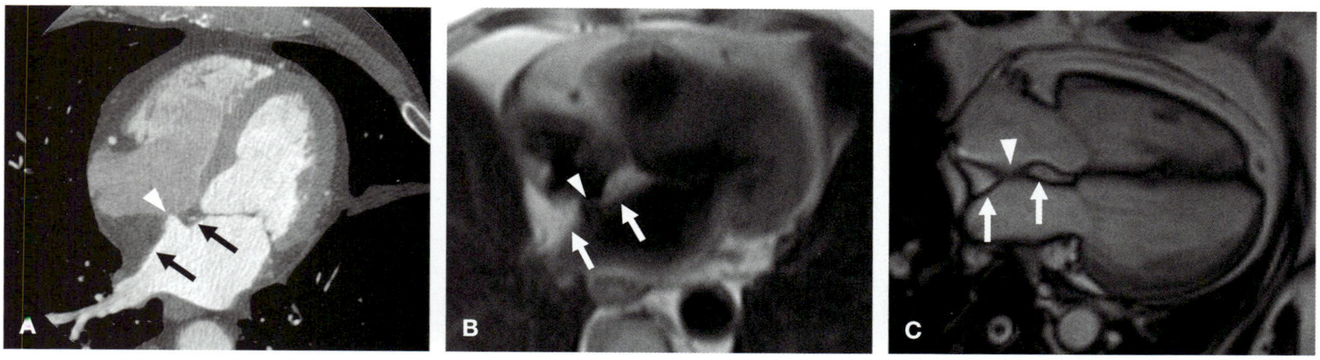

Figure 36.13. Lipomatous hypertrophy of the atrial septum. (**A**) Prospective ECG-triggered cardiac CT with contrast demonstrates thickening of the atrial septum by fat (arrows). Note its dumbbell shape due to sparing of the fossa ovalis (arrowhead). (**B**) Axial half-Fourier acquisition single-shot turbo spin-echo cardiac magnetic resonance image and (**C**) 4-chamber steady-state free precession cine image in different patients show the characteristic sparing of the fossa ovalis (arrowhead) and the septal thickening (arrows) has the same signal intensity as the epicardial and pericardial fat.

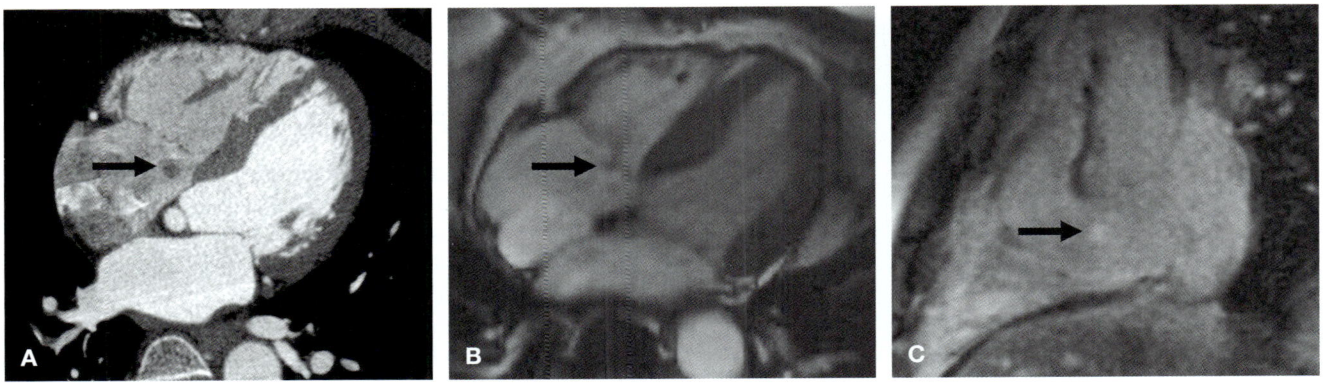

Figure 36.14. Papillary fibroelastoma. Prospective ECG-triggered cardiac CT with contrast (**A**) and 4-chamber steady-state free precession cine (**B**) images reveal a <1 cm nodular lesion in the right atrium attached to the septal tricuspid valve leaflet, which demonstrates enhancement on the short-axis late gadolinium-enhanced image (arrow) (**C**).

arises within the myocardial walls. Unlike most other primary cardiac tumors, fibromas do not usually display cystic changes, hemorrhage, or focal necrosis, but dystrophic calcification is common. Fibromas may cause arrhythmias and have been reported to be associated with sudden death. Approximately 30% of these tumors remain asymptomatic and may be discovered incidentally because of heart murmurs, ECG changes, or abnormalities on chest radiographs Fibromas occur most often within the septum or anterior wall of the RV and can reach a large size (Figs 36.15 and 36.16). On T2-weighted CMR images, they are characteristically hypointense to the surrounding myocardium because of the short T2 relaxation time of fibrous tissue. On T1-weighted images, they may appear isointense to the myocardium. Fibromas show hyperenhancement of the periphery of the tumor early after the administration of gadolinium-based contrast media. Administration of contrast has been effective for demarcating these intramural tumors more clearly from normal myocardium (see Figs. 36.15 and 36.16). Hyperenhancement of compressed myocardium at the margin of the tumor facilitates delineation of the borders of the tumor. Late enhancement of the entire mass has also been observed on the inversion recovery turbo field-echo sequence.

The differential diagnosis for intramural masses in children is rhabdomyoma versus fibroma. If the tumor is solitary and has low signal intensity on T2-weighted images, fibroma is more likely. If multiple tumors are present with high intensity on T2-weighted images, rhabdomyomas are the likely diagnosis.

Paraganglioma

Paragangliomas arise from neuroendocrine cells clustered in the visceral paraganglia in the aortopulmonary groove, in the wall of the left atrium, in the roof of the right and left atrium, in the atrial septum, behind the ascending aorta, and along the coronary arteries. Hypertension, the most common symptom, is related to catecholamine overproduction by the mass. The average age at diagnosis is 30 to 50 years.

Pheochromocytomas can be found at each of the above locations but are predominantly encountered in and around the left atrium, typically in the aortopulmonary groove (Fig. 36.17). Most are located outside of the cardiac chamber. They usually have a broad interface with the heart. Cardiac pheochromocytomas are usually benign. They are generally highly vascularized. The average size ranges from 3 to 8 cm at diagnosis. Pheochromocytomas are hyperintense to the myocardium on T2-weighted images and isointense or hyperintense on T1-weighted images (Fig. 36.17). After gadolinium-based contrast administration, they show strong signal enhancement because of their high vascularity. Enhancement may be heterogeneous, with central nonenhancing areas, related to tumor necrosis. The combination of imaging findings, clinical symptoms, and biochemical evidence of catecholamine overproduction usually permits a confident diagnosis.

Hemangioma

Cardiac hemangiomas are composed of endothelial cells that line interconnecting vascular channels. These vascular cavities are separated by connective tissue. According to the size of the vascular channels, hemangiomas are divided into capillary, cavernous, or venous types. Calcification, which can easily be identified on CT, is often present in these tumors. Hemangiomas may involve the endocardium, myocardium, or epicardium. They have been found in all chambers, and also in the pericardium, but they are most frequently seen in the ventricular free wall. On T2-weighted images, hemangiomas are hyperintense. On T1-weighted images, they are of intermediate signal intensity but can have higher intensity than myocardium (Fig. 36.18). Because of interspersed calcifications and possible flow voids at areas of blood flow in the channels of hemangiomas, they may have inhomogeneous signal intensity. They usually show intense early

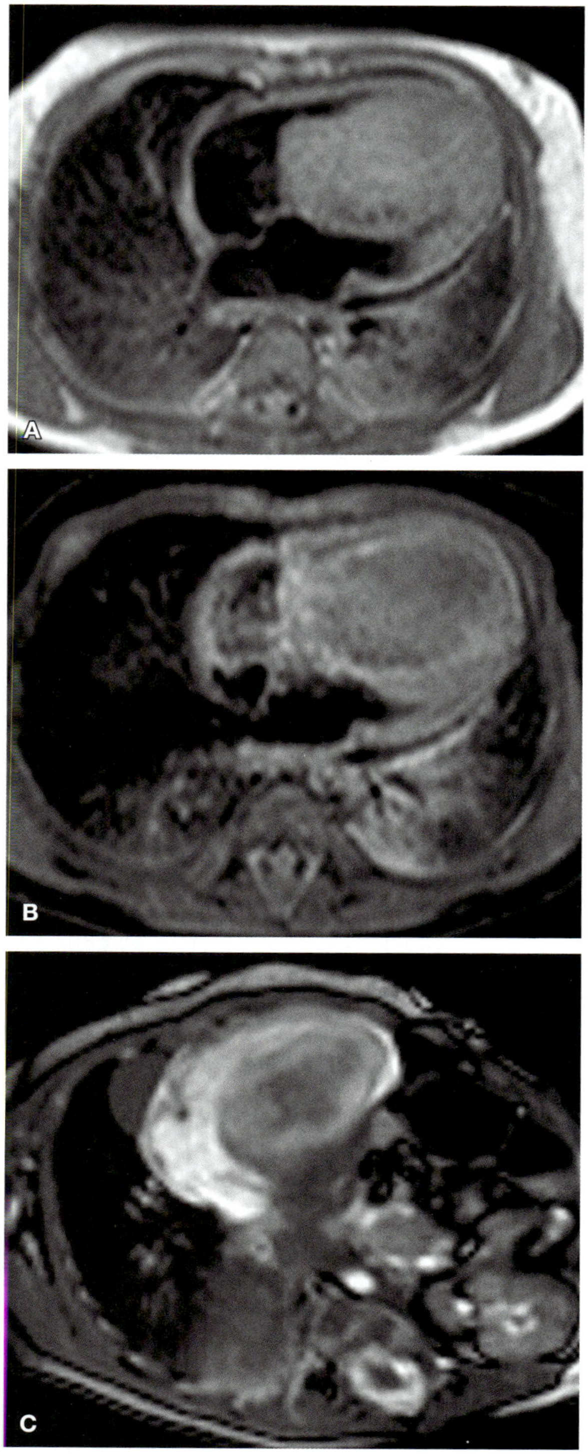

Figure 36.15. Fibroma. A large fibroma in the ventricular septum has low intensity on T1-weighted spin-echo image (**A**). After gadolinium injection on T1 spin-echo image (**B**), the periphery of tumor is enhanced left, but the center remains low intensity. Cine MR image also shows only enhancement of the peripheral part of the tumor (**C**).

enhancement after the administration of gadolinium contrast because of their rich vascularity.

MALIGNANT PRIMARY CARDIAC TUMORS

One-fourth of primary cardiac tumors are malignant; sarcomas represent the largest number, followed by primary cardiac lymphomas. The types of malignant cardiac tumor are indicated in Table 36.3. The imaging features that suggest the diagnosis of a malignant cardiac tumors (Figs. 36.2, 36.19, and 36.20) are the following: involvement of more than one cardiac chamber (Fig. 36.19); extension into pulmonary veins, pulmonary arteries, or vena cavae; wide point of attachment to the wall of a chamber or chambers (Figs. 36.19, 36.21-36.23); necrosis within the tumor (Fig. 36.22); extension outside the heart (Figs. 36.20 and 36.22); and hemorrhagic pericardial effusion. A combined intramural and intracavitary location is another suggestive feature of malignant tumors (Figs. 36.2, 36.23, and 36.24). MRI and CCT are effective for demonstrating invasion of the pericardium and extension into the pericardial fat (Figs. 36.3, 36.25, and 36.26). Pericardial infiltration is displayed on MRI and CT as a disruption, thickening, or nodularity of the pericardium, often combined with pericardial effusion. Cardiac tamponade may be a consequence of hemorrhagic pericardial effusion and can be suspected when diastolic indentation of the right atrial free wall is noted. Features of malignant tumors are summarized in Table 36.4.

Extension into the adjacent mediastinum and metastases (Figs. 36.27 and 36.28) are also clear signs of malignancy. The organs most frequently involved are the lungs, pleura, mediastinal lymph nodes, and liver. The rapid growth of malignant cardiac tumors may cause focal necrosis in the central part of the tumor. Necrotic areas are delineated as regions of lower signal intensity within a hyperenhancing mass early after the administration of gadolinium–diethylenetriamine pentaacetic acid (Gd-DTPA).

Angiosarcoma

Angiosarcomas are the most common primary malignant cardiac tumors in adults representing approximately one-third of malignant cardiac tumors (Figs. 36.3, 36.22, and 36.23). They occur predominantly in men between 20 and 50 years of age. Most frequently, angiosarcomas are found in the right atrioventricular groove and right atrium (Figs. 36.3, 36.22, and 36.23). Angiosarcomas consist of ill-defined anastomotic vascular spaces that are lined by endothelial cells and avascular clusters of moderately pleomorphic spindle cells surrounded by collagen stroma. On MRI, T1-weighted SE imaging usually demonstrates heterogeneous signal intensity of the tumor with focal areas of high signal intensity, which presumably represent hemorrhage. However, angiosarcomas can also have homogeneous signal intensity. Some of the tumors show regions of low signal intensity on both T1- and

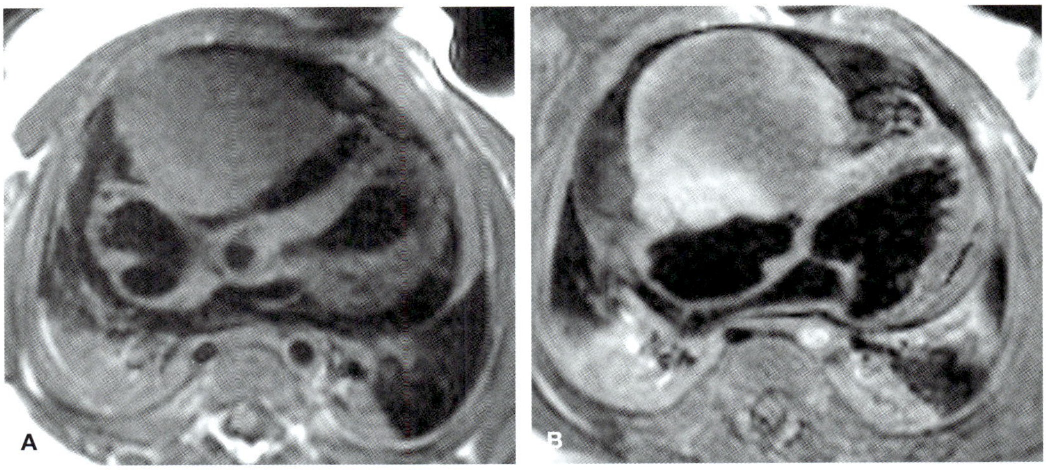

Figure 36.16. Fibroma. ECG-gated T1-weighted spin-echo transaxial images before (**A**) and after (**B**) gadolinium chelate administration in an infant. The periphery of the huge mass shows hyperenhancement. The center of the mass shows low intensity on the cine MR image. The mass bulges off the free wall of the right ventricle.

T2-weighted images. These central regions have high signal intensity on cine gradient-echo images and represent vascular channels. This finding is often described as a "cauliflower" appearance. Cases with diffuse pericardial infiltration have been found to show linear hyperenhancement along vascular spaces. After contrast administration, angiosarcomas show inhomogeneous early and late hyperenhancement, which can be seen in both CT and MRI (Fig. 36.22D). CT may depict encasement of the right coronary artery by the mass (Fig. 36.23).

Rhabdomyosarcoma

Rhabdomyosarcomas are the most common malignant cardiac tumor in children. They can arise anywhere in the myocardium and are often multiple. Their signal intensity on MRI is variable. Rhabdomyosarcomas may be isointense to the myocardium on T1- and T2-weighted images, but areas of necrosis can exhibit heterogeneous signal intensity and patchy hyperenhancement soon after Gd-DTPA administration. Extracardiac extension into the pulmonary arteries and descending aorta can be clearly delineated with MRI or CT.

Other Sarcomas (Liposarcoma, Undifferentiated Pleomorphic Sarcoma, and Others)

Beyond angiosarcoma, the most common primary sarcomas are liposarcomas and undifferentiated pleomorphic sarcoma. Other sarcomas like fibrosarcoma, osteosarcoma, and leiomyosarcoma have also been rarely seen. These all are rare tumors. The MR signal intensity characteristics of these entities are nonspecific. Most of these tumors show signal intensity isointense to normal myocardium on T1-weighted images and hyperintense

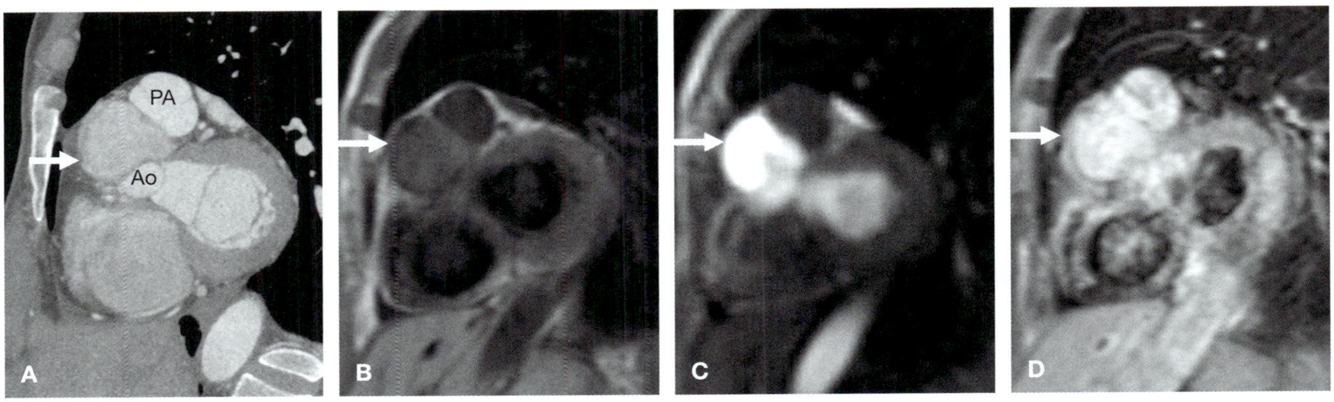

Figure 36.17. Paraganglioma. **A:** Short-axis images from a prospective ECG-triggered cardiac CT angiogram avidly enhancing mass (arrow) between the aortic root (Ao) and main pulmonary artery (PA) at the level of the pulmonic valve. It is isointense to myocardium on the precontrast ECG-gated T1-weighted MR image (**B**) and shows avid enhancement on dynamic perfusion MR image (**C**); postcontrast ECG-triggered T2-weighted fat-saturated MR image (**D**).

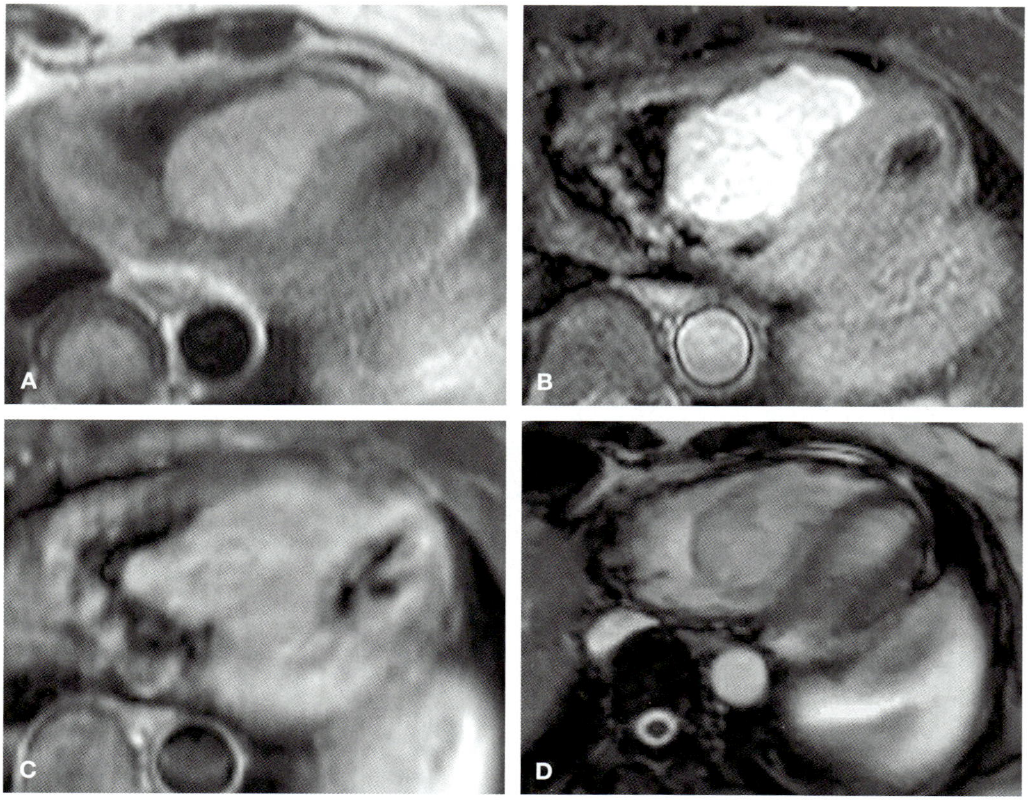

Figure 36.18. Hemangioma. T1-weighted (**A**), T2-weighted fat saturation (**B**), and T1-weighted after gadolinium chelate administration (**C**) spin-echo images and a gradient-echo cine MR image (**D**) demonstrate a large mass originating in the septum and bulging into the right ventricular cavity. The mass has high signal on all sequences.

on T2-weighted images. Most of these tumors show enhancement after contrast administration, so the lesions are more conspicuous and the delineation of the tumor margins is increased in both CT and MRI when intravenous contrast is used.

Lymphoma

Primary cardiac lymphoma is less common than secondary lymphoma involving the heart, which usually represents the spread of non-Hodgkin lymphoma. Primary lymphoma of the heart most often occurs in immunocompromised patients and is highly aggressive. Almost all (approximately 80%) primary cardiac lymphomas are diffuse large B-cell lymphoma. Although primary cardiac lymphoma is rare, it is mandatory to consider this entity in the diagnosis of malignant cardiac tumors because early chemotherapy is usually effective. These tumors arise most often on the right side of the heart (Fig. 36.24), especially in the right atrium, but have also been found in the other chambers. A large pericardial effusion is frequently present. Variable morphology of the masses has been described; both circumscribed polypoid and ill-defined infiltrative lesions have been reported. Lymphomas may appear hypointense to the myocardium on T1-weighted images and hyperintense on T2-weighted images. After Gd-DTPA administration, homogeneous or heterogeneous enhancement of the tumor, depending on the presence of necrosis, may be seen. Some lymphomas consist of a large extracardiac mediastinal mass as well as an invasive mass in the cardiac chambers.

Table 36.3 Primary Malignant Cardiac Tumors
Angiosarcoma (most frequent in adults)
Rhabdomyosarcoma (most frequent in pediatric patients)
Lymphoma
Leiomyosarcoma
Fibrosarcoma
Liposarcoma
Undifferentiated pleomorphic sarcoma

SECONDARY CARDIAC TUMORS

Secondary tumors of the heart and pericardium are about 40-fold more frequent than primary tumors. Most pericardial metastases spread through hematogenous (Fig. 36.25) or direct invasion (Fig. 36.26). Three routes of spread to the heart can be discerned: (1) direct extension from intrathoracic tumors (mediastinum and lungs), (2) extension of abdominal malignancies through the inferior vena cava into

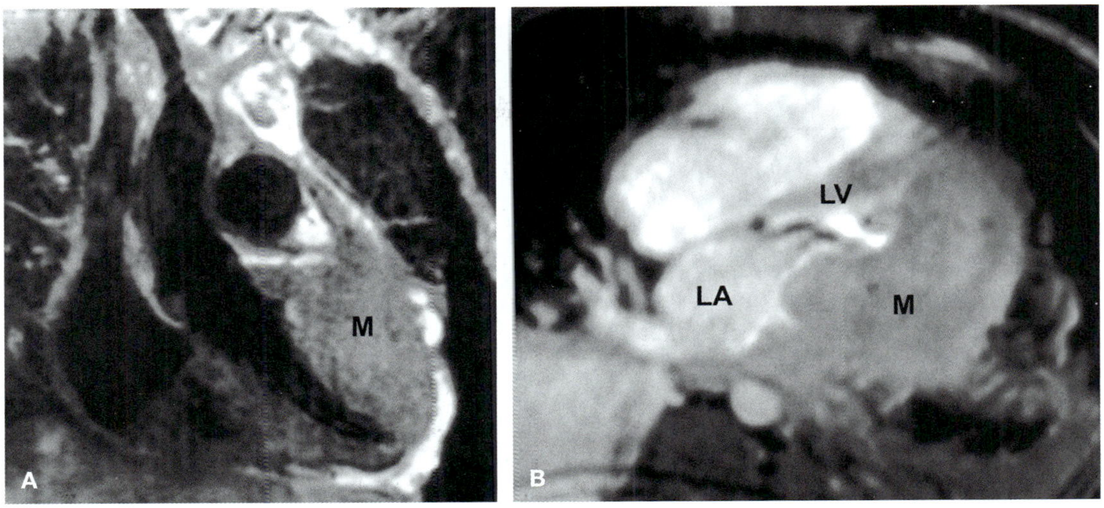

Figure 36.19. Lymphoma. Coronal spin-echo (**A**) and gradient-echo (cine MR; **B**) images demonstrate a large mass (*M*), which involves the lateral wall of the left ventricle and extends into the left ventricular (*LV*) and atrial (*LA*) cavities.

the right atrium (renal, adrenal, and hepatic carcinomas), and (3) metastases (Table 36.5).

Direct Extension From Adjacent Tumors

Tumors of the lung, pleura, and mediastinum can infiltrate the pericardium and heart directly (Fig. 36.26). It is important to recognize invasion of the heart because such a tumor is usually nonresectable. In mediastinal lymphoma, possible invasion of the pericardium can change the staging of the tumor. CT and MRI are effective for delineating paracardiac tumors and possible extension into the heart because of its wide field of view compared to echocardiography. CT and MRI clearly show extension of these tumors to the cardiac structures (Figs. 36.2 and 36.27) and possible evidence of hemorrhagic or nonhemorrhagic pericardial effusion (Fig. 36.26). These modalities are effective in demonstrating invasion of the pericardium and myocardium in advanced lung cancer.

Metastasis

Melanomas, leukemias, and lymphomas are the tumors that most frequently metastasize to the heart, but cardiac metastases can arise from almost any malignant tumor in the body. Melanomas have the highest frequency of seeding into the heart and are frequently found in the heart at autopsy. The mechanism of metastatic spread of tumors to the heart is direct seeding to the endocardium, passage of tumor emboli through the coronary arteries, or retrograde lymphatic

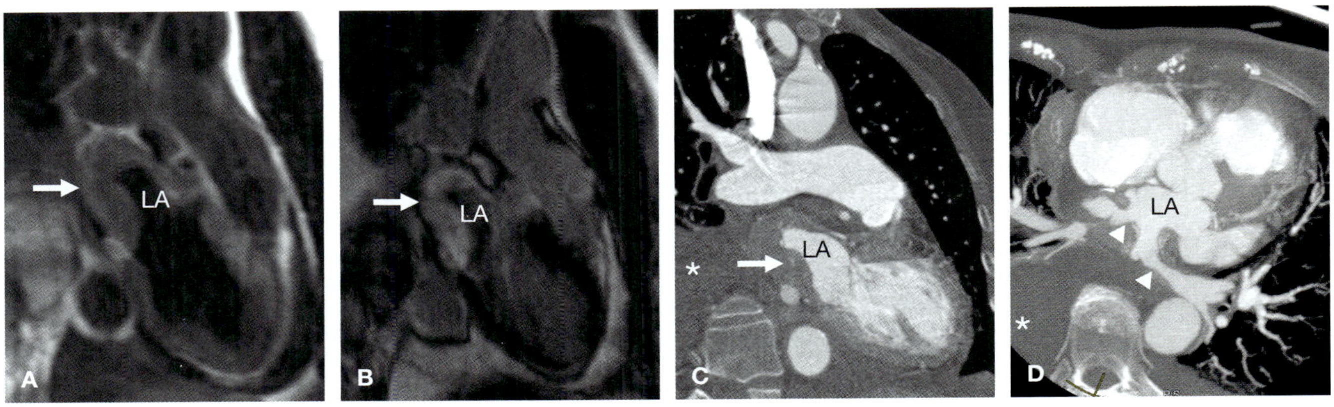

Figure 36.20. Undifferentiated pleiomorphic sarcoma of the left atrium (LA). **A:** 2-chamber T1-weighted spin-echo image depicts a mass lining the inner wall of the left atrium (arrow). **B:** It demonstrates avid enhancement on the late gadolinium-enhanced 2-chamber view (arrow). **C:** Cardiac computed tomography 2-chamber reformat confirms the left atrial mass with very small foci of arterial enhancement (arrow). **D:** An oblique off-axis maximum intensity image reveals significant narrowing of the pulmonary vein ostia (arrowheads). Note the large right pleural effusion (*).

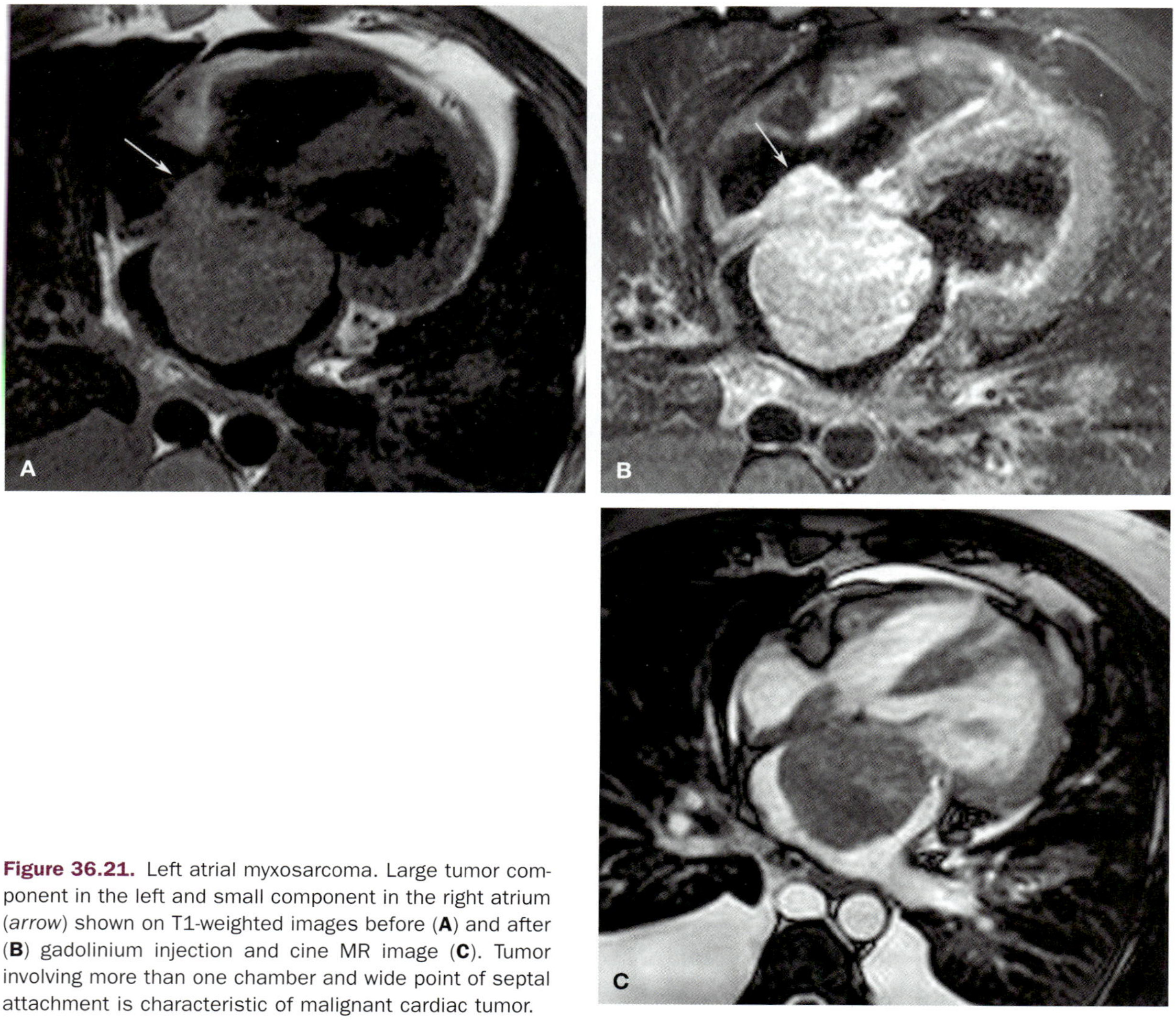

Figure 36.21. Left atrial myxosarcoma. Large tumor component in the left and small component in the right atrium (*arrow*) shown on T1-weighted images before (**A**) and after (**B**) gadolinium injection and cine MR image (**C**). Tumor involving more than one chamber and wide point of septal attachment is characteristic of malignant cardiac tumor.

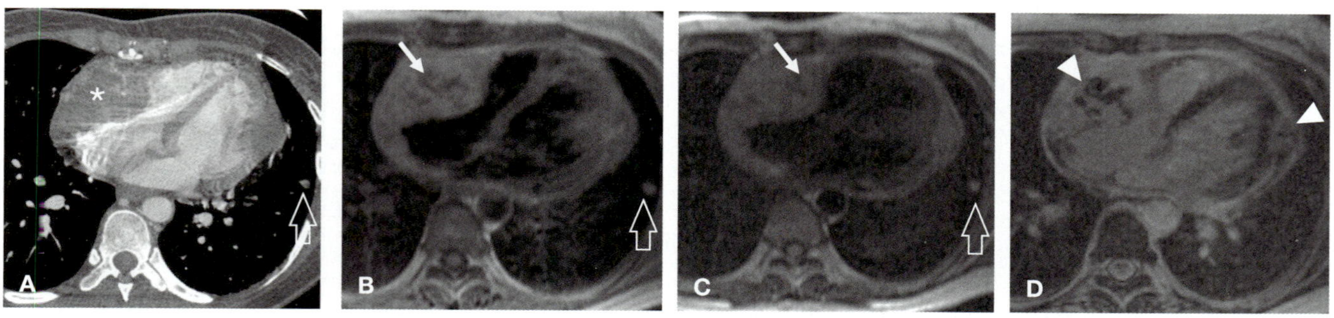

Figure 36.22. Cardiac angiosarcoma (*). Axial prospective ECG-triggered cardiac CT angiogram (**A**), T1-weighted spin-echo (**B**), T2-weighted spin-echo (**C**), and late gadolinium-enhanced (LGE) (**D**) images demonstrate a heterogeneous mass involving the right atrial and ventricular wall. It is slightly hyperintense to myocardium on T1 and isointense on T2. Foci of low signal within the mass are most in keeping with necrosis (arrows). There is avid heterogeneous enhancement of the mass and a pericardial deposit on the LGE image (arrowhead). Note the metastatic deposit in the left lower lobe (open arrow). The pericardial deposit and left lower lobe metastasis are also depicted on CT.

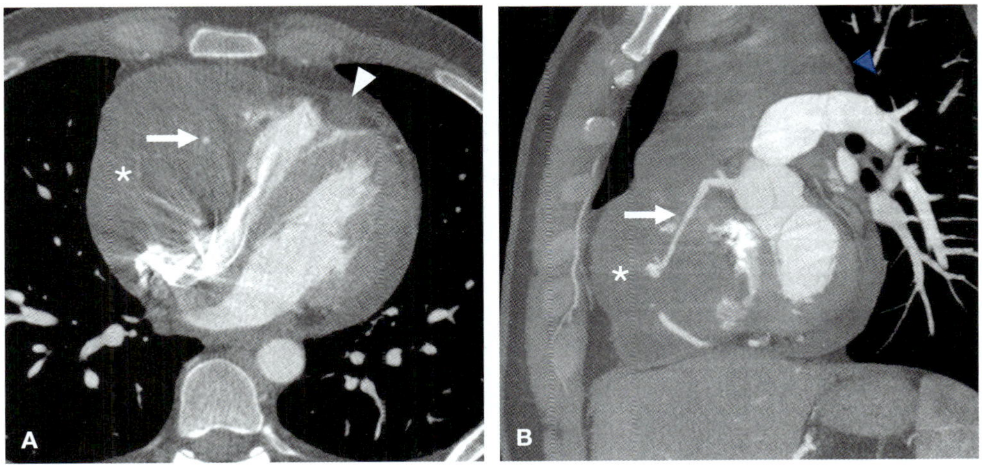

Figure 36.23. Cardiac angiosarcoma. Axial image from a prospective ECG-triggered cardiac CT angiogram (**A**) and sagittal oblique maximum-intensity image (**B**) depict a large mass (*) invading the right atrium and ventricle. The right coronary artery courses through the mass (arrow) and there is a separate pericardial deposit (arrowhead).

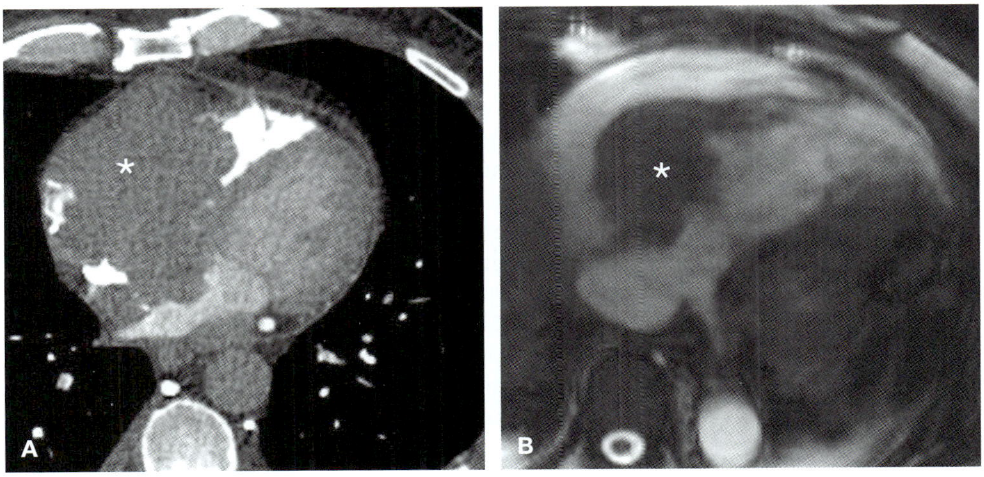

Figure 36.24. Cardiac lymphoma. Axial prospective ECG-triggered cardiac CT angiogram (**A**) and axial steady-state free precession cine image (**B**) in two different patients with primary diffuse B-cell lymphoma showing a large homogeneous mass (*) almost completely filling the right atrium and ventricle (**A**) and centered on the atrioventricular groove. These did not enhance with contrast.

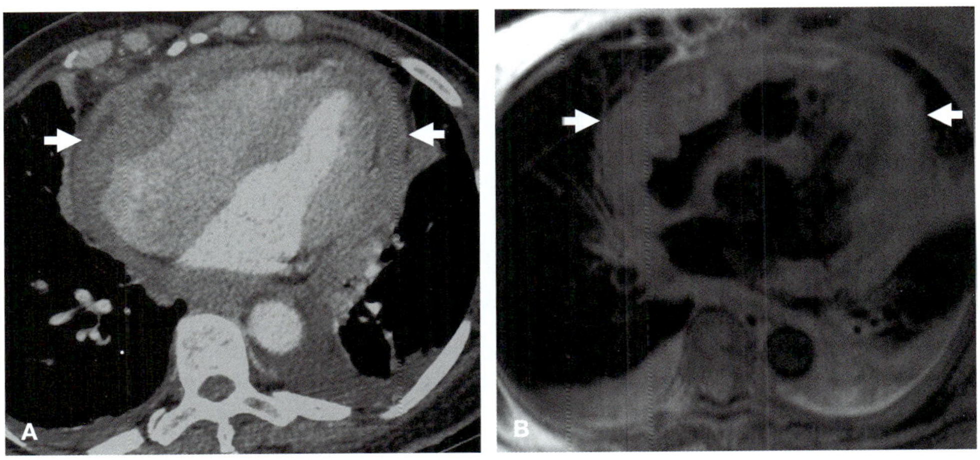

Figure 36.25. Pericardial metastases. **A:** Axial CT angiogram and (**B**) axial T1-weighted cardiac magnetic resonance images depict nodular thickening of the pericardium (white arrows).

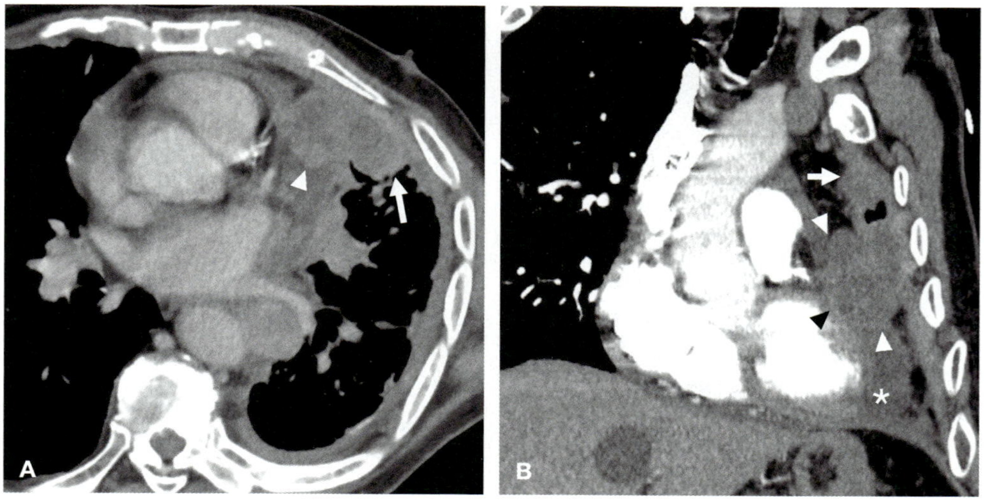

Figure 36.26. Direct invasion of mesothelioma into the pericardium. **A**: Axial CT and (**B**) coronal oblique CT reformat reveal nodular left-sided pleural thickening (arrow) directly invading the pericardium (arrowheads). Note the small associated pericardial effusion (*).

spread through bronchomediastinal lymphatic channels. MRI is highly effective for delineating the location and extent of metastatic tumors in cardiac chambers (Figs. 36.27 and 36.28) and assessing potential respectability. Cardiac metastases are frequently first detected on CT or PET-CT studies for tumor staging purposes.

Transvenous Extension Into the Heart

Another site for the entry of secondary tumors into the heart is tumor extension through the large veins connecting with cardiac chambers. Tumor thrombus arising from carcinoma of the kidney, liver, or adrenal gland can extend through the inferior vena cava into the right atrium (Fig. 36.29), and primary carcinoma of the lung and malignant thymic tumors can extend through the superior vena cava (Fig. 36.30). Lung cancer can extend into the left atrium through a pulmonary vein (Fig. 36.31). The evaluation of the possible attachment of such tumors to the atrial wall is mandatory for surgical planning and can be assessed with cine MRI images. If the atrial walls are not infiltrated, complete resection of the tumor may still be possible.

Table 36.4 Imaging Features of Malignant Cardiac Tumors

1. Involvement of more than one cardiac chamber or chamber and attaching vessel
2. Extension into pulmonary veins, vena cava; pulmonary artery or aorta
3. Wide point of attachment to wall of cardiac chamber(s)
4. Combined intramural and intracavitary components
5. Necrosis within tumor
6. Extension outside a cardiac chamber
7. Hemorrhagic pericardial effusion
8. Pulmonary metastasis(es)

INTRACARDIAC THROMBUS

Thrombus is the most common intracardiac mass, involving most frequently the left ventricle (LV) or left atrium. Atrial thrombus is encountered in patients with mitral valve disease or atrial fibrillation. LV mural thrombus is associated with akinetic or dyskinetic regions of the ventricle. It is most often located in the LV at the site of myocardial infarction (Figs. 36.32 and 36.33) or at the apex in dilated cardiomyopathy. However, any region of the ventricular cavity with static blood is prone to thrombus formation. A frequent indication for cardiac imaging is to exclude the presence of left atrial appendage (LAA) thrombus before intervention. Although cardiac MRI can be used for that purpose, cardiac CT with delayed images is especially advantageous for detecting thrombus in the LAA, which may be difficult to assess using transthoracic echocardiography. An apparent LAA filling defect on arterial phase of cardiac CT can be seen in large atria with slow flow, but filling defect due to real thrombus persists on delayed images (Fig. 36.34).

The most useful MRI sequences for detection of cardiac thrombus are SSFP cines and late gadolinium enhancement. Thrombus usually shows signal intensity lower than normal myocardium on SSFP cine, and very low signal on LGE images with long inversion time. On SE images, the signal intensity of thrombus can vary with time since it is influenced by paramagnetic hemoglobin breakdown products. Fresh thrombus usually shows high signal intensity, whereas older thrombus has low signal intensity on T1- and T2-weighted SE images.

DIFFERENTIATION BETWEEN TUMOR AND BLOOD CLOT

The distinction between clot and tumor is usually made with SSFP cine images. As the various blood degeneration products pass through the different stages of magnetic susceptibility, they cause shortening of $T2^*$ relaxivity. The result

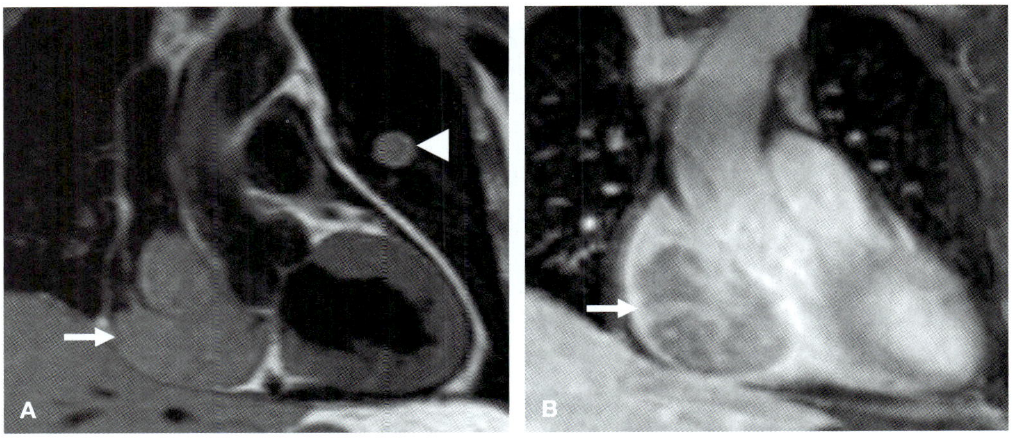

Figure 36.27. Metastasis to the right atrium (arrows) and left upper lobe (arrowhead). ECG-gated coronal oblique T1-weighted spin-echo (**A**) and postcontrast fat-saturated volumetric interpolated breath-hold examination (**B**) MR images.

is low signal intensity of the thrombus on cine MR images (Fig. 36.32, Table 36.6). An exception to this generalization is fresh thrombus, which can have high signal intensity. Tumor tissue is usually iso- or hyperintense compared to myocardium on SSFP cine images. However, some myxomas containing substantial iron produce low signal and mimic thrombus. Another method for differentiating between tumor and clot is to use Gd-DTPA–enhanced T1-weighted SE images. Thrombus does not enhance after the administration of Gd-DTPA, whereas tumors show enhancement (Figs. 36.8 and 36.11). Another approach is using the late gadolinium-enhanced sequence. At an inversion delay that nulls myocardial signal, the thrombus has even lower signal than myocardium (Figs. 36.32 and 36.33). When a long inversion time is used (like 500 ms), the myocardial signal will show recovery, whereas the thrombus will remain dark.

A rare cardiac mass that resembles an intracardiac thrombus is a calcified amorphous mass of the heart. It is unclear whether this represents a chronic organized clot, which has become calcified, or a true cardiac tumor (Fig. 36.35).

DIFFERENTIATION OF CARDIAC MASSES FROM NORMAL ANATOMIC VARIANTS

A potential pitfall in the evaluation of intracardiac masses may arise from the misdiagnosis of normal anatomic variants, such as a prominent crista terminalis, eustachian valve, or Chiari network. The crista terminalis, a fibromuscular band extending between the ostia of the superior and inferior vena cavae on the posterior right atrial wall, represents a residuum of the septum spurium where the sinus venosus was incorporated into the right atrial

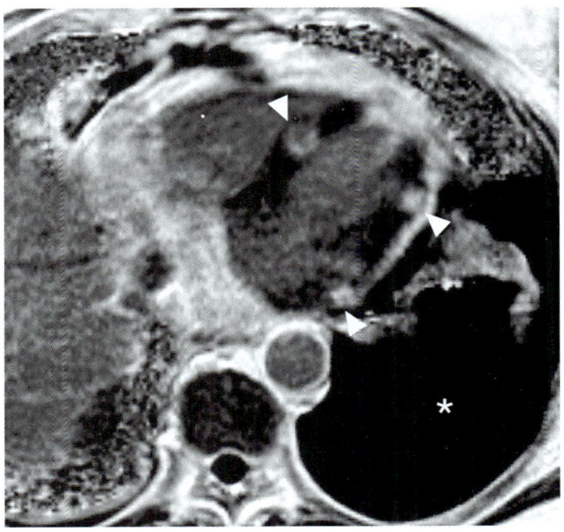

Figure 36.28. Phase contrast inversion recovery axial image depicts multiple enhancing left ventricular intramural nodules from metastatic renal cell cancer (arrowheads). There is also a large left pleural effusion (*).

Table 36.5 Secondary Cardiac Tumors

Direct extension from primary lung and mediastinal malignancy
Lung cancer
Malignant thymoma
Malignant mesothelioma
Inferior vena caval extension of abdominal malignancy
Hepatocellular carcinoma
Renal cell carcinoma
Adrenal carcinoma
Metastasis
Lung cancer
Breast cancer
Malignant melanoma
Lymphoma, leukemia
Sarcoma
Others

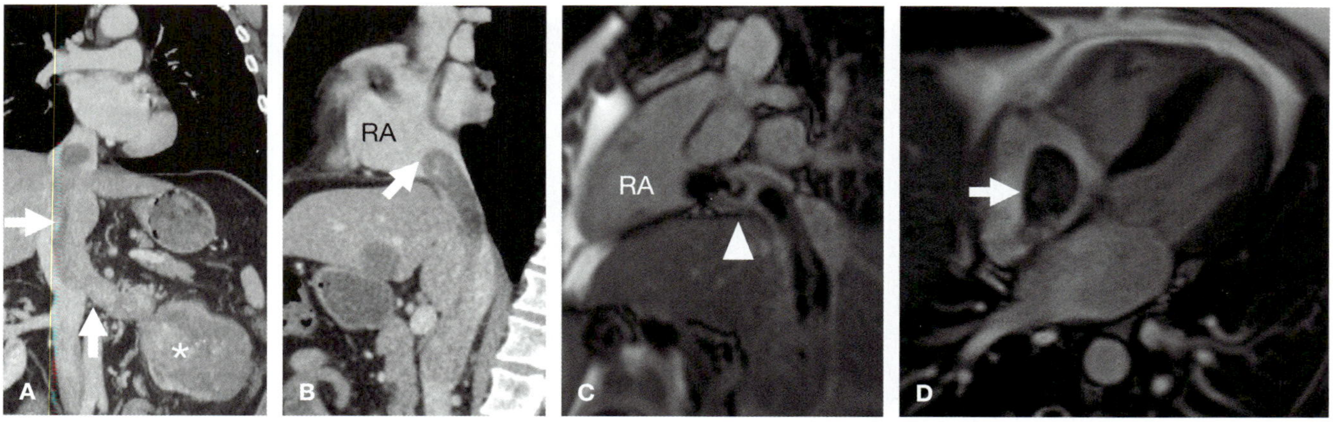

Figure 36.29. Renal cell cancer invading the inferior vena cava (IVC) into the right atrium. **A:** Coronal reformat from a contrast-enhanced CT depicts a large left renal tumor (*) invading the left renal vein and IVC (arrows). **B:** Sagittal oblique reformat from a contrast-enhanced CT reveals extension of the tumor/thrombus into the right atrium (RA) (arrow). **C:** Late gadolinium-enhanced sagittal oblique MR image shows enhancement of a portion of the mass (arrowhead). **D:** 4-chamber steady-state free precession cine MR image illustrates the tumor/thrombus in the right atrium (arrow).

wall. The Chiari network, a reticulum situated in the right atrium, is attached to the region of the crista terminalis and extends to the valves of the inferior vena cava and coronary sinus, or sometimes to the floor of the right atrium near the ostium of the coronary sinus. The Chiari network is derived from the valvulae venosi. These structures regress to variable degrees, and a nodule-like residue in the right atrium is visible on MRI and CT in some patients (Fig. 36.36). Awareness of these variants can prevent misinterpretation as mass lesions.

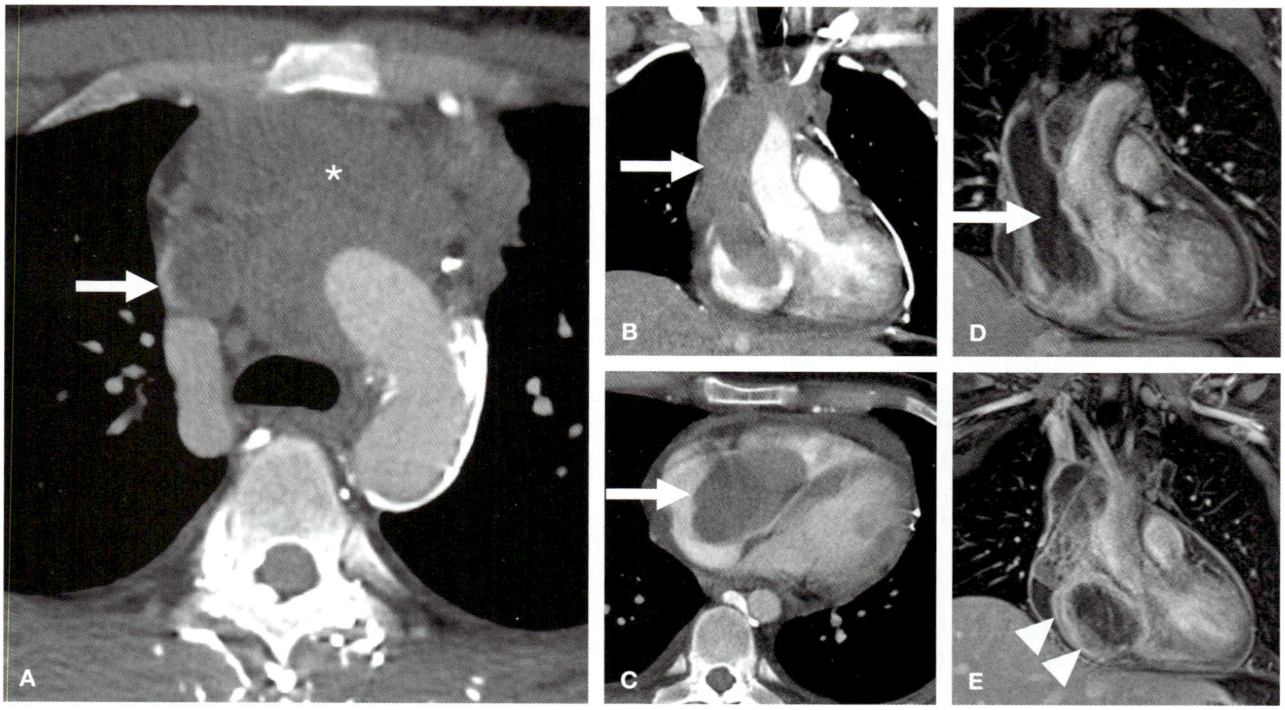

Figure 36.30. Germ cell tumor in the anterior mediastinum (*). Axial CT chest with contrast (**A** and **C**), and coronal reformat (**B**) as well as coronal fat-saturated volumetric interpolated breath-hold examination MR images postcontrast (**D** and **E**) show the tumor invading the superior vena cava into the right atrium (arrows). The periphery of the mass in the right atrium enhances (arrowheads) in **E** but the remainder is dark on MR in keeping with viable tumor at the periphery and thrombus in the center (arrow in **D**).

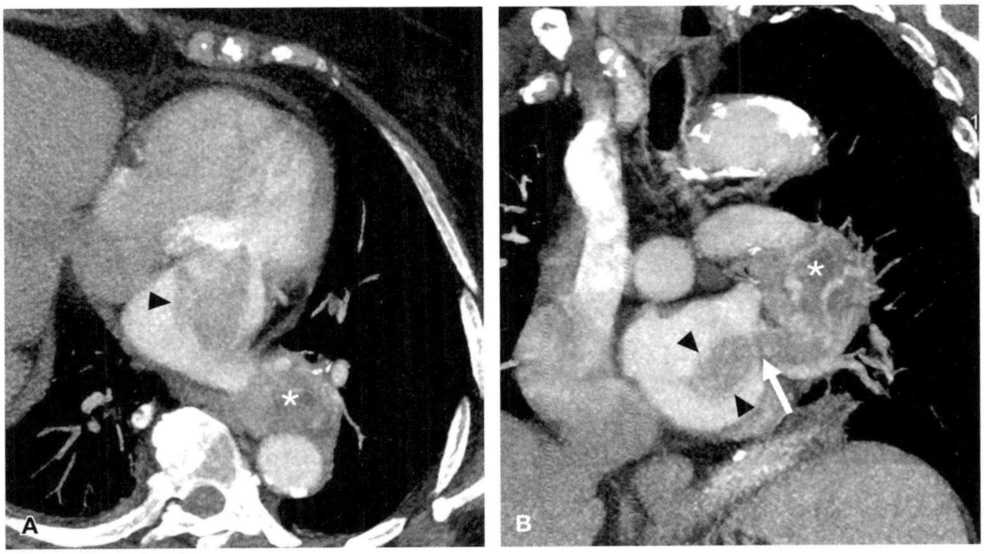

Figure 36.31. Direct extension of tumor through pulmonary veins. **A:** Axial maximum intensity projection (MIP) from a prospectively gated CT angiogram demonstrates left hilar (*) and left atrial masses (arrowhead). **B:** A coronal oblique MIP shows the hilar mass (*) extending through the left inferior pulmonary vein (arrow) into the left atrium (arrowheads).

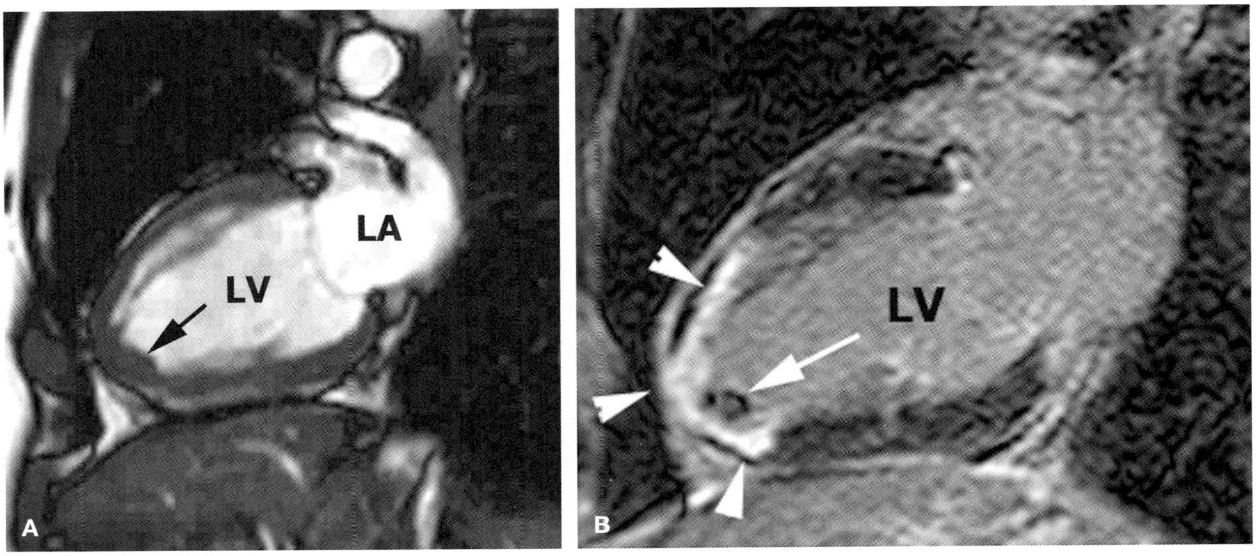

Figure 36.32. **A:** Cine MR mage in the vertical long-axis plane shows apical wall thinning and mural thrombus (*arrow*). **B:** Delayed-enhancement image in the same plane shows transmural hyperenhancement (*arrowheads*) consistent with prior myocardial infarction and a low-intensity mural thrombus (*arrow*). *LA*, left atrium; *LV*, left ventricle. (Compliments of H. Sakuma, Mie, Japan.)

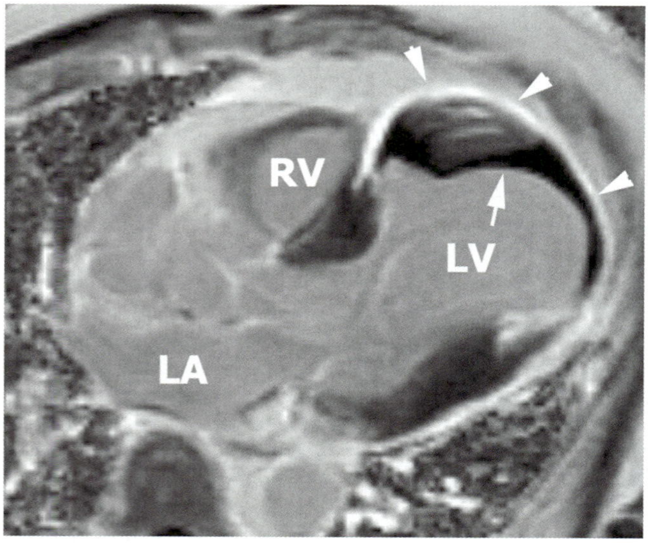

Figure 36.33. Delayed-enhancement image in the axial plane shows a low signal intensity multilayered organized thrombus in the left ventricular apex (*arrow*). Note the transmural area of delayed enhancement in the apical and apical-septal regions (*arrowheads*). *LA*, left atrium; *LV*, left ventricle; *RV*, right ventricle.

Table 36.6 Distinguishing MR Imaging Features of Tumors Versus Clot

Tumor
Intermediate signal on T1 and high signal on T2 SE
Early enhancement after gadolinium chelate on T1 SE
Shorter T1 nulling time than myocardium on delayed gadolinium-enhanced sequence (IRGRE)
Higher signal than myocardium on cine GRE or cine SSFP
Clot
Variable signal on SE depending on age
No early enhancement after gadolinium chelate on T1 SE
Longer T1 nulling time than myocardium on delayed gadolinium-enhanced sequence
Lower signal than myocardium or cine GRE and cine SSFP

GRE, gradient-recalled echo; MR, magnetic resonance; SE, spin-echo; SSFP, steady-state free precession.

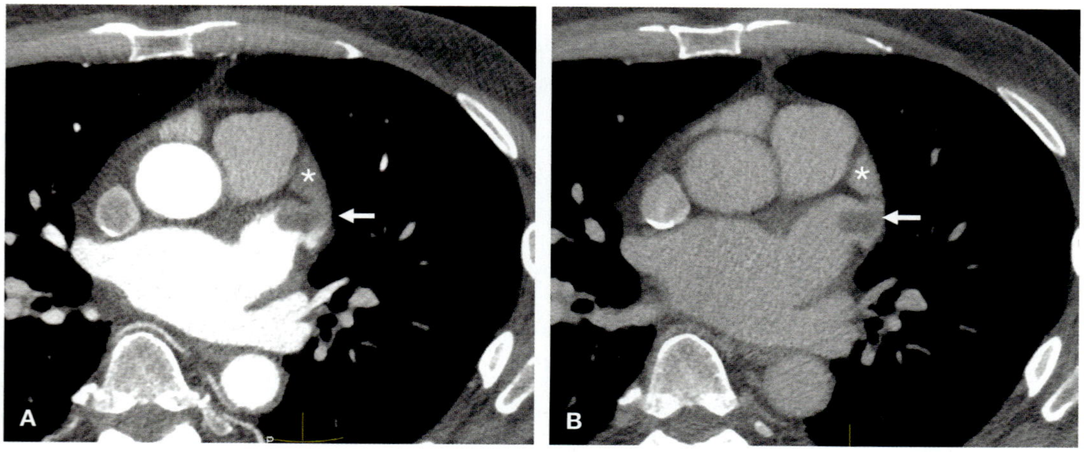

Figure 36.34. Left atrial appendage thrombus. **A:** Axial cardiac computed tomography angiogram depicts an apparent filling defect (arrow) in the left atrial appendage. **B:** A delayed acquisition obtained 60 seconds later depicts a persistent filling defect (arrow) consistent with a thrombus. However, it is much smaller than on the arterial phase (*) as the tip of the left atrial appendage was not opacified due to slow filling.

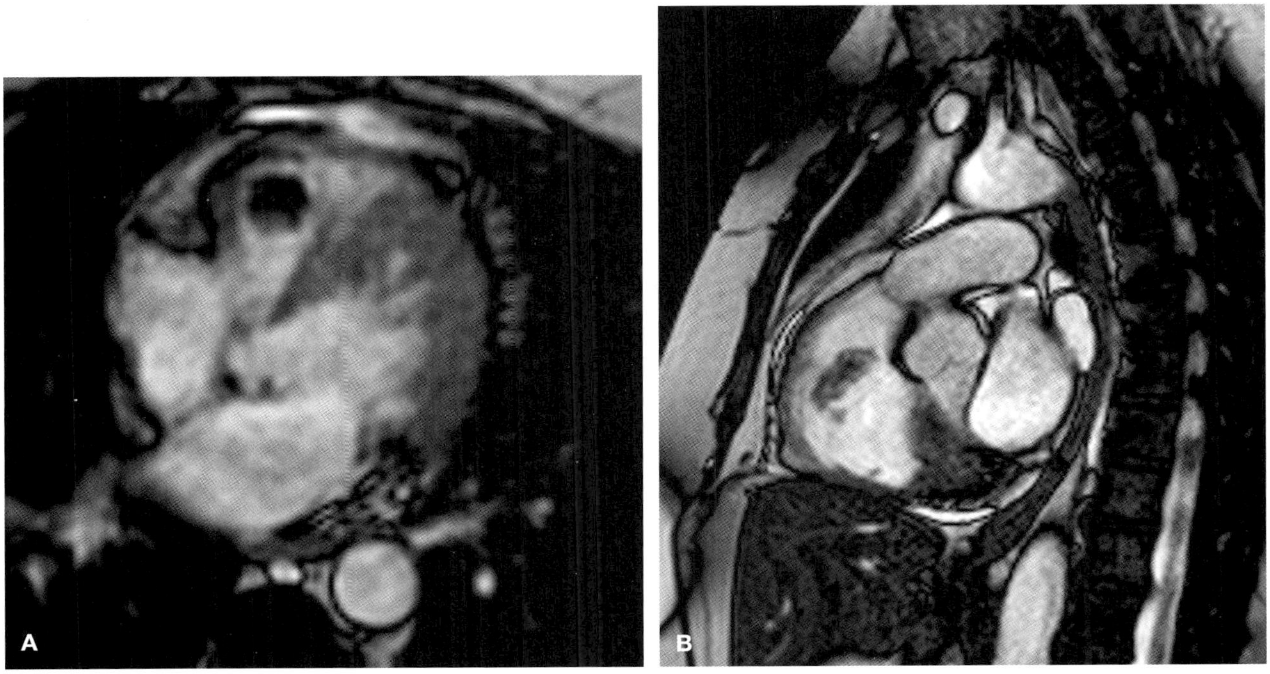

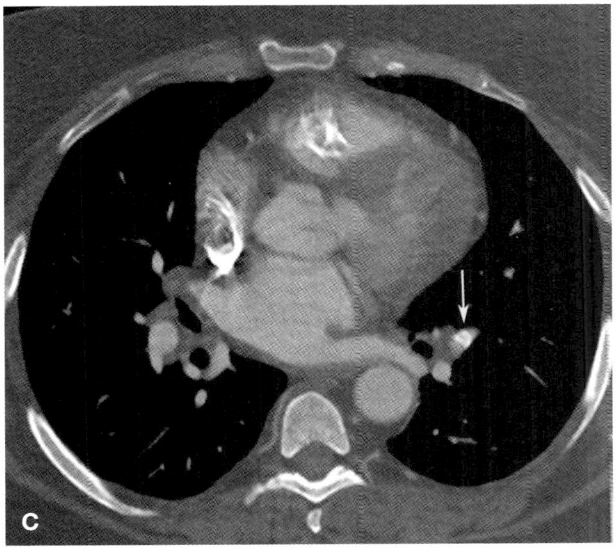

Figure 36.35. Calcified amorphous tumor (organized calcified thrombus) of the right ventricle. The mass is shown in the right ventricle on cine MR images in the axial (**A**) and right ventricular outlet (**B**) planes. Very low intensity is consistent with clot or calcified tumor. CT scan (**C**) shows mass contains calcium and also shows calcified embolism in left lower lobe pulmonary artery (arrow).

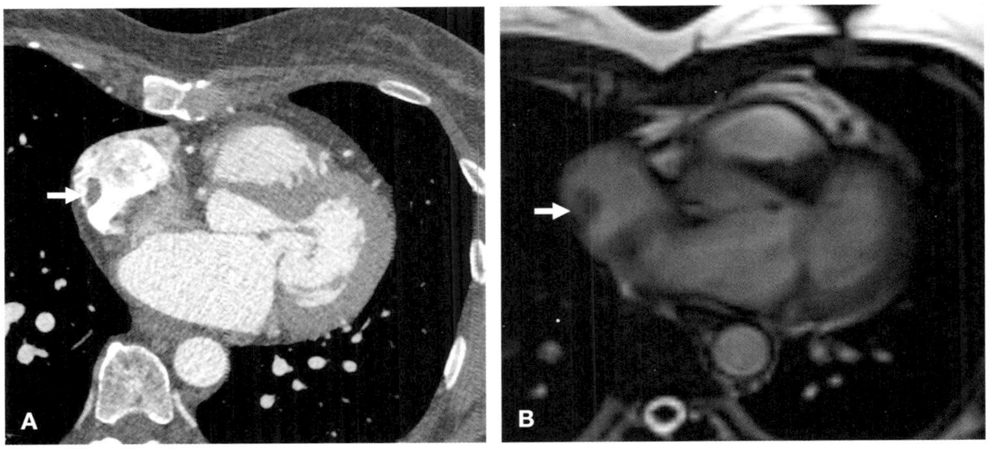

Figure 36.36. Crista terminalis (arrows). **A:** Axial prospective ECG-triggered cardiac CT and (**B**) axial steady-state free precession cine MR images show a nodular filling defect along the posterolateral wall of the right atrium.

SUGGESTED READINGS

Maleszewski JJ, Basso C, Bois MC, et al. The 2021 WHO classification of tumors of the heart. *J Thorac Oncol.* 2022;17(4):510-518. doi:10.1016/j.jtho.2021.10.021

Motwani M, Kidambi A, Herzog BA, Uddin A, Greenwood JP, Plein S. MR imaging of cardiac tumors and masses: a review of methods and clinical applications. *Radiology.* 2013;268(1):26-43.

Mousavi N, Cheezum MK, Aghayev A, et al. Assessment of cardiac masses by cardiac magnetic resonance imaging: histological correlation and clinical outcomes. *J Am Heart Assoc.* 2019;8(1):e007829.

Ordovas KG, Higgins CB. Cardiac and paracardiac masses. In: Higgins CB, de Roos A, eds. *MRI and CT of Cardiovascular System.* 3rd ed. Lippincott Williams & Wilkins; 2013:176.

Patel R, Lim RP, Saric M, et al. Diagnostic performance of cardiac magnetic resonance imaging and echocardiography in evaluation of cardiac and paracardiac masses. *Am J Cardiol.* 2016;117(1):135-140.

Schvartzman PR, White RD. Imaging of cardiac and paracardiac masses. *J Thorac Imaging.* 2000;15(4):265-273.

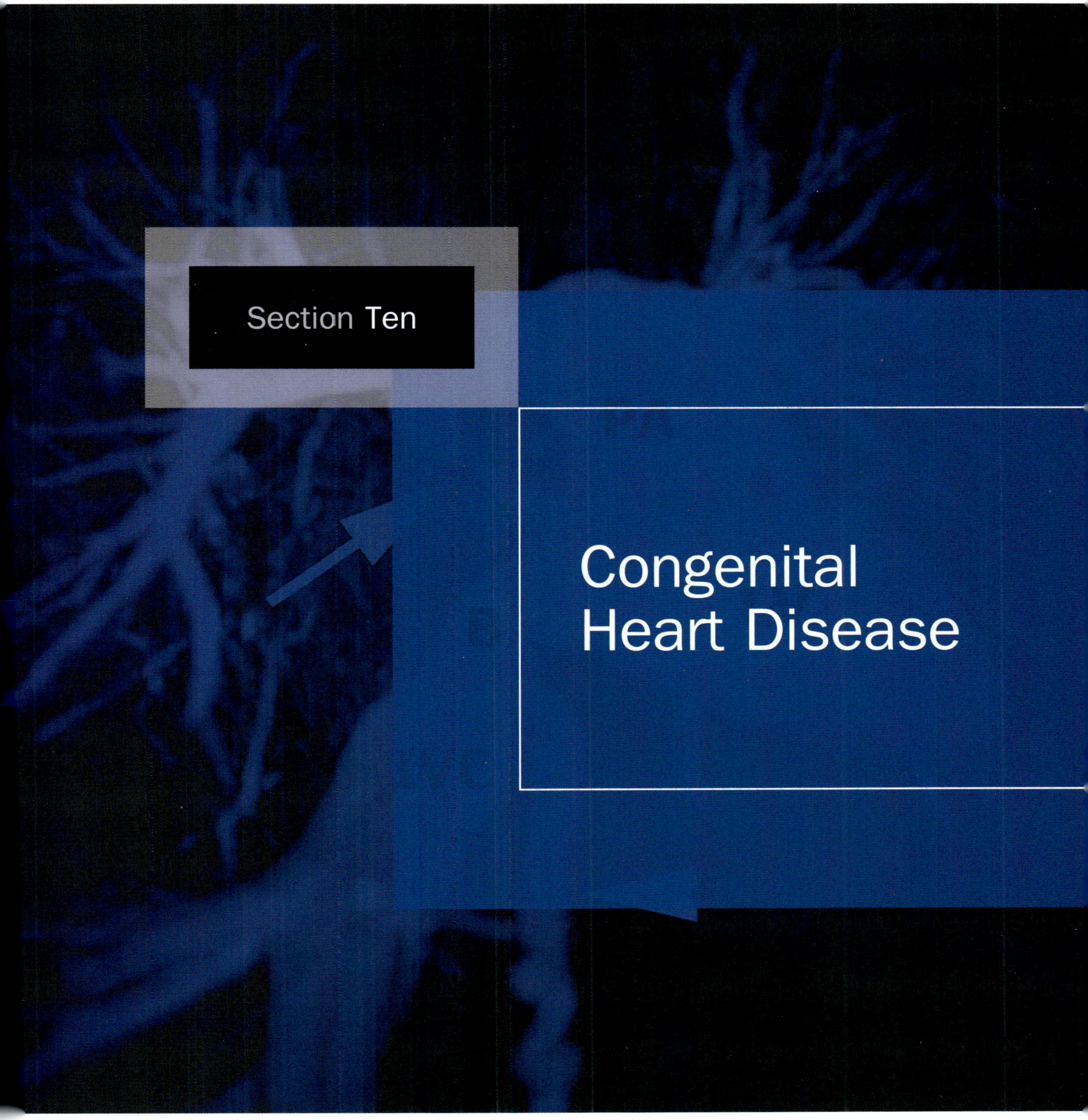

Section Ten

Congenital Heart Disease

Chapter 37

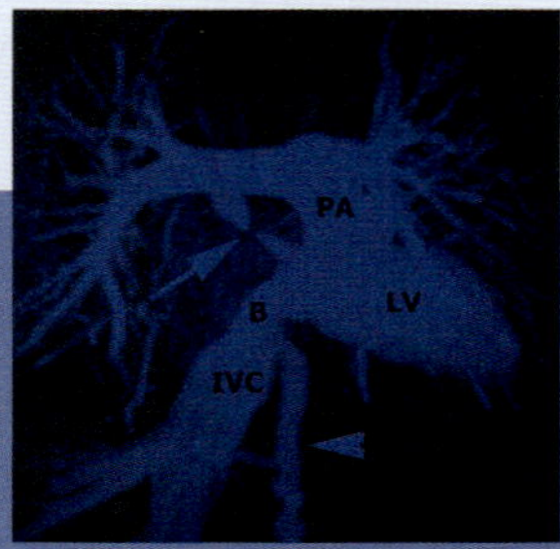

Dianna M. E. Bardo • Andrada R. Popescu • Felipe S. Torres • Cintia A. Melo • Victor Billy Guerra

Computed Tomography Angiography of Congenital Heart Disease

INTRODUCTION

Imaging in congenital heart disease (CHD) has evolved to include nearly every imaging modality. Noninvasive CHD imaging using cardiac computed tomography angiography (CCTA) has replaced most of the indications for invasive high-resolution imaging once performed using invasive cardiac catheterization.

Although echocardiography remains the primary noninvasive imaging technique in patients of all ages, CCTA enables optimal definition of cardiovascular anatomy that may not be completely visible on echo.

MAJOR CLINICAL INDICATIONS

The major indications for CCTA in CHD differ by age, primary diagnosis, secondary or interstage diagnosis, and in some instances the clinical condition of the patient. In this chapter each of five CHD anatomic areas that benefit from CCTA imaging, coronary artery anomalies, aortic arch anomalies, conotruncal malformations, single ventricle anomalies, and anomalies of pulmonary venous drainage, will be presented in three distinct age groups, newborns and infants, young children and early teens, and adolescents and adults, to direct the readers' attention to disease-specific CCTA findings. CCTA is useful in revealing cardiovascular anatomy at initial diagnosis for presurgical planning, for complete repair or at every level of staged palliation early and late postsurgical complications, and for long-term surveillance.

Newborns and infants with a primary diagnosis of CHD are often imaged using CCTA. The most common diagnoses of CHD include:

- Aortic arch anomalies
  - Coarctation of the aorta
  - Hypoplasia of the aortic arch (HAA)
  - Interrupted aortic arch
  - Vascular ring
    - Tracheal narrowing, complete tracheal rings
  - Pulmonary artery sling (not really an aortic arch anomaly but often grouped together as symptoms may be similar)
    - Tracheal narrowing, complete tracheal rings, and anomalies of bronchial branching
- Conotruncal malformations
  - Tetralogy of Fallot (TOF)
    - Pulmonary artery anatomy and stenoses
    - Major aortopulmonary collateral arteries (MAPCAs)
  - Pulmonary atresia with intact ventricular septum
    - Pulmonary artery anatomy and stenoses
  - Double outlet right ventricle (DORV)
  - Transposition of the great arteries (TGA)
    - Coronary artery origins
  - Truncus arteriosus (TA)
- Single ventricle anomalies
  - Hypoplastic left heart syndrome (HLHS)
  - Hypoplastic right heart syndrome
  - Shone syndrome
- Anomalies of pulmonary venous drainage
  - Partial anomalous pulmonary venous connection (PAPVC)
  - Total anomalous pulmonary venous connection (TAPVC)
- Coronary artery origin anatomy in complex CHD
  - TGA
    - Right and left main coronary arteries from right- and left-facing sinuses of Valsalva
    - Right or left main coronary arteries from the nonfacing sinus of Valsalva
    - Single coronary artery

- TOF
  - Dual supply of the left anterior descending (LAD) coronary artery

Young children, adolescents, and adult patients with primary diagnoses of CHD or who are interstage, after, or between staged palliative surgical procedures, or those with surgical complications that need to be investigated may also be imaged preferentially using CCTA.

- Late primary diagnosis of CHD
  - While most patients with CHD present before their first birthday, many types of CHD listed in the previous section may present in children, adolescents, and adults
- Follow-up and surveillance imaging
  - Aortic dilation
  - Pulmonary artery dimensions—stenosis, dilation, obstruction
- Interstage imaging—between stages of palliative surgical procedures
  - Patency of shunts, conduits, etc.
  - Anatomy of surgical changes prior to proceeding to the next stage
- Imaging of complications
  - Shunt, stent, conduit stenosis
  - Recoarctation of the aorta
  - Pulmonary vein stenosis

TECHNICAL ASPECTS OF CCTA

CCTA studies are performed using electrocardiographic triggering or gating techniques with time image acquisition with the R-R interval, which enables high-resolution definition of cardiovascular anatomy in patients with CHD. The properties of CCTA imaging important for producing high-quality images include the following:

Spatial Resolution

Imaging very small vascular structures requires using pixels and voxels that are smaller than the structure being imaged. Most current multidetector and volume computed tomography (CT) scanners produce images using multiple detectors measuring 0.5 to 0.625 mm. The small-caliber vessels of patients with CHD can therefore be imaged depicting

- the origins and proximal course of the coronary arteries,
- the origin and distribution of MAPCA in patients with pulmonary atresia,
- severe coarctation of the aorta (CoA) and aortic collaterals, and
- the fine trabeculations of the left ventricle (LV), pectinate muscles in atrial appendages and, to a limited extent, valve leaflet morphology.

Temporal Resolution

Imaging cardiac structures requires effectively "stopping" normal cardiac motion as well as respiratory motion. A combination of gantry rotation speed, 0.25 to 0.325 milliseconds (ms), and percentage of a 360° gantry rotation allows for high temporal resolution image acquisition. Current CT scanners are capable of 66- to 125-ms temporal resolution at heart rates (HRs) optimized to 60 beats per minute. HR control may or may not be possible or achievable in patients with CHD, particularly in infants and young children, who may have HR of 140 to 200 bpm.

- Reducing or eliminating cardiac and respiratory motion artifacts
- Ability to separate end systole and end diastole phases of the R-R interval
- Two-dimensional (2D) planar and three-dimensional (3D) volumetric reformations
- Wall motion, physiology of cardiac function, including emerging technologies for strain analysis
- Surgical planning, teaching

Speed of Imaging

Rapid imaging is critical for many reasons in patients with CHD. Patients with CHD may be in critical condition, unable to comply with remaining immobile, suspend respirations, or comply with other requirements for the imaging examination, or they may suffer from claustrophobia. Modern CT scanners are capable of performing CCTA examination image acquisition typically in the range of less than a second (a single heartbeat) to a few seconds (a few heart beats).

CCTA Radiation Dose

The radiation dose required to produce CCTA images is markedly reduced with contemporary CT scanner technology compared with old-generation scanners. Using prospective electrocardiography (ECG) triggering, CCTA examinations are routinely performed with doses less than 1 mSv in infants, children, and even many adolescents and adults. Retrospective ECG-gated CCTA examinations are not often performed, particularly in newborns and children, but may provide mostly qualitative information regarding wall motion and function, due to limitations in temporal resolution.

Intravascular Contrast

Iodinated contrast material, usually delivered via a peripheral intravenous catheter, may be timed with CCTA image acquisition to arterial (aorta or pulmonary), venous, or combined arterial and venous phases of vascular enhancement, depending on the cardiovascular structures of interest. In patients with CHD, presence of intracardiac atrial or ventricular level shunts is likely, which enables homogenous opacification of both systemic and pulmonary circulation. A delayed phase of imaging or a dual phase of contrast injection may be helpful for imaging complex CHD anatomy such as obstructed pulmonary veins or surgical anatomies such as Fontan circuits in patients with single ventricle anatomy or atrial level switches in patients with L-loop transposition of the great arteries (L-TGA).

Technologic Advances in CT Scanners

In the past 2 decades, the development of dual-energy CT scanners, wide area detectors, and new detector materials, combined with iterative reconstruction and, more recently, artificial intelligence (AI)-based reconstruction, allowed systematic acquisition of high spatial and temporal resolution images at low radiation doses, greatly benefiting patients with CHD.

Prior to approximately 2017, CT scanners produced images using one energy setting, single-energy CT. Some newer CT scanners produce images using more than one or a spectrum of energy settings, commonly referred to as dual-energy CT. The most recent addition to CT scanner technology is photon counting CT (PCCT). PCCT scanners use smaller detector elements, a technical advancement that is beneficial for two reasons in CCTA of CHD—increasing spatial resolution of tiny cardiac structures at a similar radiation dose and noise level and enabling radiation dose reduction with similar spatial resolution.

3D Models

CCTA image postprocessing is an important factor for diagnosis of CHD. Virtual 3D images may be reconstructed using numerous algorithms and colorization schemes and provide an opportunity to understand complex cardiovascular anatomy and are shown throughout this chapter. 3D printing technology is now being used to characterize the morphologic details of all types of CHD and is especially important in complex CHD. Because the quality of source images determines the quality of 3D printed heart models, high–spatial resolution CCTA is the most commonly used imaging modality in 3D printing for CHD (Fig. 37.1A-C).

A 3D printed model provides unique insight into surface spatial orientation and intracardiac anatomy compared with conventional imaging; the tactile and visual experience

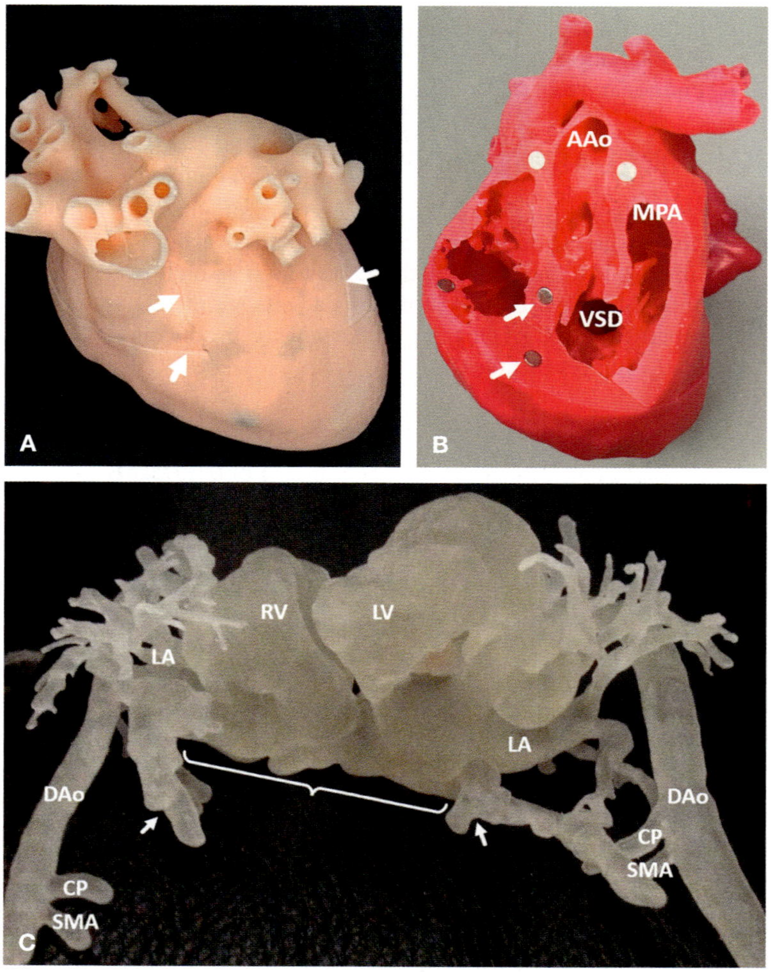

Figure 37.1. Applications of 3D printing. **A:** Infant with double outlet right ventricle (DORV). 3D printed model derived from CCTA image data provides opportunity for studying intracardiac anatomy for surgical planning or for education of trainees, patients, and parents. After printing the model has been sliced (white arrows) so that the model can be viewed as a whole or disassembled to reveal the internal cardiac anatomy. **B:** Infant with DORV, D-transposition of the great arteries and a noncommitted ventricular septal defect (VSD). 3D printed model derived from CCTA image data shows the relationship of the aortic and main pulmonary artery outflow from the right ventricle to the ascending aorta (AAo) and the main pulmonary artery (MPA) and the position of the noncommitted VSD. After printing the model has been sliced and tiny magnets (white arrows) are inserted into the model so that the model can be viewed as a whole or disassembled to reveal the internal cardiac anatomy. **C:** 3D print created from CCTA image data. 3D prints are especially valuable for understanding complex congenital heart disease anatomy as in this pair of neonatal thoroacopagus conjoined twins who share parts of their cardiac chambers. The hepatic veins (white arrows) drain to shared right atriums (bracket). The left atriums (LA), right (RV) and left (LV) ventricles are separate chambers. The celiac plexus (CP) and superior mesenteric artery (SMA) origins arise from the descending aorta (DAo).

increases a surgeons' understanding of anatomy and spatial relationships and is an outstanding teaching tool. Models are useful adjuncts in preoperative assessment of complex CHD such as DORV. A 3D printed model enables better understanding of the spatial orientation of the heart in the thorax, the size and location of the ventricular septal defect (VSD), the relationships of the great arteries and the semilunar valves, and the anticipated dimensions and orientation of the surgically planned interventricular baffle.

AORTIC ANOMALIES

Aortic Arch Anomalies

An early embryonic structure, the conotruncus, divides into the two great arteries, the aorta and the main pulmonary artery (MPA). The complex process of development and regression of six pairs of branchial arches leads to formation of the brachiocephalic arteries, the ductus arteriosus, and branch pulmonary arteries. Most commonly the aortic arch is left-sided, with brachiocephalic arteries branching in the following order: right brachiocephalic artery (divides to the right common carotid artery [CCA] and right subclavian artery), left CCA, and left subclavian artery.

Anomalies of the aortic arch are not uncommon, occurring in 1% to 2% of live births, and may be associated with complex CHDs such as TOF and TGA, CoA, aortic arch hypoplasia, aortic arch interruption, vascular rings, branching artery anomalies, and isolated aortic arch sidedness. Symptoms of aortic arch anomalies arise due to diminished or obstructed blood flow or extrinsic narrowing of the adjacent trachea and/or esophagus. Chromosomal deletions such as 22q11 are important to recognize as up to 24% have anomalies of the aortic arch. In TOF the left aortic arch regresses, with persistence of the right aortic arch, in approximately 25%, and approximately 10% will have other aortic arch anomalies including vascular rings, cervical aortic arch, interrupted aortic arch, or anomalies of aortic arch branching.

Coarctation of the Aorta

CoA accounts for 6% to 8% of all CHDs and occurs with an incidence of three to four cases of 10,000 live births with a male predominance of 2:1.2. CoA is a complex disease in which the most apparent anatomic abnormality is discrete, hemodynamically significant narrowing of the aortic isthmus, restricting blood flow to the abdominopelvic viscera and lower extremities, resulting in relative upper extremity and intracranial hypertension. Old classification terminology that attempted to differentiate infantile CoA (preductal) from adult CoA (postductal) is irrelevant and is no longer used.

CoA is often found with associated findings of bicuspid aortic valve (60%), HAA (32%), and other aortic arch anomalies (18%) such as widely spaced brachiocephalic artery origins, VSD (13%), mitral valve abnormalities (8%), and subaortic stenosis (6%). Shone syndrome is a constellation of left-sided obstructive defects, including supramitral ring, parachute mitral valve, subaortic stenosis, along with CoA, which suggests a common developmental process. Intrinsic aortopathy in CoA results in dilation of the ascending aorta (AAo) through processes of cystic medial necrosis, vascular inflammation, and epithelial dysfunction due to abnormalities of fibrin and the elastic properties of the aortic wall, which persist even after repair.

CCTA is the preferred diagnostic imaging modality as a compliment to echo for accurate imaging of the aortic arch in patients with CoA as it enables superb depiction of the vascular anatomy, including severity of the CoA narrowing, morphology of the aortic arch, widely spaced origins of the brachiocephalic arteries, detailed depiction of the ductal insertion, and presence of the aortic collaterals, and accurate orthogonal measurements are optimized. Furthermore, the spatial relationship between the transverse aortic arch, ductus arteriosus morphology, and adjacent mediastinal structures including the airways and esophagus, important considerations for preoperative planning, is readily viewed in CCTA images.

CoA and HAA are treated surgically or using interventional techniques. Recoarctation of the aorta, recurrence of narrowing at the repaired site, may require repeat imaging. If CoA was primarily treated with placement of a stent or if other surgical materials such as clips or sutures involving the ductus arteriosus are present, CCTA may be preferred over magnetic resonance imaging (MRI) due to presence of artifact, which could obscure anatomy or hinder accurate measurements.

Newborns and Infants

Prenatal diagnosis of CoA by fetal echo is difficult as CoA may develop over time and may not be entirely present at birth, worsening as the ductus arteriosus closes. Tissue of the ductus arteriosus may extend into the tissue of the aortic isthmus, presumably resulting in narrowing of the aortic isthmus as ductal tissue contracts, the normal process that leads to closure of the ductus as pulmonary vascular resistance falls postnatally. In the setting of a small-caliber hypoplastic transverse arch, in the presence of a large tortuous ductus arteriosus, CCTA is predictive of development of aortic coarctation (Fig. 37.2A and B).

Young Children and Adolescents

It is not uncommon for CoA to be discovered after infancy, in a child, in an adolescent, or even into late adulthood. In older patients, late diagnosis may be accompanied by left ventricular dysfunction, myocardial hypertrophy, aortic dilation/aneurysms, and the presence of well-developed aortic collaterals, which are readily diagnosed on CCTA images. CCTA may be used to view potential recoarctation or potential surgical complications (Figs. 37.3A-D and 37.4A and B).

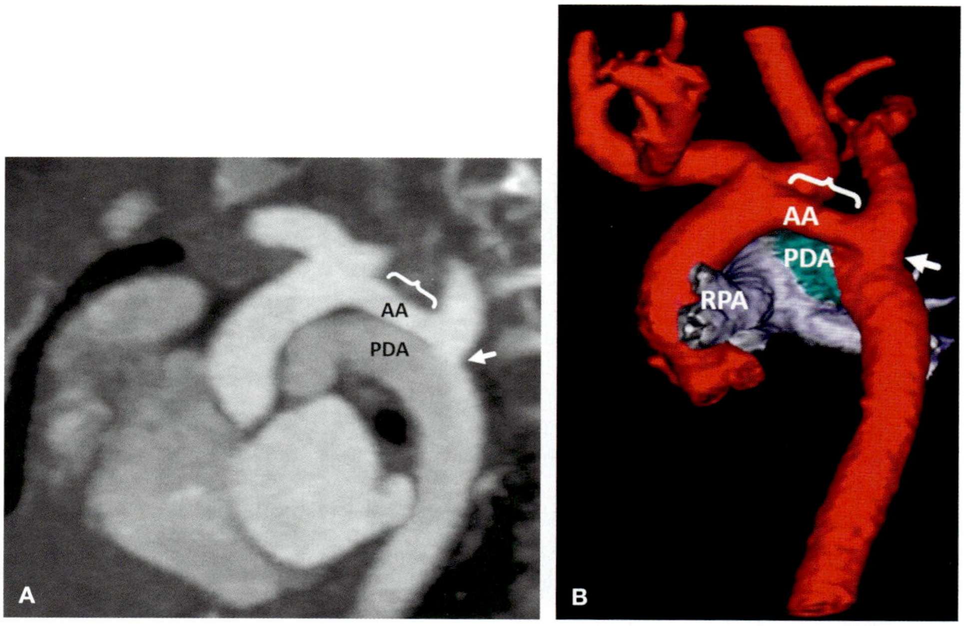

Figure 37.2. Infant with coarctation of the aorta. **A:** Sagittal oblique MIP CCTA image of the aortic (AA) and ductal (PDA) arches. The aortic arch is mildly hypoplastic, smaller caliber than the ductal arch and the brachiocephalic arteries are widely spaced (bracket). **B:** 3D CTTA reconstruction of the aortic (AA) and ductal (PDA) arches confirms mildly hypoplasia of the aortic arch, smaller caliber than the ductal arch and wide spacing of the brachiocephalic artery origins (bracket). The isthmus (white arrow) is narrowed, and a posterior shelf was present, a common finding when PDA is large caliber. PDA, patent ductus arteriosus; RPA, right pulmonary artery.

Adolescents and Adults

While young adults may present with CoA de novo, it is more often that an adult with prior history of CoA or known associated palliated complex CHD will present with recurrent narrowing of the aortic isthmus, recoarctation, versus findings of tortuous appearance of the repaired CoA, often with caliber change compared with the adjacent aortic segments, or pseudocoarctation. CCTA is the imaging modality of choice to delineate anatomy and define pathology (Figs. 37.5A-D, 37.6A-D, 37.7A and B, 37.8A-C).

Hypoplasia of the Aortic Arch and Interrupted Aortic Arch

Localized HAA not associated with CoA and interruption of the aortic arch (IAA) may occur along a spectrum of disease severity. With complete interruption the location of the interrupted segment is assigned type A, B, or C; type A (IAA distal to the left subclavian artery) seen in 30% to 45% (Fig. 37.9A-C) is less common than type B (IAA between the L CCA and the L subclavian artery), which occurs in 50% to 70% (Fig. 37.10A-D), and type C (IAA between the brachiocephalic artery and the left CCA) (Fig. 37.11A-E) is rare.

CCTA enables excellent visualization of the aortic arch anatomy and confident diagnosis of IAA. It is important to describe the anatomy of the IAA and the distance between the interrupted segments. This information is important to guiding the surgical approach, either left thoracotomy or median sternotomy.

Newborns and Infants

Diagnosis of HAA and IAA are almost always made in newborns and infants because both are blood flow limiting lesions that result in murmurs, desaturation, and poor or absent blood flow to the abdominopelvic organs and lower extremities. IAA is a ductal-dependent lesion that may result in severe or complete loss of blood flow to the descending aorta and distal organs as the ductus arteriosus closes.

Young Children, Adolescents, and Adults

Once the condition has been repaired, patients with HAA and IAA may undergo CCTA if there is clinical concern for restenosis or for imaging of concomitant CHD (Fig. 37.12A-D).

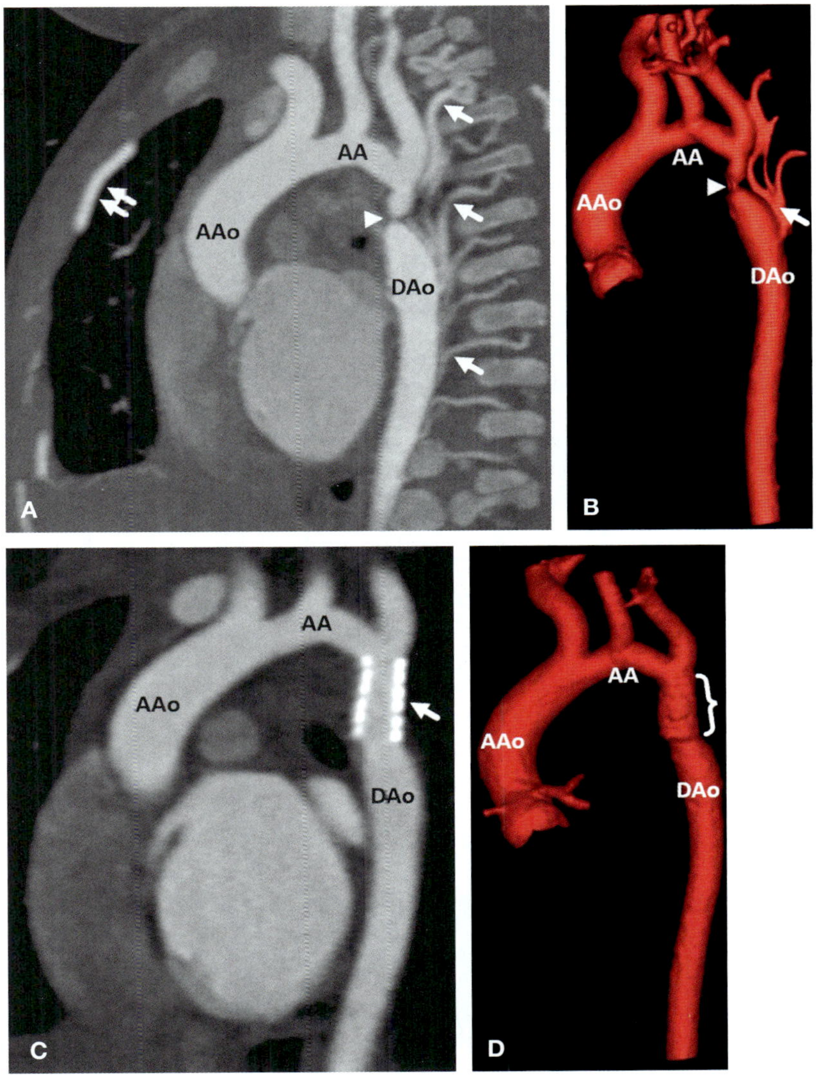

Figure 37.3. Advanced reformations in coarctation of the aorta, before and after treatment. **A:** Infant with cardiomegaly with a dilated and hypertrophied left ventricle showed poor function on echocardiography. Sagittal oblique maximum intensity projection (MIP) CCTA image of the aortic arch (AA). The ascending (AAo) and descending aorta (DAo) are normal caliber, the aortic arch is mildly hypoplastic, and severe coarctation of the aorta (arrowhead) is seen. Numerous intercostal (white arrows) and internal mammary (double white arrows) arterial collaterals have developed as means of supplying blood distal to the coarctation. **B:** 3D surface rendered CCTA reconstruction of the aortic arch (AA) for the same patient. The AAo and DAo are normal caliber, the aortic arch is mildly hypoplastic, and severe coarctation of the aorta (arrowhead) is confirmed. Numerous intercostal (white arrow) and internal mammary arterial collaterals have developed as means of supplying blood distal to the coarctation. **C:** Same patient was treated with percutaneous stenting of the coarctation in the catheterization laboratory. Sagittal oblique MIP CCTA image of the aorta shows the caliber of the AAo and DAo and AA are unchanged. The isthmus of the aorta is now normal caliber. Stent placement may be a temporizing measure before definitive surgical arch repair to allow improvement of left ventricular (LV) function. **D:** 3D surface rendered CCTA reconstruction of the same patient shows normal caliber of the isthmus (bracket).

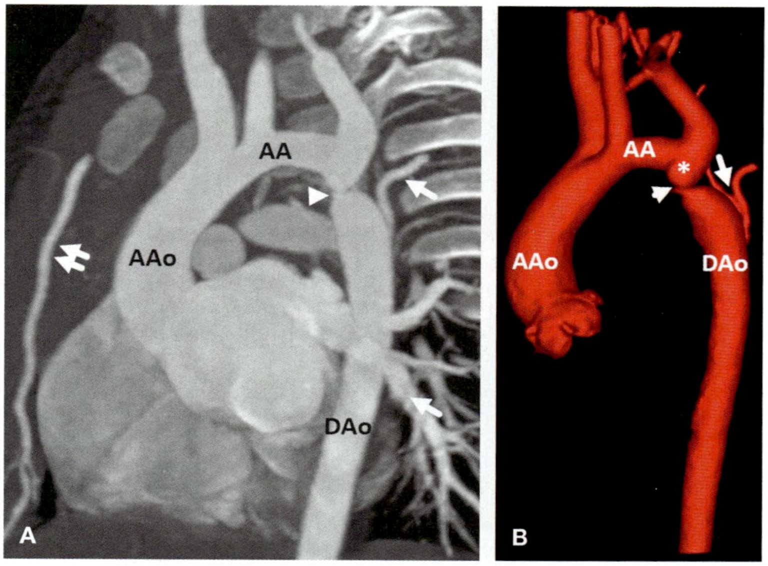

Figure 37.4. Young child with upper extremity hypertension. **A:** Sagittal oblique maximum intensity projection CCTA image of the aortic arch (AA) shows coarctation of the aortic isthmus (arrowhead). The ascending (AAo) and descending aorta (DAo) are normal caliber, the aortic arch is mildly hypoplastic. Intercostal (white arrows) and internal mammary (double white arrows) arterial collaterals have developed as means of supplying blood distal to the coarctation. **B:** 3D surface rendered CCTA reconstruction of the AA shows coarctation of the aortic isthmus (arrowhead). The AAo and DAo are normal caliber, the aortic arch is mildly hypoplastic. Intercostal (white arrow) arterial collaterals have developed as means of supplying blood distal to the coarctation. Focal outpouching of the aorta is at the insertion site of the ductal ligament (asterisk).

Vascular Ring

A vascular ring completely encircles the trachea and esophagus. Vascular rings are composed of segments of the left and/or right aortic arches, a patent ductus arteriosus (PDA), ligament of the ductus arteriosus, or an aberrant right or left subclavian artery, with the AAo anterior and the descending aorta posterior. All segments of the vascular ring do not have to remain patent; the ligament of the closed ductus arteriosus or an atretic segment of an aortic arch may complete the ring.

Anatomic variations of a vascular ring include double aortic arch (Fig. 37.13A-E), right aortic arch without or with an aberrant left subclavian artery and left PDA or ductal ligament (Fig. 37.14A and B), and, very rarely, left aortic arch without or with an aberrant right subclavian artery and right

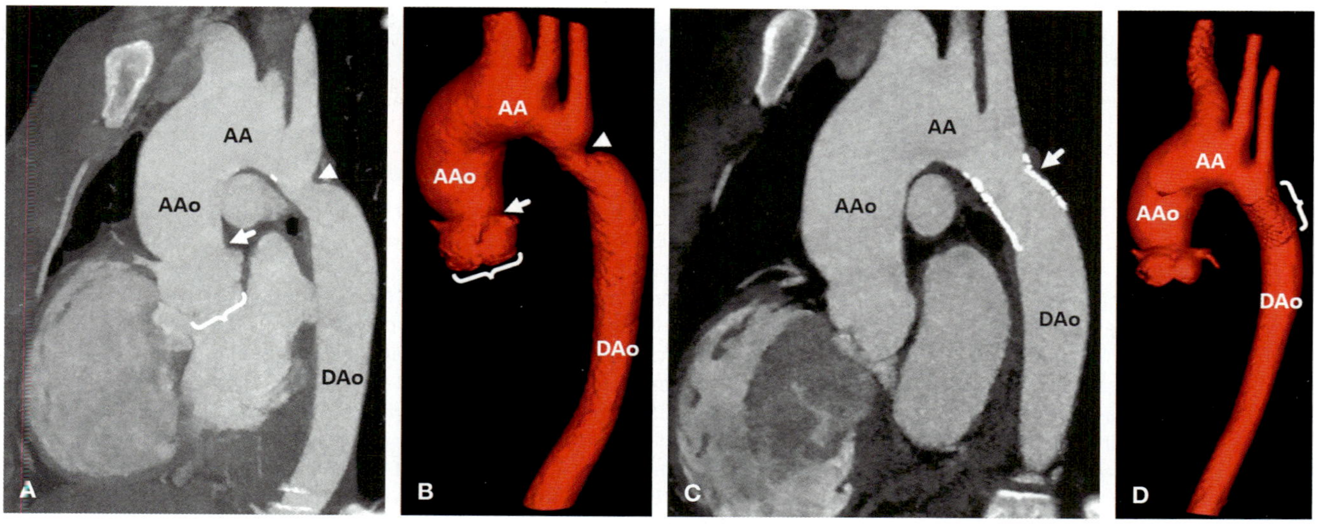

Figure 37.5. Adolescent with Shone syndrome, ventricular septal defect, VSD and coarctation repair in infancy. **A:** Sagittal oblique maximum intensity projection CCTA image of the aorta shows mild hypoplasia of the distal aortic arch (AA), which tapers to narrowing of the aortic isthmus (white arrow), or recoarctation (arrowhead). The ascending aorta (AAo) and AA are moderately dilated, definition of the sinotubular junction is maintained (white arrow), and the aortic valve annulus is normal caliber (bracket). **B:** 3D surface rendered CCTA reconstruction of the AA shows recoarctation of the aortic isthmus (arrowhead). The AAo and AA are moderately dilated, tapering to the recoarctated isthmus. Definition of the sinotubular junction is maintained (white arrow) and the aortic valve annulus is normal caliber (bracket). **C:** Sagittal oblique MIP CCTA image of the aorta shows the stent at the site of recoarctation and now normal caliber of the aortic isthmus (arrow). The AAo and AA remain moderately dilated. **D:** 3D surface rendered CCTA reconstruction of the AA shows the stent at the site of recoarctation (bracket) and now normal caliber of the aortic isthmus. The AAo and AA remain moderately dilated.

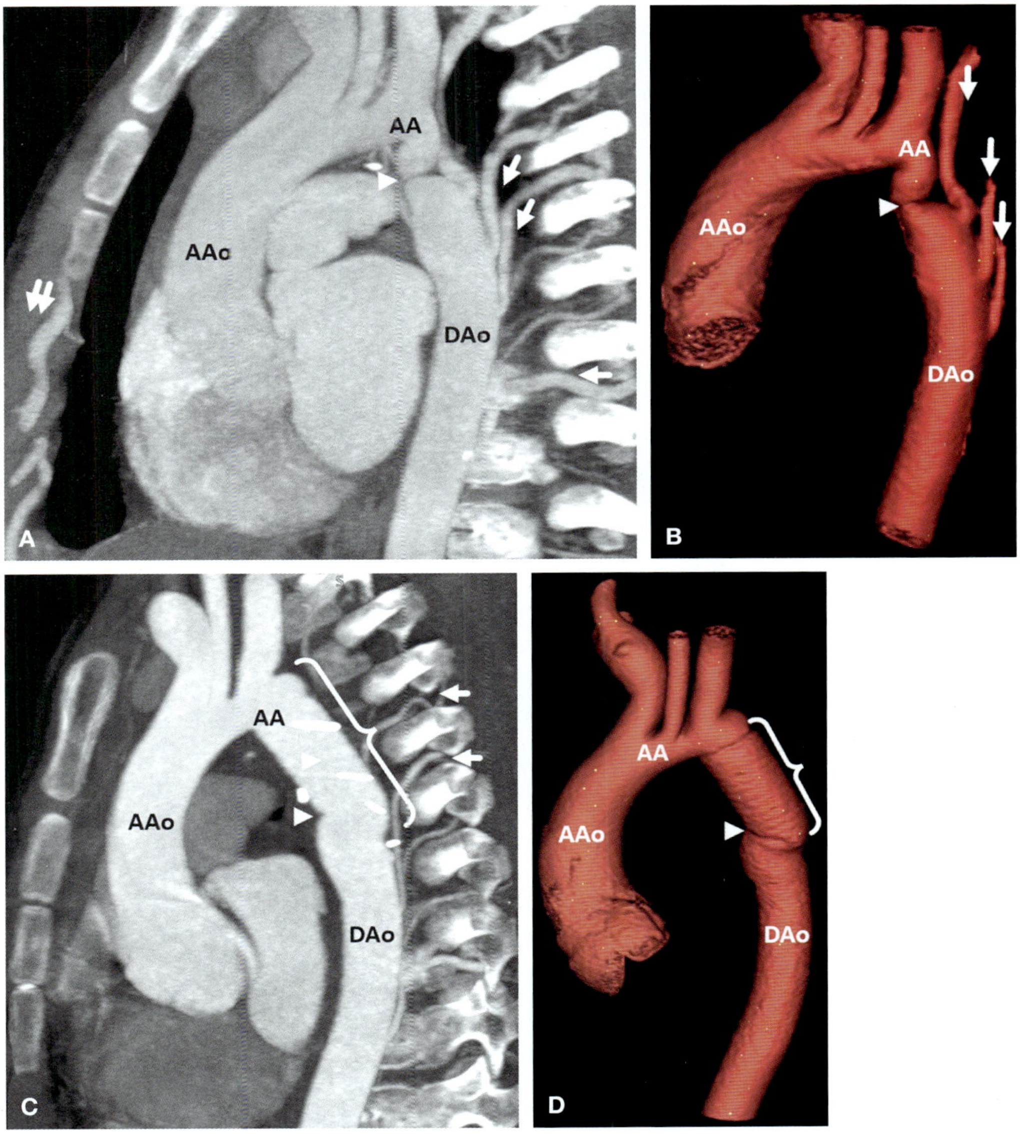

Figure 37.6. CTA for pre- and postoperative assessment of the aorta. **A:** Preteen with upper extremity hypertension. Sagittal oblique maximum intensity projection (MIP) CCTA image of the aortic arch shows severe coarctation of the aortic isthmus (arrowhead) with posterior shelf of tissue, but no poststenotic dilation of the descending aorta (DAo). The ascending aorta (AAo) and DAo are normal caliber. Intercostal (white arrows) and internal mammary (double white arrows) arterial collaterals have developed as means of supplying blood distal to the coarctation, blood flow direction is in the direction of the arrows. **B:** 3D surface rendered CCTA reconstruction of the aortic arch (AA) of the same patient confirms the severe coarctation of the aortic isthmus (arrowhead) with posterior shelf of tissue, mild hypoplasia of the distal AA, but no poststenotic dilation of the DAo. The AAo and DAo are normal caliber. Intercostal (white arrows) and internal mammary arterial collaterals have developed. **C:** Adult with history of surgical repair with interposition graft. Sagittal oblique MIP CCTA image of the aortic arch after surgical repair of coarctation. After ligation and division of the aortic isthmus an interposition graft (bracket) is in place. Mild contour irregularity at the proximal and distal interposition graft anastomoses and mild folding of the contour of the graft anteriorly near the distal anastomosis (arrowhead) are expected postoperative changes, which are not hemodynamically significant and do not represent recoarctation. The AAo and DAo are normal caliber, the AA remains mildly hypoplastic. Notice the intercostal (white arrows) arteries are now normal caliber. Streaks of hyperattention overlying the surgical graft site represents artifact from surgical clips and sutures. **D:** 3D surface rendered CCTA reconstruction of the AA for the same patient after ligation and division of the aortic isthmus and placement of an interposition graft (bracket). Mild contour irregularity at the proximal and distal interposition graft anastomoses (arrowhead) are again shown.

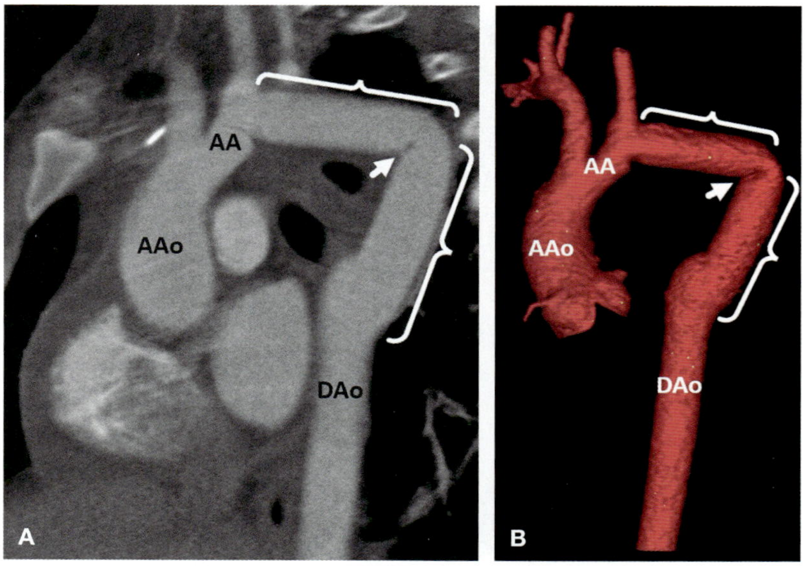

Figure 37.7. Adolescent with history of coarctation repair using an interposition graft, now with recurrent arch obstruction. **A:** Sagittal oblique maximum intensity projection CCTA image of the aortic arch (AA) and the interposition graft (brackets) shows acute angulation and kinking of the mid graft (white arrow). The ascending (AAo) and descending (DAo) aortas are normal caliber, and the AA is mildly hypoplastic. **B:** 3D surface rendered CCTA reconstruction of the AA and the interposition graft (brackets) confirms acute angulation and kinking of the mid graft (white arrow). The AAo and DAo are normal caliber, and the AA is mildly hypoplastic.

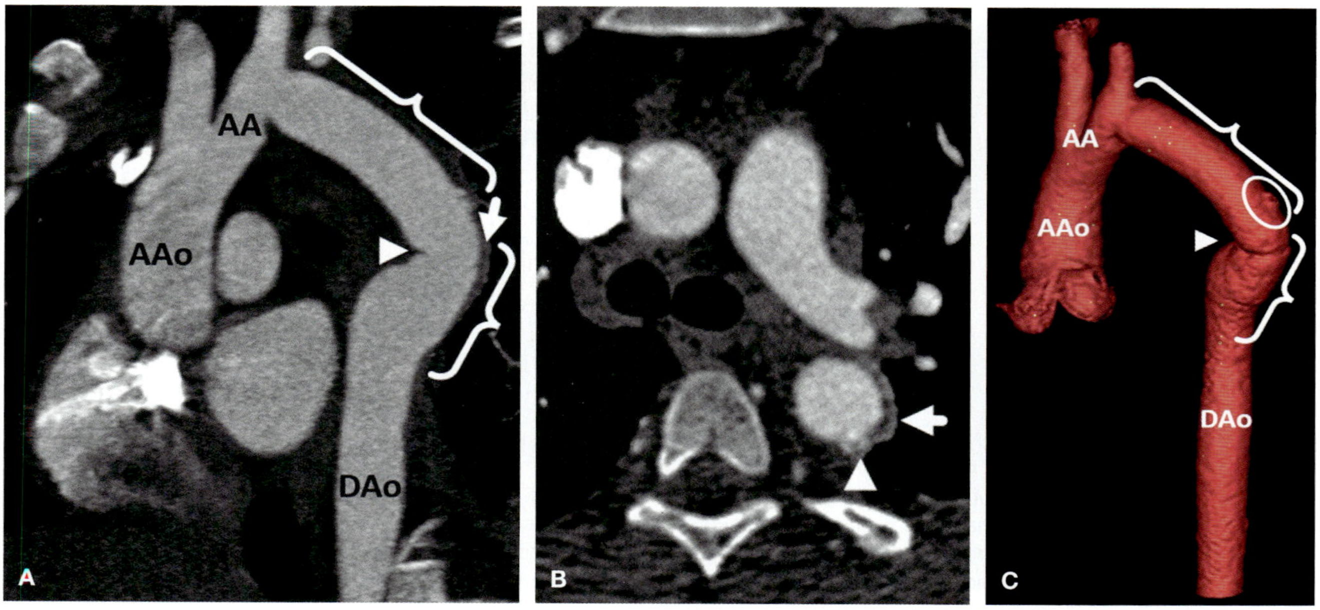

Figure 37.8. Same patient as in Figure 37.7 has undergone revision of his aortic interposition graft. **A:** Sagittal oblique maximum intensity projection (MIP) CCTA image of the aortic arch (AA), the revised interposition graft (brackets) continues to show mild kinking (arrowhead). The ascending (AAo) and descending (DAo) aortas are normal caliber, and the AA remains mildly hypoplastic. On the posterior surface of the distal graft there is a crescent of hypoattenuating material (white arrow). **B:** Axial oblique MIP CCTA image of the distal interposition graft confirms the crescent of hypoattenuating tissue (white arrow), which is perigraft hematoma and focal hyperattenuating endoleak (arrowhead). **C:** 3D surface rendered CCTA reconstruction of the AA and the revised interposition graft (brackets) confirms mild persistent kinking (arrowhead). The AAo and DAo are normal caliber, and the AA remains mildly hypoplastic. On the posterior surface of the distal graft irregularity of the graft lumen (white ellipse) corresponds to the endoleak on the axial image.

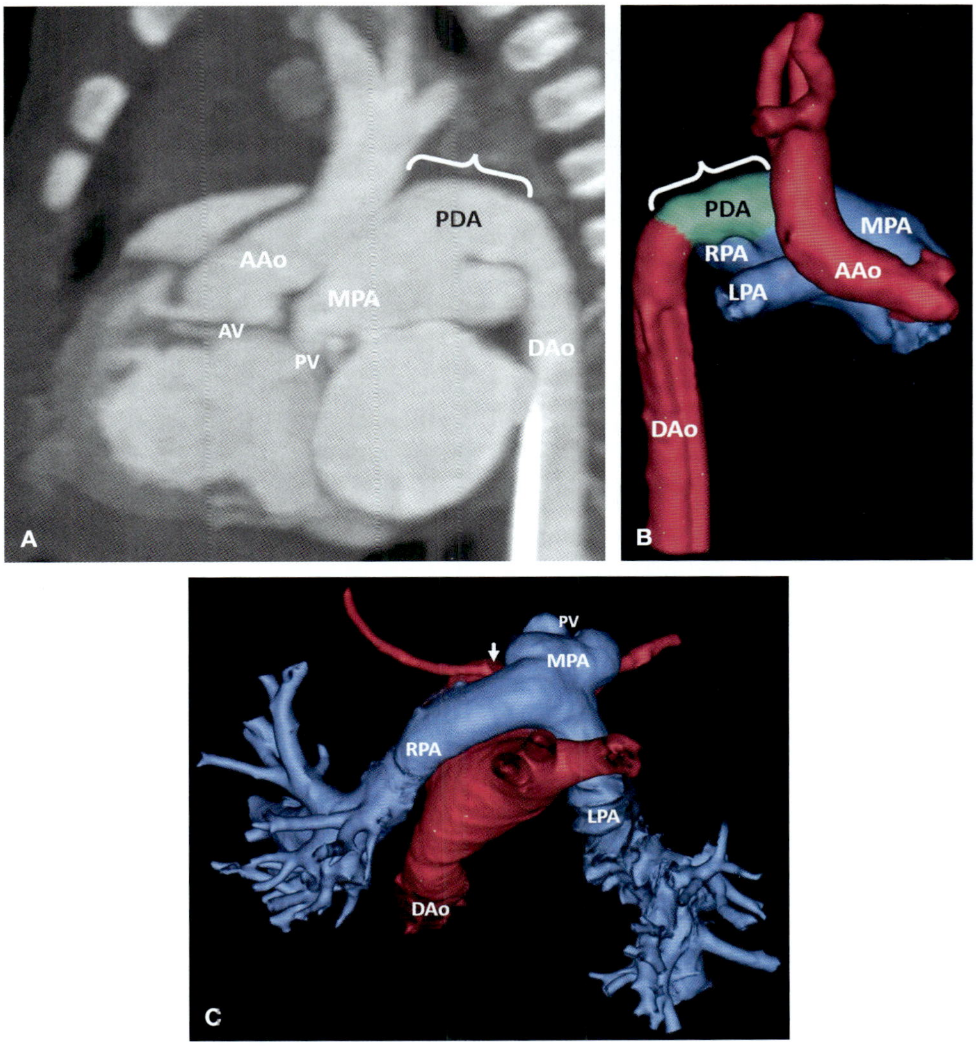

Figure 37.9. CTA of interrupted aortic arch. **A:** Newborn with interrupted aortic arch type A. Sagittal oblique 2D maximum intensity projection (MIP) CCTA image of the great vessels and patent ductus arteriosus. The great vessel origins are dextroposed, with the aortic valve (AV) anterior and rightward of the pulmonic valve (PV). The ascending aorta (AAo) is normal caliber. The aortic arch is interrupted between the origin of the left subclavian artery and the aortic isthmus (bracket). The patent ductus arteriosus spans the interrupted segment, connecting the main pulmonary artery (MPA) to the descending aorta (DAo). The arterial circulation of the lower thorax, abdomen, pelvis, and lower extremities is dependent on the patency of the ductus arteriosus. **B:** 3D surface rendered and colorized CCTA reconstruction image of the great vessels and patent ductus arteriosus for the same patient. The AAo is normal caliber. The aortic arch is interrupted between the origin of the left subclavian artery and the aortic isthmus (bracket). The patent ductus arteriosus spans the interrupted segment, connecting the MPA to the DAo. The right (RPA) and left (LPA) branch pulmonary arteries are normal caliber. The arterial circulation of the lower thorax, abdomen, pelvis, and lower extremities is dependent on the patency of the ductus arteriosus. C. Newborn with interrupted aortic arch type A and dextroposed great arteries, now status post arterial switch with LeCompte maneuver and end-to-side anastomosis of the AAo to DAo. 3D surface rendered and colorized CCTA reconstruction image of the great vessels. The PV position is now anterior to the aortic valve position (white arrow).

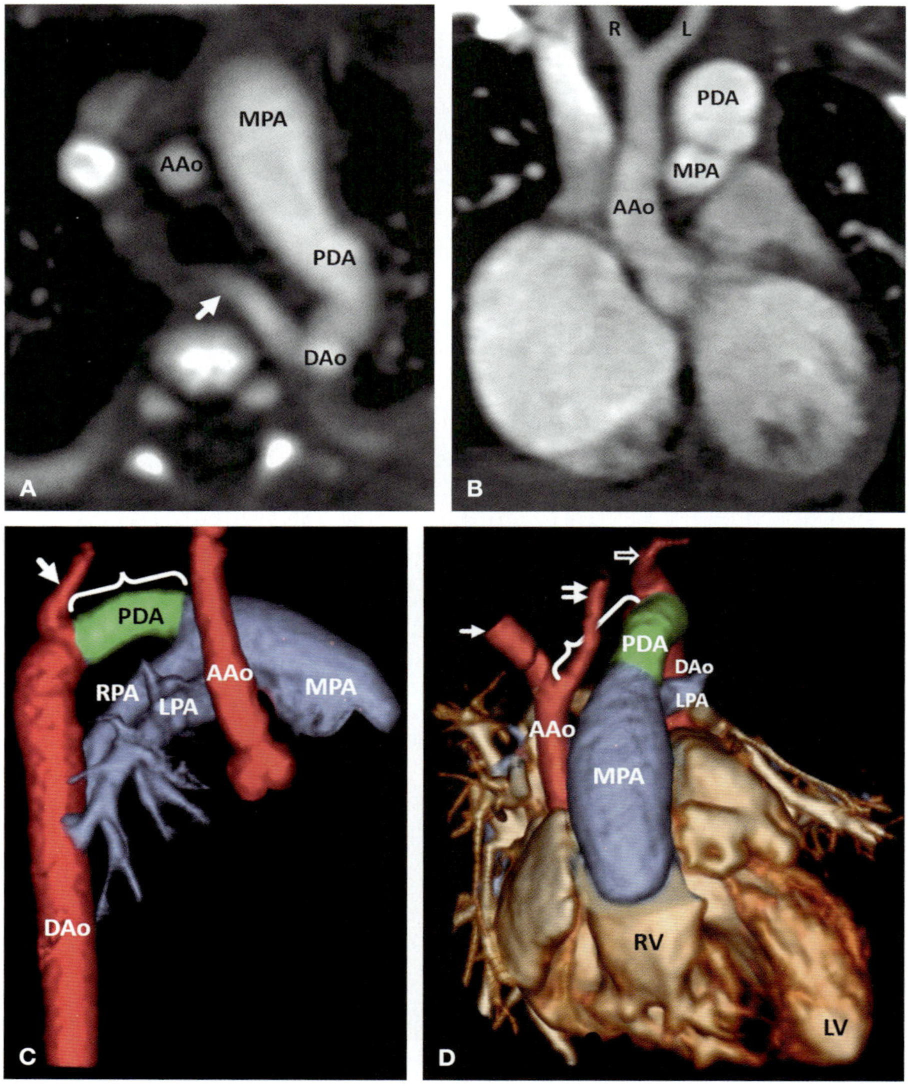

Figure 37.10. Newborn with interrupted aortic arch type B and aberrant origin of the right subclavian artery. **A:** Axial oblique 2D maximum intensity projection (MIP) CCTA image shows the hypoplastic ascending aorta (AAo), main pulmonary artery (MPA), patent ductus arteriosus (PDA), and origin of the right subclavian artery (white arrow). **B:** Coronal oblique 2D MIP CCTA image shows the hypoplastic AAo, distal MPA, and PDA. The origins of the right (R) and left (L) common carotid arteries arise from the proximal segment of the interrupted aortic arch. **C:** 3D surface rendered and colorized CCTA image reconstruction of the great vessels and patent ductus arteriosus. The AAo is mildly hypoplastic. The aortic arch is interrupted between the origin of the left common carotid artery and the origin of the left subclavian arteries (bracket). The patent ductus arteriosus spans the interrupted segment, connecting the MPA to the descending aorta (DAo). The right (RPA) and left (LPA) branch pulmonary arteries are normal caliber. The arterial circulation of the lower thorax, abdomen, pelvis, and lower extremities is dependent on the patency of the ductus arteriosus. **D:** 3D surface rendered and colorized CCTA image reconstruction of the great vessels and PDA. The AAo is mildly hypoplastic. The aortic arch is interrupted (bracket) between the common origin of the right brachiocephalic (white arrow) and left common carotid (double white arrow) arteries and the origin of the left subclavian artery (open white arrow). The patent ductus arteriosus spans the interrupted segment, connecting the MPA to the DAo. The LPA is normal caliber. The arterial circulation of the lower thorax, abdomen, pelvis, and lower extremities is dependent on the patency of the ductus arteriosus.

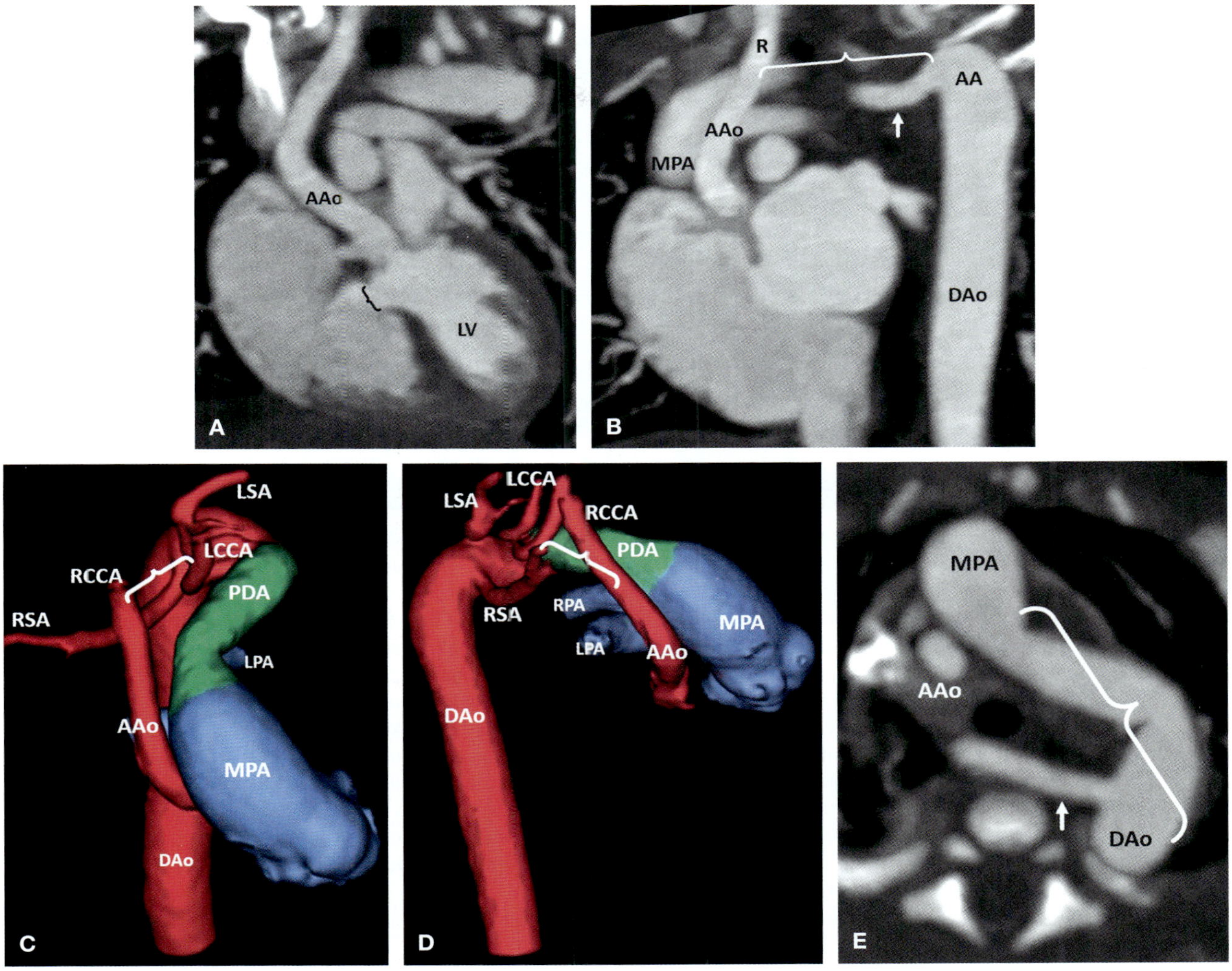

Figure 37.11. CTA interrupted aortic arch type C. **A:** Newborn with interruption of the aortic arch, type C and aberrant origin of the right subclavian artery. Coronal maximum intensity projection (MIP) CCTA image of the heart shows diffuse hypoplasia of the ascending aorta (AAo) arising from the left ventricle (LV) and a small membranous ventricular septal defect (bracket). **B:** Sagittal MIP CCTA image of the heart for the same patient shows diffuse hypoplasia of the AAo, which ends as the right common carotid artery (R). The aortic arch is interrupted between the right common carotid artery and the aberrant origin of the right subclavian artery (white arrow) arising from the distal aortic arch/isthmus (AA). The descending aorta (DAo) is normal caliber. Providing a measurement of the distance between the interrupted segments is an important point for the CCTA report. **C:** Newborn with interrupted arch type C (bracket) and aberrant origin of the right subclavian artery. Hypoplastic AAo with interruption of the aortic arch between the right (RCCA) and left (LCCA) common carotid arteries. The left (LSA) and the aberrant origin of the right (RSA) subclavian arteries are from the distal aortic arch and proximal DAo. Unusual tortuous appearance of the ductus arteriosus and the distal aortic arch with almost a 90° turn at the aortic isthmus. The main pulmonary artery (MPA) is moderately dilated. **D:** Additional 3D reformation shows normal-caliber right (RPA) and left (LPA) branch pulmonary arteries and a crisscrossed arrangement. **E:** Repaired type C interruption of the aortic arch. Axial CCTA image of the patent ductal arch (bracket), which spans the distance between the MPA and the DAo. The AAo is small caliber as it continues only as the right common carotid artery. The aberrant origin of the right subclavian artery (white arrow) arises from the distal aortic arch.

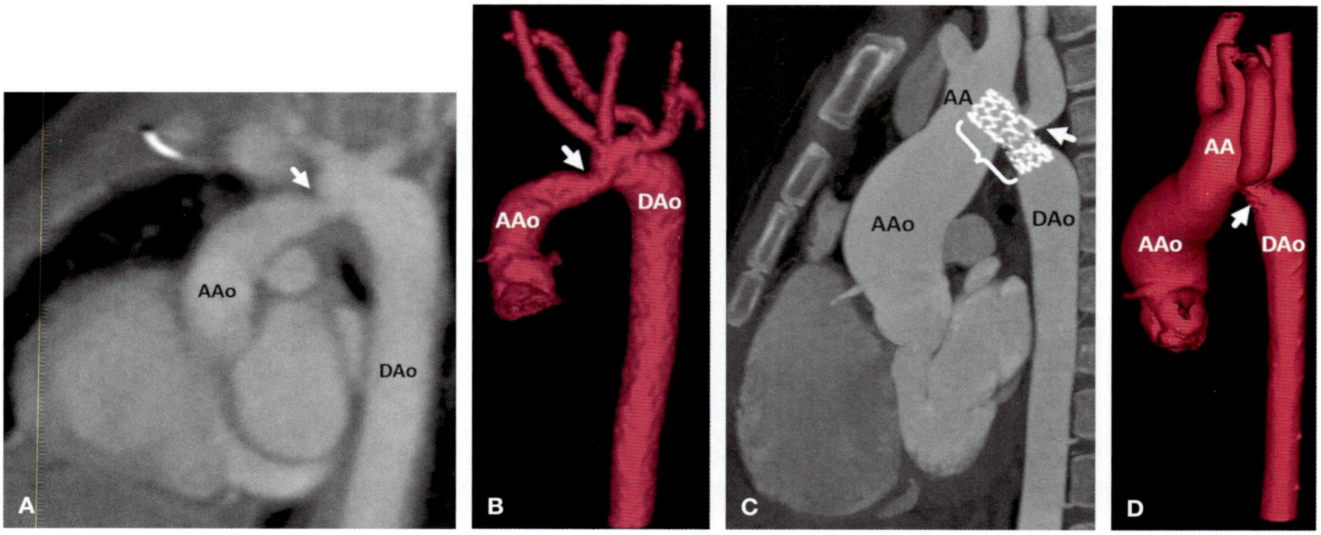

Figure 37.12. Posttreatment appearance of interrupted aortic arch (AA) type B. **A:** Infant with interrupted AA type B and aberrant origin of the right subclavian artery, status post AA advancement. Sagittal oblique 2D maximum intensity projection (MIP) CCTA image reconstruction of the reconstructed AA shows tapering of the ascending aorta (AAo) with focal narrowing/kink at anastomosis (white arrow) proximal to the origin of the brachiocephalic arteries. The AAo and descending aorta (DAo) are normal caliber. **B:** 3D surface rendered and colorized CCTA image reconstruction of the AA for the same patient shows tapering of the AAo and focal narrowing/kink at the anastomosis site (white arrow) proximal to the origin of the brachiocephalic arteries. The AAo and DAo are normal caliber. **C:** Preteen with history of interrupted left AA type B, perimembranous VSD, ASD, subaortic valve stenosis, and anomalous RCA from the left sinus of Valsalva. Status post IAA repair with residual coarctation at anastomosis site and stent placement. Sagittal 2D MIP CCTA image of the AA shows mild dilation of the AAo, intraluminal aortic stent (bracket) at the distal AA and aortic isthmus and mild stenosis of the left subclavian artery (arrow). **D:** 3D surface rendered and colorized CCTA image reconstruction of the AA for the same patient shows mild dilation of the AAo and intraluminal portion of the aortic stent (white arrow) at the distal AA and aortic isthmus.

PDA or ductal ligament. Patients with rare cardiovascular anatomies such as bilateral PDA and cervical or circumflex aortic arches may also have a complete vascular ring or may present with symptoms identical to those with vascular ring due to tracheal and esophageal compression (Figs. 37.15A-E and 37.16A-C).

Patients without a complete vascular ring may also present with symptoms that mimic those of a complete ring. In a patient with a left aortic arch Kommerell described a retroesophageal diverticulum from which the right subclavian artery arises with an aberrant origin. A complete ring may be present in these patients if completed by a rare finding, a right PDA, or the ligament of the ductus arteriosus. The eponym "diverticulum of Kommerell" is also frequently used to describe a similar situation in a patient with a right aortic arch and an aberrant left subclavian artery arising from a retroesophageal diverticulum (Fig. 37.17A and B). Although this terminology is a slight misnomer in a patient with a right aortic arch, Kommerell's original description was in patients with a left aortic arch, the clinical symptoms are often identical, and a vascular ring completed by a left-sided PDA or ductal ligament is more common.

In fetuses with a right aortic arch a right ductus arteriosus occurs 10% of the time, and more importantly, >90% of those are characterized as a normal variant and close spontaneously. Even without a complete ring, a diverticulum of Kommerell, from a right or a left aortic arch, may be symptomatic, so a description and measurement of the diameter and length of the diverticulum are important components to describe in CCTA reports. The diverticulum may cause extrinsic compression of the posterior surface of the esophagus and, even when a complete ring is divided, may remain a cause of dysphagia (Fig. 37.18A-C). Surgical techniques may include resection of the diverticulum and reimplantation of aberrant subclavian artery to its ipsilateral CCA versus ligation and division of the ligamentum, to eliminate posterior esophageal compression (Fig. 37.19).

Pulmonary artery sling, although not an aortic arch anomaly, and not a true vascular ring, often presents with symptoms similar to those in patients with a complete vascular ring. Pulmonary artery sling is almost exclusively a phenomenon in which the left pulmonary artery arises from the right branch pulmonary artery, courses between the trachea

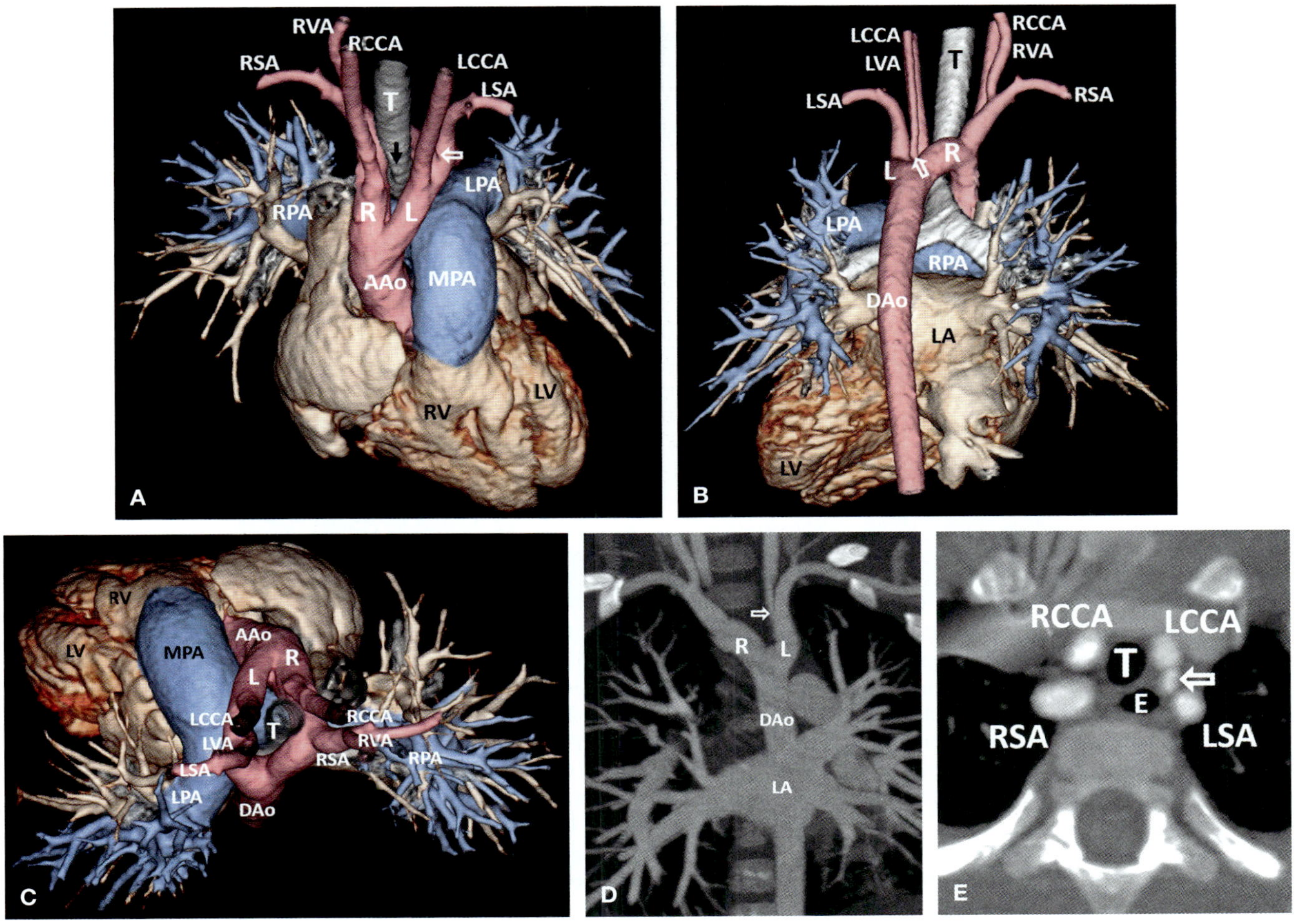

Figure 37.13. Infant with chronic respiratory issues and dysphagia to solids. **A:** 3D color segmented CCTA reconstruction of the heart shows a double aortic arch encircling the trachea (T); the esophagus is not seen. The trachea (black arrow) is narrowed as it courses through the vascular ring. The left subclavian (LSA), vertebral (LVA; open white arrow), and common carotid (LCCA) arteries arise from the left aortic arch (L). The right subclavian (RSA) and common carotid (RCCA) arteries arise separately from the right aortic arch (R). The right vertebral artery (RVA) arises from the RSA. **B:** 3D color segmented CCTA reconstruction of the heart (posterior view) shows a double aortic arch encircling the trachea (T); the esophagus is not seen. The LSA, LVA (open white arrow), and LCCA arise from the left aortic arch (L). The RSA and RCCA arise separately from the right aortic arch (R). The RVA arises from the RSA. **C:** 3D color segmented CCTA reconstruction of the heart (superior view) shows a double aortic arch encircling the trachea (T); the esophagus is not seen. The LCCA, LVA, and LSA arise from the left aortic arch (L) The RCCA and RSA arise separately from the right aortic arch (R). The RVA arises from the RSA. **D:** Coronal 2D maximum intensity projection (MIP) CCTA reconstruction shows the posterior aspect of the right (R) and left (L) aortic arches as they connect to the descending aorta (DAo). As seen in the 3D reconstructed images the left vertebral artery (white open arrow) arises anomalously from the left aortic arch. **E:** Axial 2D MIP CCTA reconstruction of the brachiocephalic arteries just above their origin from a double aortic arch shows the typical arrangement of the four brachiocephalic vessels, the RCCA and RSA and the LCCA and LSA. As seen in the 3D reconstructed images the LVA (white open arrow) arises anomalously from the left aortic arch. LA, left atrium).

and esophagus to the left hilum, and may cause extrinsic narrowing of the anterior surface of the esophagus and tracheal abnormalities including posterior extrinsic tracheal narrowing, tracheomalacia, and complete tracheal rings and may be associated with anomalous branching of the trachea and main bronchi (Fig. 37.20A and B).

Newborns and Infants

Symptoms of a vascular ring are due to extrinsic narrowing of the trachea and esophagus. Tracheal narrowing may be complicated by tracheomalacia and in a few patients by complete cartilaginous tracheal rings (Fig. 37.21A and B). The severity of tracheal disease varies, and patients with

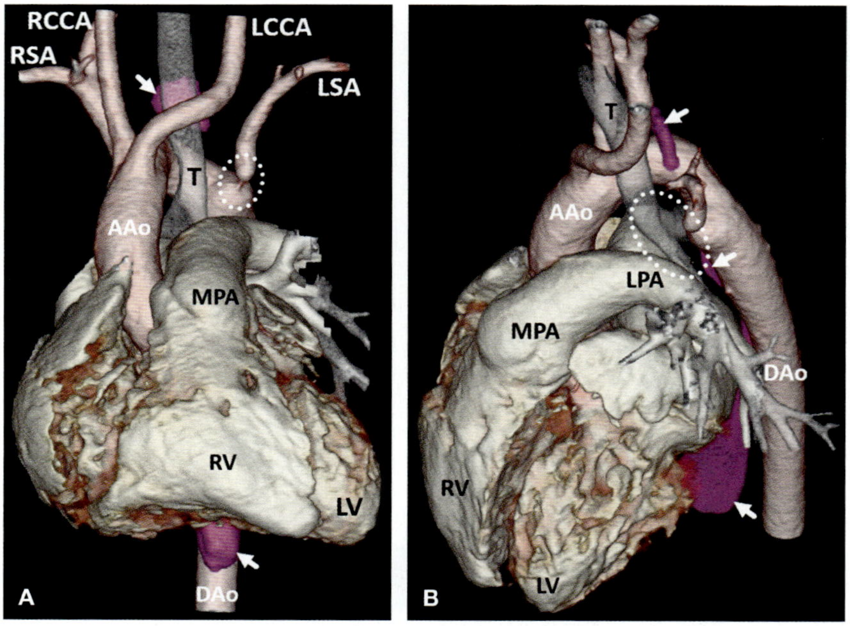

Figure 37.14. Older child with chronic respiratory issues and dysphagia to solids. **A:** 3D color segmented CCTA reconstruction of the heart shows a right aortic arch, which causes a mild degree of extrinsic narrowing on the right side of the trachea (T); the esophagus has been colorized bright pink (white arrows). The anomalous origin of the left subclavian artery (LSA) is severely narrowed (dotted ellipse). This finding is suspicious for the presence of tissue from the ductus arteriosus in the origin of the LSA, which is the cause of the stenosis. The left (LCCA) and right (RCCA) common carotid and right subclavian (RSA) arteries arise separately from the right aortic arch. **B:** 3D color segmented CCTA reconstruction of the heart from the left oblique projection shows a right aortic arch. There is moderate narrowing on the left main bronchus (dotted ellipse) and marked narrowing of the esophagus (white arrows). The anomalous origin of the left subclavian artery (LSA) is severely narrowed (dotted ellipse) by mass effect between the left pulmonary artery (LPA) and the stenosed origin of the LSA. The mild degree of anterior displacement of the LSA origin is another clue that a ligament of the ductus arteriosus is attached at this site. Although the ductal ligament is usually not visible on CCTA, the imaging findings are very likely due to a complete vascular ring.

complete tracheal rings typically present early, particularly when accompanied by intracardiac findings of CHD.

Young Children, Adolescents, and Adults

When symptoms of tracheomalacia related to vascular ring are mild, a clinical diagnosis such as "asthma" may mask the true diagnosis. Esophageal narrowing due to a vascular ring may present in childhood as dysphagia to solid foods, retained food items, or sometimes a retained esophageal foreign body, above the level of the aortic arch. Children, adolescents, and adults with a history of vascular ring repair or with persistent Kommerell diverticulum after repair may experience continued symptoms and even require additional surgery to reduce the size of the diverticulum or reimplant the aberrant subclavian artery to the ipsilateral CCA. After reimplantation of the LPA in patients with a sling, CCTA may be useful for monitoring vascular anatomy (Fig. 37.22A and B). It is unusual for an adolescent or adult to present primarily with a complete vascular ring.

CONOTRUNCAL MALFORMATIONS

Tetralogy of Fallot

TOF is the most common cyanotic CHD with an estimated incidence of approximately 1:2500 to 3000 live births. The conotruncus normally divides symmetrically to the ventricular outflow tracts, the AAo, and MPA. In TOF the conus divides in an asymmetric manner due to anterosuperior deviation of the outlet septum, leading to the four (tetralogy) major abnormal findings in patients with TOF (Fig. 37.23A and B):

- right ventricular outflow obstruction, which may involve the right ventricular outflow tract (RVOT), pulmonary valve stenosis or atresia, or main or branch pulmonary artery stenosis
- right ventricular hypertrophy, which occurs due to the right ventricle (RV) working harder to pump blood through the obstructed RVOT/pulmonary arteries

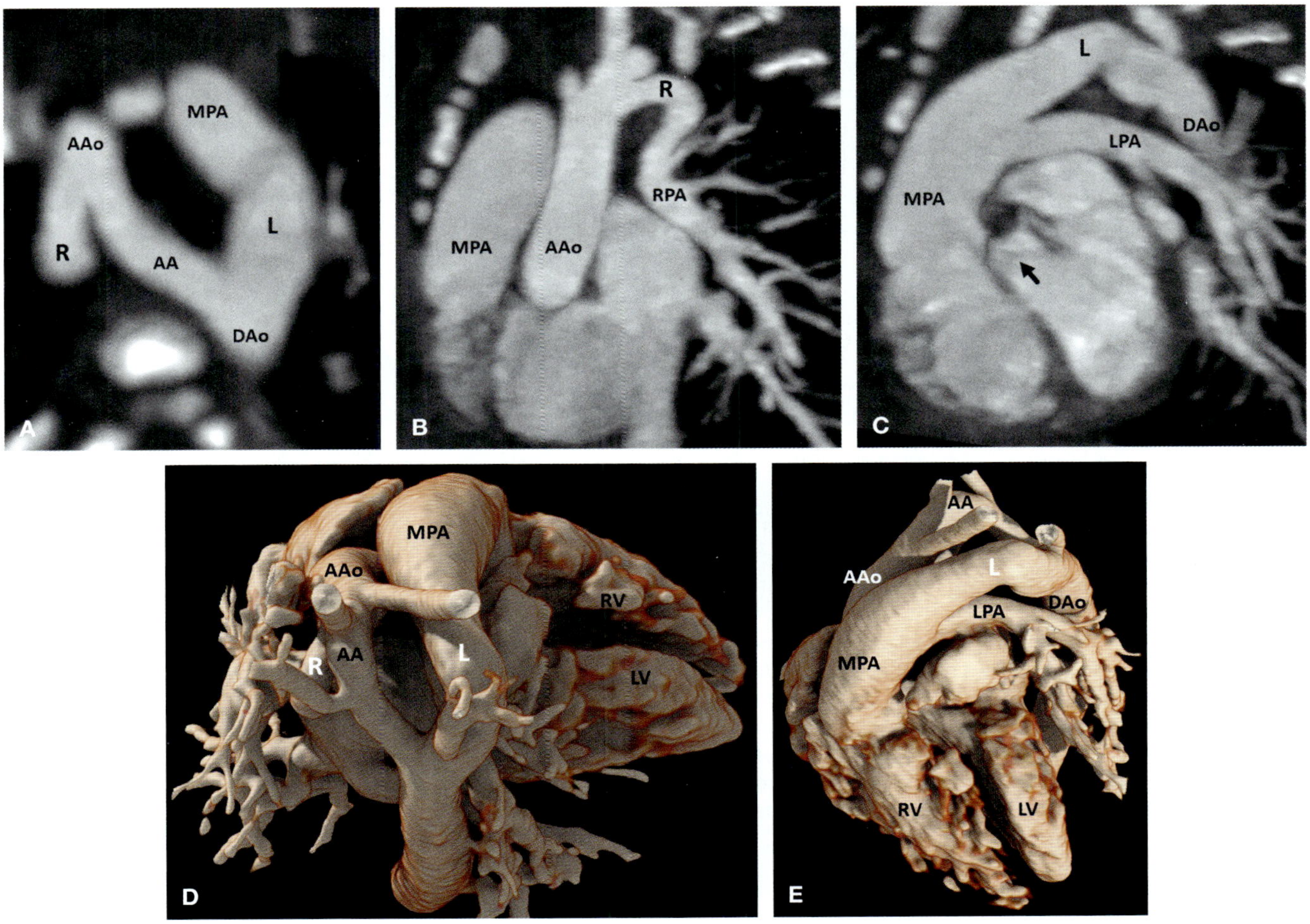

Figure 37.15. CTA complete vascular ring. **A:** Axial oblique maximum intensity projection (MIP) CCTA view of the complete vascular ring arterial segments; the ascending aorta (AAo), aortic arch (AA), main pulmonary artery (MPA), left patent ductus arteriosus (L), and proximal descending thoracic aorta (DAo). The right patent ductus arteriosus (R) arises from the underside of the AA and does not connect to the pulmonary artery. **B:** Sagittal oblique MIP CCTA view of the AAo. A right-sided patent ductus arteriosus (R) continues as the right pulmonary artery (RPA), which is isolated as the usual connection with the MPA is not present. **C:** Sagittal oblique MIP CCTA view shows the MPA and left patent ductus arteriosus (L), which continues as the DAo. The origin of the left pulmonary artery (LPA) is normal, and it shows the usual connection with the MPA. The aortic valve (arrow) is partially depicted. **D:** Cinematic rendered 3D reconstructed CCTA image of the complete vascular ring arterial segments; the AAo, AA, MPA, left patent ductus arteriosus (L), and proximal DAo. The right patent ductus arteriosus (R) origin is obscured, arising from the underside of the AA and, as seen in the 2D MIP image, does not connect to the pulmonary artery. **E:** Cinematic rendered 3D reconstructed CCTA image shows segments of the complete vascular ring, AAo, AA, MPA, and left patent ductus arteriosus (L), which continues as the DAo. The origin of the LPA is normal, and it shows the usual connection with the MPA.

- VSD, which serves as a "pop-off" for elevated RV pressure
- aortic valve overrides the VSD (overriding aorta) because the outlet septum is more anterior than normal

Most patients with are cyanotic at birth, a consequence of RVOT obstruction and right-to-left shunting of deoxygenated blood from the RV to the systemic circulation through the VSD. The severity of RVOT obstruction, ranging from complete atresia of the pulmonary valve to mild to severe main and branch pulmonary artery stenosis, dictates the severity of cyanosis. When RVOT or pulmonary artery stenosis is mild and the VSD is large, cyanosis may not be a presenting symptom of patients referred to as "pink TOF."

Pulmonary flow may be dependent on a PDA and/or on the presence of collateral pulmonary arterial blood supply from pleuroparenchymal and bronchial arteries and major aortopulmonary collaterals (MAPCAS). Associated anomalies include right aortic arch (approximately 25%),

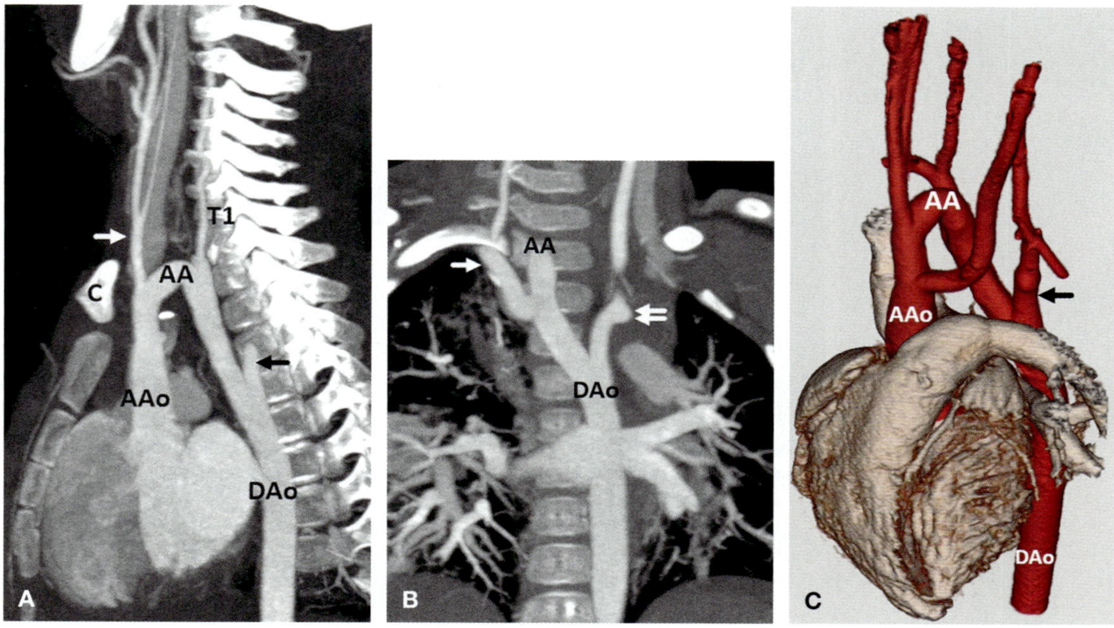

Figure 37.16. Persistent dysphagia to solids and long history of asthma. **A:** Sagittal oblique maximum intensity projection (MIP) CCTA image of the neck and chest shows a right aortic arch (AA) which is high in cephalad positions at T2-T3, just posterior to the clavicular head (C), a cervical aortic arch. Ascending aorta (AAo) and descending aorta (DAo) are shown. Origins of the right common carotid artery (white arrow) and the aberrant left subclavian (black arrow) are noted. **B:** Coronal oblique MIP CCTA image shows similar findings of a high right aortic arch (AA) and aberrant origin of the left subclavian artery (arrows) from the descending aorta (DAo). **C:** 3D surface rendered and colorized CCTA image of the neck and chest shows the AAo, right AA, which is more cephalad in position than normal, and the aberrant origin of the left subclavian artery (black arrow).

anomalous coronary artery origins and course (up to 10%), atrial septal defect (pentalogy of Fallot), anomalous pulmonary venous connections, and DORV.

Newborns and Infants

CCTA is an excellent imaging modality to provide anatomic details of TOF, in particular the degree and level of RV outflow and pulmonary artery atresia or stenosis, MAPCAS and other pulmonary artery collaterals (bronchial, subclavian, coronary), and coronary artery origins that may be anomalous in patients with TOF (up to 10%) (Fig. 37.24A and B). CT can provide important information related to the origin and course of the coronary arteries, side and diameter of the aortic root and thoracic aorta, and presence of a PDA (Fig. 37.25A-C and 37.26A-D).

Relief of RVOT, pulmonary valve or artery obstruction, and VSD closure is the primary goal of early surgical

Figure 37.17. Diverticulum of Kommerell from a right aortic arch, with aberrant left subclavian artery. **A:** Axial CCTA at the level of the aortic arch. The aortic arch is right sided (R). A diverticulum of Kommerell (bracket) is dorsal to the trachea (T) and the markedly narrowed esophageal lumen (white arrow). **B:** Coronal maximum intensity projection CCTA image of the distal right aortic arch (R) shows an aberrant left subclavian artery (double arrow) that arises from a diverticulum of Kommerell (bracket). A surgical clip is present at the site of a surgically occluded left ductus arteriosus (white arrow).

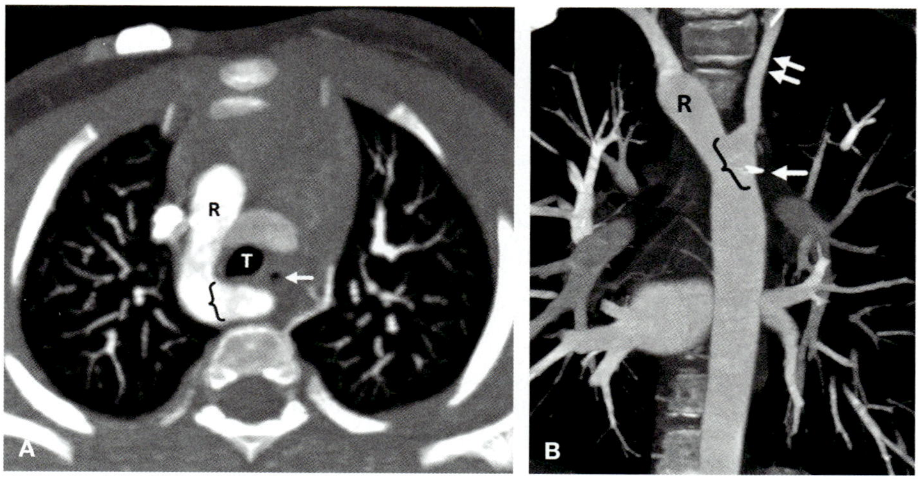

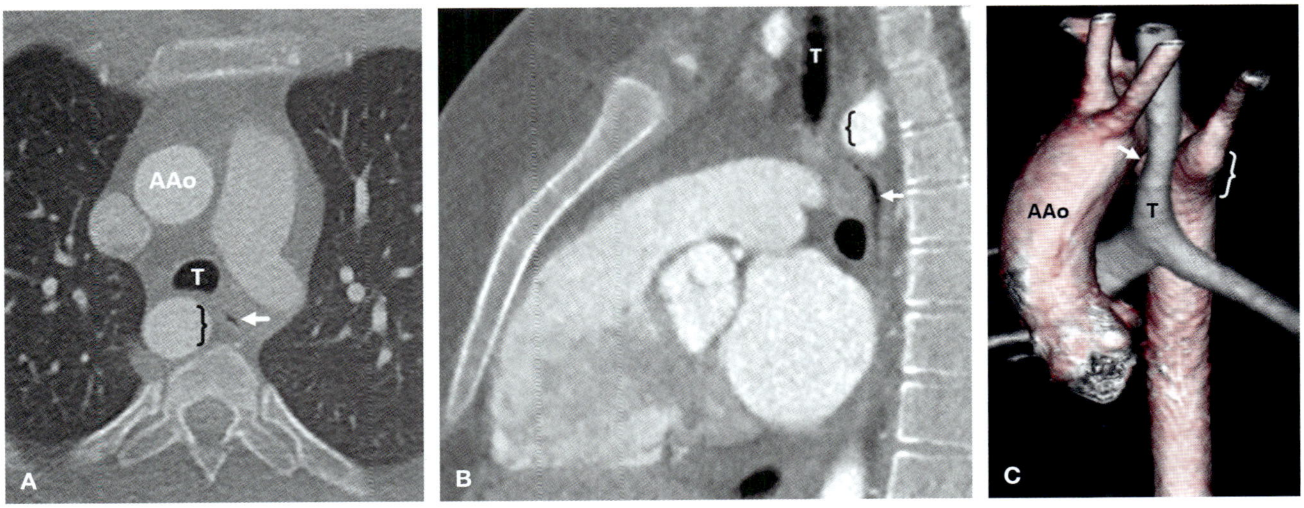

Figure 37.18. An adolescent patient with chronic respiratory problems, asthma, and dysphagia was found to have a right aortic arch and Kommerell diverticulum, which with a ductal ligament complete a vascular ring. **A:** Axial CCTA at the level of the Kommerell diverticulum (bracket) shows the esophageal lumen (white arrow) is markedly narrowed. The posterior surface of the trachea (T) is mildly flattened. **B:** Sagittal CCTA at the level of the Kommerell diverticulum (bracket) shows moderate extrinsic mass effect on the esophageal lumen (white arrow). **C:** 3D CCTA reconstruction of the aorta and trachea shows localized mild narrowing (white arrow) of the trachea (T) between the Kommerell diverticulum (bracket) and aortic arch.

palliation of TOF and depends on the native anatomy and is ideally performed as a single-staged procedure, transannular patch, in the first year of life, particularly in patients with mild RVOT or pulmonary artery stenosis. A transannular

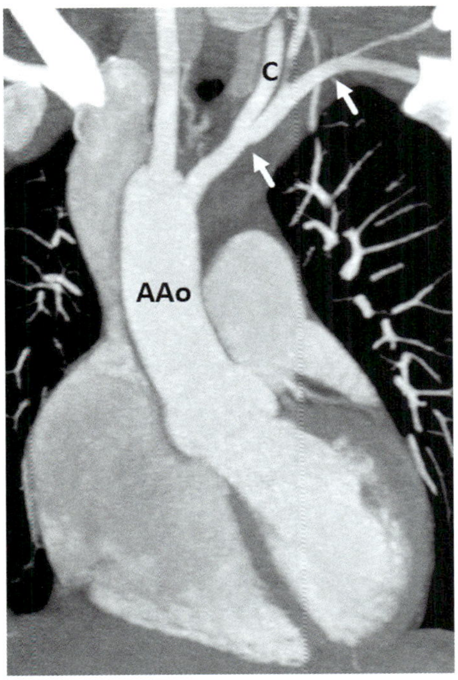

Figure 37.19. Postoperative appearance of right aortic arch with Kommerell diverticulum. Coronal CCTA of the heart and ascending aorta (AAo) shows the surgical change after the aberrant left subclavian artery (white arrow) has been reimplanted to the left common carotid artery (C).

patch of synthetic material or bovine pericardium is used to open the stenotic RV outflow and placed across the RVOT and pulmonic valve (Fig. 37.27). Multiple staged procedures may be required, particularly for patients with TOF with pulmonary atresia and multifocal and branch pulmonary artery stenosis, to ensure adequate pulmonary blood flow as the child grows. In these patients a palliative systemic-to-pulmonary Blalock-Taussig-Thomas shunt (BTTS) in the neonatal period may be performed as a first stage, in preparation for a later complete repair.

Children

Second-stage surgical intervention with takedown of the arterial pressure BTTS in favor of a venous pressure Glenn shunt or placement/replacement of an RV/PA conduit to supplement or increase pulmonary blood flow may be required as a child outgrows initial surgical palliation procedures (Fig. 37.28).

Adolescents and Adults

Early survival of TOF nears 98%, and patients with repaired TOF are known to survive into the seventh and eighth decades. Late complications are common, however, negatively impacting late survival of patients with repaired TOF, when compared with the general population. Throughout their lifetime, patients with TOF undergo surveillance imaging, and surgical and/or interventional cardiac catheterization procedures are common. Surveillance imaging beyond echocardiography is most often performed with

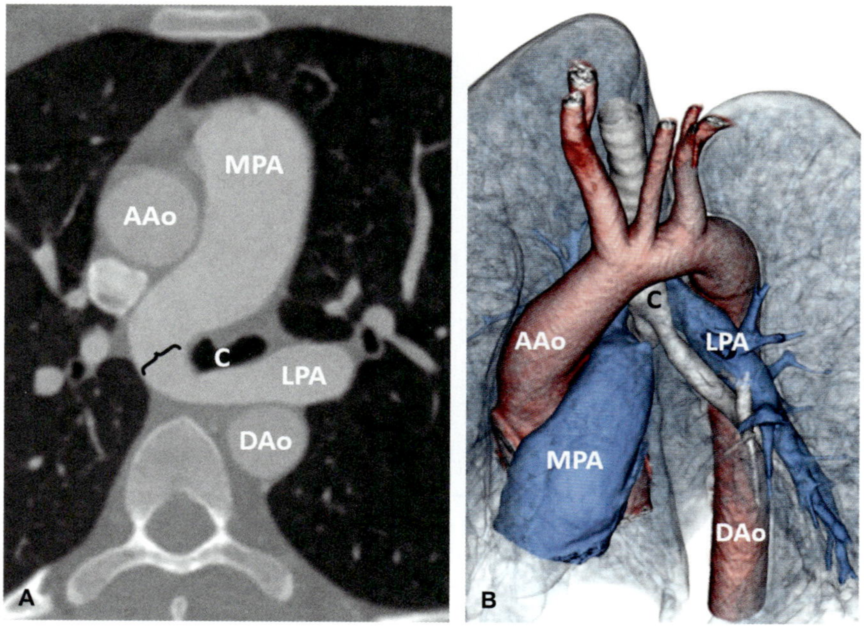

Figure 37.20. Left pulmonary artery (LPA) sling. **A:** Axial CCTA at the level of the carina shows the main pulmonary artery (MPA) in normal position to the left and slightly anterior to the ascending aorta (AAo). The LPA origin (bracket) is from the right pulmonary artery, and the vessel courses around the distal trachea, flattening the posterior surface of the carina (C) and anterior to the descending aorta (DAo). **B:** 3D colorized reconstruction CCTA image shows the MPA in normal position to the left and slightly anterior to the AAo. The LPA origin is obscured, the course of the LPA is behind the distal trachea and carina (C) and anterior to the DAo.

MRI. CCTA is an important contributor to imaging particularly in patients who have pulmonary artery or conduit stents and calcifications, when MRI is contraindicated or degraded by presence of pacemaker/defibrillator devices or extensive surgical material, or for planning for percutaneous pulmonary valve prosthesis procedures (Fig. 37.29A-D).

Patients with TOF who have undergone transannular patch or have had RV/PA conduits (without or with a valve) constructed to provide adequate pulmonary arterial blood flow may have withstood long-term pulmonary insufficiency, which leads to eventual RV dilation. As adolescents and adults, many patients with TOF will have undergone multiple surgeries requiring median sternotomy, which

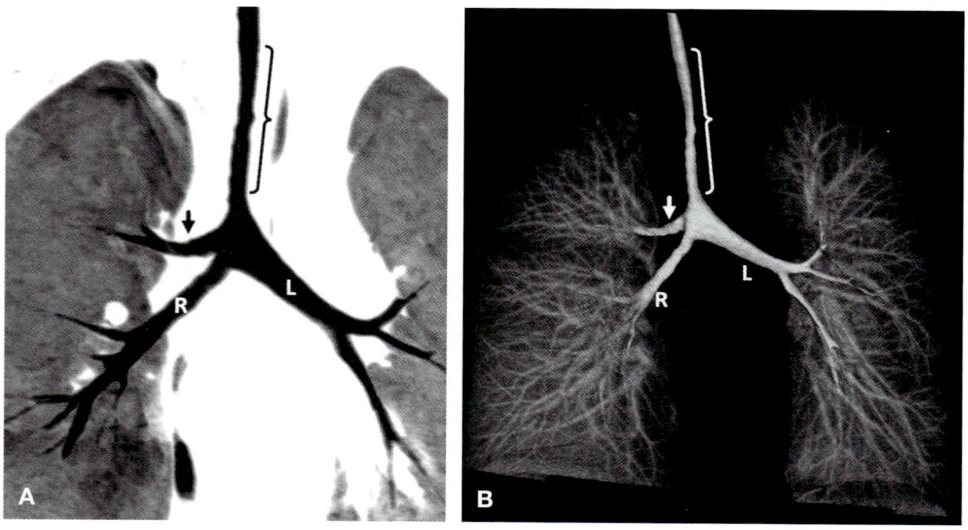

Figure 37.21. Complete tracheal rings. **A:** A coronal oblique minimum intensity projection image of the trachea shows diffuse narrowing of the mid to distal trachea (bracket). The proximal branch of the right main bronchus is a variant of normal, a pre-eparterial bronchus (black arrow) to the right upper lobe. The right bronchus intermedius (R) and left main bronchus (L) are normal caliber. **B:** A 3D reconstructed CT image of the trachea confirms diffuse narrowing of the trachea (bracket). The proximal branch of the right main bronchus is a variant of normal, a pre-eparterial bronchus (white arrow) to the right upper lobe. The right bronchus intermedius (R) and left main bronchus (L) are normal caliber.

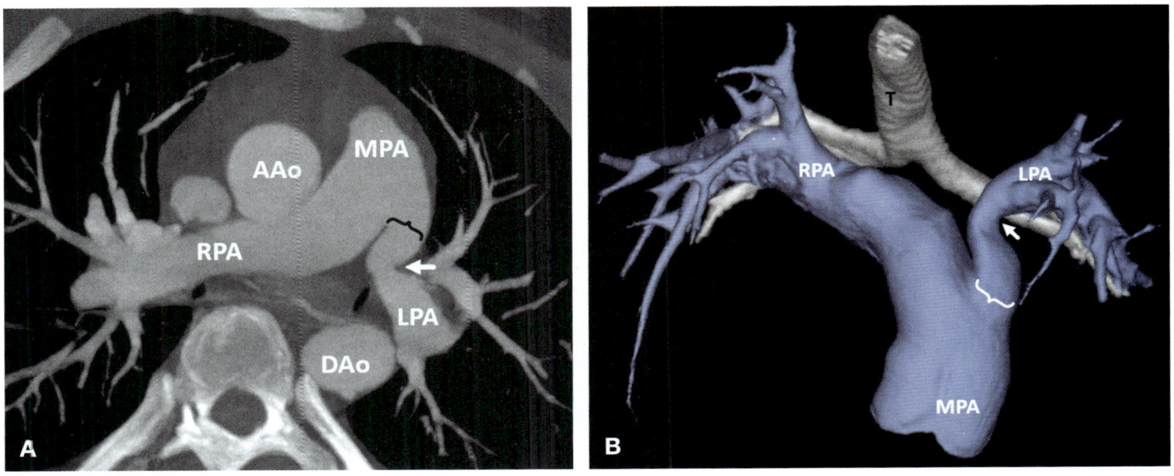

Figure 37.22. CTA post pulmonary sling repair. The patient in Figure 37.20 underwent reimplantation (bracket) of the left pulmonary artery (LPA) to the left side of the main pulmonary artery (MPA). **A:** Axial CCTA of the chest shows mild kinking (arrow) and diffuse mild narrowing of the LPA. **B:** 3D colorized CCTA reconstruction of the pulmonary arteries and the trachea shows the mild kinking of the LPA (arrow) and diffuse narrowing of the vessel.

makes continued surgical interventions less and less desirable for the cardiothoracic surgeon, especially if the patient has previously suffered surgical complications such as infection/mediastinitis. For this reason, percutaneous, transcatheter pulmonary valve insertion is a favored option for many patients with TOF. CCTA is used to assess RVOT and pulmonary artery anatomy and to produce precise measurements of the pulmonary artery and the intended implantation site, information that guides appropriateness and specifics of device selection (Fig. 37.30).

As the RV dilates secondary to long-standing pulmonary insufficiency it is important to assess ventricular function, remodeling of the RV, and signs of ventricular failure. Although most often examined using MRI for the highest degree of accuracy and reproducibility, when necessary, an estimation of RV and LV function can be made using CCTA (Fig. 37.31).

Additional abnormalities that can negatively influence the clinical course of patients with TOF include RVOT and pulmonary valve stenosis, severe branch pulmonary artery

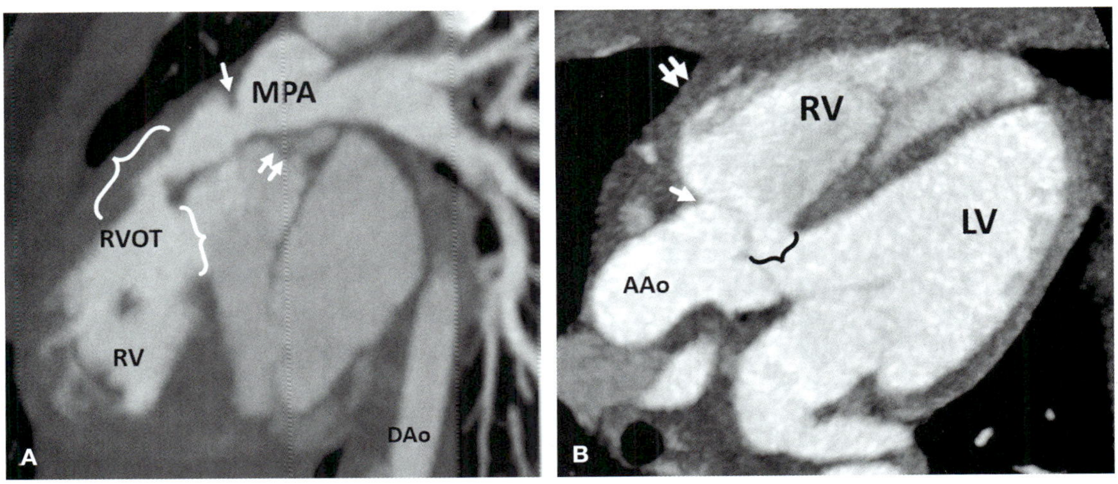

Figure 37.23. Newborn with tetralogy of Fallot. **A:** Sagittal oblique maximum intensity projection (MIP) CCTA image of the right ventricular outflow tract (RVOT) shows stenosis of the outflow tract (white bracket) and the pulmonary valve (white arrow). The ventricular septal defect (smaller bracket) underlies the partially visualized aortic valve (white double arrows). **B:** Axial oblique MIP CCTA image of the ventricles shows the aortic valve (white arrow) overrides the small ventricular septal defect (bracket). The right ventricle (RV) myocardium shows mild hypertrophy (white double arrows).

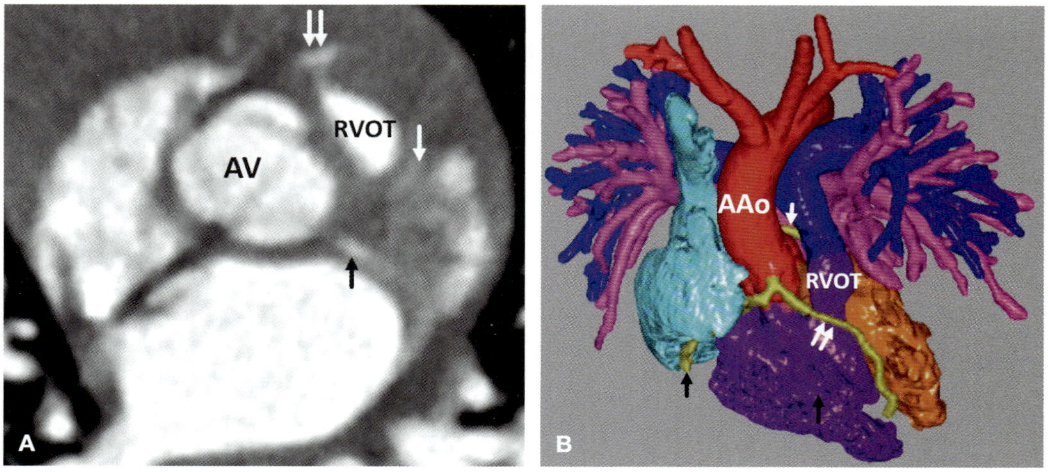

Figure 37.24. Newborn with tetralogy of Fallot with coronary artery anomaly. **A:** Axial oblique maximum intensity projection CCTA image of the aortic valve (AV) just below the level of the coronary artery origins shows the proximal segments of dual left anterior descending coronary arteries leftward (white arrow) of the stenotic right ventricular outflow tract (RVOT) and a larger-caliber artery anterior to the MPA (white double arrows). The left circumflex coronary artery is in normal position in the left atrioventricular groove (black arrow). **B:** 3D colorized reconstruction of CCTA image of the heart shows anomalous origin of a left anterior descending (LAD) coronary artery origin from the right sinus of Valsalva, courses anterior to the right ventricular outflow tract (RVOT) to the anterior interventricular groove (white double arrows). The left main coronary artery (white arrow) branches to a small-caliber LAD and left circumflex coronary are hidden from view. The right coronary artery is in normal position in the right atrioventricular groove (black arrow).

stenosis, RVOT aneurysm, tricuspid regurgitation, residual VSD, left ventricular dysfunction, dilatation of the aortic root, and aortic valve regurgitation (Fig. 37.32A-D).

Double Outlet Right Ventricle

DORV represents a complex CHD in which both great vessels, the aorta and MPA, arise entirely or predominantly from the RV, secondary to abnormal development of the conus. In DORV, the valve of one great artery and more than half of the circumference of the other semilunar valve annulus, the so-called 150% rule, originates from the morphologic RV (Fig. 37.33).

The discordant ventriculoarterial alignment of the semilunar valves and great arteries is variable in patients with DORV. The semilunar valves and great artery origins may be in normal position (the aortic valve posterior and inferior and to the right of the pulmonary valve), side by side (the aortic valve directly to the right of the pulmonic valve at near the same level), or malposed position (dextroposed, with the aortic valve lying directly anterior and rightward of the pulmonary valve, or levoposed with the aortic valve positioned anterior or posterior and to the left of the pulmonary valve). Pulmonary stenosis (PS) is another common feature of DORV, present in approximately 75% of cases.

A VSD is almost always present in DORV and is categorized based on its location in relation to the semilunar valves, in order of prevalence:

- Subaortic VSD: the outlet septum is fused to the left margin of the VSD (Fig. 37.34)
- Subpulmonic VSD: the outlet septum is fused to the right margin of the VSD (Fig. 37.35A and B)
- Noncommitted or remote VSD: the distance between the VSD and the semilunar valves is more than the diameter of the aortic valve (Fig. 37.36A and B)
- Doubly committed VSD: the VSD is related to both semilunar valves and the infundibulum is absent (Fig. 37.37A and B)

The anatomic spectrum of DORV is enormously diverse; based on the relationship of the VSD to the semilunar valves, abnormalities of atrial arrangement, atrioventricular connection, ventricular morphology, and PS, patients with DORV are categorized into four anatomical-physiological variants that hemodynamically mimic other forms of CHD, in order of decreasing frequency:

- VSD type: DORV with a subaortic VSD, without PS (Fig. 37.38A-C)
- TOF: DORV with a subaortic VSD, with PS (Fig. 37.39A-C)

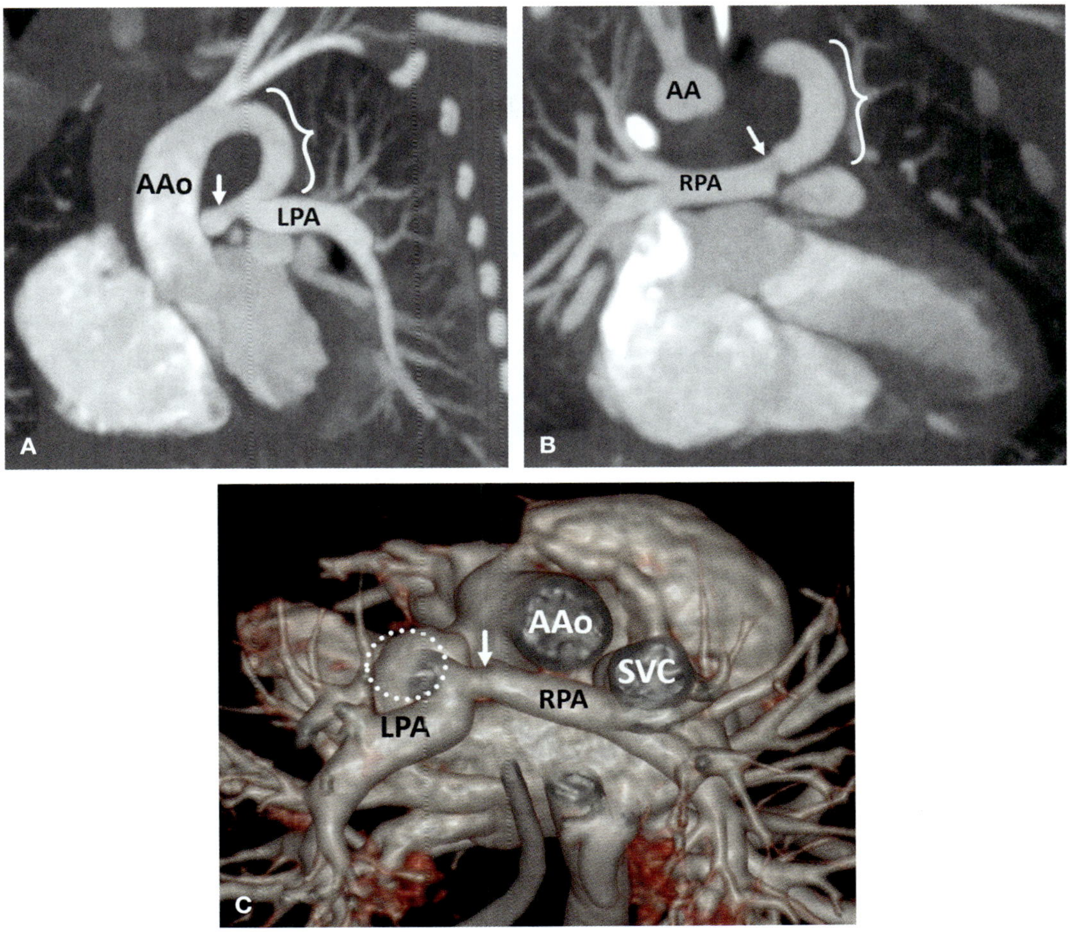

Figure 37.25. Newborn with tetralogy of Fallot with pulmonary valve atresia and ductal dependent pulmonary artery circulation. **A:** Sagittal oblique maximum intensity projection (MIP) CCTA image of the ascending aorta (AAo) and the patent ductus arteriosus (bracket). The branch left (LPA) and right (white arrow) pulmonary arteries arise from the ductus rather than from the main pulmonary artery, which was absent in this baby with pulmonary valve atresia. **B:** Sagittal oblique MIP CCTA image of the patent ductus arteriosus (bracket) and branch right pulmonary artery (RPA) shows mild stenosis at the origin (white arrow). **C:** 3D colorized reconstruction of CCTA from the superior perspective shows the right (RPA) and left (LPA) branch pulmonary arteries and mild stenosis at the RPA origin (white arrow). The position of the AAo and superior vena cava (SVC) are as expected. The pulmonary valve and main pulmonary artery are absent (dotted ellipse).

- TGA: DORV with a subpulmonic VSD, without PS
  - commonly called Taussig-Bing anomaly (Fig. 37.40A-C)
- functional single ventricle type: DORV with mitral valve atresia, unbalanced atrioventricular septal defect, or hypoplasia of one ventricle (Fig. 37.41A-C)

Newborns and Infants

The goal of imaging newborns with DORV is to provide detailed anatomy of the VSD including the spatial relationship between the VSD, the semilunar valves, and the tricuspid annulus and its septal leaflet; qualitative and relative size of ventricle size; and extracardiac anatomy, all of which are essential diagnostic information for determining an optimal surgical strategy. Echocardiogram may not adequately show the relationship between VSD and the great arteries or may be limited by acoustic window. The multiplanar reconstruction capabilities of CCTA images are useful to accurately depict the anatomic features of the VSD and its relationship to the semilunar valves. A muscular VSD is also often present in DORV; CCTA acquired in the diastolic phase is best for the most accurate depiction of muscular VSD.

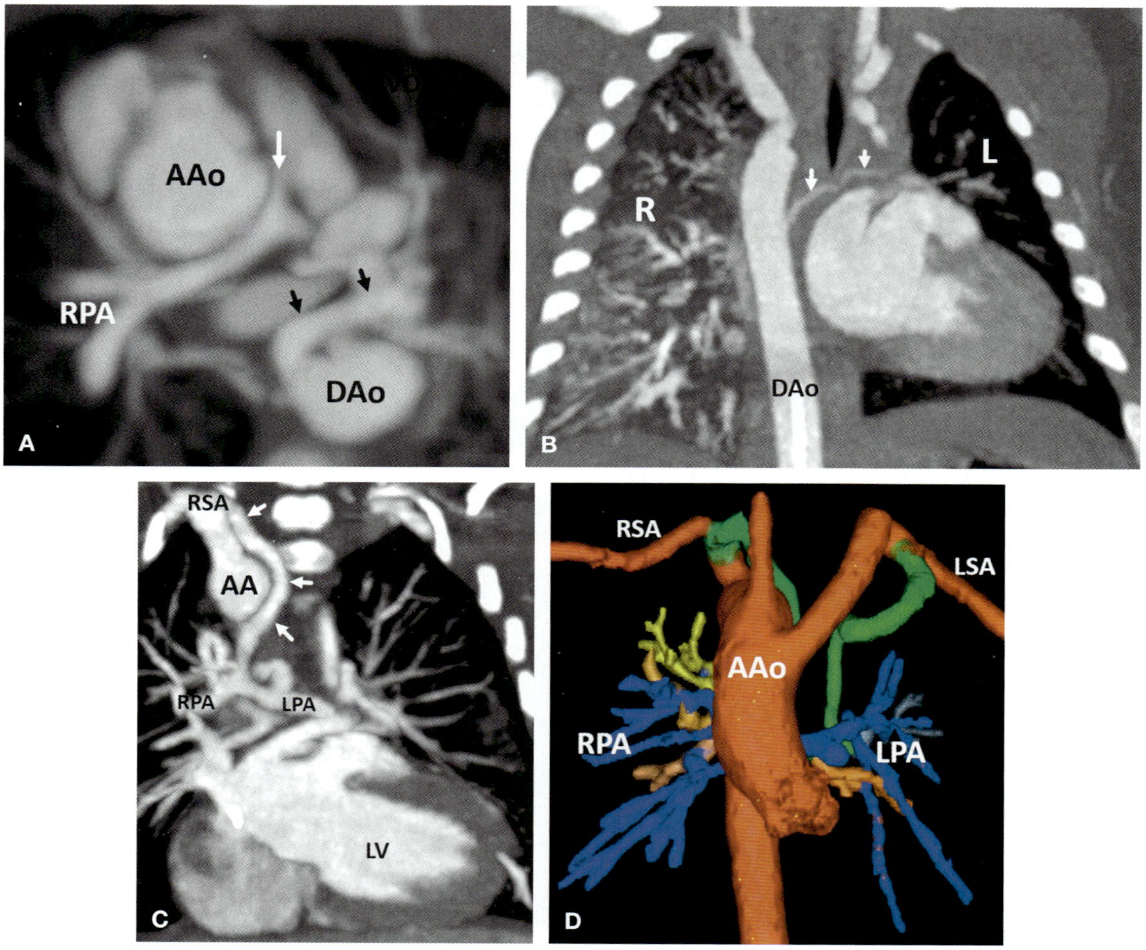

Figure 37.26. Newborn with tetralogy of Fallot with pulmonary artery atresia and major aortopulmonary artery collaterals (MAPCAs) to the left lung. **A:** Axial oblique maximum intensity projection (MIP) CCTA image at the level of the branch pulmonary arteries shows a beak-like shape of the distal main pulmonary artery (white arrow) and a small-caliber right pulmonary artery (RPA). The left pulmonary artery (LPA) was absent; the left lung arterial supply is from multiple MAPCAs arising from the descending aorta (DAo) (black arrows). **B:** Coronal MIP CCTA image of the chest shows the DAo and one of several MAPCAs (white arrow) extending leftward. The patent RPA is not seen in the plane of this image. Notice the asymmetry of the pulmonary vasculature between the right (R) and left (L) lungs. **C:** Coronal MIP CCTA image of the chest shows the aortic arch (AA) and a large-caliber collateral artery (white arrows) arising from the right subclavian artery (RSA) supplies secondary branches of the RPA and LPA pulmonary arteries. **D:** 3D colorized reconstruction of CCTA image of the heart shows the ascending aortic (AAo) and large-caliber collateral arteries (green colorized vessels) arising from the right (RSA) and left (LSA) subclavian arteries, which supply secondary branches of the RPA and LPA.

A precise understanding of the VSD and intracardiac and semilunar valve anatomy is critical, as the anatomy shown with CCTA directs the surgical approach:

- Subaortic: intraventricular tunnel diverts blood from the VSD to the aorta (Fig. 37.42)
- Subpulmonic: arterial switch operation and aorta to ventricular tunnel (Fig. 37.43)
- Noncommitted: an intraventricular baffle is constructed (Fig. 37.44)
- Doubly committed VSD: intraventricular tunnel diverts blood from the VSD to the aorta (Fig. 37.45)
- Pulmonic stenosis: a conduit may be constructed to direct blood flow to the branch pulmonary arteries (Fig. 37.46)

CT imaging is also helpful in simultaneous assessment of various anomalies associated with DORV (ie, atrioventricular valve stenosis and atresia, supravalvar or infundibular PS, complete AV canal defect, anomalies of pulmonary venous drainage, coronary artery anomalies, and aortic arch anomalies) (Fig. 37.47A and B).

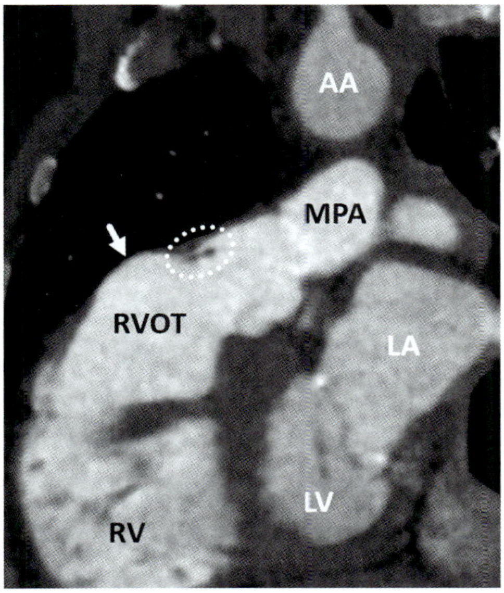

Figure 37.27. Adult with tetralogy of Fallot, status post transannular patch palliation of right ventricular outflow tract (RVOT) stenosis, as an infant. 2D sagittal oblique view of the RVOT at end diastole shows localized outpouching (white arrow) of the surgical site due to presence of a transannular patch used to relieve RVOT stenosis. The pulmonary valve leaflets are at least partially seen (white ellipse) but may be completely absent in other patients, depending upon the native anatomy. The pulmonary valve insufficiency results, allowing free pulmonary valve regurgitation. The patch material is typically bovine pericardium or other synthetic material that does not contract and expand like myocardial muscle.

Children, Adolescents, and Adults

CCTA is used to assess both palliative and corrective postoperative anatomy and surgical complications in patients with DORV. Postoperative complications related to a VSD closure in patients with DORV include residual VSD; intraventricular tunnel stenosis, leak, or aneurysm; conduit calcification, stenosis, or thrombosis; and complications in outflow tracts (RVOT obstruction, left ventricular outflow tract [LVOT] obstruction), pulmonary arteries (stenosis, aneurysm), and aorta (coarctation and recoarctation) (Fig. 37.48A-F).

Transposition of the Great Arteries

TGA describes the conotruncal abnormality with ventriculoarterial discordance, the aorta from the RV and the pulmonary artery from the LV. TGA occurs in two types, depending on the relative positions of the aortic and pulmonary valves.

- D-loop transposition of the great arteries (D-TGA) (Fig. 37.49A and B)
  - Atrioventricular relationships are normal (concordance)
  - Ventriculoarterial relationships are abnormal (discordance)

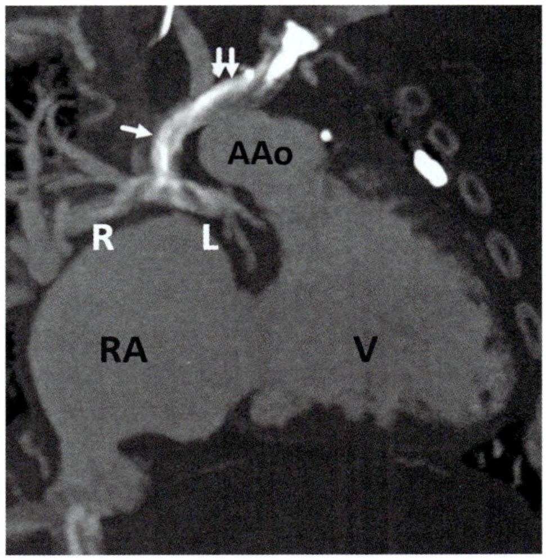

Figure 37.28. Child with tetralogy of Fallot and single ventricle physiology. Coronal oblique maximum intensity projection CCTA image of the Glenn shunt (white arrow); receives contrast injected via the left upper extremity to the left brachiocephalic vein (double arrow) and drains to the right (R) and left (L) confluent branch pulmonary arteries.

  - D-looping of the cardiac tube is normal, the RV is to the right of the LV
  - Often termed "complete" TGA. This terminology is nondescriptive and is not relevant.
- L-loop transposition of the great arteries (L-TGA) (Fig. 37.50A and B)
  - Atrioventricular relationships are abnormal (discordance)
  - Ventriculoarterial relationships are abnormal (discordance)
  - L-looping of the cardiac tube is abnormal, the RV is to the left of the LV
  - Often termed "corrected" TGA—is misleading in that it seems to imply that surgical palliation is not required. This terminology and implication are not correct!

D-TGA is more common (7% of cyanotic CHD) than L-TGA, which is very rare (less than 1% of all CHD). The key identifying relationship for diagnosis on CCTA is the relative position of the aortic and pulmonary valves. Normally the aortic valve is posterior to and rightward of the pulmonary valve on an axial image. In patients with D-TGA the aortic valve is anterior to and rightward of the pulmonary valve. In patients with L-TGA the aortic valve is anterior to and leftward of the pulmonary valve. The relative position of the aortic and pulmonary valves in TGA is quite variable, ranging from nearly side by side in the form of TGA in which both semilunar valves arise from the RV (DORV) to a direct anterior-posterior relationship of the valves.

Approximately 60% of patients with TGA have an intact intraventricular septum; 40% have VSDs (perimembranous type or muscular type) or more complex (malalignment type with associated outflow tract obstruction, doubly

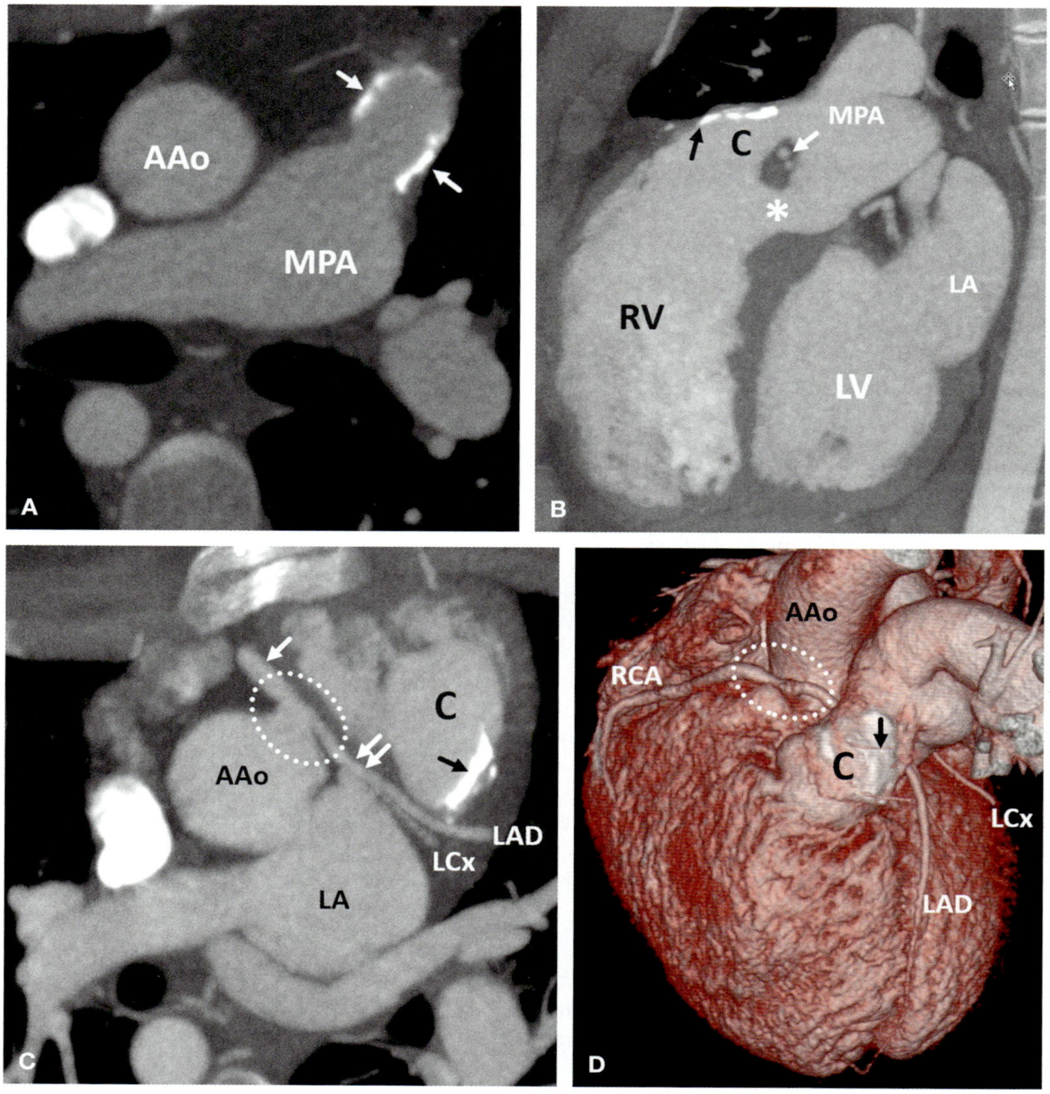

Figure 37.29. **A:** Adult with tetralogy of Fallot (TOF) with previous right ventricular outflow tract (RVOT) reconstruction using a right ventricle (RV) to main pulmonary artery (MPA) conduit. Axial CCTA image at the level of the MPA shows extensive calcification of the distal RV to pulmonary artery (PA) conduit (white arrows) as it joins the MPA. **B:** Different adult with TOF and anomalous coronary artery origin with history of RV to MPA conduit as a child. Sagittal oblique maximum intensity projection (MIP) CCTA image shows the RV to MPA conduit (C) and the stenotic native RVOT (asterisk) encircling the proximal course of the left anterior descending (LAD) and the smaller-caliber left circumflex (LCx) coronary artery (white arrow). The RV to PA conduit is partially calcified (black arrow). **C:** Axial oblique MIP CCTA image shows the common origin (dotted circle) of the left main (white double arrow) and right (white arrow) coronary arteries from the right sinus of Valsalva. The anomalous proximal course of the LAD and LCx coronary arteries is seen between the RV to pulmonary artery conduit (C) and the left atrium (LA). A segment of the conduit is calcified (black arrow). **D:** 3D surface rendered CCTA image shows the common origin (dotted circle) of the left main and right coronary arteries from the right sinus of Valsalva. The distal course of the LAD and LCx coronary arteries is normal. A segment of the RV to MPA conduit (C) is calcified (black arrow).

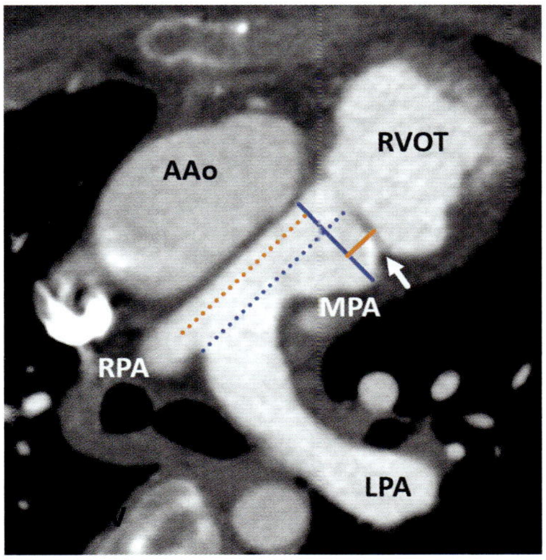

Figure 37.30. Adult with tetralogy of Fallot status post transannular patch as a neonate and long-standing free pulmonary insufficiency is now undergoing evaluation for percutaneous pulmonary valve replacement. Axial oblique CCTA image is optimized to show the long axis of the right ventricular outflow tract (RVOT), the native pulmonary valve plane (white arrow), and main pulmonary artery (MPA) to the origins of the right (RPA) and left (LPA) branch pulmonary arteries. Notice the following required measurements: widest width of the MPA sinuses (solid blue line); distance from the widest width of the MPA sinuses to the native pulmonary valve plane (solid orange line); middle of the native pulmonary valve plane to the distal division of the MPA to the branch pulmonary arteries (blue dotted line); distance from the widest plane of the MPA sinuses to the distal division of the MPA to the branch pulmonary arteries (dotted orange line).

committed sub-arterial type, or inlet type). The type of VSD often dictates the surgical options required to palliate TGA: an arterial switch operation (ASO) that necessitates reimplantation of coronary artery origins, VSD closure, baffle of the LV blood flow through the VSD to the native aortic valve, or RV/PA conduit construction when PS is an accompanying feature. Coronary artery abnormalities are present in up to 33% and can be a determinant of long-term prognosis.

Newborns, Infants, and Children

CCTA is a useful imaging technique to complement echocardiography findings in newborns, especially for evaluation of PS and confirmation of great artery anatomy and coronary artery origin anatomy (Fig. 37.51A-C). In patients with atypical VSD anatomy the multiplanar and 3D postprocessing techniques applied to CCTA image datasets is helpful in guiding surgical approach to closure.

In patients with D-TGA the favored first surgical palliation procedures include an ASO in which the AAo and MPA are transected and their position is switched to reside above the correct ventricular chamber. The coronary arteries are removed from their original position and reimplanted into the neoaortic valve position. If present, the VSD is closed with patch material.

In patients with D-TGA with posterior malalignment of the conus the interventricular septum is displaced posteriorly, resulting in subpulmonary outflow tract obstruction and VSD. Most patients with posterior malalignment VSDs have hypoplastic pulmonary valves with thickened leaflets and subpulmonary narrowing. The typical operation performed in this setting is the Rastelli procedure in which a tunnel is created from the LV through the VSD, directing blood from the LV to the aorta. A conduit from the free wall of the RV to the pulmonary artery completes the procedure. The pulmonary artery conduit typically becomes stenotic and will require periodic replacement (Fig. 37.52).

For patients with L-TGA a double switch procedure is the favored palliative surgical approach, but it is not likely to be performed in the newborn period as patients are usually not cyanotic and unless there are associated abnormalities VSD (80%), PS (40%-50%), LVOT obstruction (30%), Ebstein anomaly (30%), situs inversus, dextrocardia, complete heart block, and reentrant tachycardias, patients may not be discovered to have L-TGA until the fifth or sixth decade of life. A double switch is an ASO and an atrial level switch using the Senning or Mustard technique to baffle pulmonary venous return to the left atrium and systemic venous return to the right atrium (Fig. 37.53).

After Rastelli procedure, stenosis of the RV-PA conduit is the main complication that may require a reintervention in the first decade of life. Calcification, kinking, aneurysm, and conduit (pulmonary) regurgitation may also be seen. Obstruction, stenosis, leakage, or aneurysm may also develop in the aortic baffle.

Adolescents and Adults

CCTA is useful for follow-up and surveillance of palliation of PS, intracardiac conduits and baffles (stenosis, leak, thrombosis), residual or recurrent VSD, and coronary artery origin anatomy, mapping of collateral vessels, and planning for transcatheter procedures and interventions such as valve replacement and pulmonary artery stenting.

After ASO the native aortic valve remains the outflow from the RV and the native pulmonic valve remains the outflow from the LV, albeit to the appropriate great artery. Surveillance imaging of the "root" of the native pulmonic valve is important as the native pulmonic tissue often becomes dilated in the face of systemic arterial pressures. The valve annulus may also dilate, resulting in semilunar valve insufficiency. Reimplanted coronary arteries in the neoaortic valve are of interest on follow-up CCTA as stenosis at the surgical site is a known complication.

The ASO palliation may be performed using a technique described by LeCompte, in which the MPA is anterior and the branch pulmonary arteries are draped over the AAo, a

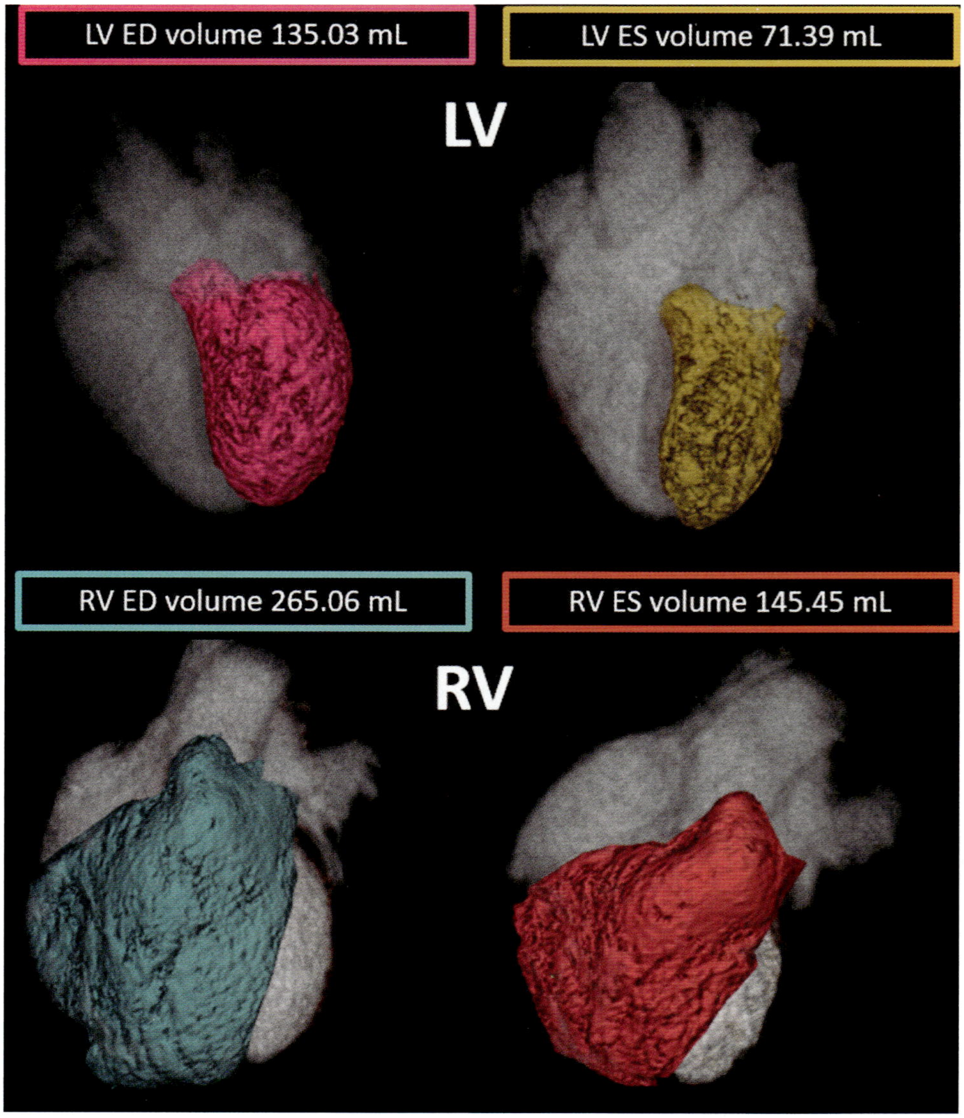

Figure 37.31. Adult with tetralogy of Fallot. Retrospectively ECG-gated CCTA enables acquisition of imaging data throughout the R-R interval. The temporal resolution, dependent on dividing that image data into distinct phases of the cardiac cycle, is typically limited to 10 phases per heart beat, lower than the temporal resolution of magnetic resonance imaging (MRI). However, when patients with contraindications to MRI, including pacemakers, defibrillators, or surgical materials that produce artifact obscuring anatomy, are examined with CCTA, a reasonably accurate estimation of ventricular volume and function may be made. 3D segmented CCTA images at end systole (ES) and end diastole (ED) are colorized to indicate the right (RV) and left (LV) ventricles. The ventricular volume, stroke volume, and ejection fracture may be calculated using CCTA data.

maneuver used to avoid distortion of the branch pulmonary arteries in the process of switching the great vessels (Fig. 37.54A-C).

Legacy procedures such as atrial level switch, described nearly simultaneously by Mustard and Senning, use pericardial tissue or native atrial tissue, respectively, to construct baffles to redirect blood flow toward the anatomically correct atrioventricular valve and ventricle (Fig. 37.55). This palliative procedure is usually seen only in adults with corrected D-TGA, as it is more technically difficult than ASO and is not physiologically effective. Atrial switch surgical anatomy is commonly seen in patients of all ages with L-TGA as a double switch palliation approach is required, an atrial level switch and ASO, to make blood flow patterns physiologic. Recognition of the anatomy and the common postsurgical complications, related to baffle leak or obstruction, is important.

CT is typically performed for evaluation of indeterminate coronary arterial anatomy at echocardiography. CT is also useful for the assessment of the coronary arteries, mapping of collateral vessels, and preprocedural planning for transcatheter interventions such as valve replacement and pulmonary stenting (Fig. 37.52b).

Truncus Arteriosus

TA is a congenital cardiac anomaly that occurs when the conotruncus, a common vascular trunk that develops into the aorta and the MPA, and coronary artery origins fail to divide normally and has a reported incidence of 2%. TA may be associated with additional anomalies of the great arteries

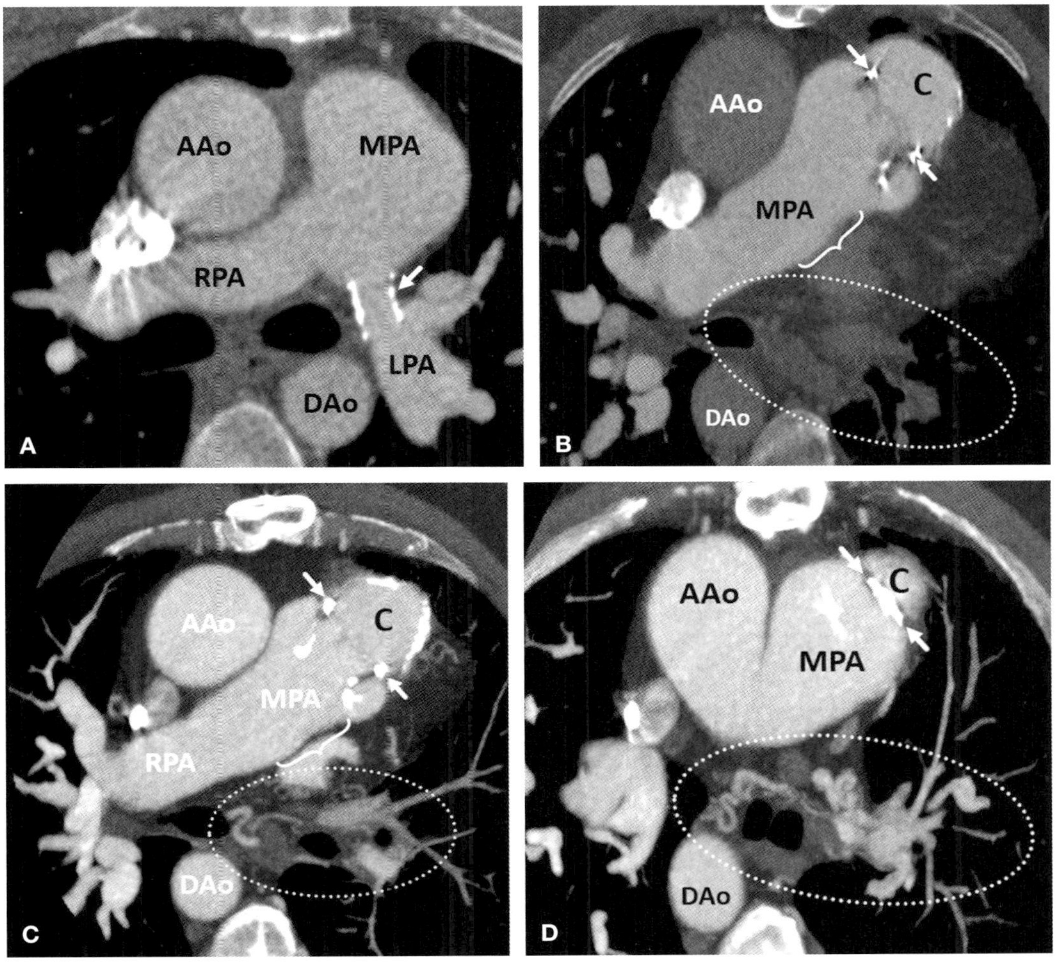

Figure 37.32. Posttreatment appearance of tetralogy of Fallot (TOF). **A:** Adult with TOF and history of left pulmonary artery stent to treat focal stenosis. Axial CCTA image at the level of the branch pulmonary arteries shows a hyperdense stent (white arrow) in the proximal left pulmonary artery (LPA). The main (MPA) and right (RPA) pulmonary arteries are normal caliber. **B:** Adult with TOF, right aortic arch, and right ventricle (RV) to pulmonary artery (PA) conduit (C) with a prosthetic valve. Axial maximum intensity projection (MIP) CCTA shows the proximal LPA (bracket) is absent and the distal LPA does not enhance in the early phase (dotted ellipse). **C:** Axial MIP CCTA image for the same patient shows the valve ring of the prosthetic valve (white arrows) between the partially calcified RV/PA conduit (C). The origin of the LPA is not seen (bracket). The distal LPA branches (dotted ellipse) enhance on the later phase, reconstituted by collaterals. **D:** Axial MIP CCTA at a higher level shows multiple collateral vessels to the distal LPA (dotted ellipse). The prosthetic valve is partially visualized (arrows).

and intracardiac defects and is associated with genetic syndromes in the spectrum of 22q11 deletion syndrome. Van Praagh described the most often used classification system, but this may not completely describe all variations:

- Type A—With associated VSD
  - Type A1—Incompletely formed aortopulmonary septum—partial separation of the MPA from the AAo (Fig. 37.56A and B)
  - Type A2—Absent aortopulmonary septum—solitary aortic trunk, right and left branch pulmonary arteries arise directly from the ascending truncus, no discrete MPA (Fig. 37.57)
  - Type A3—Absent aortopulmonary septum—solitary branch pulmonary artery branch—descending aortopulmonary collaterals supply the contralateral lung (Fig. 37.58A and B)
  - Type A4—Absent aortopulmonary septum—underdeveloped aortic arch (interruption, atresia, coarctation, or severe hypoplasia) (Fig. 37.59A-C)
- Type B—intact ventricular septum (VSD), is extremely rare

Echocardiography is the first imaging study, diagnostic even during fetal life, although there may be limitations in complete diagnosis. Definitive diagnosis of the TA vascular

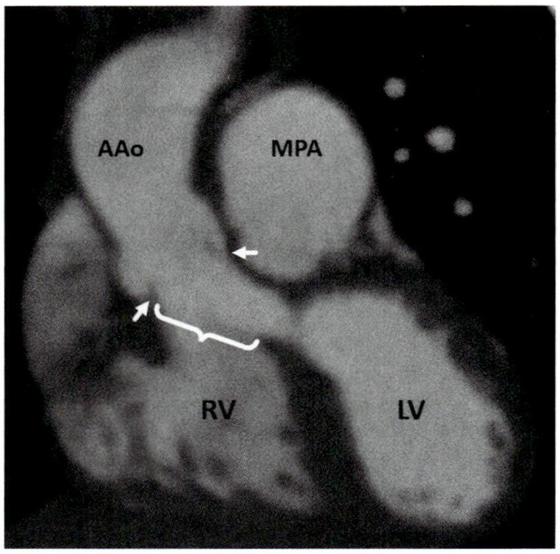

Figure 37.33. Infant with double outlet right ventricle (DORV). Coronal oblique CCTA view of the left ventricular outflow tract shows that more than 50% of the aortic semilunar valve annulus (white arrows) originates from the right ventricle (RV), satisfying the 150% rule of DORV. The ventricular septal defect (bracket) is the subaortic type.

abnormalities and intracardiac defects is most accurately revealed using cross-sectional imaging techniques such as CCTA, with high spatial resolution definition of anatomic detail in newborns with high heart rates, children in whom postsurgical evaluation is needed, and patients for whom long-term surveillance imaging is required. CCTA enables 2D multiplanar and 3D volumetric image reconstruction, which aids in guidance for surgical management.

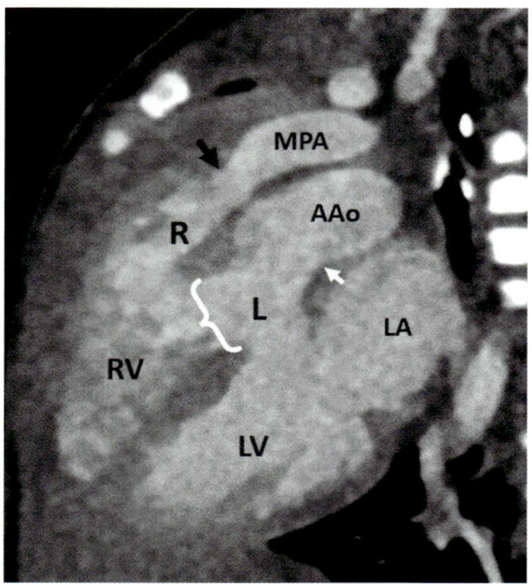

Figure 37.34. Infant with double outlet right ventricle (DORV). Sagittal oblique CCTA view of the right (R) and left (L) ventricular outflow tracts shows that more than 50% of the aortic semilunar valve annulus (white arrow) originates from the right ventricle (RV), satisfying the 150% rule of DORV. The aortic valve overrides the ventricular septal defect (bracket). The pulmonic semilunar valve (black arrow) arises solely from the right ventricle.

Newborns

Truncus arteriosus is ideally repaired in the neonatal period with low morbidity and mortality. Definition of the anatomy of the conotruncus, intraventricular septum, and the caliber of the branch pulmonary arteries is crucial for planning and prospectively anticipating postoperative complications.

Goals of the initial surgical repair in a newborn are repair of the truncal valve while maintaining competency, reconstruction of the MPA, repair of associated aortic arch, and possible reimplantation of coronary artery anomalies.

Children, Adolescents, and Adults

In postsurgical patients the size of the AAo, main and branch pulmonary arteries, and intracardiac anatomy are well defined by CCTA images (Fig. 37.60A and B). Palliation in some patients includes construction of a conduit between the RV and the branch pulmonary arteries (PAs), an RV-PA conduit. Stenosis of a conduit or the branch pulmonary arteries are the single most important factor for reoperation and catheter-based reintervention. Lifelong imaging surveillance is needed to monitor effects of somatic growth of a child in relation to a homograft or conduit that does not grow in

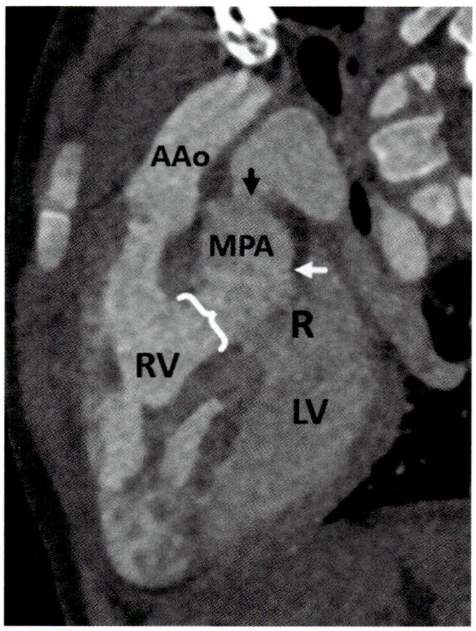

Figure 37.35. Infant with double outlet right ventricle (DORV) and D-transposition of the great arteries. Sagittal oblique CCTA view of the right (R) and left (L) ventricular outflow tracts shows the dextroposed position of the aortic and pulmonic valves, the ascending aorta (AAo) is anterior to the main pulmonary artery (MPA). In this type of DORV pulmonic stenosis is not seen. A band has been surgically placed on the MPA (black arrow) to limit pulmonary blood flow. More than 50% of the pulmonic semilunar valve annulus (white arrow) originates from the right ventricle (RV), satisfying the 150% rule of DORV. The pulmonic valve overrides the ventricular septal defect (bracket). The aortic semilunar valve arises solely from the right ventricle.

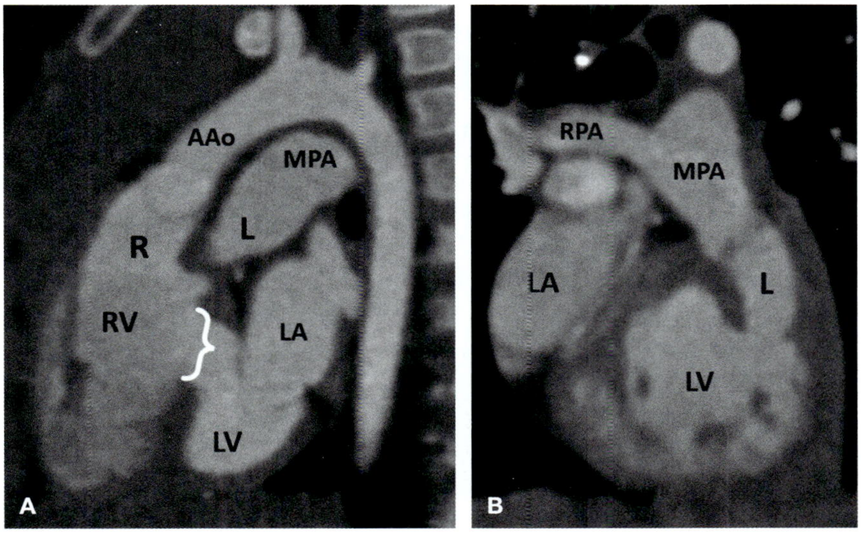

Figure 37.36. Infant with double outlet right ventricle, D-transposition of the great arteries, and a noncommitted ventricular septal defect (VSD). **A:** Sagittal oblique maximum intensity projection (MIP) CCTA image of the right (R) and left (L) ventricular outflow tracts shows the dextroposed position of the aortic and pulmonic valves, the ascending aorta (AAo) is anterior to the main pulmonary artery (MPA). The VSD (bracket) is remote from both semilunar valves. **B:** Sagittal oblique MIP CCTA image of the left ventricular outflow tract in the same patient does not show the noncommitted VSD. The left ventricular outflow tract (L) drains to the MPA.

proportion to the physiologic requirements of a child, into adolescence and adulthood (Fig. 37.60C).

CCTA is best used in the initial diagnosis and in long-term follow-up of these patients and can guide further decisions on surgical versus catheter-based intervention on the RV-PA conduit and/or truncal valve.

SINGLE VENTRICLE CONGENITAL HEART ANOMALIES

Single ventricle CHD anomalies involve marked or severe hypoplasia of the left or right ventricular chamber and often involve the atrioventricular valve, semilunar valve, and the arterial outflow of the affected ventricle. The hypoplastic ventricle is not capable of pumping the volume of blood required to support the systemic left or the pulmonic right-sided circulation. Patients with single ventricle physiology have severe, complex CHD, which requires multimodality imaging and numerous staged palliative surgical procedures throughout infancy, childhood, and often as adolescents and adults in order to shunt blood flow to the systemic and pulmonic circulations, to manage systemic venous return to the heart, and to treat or repair cardiac valve insufficiency and surgical complications. Owing to complexity of the surgical palliation procedure many of these patients will acquire heart block or present early after surgery with arrhythmias and often time will require permanent epicardial leads and pacemaker.

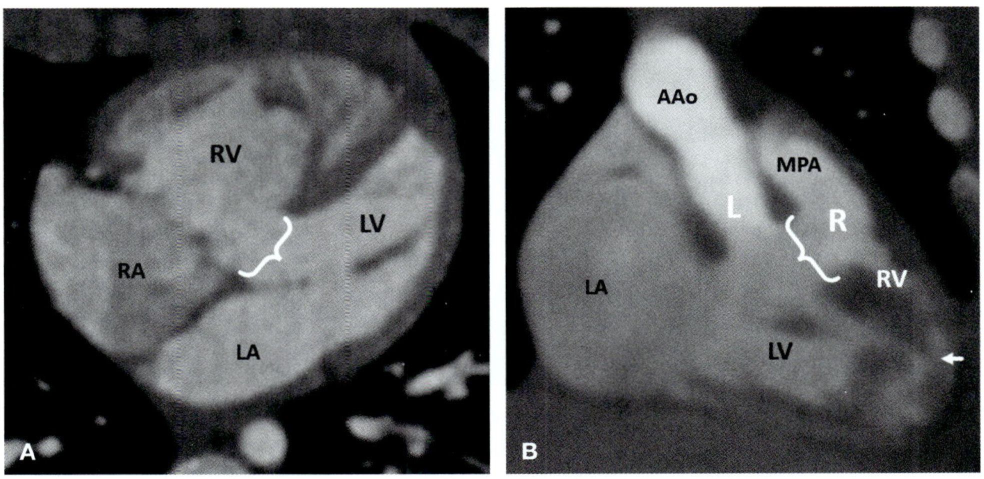

Figure 37.37. Infant with double outlet right ventricle (DORV), D-transposition of the great arteries, and a noncommitted ventricular septal defect (VSD). **A:** Axial oblique 4-chamber maximum intensity projection (MIP) CCTA image shows the noncommitted VSD (bracket), which is remote from the ventricular outflow tracts. B. A coronal oblique MIP CCTA view of the right (R) and left (L) ventricular outflow tracts. The VSD (bracket) underlies both outflow tracts symmetrically; the left ventricular outflow tract (L) is elongated. A distal muscular VSD is located toward the apex (white arrow).

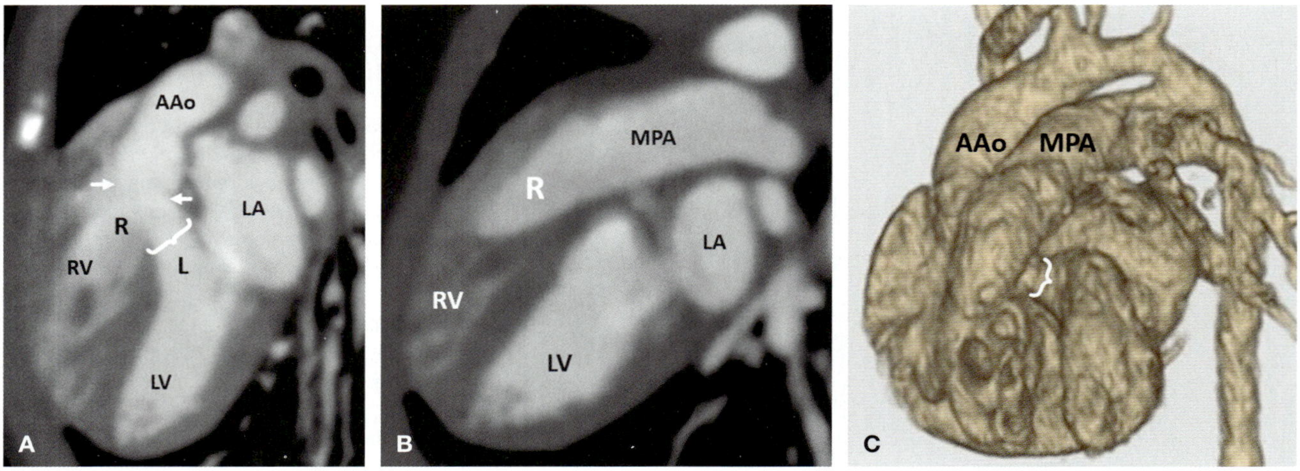

Figure 37.38. Infant with double outlet right ventricle (DORV) with subaortic ventricular septal defect (VSD). **A:** A nearly 3-chamber oblique maximum intensity projection (MIP) CCTA view of the right (R) and left (L) ventricular outflow tracts shows that more than 50% of the aortic semilunar valve annulus (white arrows) originates from the right ventricle (RV), satisfying the 150% rule of DORV. The ventricular septal defect (VSD) (bracket) is the subaortic type. **B:** A sagittal oblique MIP CCTA view of the right ventricular outflow tract (R) does not show the VSD, which is known to be subaortic. **C:** 3D volume rendered CCTA view of the heart shows normal arrangement of the right and left ventricular outflow tracts and the VSD (bracket), which in a 3D rendering is seen as a communication between the ventricles.

CCTA is important for imaging patients at many times through their lives, most importantly in follow-up of surgical anatomy and often surgical palliation complications.

Hypoplastic Left Heart Syndrome

HLHS is a spectrum of left heart underdevelopment, involving the mitral valve, LV, aortic valve, and AAo in which stenosis or atresia of the mitral and/or aortic valve limits flow of blood into the LV and AAo, severely limiting growth of the LV with resultant severe hypoplasia of the AAo. The LV is unable to support the systemic circulation; the aortic arch and descending aorta grow in utero because of adequate blood flow via the PDA, and the AAo receives retrograde blood flow from the ductus arteriosus to supply the coronary arteries (Fig. 37.61A-E).

Occurring in around 1% to 2% of patients with CHD, HLHS is universally fatal without surgical intervention performed in 3 palliative stages:

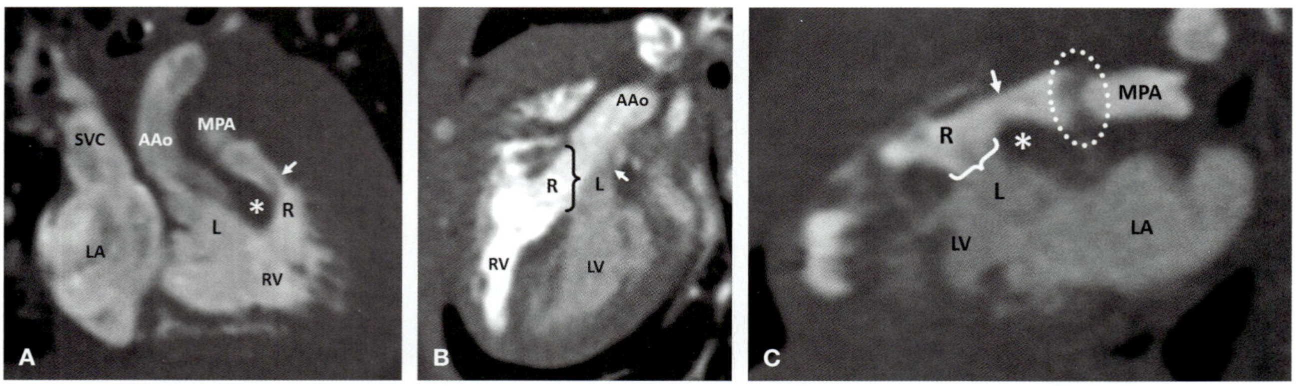

Figure 37.39. Infant with tetralogy of Fallot–type double outlet right ventricle, subpulmonic right ventricular outflow tract obstruction, and pulmonic valve stenosis. **A:** Coronal oblique maximum intensity projection (MIP) CCTA view of the right (R) and left (L) ventricular outflow tracts shows prominent myocardial conal tissue (asterisk), which contributes to narrowing of the right ventricular outflow tract. The subaortic VSD is out of plane. **B:** Coronal oblique MIP CCTA view of the right (R) and left (L) ventricular outflow tracts shows the aortic semilunar valve (white arrow) overriding the VSD. Note the narrowing of the right ventricular outflow tract (bracket). The pulmonic valve is out of plane. **C:** Sagittal oblique MIP CCTA view shows narrowing (white arrow) of the right ventricular outflow tract by the prominent myocardial conal tissue (asterisk) and thickened pulmonic valve leaflets (dotted ellipse). The subaortic VSD (bracket) is partially included in the image. The aortic valve is out of plane.

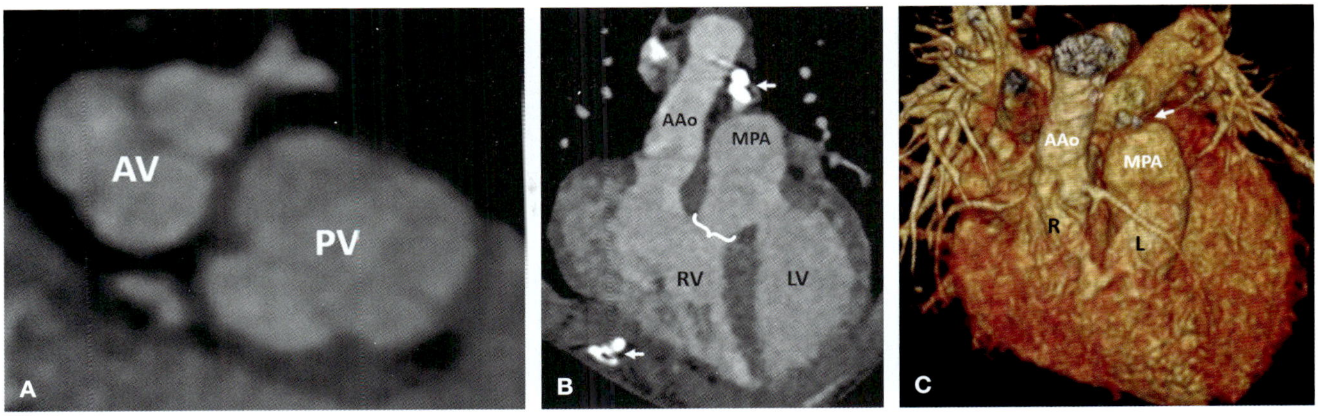

Figure 37.40. Infant with Taussig-Bing type double outlet right ventricle (DORV) with transposition of the great ventricles and subpulmonic ventricular septal defect (VSD). **A:** Axial oblique maximum intensity projection (MIP) CCTA view of the aortic (AV) and pulmonic (PV) valve planes, which are nearly side by side, the expected position of the semilunar valves in DORV. **B:** A coronal oblique MIP CCTA view of the right (R) and left (L) ventricular outflow tracts shows the dextroposed positions of the aortic and pulmonic valves and the great vessels. The VSD (bracket) is subpulmonic. Surgical clips and sutures create streak artifacts (white arrows). **C:** 3D volume rendered CCTA view of the heart shows the right (R) and left (L) ventricular outflow tracts the dextroposed positions of the aortic and pulmonic valves and the great vessels, the aortic valve and ascending aorta (AAo) are to the right of the pulmonic valve and the main pulmonary artery (MPA). Streak artifact (arrow) from surgical clips are seen.

Stage 1—Norwood or hybrid procedure establishes systemic blood flow, while maintaining pulmonary arterial blood flow is performed in the first few days of life.

- Norwood procedure: Side-to-side anastomosis of the aortic arch to the MPA to provide systemic blood flow from the morphologic RV, which is the single pumping chamber of the heart. An arterial pressure modified BTTS (Fig. 37.62A and B) or a right ventricular to branch pulmonary artery conduit (Sano modification) supplies the confluent branch pulmonary arteries. An atrial septostomy is performed to allow mixing of systemic and venous return before it enters the single ventricle (Fig. 37.63A-D).

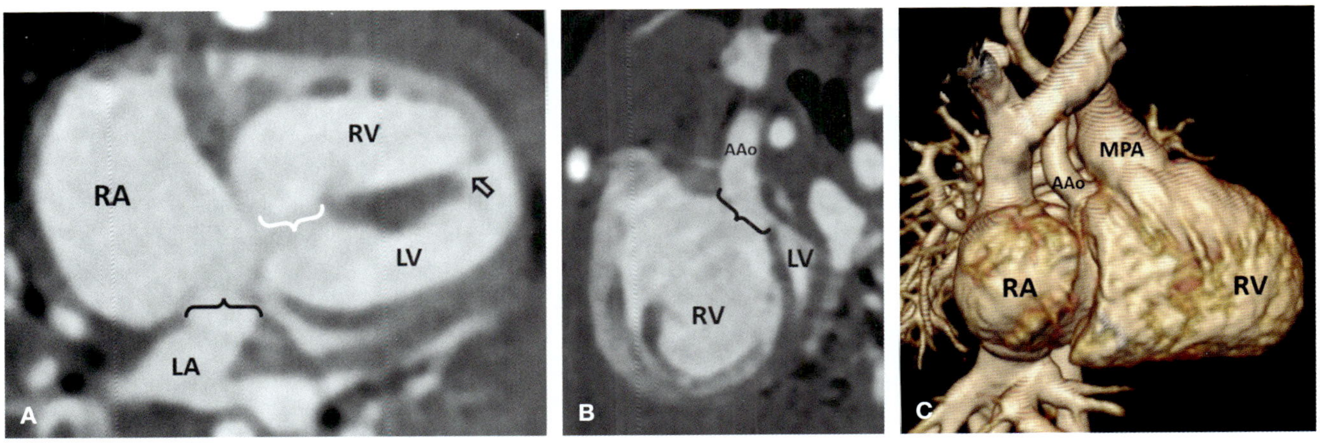

Figure 37.41. CCTA Hypoplastic left ventricle. **A:** Infant with unbalanced atrioventricular septal defect with hypoplastic left ventricle, resulting in double outlet right ventricle (DORV). Axial oblique maximum intensity projection (MIP) CCTA view of the heart shows marked dilation of the right atrium (RA), an atrial septal defect (black bracket), ventricular septal defect (VSD) below the common atrioventricular valve (white bracket), and an apical VSD (open black arrow). **B:** Infant with DORV and severely hypoplastic left ventricle. Coronal oblique CCTA view of the aortic outflow tract shows that almost 100% of the aortic semilunar valve annulus (bracket) originates from the right ventricle (RV) and the severely hypoplastic left ventricle (LV) and the RV is markedly dilated. The VSD is subaortic (bracket). **C:** Infant with unbalanced atrioventricular septal defect with hypoplastic left ventricle, resulting in DORV. 3D surface rendered CCTA view of the heart shows marked dilation of the RA and RV. The main pulmonary artery (MPA) and the small-caliber ascending aorta (AAo) arise from the RV.

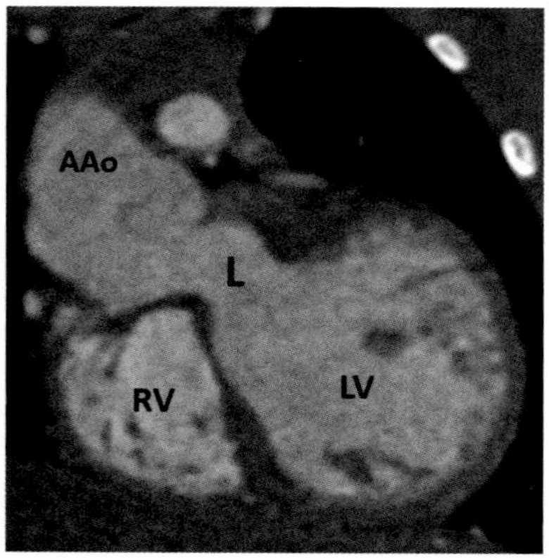

Figure 37.42. Child with double outlet right ventricle with subaortic ventricular septal defect (VSD), status post closure using a subaortic intraventricular tunnel technique. This technique diverts left ventricle (LV) blood flow to the left ventricular outflow tract (L) and aortic valve. Coronal oblique maximum intensity projection CCTA view of the left ventricular outflow tract (L) shows prominent myocardial conal tissue, which contributes to narrowing of the right ventricular outflow tract. The subaortic VSD is out of plane.

- Damus-Kaye-Stansel (DKS): An end-to-side anastomosis of the AAo to the MPA is now more often used as an alternative to the Norwood side-to-side aortic arch to MPA anastomosis (Fig. 37.64A-C).
- Hybrid procedure: This procedure utilizes surgical and interventional techniques and was developed as a lower-risk alternative, as it avoids cardiopulmonary bypass. Prostaglandin infusion or a stent in the PDA maintains blood flow to the systemic circulation, bands are placed on the main or branch pulmonary arteries to restrict high-pressure arterial blood flow to the pulmonary vascular bed, and atrial septostomy may be performed (Fig. 37.65A-C).

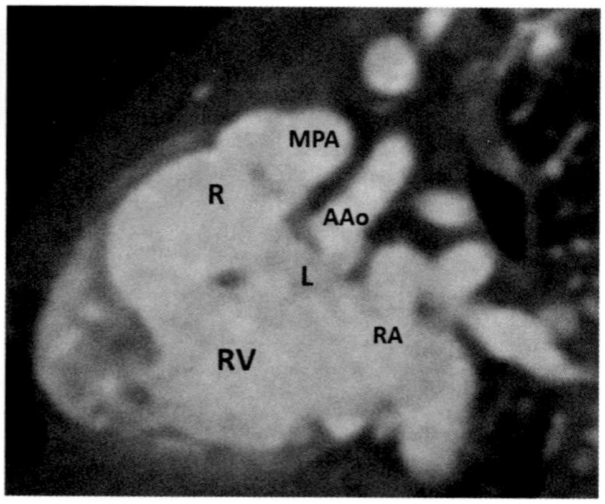

Figure 37.43. Infant with double outlet right ventricle and severely hypoplastic left ventricle. Sagittal oblique CCTA view of the right (R) and left (L) ventricular outflow tract shows normal arrangement, with anterior position of the pulmonic valve and the main pulmonary artery relative to the aortic valve and the ascending aorta (AAo). Both great arteries arise from the right ventricle (RV). The ventricular septal defect is subaortic.

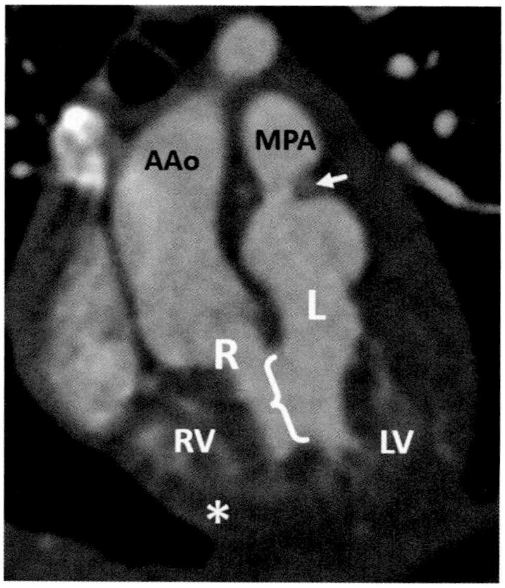

Figure 37.44. Child with double outlet right ventricle, D-transposition of the great arteries, with noncommitted ventricular septal defect (VSD), status post closure using a subaortic intraventricular tunnel technique. Coronal oblique maximum intensity projection CCTA view of the right (R) and left (L) ventricular outflow tracts show the muscular VSD (bracket), which is neither subaortic or subpulmonic. The main pulmonary artery (MPA) shows focal narrowing from a band placed to limit pulmonary blood flow. Right ventricular hypertrophy (asterisk) is present.

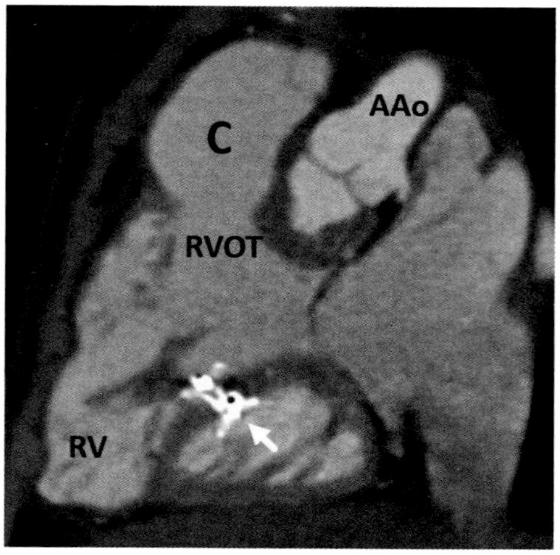

Figure 37.45. Adolescent with double outlet right ventricle, D-transposition of the great arteries type, status post Rastelli procedure tunneling of the left ventricular outflow directed through a ventricular septal defect. Sagittal oblique maximum intensity projection CCTA image shows the right ventricular outflow tract from the right ventricle (RV) to the conduit (C) which is dilated, a postsurgical complication. High-attenuation material (white arrow) in the intraventricular septum used to close a small muscular ventricular septal defect.

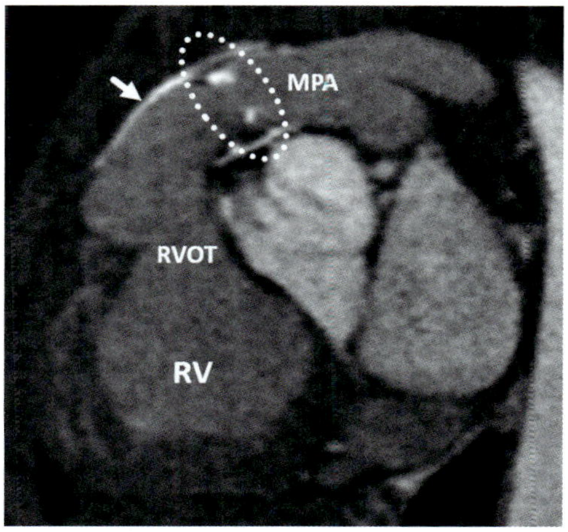

Figure 37.46. Child with double outlet right ventricle, after right ventricle to pulmonary artery (RV-PA) conduit construction. Sagittal oblique CCTA image of the right ventricular outflow tract (RVOT) and the conduit with (white arrow) shows a valve apparatus in the conduit (dotted ellipse). Right and left ventricular outflow tracts show side-by-side position of the great arteries, the ascending aorta (AAo), and narrowing of the main pulmonary artery lumen by a surgically placed band.

Stage 2—As pulmonary vascular resistance drops, around 3 to 6 months of age, before the arterial pressure BTTS leads to pulmonary hypertension it is exchanged for a venous pressure shunt.

- Superior cavopulmonary shunt or Glenn shunt is constructed to direct systemic venous blood from the upper extremities, head, and neck through the superior vena cava (SVC) to the branch pulmonary arteries (Fig. 37.66A and B).
- Norwood or DKS conversion and Glenn shunt: patients who have previously undergone the less invasive hybrid procedure now undergo a combined construction of the ventricular outflow to the systemic arterial blood flow, the venous pressure redirection of SVC drainage to the branch pulmonary arteries, and removal of pulmonary artery bands.

Stage 3—After the second stage palliation, deoxygenated visceral and lower extremity systemic venous return continues to drain to the heart. By 4 years of age, children typically undergo total cavopulmonary connection surgery or completion of a Fontan circuit.

Fontan: Blood flow from the inferior vena cava is directed to the branch pulmonary arteries, completing the direction of all systemic flow to the pulmonary arterial circulation. The IVC attachment to the branch pulmonary arteries is performed with a conduit or shunt that may be in the right atrium,or may be extra-atrial, and may be fenestrated to allow communication with the right atrium (Fig. 37.67A and B).

CCTA is a valuable imaging tool used for interventional and surgical decision making throughout the palliative surgical care of patients with HLHS, particularly for assessment of the caliber of branch pulmonary arteries, pulmonary venous drainage, and patency of BTTS and Glenn shunts and the Fontan circuit.

Neonates and Infants

CCTA is performed in newborns to assess ductal morphology, accompanying aortic arch anomaly, branch pulmonary arteries size and appearance, or if visceral abnormalities such

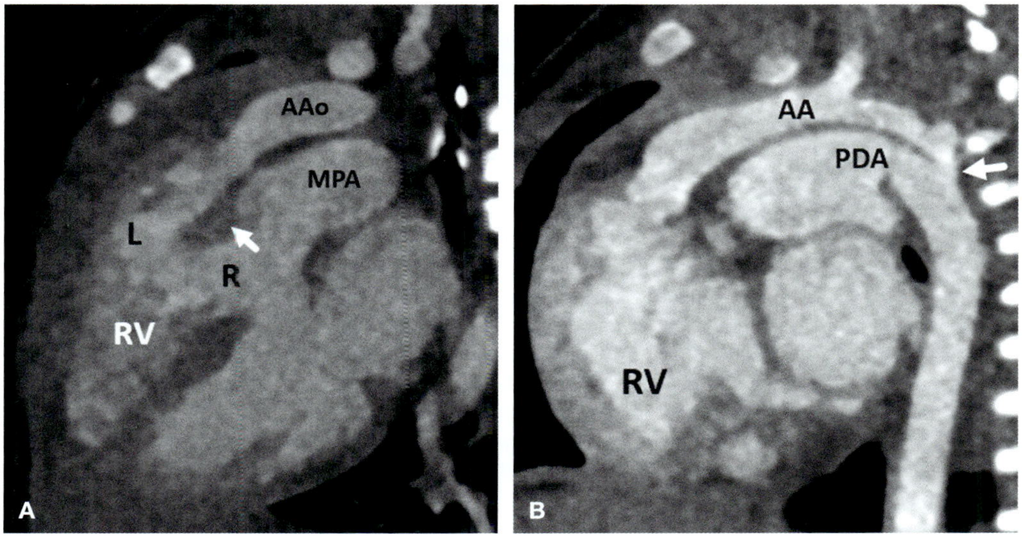

Figure 37.47. Child with double outlet right ventricle, subaortic stenosis, hypoplastic aortic arch and coarctation of the aorta. **A:** Sagittal oblique CCTA image of the right (R) and left (L) ventricular outflow tracts arising form the right ventricle (RV). The infundibular septum (white arrow) contributes to subaortic stenosis. AAo, ascending aorta; MPA, main pulmonary artery. **B:** Sagittal oblique CCTA image shows the hypoplastic aortic arch (AA), patent ductus arteriosus (PDA), and coarctation of the aorta (white arrow). RV, right ventricle.

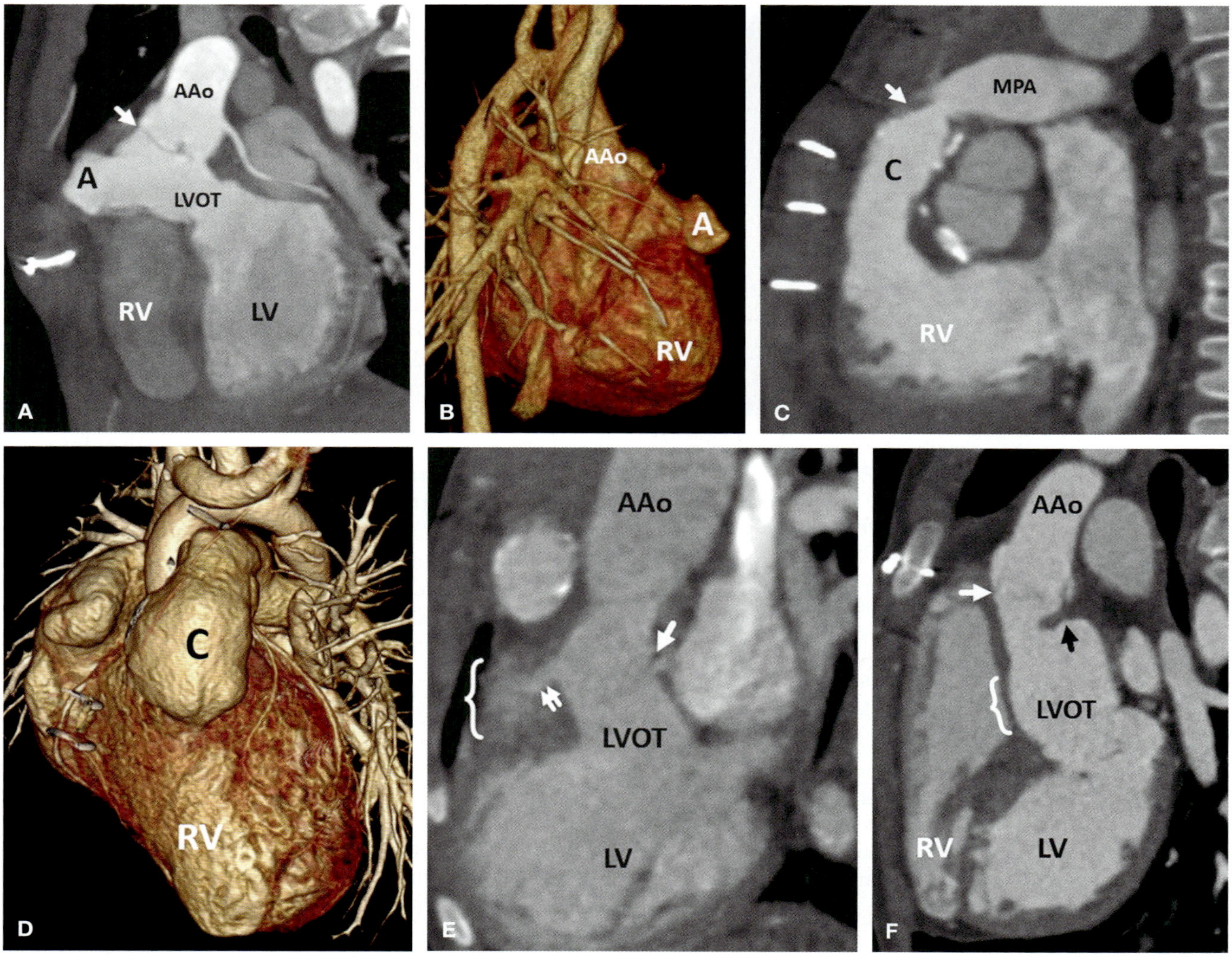

Figure 37.48. **A:** Child with double outlet right ventricle (DORV), D-transposition of the great arteries (D-TGA) type, status post Rastelli procedure tunneling of the left ventricular outflow directed through a ventricular septal defect. Sagittal oblique maximum intensity projection (MIP) CCTA image from same patient shows the left ventricular outflow tract (LVOT) from the left ventricle (LV) to the aortic valve (white arrow) and ascending aorta (AAo). Aneurysm (A) of the LVOT is a surgical complication. **B:** Sagittal oblique 3D surface rendered reconstruction CCTA image shows aneurysm (A) of the LVOT projecting from the anterior surface of the heart. **C:** Child with DORV tetralogy of Fallot type, placement of a right ventricle to pulmonary artery (RV-PA) conduit to augment pulmonary blood flow. Sagittal oblique MIP CCTA image shows the right ventricle (RV), conduit (C), and main pulmonary artery (MPA). The distal conduit shows focal stenosis (white arrow). **D:** Adolescent with DORV D-TGA type, status post Rastelli procedure tunneling of the left ventricular outflow directed through a ventricular septal defect. Coronal oblique 3D surface rendered reconstruction CCTA image shows dilation of the RV to pulmonary artery conduit (C), a postsurgical complication. **E:** Child with DORV D-TGA type, status post Rastelli procedure tunneling of the left ventricular outflow directed through a ventricular septal defect. Sagittal oblique MIP CCTA image shows the LVOT from the LV to the aortic valve (white arrow) and AAo. Surgical complication of ventricular septal defect leak has occurred at two points, a tiny leak on the posterior surface (white arrow) and a larger leak anterior (double white arrow) shows a small collection of contrast (bracket). **F:** Adolescent with DORV D-TGA type, status post Rastelli procedure tunneling of the left ventricular outflow directed through a ventricular septal defect. Sagittal oblique MIP CCTA image shows the LVOT from the LV to the aortic valve (white arrow) and AAo. Just below the aortic valve a subaortic membrane (black arrow) has formed, resulting narrowing of the LVOT and blood flow turbulence on echocardiography and a murmur on physical examination. The ventricular septal defect (bracket) has been patched.

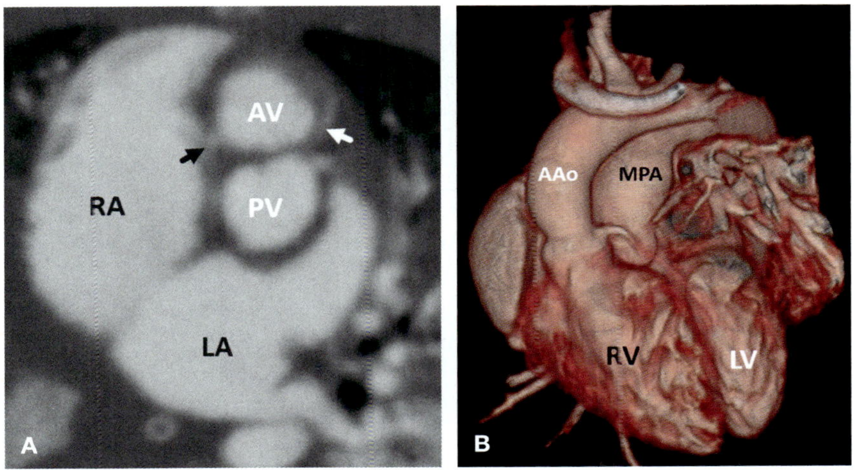

Figure 37.49. Child with D-transposition of the great arteries. **A:** Axial oblique maximum intensity projection (MIP) CCTA image at the aortic (AV) and pulmonary (PV) valve level shows the AV anterior to the PV and right (black arrow) and left main (white arrow) coronary artery origins from sinuses "facing" the PV. The right (RA) and left (LA) atria, identifiable by the morphology of the atrial appendages are in normal position. **B:** 3D reconstructed CCTA of the heart shows the ascending aorta (AAo) arises from the right ventricle (RV) and the main pulmonary artery (MPA) arises from the left ventricle (LV).

as lungs abnormalities (lymphangiectasia) or heterotaxy are raised.

CCTA is not often performed to investigate coronary artery anatomy of patients with HLHS unless myocardial ischemia is suspected, and the coronary arteries are not visualized by echocardiography. Coronary artery anatomy is usually normal in patients with HLHS, arising from the severely hypoplastic AAo, and supplied in utero and postnatally via retrograde blood flow from the ductus arteriosus. Coronary artery blood flow is therefore "ductal dependent"; if the ductus is allowed to close, coronary blood flow would cease, resulting in myocardial ischemia (Fig. 37.68).

After stage I palliation (Norwood or DKS and BTTS or Sano shunt) surgical complications stenosis or thrombosis of the shunt, AAo, and branch pulmonary arteries are readily shown with the high-spatial resolution CCTA (Fig. 37.69A and B).

Infants and Young Children

Prior to the second stage palliation of HLHS, converting BTTS to a Glenn shunt, CCTA is the optimal imaging modality used for anatomic definition of the cardiovascular anatomy. Cardiac catheterization is performed when intracardiac pressures or interventions are required. CCTA is ideal for evaluation of branch pulmonary artery diameter and BTTS shunt patency prior to transformation to a Glenn shunt, particularly in patients with echo findings of blood flow acceleration raising suspicion for luminal narrowing (Fig. 37.70A and B).

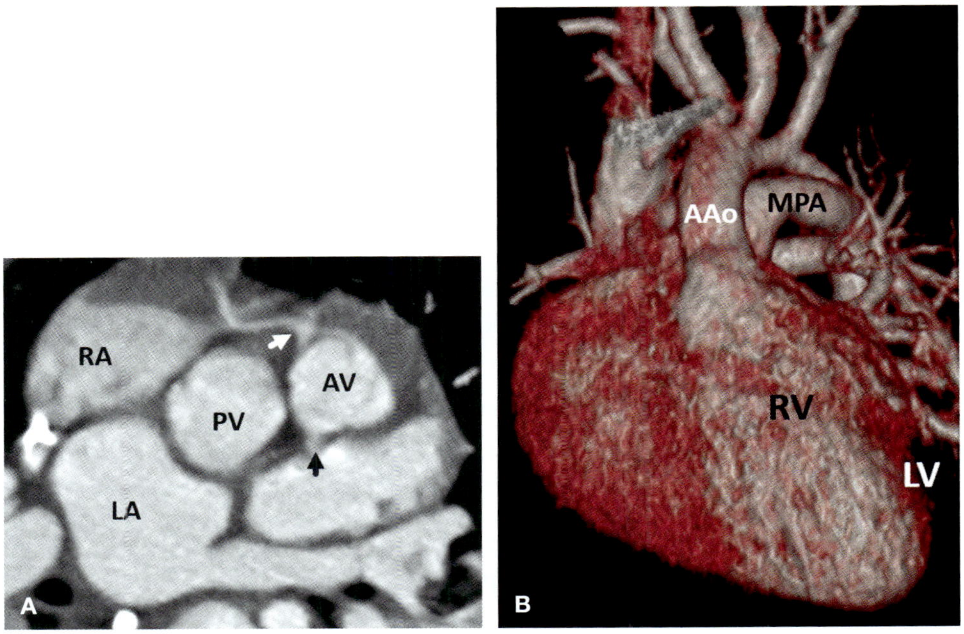

Figure 37.50. Child with L-transposition of the great arteries. **A:** Axial oblique maximum intensity projection (MIP) CCTA image at the aortic (AV) and pulmonary (PV) valve level shows the AV to the left of the PV and right (white arrow) and left main (black arrow) coronary artery origins from sinuses "facing" the PV. **B:** 3D reconstructed CCTA of the heart shows the ascending aorta (AAo) arises from the right ventricle (RV), anterior and leftward of the main pulmonary artery (MPA), which arises from the left ventricle (LV).

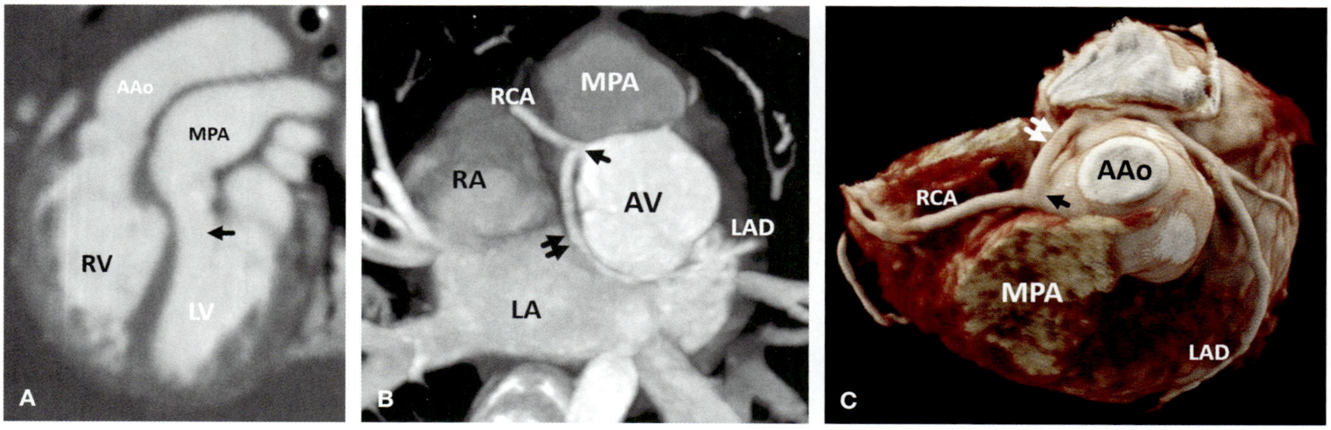

Figure 37.51. Child with D-transposition of the great arteries (D-TGA). **A:** Sagittal oblique maximum intensity projection (MIP) CCTA image shows the ascending aorta (AAo) arising from the right venricle (RV), directly anterior to the main pulmonary artery (MPA) that arises from the left ventricle (LV). The intraventricular septum is intact. The subpulmonic region is mildly narrowed (black arrow). **B:** Adult with D-transposition of the great arteries (D-TGA). History of arterial switch operation, reimplantation of a single coronary artery origin, and LeCompte maneuver. Axial oblique MIP CCTA image at the level of the aortic valve (AV) and anterior position of the MPA shows the reimplanted single coronary artery origin (black arrow), which divides to the right coronary artery (RCA) with a normal proximal course and the anomalous retroaortic couse of the left main coronary artery (black double arrows), which continues to the left anterior descending coronary artery (LAD). **C:** 3D reconstructed CCTA of the heart from same patient shows ascending aorta (AAo) and anterior position of the MPA, which has been cut away to reveal the reimplanted single coronary artery origin (black arrow), which divides to the RCA with a normal proximal course and the anomalous retroaortic couse of the left main coronary artery (white double arrows), which continues to the left anterior descending coronary artery (LAD).

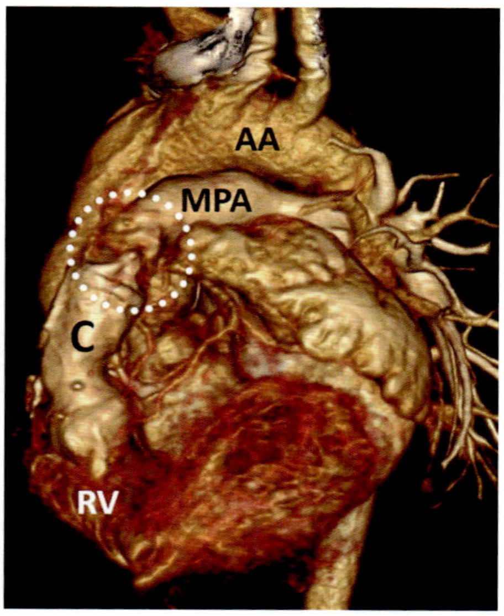

Figure 37.52. Child with double outlet right ventricle D-transposition of the great arteries type, status post arterial switch operation and RV-PA conduit. Sagittal oblique 3D surface rendered reconstruction CCTA image shows the conduit (C) arising from the right ventricle (RV) and focal narrowing (dotted ellipse) of the distal conduit as it joins the main pulmonary artery (MPA). AA, aortic arch.

After Glenn shunt, patients with HLHS continue to be monitored with echocardiograms for growth of the branch pulmonary arteries and evaluation of the aortic arch; however, CCTA remains the ideal imaging modality to provide the cardiac interventionalist with a vascular road map and enable accurate measurement of stenoses of the branch pulmonary arteries or aortic arch (Fig. 37.71).

After the third stage palliation of HLHS (Fontan circuit completion) the connection of all systemic blood flow returning to the pulmonary arteries is passive, as it does not flow through a ventricular pumping chamber. Passive flow raises concern for stagnant blood and risk of thrombus in the Fontan circuit; CCTA is often used to evaluate for filling defects or thrombi in the Fontan or, in some cases, pulmonary embolus (Figs. 37.72A and B, 37.73 and 37.74A and B).

Adolescents and Young Adults

It is a relatively recent advancement in CHD that patients with HLHS are surviving into adolescents and young adulthood, as this group of patients benefits from improvements in clinical, surgical, and imaging care. In younger patients, complications of the Fontan circuit connection, stagnant blood, risk of thrombus in the Fontan circuit, and

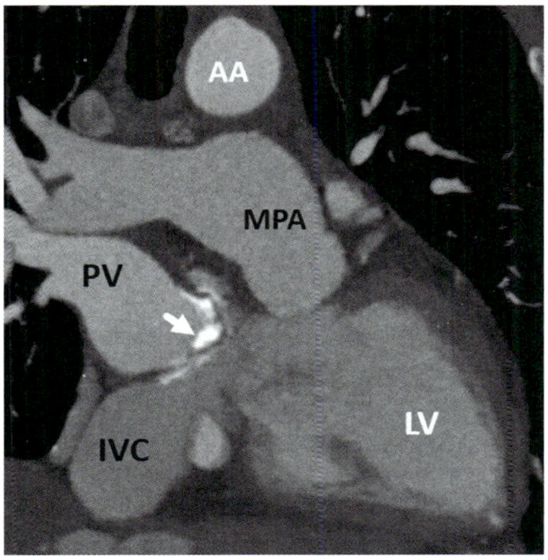

Figure 37.53. Adult with D-transposition of the great arteries, status post atrial level switch. Coronal oblique maximum intensity projection CCTA image shows the partially calcified surgical material (white arrow) used to direct pulmonary vein (PV) and inferior vena cava (IVC) flow toward the systemic and pulmonic circulations.

pulmonary embolus and branch pulmonary artery stenosis may be optimally imaged using CCTA (Figs. 37.75A and B) (Fig. 37.76A-C).

- Hypoplastic right heart syndrome in which all right-sided heart structures are affected. The tricuspid and pulmonic valves may be atretic or hypoplastic, and the right atrium and ventricle are hypoplastic.
- Double inlet left or right ventricle, in which both atrioventricular valves empty to the same ventricular chamber and the other ventricle is hypoplastic.
- Unbalanced atrioventricular canal defect in which the atrioventricular valve is dedicated to one ventricle and the other ventricle is hypoplastic.

Each single ventricle CHD type is treated using a similar palliative surgical approach, enabling the single ventricle to pump to the systemic circulation and the branch pulmonary artery blood flow established by a shunt, eventually completing the venous drainage pattern through a Fontan circuit. Therefore, patients require imaging to monitor vascular anatomy and develop similar complications for which CCTA is often the optimal imaging modality (Fig. 37.77).

ANOMALIES OF PULMONARY VENOUS DRAINAGE

The pulmonary veins form via a complex process of heart and lung formation beginning in the fourth and fifth weeks of gestation at the same time systemic veins are forming and are becoming a separate venous system. The pulmonary veins carry oxygenated blood from the lungs to the left atrium and show common anatomic variation in number and arrangement. When this process does not proceed normally pulmonary veins may communicate with systemic venous structures rather than to the left atrium, draining to supracardiac (left brachiocephalic vein or SVC) or infracardiac (inferior vena cava or portal vein) systemic veins, the

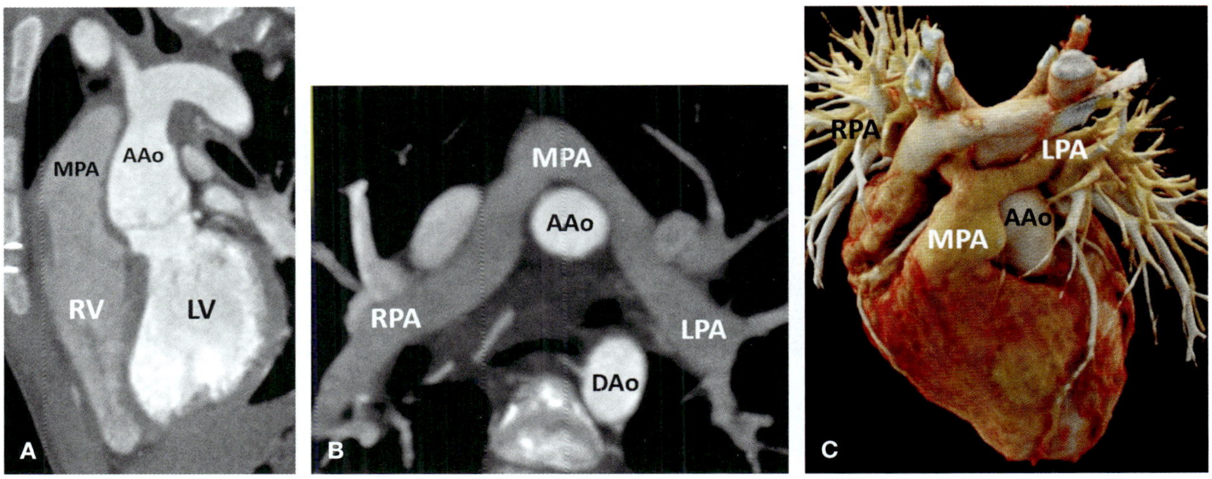

Figure 37.54. Adolescent with D-transposition of the great arteries. History of arterial switch operation with LeCompte maneuver. **A:** Sagittal oblique maximum intensity projection (MIP) CCTA image shows the ascending aorta (AAo) arising from the left venricle (LV), directly anterior to the main pulmonary artery (MPA) that arises from the right ventricle (RV). **B:** Axial oblique MIP CCTA image at the level of the AAo and anterior position of the MPA. The LeCompte maneuver leaves the right (RPA) and left (LPA) branch pulmonary arteries draped over the AAo. **C:** 3D reconstructed CCTA image of the heart shows the AAo posterior to the MPA. The LeCompte maneuver leaves the right (RPA) and left (LPA) branch pulmonary arteries draped over the AAo.

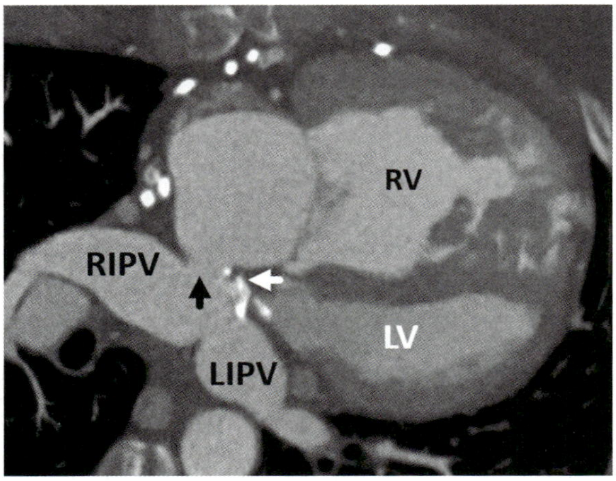

Figure 37.55. Adult with D-transposition of the great arteries, status post atrial level switch. Axial oblique maximum intensity projection CCTA image of the heart shows the partially calcified surgical material (white arrow) used to direct pulmonary vein and inferior vena cava flow toward the systemic and pulmonic circulations. The baffle draining pulmonary vein flow is narrowed (black arrow), and the right (RIPV) and left (LIPV) inferior pulmonary veins are dilated.

coronary sinus, or the right atrium. One, more than one, or all pulmonary veins may have abnormal connections, termed partial (PAPVC) or total anomalous pulmonary venous connection (TAPVC). The term "connection" is sometimes referred to as return or drainage.

PAPVC or TAPVC occurs either as an isolated condition, in less than 1% of the population, or in up to 2% of patients with other CHD diagnoses and results in a left to right shunt. An atrial septal defect or patent foramen ovale is essential for mixing of oxygenated and nonoxygenated blood for early postnatal survival, especially when a large-volume left-to-right shunt is present. Depending on the volume of blood draining to the right atrium from the anomalous pulmonary vein(s) (ie, volume of the left-to-right shunt), increased volume may result in enlargement of the right-sided heart chambers and the pulmonary arteries and pulmonary hypertension.

Anomalous pulmonary veins may or may not be obstructed, due to focal or diffuse narrowing of a vein or its outflow or unobstructed distal drainage to systemic venous structures. When obstruction is present, pulmonary edema and congestion may be the presenting symptom.

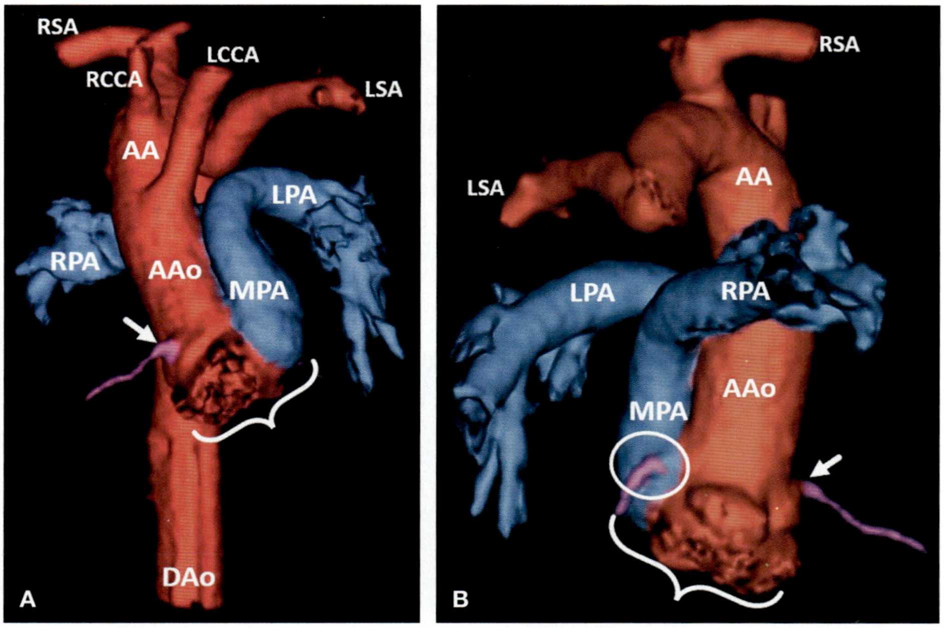

Figure 37.56. Newborn with common arterial trunk (Van Praagh type A1). **A:** 3D colorized reconstruction of CCTA from the anterior perspective shows dilation of the truncal valve (bracket), which is the combined aortic and pulmonic valves. The right coronary artery arises from the right sinus of the truncal valve (white arrow). The aortic arch (AA) is right sided. The left common carotid (LCCA), right common carotid (RCCA), right subclavian (RSA), and aberrant left subclavian (LSA) arteries branch from the AA. The main pulmonary artery (MPA) arises from the left side of the truncal valve and divides to confluent left (LPA) and right (RPA) branch pulmonary arteries. **B:** 3D colorized reconstruction of CCTA from the posterior perspective shows dilation of the truncal valve (bracket) which is the combined aortic and pulmonic valves. The main coronary artery arises from the right sinus of the truncal valve (white arrow). The left main coronary artery arises from a pulmonic sinus of the truncal valve (white ellipse). The AA is right sided. The LCCA, RCCA, RSA, and the aberrant LSA branch from the AA. The MPA arises from the left side of the truncal valve and divides to confluent left (LPA) and right (RPA) branch pulmonary arteries.

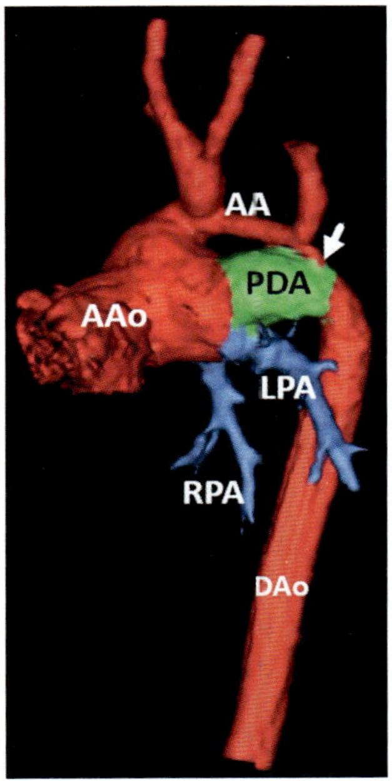

Figure 37.57. Newborn with common arterial trunk (Van Praagh type A2), but with moderate hypoplasia of the aortic arch and severe coarctation of the aorta. 3D colorized volume rendered CCTA image shows mild dilation of the truncal valve and ascending aorta (AAo). The aortic arch (AA) is moderately hypoplastic, and severe coarctation is seen at the ductus insertion (white arrow) versus near interruption. The patent ductus arteriosus (PDA) is large caliber. The right (RPA) and left (LPA) branch pulmonary arteries arise from the posterolateral aspect of the truncus at approximately the same level.

CCTA is an excellent imaging modality for delineation of normal and abnormal pulmonary venous anatomy due to its high spatial resolution, multiplanar reformat capabilities, and 3D reconstructions, particularly in CHD. ECG gating or triggering is not required for a general overview of the pulmonary venous anatomy but is especially useful when detailed anatomy of the pulmonary veins course and ostia is necessary, particularly when pulmonary vein stenosis is suspected.

Newborns and Infants

Neonates with obstructed TAPVC present within the first few days of life with a murmur, desaturation, and pulmonary vascular congestion. Before performing CCTA to assess anatomy it is vital to understand echo findings regarding known or expected anatomy of supracardiac (most common) (Fig. 37.78A-D), infracardiac, intracardiac, or mixed pulmonary venous connections (Fig. 37.79A-C). CCTA in neonates and infants is most often performed to fully delineate the anatomy and to clearly visualize focal obstructive lesions and the adjacent cardiac and mediastinal structures. The imaging field of view is an important aspect of CCTA because the lower neck must be included in patients with supracardiac PAPVC or TAPVC to view the entire SVC and innominate veins and the upper to mid abdomen to include the portal vein must be included when infracardiac PAPVC or TAPVC is known or suspected.

When PAPVC is suspected in neonates and infants CCTA is a valuable imaging modality for complete definition of anatomy.

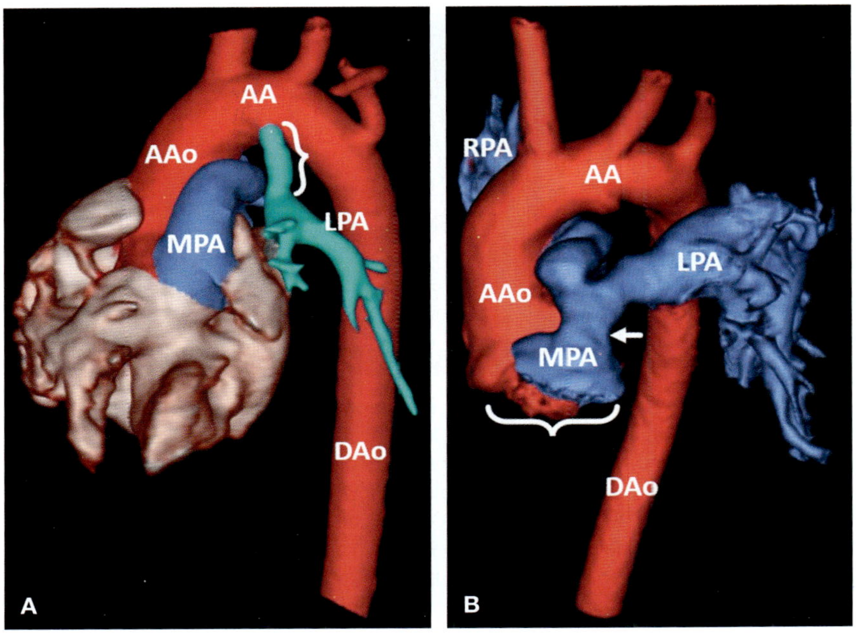

Figure 37.58. A: Newborn with common arterial trunk (Van Praagh type A3). 3D volume rendered colorized CCTA shows asymmetry in the great artery caliber, the ascending aorta (AAo) is mildly dilated compared with the main pulmonary artery (MPA). The left pulmonary artery (LPA) is isolated, arising from the patent ductus arteriosus (bracket). **B:** Young child, now with repaired common arterial trunk (Van Praagh type A3). 3D colorized volume rendered CCTA shows the postoperative findings of the surgically divided conus (bracket). Diffuse mild narrowing (white arrow) of the MPA homograft conduit with normal right (RPA) and left (LPA) branch pulmonary artery caliber.

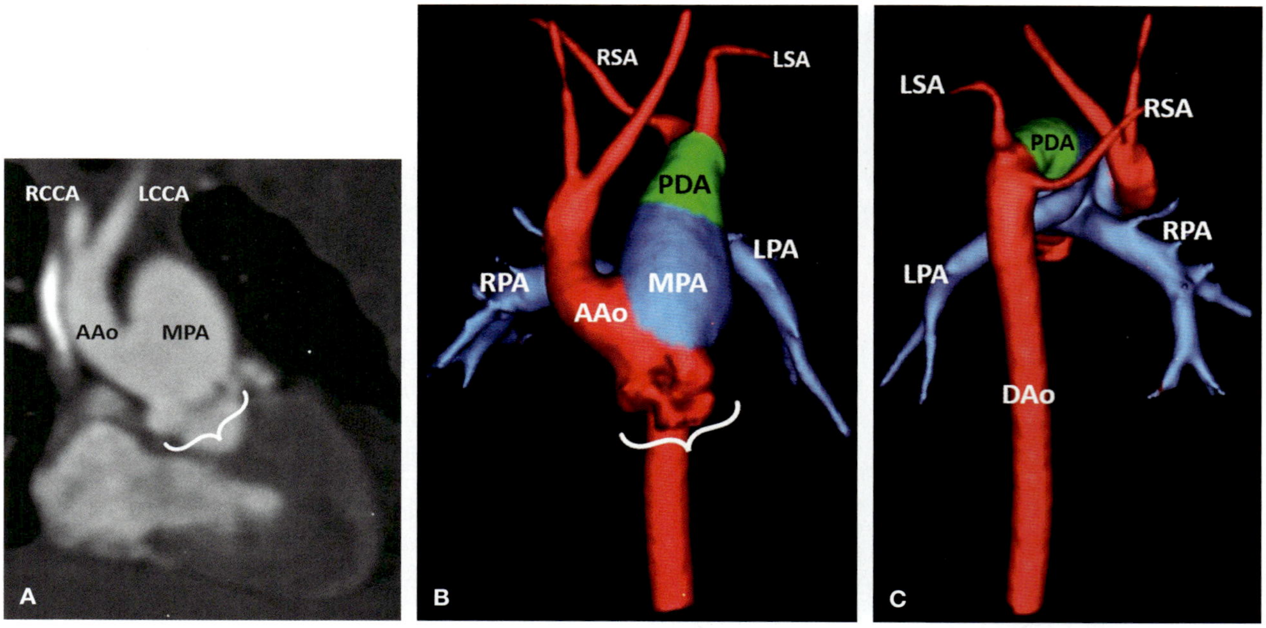

Figure 37.59. Newborn with common arterial trunk (Van Praagh type A4) and interrupted aortic arch, type B. **A:** Coronal CCTA image of the common truncus shows the truncal valve and mildly dilated, short truncal root (bracket) that divides to the ascending aorta (AAo) and the main pulmonary artery (MPA). The aortic arch is interrupted. The right (RCCA) and left (LCCA) common carotid arteries arise from the AAo. **B:** 3D colorized volume rendered CCTA shows mild to moderate dilation of the truncal root (bracket) and short common truncus giving rise to the AAo and the MPA. The MPA continues as the patent ductus arteriosus (PDA) to the distal aortic arch. The left (LSA) and aberrant right (RSA) subclavian artery origins arise from the distal aortic arch. **C:** 3D colorized volume rendered CCTA shows separate origins of the normal-caliber left (LPA) and right (RPA) pulmonary arteries from the common truncus; the LPA origin is superior to the RPA. The left (LSA) and aberrant right (RSA) subclavian artery origins arise from the distal aortic arch.

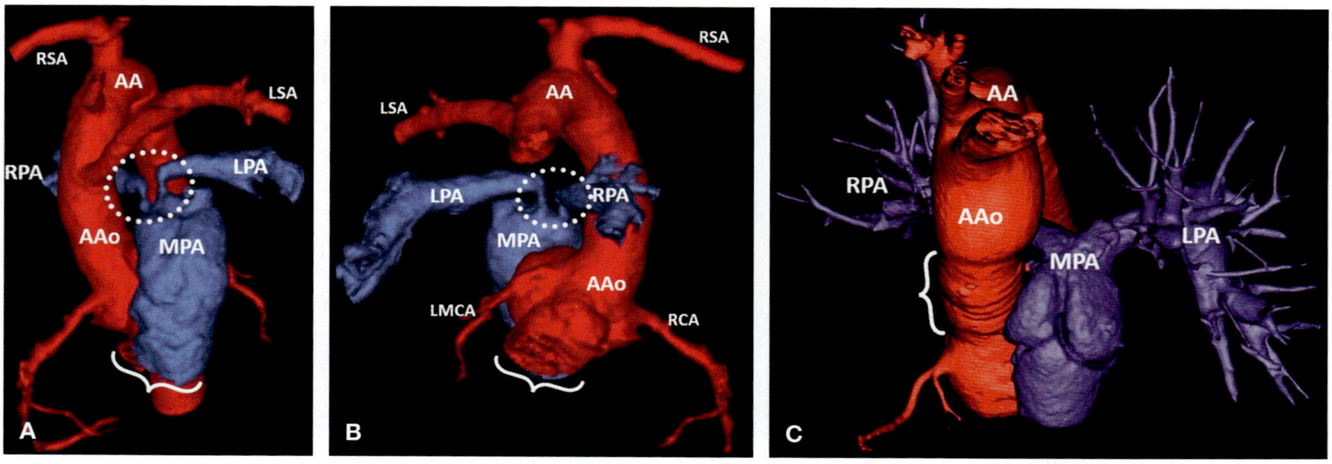

Figure 37.60. **A:** Newborn with common arterial trunk (Van Praagh type A1), status post surgical separation of truncal elements with reimplantation of the branch pulmonary arteries. 3D colorized reconstruction CCTA image shows severe focal stenosis of the right (RPA) and left (LPA) pulmonary artery origins (dotted ellipse). Note the postoperative appearance of the main pulmonary artery (MPA) and the outflow tract (bracket). **B:** 3D colorized volume rendered image from the same patient with a posterior projection. The right coronary artery (RCA) arises from the right-sided neoaortic sinus. The left main coronary artery (LMCA) arises from the posterior aspect of the left neoaortic sinus (bracket). **C:** Adolescent with native anatomy of common arterial trunk (Van Praagh type A1), status post truncal valvuloplasty, and branch pulmonary arterioplasty, ascending aorta graft. 3D colorized volume rendered CCTA shows postoperative findings of separation of the truncal elements and the conduit (bracket) and mild dilation of the distal ascending aorta (AAo). The aortic arch (AA) is right sided with mirror image arch branching.

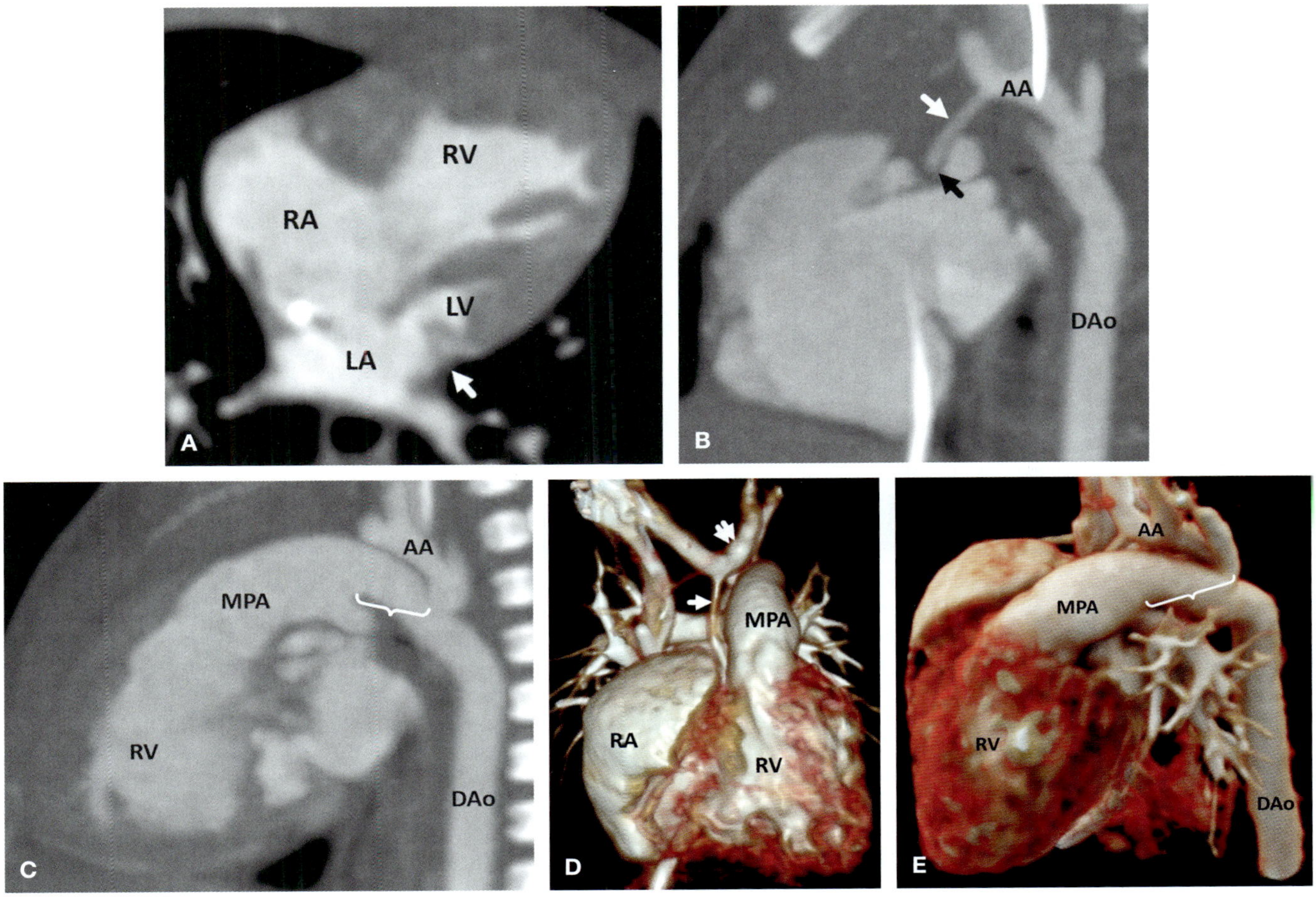

Figure 37.61. Newborn with hypoplastic left heart syndrome. **A:** Axial oblique 4-chamber CCTA view of the heart shows a markedly hypoplastic mitral valve annulus (white arrow) and severly hypoplastic left ventricle (LV).The right ventricle (RV) is normal volume. A secundum interatrial defect allows mixing of oxygenated and deoxygenated blood between the left (LA) and right (RA) atria. **B:** Sagittal oblique CCTA maximum intensity projection (MIP) reformatted image shows the marked degree of hypoplasia of the ascending aorta (white arrow) and that the ascending aorta does not connect with a cardiac chamber in this patient with aortic valve atresia (black arrow). The aortic arch (AA) is hypoplastic, and the descending thoracic aorta (DAo) is normal caliber. **C:** Sagittal oblique CCTA MIP reformatted image shows the patent ductus arteriosus (bracket) between the normal-caliber main pulmonary artery (MPA) and the hypoplastic AA. It is crucial to maintain patency of the ductus arteriosus in order to maintain blood supply to hypoplastic ascending aorta and coronary arteries. **D:** 3D volume rendered image of heart shows the severely hypoplastic ascending aorta (white arrow) and hypoplastic AA (double white arrow). Right-sided heart structures, right atrium (RA), RV, and the MPA are normal size. **E:** A 3D cinematic rendered CCTA image of the heart shows the patent ductus arteriosus (bracket) between the normal-caliber MPA and the distal hypoplastic AA.

Children, Adolescents, and Adults

Although it is less likely for a child or an adult patient to present with previously undiagnosed CHD, it is not uncommon that a child or adult patient with a single anomalously draining pulmonary vein is first diagnosed on a routine CT examination or a dedicated CCTA to be performed to confirm a diagnosis based on an enlarged cardiac silhouette seen on chest radiographs or an echocardiography performed for other indications. When late diagnosis is made the most common anomalies of pulmonary venous connection diagnoses include forms of PAPVC. The volume of the left-to-right shunt of PAPVC may or may not warrant surgical repair in older children and adults.

Patients without or with history of previous surgical repair of PAPVC or TAPVC may undergo CCTA imaging follow-up of the known diagnosis for further anatomic definition, complications of the disease such as pulmonary vein stenosis, or prior to redo or the next stage of surgical palliation.

PAPVC anatomy is variable. When undiagnosed beyond infancy, the most often encountered anatomical variations include a defect in the superior sinus venosus (Fig. 37.80A and B) or, less commonly, an inferior sinus venosus defect

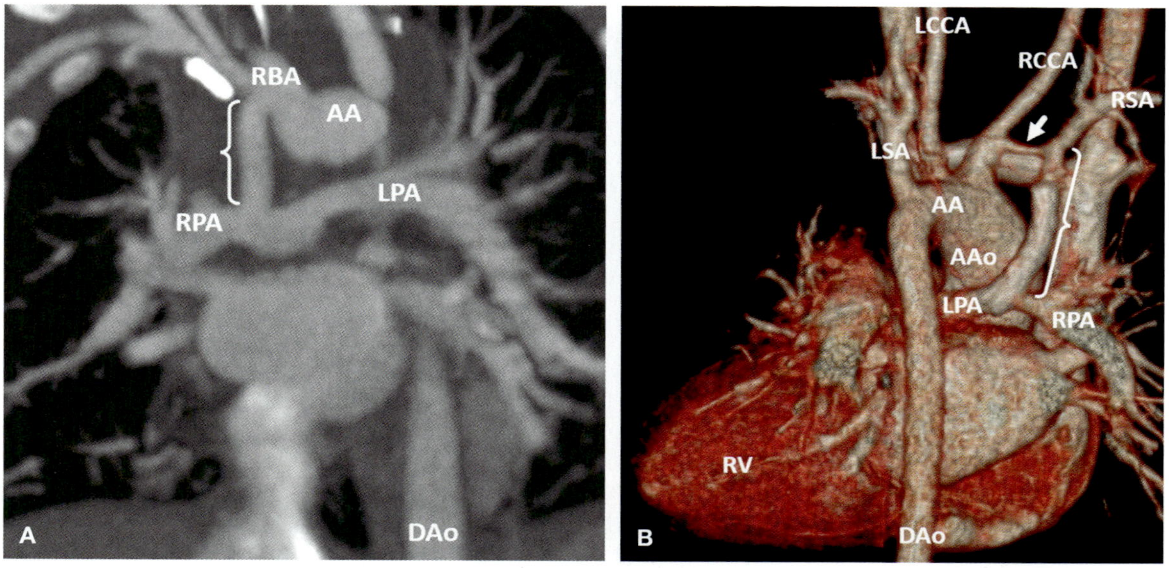

Figure 37.62. Infant with hypoplastic left heart syndrome, status post. Norwood procedure and Blalock-Taussig-Thomas shunt (BTTS). **A:** Coronal oblique 2D maximum intensity projection (MIP) CCTA image of the mediastinum in a patient with hypoplastic left heart syndrome, after Norwood procedure and BTTS. The BTTS (bracket) courses between the right brachiocephalic artery (RBA) and the confluent right (RPA) and left (LPA) pulmonary arteries. **B:** 3D volume rendered CCTA image of the heart in a patient with hypoplastic left heart syndrome, after Norwood procedure and BTTS. From a posterior view the BTTS (bracket) courses between the right subclavian artery (RSA) and the confluent RPA and LPA. Stenosis of the proximal RSA (arrow) may be a complication of the surgical procedure. The neo–ascending aorta (AAo) was created in the Norwood manner with a side-to-side anastomosis of the hypoplastic native AAo and the main pulmonary artery.

(SVD) (Fig. 37.81A and B). The sinus venosus is an embryologic posterior connection between the right and left atrium and in up to 90% of patients is associated with PAPVC. An SVD is not a true atrial septal defect but is often inaccurately referred to as such. PAPVC in SVD typically involves drainage of one or two right pulmonary veins to the SVC or the IVC/RA junction; the degree of left-to-right shunting in patients with an SVD is usually substantially larger when compared with single isolated PAPVC. In other forms of PAPVC, a single or multiple right pulmonary veins drain to the IVC, a right or less commonly a left scimitar vein drains to the IVC (Figs. 37.82A-D and 37.83A-C), or a left-sided pulmonary vein drains via a vertical vein to the left innominate/brachiocephalic vein (Fig. 37.84A and B).

PULMONARY VEIN STENOSIS OR ATRESIA

Congenital pulmonary vein stenosis and atresia are very rare, estimated to occur in 0.03% of newborns with CHD and is more often associated with prematurity and poor prognosis (Fig. 37.85A-C).

Cor Triatriatum

Cor triatriatum occurs as a result of stenosis of the common pulmonary vein, which does not incorporate normally into the left atrium, resulting in a septated appearance of the left atrium as the pulmonary veins connect to a chamber that is separated from the left atrium by a membrane. The degree of communication between the left atrium (cor triatriatum sinister) or rarely the right atrium (cor triatriatum dexter) and the confluence of pulmonary veins is variable (Fig. 37.86A and B).

CCTA is also an ideal imaging modality for delineating the anatomy of other types of pulmonary vein anomalies, including pulmonary varix or aneurysm of a pulmonary vein, meandering pulmonary vein (a rare congenital pulmonary venous anomaly with an single pulmonary vein taking a tortuous/ meandering route in the lung and draining to the left atrium), levoatrial cardinal vein (an embryologic remnant of a cardinal vein which connects a systemic vein , usually brachiocephalic vein, to the left atrium), and pulmonary arteriovenous malformation (Fig. 37.87).

CORONARY ARTERY ANOMALIES

The coronary arteries are believed to form through a complex process of cellular interactions of the sinus venosus, ventricular endocardium, and epicardial cells, almost always resulting in coronary artery origins arising from the left and right sinuses of Valsalva and follow a predictable branching pattern:

- Left main coronary artery (LMCA) to the LAD and the left circumflex (LCx)

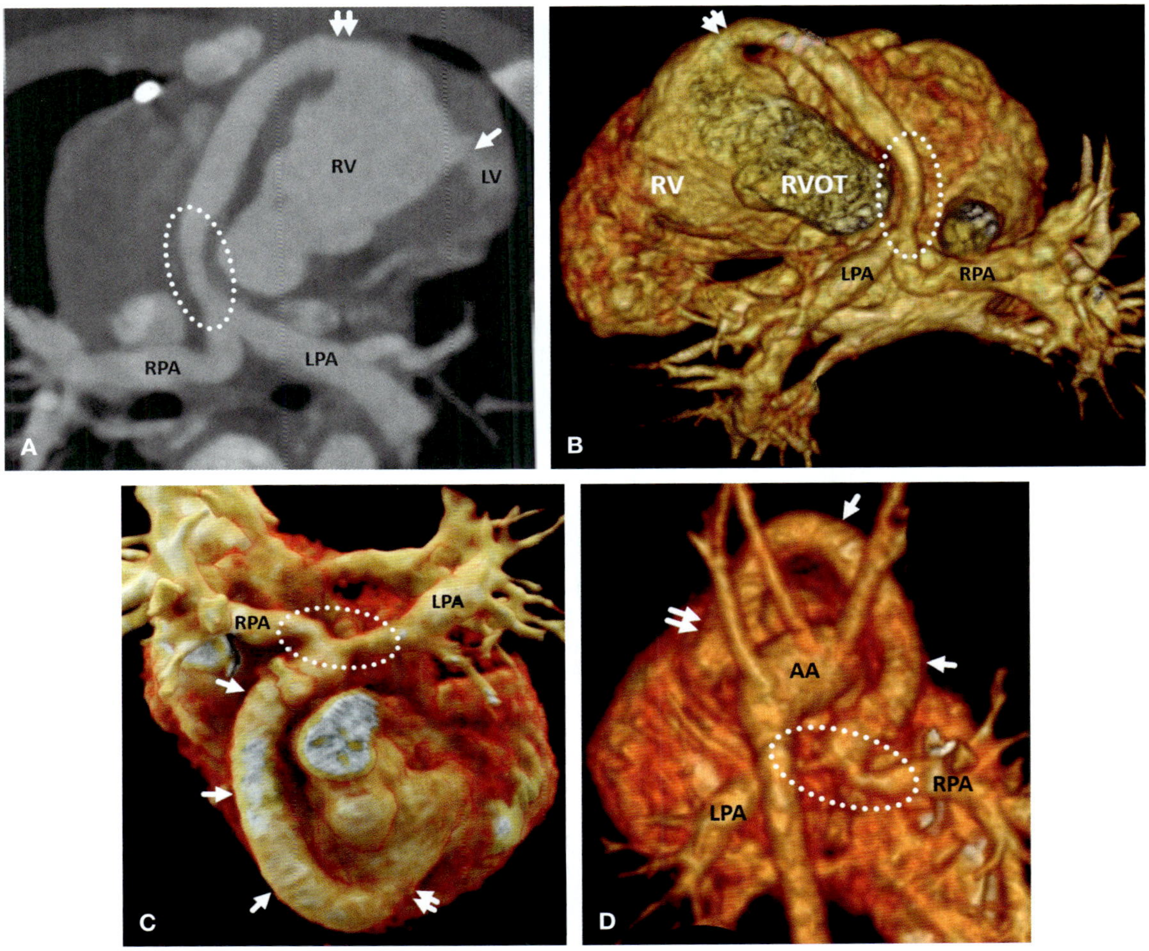

Figure 37.63. A: Young child with hypoplastic left heart syndrome, status post Damus-Kaye-Stansel (DKS) and Sano shunt. Axial oblique maximun intensity projection (MIP) shows a Sano shunt extending from the right ventricle (RV) (double arrows) to confluent right (RPA) and left (LPA) branch pulmonary arteries. The distal shunt shows at least mild narrowing (dotted elipse). The left ventricle (LV) is markedly hypoplastic and communicates via a muscular ventricular septal defect (VSD) (arrow) to the RV. **B:** 3D volume rendered CCTA view of the heart for the same patient shows the Sano shunt extending from the RV (double arrows) to confluent right (RPA) and left (LPA) branch pulmonary arteries. The distal shunt shows at least mild narrowing (dotted elipse). The RV and the right ventricular outflow tract (RVOT) has been cut away to show the course of the Sano shunt. **C:** Child with hypoplastic left heart syndrome, status post Norwood procedure and Sano shunt. 3D cinematic volume rendered CCTA reconstruction of the heart after Sano shunt shows mild to moderate stenosis at the origins of the of the right (RPA) and left (LPA) branch pulmonary arteries (dotted elipse). The Sano shunt from its origin from the RV (double arrows), throughout its course (white arrows) is widely patent. **D:** 3D volume rendered CCTA reconstruction of the heart for the same patient from the posterior view after Sano shunt shows mild to moderate stenosis at the origins of the right (RPA) and left (LPA) branch pulmonary arteries (dotted elipse). The Sano shunt from its origin from the RV (double arrows), throughout its course (white arrows), is widely patent. The neo–aortic arch (AA) is now larger caliber.

- Right coronary artery (RCA), commonly continuing as the posterior descending coronary artery

Anomalous coronary artery origins are believed to occur in approximately 1.3% of the population based on cardiac catheterization coronary angiography imaging examinations in large population studies, but it may be more prevalent, in some studies discovered in 2.33% of patients undergoing CCTA. Although a true estimate is unknown, coronary artery anomalies are believed to be more common in patients with complex CHD, the best known of these anomalies are found in patients with TGA and TOF.

Anomalous coronary artery course may lead to life-threatening events due to diminished blood flow to the myocardium. Approximately 20% of anomalous coronary arteries are the proximate cause of lethal arrhythmia, myocardial infarction, or sudden cardiac death or non-life-threatening syncope or chest pain due to narrowing of the coronary

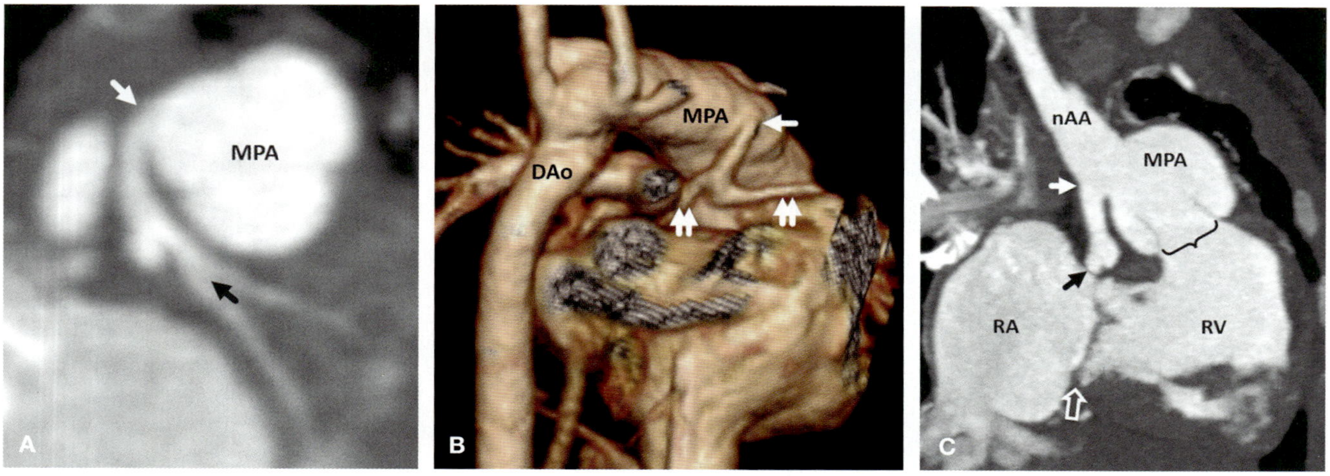

Figure 37.64. **A:** Young child with hypoplastic left heart syndrome, status post Damus-Kaye-Stansel (DKS) and Blalock-Taussig-Thomas shunt (BTTS). DKS is an end-to-side anastomosis (white arrow) of the hypoplastic ascending aorta to the main pulmonary artery (MPA). Axial oblique CCTA view just above the pulmonic valve, in the proximal MPA. The markedly hypoplastic ascending aorta (AAo) is anastomosed to the MPA (white arrow). The coronary arteries (black arrow) are approximately the same caliber as the AAo. **B:** 3D volume rendered reconstruction from the same patient shows the DKS anastomosis site (white arrow) and the bifurcation of the AAo to the coronary arteries (double arrows). The MPA remains contiguous with the descending aorta (DAo) as the ductus arteriosus is patent by infusion of prostaglandin, stenting, or reconstruction with a conduit. **C:** Infant with hypoplastic left heart syndrome, status post DKS and BTTS. The atretic aortic valve (black arrow) does not communicate with a cardiac chamber. The markedly hypoplastic AAo is anastomosed to the MPA (white arrow) in an end-to-side DKS manner. Distal to this anastomosis the MPA is now the neo–ascending aorta (nAA). The right-sided heart structures are normal size, the right atrium (RA), tricuspid valve (open arrow), right ventricle (RV), and pulmonary valve plane (bracket).

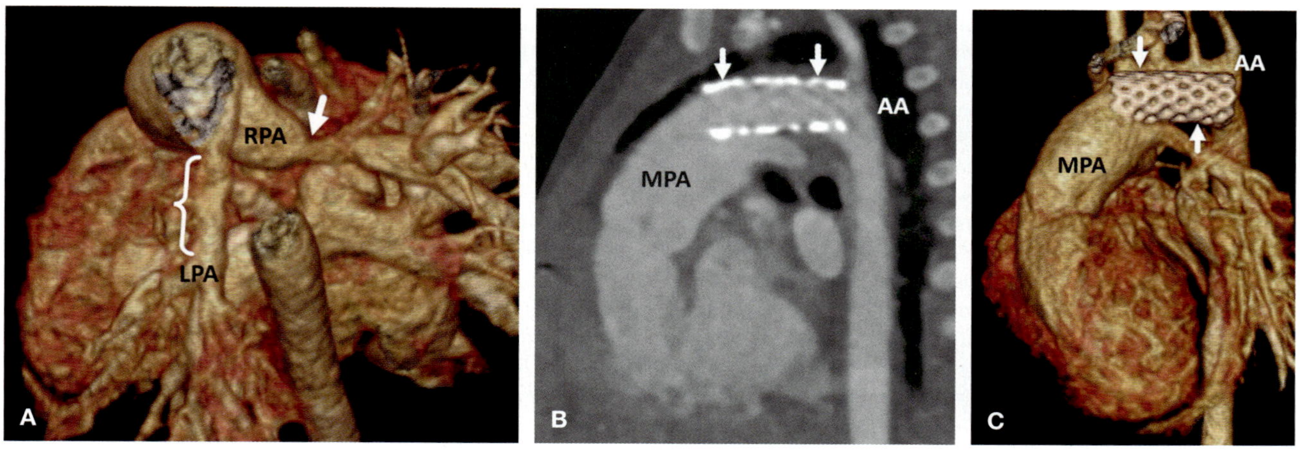

Figure 37.65. Child with hypoplastic left heart syndrome, status post hybrid procedure. **A:** 3D volume rendered CCTA shows focal narrowing of the branch right pulmonary artery (RPA) (white arrow), which also shows mild proximal dilation. The band location and narrowing of the left pulmonary artery (LPA) are not obvious (bracket). **B:** Sagittal oblique maximum intensity projection (MIP) CCTA image of the ductus arteriosus between the main pulmonary artery (MPA) and the distal aortic arch (AA) shows the stent placed to maintain ductal patency (arrows). **C:** 3D volume rendered CCTA image of the heart shows the stent (white arrows) in the ductus arteriosus between the MPA and the partially obscured distal AA.

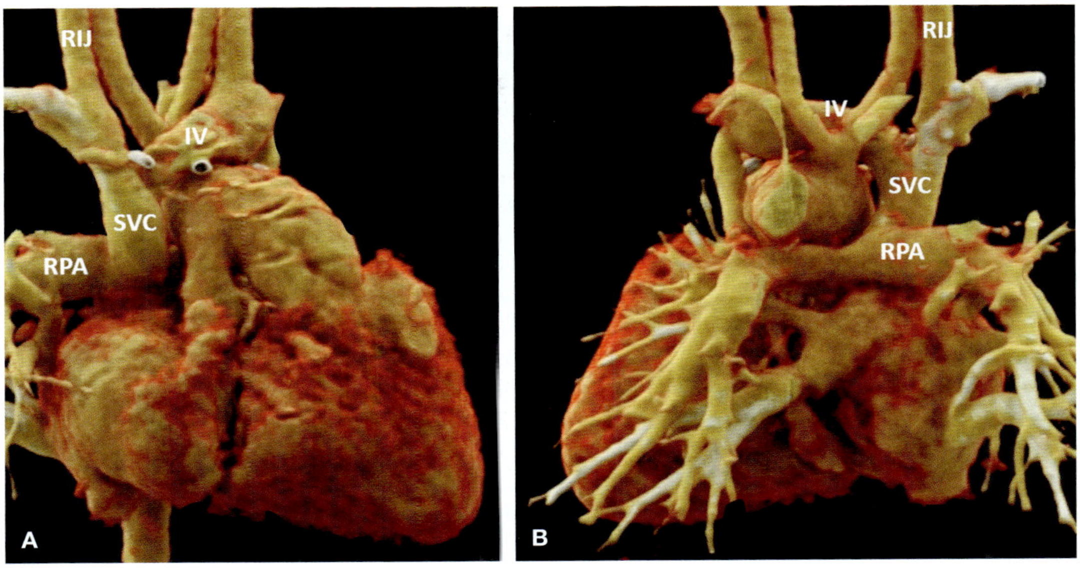

Figure 37.66. Child with hypoplastic left heart syndrome, status post Damus-Kaye-Stansel anastomosis, now status post Blalock-Taussig-Thomas shunt takedown and Glenn shunt. **A:** 3D cinematic volume rendered CCTA of the heart shows the right internal jugular (RIJ) vein and the innominate vein (IV) drain to the superior vena cava (SVC), which has been anastomosed with the right pulmonary artery (RPA), the Glenn shunt. **B:** 3D cinematic volume rendered CCTA of the heart from posterior shows the RIJ vein and the IV drain to the SVC, which has been anastomosed with the RPA, the Glenn shunt.

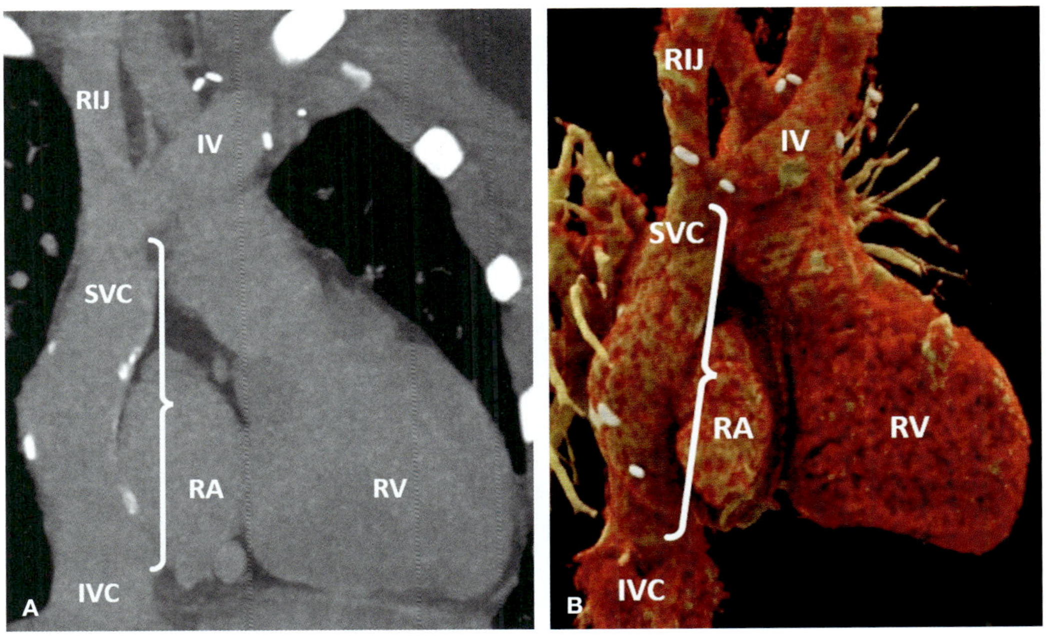

Figure 37.67. Preteen with hypoplastic left heart syndrome, status post Norwood procedure, now extracardiac Fontan. **A:** Coronal CCTA maximum intensity projection shows an extra cardiac conduit (bracket) from the superior vena cava (SVC) to the inferior vena cava (IVC), the Fontan circuit, which delivers deoxygenated blood to the pulmonary arteries, which are out of view. The conduit material shows foci of calcification, a common finding, and no stenosis. In this patient with hypoplastic left heart syndrome the right ventricle (RV) is the single ventricle that delivers blood to the systemic circulation. **B:** 3D cinematic volume rendered CCTA of the heart shows an extra cardiac conduit (bracket) from the SVC to the IVC, the Fontan circuit, which delivers deoxygenated blood to the pulmonary arteries, which are out of view. The RV is the single ventricle that delivers blood to the systemic circulation.

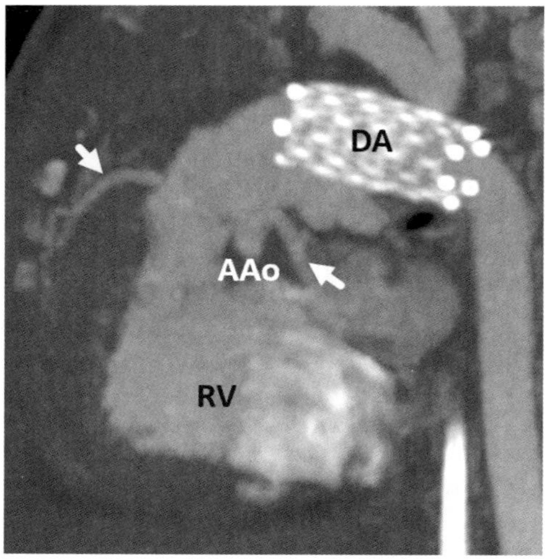

Figure 37.68. Preteen with hypoplastic left heart syndrome, status post Damus-Kaye-Stansel anastomosis and stenting of the ductus arteriosus, now with extracardiac Fontan. Sagittal oblique CCTA maximum intensity projection image shows a metallic stent in the ductus arteriosus (DA), used to maintain patency of the ductus, which is vital to maintain retrograde flow to supply the hypoplastic ascending aorta (AAo) and the coronary arteries (white arrows). In this patient with hypoplastic left heart syndrome the right ventricle (RV) is the single ventricle that delivers blood to the systemic circulation.

artery lumen leading to reduction in antegrade blood flow. The proximal course of an anomalous RCA, LMCA, or LAD from its contralateral sinus is important as the coronary artery may travel within the wall of the AAo (intramural) or course in the space between the AAo and the MPA (extramural). Historical terminology to describe the course of the proximal segment of a coronary artery with an anomalous origin as "benign" or "malignant" is no longer germane. By describing the anomalous course of the coronary artery as intramural or extramural we provide important diagnostic information, indicating that an intramural coronary artery is likely to lead to diminished blood flow to the myocardium as an intramural coronary segment becomes stretched and narrowed in the wall of the AAo resulting in restricted blood flow, while an extramural coronary artery segment will not experience blood flow restriction.

ECG triggering and timing of CCTA image acquisition of the coronary arteries is best performed in diastole at low heart rates. In infants and young children who have high heart rates (≥120 beats per minute), the length of the diastasis period shortens and the systolic period of isovolumetric contraction lengthens, which makes end-systole the more desired phase of image acquisition. When appropriate, heart rate control with beta blockers can be helpful for decreasing the heart rate to the desired rate of 60 to 70 beats per minute in older children, adolescents, and adults. This low heart rate is not a realistic goal in newborns, infants, and young children, however.

Newborns and Infants

When associated with complex CHD such as TGA, TOF, or truncus arteriosus, CCTA may be used to confirm the native coronary artery origin anatomy in newborns and infants prior to surgery (Fig. 37.88A and B). In 99% of patients with TGA the RCA and LMCA arise from sinuses of Valsalva that "face" the MPA (Fig. 37.89). It is important to the surgeon to know that the coronary artery anatomy is as expected because reimplantation of coronary artery origins from

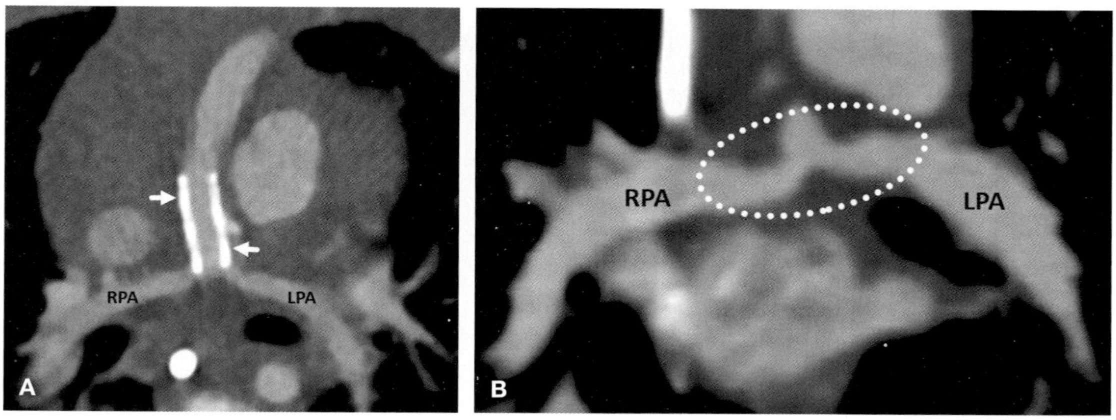

Figure 37.69. A: Child with hypoplastic left heart syndrome, status post Norwood procedure and Sano shunt. Axial oblique maximum intensity projection reconstruction of a patient with treated Sano shunt stenosis. A stent (white arrows) has been placed in the distal Sano shunt. At least mild stenosis of the origins of the branch right (RPA) and left (LPA) pulmonary arteries is seen. **B:** Young child with hypoplastic left heart syndrome, status post Damus-Kaye-Stansel and Sano shunt. Axial oblique curved planar CCTA reconstruction of the branch pulmonary arteries after Sano shunt shows ostium stenosis of the right (RPA) and left (LPA) branch pulmonary arteries (dotted ellipse).

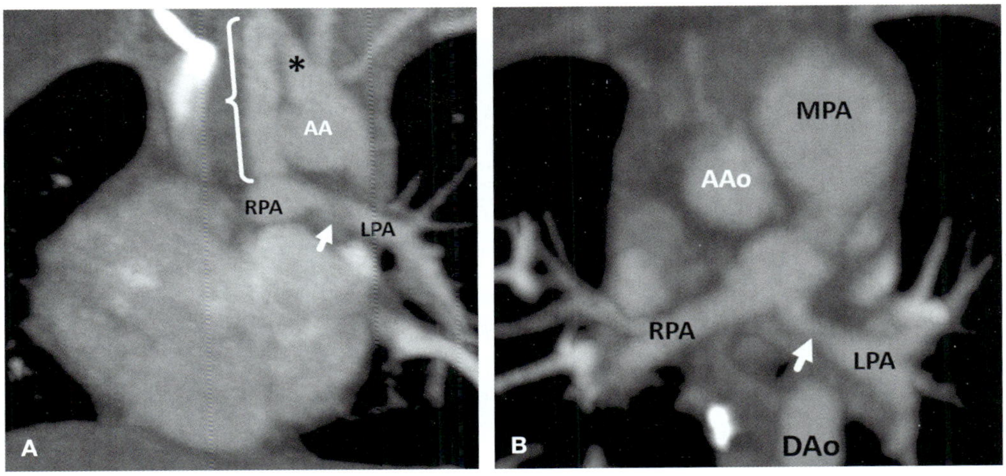

Figure 37.70. Infant with hypoplastic left heart syndrome, status post Damus-Kaye-Stansel side-to-side anastomosis of the ascending aorta to the main pulmonary artery and Blalock-Taussig-Thomas shunt (BTTS), left pulmonary artery (LPA) stenosis. **A:** Coronal CCTA maximum intensity projection (MIP) image of the BTTS shows mild narrowing of the proximal LPA lumen (white arrow). The BTTS (bracket) connecting the right brachiocephalic artery (asterisk) and the origin of the right pulmonary artery (RPA). **B:** Axial CCTA MIP image confirms mild narrowing of the proximal LPA lumen (white arrow). The RPA is normal caliber.

the native AAo to the native MPA (nee, the neoascending aorta) is performed in the most common surgical palliation of TGA, the ASO (Jatene). Coronary artery origin and proximal course in patients with TOF is crucial as approximately 0.7% of patients with TOF will have a dual LAD or a segment of the LAD coronary artery that arises from the RCA, which then courses across the RVOT to the anterior intraventricular septum. When present, an anomalous LAD segment overlying the RVOT may interfere in performing a commonly used procedure for palliation of TOF, transannular patch, which opens the stenotic pulmonary valve and MPA. When an anomalous LAD is present, an alternative procedure, RV to branch pulmonary artery shunt (RV to PA conduit) may be performed.

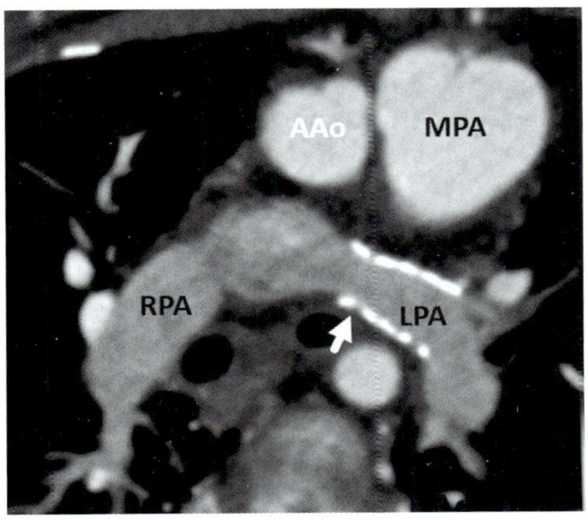

Figure 37.71. Preteen with hypoplastic left heart syndrome, status post Damus-Kaye-Stansel (DKS) side-to-side anastomosis of the ascending aorta to the main pulmonary artery and Blalock-Taussig-Thomas shunt (BTTS), left pulmonary artery (LPA) stenosis. Axial CCTA maximum intensity projection shows a metallic stent (arrow) in the LPA, used to maintain patency of the ductus, which is vital to maintain retrograde flow to supply the hypoplastic ascending aorta (AAo) and the coronary arteries.

Neonates and newborns with complex, acyanotic CHD, pulmonary valve atresia with intact ventricular septum, may present with RV-dependent coronary artery circulation, a phenomenon of abnormal coronary artery development in which the coronary arteries form sinusoids, coursing through the myocardium, communicate with the RV chamber. CCTA is not a reliable imaging modality for diagnosis or confirmation of this diagnosis, but the condition may be partially visible as abnormal enhancement of the myocardium.

A very rare type of coronary artery origin anomaly of the LMCA, arising from the pulmonary artery (ALCAPA), also known by the eponym Bland-White-Garland syndrome, or RCA arising from the pulmonary artery (ARCAPA) may be discovered on echo and confirmed using CCTA, typically during an investigation of cardiomegaly and heart failure in neonates and young children (Fig. 37.90A-D). It is unusual to discover ALCAPA in older patients as survival of this coronary anomaly is poor (Fig. 37.91A-D).

Young Children, Early Teens, and Adults

Symptoms of coronary artery anomalies, those of anomalous origin and course, usually do not become evident until late childhood or adolescence, when a child's level of physical activity, often in competitive sports activities, increases. Therefore, unless there is a reason to image the coronary arteries based on a known underlying diagnosis of CHD or discovered or

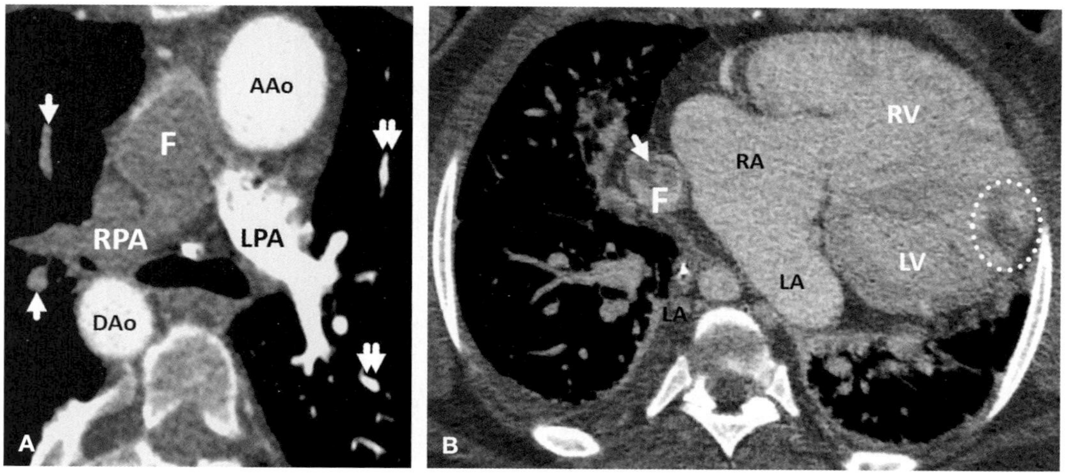

Figure 37.72. Complications are not uncommon in patients with Fontan physiology. **A:** Adult with Fontan physiology, known anatomy of persistent left superior vena cava, right aortic arch, and suspected pulmonary artery embolism. Axial CCTA was performed following peripheral injection of contrast in the left upper extremity. At the level of the upper mediastinum concentrated contrast material is in the left pulmonary artery (LPA). The Fontan circuit (F) and the right pulmonary artery (RPA) show no intraluminal enhancement secondary to thrombosis. Pulmonary artery embolization is seen in peripheral branches of the RPA (white arrows). Peripheral branches of the LPA enhance normally (double white arrows). **B:** Adult with Fontan physiology was found to have partial thrombosis of the Fontan circuit. Axial CCTA was performed following peripheral injection of contrast, at a 120-second delay in order to allow for circulation of contrast to the Fontan circuit. The level of the lower margin of the extracardiac Fontan circuit (F) shows filling defect within the lumen, indicating partial thrombosis (white arrow). Thrombus is also in the left ventricle (LV) apex (dotted ellipse).

suspected on echocardiography performed for other reasons, a coronary artery anomaly that is not symptomatic may not be discovered until childhood, the teenage years, or adulthood.

The anatomy of the coronary artery origin and course anomalies most often found in symptomatic patients include

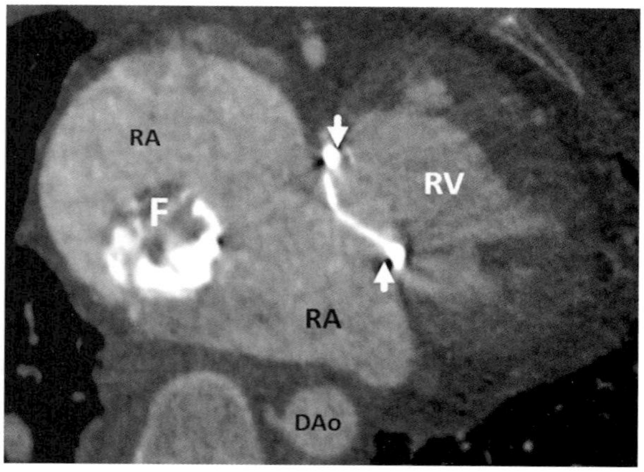

Figure 37.73. Complications are not uncommon in patients with Fontan physiology. Adult with Fontan physiology, atrioventricular valve prosthesis, and suspected pulmonary artery embolism. Axial CCTA was performed following dual contrast injection, peripheral upper extremity and centrally through femoral vein access. At the level of the heart the intracardiac Fontan circuit (F) shows incomplete enhancement of the lumen secondary to partial thrombosis. The St. Jude valve prosthesis is at the atrioventricular valve position (arrows).

RCA from the left sinus of Valsalva and left main (LM) or LAD from the right sinus of Valsalva and are associated with an intramural course of the proximal segment of the coronary artery arising from an anomalous position. Symptoms are typically related to ischemia, chest pain (usually exertional), arrhythmia resulting from conduction abnormalities, and atrioventricular valve regurgitation related to myocardial ischemia, damage to conduction pathways, and/or papillary muscle involvement (Figs. 37.92A-C and 37.93A-C).

Anomalies of coronary artery termination in young children and children in early teenage years may be known because of previous imaging such as survivors of TGA, TOF, or pulmonary artery atresia with intact ventricular septum but may also be discovered.

- Anomalies of coronary artery origin
  - RCA from the left sinus of Valsalva
  - LMCA from the right sinus of Valsalva
  - Right or left main coronary artery from the noncoronary sinus of Valsalva
  - Right or left main coronary artery from the AAo (above the sinus of Valsalva)
  - Right or left main coronary artery from the pulmonary artery
  - Dual LAD coronary artery
  - Single coronary artery
  - Coronary artery origins in TGA
    - Right and left main coronary arteries from right- and left-facing sinuses of Valsalva

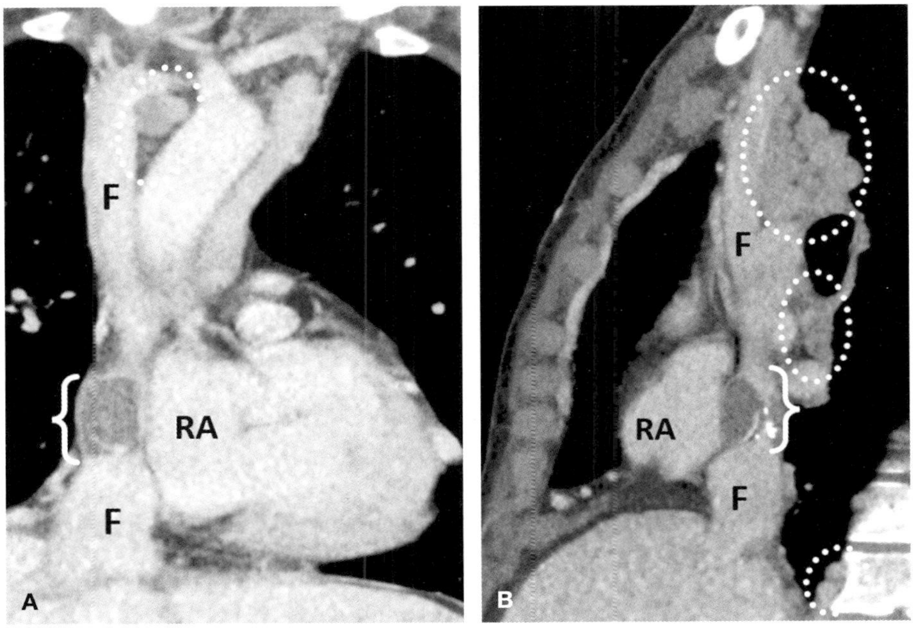

Figure 37.74. Adult with Fontan physiology and suspected Fontan circuit thrombus on echocardiography. **A:** Coronal CCTA was performed following peripheral upper extremity contrast injection.The Fontan circuit (F) shows a filling defect (bracket) in the circuit at the level of the right atrium (RA), representing partial thrombosis. Nodular enhancing densities in the superior mediastinum (dotted ellipse) are prominent venoveno collaterals that were seen throughout the mediastinum. **B:** Sagittal CCTA shows nodular enhancing densities at multiple locations in the mediastinum (dotted ellipses) are prominent venoveno collaterals, seen throughout the mediastinum.

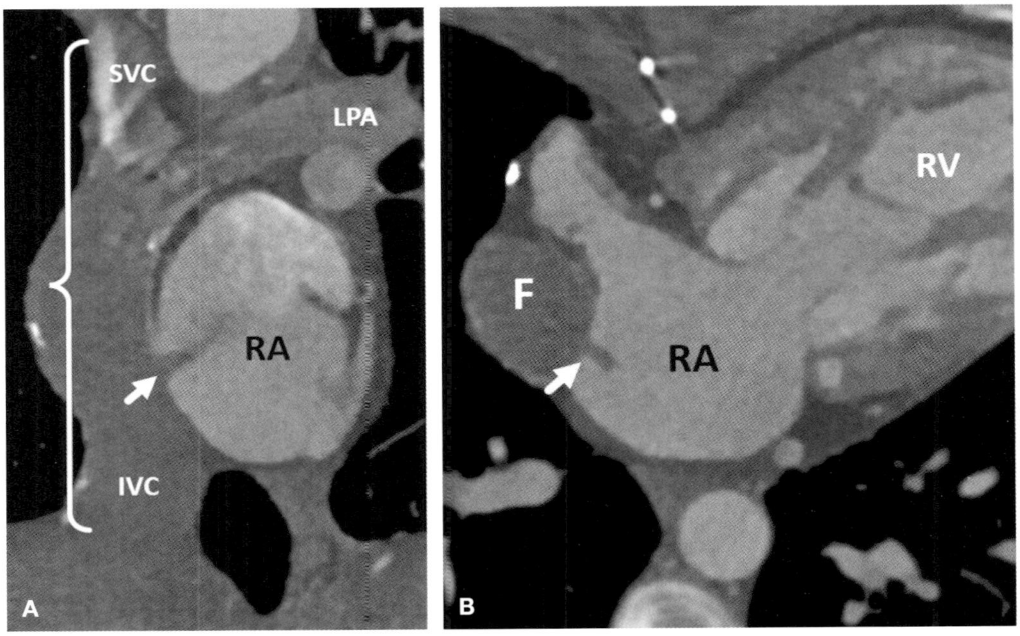

Figure 37.75. Preteen with hypoplastic left heart syndrome, status post Damus-Kaye-Stansel side-to-side anastomosis of the ascending aorta to the main pulmonary artery and fenestrated Fontan. **A:** Coronal CCTA image of the Fontan circuit (bracket) shows the superior (SVC) and inferior vena cavae (IVC) and left pulmonary artery (LPA) connections of the circuit. Non-contrast-enhanced blood decompresses pressure in the Fontan circuit, into the right atrium (RA), through a surgically created fenestration (arrow). **B:** Axial CCTA image of heart shows the extracardiac position of the Fontan circuit (F). Non-contrast-enhanced blood in the Fontan circuit decompresses pressure into the right atrium (RA), through a surgically created fenestration (arrow) that is performed to allow a "pop-off valve" to relieve pressure in the Fontan circuit and downstream venous structures.

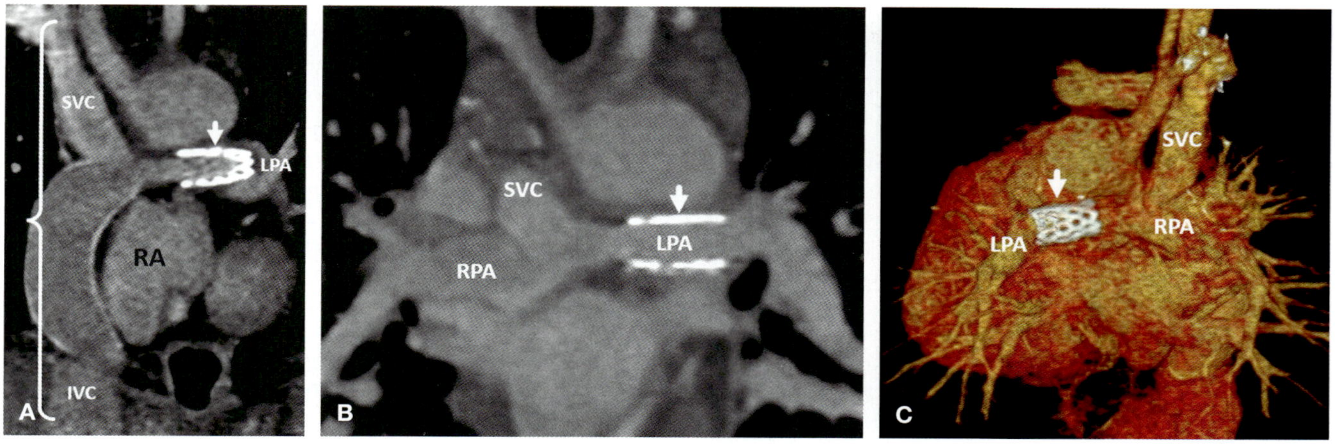

Figure 37.76. Left pulmonary artery (LPA) stenosis after Fontan. **A:** Adolescent with hypoplastic left heart syndrome, status post Fontan, and LPA stenosis stent. Coronal CCTA image of the Fontan circuit (bracket) shows the superior (SVC) and inferior vena cavae (IVC) and LPA connections of the circuit, and the metallic stent (white arrow) placed to treat LPA stenosis. **B:** Child with hypoplastic left heart syndrome, status post Glenn shunt, and LPA stenosis, now stented. Coronal oblique CCTA image shows the SVC and right (RPA) and left (LPA) pulmonary artery connections with the SVC. The metallic stent (white arrow) was placed to treat LPA stenosis. **C:** Child with hypoplastic left heart syndrome, status post Glenn shunt, and LPA stenosis, now stented. 3D reconstructed CCTA of the posterior view of the heart shows the SVC and right (RPA) and left (LPA) pulmonary artery connections with the SVC. The metallic stent (white arrow) was placed to treat LPA stenosis.

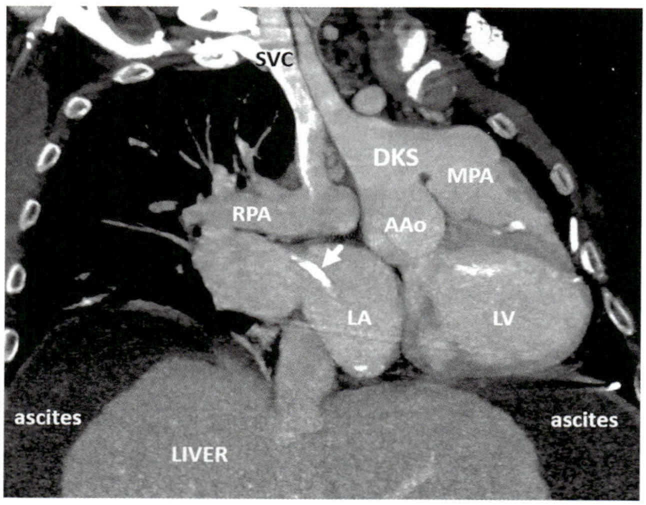

Figure 37.77. Adult with history of double inlet left ventricle, another form of congenital heart disease in which a single ventricle is present, status post Damus-Kaye-Stansel (DKS) and Fontan. Coronal oblique maximum intensity projection CCTA image of the heart, mediastinum, and upper abdomen shows the superior vena cava (SVC) and right pulmonary artery (RPA). The left pulmonary artery (LPA) and the rest of the Fontan circuit are out of the image plane. The DKS anastomosis of the main pulmonary artery (MPA) and ascending aorta (AAo) is patent. High-attenuation artifacts (white arrow) are due to pacemaker wires. In the upper abdomen, the liver is small and has a nodular surface due to cirrhosis and a large volume of ascites surrounds the liver.

    - Right or left main coronary arteries from the nonfacing sinus of Valsalva
- Anomalies of coronary artery course
    - Extramural—between or around the great arteries
    - Intramural—in the wall of the AAo
    - Intramyocardial (Fig. 37.94A-D)
- Anomalies of coronary artery termination
    - Coronary artery fistula
    - RV-dependent coronary artery circulation

Important diagnostic imaging features of these coronary origin anomalies from the sinuses of Valsalva are shown in the following figures:

- Origin—RCA from left sinus of Valsalva, LMCA from right sinus of Valsalva, acute angle, not such an acute angle
- Course—intramural, extramural
- Lumen shape—round, elliptical
- Dominance—right dominance from an anomalous RCA origin (controversy regarding need for surgical intervention), left dominance from an anomalous LMCA origin, left dominance when the RCA origin is anomalous from left sinus of Valsalva

Very rarely, the LMCA or RCA origin arises from a pulmonary artery. The vessel then courses to the expected epicardial distribution, and the caliber of the artery is larger

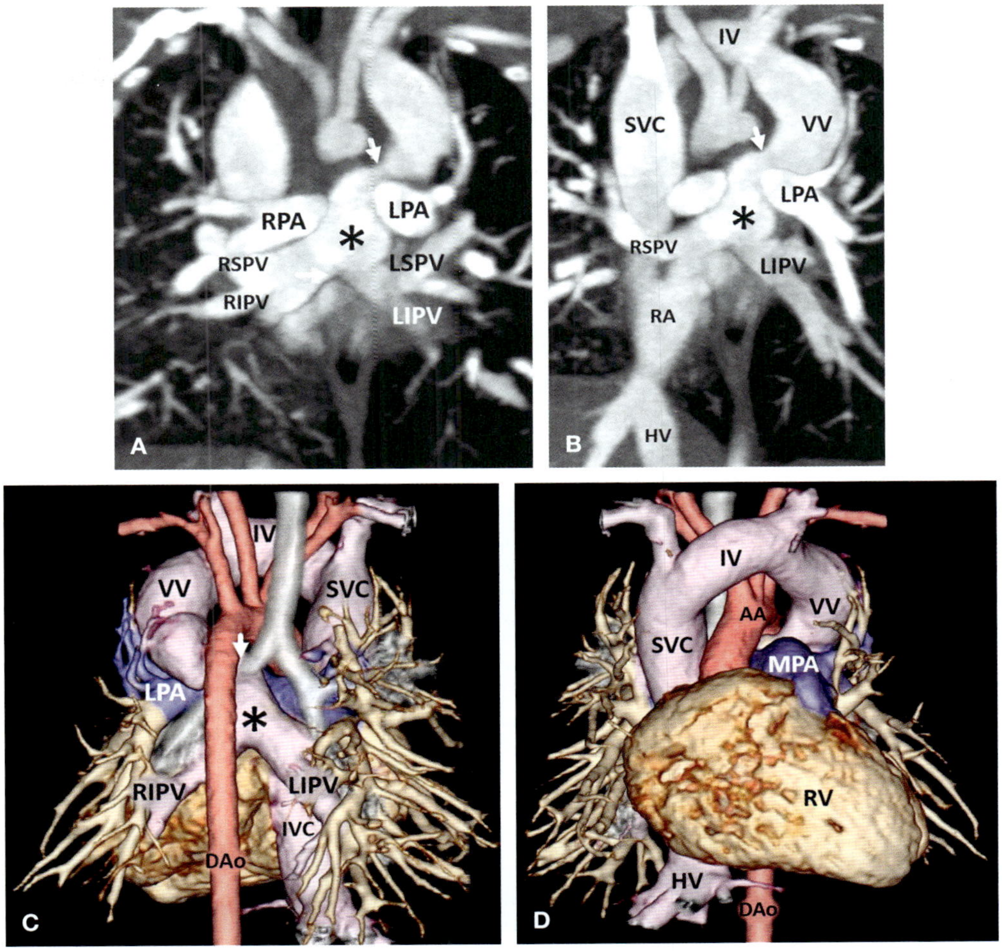

Figure 37.78. Newborn with supracardiac, obstructed, total anomalous pulmonary venous drainage. **A:** Coronal oblique maximum intensity projection (MIP) CCTA image of the heart shows the right (RSPV) and left (LSPV) superior pulmonary vein and the right (RIPV) and left (LIPV) inferior pulmonary vein drainage pattern to a confluence (asterisk), which is too small to be the left atrium. The confluence drains cephalad, narrows to a marked degree (white arrow) as it courses over the left pulmonary artery (LPA). **B:** Coronal oblique MIP CCTA image of the heart shows the RSPV and LIPV drainage pattern to a confluence (asterisk), which is too small to be the left atrium. The confluence drains cephalad, narrows to a marked degree (white arrow) as it courses over the LPA, to a left-sided vertical vein (VV), to the left innominate vein (IV), to the superior vena cava (SVC), to the right atrium (RA) along with the hepatic veins (HV). The result is drainage of all oxygenated blood to the systemic venous return rather than to the left atrium and the systemic arterial supply. An atrial or ventricular septal defect is needed in order to allow mixing of oxygenated and deoxygenated blood. **C:** 3D volume rendered CCTA view of the heart from a posterior perspective shows the RIPV and LIPV drainage pattern to a confluence (asterisk), which is too small to be the left atrium. The confluence drains cephalad, coursing over the LPA, to a left-sided VV, to the left IV and SVC. The inferior vena cava is seen, but the RA is out of view. Severe stenosis of the left main bronchus (white arrow) is due to extrinsic mass effect between the confluence drainage and the descending thoracic aorta (DAo). **D:** 3D volume rendered CCTA view of the heart shows the left-sided VV, left IV, and SVC, which joins the HVs to drain to the RA, which is out of view, hidden by the right ventricle (RV). The aortic arch (AA) and the descending thoracic aorta (DAo) are normal.

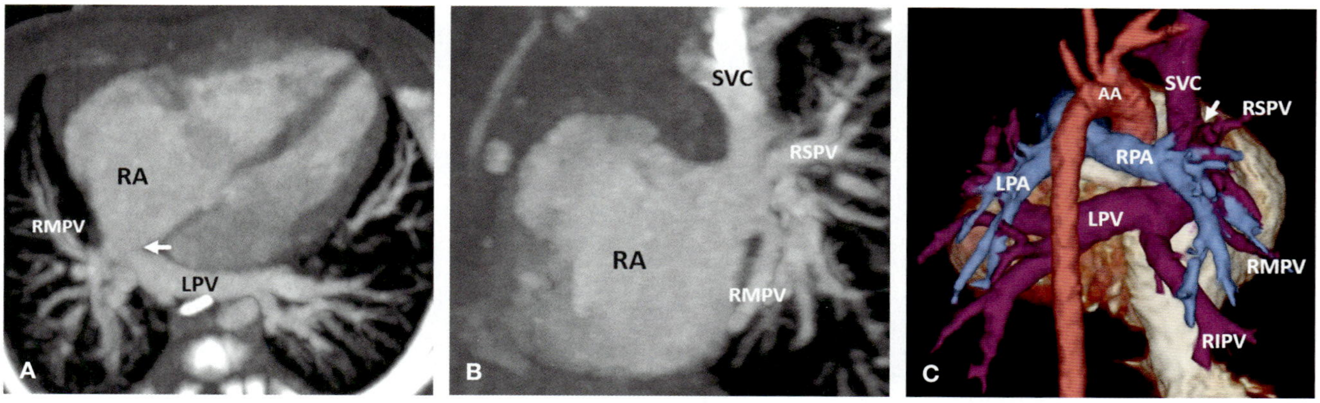

Figure 37.79. Newborn with mixed, partially obstructed, total anomalous pulmonary venous drainage. **A:** Axial oblique maximum intensity projection (MIP) CCTA image of the heart shows the left pulmonary veins (LPVs) coursing across the posterior mediastinum to a narrow opening (white arrow) to the right atrium (RA). The right middle pulmonary vein (RMPV) also drains to the RA. **B:** Sagittal oblique MIP CCTA image of the heart at the level of the superior vena cava (SVC). The right superior pulmonary vein (RSPV) drains to the SVC. **C:** 3D colorized reconstruction CCTA image of the heart shows the LPVs coursing across the posterior mediastinum and joining with the right inferior (RIPV) and right middle (RMPV) pulmonary veins before draining to the RA. The right superior pulmonary vein (RSPV) drains to the SVC (white arrow).

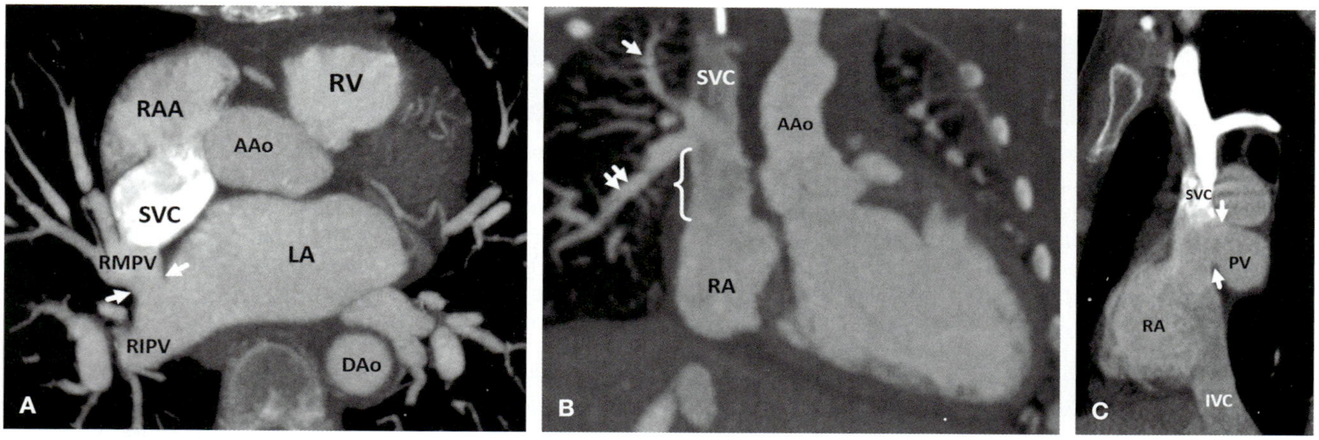

Figure 37.80. Adolescent with a murmur and desaturations has a superior sinus venosus defect on echocardiography. **A:** Axial maximum intensity projection (MIP) CCTA image of the heart shows a defect in the superior sinus venosus, which allows abnormal communication (white arrows) between the superior vena cava (SVC), right atrium (RA), which is out of the image plane, and left atrium (LA). The right atrial appendage (RAA) is dilated. Partial anomalous venous drainage of right middle (RMPV) and inferior (RIPV) pulmonary veins is associated. A defect of the superior sinus venosus is often inaccurately termed a defect of the interatrial septum, allows mixing of oxygenated and deoxygenated blood at the atrial level. **B:** Coronal MIP CCTA image of the heart shows a right upper lobe (white arrow) and right middle lobe (white double arrows) pulmonary veins draining to the SVC. A finding commonly associated with a superior sinus venosus defect. A measurement between the pulmonary veins and the cavoatrial junction (bracket) should be included in CCTA reports. C. Sagittal MIP CCTA image of the SVC shows a defect of the superior sinus venosus (white arrows), which allows abnormal communication between the SVC, RA, and right-sided pulmonary veins (PVs). A defect of the superior sinus venosus is often inaccurately termed a defect of the interatrial septum, allows mixing of oxygenated and deoxygenated blood at the atrial level.

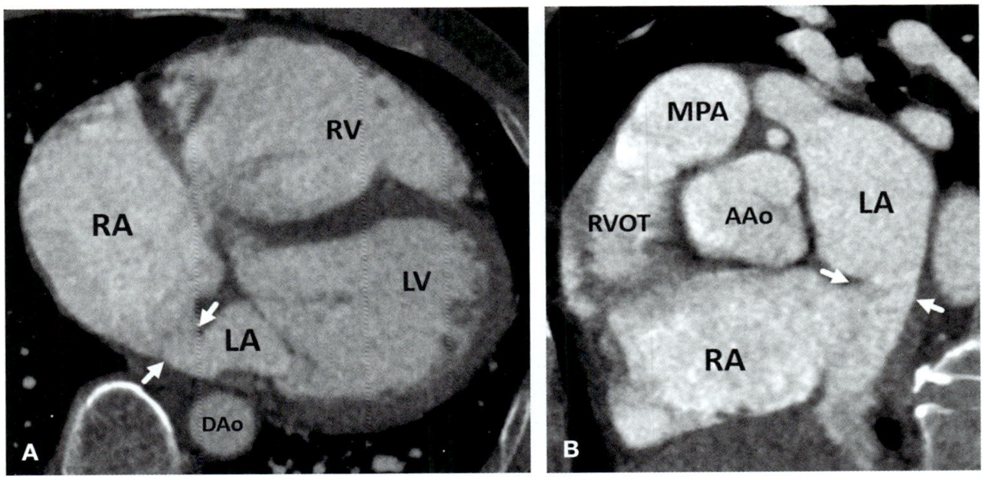

Figure 37.81. Child with a murmur and desaturations has an inferior sinus venosus defect. **A:** Axial maximum intensity projection (MIP) CCTA image of the heart shows a defect in the inferior sinus venosus that allows abnormal communication (white arrows) between the right (RA) and left (LA) atria. Left-to-right shunting through the defect results in enlargement of the right-sided heart chambers, the RA, and right ventricle (RV). The inferior sinus venosus extends from the left portal vein to the inferior vena cava, draining to the right atrium. A defect of the sinus venosus allows mixing of oxygenated and deoxygenated blood at the atrial level. **B:** Sagittal MIP CCTA image of the heart shows the defect in the inferior sinus venosus that allows abnormal communication (white arrows) between the RA and LA. Left-to-right shunting through the defect results in enlargement of the right-sided heart chambers. The inferior sinus venosus extends from the left portal vein to the inferior vena cava, draining to the right atrium. A defect of the sinus venosus allows mixing of oxygenated and deoxygenated blood at the atrial level.

than a normal coronary artery as blood flow is reversed away from the myocardium to the lower pressure pulmonary vascular system, ie, a steal of oxygenated blood from the myocardium is the pathophysiology that leads to arrhythmias, myocardial ischemia, and chest pain.

Diagnostic findings of anomalous coronary artery origin from a pulmonary artery are shown in the following figures:

- Anomalous coronary artery origin from the left pulmonary artery (ALCAPA)
- Anomalous coronary artery origin from the right pulmonary artery (ARCAPA)

Other anomalies of coronary artery origin are frequently seen on CCTA examinations but are not considered to be the cause of chest pain, arrhythmia, or myocardial ischemia. Although seen in patients without CHD, these are also more prevalent in patients with CHD. CCTA images show these features:

- LMCA or RCA from the noncoronary sinus of Valsalva, with retroaortic course to the usual epicardial distribution
- Anomalous origin of the LMCA with transseptal course to the epicardial surface and division to the LAD and LCx
- Origin of the LMCA or RCA from the AAo, above the sinuses of Valsalva, and expected course to the usual distribution
- Side-by-side separate origins of the LAD and LCx from the left sinus of Valsalva

ARTIFICIAL INTELLIGENCE

AI can be defined as a computer system that can extract information from the environment and use it to achieve a specific goal in a process that mimics the cognitive function of humans, but without human intervention. Machine learning is the subfield of AI in which an agent (a program or algorithm) learns from data without being explicitly programmed to do so. Deep learning is one of such algorithms that uses neural networks, and it is the basis of most AI tools for image interpretation.

AI is a field that has expanded rapidly in the past decade, with multiple applications in medical imaging, including in CT imaging for CHD. For example, segmentation of vessels and cardiac structures is a labor-intensive and time-consuming process for postprocessing CT images. Automatic segmentation of structures is a task suitable for AI applications, with intensive research currently being performed in medical and nonmedical imaging fields. In addition to automatic image segmentation,

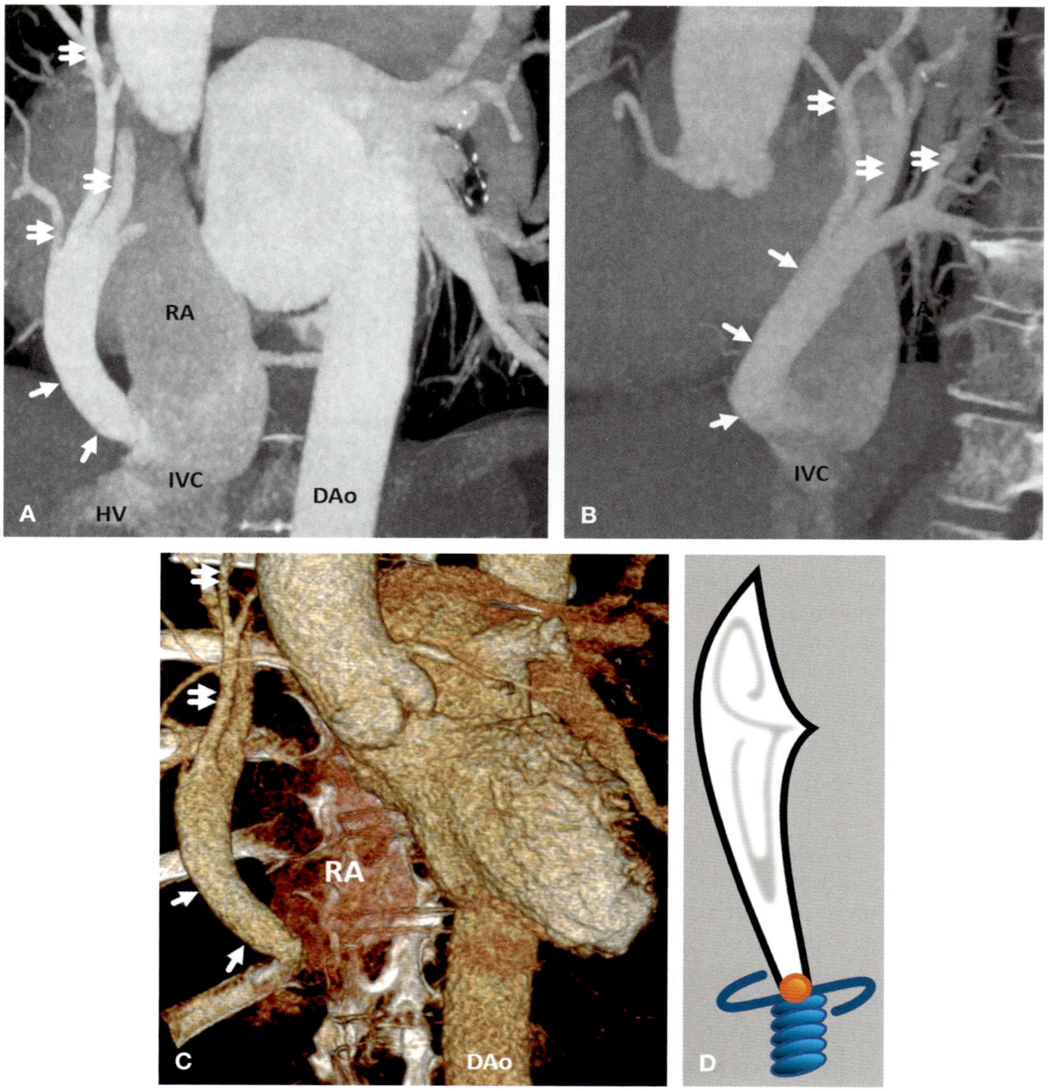

Figure 37.82. Adolescent with right-sided scimitar vein, partial anomalous pulmonary venous connection. **A:** Coronal oblique maximum intensity projection (MIP) CCTA image of the chest shows right pulmonary veins (white double arrows) draining via an anomalous venous connection (white arrows) to the hepatic vein (HV)/ inferior vena cava (IVC) junction, which subsequently drains to the right atrium (RA). **B:** Sagittal oblique MIP CCTA image of the chest shows right pulmonary veins (white double arrows) draining via an anomalous venous connection (white arrows) to the HV/IVC junction, which subsequently drains to the RA. **C:** 3D volume rendered CCTA view of the heart shows right pulmonary veins (white double arrows) draining via an anomalous venous connection (white arrows) to the HV/IVC junction, which subsequently drains to the RA, which is out of view. **D:** Illustration of a scimitar, a short sword with a curved blade. An anomalous pulmonary vein, draining to the HVs and IVC has a curvature that is similar to the curved blade of a scimitar.

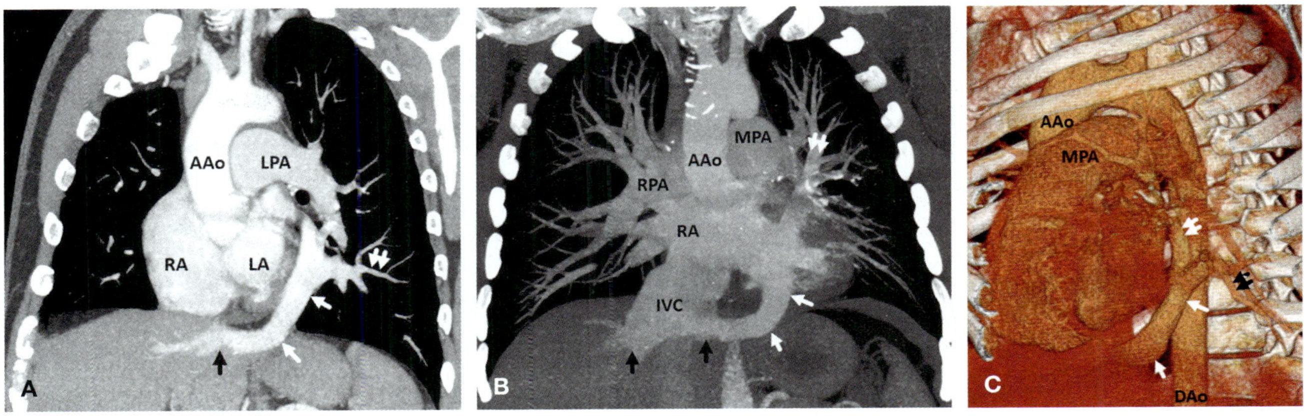

Figure 37.83. Adolescent with left-sided scimitar vein, partial anomalous pulmonary venous connection. **A:** Sagittal oblique maximum intensity projection (MIP) CCTA image of the chest shows a left lower lobe pulmonary vein (white double arrows) draining to an anomalous venous connection (white arrows) to a hepatic vein (black arrow), which subsequently drained to the right atrium (RA). The left pulmonary artery (LPA) and ascending aorta (AAo) anatomy is normal. **B:** Coronal oblique MIP CCTA image of the chest shows a left lower lobe pulmonary vein (white double arrows) draining from the apical segment to an anomalous venous connection (white arrows) to hepatic veins (black arrows), and subsequently to the RA. The main (MPA) and right pulmonary artery (RPA) and AAo anatomy is normal. **C:** Left anterior oblique MIP CCTA image of the chest shows a left lower lobe pulmonary vein (black double arrows) and a vein draining from the apical segment (white double arrows) to an anomalous venous connection (white arrows) to below the diaphragm. The MPA and the ascending (AAo) and descending (DAo) aorta anatomy is normal.

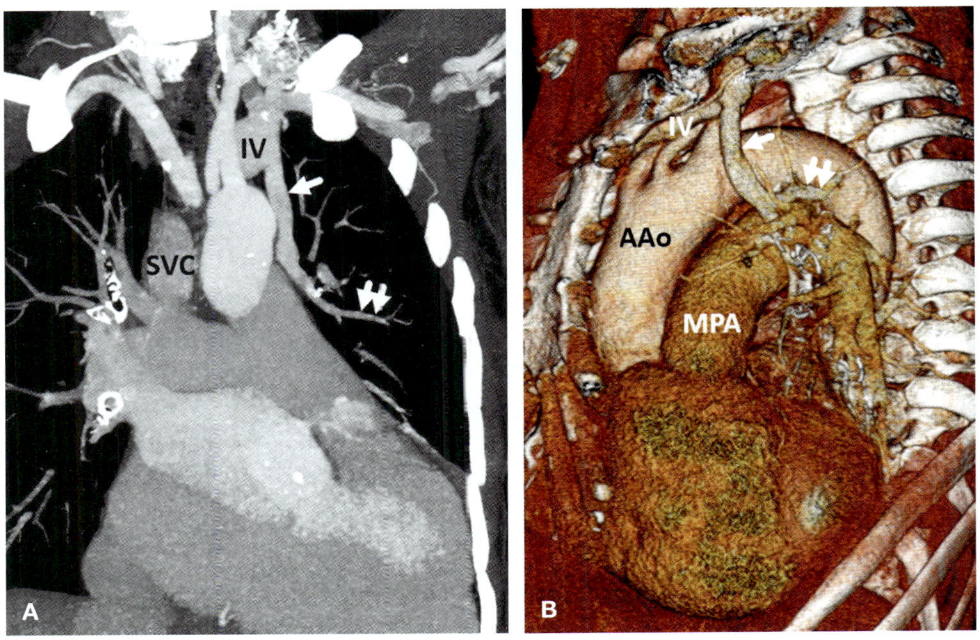

Figure 37.84. Adult with no known congenital cardiac history was found to have an abnormal vein, partial anomalous pulmonary venous connection, on echocardiography. CCTA was performed to investigate this further. **A:** Coronal maximum intensity projection CCTA image of the heart shows a vein draining from the left upper lobe (white double arrow) via a vertical vein (white arrow) to the left innominate vein (IV), and eventually to the superior vena cava (SVC) and right atrium. **B:** 3D volume rendered CCTA left anterior oblique view of the heart shows a vein draining from the left upper lobe (white double arrow) via a vertical vein (white arrow) to the left IV, which courses over the aortic arch and brachiocephalic arteries. The ascending aorta (AAo) and main pulmonary artery (MPA) anatomy is normal.

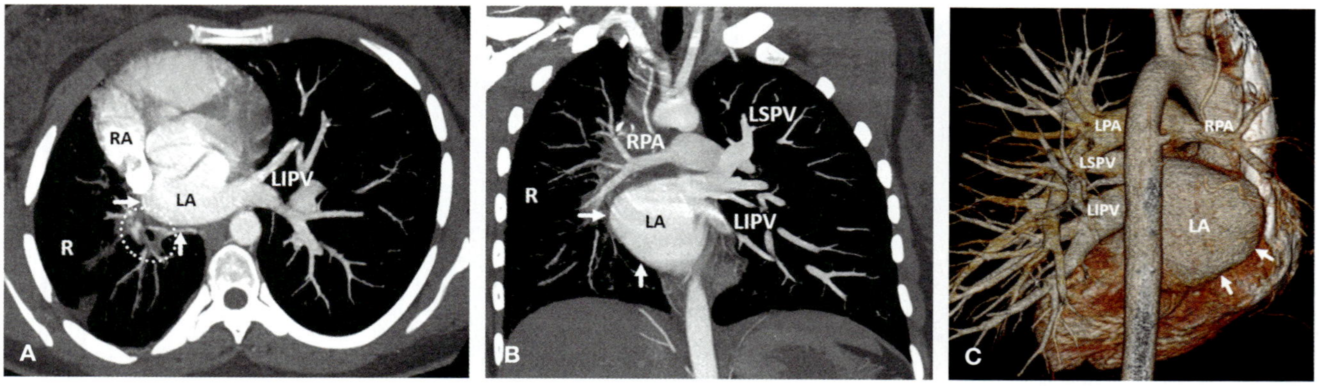

Figure 37.85. Adult with unilateral left pulmonary veins, absent right pulmonary veins, and hypoplasia of the right pulmonary artery (RPA) and right lung. **A:** Axial maximum intensity projection (MIP) CCTA image of the heart shows the normal left inferior pulmonary vein (LIPV) draining to the left side of the left atrium (LA) and absence of right pulmonary veins (white arrows) on the rightward, posterior wall of the LA. The tiny-caliber vessels behind the LA may represent anomalous veins draining the right lung (dotted ellipse). The heart is dextroposed to the right, and the right lung (R) is hypoplastic. **B:** Coronal MIP CCTA image of the heart shows the normal left superior (LSPV) and inferior (LIPV) pulmonary veins draining to the left side of the LA and absence of right pulmonary veins (white arrows) on the rightward, posterior wall of the LA. The RPA is small caliber, and the right lung (R) is hypoplastic. **C:** 3D volume rendered CCTA view of the heart from a posterior perspective shows the normal LSPV and LIPV draining to the left side of the LA and absence of right pulmonary veins (white arrows) on the rightward, posterior wall of the LA. The RPA is small caliber compared with the normal left pulmonary artery (LPA).

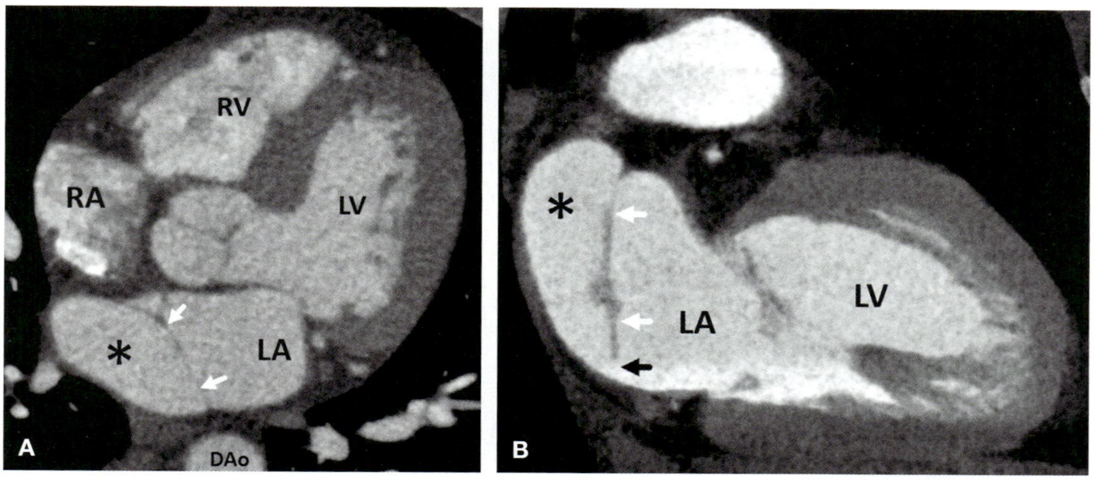

Figure 37.86. Cor triatriatum sinister. An adolescent with an abnormality seen on echocardiography for an unrelated reason was found to have a septation dividing the left atrium (LA). **A:** Axial CCTA image of the heart shows a thin membrane (white arrows) separating the portion of the LA (asterisk) that receives pulmonary venous drainage, from the portion of the LA that drains through the mitral valve to the left ventricle (LV). The right atrium (RA) and right ventricle (RV) are normal. **B:** Sagittal CCTA image of the heart shows a thin membrane (white arrows) separating the portion of the LA (asterisk) that receives pulmonary venous drainage from the rest of the LA. A defect in the membrane (black arrow) allows drainage of pulmonary venous blood into the rest of the LA and through the mitral valve to the LV.

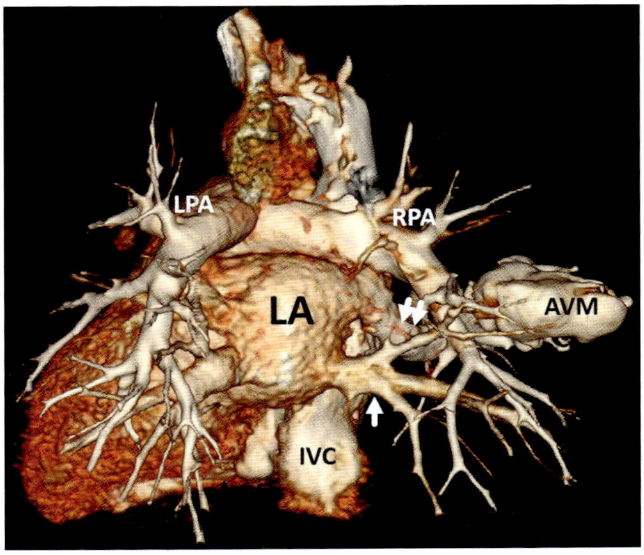

Figure 37.87. Adolescent with desaturation and positive bubble study on echocardiography. 3D reconstructed CCTA image of the heart from a posterior view with the descending aorta cut away to optimally show the left atrium (LA) and the pulmonary veins. The right (RPA) and left (LPA) branch pulmonary arteries are symmetric. Branches of the RPA supply a nidus of a pulmonary arteriovenous malformation (AVM). The venous drainage of the AVM is to the left superior pulmonary vein (white double arrows), which is large caliber. The left inferior pulmonary vein (white arrow) is normal caliber.

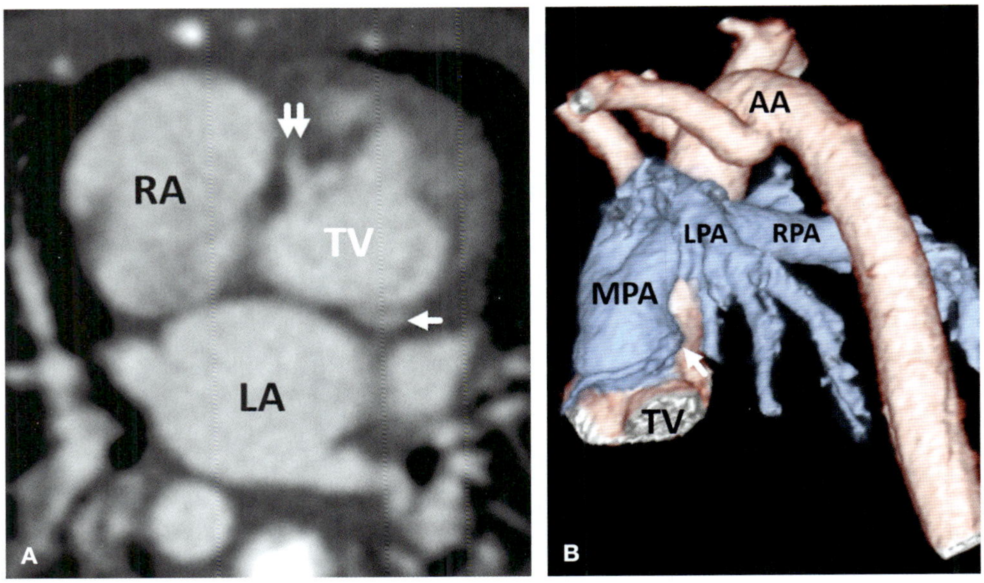

Figure 37.88. Newborn with truncus arteriosus type 1. **A:** Axial oblique maximum intensity projection CCTA image of the heart shows the heart at the truncal valve (TV) stradling the interatrial septum between the right (RA) and left (LA) atria, and the right (white double arrows) and left main (white arrow) coronary artery origins. **B:** 3D volume rendered CCTA reconstruction of the TV, main (MPA) and branch right (RPA) and left (LPA) pulmonary arteries, and aortic arch (AA) shows the origin of the left main coronary artery (white arrow) arising from the pulmonary cusp of the TV. The origin of the right coronary artery from the aortic side of the TV is not seen.

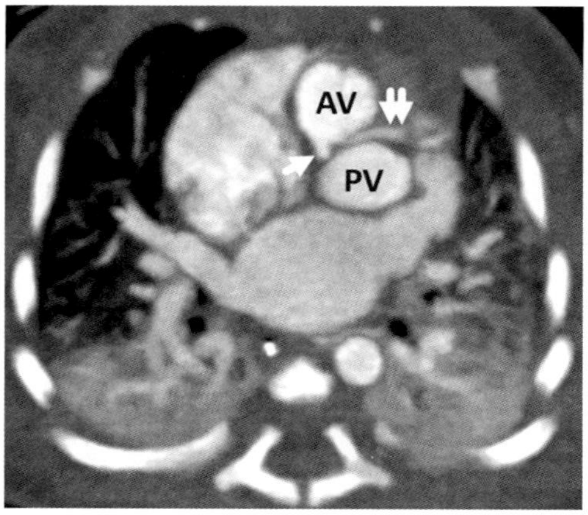

Figure 37.89. Neonate with D-transposition of the great arteries. Axial oblique maximum intensity projection (MIP) CCTA image at the aortic (AV) and pulmonary (PV) valve level shows the AV anterior to the PV. The left main (double white arrow) and right (white arrow) coronary artery origins arise from the posterior sinus of Valsalva which is "facing" the PV.

several potential use cases of AI in CT of CHD can be listed, including:

- Automatic measurement of the size and length of vessels, baffles, and conduits, as well as volumetric assessment of cardiac chambers
- Automated detection of abnormalities
- Prediction of outcomes
- Image quality control
- Personalized treatment planning

Despite the recent increase in applications of AI in medical imaging, many barriers still exist that prevent broader implementation of this technology, particularly for CHD studies. For example, the variability of cardiovascular structures and the lack of labeled datasets in CHD create layers of complexity for the development of automatic segmentation models. Nonetheless, there are great expectations for future applications of AI in CHD, given the potential to improve the accuracy and efficiency of CT imaging in the diagnosis and management of these patients.

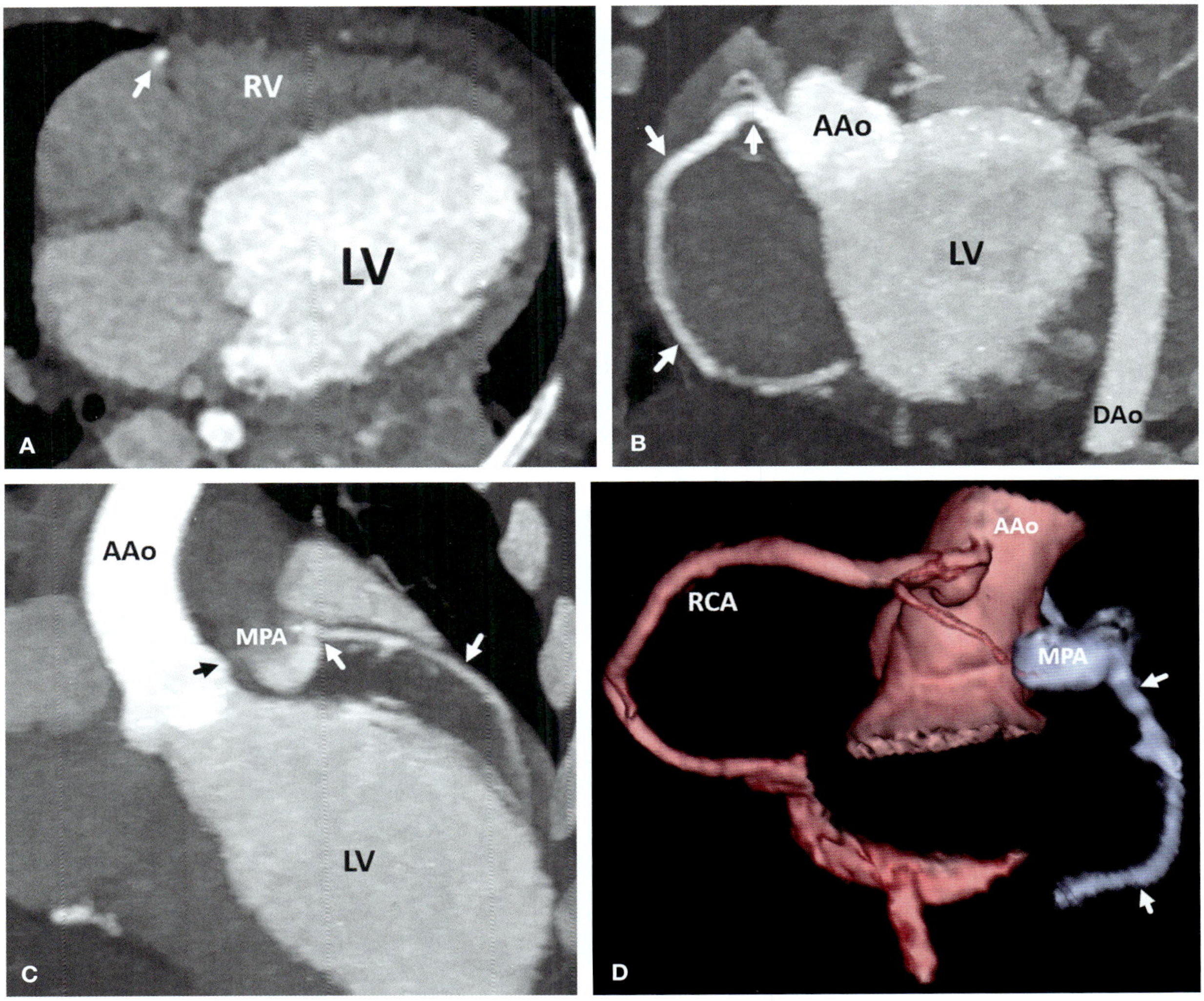

Figure 37.90. Newborn with dilated cardiomyopathy with echocardiogram findings suspicious for abnormal blood flow direction in the left main coronary artery. **A:** Axial oblique 4-chamber maximum intensity projection (MIP) CCTA view of the heart shows the markedly dilated left ventricle (LV) and the normal right ventricle (RV) chambers. The right coronary artery (RCA) (white arrow) is seen in the right arterioventricular groove. **B:** Sagittal oblique short-axis MIP CCTA view of the heart at the level of the right atrioventricular groove shows the dilated RCA (white arrows) arises from the right sinus of Valsalva and courses in the right arterioventricular groove. Although usually the left main coronary artery would be seen in this view, it is not present. **C:** Coronal oblique MIP CCTA view of the heart at the level of the aortic sinuses of Valsalva. The left main coronary artery does not arise from the left sinus of Valsalva at the expected location (black arrow). The left main and anterior descending coronary arteries (white arrows) drain to the main pulmonary artery (MPA), which shows a blush of contrast beginning to fill the vessel at this arterial phase examination. The RCA is supplying all of the oxygenated blood to the myocardium, while the left coronary artery system is stealing blood and draining to the MPA, a lower-pressure system than the aorta. **D:** 3D colorized reconstruction CCTA view of the coronary artery origins shows the dilated RCA arises normally from the aortic right sinus of Valsalva. The left main coronary artery (white arrows) drains to the MPA.

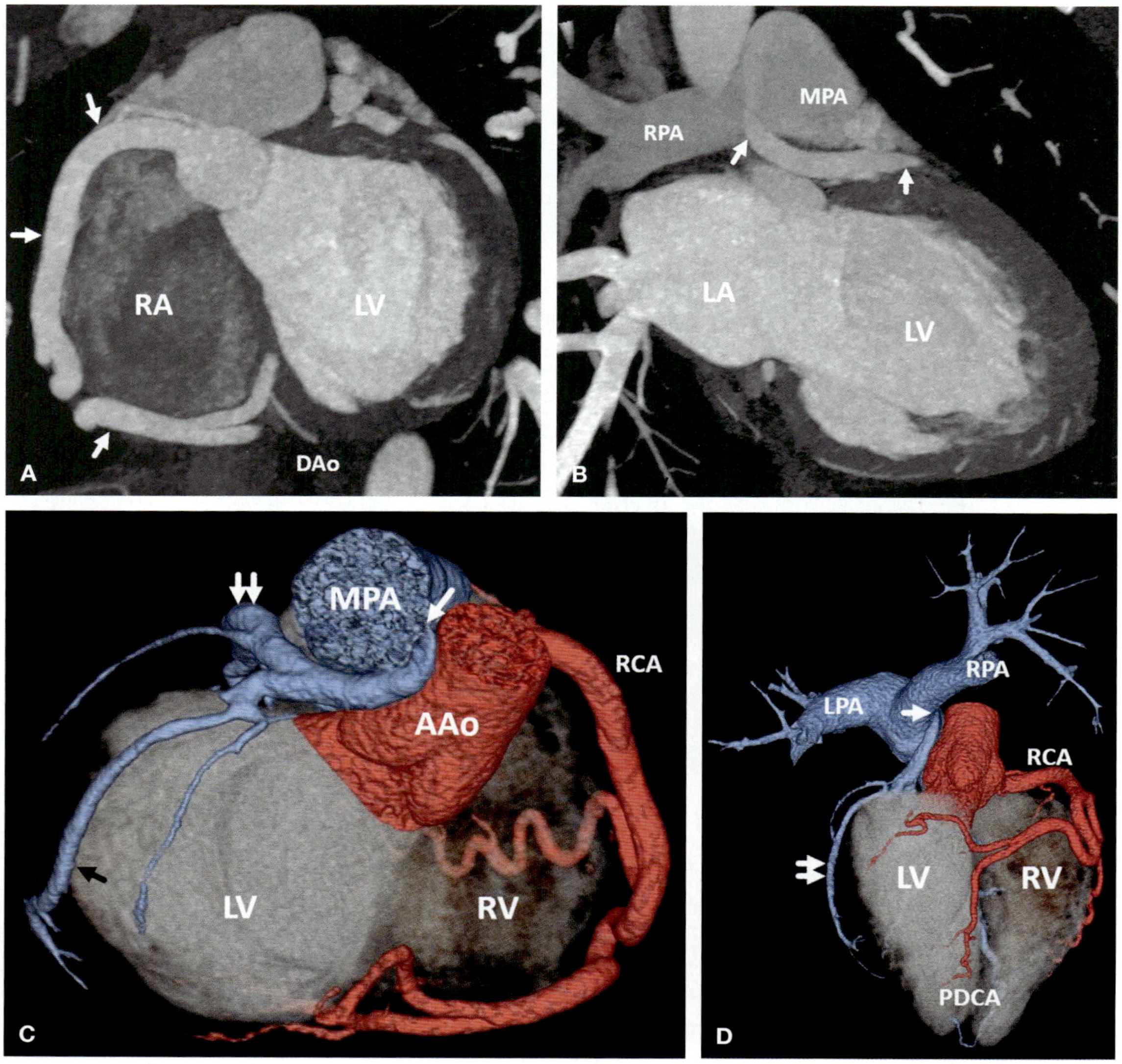

Figure 37.91. Adolescent with recent syncopal episode, now also reports exertional chest pain. Echocardiogram findings show reversed blood flow direction in the left main coronary artery. **A:** Sagittal oblique short-axis maximum intensity projection (MIP) CCTA view of the heart at the level of the right atrioventricular groove shows the markedly dilated right coronary artery (white arrows) arises from the right sinus of valsalva and courses in the right arterioventricular groove. **B:** Coronal oblique MIP CCTA view of the heart at the level of the distal main (MPA) and right (RPA) pulmonary arteries shows the markedly dilated left coronary artery (white arrows) draining contrast-enhanced blood into the pulmonary artery. **C:** 3D colorized reconstruction CCTA view of the coronary artery origins shows the dilated right coronary artery (RCA) arises normally from the aortic right sinus of Valsalva. The left anterior descending (double white arrows), the left circumflex (black arrow), and the left main (white arrow) cornary arteries drain to the MPA. **D:** 3D colorized reconstruction CCTA view of the coronary artery origins shows the dilated RCA arises normally from the aortic right sinus of Valsalva. A dilated oblique marginal branch of the left anterior descending (double white arrows) and the left main (white arrow) cornary arteries drain to the MPA. The RCA and its posterior descending (PDCA) are dilated.

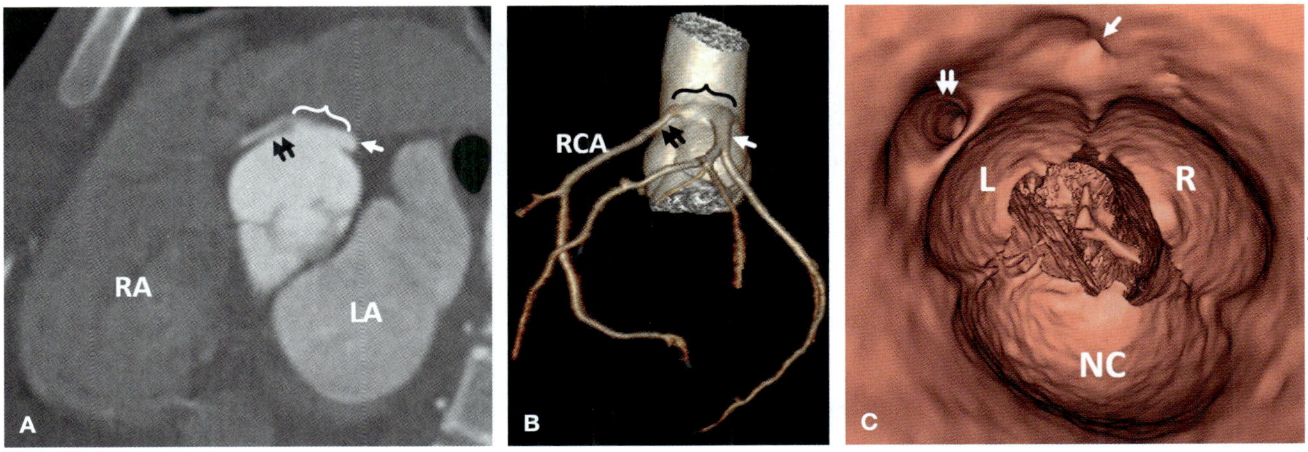

Figure 37.92. Adolescent with exertional chest pain found to have abnormal coronary artery origins on echocardiography. **A:** Short-axis maximum intensity projection CCTA image of the aortic sinuses of Valsalva shows the anomalous common origin (bracket) of the left main (white arrow) and right coronary arteries arising from the sinotubular junction, above the left sinus. The first several millimeters of the right coronary artery are intramural (double black arrows). **B:** 3D reconstructed CCTA image of the aortic sinuses of Valsalva shows the anomalous common origin (bracket) of the left main (white arrow) and right coronary arteries arising from the sinotubular junction, above the left sinus. The first several millimeters of the right coronary artery are intramural (double black arrows). **C:** 3D endoluminal CCTA reconstruction view looking into the aortic sinuses of Valsalva from above shows the round shape of the origin of the left main coronary artery (white double arrows) and the slit-like origin of the right coronary artery (white arrow) also from the right, just above the commissural post, superior to its normal location, at the level of the sinotubular junction.

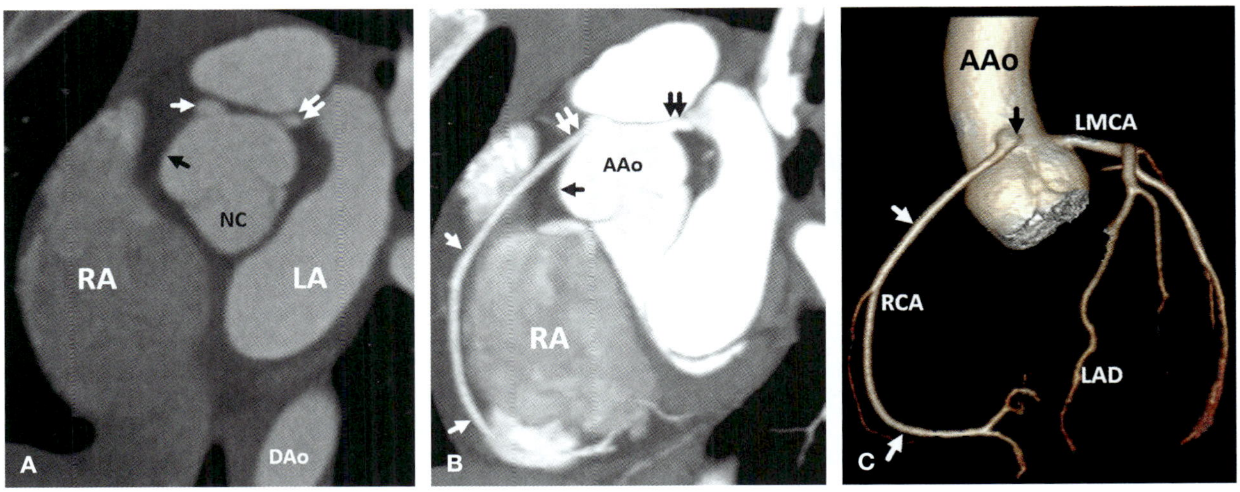

Figure 37.93. Young adult with syncopal episode and abnormal coronary artery origins suspected on echocardiography. **A:** Short-axis maximum intensity projection (MIP) CCTA image of the aortic sinuses of Valsalva shows the origins of the left main (double white arrows) arising from the left sinus and the right (white arrow) coronary artery origin arising more to the left of midline than expected (black arrow). Note the position of the interatrial septum between the right (RA) and left (LA) atria. The aortic sinus that straddles the interatrial septum is always the noncoronary sinus of Valsalva (NC). **B:** Short-axis MIP CCTA image of the aortic sinuses of Valsalva shows the origins of the left main (double black arrows) arising high from the left sinus and the right coronary artery origin arising more to the left of midline than its expected origin (black arrow). The proximal right coronary artery (double white arrows) arises at an acute angle and is in very close approximation to the aortic wall, therefore may be intramural. The course of the remainder of the right coronary artery (single white arrows) in the right atrioventricular groove is normal. **C:** 3D reconstructed CCTA image of the aortic sinuses of Valsalva shows the left main coronary artery arising high from the left sinus and the right coronary artery origin arising more to the left of midline, just above the commissural post (black arrow). The proximal right coronary artery arises at an acute angle and is in very close approximation to the aortic wall, the course of right coronary artery (single white arrows) in the right atrioventricular groove is normal.

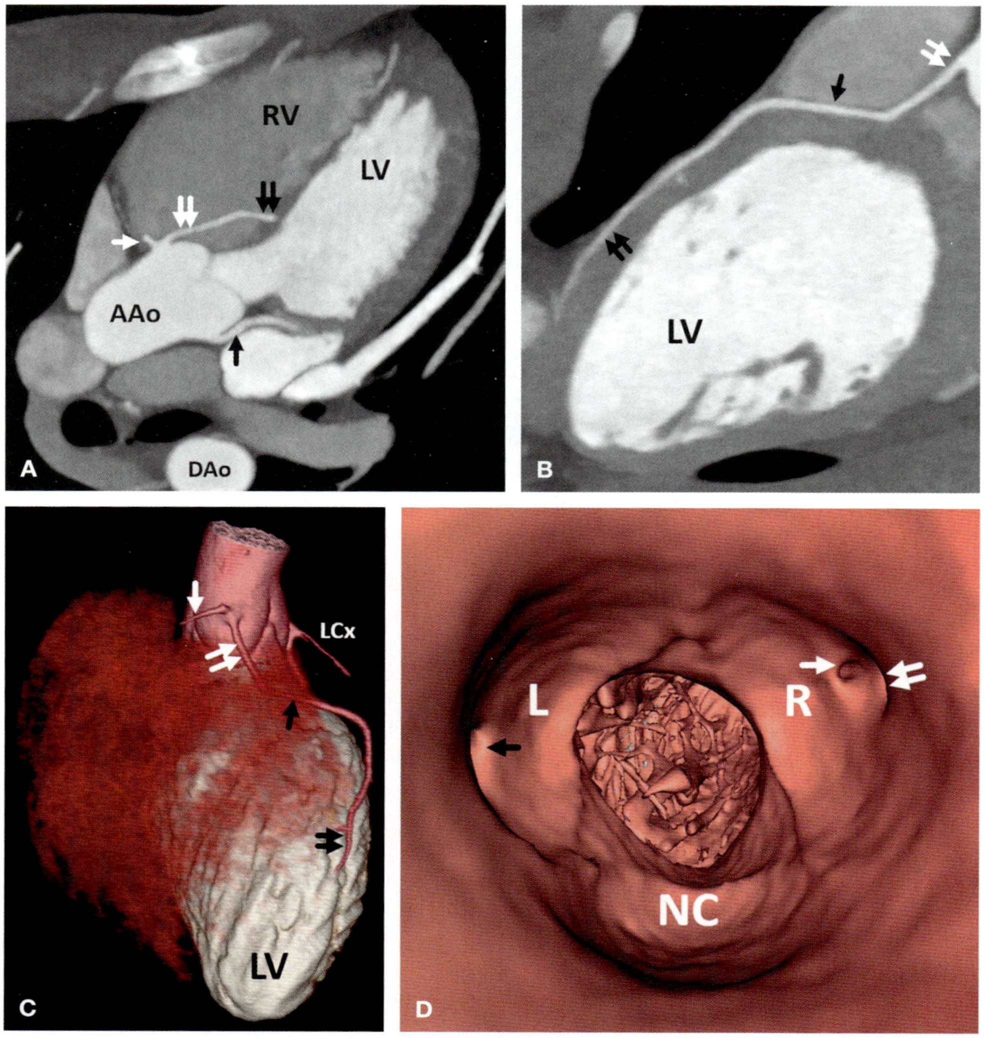

Figure 37.94. Adolescent with abnormal coronary artery origins on echocardiography performed for sports physical examination. **A:** 2D maximum intensity projection (MIP) image of the heart in an axial oblique plane of the aortic root shows the common origin of the left main (white double arrows) and right (white arrow) coronary arteries from the right sinus of Valsalva. Distally the left main continues as the left anterior descending coronary artery, which courses initially in the intraventricular descending coronary artery (black double arrows). The left circumflex coronary artery from the left sinus of Valsalva (black arrow). **B:** 2D MIP image of the heart in a coronal oblique plane of the aortic root shows the origin of the left main (white double arrows) coronary artery from the right sinus of Valsalva. Distally the left main continues as the left anterior descending coronary artery, which courses initially in the intraventricular descending coronary artery (black arrow) and distally in the epicardial intraventricular septum (black double arrows). **C:** 3D surface rendered and colorized CCTA image of the heart shows the origin of the left main (white double arrows) and right (white arrow) coronary arteries from the right sinus of Valsalva. Distally the left main continues as the left anterior descending coronary artery, which courses initially in the intraventricular septum as the left anterior descending coronary artery (black arrow) and distally, along the epicardial anterior intraventricular septum (black double arrows). **D:** 3D endoluminal CCTA reconstruction view looking into the aortic sinuses of Valsalva from above shows the origin of the left main (white double arrows) and right (white arrow) coronary arteries from the right sinus of Valsalva (R). The left circumflex coronary artery origin (black arrow) arises from the left sinus of Valsalva (L).

SUGGESTED READINGS

Agarwal PP, Mahani MG, Lu JC, Dorfman AL. Levoatriocardinal vein and mimics: spectrum of imaging findings. *AJR Am J Roentgenol.* 2015;205(2):W162-W171. doi:10.2214/AJR.15.14365

Ahmed Z, Campeau D, Gong H, et al. High-pitch, high temporal resolution, multi-energy cardiac imaging on a dual-source photon-counting-detector CT. *Med Phys.* 2023;50(3):1428-1435. doi:10.1002/mp.16124

Backer CL, Mavroudis C. Congenital Heart Surgery Nomenclature and Database Project: patent ductus arteriosus, coarctation of the aorta, interrupted aortic arch. *Ann Thorac Surg.* 2000;69(4 suppl l):S298-S307. doi:10.1016/s0003-4975(99)01280-1

Bae SB, Kang EJ, Choo KS, et al. Aortic arch variants and anomalies: embryology, imaging findings, and clinical considerations. *J Cardiovasc Imaging.* 2022;30(4):231-262.

Bardo DME, Frankel DG, Applegate KE, Murphy DJ, Saneto RP. Hypoplastic left heart syndrome. *Radiographics.* 2001;21(3):705-717. doi:10.1148/radiographics.21.3.g01ma09705

Barrera CA, Saul D, Rapp JB, et al. Diagnostic performance of CT angiography to detect pulmonary vein stenosis in children. *Int J Cardiovasc Imag.* 2020;36(1):141-147. doi:10.1007/s10554-019-01693-8

Bravo C, Gámez F, Pérez R, Álvarez T, De León-Luis J. Fetal aortic arch anomalies key sonographic views for their differential diagnosis and clinical implications using the cardiovascular system sonographic evaluation protocol. *J Ultrasound Med.* 2016;35(2):237-251. doi:10.7863/ultra.15.02063

Bronshtein M, Zimmer EZ, Blazer S, Blumenfeld Z. Right ductus arteriosus: facts and theory. *Eur J OB Gyn Repro Bio.* 2011;159(2):282-288.

Chikkabyrappa SM, Loomba RS, & Tretter JT. Pulmonary atresia with an intact ventricular septum: preoperative physiology, imaging, and management. *Semin CardioThorac Vasc Anesth.* 2018;22(3):245-255.

Dillman JR, Yarram SG, Hernandez RJ. Imaging of pulmonary venous developmental anomalies. *AJR Am J Roentgenol.* 2009;192(5):1272-1285. doi:10.2214/AJR.08.1526

DiLorenzo MP, Santo A, Rome JJ, et al. Pulmonary vein stenosis: outcomes in children with congenital heart disease and prematurity. *Semin Thoracic Surg.* 2019;31(2):266-273. doi:10.1053/j.semtcvs.2018.09.027

Dodge-Khatami J, Adebo DA. Evaluation of complex congenital heart disease in infants using low dose cardiac computed tomography. *Int J Cardiovasc Imag.* 2021;37(4):1455-1460. doi:10.1007/s10554-020-02118-7

Douglas YL, Jongbloed MR, Deruiter MC, Gittenberger-de Groot AC. Normal and abnormal development of pulmonary veins: state of the art and correlation with clinical entities. *Int J Cardiol.* 2011;147(1):13-24. doi:10.1016/j.ijcard.2010.07.004

Dyer KT, Hlavacek AM, Meinel FG, et al. Imaging in congenital pulmonary vein anomalies: the role of computed tomography. *Pediatr Radiol.* 2014;44(9):1158-1157; quiz 1155-7. doi: 10.1007/s00247-014-3044-7.

Edwards JE. Anomalies of the derivatives of the aortic arch system. *Med Clin North Am.* 1948;32:925-949. doi:10.1016/s0025-7125(16)35662-0

Goldmuntz E. 22q11.2 deletion syndrome and congenital heart disease. *Am J Genet.* 2020;184(1):64-72. doi:10.1002/ajmg.c.31774

Gould SW, Rigsby CK, Donnelly LF, McCulloch M, Pizarro C, Epelman M. Useful signs for the assessment of vascular rings on cross-sectional imaging. *Pediatr Radiol.* 2015;45(13):2004-2003. doi:10.1007/s00247-015-3424-7

Graidis C, Dimitriadis D, Karasavvidis V, et al. Prevalence and characteristics of coronary artery anomalies in an adult population undergoing multidetector-row computed tomography for the evaluation of coronary artery disease. *BMC Cardiovasc Disord.* 2015;15:112. doi:10.1186/s12872-015-0098-x

Hanneman K, Newman B, Chan F. Congenital variants and anomalies of the aortic arch. *Radiographics.* 2017;37(1):32-51. doi:10.1148/rg.2017160033

Hassani C, Saremi F. Comprehensive cross-sectional imaging of the pulmonary veins. *Radiographics.* 2017;37(7):1928-1954. doi:10.1148/rg.2017170050

Howard JP, Francis DP. Machine learning with convolutional neural networks for clinical cardiologists. *Heart.* 2022;108(12):973-981. doi:10.1136/heartjnl-2020-318686

Johnson KW, Torres Soto J, Glicksberg BS, et al. Artificial intelligence in cardiology. *J Am Coll Cardiol.* 2018;71(23):2668-2679. doi:10.1016/j.jacc.2018.03.521

Karaosmanoglu AD, Khawaja RDA, Onur MR, Kalra MK. CT and MRI of aortic coarctation: pre- and postsurgical Findings. *AJR Am J Roentgenol.* 2015;204(3) W224-W233. doi:10.2214/AJR.14.12529

Kim YY, Andrade L, Cook SC. Aortic coarctation. *Cardiol Clin.* 2020;38(3):337-351. doi:10.1016/j.ccl.2020.04.003

Kische S, Schneider H, Akin I, et al. Technique of interventional repair in adult aortic coarctation. *J Vasc Surg.* 2010;51(6):1550-1559. doi:10.1016/j.jvs.2009.12.063

Krittanawong C, Johnson KW, Rosenson RS, et al. Deep learning for cardiovascular medicine: a practical primer. *Eur Heart J.* 2019;40(25):2058-2073. doi:10.1093/eurheartj/ehz056

Kubota H, Endo H, Ishii H, et al. Adult ALCAPA: from histological picture to clinical features. *J Cardiothorac Surg.* 2020;15(1):14. doi:10.1186/s13019-020-1048-y

Kumar P, Bhatia M. Role of CT in the pre- and postoperative assessment of conotruncal anomalies. *Radiol Cardiothorac Imaging.* 2022;4(3):e210089.

Manlhiot C, van den Eynde J, Kutty S, Ross HJ. A primer on the present state and future prospects for machine learning and artificial intelligence applications in cardiology. *Can J Cardiol.* 2022;38(2):169-184. doi:10.1016/j.cjca.2021.11.009

Martín de Miguel I, Jain CC, Egbe AC, Hagler DJ, Connolly HM, Miranda WR. Surgical repair of truncus arteriosus: a long-term hemodynamic assessment. *World J Pediatr Congenit Heart Surg.* 2022;13(6):716-722. doi:10.1177/21501351221114779. PMID: 36300270

McElhinney DB, McDonald-McGinn D, Zackai EH, Goldmuntz E. Cardiovascular anomalies in patients diagnosed with a chromosome 22q11 deletion beyond 6 months of age. *Pediatrics.* 2001;108(6):E104. http://www.pediatrics.org/cgi/content/full/108/6/e104

Mery CM, Lawrence SM, Krishnamurthy R, et al. Anomalous aortic origin of a coronary artery: toward a standardized approach. *Semin Thorac Cardiovasc Surg.* 2014;26(2):110-122. doi:10.1053/j.semtcvs.2014.08.001

Momma K, Matsuoka R, Takao A. Aortic arch anomalies associated with chromosome 22q11 deletion (CATCH 22). *Pediatr Cardiol.* 1999;20(2):97-102..

Peña E, Nguyen ET, Merchant N, Dennie C. ALCAPA syndrome: not just a pediatric disease. *Radiographics.* 2009;29(2):553-565.

Pérez-Pomares JM, de la Pompa JL, Franco D, et al. Congenital coronary artery anomalies: a bridge from embryology to anatomy and pathophysiology—a position statement of the development, anatomy, and pathology ESC Working Group. *Cardiovasc Res.* 2016;109(2):204-216. doi:10.1093/cvr/cvv251

Prabhu S, Kasturi S, Mehra S, et al. The aortic arch in tetralogy of Fallot: types of branching and clinical implications. *Cardiol Young.* 2020;30(8):1144-1150. doi:10.1017/S1047951120001705

Restivo A, di Gioia C, Marino B, Putotto C. Transpositions of the great arteries versus aortic dextropositions. A review of some embryogenetic and morphological aspects. *Anat Rec.* 2023;306(3):502-514. doi:10.1002/ar.25129

Rodefeld MD, Hanley FL. Neonatal truncus arteriosus repair: surgical techniques and clinical management. *Semin Thorac Cardiovasc Surg Pediatr Card Surg Annu.* 2002;5:212-217. doi:10.1053/pcsu.2002.31497

Saran N, Dearani J, Said S, et al. Vascular rings in adults: outcome of surgical management. *Ann Thorac Surg.* 2019;108(4):1217-1227.

Sharma A, Neupane NP, Dhakal P, Sharma S, Sitaula A, Rajlawot K. Complete interruption of aortic arch diagnosed in adulthood: a case report. *Radiol Case Rep.* 2022;17(10):3963-3965.

Song MK, Bae EJ, Jeong SI, et al. Clinical characteristics and prognostic factors of primary pulmonary vein stenosis or atresia in children. *Ann Thorac Surg.* 2013;95(1):229-234.

Steeden JA, Muthurangu V, Secinaro A. Artificial intelligence-based evaluation of congenital heart disease. In: De Cecco CN, van Assen M, Leiner T, eds. *Artificial Intelligence in Cardiothoracic Imaging. Contemporary Medical Imaging.* Humana; 2022. doi:10.1007/978-3-030-92087-6_36

Szmigielska A, Roszkowska-Blaim M, Gołąbek-Dylewska M, Tomik A, Brzewski M, Werner B. Bland-White-Garland syndrome - a rare and serious cause of failure to thrive. *Am J Case Rep.* 2013;14:370-372. doi:10.12659/AJCR.889112

Türkvatan A, Güzeltaş A, Tola HT, Ergül Y. Multidetector computed tomographic angiography imaging of congenital pulmonary venous anomalies: a pictorial review. *Can Assoc Radiol J.* 2017;68(1):66-76. doi:10.1016/j.carj.2016.05.003

Valente AM, Geva T. How to image repaired tetralogy of Fallot. *Circ Cardiovasc Imaging.* 2017;10(5):e004270.

Van Praagh R. Truncus arteriosus: what is it really and how should it be classified? *Eur J Cardio Thorac Surg.* 1987;1(2):65-70. doi:10.1016/1010-7940(87)90014-5

Xiong L, Patel MD, Biliciler-Denktas G, Dodge-Khatami A, Salazar J, Adebo DA. Perioperative anomalous pulmonary venous return evaluation with low-dose cardiac computed tomography. *World J Pediatr Congenit Heart Surg.* 2021;12(4):529-534. doi:10.1177/21501351211010115

Yamanaka O, Hobbs RE. Coronary artery anomalies in 126,595 patients undergoing coronary arteriography. *Cathet Cardiovasc Diagn.* 1990;21(1):28-40. doi:10.1002/ccd.1810210110

Yun G, Nam TH, Chun EJ. Coronary artery fistulas: pathophysiology, imaging findings, and management. *Radiographics.* 2018;38(3):688-703. doi:10.1148/rg.2018170158

Zucker EJ. Computed tomography in tetralogy of Fallot: pre- and postoperative imaging evaluation. *Pediatr Radiol.* 2022;52(13):2485-2497.

Chapter 38

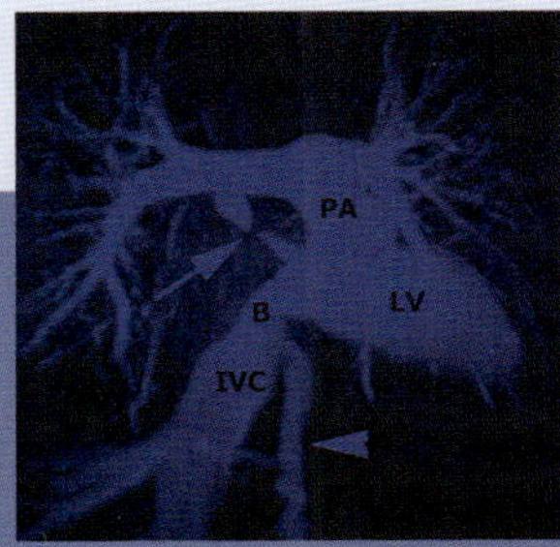

Eric Krieger • Sadaf Bhutta • Charles B. Higgins •
Karen G. Ordovas

Magnetic Resonance Imaging of Congenital Heart Disease

INTRODUCTION

The overall objectives of imaging in congenital heart disease (CHD) are the precise delineation of cardiovascular anatomy and the quantitative assessment of function. The evaluation of CHD was one of the first applications of cardiac magnetic resonance imaging (MRI) and continues to be one of its most important indications. MRI has significant advantages over other modalities, including echocardiography and angiography, for the definitive assessment of congenital cardiovascular anomalies. MRI does not require the use of a contrast agent or ionizing radiation. The absence of ionizing radiation is a major advantage of MRI in children, who in the past have been exposed to large doses of radiation during cine angiography for initial diagnosis and postoperative monitoring which has been associated with increases in cancer incidence in adults with CHD.

The role of MRI has been influenced by the success of echocardiography as the primary noninvasive imaging technique in CHD. The major applications have been for lesions incompletely evaluated by echocardiography. However, substantial technological improvements, especially fast cine MRI using steady-state free precession (SSFP) and non–contrast- and contrast-enhanced magnetic resonance angiography (MRA), make MRI at least equal to echocardiography in the diagnosis of most types of CHD in children and adults. Echocardiography is still considered to be the primary imaging modality for infants and young children with CHD. However, in adolescents and adults, MRI is a critical component of the longitudinal follow-up for a variety of native and corrected forms of CHD.

MAJOR CLINICAL INDICATIONS

The major indications for MRI are diagnosis, severity assessment, and pre and postoperative management of the following congenital heart defects:

1. Thoracic aortic anomalies, such as coarctation and arch anomalies
2. Pulmonary arterial anomalies
3. Cyanotic heart diseases, such as tetralogy of Fallot, transposition of great arteries, and single ventricle
4. Cardiac and extra-cardiac shunts
5. Coronary arterial anomalies

TECHNIQUES

MRI studies are directed toward precise display of the cardiovascular anatomy and quantification of ventricular function and blood flow. An advantage of MRI in CHD is measurement of ventricular volumes and function using cine MRI and velocity-encoded cine MRI (VEC-MRI).

For children younger than 8 to 10 years and children unwilling or unable to remain immobile and cooperative during imaging, light anesthesia without intubation is used. This is usually under the control of an anesthesiologist. Blood pressure, heart rate, and oxygen saturation are monitored during the procedure.

Anatomy

Assessment of anatomy can be performed with balanced SSFP (white blood), and non–contrast- and contrast-enhanced three-dimensional (3D) MRA. The latter technique is usually applied for the evaluation of anomalies of the great arteries, pulmonary veins, and surgical shunts. ECG-gated multislice double inversion-recovery spin-echo images (black-blood) are less commonly required in contemporary practice as it may be time-consuming. The main role of this sequence is to delineate anatomy when stents and surgical clips are present, as it is less affected by susceptibility artifacts than SSFP and MRA images.

Function

The techniques used in the evaluation of right and left ventricular function are generically called cine MRI. There are a multitude of cine MRI sequences; the most frequently applied one now is a balanced SSFP sequence because of optimized homogeneous contrast between cavitary blood and myocardium. The so-called real-time cine sequence may be advantageous in infants and young children who cannot hold their breath but has a lower signal-to-noise ratio.

Cine MR images are used to quantify ventricular volumes and function. Right and left ventricular volumes are indexed to body surface area (BSA). For example, left ventricular end-diastolic volume index (LEDVi; mL/m^2) is calculated by dividing the end-diastolic volume (LVEDV; mL) by the BSA (m^2). A distinct advantage of MRI compared to echocardiography is its precision and reproducibility for quantifying right ventricular volume and function. For ventricular volumetrics, images are usually acquired in the cardiac short-axis plane. Right ventricular volumes can alternatively be analyzed in the horizontal long-axis plane.

Cine MR images are also used to evaluate valvular function. Planes approximately parallel to the valve leaflet or cusps can demonstrate valve motion, such as the horizontal long-axis plane for assessing mitral valve motion and RV outlet plane for visualizing infundibular and pulmonary valvular stenosis. The high-velocity jet caused by valvular stenosis and regurgitation may be identified on cine MR images as a flow void (Fig. 38.1).

Volume and Velocity of Blood Flow

Quantification of blood flow is done using velocity-encoded (VEC; phase-contrast) MRI. In phase-contrast imaging, the signal intensity signifies the velocity of blood at each pixel. ECG-gated phase-contrast images can be produced in which each image shows the velocity at a different time in the cardiac cycle. Because these are cine images, they can be referred to as VEC cine MRI. A region of interest drawn around a blood vessel will give the mean velocity within the vessel at that point in the cardiac cycle. The cross-sectional area of the vessel can be multiplied by the spatial mean velocity to obtain the flow in the blood vessel.VEC cine MRI is used to measure valvular regurgitant volume (Fig. 38.2), differential flow in central pulmonary arteries, systemic to pulmonary shunt flow, flow through surgical conduits, and collateral flow in coarctation. By determining the voxel with the peak velocity just beyond a stenosis, this technique can estimate the peak gradient across a valvular or conduit stenosis.

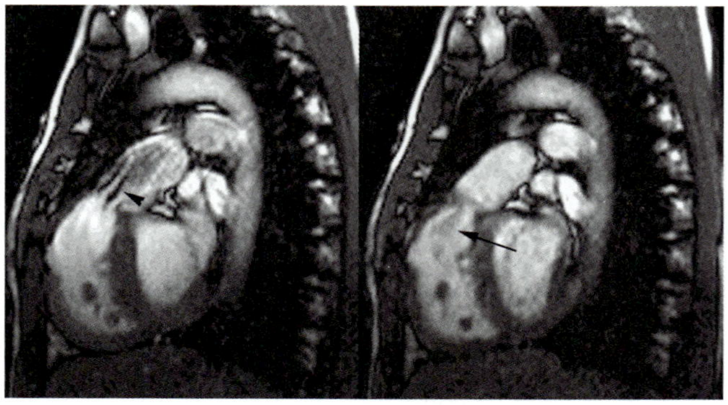

Figure 38.1. Postoperative tetralogy of Fallot. Sagittal cine MR images in systole (**left**) and diastole (**right**), and associated movie file, demonstrate a signal void (*arrowhead*) projected into the pulmonary artery (pulmonary stenosis) and a signal void (*arrow*) into the right ventricle (pulmonary regurgitation).

ACYANOTIC LESIONS

Left-to-Right Shunts

MRI is useful in patients with left-to-right shunts and can provide important information about the location, direction, and magnitude of shunt in patients with atrial septal defect (ASD), ventricular septal defect (VSD), partial anomalous pulmonary venous connection (PAPVC), patent ductus arteriosus (PDA). MRI can be used to determine the size of a defect to help plan for transcatheter or surgical closure. VEC cine MRI is used to measure the systemic-to-pulmonary flow ratio.

Atrial Septal Defect

There are four major types of ASD: Ostium secundum ASD, ostium primum ASD, sinus venosus ASD (superior or inferior), and unroofed coronary sinus (coronary sinus septal defects) (Fig. 38.3). Although the first two types are easily identifiable on echocardiogram, sinus venosus ASD and unroofed coronary sinus may be only visible on cross-sectional imaging, and can be demonstrated on CMR. ASDs will cause dilation of the right atrium, right ventricle, and pulmonary artery. Cine MR images in the transaxial or four-chamber planes demonstrate the site of the ASD (Fig. 38.4A). Short-axis cine image can also be helpful to delineate the edges of the defect (Fig. 38.4B).

MRI can clearly depict a defect in the portion of the septum separating the superior vena cava from the right pulmonary vein and left atrium, which is called superior sinus venosus ASD (Fig. 38.5). It also shows the anomalous connection of the right upper lobe pulmonary vein to the superior vena cava adjacent to the septal defect, which is seen in the majority of cases. A rare ASD is the inferior type of sinus venosus ASD. This defect is at the portion of the septum separating the inferior vena cava from the left atrium. Usually, the right inferior pulmonary veins drain anomalously to the upper inferior vena cava. Secundum ASD is situated in the middle of the atrial septum in the region of the

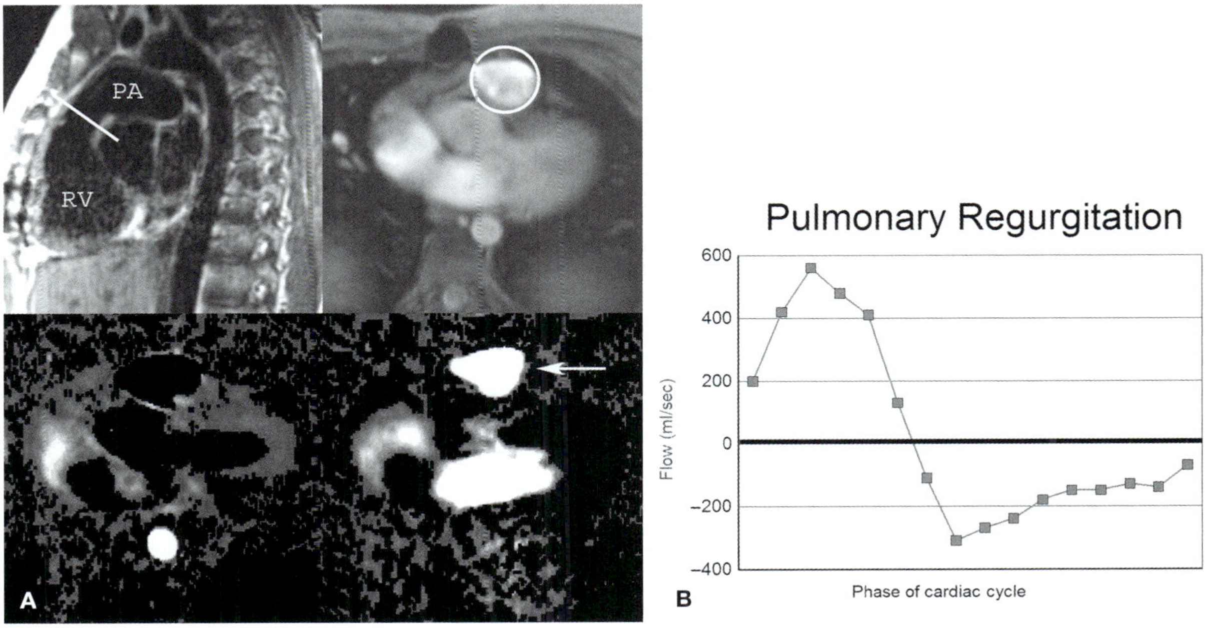

Figure 38.2. A: Postoperative tetralogy of Fallot. Sagittal spin-echo image (**top left**), axial magnitude image (**top right**), and phase images in systole (**bottom left**) and diastole (**bottom right**). Phase-contrast images and associated video show forward flow in systole (dark voxels) and retrograde flow in diastole (bright voxels; *arrow*). Region of interest for flow measurements is shown on the pulmonary artery. **B:** Flow versus time curve displays the forward and retrograde flow in the pulmonary artery. Area under negative component of the curve yields a direct quantification of the volume of regurgitation.

fossa ovalis (Fig. 38.3). If large, it may approach the aortic or mitral valve annulus. Thin fossa ovalis can be mistaken for an ASD. To avoid this error, the defect should be evident at two adjacent anatomic levels or confirmed by a flow jet (void) across the defect on cine MRI. Primum ASD is situated just adjacent to the atrioventricular valves (Fig. 38.6. A diagnostic characteristic of primum ASD is that the mitral and tricuspid valves are at the same level (distance) from the cardiac apex (Fig. 38.6). The demonstration of the location and size of an ASD is facilitated by cine MRI in the horizontal long-axis (four-chamber) plane. Ostium primum ASD is typically associated with abnormal atrioventricular valve formation (cleft mitral valve) and an inlet-type VSD. Finally, an unroofed coronary sinus is a defect in the superior aspect of the coronary sinus as it courses under the left atrium, as is best seen in the vertical long-axis plane (Fig. 38.7).

VEC (phase-contrast) cine in a plane parallel to the ASD can be used to determine the dimensions of the defect and help determine if it is amenable to closure with an ASD closure device (Fig. 38.8). For this purpose, a low-velocity encoding value (40 cm/s) is used in order to include flow at the margins of the defect. For placement of a closure device, the defect

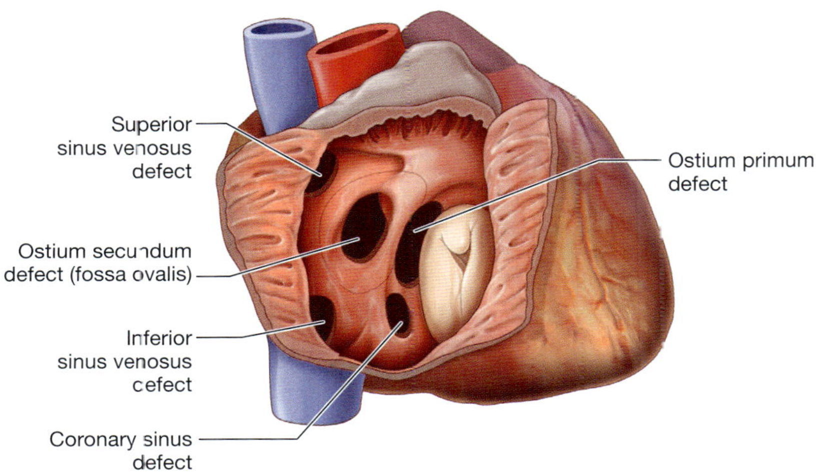

Figure 38.3. Illustration from the right atrial side showing the locations of atrial level shunts.

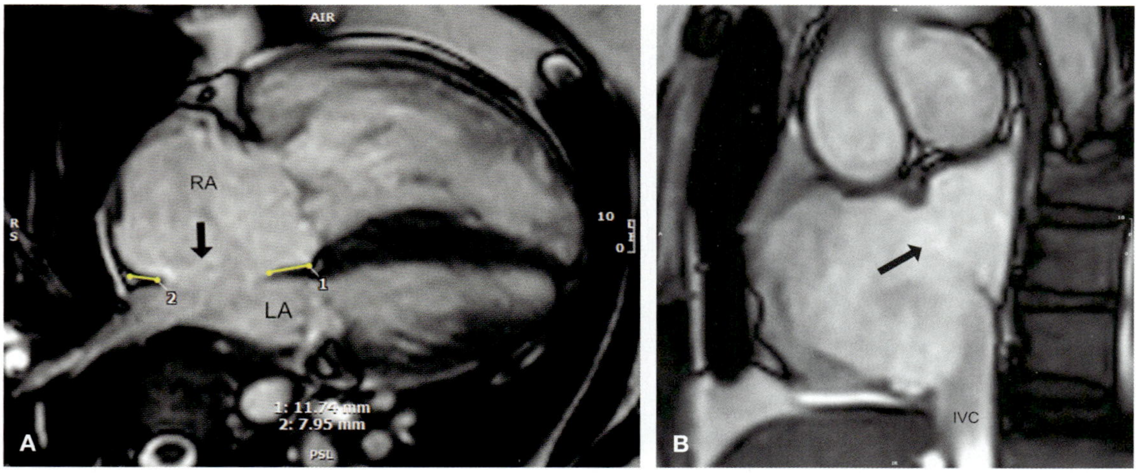

Figure 38.4. Secundum atrial septal defect. Cine MR image in the horizontal long-axis plane **(A)** and short-axis plane **(B)**, and associated video, demonstrate the defect in the atrial septum (black *arrows*). Measurements of the superior and inferior rims are displayed in yellow. IVC, inferior vena cava; LA, left atrium; RA, right atrium.

should be less than 3.5 cm in diameter. Only secundum ASDs can be routinely closed with a closure device; other types of defects typically require surgery. Cine MRI is also used to measure the distance of the margins of the defect from the mitral and aortic valves and pulmonary veins.

VEC cine MRI measurement in the main pulmonary artery and proximal ascending aorta can be used to calculate pulmonary-to-systemic flow ratio (Qp/Qs) (Fig. 38.9). The imaging planes are placed perpendicular to the direction of blood flow in each artery using sagittal images to identify their planes. Good correlations have been found for Qp/Qs, measured by VEC cine MR and oximetric samples acquired at cardiac catheterization.

Partial Anomalous Pulmonary Venous Connection

MRI and MRA are the procedures of choice for identifying PAPVC. PAPVC produces volume overload of right-sided cardiac chambers. The hemodynamics are identical to ASD.

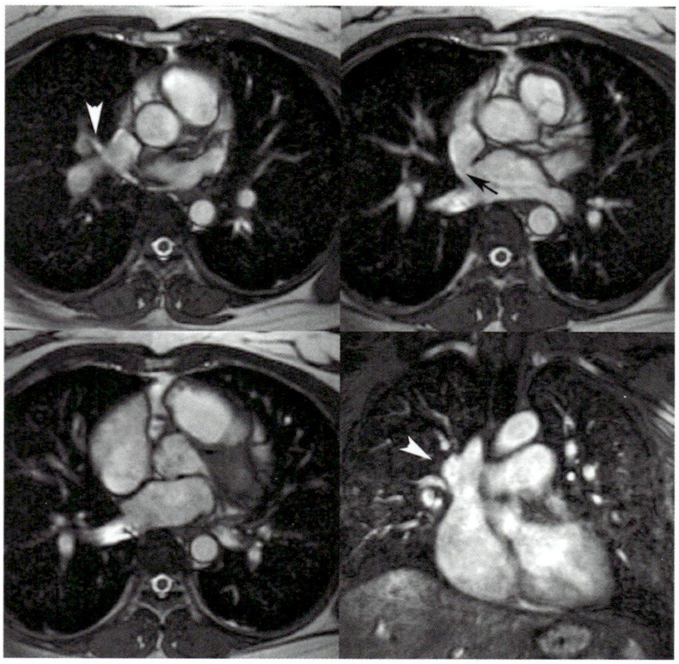

Figure 38.5. Sinus venosus atrial septal defect. Cine MR images in three axial planes (**top row and bottom left**) and the coronal plane (**bottom right**) show the defect (*arrow*) in the portion of the atrial septum between the superior vena cava and the left atrium. The right upper lobe pulmonary vein (*arrowheads*) connecting at the junction of the superior vena cava (*SVC*) with the right atrium is associated with the sinus venosus defect. Coronal image shows the dilatation of the SVC at the site of connection of the anomalous pulmonary vein.

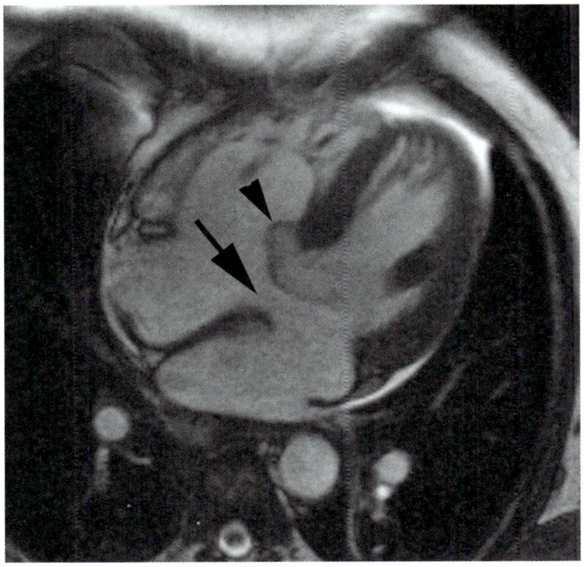

Figure 38.6. Primum atrial septal defect. Axial cine MR image shows a defect in the primum atrial septum (*arrow*). The atrioventricular valve is attached to the foreshortened ventricular septum (*arrowhead*).

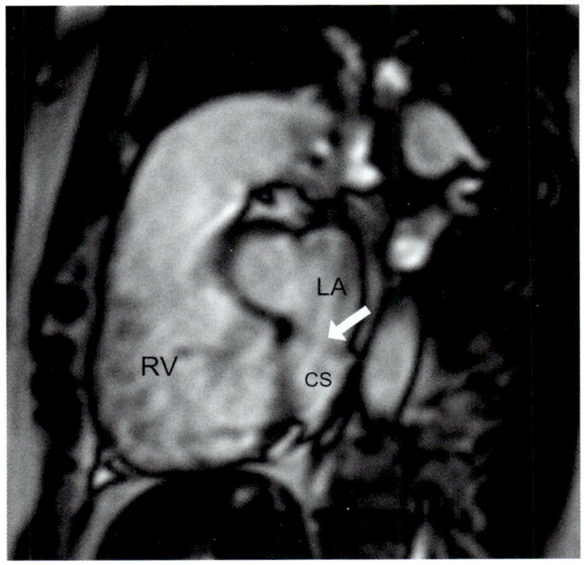

Figure 38.7. Unroofed coronary sinus. Cine steady-state free precession in an oblique sagittal plane shows a connection (arrow) between the superior aspect of the coronary sinus (CS) and the left atrium (LA). RV, right ventricle.

The most common type is connection of right upper lobe pulmonary vein to superior vena cava. This type of connection can occur alone (Fig. 38.10A) or accompany sinus venosus ASD (Fig. 38.5). Nearly equally frequent is left upper lobe vein drainage via a vertical vein to the left innominate vein (Fig. 38.10B). There is an increased incidence of secundum ASD as well as sinus venosus ASD in patients with PAPVC. The connection of the right-sided pulmonary veins to one or more veins that connect to the inferior vena cava (IVC) can be displayed in the scimitar syndrome (Fig. 38.11), which is associated with ipsilateral pulmonary hypoplasia.

Cine MR is done in the horizontal long-axis plane to exclude a concomitant ASD. Cine MRI is also performed in the short-axis plane in order to document the degree of right ventricular enlargement. VEC cine MR is performed perpendicular to the direction of flow in the proximal pulmonary artery and aorta in order to calculate pulmonary-to-systemic flow ratio (Qp/Qs) (Fig. 38.9).

Ventricular Septal Defect

The types of ventricular septal defects are membranous (or perimembranous), muscular, inlet, and supracristal (or outlet) (Fig. 38.12). MRI in the transaxial, horizontal long-axis, or four-chamber plane can precisely demonstrate the site of single or multiple VSDs. Membranous VSDs are the most common form of VSD in adults and are located between the aortic valve and the septal leaflet of the tricuspid valve (Fig. 38.13). Muscular VSDs are located in the muscular or trabeculated septum (Fig. 38.14). Inlet VSD is situated just beneath the atrioventricular valves (Fig. 38.15). The tricuspid and mitral valves are equidistant from the cardiac apex. This relationship and the defect are displayed optimally on cine MR in the horizontal long-axis plane. The supracristal VSD, also called doubly committed, is characterized by a defect that lies between the right ventricular outlet and the base of the aorta (Fig. 38.16A). On cine MR, a flow void apparently passes

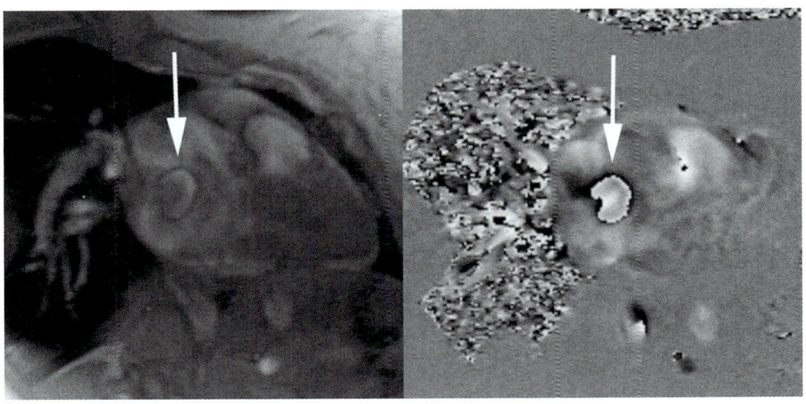

Figure 38.8. Magnitude (**left**) and phase (**right**) images from velocity-encoded cine MR sequence with low encoding velocity acquired parallel to the atrial septum (en face) delineates the flow through the defect (white *arrows*) allowing precise measurement of the defect dimensions.

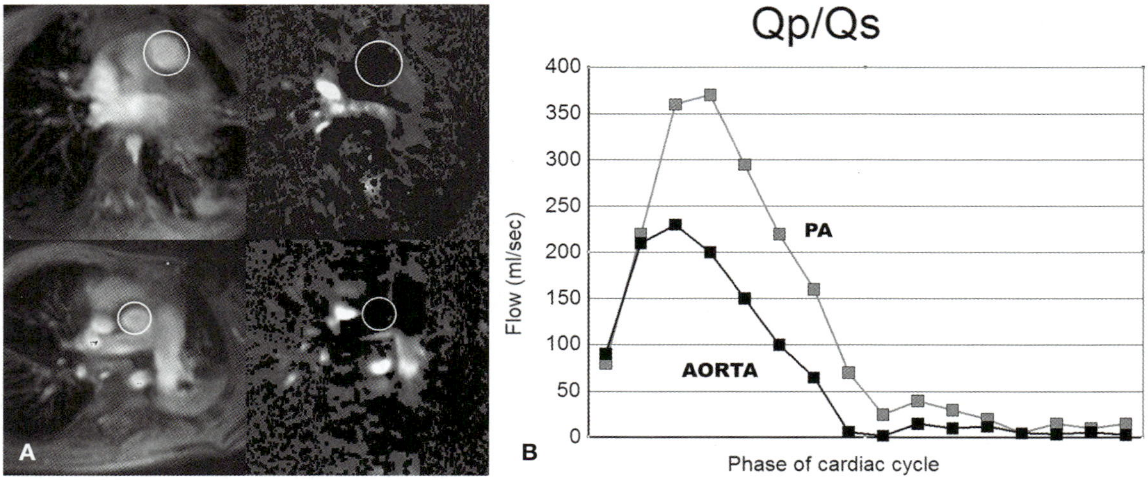

Figure 38.9. A: Atrial septal defect. Magnitude (**left**) and phase (**right**) images from velocity-encoded cine MR in planes perpendicular to the long axis of the pulmonary artery (**top**) and the proximal ascending aorta (**below**). Regions of interest surround the aorta and pulmonary artery. **B:** Flow versus time curves for the aorta and pulmonary artery. Because of the left-to-right shunt, the area under the pulmonary artery curve is greater. The area under each curve provides a direct measurement of the pulmonary-to-systemic flow ratio (2.1:1).

from the base of the aorta (it actually passes from just below the aortic valve) to the right ventricular outlet region and into the proximal pulmonary artery (Fig. 38.16B). VEC cine MRI can be used to calculate Qp/Qs and quantify the left-to-right shunt. Unlike ASDs and PAPVC which cause right heart enlargement, VSDs cause dilation of the left atrium and left ventricle.

Aorta to Right-Sided Shunts

MRI can demonstrate a PDA or aorticopulmonary window (Fig. 38.17). With recent improvements in coronary MRA, it is effective for demonstrating the presence and sites of emptying of coronary arteriovenous fistulas. MRI and MRA are very effective for demonstrating sinus of Valsalva aneurysms and fistulas.

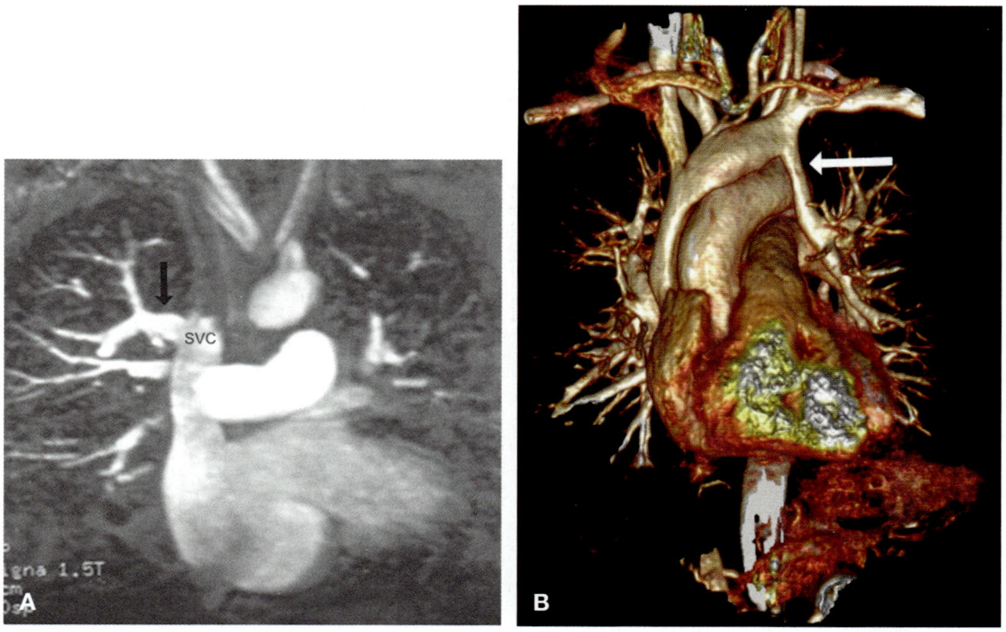

Figure 38.10. Partial anomalous pulmonary venous connection. **A:** Contrast-enhanced 3D MRA shows anomalous connection of the right upper pulmonary vein (black *arrow*) to the superior vena cava (SVC). **B:** Volume rendering reformation of 3D MRA shows left upper lobe anomalous vein (white arrow) draining to the left brachiocephalic vein. MRA, magnetic resonance angiography.

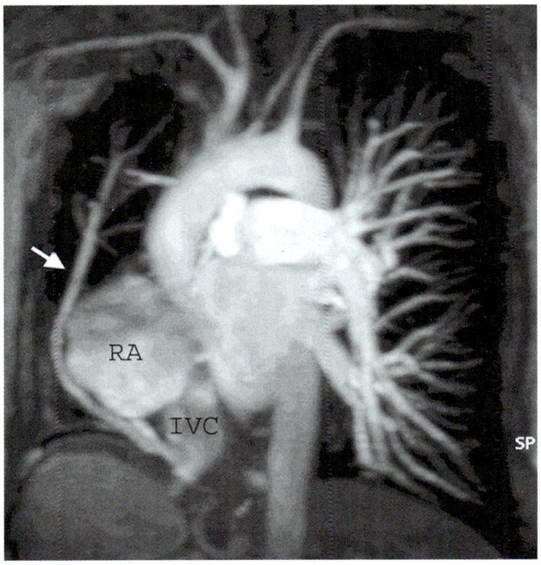

Figure 38.11. Scimitar syndrome—magnetic resonance angiography of the chest shows an anomalous vein (arrow) draining the entire right lung blood flow into the inferior vena cava (*arrowhead*) in a patient with scimitar syndrome. Note the small size of the right lung and its vessels compared to the left lung.

Atrioventricular Septal Defect/Atrioventricular Canal (Endocardial Cushion Defect)

These terms denote a spectrum of abnormalities that have in common an abnormal septation between the atria and ventricles. They are also called endocardial cushion defects because the defects are considered to be abnormalities of the embryologic endocardial cushions, which grow together in the center of the heart and divide the atria from the ventricles.

In the normal heart, the atrioventricular septum separates the right atrium from the left ventricle. The atrioventricular septum lies between the more apically located normal tricuspid valve and the mitral valve (Fig. 38.18). In all cases of atrioventricular septal defect, the tricuspid and mitral valves lie at the same level, and the atrioventricular septum is defective. This abnormal relationship can be shown on MRI in the transaxial or horizontal long-axis plane. A partial atrioventricular septal defect involves a primum ASD and a cleft mitral valve but no VSD. In a complete atrioventricular septal defect both the atrial and ventricular portions of the septum around the valve origins are absent and can be seen in the same axial image as the atrioventricular valve or valves (Fig. 38.19). This creates a common atrioventricular valve orifice with continuous, common atrioventricular valve leaflets (Fig. 38.20).

Coarctation of the Aorta

MRI is the procedure of choice for definitive diagnosis and assessment of the severity of coarctation. MRI has been shown to be effective for preoperative assessment of coarctation and for postoperative evaluation of recurrent or persistent hypertension. To evaluate coarctation, black blood spin-echo or cine MR sequences can be obtained in an oblique sagittal plane which show the diameter of the stenosis and provide an accurate measurement of its length (Fig. 38.21).

Gadolinium-enhanced 3D MRA can display the entire thoracic aorta on a single image with the use of maximum intensity projection or volume-rendering reconstruction techniques (Fig. 38.22). Gadolinium-enhanced MRA is also effective for demonstrating collateral vessels (Fig. 38.23).

VEC cine MRI can be applied to demonstrate the presence of and estimate the volume of collateral circulation to the descending aorta below the coarctation site (Fig. 38.24). This is accomplished by using two imaging planes perpendicular to the aorta; one is about 2 cm beyond the coarctation and the other at the level of the diaphragm. In the normal aorta, volume flow is greater (about 5%-7% higher) at the proximal site. On the other hand, in a hemodynamically significant coarctation, volume flow is greater at the diaphragm because of retrograde flow through the intercostal and mammary arteries and other collaterals into the distal aorta. The presence of greater flow at the diaphragmatic level is considered a functional indicator

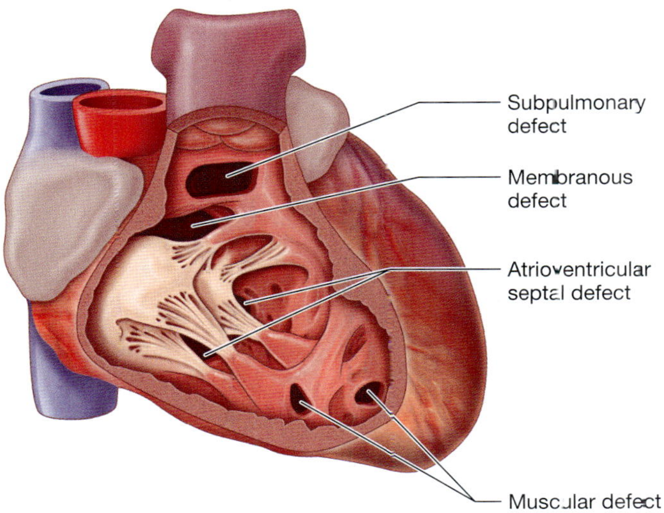

Figure 38.12. Ventricular septal defect diagram.

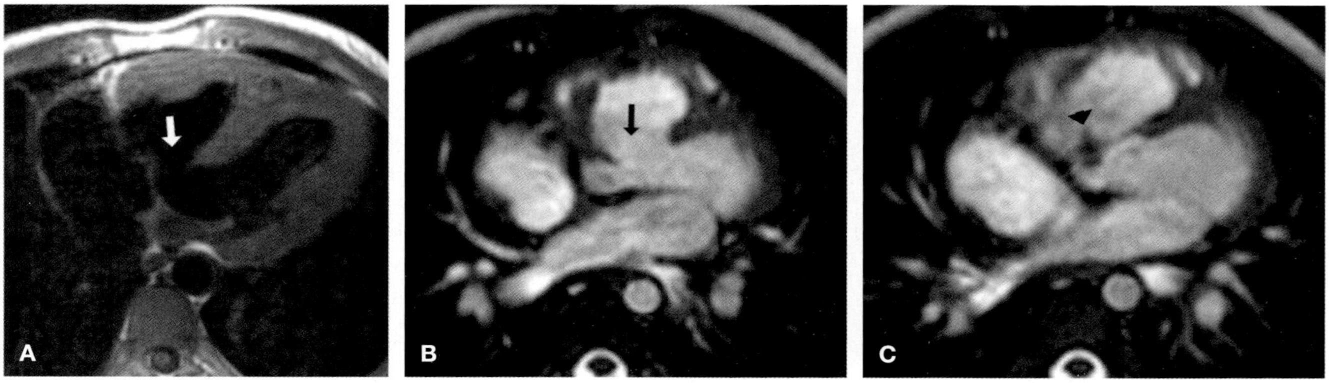

Figure 38.13. Ventricular septal defect. Spin-echo **(A)** and steady-state free-precession in diastole **(B)** and systole **(C)** axial images show a defect in the perimembranous ventricular septum (*arrows*). A signal void at the defect is projected into the right ventricle during systole (*arrowhead*).

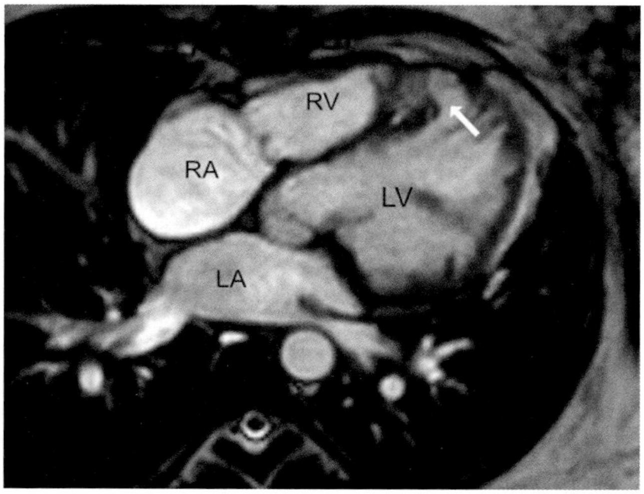

Figure 38.14. Muscular VSD. Axial cine MR image shows a defect in the muscular ventricular septum (*arrow*). LA, left atrium; LV, left ventricle; RA, right atrium; RV, right ventricle.

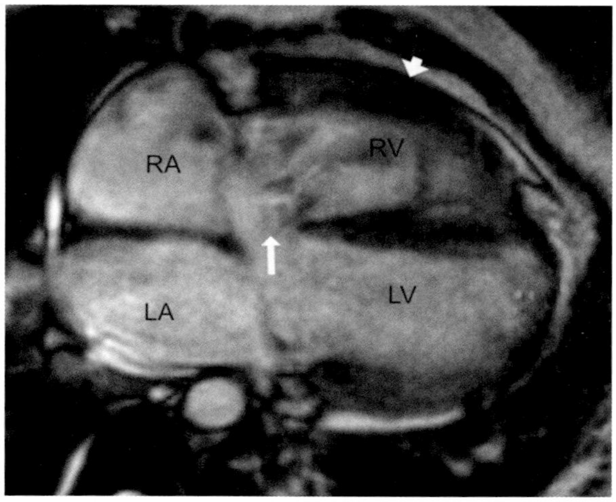

Figure 38.15. Inlet ventricular septal defect. Horizontal long-axis cine image shows a ventricular septal defect (*arrow*) just beneath the atrioventricular valves. LA, left atrium; LV, left ventricle; RA, right atrium; RV, right ventricle.

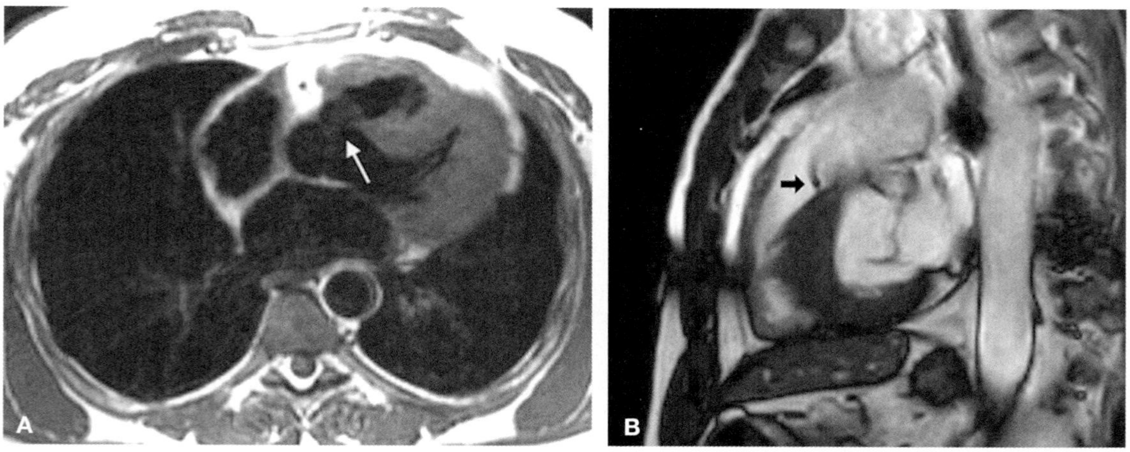

Figure 38.16. Supracristal (doubly committed) ventricular septal defect. Spin-echo image in the axial plane **(A)** and cine MR image in the right ventricular outflow tract plane **(B)**, from a different patient, demonstrate a defect (*white arrow*) in the outlet portion of the septum. A flow void (*black arrow*) projects into the upper region of the right ventricular outflow region.

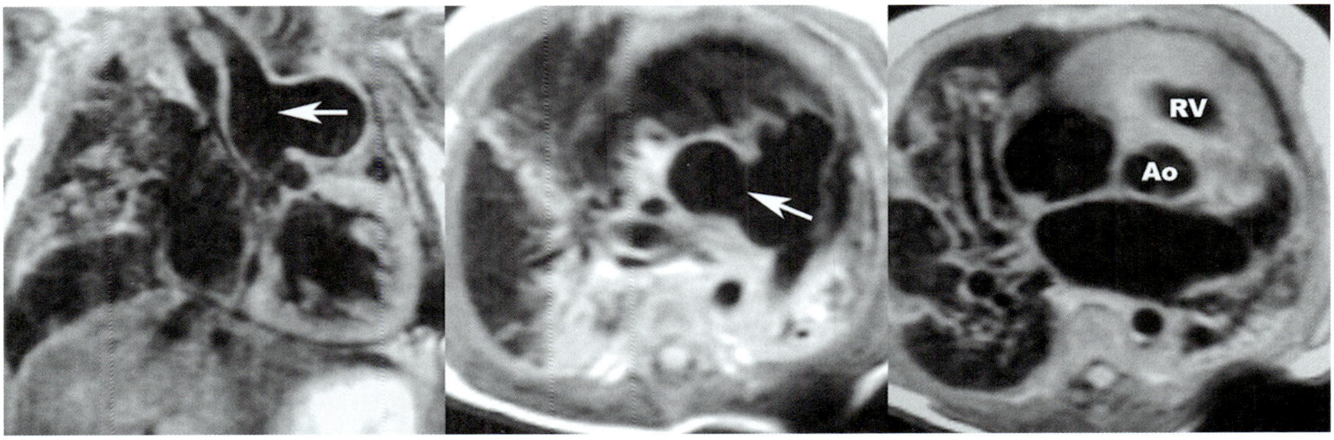

Figure 38.17. Aorticopulmonary window. Coronal (**left**) and axial (**center and right**) spin-echo images demonstrate a defect (*arrows*) between the proximal ascending aorta and the pulmonary artery. Ao, aorta; RV, right ventricular outlet region.

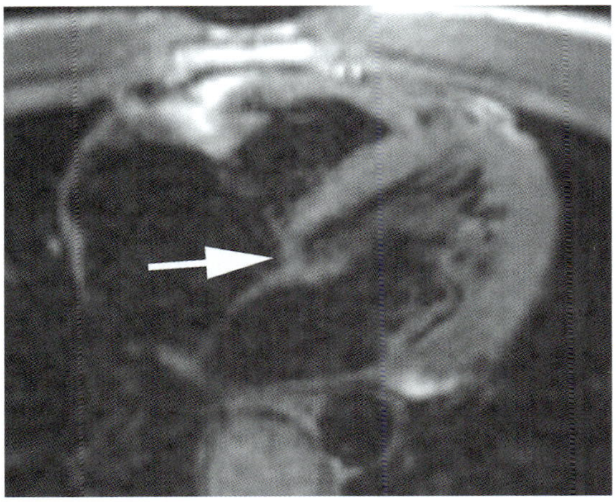

Figure 38.18. Atrioventricular septum. Axial spin-echo image shows the small portion (*arrow*) of ventricular septum separating the left ventricle and the right atrium. Note the more ventral position of the tricuspid valve relative to the mitral valve.

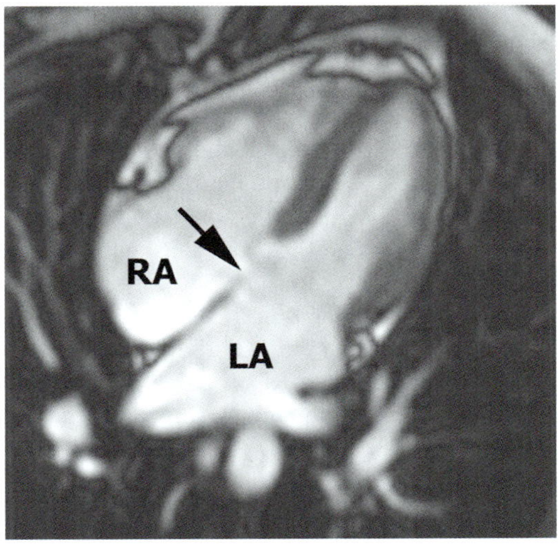

Figure 38.19. Primum atrial septal defect. Cine MR image in the horizontal long-axis plane shows a defect at the level of the septum primum (*arrow*). LA, left atrium; RA, right atrium.

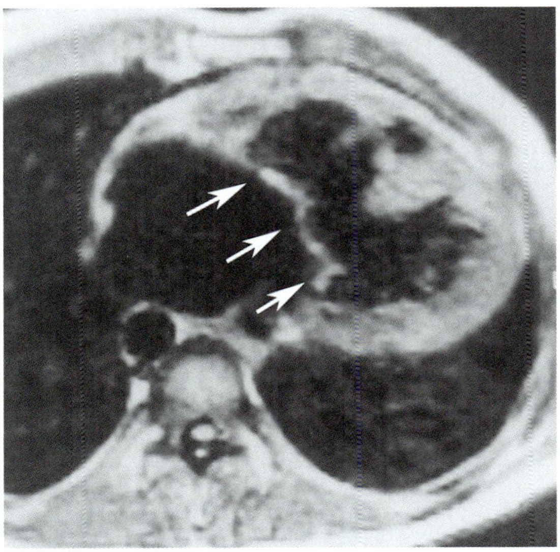

Figure 38.20. Atrioventricular canal (endocardial cushion) defect. Axial spin-echo image shows a large defect in the inlet portion of the ventricular septum. A single atrioventricular valve (*arrows*) spans the inlet of both ventricles.

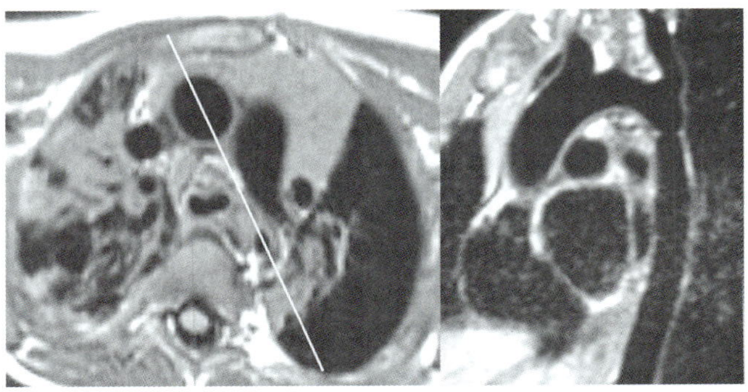

Figure 38.21. Coarctation of the aorta. Axial (**left**) and oblique sagittal (**right**) spin-echo images. A line bisecting the ascending and descending aorta at the coarctation prescribes the oblique sagittal plane (long-axis plane of the thoracic aorta). This latter image displays the coarctation site along with the arch.

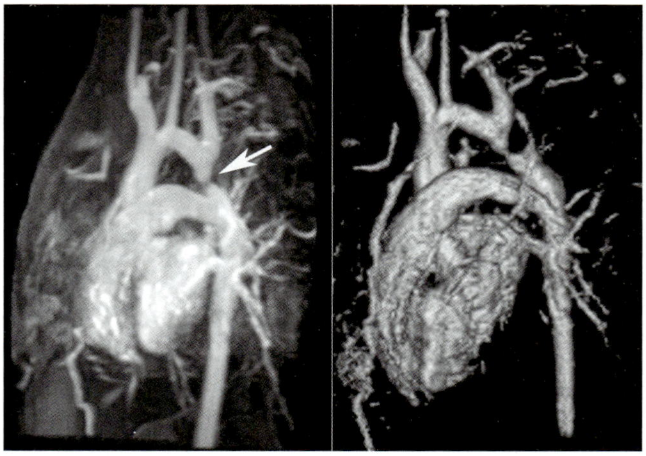

Figure 38.22. Coarctation of the aorta. Contrast-enhanced 3D magnetic resonance angiography in the sagittal plane shows a discrete juxtaductal coarctation (*arrow*) on the maximum intensity projection (**left**) and the volume-rendered 3D reconstruction (**right**).

of hemodynamic significance of the coarctation. There is a rough linear relationship between the percentage of stenosis and the volume of collateral circulation. After stenting of the coarctation, VEC cine MRI has demonstrated a reversal of the collateral flow since flow at the proximal site becomes greater than at the distal one. Another flow indication of a hemodynamically significant coarctation is forward flow throughout the diastole in the distal descending aorta.

Theoretically, VEC cine MRI can also be used to estimate the gradient across the coarctation. Using planes perpendicular and parallel to the coarctation, the peak velocity of flow can be estimated. Applying the modified Bernoulli formula (peak pressure gradient = 4 × [peak velocity]^2), the peak gradient is estimated. The voxel (s) with highest velocity in systole can be identified on phase images in both planes. The highest in either plan is considered the peak velocity (Fig. 38.25).

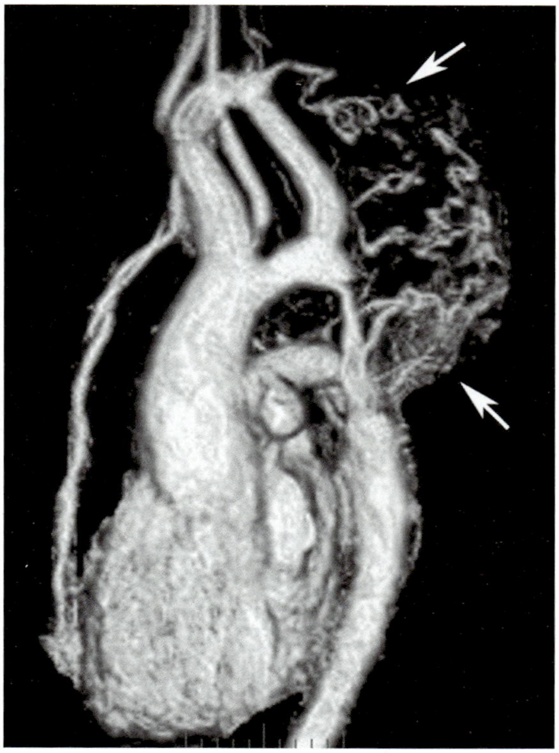

Figure 38.23. Coarctation of the aorta. Contrast-enhanced 3D magnetic resonance angiography in the sagittal plane shows long-segment coarctation caused by Takayasu's arteritis. Note the abundant collateral arterial connections (*arrows*).

Arch Anomalies

There are numerous types of arch anomalies resulting from abnormal resorption of the anterior or posterior segments of the embryonic double-arch configuration. However, the only ones encountered with greatest frequency are complete (patent) double arch, double arch with atretic posterior

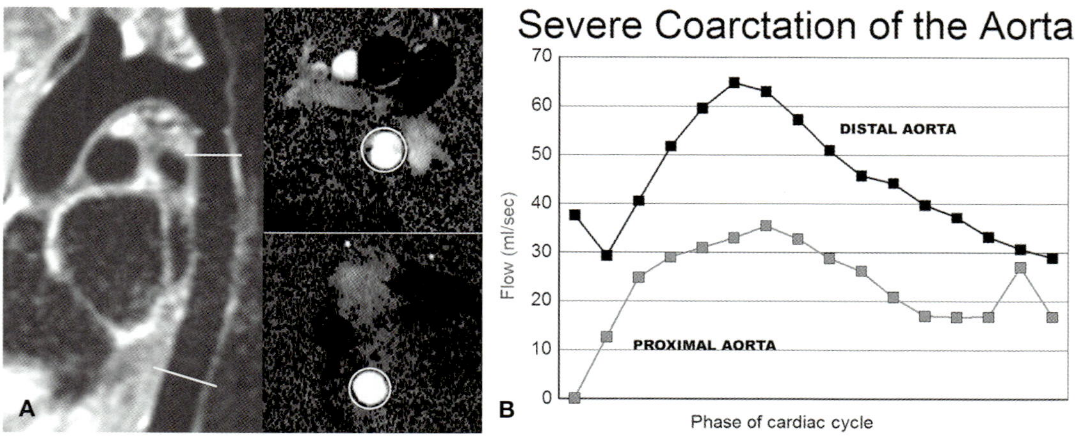

Figure 38.24. **A:** Coarctation of the aorta. Sites of planes for magnitude and phase images in the proximal (**top**) and distal aorta (**bottom**) used to estimate the volume of collateral flow. **B:** Flow versus time curves for the proximal and distal descending aorta show a larger flow volume in the distal compared with the proximal aorta caused by retrograde flow in aortic branches below the coarctation. The volume of collateral flow is estimated as the difference in flow volumes (areas under the curves) at the two sites.

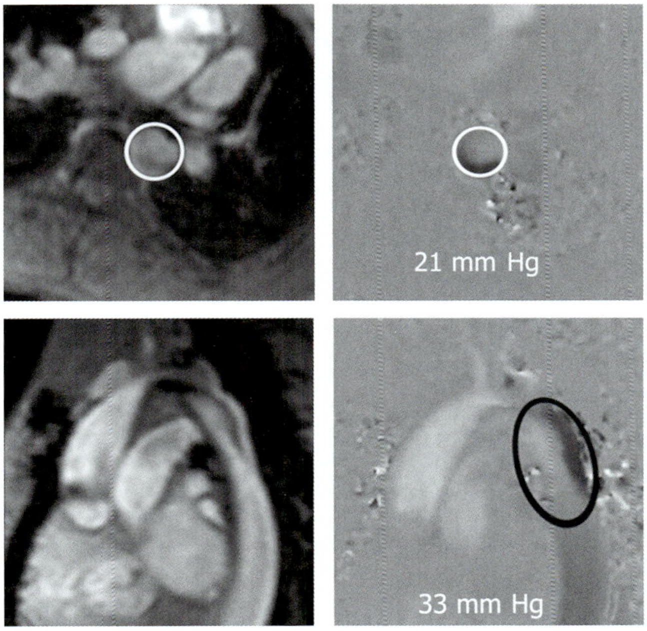

Figure 38.25. Pressure gradient in aortic coarctation. Magnitude (**top left**) and phase (**top right**) images from VEC-MR acquisition perpendicular to the descending aorta in a level distal to the coarctation demonstrate an estimated pressure gradient of 21 mm Hg. Magnitude (**bottom left**) and phase (**bottom right**) images from an in-plane VEC-MR aligned to the descending aorta show an estimated pressure gradient of 33 mm Hg. VEC-MR, velocity-encoded cine-MR.

component of the left arch (Fig. 38.26), right arch with aberrant (retroesophageal) left subclavian artery (Fig. 38.27), and left arch with aberrant right subclavian artery. The first three produce complete vascular rings that may narrow the trachea and esophagus; a left arch with aberrant right subclavian artery usually is without physiologic consequence. In vascular rings, compression of the trachea is by the aortic component situated between the vertebral body and the esophagus. The vascular ring with right arch and aberrant left subclavian artery is completed by the posterior component that is tethered anteriorly by a left-sided ligamentum arteriosum. With mirror-image right aortic arch, the ligamentum courses between the left innominate artery and the proximal left pulmonary artery. On the other hand, with right aortic arch and aberrant left subclavian aretery, the ligamentum courses between the descending aorta and the proximal left pulmonary artery. At the site of attachment of the ligamentum, there is an enlargement or diverticulum of the descending aorta. This localized dilatation tethered anteriorly by the posterior left-sided ligamentum is the structure that compresses the trachea and esophagus rather than the left subclavian artery itself. These anatomic arrangements can be readily discerned on MR images in the transaxial plane and 3D MRA.

For the evaluation of arch anomalies, spin-echo images can be acquired in sagittal (5-mm slice thickness) and transaxial (3-mm slice thickness) planes. These images display the aortic anomaly and verify that the anomalous component produces airway compression. Cine MR images may be used to display the pulsatile nature of the airway obstruction. In some cases, the site of maximal airway compression is at the carina or even involves a proximal bronchus.

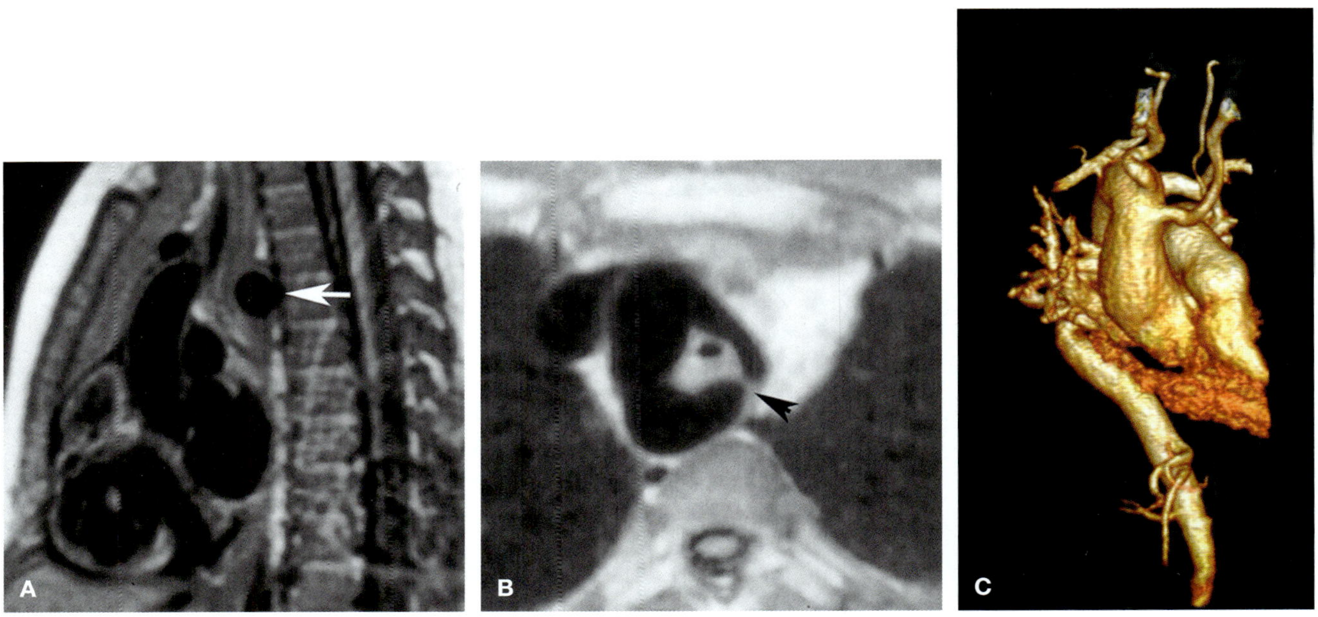

Figure 38.26. Double aortic arch. Spin-echo images in sagittal **(A)** and axial **(B)** planes display posterior compression of the trachea by a retroesophageal component (*arrow*) of a double arch. The axial plane shows that the right arch is the larger of the two and also shows a short atretic posterior segment (*arrowhead*) of the left arch. Volume-rendered reformation of a magnetic resonance angiography **(C)** from a different patient with a double aortic arch shows a similar ring configuration atretic segment of the left arch.

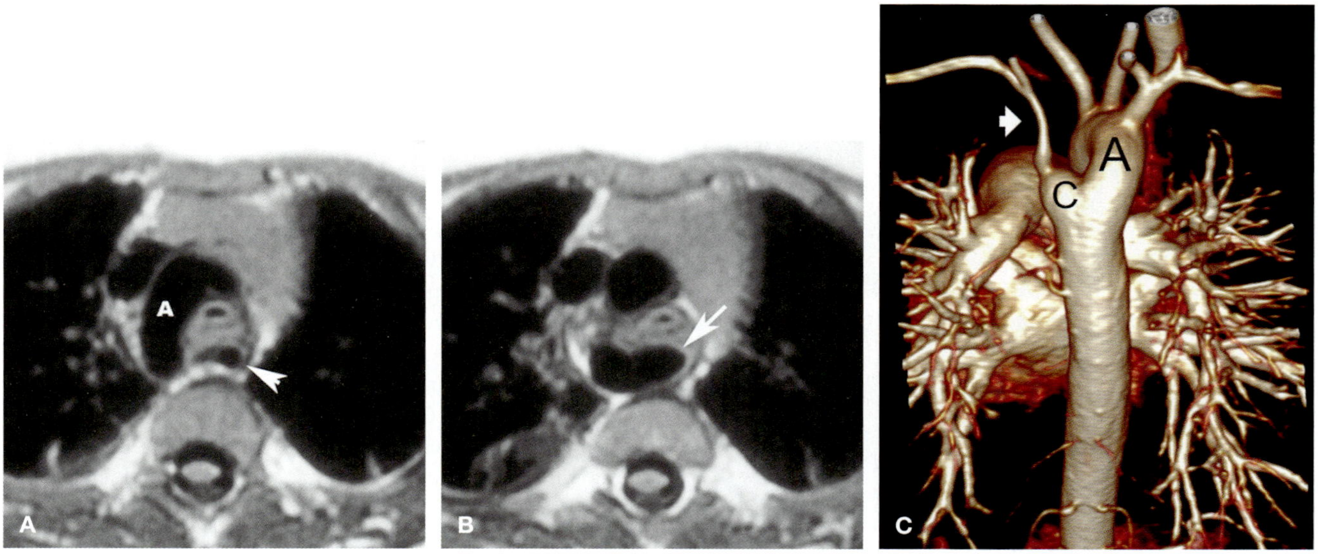

Figure 38.27. Right aortic arch with aberrant left subclavian artery. Spin-echo axial images **(A)** show the right arch (*A*) and aberrant left subclavian artery (*arrowhead*). Adjacent axial image **(B)** shows the diverticulum (*arrow and C*) of the descending arch, which is the site of origin of the left subclavian artery. Volume-rendered reformation of an MRA **(C)** for different patient shows a posterior projection of the abnormality.

Contrast-enhanced 3D MRA is more efficient to demonstrate the arch anomaly given shorter acquisition time compared to spin echo images. The MRA acquisition is done in either the sagittal or coronal planes and can be reformatted in any plane that best displays the abnormality.

Pulmonary Arterial Anomalies

Pulmonary arterial anomalies can be evaluated with contrast-enhanced 3D MRA (Fig. 38.28), and can also be identified on spin-echo and cine MRI images. Contrast-enhanced 3D MRA is usually acquired in the coronal plane; a short acquisition period is optimal to depict the pulmonary arteries before enhancement of the left heart and aorta. VEC-MRI cine sequences are obtained perpendicular to the long axis of the right, left, and main pulmonary arterial segments. VEC-MRI can be used for measuring blood flow and calculating the differential pulmonary flow to the right and left lungs (Fig. 38.29).

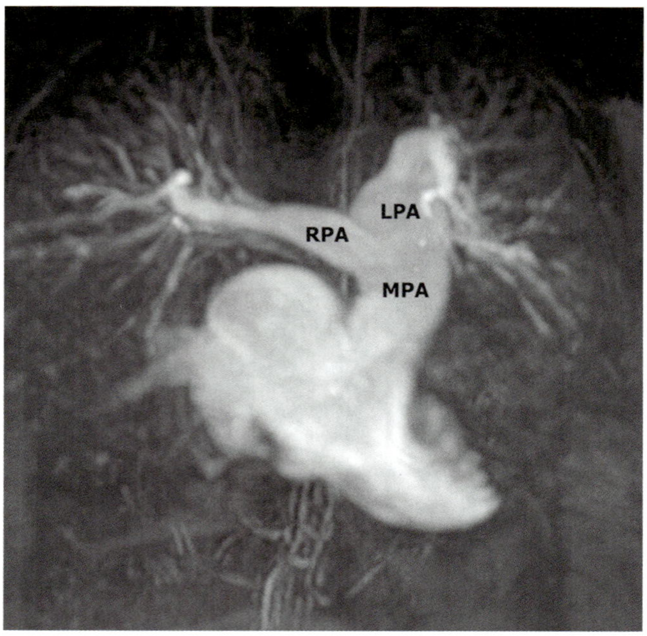

Figure 38.28. Pulmonary valvular stenosis. 3D reconstructions from a magnetic resonance angiography demonstrate enlargement of the main (*MPA*) and left (*LPA*) pulmonary arteries, with normal dimension of the right pulmonary artery (*RPA*).

Compared to echocardiography, MRI is more useful for examining the right and left pulmonary arteries, as well as the lobar and segmental arteries. MRI is especially useful for demonstrating central and peripheral pulmonary artery stenoses (see Fig. 38.30), absent pulmonary artery (Fig. 38.31), and pulmonary artery sling (Fig. 38.32). MRI and MRA are the preferred techniques for the evaluation of residual pulmonary arterial stenoses after repair of tetralogy of Fallot (Fig. 38.28).

The hemodynamic significance of branch pulmonary arterial stenoses is assessed by VEC cine MRI measurement of blood flow separately for each pulmonary artery (Fig. 38.29). Since flow is also measured for the main pulmonary artery, the values can be expressed as the percentage of total pulmonary blood flow to each lung. The measurement can be done before and after angioplasty to document therapeutic benefit, although such measurements may not be possible in the presence of stainless steel stents.

Pulmonary Valvular Stenosis

Pulmonary valvular stenosis is characterized morphologically on MR as enlargement of the main and left pulmonary arteries (Figs. 38.28 and 38.33). There is a systolic high-velocity flow jet across the valve on cine MRI. Cine MRI also displays hypertrabeculation and hypertrophy of the infundibulum. Cine MRI in the right ventricular outflow track (RVOT) plane can be used

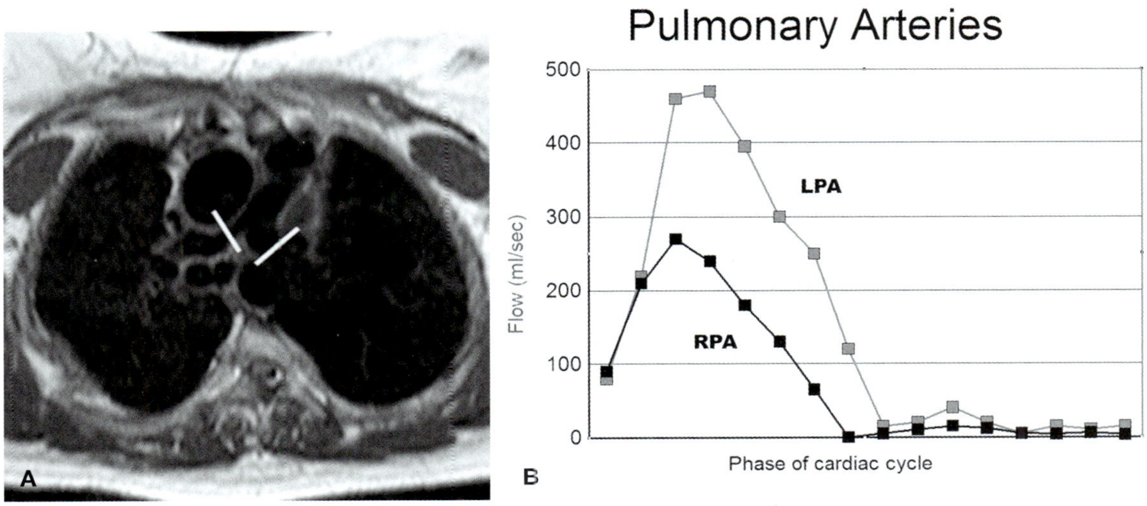

Figure 38.29. **A:** Sites of acquisition of velocity-encoded (phase-contrast) cine MR sequence for the right and left pulmonary arteries. **B:** Flow versus time curves for the right and left pulmonary arteries demonstrate drastically impaired flow in the right pulmonary artery.

to exclude or determine the severity of any concomitant infundibular stenosis. This plane is also used to measure the diameter of the annulus. Velocity-encoded cine MRI sequences in planes both parallel (RVOT plane) and perpendicular to flow across the valve are used to determine peak velocity of flow in order to estimate transvalvular gradient (Fig. 38.34).

After pulmonary valvuloplasty, cine MRI and VEC MR are applied for quantifying any resultant pulmonary regurgitation. For this purpose, VEC MR is acquired in a plane perpendicular to flow in the proximal pulmonary artery. Cine MRI in the short-axis plane is used to measure RV volumes and ejection fraction.

Congenital Aortic Stenosis

MRI is not used typically to evaluate aortic stenosis severity; this is done with echocardiography. The major role of MRI is to evaluate the severity of poststenotic dilatation of the ascending aorta and secondary left ventricular hypertrophy or dysfunction. Severe aortoannular ectasia of the proximal ascending aorta in association with aortic stenoses or even nonobstructive bicuspid valve can occur in childhood. MRI and MRA in the sagittal plane are optimal for demonstrating the dimensions of the aorta (Fig. 38.35). VEC cine MRI may be used to quantify concomitant aortic regurgitation.

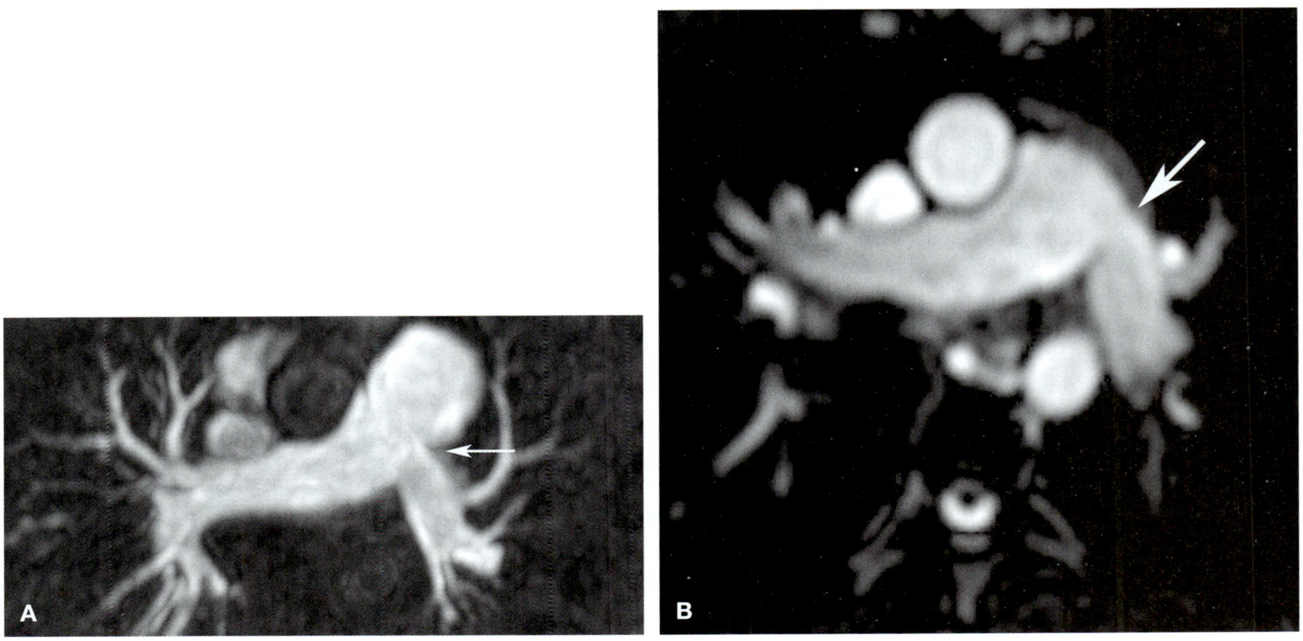

Figure 38.30. Coronal multisectional maximum intensity projection (MIP) of contrast magnetic resonance angiography (**A, left**) and axial cine MR (**B, right**) in postoperative tetralogy of Fallot shows residual stenosis (*arrow*) in proximal left pulmonary artery.

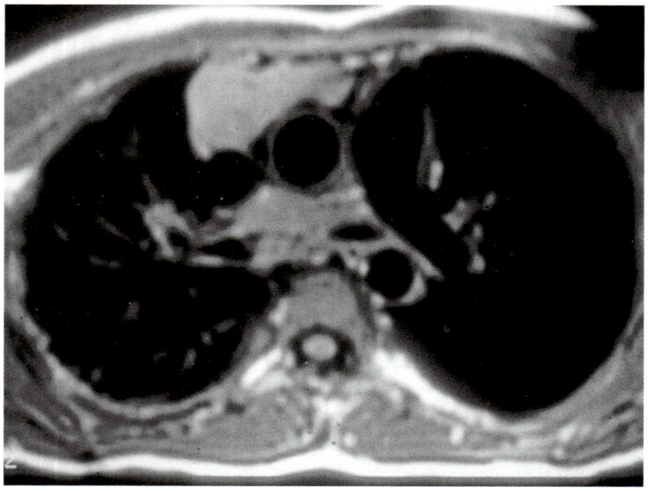

Figure 38.31. Absent pulmonary artery. Spin-echo axial image shows absence of the right pulmonary artery. There is no pulmonary artery coursing between the ascending aorta and the right bronchus.

Coronary Artery Anomalies

Coronary MRA can be used to demonstrate anomalies in the origin and course of the coronary arteries. Coronary anomalies may occur as isolated lesions or in association with other congenital cardiac anomalies, such as tetralogy of Fallot or transposition of the great arteries.

The most common clinically relevant coronary anomalies involve an anomalous aortic origin of a coronary artery, often from the opposite aortic sinus. Anomalous aortic origin may be innocuous (Fig. 38.36) or potentially lethal (Fig. 38.37). The potentially lethal anomalies have a proximal course between the base of the aorta and the proximal pulmonary artery (interarterial course). With innocuous ectopic origin, the proximal coronary courses behind the aorta (retroaortic course) or anterior of the pulmonary artery. A coronary artery can also pass through the right ventricular outlet region (transseptal course), the clinical significance of this finding is less well-known. While selective (x-ray) coronary arteriography can demonstrate ectopic origin, it can be challenging to define the proximal course of the artery so noninvasive imaging with coronary MRA (or coronary CT angiography) is preferred.

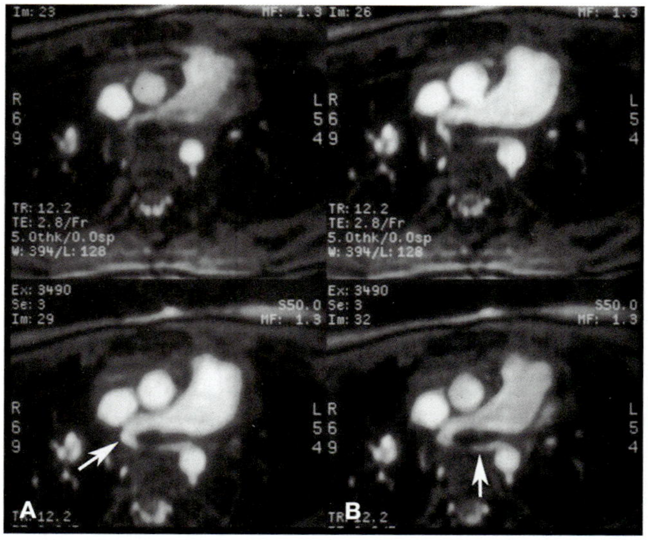

Figure 38.32. Pulmonary artery sling. Spin echo image in the axial plane **(A)** and maximum intensity projection reconstruction of magnetic resonance angiography **(B)** show the left pulmonary artery (*arrowhead*) taking off from the right pulmonary artery. The left pulmonary artery curves around and posterior to the right bronchus as it courses to the left side. Note the narrowing of the right bronchus (*arrow*).

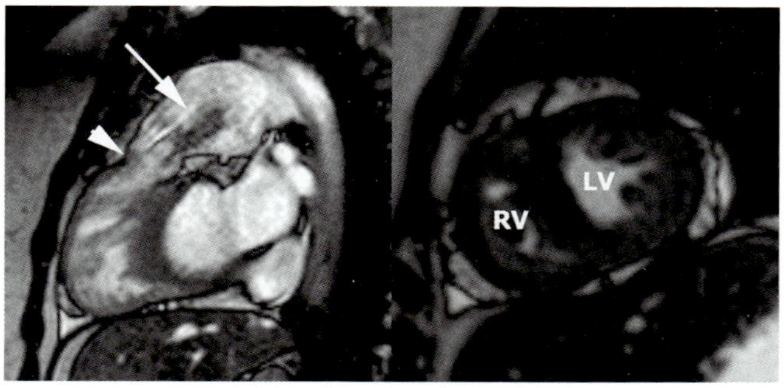

Figure 38.33. Pulmonary valve stenosis. Cine MR image during early systole in the right ventricular outflow tract plane (**left**) and during end systole in the short-axis plane (**right**). Note the poststenotic flow jet (*arrow*) emanating from the pulmonary valve (*arrowhead*). Right ventricular hypertrophy is seen as almost complete cavity obliteration during end systole. LV, left ventricle; RV, right ventricle.

Rarely the right or left coronary artery can arise anomalously from the pulmonary artery (Fig. 38.38). In this configuration the coronary artery which arises normally from the aorta will receive anterograde flow and feed the anomalous coronary artery via dilated collaterals. The anomalous coronary will flow retrograde and *drain* into the pulmonary artery. Both coronary arteries are typically dilated.

Coronary MRA employs a respiratory navigator-compensated ECG-gated 3D free-breathing technique.

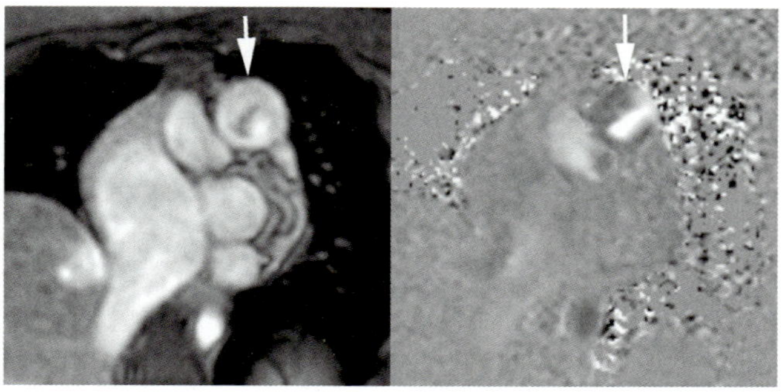

Figure 38.34. Pulmonary valve stenosis. Magnitude (**left**) and phase (**right**) images from velocity-encoded cine-MR sequence perpendicular to the blood flow in the main pulmonary artery. Note the flow jet (*arrows*) representing high-velocity flow distal to the stenotic pulmonary valve.

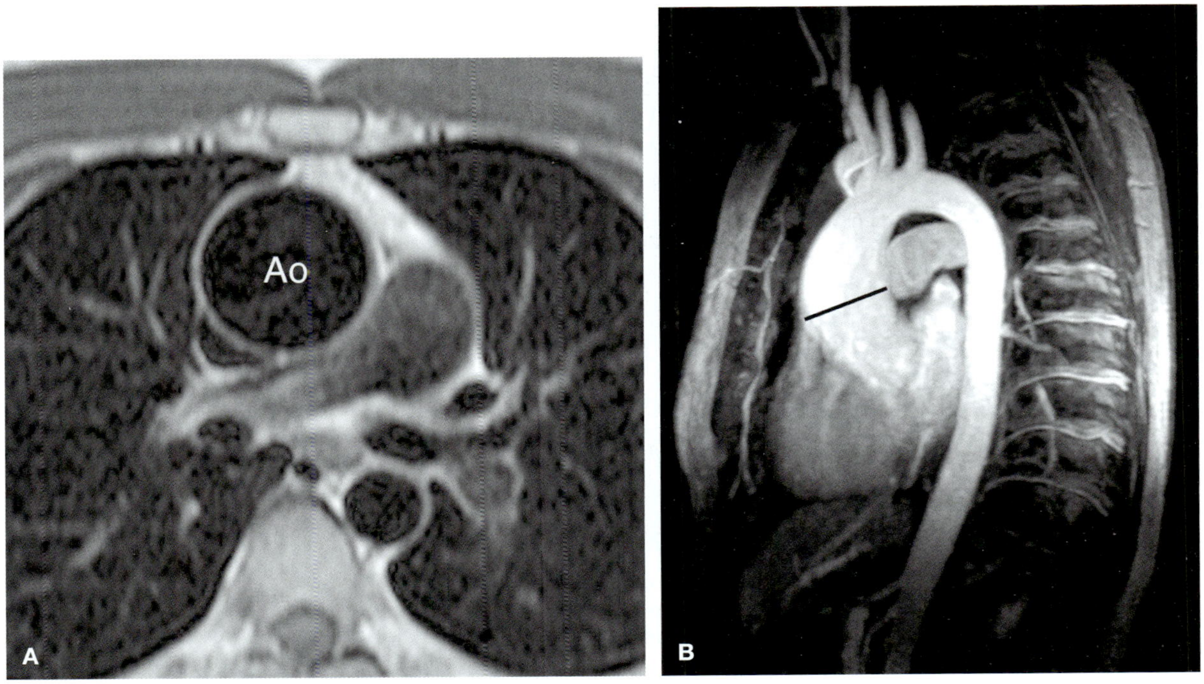

Figure 38.35. Spin-echo image in axial plane (**A, left**) and contrast magnetic resonance angiography in sagittal plane (**B, right**) show aneurysmal ascending aorta in patient with bicuspid aortic valve. Maximum diameter (line) in the ascending aorta is 5.6 cm.

This technique displays clearly the origin of the coronary artery from the sinus of Valsalva and its proximal course. A single coronary artery may arise from either the right or left sinus of Valsalva, or both coronary arteries may arise individually from one sinus of Valsalva (Fig. 38.37). In a child with chest pain or syncope during exercise or aborted sudden death, coronary MRA can be used to exclude a proximal interarterial course.

CYANOTIC LESIONS

Analysis of Complex Congenital Heart Disease Using MRI: Segmental Approach

The analysis of complex CHD requires a systematic approach. The approach most widely used today is the segmental one, in which the heart is partitioned into three main segments (atria, ventricles, and great vessels) and the connections

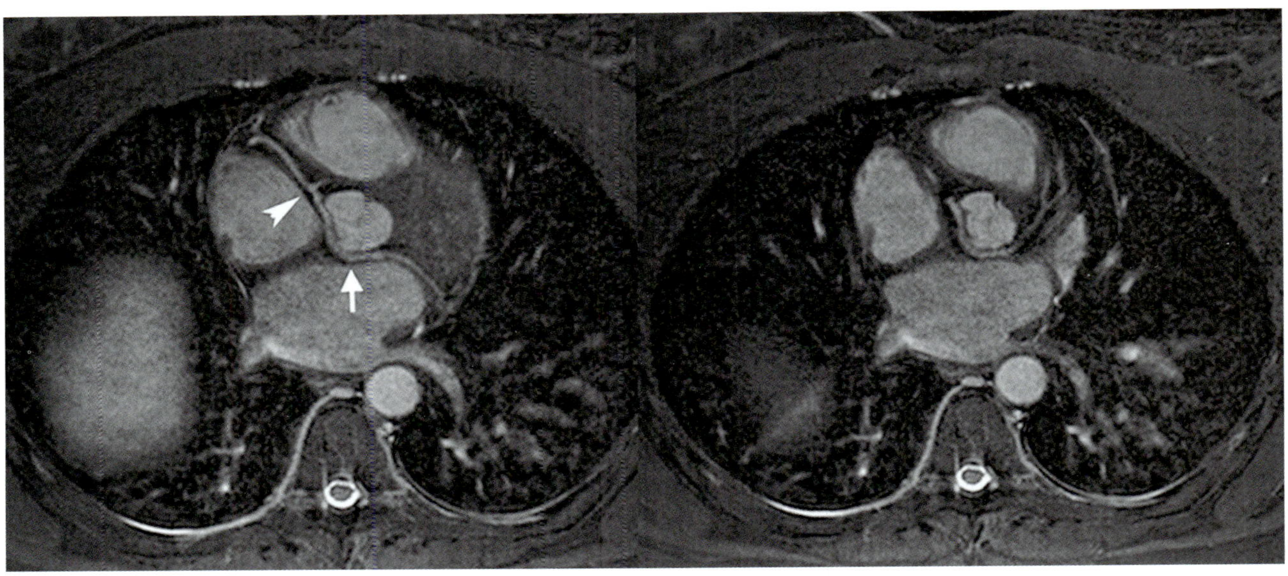

Figure 38.36. Anomalous origin of the left coronary artery from the right coronary artery with a retroaortic course. Two adjacent sections from coronary magnetic resonance angiography display the ectopic origin of the left coronary artery from the right coronary (*arrowhead*) and passage of the left artery behind the aorta (*arrow*).

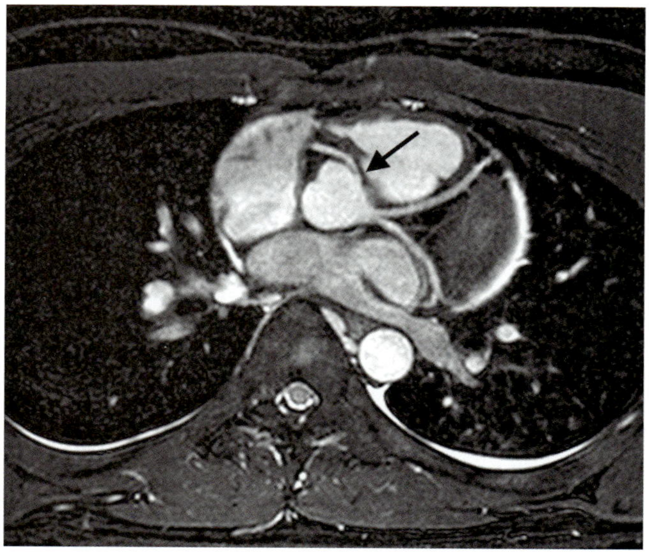

Figure 38.37. Ectopic origin of the right coronary artery with an interarterial course. Coronary magnetic resonance angiography shows the origin of the right coronary artery (*arrow*) from the right end of the left sinus of Valsalva in a position where the proximal portion of the artery is compressed between the aorta and the main pulmonary artery.

between them (atrioventricular and ventriculoarterial connections). Transaxial images from the aortic arch to the upper abdomen clearly demonstrate the segmental cardiovascular anatomy and connections of one segment to the other (atrioventricular connections and ventriculoarterial connections) and the types of situs.

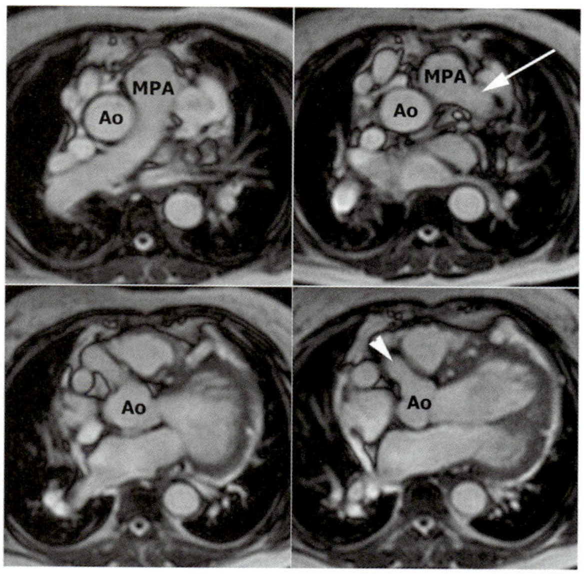

Figure 38.38. Anomalous origin of the left coronary artery. Axial cine MR images from the base of the heart (**bottom right**) to the level of the great vessels (**top left**) demonstrate anomalous origin of the left coronary artery (*arrow*) from the main pulmonary artery (*MPA*). Note the dilated right coronary artery (*arrowhead*) connecting normally to the aorta (*Ao*).

Table 38.1 Identification and Position of Atria
Left atrium
"Finger-shaped" appendage
Narrow orifice of appendage
Right atrium
Triangular-shaped appendage
Wide orifice of appendage
Connects to inferior vena cava
Right atrium on the right side—situs solitus
Right atrium on the left side—situs inversus
Bilateral morphologic right atria—right sidedness (frequently asplenia)
Bilateral morphologic left atria—left sidedness (frequently polysplenia)

Visceroatrial Situs

The right atria and left atria are described by their morphologic structure and not their position (Table 38.2). An atrium with the morphologic features of a left atrium, which may be located to the right of midline, is called a morphologic left atrium. Cine MR images can clearly depict the characteristic morphologic features of the atria.

The most definite features of the atria are the appendages. On an axial MR image, the right atrial appendage appears as a triangular structure with a broad-based opening into the right atrium. This is in distinction to the left atrial appendage, a long, narrow, finger-like projection with a narrow orifice. The atrial appendages are the most constant part of the atria, even in complex abnormalities. If the atrial appendages are difficult to identify, the next most reliable structure is the drainage of the IVC. The atrium connecting to the IVC is considered the morphologic right atrium. Superior vena caval and pulmonary venous drainage are variable and are not used to identify atrial morphology. The ostium of the coronary sinus drains into the

Table 38.2 Morphologic Features of Ventricles
Right ventricle
Infundibulum
No fibrous continuity between atrioventricular and semilunar valves
Moderator band
Corrugated surface of ventricular septum near apex
Left ventricle
No infundibulum
Fibrous continuity between atrioventricular and semilunar valves
Papillary muscles
Smooth septal surface near apex

right atrium but may be difficult to identify, particularly in cases when it is unroofed. The thin flap of septum primum belongs to the left atrium while the thicker folds of septum secundum are on the right atrial side.

Ventricular Loop

Several morphologic features identify right versus left ventricle (Table 38.2). Identification of these characteristics is readily accomplished using cine images. The right ventricle has a muscular infundibulum (tunnel of myocardium) separating the atrioventricular and semilunar valves, a moderator band, and trabeculated surface of the right ventricular aspect of the septum (Fig. 38.39). The left ventricle shows direct fibrous continuity between the mitral and aortic valves (in patients with normally related great arteries), two distinct papillary muscles that attach to the free wall, fine apical trabeculations, and the smooth surface of the left ventricular aspect of the septum.

The normal rightward bending of the primitive cardiac tube places the morphologic right ventricle on the right side of the heart. This rightward bending is called D-looping (D for dextro, right). If the primitive heart tube bends to the left, the result is called L-looping (L for levo, left), in which the morphologic right ventricle is placed on the left side of the heart. A heart with the morphologic right ventricle on the left side usually has an L-ventricular loop. In situs solitus, a D-loop is normal. In situs inversus, L-loop is normal.

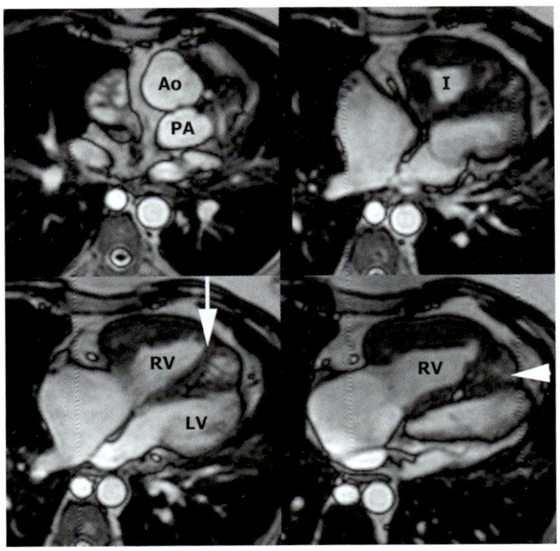

Figure 38.39. Right ventricular characteristics. Axial cine MR images from the level of the great vessels (**top left**) to the midventricular level (**bottom right**) show a hypertrophied systemic right ventricle (*RV*) in a patient with transposition of the great arteries. Note the muscular infundibulum (*I*), moderator band (*arrow*), and irregular surface of the ventricular septum (*arrowhead*) at the apical level. Ao, aorta; LV, left ventricle; PA, pulmonary artery.

Atrioventricular connections can be concordant or discordant. In normal, concordant atrioventricular connections, the right atrium is connected to the right ventricle and the left atrium to the left ventricle. The atrioventricular valves remain with their respective ventricles, regardless of the type of ventricular loop: The mitral valve resides with the left ventricle, and the tricuspid valve is part of the right ventricle.

Discordant atrioventricular connections are right atrium to the left ventricle and left atrium to the right ventricle. Congenitally corrected transposition of the great arteries (TGA) is an example of an anomaly with atrioventricular discordance.

Great Artery Relationships

MRI images at the base of the heart clearly define the normal relationship of the pulmonary artery anterior and to the left of the aorta. Such images also identify concordant (aorta connected to the left ventricle and pulmonary artery connected to the right ventricle) and discordant (aorta connected to the right ventricle and pulmonary artery connected to the left ventricle) ventriculoarterial connections.

Complete TGA is an example of atrioventricular concordance and ventriculoarterial discordance. Corrected TGA is an example of atrioventricular and ventriculoarterial discordance. Double discordance results in blood flowing serially through the pulmonary and systemic circulation and therefore is a non-cyanotic congenital heart defect.

Tetralogy of Fallot

Tetralogy of Fallot consists of obstruction to the right ventricular outlet region (usually multilevel), malalignment outlet VSD, enlarged aorta overriding the VSD, and a hypertrabeculated, hypertrophied right ventricle. These features are clearly defined on spin-echo and cine MR images (Fig. 38.40). Transaxial and oblique coronal images demonstrate the VSD and the position of the aorta overriding the defect. Cine MRI in the RVOT plane defines the narrowed infundibulum and in most cases a stenotic pulmonic annulus and/or valve. Sagittal and transaxial images are used to assess the size of the main and central pulmonary arteries and to display focal stenoses which are better demonstrated on MRA. Imaging oriented in a plane parallel to the long axis of the right (oblique coronal plane) and left (oblique sagittal plane) pulmonary arteries is used to assess the severity of central pulmonary arterial stenoses, which are common in this anomaly. Contrast-enhanced 3D MRA is employed to demonstrate pulmonary arterial stenoses and the systemic source of collateral flow to the lungs (Fig. 38.41). VEC cine MRI can be used to define differential blood flow to the two lungs and measure pulmonic valve stenosis or regurgitation.

Tetralogy of Fallot is usually repaired by relieving the pulmonic stenosis and closing the VSD. Stenosis of the main or branch arteries, the size of the right ventricle outflow tract, and the size and function of the right ventricle are important

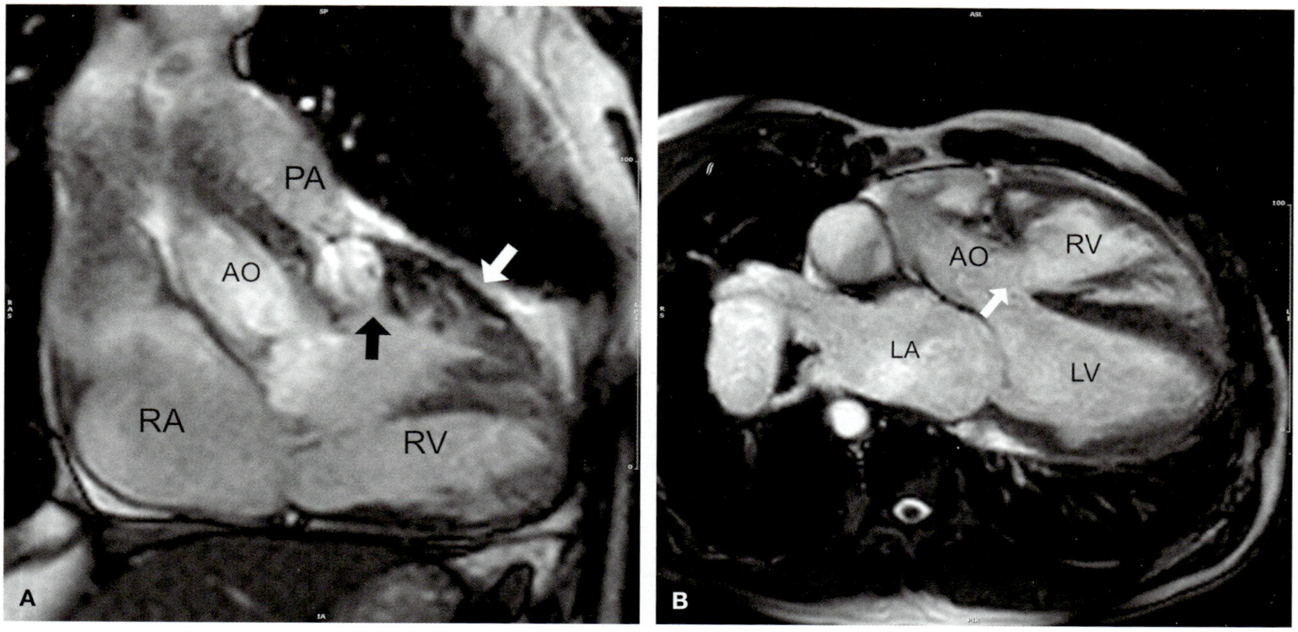

Figure 38.40. Unrepaired tetralogy of Fallot. Oblique coronal **(A)** SSFP cine MR image shows right ventricular (RV) hypertrophy (white arrow), and subvalvular pulmonary stenosis (black arrow). SSFP image in the axial plane **(B)** shows a perimembranous venricular septal defect (white arrow), and the aorta (AO) overriding the defect. LA, left atrium; LV, left ventricle; PA, pulmonary artery; RA, right atrium; RV, right ventricle.

to assess in preoperative planning and are well defined by MRI. Coronary anomalies may occur in patients with tetralogy of Fallot. The most important is the origin of the left anterior descending coronary artery from the right coronary artery with anomalous artery passing anterior to the right ventricle outflow tract. This configuration may prevent an incision along the RVOT and require repair with a right ventricle to pulmonary artery conduit.

Tetralogy of Fallot With Pulmonary Atresia

Tetralogy of Fallot with pulmonary atresia is a severe form of tetralogy of Fallot in which a direct connection from the right ventricle to the pulmonary arteries is absent. On axial or RVOT MRI, a solid layer of muscle in the region of the right ventricle outflow tract indicates an infundibulum with a blind end. No connection between the right ventricle and the pulmonary artery confluence (if present) can be demonstrated (Fig. 38.42). The atresia can be focal, limited to the valve level, or more extensive. The length of the atresia can be determined by inspecting sequential axial images. Focal membranous pulmonary atresia may be indistinguishable from severe stenosis on axial MR images because of partial volume averaging. The use of 3-mm-thick spin-echo images reduces partial volume effects. Cine MRI in RVOT plane can establish the presence or absence of flow across the valve. An enlarged aorta is seen overriding the VSD (Fig. 38.42). Blood is usually delivered to the lungs via a PDA or via systemic to pulmonary collateral channels, which can be seen as abnormal vessels originating from the descending aorta and traveling toward the lungs or connecting with the pulmonary arteries. These are shown best on contrast-enhanced 3D MRA (Fig. 38.41).

The surgical correction of tetralogy of Fallot with pulmonary atresia usually consists of placing a conduit from the right ventricle to the central pulmonary arteries (if present) or to a surgically created confluence of pulmonary arteries. In patients where the pulmonary blood flow is via extensive

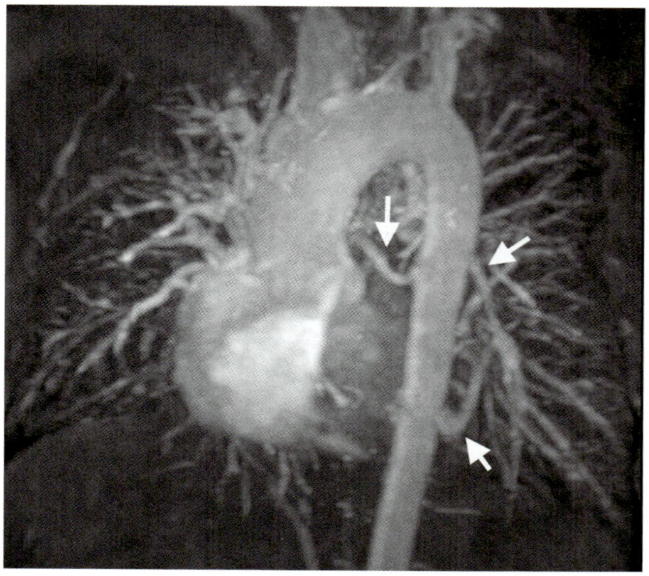

Figure 38.41. Pulmonary atresia with ventricular septal defect. Contrast-enhanced 3D magnetic resonance angiography in the coronal plane displays several large systemic to pulmonary artery collaterals (*arrows*) arising from the descending aorta.

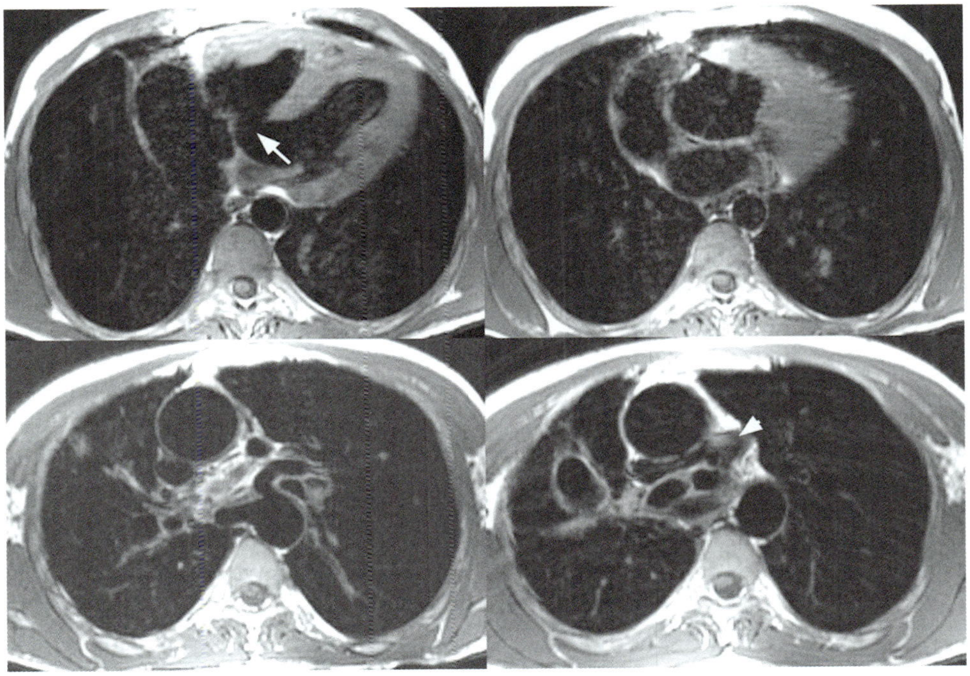

Figure 38.42. Pulmonary atresia with ventricular septal defect. Spin-echo axial images arranged from caudal (**top left**) to cranial (**bottom right**) demonstrate a single large artery (aorta) at the base of the heart, which overlies the ventricular septal defect (*arrow*). Right ventricular wall is hypertrophied. Note the central confluence (*arrowhead*) of the right and left pulmonary arteries distal to the atretic segment.

aorticopulmonary artery collaterals, a unifocalization procedure is performed. Therefore, it is important for the surgeon to know whether a native confluence of the pulmonary arteries is present, its size, and the number and size of collateral vessels, which may be not opacified on MRA images. In that instance, spin echo MRI has the unique capability to delineate the vessel and its relationship with the bronchi. The pulmonary arteries are frequently hypoplastic, or the central or peripheral arteries may contain one or more stenoses.

Cine MRI and contrast-enhanced MRA can be used to identify the blood supply to the lungs. Pulmonary and bronchial arteries have bright signal on cine MRI. On transaxial images at the level of the carina, pulmonary arteries can be differentiated from bronchial arteries. Bronchial arteries or systemic to pulmonary artery collaterals arise from the aorta or its branches and are usually located dorsal to the bronchi, whereas pulmonary arteries are ventral to the bronchi. On occasion, a bronchial artery originating from a subclavian artery is seen ventral to the bronchi.

Pulmonary Atresia With Intact Ventricular Septum

In pulmonary atresia with intact ventricular septum, a VSD is not present. MRI is effective for demonstrating the size of the RV, which varies from markedly hypoplastic to dilated. The tricuspid annulus may be hypoplastic and the tricuspid valve may be dysplastic. The pulmonary arteries are usually normal or nearly normal in size and rarely are stenotic.

Cine MR images can be acquired in the short-axis plane to quantify the volumes of the right and left ventricles. The size of the right ventricle and tricuspid annulus is critical for the determination of the surgical approach. A right ventricle and tricuspid annulus of adequate size are necessary to consider a biventricular repair. Exit of blood from the right ventricle in this anomaly is by tricuspid regurgitation or retrograde flow through myocardial sinusoid and coronary arteries into the aorta. Cine MR can demonstrate and give some insight into the severity of tricuspid regurgitation.

Abnormalities of Ventriculoarterial Connections

These abnormalities consist of complete TGA, congenitally corrected TGA (ccTGA), double-outlet right ventricle (DORV), and double-outlet left ventricle (DOLV) (Table 38.3). The last anomaly is exceedingly rare. Truncus arteriosus will also be considered under this heading.

Discordant ventriculoarterial connections occur in a diverse group of anomalies in which the great arteries are inverted (transposition), or both great arteries arise predominantly from one of the ventricles (double-outlet ventricle). The ventriculoarterial connections and the arterial relationships are depicted on oblique coronal and transverse MR images.

A great artery is considered connected to a ventricle if more than half of its orifice arises from that ventricle. The initial determination is to identify the aorta unequivocally by following one of the great arteries to the arch. If this great artery (aorta) connects to the right ventricle and the pulmonary artery to the left ventricle, then the diagnosis of complete TGA is established (Figs. 38.43 and 38.44).

Table 38.3 Summary of Anatomy of Ventriculoarterial Connection Abnormalities

Complete transposition
Situs solitus (right atrium on the right side of the chest)
D-ventricular loop (right ventricle to the right of the left ventricle)
D-TGA (aorta anterior and to the right of pulmonary artery)
Corrected transposition
Situs solitus
L-ventricular loop (right ventricle to the left of the left ventricle)
L-TGA (aorta anterior and to the left of pulmonary artery)
Double-outlet right ventricle
Aorta orifice >50% overlies the right ventricle
Pulmonary orifice >50% overlies the right ventricle
Subaortic, subpulmonary, doubly committed or noncommitted VSD
Double-outlet left ventricle
Aorta orifice >50% overlies the left ventricle
Pulmonary orifice >50% overlies the left ventricle
Truncus arteriosus
One enlarged great artery (truncus) overlies VSD immediately beneath orifice of truncus

TGA, transposition of the great arteries.

There are two main forms of TGA. The most common form involves atrial situs solitus, normal atrioventricular alignment (right atrium connects to the right ventricle and the left atrium connects to the left ventricle). However, the aorta arises from the right ventricle and is anterior and to the right of the pulmonary artery and is called d-TGA.

In the second, less common form of TGA, there is ventricular inversion as well as TGA. The right atrium connects to a right-sided left ventricle and the left atrium connects to a left-sided right ventricle. There is TGA and the aortic valve is typically anterior and leftward of the pulmonic valve. This is termed l-TGA or ccTGA (Fig. 38.45). This anomaly is considered to be physiologically corrected in terms of blood flow since systemic venous blood flows from the right atrium into the left ventricle and out to the pulmonary artery for normal oxygenation, precluding obligatory cyanosis. Occasionally, l-TGA can be associated with mirror-image dextrocardia. Cine MR images also demonstrate anomalies frequently associated with complete and corrected transposition, such as ASD, VSD, subvalvular and valvular pulmonic stenosis, tricuspid atresia, and Ebstein-like anomaly of the tricuspid valve. Note that in both uncorrected forms of TGA the tricuspid valve, which is associated with the right ventricle is the systemic atrioventricular valve.

In DORV, both great arteries are connected to the right ventricle. There are multiple subtypes of DORV defined by

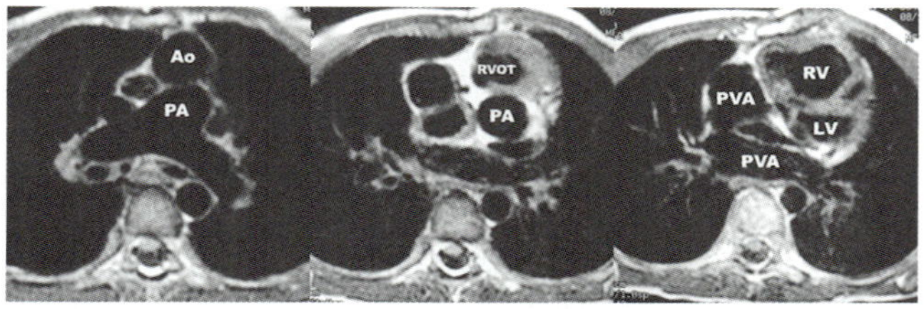

Figure 38.43. D-Transposition of great arteries. Spin-echo images arranged from cranial (**left**) to caudal (**right**) show the aorta (*Ao*) ventral and slightly to the right of the pulmonary artery (*PA*). The aorta is shown connecting to the right ventricle (*RV*) and the pulmonary artery to the left ventricle (*LV*). There is a baffle (Mustard procedure) in the atrium, separating the mitral valve from the pulmonary venous atrium (*PVA*). *RVOT*, right ventricular outflow track.

the relationship of the VSD to the outflow tracts. Cine and spin echo images are very effective for demonstrating the relationship of the obligatory VSD to the great arteries in DORV (Fig. 38.46). The defect may be just below the aortic orifice (subaortic VSD) or pulmonary artery orifice (subpulmonary VSD), beneath both orifices (doubly committed VSD), or removed some distance from both (noncommitted VSD). Rarely, both great arteries connect to the anatomic left ventricle, indicating DOLV.

Truncus Arteriosus

Truncus arteriosus was classified by Collet and Edwards based on the origin of the pulmonary artery from the

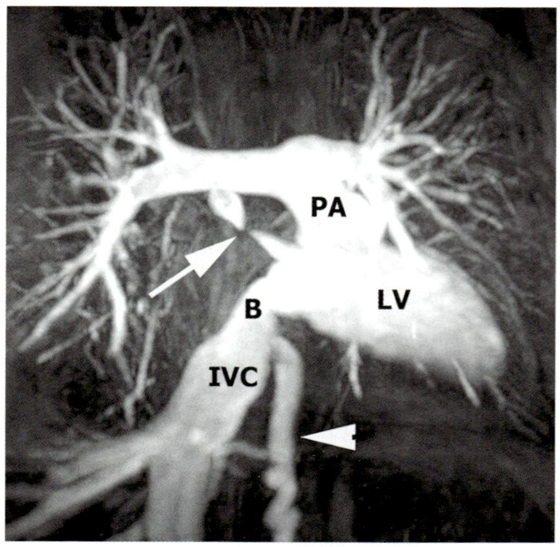

Figure 38.44. Magnetic resonance angiography status post atrial switch procedure. Gadolinium-enhanced MR angiography in the coronal plane is shown in a patient status post atrial switch procedure for correction of transposition of great arteries. The inferior vena cava (*IVC*) is dilated and connects to the inferior limb of the baffle (*B*), which is then attached to the mitral valve. The superior limb of the baffle is occluded (*arrow*). Note an enlarged azygos vein (*arrowhead*). LV, left ventricle; PA, pulmonary artery.

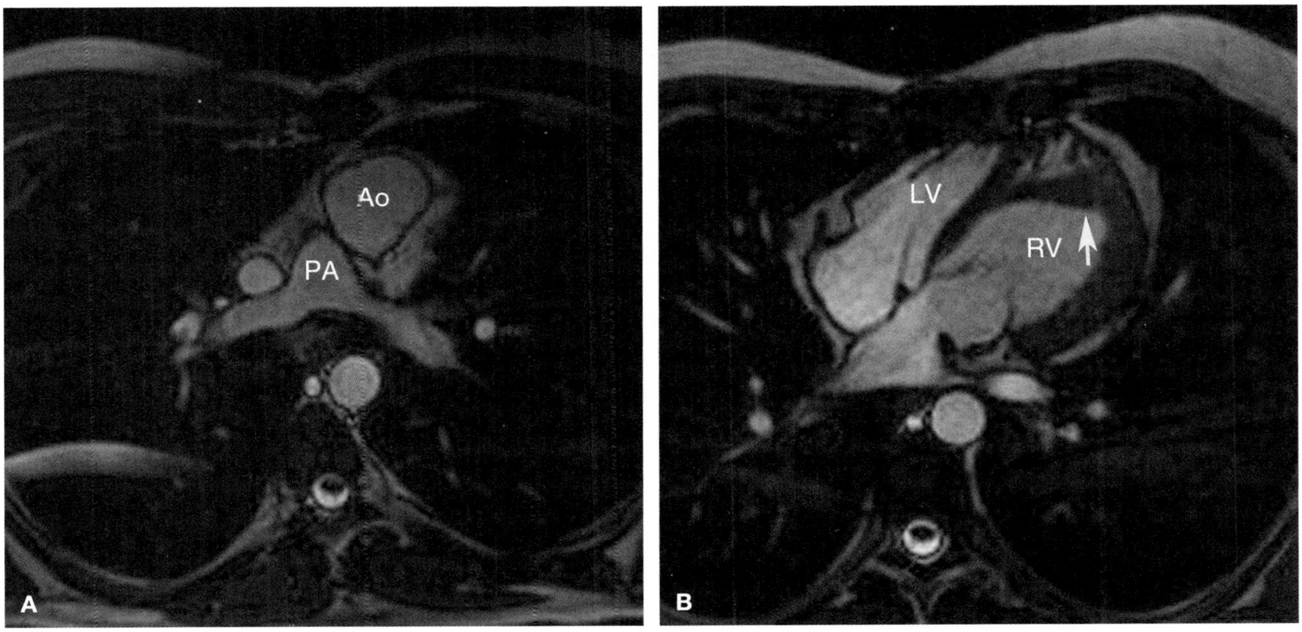

Figure 38.45. ccTGA: Axial cine MR at level of great arteries (**A, left**) and ventricles (**B, right**) in a patient with corrected transposition (L-transposition with L-ventricular loop). ccTGA, congenitally corrected transposition of the great arteries. Ao, aorta; LV, left ventricle; PA, pulmonary artery; RV, right ventricle; arrow, moderator band of the right ventricle.

common arterial trunk. In type I, a septum divides the origin of the aorta and pulmonary trunk. In type II, the right and left pulmonary arteries are close to each other but arise separately from the pulmonary trunk. In type III, right and left pulmonary arteries arise further laterally. The lesion labeled type IV truncus is in fact pulmonary atresia with VSD rather than truncus arteriosus.

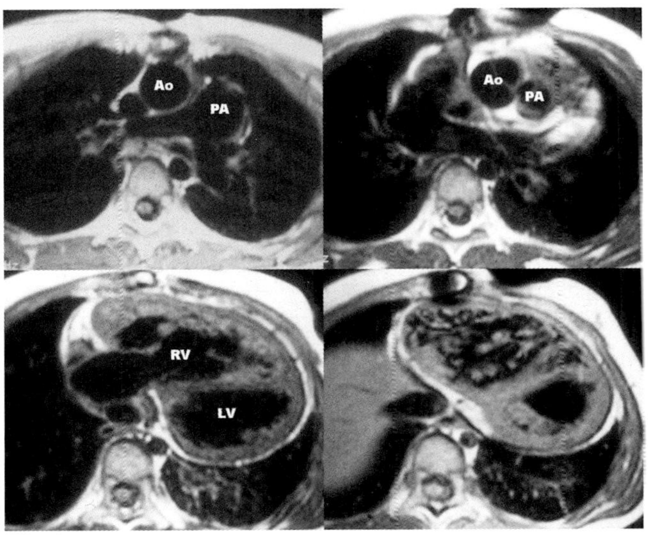

Figure 38.46. Double-outlet right ventricle. Cine MR image and associated video in an oblique sagittal view show the aorta (AO) anteriorly and the pulmonary artery (PA) connected to the right ventricle (RV).

MR images at the base of the heart in multiple planes can show the truncus arteriosus aligned over the VSD (Fig. 38.47). The origins of the main pulmonary artery from the truncus in type I can be delineated with MRI. Cine MR images can show the relative sizes of the ventricles. Because it can demonstrate a small infundibular chamber in pulmonary atresia, MRI can be used to distinguish truncus arteriosus from pulmonary atresia.

It is important to define the relative sizes and confluence of the pulmonary arteries because surgical treatment involves excision of the pulmonary arteries from the common trunk and the creation of a conduit from the right ventricle to the pulmonary arteries. Also important is the demonstration of

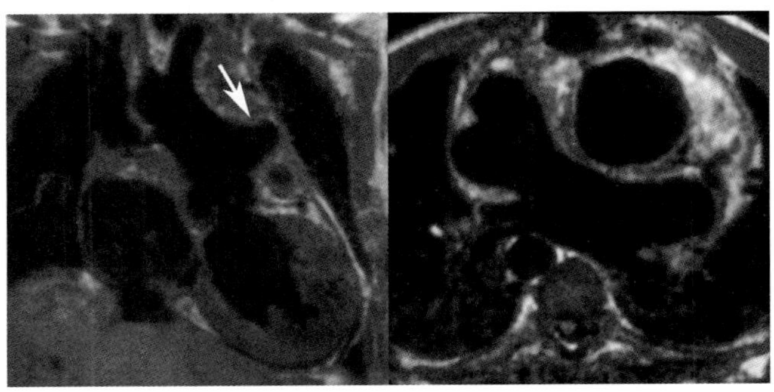

Figure 38.47. Truncus arteriosus, type I. Spin-echo images in the coronal (**left**) and axial (**right**) planes demonstrate a large single artery arising from the heart. The pulmonary artery (*arrow*) arises from the left side of the truncus, and the aortic arch is right-sided.

a right aortic arch (35%) or other arch anomalies. Cine MRI and VEC cine MRI can be employed to identify and quantify the severity of truncal valve regurgitation. Cine MRI can also be used to quantify the volume and mass of the two ventricles.

ABNORMALITIES OF ATRIOVENTRICULAR CONNECTIONS

Discordant Atrioventricular Connections

The right atrium connects with the left ventricle and the left atrium connects with the right ventricle, constituting discordant connections, as is seen in ccTGA. When this occurs with situs inversus, the anatomic right atrium (situated left of midline) connects discordantly to the left ventricle and the anatomic left atrium (situated right of midline) connects to the right ventricle (Fig. 38.48).

Double-Inlet Ventricle (Single Ventricle; Univentricular Heart)

This complex anomaly consists of one adequate-size ventricle and one rudimentary ventricle. The most frequent type is double-inlet left ventricle: both atrioventricular valves connect to the morphologic left ventricle. The dominant left ventricle is attached to a rudimentary right ventricular outlet via a bulboventricular foramen. In most instances, L-TGA is present.

Cine MRI can provide a set of end-diastolic and end-systolic images encompassing the entire heart; consequently, it is the optimal method for quantifying the volumes, mass, and function of the dominant and rudimentary ventricles. Volumetric data may be essential for surgical planning. After repair with the Fontan procedure, cine MR is used to monitor the volumes and ejection fraction of the dominant ventricle.

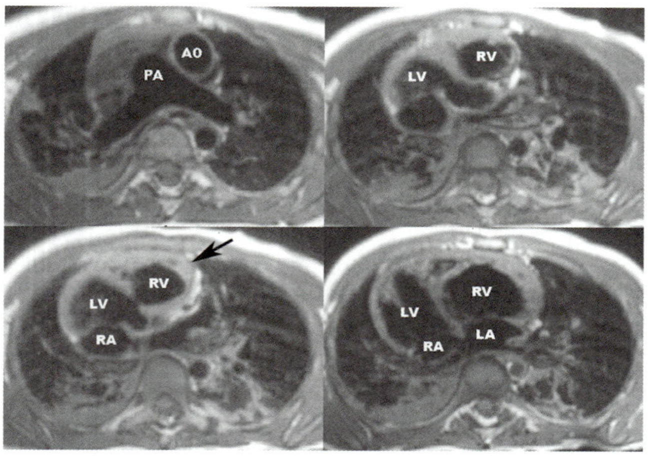

Figure 38.48. Situs solitus with corrected transposition and isolated dextrocardia. Spin-echo axial images arranged from cranial (**top left**) to caudal (**bottom right**). The right atrium (*RA*) is right sided, and the left atrium (*LA*) is left sided, indicating situs solitus. The right ventricle (*RV*) is positioned to the left of the left ventricle (*LV*). The aorta (*AO*) is anterior and leftward to the pulmonary artery (*PA*). Note the conus (*arrow*) and moderator band on the left-sided ventricle, indicating it is a morphologic right ventricle in an L-ventricular loop. Thus, this arrangement of connections is situs solitus, L-ventricular loop, L-transposition, which constitutes corrected transposition of the great arteries. The cardiac apex is right sided, which indicates isolated dextrocardia.

Atresia of Atrioventricular Valve

Either the tricuspid or mitral valves can be atretic; tricuspid atresia is more frequent. In tricuspid atresia, D-TGA is present in nearly 50% of patients and a VSD is often present. It is also frequently associated with valvular or subvalvular pulmonary stenosis or atresia. The right ventricle is invariably hypoplastic. Transaxial MR images demonstrate a band of muscle and fat across the atrioventricular inlet of the right ventricle (Figs. 38.49-38.51). Cine MR images display the degree of right ventricle hypoplasia, interatrial communication, VSD, and ventriculoarterial connections. In a few cases, a thick membrane separates the right atrium and right ventricle (imperforate tricuspid valve). The atrial septal defect permits systemic venous blood to flow into the ventricles.

MR is frequently used to evaluate tricuspid atresia after various stages of surgical correction. Cine MR images and

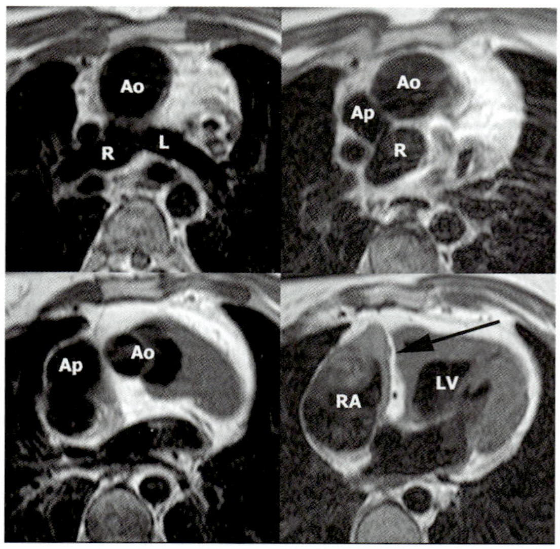

Figure 38.49. Classic Fontan procedure. Axial black-blood images from the level of the great vessels (**top left**) to the midventricular level (**bottom right**) in a patient with tricuspid atresia status post classic Fontan operation. The right pulmonary artery (*R*) connects to the right atrial appendage (*Ap*). A dominant left ventricle (*LV*) is seen. Note the fatty replacement of the right atrioventricular grove (*arrow*). Ao, aorta; L, left pulmonary artery; RA, right atrium.

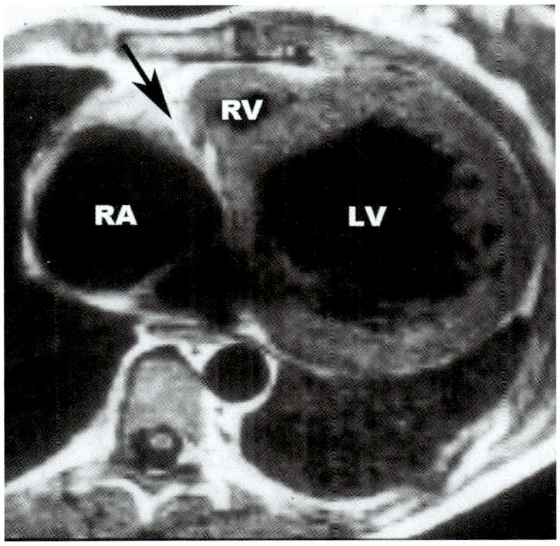

Figure 38.50. Tricuspid atresia. Spin-echo axial image shows a bar of fat and muscle (*arrow*) separating the right atrium (*RA*) from the hypoplastic right ventricle (*RV*). The left ventricle (*LV*) is enlarged.

3D contrast-enhanced MRA are effective for displaying the anatomy of the Glenn anastomosis (Figs. 38.51 and 38.52) and the Fontan procedure and the status of the central pulmonary arteries (Figs. 38.51-38.53). VEC cine MR may be employed to quantify blood flow in the Glenn shunt (superior vena cava), Fontan conduit (IVC to pulmonary artery conduit), and pulmonary arteries.

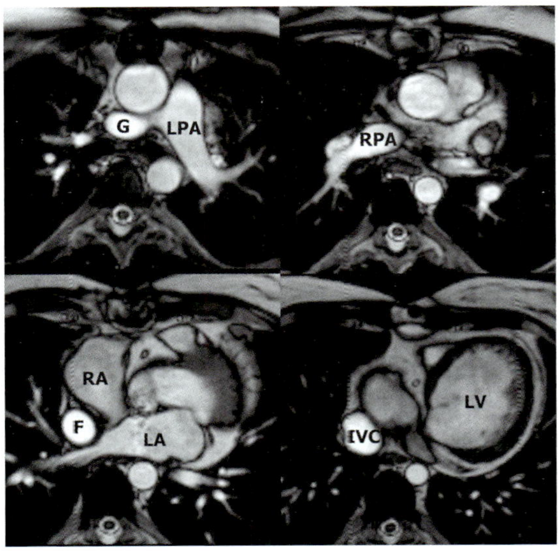

Figure 38.51. Tricuspid atresia with Fontan. Axial images, from the ventricular level (**bottom right**) to the level of the great vessels (**top left**), show a Fontan conduit (*F*) connecting the inferior vena cava (*IVC*) to the right pulmonary artery (*RPA*). A Glenn shunt (G) connects the superior vena cava to the RPA. A dominant left ventricle (*LV*) is seen. *LA*, left atrium; *LPA*, left pulmonary artery; *RA*, right atrium.

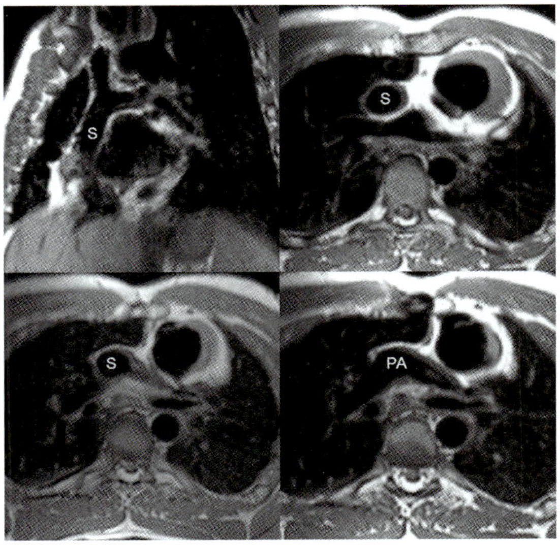

Figure 38.52. Glenn shunt. Oblique coronal MR angiogram of a patient who is status post Glenn procedure (superior cavo-pulmonary anastomosis). LPA, left pulmonary artery; RPA, right pulmonary artery; SVC, superior vena cava.

Ebstein's Malformation

Ebstein's malformation is a primary abnormality of the tricuspid valve in which the septal and posterior leaflets of the valve adhere to the right ventricle wall. The leaflets become free at a variable distance, at a location more apical than usual, so that the tricuspid valve orifice is displaced toward the apex. The tricuspid annulus still defines the border of the anatomic right ventricle; however, because the valve orifice is more apical than usual, the functional part of the right ventricle is truncated. The portion of the right ventricle that is basal to the valve orifice becomes

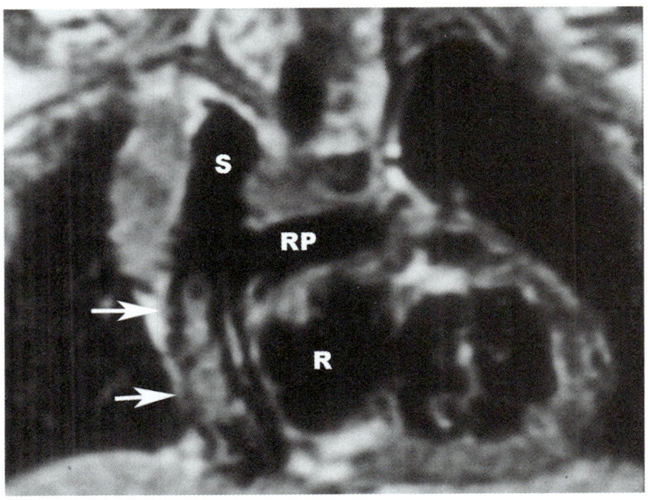

Figure 38.53. Fontan procedure. Steady-state free precession (bright-blood cine) image in the 4-chamber plane of a patient with tricuspid atresia who has undergone an extracardiac Fontan operation. Asterisk denotes Fontan, LA, left atrium; LV, left ventricle.

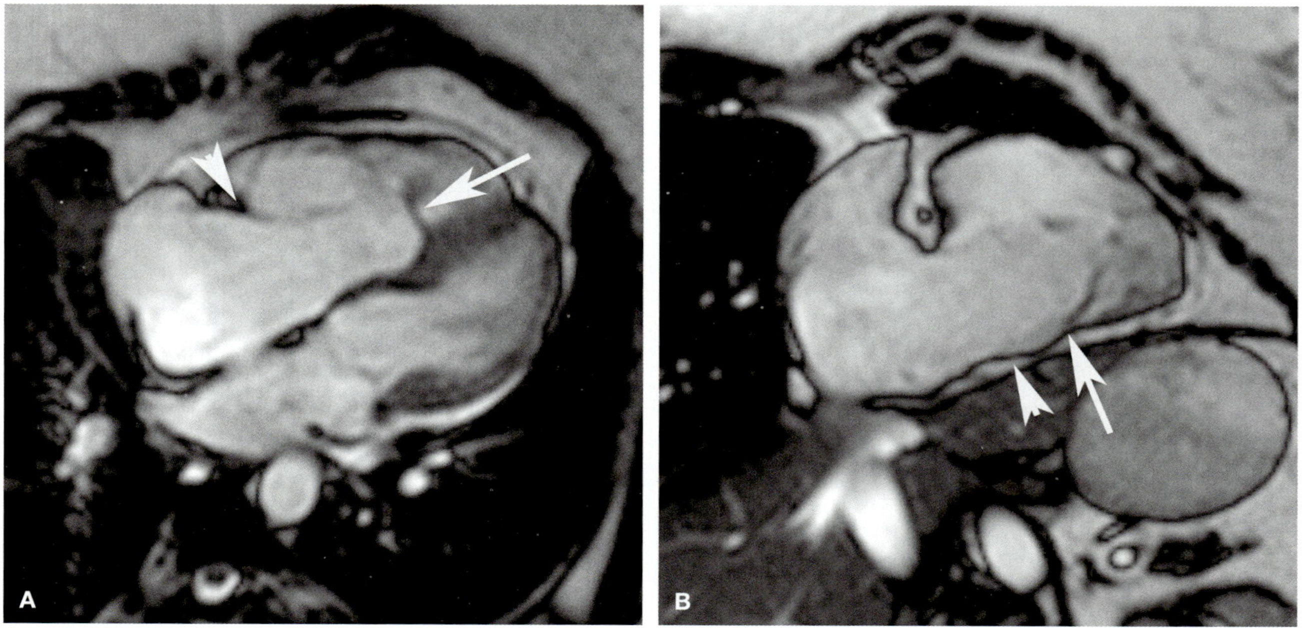

Figure 38.54. Ebstein's anomaly. Horizontal long-axis (**A, left**) cine MR shows displacement of the sepal leaflet of tricuspid valve toward apex (*arrow*) and normal attachment of the anterior leaflet at the right atrioventricular groove (*arrowhead*). Vertical long-axis cine MR through the right ventricle (**B, right**) shows transition (*arrow*) between the atrialized (*arrowhead*) and ventricularized portions of the right ventricle.

"atrialized," meaning that it functions as part of the atrium rather than as part of the right ventricle. The atrialized portion of the right ventricle is thin-walled and nontrabeculated, and it may become dilated. Right ventricular function may be abnormal. Ebstein's anomaly is frequently associated with ASD.

MRI can demonstrate the position of the tricuspid valve (Fig. 38.54), and cine MRI can be used to quantify chamber size and the ejection fraction of the functional right ventricle. Cine MR in the vertical long-axis plane is best for demonstrating the extent of atrialization of the right ventricular inlet region (Fig. 38.54). Cine MR also demonstrates the systolic signal void projected into the right atrium, indicating tricuspid regurgitation, which is invariably present with this anomaly.

Hypoplastic Left Heart Syndrome

The term *hypoplastic left heart syndrome* refers to hypoplasia or atresia of the mitral and aortic valves leading to underdevelopment of the left ventricle and ascending aorta. It is caused by aortic stenosis or atresia, mitral stenosis or atresia, or both. As in tricuspid atresia, the degree of ventricular hypoplasia varies, depending on the location and severity of the obstruction. For example, in mitral atresia the left ventricle may be a small mass of muscle with no visible lumen (Fig. 38.55). The right atrium tends to be enlarged and the right ventricle to be dilated and hypertrophied. Axial MRI can readily depict the chamber enlargement and ventricular hypertrophy.

In most cases of hypoplastic left heart syndrome, little blood flows through the ascending aorta. Blood tends to flow from the pulmonary artery through the ductus arteriosus into the aorta and then in retrograde fashion to the aortic root to supply the coronary arteries. As a result, the ascending aorta is usually very small and the main pulmonary artery, which receives most of the cardiac output, is large. The diameters of the great arteries are clearly defined on axial MR images.

Hypoplastic left heart syndrome is treated by a staged procedure that culminates in a Fontan operation and a right ventricle that pumps blood to the systemic circulation. The first stage includes transecting the main pulmonary artery

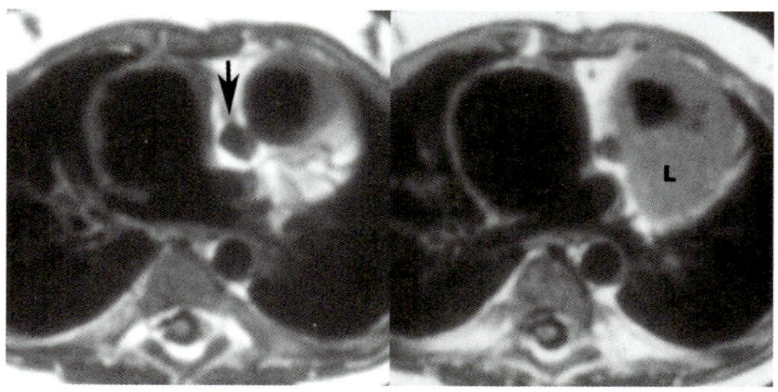

Figure 38.55. Hypoplastic left heart syndrome. Spin-echo axial images demonstrate the severely hypoplastic ascending aorta (*arrow*) and lack of cavitation of the left ventricle (*L*) at the level displayed.

and using this tissue to augment the ascending aorta. The pulmonary circulation is reestablished by routing systemic blood into the pulmonary circulation with a systemic-to-pulmonary shunt. In the second stage, a superior cavo-pulmonary anastomosis is created (bidirectional Glenn procedure) and the previously placed shunt is taken down. In the final stage, the Fontan circulation is completed. An important role for MRI in hypoplastic left heart syndrome has been the evaluation of the morphology and function of the various stages of the repair.

Total Anomalous Pulmonary Venous Connection

In the embryo, the pulmonary veins grow from the lung buds and come together to form a confluence, which normally is incorporated into the posterior wall of the left atrium. However, if this confluence joins the circulatory system elsewhere, a situation is created in which the entire pulmonary venous return is anomalous: total anomalous pulmonary venous connection (TAPVC). TAPVC is usually classified according to the location of the venous insertion. It may be supracardiac (type I), in which the pulmonary venous confluence usually drains into the superior vena cava or an anomalous left-sided "vertical vein," which in turn drains into the left brachiocephalic vein. TAPVC at the cardiac level (type II) usually drains into the right atrium. In type III TAPVC, the pulmonary venous confluence drains below the diaphragm into the truncus venous or the portal venous or hepatic venous system. As the pulmonary veins pass below the diaphragm, obstruction to flow frequently results in pulmonary venous hypertension. Patients can also have mixed connections with a combination of the above (type IV).

MRI is accurate for the diagnosis of anomalous pulmonary venous connection. TAPVC can be diagnosed when an MRI demonstrates that no pulmonary veins drain into the left atrium. Transaxial MRI and gadolinium-enhanced MRA can demonstrate the location of the anomalous connection along with enlargement of the superior vena cava or coronary sinus or the presence of a common pulmonary vein posterior to or above the left atrium.

Situs Abnormalities

The right-sided abdominal and thoracic structures are usually on the same side as the morphologic right atrium; likewise, the left-sided organs are usually on the same side as the morphologic left atrium. In a developmental anomaly in which both atria have morphologic features of a right atrium (RA isomerism), the visceral and thoracic structures tend to be right-sided. Likewise, bilateral left atria (LA isomerism) are associated with bilateral left-sided visceral and thoracic structures.

The bronchi and pulmonary arteries have a characteristic relationship in isomerism syndromes. In RA isomerism, both

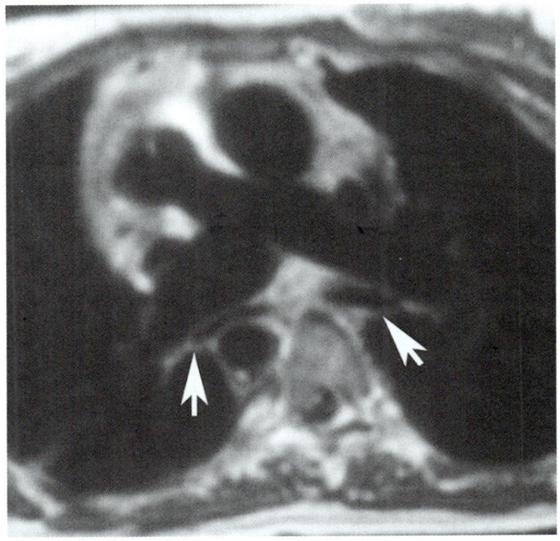

Figure 38.56. Right-sided isomerism. Spin-echo axial image at the level of the main bronchi (*arrows*) shows that both pulmonary arteries are situated ventral to the bronchi.

lungs usually have three lobes and both bronchi have the pattern of a right bronchus—that is, the pulmonary artery runs in front of and beneath the main bronchus (a type of bronchus known as an eparterial bronchus) (Fig. 38.56). Right-sided isomerism is often associated with asplenia syndrome. The liver is large and crosses the midline, and the spleen is often absent.

In left-sided isomerism, both lungs have two lobes, and both the right and left pulmonary arteries pass over their respective bronchi. This type of bronchial pattern is known as hyparterial because the bronchus passes below the pulmonary artery (Fig. 38.57). Left-sided isomerism is associated with polysplenia syndrome, characterized by multiple spleens. The IVC is frequently interrupted, with azygous continuation (Fig. 38.57).

Coronal and transaxial MR images are very effective for showing the anatomy of the pulmonary arteries in order to establish the diagnosis of isomerism. MRI also clearly defines the systemic, pulmonary venous anatomy and the morphology of the atrial appendages. Patients with isomerism often have complex congenital heart disease.

Postoperative Evaluation

MRI is excellent for the postoperative evaluation of CHD. The wide field of view permits effective depiction of complex repairs used to correct complex lesions.

Contrast-enhanced 3D MRA and tomographic images demonstrate surgical anastomoses, conduits, and shunts. Moreover, the 3D data set available from contiguous cine MR images at multiple phases in the cardiac cycle permits precise quantification of left and right ventricular volumes, mass, and function. Since cine MRI has high interstudy reproducibility,

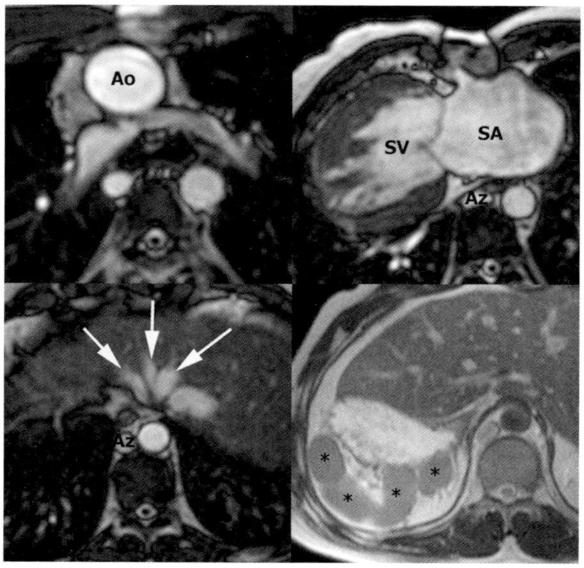

Figure 38.57. Polysplenia with interrupted inferior vena cava (IVC). Multiple axial cine MR images from the great vessels (**top left**) to the liver (**bottom left**) demonstrate a single ventricle (*SV*) and single atrium (*SA*). Note multiple hepatic veins (*arrows*) without an intrahepatic inferior vena cava (IVC). Azygos vein (*Az*) is dilated. Bilateral morphologic left pulmonary arteries (**top left**). Multiple spleens (*asterisks*) are seen in the axial black-blood image (**bottom right**). Ao, aorta.

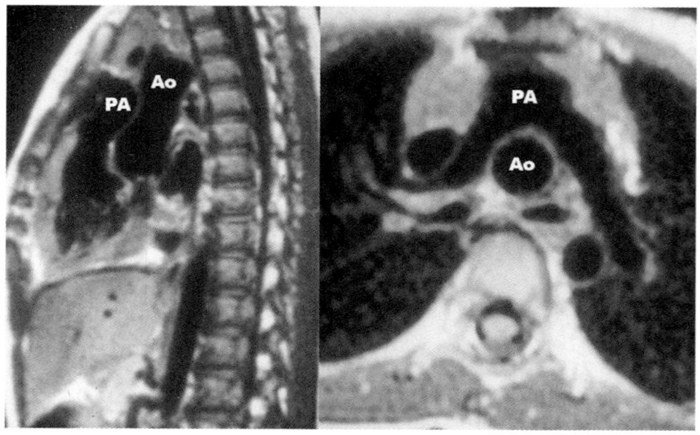

Figure 38.59. Jatene procedure. Spin-echo images in the sagittal (**left**) and axial (**right**) planes show the arterial correction. The aorta (*Ao*) above the anastomosis is situated between the right and left pulmonary arteries. This position can cause narrowing of the branch pulmonary arteries. *PA*, pulmonary artery.

it is the best technique available for serial monitoring of ventricular volumes, mass, and function after surgery.

Spin-echo MRI, cine MRI, and 3D contrast-enhanced MRA have demonstrated the anatomy of complex repairs such as the Norwood procedure for hypoplastic left heart (Fig. 38.58), the Jatene procedure (arterial switch) for TGA (Fig. 38.59), Senning and Mustard procedures (atrial baffle redirection of venous flow) for TGA (Fig. 38.44), the Fontan procedure for functional single ventricle (Figs. 38.49 and 38.51), the Rastelli procedure for pulmonary atresia (Fig. 38.60), and various repairs of tetralogy of Fallot (Figs. 38.1, 38.2, 38.61, 38.62).

VEC cine MRI is employed for quantification of the volume and fraction of pulmonary regurgitation (Fig. 38.2), flow through various components of the Fontan repair, and differential flow in the central pulmonary arteries (Fig. 38.30). After various surgical procedures in cyanotic CHD, residual stenosis of the central pulmonary arteries is frequent. VEC cine MRI can be used to demonstrate disparity in flow between the right and left pulmonary arteries and changes after angioplasty.

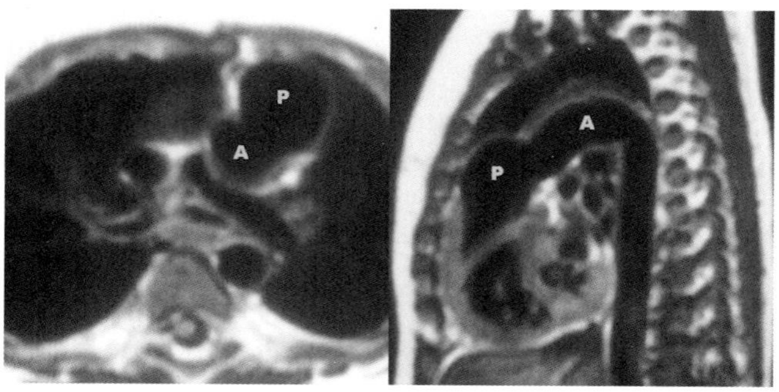

Figure 38.58. Norwood procedure. Spin-echo axial (**left**) and sagittal (**right**) images show the anastomosis of the proximal pulmonary artery (*P*) to the ascending aorta (*A*). Sagittal view shows the pulmonary artery (*P*) connected to a reconstructed distal ascending aorta (*A*) and arch. Blood flow to the distal pulmonary artery is reconstituted with a central shunt (not shown).

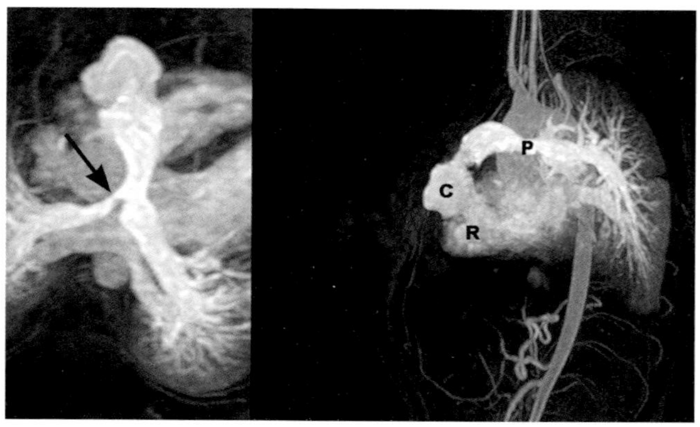

Figure 38.60. Rastelli procedure. Contrast-enhanced 3D magnetic resonance angiography in oblique axial (**left**) and sagittal (**right**) planes shows a conduit (*C*) between the right ventricle (*R*) and the pulmonary artery (*P*). The oblique axial plane depicts a stenosis (*arrow*) of the right pulmonary artery.

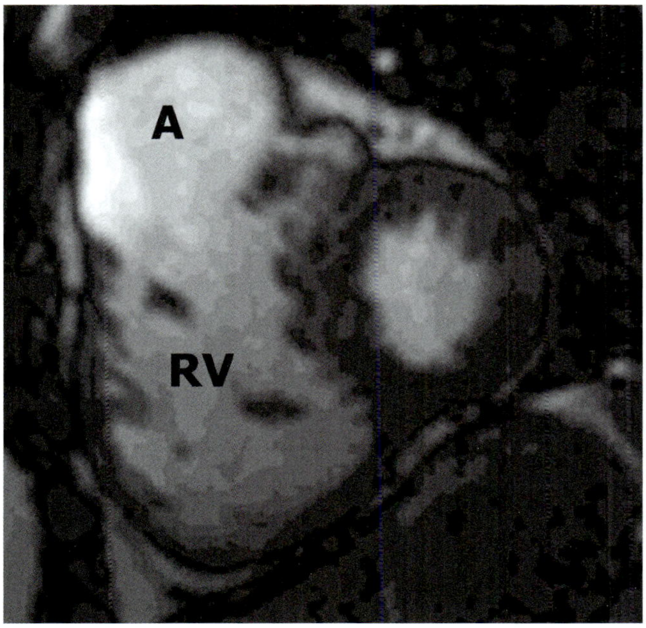

Figure 38.61. Tetralogy of Fallot with right ventricular outflow tract aneurysm. Short-axis cine MR image at end-diastole demonstrates aneurysm (*A*) of the right ventricular outflow tract and an overall enlarged right ventricle (*RV*).

Monitoring of Ventricular Function and Pulmonary Regurgitation in Postoperative Tetralogy of Fallot (T of F)

Several surgical procedures are employed in total correction of tetralogy of Fallot. Correction may be preceded by a surgical shunt between the aorta and pulmonary artery for palliation. If the shunt originates in the ascending aorta, it is called a central shunt. If the shunt is between a subclavian artery and a pulmonary artery, it is called a modified Blalock-Taussing-Thomas shunt. Historically, the subclavian artery contralateral to the aortic arch was directly anastomosed to the central pulmonary artery, referred to as a classic Blalock-Taussig-Thomas shunt. At definitive correction, the shunt is closed and the VSD is closed. The RVOT obstruction is removed using one or more of several techniques: infundibulectomy, transannular patch, or conduit from right ventricular to the main or bifurcation of the pulmonary artery (Figs. 38.1, 38.2, 38.60, 38.61).

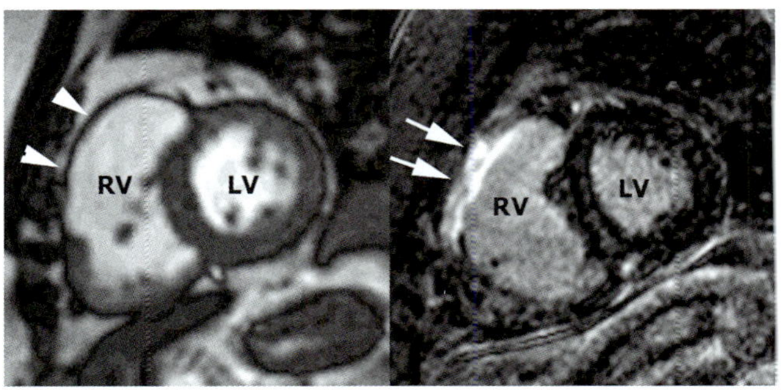

Figure 38.62. Tetralogy of Fallot after transannular patch. Cine MR (**left**) and delayed enhancement (**right**) images in the short-axis plane show thinning of the right ventricular free wall (*arrowheads*) with associated delayed enhancement (*arrows*). These findings are consistent with myocardial scar related to the surgical procedure. LV, left ventricle; RV, right ventricle.

MRI is now used to identify, assess the severity, and monitor any residual abnormalities, and to quantify RV function. A typical study involves the following: cine MR images to evaluate anatomy; cine MR in the short-axis plane to quantify RV volumes and ejection fraction; cine MR in the RVOT plane to identify sites of RV infundibular, valvular, or supravalvular stenosis(es); contrast-enhanced MRA in coronal plane to evaluate stenosis of main, central, or branch pulmonary arteries or in conduits; and VEC (phase-contrast) cine MR perpendicular to direction of flow in main, right, and left pulmonary arteries to quantify pulmonary regurgitation and differential pulmonary flow to the lungs. Delayed contrast-enhanced inversion recovery gradient echo sequence may be done to identify fibrosis (scar) (Fig. 38.62).

The most frequent residual abnormality following repair of tetralogy of Fallot is pulmonary regurgitation. This nearly always presents after repair by transannular patch. Severity of regurgitation is stated as follows using regurgitation fraction: in general, less than 20% is considered mild, 20% to 40% is moderate, and greater than 40% is severe. Moderate and severe regurgitation is typically associated with right ventricular dilation(Fig. 38.63). End-diastolic volumes greater than 150 to 160 mL/m^2 and/or end-systolic volume greater than 90 to 100 mL/m^2 or presence of a reduced right ventricular ejection fraction (<40%) and may prompt consideration of pulmonary valve replacement.

Residual or recurrent stenosis of the RV infundibulum, pulmonary valve, or valved conduit is also common following the repair of tetralogy of Fallot. There may also be both residual stenosis and regurgitation. If stenosis is the dominant lesion, then the RV shows hypertrabeculation and hypertrophy. Moreover, the combination of stenosis and regurgitation produces less severe RV enlargement and better preservation of RV ejection fraction.

Regional contraction abnormalities of the RV are frequent after the repair of tetralogy. Akinesis or dyskinesis of the RV outlet region can be displayed on cine MR images in the sagittal or RVOT planes. After placement of a large outflow tract patch, there may be an aneurysm of this region (Fig. 38.61). The inlet and body portions of the RV typically show less severe contractile dysfunction.

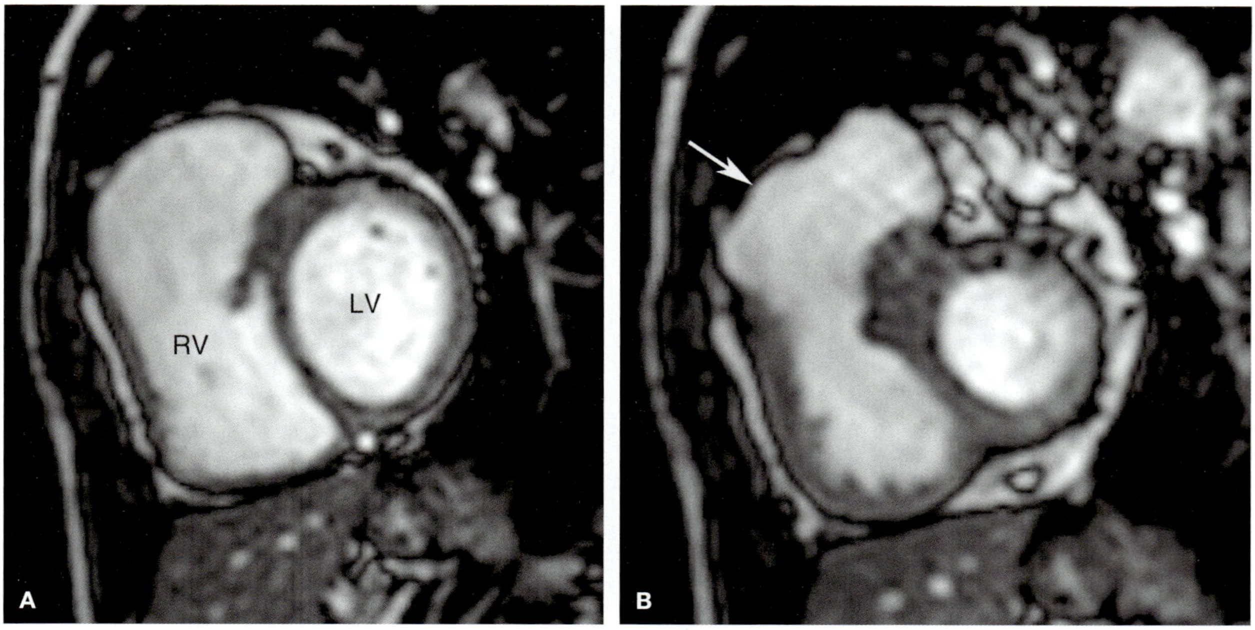

Figure 38.63. Postoperative tetralogy of Fallot with severely dilated right ventricle. Cine MR in short-axis plane at end-diastole (**A, left**) and end-systole (**B, right**) shows dyskinesis of the right ventricular outlet region (*arrow*). LV, left ventricle; RV, right ventricle.

SUGGESTED READINGS

Bemerich J, Wyttenbach R, Buser P, Higgins CB. Cardiovascular MR in complex congenital heart disease. In: Manning WJ, Pennell DJ, eds. *Cardiovascular MR*. 2nd ed. Saunders Publishing; 2010:408.

Fogel MA, Anwar S, Broberg C, et al. Society for Cardiovascular Magnetic Resonance/European Society of Cardiovascular Imaging/American Society of Echocardiography/Society for Pediatric Radiology/North American Society for Cardiovascular Imaging guidelines for the use of cardiovascular magnetic resonance in pediatric congenital and acquired heart disease: endorsed by the American Heart Association. *J Cardiovasc Magn Reson*. 2022;24(1):37.

Geva T, Dorfman AL, Powell AJ. Complex congenital heart disease: infant and pediatric patients. In: Manning WJ, Pennell DJ, eds. *Cardiovascular MR*. 2nd ed. Saunders Publishing; 2010:410.

Higgins CB, Ordovas KG. Congenital heart disease: magnetic resonance imaging of morphology and function. In: Higgins CB, de Roos A, eds. *MRI and CT of the Cardiovascular System*. 3rd ed. Lippincott Williams & Wilkins; 2013:433.

Knauth Meadows A, Ordovas K, Higgins CB, Reddy GP. Magnetic resonance imaging in the adult with congenital heart disease. *Semin Roentgenol*. 2008;43(3):246-258.

Ordovas KG, Muzzarelli S, Hope MD, et al. Cardiovascular MR imaging after surgical correction of tetralogy of Fallot: approach based on understanding of surgical procedures. *Radiographics*. 2013;33(4): 1037-1052.

Roest AAW, Croft LJM, de Roos A. Magnetic resonance imaging of function and flow in postoperative congenital heart disease. In: Higgins CB, de Roos A, eds. *MRI and CT of the Cardiovascular System*. 3rd ed. Lippincott Williams & Wilkins; 2013:471.

Section Eleven

Ischemic Heart Disease

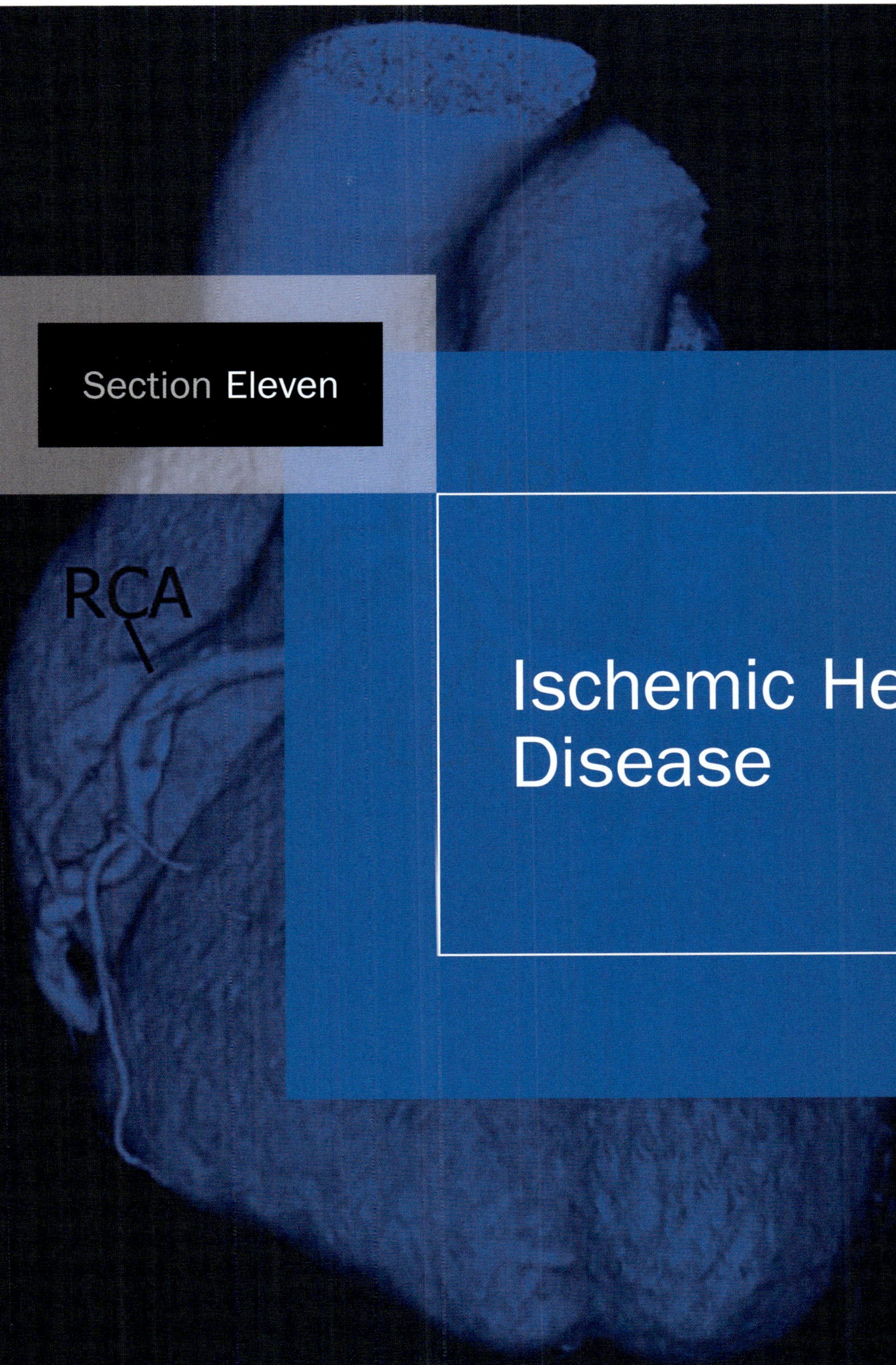

Chapter 39

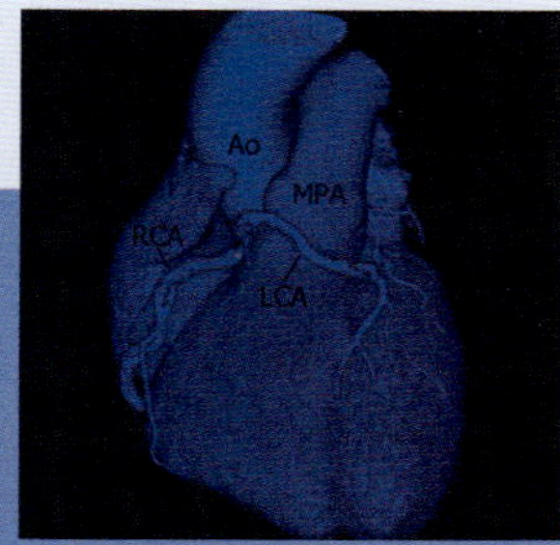

Benedikt Bernhard • Raymond Kwong • Karen G. Ordovas

Magnetic Resonance Imaging of Ischemic Heart Disease

Abbreviations

CABG coronary artery bypass graft
CMR cardiovascular magnetic resonance imaging
IHD ischemic heart disease
LV left ventricle

INTRODUCTION

Cardiovascular magnetic resonance imaging (CMR) has emerged as a cornerstone in the noninvasive evaluation of ischemic heart disease (IHD) and provides complementary information to mainstay investigations such as invasive angiography, nuclear imaging, and echocardiography. The detection of IHD has become the most common indication for CMR, and a large body of evidence and several randomized controlled trials support its role in this setting. In addition to the detection of IHD and definition of its severity, CMR inherits the capability to determine myocardial viability, diagnose complications of myocardial infarction, guide therapeutic management after revascularization, and allow for a risk stratification in patients with IHD. If CMR can rule out IHD, its capability to elucidate the underlying etiology of chest pain symptoms is superior to any other imaging modality. Several techniques are available to obtain information not only on myocardial perfusion and wall motion but also on ventricular dimensions and tissue characteristics without the need for ionizing radiation. The various sequences for accomplishing these tasks will be described in the following.

DETECTION OF ISCHEMIC HEART DISEASE

If IHD is suspected, CMR is one of several diagnostic imaging modalities or invasive strategies with overlapping indications. To select the appropriate diagnostic test, the estimation of the pretest probability for the presence of significant coronary artery stenosis is recommended by current international practice guidelines.[1] While invasive strategies are preferred in patients with high pretest probability for IHD, the ability of CMR to accurately detect and define the severity of IHD renders it the modality of choice in patients with moderate to high pretest probability and to assess the need for revascularization in these patients.[2] The detection and characterization of IHD by CMR employs two approaches: stress testing and tissue characterization with delayed enhancement images and T1- or T2-weighted images or mapping. Stress CMR can be further subcategorized to stress function and stress perfusion CMR. Both techniques are functional tests that can only detect coronary lesions with hemodynamic significance under resting or stress conditions. In contrast to coronary computed tomography, nonsignificant lesions cannot be identified with appropriate accuracy, the detection of which might support the decision to prescribe antiplatelets or statins. In CMR, the visually detected site of myocardial ischemia is assigned to a major coronary artery based on anatomic considerations using the American Heart Association 17 segment model (Fig. 39.1). The 17 segments are evaluated in multiple short-axis planes and the vertical long-axis plane. The apical segment (segment 17) of the left ventricle (LV) is assessed in the vertical long-axis plane, while the other 16 segments are inspected in three short-axis planes at the height of the left ventricular base, the papillary muscles (mid-ventricle), and the apex.

Stress Function CMR

The rationale for stress CMR to identify a hemodynamically significant coronary arterial stenosis is that patients with

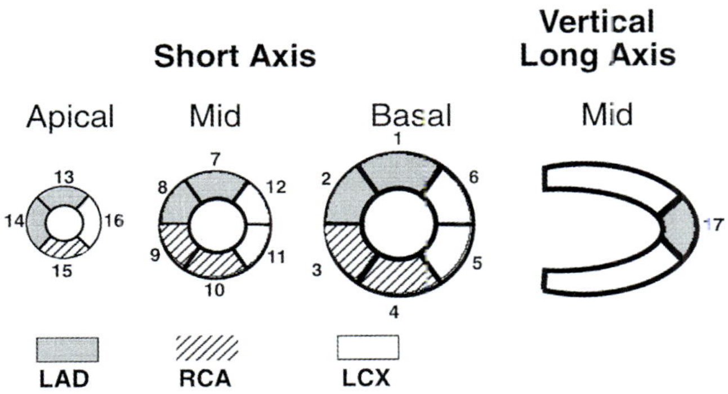

Figure 39.1. Seventeen-segment model suggested by the American Heart Association. The coronary artery territories are shown in the graph.

such lesions have adequate blood flow under resting conditions but not after application of a pharmacological stressor. A pharmacologically provoked increase of myocardial contractility and heart rate amplifies myocardial oxygen consumption (demand) and comes with the need for increased coronary blood flow. In nondiseased coronary arteries, blood flow may increase three-to fivefold when pharmacologic stress is applied. In contrast, flow cannot increase to the appropriate level in a stenotic artery, which results in regional demand/supply mismatch and causes contractile dysfunction. Significant coronary artery stenosis can be suspected if a segmental decrease in wall thickening, wall motion, or both are observed under stress but not under resting conditions in the left ventricular myocardium.

The pharmacologic stressor is usually an infusion of dobutamine. Dobutamine is a secondary coronary vasodilator and increases myocardial contractility and heart rate by beta-sympathomimetic stimulation. The dose is gradually increased to stimulate intermediate stress (20 μg/kg/min) and then peak stress (40 μg/kg/min).[3] At peak stress, a heart rate equal to 85% of the maximum heart rate predicted for age (0.85 × 220 – age in years) should be achieved. Atropine may be administered to attain the targeted heart rate. As an alternate to inotropic stress testing with dobutamine, the administration of a primary vasodilator such as dipyridamole, adenosine, or the more coronary-specific A2A receptor agonist regadenoson increases coronary flow by dilating coronary arterioles (resistance vessels). In the presence of a hemodynamically significant stenosis, resistance vessels in the myocardium served by the coronary artery (conductance vessel) are already maximally dilated. Consequently, the primary vasodilator only increases flow to myocardium served by nonstenotic arteries and flow is stolen from the stenotic region, inducing regional myocardial ischemia (coronary arterial steal). The failure of coronary flow to meet the appropriate demand may be reflected in a regional contraction abnormality. Regional wall-motion abnormalities are, however, less pronounced after application of primary vasodilators compared with dobutamine stress CMR, wherefore these techniques are frequently combined with stress perfusion CMR (see later discussion).

Image acquisition for stress function encompasses cine CMR in a short-axis plane at multiple levels and vertical long-axis plane in the baseline state, at intermediate stress, and at peak stress using a balanced steady-state free precession sequence, variably named by the manufacturers as balanced fast field echo, true fast imaging with steady precession, or fast imaging employing steady-state acquisition. With these sequences, cine magnetic resonance (MR) images consisting of 16 to 40 phases can be acquired at three anatomic locations in a breath-hold of 10 to 20 seconds. Since myocardial ischemia is provoked by this test, careful patient monitoring is essential during and after the scan and several contraindications have to be considered,[3] although the rate of relevant adverse events is below 0.1%.[4]

Stress Perfusion CMR

Stress perfusion CMR is based on the same technique used for nuclear scintigraphy and the coronary artery steal phenomena described earlier. Contrary to stress function, it is a contrast-based method with higher specificity for IHD, shorter acquisition times, and a lower arrhythmic risk compared with dobutamine stress. Pharmacologic stress is used to provoke a perfusion deficit in the myocardium supplied by a coronary artery with a hemodynamically significant stenosis. The pharmacologic agents used are dipyridamole, adenosine, and regadenoson, as described earlier. In addition to the visual assessment of wall-motion abnormalities performed in stress function CMR, in perfusion CMR the induced ischemia is demasked by additional gadolinium-based contrast agent application. Relevant perfusion deficits appear with delayed wash-in and wash-out of the contrast agent (Figs. 39.2 and 39.3) and typically originate from the subendocardial layer. Additional quantitative analysis of the regional intensity-time curve during initial passage of the contrast might improve the diagnostic accuracy. Healthy myocardium, on the other hand, is visually perceived bright with homogeneous rapid contrast agent uptake starting at the anteroseptal wall in the epicardial layer. No clear cutoff level for the extent of ischemia exists at which invasive revascularization has proven to be superior to medical treatment alone. Observational data from scintigraphy suggest a proportion of >10% of ischemic myocardium at which revascularization might reduce the rate of adverse events; however, the patient's symptoms and medical history often outweigh predefined cutoff levels in the decision pathway. Other more practice—than evidence—oriented cutoff levels to define relevant ischemia in CMR are the presence of ischemia in at least two corresponding American Heart Association segments or transmural ischemia.

For stress perfusion CMR, images are acquired in the short-axis plane at three to five anatomic levels (base to apex) and a vertical long-axis plane after application of

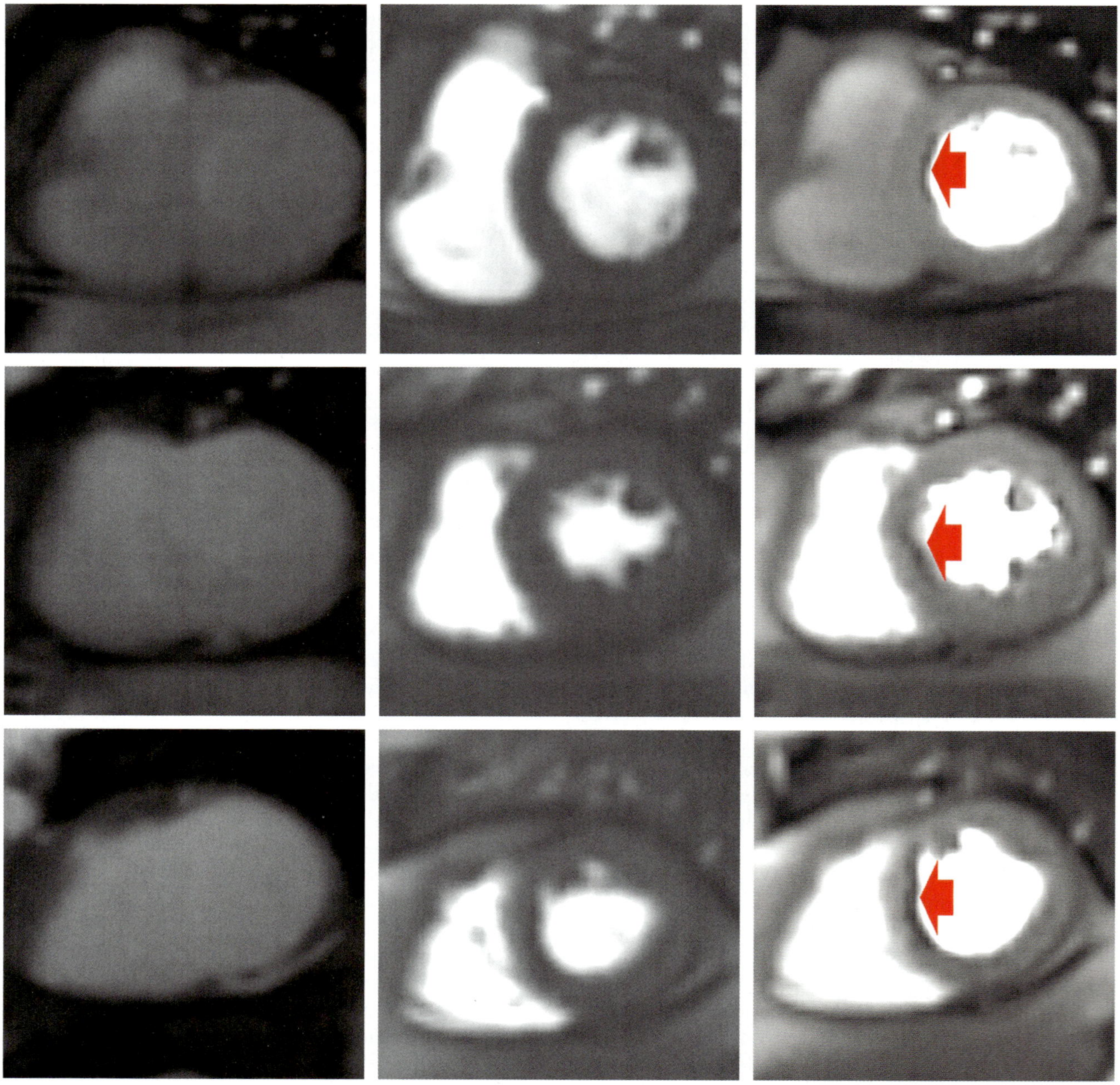

Figure 39.2. Inversion recovery short-axis images before (**left**) and after the arrival of gadolinium chelate in the left ventricular cavity (**center**) and myocardium (**right**) demonstrate an epicardial perfusion deficit in the ventricular septum (red *arrows*).

the vasodilating agent. While regadenoson has a three- to five-minute half-life and can therefore be applied as a single dose, adenosine requires continuous administration through a second intravenous line. A saturation recovery or inversion recovery fast gradient-echo sequence is used to diminish the signal of myocardium and blacken the background signal prior to the first passage of intravenously injected gadolinium chelate (0.03-0.1 mmol/kg). The images at each anatomic level are acquired at a rate of about one per second for about 30 to 60 seconds depending on heart rate.

Compared against the diagnostic gold standard, the assessment of fractional flow reserve in invasive angiography, several studies validated the high accuracy of stress perfusion CMR in the detection of significant coronary artery stenosis and demonstrated a sensitivity and specificity of >85%, depending on the cohort studied.[5,6] Compared with single-photon emission tomography and positron emission tomography, the diagnostic accuracy of stress perfusion CMR has been found to be equal or better. The higher spatial resolution of CMR can help to identify small subendocardial

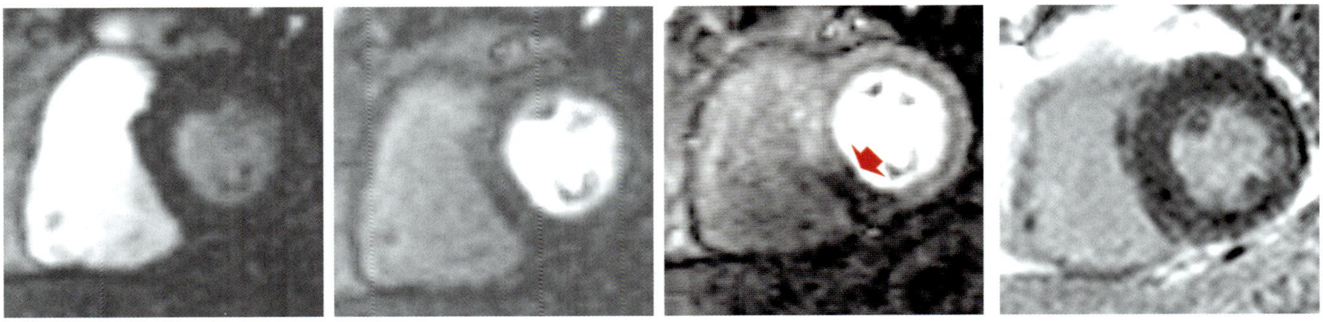

Figure 39.3. Inversion recovery short-axis images at several time frames after administration of gadolinium chelate under regadenoson stress demonstrate a transmural perfusion deficit (red *arrow*) in the inferoseptal wall of the left ventricle suggestive of ischemia in the territory of the right coronary artery. Absence of late gadolinium enhancement in the inversion recovery sequence (**right**) indicates viability without prior myocardial infarction.

perfusion deficits (Fig. 39.2) and to detect triple vessel disease with diffuse myocardial ischemia (Fig. 39.4). If screening for IHD is made by stress perfusion CMR in intermediate- to high-risk patients, the number of patients referred for revascularization can be reduced without impacting the rate of major adverse cardiac events compared with an invasive strategy.[7] Accordingly, the prognostic capability of stress function and perfusion CMR was demonstrated in several studies, and the rate of adverse events in patients with no ischemia and no delayed enhancement is below 1% within the first 5 years after the scan.[8] Not only the proof of ischemia but also its severity (eg, the number of segments with ischemia) is directly linked to the occurrence of adverse events and may support therapeutic decision.[9]

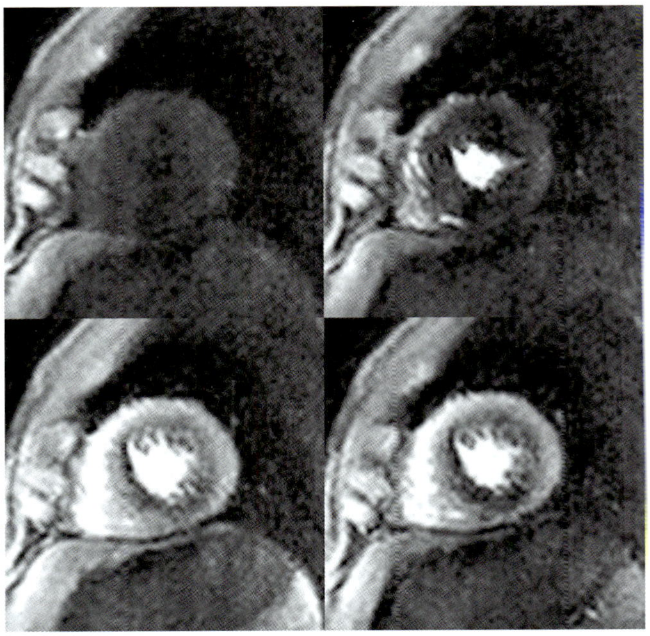

Figure 39.4. Inversion recovery short-axis images before and at three time intervals after arrival of gadolinium chelate in the left ventricle show perfusion deficits around the entire circumference of the myocardium, indicating the likelihood of triple vessel disease. (Courtesy of Hajime Sakuma, M.D., Mie, Japan.)

CMR Tissue Characterization

Although several findings in CMR tissue characterization can be highly suggestive of IHD, most features are not specific for IHD, and additional sequences, combination with other modalities, or an appropriate clinical context is required to obtain the diagnosis.

LGE CMR uses gadolinium to contrast fibrotic tissue based on the contrast-induced shortening of T1 relaxation times. Regional variations in the uptake and washout patterns of gadolinium are identified by employment of an inversion recovery gradient-echo sequence with an inversion time set to attenuate the signal of normal myocardium at 10 to 15 minutes after intravenous contrast medium administration (0.1-0.2 mmol/kg gadolinium). At this time, the contrast is substantially cleared from viable myocardium, which appears black. In nonviable myocardium (necrotic or fibrotic) or in the presence of myocardial edema, contrast agent is trapped in the interstitial space, which translates to LGE (Fig. 39.5). LGE in IHD corresponds to the distribution of one or more coronary arteries or branch arteries and always involves at least the subendocardial layer of the myocardium where myocardial ischemia is most severe. LGE in a distribution that does not include the subendocardium suggests a nonischemic etiology. A midwall distribution might suggest idiopathic dilated cardiomyopathy, while subepicardial distribution suggests myocarditis (see Chapter 34). Ischemic cardiomyopathy invariably shows some region(s) with at least subendocardial LGE. LGE with a central zone of attenuation (lack of enhancement) in the subendocardium is indicative of myocardial infarction with microvascular obstruction (Fig. 39.6). Microvascular obstruction occurs after prolonged occlusion or incomplete restoration of blood flow after myocardial infarction and is associated

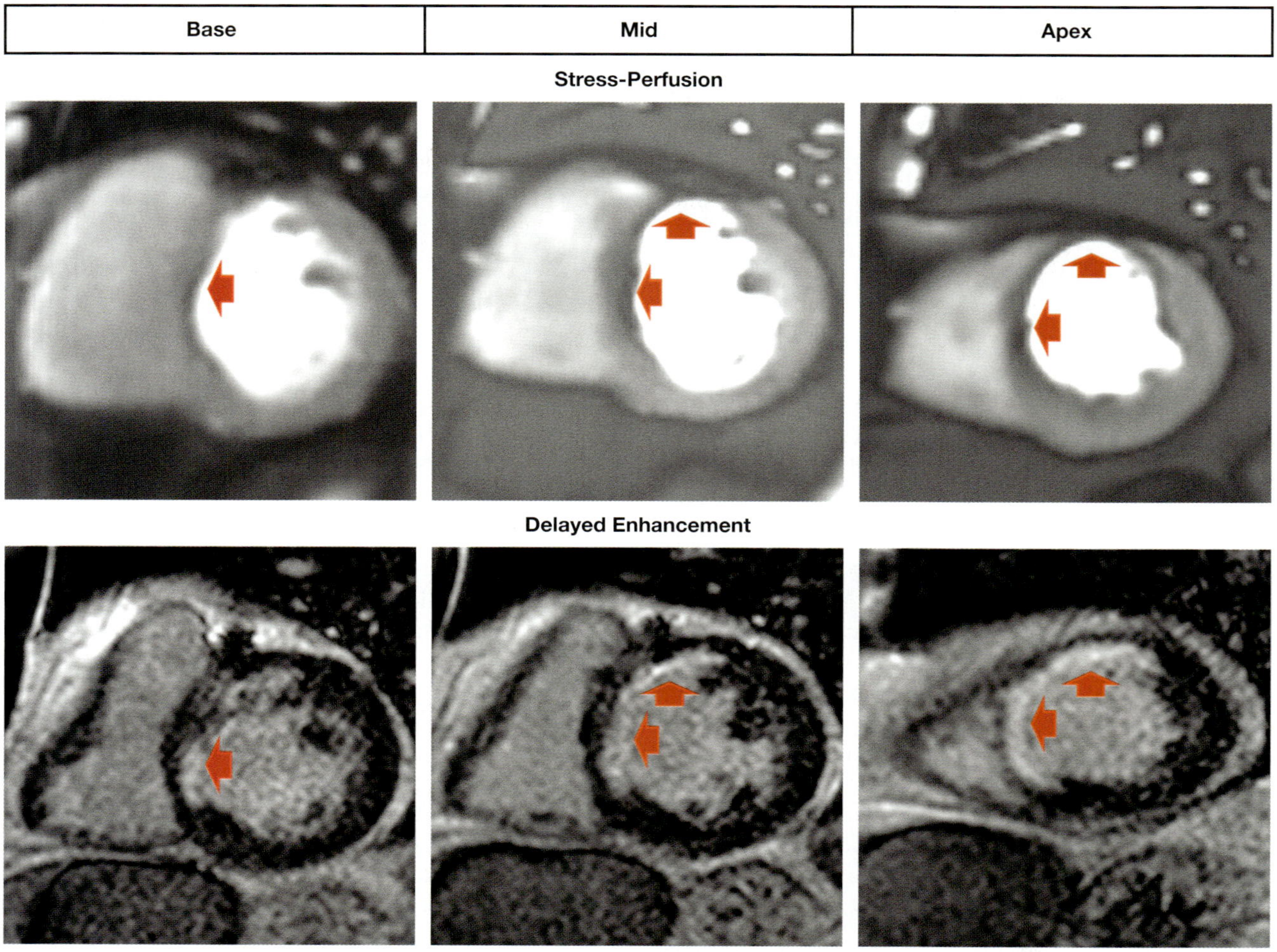

Figure 39.5. Regadenoson stress perfusion and delayed enhancement images in the short-axis plane. The late gadolinium enhancement images were acquired 15 minutes after intravenous administration of gadolinium chelate using an inversion time, which attenuates the signal of normal myocardium. There is induced first-pass myocardial perfusion defect in the territory of the left anterior descending coronary artery within the myocardial extent of late gadolinium enhancement, indicating no peri-infarct ischemia (red *arrows*). Transmurality of late gadolinium enhancement >50% in the midventricular and apical septum indicates a lack of viability.

with adverse outcomes. The extent of LGE is also linked to outcomes and particularly to the occurrence of ventricular tachycardia and sudden cardiac death.[10] Therefore, in patients with reduced LV ejection fraction, the presence and extent of LGE should be considered in the evaluation of sudden cardiac death prophylaxis with an implantable cardioverter defibrillator.

T1-weighted imaging and quantitative parametric T1 mapping are complementary to LGE MR imaging in the identification of fibrosis. Native (without contrast) T1 relaxation times can be assessed qualitatively (T1-weighted imaging) or quantitively with definition of a scanner-specific T1 time in each voxel (T1 mapping). Native T1 relaxation times are increased in acute and chronic myocardial infarction in the ischemic regions, and also in inflammation and edema (myocarditis), and in infiltrative cardiac diseases like cardiac amyloidosis. In contrast to LGE imaging, it can also identify diffuse changes in myocardial structure resulting from adverse remodeling after myocardial infarction. Native T1 is a contrast-free method that can be particularly helpful to identify localized or diffuse fibrosis in patients with chronic kidney disease (glomerular filtration rate <30 mL/m^2), when gadolinium is relatively contraindicated due to the low potential risk of contrast-induced nephrogenic fibrosing sclerosis.

The combination of native T1 with postcontrast T1 mapping enables the quantitative evaluation of the extracellular volume fraction (ECV). Retained contrast in the myocardium as described earlier decreases postcontrast T1 times and increases ECV, which is calculated from the relation of myocardial and blood pool native and postcontrast T1 times and the patient's hematocrit. As described previously, the extent of fibrosis is linked to outcomes, and also the ECV and native T1 of the noninfarcted remote myocardium was

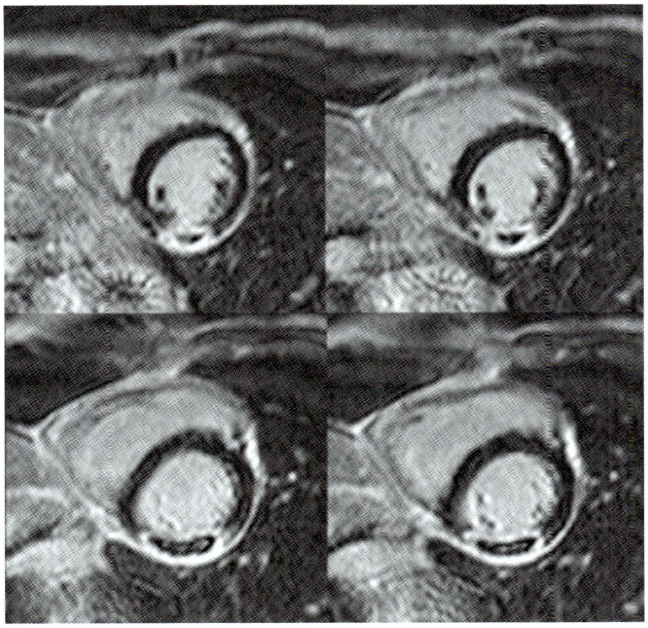

Figure 39.6. Multilevel short-axis late gadolinium enhancement images showing an acute inferior myocardial infarction with microvascular obstruction. There is hyperenhancement of the periphery of the infarction. The endocardial center shows no enhancement due to microvascular obstruction. (Courtesy of H. Sakuma, Mie, Japan.)

demonstrated to be an important predictor of outcomes in patients with IHD.[11]

T2-weighted images or T2 mapping can be used to identify myocardial edema related to myocardial infarction, which provides information on temporality of the infarction, as regions of acute myocardial infarction will typically show elevated T2 signal.

ASSESSMENT OF MYOCARDIAL VIABILITY

In the setting of IHD a continuum of several types of myocardial dysfunction can be present. Below a critical supply/demand threshold, ischemia results in myocardial infarction with inflammation, necrosis, replacement-fibrosis, and irreversible scarring, whereas the mismatch between blood supply and demand is often less severe in the surrounding tissue. This so-called hibernating myocardium presents a persistently decreased contractility but might still be viable. Since dysfunction is potentially reversible after restoration of the blood supply, these patients may benefit from coronary revascularization. Additionally, the assessment of viability can inform on the risk of sudden cardiac death.[12] However, in standard echocardiography or CMR cine images transient hibernating myocardium cannot be accurately differentiated from scarring. It is the ability to compare the results of functional testing against tissue characteristics that makes CMR the gold standard for the detection of viability. Highest diagnostic accuracy is achieved if perfusion defects identified by stress CMR are evaluated in the LGE sequences (Table 39.1). Stunned and hibernating myocardium shows regional contractile dysfunction but no LGE. In contrast, acute and chronic infarction without viability is characterized by regional dysfunction and LGE. Moreover, the transmurality of LGE can predict the likelihood for the recovery of regional contractile function after myocardial revascularization. Segments with LGE with >50% transmurality are unlikely to recover function after restoration of blood flow (Figs. 39.5, 39.7, and 39.8).

Another approach to test for viability is the assessment of the contractile reserve of a dysfunctional LV segment by dobutamine application (5-10 µg/kg/min). Viable myocardium with contractile dysfunction under resting conditions can increase contractility under stimulation with

Table 39.1 Types of Myocardial Injuries

Type	Regional Function	Late Gadolinium Enhancement	Perfusion
Normal myocardium	Normal	No	Normal
Stunned myocardium	Dysfunction	No	Acute transient decrease
Hibernating myocardium (ischemic cardiomyopathy)	Dysfunction (regional or global)	No	Chronic decrease
Acute infarction (necrosis)	Dysfunction	Yes	Decreased until reperfusion
Chronic infarction	Dysfunction (wall thinning)	Yes	Decreased until reperfusion
Nonischemic cardiomyopathy	Global dysfunction	Possible—not subendocardial	Normal

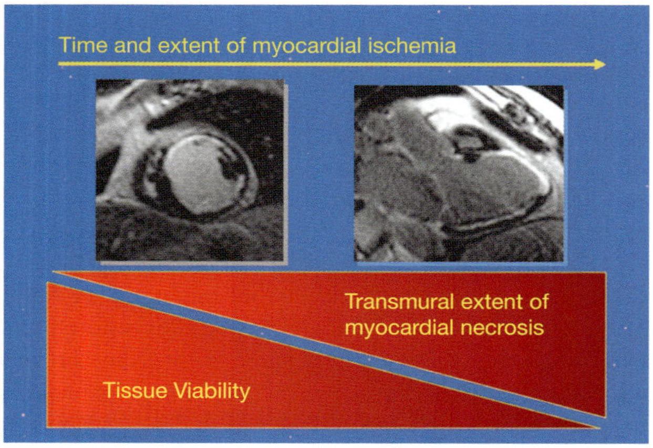

Figure 39.7. Short-axis and vertical long-axis late gadolinium enhancement images demonstrate a transmural infarction of the anterior region and a subendocardial infarction in the diaphragmatic posterolateral region of the left ventricle. Time and extent of myocardial ischemia determines the transition from some degree of viability to transmural necrosis. (MR images are courtesy of S. Wolff, New York.)

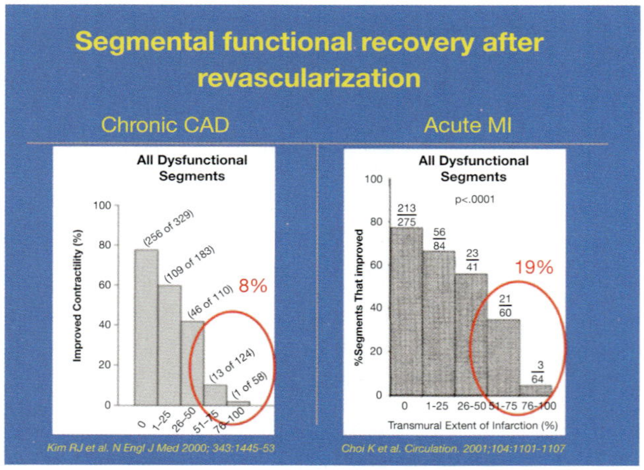

Figure 39.8. Left: Graph showing the percent of dysfunctional segments with recovery in regional contractility versus transmural extent of late gadolinium enhancement after revascularization for chronic myocardial infarction. **Right:** Graph showing the percent of dysfunctional segments with recovery in regional contractility versus transmural extent of late gadolinium enhancement at late follow-up after acute myocardial infarction. If there is greater than 50% transmurality, recovery occurred in 8% of chronic infarcts and 19% of acute infarcts. CAD, coronary artery disease; MI, myocardial infarction. **(Left:** From Kim RJ, Wu E, Rafael A, et al. The use of contrast-enhanced magnetic resonance imaging to identify reversible myocardial dysfunction. *New Engl J Med*. 2000;343:1445-1453, with permission; **Right:** From Choi K, Kim RJ, Gubernikoff G, Vargas JD, Parker M, Judd RM. Transmural extent of acute myocardial infarction predicts long-term improvement in contractile function. *Circulation*. 2001;104:1101-1107, with permission.)

dobutamine. Not only an improvement in wall motion and wall thickening (more than 2 mm) during systole but also an end-diastolic wall thickness greater than 5.5 mm can predict response to coronary revascularization.

EVALUATION OF MYOCARDIAL REVASCULARIZATION BY CMR

In patients after myocardial infarction with implantation of coronary stents or after coronary artery bypass graft (CABG) operation, anatomical imaging like cardiac computed tomography has limitations in the capability to assess graft patency and progression of coronary artery disease. After surgical revascularization, contrast kinetics are challenging to analyze and often subject to individual vessel anatomy and bypass type, also leading to lower diagnostic accuracy of stress CMR.[13] Nevertheless, if performed by experienced readers, stress perfusion CMR can reliably discriminate inducible ischemia following CABG and inherits high prognostic value in this setting.[14] CMR is an excellent modality to noninvasively exclude a progression in IHD after CABG in patients with suggestive symptoms and also to identify silent ischemia in asymptomatic patients in 5-year intervals following CABG. Patency of the graft(s) supplying the territory of the left anterior descending coronary artery is of particular importance and strongly linked to survival.

The assessment of the coronary flow reserve in patients with known IHD by noncontrast phase-contrast cine MR imaging of the coronary sinus blood flow is another method that also inherits prognostic value after CABG.[15] The coronary sinus conducts about 90% of the left ventricular myocardial flow, and its blood flow can be extrapolated to the coronary flow at rest and the flow reserve at stress. Velocity-encoded phase contrast cine CMR provides a pair of images at approximately 12 to 16 phases of the cardiac cycle. The pair consists of magnitude and phase images acquired perpendicular to the direction of blood flow in the coronary sinus. A set of images is acquired under resting conditions and under pharmacologically induced stress. Total coronary flow is normalized to LV mass to express the flow in mL/min/g myocardium. LV mass is measured from a stack of cine MR images encompassing the entire LV. The velocity-encoded images are acquired in the basal and vasodilated states to calculate peak velocity of flow and to derive coronary flow reserve as the ratio of maximal flow to basal flow. A normal value is designated as a ratio greater than 2.3 to 2.5. In the presence of a hemodynamically significant stenosis (more than 50% reduction in luminal diameter), it is lower than 2.3. Abnormal coronary flow and flow reserve may occur in not only IHD but also in patients with heart transplants, heart failure with preserved ejection fraction, hypertrophic cardiomyopathy, and dilated cardiomyopathy. Owing to the lack of specificity, this method is mostly used after CABG[15] or to demonstrate a hemodynamic stenosis before treatment. After stent placement, measurement of coronary flow reserve with CMR can be used to monitor the coronary functional status in order to detect recurrence of stenosis. Furthermore, it can be used as amendment to stress perfusion CMR to refine prognostication in known or suspected IHD.[16,17]

Contrast-enhanced 3D MR angiography or coronary MR angiography may be used to demonstrate the blood flow in revascularization conduits and internal mammary arterial and saphenous vein grafts. However, this technique never made into routine practice and cannot provide a satisfactory level of diagnostic accuracy for the detection of significant stenosis.

MYOCARDIAL INFARCTION AND ITS COMPLICATIONS

If there is evidence for acute myocardial infarction, CMR is not part of the recommended approach at first line. However, if mechanical complications are suspected, if revascularization is not possible, or in myocardial infarction with non-obstructive coronary arteries, CMR has an important role to manage these patients and provide better risk stratification.

T2-weighted images or T2-parametric mapping can identify interstitial and intracellular edema associated to infarction and consecutively increased myocardial cellular permeability. Triple inversion recovery spin-echo sequences with inversion pulses for suppression of the signal intensity of fat and blood are used to provide improved contrast between normal and edematous myocardium with attenuated respiratory and blood flow signal artifacts. The edematous myocardial region (increased T2 signal) has been shown to correspond to the region rendered ischemic (ischemic jeopardy zone) after coronary occlusion. Usually, the area of LGE (infarction) is smaller than the T2-hyperintense

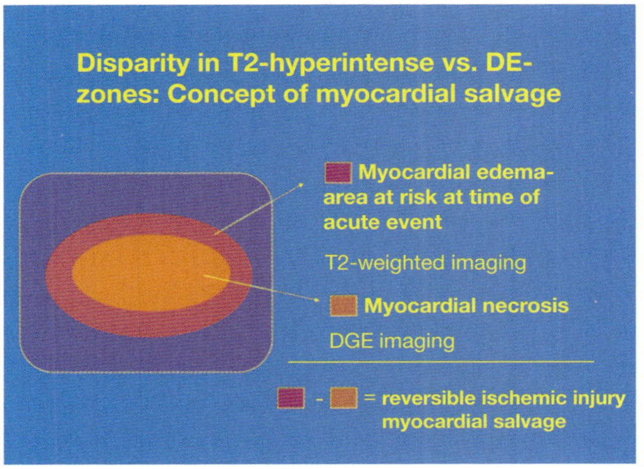

Figure 39.9. Diagram showing relationship between area of hyperintensity of ischemic region on T2-weighted image (myocardial edema) and area of delayed gadolinium enhancement (DGE) (myocardial necrosis) of the infarcted region. In the event of early reperfusion, the difference between the areas represents salvage of ischemic myocardium (salvage area or salvage index). DE, delayed enhancement.

region (ischemic jeopardy zone). In patients who undergo early interventions (within 90 minutes) to open the occluded artery, there may be a much smaller infarct area compared with the jeopardy zone. The difference between the two has been called the myocardial salvage index (Fig. 39.9).

Cine CMR or electrocardiogram-gated spin-echo images can demonstrate the mechanical complications that may result from myocardial infarction, such as true and false LV aneurysms (Figs. 39.10 and 39.11), mural thrombus

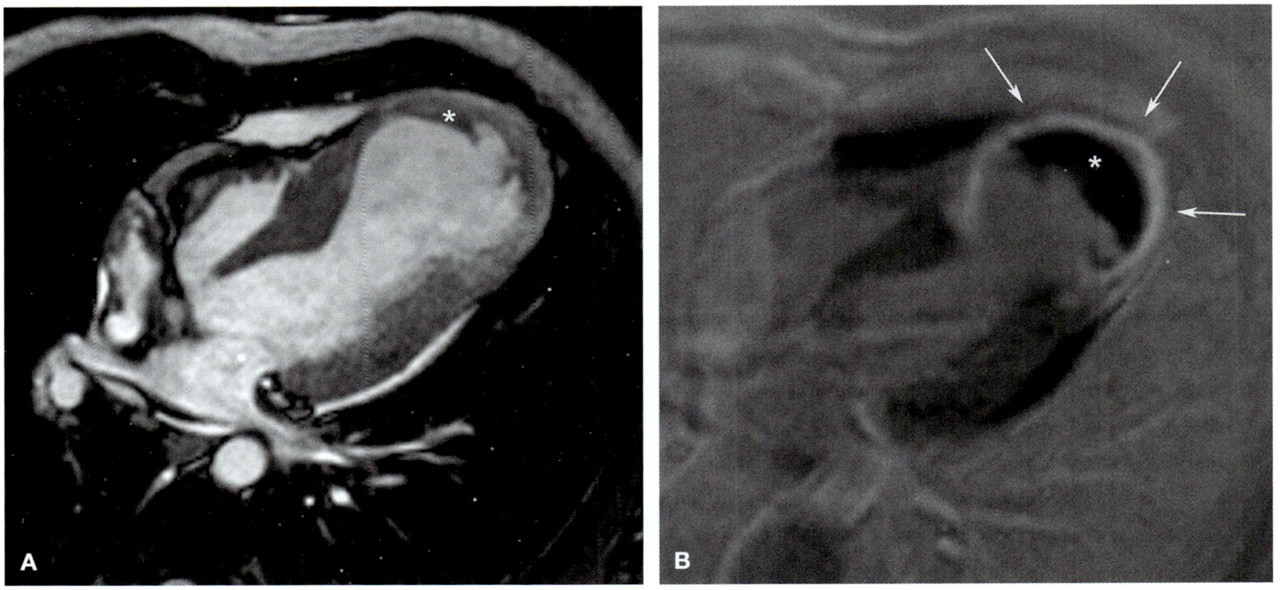

Figure 39.10. LV apical true aneurysm and clot. **A:** Cine MR in horizontal long-axis plane. **B:** Late enhanced image in the same plane shows transmural late enhancement of the infarction (*arrows*). Apical clot (*asterisk*) is delineated best on the late enhanced image.

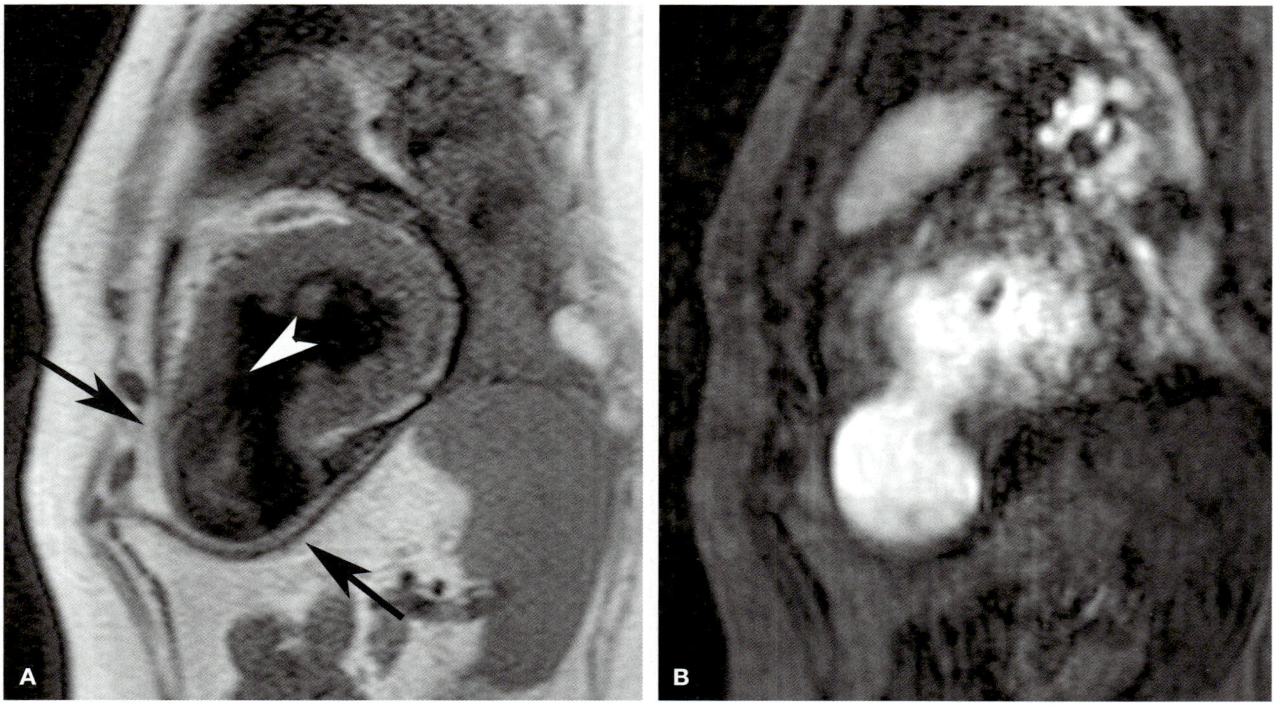

Figure 39.11. LV apical false aneurysm. **A:** A spin-echo image in sagittal plane shows that the widest diameter (*arrows*) of aneurysm is much wider than the ostium. **B:** MR angiograms in the sagittal plane show narrow ostium (*arrowhead*).

(Fig. 39.12), and mitral regurgitation due to papillary muscle dysfunction or rupture. CMR is particularly effective for demonstrating the narrow ostium between the LV cavity and the false aneurysm (Fig. 39.11). With increasing extent of ischemia, LV adverse remodeling with LV hypertrophy and dilatation can be observed. CMR is the diagnostic gold standard to detect increased LV volumes, reduced ejection fraction, and decreased longitudinal strain in ischemic dilated cardiomyopathy (Fig. 39.13).

ARTIFICIAL INTELLIGENCE APPLICATIONS IN CMR FOR IHD

Recent advances in imaging postprocessing using artificial intelligence (AI) may aid in the detection of CMR abnormalities in patients with IHD. Current postprocessing software already use AI tools for interpolation of cine images and perfusion maps and for semiautomatic detection of areas of LGE and perfusion defects.

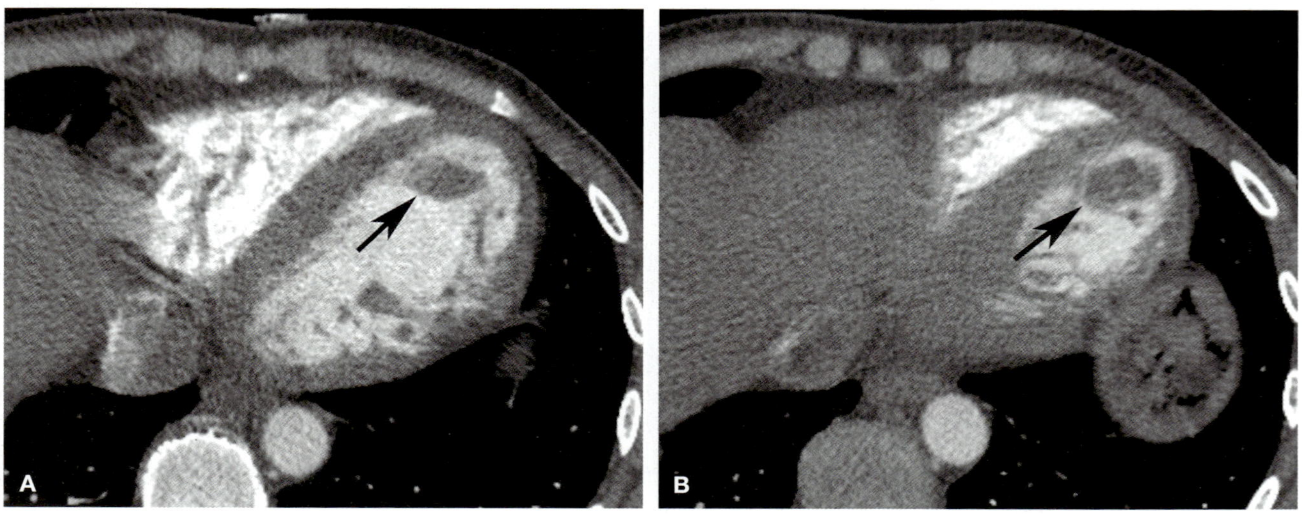

Figure 39.12. Left ventricular thrombus. Axial scans of middle of left ventricle (**A**) and at apex (**B**). Contrast-enhanced computed tomography scan shows thrombus (*arrow*) on site of anteroapical myocardial infarction.

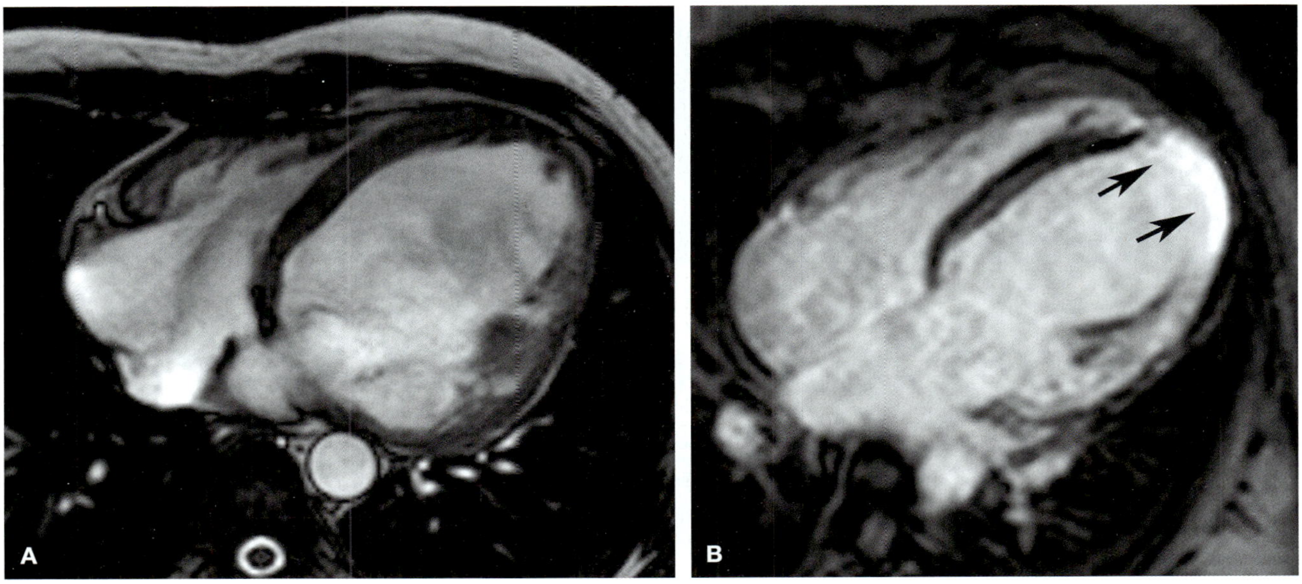

Figure 39.13. Ischemic dilated cardiomyopathy with heart failure with reduced ejection fraction. Cine MR (**A**) and late gadolinium enhancement (**B**) images in the axial plane show severely dilated left ventricle with transmural late enhancement (*arrows*) at the apex.

REFERENCES

1. Knuuti J, Wijns W, Saraste A, et al; ESC Scientific Document Group. 2019 ESC Guidelines for the diagnosis and management of chronic coronary syndromes. *Eur Heart J.* 2020;41(3):407-477. doi:10.1093/eurheartj/ehz425
2. Knuuti J, Ballo H, Juarez-Orozco LE, et al. The performance of non-invasive tests to rule-in and rule-out significant coronary artery stenosis in patients with stable angina: a meta-analysis focused on post-test disease probability. *Eur Heart J.* 2018;39(35):3322-3330. doi:10.1093/eurheartj/ehy267
3. Kramer CM, Barkhausen J, Bucciarelli-Ducci C, Flamm SD, Kim RJ, Nagel E. Standardized cardiovascular magnetic resonance imaging (CMR) protocols: 2020 update. *J Cardiovasc Magn Reson.* 2020;22(1):17. doi:10.1186/s12968-020-00607-1
4. Bruder O, Wagner A, Lombardi M, et al. European Cardiovascular Magnetic Resonance (EuroCMR) registry—multi national results from 57 centers in 15 countries. *J Cardiovasc Magn Reson.* 2013;15(1):9. doi:10.1186/1532-429x-15-9
5. Watkins S, McGeoch R, Lyne J, et al. Validation of magnetic resonance myocardial perfusion imaging with fractional flow reserve for the detection of significant coronary heart disease. *Circulation.* 2009;120(22):2207-2213. doi:10.1161/circulationaha.109.872358
6. Takx RA, Blomberg BA, El Aidi H, et al. Diagnostic accuracy of stress myocardial perfusion imaging compared to invasive coronary angiography with fractional flow reserve meta-analysis. *Circ Cardiovasc Imaging.* 2015;8(1):e002666. doi:10.1161/circimaging.114.002666
7. Nagel E, Greenwood JP, McCann GP, et al; MR-INFORM Investigators. Magnetic resonance perfusion or fractional flow reserve in coronary disease. *N Engl J Med.* 2019;380(25):2418-2428. doi:10.1056/NEJMoa1716734
8. Kwong RY, Ge Y, Steel K, et al. Cardiac magnetic resonance stress perfusion imaging for evaluation of patients with chest pain. *J Am Coll Cardiol.* 2019;74(14):1741-1755. doi:10.1016/j.jacc.2019.07 074
9. Pezel T, Unterseeh T, Garot P, et al. Long-term prognostic value of stress cardiovascular magnetic resonance-related coronary revascularization to predict death: a large registry with >200 000 patient-years of follow-up. *Circ Cardiovasc Imaging.* 2021;14(10):e012789. doi:10.1161/circimaging.121.012789
10. Kwon DH, Halley CM, Carrigan TP, et al. Extent of left ventricular scar predicts outcomes in ischemic cardiomyopathy patients with significantly reduced systolic function: a delayed hyperenhancement cardiac magnetic resonance study. *JACC Cardiovasc Imaging.* 2009;2(1):34-44. doi:10.1016/j.jcmg.2008.09.010
11. Puntmann VO, Carr-White G, Jabbour A, et al; International T1 Multicentre CMR Outcome Study. Native T1 and ECV of noninfarcted myocardium and outcome in patients with coronary artery disease. *J Am Coll Cardiol.* 2018;71(7):766-778. doi:10.1016/j.jacc.2017.12.020
12. Garcia MJ, Kwong RY, Scherrer-Crosbie M, et al; American Heart Association Council on Cardiovascular Radiology and Intervention and Council on Clinical Cardiology. State of the art: imaging for myocardial viability—a scientific statement from the American Heart Association. *Circ Cardiovasc Imaging.* 2020;13(7):e000053. doi:10.1161/hci.0000000000000053
13. Bernhardt P, Spiess J, Levenson B, et al. Combined assessment of myocardial perfusion and late gadolinium enhancement in patients after percutaneous coronary intervention or bypass grafts: a multicenter study of an integrated cardiovascular magnetic resonance protocol. *JACC Cardiovasc Imaging.* 2009;2(11):1292-1300. doi:10.1016/j.jcmg.2009.05.011
14. Kinnel M, Sanguineti F, Pezel T, et al. Prognostic value of vasodilator stress perfusion CMR in patients with previous coronary artery bypass graft. *Eur Heart J Cardiovasc Imaging.* 2021;22(11):1264-1272. doi:10.1093/ehjci/jeaa316
15. Seraphim A, Dowsing B, Rathod KS, et al. Quantitative myocardial perfusion predicts outcomes in patients with prior surgical revascularization. *J Am Coll Cardiol.* 2022;79(12):1141-1151. doi:10.1016/j.jacc.2021.12.037
16. Indorkar R, Kwong RY, Romano S, et al. Global coronary flow reserve measured during stress cardiac magnetic resonance imaging is an independent predictor of adverse cardiovascular events. *JACC Cardiovasc Imaging.* 2019;12(8 pt 2):1686-1695. doi:10.1016/j.jcmg.2018.08.018
17. Kato S, Saito N, Nakachi T, et al. Stress perfusion coronary flow reserve versus cardiac magnetic resonance for known or suspected CAD. *J Am Coll Cardiol.* 2017;70(7):869-879. doi:10.1016/j.jacc.2017.06.028

SUGGESTED READINGS

El Aidi H, Adams A, Moons KGM, et al. Cardiac magnetic resonance imaging findings and the risk of cardiovascular events in patients with recent myocardial infarction or suspected or known coronary artery disease: a systematic review of prognostic studies. *J Am Coll Cardiol.* 2014;63:1031-1045. doi:10.1016/j.jacc.2013.11.048.

Velazquez EJ, Lee KL, Jones RH, Al-Khalidi HR, Hill JA, Panza JA, Michler RE, Bonow RO, Doenst T, Petrie MC, Oh JK, She L, Moore VL, Desvigne-Nickens P, Sopko G, Rouleau JL; STICHES Investigators. Coronary-artery bypass surgery in patients with ischemic cardiomyopathy. *N Engl J Med.* 2016;374(16):1511-1520. doi:10.1056/NEJMoa1602001.

Chapter 40

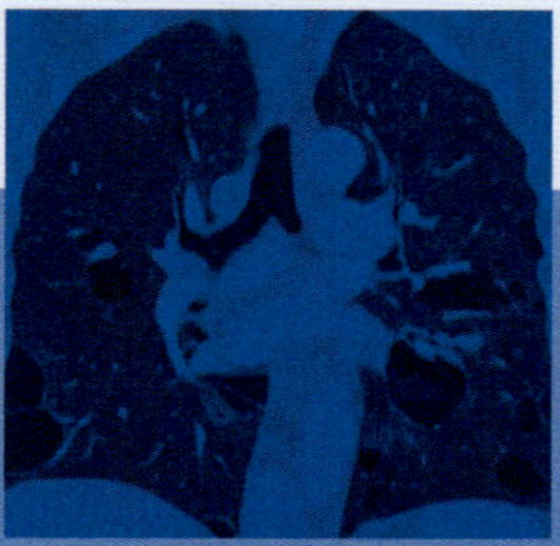

Nicola Fink • Akos Varga-Szemes • U. Joseph Schoepf • Tilman Emrich

Computed Tomography of Coronary Arteries and Ischemic Heart Disease

INTRODUCTION

With changing living standards over the last centuries, cardiovascular diseases (CVDs), especially ischemic heart disease (IHD), became the leading cause of mortality in the United States and worldwide. Nevertheless, simultaneous improvements in medical care have led to a better prognosis of myocardial infarction and a consequent rise in individual morbidity and overall health care costs. Thus, coronary artery disease (CAD) increases the individual and the socioeconomic disease burden. With the introduction of specific drugs (eg, statins) and procedures (eg, coronary angioplasty, stenting, and coronary bypass surgery), preventive and therapeutic options became available. However, to maximize the benefit of these options for primary and secondary prevention of major adverse cardiac events (MACE), methods to identify patients at risk are crucial.

The visualization of coronary arteries using computed tomography (CT) remains challenging, as it requires both high temporal resolution to freeze cardiac motion and high spatial resolution to visualize the relatively small-caliber vessels. Owing to recent technical developments addressing such requirements and the growing clinical evidence, cardiac CT has evolved into being a robust method in the assessment of CAD. While coronary artery calcium scoring (CACS) has already been feasible in the early 1980s using electron beam CT, the introduction of multidetector CT (MDCT) in the 1990s was the first to enable accurate visualization of the coronary arteries. However, this was not the final destination in CT technology development. In addition to the evolution of 256- and 320-MDCT systems in the 2000s, new developments, such as dual-energy and dual-source, as well as photon-counting detector (PCD) CT systems have become available and revolutionized cardiac CT. Meanwhile, cardiac CT plays an important role in the evaluation and management of patients with known or suspected CAD. In current guidelines, it is recommended as strategy to exclude obstructive CAD and to detect nonobstructive CAD depending on the individual cardiovascular risk, thus guiding further risk classification and clinical decision making.

INDICATIONS

Driven by the growing evidence demonstrating similar or better results regarding outcome and cost compared with functional testing, the clinical use of coronary CT angiography (CTA) has been increasing worldwide. The main clinical applications of coronary CT can be summarized under the following indications:

1. Screening in asymptomatic patients (ie, primary prevention of MACE)
2. Assessment of CAD in symptomatic patients with stable or acute chest pain

Other indications include planning before cardiac surgery, assessment of coronary stents and bypass grafts, and risk evaluation before liver or lung transplantation.

Asymptomatic Patients

Owing to the high individual and socioeconomic disease burden of CAD, adequate primary prevention strategies, including risk stratification in asymptomatic patients, are important. Common risk stratification tools include the Framingham risk score and the atherosclerotic CVD

(ASCVD) risk factors. Both methods aim to estimate the 10-year risk of a first MACE by using pooled cohort equations based on clinical and laboratory risk factors such as age, sex, race, smoking history, history of diabetes mellitus, systolic blood pressure, and serum cholesterol level.

Multiple studies demonstrated that CACS is a strong predictor of MACE in asymptomatic patients. However, despite the predictive strength of a CACS screening, the benefits of a screening test must be weighed against the cost, as well as the risk of exposing asymptomatic patients to radiation. Therefore, CACS is not recommended as a screening tool for every asymptomatic patient. The 2019 American College of Cardiology/American Heart Association (ACC/AHA) Guideline on the Primary Prevention of CVD suggests CACS as a reasonable method only in patients with borderline (5% to <7.5%) or intermediate (≥7.5% to <20%) 10-year ASCVD risk and uncertainty about the benefit of preventive therapy, in order to reclassify risk as part of improved clinical decision making, eg, regarding a statin therapy.

Although coronary CTA (CCTA) has also been shown to have a predictive value for MACE in recent randomized clinical trials, it is not explicitly part of primary prevention strategies in asymptomatic patients. However, according to the Society of Cardiovascular Computed Tomography (SCCT) 2021 Expert Consensus Document on CCTA, it may be reasonable to perform CCTA in selected asymptomatic patients with high risk, especially if predominantly noncalcified plaques are suspected and the individual risk and benefit of therapy are uncertain.

Symptomatic Patients

The ISCHEMIA (International Study of Comparative Health Effectiveness with Medical and Invasive Approaches) trial compared invasive versus conservative initial strategy in over 5000 patients with at least moderate ischemia on a stress test and demonstrated no benefit of initial invasive coronary angiography (ICA) regarding the occurrence of MACE. Another registry study (CathPCI [percutaneous coronary intervention] Registry of the National Cardiovascular Data Registry), including 398,978 patients without known CAD who underwent elective ICA, demonstrated that only about one-third of them had an obstructive CAD. The remaining two-thirds were diagnosed with nonobstructive CAD without the need for revascularization, meaning that they received unnecessary invasive assessment. These results highlight the need for a strategy that reliably identifies those patients who will benefit from invasive diagnostics and subsequent therapy: a gatekeeper for ICA.

Several clinical studies evaluated the diagnostic accuracy of CCTA and its role in the management of symptomatic patients with suspected CAD. The DISCHARGE (Diagnostic Imaging Strategies for Patients With Stable Chest Pain and Intermediate Risk of Coronary Artery Disease) trial confirmed the results of the ISCHEMIA trial with a similar risk of MACE when comparing invasive strategy (ICA) with CCTA as the initial diagnostic test. At the same time, major procedure-related complications were more frequent in the ICA group than in the CCTA group (1.9% vs 0.5%). In the SCOT-HEART (Scottish Computed Tomography of the HEART) trial, over 4000 patients with stable chest pain were randomly assigned to standard of care combined with CCTA or standard of care alone. According to this multicenter study, the addition of CCTA to standard of care resulted in a significant reduction of death from CAD or myocardial infarction at 5 years without increasing the rate of ICA or coronary revascularization. At the same time, the use of preventive therapy was more frequent in the CCTA group, which may be the reason for the lower rate of MACE. These results indicate that patients also benefit from the early detection of nonobstructive CAD. The latter was confirmed by the PROMISE (Prospective Multicenter Imaging Study for Evaluation of Chest Pain) trial in which CCTA outperformed functional testing in terms of identifying patients at risk for MACE, probably due to the detection of nonobstructive CAD. From a clinical perspective, the ability not only to assess the vessel lumen but also to detect the overall atherosclerotic burden of the heart including nonobstructive CAD is one of the advantages of CCTA over ICA. In addition, several studies analyzed CCTA regarding its cost-effectiveness. For example, the BEACON (Better Evaluation of Acute Chest Pain with Coronary Computed Tomography Angiography) trial demonstrated the use of CCTA as a safe workup strategy and associated it with fewer outpatient testing and lower cost.

All these studies have reinforced the value of CCTA in the management of patients with CAD and led to the revision of national and international guidelines. Recently, the new US multisociety Guideline for the Evaluation and Diagnosis of Chest Pain has been published including clinical recommendations for the use of CCTA in patients with stable and acute chest pain.

Patients With Stable Chest Pain

In patients with stable chest pain, the guideline distinguishes between patients with no known CAD and those with known CAD.

Patients with stable chest pain and no known CAD should first undergo clinical risk assessment to determine the pretest probability of obstructive CAD. In low-risk patients (<15% pretest probability) CACS or exercise testing may be reasonable for excluding coronary plaques or myocardial ischemia. For intermediate- to high-risk (≥7.5%) patients without known CAD, CCTA is recommended as a class I strategy to rule out obstructive CAD, to detect nonobstructive CAD, and to guide further risk stratification and decision making, especially in patients under 65 years of age. In corresponding patients above 65 years of age, stress testing is preferred over CCTA due to their higher risk for ischemia and obstructive CAD. However, in these patients, additional CACS can be useful. In case of a stenosis of 40% to 90% in a proximal or middle coronary segment on CCTA, CT-based fractional flow reserve (FFR) assessment can help to determine the hemodynamic significance of the stenosis and to guide further decision making. In patients with high-risk CAD (left main stenosis ≥50%; 3-vessel disease ≥70%), ICA is recommended.

In patients with stable chest pain and known CAD, CCTA may be useful to characterize disease progression of a known nonobstructive CAD or to evaluate bypass graft or stent patency in case of known previous revascularization.

Patients With Acute Chest Pain

Patients with acute chest pain should also primarily undergo clinical risk classification to guide further management. Patients with low risk (<1% 30-day risk for death or MACE) are reasonable to be discharged without urgent cardiac testing. In intermediate-risk patients (≥7.5%) with acute chest pain, CCTA can be useful to exclude plaques or obstructive CAD in case of no known CAD after negative or inconclusive clinical evaluation for acute coronary syndrome or to characterize progression of known CAD. For high-risk patients, ICA is recommended.

ACQUISITION TECHNIQUES

With the ongoing evolution of CT technology, coronary CT has developed into a well-established and robust modality with high accuracy in detecting CAD. The initial concerns regarding high radiation and contrast media exposure when performing coronary CT have decreased as CT technology significantly evolved, especially with regards to temporal and spatial resolution, enabling high-quality imaging at relatively low radiation and contrast media doses.

Cardiac Gating

To minimize motion artifacts, cardiac CT is performed using electrocardiography (ECG) gating, which enables reconstructions at defined time points of the cardiac cycle (Fig. 40.1).

Retrospective Gating

With retrospective gating, images are continuously acquired throughout the entire cardiac cycle and the ECG is recorded simultaneously, which allows for individual reconstructions with the lowest motion artifacts even after image acquisition. This is especially beneficial in patients with irregular heart rhythm or high heart rates that cannot be adequately addressed with premedication. In addition, recording the entire cardiac cycle offers the ability to evaluate ventricular or valvular function. The main disadvantage of this gating technique is the relatively high radiation dose compared with prospective gating. Thus, ECG-controlled tube current modulation ("pulsing") should always be considered when using the retrospective gating technique.

Prospective Gating

With prospective gating, images are acquired during a predefined phase of the cardiac cycle, determined by the ECG signal. There are two approaches for prospective ECG gating: (1) sequential ("step-and-shoot") acquisition and (2) spiral, high-pitch acquisition.

In sequential scanning mode, there are no table movements during but only between image acquisitions. Owing to the lower radiation exposure, sequential prospective gating should be the scanning approach of choice in patients

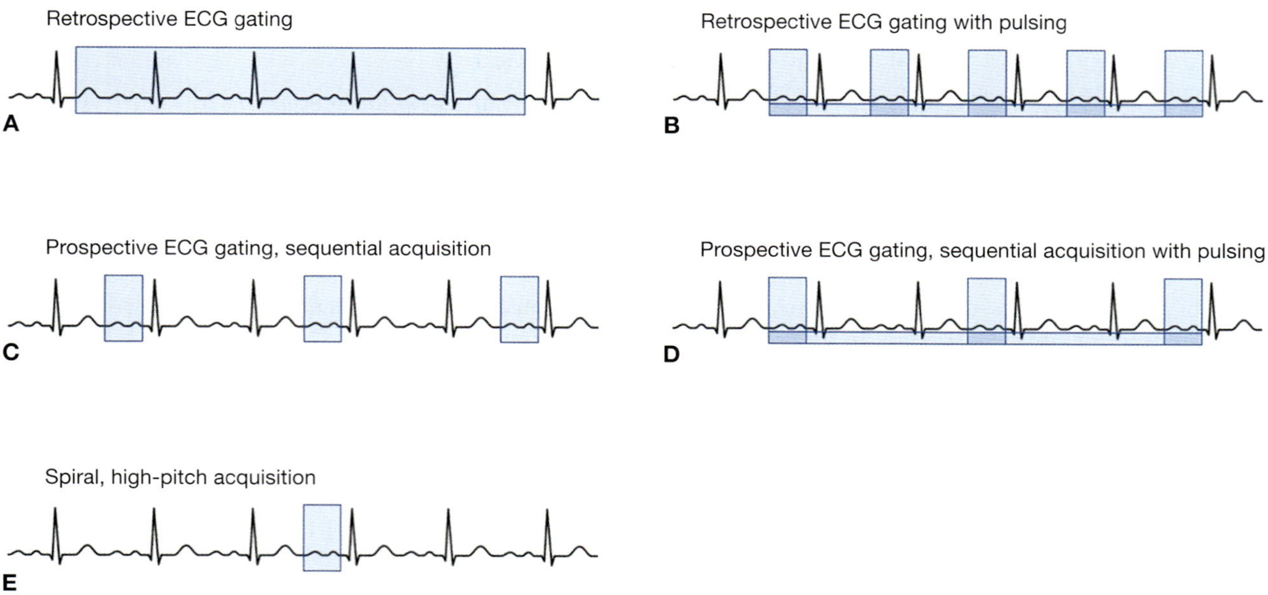

Figure 40.1. Coronary CT angiography acquisition protocols. **A:** Retrospective ECG gating. **B:** Retrospective ECG gating with pulsing. **C:** Prospective ECG gating, sequential acquisition. **D:** Prospective ECG gating, sequential acquisition with pulsing. **E:** Spiral, high-pitch acquisition.

with regular heart rhythm and heart rates up to 60 beats per minute (bpm). One disadvantage compared with retrospective gating is that suboptimal acquisition timing cannot be compensated afterward due to the limited ability of reconstructing different cardiac phases. However, the risk of a nondiagnostic scan can be reduced by using so-called padding. With this technique, the temporal scan interval is stretched while aiming for an optimal compromise between reconstruction flexibility and radiation exposure.

Radiation exposure can be further reduced by using prospective gating in a spiral, high-pitch mode in which the entire heart is scanned within one cardiac cycle. This technique requires a dual-source CT system since this enables gapless scanning at higher pitch values compared with single-source systems. Its main advantage is the ability of performing very low-dose examinations. However, since only one cardiac phase is acquired, this technique should only be considered in nonobese patients with optimal control of heart rhythm and rate, eg, when radiation dose is to be minimized, particularly in young patients.

Premedication

Heart Rate Control

Owing to temporal and spatial resolution considerations, adequate heart rate management is crucial in coronary CT imaging. A slow and rhythmic heartbeat offers the benefit of higher image quality and the ability to perform dose reduction acquisition techniques. In clinical practice, the target heart rate for CCTA is usually set at 60 bpm. The maximum acceptable heart rate may differ individually depending on the scanner (or its temporal resolution) and the acquisition protocol. In general, however, heart rate control should be administered in patients with a heart rate above 60 bpm, a high heart rate variability, and the absence of contraindications. In this context, beta-blockers are considered the medication of choice, typically starting with an oral premedication (eg, metoprolol 50-100 mg, depending on the individual heart rate) 1 hour prior to the examination, followed by supplemental intravenous administration (metoprolol, 5 mg, repeated as needed), in case of persistently high heart rates, immediately before scanning. Alternatively, oral premedication may be omitted and only intravenous administration performed immediately prior to the examination (maximum of 30 mg metoprolol as needed), as this heart rate control method is usually more efficient and faster. In both ways, continuous cardiac monitoring should be used during administration and scanning. Furthermore, prior to the administration, the following absolute contraindications of beta-blockers must be excluded:

- Bronchial asthma or chronic obstructive pulmonary disease
- Bradycardia (<50 bpm)
- Atrioventricular block
- Hypotension (systolic <100 mm Hg)
- Cardiac decompensation or end-stage heart failure
- Untreated pheochromocytoma
- Prior administration of calcium channel antagonists (verapamil- and diltiazem-class)

Nitrates

To further improve the visualization of the coronary arteries, nitrates should be applied about 5 minutes prior to CCTA to induce coronary vasodilatation. Since this can lead to a drop in blood pressure, among other side effects, contraindications should be carefully considered before administration. A common protocol contains sublingual application of 0.4 to 0.8 mg nitroglycerin (tablet or spray). Absolute contraindications for nitrates are:

- Severe aortic stenosis
- Hypotension
- Prior intake of phosphodiesterase inhibitors (eg, sildenafil)

The Protocol

In clinical practice, cardiac CT scans are usually acquired as a combination of a nonenhanced acquisition for CACS and a contrast-enhanced scan for the visualization of the coronary arteries. In order to minimize artifacts due to respiratory motion, examinations should be performed during breath-hold at end-inspiration. Especially in case of CCTA, a test breath-hold should be performed prior to the actual scan to ensure appropriate performance and compliance and to detect possible breath-dependent fluctuations of the heart rate and rhythm that may require adjustment of heart rate control measures or acquisition technique.

Calcium Scoring

CACS can be performed using electron-beam CT or MDCT. Since the spatial resolution of MDCT is superior to electron-beam CT, the latter is usually not used in clinical practice. The standard acquisition protocol consists of an axial, nonenhanced scan with prospective gating and a tube voltage of 120 kVp at end-inspiration. The optimal cardiac phase depends on the heart rate and ranges between 65% and 80% (usually 75%) of the R-R interval. Images are typically reconstructed with a slice thickness of 2.5 to 3.0 mm and a small field of view of 200 to 250 mm^2.

Coronary CT Angiography

Compared with CACS, the visualization of the coronary arteries requires higher spatial resolution and therefore requires an MDCT system with 64 slices or higher. CCTA is performed as a contrast-enhanced scan with prospective or retrospective gating and breath-hold at end-inspiration. Images are reconstructed with the smallest available slice thickness (varies depending on the CT system) and a field of view of 200 to 250 mm^2. The convolution kernel chosen influences the image noise. A smooth kernel reduces image noise, which may facilitate the assessment of the vessel lumen. In patients with heavy calcifications or stents, however, a sharper kernel is recommended in order to reduce blooming artifacts.

Contrast Injection

The application of contrast media is necessary to ensure proper evaluation of the coronary arteries. Previous studies demonstrated that an intraluminal attenuation of at least 200 to 350 Hounsfield units (HU) is required for optimal assessment. At the same time, too high attenuation (>500 HU) may lead to a significant underestimation of stenosis due to a partial volume effect of the contrast media on the plaque. This highlights the need for optimal protocols for intravenous contrast injection. Contrast media should be applied using either a biphasic or a triphasic protocol, each typically with an injection rate of 5 mL/s. In a biphasic protocol, the application of contrast media is followed by the application of saline. The advantage of this protocol is the washout of dense contrast in the right atrium and the superior vena cava resulting in less artifacts. However, in some cases, depending on the scan indication, it might be necessary to evaluate the right-sided heart chambers. In such cases, a triphasic protocol is preferred consisting of an initial application of contrast media alone, followed by a mixture of contrast media and saline, followed by saline alone.

There are two main methods to ensure accurate timing of image acquisition to contrast media administration: the bolus tracking and the test bolus techniques. In bolus tracking, a region of interest (ROI) is placed in a predefined anatomic location (typically the ascending aorta) to continuously monitor the arrival of contrast media. The scan is automatically started with a preset delay time when the attenuation measured within the ROI exceeds a certain HU threshold. The test bolus technique involves a test injection of a small amount of contrast media, followed by a saline bolus, prior to the actual examination to further optimize scan timing. While bolus tracking allows for shorter scan time and lower contrast media and radiation doses, the test bolus technique provides the ability to identify factors that may affect scan timing and image quality prior to the actual scanning.

Strategies for Contrast Media Dose Reduction

Lowering the tube voltage, eg, to 70, 80, or 90 kVp, is an option to reduce not only radiation but also contrast media doses by increasing the in-vessel attenuation. Furthermore, the introduction of dual-energy CT systems enabled the generation of virtual monoenergetic image reconstructions at different energy levels. Reconstructions at low kiloelectron volt levels increase the iodine attenuation closer to its k-edge (33.2 keV; highest X-ray photon absorption of iodine), reducing the amount of contrast agent required for diagnostic vascular attenuation (Fig. 40.2).

RADIATION DOSE–REDUCTION TECHNIQUES

One concern that remains with CCTA is exposing patients to ionizing radiation. Therefore, risk-benefit assessment should always be conducted prior to the scan, in accordance with guidelines and recommendations. Even with reasonable indication, examinations should be performed with a radiation dose that is "as low as reasonably achievable" while maintaining diagnostic image quality. In the last years, technical advances led to a significant reduction of radiation dose in CCTA. Before the introduction of radiation dose–reduction techniques CCTA studies reached an effective dose up to 20 mSv, whereas the corresponding value now averages at 4.5 mSv, with potential further reduction even to less than 1 mSv, under optimal scanning conditions.

Monitoring of Radiation Dose Exposure

The individual radiation exposure of the patient should be monitored using volumetric CT dose index ($CTDI_{Vol}$; mGy) and dose-length product (mGy*cm) since effective dose (mSv) requires a conversion factor that is not unique to CCTA.

Scan Coverage

Since the total radiation dose is directly proportional to the scan coverage, limiting the scan range to the extent necessary is a simple and effective parameter to reduce individual radiation exposure without compromising image quality. In clinical practice, a localizer scan ("topogram") is usually performed prior to the actual examination, which is used to accurately plan the scan length required for the individual clinical question without scanning structures that do not add diagnostic value. If a nonenhanced CACS scan is performed prior to CCTA, this can be used for detailed planning of the contrast-enhanced scan. Typically, the optimal cardiac scan length ranges from the tracheal bifurcation (carina) to the lower cardiac border. However, depending on the individual clinical question, an extension of the scanned volume may be required, eg, when assessing coronary bypass grafts.

Optimal Mode of Data Acquisition

The choice of the scanning mode also influences the individual radiation dose. As mentioned in the section "Acquisition Techniques," the radiation exposure is significantly lower with prospective compared with retrospective ECG gating. However, since this technique is less flexible in terms of subsequent reconstructions, it should only be performed in patients with adequate heart rate and rhythm control. In case of an irregular rhythm or high heart rates, retrospective ECG gating should be used, but then with ECG-based tube current modulation.

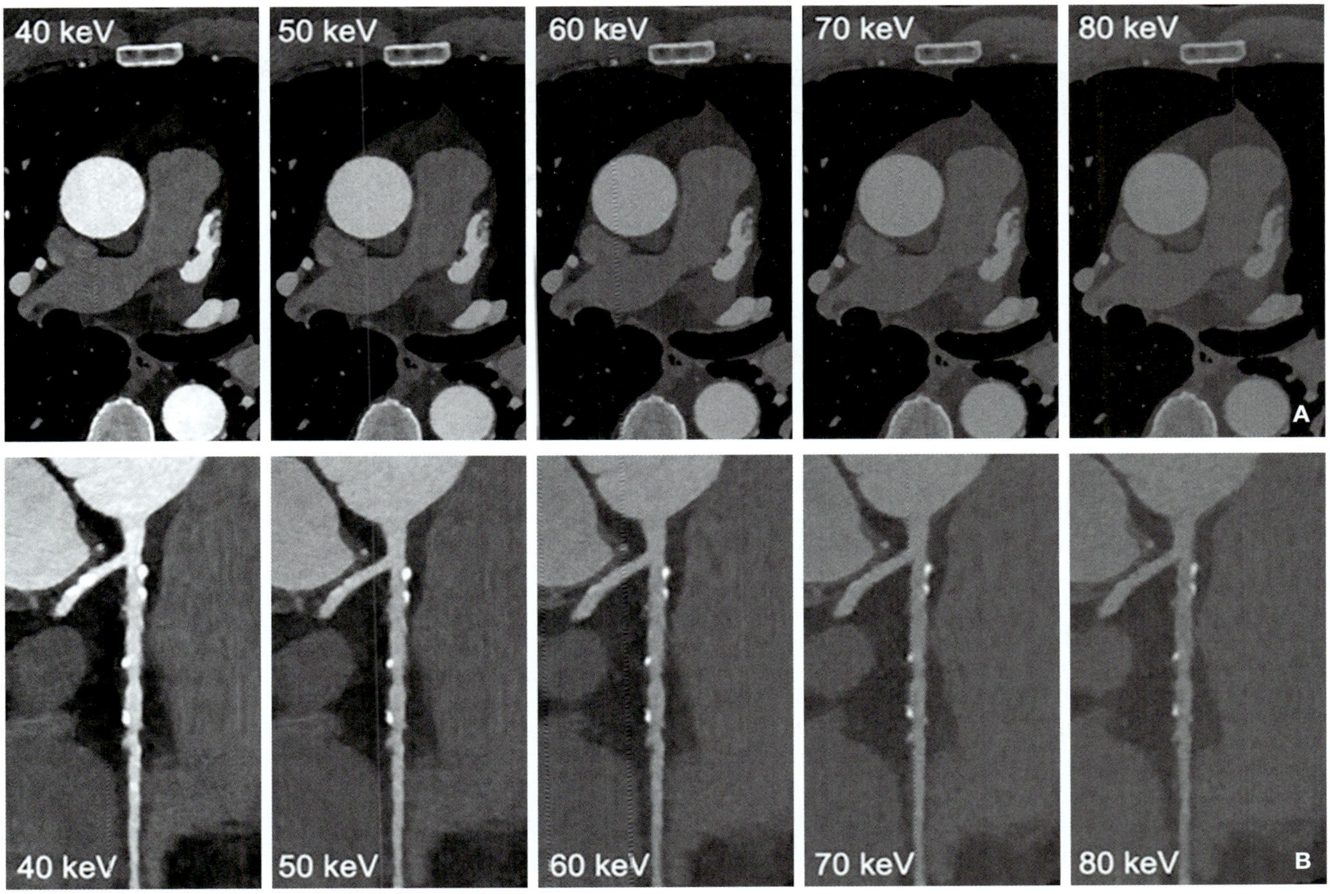

Figure 40.2. **A:** Axial and **B:** curved multi-planar reformatting (MPR) reconstructions of a contrast-enhanced coronary CT angiography at different virtual monoenergetic image levels (40-80 keV, in 10-keV-intervals) illustrating an increasing in-vessel attenuation with decreasing keV level.

ECG-Based Tube Current Modulation ("Pulsing")

Within the cardiac cycle, there are specific phases where motion artifacts are expected to be lowest, usually the diastolic phase, which most likely provides the highest image quality. In ECG-based tube current modulation, the full radiation dose is applied during this phase and reduced during the more motion-prone phases, as this is where the probability of nondiagnostic images is higher.

Anatomic-Based Tube Current Modulation

Some scanners have the ability to adjust the tube current automatically during image acquisition depending on the tissue density scanned, which is usually estimated from the localizer scan and determined by an image noise target.

Tube Voltage

The tube voltage defines the energy of emitted X-ray, thus the degree of tissue penetration. Lowering the tube voltage to 100 or 80 kVp can substantially reduce individual radiation exposure, since the radiation dose increases approximately with the square of the tube voltage and also has an impact on image quality due to an increase of image noise. Therefore, this technique should only be performed in nonobese patients or children in order to maintain diagnostic contrast-to-noise ratio. In patients with body mass index >30 kg/m^2, however, it might even be necessary to increase the tube voltage to 140 kVp—despite the increasing radiation dose—to receive diagnostic image quality.

Iterative Reconstructions

By reducing image noise, iterative reconstructions can be used to maintain or even improve image quality (Fig. 40.3), eg, at lower tube voltage and/or tube current. Furthermore, the use of iterative reconstructions enables noise reduction in obese patients.

IMAGE POSTPROCESSING

Coronary Artery Calcium Scoring

CACS is performed using a vendor-provided software that automatically identifies calcified lesions with a threshold of

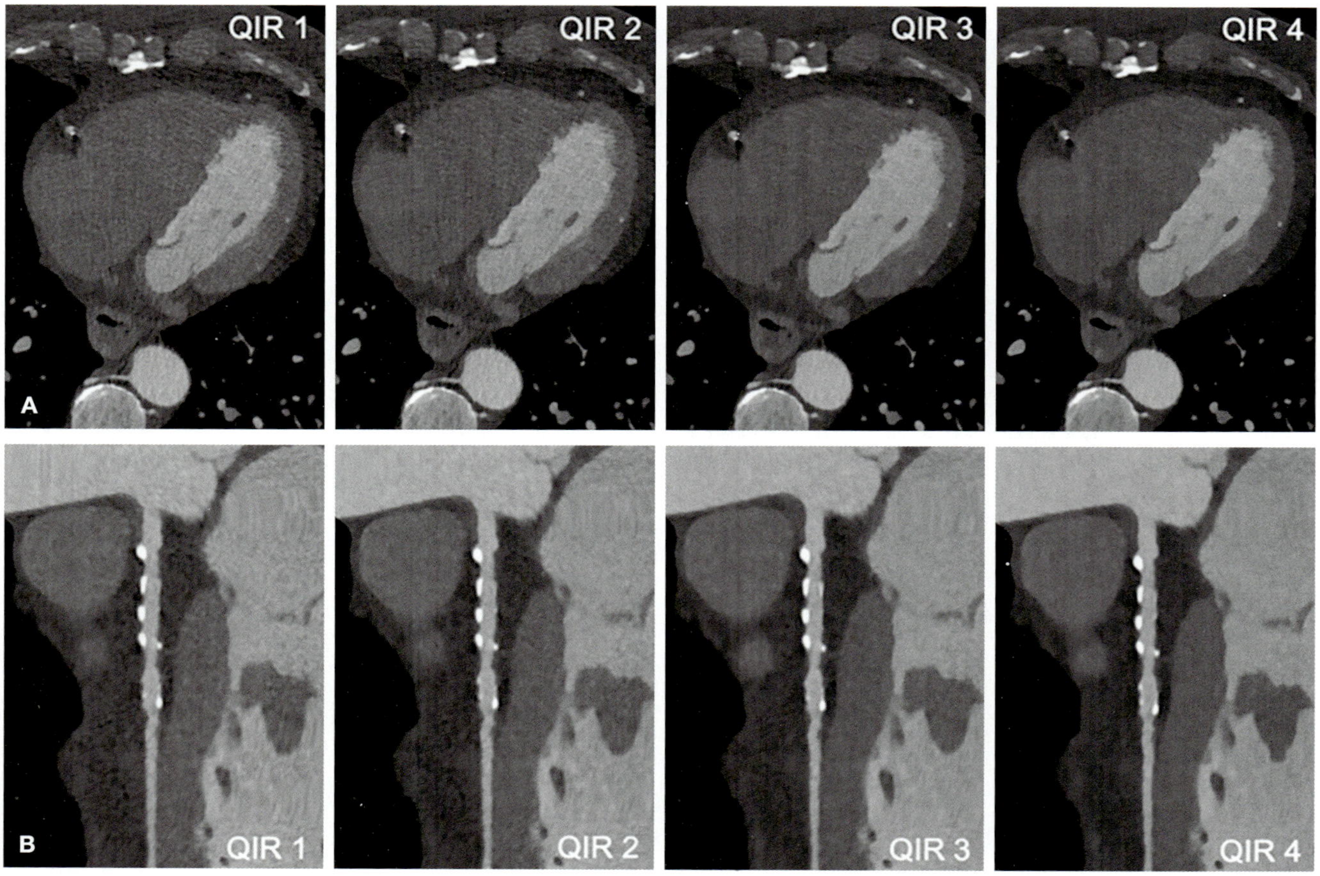

Figure 40.3. **A**: Axial and **B**: curved multi-planar reformatting (MPR) reconstructions of a contrast-enhanced coronary CT angiography at different quantum iterative reconstruction (QIR; iterative reconstruction algorithm for photon-counting detector CT data) levels (strength 1-4) illustrating the noise reduction with rising QIR level.

130 HU and an area of at least 1 mm^2. Currently, the methods to express CACS, typically reported as per vessel and as total score, are as follows: calcium volume, calcium mass, and the Agatston score. The calcium volume is estimated using plaque diameter and thickness (mm^3), and the calcium mass is a calculation of calcium hydroxyapatite (mg) based on plaque volume and attenuation using a calibration factor considering the attenuation of water. The Agatston score represents a standardized score that accounts for the total area and density of the detected calcifications. Figure 40.4 shows two sample cases for calcium scoring, one with a score of zero and one with coronary calcifications.

Coronary CT Angiography

With retrospective image acquisition, reconstructions can be performed at different time points of the cardiac cycle. These time points are usually expressed as percentage of the cardiac cycle (% of the R-R interval) or as absolute time after the R-peak (ms). In order to obtain high-quality and diagnostic CCTA images, it is crucial to select reconstructions at a cardiac phase with minimal motion artifacts (Fig. 40.5). The extent of cardiac motion changes during the cardiac cycle and depends on the heart rate. In patients with lower heart rates, end-diastole (approximately 75% of the R-R interval) is considered to be optimal, whereas end-systole is better in patients with higher heart rates. Algorithms are available that automatically select the reconstruction with the fewest motion artifacts. This flexibility in reconstructing different phases of the cardiac cycle is limited with the prospective acquisition technique, as mentioned earlier.

Furthermore, the simultaneously recorded ECG signal should be reviewed for misregistration of the R wave or too short R-R intervals that may cause a lack of image data. These errors especially occur in patients with an irregular heart rhythm and should be edited by adjusting the R-detection or deleting the affected R-R interval and adding additional reconstruction windows in the next heartbeat.

IMAGE INTERPRETATION

Coronary Artery Calcium Scoring

By comparing the individual Agatston score with an age- and gender-matched cohort based on the Multi-Ethnic Study of Atherosclerosis (MESA) or other large cohort studies, percentiles can be calculated. These results can then be used, along with clinical risk assessment, to estimate the 10-year

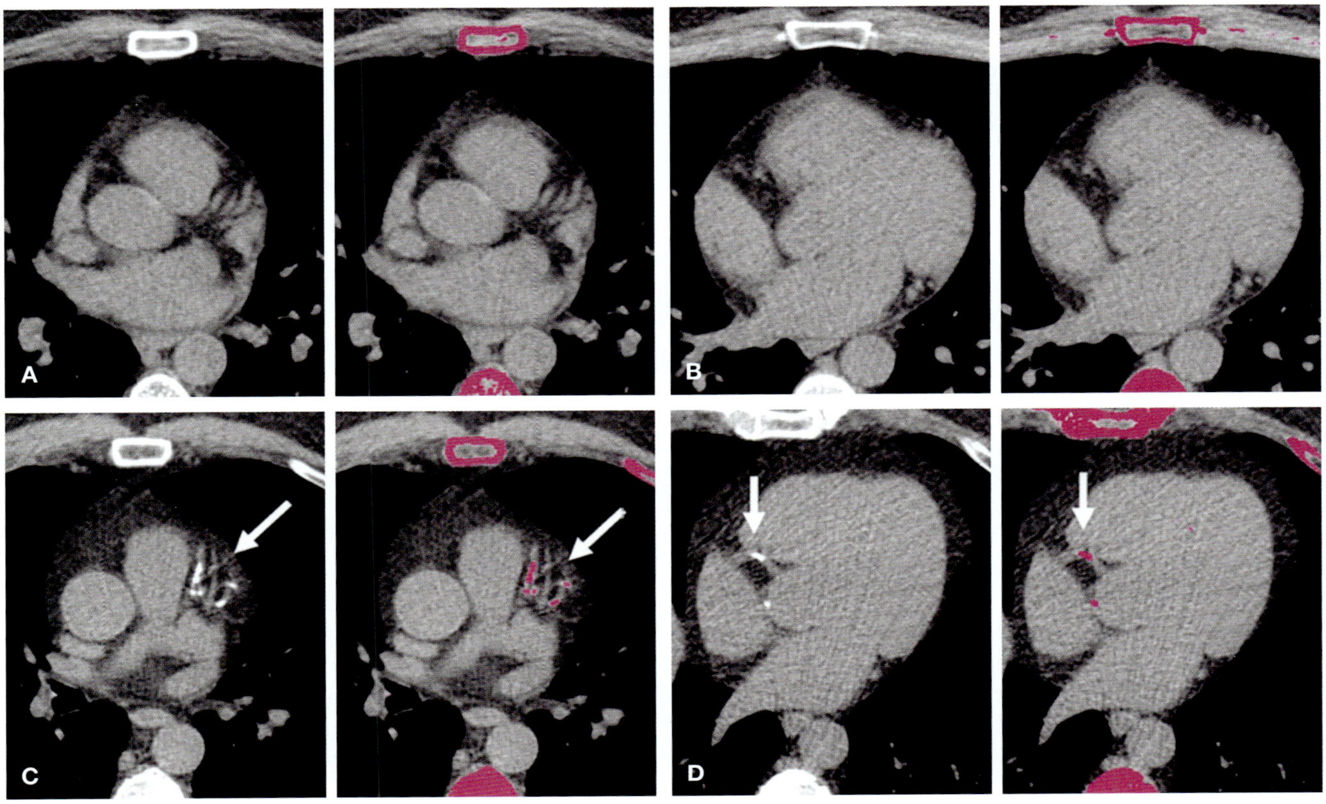

Figure 40.4. Coronary artery calcium scoring. Axial nonenhanced CT scans in a patient with no coronary calcifications (**A** and **B**; calcium score zero) and in a patient with coronary calcifications (arrows) (**C** and **D**; total Agatston score 470).

risk of MACE. According to guidelines, CACS can be used for reclassification especially in patients with intermediate risk and selected patients with borderline risk for MACE when decision making remains uncertain after clinical risk evaluation.

The Society of Cardiovascular Computed Tomography recently published the "Coronary Artery Calcium Data and Reporting System" (CAC-DRS) that aims for standardized reporting of CACS, subsequent risk assessment, and treatment recommendation (Table 40.1).

Coronary Artery Assessment

Most findings on a cardiac CT can usually be assessed in the axial dataset. However, especially in the evaluation of the coronary arteries, there are several reconstructions that may improve the assessment, such as the multiplanar reformatting (MPR, cross-sectional and curved or stretched) and the 3D volume rendering technique (VRT) reconstructions. Cross-sectional MPRs are typically reconstructed in the standard long- and short-axis planes (Fig. 40.6A-C). Depending on the clinical question, further reconstructions,

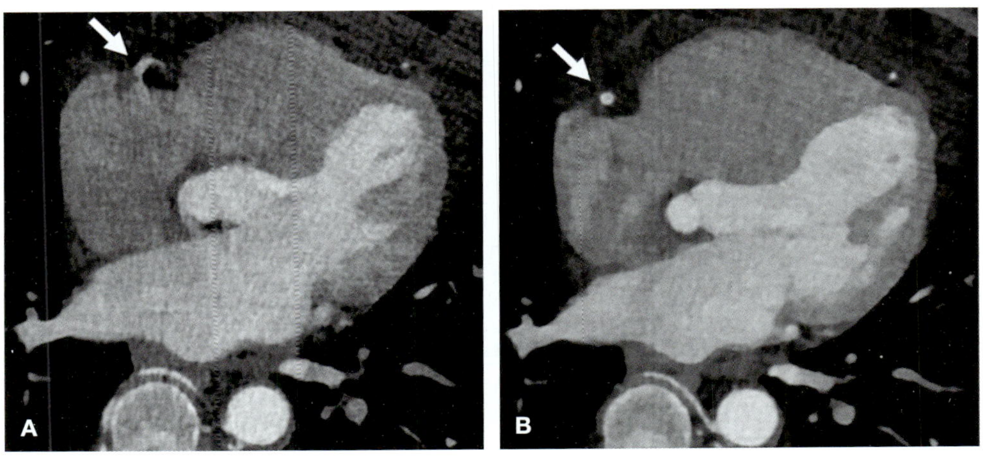

Figure 40.5. Selection of the cardiac phase with the least cardiac motion. Panel **A** shows an axial coronary CT angiography image reconstructed at 37% of the R-R interval with motion artifacts making assessment of the right coronary artery impossible (arrow). Panel **B** shows the same patient with image reconstructions at 76% of the R-R interval resulting in good visualization of the right coronary artery (arrow).

Table 40.1 CAC-DRS (Coronary Artery Calcium Data and Reporting System) Category Based on Agatston Scores Including Corresponding Risk Classification and Treatment Recommendation

CAC-DRS	Agatston Score	Risk	Treatment Recommendation
0	0	Very low	Statin treatment not recommended. *(Exception: familial hypercholesterolemia)*
1	1–99	Mildly increased	• Moderate-intensity statin if <75th percentile • Moderate- to high-intensity statin if >75th percentile
2	100–299	Moderately increased	Moderate- to high-intensity statin + ASA 81 mg
3	≥300	Moderately to severely increased	High-intensity statin + ASA 81 mg

ASA, acetylsalicylic acid.

eg, of the valves, can be generated. Curved MPRs are used for a detailed assessment of vessels (Fig. 40.6D). Those reconstructions are created (semi-)automatically by placing a centerline in the vessel lumen resulting in projections perpendicular to this centerline as well as a 360° view of the vessel. Since a centerline outside the lumen can erroneously simulate a stenosis, it is crucial to review the segmentations prior to evaluation. Similar to curved MPRs, stretched MPRs are based on the same centerline within the vessel lumen but are virtually straightened (Fig. 40.6E). 3D VRT reconstructions (Fig. 40.6F) are mainly used for an general overview, especially in the presence of bypass grafts.

A structured report with respect to the coronary arteries should include the evaluation of coronary arterial

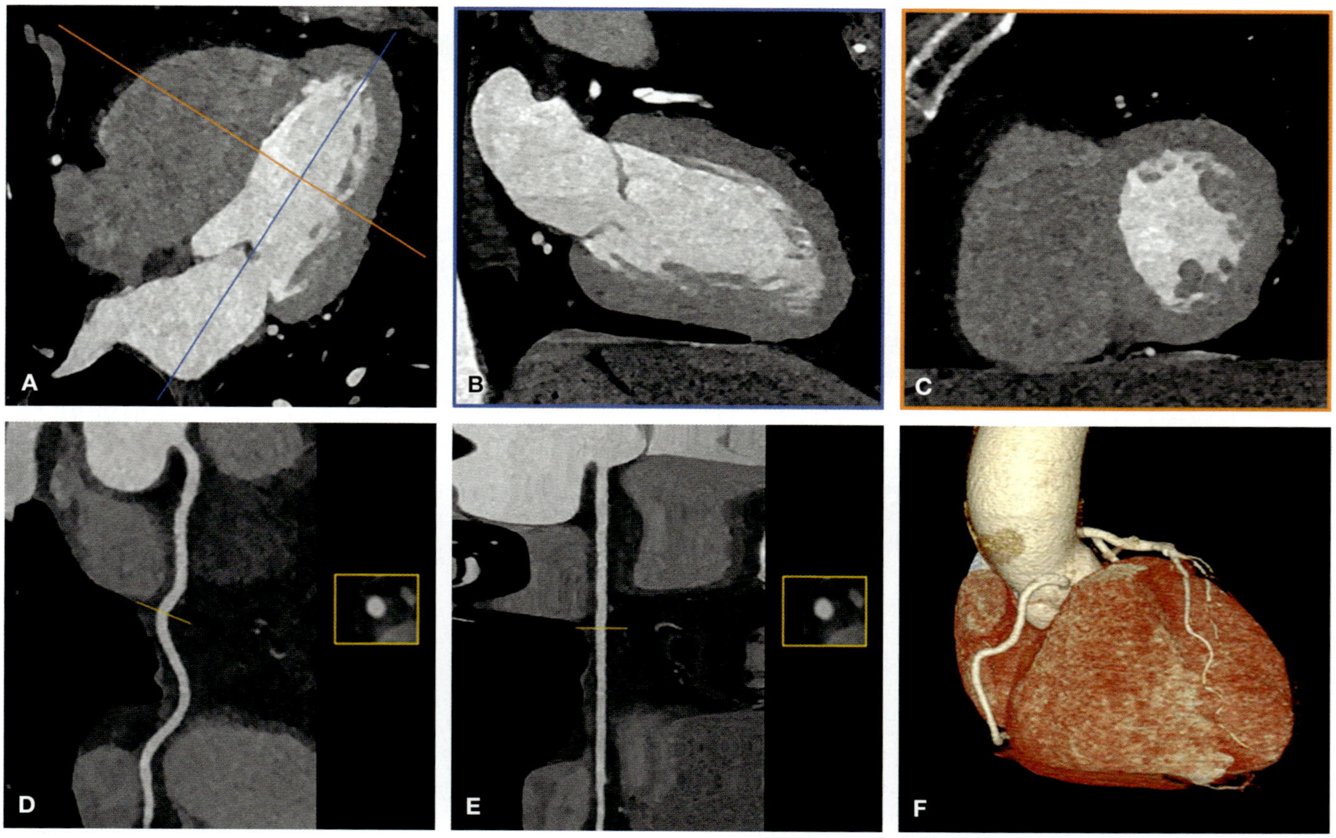

Figure 40.6. Coronary CT angiography reconstructions. Panels **A-C** show cross-sectional multiplanar reformatting (MPR) reconstructions at the standard long-axis four chamber (**A**) and two-chamber (**B**) as well as the short-axis (**C**) planes. Panels **D** and **E** show curved (**D**) as well as straightened (**E**) MPRs. Panel F illustrates a 3D volume rendering technique reconstruction.

dominance, coronary artery anatomy (normal, variants, and anomalies), atherosclerotic plaques and stenoses, coronary artery aneurysms/ectasia, and, if present, coronary bypass grafts and stents.

The coronary artery dominance is determined by which coronary artery branch gives off the posterior descending artery (PDA) and supplies the inferior wall. Most commonly the PDA originates from the right coronary artery (RCA, right dominant; 80%). Less frequently, the PDA originates from the left circumflex artery (LCX, left dominant) or both arteries (codominant).

Variants and Anomalies of the Coronary Arteries

Normally, there are two main coronary arteries: the RCA and the left coronary artery (LCA). The RCA originates from the right coronary sinus of Valsalva and gives off several smaller branches including the conus artery. The LCA originates from the left coronary sinus of Valsalva, has a common tract, the left main coronary artery (LMCA), and then divides into the left anterior descending (LAD) and the LCX arteries. In some cases, the LCA trifurcates with an additional intermediate ramus branch. There are several variations in the course and the number of the collateral branches that are not associated with MACE and are defined as normal variants (>1% of the general population). For example, the absence of the LMCA with a direct separation of LAD and LCX is considered to be a normal variant.

Coronary artery anomalies (CAAs) are congenital conditions that concern the origin, the course, or the termination of the coronary arteries (Table 40.2). They can be characterized as low risk (most common) and high risk, the latter possibly leading to life-threatening situations and sudden death.

The main CAAs are those that affect the origin or the coronary arteries. These include an origin from the wrong sinus of Valsalva (opposite or noncoronary sinus), from another coronary artery, from the pulmonary trunk (usually considered high risk), and from the aorta. An anomalous origin may also result in an abnormal course of the coronary arteries (Fig. 40.7). These anomalous courses include subpulmonic, prepulmonic, retroaortic, retrocardiac, and interarterial courses. While those mentioned first are usually not associated with MACE, an interarterial course is considered a high-risk CAA. This may also be exacerbated by an intramural course, most commonly in the wall of the aorta. Another type of an anomalous course is myocardial bridging, which means that a coronary segment completely or incompletely courses within the myocardium instead of the epicardial fat. Owing to the myocardial compression during systole, this can cause angina or even ischemia. However, the extent of the clinical association of myocardial bridging with MACE is still controversial and may depend, for example, on the length and the depth of the intramyocardial course. Anomalies of termination are primarily fistulas between a coronary artery and another vessel or cardiac chamber. The clinical severity mainly depends on the degree of shunt and the drainage site.

Table 40.2 Types of Coronary Artery Anomalies

Type of Anomaly	Variant
Anomalies of the origin	Origin from the aorta
	Origin from the wrong sinus of Valsalva (opposite or noncoronary sinus)
	Origin from the pulmonary trunk (high risk)
	Origin from another coronary artery
Anomalies of the course	Myocardial bridging
	Artery duplications
	Subpulmonic (inferior to the pulmonary trunk)
	Prepulmonic (anterior to the pulmonary trunk)
	Retroaortic (between noncoronary sinus and interatrial septum)
	Retrocardiac
	Interarterial (between ascending aorta and pulmonary trunk; high risk)
Anomalies of the termination	Coronary arteriovenous fistula

Plaque and Stenosis

One of the main clinical indications for CCTA is the exclusion of coronary stenosis. Those stenoses are usually caused by atherosclerotic plaques that can be calcified or soft, or even mixed. The following plaque characteristics are considered high-risk features for the occurrence of MACE (vulnerable plaques) and can be assessed by CCTA: (1) low CT attenuation (<30 HU), (2) positive remodeling (compensatory increase of the vessel diameter in the area of the stenosis beyond the level of the vessel wall; ratio of vessel diameter in relation to the diameter proximal/distal to the plaque >1.1), (3) napkin-ring sign (central structure of low attenuation surrounded by a thin peripheral ring of higher attenuation),

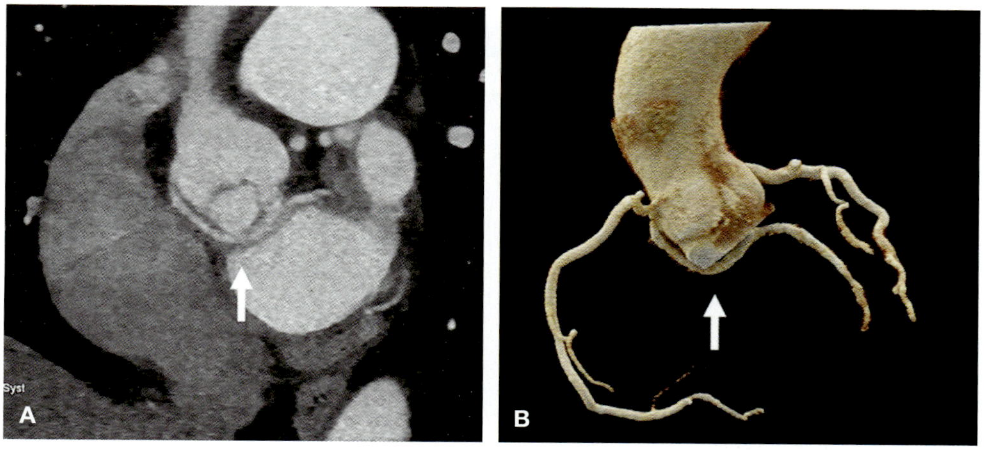

Figure 40.7. Sample case of a 60-year-old, male patient with a coronary artery anomaly: The left (**A**) main coronary artery originates from the right (**B**) sinus of Valsalva and passes between the aorta and the pulmonary trunk (arrow).

and (4) spotty calcifications within the plaque. The presence and extent of those high-risk features should be reported. Figure 40.8 shows a sample case of a high-risk plaque.

The location of coronary stenosis should be reported according to the standardized segmentation diagram that was first implemented for ICA by the AHA in 1975 and adapted into an axial diagram for CCTA by the SCCT in 2014. The severity of stenosis should be reported as the percentage luminal narrowing in relation to the vessel diameter proximal or distal to the plaque.

With the second edition of the "Coronary Artery Disease Reporting and Data System," called CAD-RADS 2.0, a standardized reporting system of coronary stenosis has been developed, using the presence, extent/severity, and composition of coronary plaques, mainly based on the highest-grade coronary lesion. The CAD-RADS score ranges from 0 (no plaque/stenosis) to 5 (total occlusion), which represents grading of stenosis severity in vessels greater than 1.5 mm and can be modified using abbreviations for a nondiagnostic study (N) or the presence of stents (S), grafts (G), and high-risk plaques (HRPs). Furthermore, this reporting system includes categories for overall plaque burden ("P") and ischemia assessment using CT-FFR or CT-Perfusion ("I") as well as a modifier "E" for exceptions to indicate nonatherosclerotic narrowing of the coronary arteries (Table 40.3).

Aneurysm and Ectasia

Coronary artery aneurysm is defined as a focal and coronary artery ectasia as a diffuse dilation of at least 1.5 times the adjacent nondilated coronary segment; a giant aneurysm is defined as a vessel diameter of more than 20 mm. Coronary aneurysms can be described as saccular (transverse exceeds longitudinal diameter) or fusiform (longitudinal exceeds transverse diameter) depending on their shape. In addition, aneurysms can be distinguished

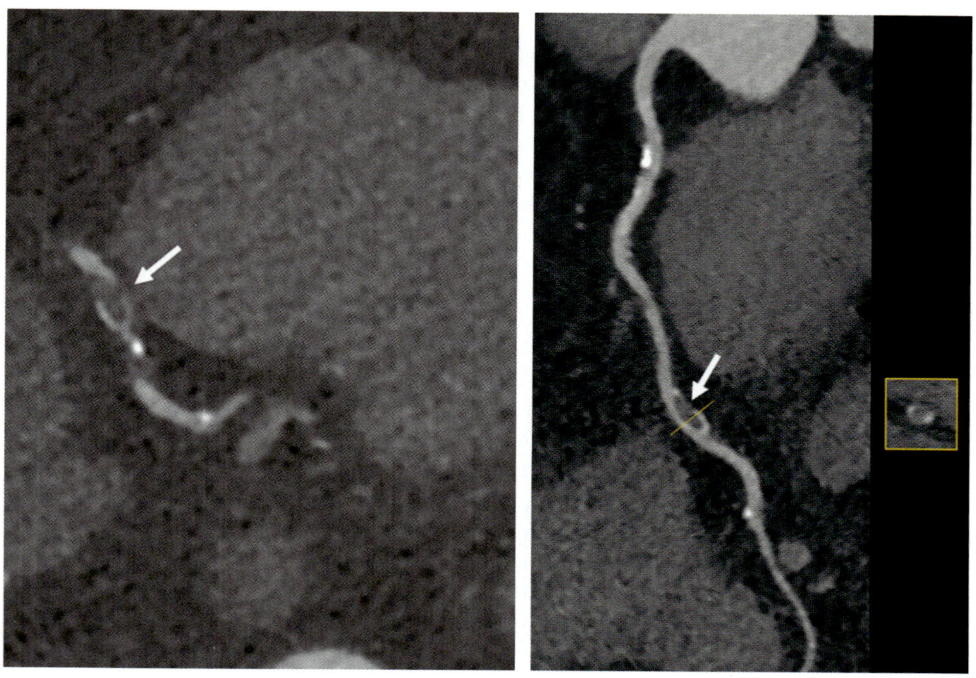

Figure 40.8. Sample case of a high-risk right coronary artery plaque (arrow) in a 74-year-old male patient with low attenuation, positive remodeling, and napkin-ring sign.

Table 40.3 CAD-RADS Classification for Patients With Stable Chest Pain and Patients With Acute Chest Pain Including Recommendations on Interpretation, Further Assessment, and Considerations

CAD-RADS	Max. Degree of Stenosis	Interpretation	Further Assessment	Considerations
Patients With Stable Chest Pain				
0	0% (no plaque)	Absence of CAD	None	Reassurance. Consider nonatherosclerotic causes of symptoms.
1	1%-24% (or plaque with no stenosis)	Minimal nonobstructive CAD	None	Consider nonatherosclerotic causes of symptoms. P1:[a] Consider risk factor modification and preventive pharmacotherapy. P2:[a] Risk factor modification and preventive pharmacotherapy. P3 or P4:[a] Aggressive risk factor modification and preventive pharmacotherapy.
2	25%-49%	Mild nonobstructive CAD	None	Consider nonatherosclerotic causes of symptoms. P1 or P2:[a] Risk factor modification and preventive pharmacotherapy. P3 or P4:[a] Aggressive risk factor modification and preventive pharmacotherapy.
3	50%-69%	Moderate stenosis	Consider functional assessment[c]	P1, P2, P3, or P4:[a] Aggressive risk factor modification and preventive pharmacotherapy. Other treatments (including antianginal therapy) should be considered per guideline-directed care. When modifier I+[b], consider ICA, especially if frequent symptoms persist after guideline-directed medical therapy.
4	A: 70%-99% B: Left main ≥50% or 3-vessel ≥70%	Severe stenosis	A: consider ICA or functional assessment[c] B: ICA recommended	P1, P2, P3, or P4:[a] Aggressive risk factor modification and preventive pharmacotherapy. Other treatments (including antianginal therapy) should be considered per guideline-directed care.
5	100%	(Sub-)total occlusion	Consider ICA, functional[c] and/or viability assessment	P1, P2, P3, or P4:[a] Aggressive risk factor modification and preventive pharmacotherapy. Other treatments (including antianginal therapy) should be considered per guideline-directed care.
N	Nondiagnostic	Obstructive CAD cannot be excluded	Consider additional/alternative evaluation	
Patients With Acute Chest Pain				
0	0%	ACS highly unlikely	No further ACS evaluation required If troponin + consider other source for increase	Reassurance.

Table 40.3 CAD-RADS Classification for Patients With Stable Chest Pain and Patients With Acute Chest Pain Including Recommendations on Interpretation, Further Assessment, and Considerations (Continued)

CAD-RADS	Max. Degree of Stenosis	Interpretation	Further Assessment	Considerations
1	1%-24%	ACS unlikely	No further ACS evaluation required If troponin + consider other source for increase	P1 or P2:[a] Referral for outpatient follow-up for risk factor modification and preventive pharmacotherapy. P3 or P4:[a] Referral for outpatient follow-up for aggressive risk factor modification and preventive pharmacotherapy.
2	25%-49%	ACS less likely	No further ACS evaluation required If clinical suspicion of ACS is high, troponin + or HRP features, consider hospital admission with cardiology consultation	P1 or P2:[a] Referral for outpatient follow-up for risk factor modification and preventive pharmacotherapy. P3 or P4:[a] Referral for outpatient follow-up for aggressive risk factor modification and preventive pharmacotherapy.
3	50%-69%	ACS possible	Consider hospital admission with cardiology consultation Consider functional assessment[c]	P1, P2, P3, or P4:[a] Preventive management, including aggressive preventive pharmacotherapy. Other treatments, including antianginal therapies, should be considered per guideline-directed care. When modifier I+[b], consider ICA.
4	A: 70%-99% B: Left main ≥50% or 3-vessel ≥70%	ACS likely	Hospital admission with cardiology consultation A: Consider ICA or functional assessment[c] B ICA is recommended	P1, P2, P3, or P4:[a] Preventive management, including aggressive preventive pharmacotherapy. Other treatments, including antianginal therapies, should be considered per guideline-directed care.
5	100%	ACS very likely	Hospital admission with cardiology consultation. Expedited ICA and revascularization if suspected acute occlusion.	P1, P2, P3, or P4:[a] Preventive management, including aggressive preventive pharmacotherapy. Other treatments, including antianginal therapies, should be considered per guideline-directed care.
N	Nondiagnostic	ACS cannot be excluded	Additional/alternative evaluation of ACS needed	

ACS, acute coronary syndrome; CAD, coronary artery disease; CAD-RADS, Coronary Artery Disease Reporting and Data System; HRP, high-risk plaque; ICA, invasive coronary angiography.

From Cury RC, Leipsic J, Abbara Set al. CAD-RADSTM 2.0-2022 coronary artery disease-reporting and data system. J Cardiovasc Comput Tomogr. *2022; 16(6):536-557.*

[a]*Grading scale for overall plaque burden: P1, mild amount; P2, moderate amount; P3, severe amount; P4, extensive amount of plaque.*

[b]*Grading scale for ischemia detection: I+ indicates that CT-FFR or CT-perfusion demonstrates lesion-specific ischemia or reversible perfusion defect; I- indicates that CT-FFR or CT-perfusion is negative for lesion-specific or reversible ischemia; I± indicates that CT-FFR or CT-perfusion is borderline.*

[c]*Functional assessment includes CT-FFR, CT-perfusion, stress testing (ETT, stress echocardiogram, SPECT, PET, cardiac MRI), or invasive FFR.*

Table 40.4 Common Causes for Coronary Artery Aneurysms

Common Cause	Examples
Genetic susceptibility (specific HLA class II genotypes)	Idiopathic coronary artery aneurysm
Atherosclerosis	Atherosclerotic coronary artery aneurysm
Autoimmune/inflammatory process	• Systemic vasculitis (eg, Kawasaki disease, Takayasu arteritis) • Lupus erythematosus • Marfan syndrome
Infectious (immune complex deposition or direct invasion of pathogens into vessel wall)	Bacterial, mycobacterial, fungal, syphilitic, Lyme, septic emboli, mycotic aneurysms
Dynamic wall stress changes	Cocaine use
Vessel wall injury	• Iatrogenic (post-balloon angioplasty, -stenting, -atherectomy) • Poststenotic coronary artery aneurysm

HLA, human leukocyte antigen.

Reproduced from Kawsara A, Nunez Gil IJ, Alqahtani Fet al. Management of coronary artery aneurysms. JACC Cardiovasc Interv. *20189; 11(13):1211-1223.*

between true (preserved vessel wall integrity) and pseudoaneurysm (damage to adventitia). Risk factors for coronary artery aneurysms are illustrated in Table 40.4. While most coronary aneurysms are incidental findings in asymptomatic patients, they can cause symptoms in other patients, eg, due to local thrombosis, concomitant obstructive CAD, massive dilation with subsequent compression of adjacent structures, or microvascular dysfunction causing myocardial ischemia. Owing to the lack of evidence, management of patients with coronary aneurysms remains challenging and usually depends on the individual case based on aneurysm localization and morphology, patient's characteristics, and clinical symptoms. Since atherosclerosis contributes to the development of coronary artery aneurysms, aggressive risk factor modification should be considered in all affected patients. Depending on the clinical presentation, patients may also undergo percutaneous intervention.

Coronary Bypass Graft Imaging

Cardiac CT can be used for the assessment of coronary artery bypass graft patency with a high diagnostic accuracy. In contrast to native coronary arteries, grafts are less prone to cardiac motion artifacts. However, blooming and beam hardening artifacts are more common due to surgical clips. Because of their course, imaging of coronary artery bypass grafts requires an adjusted CT protocol including a larger scan range. To guarantee optimal attenuation of coronary arteries and bypass grafts, bolus tracking is usually used with a threshold of 150 HU in the descending aorta and 8 to 10 seconds delay. Generating a 3D VRT reconstruction can be used for an overview in case of complicated anatomical conditions but should not be the only view for final assessment. A standardized report should include the number and type (venous or arterial) of grafts in addition to the patency assessment. Coronary artery bypass graft stenosis or occlusion is more common in venous grafts and can occur early (within 1 month) or late after bypass surgery. Early graft failure is often caused by thrombosis and late graft failure usually by compensatory wall hyperplasia with secondary thrombosis due to the exposure of a venous vessel to a high-blood-pressure environment. Arterial grafts are typically more resistant. In contrast to venous graft failure, arterial graft failure is usually caused by a progression of atherosclerotic plaques.

Stent Imaging

Percutaneous coronary intervention with stent implantation is the standard technique for coronary revascularization in case of hemodynamically significant coronary artery stenosis; however, in-stent restenosis is a common complication after intervention. CCTA enables visualization of the stent but is limited in terms of the assessment of the in-stent lumen due to blooming and beam hardening artifacts of the metallic stent. Therefore, the multisociety guideline, "2010 Appropriate Use Criteria for Cardiac Computed Tomography," classified CCTA as appropriate only for the assessment of asymptomatic patients with stenting of the LMCA and a stent diameter of at least ≥3 mm. The use was classified as uncertain in symptomatic patients with stent diameter ≥3 mm and was rated inappropriate in all patients

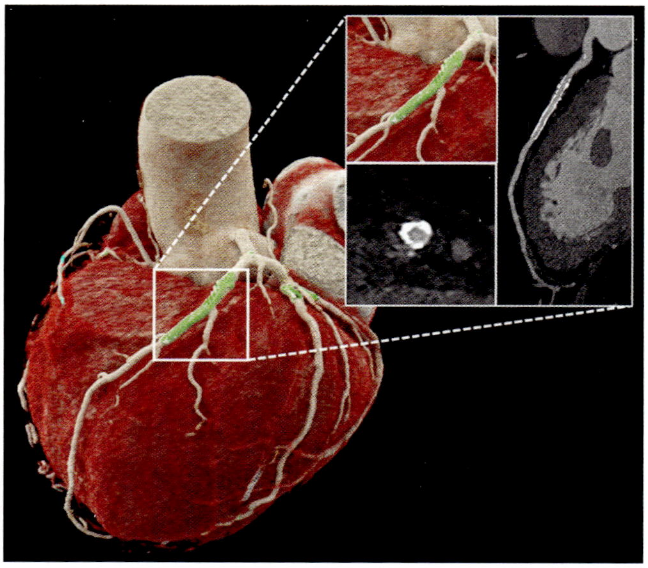

Figure 40.9. Sample case of a 68-year-old male patient with a coronary stent scanned on a clinical, first-generation PCD-CT using ultrahigh resolution with improved in-stent visibility.

with stent diameter <3 mm. However, recent advances, such as the introduction of PCD CT enabling ultra-high-resolution imaging with reduced blooming and beam hardening artifacts, have the potential to significantly improve coronary stent imaging (Fig. 40.9) and strengthen the role of CCTA as a gatekeeper for ICA.

Cardiac Findings

In addition to assessing the coronary arteries, CCTA can also be used to assess other cardiac structures including the myocardium, pericardium, cardiac chambers, cardiac valves, pulmonary arteries and veins, as well as the aorta and vena cava. As mentioned before, the ability to assess the right-sided cardiac chambers mainly depends on the contrast injection protocol chosen: while a triphasic injection protocol enables contrast-enhanced visualization of the right side of the heart, the biphasic injection protocol is suboptimal for such visualization.

Retrospective image acquisition additionally enables reconstruction of the entire cardiac cycle as cine loops allowing evaluation of left and right ventricular volumes (end-diastolic, end-systolic, and stroke volumes), ejection fraction, and left ventricular mass.

The assessment of noncoronary cardiac structures should include the following aspects:

- Myocardium:
  - Hypo-/hypertrophy, perfusion defects, fatty replacement, calcifications
  - Occurrence of aneurysms or diverticula
- Pericardium:
  - Thickening, calcifications
  - Effusion
- Cardiac chambers:
  - Morphology including size
  - Masses, thrombus
  - If available: wall motion and cardiac function including filling defects
- Cardiac valves:
  - Congenital abnormalities such as a bicuspid aortic valve
  - Thickening, calcifications, thrombus
  - If available: valve motion (complete closing and adequate opening of all leaflets), valvular regurgitation
  - If part of the clinical question (planning prior to transcatheter aortic valve replacement): diameter, area, and circumference of the aortic valve annulus and distance of the coronary arteries' origins to the aortic valve annulus plane

Extracardiac Findings

Even if the clinical question focuses on cardiac structures, it is crucial to review the entire field of view, usually including parts of the lung, airways, mediastinum, and upper abdominal organs. As there is an overlap in risk factors between patients with suspected CAD and those at risk for the development of lung cancer, such as smoking history and higher age, pulmonary nodules are the most common incidental findings. Other incidental extracardiac findings include pulmonary emboli, pneumonia, pleural effusion, lymphadenopathy, or other mediastinal masses. Although most incidental findings are clinically insignificant, it is crucial to report them since some require clinical or radiological follow-up or even direct further investigation.

COMMON ARTIFACTS

Motion Artifacts

Motion artifacts are the most common in coronary imaging and include cardiac motion, respiratory movements, and body movements of the patient.

The main challenge in cardiac imaging is cardiac motion due to the beating heart. Those artifacts mainly affect the RCA region. In order to minimize cardiac motion artifacts and to obtain high-quality diagnostic images, optimal heart rate and rhythm control as well as ECG gating including reconstructions at the ideal cardiac phase are crucial. Furthermore, as discussed earlier, editing the simultaneously recorded ECG in case of misregistration or too short R-R intervals can further improve image assessment. Owing to the acquisition of the entire cardiac cycle, retrospective ECG gating provides the greatest flexibility with regard to subsequent reconstructions.

Another cause of motion artifacts is respiration during the image acquisition. Because of this and since the heart rate may change during inspiration, a test breath-hold should be performed prior to the actual examination. Patients' body movements usually cause larger artifacts and should be addressed by clear instructions prior to the scan.

Beside smaller motion artifacts resulting in a blurring of contours, cardiac, respiratory, or patients' movements during image acquisition can also result in misregistration artifacts. A lack of data during image acquisition leads to "stair-step" artifacts and can either simulate or even hide coronary stenoses.

Streaking Artifacts

Streaking artifacts are beam hardening artifacts that look like dark bands and are typically caused by high-attenuating foreign materials such as surgical clips/markers, artificial valves, and coronary stents and also by high iodine concentrations. Beam hardening artifacts may be reduced by increasing the tube voltage due to the better penetration of structures including high-density objects or by creating virtual monoenergetic images at high kiloelectron volt levels, which requires a dual-energy CT system. The use of iterative reconstructions can also reduce beam hardening artifacts. The application of saline after the injection of contrast agent reduces artifacts caused by high iodine concentrations especially in the atrium and the superior vena cava (area of RCA course).

Blooming Artifacts

The presence of blooming artifacts means that high-attenuating structures appear larger than their actual size due to volume averaging, which is typically seen in coronary calcifications and smaller metallic foreign materials such as clips and coronary stents. This can lead to an overestimation of coronary stenoses. The use of sharper reconstructions kernels, thinner slice thickness, and iterative reconstructions and reducing the field of view can limit the occurrence of these artifacts. The spectral separation capability of dual-energy CT systems enables the subtraction of calcified lesions, and therefore also of beam-hardening artifacts. In addition, further advances especially with regard to spatial resolution, including the recent introduction of PCD CT, are promising for the overall reduction of blooming artifacts.

Reconstruction-Related Artifact

As mentioned previously, curved and stretched MPRs are prone to artifacts due to the (semi-) automatic segmentation of the coronary artery. A stenosis may be erroneously simulated if the centerline is not placed within the vessel lumen. Therefore, it is important to review the course of the centerline and, if required, adjust it prior to the final analysis.

NEW APPLICATIONS

Photon Counting CT

Recently, a PCD CT system has become clinically available offering several advantages to standard CT systems. Conventional detectors require a separation between neighboring elements to prevent incoming photons from crossing over, which limits the ability to reduce the size of conventional detectors due to a relatively high proportion of separation area. Furthermore, incoming X-rays have to be converted into visible light before an electric signal based on the total photon energy can be created. In contrast, PCD CT provides the ability to directly convert each incoming photon without separation between neighboring elements. This enables weighing each photon by its energy, lowering the detector size, improving spectral separation, and allowing for ultra-high-resolution imaging (Fig. 40.10).

CT-FFR

A common limitation of CCTA is the overestimation of coronary stenosis severity, which may cause unnecessary further invasive evaluation. Currently invasive FFR is the gold standard technique to assess the hemodynamic significance of coronary stenoses. However, new advances include CCTA-derived algorithms for noninvasive FFR assessment (CT-FFR). Several studies compared the diagnostic performance of CT-FFR with CCTA, single-photon emission CT (SPECT), and positron emission tomography (PET) and demonstrated the highest diagnostic performance for vessel-specific ischemia using CT-FFR. The ADVANCE (Assessing Diagnostic Value of Non-invasive FFRCT in Coronary Care) registry, including 5083 patients with CAD symptoms, showed that the application of CT-FFR led to a change in patient management, including less revascularization, and was associated with less negative ICA.

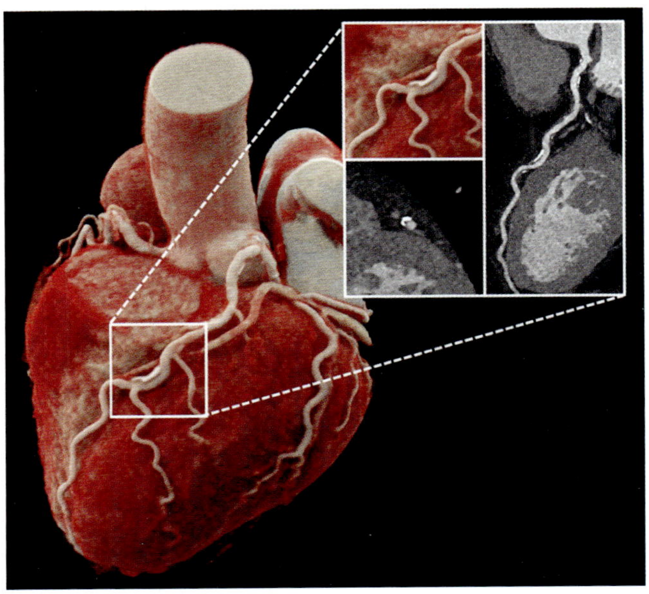

Figure 40.10. Sample case of a 74-year-old male patient with coronary artery disease scanned on a clinical, first-generation PCD-CT using ultrahigh resolution, resulting in improved in-lumen and plaque visibility.

Myocardial Perfusion

Another way to evaluate hemodynamic relevance of coronary artery stenoses is CT-based perfusion imaging, which assesses myocardial enhancement during hyperemia. Several studies demonstrated at least similar diagnostic accuracy compared with other perfusion imaging techniques. Furthermore, the combination with myocardial perfusion imaging has been shown to add diagnostic value compared with CCTA alone by improving the assessment of the hemodynamic relevance of stenoses. In general, there are two techniques used for CT myocardial perfusion imaging: static and dynamic perfusion protocols.

Static myocardial perfusion imaging is based on a single contrast-enhanced scan of the myocardium during the first pass of the contrast media and enables the identification of hypoperfused areas. In contrast to normal myocardium, ischemic myocardium enhancement is delayed resulting in lower attenuation. Since this technique consists only measurements at one timepoint, optimal timing is required. Static perfusion imaging can be performed on most CT scanners and regardless of the selected gating method. Using dual-energy CT systems for static myocardial perfusion imaging, iodine maps can be generated to improve the detection of ischemia due to better material separation.

Dynamic myocardial perfusion imaging is based on ECG-based acquisition of a series of datasets during contrast media injection. After correcting for cardiac motion, these datasets can be used to create myocardial attenuation time curves to calculate quantitative parameters such as myocardial blood flow. Several studies indicate a slightly higher accuracy of dynamic perfusion compared with static perfusion, although no study has yet conducted a direct comparison. Disadvantages of the dynamic compared with the static protocol are higher radiation doses and higher susceptibility to misalignment artifacts.

Myocardial Viability

Currently, myocardial viability assessment is mainly performed using cardiac magnetic resonance imaging (MRI). Since iodine-based contrast media, used for CT imaging, have pharmacodynamics similar to that of gadolinium, CT-based myocardial viability evaluation works on the same principle: both contrast agents accumulate in areas of nonviable tissue with high extracellular volume resulting in delayed enhancement while the normal myocardium is washed out after first-pass perfusion. Owing to better tissue characterization, MRI has been preferred over CT, despite strong correlation of CT with MRI and histological results. However, with improved spectral tissue separation, new advances including dual-energy and PCD CT systems have the potential to enable accurate myocardial viability assessment.

SUGGESTED READINGS

Abbara S, Blanke P, Maroules CD, et al. SCCT guidelines for the performance and acquisition of coronary computed tomographic angiography: a report of the society of cardiovascular computed tomography guidelines Committee—endorsed by the North American Society for Cardiovascular Imaging (NASCI). *J Cardiovasc Comput Tomogr*. 2016;10(6):435-449. doi:10.1016/j.jcct.2016.10.002

Cury RC, Leipsic J, Abbara S, et al. CAD-RADS™ 2.0-2022 coronary artery disease-reporting and data system: an expert consensus document of the Society of Cardiovascular Computed Tomography (SCCT), the American College of Cardiology (ACC), the American College of Radiology (ACR), and the North America Society of Cardiovascular Imaging (NASCI). *J Cardiovasc Comput Tomogr*. 2022;16(6):536-557. doi:10.1016/j.jcct.2022.07.002

Gentile F, Castiglione V, De Caterina R. Coronary artery anomalies. *Circulation*. 2021;144(12):983-996. doi:10.1161/CIRCULATIONAHA.121.055347

Gulati M, Levy PD, Mukherjee D, et al. 2021 AHA/ACC/ASE/CHEST/SAEM/SCCT/SCMR guideline for the evaluation and diagnosis of chest pain: a report of the American College of Cardiology/American Heart Association Joint Committee on clinical practice guidelines. *Circulation*. 2021;144(22):e368-e454. Erratum in: *Circulation*. 2021;144(22):e455. doi:10.1161/CIR.0000000000001029

Hecht H, Blaha MJ, Berman DS, et al. Clinical indications for coronary artery calcium scoring in asymptomatic patients: expert consensus statement from the Society of Cardiovascular Computed Tomography. *J Cardiovasc Comput Tomogr*. 2017;11(2):157-168.doi:10.1016/j.jcct.2017.02.010

Hecht HS, Blaha MJ, Kazerooni EA, et al. CAC-DRS: coronary artery calcium data and reporting system. An expert consensus document of the Society of Cardiovascular Computed Tomography (SCCT). *J Cardiovasc Comput Tomogr*. 2018;12(3):185-191. doi:10.1016/j.jcct.2018.03.008

Kawsara A, Núñez Gil IJ, Alqahtani F, Moreland J, Rihal CS, Alkhouli M. Management of coronary artery aneurysms. *JACC Cardiovasc Interv*. 2018;11(13):1211-1223. doi:10.1016/j.jcin.2018.02.041

Knuuti J, Wijns W, Saraste A, et al; ESC Scientific Document Group. 2019 ESC Guidelines for the diagnosis and management of chronic coronary syndromes. *Eur Heart J*. 2020;41(3):407-477. *Eur Heart J*. 2020;41(44):4242. doi:10.1093/eurheartj/ehz425

Leipsic J, Abbara S, Achenbach S, et al. SCCT guidelines for the interpretation and reporting of coronary CT angiography: a report of the Society of Cardiovascular Computed Tomography Guidelines Committee. *J Cardiovasc Comput Tomogr*. 2014;8(5):342-358. doi:10.1016/j.jcct.2014.07.003

Serruys PW, Hara H, Garg S, et al. Coronary computed tomographic angiography for complete assessment of coronary artery disease: JACC state-of-the-art review. *J Am Coll Cardiol*. 2021;78(7):713-736. doi:10.1016/j.jacc.2021.06.019

Section Twelve

Cardiac Arrhythmias

Chapter 41

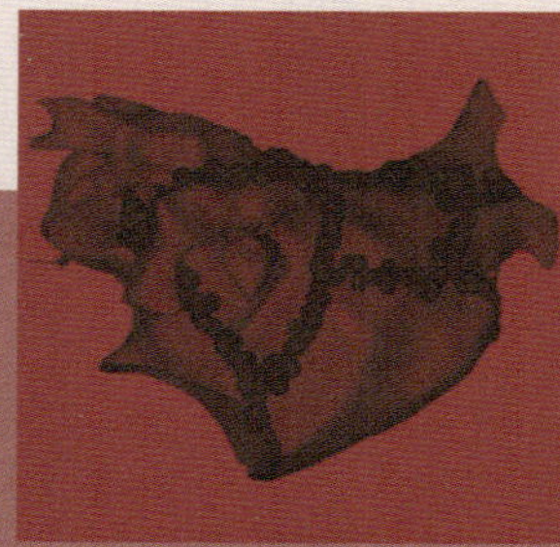

Avanti Gulhane • Harold I. Litt

Cardiac Magnetic Resonance for Guidance of Electrophysiology Procedures

INTRODUCTION

Patients with atrial and ventricular arrhythmias usually receive medical management with antiarrhythmic medications as the first line of action. Due to a high risk of major adverse cardiac events (MACE) such as sudden cardiac death (SCD), they also frequently receive cardiac implantable electronic devices (CIEDs) to treat future events. Cardiac magnetic resonance (CMR) can play an important role in the decision to treat patients with CIEDs by confirming the presence of a scar that may serve as the arrhythmogenic substrate and quantifying scar in both ischemic and nonischemic cardiomyopathy (NICM). However, the defibrillator or pacemaker only terminates the event while scar may increase over time. The increasing burden of arrhythmias can result in repeated shocks that decrease overall quality of life for these patients and may warrant ablation of the arrhythmogenic substrate guided by electrophysiologic procedures. Multiparametric CMR is valuable for guiding the implantation of defibrillators and pacemakers as well as planning of electrophysiology procedures (EP) such as atrial or ventricular ablations. The 2017 American Heart Association (AHA)/American College of Cardiology (ACC)/Heart Rhythm Society (HRS) guidelines recommend CMR as a standard imaging modality for such preprocedural planning of patients with arrhythmias and the prevention of MACE. The main applications of CMR in electrophysiology have been listed in Table 41.1.

The purpose of this chapter is to:

1. Discuss the role of CMR in EP for atrial arrhythmias
2. Describe CMR guidance of ablation procedures in ischemic and nonischemic ventricular arrhythmias.
3. Discuss CMR imaging in patients with CIEDs.
4. Discuss novel postprocessing strategies for CMR and real-time CMR-guided EP ablations.

ROLE OF CMR IN GUIDING EP FOR ATRIAL ARRHYTHMIA

Pulmonary Vein Mapping

The sinoatrial (SA) node, also known as the pacemaker of the heart, maintains normal sinus rhythm; electrical impulses from the SA node propagate to the AV node, bundle of HIS, right and left bundle branch, and into the Purkinje fibers. Arrhythmia is disruption of normal sinus rhythm, including atrial fibrillation (AF). In AF, triggers may arise within the atrial wall near the SA node, particularly at the pulmonary vein (PV) ostia, and they are responsible for the initiation of AF; the presence of fibrotic substrate is responsible for its perpetuation.

Patients with symptomatic paroxysmal and persistent AF are commonly treated by pulmonary vein isolation (PVI), a procedure involving circumferential ablation strategies to create circular lesions further from the PV ostia to block the exit of PV triggers that gives rise to AF. CMR assists in PVI by providing three-dimensional (3D) representations of the size and number of PV ostia, identification of variant anatomy, evaluation of left atrial dimensions, and the presence of atrial or atrial appendage thrombus.

Magnetic resonance angiography (MRA) is the usual sequence for delineation of left atrial and pulmonary venous anatomy, and identification of venous variants. The gadolinium-enhanced MR angiogram (MRA) with bolus tracking

Table 41.1 Main Applications of CMR in Electrophysiology

Role of CMR in Guiding Electrophysiology Procedures for Atrial Arrhythmia

1. Pulmonary vein mapping
2. CMR evaluation of persistent conduction after pulmonary vein isolation
3. Atrial scar mapping for atrial fibrillation ablation and atrial cardiomyopathy
4. Left atrial appendage ligation

CMR for Electrophysiology Procedures Guidance in Ventricular Arrhythmia

1. Indications for CMR in patients with ventricular arrhythmias
2. Functional assessment on CMR in ischemic and nonischemic ventricular arrhythmias
3. Characterization of arrhythmogenic substrate on CMR for ablation planning
4. CMR for ablation of ischemic cardiomyopathy–related ventricular arrhythmias
5. Role of CMR in electrophysiology procedures for nonischemic cardiomyopathy
    a. Nonischemic dilated cardiomyopathy
    b. Arrhythmogenic cardiomyopathy
    c. Hypertrophic cardiomyopathy
    d. Premature ventricular complex–induced cardiomyopathy

CMR Imaging in Patients With Cardioverter Implantable Electronic Devices

1. CMR protocol for pacemaker, defibrillator, and cardiac resynchronization therapy
2. Newer CMR sequences in patients with cardioverter implantable electronic devices
3. Pacing-induced cardiomyopathy

Novel Postprocessing Strategies on CMR and Feasibility of Real-Time CMR-Guided Electrophysiology Ablations

1. CMR strain
2. LGE-CMR image analysis for VT pathway identification
3. Feasibility of intraprocedural MRI

The Role of Artificial Intelligence in Cardiac Imaging to Inform Electrophysiology Procedures

1. Radiomics as cardiac imaging biomarkers
2. VT MUSIC platform
3. inHEART platform

CMR, cardiac magnetic resonance; LGE, late gadolinium enhancement; VT, ventricular tachycardia.

or timed bolus of contrast is optimized to have the highest opacification of the left atrium and the PVs, though time-resolved imaging can also be performed. In patients with contrast allergies or contraindications, noncontrast MRA can be obtained, however with a caveat of a longer acquisition time and lower signal-to-noise ratio compared to gadolinium-enhanced MRA.

A free-breathing 3D late gadolinium enhancement (LGE) sequence with navigator gating to track the motion of the diaphragm and myocardial nulling is frequently added to this protocol to identify the presence of additional atrial or ventricular scar that may contribute to the arrhythmogenic substrate. 3D LGE images help in preprocedural planning to identify the course of the esophagus and to assess for close proximity to pulmonary venous ostia, which increases risk for thermal injuries. Other sites of arrhythmias that can be evaluated on CMR include the cavotricuspid isthmus for atrial flutter and atrial wall scar. Measurements of the pulmonary venous ostia are provided using standard postprocessing tools. Cross-sectional orthogonal views are used to measure maximal and minimal diameters; ostial areas are obtained by multiplanar reconstruction (Fig. 41.1). Postprocedural complications, such as pulmonary venous stenosis, can also be defined on MRA. 3D reconstruction of the LA surface can be imported into EP navigation platforms to improve the accuracy of ablation procedures.

CMR Evaluation of Persistent Conduction After PVI

Postprocedural complications of PVI include persistent conduction of AF from residual conduction gaps in the ablation. Gaps in the ablation lines are defined as any discontinuity in the circumferential scar around the PVs and can lead to venoatrial reconnection after PVI for AF. About ~20% of patients with persistent conduction will require a second ablation procedure. Another site for persistent left atrial–PV conduction and early PV activation is the intervenous carina, an area between ipsilateral PVs that may result in persistent conduction. Repeat ablation of carina-related persistent conduction may be needed when the distance between the wide-area circumferential ablation circle and the PV ostium is greater than 8 mm (Fig. 41.2).

A standard LGE-CMR acquisition for identifying ablation gaps includes a free-breathing 3D navigator and electrocardiogram-gated inversion-recovery gradient-echo sequence in axial projection with an acquired voxel size of 1.25 × 1.25 × 2.5 mm. The typical scan time for such an acquisition is 15 min (11-18 min). It has been reported that patients who undergo LGE-CMR to identify anatomical venoatrial gaps have lower recurrence rates of AF, atrial tachycardia, and flutter after repeat PVI compared to those with conventional repeat PVI procedures.

Atrial Scar Mapping for AF Ablation and Atrial Cardiomyopathy

The European Heart Rhythm Association (EHRA)/HRS/Asian Pacific Heart Rhythm Society (APHRS)/Sociedad Latino Americana de Estimulacion Cardiaca y Electrofisiologia (SOLAECE) expert consensus document recognized atrial cardiomyopathy as a new clinical and histopathological entity in 2016. Atrial cardiomyopathy is

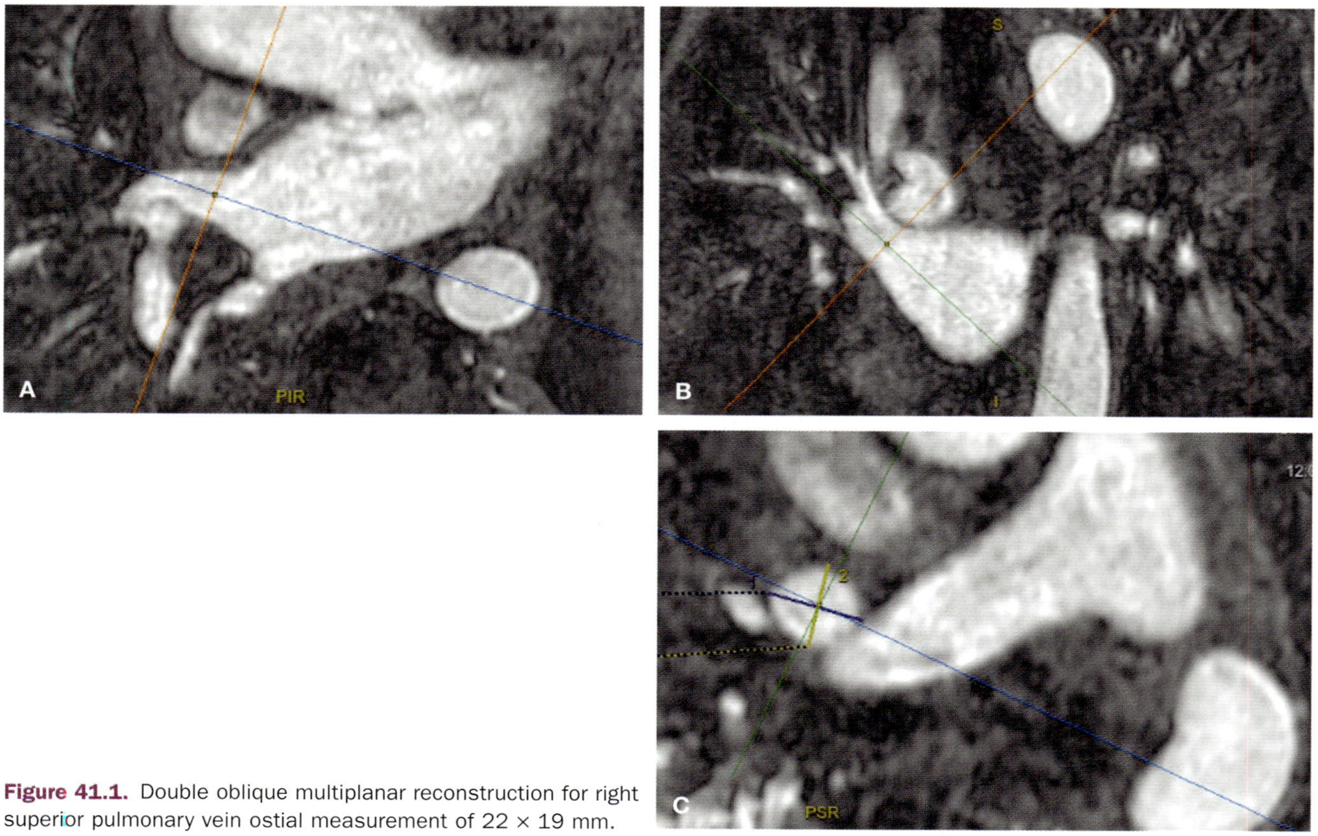

Figure 41.1. Double oblique multiplanar reconstruction for right superior pulmonary vein ostial measurement of 22 × 19 mm.

subdivided into four classes based on the different pathophysiology including genetic, fibrosis, heart failure and valvular dysfunction, and non-collagen deposition disease conditions. LGE-CMR can be used to evaluate atrial fibrosis using pixel signal intensity (PSI) maps normalized to the mean intensity of the blood pool signal. An image intensity ratio (IIR) >1.32 has been used to define dense scar areas, and an IIR between 1.2 and 1.32 is labeled as interstitial fibrosis.

Atrial scar/fibrosis has been classified on LGE-CMR in four Utah stages (I, 0%-10%; II, 10%-20%; III, 20%-30%; and IV, >30% of the atrial wall displaying fibrosis) and demonstrated to have a graded effect on arrhythmia recurrence or need for second ablation within 5 years. In patients with advanced atrial fibrosis, AF ablation is associated with a high procedural failure rate.

In a multicenter prospective study titled "Delayed Enhancement—MRI Determinant of Successful Catheter

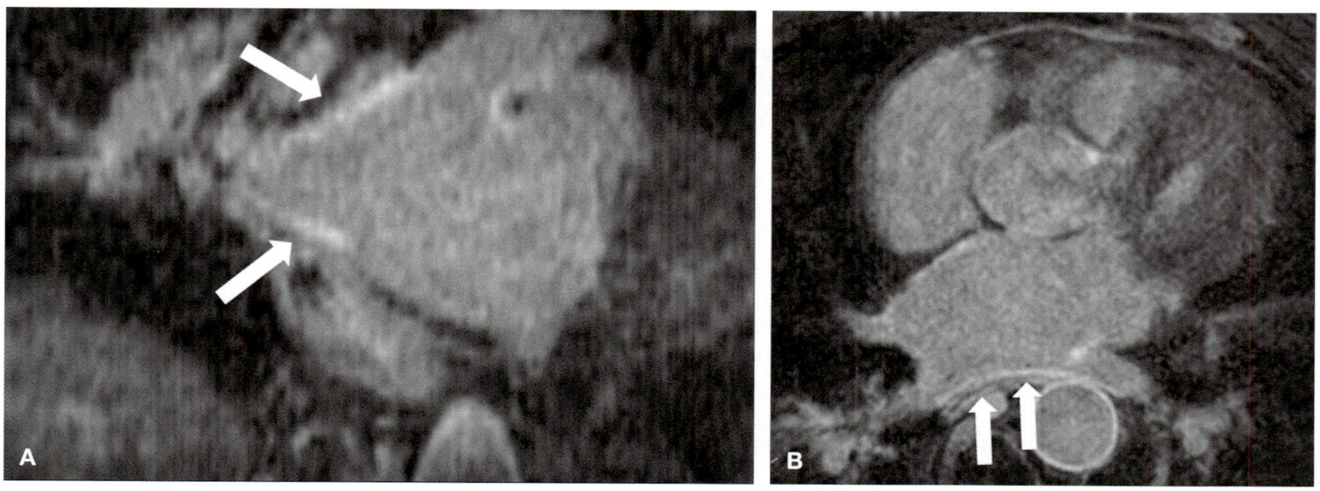

Figure 41.2. Prior atrial fibrillation ablation with radiofrequency isolation of right pulmonary vein set shows scar inferiorly and superiorly in the pulmonary vein ostium (arrows) (**A**) Additional linear roofline ablation between the right and left inferior pulmonary veins (arrows) achieved posterior wall isolation (**B**).

Ablation of Atrial Fibrillation" (DECAAF), a high degree of atrial fibrosis (Utah stage IV vs stage I) was found to be independently associated with a >fourfold increased likelihood of recurrent arrhythmia within 1 year after AF ablation. Results of the intention-to-treat analysis in the recently published DECAAF II trial including 843 patients show improved outcomes of ablation procedures when directed toward AF patients with baseline low levels of fibrotic disease (less than 20%, stage I and II). In patients with persistent AF and higher stage of fibrosis (stage III and IV), the addition of CMR-guided atrial fibrosis ablation to PVI showed no improvement in success rates compared with PVI alone.

Left Atrial Appendage Ligation

Patients with AF are at an increased risk for the development of thrombus within the atrial appendage. Transcatheter occlusion of the left atrial appendage (LAA) is routinely employed to prevent ischemic cerebral stroke and peripheral embolism and is a viable alternative to prophylactic anticoagulation. CT is commonly used in preprocedural planning of LAA ligation to assess morphology and the presence of appendage thrombus. However, when CT is contraindicated, CMR can be employed in such patients and add value by identification and quantification of left atrial scar.

CMR FOR EP GUIDANCE IN VENTRICULAR ARRHYTHMIA

Indications for CMR in Patients With Ventricular Arrhythmias

In ventricular arrhythmias, focal triggers occur when cells of the ventricles are irritated and overfire, sending extrastimuli to the ventricular conducting system, causing the ventricles to beat rapidly. Reentrant ventricular tachycardia (VT) occurs due to myocardial scar formation; dead cells disrupt normal electrical conduction and the electric current keeps going around the scar forming reentrant circuits, which sends a rapid signal to the ventricles. Patients with ischemic and NICM are at an increased risk of SCD from sustained VT, ventricular fibrillation (VF), or premature ventricular complex (PVC) due to myocardial scar formation (Fig. 41.3).

CMR is indicated in patients with ventricular arrhythmias to evaluate cardiac function, identify regional wall motion abnormalities, and localize and quantify the amount of LGE

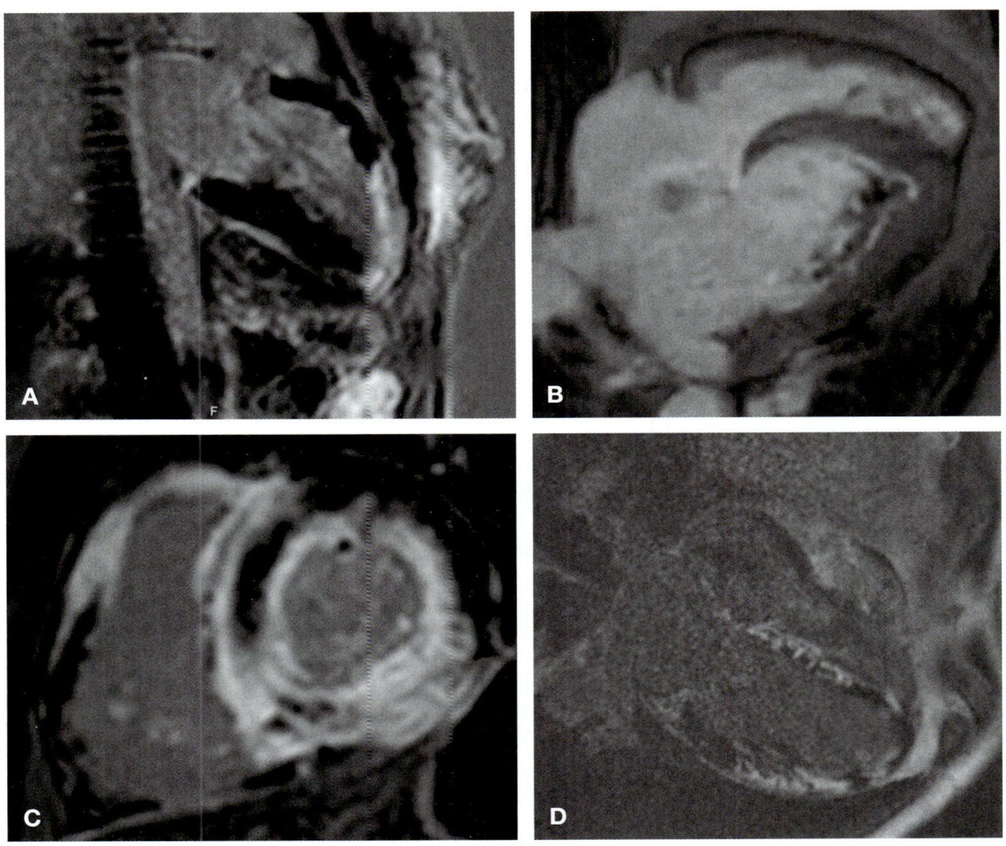

Figure 41.3. Late gadolinium enhanced cardiac magnetic resonance (LGE-CMR) images depicting classic scar patterns in various ischemic and nonischemic cardiomyopathy. **A:** Transmural left anterior descending territory infarction. **B:** Global subendocardial LGE and left ventricular apical thrombi in endomyocardial fibrosis. **C:** Global subendocardial LGE in amyloidosis. **D:** Subepicardial to midmyocardial patchy LGE in sarcoidosis.

that may represent arrhythmogenic substrate. Based on this information, a cardiologist may plan to treat patients with medications or use CIEDs such as pacemakers or defibrillators to treat the arrhythmia episodes. The electrophysiologist may decide on an epicardial versus endocardial approach for substrate-based ablation based on the location of the scar. CMR parametric mapping can identify myocardial interstitial fibrosis, edema, and inflammation that could affect the feasibility of ablation procedures. In patients who are already being treated with CIEDs, CMR is indicated to define the progression of arrhythmogenic burden that may need further repeat ablation or identify novel entities such as pacing-related cardiomyopathy.

Functional Assessment on CMR in Ischemic and Nonischemic Ventricular Arrhythmias

Patients with a ventricular arrhythmia have an increased risk of SCD if they develop severe ventricular systolic dysfunction. A left ventricular ejection fraction (LVEF) ≤35% is an established high-risk predictor of SCD. Even a mild decrease in LVEF < 50% possess an increased risk of SCD and mortality of up to 20% of such patients. Therefore, accurate functional assessment forms a cornerstone for the evaluation of the impact of ventricular arrhythmia. CMR is the current gold standard for accurate cardiac functional assessment due to higher spatial resolution and higher reproducibility. It helps to confirm the findings of echocardiography or nuclear tests such as multigated acquisition scan. Balanced steady-state free precision (bSSFP), a modification of gradient-recalled echo, is the CMR sequence used for the purpose of volumetric and functional assessment. For cine bSSFP acquisition, the transverse magnetization is refocused during each cardiac cycle to contribute to steady-state formation. ECG gated data are acquired and reconstructed retrospectively over multiple cardiac cycles as cardiac phases that can be played as a cine loop. An ongoing arrhythmia during cine imaging can impair the accuracy of the reconstruction and artifacts arise from inconsistent data of multiple heartbeats. Real-time free-breathing cine and compressed sensing sequences can be employed to mitigate the potential limitation of functional assessment in patients with arrhythmia-related artifacts. These sequences are independent of ECG gating, possess high temporal resolution, and have comparable performance to bSSFP imaging.

Characterization of Arrhythmogenic Substrate on CMR for Ablation Planning

Radiofrequency (RF) ablation is an accepted technique for treatment of VT. For purpose of ablation, electroanatomic mapping (EAM) is traditionally used to locate areas in scar tissue giving rise to VT known as arrhythmogenic substrate. Substrate-based ablation involves interruption of abnormal electrograms within the scar to terminate reentrant VT circuits. This involves point-by-point mapping of electrical voltages of the heart to create surface maps of electrical voltages in a 3D space. EAM systems use fluoroscopy guidance to locate the catheter tip in 3D space relative to electric field transmitters and create 3D surface maps of electrical voltages from multiple regions of the heart. Color coding is given based on the magnitude of the voltage potentials. At the same time, electrograms are recorded continuously; electroanatomic substrate involves abnormal electrograms such as critical isthmus, entry and exit electrograms, late potentials, and fractionated potentials from dead and necrotic myocardium aka scar core, which has a potential of <0.5 mV, border zone myocardium with a potential of 0.5 to 1.5 mV, and normal myocardium >1.5 mV. Ablation points are displayed on EAM so as to enable the creation of more elaborate ablation patterns.

LGE-CMR is being increasingly used to evaluate anatomical sites and extent of scar in patients with myocardial infarction (MI) or NICM, which harbors the arrhythmogenic substrate to guide their ablation. It also helps to decide endocardial versus epicardial approach for ablation by identifying the scar pattern.

The following sequences are used to identify replacement fibrosis and reactive/interstitial fibrosis on CMR:

- 2D LGE—phase-sensitive inversion recovery (PSIR) sequence—replacement fibrosis
- 3D LGE PSIR whole-heart navigator-gated sequence—replacement fibrosis
- T1 mapping and extracellular volume (ECV) estimation—reactive/interstitial fibrosis

A T1-weighted inversion recovery sequence, called Look-Locker or TI scout, consisting of multiple images from different inversion recovery times, is obtained before LGE PSIR to identify the nulling time of normal myocardium. This technique allows demarcation of postcontrast enhancement in the myocardial scar from the normal nulled myocardium after 10 to 15 minutes of intravenous gadolinium administration.

Myocardial scar can be quantified using different approaches available in standard clinical software such as six standard deviations, full width at half maximum, or manual delineation. Novel postprocessing software that generates PSI maps from LGE-CMR using predefined signal intensity thresholds that correlate with EAM voltage thresholds. Such image postprocessing can help to locate conducting corridors in scar tissue, which form VT substrate that corresponds to abnormal voltage potentials that define sites of entry and critical isthmuses within the arrhythmogenic substrate and critical slow conduction that form components of reentry circuits (Fig. 41.4). Ablation of such abnormal sites on CMR can help improve outcomes of substrate-based EP. LGE-CMR also helps in distinguishing irreversible injury from edema in the setting of catheter ablation.

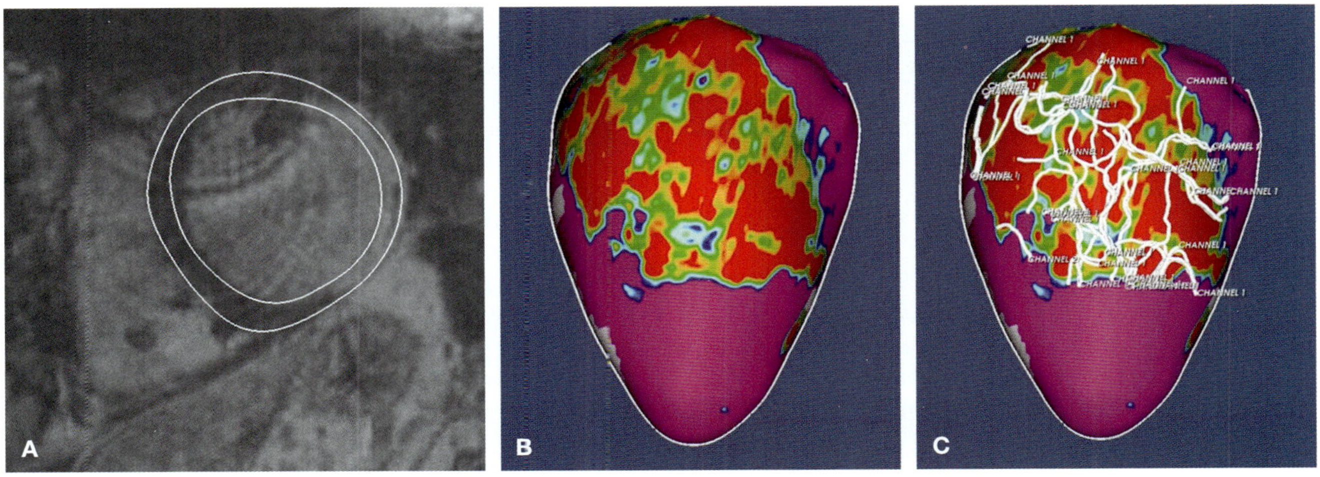

Figure 41.4. **A:** Segmentation of left ventricle on late gadolinium enhanced cardiac magnetic resonance (LGE-CMR) image to generate pixel signal intensity maps on Automatic Detection Arrhythmia Substrate software to generate 3D LGE pixel signal intensity maps (**B**) and conducting channels (**C**).

CMR for Ablation of Ischemic Cardiomyopathy–Related Ventricular Arrhythmias

As a rule of thumb, MI involves the subendocardial region and follows the coronary territory distribution. Depending on the severity of obstructive coronary artery disease, myocardial scar can be subendocardial (involving <50% of the myocardial thickness), subendocardial to mid-myocardial (up to 50%-75% of myocardial thickness), or transmural (>75% of myocardial thickness). Structural changes within the ischemic infarct and the peri-infarct border zone can lead to the formation of an arrhythmogenic substrate. The underlying strands of surviving tissue within and at the periphery of the infarct region form tortuous and slowly conducting channels that support reentry that result in inducibility of ventricular arrhythmia. Such an infarct border zone frequently has a heterogeneous signal intensity on LGE-CMR.

Areas of microvascular obstruction (MVO) from small thrombi within the subendocardial vessels in the infarcted myocardium can predispose to malignant ventricular arrhythmias. MVO is easily identified on LGE-CMR. CMR can help with identifying subacute and organized thrombi within the ventricular cavity using a long inversion time of 600 ms (Fig. 41.5)

Role of CMR in EP for NICM

The structural abnormality causing ventricular arrhythmia in patients with NICM is not clearly defined as the underlying pathology may have myriad of heterogeneous processes. Arrhythmogenic scar may be located in right ventricle or left ventricle mid-wall, in a subepicardial or diffuse subendocardial pattern, and in a noncoronary distribution. Identification of mid-wall scar is particularly challenging on EAM due to lack of adequate contact of the catheter tip with the substrate leading to erroneous voltages. This may eventually lead to poor postprocedural outcomes such as recurrent VT/VF or lack of noninducibility and need for repeat ablations.

NICM with high propensity for requiring epicardial ablation includes conditions such as arrhythmogenic right ventricular cardiomyopathy (ARVC), cardiac sarcoidosis, Chagas disease, and myocarditis. The epicardial right ventricular (RV) outflow tract may harbor substrate in patients with type I Brugada syndrome and may need ablation targeting to prevent VT/VF. CMR can help to define nonischemic scar patterns, narrow down possible nonischemic pathologies, and decide the best possible approach for ablation when needed. It has been suggested that athletes with a stria pattern LGE may present a higher risk of malignant ventricular arrhythmia than those with a spotty LGE pattern. The role of CMR in distinct NICM is described below.

Nonischemic Dilated Cardiomyopathy

CMR helps to establish the diagnosis in nonischemic dilated cardiomyopathy (DCM) and to risk stratify for adverse cardiovascular events such as malignant arrhythmia in these patients. Patients with DCM and LVEF <35% are likely to be at high risk of SCD and warrant an implantable cardioverter-defibrillator (ICD), but the positive predictive value of LVEF is low. RV involvement on CMR, often poorly visualized by echocardiography, has emerged as an important tool in DCM risk stratification. Cine CMR allows simultaneous evaluation of ventricular dyssynchrony in DCM, which commonly needs cardiac resynchronization therapy (CRT).

Acute myocarditis is another condition that can present as DCM, can be evaluated with the updated Lake Louise criteria, and can include a multiparametric approach for the diagnosis of acute myocarditis on CMR. This involves a "T1 criterion" of LGE, increased native T1 mapping or ECV

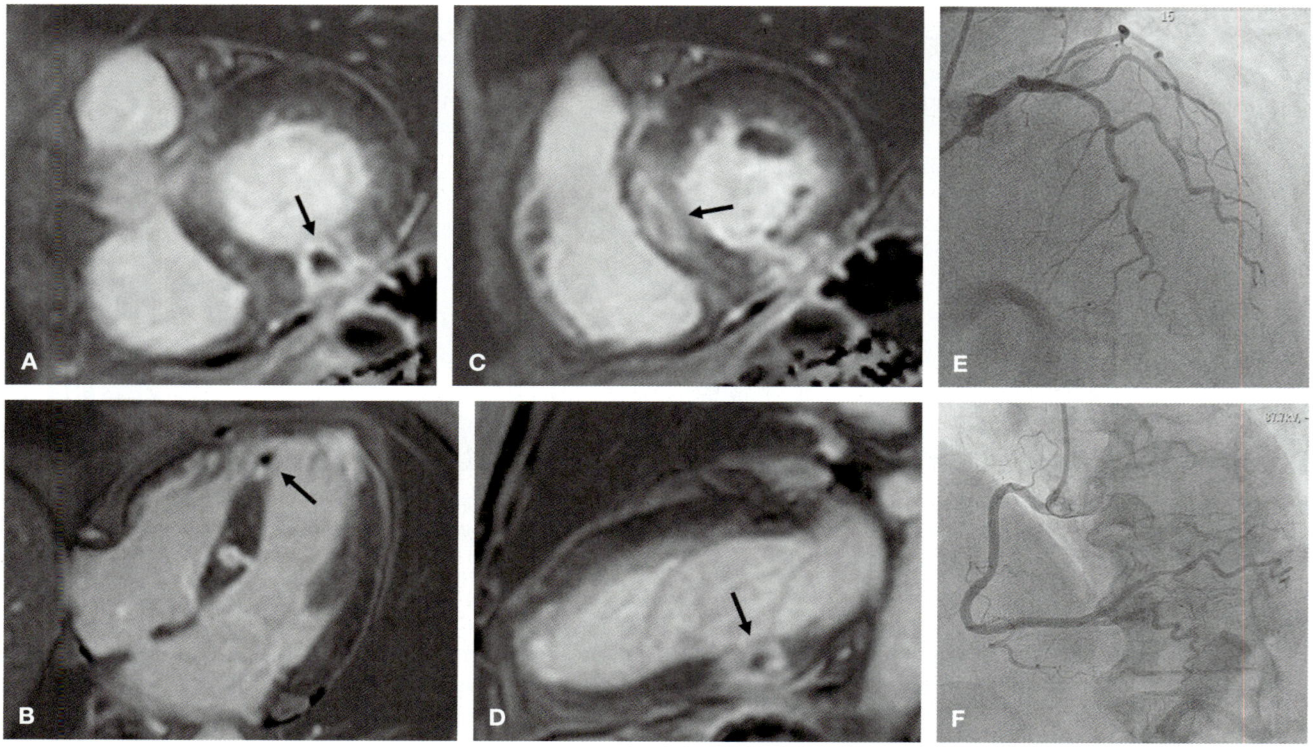

Figure 41.5. A 68-year-old woman with a history of hypertension, hyperlipidemia, rising troponins, and sudden-onset acute chest pain. Cardiac magnetic resonance (CMR) was requested to rule out stress cardiomyopathy. 1.5 T CMR showing transmural late gadolinium enhancement with microvascular obstruction in the basal interventricular septum and mid-inferior wall (arrows in **A–D**) suggestive of multivessel injury/myocardial infarctions with edema and microvascular obstruction. Differential considerations were diffuse embolic event versus multivessel spontaneous carotid arterial dissection or possibly coronary vasculitis. Findings were not consistent with stress cardiomyopathy. Coronary angiogram showing left (**E**) and right coronary arteries (**F**) without significant obstructive disease.

values, and a "T2 criterion" of hyperintensity on T2-weighted sequences or increased T2 mapping values (Fig. 41.6).

The presence of LGE is significantly associated with arrhythmic end points, such as SCD, sustained VT, and appropriate ICD therapy in DCM. Among clinical and imaging parameters, LGE is the strongest independent predictor of mortality in myocarditis, with hazard ratio of 12.8 for cardiac mortality. Another CMR marker of adverse outcomes in myocarditis is abnormal T2-weighted findings and ECV >35%. Subepicardial LGE in the lateral wall or mid-wall of the interventricular septum are common pattern of myocardial damage in patients with myocarditis. A ringlike LGE pattern involving more than three contiguous segments with subepicardial and/or mid-wall LGE in the same slice is one of the high-risk predictors for malignant arrhythmia in nonischemic DCM and chronic inflammatory cardiomyopathy. Identification of LGE on CMR helps in guiding left ventricular (LV) lead placement for CRT away from scarred tissue. Quantification of LGE on CMR also helps in predicting CRT response, which is known to have an inverse relationship with scar tissue (Fig. 41.7).

Arrhythmogenic Cardiomyopathy

Originally, ACM was described as a disease with predominant RV involvement aka ARVC. However, in the recent years, there has been increased recognition of biventricular and left-dominant phenotypic variants. This has evolved into the newer concept of arrhythmogenic cardiomyopathy (ALVC) with the 2020 Padua criteria defining its diagnostic and phenotype characterization in clinical practice. It includes modifications to the 2010 revised task force criteria to include left-sided variants and tissue characterization on LGE-CMR, especially when present without associated ventricular wall motion abnormalities.

On CMR, major criteria for RV involvement is transmural LGE in a stria pattern of ≥1 RV region in the inlet, outlet, and apex in two orthogonal views. Major criteria for LV involvement includes LV LGE in a stria pattern of ≥1 bull's-eye segment in two orthogonal views of the free wall subepicardial or mid-myocardial, septum, or both excluding septal junctional LGE. Based on imaging, ACM phenotype can be characterized in one of three different variants—classic right-dominant ARVC, biventricular ACM, or LV

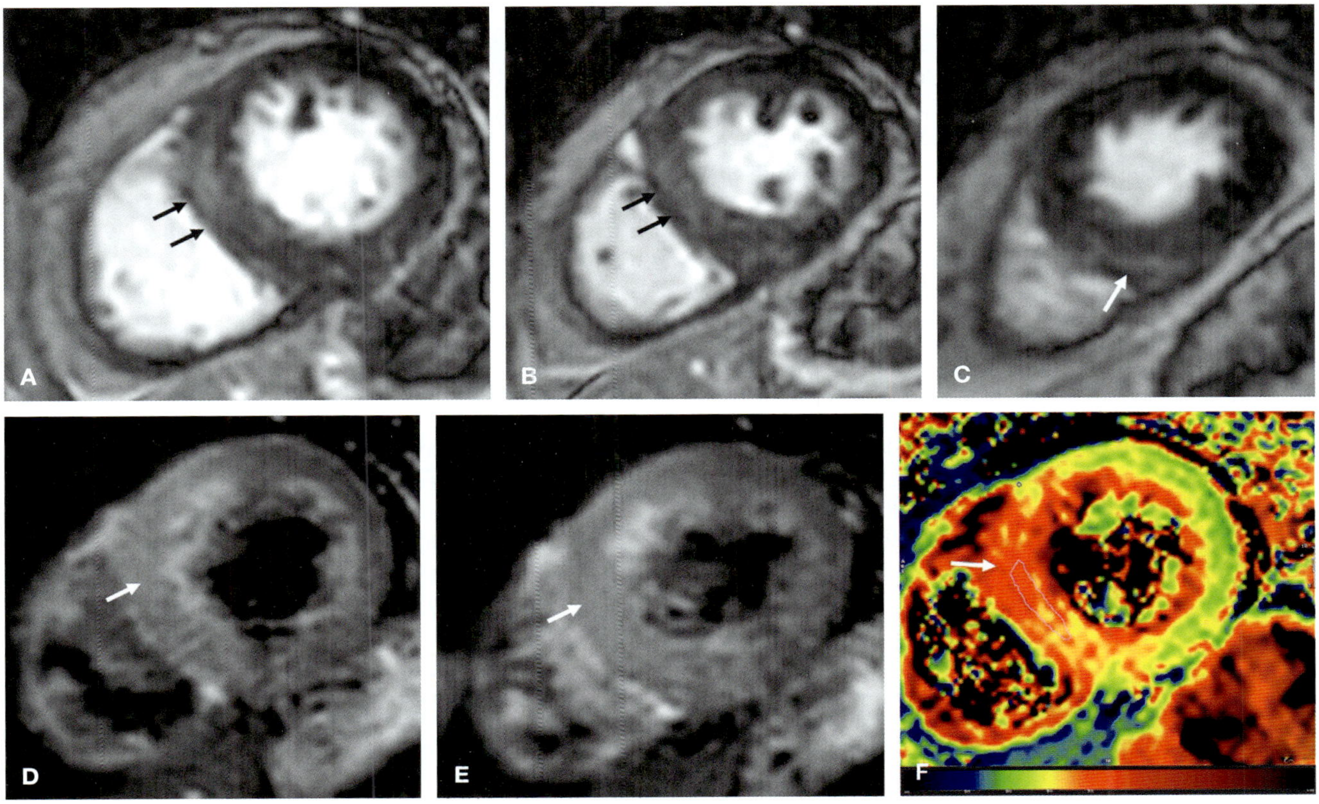

Figure 41.6. A 61-year-old female with cough, palpitations, and tachycardia. Blood work showed elevated troponin and wall motion abnormalities on echocardiography. **A–C:** Cardiac magnetic resonance (CMR) image shows midmyocardial and subepicardial late gadolinium enhancement in the basal to mid-anterior, anteroseptum, inferoseptum, and basal inferolateral segments (black arrows in **A** and **B**, white arrow in **C**.) on magnitude phase-sensitive inversion recovery sequence. **D, E:** Substantial myocardial edema in the anterior and septal wall on T2-weighted images (white arrows in **D** and **E**.). **F:** T2 map showing elevated T2 value measured as 64 ms (white arrow in **F**). CMR findings were consistent with acute myocarditis.

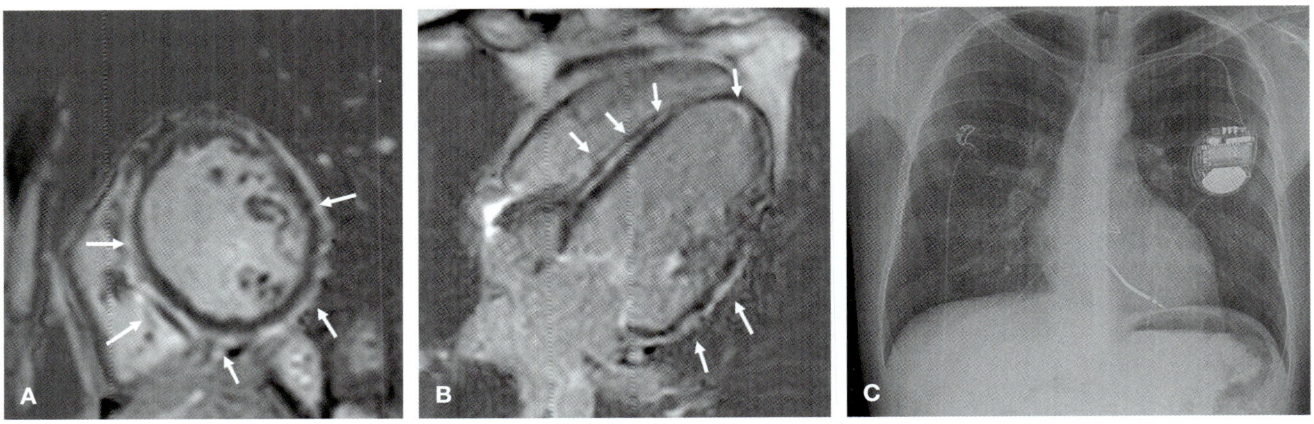

Figure 41.7. A 37-year-old man with a history of heart failure with reduced ejection fraction (LVEF 29%), recurrent ventricular tachycardia, polysubstance use, and hepatitis C infection. Cardiac magnetic resonance (CMR) was requested post implantable cardioverter-defibrillator placement (radiograph image **C**.). Ringlike enhancement was seen in the left ventricle on late gadolinium enhancement CMR on short-axis view (arrows in **A**) and 4-chamber view (arrows in **B**) Differential considerations included chronic inflammatory myocarditis, cardiac sarcoidosis, and arrhythmogenic or lamin mutation cardiomyopathy.

arrhythmogenic cardiomyopathy according to the combination of criteria.

Most tertiary care centers offer catheter ablation as a potential treatment option to ACM patients with recurrent VT refractory or intolerant to medical therapy. Exhaustive EAM ablation strategies to target CMR identify endocardial and epicardial substrate for elimination of all the abnormal electrograms and inducible VT provides long-term drug-free arrhythmia control in a large majority of these patients.

Hypertrophic Cardiomyopathy

CMR offers benefit in the comprehensive assessment of sarcomeric hypertrophic cardiomyopathy (HCM) and prognostication of SCD. The major predictors include progressive left ventricular outflow tract (LVOT) obstruction, systolic anterior motion of mitral leaflet, and LGE ≥15% of the total myocardial volume as delineated on CMR. LGE cutoff of 10% to 15% is also the most reliable CMR marker for selecting HCM patients needing ICD therapy. Additionally, high signal intensity on T2-weighted images is emerging as a predictor of arrhythmic events in the setting of HCM (Fig. 41.8).

CMR can detect subtle markers of the disease in patients with positive genotype but negative phenotype (no LV hypertrophy). These include presence of myocardial crypts, elongated anterior mitral leaflet, papillary muscle abnormalities, abnormal apical trabeculae, and smaller LV volumes. CMR can easily differentiate secondary hypertrophy based on the pattern and location of LV hypertrophy, pattern and distribution of LGE, and native T1.

CMR is useful for preoperative planning in patients undergoing septal reduction surgery. About 20% of hypertrophic obstructive cardiomyopathy patients develop AF as the most common tachyarrhythmia and associated with malignant outcomes. The current European and American guidelines provide a level IIa indication to surgical AF ablation in patients who require surgical myectomy as a potential benefit for paroxysmal or persistent AF rhythm control. A septal myectomy combined with a Maze III or Maze IV

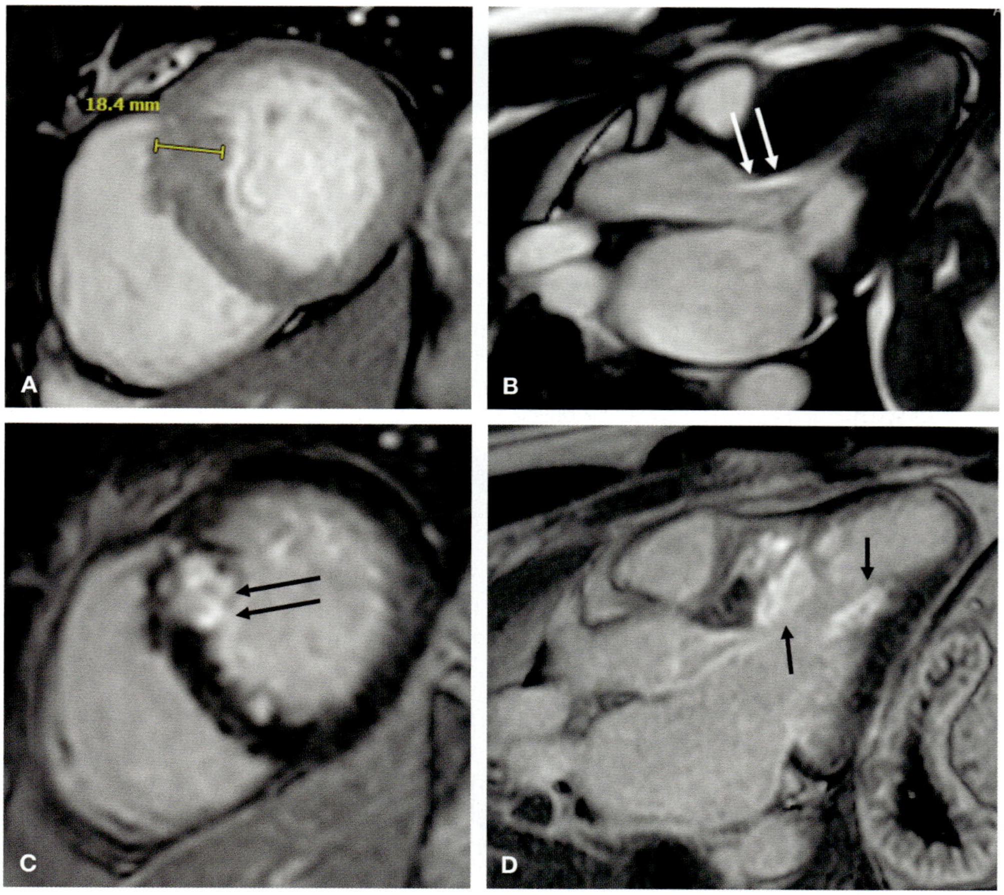

Figure 41.8. Asymmetric sigmoidal basal septal hypertrophy with maximum wall thickness of 18 mm on short-axis view (**A**). 3-chamber view showing left ventricular (LV) outflow tract flow acceleration (white arrows in **B**.) and cavity obliteration. There was no mitral systolic anterior motion at rest. Midmyocardial late gadolinium enhancement in the basal to midventricular septum comprising 21 g, which corresponds to 16% of the total LV mass using the 5-SD threshold criteria on the SAX and 3-chamber view (black arrows in **C** and **D**).

procedure for AF ablation can restore atrioventricular synchrony, improve atrial transport function, and improve the postoperative hemodynamics in these patients.

Premature Ventricular Complex–Induced Cardiomyopathy

The diagnosis of premature ventricular complex (PVC)–induced cardiomyopathy is based on the presence of frequent PVCs, an existing cardiomyopathy, and a lack of an alternative etiology for the cardiomyopathy. PVCs can contribute to LV dysfunction, cardiomyopathy, and heart failure. LVEF impairment can occur within 3 months of induced ventricular ectopy. Some explanations include increased repolarization heterogeneity, ventricular dyssynchrony similar to that of left bundle branch block, either physiological or induced by chronic RV pacing, asymmetrically increased wall thickness in the late-activated regions and altered myocardial blood flow.

PVC-induced cardiomyopathy is a potentially reversible condition but requires the exclusion of other causes of cardiomyopathy, such as infective, drug-induced, and metabolic, excess alcohol/caffeine intake, or emotional stress (Fig. 41.9). Predictors of PVC-induced cardiomyopathy include consistency in PVC burden throughout the day and PVC burden >24 % (sensitivity and specificity 79% and 78%, respectively) and presence of epicardial scar. Right ventricular outflow tract (RVOT) is the most frequent site of origin of idiopathic PVCs. Other sites include myocardial extensions to the aortic and pulmonary cusps, septum, papillary muscles, free walls, or LV fascicles. Improvement in LV function has been reported after suppressing PVCs with pharmacologic antiarrhythmic drugs or catheter ablation. The rationale that frequent PVCs could trigger VT, VF, and SCD in post-MI patients warrants PVC suppression was backed by the Cardiac Arrhythmia Suppression Trial. The 2015 European Society of Cardiology guidelines state that, in

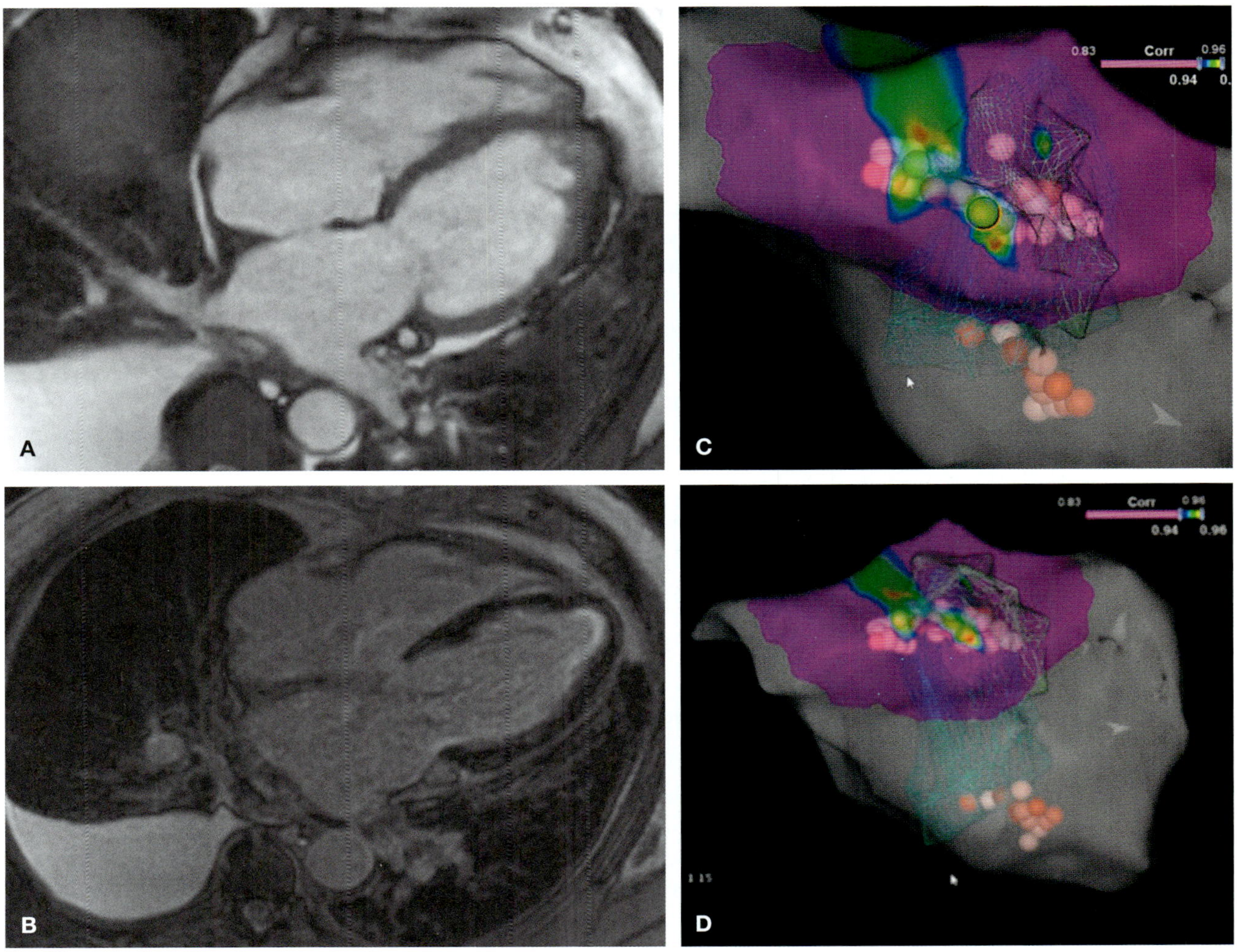

Figure 41.9. Patient with PVC-related cardiomyopathy and drug toxicity showing hypertrabeculations in the left and right ventricular apex on bright blood image (**A**) and diffuse subendocardial enhancement on late gadolinium enhancement imaging (**B**). Electroanatomic mapping with ablation of papillary muscles was performed due to high PVC burden with ablation set depicted in **C** and **D**.

patients with RVOT PVCs needing treatment, catheter ablation should be recommended as first-line treatment, whereas in patients with LVOT PVCs, catheter ablation should only be considered after failed AAD.

Markers of PVC-induced cardiomyopathy include echocardiographic findings of increased systolic and diastolic LV size, global LV systolic impairment, altered LV contractility despite normal LVEF, and functional mitral regurgitation. Cardiac MRI helps evaluate for scar and exclude infiltrative diseases. ECV evaluated in CMR T1 mapping correlates with both PVC-induced cardiomyopathy and PVC burden. A preprocedural CMR guides in planning ablation by identifying endocardial versus epicardial scar as well as extent of scar if present. Catheter ablation locations for PVC-induced cardiomyopathy are RVOT, epicardium, LV summit, intramural location, papillary muscles, and a para-Hisian origin.

CMR IMAGING IN PATIENTS WITH CARDIOVERTER IMPLANTABLE ELECTRONIC DEVICES

Recent developments in CIED engineering have led to devices that do not appear to cause significant clinical harm to patients undergoing MRI as their operation is largely resistant to electromagnetic interference in the MRI environment, particularly at 1.5 T. Radiologists do need to be aware of several underlying issues regarding MRI patients with CIEDs (Fig. 41.10). The most pertinent are a result of interactions of the device components with static and time-varying magnetic gradients or RF pulses. The deleterious effects described include translation or torque on device components due to the B0 field; induced currents in the leads resulting in oversensing, inadvertent myocardial stimulation, or heating at the lead tips; inhibition of pacing output; partial- or full-device resets including power-on resets; activation of the reed switch which can revert the device into "magnet mode"; loss of the device's programmed data; premature battery depletion; and severe image artifacts that can affect image interpretation.

It is interesting to note that many of the adverse incidents from the abovementioned complexities are not well documented and the nature of the exact interactions between the devices and MRI was often not reliably determined. These were also more common in legacy devices manufactured before the year 2000.

Recent devices manufactured include advances in technology and engineering such as reduction of the amount of ferromagnetic material for measurably reduced forces and torque in the magnetic field, improvements in circuitry, sensing/detection algorithms, and general robustness to electromagnetic interference.

New devices usually have MR conditional labeling that refers to an object or device which has been demonstrated to pose no known hazards within specified conditions of use.

The conditions of use include:

- Configuration of the device (eg, combination of generator and leads and allowed implant locations)
- Specific device programming requirements during the MRI exam
- Required staff for device programming and patient monitoring

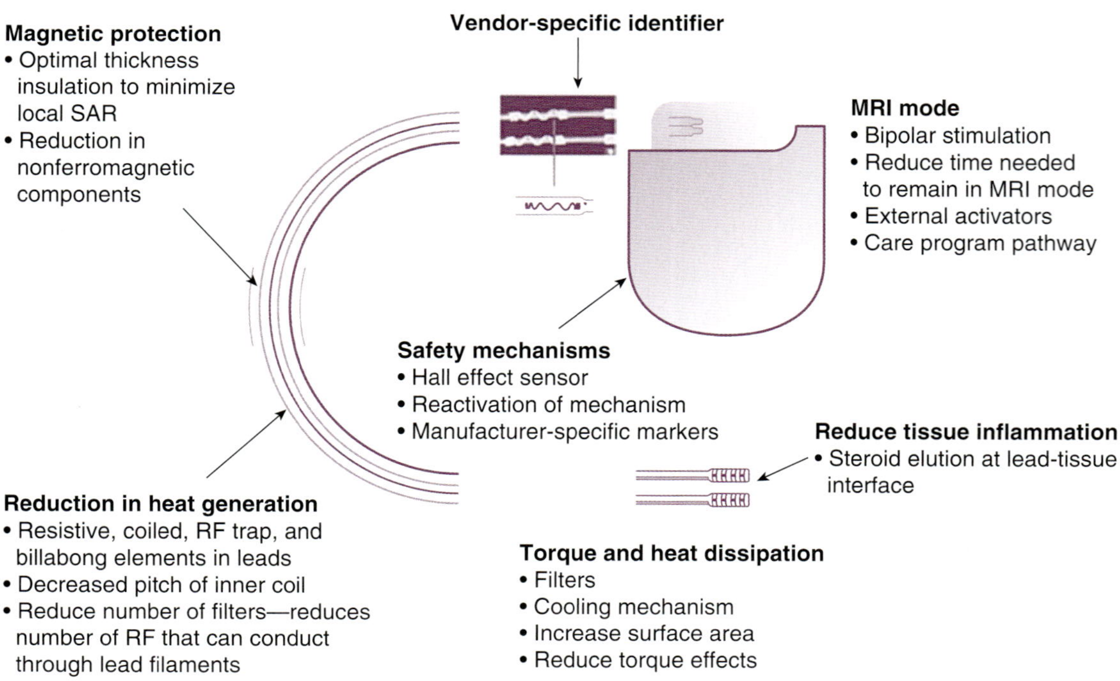

Figure 41.10. Various interactions of cardiac implantable electronic devices in MRI environment are described.

CIED systems that have not met regulatory criteria for MR conditional labeling as nonconditional. Such devices are labeled by the device manufacturer and/or MRI system manufacturer as contraindicated for MRI. These device systems do not have conforming configurations or with some components that do not have MR conditional labeling. In practice, they have often been considered MR unsafe and were manufactured before 2000. "Non-MR conditional" or "legacy" devices are now considered by many as a relative contraindication to MRI.

In 2017, the MagnaSafe Registry reported no cases of device or lead failure in 1500 nonthoracic MRI studies (1000 pacemakers and 500 ICDs) at 1.5 Tesla with nonconditional CIEDs. In view of such developments, the comprehensive consensus report from the Heart Rhythm Society for MRI, CT, and radiation therapy in the year 2017 identified class I recommendation for MRI in patients with MR conditional CIEDs and class IIa recommendation for MRI in patients with non-MR conditional CIEDs.

CMR Protocol for Pacemaker, Defibrillator, and Cardiac Resynchronization Therapy

CMR protocols depend on whether the CIED has MR conditional or MR nonconditional labeling. Any MRI for patients with a CIED that does not have FDA labeling specific for use in an MRI environment will be covered under the following conditions:

1. MRI field strength is 1.5 T or less using normal operating mode, ie, whole-body specific absorption rate is <2 W/kg
2. The implanted CIED has no epicardial, fractured, or abandoned lead

An organized institutional workflow with an established protocol involves proper patient screening, device programming, scan monitoring, and pre- and post-ICD interrogation to minimize risk in patients with conditional and nonconditional CIEDs.

Newer CMR Sequences in Patients With Cardioverter Implantable Electronic Devices

In patients with CIEDs, imaging artifacts are related to the type and proximity of the device, being more prominent in ICDs than PPMs due to the greater off-resonance induced by the battery and high-voltage transformer. The typical artifact from the device generator as well as the electrode appears as a central signal void and peripheral hyperintensity and may preclude scar assessment (Fig. 41.11).

MR acquisition strategies devised to reduce artifacts generally yield interpretable results and with a high clinical yield. The most popular strategies include:

- spoiled gradient echo cine imaging to reduce the susceptibility artifacts
- shorter echo times to reduce specific absorption ratio
- wideband inversion recovery pulses for LGE—help to reduce B0-related artifacts (Fig. 41.12)

Pacing-Induced Cardiomyopathy

Chronic conventional RV pacing with other structural abnormalities such as reduced myocardial perfusion and myofibrillar disarray is thought to lead to dyssynchronous ventricular activation and subsequent LV dysfunction and

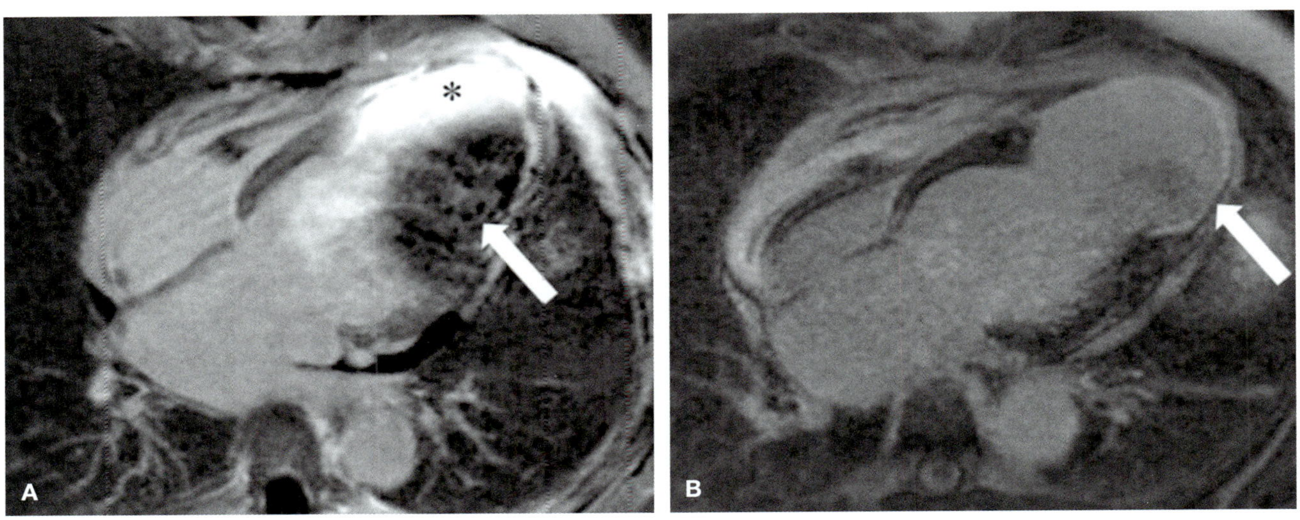

Figure 41.11. **A:** Artifact due to a cardiac implantable electronic device with central signal void (white arrow in **A**.) and peripheral hyperintensity (asterisk in **A**.) obscuring the underlying septum and lateral left ventricular (LV) wall as well as the apex. **B:** Wideband late gadolinium enhanced cardiac magnetic resonance showing a large left anterior descending infarct involving LV apical cavity and apex with aneurysmal dilation (white arrow in **B**.)

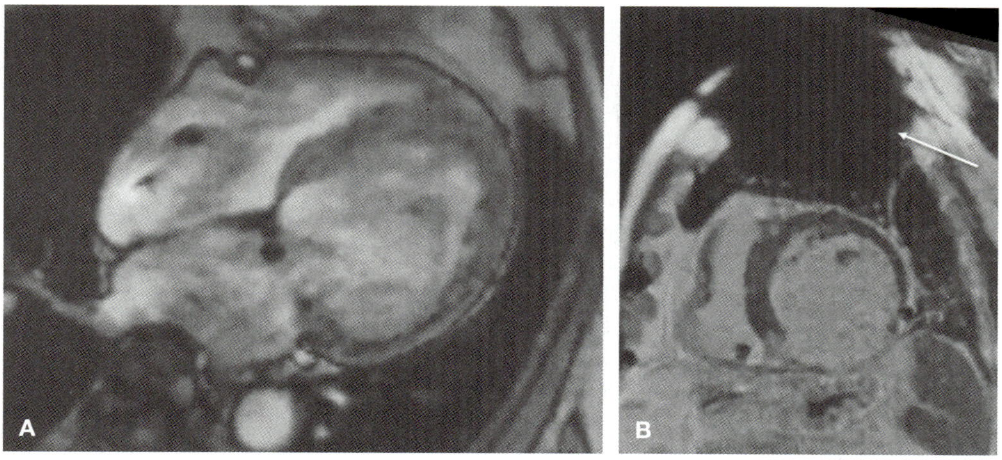

Figure 41.12. A: Four-chamber spoiled gradient-recalled echo for cine imaging. **B:** 2D late gadolinium enhanced phase-sensitive inversion recovery wideband breath-hold, motion correction, 16 averages, 6-mm spatial resolution image depicting inferior left ventricular infarct. White arrow points toward artifact from the device generator.

heart failure. Severity of baseline LV systolic dysfunction on CMR is one of the important risk factors for development of pacing induced cardiomyopathy (PIC). The most acceptable definition for PIC is LVEF of <50% or absolute decline of LVEF by ≥10% and/or new-onset HF symptoms or AF after pacemaker implantation. However, there are significant variations in the definition of PIC that includes a combination of echocardiographic, clinical features, RV pacing percentage, and paced QRS duration.

NOVEL POSTPROCESSING STRATEGIES ON CMR AND FEASIBILITY OF REAL-TIME CMR-GUIDED EP ABLATIONS

CMR Strain

Novel postprocessing strategies such as feature tracking strain show potential for risk stratification and postprocedural outcomes in patients with atrial or ventricular arrhythmias. Recently, the feasibility to assess atrial function, strain, and the burden of cardiac adipose tissue with CMR has been discussed to provide more elements for risk stratification and clinical decision-making in the setting of catheter ablation planning of AF. Reduced atrial strain in patients with heart failure has been described as a predictor of new-onset AF. Left atrial strain was also found to be associated with arrhythmia recurrence after catheter ablation. Pericardial adipose tissue burden as quantified using fat-water separation sequences, such as 3-point Dixon, is another predictor of AF recurrence following catheter ablation (Fig. 41.13).

LGE-CMR Image Analysis for VT Pathway Identification

Postprocessed 3D LGE-CMR data can be integrated into electrophysiology navigation platforms to further assist in ablation procedures. A PSI-based algorithm can characterize myocardial scar as core or border zone on 3D/2D LGE-CMR acquisitions. Infarct core is defined as a region with signal intensity greater than 50% of the peak SI of the total hyperenhanced area, gray zone/border zone as region with signal intensity between 35% and 50% of the peak SI. PSI-based thresholds are found to correlate with EAM voltage thresholds of infarct core <0.5 mV, border zone 0.5 to 1.5 m, and healthy tissue with >1.5 mV. Border zone extent on CMR is a stronger predictor of subsequent ventricular arrhythmic events compared with core extent. Scar border zone is critical for the perpetuation of the arrhythmia and its abolition forms the basis of substrate-based VT ablation. CMR conducting channels are generated topologically as border zone coursing through scar core and connecting healthy myocardium. The CMR conducting channels can identify critical isthmus, which are sites of ischemic VT in zones of tissue heterogeneity, critical slow conduction which form components of reentry circuits and to distinguish irreversible injury from edema in the setting of catheter ablation. Previous studies have reported that imaging-based channel identification and dechanneling with RF ablation have been found to render 54.4% of patients noninducible after ablation. Those who required only image-based dechanneling had shorter procedure time, fewer RF ablation lesions, and fewer intraprocedural external cardioversions/defibrillations.

Feasibility of Intraprocedural MRI

Real-time MR guidance of EPs offers the potential for enhanced arrhythmia substrate assessment, improved procedural guidance, and real-time assessment of ablation lesion formation. MR-guided EP is currently performed with limited surface electrogram data. The first human ablation procedure of the cavotricuspid isthmus was performed by a group from Würzburg, Germany, in 2012.

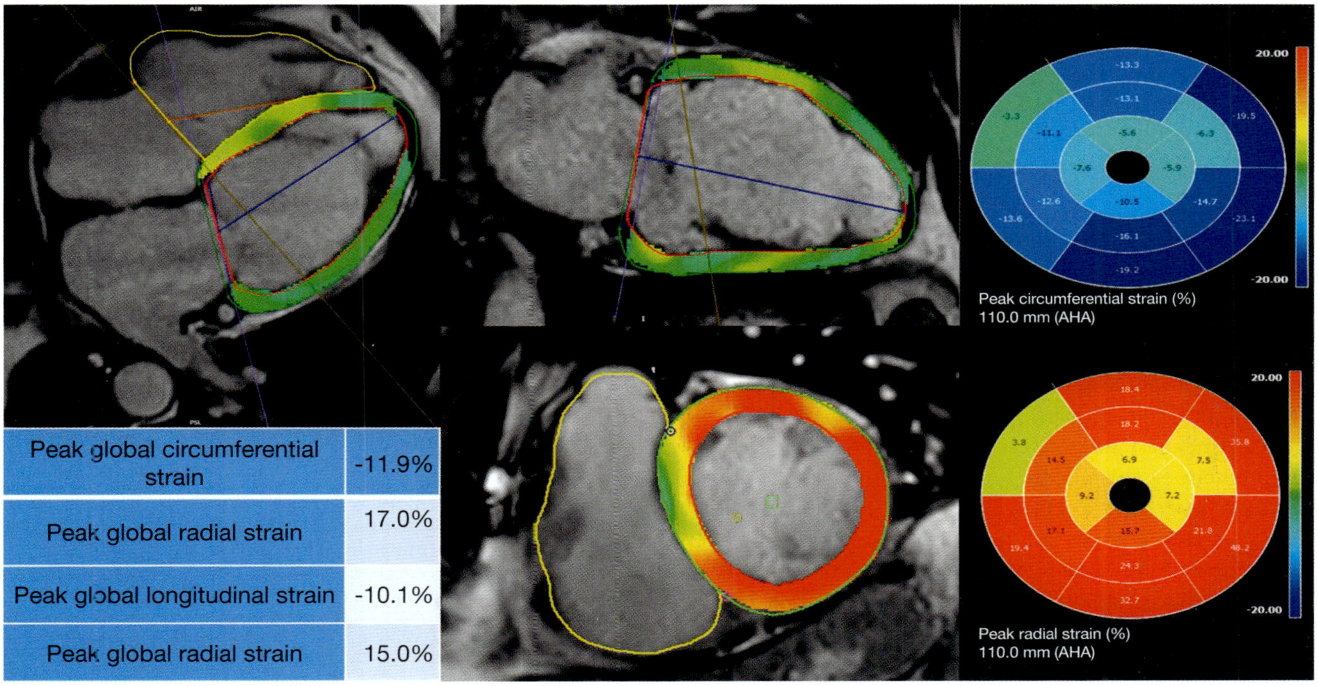

Figure 41.13. Impaired peak global longitudinal strain on cardiac magnetic resonance −10.0% (normal cutoff −13.9%) in a patient with PVC-induced cardiomyopathy.

The advent of MRI-compatible catheters and RF filters can mitigate issues such as catheter heating, current induction, image distortion, and electromagnetic interference and allow real-time MR-guided ablations. Passive or active real-time assessment of anatomy, catheter position, and lesion formation are feasible. Such an approach can limit or eliminate the need for ionizing radiation from fluoroscopy.

Passive tracking sequences have been developed for passive device tracking and identification of the device on an imaging sequence. Such a procedure currently suffers from poor contrast to noise ratio, lower spatial resolution with thicker imaging slices (>10 mm), and is highly time consuming. A relatively high-speed imaging sequence will be required to achieve imaging frame rates of at least 1 Hz. Active tracking sequences exploit the imaging gradient fields to derive device location or employ a dedicated tracking sequence, detected by microcoils within the catheter. Small receive coils detect a highly localized spatially encoded signal from the surrounding tissue. These coils are insensitive to signal arising more than ~1 mm away. High-frequency tracking sequences (>10 Hz) with a high spatial resolution (<1 mm) are behind developed that will contribute to exceptional advances in MRI technology for future developments.

THE ROLE OF ARTIFICIAL INTELLIGENCE IN CARDIAC IMAGING TO INFORM EP

Currently, there is immense interest in development of artificial intelligence (AI)-based technologies that can aid CMR guidance in EP. Clinical, standard CMR parameters and quantitative analysis can be utilized in developing several machine learning models with further potential to improve the performance of neural networks in AI models targeted in analyzing diagnostic and prognostic information in patients with myocardial diseases causing arrhythmias. Radiomics and pathomics are some examples of novel image postprocessing techniques that can help in automating clinical workflows using AI technologies.

Radiomics as Cardiac Imaging Biomarkers

Radiomics is a novel image quantification technique whereby pixel-level data are analyzed to derive multiple quantifiers of tissue shape and texture. Multiparametric imaging with addition of radiomics texture features to other conventional imaging approaches has the potential to improve the diagnostic accuracy of CMR for the diagnosis of ischemic and nonischemic myocardial diseases. Several studies have analyzed radiomics features derived from standard CMR sequences such as LGE, white and black blood imaging, and T1/T2 quantitative mapping. New radiomics morphometric markers, such as greater right carina angle, reduced anterior-posterior atrial diameter, greater atrial volume normalized to height, and steeper right inferior PV angle have been found to be associated with postablation recurrence of AF. CMR radiomics has the added potential of combining noninvasive tissue characterization on CMR with novel quantitative radiomics-derived texture maps. Such a technique can be used to generate texture maps at the scanner level and add value to CMR as a one-stop shop for patients with arrhythmias. Exploiting machine learning strategies with CMR radiomics may improve the diagnostic ability of CMR for screening, risk stratification, and treatment monitoring in patients with arrhythmias and mitigate the need for the added cost of nuclear imaging studies and its potential burden on patient costs and health care.

VT MUSIC Platform

The MUSIC platform is an innovative interface that is currently under active development to allow users to import, export, and provide AI-based modeling approaches for patient-specific VT ablation procedures. Both CMR and CT data sets can be used in the automatic pipelines for left wall thickness map extraction and ventricular arrhythmia prediction. This allows VA classification from 2D wall thickness map and a Dual-UNet segmentation classifier model. Attention maps are generated from gradient back propagation of the classification score. MRI-guided RF ablation of cardiac arrhythmias have been performed on the MUSICardio application. RF energy delivered under MRI thermometry can be used to monitor treatment progression with lesion transmurality a major parameter to assess the therapeutic success of RF ablation.

inHEART Platform

inHEART is another emerging AI-enabled digital platform for image-guided ablations to optimize VT ablation strategies. The platform provides anatomic and structural characteristics from digitally rendered 3D cardiac models using AI-based segmentations of MR and CT images. These post-processed images can be integrated with any EAM system.

CONCLUSION

CMR is an excellent tool for assisting in the management of myriad of cardiac electrophysiological processes. Its ability to identify etiopathogenesis for atrial or ventricular arrhythmias, assessment of severity of cardiac dysfunction, scar characterization, and prognostication is exceptional. Advances in CMR and device technology have enabled imaging for management of patients with CIEDs. Assessment of cardiac structure, function, and arrhythmogenic substrate is crucial for planning of atrial and ventricular ablations procedures in these patients. CMR is helpful to identify postprocedural complications such as postatrial ablation arrhythmias. In the near future, CMR-guided real-time ablations will improve procedural accuracy in a subset of patients with electrophysiological abnormalities.

SUGGESTED READINGS

Berte B, Cochet H, Dang L, et al. Image-guided ablation of scar-related ventricular tachycardia: towards a shorter and more predictable procedure. *J Interv Card Electrophysiol.* 2020;59(3):535-544. doi:10.1007/s10840-019-00686-w

Bhargava M, Di Biase L, Mohanty P, et al. Impact of type of atrial fibrillation and repeat catheter ablation on long-term freedom from atrial fibrillation: results from a multicenter study. *Heart Rhythm.* 2009;6(10):1403-1412.

Eichhorn C, Greulich S, Bucciarelli-Ducci C, Sznitman R, Kwong RY, Gräni C. Multiparametric cardiovascular magnetic resonance approach in diagnosing, monitoring, and prognostication of myocarditis. *JACC Cardiovasc Imaging.* 2022;15(7):1325-1338.

Goldberger JJ, Cain ME, Hohnloser SH, et al; American Heart Association,American College of Cardiology Foundation, Heart Rhythm Society. American Heart Association/American College of Cardiology Foundation/Heart Rhythm Society scientific statement on noninvasive risk stratification techniques for identifying patients at risk for sudden cardiac death: a scientific statement from the American Heart Association Council on Clinical Cardiology Committee on Electrocardiography and Arrhythmias and Council on Epidemiology and Prevention. *Circulation.* 2008;118(14):1497-1518.

Graziano F, Zorzi A, Cipriani A, et al. The 2020 "Padua criteria" for diagnosis and phenotype characterization of arrhythmogenic cardiomyopathy in clinical practice. *J Clin Med.* 2022;11(1):279.

Marrouche NF, Wazni O, McGann C, et al; DECAAF II Investigators. Effect of MRI-guided fibrosis ablation vs conventional catheter ablation on atrial arrhythmia recurrence in patients with persistent atrial fibrillation: the DECAAF II Randomized clinical trial. *JAMA.* 2022;327(23):2296-2305.

Priori SG, Blomstrom-Lundqvist C, Mazzanti A, et al; ESC Scientific Document Group. 2015 ESC guidelines for the management of patients with ventricular arrhythmias and the prevention of sudden cardiac death: the task force for the management of patients with ventricular arrhythmias and the prevention of sudden cardiac death of the European Society of Cardiology (ESC). Endorsed by—Association for European Paediatric and Congenital Cardiology (AEPC). *Eur Heart J.* 2015;36(41):2793-2867.

Wang H, Bo K, Gao Y, Zhou Z, Xu L. Prognosis evaluation of chronic inflammatory cardiomyopathy with ring-like late gadolinium enhancement. *ESC Heart Fail.* 2023;10(3):1735-1744.

Chapter 42

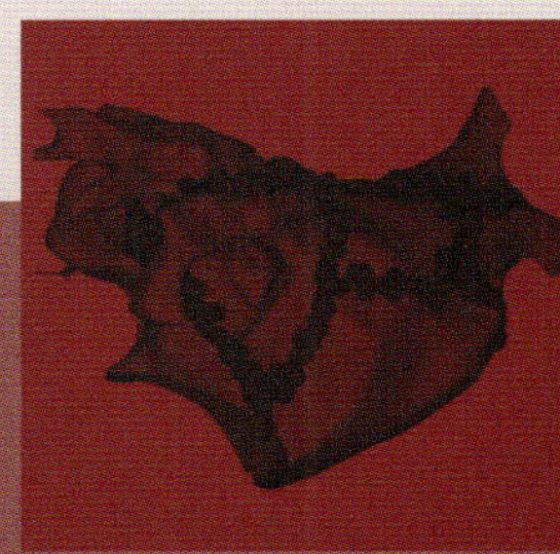

Hamid Chalian • Seyed Ali Nabipoorashrafi • Zahra Chakeri • Tushar Kumar • Eric Williamson

CTA for Guidance of Structural Heart Disease Procedures

INTRODUCTION

Cardiovascular computed tomography angiography (CTA) is a medical imaging modality utilizing X-ray technology to produce cross-sectional images of the heart and blood vessels, assisting in precise anatomical assessment, diagnostic evaluation, and procedural planning in cardiovascular medicine. Recent advancements in cardiovascular imaging and CT technologies have greatly expanded applications of CTA and its integration into medical guidelines.

The expanding applications of CTA extended from traditional coronary artery imaging to comprehensive assessments of structural heart diseases, including but not limited to evaluation of cardiac chambers, valvular structures, and vascular access routes. This broadening scope enhances CTA's applications for guidance of structural heart disease procedures (Table 42.1). Recently, several artificial intelligence algorithms have been introduced with promising applications for assessment of structural heart disease from image segmentation to estimation of outcome.

In this chapter we will focus on applications of CTA in management of aortic stenosis (transcatheter aortic valve replacement [TAVR]), mitral valve disease (transcatheter mitral valve replacement [TMVR) and left atrial appendage occlusion (LAAO). The purpose of this chapter is to:

1. Review the applications and benefits of CTA in preprocedural planning for management of the abovementioned structural heart diseases.
2. Review the imaging protocols and techniques for ideal assessment of these structural heart diseases.
3. Get familiar with the potential complications after management of these structural heart diseases, and their imaging appearance.

CTA FOR PRE- AND POSTPROCEDURAL TAVR EVALUATION

Aortic stenosis, caused by various reasons such as degenerative calcification and congenital conditions, is the primary cause of cardiac outlet obstruction. Surgical aortic valve

Table 42.1 CTA Applications in Structural Heart Disease

Structural Heart Disease	CTA Application
Aortic stenosis	Pre- and post-procedural planning, Intra-procedural navigation
Mitral valve prolapse	Pre- and post-procedural planning, Guidance for interventions
Atrial septal defect	Evaluation of cardiac chambers, Intra-procedural navigation
Coronary artery disease	Coronary anatomy visualization
LAA occlusion	Assessment of cardiac chambers, Guidance for LAA closure procedures
Ventricular Septal Defect	Cardiac chamber evaluation, Intra-procedural guidance
Pulmonary Valve Stenosis	Pre- and post-procedural planning, Intra-procedural navigation

CTA, computed tomography angiography; LAA, left atrial appendage.

replacement (SAVR) is the main treatment for aortic stenosis. More recently, the TAVR procedure was introduced as a much less invasive option for aortic valve replacement compared to SAVR in eligible patients.

The TAVR procedure was performed on humans for the first time in 2002. Although initially mostly considered an alternative to SAVR, particularly for high surgical-risk individuals, recent evidence has shown that the adverse events of this procedure in other groups of valve replacement, including low-risk patients, are significantly less than those associated with SAVR.

As the performance and safety of TAVR has been proven in different randomized control trials, the indication of using this procedure is updating constantly. TAVR is now not only indicated for high-risk or inoperable patients but also indicated in intermediate and low-risk patients with severe aortic stenosis. Based on AHA guidelines, TAVR outweighs SAVR in following all Individuals older than 80 years or younger patients with a life expectancy less than 10 years, and without anatomical contraindications to transfemoral TAVR.

For candidates for aortic valve replacement aged between 65 and 80 years, TAVR is advised for individuals experiencing symptomatic severe AS, with no anatomical contraindications to transfemoral TAVR. According to the 2021 ESC guidelines, TAVR is recommended for candidates ages 75 years and older or those considered at high risk or ineligible for surgical intervention. However, for candidates younger than 75 years old, the procedure (TAVR or SAVR) will be selected after considering patients' clinical and anatomic conditions.

Over the past two decades, several different devices have been introduced for TAVR. Table 42.2 lists the most commonly used devices with their specific characteristics.

CTA Technique and Image Acquisition

Imaging before the procedure provides interventionists with accurate anatomical and functional information about aortic stenosis and has a direct impact on the success rate of the procedure. Various imaging methods are being used for this purpose, including CTA, MRI, echocardiography, and cardiac catheterization. Although each technique has its own indications, the CTA modality is the most common imaging technique used for TAVR planning.

Various CTA acquisition protocols have been introduced for TAVR, typically involving a combination of ECG-gated and non-ECG-gated approaches. electrocardiogram (ECG)-gated CTA provides high-resolution and volumetric data that allows for specific reconstructions that provide information needed before TAVR. The usual protocols include:

A. Non-ECG-gated CTA of the abdomen and pelvis, along with a fully ECG-gated CTA of the chest.
B. Non-ECG-gated CTA of the chest, abdomen, and pelvis coupled with ECG-gated CTA of the cardiac region and aorta.

The second protocol (B) leads to less radiation exposure and IV contrast volume; therefore many institutions prefer to use this protocol for pre-TAVR assessment. Table 42.3 shows our institutional TAVR protocol.

CTA Image Postprocessing and Reporting

Information regarding anatomy of the aortic annulus and landing zone is the main goal of pre-TAVR imaging. There are several critical pieces of information that should be provided by the radiologist to increase the chance of proper deployment of the valve with the low complication rates. Measurements include size of aortic annulus, coronary origin heights, diameter of the sinus of Valsalva, sinotubular junction height, and membranous septum length. Similarly, in pre-TAVR imaging, information regarding valve morphology (bicuspid vs tricuspid), severity of leaflet calcification, or abnormalities in the aortic root should be reported.

In addition to the landing zone, CTA of the abdomen and pelvis allows for precise delineation of the entire femoral arterial approach. The morphology and luminal diameter of

Table 42.2 TAVR Devices and Their Features

Device Name	Valve Position and Expansion	Additional Features
Sapien Family	Supra-annular and self-expandable	Broad variety of annular sizes
Acurate Neo	Supra-annular and self-expandable	Balloon-expandable, low frame height, outer skirt
Allegra (NVT AG)	Supra-annular and self-expandable	Low pacemaker rates, adjustable delivery access
Centera	Supra-annular and self-expandable	Adjustable delivery access
LenaValve	Self-expandable, expands within the annulus	Less observed paravalvular bleeding and pacemaker complications
Lotus Edge	Self-expandable, expands within the annulus	Transfemoral access
Portico	Mechanically expandable within the annulus	Less observed paravalvular leakage, fully repositionable
Sapien Family	Self-expandable, expands within the annulus	Fully repositionable (less than Lotus Edge), adjustable delivery access

Table 42.3 TAVR CT Imaging Protocol

Size (DFOV)	Noise Index	kVp	Contrast Vol/Rate 30 cc Saline Chaser
Small (≤34 cm)	28 NI	80-100 kVp	80 @4 cc/s
Medium (35-41 cm)	30 NI	100-120 kVp	80 @4 cc/s
Large (≥42 cm)	33 NI	120 kVp	80 @4 cc/s
Arterial phase (ECG-gated)		***Arterial phase (non-ECG-gated)***	
Anatomy Selection		***Anatomy Selection***	
Carina to base of the heart		*Clavicle to ischial tuberosities*	
SFOV Cardiac Large		*SFOV large body*	
DFOV: Rib to Rib		*DFOV adjust to cover*	
KV and mA Control		***KV and mA Control***	
Manual 80-120 kV		*GSI manual*	
Smart/Auto mA 100-740			
Timing		***Timing***	
Smart Prep @ descending Aorta.		*Immediately after Heart scan (7.6 s delay)*	
Auto trigger scan @ 150 HU			
Scan Type		***Scan Type***	
Cardiac 0%-90% R-R		*GSI Helical*	
Coverage Speed		***Coverage Speed***	
One box 0.28 s		*One or More/SC 0.8 s*	
Primary Recon		***Primary Recon***	
0.625 mm/Std/ASIRV 50/800@100		*0.625 mm/Std 400/40/ASIRV 50/50 keV*	
ECG-gating		***ECG-gating***	
On		*off*	
Image reconstruction		***Image reconstruction***	
Scout		*0.625 mm std*	
0.625 mm std		*Full field 2.5 mm Std DLIR Medium*	
Full field 0.625 mm heart Std DLIR Medium		*Full field 0.625 mm Std DLIR Medium*	
Coronal heart		*Coronal body*	
Sagittal heart		*Sagittal body*	
Full field 0.625 mm heart Std DLIR Medium		*Chest maximum intensity projection*	
Heart navigator 75%			
Heart navigator 40%			
Full field 0.62 5 mm Std DLIR Medium			
mode 0%-90%			

ASIR-V, adaptive statistical iterative reconstruction-v; cm, centimeters; DFOV, display field of view; DLIR, deep learning image reconstruction; GSI, Gemstone spectral imaging; HU, Hounsfield units; kVp, Kilovoltage peak; mm, millimeters; NI, noise index; Sec, second; SFOV, scan field of view; Std, standard; TAVR, transcatheter aortic valve replacement.

the femoral arterial approaches are used to define eligibility for the TAVR procedure, as small and heavily calcified and tortuous vessels could lead to access complications.

Measurements, Morphology, and Access

Annulus Size

This parameter is measured in the narrowest section of the valve, forming a ring-like structure at the base of the heart between the left ventricular outlet and the root of the ascending aorta (Figure 42.1). The recommended annulus measurements are maximum and minimum diameters, area, and perimeter.

During systole, contraction force of the heart leads to larger annular size in comparison to diastole. So, measuring this parameter in the diastolic phase may lead to miscalculation and undersizing of the annulus. To prevent this error, the annular size should be measured in ECG-gated reconstructed CT during the systolic phase (30%-40% of the R-R interval), and the largest annular dimensions should be considered for device selection.

Although guidelines recommend oversizing the prosthetic valves to some degree (approximately 20%) to prevent paravalvular leak, severe oversizing, and undersizing of the annulus both may lead to TAVR complications. Considerable oversizing of the annulus and using inappropriate devices may lead to annular rupture, while undersizing the annulus may result in incomplete valve deployment, perivalvular regurgitation, valve stenosis, and valve migration.

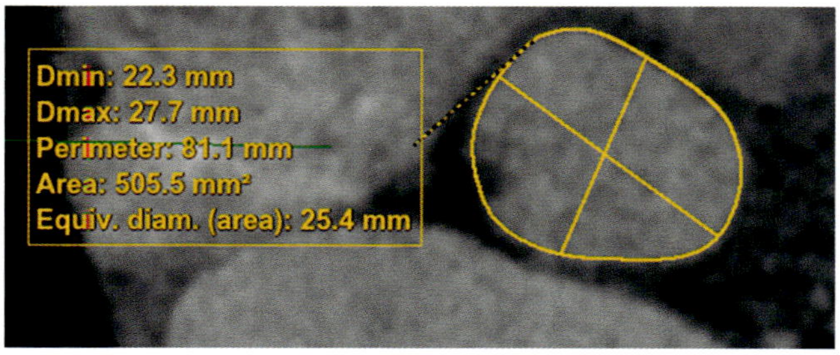

Figure 42.1. Double-oblique reformation shows cross-section of aortic annulus demonstrating minimum and maximum dimensions with perimeter and area.

Coronary Ostium Height

The length from the coronary ostium to the aortic valve annulus, referred to as coronary height, is a critical factor influencing the risk of coronary obstruction in TAVR procedures with native valves (Figure 42.2). It is measured as line from the annulus to the inferior margin of the coronary ostium, perpendicular to the annulus plane. The distance from the superior margin of the coronary ostium and the annulus plane may also be useful. The distance coronary occlusion is an infrequent yet critical complication of TAVR. While there is no specific cut-off for coronary ostium height, research has demonstrated that values above 12 mm are not associated with an increased risk of this complication. Note that this parameter is not an isolated factor for coronary occlusion risk. Other factors, such as the size of the valve, underlying diseases, and the size of the sinus of Valsalva, should be considered in the risk assessment.

Sinus of Valsalva (SV) Size

The evaluation of the sinus of Valsalva (SV) size includes measurement of diameters from the cusps to the commissures, perpendicular to the annular plane. In cases of symmetrical anatomy, the average of the measurements provides the average diameter of the SV. This measurement can be performed manually, automatically, or through a combination of both methods (semi-automated) (Figure 42.3). SV diameter less than 30 mm is associated with an increased risk of coronary occlusion.

Sinotubular Junction (STJ) Size

Sinotubular junction (STJ) sizing includes length and diameter. Length is measured as the distance between the perpendicular line from the annular plane to the lowest point of the STJ. This parameter has predictive value in the odds of contact between the valve and the STJ during TAVR deployment. The average diameter of the STJ should be provided. As a prosthetic valve diameter larger than the STJ diameter indicates a higher risk of STJ injury (particularly in balloon-expandable valves), it is important to compare the STJ diameter with the size of the anticipated prosthetic valve that will be used in the TAVR (Figure 42.4).

Membranous Septum (MS) Length

This measurement is determined by the distance between the basal aortic annulus and the point where the membranous portion of the interventricular septum transitions into the muscular segment of the interventricular septum (Figure 42.5). Although several studies have reported that membranous septum (MS) length correlates with the success of the procedure and complications, reporting MS length is not part of the assessment for all TAVR candidates in many institutions. For instance, shorter MS lengths have been linked to a greater incidence of electrical conduction issues after TAVR. there is an increased probability of encountering significant cardiac rhythm complications when the MS is short, especially when the length is less than approximately 8 mm. This risk is increased when the valve is positioned at a significant depth or when there is an underlying conduction block.

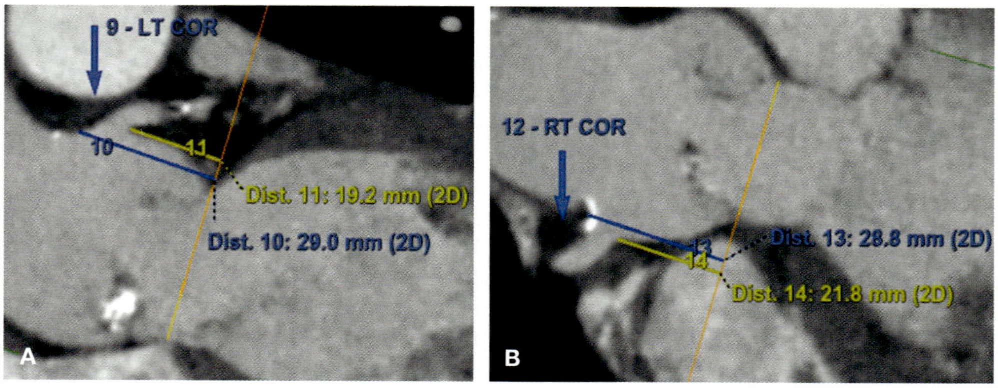

Figure 42.2. Coronary heights. **A:** Minimum (yellow line) and maximum (blue line) distance of left coronary ostium from aortic annulus (orange line). **B:** Minimum (yellow line) and maximum (blue line) distance of right coronary ostium from aortic annulus (orange line).

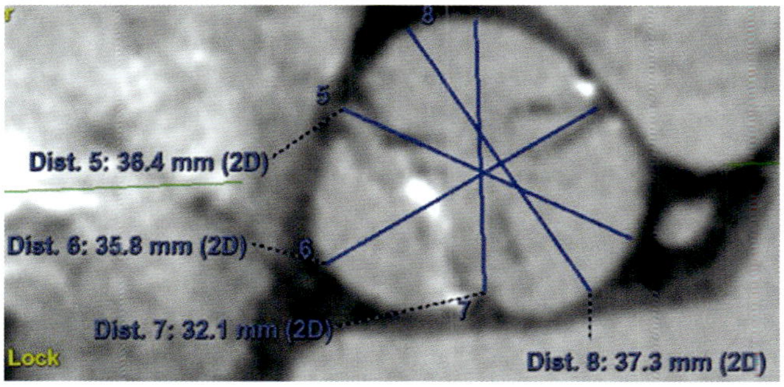

Figure 42.3. Double oblique reformation at the level of the sinus of Valsalva showing trileaflet aortic valve with cusp-to-commissure dimensions. Maximum cusp to cusp distance measures 37 mm in this 64-year-old male.

Access

A comprehensive evaluation of the arterial access is highly recommended to guarantee the smooth advancement of the delivery system to the aortic valve. As the femoral artery approach is considered the most common access site for TAVR (Figure 42.6) any anatomic variation or abnormality should be mentioned in the pre-procedural evaluation including stenosis, calcification, dissection, aneurysm, and the narrowest diameter of the vessel (Figure 42.7). The femoral arterial access assessment should include the common femoral arteries, external iliac arteries, common iliac arteries, and entire abdominal and thoracic aorta. For determining eligibility for the procedure, the narrowest site of the entire vascular approach is identified, and measurements of the minimum, maximum and average diameter at that site are obtained.

Suitability of the access for TAVR procedure depends on both the type of valve used and the specific anatomical characteristics of the patient. Generally, the implantation of balloon-expandable valves requires a smaller luminal diameter compared to self-expanding valves. It is important to note that not only does a small luminal diameter increase the risk of complications, but also a large luminal size. For instance, when the vessel lumen is less than 6 mm, there may be challenges in advancing the catheter to the aortic valve. However, a larger vessel luminal diameter, over 20 mm, increases the risk of bleeding. Alternative arterial access sites should be evaluated if the femoral arterial approach is not feasible including the subclavian artery, the carotid artery and the abdominal aorta.

Valve Morphology

Evaluating the shape of the valves is an essential component of the CTA assessment. Bicuspid aortic valve (BAV) is the most common congenital heart disease, and it is three to four times more prevalent in men than in women. Although various classifications for BAV are available, the basis for TAVR classification is to describe BAV based on the number of commissures and the presence of a raphe.

Assessing valvular calcification before the procedure can decrease the rate of TAVR complications. The most important reason is that heavily calcified valves determine the need for balloon-expandable versus self-expandable devices. In addition, it may be difficult to accurately determine the annulus size and shape in patients with heavily calcified BAV, requiring technical adjustment. It can also be challenging to differentiate mild valve calcifications from contrast (Figure 42.8). Additionally, assessing the size of the ascending aorta in patients with BAV is crucial, as there is an association between BAV and aortopathy.

Landing Zone Calcification

The landing zone for TAVR included left ventricle outflow tract, aortic annulus, and aortic leaflets. Precision in obtaining information about the landing zone before TAVR increases the success of the procedure with minimal complications and ensures accurate implantation in the designated landing zone. CT can provide various pieces of information regarding the landing zone, including calcification and anatomy.

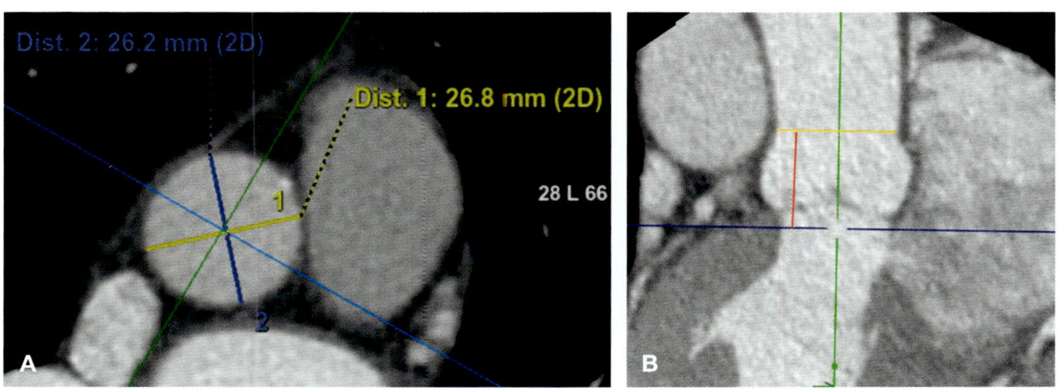

Figure 42.4. Sinotubular junction. **A:** Double oblique reformation shows cross-section of the sinotubular junction with maximum and minimum dimensions. **B:** Distance (red line) of sinotubular junction (yellow line) from aortic annulus level (blue line) measured 2.8 cm.

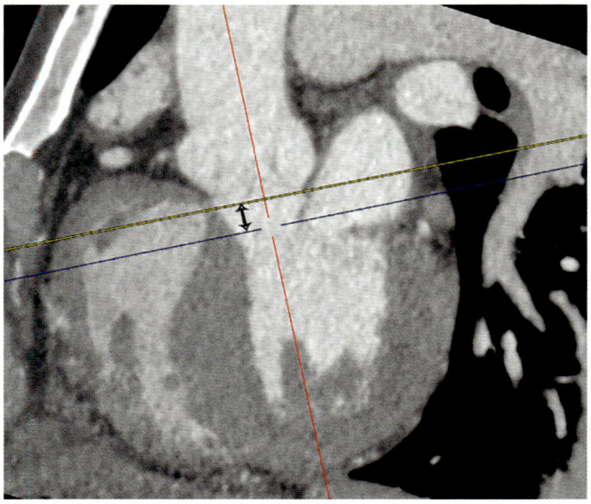

Figure 42.5. Membranous septal length. Oblique sagittal reformation of the left ventricular outflow track shows length of the membranous septum (double-headed arrow) measuring 10 mm. The membranous septum separates the aortic vestibule from lower part of right atrium and upper part of right ventricle and forms upper part of interventricular septum.

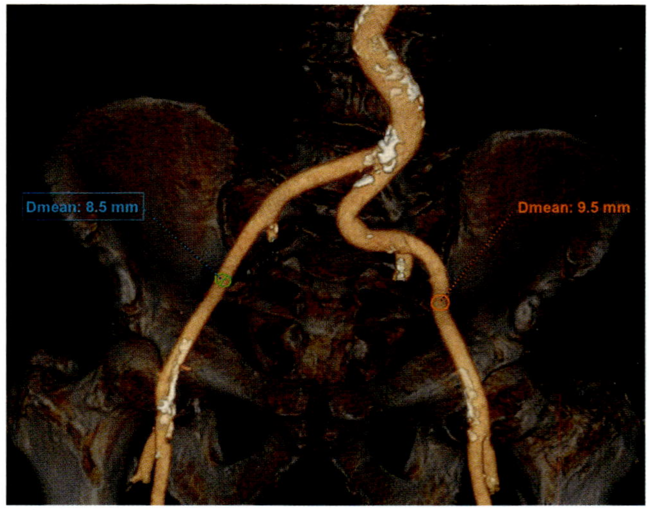

Figure 42.7. Volume rendering reformation of the pelvic and abdominal vessels demonstrating mean dimensions at the narrowest points of the femoral arterial approaches. In this patient aged 69 years old, minimum mean diameter was seen in right external iliac artery, measuring 8.5 mm (green circle).

Calcification in the landing zone poses a notable challenge in placing the valve and may impede the proper adherence of the new valve to the vessel wall. In addition, considerable and substantial calcification surrounding the annulus can result in complications like leakage, rupture of the annulus, and regurgitation.

Consequently, it is crucial to assess and understand the characteristics of calcification in the landing zone before undertaking TAVR (Figure 42.9). The shape and degree of calcification should be reported in the annular and subannular regions. For instance, deeper calcification in left ventricular outflow tract (LVOT) has been associated with complications such as rupture. Also, when comparing flat to nodular shaped calcifications, the latter is associated with a higher risk of complications. the location of calcification is another variable for TAVR complications. The degree of calcification in the sub-annular region can predict the need for pacemaker after the procedure due to conduction disturbances. Reporting this feature is particularly important for patients at risk for conduction block.

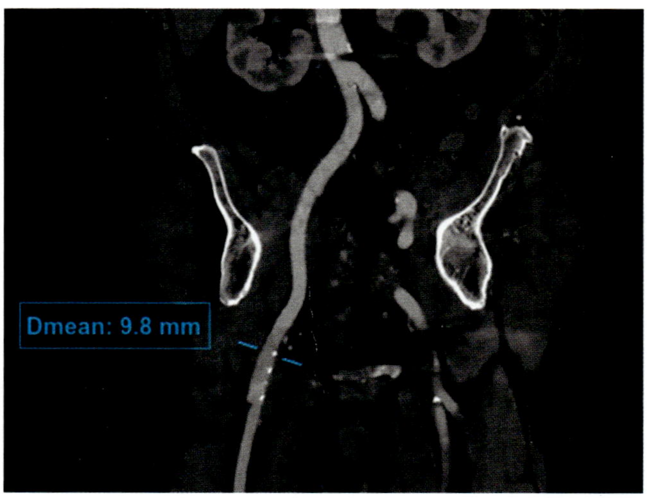

Figure 42.6. Maximum intensity projection of lower abdomen and pelvis demonstrating the vascular anatomy and morphology. Mean diameter at the common femoral artery measures 9.8 mm (blue dashed line) in this 64-year-old male.

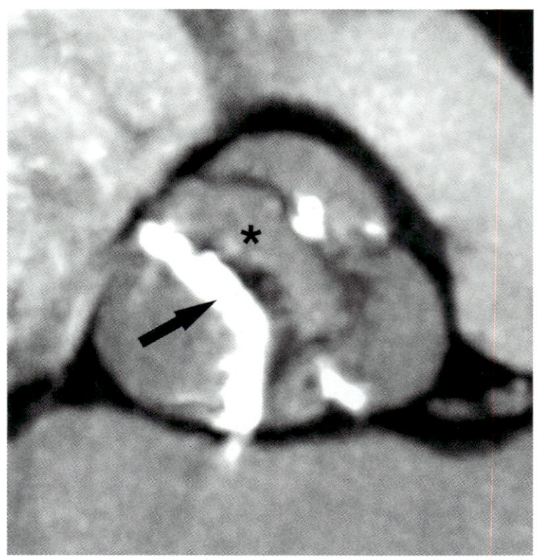

Figure 42.8. Maximum intensity projection image at the level of Sinus of Valsalva demonstrating bicuspid aortic valve with differentiation of dense calcifications (arrow) from relatively hypodense contrast (asterisk).

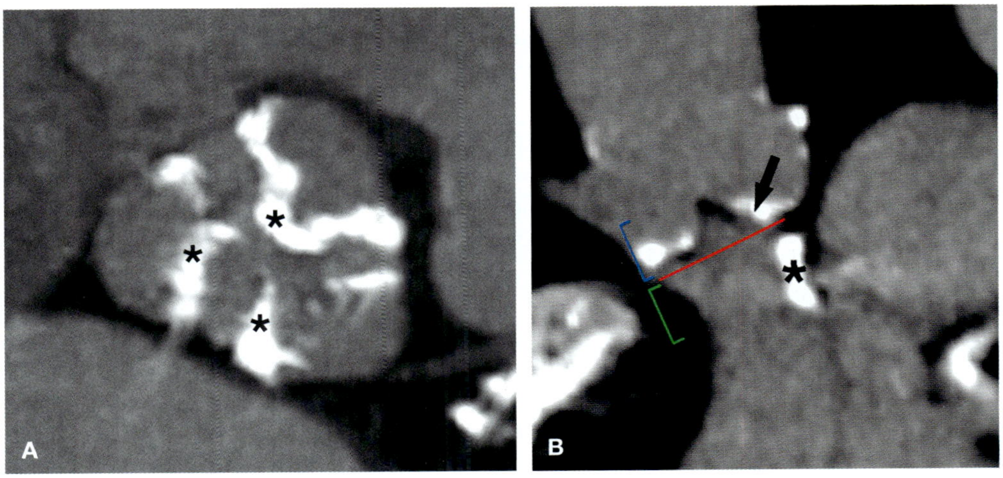

Figure 42.9. Landing zone with calcifications. **A:** Maximum intensity projection image perpendicular to the sinus of Valsalva (**A**) shows dense calcifications involving all three leaflets of aortic valve (asterisks). **B:** Double oblique reformation shows regions of landing zone, including aortic leaflet region (blue bracket), annulus (red line), and left ventricle outflow tract region (green bracket). Calcifications seen involving aortic valve leaflets (arrow) and left ventricle outflow tract wall (asterisk).

Most Common Complications

TAVR complications are divided into short-term periprocedural and long-term (postprocedural) complications. Periprocedural complications include myocardial infarction and occlusion of coronary vessels, rupture of the landing zone, cardiac tamponade, and valve embolization. Postprocedural complications encompass issues with the arterial access site, vascular closure, problems related to the replaced valve, disturbances in electrical conduction, and organ injury due to decreased blood supply. Table 42.4 summarizes type and incidence of post-TAVR complications.

Although CTA can be very useful for detection and characterization of TAVR complications, it is not routinely recommended unless the procedure was particularly challenging or there is clinical suspicion. Imaging appearance of a few post-procedural complications that may be encountered in clinical practice are described below.

Table 42.4 Most Common Post TAVR Procedure Complications

TAVR Complication	Incidence (%)
Pacemaker implantation	17.0
Perivalvular leakage	1.8
Transitory ischemic attack	2.0
Stroke	2.0
Myocardial infarction	0.5
Coronary occlusion	0.1
Vascular complication	5.4
Surgical procedure required	0.5
Bleeding	7.5
Death	1.5

TAVR, transcatheter aortic valve replacement.

Hypoattenuated Leaflet Thickening

Hypoattenuated leaflet thickening (HALT) refers to a specific finding observed in imaging studies, particularly CTA, where there is a thickening of the leaflets of a heart valve with a reduced density or attenuation compared to the surrounding structures. HALT is commonly associated with bioprosthetic aortic valves used in TAVR. It has been identified as a potential factor that may affect valve function and clinical outcomes in patients who have undergone TAVR. Approximately 10% to 12% of patients following TAVR experience HALT. HALT has been found to potentially correlate with cerebrovascular events and malfunctioning of the heart valve due to hemodynamic issues (Figure 42.10).

Complete Thrombosis of TAVR

Thrombosis or vegetation can occur on the TAVR valve. CT is a powerful technique for the assessment of the morphology and excursion of the leaflets. Given potential artifact from the metallic portions of the valve, techniques to decrease streak and blooming artifact can improve imaging assessment. Rarely, complete thrombotic occlusion of TAVR has been seen (Figure 42.11).

Valve Migration

Rare instances of valve migration have been reported that highlight the importance of accurate sizing on pre-TAVR imaging. CTA can be performed to assess for landing of a migrated valve, and potential complications (Figure 42.12).

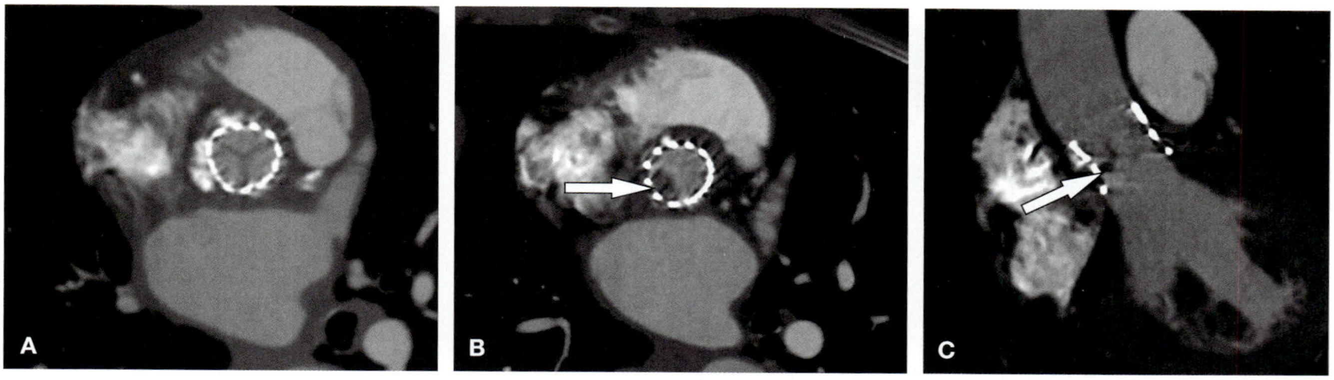

Figure 42.10. 79-year-old female status post transcatheter aortic valve replacement. Double oblique image perpendicular to the TAVR stent (**A**) shows expected post-procedure appearance. Two months after the procedure reformations perpendicular (**B**) and parallel (**C**) to the stent show development of severe hypo-attenuating leaflet thickening (arrow) involving the entire length of the noncoronary TAVR leaflet. TAVR, transcatheter aortic valve replacement.

CTA FOR LEFT ATRIAL APPENDAGE OCCLUSION

The incidence of atrial fibrillation (AF) is continuously rising globally, impacting over 50 million individuals in 2020. Strokes linked to AF have high risks of morbidity and mortality. Although the primary management to prevent stroke in the setting of AF is oral anticoagulation (OAC), OAC has its own complications, eg, intracerebral bleeding, in high-risk patients. These complications are highest in the elderly, those with previous bleeding, and patients with significant health conditions.

Percutaneous left atrial appendage occlusion (LAAO) is an alternative to OAC in patients with concomitant high risk for thromboembolism from AF and bleeding from prolonged anticoagulation therapy. Several randomized clinical trials have shown that LAAO is noninferior to OAC for stroke and systemic embolism prevention. LAAO device should be deployed in patients with an elevated risk for thromboembolic events based on commonly practiced risk stratification calculators who can tolerate short-term OAC but have absolute long-term contraindications for OAC therapy (Table 42.5).

Since the anatomy of the LAA is complex and highly variable, pre-procedural cardiac CTA plays a significant role in assessing the anatomical feasibility of transcatheter LAAO. CTA allows for precise assessment of LAA dimensions for device selection, including measurements of the landing zone and the LAA length. It is also useful for ruling out LAA thrombus, which could cause significant complications during the procedure. Various types of LAAO devices have been developed, each presenting unique morphology and landing deployment mechanism features. The most common clinically used devices are Watchman/Watchman FLX, Amplatzer Amulet, and Lariat (Table 42.6).

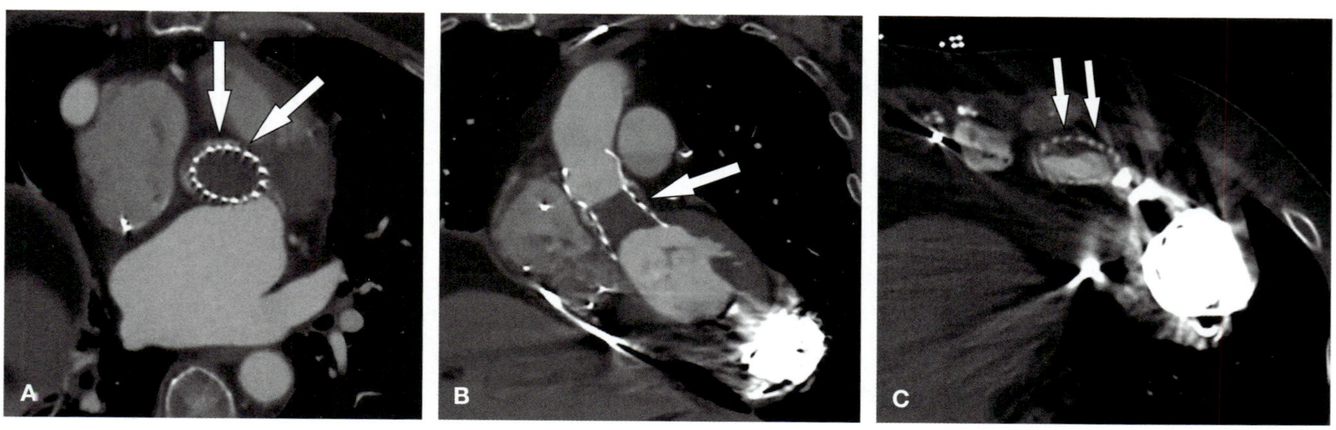

Figure 42.11. 68-year-old man with left ventricular assist device and recent transcatheter aortic valve replacement. Computed tomography angiography perpendicular (**A**) and parallel (**B**) to the stent shows total occlusion of the transcatheter aortic valve replacement orifice with hypodense thrombus. Oblique reformation along the left ventricular assist device shows an eccentric thrombus in the proximal outflow cannula (**C**).

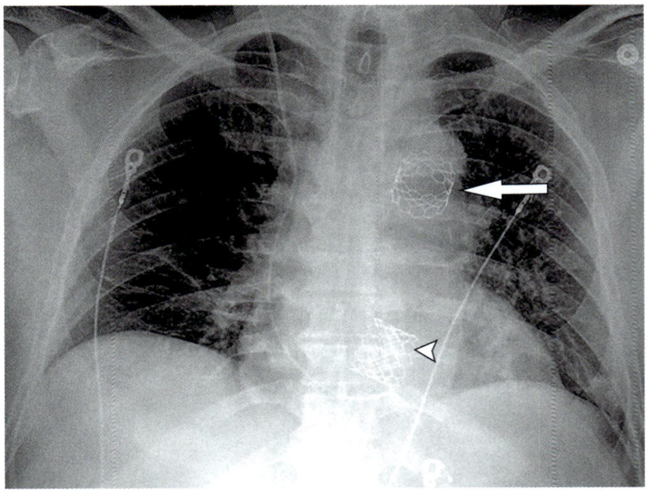

Figure 42.12. Chest radiograph showing transcatheter aortic valve replacement migration into the proximal descending thoracic aorta (arrow). A new transcatheter aortic valve replacement was deployed in the aortic root (arrowhead).

CTA Technique and Image Acquisition

Preprocedural CTA scan can be conducted with retrospective and prospective ECG-gating to capture images of the LAA. Since prospective ECG-gating has less radiation exposure, it is preferred to retrospective ECG-gating for this application. When retrospective technique is used, multi-planar cross-sectional views are reconstructed at 10% R-R intervals across the complete cardiac cycle to evaluate the LAA. A 64-slice CT platform is adequate for imaging. However, to achieve a superior image quality, higher slice counts are recommended. For example, a 128-slice CT scanner provides increased image quality with higher spatial resolution and less motion artifact. To achieve a higher specificity and sensitivity for diagnosing LAA thrombus, delayed imaging with a 60 s delay from contrast peak is obtained. Alternative protocols, such as double-contrast single-phase acquisition, have been explored, but their increased contrast load makes it suboptimal.

Contrast medium concentration of 350 mg iodine/mL, volumes between 40 and 100 mL and a dual-head power injector with saline chaser are recommended. Heart rate control medications are typically unnecessary unless patients exhibit very high heart rates. Nitroglycerin is not indicated for CTA for LAAO planning. Table 42.7 shows our institutional LAAO pre-procedural CTA protocol.

CTA Image Postprocessing and Reporting

The LAA has a complex morphologic structure divided into three main anatomical regions: (1) the ostium, (2) neck (landing zone for transcatheter devices), and (3) lobar region. Different LAA morphologies significantly influence the approach and device selected for transcatheter LAAO, which highlights the importance of a high-quality CTA to illustrate the anatomy of the LAA. LAA morphologies include chicken wing, cactus, windsock, and cauliflower (Figure 42.13). CTA images are processed and analyzed for landing zone sizing and LAA length for selection of appropriate LAAO devices.

Measurements

The Ostium and Landing Zone Sizing

The ostium is typically a well-defined plane that forms the opening from the left atrium to LAA. It is generally oval shaped with a thin wall (Figure 42.14). The LAAO device landing zone is determined and measured during maximal LAA diastole or mid to late left ventricular systole, precisely when the LAA exhibits maximum end-diastolic filling (when the LAA is the largest). The area between the main lobe of the LAA and the left circumflex artery defines the LAA planned landing zone. The device landing zone dimensions allows for selection of proper LAAO device. The goal is to place the device below trabeculations, as it could leave a residual nidus

Table 42.5 Indications for LAAO Procedure

Indication	Reason	Example
Patient not eligible for long-term OAC therapy (absolute contraindications to OAC).	High risk for bleeding	• Intracranial bleeding • GI bleeding • Recurrent falls with head trauma and significant musculoskeletal injury • Bowel angiodysplasia
	Inability to take OACs for reasons other than high risk for bleeding.	• Intolerance • Documented poor adherence to medication
Thromboembolic event or documented presence of thrombus in the LAA despite adequate OAC therapy.	• Documented thrombus formation in the LAA on adequate OAC therapy • Embolic stroke or other systemic thromboembolism on adequate OAC therapy with evidence for thrombus origin from the LAA.	

GI, gastrointestinal; LAA, left atrial appendage; LAAO, left atrial appendage occlusion; OAC, oral anticoagulation.

Table 42.6 Different Devices for LAAO and Their Features

Device	Approach	Implantation	Mechanism	Size (mm)	Indication	FDA Approval	Description
Watchman	Endocardial	Transseptal, Implantable	LAA closure	21, 24, 27, 30, 33	Stroke risk reduction	YES	Self-expanding nickel titanium device with a polyester covering and fixation barbs.
Watchman FLX	Endocardial	Transseptal, Implantable	LAA closure	20, 24, 27, 31, 35	Stroke risk reduction	YES	Self-expanding nickel titanium device with a polyester covering and fixation barbs.
Amplatzer Amulet	Endocardial	Transseptal, Implantable	LAA closure	16, 18, 20, 22, 25, 28, 31, 34	Stroke risk reduction	YES	Self-expanding nitinol device with a distal lobe and a proximal disc.
Lariat	Epicardial	Endoepicardial, non-implantable	Closure of LAA orifice	40 (W) × 20 (H) × 70 (L)	Adjunct to AF ablation	NO	Multicomponent device with balloon catheter, magnet tipped and suture delivery system.

FDA, food and drug administration; H, height; L, length; LAA, left atrial appendage; LAAO, left atrial appendage occlusion; mm, millimeter; W, weight.

Table 42.7 Example of CT Imaging Protocol for LAAO Planning

CONTRAST ADMINISTRATION		
Rate	Concentration	Volume
4 cc/s	*100% contrast*	*80 cc*
3 cc/s	*Saline*	*30 cc*

ARTERIAL PHASE	**DELAYED PHASE (60s)**
Anatomy Selection	***Anatomy Selection***
2 cm above Carina to base of heart	*2 cm above Carina to base of heart*
SFOV Cardiac Large	*SFOV Cardiac L*
DFOV 20-25 cm Heart only	*DFOV 20-25 cm Heart Only*
kV and mA Control	***kV and mA Control***
Manual 80-100 kV	*Manual 80-100 kV*
Smart/Auto mA 80-740/NI	*Smart/Auto mA 80-740/NI*
Timing	
smart prep @ left atrium	
Scan Type	***Scan Type***
Cardiac- ***30%-60% R-R***	*Cardiac-* ***45% R-R***
Coverage Speed	***Coverage Speed***
One or More/SC 0.28 s	*One or More/SC 0.28 s*
Primary Recon	***Primary Recon***
0.625 mm/Std/ASIRV 50/800@100	*0.62 mm/Std/ASIRV 50/800@100*
ECG-gating	***ECG-gating***
On	*On*

ASIR-V, adaptive statistical iterative reconstruction-v; cm, centimeters; cc, cubic centimeter; DFOV, display field of view; DLIR, deep learning image reconstruction; GSI, Gemstone spectral imaging; kVp, Kilovoltage peak; LAAO, left atrial appendage occlusion; mA, milliampere; mm, millimeters; MIP, maximum intensity projection; NI, noise index; sec, second; SFOV, scan field of view; Std, standard; TAVR, transcatheter aortic valve replacement.

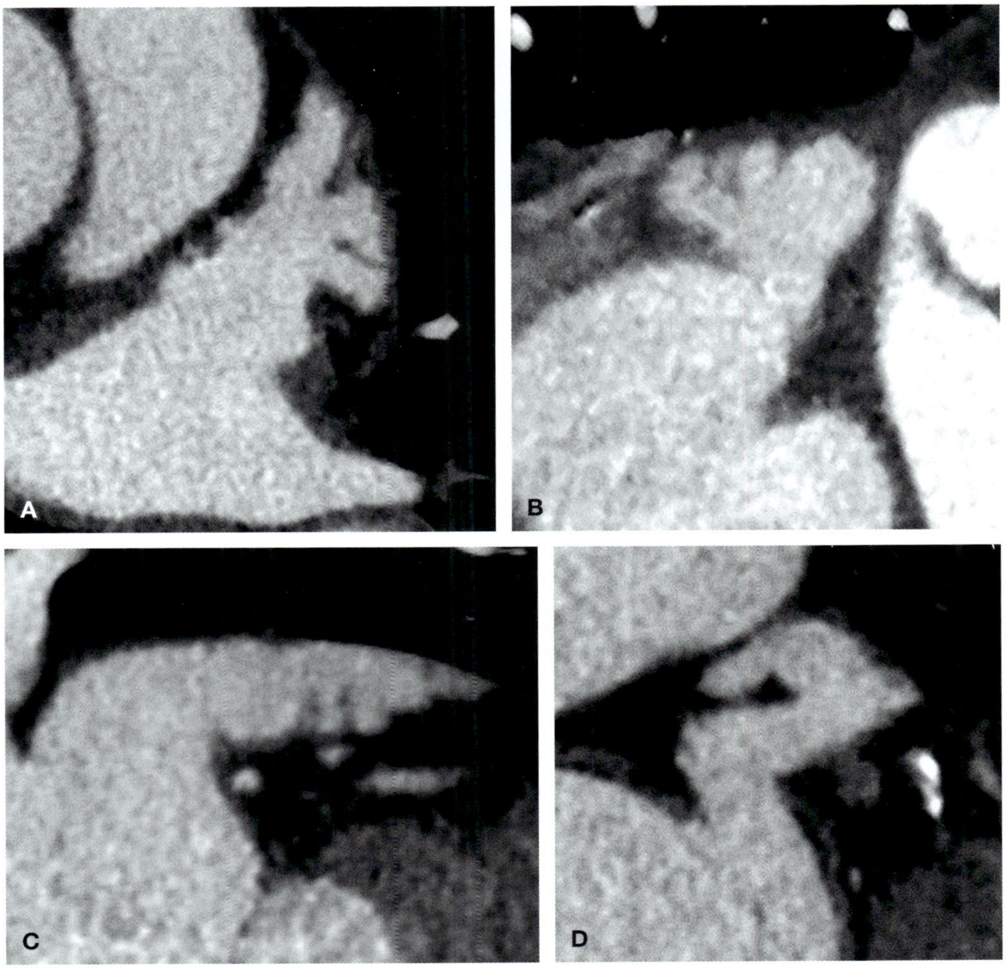

Figure 42.13. Shapes of left atrial appendage. Oblique reformations of computed tomography angiography along the left atrial appendage show a cauliflower-shaped (**A**), a cactus-shaped (**B**), a windsock-shaped (**C**), and a chicken wing-shaped (**D**) structure.

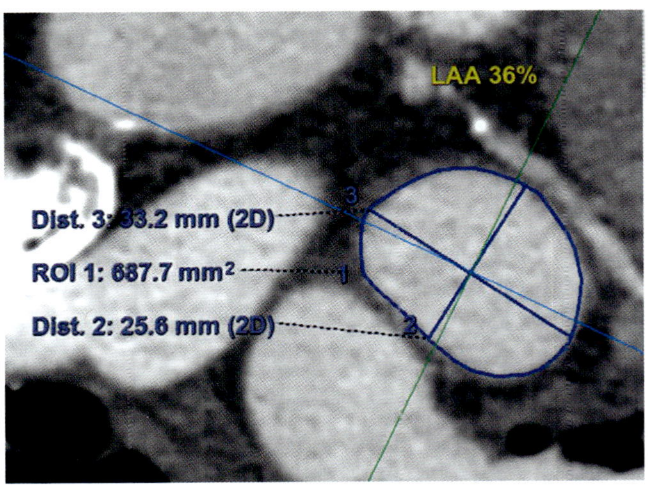

Figure 42.14. Left atrial appendage ostial dimensions. Double-oblique reformation aligned to an oval-shaped left atrial appendage ostium with measurements of minimum and maximum dimensions (Dist.) and area (ROI 1).

for thromboembolism if placed above it (Figure 42.15). For ostium and landing zone sizing, various measurements are suggested such as maximal, minimal, and average diameters, area, and perimeter. The widest dimensions are used to determine device size.

Depth

The depth of LAA is defined as the distance between the landing zone to the apex of LAA. Oblique sagittal and coronal views are used to measure the depth of the LAA (Figure 42.16). The depth of the LAA must be at least longer than the width of the ostium for optimal device placement and closure of the LAA.

Most Common Complications

Transcatheter LAAO complications may occur during or after the procedure. In general, LAAO procedure complications can be divided into access-related, device

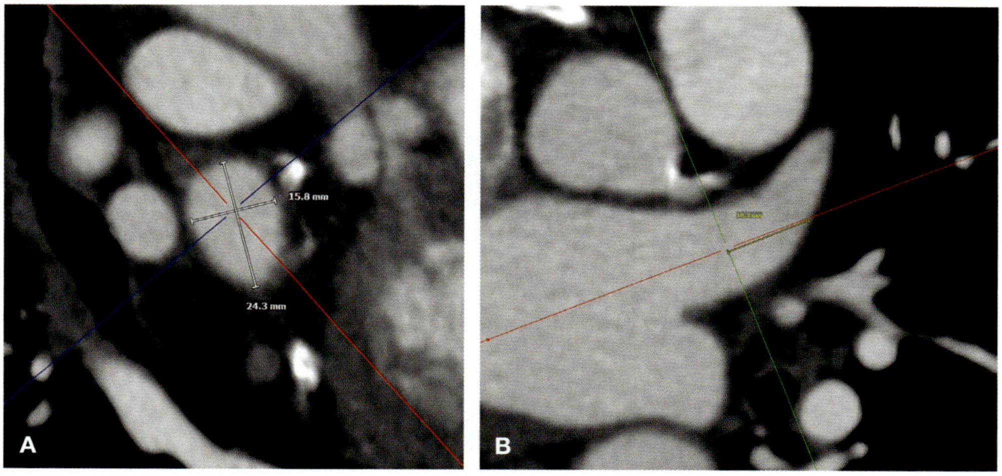

Figure 42.15. Landing zone. Cross-sectional image of the landing zone (**A**) shows maximum and minimum diameters (white lines). Longitudinal reformation along the landing zone (**B**) shows measurement of the distance between the landing zone (red line) and the anterior wall of the left atrial appendage (yellow line).

implantation-related, and antithrombotic treatment-related. Most common complications include cardiac perforation, pericardial effusion, tamponade, device embolization, device-related thrombosis (DRT), peri-device leak, systemic thromboembolism, and injury related to vascular access (Table 42.8).

Post-procedure CTA may be obtained to assess patients for a range of LAAO complications, especially when suspected on transesophageal echocardiography. a few examples of post-procedural complications that may be encountered in clinical practice are illustrated.

Device Related Thrombus

DRT formation is a major issue in LAAO procedure. Its incidence and timing have been documented in many studies. For example, its incidence in Watchman RCT was reported 3.74%. In the Amulet IDE trial, the Amulet device had a slightly lower DRT incidence (3.3%) than the Watchman device (4.5%) at 18 months. Among the FDA-approved devices, the Watchman FLX device has the lowest DRT incidence (1.7%). Three-fold increased risk for stroke and systemic embolism has been found in patients with device-related thrombosis (Figure 42.17).

Peri-Device Leak

Percutaneous LAAO devices sometimes do not result in complete occlusion of the appendage. As an accepted clinical practice, a CT examination with delayed phase 45 days post device implantation can help assessment of the device and possible peri-device leak (PDL). A mismatch between circular geometry of LAAO devices and elliptical shape of ostium may lead to incomplete LAAO and PDL which is defined by residual flow of any size. The cutoff to determine the significance of PDL differs between studies and it is often

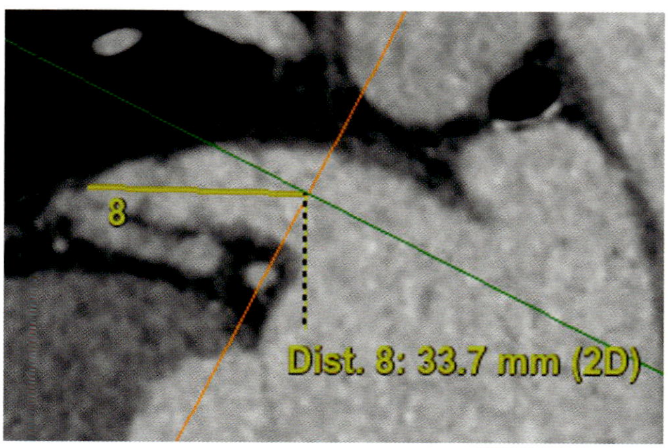

Figure 42.16. Depth of left atrial appendage (yellow line) measured from the landing zone (orange line).

Table 42.8 Complications Related to LAAO

Complication	Incidence
Pericardial effusion/tamponade	1.2%-5%
Device embolization	0%-3.7%
Device related thrombus	1.5%-14%
Persistent ASD	11% at 6 mo and 7% at 12 mo
Cardiac perforation	0.4%
Procedure related stroke	1.1%
Implant displacement	0.07%
Peri-device leak	0.01%
Major bleeding	1.4%
Death	0.15%

ASD, atrial septal defect; LAAO, left atrial appendage occlusion.

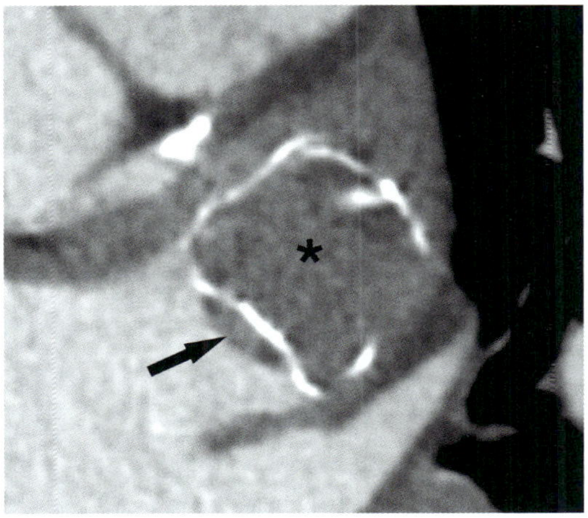

Figure 42.17. Device-related thrombus. Oblique reformation along the left atrial appendage shows a small device-related thrombus (arrow) protruding into the left atrium. Normal thrombus within the left atrial appendage occlusion device (asterisk) is also seen.

set arbitrarily. For example, current guidelines use an arbitrary cutoff of >5 mm to classify leaks as significant. Contrast in and beyond the device does not necessarily mean there is peri-device leak as endothelialization does not happen immediately after the procedure. Detailed three-dimensional (3D) assessment of the presence of contrast connection around the device to the contrast pool beyond the device (Figure 42.18) can be performed with CTA. "En face" view can be very helpful for such assessment (Figure 42.19). Significant PDL can be treated by additional transcatheter procedure to deploy coils, plugs, and occluders (Figure 42.20).

CTA FOR PRE- AND POSTPROCEDURAL TMVR EVALUATION

TMVR is a minimally invasive catheter-based interventional technique for treating severe mitral valve disease in patients who fail medical treatment, do not have favorable anatomy for transcatheter mitral valve repair with MitraClip, and are deemed high risk for traditional open mitral valve surgery.

Over 30 devices with distinct sizes, implantation approaches, and anchoring mechanisms have been introduced for TMVR. Transapical and transseptal routes are the most common approaches for the delivery of various TMVR devices. The transapical approach is preferred to the arterial femoral approach considering the larger TMVR device profiles compared to TAVR devices (Table 42.9).

The first-line imaging for characterizing and quantifying mitral valve disorders is achieved through transthoracic echocardiography. However, echocardiography has several limitations for precise delineation of the mitral valve annulus for pre-procedure including lower resolution and increased subjectivity compared to CTA. CTA plays a crucial role in preprocedural planning and offers numerous advantages, including high isotropic spatial and temporal resolution, a broad field of view, ability to perform virtual prosthesis modeling, neo-LVOT evaluation and multiplanar reconstruction. CTA is also highly valuable for post-TMVR assessment. Follow-up CTA can be helpful in identifying complications such as DRT, device malpositioning/embolization, pseudoaneurysm, LVOT obstruction, and paravalvular leak.

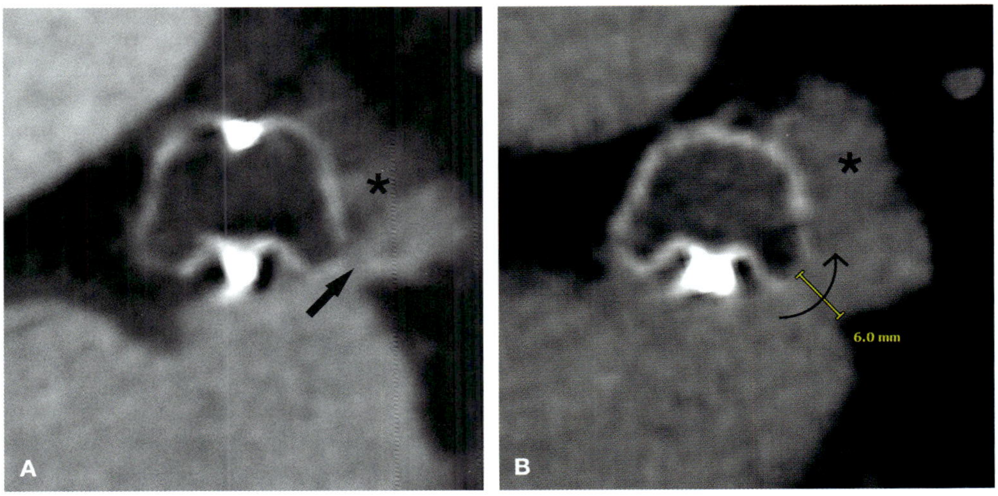

Figure 42.18. Peri-device leak. **A:** Post-Watchman early phase contrast CTA perpendicular to the device shows small communication (arrow) between left atrium and excluded left atrial appendage along the Watchman device, with contrast filling the distal left atrial appendage seen (asterisk). **B:** Delayed phase CTA image in the same plane shows better visualization of the column of contrast (curved arrow) adjacent to the rim of the device, with a thickness of 6 mm. Increased opacification of distal left atrial appendage seen is noted (asterisk). CTA, computed tomography angiography.

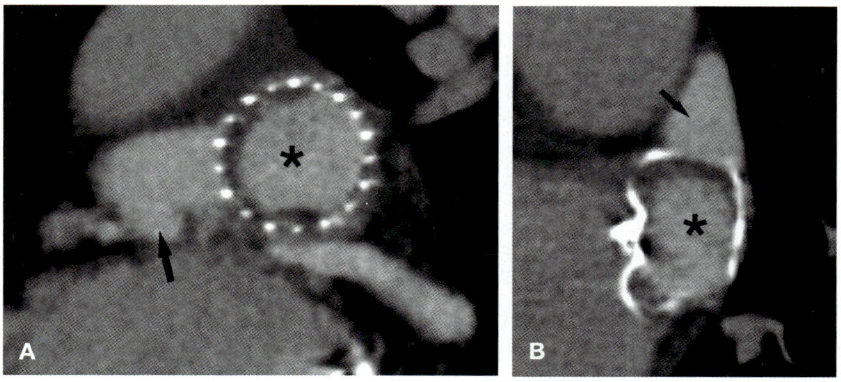

Figure 42.19A. En-face view of the LAAO device (**A**) with normal contrast within the device (asterisk) and into the distal left atrial appendage beyond the device (arrow) with no peri-device leak. Longitudinal view along the device (**B**) shows contrast into the left atrial appendage beyond the LAAO device in (arrow) with normal contrast leakage into the device (asterisk). LAAO, left atrial appendage occlusion.

CTA Technique and Image Acquisition

CTA imaging protocol for TMVR is not different than TAVR protocol in most institutions. Please refer to the CT imaging protocol subsection of the TAVR section and Table 42.3. However, there are several important postprocessing simulations and measurements that need to be considered specifically for TMVR procedure, as discussed below.

CTA Image Postprocessing and Reporting

CTA is a precise technique for TMVR preprocedural planning. CTA imaging can provide precise assessment of unique parameters such as mitral annulus area, perimeter, trigone-trigone (TT) distance, intercommissural (IC) distance, and septolateral (SL) distance.

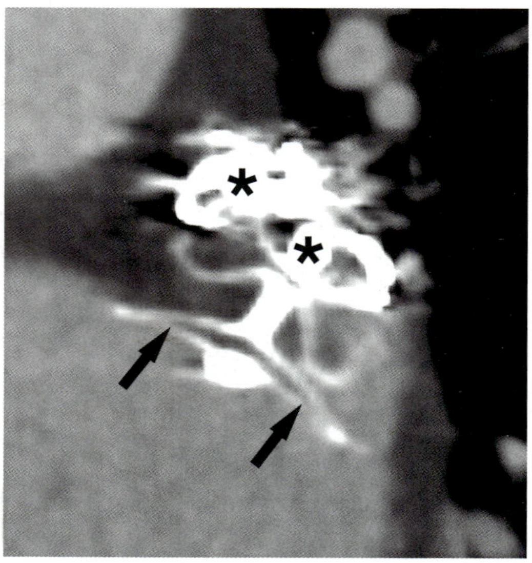

Figure 42.20. Post-operative computed tomography angiography scan of left atrial appendage of a 63-year-old man with peri-device leak around the left atrial appendage occlusion. A 25 mm amulet occluder device (arrows) was used to close the leak and is well-seated in the left atrial appendage with no device-related thrombus. Vascular coils (asterisks) are seen in the distal left atrial appendage.

Annulus Measurement

Precise measurement of the mitral valve annulus is critical for TMVR device sizing. Oversizing of the annulus can result in annular rupture while undersizing of the annulus can result in device migration.

Anatomically, the mitral annulus has a 3D saddle shape with an anterior horn extending between the trigones along the aortomitral continuity. For measurement of the mitral annulus, A D-shaped annulus can be obtained from the saddle-shaped annulus by drawing a virtual line between the medial and lateral trigones and eliminating the anterior horn (Figure 42.21).

Because the mitral valve is dynamic and changes in size during the heart cycle, mitral annular measurements should be obtained at the phase the annulus is largest. The mitral annulus is usually largest at the end of diastole (70%-90% R-R interval). However, since the mitral annulus can occasionally be Larger at the end-systole phase (30%-40% R-R interval), it is ideal to also measure the mitral annulus at the end-systolic phase (Figure 42.22).

Mitral annular measurements can be performed manually, or semi-automatically. D-shaped annulus can be created by manipulation of multiplanar reformats across different axes. There are several commercially available software packages with platforms automating or facilitating mitral annulus measurements. The way that most of these software platforms work is by manual placement of several seed points at the insertion of the mitral valve leaflets to the adjacent myocardium to achieve a 360° boundary coverage. The 3D perimeter of the saddle-shaped annulus will then be created by cubic spline interpolation using the seed points after excluding the anterior horn by drawing a line across the trigones. The two-dimensional D-shaped annulus will be created by

Table 42.9 TMVR Devices and Their Features

Device	Implantation Approach	Expansion	Access Size Sheath	Anchoring Mechanism	Valve Size	Valve Position	Shape	Leaflets	Required Measurements
Sapien 3	Transseptal	Balloon expandable	20 Fr.	Radial force, requires MAC	20, 23, 26, 29 mm	Intra-annular	Circular	Bovine pericardium, trileaflet	Maximum diameter, perimeter
Tendyne	Transapical	Self-expandable	34 Fr.	Apical tether	30-43 mm in the SL dimension and 34-50 in the IC dimension	Intra-annular	D-shaped (outer stent) Circular (inner frame)	Porcine pericardium, trileaflet	IC and SL distance
Intrepid	Transapical	Self-expandable	33 Fr	Radial force and sub-annular cleats	Inner stent–27 mm (Outer stent–43, 46, and 50 mm)	Intra-annular	Circular	Bovine pericardium, trileaflet	IC and SL distance, perimeter
HighLife	transseptal	Self-expandable	39 Fr	External anchor; valve in sub-annular mitral ring	31 mm	Intra-annular	Circular	Bovine pericardium, trileaflet	Maximum diameter, perimeter
CardiaQ	Transapical, transseptal	Self-expandable	33 Fr	Annulus and native leaflet engagement	30 mm	Supra-annular	Circular	Bovine pericardium, trileaflet	Maximum diameter
TIARA	Transapical	Self-expandable	32, 36 Fr	Onto the fibrous trigone and atrioventriular shelf	35 and 40 mm	Intra-annular	D-shaped	Bovine pericardium, trileaflet	IC distance and perimeter
Caisson	Transseptal	Self-expandable	31 Fr	4 sub-annular anchoring feet 3 atrial holding features	36 and 42 mm	Supra-annular	D-shaped	Porcine Pericardium, trileaflet	IC and SL distance, perimeter
CardioValve	Transseptal	Self-expandable	28 Fr	24 focal "sandwiching" points	Three sizes (range 40-40 mm)	Intra-annular	Circular	Bovine pericardium, trileaflet	Maximum diameter, perimeter
Evoque	Transseptal	Self-expandable	28 Fr	External anchor	Three sizes (44 and 48 mm)	Intra-annular	Circular	Bovine pericardium, trileaflet	Maximum diameter, perimeter

Fr, French; IC, intercommissural distance; SL, septolateral distance; TMVR, transcatheter mitral valve replacement.

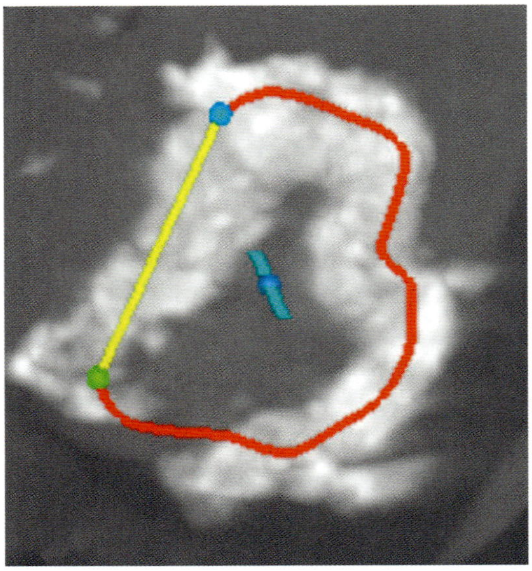

Figure 42.21. D-shaped mitral annulus with severe annular calcifications. Reformation parallel to the annulus shows calcifications along the mitral annulus (red line), and the trigone to trigone distance (yellow line), whereas blue dot marks the medial trigone, and green dot marks the lateral trigone.

projecting the 3D annulus onto the short-axis view of the heart. Annular measurements will then be obtained using this two-dimensional D-shaped annulus.

The most common measurements for TMVR planning are the perimeter and area of the mitral valve annulus (Figure 42.23). Other useful measurements include the TT, IC, and SL measurements. Different TMVR devices use different measurements for sizing. For example, the Tendyne device uses SL and IC distances while the Sapien valve uses the annulus area for sizing (Table 42.3). The TT is the straight distance between the trigones. The IC distance is the maximum diameter of the mitral annulus parallel to the TT. The SL measurement is the maximum mitral annulus distance perpendicular to the TT. As expected, the TT and IC distances are the same for the saddle-shaped and D-shaped annulus while the SL distance is shorter for the D-shaped annulus compared to the saddle-shaped annulus (Figure 42.24).

Landing Zone Assessment

CTA is an excellent tool for providing the information needed to assess the landing zone. In general, 20% atrial offset and 80% ventricular offset is expected for most TMVR devices. There are four major features that need to be assessed for ideal assessment of the landing zone. These include mitral annular calcification (MAC), atrioventricular shelf, Mitral prolapse, and mitral annular disjunction (MAD).

CTA is an excellent tool for assessment of the severity, extension, and density of MAC. MAC is essential for devices using radial force mechanism for anchoring such as the Sapien valve. A shot axis multiplanar reformatted image or maximum intensity projection reconstruction of the mitral annuls provides good assessment of the extension of MAC (Figure 42.25). A caseous MAC with a liquefactive core provides less support for anchoring when compared to a solid MAC. Some ongoing clinical trials such as SUMMIT and APOLLO evaluating TMVR devices have added a MAC subgroup to better understand the importance of MAC. Please note that MAC is considered a contraindication for some TMVR devices.

It is not uncommon for patients with mitral regurgitation to have an atrioventricular shelf of the left ventricle myocardium on the ventricular side of the mitral valve posterior leaflet insertion point. The atrioventricular shelf is larger in diastole and smaller or absent in systole (Figure 42.26). Some TMVR devices such as Tiara are using the inferolateral basal myocardium for anchoring, therefore a persistent atrioventricular shelf is important for using these devices.

Above 2 cm protrusion of a mitral leaflet beyond the mitral valve annulus into the left atrium in systole defines mitral valve prolapse (Figure 42.27). Detachment of the mitral annulus from the left ventricle myocardium at the atrioventricular junction is called MAD (Figure 42.28). MAD may be seen is seen in patients with severe mitral prolapse, or in isolation. It is essential to exclude mitral valve

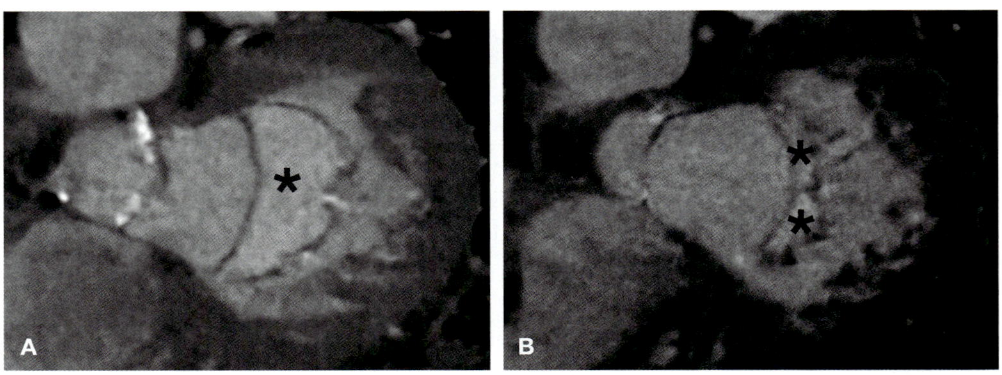

Figure 42.22. Mitral valve orifice. Short axis computed tomography angiography images at the level of the mitral valve orifice in diastole (**A**) and systole (**B**), with asterisk showing the orifice area.

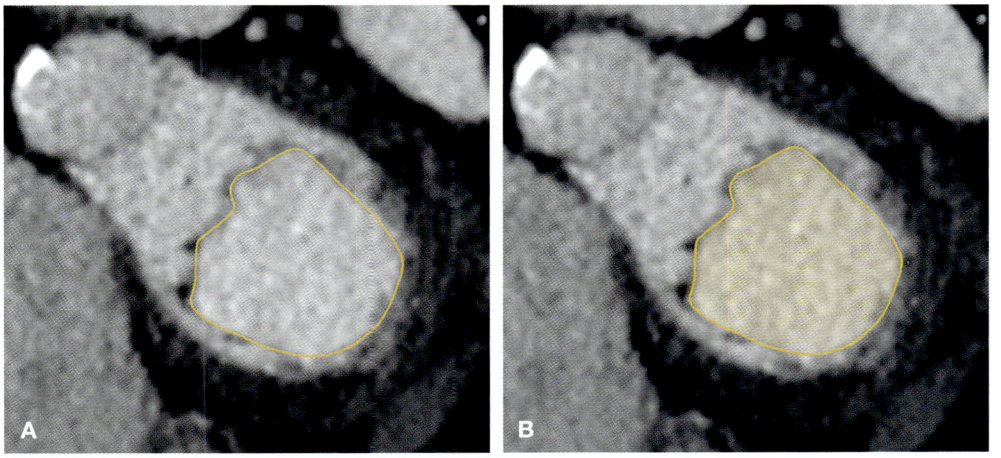

Figure 42.23. Mitral valve annulus measurements. Computed tomography angiography images during end-diastole in the short axis plane show the perimeter (**A**) of mitral valve measuring 133 mm, and the area of mitral valve measuring (**B**) measuring 13.3 cm^2.

prolapse and MAD before using TMVR devices that anchor onto the mitral valve leaflets. These devices also need adequate mitral valve leaflet length (Figure 42.29).

Adjacent Structures Assessment

Some adjacent structures such as the coronary sinus and the left circumflex coronary artery are potentially at risk of compression particularly in case of TMVR device oversizing. This highlights the importance of adequate mapping of the anatomy of these structures before procedure. Lack of a fluoroscopic landmark showing the mitral annulus makes TMVR deployment challenging. CTA provides excellent anatomical information on the adjacent structures in relation to the mitral valve annulus. CTA data can be used to simulate the course of the left circumflex coronary artery and/or the coronary sinus relative to the mitral annulus and guide deployment of the TMVR devices (Figure 42.30).

The distance between the mitral valve annulus and the ostium of the left atrial appendage is important for planning transcatheter procedures for devices with supravalvular seating. There is no specific eligibility cut-off to be used for assessment of this distance. In general, the shorter this distance, the higher the chance of occluding the left atrial appendage ostium (Figure 42.31).

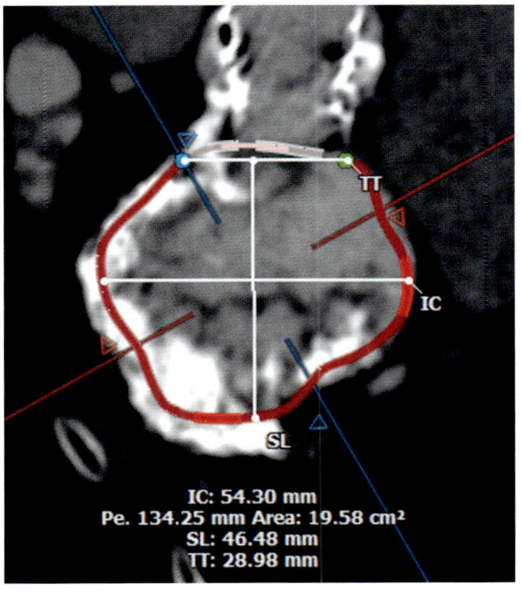

Figure 42.24. Measurements of mitral annulus derived from computed tomography angiography reformation: TT = distance between trigones. IC = maximum diameter of mitral annulus bilateral to TT. SL = maximum mitral annulus distance perpendicular to TT. Severe mitral annular calcifications also seen.

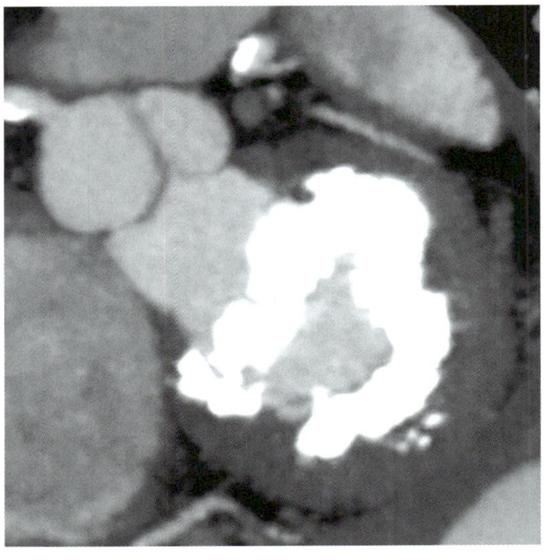

Figure 42.25. Maximum intensity projection image of mitral valve demonstrating severe mitral annular calcifications involving anterior leaflet, posterior leaflet, and medial trigone.

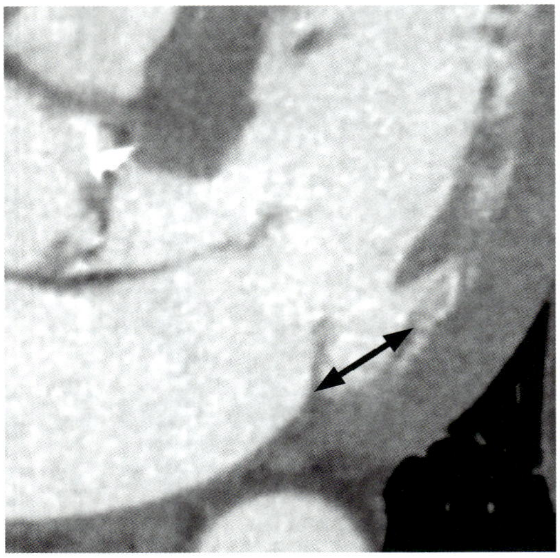

Figure 42.26. Atrioventricular shelf. Computed tomography angiography in the left ventricular outflow tract plane shows the atrioventricular shelf distance (double headed arrow) of the left ventricle myocardium on the ventricular side of the mitral valve posterior leaflet insertion point.

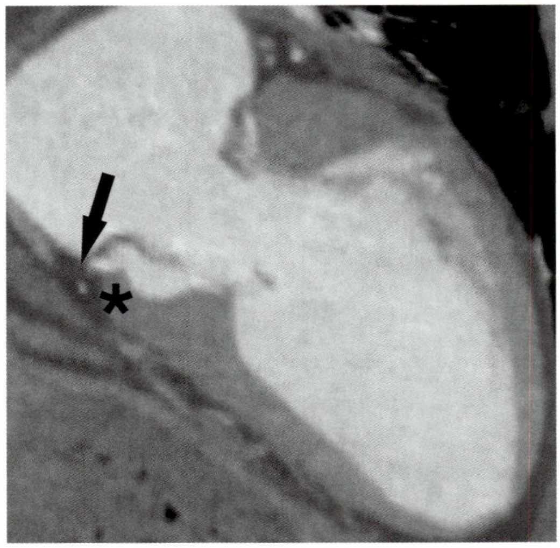

Figure 42.28. Mitral annular disjunction. Computed tomography angiography reformation in the vertical long axis plane showing the attachment of mitral valve leaflet (arrow) above the superior extent of left ventricular myocardium (asterisk).

TMVR devices with extension to the left ventricle may interfere with the papillary muscles and chordae tendinea. Use of these devices necessitates close attention to some measurements such as the distance between the papillary muscles and the mitral valve annulus, and the distance between the papillary muscles and the left ventricle wall (Figures 42.32-42.34). The presence of a dilated ventricle [>7.0 cm inner diameter] or a small ventricle [<4.0 cm inner diameter] may also limit utilization of some TMVR devices.

Most Common Complications

Most common complications post-TMVR include device thrombosis, device malposition, device migration or embolization, acute valvular dysfunction, pseudoaneurysm, LVOT obstruction, stroke, device hemolysis, and endocarditis. These complications can be categorized into short-term (within 30 days), mid-term (>30 days), and long-term complications. Incidence of Long-term complications is not well reported given the fact that TMVR is a relatively novel treatment procedure. Table 42.10 summarizes post-TMVR complications with postprocedural timing and their incidence rate.

ARTIFICIAL INTELLIGENCE (AI) APPLICATIONS

It has been shown that the field of imaging can significantly benefit from the integration of artificial intelligence algorithms and technologies. Pre- and poststructural heart

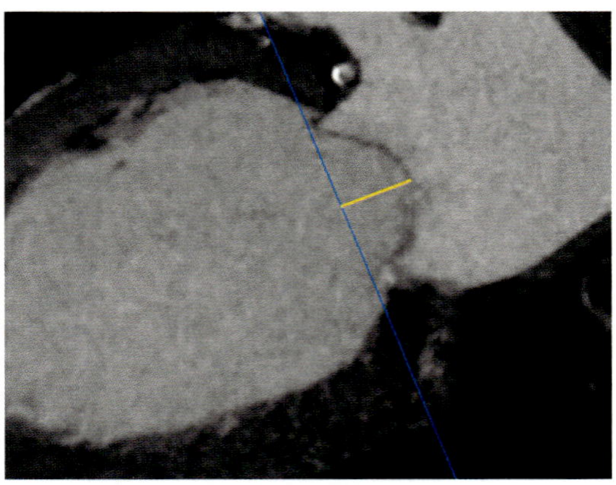

Figure 42.27. Mitral valve prolapse. Computed tomography angiography in the vertical long axis plane during systole shows bulging of mitral valve leaflet measuring 2 cm (yellow line) above the level of mitral annulus (blue line).

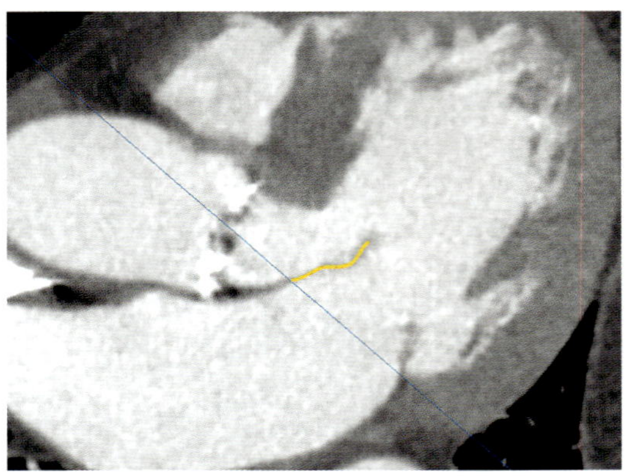

Figure 42.29. Length of mitral valve leaflet. Computed tomography angiography reformation in the left ventricular outflow tract plane shows measurement of the anterior mitral valve leaflet (yellow curve) extending from the level of mitral annulus (blue line) measuring 1.7 cm.

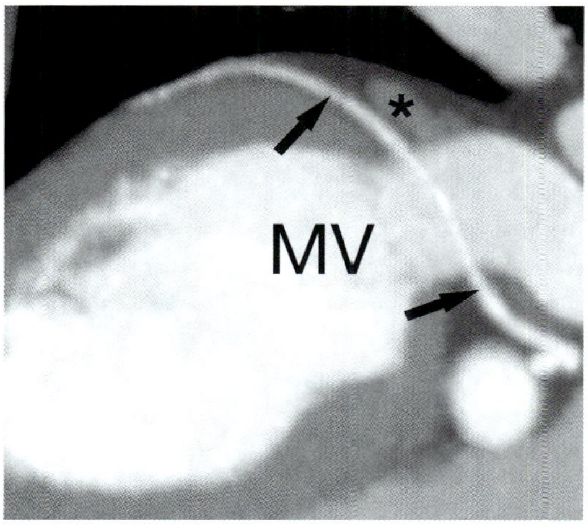

Figure 42.30. Maximum intensity projection reformation in an oblique sagittal plane showing close association of left circumflex artery (arrows) and coronary sinus (asterisk) to the mitral valve.

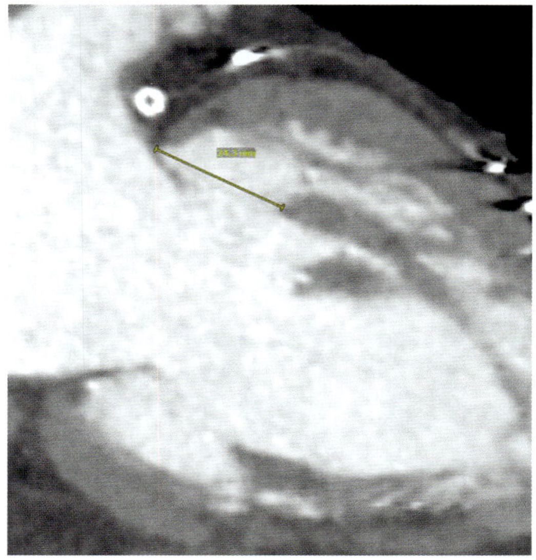

Figure 42.32. Left atrial appendage occlusion pre-procedure planning. Computed tomography angiography reformation along the vertical long axis plane shows measurement of the distance between tip of antero-lateral papillary muscle and mitral valve annulus (yellow line).

disease (TAVR, TMVR, and LAAO) assessment is not an exception. AI algorithms have been introduced with promising results to facilitate selection of these patients, automate image analysis, and even provide postprocedure risk assessment. Most of the studies in this field are focused on TAVR as there is larger data available for this procedure.

Deep learning algorithms that automatically segment and score aortic valve calcification have been introduced and can help with selection of patients with severe aortic stenosis. AI algorithms can also help automating TAVR CTA analysis by determining the aortic valve annulus and access routes. Several vendors provide automated or semiautomated algorithms that can even perform required measurements for TAVR planning and facilitate device sizing with minimizing human error. Another potential application of AI in management of patients with structural heart disease is predicting post-procedure outcome and mortality risk. For example, AI algorithms have shown promising results in predicting mortality risk post-TAVR by analyzing patients' medical records and imaging data. Some AI algorithms even claim to outperform the traditional risk assessment models such as TAVI2-SCORE and CAPRI models.

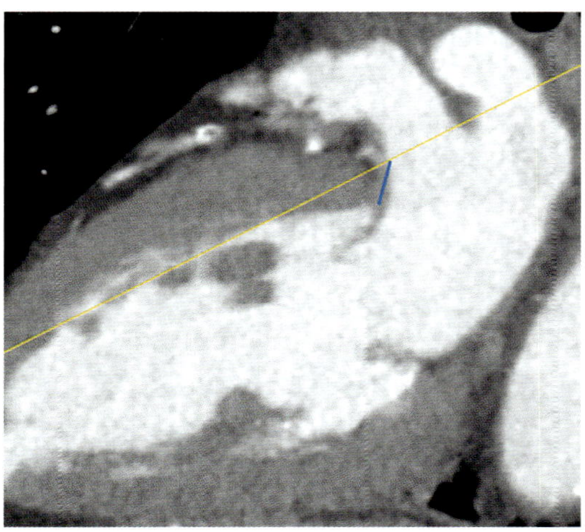

Figure 42.31. Left atrial appendage occlusion pre-procedure planning. Computed tomography angiography reformation along the vertical long axis plane shows the measurement of distance between ostium of the left atrial appendage (yellow line) and mitral annulus measuring 11 mm (blue line).

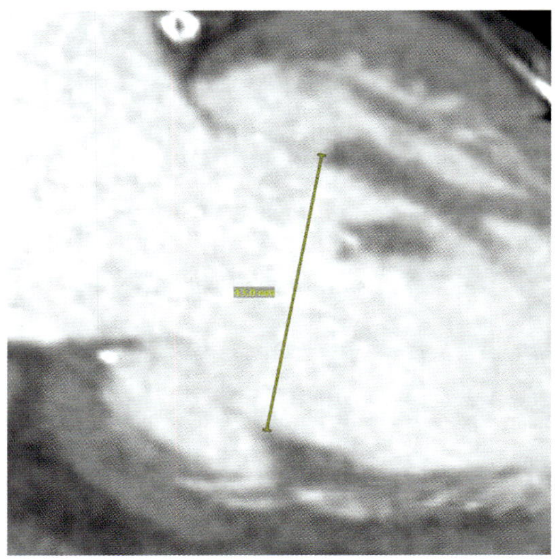

Figure 42.33. Left atrial appendage occlusion pre-procedure planning. Computed tomography angiography reformation along the vertical long axis plane shows measurement of the distance between upper ends of antero-lateral and postero-medial papillary muscles (yellow line).

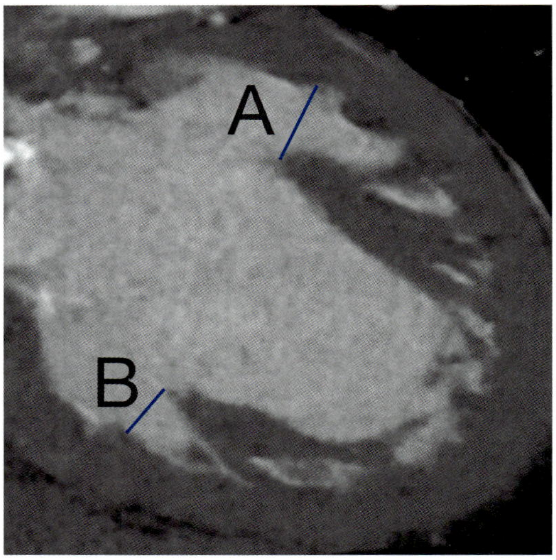

Figure 42.34. Left atrial appendage occlusion pre-procedure planning. Computed tomography angiography reformation along the vertical long axis plane shows measurement of the distance between anterolateral papillary muscle and left ventricular wall (**A**) measuring 11 mm and between posteromedial papillary muscle and left ventricular wall (**B**) measuring 9 mm.

Although artificial intelligence offers significant promise for enhancing management of structural heart diseases at different levels of care, it's crucial to tackle challenges for its safe and ethical incorporation. Careful consideration is necessary concerning publication bias in AI research, as there's a risk that studies with favorable results might receive preferential publication, potentially inflating perceptions of the technology's effectiveness and suitability.

Table 42.10 Post-TMVR Complications

Short-Term (30 d) Complications	
Device malposition	3.4%
Device migration/embolization	0.8%
Valve thrombosis	1.7%
LVOT obstruction	0.4%
MR (moderate or severe)	1.5%
Conversion to open heart surgery for complications	4.0%
Mid-Term (>30 d) Complications	
Stroke	4.5%
Device-related thrombosis	3.0%
Device-related hemolysis	4.0%
Endocarditis	4.0%
Mitral valve dysfunction requiring reintervention	2.3%

LVOT, left ventricular outflow tract; MR, mitral regurgitation; TMVR, transcatheter mitral valve replacement.

SUGGESTED READINGS

Ranganath P, Moore A, Guerrero M, et al. CT for pre- and postprocedural evaluation of transcatheter mitral valve replacement. *Radiographics.* 2020;40(6):1528-1553. doi:10.1148/rg.2020200027

Del Val D, Ferreira-Neto AN, Wintzer-Wehekind J, et al. Early experience with transcatheter mitral valve replacement: a systematic review. *J Am Heart Assoc.* 2019;8(17):e013332. doi:10.1161/JAHA.119.013332

Kaafarani M, Saw J, Daniels M, et al. Role of CT imaging in left atrial appendage occlusion for the WATCHMAN™ device. *Cardiovasc Diagn Ther.* 2020;10(1):45-58. doi:10.21037/cdt.2019.12.01

Alkhouli M, Ellis CR, Daniels M, Coylewright M, Nielsen-Kudsk JE, Holmes DR. Left atrial appendage occlusion. *JACC (J Am Coll Cardiol): Adv.* 2022;1(5):1-18. doi:10.1016/j.jacadv.2022.100136

Beigel R, Wunderlich NC, Ho SY, Arsanjani R, Siegel RJ. The left atrial appendage: anatomy, function, and noninvasive evaluation. *JACC Cardiovasc Imaging.* 2014;7(12):1251-1265. doi:10.1016/j.jcmg.2014.08.009

Gheorghe L, Brouwer J, Wang DD, et al. Current devices in mitral valve replacement and their potential complications. *Front Cardiovasc Med.* 2020;7:531843. PMID: 33330637; PMCID: PMC7728606. doi:10.3389/fcvm.2020.531843

Blanke P, Weir-McCall JR, Achenbach S, et al. Computed tomography imaging in the context of Transcatheter Aortic Valve Implantation (TAVI)/Transcatheter Aortic Valve Replacement (TAVR): an expert consensus document of the society of cardiovascular computed tomography. *JACC Cardiovasc Imaging.* 2019;12(1):1-24. doi:10.1016/j.jcmg.2018.12.003

Tully A, Tom S, Xie J, O'Brian C, Gleason P, Grubb KJ. Evolving computed tomography angiography for aortic valve replacement: optimizing transcatheter and surgical therapies. *J Card Surg.* 2022;37(12):4124-4132. doi:10.1111/jocs.16977

Index

Note: Page numbers followed by '*f*' indicate figures and '*t*' indicate tables.

A

B

C

E

I

K

L

M

N